Paediatric Ophthalmology

Paediatric Ophthalmology

EDITED BY

DAVID TAYLOR FRCS FRCP FRCOphth
Consultant Paediatric Ophthalmologist,
The Hospital for Sick Children,
Great Ormond Street, London

FOREWORD BY
MARSHALL M. PARKS

SECOND EDITION

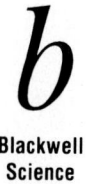

Blackwell
Science

© 1990, 1997 by
Blackwell Science Ltd
Editorial Offices:
Osney Mead, Oxford OX2 0EL
25 John Street, London WC1N 2BL
23 Ainslie Place, Edinburgh EH3 6AJ
350 Main Street, Malden
  MA 02148-5018, USA
54 University Street, Carlton
  Victoria 3053, Australia

Other Editorial Offices:
Arnette Blackwell SA
  224, Boulevard Saint Germain
  75007 Paris, France

Blackwell Wissenschafts-Verlag GmbH
  Kurfürstendamm 57
  10707 Berlin, Germany

  Zehetnergasse 6
  A-1140 Wien
  Austria

First published 1990
Second edition 1997

Set by Excel Typesetters Co., Hong Kong
Printed and bound in Italy
by Rotolito Lombarda SpA, Milan

The Blackwell Science logo is a
trade mark of Blackwell Science Ltd,
registered at the United Kingdom
Trade Marks Registry

DISTRIBUTORS

Marston Book Services Ltd
PO Box 269
Abingdon
Oxon OX14 4YN
(*Orders*: Tel: 01235 465500
           Fax: 01235 465555)

USA
Blackwell Science, Inc.
Commerce Place
350 Main Street
Malden, MA 02148-5018
(*Orders*: Tel: 800 759 6102
               617 388 8250
           Fax: 617 388 8255)

Canada
Copp Clark Professional
200 Adelaide St, West, 3rd Floor
Toronto, Ontario M5H 1W7
(*Orders*: Tel: 416 597-1616
               800 815-9417
           Fax: 416 597-1617)

Australia
Blackwell Science Pty Ltd
54 University Street
Carlton, Victoria 3053
(*Orders*: Tel: 03 9347 0300
           Fax: 03 9349 3016)

A catalogue record for this title
is available from the British Library

ISBN 0-86542-831-X

Library of Congress
Cataloging-in-publication Data

Paediatric ophthalmology/[edited by]
   David Taylor.—2nd ed.
       p.   cm.
   Includes bibliographical references
and index.
   ISBN 0-86542-831-X
   1. Pediatric ophthalmology.
I. Taylor, David, 1942–
   [DNLM: 1. Eye Diseases–in infancy &
childhood.   2. Vision Disorders– in
infancy & childhood.   WW 600   P3713
1996]
RE48.2.C5P432   1996
618.92'0977– dc20
DNLM/DLC
for Library of Congress   96-24809
                                         CIP

Contents

v

vi   *Contents*

List of Contributors

Michael Baraitser Consultant in Clinical Genetics, Great Ormond Street Hospital for Children, London WC1N 3JH, UK.

Donal Brosnahan Consultant Ophthalmologist, Department of Ophthalmology, The Royal Hallamshire Hospital, Glossop Road, Sheffield S10 2JF, UK.

Nicholas Cavanagh Consultant Paediatric Neurologist, Chelsea and Westminster Hospital, 369 Fulham Road, London SW10 9NH, UK.

J. Richard Collin Consultant Ophthalmologist, Moorfields Eye Hospital, City Road, London EC1V 2PD, UK.

Susan H. Day Ophthalmologist, 2340 Clay Street, Suite 100, San Francisco, California 94115, USA.

John Elston Consultant Ophthalmologist, The Radcliffe Infirmary, Woodstock Road, Oxford OX2 6HE, UK.

Kevin Evans Senior Registrar, Moorfields Eye Hospital, City Road, London EC1V 2PD, UK.

Alistair Fielder Professor of Ophthalmology, Western Eye Hospital, Imperial College School of Medicine at St Mary's, Marylebone Road, London NW1 5YE, UK.

Allen Foster Department of Epidemiology, Institute of Ophthalmology, Bath Street, London EC1V 9AL, UK.

Brenda Gallie Professor of Ophthalmology Department of Ophthalmology, Hospital for Sick Children, The University of Toronto, 555 University Avenue, Toronto, Canada M5G 1X8.

Clare Gilbert Department of Preventative Ophthalmology, Institute of Ophthalmology, Bath Street, London EC1V 9EL, UK.

William V. Good University of Cincinnati, Department of Ophthalmology, 350 Health Professions Building, Cincinnati, Ohio 45267-0527, USA.

Christopher Harris Senior Lecturer, Institute of Child Health, and Great Ormond Street Hospital for Children, London WC1N 3JH, UK.

Creig S. Hoyt Professor of Ophthalmology, Department of Ophthalmology, University of California, 400 Parnassus Avenue, Room 702-A, San Francisco, California 94143, USA.

Hanne Jensen Department of Ophthalmology, Herlew Hospital, Öjenklinikhen, Bank Mikkelsensug 1, 2820 Gentofte, Denmark.

Anthony Kriss Department of Ophthalmology, Great Ormond Street Hospital for Children, London WC1N 3JH, UK.

Scott Lambert Associate Professor, The Emory Eye Centre, Emory University, 1365B Clifton Road NE, Atlanta, Georgia 30322, USA.

R. Jane Leitch Consultant Ophthalmologist, Sutton Hospital, Cotswold Road, Sutton, Surrey SM2 5NF, and honorary consultant Great Ormond Street Hospital, London WC1N 3JH, UK.

Jean-Pierre Lin Paediatric Neurologist, Newcomen Centre and Gait and Movement Laboratory, Guy's Hospital, St Thomas's Street, London SE1 9RT, UK.

Christopher Lyons Consultant Ophthalmologist, Department of Ophthalmology, BC Children's Hospital, 4480 Oak Street, Vancouver, British Columbia, Canada V6H 3V4.

Hans Ulrik Møller Consultant Ophthalmologist, Eye Department, University Hospital, DK 8000 Århus, Denmark.

Anthony Moore Consultant Ophthalmic Surgeon, Ophthalmology Department, Addenbrooke's Hospital, Hills Road, Cambridge CB2 2QQ, UK.

Robert Morris Consultant Ophthalmologist, Southampton Eye Unit, Tremona Road, Southampton, Hampshire SO16 6YD, UK.

Andrew S. Narita Consultant Ophthalmologist, The Royal Children's Hospital, Melbourne 3052, Australia.

R. David Reynolds Attending Physician, Wills Eye Hospital, Philadelphia, Pennsylvannia 19107, USA.

Jack Rootman Professor of Ophthalmology and Pathology, Department of Ophthalmology and Pathology, University of British Columbia, 2550 Willow Street, Vancouver, British Columbia V52 3N9, Canada.

Isabelle Russell-Eggitt Consultant Ophthalmologist, Great Ormond Street Hospital for Children, London WCIN 3JH, UK.

Martin Snead Consultant Ophthalmic Surgeon, Addenbrooke's Hospital, Hills Road, Cambridge CB2 2QQ, UK.

Lynne Speedwell Senior Optometrist, Great Ormond Street Hospital for Children, London WC1N 3JH, UK.

Ann Stout Assistant Professor of Ophthalmology and Pediatrics, USC School of Medicine, Children's Hospital of Los Angeles, 4650 Sunset Boulevard, Los Angeles, California 90027, USA.

David Taylor Consultant Ophthalmic Surgeon, Great Ormond Street Hospital for Children, London WC1N 3JH, UK.

Dorothy Thompson, Clinical Vision Scientist and Honary Lecturer, Great Ormond Street Hospital for Children, London WC1N 3JH, UK.

Elizabeth Thompson Consultant Clinical Geneticist, Centre for Medical Genetics, Women's and Children's Hospital, 72 King William Road, North Adelaide, South Australia 5006, Australia.

Andrew Webster Specialist Registrar, Department of Ophthalmology, Addenbrooke's Hospital, Cambridge CB2 2QQ, UK.

Foreword to the First Edition

Many years ago my 6-year-old son and his classmates attended their first performance of the Washington Symphony Orchestra; an extracurricular activity intended to introduce children to classical music. That evening in response to my inquiry about his day's unique experience he looked at me with sadness in his eyes and replied, 'But dad, they play such long songs.' Were this lad asked to comment about this text authored by Taylor and colleagues I suspect a similar response would be evoked perhaps — 'it is such a long story.'

Nearly all specialties in medicine and surgery share a natural division of their discipline into pediatric and geriatric portions. Ophthalmology is no exception to this generalization since the bulk of its pathology occurs either in pediatric or geriatric patients. Moreover, each age group has special ophthalmic care delivery needs with a special type of support from the physician and technical personnel in the specialties surrounding ophthalmology and unique facilities to render appropriate diagnostic and therapeutic methods. Also texts written for one group must differ from texts written for the other in order to include the relevant material and exclude the irrelevant. But the range and volume of material to be included in a text written either for pediatric ophthalmology or geriatric ophthalmology are comparable. A relatively complete text in either by necessity must be a long story.

The first text I recall written exclusively for pediatric ophthalmology was thirty years ago (Doggart 1959). Since then, as the subspecialties became established, the pace of new pediatric ophthalmology texts appearing on the market has broken into full stride. This is good, for the ultimate beneficiaries of this trend are our patients. This trend provides maximal opportunity to us who must learn or constantly review the multitude of details required for delivering quality care. We are fortunate to be surrounded by such a plethora of excellent minds with so many motivated physicians willing to collect and organize all the material for us.

The contrast is striking between Doggart's text (1959) and Taylor *et al.*'s (1990) text on pediatric ophthalmology. One is thin, the other is thick. The quantity of information imparted in the thick one is amazing. Is this difference in thickness between the two texts due solely to the amount of new knowledge that has been revealed during the past thirty years? I am afraid the answer is yes. At the time of my entry into pediatric ophthalmology in 1947, the total knowledge developed in this subspecialty was even less than that contained in Doggart's thin text. Prior to 1950 only a very few ophthalmologists had any idea that the subspecialty was needed and none appreciated the importance of the role it was destined to play in relationship to the flowering of the multiple subspecialties in either pediatrics or ophthalmology.

During the century prior to 1950 every advanced nation evolved special care facilities and health care delivery systems for their children. Eventually ophthalmology would certainly become a part of this scheme. The start of ophthalmology's involvement was slow, but by 1959 the pace had quickened; training in the subspecialty had become structured and was sought. A text was needed and Doggart, an Englishman, delivered it.

The task of producing a text today which provides the reader with the entire knowledge relevent to our field has become almost insurmountable. The array of diseases that affect the visual system and the anatomy surrounding the eye is enormous. Add to this the advent of the rapidly advancing field of genetics, its annual revelations of new basic facts and newly categorized diseases and now one can sense the magnitude of the onrushing front of new knowledge that has to be cataloged and disseminated. From such a crowded knowledge base, the first decision an editor of a comprehensive text in our subspecialty must face is what to include and exclude. It would be much easier to continue the trend of publishing theme texts which focus on only one facet, such as genetics, strabismus, pediatric ocular oncology, pediatric glaucoma, etc. Such limited texts serve a purpose, but there is always the need for a comprehensive text covering the entire breadth of our specialty. To accomplish this mission in 1990 requires a thick book. Taylor and his associate authors have succeeded in this mission by bringing us their monumental treatise on pediatric ophthalmology.

The text is divided into seven parts using 84 chapters to record this long list of subjects. Almost every statement is

xi

backed up by a total of 3688 references spotted throughout this book and the comprehensive coverage of this broad subspecialty deserves a note of gratitude from each reader to each of the authors. It is a thick book with the melodious appeal of a symphony. It is a long song.

Marshall M. Parks MD

Reference

Doggart JH. *Diseases of Children's Eyes*. The CV Mosby Co., St Louis, 1959

Preface to the Second Edition

The success of the first edition was a surprise and a pleasure to all of its contributors, particularly because 'the Green Book' was often kept in the clinic as a source of immediate reference, to compare patients' conditions with those in the book and to demonstrate pictures of abnormalities to patients and parents.

In this edition we have increased the width and depth of coverage of our subject by adding several new chapters, many new illustrations and completely rewriting virtually all the chapters. Because of the importance of cerebral palsy in our society, and the frequency of eye complaints in affected children there is a chapter devoted to this subject alone, in order to give ophthalmologists, should they wish, a grounding in this vital area.

We have again tried to highlight the paramountcy of clinical skills and the importance of first making a clinical diagnosis, whilst further emphasizing the power and usefulness of the new investigations. The primacy of a clinical approach to patients' problems, which are such subtle and complex interactions of disturbances of physiology, anatomy and psychology, must become more, rather than less, compelling as the investigations become more powerful.

The English language, and the spelling and grammar of the American and English forms of it, has given us some cause for thought. We have tried to avoid clearly unacceptable Anglicisms such as 'screwing up the eyes' (to think that we nearly had a chapter with that title in the first edition!), or Americanisms such as 'patient in the pediatric age group' (Child?) or OD, OU and OS (what's wrong with RE, BE, LE?). We feel that the readers of this book are likely to be able to accept easily an amalgam.

So many people have given generously of their time and skills to this edition that I cannot mention them all, but some deserve special thanks. Angela Tank and Jo Wilby gave invaluable advice and assistance with the manuscript and they honed-up my wordprocessing skills to their current still tenuous level. Simon Brown, and more recently Jeremy Nayler and the team in the medical illustration department at Great Ormond Street Hospital continued cheerfully to provide the excellent work that forms the vast majority of the illustrations. Kling Chong, Brian Lake, Hans Møller, Tony Vivian, Isabelle Russell-Eggitt and many others helped with advice, and Colin Richardson drew the cover figure which originally was the logo for 'Help a Child to See'. Many people contributed to Chapter P30, Support Groups, and I am especially grateful to them; without their work the accurate compilation of this type of international chapter would have been impossible.

Our work at Great Ormond Street, which drew our attention to the need for this book, has been generously supported by The Iris Fund, The Ulverscroft Foundation and Help a Child to See, amongst many others.

As time goes by one inevitably collects more friends and mentors and I would like to acknowledge particularly Michael Sanders, June Lloyd and Roland Levinsky. I cannot fail to mention my colleagues at Great Ormond Street and the many others who have referred the patients who were the inspiration for this book.

I must especially thank Rebecca Huxley of Blackwell Science: she has again made my load light by the speed, precision and style of her work and the good humour with which she does it! I would also like to thank David Gardner for the reproduction of the illustrations, Karen Anthony and Robert Hine for their meticulous work on the manuscript and proofs, and Karin Woodruff for her endless patience when compiling the index.

The second edition has taken 3 years of my weekends, evenings and some holidays; this has given me a great deal of interest and some pleasure but has been dependent on the generosity of my friends and family — Matt (who also guided my fumblings with computers and word processing) and Nick, but mostly my lifelong love and friend Anna.

DAVID TAYLOR

Preface to the First Edition

We have aimed to make this book a combination of a useful referenced text for referral and a practical clinical guide to paediatric ophthalmology.

Paediatric ophthalmology has changed greatly in ten years and this book aims to reflect the change. The thrust of the change has been due to the greater interest that ophthalmologists have developed in the care of the whole child and in medical as well as surgical care. In my experience this worldwide change has been spurred by demand from paediatricians with sick children with eye problems and where eye signs form vital diagnostic clues. The ophthalmologist has responded by arming himself with not only vital knowledge about strabismus, cataracts and other eminently treatable eye conditions but also with the wider fields of medicine which have expanded so much in the decade. This has the dual benefit to the paediatric ophthalmologist that he has become highly specialized in the care of a tiny, but vital, organ and he is one of the few ophthalmologists who can justify being a real generalist dealing with conditions as widely diverse as orbital disease and metabolic disease, strabismus and neuroophthalmology. We also have to thank our paediatrician colleagues for showing us how to approach the child and his problems. I believe that the child has benefited from these changes.

We have achieved an international flavour by close Anglo-American and Russian collaboration. This has been very rewarding and reflects the nature of post-graduate education that was achieved by the imagination and effort of the contributors, not by government sponsorship—long may we be able to continue to help each others' apprentices for the widening and deepening of their training!

We have tried to avoid overlap of subjects by careful planning, editing and indexing but some overlap is inevitable and deliberate to avoid the need to jump around the book too much. Individual subjects have not been treated in excessive depth in most areas, but references have been provided for the reader with greater curiosity.

The problems in the appendix have been included to help the clinician to find a way through the process of diagnosis. Most of the sections provide only guidelines and their use should be supplemented by reading appropriate areas of the main text.

Sexism creeps into any publication and we have not done much to avoid it other than by using a liberal mix of him and her when referring to babies. We were unable to stomach the use of generic pronouns (shem, shim, thon, na, per, hir, himorher, himmer) although we endorse Burkhart's (1987) principles of non-sexist writing!

The spelling of the title of this book is a pragmatic response to a majority view; we expect that anyone who has been so meticulous as to read the Preface as far as this will judge the work more on its content than its packing!

The photographs have come mainly from my own collection with occasional ones lent by kind colleagues who are acknowledged in the legends. The purpose has been to illustrate pertinent points in the text rather than to form an all-encompassing collection, on the one hand, or to initiate the beginner in the basics of paediatric ophthalmology, on the other hand.

Surgery is not learnt from books and we have confined ourselves to surgical principles and indications. The best place to learn surgery is in the operating room or theatre guided by surgical texts and papers.

Aspects of genetics have been dealt with in a general section by Baraitser and Thompson and some details are given in each relevant section. In genetics lies not only the future of so much paediatric ophthalmology but it is also a fascinating and rewarding area for study with enormous benefits to families.

I would like to express my personal gratitude to my friends and mentors, particularly to Bill Hoyt, Kenneth Wybar, Marshall Parks, Otto Wolff and Stephen Miller who have enriched and enlarged my view of ophthalmology.

DAVID TAYLOR

Reference

Burkhart S. Sexism in medical writing. *Br Med J* 1987; **295**: 1585.

Section 1
Epidemiology, Growth
and Development

1: Epidemiology of Visual Impairment in Children

Allen Foster and Clare Gilbert

Epidemiology is defined as the quantitative assessment of the distribution, determinants and control of disease in populations. In this chapter four questions will be asked in order to discuss the epidemiology of visual impairment in children. These questions are:

1 What is the definition of visual impairment in children?
2 How many children have visual impairment — prevalence and incidence?
3 What are the causes of visual impairment in children?
4 How can the number of children with visual impairment be reduced?

Before addressing these questions, however, it is relevant to consider some of the difficulties encountered when collecting data on visual loss in children.

Methodological difficulties in data collection

Definitions

In various studies different definitions have been used, not only for the term 'visual impairment' but also for 'childhood'. The World Health Organization (WHO) defines childhood as 0–15 years inclusive. Some population-based studies have only examined preschool children, and other studies on the causes of childhood blindness have included children up to the age of 18 years.

The definition of what constitutes visual impairment in children also varies from study to study and country to country. WHO defines five categories of visual impairment (Table 1.1). In this chapter emphasis is placed on the epidemiology of severe visual impairment and blindness by WHO categories. It should be noted, however, that lesser degrees of visual loss, visual field defects or unilateral blindness can also result in significant visual disability to the individual child.

Assessment of visual function

There are difficulties in accurate assessment of visual function in children, particularly under the age of 2 years. A variety of methodologies have been used to assess the vision in very young children but there is need for further work on how these methodologies equate with visual function in later years. A significant proportion of children with severe visual impairment also suffer from other disabilities which complicates the accurate assessment of visual function.

Sources of data

Different methods of collecting data on the causes of severe visual impairment in children have been used. Each of these methods has its own disadvantages. Registration data, which are commonly used in industrialized countries, are often incomplete with underreporting (Wormald & Evans 1994). Registration data also have the problem of interobserver error as many different ophthal-

Table 1.1 WHO categories of visual impairment. Adapted from the 1975 revised edition of the WHO International Classification of Diseases, World Health Organization (1977).

Category of visual impairment	Visual acuity in better eye after correction
1 Visual impairment	<6/18–6/60
2 Severe visual impairment	<6/60–3/60
3 Blind	<3/60–1/60
4 Blind	<1/60–PL
5 Blind	NPL

PL: Light perception; NPL: No light perception.

mologists are involved in collecting the data. Population-based surveys are the best means of collecting accurate prevalence data. Few such surveys have, however, been conducted. Large samples are required for these studies because the prevalence of severe visual impairment in childhood is low. These studies are therefore expensive. For incidence data longitudinal cohort studies are required, which are again expensive and time-consuming.

Studies of children in blind schools have been used to investigate the causes of visual impairment. These studies allow a large number of severely visually impaired children to be examined in a short time by one observer, but they suffer from being non-representative as not all socioeconomic groups are equally represented. Children with additional handicap and preschool age children may also be underrepresented.

Definition

In this chapter childhood is defined as 0–15 years (unless otherwise stated) and emphasis is placed on the magni-tude and causes of severe visual impairment and blindness (corrected vision in the better eye of less than 6/60).

Magnitude

Prevalence

A report by WHO in 1992 on the prevention of childhood blindness estimated that worldwide there are 1.5 million severely visually impaired and blind (SVI/BL) children of whom approximately 1 million live in Asia, 300 000 in Africa, 100 000 in Latin America and 100 000 in the rest of the world (WHO 1992).

The prevalence of SVI/BL in different countries is given in Table 1.2. Although different methodologies and age groups have been used, one can see that the prevalence in children in European countries varies from 0.1 to 0.41 per 1000 children. Studies in Asia give prevalence figures of 0.63–1.09, and in Africa from 0.3 to 1.1 per 1000 children.

The prevalence of low vision (i.e. <6/18–3/60) is likely to be five to 10 times the figure for blindness. This has been demonstrated in various studies, for example, in Morocco the prevalence of blindness (<3/60) was 0.3 per 1000 children and the prevalence of low vision (<6/18–3/60) 3.8 per 1000 (WHO 1994).

Incidence

The incidence of severe visual impairment in children is unknown. The WHO report gave an estimated figure of 500 000 new cases per year of which at least 50% are believed to die in childhood because of the diseases causing loss of vision or because of the visual handicap itself. In England there are between 200 and 250 new blind regis-

Table 1.2 Prevalence of blindness and severe visual impairment in children in different countries.

Region	Country	Reference	Year	Prevalence per 1000 children	Age group (years)	Source of data
Europe	Iceland	Halldorsson & Bjornsson	1980	0.36	0–14	Survey
	England	RNIB	1985	0.10	0–4	Registration
	England	RNIB	1985	0.22	5–9	Registration
	England	RNIB	1985	0.23	10–14	Registration
	UK	Stewart-Brown & Haslum	1988	0.34	10	Cohort study
	Eire	Goggin & O'Keefe	1991	0.20	0–16	Estimate
	Scandinavia	Riise *et al.*	1992	0.15–0.41	0–15	Registration
Asia	Nepal	Brilliant	1981	0.63	0–14	Survey
	Bangladesh, rural	Cohen *et al.*	1985	0.64	0–5	Survey
	Bangladesh, urban	Cohen *et al.*	1985	1.09	0–5	Survey
Africa	Malawi	Chirambo *et al.*	1983	1.10	0–5	Survey
	The Gambia	Faal *et al.*	1986	0.70	0–19	Survey
	Benin	WHO	1991	0.60	0–15	Survey
	Morocco	WHO	1994	0.30	0–15	Survey

trations per year in the age group 0–15 years (Royal National Institute for the Blind 1985). In Canada the incidence of congenital blindness is reported as 3 per 10 000 live births (Robinson 1987).

Causes of severe visual loss in childhood

Different classifications have been used to describe the causes of visual loss in children. The anatomical classification defines the part of the eye which has been damaged leading to visual loss. Classification based upon the time of insult — prenatal (hereditary and intrauterine factors), perinatal and postnatal—has been used by some authors. This classification can be further subdivided giving specific known aetiological causes, e.g. rubella infection in the intrauterine period, vitamin A deficiency in the postnatal period, and so on.

A standard reporting form for SVI in childhood has recently been developed and published by the International Centre of Eye Health, London, and the WHO's Programme for the Prevention of Blindness (Gilbert *et al.* 1993). This form, together with its coding instructions, allows for standardized data collection on the causes of childhood blindness by anatomical and aetiological classifications. Studies using this form have shown marked geographical variations in the causes of visual loss in children in different parts of the world.

Europe and North America

Studies from the UK, Eire, Scandinavian countries and North America document the main anatomical causes of childhood visual loss to be retinal disease, optic atrophy and lesions of the higher visual pathways (Table 1.3). Hereditary retinal dystrophies and perinatal retinopathy of prematurity (ROP) account for the majority of the retinal causes. Lesions of the central nervous system are often associated with other handicaps and are due to a variety of causes, some of which are prenatal, and others which are caused by cerebral hypoxia and/or intracranial haemorrhage at or early after birth. Cataract is responsible for approximately 10% of cases. A variety of malformations and anomalies of the eye due to unknown aetiological factors are responsible for approximately one-third of cases. Genetic factors account for half of all cases with perinatal factors being responsible for at least one-quarter (Table 1.4).

Robinson has documented the trends in congenital and acquired blindness in children in Canada between 1945 and 1989 (Robinson *et al.* 1987; Robinson & Jan 1993). Congenitally acquired rubella has declined as a cause of childhood blindness in Canada since the early 1960s, probably due to the introduction of a rubella immunization programme. Lesions of the optic nerve, including optic atrophy and optic nerve hypoplasia, are becoming relatively more important. During the early 1950s ROP was the single most common cause, accounting for up to 50% of childhood blindness. There was a decline in the incidence of blinding ROP from 1955 to 1975 due to awareness of the risk of high oxygen levels. A gradual increase is again now being reported due to the increased survival of neonates with a birth weight of less than 1000 g.

Latin America

There are no data from population-based studies or registers in Latin American countries. The available data on causes are summarized in Tables 1.5 and 1.6. In the lower income countries of Latin America (e.g. Bolivia, Peru and Ecuador) visual loss from corneal scarring is an important cause, representing approximately 20% of all causes. However, in the more prosperous countries of the continent (e.g. Argentina, Chile and Uruguay) corneal blindness is rare, being similar to the proportion found in

Table 1.3 Anatomical classification of blindness and severe visual impairment in children in Europe and North America (%).

Country	Reference	Year	n	Cornea	Lens	Retina	Optic nerve	Glaucoma	Other
USA	Kahn & Moorhead	1973	*	2	13	33	9	0	43
Canada	Pearce	1975	1046	2	15	28	17	2	36
The Netherlands	Henkes	1975	735	1	13	39	20	3	24
Denmark	Rosenberg	1987	150	0	6	21	26	1	46
Scotland	Phillips *et al.*	1987	99	1	12	40	21	2	24
England	Dpt. Health	1991	235	0	4	28	20	1	47
Eire	Goggin & O'Keefe	1991	172	1	4	23	44	2	26
Nordic	Hansen *et al.*	1992	1059	1	5	36	30	0	28
Canada	Robinson	1987	576†	1	15	32	29	2	21
Canada	Robinson & Jan	1993	156‡						

* Blind registrations in 16 states 1970.

† 576 cases of 'congenital' blindness between 1945 and 1984.

‡ 156 cases of 'acquired' blindness between 1960 and 1989.

Table 1.4 Aetiological categories of blindness and severe visual impairment in children in Europe (%).

Country	Reference	Year	n	Hereditary	Intrauterine	Perinatal	Childhood	Unclassified
UK	Fraser & Friedman	1967	776	50	6	33	11	0
N Ireland*	Bryars & Archer	1977	486	51	11	11	5	22
Denmark	Rosenberg	1987	150	30	7	16	19	28
Scotland	Phillips et al.	1987	99	48	1	21	11	19
Eire	Goggin & O'Keefe	1991	172	16	4	27	13	40

* Individuals aged less than 20 years with visual acuity < 6/18.

Table 1.5 Anatomical classification of blindness and severe visual impairment in children attending schools for the blind in Latin America (%).

Country	Reference	Year	n	Cornea	Lens	Retina	Optic nerve	Glaucoma	Other
Uruguay*	(Martinez A)	(1986)	220	1	25	33	12	9	22
Jamaica	Moriarty	1988	108	5	39	15	18	15	8
Bolivia	Foster	1988	78	23	21	23	10	10	13
Peru	Rojas et al.	1990	202	18	12	25	8	12	15
Dominican Republic*	(Duerkson R)	(1991)	51	18	31	10	8	18	15
Argentina*	(Muriz S)	(1993)	573	1	8	51	10	6	24
Ecuador*	(Gilbert C)	(1994)	142	16	8	42	15	3	16
Chile	Gilbert et al.	1994	267	6	9	47	13	8	17
Columbia*	(Gilbert C)	(1994)	94	5	5	35	14	12	29

* Unpublished data.

Table 1.6 Aetiological categories of blindness and severe visual impairment in children attending schools for the blind in Latin America (%).

Country	Reference	Year	n	Hereditary	Intrauterine	Perinatal	Childhood	Unclassified
Chile	Gilbert et al.	1994	267	30	8	23	11	28
Ecuador*	(Gilbert C)	(1994)	142	39	4	17	15	25
Colombia*	(Gilbert C)	(1994)	94	22	11	14	10	42

* Unpublished data.

Europe. Retinal disease is an important cause, particularly in the more developed countries where ROP is increasingly emerging as an important problem (Gilbert et al. 1994). Other significant causes are cataract (10–20% of cases), and congenital glaucoma (10%). Moriarty, working in Jamaica, found that many cases of cataract and glaucoma were due to congenital rubella syndrome, which he estimated to be responsible for 22% of all cases of childhood blindness (Moriarty 1988).

Middle East

The results of studies conducted in the Middle East are summarized in Tables 1.7 and 1.8. Genetic diseases are particularly important (47–80%) in this part of the world where consanguinity is common. A changing pattern in childhood blindness has been documented in Saudi Arabia over the last 30 years with a reduction in the proportion of blindness due to corneal scarring from vitamin A deficiency and infections and a consequent increase in the proportion of childhood blindness from retinal diseases due to hereditary factors (Tabbara & Badr 1985). Cataract is responsible for 7–21% of cases and congenital glaucoma 0–19%. The reason for this wide variation is unknown.

Asia

A large study in India has documented that approximately 20% of childhood blindness is due to vitamin A deficiency (Rahi et al. 1995a) although there are marked variations from state to state. Congenital anomalies of the eye, particularly anophthalmos and microphthalmos, were found to be common and accounted for approximately 20% of cases. Other major causes were retinal dystrophies and cataract (Eckstein et al. 1995). ROP accounted for only three out of more than 1000 cases.

Within Asia the causes of childhood blindness differ

Table 1.7 Anatomical classification of blindness and severe visual impairment in children attending schools for the blind in the eastern Mediterranean region (%).

Country	Reference	Year	n	Cornea	Lens	Retina	Optic nerve	Glaucoma	Other
Cyprus	Merin *et al.*	1972	112	6	12	39	4	5	34
Lebanon	Baghdassarian & Tabbara	1975	203	5	18	32	18	6	21
Saudi Arabia	Tabbara & Badr	1985	170	26	21	20	11	0	22
Jordan	Al-Salem & Rawashdeh	1992	260	15	19	28	11	3	24
West Bank	Elder & de Cock	1993	173	3	7	52	9	12	17
Tunisia*	(Trabelsi A)	(1993)	73	4	21	37	8	19	11

* Unpublished data.

Table 1.8 Aetiological categories of blindness and severe visual impairment in children attending schools for the blind in the eastern Mediterranean region (%).

Country	Reference	Year	n	Hereditary	Intrauterine	Perinatal	Childhood	Unclassified
Cyprus	Merin *et al.*	1972	112	80	4	2	12	2
Lebanon	Baghdassarian & Tabbara	1975	203	77	1	2	20	0
Saudi Arabia	Tabbara & Badr	1985	170	60	2	1	30	7
Jordan	Al-Salem & Rawashdeh	1992	260	74	4	6	16	0
West Bank	Elder & de Cock	1993	173	55	1	2	5	37
Tunisia*	(Trabelsi A)	(1993)	73	47	0	1	16	36

* Unpublished data.

Table 1.9 Anatomical classification of causes of blindness and severe visual impairment in children attending schools for the blind in Asia (%).

Country	Reference	Year	n	Cornea	Lens	Retina	Optic nerve	Glaucoma	Other
India	Rahi	1995	1623	29	11	21	6	3	30
Sri Lanka	Eckstein	1995	226	11	17	22	7	6	37
Thailand/Philippines	Gilbert & Foster	1993a	244	22	15	20	7	6	30

Table 1.10 Aetiological categories of blindness and severe visual impairment in children attending schools for the blind in Asia (%).

Country	Reference	Year	n	Hereditary	Intrauterine	Perinatal	Childhood	Unclassified
India	Rahi	1995	1623	24	2	1	30	43
Sri Lanka	Eckstein	1995	226	35	4	0	5	56
Thailand/Philippines	Gilbert & Foster	1993a	244	16	2	16	26	40

from place to place depending on socioeconomic conditions and the availability of health-care services. Vitamin A deficiency and infections of the eye are more common in poorer areas, with hereditary conditions being important in those situations where consanguinity is common. ROP will probably be increasingly seen in the large cities as demonstrated in the study from Thailand and the Philippines (Gilbert 1993a). This is probably due to improvements in neonatal care resulting in higher survival rates of low birth weight babies. Tables 1.9 and 1.10 summarize recent studies from different countries in Asia.

Africa

The pattern of causes of childhood blindness in Africa is changing over time. Twenty years ago corneal scarring from vitamin A deficiency and measles was responsible for more than 70% of childhood blindness in East Africa. Recent data suggest that this figure is decreasing probably due to measles immunization although vitamin A deficiency still remains the important cause in many areas (Foster & Yorston 1992). In coastal West Africa where red palm oil (which is rich in vitamin A) is commonly used in cooking, corneal blindness is seen less commonly, with

Table 1.11 Anatomical classification of causes of blindness and severe visual impairment in children attending schools for the blind in Africa (%).

Country	Reference	Year	n	Cornea	Lens	Retina	Optic nerve	Glaucoma	Other
West Africa									
Nigeria	Sandford-Smith & Whittle	1979	104	69	3	11	5	4	8
Ghana/Togo/Benin	Gilbert & Foster	1993b	284	36	16	20	6	13	9
East/Southern Africa									
Ethiopia	Foster	1988	195	72	6	3	10	0	9
Tanzania	Foster	1984	72	67	18	4	3	1	7
Kenya*	(Wood M)	(1989)	783	24	12	26	14	4	20
Zimbabwe†	Schwab & Kagame	1993	430	67	7	5	4	2	15
Malawi*	(Gilbert C)	(1994)	218	56	11	8	5	9	11

* Unpublished data.
† Includes 31 children with visual acuity of better than 6/60.

Table 1.12 Aetiological categories of blindness and severe visual impairment in children attending schools for the blind in Africa (%).

Country	Reference	Year	n	Hereditary	Intrauterine	Perinatal	Childhood	Unclassified
West Africa								
Ghana/Togo/Benin	Gilbert	1993b	284	21	8	3	34	34
East/Southern Africa								
Malawi*	(Gilbert C)	(1994)	218	11	1	1	60	27

* Unpublished data.

cataract and glaucoma being proportionally more important. It is interesting to note that the proportion of childhood blindness due to cataract and glaucoma is highest in West Africa and in the Caribbean Islands (Jamaica and Dominican Republic). This may be due to hereditary factors. Retinal diseases and optic atrophy are less important causes of childhood blindness in Africa (Tables 1.11 and 1.12).

Overview

In summary therefore there are marked variations in the magnitude and causes of SVI/BL among regions of the world, and among places within individual countries of those regions. Also the relative importance of different causes changes over time as the socioeconomic condition of the country, and particularly the delivery of primary health care improves.

In the poorest countries of the world vitamin A deficiency, often in association with measles and diarrhoea, remains the single most important cause of childhood blindness (WHO 1992). In the intermediate countries corneal blindness is still seen but is relatively less important and cataract and glaucoma become proportionately more significant. In the urban centres of these inter-

mediate countries ROP is increasingly seen, as neonatal services improve with a consequent increase in the survival rate of low birth weight babies. In the developed world genetic causes are the most important cause of registration in children. Optic atrophy and lesions of the higher visual pathways due to perinatal cerebral hypoxia and other causes are often associated with multiple disabilities as well as visual loss.

Control of childhood visual impairment

The prevention of visual loss in children can be considered at three levels. Primary prevention involves preventing the occurrence of diseases which may lead to loss of vision, e.g. measles immunization, or nutrition education to avoid vitamin A deficiency. Secondary prevention involves the management of established disease in order to prevent the development of visual loss. Examples are the treatment of ophthalmia neonatorum to prevent corneal ulceration and scarring, the diagnosis and management of threshold ROP. Tertiary prevention of blindness involves the management of diseases causing visual loss in children with a view to restoring vision. Examples include cataract surgery and correction of aphakia, and the provision of low vision devices and services.

In order to prevent visual impairment in children it is necessary to identify at an early stage those children at high risk in order to take appropriate early action to manage the condition.

Screening

The term 'screening' should strictly be used to describe programmes which use a simple, non-invasive and inexpensive test to identify individuals with subclinical disease who can benefit from specific interventions. Screening programmes are usually targeted at high-risk groups. However, the term is often used loosely to describe other methods of detecting disease.

Early identification of infants and children with ocular abnormalities and visual impairment is important. First, because early management of treatable conditions such as congenital cataract and glaucoma favourably influences the visual outcome; and second, because appropriate intervention can prevent or minimize the psychomotor developmental delay which often accompanies severe visual loss of early onset.

To detect ocular abnormalities and visual impairment in children the following steps are recommended.

Examination of the newborn

The eyes and adnexa of all newborn babies should be examined shortly after birth. A simple examination with an ophthalmoscope to examine the external eye, pupillary reflexes and the red reflex may detect obvious structural abnormalities such as microphthalmos, congenital cataract, buphthalmos and iris coloboma. These examinations are usually undertaken by paediatricians and neonatologists and clear guidelines need to be given on which cases to refer, and to whom the child should be referred.

Screening of low birth weight babies for retinopathy of prematurity

As cryotherapy has recently been shown to favourably influence the anatomical and functional outcome of stage 3+ ROP, low birth weight babies should be screened for treatable, threshold disease (Cryotherapy for ROP Cooperative Group 1990). The aim of screening is to detect stage 3 ROP which may require treatment, or ROP which has the potential to reach stage 3. Babies at risk of severe ROP are those weighing less than 1500 g at birth and those born at less than 32 weeks gestation (College of Ophthalmologists 1990). The first examination should take place 5–7 weeks after birth and examination should be repeated every 1–2 weeks until the infant has reached 36 weeks gestational age; or until there are definite signs of regression; or until the nasal retinal periphery is completely vascularized. Infants with threshold disease should have laser photo-coagulation or cryotherapy to the avascular retinal periphery (see Chapter 43).

Examination of high-risk groups

Children born to families with genetic disease, such as retinoblastoma, familial cataract or aniridia, should be examined and investigated so that appropriate interventions can be initiated early. Identification is also important for the parents, so that they can be informed of the likely prognosis, and for the children themselves so that they can receive genetic counselling at an appropriate age.

Children with certain systemic diseases where there is a high risk of eye disease (such as uveitis in children with Still's disease) should also be examined on a regular basis.

Preschool screening

In countries with good primary health-care systems it is likely that children with major structural abnormalities and/or severe visual impairment will already have been identified by the age of 2–3 years. This is because either those responsible for their care noticed a problem, or because the abnormality was detected by health-care workers during routine examination in well baby or child clinics (Yu-Dong *et al.* 1990).

Accurate measurement of visual acuity in preschool age children is difficult and unreliable, leading to difficulties in the identification of children with unilateral or bilateral visual impairment due to refractive errors, amblyopia or less obvious structural abnormalities (such as retinal lesions, optic nerve disease or media opacities). Screening of preschool age children, although desirable as early identification and treatment of amblyogenic factors may favourably influence the final outcome, raises several contentious issues. One area of debate concerns the lack of agreement on an appropriate methodology for detecting amblyogenic factors. For children aged 3–4 years visual acuity measurement may be possible, but for younger children other methods are needed. Refraction (Hopkisson *et al.* 1992), cover tests, tests of stereopsis, and a variety of photorefractive methods have all been evaluated. In order not to miss true positive cases, and not to overload referral centres with false positives the screening test must have high levels of sensitivity and specificity. The issues over who should undertake the screening, and the cost-effectiveness of preschool age screening programmes have not yet been resolved.

School screening

Most industrialized countries have vision screening programmes for 5–6 year olds which forms part of a general assessment. These programmes provide a valuable safety net to identify children with visual or refractive problems although the skill of the tester and the uptake may reduce the effectiveness of the programme (Allen & Bose 1992; Jewell *et al.* 1994). In developing countries, or in situations with poor primary health care, visual acuity screening of school age children assumes greater importance. Vision screening programmes, often undertaken by teachers trained for the task, are being introduced in some developing countries, such as India.

Overview of screening

The purpose of any screening programme is to detect disease early, using simple tests. Those who fail the screening test must be referred for confirmation of the diagnosis so that effective treatment can be instituted. The following all need to be considered:

1 the seriousness and frequency of the disease in the population;

2 the consequences of a delay in treatment;

3 the risks and benefits of the screening procedure and the intervention; and

4 the feasibility and cost-effectiveness of the screening programme.

The following criteria should be fulfilled for screening programmes:

1 The condition must be a significant health problem to the individual or community.

2 The natural history of the condition must be known.

3 A latent or preclinical phase must exist.

4 An effective treatment must be available.

5 The screening test should be simple, inexpensive, non-invasive and acceptable.

6 The screening test must be valid, with reasonable levels of specificity and sensitivity.

7 Full diagnostic and therapeutic services must be available.

8 Early intervention must favourably influence the outcome.

9 The screening programme should be cost-effective.

10 The screening programme should be continuous.

Although a screening programme may seem to be worthwhile (Fulton 1992; Lichter 1992; Stayte *et al.* 1993) it must be remembered that it is screening, not the full examination of children. Thus cases are bound to be missed by the very nature of the diseases screened for, the training of the screeners and the tests employed (De Becker *et al.* 1992). Factors such as who does the screening, the availability of local resources for the cases detected and what tests are used all have a significant bearing on making the programme cost-effective.

Table 1.13 Avoidable causes of severe visual impairment and blindness in children attending schools for the blind in different regions of the world (%).

	Africa		Asia			Latin America	
Country	Malawi	W. Africa	Thailand/Philippines	India	Sri Lanka	Chile	Ecuador
n	218	284	244	1318	226	267	142
Reference	(Gilbert C)*	Gilbert	Gilbert	Rahi	Eckstein	Gilbert	(Gilbert C)*
Year	(1994)	1993b	1993a	1995	1995	1994	(1994)
Preventable conditions							
M/VAD/TEM	51	29	19	23	2	0	2
Rubella	0.5	7	2	1	3	6	0
Toxoplasmosis	0	0	0	0	0	0	2
Cerebral malaria/meningitis	2	0	0	4	1	0	0
Ophthalmia neonatorum	0.5	3	6	1	0	2	2
Others	5	0	6	2	6	9	3
Subtotal	58%	39%	33%	31%	12%	17%	9%
Treatable conditions							
ROP	0	0	11	0	0	18	14
Cataract	10	10	8	12	12	7	8
Glaucoma	4	13	6	3	6	6	3
Others	0	8	2	1	0	0	0
Subtotal	14%	31%	27%	16%	18%	31%	25%
Total avoidable	72%	70%	60%	47%	30%	48%	34%

* Unpublished data.

M/VAD/TEM, measles/vitamin A deficiency/traditional eye medicines; ROP, retinopathy of prematurity.

Avoidable causes of visual impairment in children

The term avoidable is used to encompass those conditions which are readily preventable or treatable. Table 1.13 summarizes the major avoidable causes of childhood blindness in different parts of the world. Between 30 and 75% of all childhood blindness is avoidable. The major preventable conditions are vitamin A deficiency, measles, ophthalmia neonatorum and certain autosomal dominant conditions. The important surgically treatable conditions are congenital cataract, ROP and glaucoma.

Besides these avoidable causes many children with SVI/BL can be helped to read normal print using low vision devices, for example stand magnifiers. The ability to read print instead of learning Braille is important, enabling full integration into educational and vocational training programmes, and in improving the independence and quality of life of the child with visual handicap. The assessment, prescription and motivation of children to use low vision devices is a specialized area which needs more attention and development, not only in industrialized countries but particularly in the poorer countries of the developing world.

Conclusion

Of the estimated 1.5 million children with SVI/BL in the world approximately one-third is due to corneal scarring from preventable conditions such as vitamin A deficiency, measles, the use of harmful traditional eye medicines and ophthalmia neonatorum. Treatable congenital cataract is responsible for 10–20%. ROP is an increasingly important cause in the large cities of the intermediate and newly industrialized countries of the world. Hereditary disease and factors operating in the perinatal period are the major causes in Europe and the Western world. It is estimated that at least 50% of all cases of childhood blindness are avoidable through the provision of preventive services at the community level, specialized surgical services in paediatric ophthalmic units and the provision of low vision devices and services to those children with established visual loss.

References

Allen J, Bose B. An audit of preschool vision screening. *Arch Dis Child* 1992; **67**: 1292–3.

Al-Salem M, Rawashdeh N. Pattern of childhood blindness and partial sight among Jordanians in two generations. *J Paediatr Ophthalmol Strabismus* 1992; **29**: 361–365.3.

Baghdassarian SA, Tabbara KT. Childhood blindness in the Lebanon. *Am J Ophthalmol* 1975; **79**: 827–30.

Brilliant GE (ed.). *The Epidemiology of Blindness in Nepal. Report of the 1981 Nepal Blindness Survey.* Seva Foundation, 1981.

Bryas JH, Archer DB. Aetiological survey of visually handicapped children in Northern Ireland. *Trans Ophth Soc UK* 1977; **97**: 26–30.

Chirambo MC, Tielsch JM, West KP *et al.* Blindness and visual impairment in southern Malawi. *Bull WHO* 1986; **64**: 567–72.

Cohen N, Rahman H, Sprague J, Jahl M, Leambujis E, Mitra M. Prevalence and determinants of nutritional blindness in Bangladeshi children. *World Health Statistics Q* 1985; **38**: 317–29.

College of Ophthalmologists. *Screening for Retinopathy of Prematurity. Report of Working Group, 1990.* College of Ophthalmologists, 1990.

Cryotherapy for Retinopathy of Prematurity Cooperative Group. Multicenter trial of cryotherapy for retinopathy of prematurity. One year outcome—structure and function. *Arch Ophthalmol* 1990; **108**: 1408–16.

De Becker I, MacPherson H, LaRoche G *et al.* Negative predictive value of a population-based preschool vision screening program. *Ophthalmology* 1992; **99**: 998–1003.

Department of Health. *Causes of Blindness among New Registrations Aged under 16 years, April 1987 to March 1990.* Statistical Bulletin, Vol. 3, No. 5. London: Department of Health, 1991.

Eckstein M, Foster A, Gilbert C. Causes of childhood blindness in Sri Lanka. *Br J Ophthalmol* 1995; **79**: 633–6.

Elder MJ, de Cock R. Childhood blindness in the West Bank and Gaza Strip: prevalence, aetiology and hereditary factors. *Eye* 1993; **7**: 580–3.

Faal H, Minassian D, Sowa S, Foster A. National survey of blindness and low vision in the Gambia: results. *Br J Ophthalmol* 1986; **73**: 82–7.

Foster A. Patterns of blindness. In: Duane TD, ed. *Clinical Ophthalmology*, Vol. 5. Harper & Row, 1984.

Foster A. Childhood blindness. *Eye* 1988; **2** (Suppl.): S27–36.

Foster A, Yorston D. Corneal ulceration in Tanzanian children: relationship between measles and vitamin A deficiency. *Trans Roy Soc Trop Med Hyg* 1992; **86**: 454–5.

Fraser GR, Friedman AI. *The Causes of Blindness in Childhood: a Study of 776 children with Severe Visual Handicaps.* Baltimore: Johns Hopkins, 1967.

Fulton A. Screening preschool children to detect visual and ocular disorders. *Arch Ophthalmol* 1992; **110**: 1553–4.

Gilbert C, Foster A. Causes of blindness in children attending four schools for the blind in Thailand and the Philippines—a comparison between urban and rural blind school populations. *Int Ophthalmol* 1993a; **17**: 229–34.

Gilbert C, Foster A, Negrel D, Thylefors B. Childhood blindness: a new form for recording causes of visual loss in children. *WHO Bull* 1993; **71**: 485–9.

Gilbert CE, Canovas R, Kocksch R, Foster A. Causes of blindness and severe visual impairment in children in Chile. *Dev Med Child Neurol* 1994; **36**: 334–43.

Gilbert CE, Foster A. Causes of childhood blindness: results from West Africa, South India and Chile. *Eye* 1993b; **7**: 184–8.

Goggin M, O'Keefe M. Childhood blindness in the Republic of Ireland: a national survey. *Br J Ophthalmol* 1991; **75**: 425–9.

Halldorsson S, Bjornsson G. Childhood blindness in Iceland. A study of legally blind and partially seeing children in Iceland 1978. *Acta Ophthalmol* 1980; **58**: 237–42.

Hansen E, Flage T, Rosenberg T, Rudanko S-L, Viggosson G, Riise R. Visual impairment in Nordic children. III Diagnoses. *Acta Ophthalmol* 1992; **70**: 597–604.

Henkes HE. Causes of severe visual impairment in children and their prevention. *Documenta Ophthalmol* 1975; **39**: 213–48.

Hopkisson B, Arnold P, Billingham B, McGarrigle M, Shribman S. Can retinoscopy be used to screen infants for amblyopia? A longitudinal study of refraction in the first year of life. *Eye* 1992; **6**: 607–9.

Jewell G, Reeves B, Saffin K, Crofts B. The effectiveness of vision screening by school nurses in secondary school. *Arch Dis Child* 1994; **70**: 14–18.

Kahn HA, Moorhead HB. *Statistics on Blindness in the Model Reporting Area, 1960–1970*, Public Health No. NIH 73-427. Washington DC: US Department of Public Health, 1973.

Lichter P. Editorial: vision screening and children's access to eye care. *Ophthalmology* 1992; **99**: 843–5.

Merin S, Lapithis AG, Horovitz D, Michaelsonn IC. Childhood blindness in Cyprus. *Am J Ophthalmol* 1972; **74**: 538–42.

Moriarty BJ. Childhood blindness in Jamaica. *Br J Ophthalmol* 1988; **72**: 65–7.

Pearce WG. Causes of blindness in 1046 children registered with the Canadian National Institute for the Blind 1970–1973. *Canad J Ophthalmol* 1975; **10**: 469–72.

Phillips CI, Levy AM, Newton M, Stokoe NL. Blindness in schoolchildren; importance of heredity, congenital cataract, and prematurity. *Br J Ophthalmol* 1987; **71**: 578–84.

Rahi J, Sripathi S, Gilbert C, Foster A. Causes of childhood blindness due to vitamin A deficiency in India. *Arch Dis Child* 1995a; **72**: 330–4.

Rahi J, Sripathi S, Gilbert CE, Foster A. Childhood blindness in India: causes in 1318 blind school students in 9 states. *Eye* 1995b; **9**: 545–50.

Riise R, Flage T, Hansen E, Rosenberg T, Rudanko S-L, Viggosson G. Visual impairment in Nordic children IV. Sex distribution. *Acta Ophthalmol* 1992a; **70**: 605–9.

Riise R, Flage T, Hansen E *et al.* Visual impairment in Nordic children 1. Nordic registers and prevalence data. *Acta Ophthalmol* 1992b; **70**: 145–54.

Robinson CG, Jan JE. Acquired ocular visual impairment in children 1960–1989. *Am J Dis Child* 1993; **147**:325–8.

Robinson CG, Jan JE, Kinnis C. Congenital ocular blindness in children, 1945–1984. *Am J Dis Child* 1987; **141**: 1321–34.

Rojas JR, Lavado L, Echegaray L. Childhood blindness in Peru. *Ann Ophthalmol* 1990; **22**: 423–5.

Rosenberg T. Visual impairment in Danish children. *Acta Ophthalmol* 1987; **65**: 110–17.

Rosenberg T, Flage T, Hansen E, Rudankio S-L, Viggosson G, Riise R. Visual impairment in Nordic children 11. Aetiological factors. *Acta Ophthalmol* 1992; **70**: 155–64.

Royal National Institute for the Blind. *Initial Demographic Study 1985. A Review of the Available Data on the Visually Disabled Population (by Shankland Cox)*. London: RNIB, 1985.

Sandford-Smith J, Whittle HC. Corneal ulceration following measles in Nigerian children. *Br J Ophthalmol* 1979; **63**: 720–4.

Schwab L, Kagame K. Blindness in Africa: Zimbabwe schools for the blind survey. *Br J Ophthalmol* 1993; **77**: 410–12.

Stayte M, Reeves B, Wortham C. Ocular and vision defects in preschool children. *Br J Ophthalmol* 1993; **77**: 228–32.

Stewart-Brown SL, Haslum MN. Partial sight and blindness in children of the 1970 birth cohort at 10 years of age. *J Epidemiol Comm Health* 1988; **42**: 17–23.

Tabbara KT, Badr IA. Changing pattern of childhood blindness in Saudi Arabia. *Br J Ophthalmol* 1985; **69**: 312–15.

World Health Organization. *Manual of the International Statistical Classification of Disease, Injuries, and Causes of Death*, Vol. 1. Geneva: WHO, 1977.

World Health Organization. Prevalence and causes of blindness and low vision, Benin. *Weekly Epidemiol Record* 1991; **66**: 337–44.

World Health Organization. *Prevention of Childhood Blindness*. Geneva: WHO, 1992.

World Health Organization. Prevalence and causes of blindness and low vision, Morocco. *Weekly Epidemiol Record* 1994; **69**: 129–31.

Wormald R, Evans J. Registration of blind and partially sighted people. *Br J Ophthalmol* 1994; **78**: 7334.

Yu-Dong W, Thompson JR, Goulstine DB, Rosenthal AR. A survey of the initial referral of children to an ophthalmology department. *Br J Ophthalmol* 1990; **74**: 650–3.

2: Normal and Abnormal Visual Development

Susan Day

The development of vision in infants is a difficult area to study since the process of seeing, as well as the evaluation of this process, encompasses ocular, central nervous system, and behavioural development. A baby's eyesight nevertheless represents the most important source of information about his or her new environment and is of vital developmental significance. Indeed, general development may be severely affected when visual perception is impaired.

The reader is referred to an excellent text which discusses visual development in exquisite detail: *Early Visual Development, Normal and Abnormal*, edited by Kurt Simons. This textbook includes contributions from both clinicians and basic scientists which detail the rapidly expanding knowledge in this field.

Neonatal vision

The visual system is relatively mature at birth. The first year of life represents a very dynamic period in vision development, and any pathology which impairs visual development has a long-standing impact. The visual system remains malleable at least for the first decade, and attention to this visual plasticity is paramount in the management of childhood eye problems.

When questioned, parents are usually aware of their baby's visual development. Although traditional teaching suggests that the fixation and following reflexes are present at the age of 6 weeks, many parents will report that their baby sees at a much younger age. Parents will also observe a baby's fascination with brightly coloured objects, such as mobiles, rapidly moving objects such as fans, and fascination simply with the human face. In the event that their baby has poor vision, many parents are almost intuitive in their ability to discern that a problem exists.

Various anatomical and physiological factors influence the developing vision of an infant. Not only the eye's maturation, but also the central nervous system's growth and maturation must be considered.

Anatomical aspects

Prenatal development of the eye and brain occurs relatively early in comparison to other systems. By 6 weeks of gestation, the ocular structures and differentiation of the brain are fairly well developed. Teratogenic factors occurring within the first trimester commonly result in ocular defects. At birth, the anteroposterior diameter of the infant's eye is 70% that of an adult, measuring approximately 17 mm. The volume of the infant's eye, in contrast, is only 50% that of an adult's eye. Thus, differential growth of the eye occurs after birth. The anterior structures consisting of cornea, lens and iris are generally more completely developed than the posterior segment of the eye (Swan & Wilkins 1984).

Periorbital tissue also is relatively well developed at birth although some growth does occur after birth. The muscle insertions and their relationships to the limbus and equator change dramatically within the first year of life; such knowledge must be considered with regards to timing of strabismus surgery. It has been recommended that strabismus surgery not be performed prior to the age of 6 months because of the changing relative anatomical relationships (Swan & Wilkins 1984).

The inner layers of the eye also undergo further growth and differentiation after birth. Examination of neonatal monkeys has shown that differentiation of the fovea occurs relatively late in comparison to other regions of the retina (Hendrickson & Kupfer 1976; Hendrickson 1992) and may be incomplete until 4 months after birth in monkeys (Hendrickson & Kupfer 1976; Abramov *et al.* 1982; Hendrickson & Yuodelis 1984) and at 11–15 months in humans, continuing to 5 years (Hendrickson 1992). Clinically, one often sees a relatively dull foveal reflex which gains an added sense of dimension presumably due to thickening and the development of the internal limiting membrane within the first few months. The peripheral temporal retina does not achieve complete vascularization until 44 weeks of gestation. Due to the greater length between the optic nerve and temporal ora serrata compared to the nasal ora serrata, there is a predilection for abnormal vascularization in the temporal retina as in retinopathy of prematurity.

The optic nerve head itself is relatively full size at birth although there may be minimal postnatal growth. Clinical evidence of severe optic nerve hypoplasia implies a severe early insult occurring at 6–10 weeks gestational age; such a hypoplastic nerve has no significant potential for postnatal growth. Minor degrees of optic nerve hypoplasia may result from later prenatal influences.

In addition to the growth of the eye postnatally, the central nervous system is also maturing. Within the visual cortex the ocular dominance columns essential for the cortical integration of inputs from the two eyes are completely segregated at birth in both humans and monkeys (LeVay *et al.* 1978, 1980; Hickey & Peduzzi 1987) until 6 weeks postnatally (LeVay *et al.* 1980). Human anatomical studies have demonstrated an ongoing change in the number of visual cortex synapses until up to 8 months postnatally (Huttenlocher *et al.* 1982). The myelination of visual pathways, for instance, is not complete until 2 years of age (Magoon & Robb 1981). Control of eye movements may also be influenced by the development of supranuclear eye movement systems involving the cerebellar, brain stem, and vestibular input. It is probable that there are two pathways or streams through which information is taken from the retina through the occipital cortex (Atkinson 1992). The 'parvocellular' pathway carries colour, form and object discrimination through to the temporal lobes, and is active early in postnatal life. The magnocellular pathway is involved with disparity detection, fine discrimination of orientation and relative direction; it projects through to the parietal and frontal lobes.

Even before birth, the template for binocular vision is developing. This template has been experimentally interrupted in monkeys and cats by prenatal enucleation of one eye so that a comparison can be made to normal prenatal development and its influences on the anatomy of the visual system. Anatomical abnormalities at many levels have been found when prenatal binocularity is eliminated. First, the remaining eye retains more ganglion cells with their projections to the lateral geniculate nuclei (LGN) (Williams & Chalupa 1983; Rakic 1988). Second, the LGN shows only two rather than six laminae (Chalupa & Williams 1984). Third, the visual cortex receives expanded projections from the remaining eye (Rakic 1982; Williams & Chalupa 1983). These prenatal experiments show the importance of the presence of two eyes for the normal development of the pathways subserving binocular vision.

Physiological aspects

The development of normal function of the visual system, both sensory and motor, in large part parallels anatomical development. It is not surprising, for instance, that visual evoked potential (VEP) and forced preferential looking (FPL) data show rapid improvement of grating resolution in the first months of life when we recognize that foveal differentiation is incomplete at birth (Banks *et al.* 1988). The variation of binocular alignment (Nixon *et al.* 1985) during the first months of life may reflect orbital growth, ocular growth, and maturation of supranuclear eye movement control as well as improved acuity and binocular function. To isolate one particular system and study its role in changing functions becomes a very difficult task. Increasingly, this 'co-development' of sensory and motor functions has been acknowledged among infant vision researchers (Day & Norcia 1990).

Extrageniculostriate vision

A non-striate visual system seems to exist in non-human primates (Humphrey & Weiskrantz 1967), possibly via the lateral geniculate body (Weiskrantz *et al.* 1974) and this subcortical system may predominate in neonatal vision (Bronson 1974).

Clinical examples are often complicated by the necessary inexactness of defining the lesion, but some examples are interesting and may be convincing. Jan *et al.* (1986) described two cases in one of whom collicular vision provided enough for navigation and detection to make up for occipital loss. The other, who had more damage to association areas than primary visual areas, had good acuity but defective spatial and navigational skills.

Dubowitz *et al.* (1986) suggest that in early neonatal

vision, subcortical regions may play a significant role in vision behaviour. Premature infants were assessed behaviourally by their ability to track a red ball as well as with visual evoked responses (VER) and a version of preferential looking (PL). Infants were also assessed neurologically; cranial ultrasound and computed tomographic (CT) scans were also performed. Curiously, some infants with ultrasound or radiological evidence of occipital cortex abnormality had good initial visual function behaviourally as well as in the presence of a VER. One infant appeared to see initially despite postmortem documentation of an absent occipital cortex.

This occurrence of some, albeit abnormal, vision in infants with tomographic evidence of visual cortical absence or damage should make the clinician wary of making too dogmatic a prognosis in these cases (Summers & MacDonald 1990).

Normal visual development

The development of visual acuity in infants has been measured in various ways. The standard clinical techniques of 'fix and follow' response and the CSM (central, steady and maintained fixation) classification rely upon interpretation of motor responses. Early attempts to quantify visual acuity were made with optokinetic nystagmus testing in which stripes of varying size were passed in front of an infant's eye (Gorman *et al.* 1957; Dayton *et al.* 1964). The presence of induced optokinetic nystagmus implied the infant's ability to see the stripes. More recent efforts to quantify infant vision fall into two basic categories, psychophysical testing and electrophysiological techniques.

Psychophysical measurement

The most common psychophysical test is some variant of PL; it is often described as FPL. With psychophysical testing, interpretation of a child's ability to see is dependent upon a child's motor response. A child is given a choice of looking at a homogeneous target or at a target with gratings. When the child appears to see a large grating, subsequent test samples are performed with progressively finer grating size.

Measurements with this technique have suggested that an ability to resolve 20/100 equivalent gratings is present by the age of 1 year and 20/20 equivalent gratings by the age of 3 years (Teller *et al.* 1986) (Fig. 2.1). FPL techniques have been applied clinically to patients with strabismus, amblyopia and aphakia (Catalano *et al.* 1987). The 1–2-year age group appears to be most easily tested with this technique, but one must remember that the responses to the FPL test are always dependent on a movement, and may be defective for motor as well as visual reasons. Strictly speaking, there is no direct equivalence between

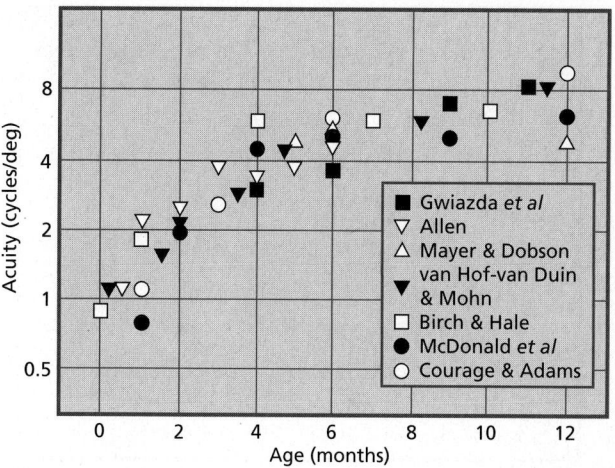

Fig. 2.1 PL: development of grating visual acuity as determined by PL techniques. Similar acuities are found across seven studies. Acuities are expressed in cycles per degree. From Dobson (1994).

Snellen acuity and FPL gratings which are measured in cycles per degree.

Electrophysiological measurement

The second method of measurement, electrophysiological testing, records infants' VEPs to projected gratings of various sizes; it is not dependent on eye movements. Both checker-board and stripe gratings have been used. The techniques of acuity estimation vary, and include reliance upon a signal generated by a series of quickly projected samples (Sokol 1978). Extrapolation of visual acuity on the basis of the VER to a rapidly changing grating size is known as the 'sweep' technique (Tyler *et al.* 1979), it is direct measurement in which acuity is estimated on the basis of responses. This technique implies the ability to resolve 20/20 gratings by the age of 6–8 months (Fig. 2.2).

The apparent difference in visual acuities between VEP and FPL quantification arises from the basic differences between electrophysiological and psychophysical testing. Application of both the FPL and the VER in infants has been helpful in establishing normal vision development. Application of either of these techniques to pathological conditions is far more difficult; the limitations are greatest in the very children in which we need this information. Bane and Birch (1992) found that FPL was more successful in bilateral moderate to severe visual impairment, but it must be emphasized that the skill and patience of the tester is paramount whatever the technique used.

Clinical application of preverbal vision quantification

Thus far, both PL and VEP quantification techniques have

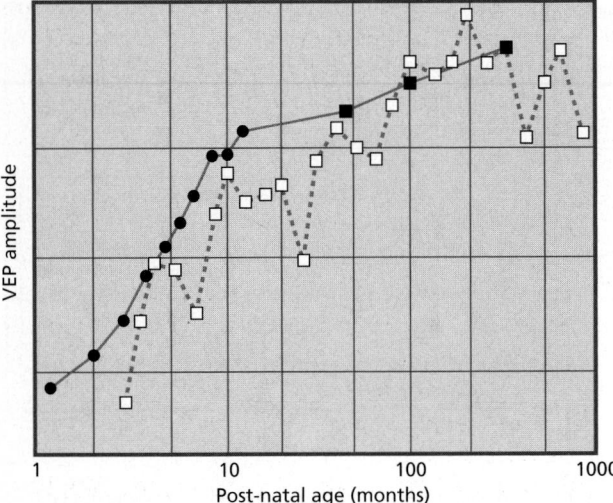

Fig. 2.2 VEP: development of grating visual acuity determined by sweep VEP techniques. Consistency of acuities is found in two studies, represented by filled versus open symbols. Development is rapid from birth to 8 months; a second slower growth phase persists through late childhood. From Norcia (1994).

assisted our knowledge of normal vision development in infant and preverbal toddlers. In centres where a large experience in these techniques has been gained, application has also been made to clinical circumstances such as the aphakic infant, the infant with retinopathy of prematurity, and the multiply handicapped child. Great caution should be exercised, however, in extrapolating this information, since these techniques are not equivalent to the task required for reading a Snellen chart. When levels of function are reported to referring physicians or to anxious parents, it is imperative to stress the difference inherent in the techniques. Declaration, for instance, of 'legal blindness' on the basis of techniques such as PL and VEP is inappropriate and inaccurate.

Other techniques have been used to measure maturity of the visual system in infants, including vernier visual acuity (Shimojo & Held 1987) and contrast sensitivity (Fig. 2.3). It should be emphasized that each of these techniques measures a very precise function. Attempts to correlate acuities obtained with these techniques directly to Snellen acuities are not appropriate. Thus, a mother who is told that her baby is seeing 20/80 by any given technique should not be led to believe that this will necessarily be the level obtained when her child is 15 years old. Rather than providing us with the precise number, these techniques have been helpful in research settings in documenting differences between the two eyes, improvement or worsening of vision, and an estimate of severe versus mild visual loss in comparison to other age-matched controls.

Binocular functions

Binocular visual development has been carefully assessed by research scientists. Its development has been assessed as individual functions, including stereopsis, fusion and ocular rivalry. Stereopsis relates to the visual system's ability to process information about depth perception as a consequence of simultaneous but slightly disparate images present to the two eyes. Fusion relates to the visual system's ability to combine similar and perhaps non-identical information from the two eyes into one image.

Stereopsis

Our understanding of the development of stereopsis was gained in early studies that assessed an infant's response to either real or illusory indicators of depth, or to an infant's ability to reach for an object (Bower 1971; Walters & Walker 1974). More recent studies for assessing stereopsis have adapted PL techniques (Held *et al.* 1980; Atkinson *et al.* 1982; Birch *et al.* 1982), eye movement analysis (Fox *et al.* 1980), and VEP techniques (Petrig *et al.* 1981; Norcia *et al.* 1985; Eizenman *et al.* 1989). Consistent findings, regardless of testing technique, place the development of stereopsis between 2 and 6 months of age. Interestingly,

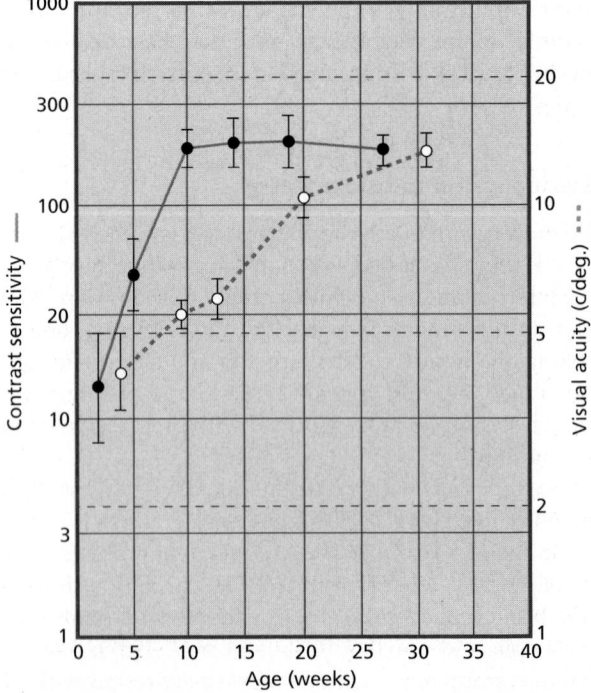

Fig. 2.3 Contrast sensitivity: development of contrast sensitivity (closed circles) as compared to visual acuity, using sweep VEP technology. Development is more rapid than that of acuity. From Norcia (1994).

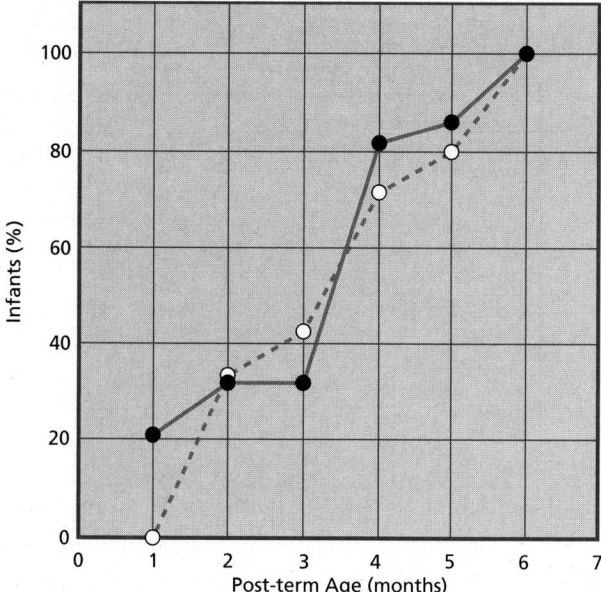

Fig. 2.4 Development of stereopsis (closed circle) and fusion (open circle) using PL techniques that provide one disparate image (stereogram) and one without disparity. Each system develops rapidly within the first 6 months. From Birch (1993).

this development is quite abrupt, with little maturation of the system occurring after the age of 6 months (Fig. 2.4).

Fusion

Our understanding of the development of fusion has also been expanded by tests employing PL (Birch *et al.* 1991) and VEP techniques (Petrig *et al.* 1981; Atkinson *et al.* 1991). Even though these functions are different from the cortical task for stereopsis, the timing of their development is very similar with the exception of one study, which found fusion to develop earlier than stereopsis (Eizenman *et al.* 1989). This parallel development has been regarded as a function of the development of the visual cortex (Birch *et al.* 1991). Accommodation and associated neurological reflex of convergence also deserve consideration. The ability of the lens to increase its power is very limited at birth but improves rapidly over the first 6 months of life (Haynes *et al.* 1965; Banks 1980; Brookman 1983) (Fig. 2.5). Convergence, whose function is to maintain bifoveal fixation on an object as its distance to the observer is reduced, increases in accuracy by the age of 6 months (Aslin 1977). The development of vergence, although a factor, does not appear to be the sole limiting factor for the development of binocular vision (Birch *et al.* 1982).

The final prerequisite for binocular vision relates to eye alignment. Without bifoveal fixation, binocular visual functions are impaired. Bifoveal fixation can be present only when the eyes are manifestly orthotropic. The

natural progression toward orthotropia has been ascertained in a large longitudinal study (Archer *et al.* 1989). Most normal infants are orthotropic by 3 months of age, but some do not achieve this until 6 months of age (Fig. 2.6).

Clinical assessment

Establishing normal levels of visual function is, despite research efforts to quantify them, still primarily one of observation of behaviour. Guidebooks for new parents will rightly tell them the baby should steadily fix on an object (such as their faces) by 6 weeks. In fact, many parents will volunteer that their babies were able to fix steadily within the first few days.

Specific guidelines for the neonatal examination have been made to help in the assessment of a baby's development. Although some tests are directly intended to assess a baby's vision, others designed to assess motor development are in fact vision-dependent, highlighting the key role that vision plays in the normal general development of a child. By 2 months, a following response should be present, and the baby should smile responsively to a parent. At 4 months, a child should reach for an object. At 6 months, a child plays with an object in his or her hand. Shortly after 1 year of age, a child begins to scribble with a crayon and point to desired objects (Swaiman & Wright 1975).

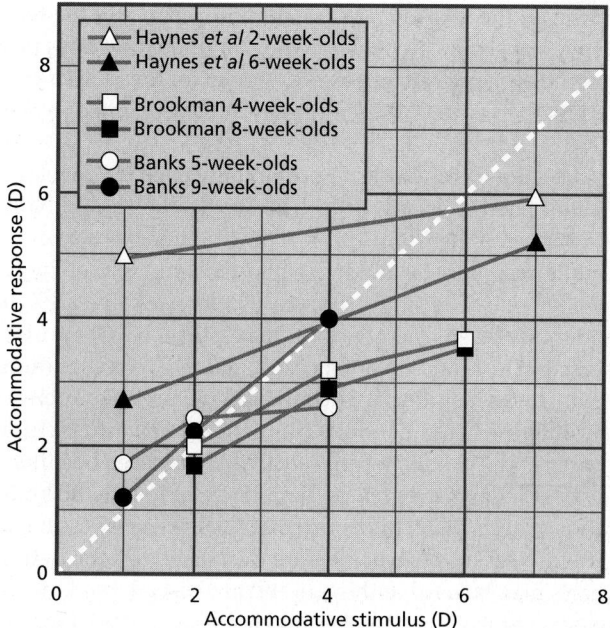

Fig. 2.5 Development of accommodation as determined by retinoscopy in three accommodation studies. Data suggest rapid development of this function by the age of 6 months. From Aslin (1993).

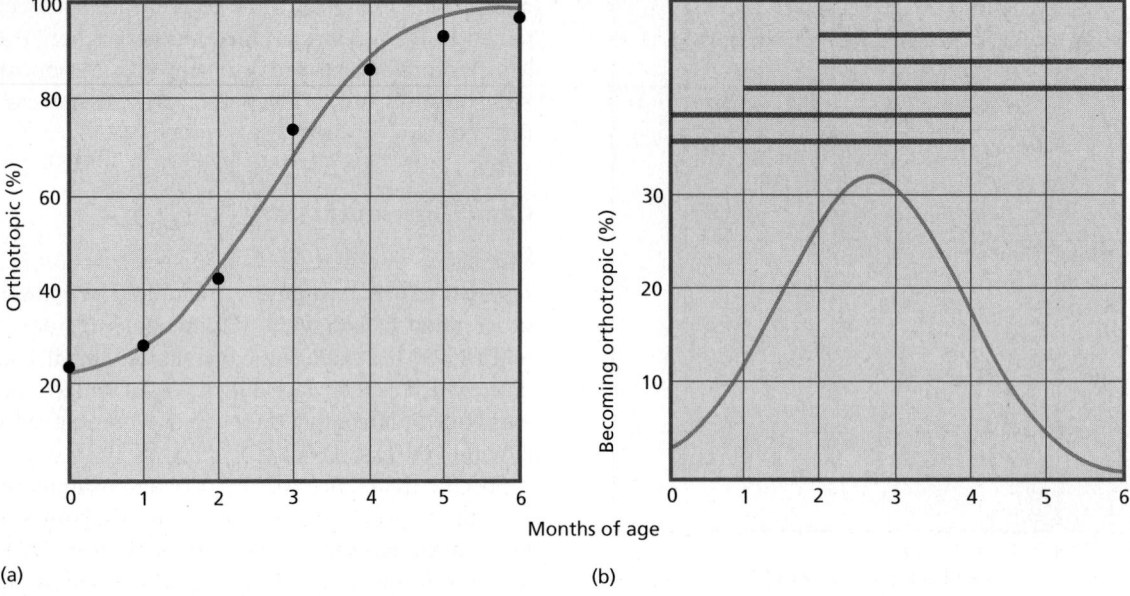

(a)

(b)

Months of age

Fig. 2.6 Development of orthotropia. (a) Percentage of infants with orthotropia at a given age; (b) age distribution for onset of orthotropia. Variation in onset of esotropia which was confirmed by examination of Archer is signified by horizontal bars depicting possible time course of onset for given individuals. From Archer (1994).

Assessment of vision in toddlers (McDonald 1986) becomes easier due to the child's ability to communicate. Although many clinicians rely too simply on fix and follow or CSM criteria (see Chapter 8) vision can be quantified without research techniques. One must remember, however, the shortness of the attention span and the tendency to become quickly bored by anything that does not resemble a game. Acuity tests designed for the toddler can be regarded as to the task which must be performed by the child.

Detection acuity tasks are commonly used by developmental paediatricians, especially the Stycar graded balls vision test (Sheridan 1973). The examiner observes a child's response to moving white balls of progressively smaller size. The Catford drum (Catford & Oliver 1973) and the dot visual acuity test (Kirschen *et al.* 1983) are also detection tests and do not measure acuity. The recognition acuity tasks include: (i) direction-orientated tasks such as the illiterate E and Landolt C; (ii) letter charts; (iii) picture charts; and (iv) Bailey–Hall cereal test. Of these, the illiterate E test enjoys the greatest popularity, although the limitation placed by a child's orientational skill makes this a difficult test to rely upon before the age of 3 years. Letter charts may be used at this age and are best adapted into a matching format where the child holds a key card. Picture charts including the lighthouse test (Grier 1973) and the Allen picture cards (Allen 1957) each have some limitation as a consequence of cultural and social differences among children. The Bailey–Hall cereal test uses breakfast cereal-like objects to entice a child's response (Bailey 1983).

Visual acuity norms in the 18-month to 3-year old child have been highly variable, depending not only on the type of testing (detection versus recognition versus resolution) but also on the particular research centre. Regardless of the type of test, there is a variation of one octave, that is a halving or doubling of spatial frequency, such as from 10′ arc to 5 or 20′ of arc: comparable to the difference between 20/20 and 20/40 and 20/80 vision (McDonald 1986). To the busy clinician, it appears that the best advice regarding norms in this age group is to gain familiarity with one or two of the available tests, gather one's own sense of what is normal, and pursue equivocal results with further testing and careful follow-up. Above all, any specific number obtained for a toddler's vision must be matched with the clinical story to give an interpretation of testing results.

Visual acuity norms in children aged 3–6 years have received attention from Simons (1983). He recommends the use of a single optotype test (such as Landolt C or HOTV) with a constant surround which is non-memorizable. Particular attention must be paid to the child's difficulty lateralizing, i.e. distinguishing between right and left, if an E optotype is used. A further recommendation is made to perform distance testing at 3 rather than 6 m. Specific visual acuity norms are largely dependent upon the type of optotype used (Simons 1983).

At the age of 4 years, most researchers have found 'normal' vision by Snellen testing to be between 20/20 and 20/40 (Slataper 1950; Romano *et al.* 1975; Simons 1983). A visual acuity of 20/20 is not reached by more than 70% of those tested until the age of 7 years (Simons 1983). The National Society to Prevent Blindness (1976) has established the following criteria for referral: (i) in 3–4 year olds 20/50 or less in either or both eyes by isolated symbols;

and (ii) in 5–6 year olds 20/40 or less in either or both eyes and/or an interocular acuity difference of one line on isolated symbols or two lines on linear presentations. Further guidelines for ophthalmological assessment as well as a review of current screening practices are given by Ehrlich *et al.* (1983).

Abnormal visual development

Critical period

The period of development in which experience plays an influential role has been termed by some as the 'sensitive' period (Blakemore & Van Sluyters 1974; Banks *et al.* 1975; Gottlieb 1976; Aslin 1981) and by others as the 'critical' period (Hubel & Livingstone 1987; Tychsen 1994). Historically, an understanding of the critical time period for visual development has been gained through observation of abnormal circumstances, be they experimental or clinical observation. Abnormal binocular vision development has served as a model for assessing developmental issues, in large part due to the classic experimentation in which monocular suturing of kitten lids resulted in a marked reduction of cortical cells that could subsequently be driven by a stimulus presented to the deprived eye (Wiesel & Hubel 1963a, b, 1965). These authors found the LGN response to be relatively normal, prompting them to suspect the geniculocortical pathways or the cortex itself to be the site of pathology (Wiesel & Hubel 1963a). In anticipation of more extensive physiological abnormalities as a consequence of doubling the amount of deprivation, the authors sutured the lids of both eyes over the same time course as the monocularly sutured kittens. To their surprise, the cortical recordings were far more accessible than anticipated (Wiesel & Hubel 1965). The responses had been altered from the norm, but not to the extent associated with unilateral closure. They concluded that 'at the cortical level the results of closing one eye depend upon whether the other eye is also closed. The damage produced by monocular closure may therefore not be caused simply by disuse, but may instead depend to a large extent on *interaction* of the two pathways' (Hubel & Wiesel 1965; emphasis added).

This early powerful research and its conclusions provided enthusiasm and a focus for the next generation of vision investigators. As so pointedly discussed by Jampolsky (1978), there unfortunately was a proliferation of laboratory research and conclusions that failed to pay attention to the methodology of the Wiesel and Hubel research. The kitten lid suture model provided a model for deprivation or diffusion of light to one eye which resulted in imbalanced inputs from the two eyes. Enough light could pass through the closed lid to create a diffused image for the 'deprived' retina. This was often accepted by others to be equivalent to the model of occlusion, or

absence of any input. The importance of this differentiation was most evident in the clinical model of occlusion for the treatment of amblyopia and in the reverse extrapolation of the clinical model of occlusion into animal studies in which lid suturing was used to simulate occlusion. Lid suturing is a dissimilar stimulus to the visual cortex than occlusion.

That a critical period exists for normal visual development is demonstrated clinically by studies of the child born with cataract and operated upon at several years of age. Despite clearing of the media, and even with proper optical correction, such a child has a permanent profound visual deficit.

The critical time period for development of normal infant vision when the insult is binocular appears to be within the first 3 months of life, i.e. with failure of a focused image such as with complete congenital cataracts. Clearing of the media and optical correction should be in place within the first few months of life in order to ensure vision which will allow a relatively normal life (Vaegan & Taylor 1979). From a practical standpoint, however, the clinician is rarely completely assured of what an infant's past visual experience has been. The benefit of the doubt must be given to the infant presenting with this clinical circumstance and treatment rendered as promptly as possible.

Before the infant becomes sensitive to deprivation there may be a brief 'period of grace' when events that would give rise to amblyopia in older children may leave the very young baby, less than a very few days or weeks old, unscathed. Thus neonatal macular haemorrhages may not lead to amblyopia (von Noorden & Khodadoust 1973), whereas later onset haemorrhages occurring in the sensitive period are often associated with reduced vision beyond that expected from any organic defect. This 'period of grace' may give the doctor and the parents of a neonate with cataract a few days before surgery is mandatory to achieve the best eventual vision, although a general rule is—the earlier the better.

In the most severe example of deprivation, a child with unilateral congenital cataract, it appears that the window of opportunity for successful treatment may be as short as from shortly after birth to 6 weeks. In long-term follow-up of children with congenital cataracts, acuity better than 20/40 is rarely obtained when surgery and optical correction is delayed beyond 2 months (Vaegan & Taylor 1979), although other reports have been far more encouraging (Beller *et al.* 1981; Robb *et al.* 1987). Epelbaum *et al.* (1993) reviewed the sensitive period for strabismic amblyopia in 407 children; the improvement in acuity was best before 3 years and zero after 12 years. Conversely, Klaeger-Manzanell *et al.* (1994) described a patient who underwent a two-stage improvement in acuity after loss of the 'good' eye—from 6/60 to 6/9!

At the centre of abnormal binocular visual development

is a difference between the two eyes which is present during the sensitive period for binocular vision development. Commonly, this difference is related to infantile esotropia. The difference between the two eyes is that the object of regard does not simultaneously stimulate the two foveas. Although each fovea is receiving some stimulus, the object of regard stimulates one fovea, a more peripheral object (in relationship to the object of regard) the other. Other abnormal, unequal inputs are related to the anisometropia (Donzis *et al.* 1983; Lovasik & Szymkiw 1985) or deprivation such as with a unilateral congenital cataract (Beller *et al.* 1981).

Plasticity of the visual system

The infant with a window of critical vision development is replaced by an individual with a more mature visual system. Its fragility, however, remains, and any new insult has the potential for impairing good vision (Von Noorden 1985). The plasticity of the visual system extends up to 12 years after birth. Any acquired abnormality such as strabismus or a traumatic cataract can result in altered visual development. Most clinicians have established a cut-off at 10–12 years in terms of any possible response to treatment aimed at recovering vision.

Abnormal visual development occurs whenever a clearly focused image on the retina is not maintained during the first months to years of life. The type of insult, be it poor focus (ametropia), poor 'aim' (strabismus) or media opacity, does not seem to be nearly as important as other critical factors including: (i) the age of onset; (ii) the severity of the insult; (iii) the age of initiation of treatment; (iv) compliance with treatment; and (v) the health of the fellow eye.

In general, the younger the onset, the more severely damaging is the insulting factor. This is especially true if the insult occurs within the first few months of life during the critical time period. For instance, a child with bilateral congenital cataracts must receive attention within the first few months of life if vision better than 20/40–20/60 is to be achieved. Clinically, the most difficult feature in this regard is determining the age of onset: parental observation, the position of the cataract, and the degree to which the media are opaque are indicators of a true congenital onset of the visual defect. A postnatal assessment of an abnormal red reflex or the presence of a microphthalmic eye are stronger indicators of an early onset visual defect. A congenital cataract, though present at birth, is not necessarily associated with a significant visual defect from birth (such as with a small anterior polar cataract) or at least not at all stages of its development; it is the onset of the visual defect that is the important factor and the most difficult to determine. As the child grows older the chances of developing amblyopia reduce, becoming very small after 6 years of age (Keech & Kutschke 1995). Amblyopia, of

varying but less severity, can develop in older children.

The severity of the insult also contributes to the prognosis. Significance is in part related to the location of the abnormality. An anterior polar cataract, far away from the nodal point of the eye, is unlikely to result in any significant visual disturbance whilst an opacity of similar size which is posteriorly placed may impair vision significantly.

The earlier appropriate treatment is started, the better the prognosis; compliance with treatment, such as with occlusion therapy, is also important. Finally, the status of the fellow eye appears to be a significant feature relating to permanent visual loss. Large differences between the two eyes appear to evoke a more extensive visual loss in the poorer eye. Some clinicians have argued that in conditions which are essentially unilateral such as monocular congenital cataract, treatment should include bilateral occlusion prior to completion of surgery and optical correction of the pathological eye so that asymmetrical development of vision does not occur (Cynader *et al.* 1976).

Amblyopia

Definition

When significant interruption of normal visual development occurs, then amblyopia is the term used to describe this loss of vision. Amblyopia, derived from the Greek word for 'dullness of vision', is usually unilateral; rarely bilateral amblyopia may occur and always implies a deprivation during the early months or years of life. Amblyopia is significant in that it is a potentially reversible condition. Although classic definitions stress that amblyopia is visual loss 'with no associated organic defect', in fact there is always an abnormality, be it strabismus, or isoametropia, anisometropia media opacity, which predisposes the eye or eyes to amblyopia.

Classification

Amblyopia is usually classified as to the type of associated pathology: most commonly the pathology occurs in one eye only. The most common type of unilateral amblyopia is strabismic amblyopia. Strabismic amblyopia is most commonly associated with esotropia although it can occasionally occur with exotropia as well. The amount of deviation cannot be correlated with the degree of amblyopia.

The second most common form of unilateral amblyopia is anisometropic amblyopia, in which a difference in refractive error in the two eyes results in poor visual development in one eye. Hypermetropic anisometropic amblyopia may occur when a difference of greater than 1 dioptre is present. Myopic anisometropia must be considered as a potential amblyogenic factor if a difference in excess of −3 dioptres is present. Astigmatic amblyopia, far less common, should be considered in terms of the sphere-equivalent of the two eyes. The resultant amblyopia may be meridional, i.e. at only one axis.

Deprivational amblyopia occurs monocularly whenever any imbalance in media clarity occurs between the two eyes, such as cataract, ptosis, corneal opacity, hyphaema, vitreous haze, occlusion amblyopia, or even the prolonged use of atropine.

Bilateral amblyopia occurs much more rarely. Deprivational amblyopia is the classic example, as in the infant with bilateral congenital cataracts. Isoametropic amblyopia occurs with bilateral refractive errors which are so severe as to prevent any clear image from forming on the developing retina. Hypermetropic isoametropia is of concern whenever the refractive error exceeds 4 dioptres, but is usually clinically relevant with refractive errors of 6 dioptres or more (Schoenleber & Crouch 1987). Myopic isoametropic amblyopia may occur with refractive errors exceeding 8–10 dioptres.

The classification of amblyopia has more recently been attempted not on the basis of underlying predisposing factor but rather on a functional basis. Such classification is dependent upon the use of both psychophysical and oculomotor tests available to the serious laboratory researcher (McKee *et al.* 1992). Psychophysical research has highlighted differences in contrast sensitivity function between predominantly strabismic and predominantly anisometropic amblyopia (Bradley & Freeman 1985; Hess & Pointer 1985). Ocular motility research has shown abnormalities of fixation (Schor & Flom 1975), saccades and pursuits (Schor 1975), and optokinetic nystagmus (Schor & Levi 1980). Further research will be required to more fully understand the sensory and motor abnormalities associated with amblyopia, as well as an attempt to understand whether these associated abnormalities are a cause or an effect of the amblyopia. With better understanding of these mechanisms better treatment of amblyopia might be rendered.

Incidence

Amblyopia affects between 2 and 5% of the general population. The vast majority of amblyopia occurs in one eye only. Strabismus is by far the most common cause of amblyopia, followed by anisometropia and media opacities such as congenital cataract.

Anisometropic amblyopia can be a difficult condition to detect in the absence of obvious strabismus. The better seeing eye provides vision which allows the child to function normally. Routine primary care physician screening tests do not in general include an examination for refractive errors although assessment of the Bruckner reflex (Tongue & Cibis 1981) or photorefraction has been advocated to assess for amblyogenic factors including anisometropic amblyopia (Atkinson & Braddick 1983; Day & Norcia 1986). Before photorefraction is instituted in mass screening, careful attention must be paid to the following:

1 the age of the child to be screened;
2 the normal refractive error for age-specific considerations;
3 specificity and sensitivity measurement for a specific device;
4 validation of the device for a specific age;
5 cost-efficiency analysis; and
6 scientific data which verify treatment effectiveness for a specific issue (such as anisometropia).

The degree of anisometropia which is sufficient to induce amblyopia seems to vary greatly from individual to individual. Nevertheless, any child with a difference of 1 dioptre of hyperopia or 3 dioptres of myopia must be carefully followed to exclude the possibility of amblyopia. The optical correction of anisometropic amblyopia at times warrants a monocular contact lens to eliminate concerns about aniseikonia.

Media opacities of various types can also cause unilateral amblyopia. Some conditions are obvious such as a near complete ptosis of one eye. Others, such as a posterior capsular cataract, can only be detected with careful screening. Teaching primary care physicians to use the direct ophthalmoscope to screen for this condition at birth, 6 weeks and 6 months is essential.

Significance

Although an adult with unilateral amblyopia usually has no significant limitations of day-to-day life, prevention of amblyopia is in large part warranted to guard the devastating effect of loss of the good eye at an age where amblyopia can no longer be treated. One study cites the risk of blindness as being greater when amblyopia is present (Tommila & Tarkkanen 1981). Although some authors have claimed that in adulthood the use of an amblyopic eye can improve in the event of loss of the good eye (Rabin 1984), most clinicians have observed that profound amblyopia is not reversible during adulthood.

Strabismic amblyopia occurs when in association with strabismus, a strong fixation preference for one eye is made. Although the visual loss often follows the onset of strabismus, the strabismus can be a consequence of poor vision in one eye. The presence of amblyopia does not appear to have any correlation with the angle of deviation although amblyopia is far more commonly associated with esotropia than exotropia. In the management of strabismus, one must traditionally reverse the amblyopia as best as possible before proceeding with strabismus surgery.

Bilateral amblyopia

Bilateral amblyopia is a far less common condition, although its effects on any individual are potentially far more serious than unilateral amblyopia. The most severe type of bilateral amblyopia occurs in instances where the management of media opacities has been delayed. In many children with bilateral severe congenital cataracts who have had surgery at the age of 1 year, despite the clearing of the media the best visual acuity may be in the 20/400 range. A similar visual level also results if the child has had surgery at 1 month but did not receive optical correction of the resultant hyperopia until the age of 1 year. It must also be appreciated that the ultimate vision achieved in these cases is not simply dependent on timing or on anatomical factors. There are still several cases in which, despite 'perfect' management and no complications, the visual results are still poor. Although it is probably not correct to ascribe all of the deficit to amblyopia, it is likely that bilateral amblyopia plays a significant role in these cases.

More mild forms of bilateral amblyopia occur when refractive errors prevent a clearly focused image on both retinas at all times. This condition, isoametropic amblyopia, most commonly occurs with hyperopia. No specific refractive error can be regarded as the exact cut-off for susceptibility to this condition, although most clinicians feel that any refractive error in excess of 4 dioptres of hyperopia, 8 dioptres of myopia or 2 dioptres of astigmatism potentially creates a condition which could lead to bilateral amblyopia. The majority of people with isoametropic amblyopia have hyperopia in excess of 6 dioptres. Detection of this condition may often not be made until visual acuity tests are performed at school. When the refractive error is symmetrical in the two eyes, strabismus may not develop, since additional accommodative effort still results in a blurred image and accommodative convergence is not used because it does not result in clearing of the image.

Any patient who has hyperopic isoametropia must be regarded as possibly having other pathology. Retinal dystrophies, especially Leber's congenital amaurosis, may have a high incidence of hyperopia. The proper management of hyperopic isoametropia includes either spectacles or contact lenses. Contact lenses provide a greater drive to peripheral fusion since the peripheral visual field is enhanced with lens wear. The ability of young children to wear contact lenses is highly variable, and the child's motivation as well as parental support must be excellent.

Bilateral myopic isoametropic amblyopia is far less common since bilateral myopia still allows for a focused image to develop at near; thus, bilateral amblyopia is unlikely unless the myopia exceeds 8 dioptres. High degrees of myopia in a child warrant concern about systemic health (see Chapter 7).

Treatment

The treatment of abnormal visual development rests on simple principles. Initially, attention must be directed to the amblyogenic factor. If significant refractive error exists, then optical correction must be made. If significant media opacities are present, then these must be dealt with, usually surgically. If strabismus is present, then amblyopia must first be reversed with occlusion therapy prior to any surgical treatment. Occlusion therapy itself is not innocuous. In general, total full-time occlusion should not be prescribed in excess of 1 week of occlusion per year of age. A 2-year-old child, for instance, should be given 2 weeks of occlusion therapy with a follow-up appointment at 2 weeks. Conversely, a 6-month-old baby can only be occluded safely for a few days before repeat assessment is indicated. To ensure the best possible compliance, it is best to initially recheck vision after 3 weeks of patching, with longer gaps in older children. Also, occlusion appears to work best when a concentrated effort is made so that therapy is nearly full time. Reports of occlusion amblyopia (amblyopia in the eye that is being occluded) have cautioned us in ensuring that any patient who is patched must be followed carefully. Compliance with patching is a major problem in the management of amblyopia, depending on the child's and the parents' personality, social circumstances, and so on (Woodruff *et al.* 1994).

Alternatives to occlusion therapy include optical and pharmacological penalization (Repka & Ray 1993) such as atropine 1% eye drops once a week to the fixing eye, or homatropine 2% twice a week. It is probably less effective than occlusion especially when the interocular difference in vision is great.

When amblyopia is associated with an organic lesion such as optic nerve hypoplasia (Kushner 1984), myelinated nerve fibres (Summers *et al.* 1991), media opacities, and macular abnormalities (Bradford *et al.* 1992) appropriately vigorous occlusion may give useful improvement in vision. Even the presence of a relative afferent defect does not preclude a good result (Bradford *et al.* 1992). If, however, occlusion fails to result in an improved function, care must be taken not to overdo such treatment.

When strabismic amblyopia is present, conventional treatment is to reverse the amblyopia with occlusion therapy prior to realignment attempts although others (Lam *et al.* 1993) have argued to straighten the eyes first.

Some debate has been raised as to the 'healthiness' of the good eye in conditions of amblyopia; confusingly both 'supernormal' function (Bradley & Freeman 1981; Rentschler & Hitz 1985) and 'subnormal' function (Kandel *et al.* 1986) have been found in research settings. In congenital cataract, especially monocular, careful occlusion regimes are mandatory if good vision is to be obtained in both eyes: anomalous vision in the occluded eye may be obtained by excessive occlusion, although fortunately the defects are mostly subclinical (see Chapter 39).

Treatment limitations must be recognized, particularly when underlying pathology is overwhelmingly evident. As much as we must recognize the plasticity of a young child's system, their general developmental needs must also be recognized. If a good series of trials of occlusion has been attempted and vision is not improving, a restructuring of goals may be in order.

The neural substrate

Wiesel and Hubel (1963a) from single-unit recordings of kitten striate cortex found abnormal cortical cells firing when driven by the deprived eye; this abnormal recording was accompanied by behaviourally poor vision. These abnormal recordings could not be reproduced when deprivation was imposed upon an adult cat. They concluded that the affected pathways had been normal at birth but were then influenced by the deprivation. Von Noorden *et al.* (1970a, b; Von Noorden 1973) produced experimental esotropia in infant monkeys and created deprivation amblyopia with lid suturing. Both behavioural studies (Von Noorden *et al.* 1970a, b; Von Noorden 1973) and neurophysiological recordings (Baker *et al.* 1974) demonstrated findings similar to the previous animal experiments: deprivation resulted in abnormal responsiveness in cortical cells driven by the amblyopic eye or in cortical cells which required binocular input.

In monkeys there may be two distinct sensitive periods (Sloper 1993). The first period occurs between birth and 8 weeks when there is 'competitive interaction' between the pathways from the two eyes such that reopening a sutured eye produces no improvement but reverse suture is effective in reversing the shrinkage of lateral geniculate body cells. The second period is from 8 weeks to 7–18 months, and involves 'co-operative interaction' between the pathways between the two eyes: reopening an eye during this period allows recovery of affected lateral geniculate cells to normal size. This has interesting implications for human amblyopia.

A search for the histopathological correlate, seemingly a simple task given the prevalence of this condition, has yielded sparse findings. Weisel and Hubel (1963a) demonstrated shrinkage in regions of the lateral geniculate body in kittens with one sutured eye. A single report of similar LGN pathology in one human with anisometropic amblyopia has been made (Von Noorden *et al.* 1983). Ikeda and Tremain (1979), because of changes they found in ganglion cells, have argued that a site for amblyopia is within the retina on the basis of studies in kittens with strabismus. Von Noorden contests the clinical relevance of this research by arguing that with strabismic amblyopia (as opposed to deprivation amblyopia), the fovea of the deviating eye does in fact receive a clear image but that the

brain is unable to process the conflicting information from the two eyes (Von Noorden 1985).

In general, relative afferent pupillary defects, or Marcus Gunn pupils, are not clinically apparent in patients with amblyopia. However, clinical observation (Greenwald & Folk 1983) and more sophisticated testing have indicated more subtle pupillary abnormalities in some of these patients, supporting the possibility for a very anteriorly located abnormality in these patients (Ikeda 1980).

Future directions

Considering that Hippocrates in 400 BC defined amblyopia as 'when the doctor and the patient see nothing', and that the grandfather of Charles Darwin was one of the first to advocate occlusion therapy, our understanding of the complexities of amblyopia may have improved, but our understanding of the effective management has not changed significantly. Several avenues of investigation have suggested a potential next step in the neurobiochemical direction. Experimentally, amblyopia has been reversed with bicuculline in animals, as evidenced by neurophysiological recordings (Duffy *et al.* 1985). Unfortunately, a constant side-effect of seizures accompanies the 'cure', and thus human studies have not been performed. A second avenue of research centres on a better understanding of the plasticity of the central nervous system. The use of levodopa partially to reverse amblyopia has been studied both in laboratory animals and in human subjects (Leguire *et al.* 1993). Levodopa appears to be successful in improving the results of part-time occlusion treatment in older children (Leguire *et al.* 1995) but its clinical role is not established. It has been postulated that certain other biochemicals may prolong plasticity so that the effective window for treatment of amblyopia might be prolonged.

Colour vision

Normal development

When does a baby develop colour vision? As with visual acuity testing, quantification is an awesome task. Simple observation was used by Charles Darwin who reported that his newborn son could see a candle at 9 days but could not appreciate colour until 48 days (Darwin 1877). Parents often decorate infants' rooms with brightly coloured, highly colour-saturated toys, mobiles and furniture. Tutors of poorly sighted infants suggest the use of brightly coloured objects to encourage vision development.

Scientific understanding of infant colour vision has relied initially on behavioural tests, in ways analogous to preferential visual acuity testing. One aspect of colour vision testing has been to determine which colours were most interesting to children. Using preferential grabbing as an indicator, several observers found yellow to be the most appealing colour (Valentine 1914; Shirley 1933). An ability to match colours is present by 2 years (Cook 1931).

More recent studies have isolated different aspects of colour vision development into spectral sensitivity and brightness determinators, and chromatic vision discrimination (Bornstein 1978). Although one such study showed relatively depressed blue sensitivity (Trincken 1955) in infants 3 months old and younger, other behavioural tests show spectral sensitivity identical to adults (Peeples & Teller 1978). Electrophysiological recordings have shown better sensitivity in wave lengths shorter than 550 nm. A similar study performed longitudinally agreed that infants do have such developmental differences when compared to adult spectral sensitivity (Moskowitz-Cook 1979). These differences have been explained on the basis of differing absorption characteristics of the infant lens and macular pigment (Dobson 1976) and on developmental factors involving the infant's rods and cones (Moskowitz-Cook 1979) in the parafoveal and foveal regions.

The routine testing of children for colour vision is included in many screening systems for childrens' eyes (Ehrlich *et al.* 1983).

Recently, infant toys and targets have been developed with black and white patterns, as if this design would improve the child's vision development. Such objects are even found in intensive care units for premature infants. The 'attraction' for these objects may well be the total contrast between black and white and should not be construed as an inability of an infant to see colours.

Abnormal colour vision

Abnormal colour vision is a common condition which has an impact on individuals and society (Fletcher & Voke 1985). Defective colour vision can be defined as congenital or acquired on the basis of response to colour vision testing.

Congenital colour vision abnormalities affect approximately 5–6% of males in Western Europe and North America (Waardenberg *et al.* 1963) due to their X-linked inheritance pattern. Their classification is based on the presence of three colour classes of cones: red-, green-, and blue-sensitive systems. A person is termed trichromatic if all systems are present, dichromatic if one is absent, and monochromatic if two are absent. The abnormal system is indicated by the terms protanomaly (red defect), deuteranomaly (green defect), and tritanomaly (blue defect). If function is completely absent (as opposed to defective) the suffix '-anopia' is used (hence: protanopia, deuteranopia, and tritanopia).

Deuteranomaly represents the most common inherited abnormality; other X-linked inherited abnormalities are deuteranopia and protanopia. Tritanomaly and tritanopia are inherited as autosomal dominant conditions but affect only a tiny proportion of the population (Verriest 1974). The impact of inherited colour vision, referred to loosely as colour blindness and sometimes in the UK as Daltonism, has been studied extensively. From an educational standpoint, children with congenital defects do not appear to have any difficulty during elementary school (Lampe *et al.* 1973). Children themselves may report limits in appreciation of colour television or food appearance, or difficulty seeing car rear lights (Voke 1984). The greatest impact of defective colour vision appears to be on career choice. Although understandably difficult to compile, a list of vocations in which colour vision defects are possible handicaps or career limitations is available (Voke 1980). Strict requirements limiting military careers, particularly with regards to flying aeroplanes, still exist.

Acquired colour vision defects imply an entirely different set of underlying conditions. Testing for these defects centres not on defining a particular spectral sensitivity which is defective, but rather on defining loss of brilliance, or desaturation of colours. Such colour vision loss is often termed dyschromatopsia.

Acquired colour vision defects can occur with media opacity, optic nerve or retinal disorder with central nervous system pathology. Amblyopia typically does not cause a colour vision deficit although subtle abnormalities may be present (Marre & Marre 1978; Bradley *et al.* 1986). A review of the specific defect in these abnormalities indicates defects predominantly in the blue–yellow distribution (Fletcher & Voke 1985).

Impact of abnormal vision on general child development

Abnormal visual development begets abnormal child development. Vision is the most important sense for general development and education (Jan *et al.* 1977). Babies learn by imitating, by becoming aware of their own hands and feet through vision, and by eye contact with parents which provides clues about their performance. The blind or partially sighted baby is deprived, in varying degrees, of these ingredients of normal development.

Stereotyped behaviour or 'blindisms' are repetitive, purposeless, movements made by children with poor vision (Jan *et al.* 1977). They include eye-rubbing or eye-poking, rocking, hand flapping, head movements, thumb- or finger-sucking, hand gnawing, or repetitive noise making. They may be adaptations to understimulation, overstimulation, stress, or to neurological or ocular disease (Good 1991).

Blindness may also detrimentally affect behaviour, and development; autism (Rogers & Newhart-Larson 1989), impaired intellectual potential, and learning disorders

(Black & Sonksen 1992) have been noted in children with Leber's amaurosis. The developmental setback may occur after the first year of life (Cass *et al.* 1994), and is most severe in children who are blind as opposed to those who have some residual sight: this emphasizes the importance of early intervention to promote the best use of residual vision and general development (Sonksen *et al.* 1991).

Blindness has a profound effect on motor development, and developmental milestones are delayed. Sighted babies will raise their heads and look about at 12 weeks of age; blind babies are unhappy in this position, and prefer to be on their backs (Jan *et al.* 1977) which causes a delay in control of the head and trunk. The ability to grasp an object, usually present at 5–6 months, is often delayed until 1 year. Conversely, walking readiness is not retarded, whereas crawling is more difficult. The physiotherapist can play an important role in helping the parents to pace the motor development of the blind child and to develop postural position which will enhance mobility (Siegal & Murphy 1970).

In contrast to motor development, speech development commences at about the same age 6—8 weeks in sighted and unsighted children. However, lack of visual input slows progress, as words are less meaningful without the corresponding visual symbol.

Typically, blind children repeat words (echolalia) much more commonly than sighted children (Fay 1973). Finally, non-verbal communication, such as a smile in response to others is understandably delayed.

Does blindness enhance the other senses, such as hearing or touch? Although it is much talked about, infant research has disproved this theory. Rather, educational efforts are enhanced in other disciplines such as tactile sense. The limitations in playing certain sports may, for instance, result in opportunities to undertake music lessons at an earlier age (Jan *et al.* 1977).

Some physiological functions of the blind child are, however, influenced by blindness. These changes exist even when other congenital abnormalities are not present. Electroencephalograms show altered recordings, such as an absence of rapid eye movement (REM) recordings (Berger *et al.* 1962). The response to caloric testing of the vestibular system is reduced (Forssman 1964). Altered growth patterns, circadian rhythms and sleep patterns also occur in blind children (Jan *et al.* 1977).

As the child grows older, mobility skills and educational needs become increasingly important. Mobility is greatly enhanced by the slightest of remaining vision, not only in getting about but also in awareness of his or her own body parts. Mobility education of such children must be tailored to the individual due to the multiple factors involved with this skill (Garry & Ascarelli 1960). Schools for the blind concentrate teaching resources on dealing with issues such as maximum use of remaining vision, special technology providing education means (such as magnifying book print) and practical vocational counselling. A major effort is made to allow contact with sighted individuals and encourage incorporation of the blind child into the sighted society (Lowenfeld 1973). Undoubtedly the blind child's general development is heavily influenced by other congenital limitations. Mental retardation is present in 25–80% of blind children, depending on one's definition of blindness and mental retardation (Graham 1968). Cerebral palsy, present in 6–15% of blind children, represents a particular impact on the blind child when the hands are spastic (Jan *et al.* 1977). Varied degrees of hearing loss are found in 10% of blind children (Robinson 1974). The combination of deafness and blindness necessitates particularly creative efforts in education and socialization (Van Dijk 1971).

Finally, the responsibility of the blind child's general development and incorporation rests not only with the blind child and the family, but also with the attitudes of the sighted towards the child (ophthalmologists included!). Helen Keller reflected that 'not blindness, but the attitude of the seeing to the blind is the hardest burden to bear' (Jan *et al.* 1977).

References

Abramov I, Garden J, Hendrickson A *et al.* The retina of the newborn infant. *Science* 1982; **217**: 265–7.

Allen H. A new picture series for preschool vision testing. *Am J Ophthalmol* 1957; **44**: 38–41.

Archer SM. Detection and treatment of congenital esotropia. In: Isenberg SJ, ed. *The Eye in Infancy*, 2nd edn. St Louis: CV Mosby, 1994: 352.

Archer SM, Sondhi N, Helveston EM. Strabismus in infancy. *Ophthalmology* 1989; **96**: 133–7.

Aslin RN. Development of binocular fixation in human infants. *J Exp Child Psychol* 1977; **23**: 133–50.

Aslin RN. Experiential influences and sensitive periods in perceptual development: a unified model. In: Aslin RN, Alberts JR, Peterson MR, eds. *Development of Perception*, Vol. 2. San Diego: Academic Press, 1981: 45–93.

Aslin RN. Infant accommodation and convergence. In: Simons K, ed. *Early Visual Development, Normal and Abnormal*. New York: Oxford, 1993: 30–8.

Atkinson J. Early visual development: differential functioning of parvocellular and magnocellular pathways. *Eye* 1992; **6**: 129–35.

Atkinson J, Braddick O. The use of isotropic photorefraction for vision screening in infants. *Acta Ophthalmol (Copenh)* 1983; **157** (Suppl.): 36–45.

Atkinson J, Braddick O, Pimm-Smith E. Preferential looking for monocular and binocular testing of infants. *Br J Ophthalmol* 1982; **66**: 264–8.

Atkinson J, Smith J, Anker S *et al.* Binocularity and amblyopia before and after early strabismus surgery. *Invest Ophthalmol Vis Sci* 1991; **32**: 820.

Bailey I. *Bailey–Hall Cereal Test*. California: University of California, Berkeley, 1983.

Baker F, Griggs P, Von Noorden G. Effects of visual deprivation and strabismus on the response of neurons in the visual cortex of the monkey, including studies on the striate and prostrate cortex in the normal animal. *Brain Res* 1974; **66**: 185.

Bane M, Birch E. VEP acuity, FPL acuity and visual behaviour of visually impaired children. *J Pediatr Ophthalmol Strabismus* 1992; **29**: 202–9.

Banks MS. The development of visual accommodation during early infancy. *Child Dev* 1980; **51**: 646–9.

Banks MS, Aslin RN, Letson RD. Sensitive period for the development of human binocular vision. *Science* 1975; **190**: 675–7.

Banks MS, Bennett PJ, Schefrin B. Inefficient cones limit infants' spatial and chromatic vision. *Invest Ophthalmol Vis Sci* 1988; **29**: 59.

Beller R, Hoyt CS, Marg E, Odom JV. Congenital monocular cataracts: good visual function with neonatal surgery. *Am J Ophthalmol* 1981; **91**: 559–67.

Berger R, Olley P, Oswald I. The EEG, eye movements, and dreams of the blind. *Q J Exp Psychol* 1962; **14**: 183–6.

Birch EE. Stereopsis in infants and its developmental relation to visual acuity. In: Simons K, ed. *Early Visual Development, Normal and Abnormal.* Oxford University Press, Oxford, New York, 1993: 224–36.

Birch EE, Gwiazda J, Held R. Stereoacuity development for crossed and uncrossed disparities in human infants. *Vision Res* 1982; **22**: 507–13.

Birch EE, Shimojo S, Held R. Preferential looking assessment of fusion and stereopsis in infants aged 1–6 months. *Invest Ophthalmol Vis Sci* 1991; **32**: 820.

Black M, Sonksen P. Congenital retinal dystrophies: a study of early cognitive and visual development. *Arch Dis Child* 1992; **67**: 262–5.

Blakemore C, Van Sluyters RC. Reversal of the physiological effects of monocular deprivation in kittens: further evidence for a sensitive period. *J Physiol (Lond)* 1974; **237**: 195–216.

Bornstein M. Chromatic vision in infancy. In: Reese H, Lipsett L, eds. *Advances in Child Development* and *Behaviour,* Vol. 12. New York: Academic Press, 1978: 117–82.

Bower TGR. The object in the world of the infant. *Sci Am* 1971; **225**: 30–8.

Bradford G, Kutschke P, Scott W. Results of amblyopia therapy in eyes with unilateral structural abnormalities. *Ophthalmology* 1992; **99**: 1616–21.

Bradley A, Dahlman C, Switkes E, De Valois K. A comparison of colour and luminance discrimination in amblyopia. *Invest Ophthalmol Vis Sci* 1986; **27**: 1404–9.

Bradley A, Freeman RD. Contrast sensitivity in anisometropic amblyopia. *Invest Ophthalmol Vis Sci* 1981; **24**: 467–76.

Bradley A, Freeman RD. Temporal sensitivity in amblyopia: an explanation of conflicting reports. *Vision Res* 1985; **25**: 39–46.

Bronson GW. The postnatal growth of visual capacity. *Child Dev* 1974; **45**: 873–90.

Brookman KE. Ocular accommodation in human infants. *Am J Optom Physiol Opt* 1983; **60**: 91–9.

Cass H, Sonksen P, McConachie H. Developmental setback in severe visual impairment. *Arch Dis Child* 1994; **70**: 192–6.

Catalano RA, Simon JW, Jenkins PL, Kandel GL. Preferential looking as a guide for amblyopia therapy in monocular infantile cataracts. *J Pediatr Ophthalmol Strabismus* 1987; **24**: 56–63.

Catford G, Oliver A. Development of visual acuity. *Arch Dis Child* 1973; **48**: 47–50.

Chalupa LM, Williams RW. Organisation of the cat's lateral geniculate nucleus following interruption of prenatal binocular competition. *Hum Neurobiol* 1984; **3**: 103–7.

Cook W. Ability of children in colour discrimination. *Child Dev* 1931; **2**: 303–20.

Cynader M, Berman N, Hein A. Recovery of function in cat visual cortex following prolonged deprivation. *Exp Brain Res* 1976; **25**: 139–56.

Darwin C. A biographical sketch of an infant. *Mind* 1877; **2**: 285–94.

Day SH, Norcia AM. Infantile esotropia and the developing visual system. In: Greenwald MJ, ed. *Ophthalmology Clinics of North America: Pediatric Ophthalmology.* Philadelphia: WB Saunders, 1990: 3: 281–7.

Day SH, Norcia AM. Photographic detection of amblyogenic factors. *Ophthalmology* 1986; **93**: 25–8.

Dayton G, Jones M, Ain P *et al.* Developmental study of coordinated eye movements in the human infant I. Visual acuity in the newborn human: a study based on induced optokinetic nystagmus recorded by electro-oculography. *Arch Ophthalmol* 1964; **71**: 865–70.

Dobson V. Spectral sensitivity of the 2-month old infant as measured by the visual evoked cortical potential. *Vision Res* 1976; **16**: 367–74.

Dobson V. Visual acuity testing by preferential looking technique. In: Isenberg SJ, ed. *The Eye in Infancy,* 2nd edn. St Louis: CV Mosby, 1994: 139.

Donzis PB, Rappazzo JA, Burde RM *et al.* Effect of binocular variations of Snellen's visual acuity on Titmus stereoacuity. *Arch Ophthalmol* 1983; **101**: 930–2.

Dubowitz L, de Vries L, Mushin J, Arden G. Visual function in the newborn infant: is it cortically mediated? *Lancet* 1986; **i**: 1139–41.

Duffy FH, Burchfiel JL, Maver GD, Joy RM, Snodgrass SR. Comparative pharmacological effects on visual cortical neurones in monocularly deprived cats. *Brain Res* 1985; **339**: 257–64.

Ehrlich M, Reinecke R, Simons K. Preschool vision screening for amblyopia, strabismus. Programs, methods, guidelines. *Surv Ophthalmol* 1983; **28**: 145–63.

Eizenman M, Skarf B, McCulloch D. Development of binocular vision in infants. *Invest Ophthalmol Vis Sci* 1989; **30** (Suppl.): 313.

Epelbaum M, Milleret C, Buisseret P, Dufier JL. The sensitive period for strabismic amblyopia in humans. *Ophthalmology* 1993; **100**: 323–7.

Fay W. On the echolalia of the blind and the autistic child. *J Speech Hear Dis* 1973; **38**: 478–89.

Fletcher R, Voke J. *Defective Colour Vision. Fundamentals, Diagnosis and Management.* Bristol: Adam Hilger, 1985.

Forssman B. Vestibular reactivity in cases of congenital nystagmus. *Otolaryngology* 1964; **57**: 539–55.

Fox R, Aslin RN, Shea SL *et al.* Stereopsis in human infants. *Science* 1980; **207**: 323–4.

Garry R, Ascarelli A. Teaching typographical orientation and spatial orientation to congenitally blind children. *J Educ* 1960; **143**: 1–49.

Good WV. Behaviour of visually impaired children. *Semin Ophthalmol* 1991; **6**: 158–60.

Gorman J, Cogan D, Gellis S. An apparatus for grading the visual acuity of infants on the basis of optokinetic nystagmus. *Pediatrics* 1957; **19**: 1088–92.

Gottlieb G. The role of experience in the development of behavior and the nervous system. In: Gottlieb G, ed. *Neural and Behavioral Specificity.* New York: Academic Press, 1976:

Graham M. *Multiply Impaired Blind Children: a National Problem.* New York: American Foundation for the Blind, 1968.

Greenwald MJ, Folk ER. Afferent pupillary defect in amblyopia. *J Pediatr Ophthalmol Strabismus* 1983; **20**: 63–7.

Grier T. Visual acuity development and evaluation in the preschool child. *Optom Weekly* 1973; **64**: 370–4.

Haynes H, White BL, Held R. Visual accommodation in human infants. *Science* 1965; **148**: 528–30.

Held R, Birch EE, Gwiazda J. Stereoacuity in human infants. *Proc Natl Acad Sci USA* 1980; **77**: 5572–4.

Hendrickson A. A morphological comparison of foveal development in man and monkey. *Eye* 1992; **6**: 136–44.

Hendrickson A, Kupfer C. The histogenesis of the fovea in the macaque monkey. *Invest Ophthalmol Vis Sci* 1976; **15**: 746–56.

Hendrickson AE, Yuodelis C. The morphological development of the human fovea. *Ophthalmology* 1984; **91**: 603–12.

Hess RF, Pointer JS. Differences in the neural basis of human amblyopia: the distribution of the anomaly across the visual field. *Vision Res* l985; **25**: 1577–94.

Hickey JL, Peduzzi JD. Structure and development of the visual system. In: Salapatek P, Cohen L, eds. *Handbook of Infant Perception*. Orlando: Academic Press, 1987: 1–42.

Hubel D, Livingstone MS. Segregation of form, color, and stereopsis in primate area 18. *J Neurosci* 1987; **7**: 3378–415.

Hubel D, Wiesel T. Binocular interaction in striate cortex of kittens reared with artificial squint. *J Neurophysiol* 1965; **28**: 1041–59.

Humphrey NK, Weiskrantz L. Vision in monkeys after removal of the striate cortex. *Nature* 1967; **215**: 595–7.

Huttenlocher PR, de Courten C, Garey L *et al.* Synaptogenesis in human visual cortex — evidence for synapse elimination during normal development. *Neurosci Lett* 1982; **33**: 247–52.

Ikeda H. Visual acuity, its development and amblyopia. *J Roy Soc Med* 1980; **573**: 546.

Ikeda H, Tremain K. Amblyopia occurs in retinal ganglion cells in cats reared with convergent squint without alternating fixation. *Exp Br Res* 1979; **35**: 559.

Jampolsky A. Unequal visual inputs and strabismus management: a comparison of human and animal strabismus. In: *Symposium on Strabismus. Transactions of the New Orleans Academy of Ophthalmology*. St Louis: CV Mosby, 1978: 358.

Jan J, Freeman R, Scott E. *Visual Impairment in Children and Adolescents*. New York: Grune & Stratton, 1977.

Jan J, Wong PKH, Groenveld M, Flodmark O, Hoyt CS. Travel vision: 'collicular visual system'? *Pediatr Neurol* 1986; **2**: 359–62.

Kandel GL, Simon JW, Drylewski A. Acuities of dominant eyes of infant amblyopes are subnormal before treatment. *Invest Ophthalmol Vis Sci* 1986; **27**: 2.

Klaeger-Manzanell C, Hoyt C, Good W. Two-step recovery of vision in the amblyopic eye after visual loss and enucleation of the fixing eye. *Br J Ophthalmol* 1994; **78**: 506–7.

Keech RV, Kutschke PJ. Upper age limit for the development of amblyopia. *J Pediatr Ophthalmol Strabismus* 1995; **32**: 89–93.

Kirschen D, Rosenbaum A, Ballard C. The dot visual acuity test — a new acuity test for children. *J Am Optom Assoc* 1983; **54**: 1055–9.

Kushner BJ. Functional amblyopia associated with abnormalities of the optic nerve. *Arch Ophthalmol* 1984; **102**: 683–5.

Lam G, Repka M, Guyton D. Timing of amblyopia therapy relative to strabismus surgery. *Ophthalmology* 1993; **100**: 1751–6.

Lampe J, Doster M, Beal B. Summary of a three-year study of academic and school achievement between colour defective and normal primary age pupils. *J School Health* 1973; **43**: 309–11.

Leguire LE, Walson P, Rogers G *et al.* Longitudinal study of levodopa/carbidopa for childhood amblyopia. *J Pediatr Ophthalmol Strabismus* 1993; **30**: 354–60.

Leguire LE, Walson PD, Rogers GL, Bremer DL, McGregor ML. Levodopa/carbidopa treatment for amblyopia in older children. *J Pediatr Ophthalmol Strabismus* 1995; **32**: 143–51.

LeVay S, Stryker MP, Schatz CJ. Ocular dominance columns and their development in layer IV of the cat's visual cortex: a quantitative study. *J Comp Neurol* 1978; **179**: 223–44.

LeVay S, Wiesel TN, Hubel DH. The development of ocular dominance columns in normal and visually deprived monkeys. *J Comp Neurol* 1980; **191**: 1–51.

Lovasik JV, Szymkiw M. Effects of aniseikonia, anisometropia, accommodation, retinal illuminance and pupil size on stereopsis. *Invest Ophthalmol Vis Sci* 1985; **26**: 741–50.

Lowenfeld B (ed.). *The Visually Handicapped Child in School*. New York: John Day, 1973.

McDonald M. Assessment of visual acuity in toddlers. *Surv Ophthalmol* 1986; **31**: 189–210.

McKee SP, Schor CM, Steinman SB *et al.* The classification of amblyopia on the basis of visual and oculomotor performances. *Trans Am Ophthalmol Soc* 1992; **90**: 123–44.

Magoon EH, Robb RM. Development of myelin in human optic nerve and tract, a light and electron-microscopic study. *Arch Ophthalmol* 1981; **99**: 655–9.

Marre M, Marre E. Colour vision in squint amblyopia. *Mod Probl Ophthalmol* 1978; **19**: 308.

Moskowitz-Cook A. The development of spectral sensitivity in human infants. *Vision Res* 1979; **19**: 1133–42.

Nixon RB, Helveston EM, Miller K *et al.* Incidence of strabismus in neonates. *Am J Ophthalmol* 1985; **100**: 798–801.

Norcia AM. Vision testing by visual evoked potential techniques. In: Isenberg SJ, ed. *The Eye in Infancy*, 2nd edn. St Louis: CV Mosby, 1994: 157–73.

Norcia AM, Sutter EE, Tyler CW. Electrophysiological evidence for the existence of coarse and fine disparity mechanisms in humans. *Vision Res* 1985; **25**: 1603–11.

Peeples D, Teller D. White-adapted photopic spectral sensitivity in human infants. *Vision Res* 1978; **18**: 49–53.

Petrig B, Julesz B, Kropfl W *et al.* Development of stereopsis and cortical binocularity in human infants: electrophysiological evidence. *Science* 1981; **213**: 1402–5.

Rabin J. Visual improvement in amblyopia after visual loss in the dominant eye. *Am J Optom Physiol Optics* 1984; **61**: 334–7.

Rakic P. Development of visual centers in the primate brain depends on binocular competition before birth. *Science* 1982; **214**: 928–31.

Rakic P. Specification of cerebral cortical areas. *Science* 1988; **241**: 170–6.

Rentschler I, Hitz R. Amblyopia processing of positional information. Part 1: vernier acuity. *Exp Brain Res* 1985; **60**: 270–8.

Repka M, Ray J. The efficacy of optical and pharmacological penalization. *Ophthalmology* 1993; **100**: 769–75.

Robb RM, Mayer DL, Moore BD. Results of early treatment of unilateral congenital cataracts. *J Pediatr Ophthalmol Strabismus* 1987; **24**: 178–81.

Robinson G. *Epidemiological Studies of Congenital and Acquired Blindness in Blind Children Born in British Columbia 1944–1973*. First National Multi-Disciplinary Conference on Blind Children, Canadian Medical Association, Vancouver, Canada. 1974: 1–91.

Rogers SJ, Newhart-Larson S. Characteristics of infantile autism in five children with Leber's congenital amaurosis. *Dev Med Child Neurol* 1989; **31**: 598–607.

Romano P, Romano J, Puklin J. Stereoacuity development in children with normal binocular single vision. *Am J Ophthalmol* 1975; **79**: 966–71.

Schoenleber DB, Crouch ER. Bilateral hypermetropic amblyopia. *J Pediatr Ophthalmol Strabismus* 1987; **75**: 77–9.

Schor CM. A directional impairment of eye movement control in strabismic amblyopia. *Invest Ophthalmol Vis Sci* 1975; **14**: 692–7.

Schor CM, Flom MC. Eye position control and visual acuity in strabismus amblyopia. In: *Basic Mechanisms of Ocular Motility and their Clinical Implications*. Oxford: Pergamon Press, 1975: 555–69.

Schor CM, Levi D. Disturbances of small field horizontal and vertical optokinetic nystagmus in amblyopia. *Invest Ophthalmol* 1980; **19**: 668–83.

Sebris SL, Dobson V, McDonald MA, Teller DV. Acuity cards for visual acuity assessment of infants and children in clinical settings. *Clin Vis Sci* 1987; **9**: 45–58.

Sheridan M. The stycar graded balls vision test. *Dev Med Child Neurol* 1973; **15**: 423–32.

Shimojo S, Held R. Vernier acuity is less than granting acuity in 2- and 3-month olds. *Vision Res* 1987; **27**: 77–86.

Shirley M. *The First Two Years. Intellectual Development.* Minneapolis: University of Minnesota Press, 1933.

Siegel I, Murphy T. *Postural Determinants in the Blind. Final Project Report.* Washington DC: Division of Research and Demonstration Grants, Social Rehabilitation Service, DHEW, 1970.

Simons K. Visual acuity norms in young children. *Surv Ophthalmol* 1983; **28**: 84–92.

Simons K, ed. *Early Visual Development, Normal and Abnormal.* New York: Oxford University Press, 1993.

Slataper F. Age norms of refraction and vision. *Arch Ophthalmol* 1950; **43**: 466–79.

Sloper J. Edridge-Green lecture. Competition and co-operation in visual development. *Eye* 1993; **7**: 319–31.

Sokol S. Measurement of infant visual acuity from pattern reversal evoked potentials. *Vision Res* 1978; **18**: 33–9.

Sonksen P, Petrie A, Drew K. Promotion of visual development of severely visually impaired babies: evaluation of a developmentally based programme. *Dev Med Child Neurol* 1991; **33**: 320–35.

Summers C, MacDonald J. Afterimages. Vision despite tomographic absence of the occipital cortex. *Surv Ophthalmol* 1990; **35**: 188–91.

Summers CG, Romig L, Lavoie JD. Unexpected good results after therapy for anisometropic amblyopia associated with unilateral peripapillary myelinated nerve fibres. *J Pediatr Ophthalmol Strabismus* 1991; **28**: 134–7.

Swaiman K, Wright F. The neurologic examination in children. In: *The Practice of Pediatric Neurology.* St Louis: CV Mosby, 1975.

Swan KC, Wilkins JH. Extraocular muscle surgery in early infancy— anatomical factors. *J Pediatr Ophthalmol Strabismus* 1984; **21**: 44–9.

Teller D, McDonald M, Preston K, Sebris S, Dobson V. Assessment of visual acuity in infants and children: the acuity card procedure. *Dev Med Child Neurol* 1986; **28**: 770–90.

Tommila V, Tarkkanen A. Incidence of loss of vision in the healthy eye in amblyopia. *Br J Ophthalmol* 1981; **65**: 575–7.

Tongue AC, Cibis GW. Bruckner test. *Ophthalmology* 1981; **88**: 1041–4.

Trincken D. Die ontogenetische entwicklung des helligkeitsund forbensehens bein menschen. I. Die entwicklung des helligketissehens. *Albrecht Gruefes Arch Clin Exp Ophthalmol* 1955; **156**: 519–43.

Tychsen L. Development of vision. In: Isenberg SJ, ed. *The Eye in Infancy*, 2nd edn. St Louis: CV Mosby, 1994: 121–30.

Tyler C, Apkarian P, Levi D, Nakayama K. Rapid assessment of visual function: an electronic sweep technique for the pattern visual evoked potential. *Invest Ophthalmol Vis Sci* 1979; **18**: 703–13.

Vaegan, Taylor D. Critical period for deprivation amblyopia in children. *Trans Ophthalmol Soc UK* 1980; **99**: 432–439.

Valentine C. The colour perception and colour preference of an infant during its fourth and eighth months. *Br J Psychol* 1914; **6**: 363–86.

Van Dijk J. Educational approaches to abnormal development. In: *Deaf–Blind Children and Their Education. Proceedings of the 1970 International Conference on the Education of Deaf–Blind Children.* Rotterdam: Rotterdam University Press, 1971.

Verriest M. Recent progress in the study of acquired deficiencies of colour vision. *Bull Soc Ophthalmol Fr* 1974; **74**: 595–621.

Voke J. *Colour Vision Testing in Specific Industries and Professions.* London: Keeler, 1980.

Voke J. But spinach is black. *Optician* 1984; **187**: 35–6.

Von Noorden G. Experimental amblyopia monkeys. Further behavioural observation and clinical correlations. *Invest Ophthalmol* 1973; **12**: 721.

Von Noorden G. Amblyopia: a multi-disciplinary approach (Proctor lecture). *Invest Ophthalmol Vis Sci* 1985; **26**: 1704–16.

Von Noorden G, Crawford M, Levery R. The lateral geniculate nucleus in human amnisometropia amblyopia. *Invest Ophthalmol* 1983; **24**: 788–90.

Von Noorden G, Dowling J, Ferguson D. Experimental amblyopia in monkeys II. Behavioural studies in strabismus amblyopia. *Arch Ophthalmol* 1970a; **84**: 215.

Von Noorden G, Dowling J, Ferguson D. Experimental amblyopia in monkeys I. Behavioural studies of stimulus deprivation amblyopia. *Arch Ophthalmol* 1970b; **84**: 206.

Von Noorden G, Khodadoust A. Retinal hemorrhage in newborns and organic amblyopia. *Arch Ophthalmol* 1973; **89**: 91–3.

Waardenberg P, Franceschetti A, Klein D. *Genetics and Ophthalmology.* Illinois: Thomas Springfield, 1963.

Walters CP, Walker RD. Visual placing by human infants. *J Exp Child Psychol* 1974; **18**: 34–40.

Weiskrantz L, Warrington EK, Sanders MD, Marshall J. Visual capacity in the hemianopic field following a restricted occipital ablation. *Brain* 1974; **97**: 709–28.

Wiesel T, Hubel D. Effects of visual deprivation of morphology and physiology of cells in the cat's lateral geniculate body. *J Neurophysiol* 1963a; **96**: 578–85.

Wiesel T, Hubel D. Single cell response in striate cortex of kittens deprived of vision in one eye. *J Neurophysiol* 1963b; **26**: 1003–17.

Wiesel T, Hubel D. Comparison of the effects of unilateral and bilateral eye closure on cortical unit response in kittens. *J Neurophysiol* 1965; **28**: 1029–40.

Williams RW, Chalupa LM. Expanded retinogeniculate projections in the cat following prenatal unilateral enucleation: functional and anatomic analyses of an anomalous input. *Soc Neurosci Abst* 1983; **9**: 701.

Woodruff G, Hiscox F, Thompson JR, Smith LK. Factors affecting the outcome of children treated for amblyopia. *Eye* 1994; **8**: 627–31.

3: Delayed Visual Maturation

Creig S. Hoyt

When a baby is referred because the parents are worried about its vision, the cause is usually evident to the ophthalmologist on the first examination. At the very least there is usually a strong suspicion about the site of the problem in the visual or neurological system. In some babies, no apparent cause can be found; their vision just seems worse for their chronological age than it should be, and their estimated or measured visual function is worse than expected. In many of these infants, however, vision improves over time, without specific treatment.

This phenomenon has been recognized for many years. Illingworth (1961) first introduced the term 'delayed visual maturation' to describe it. He described two children who had been visually unresponsive as infants, but at 6 months of age began to be attentive to visual stimuli. It is noteworthy that one child was considerably late in walking. In all other regards, however, Illingworth's first two patients were not developmentally delayed, except with regard to their visual function.

It should be noted that although Illingworth introduced the term, similar cases had previously been described using other terms. Beauvieux (1926, 1947) noted the anomalous appearance of optic discs in infants whom they referred to as having 'temporary visual inattention'. With time the discs appeared to assume a normal adult appearance, and the visual function improved. Believing this problem to be due to a defect in the myelination of the optic nerve, the authors coined the term 'pseudo-atrophie optique dysgenesie myelinique'. Beauvieux (1947), however, appreciated that the situation could be more complex, and might be compounded by neurodevelopmental or ocular anomalies that might influence eventual visual outcome. He considered that there were two distinct categories of affected infants. In the first, delayed visual maturation is an isolated anomaly, with rapid and complete recovery within 4–6 months. In the second, because of associated problems such as strabismus, high refractive errors or mental retardation, visual improvement is slower and less complete.

Clinical presentation

Most parents and many doctors do not expect the newborn baby to see well, so it is only when the child is not fixing and following by 2–4 months of age that they are referred by the parents themselves, or their advisors, to the ophthalmologist or paediatrician. The diagnosis of delayed visual maturation is really done retrospectively, and by exclusion of visual system disease as far as that is possible. It is essential for the diagnosis that the vision should improve with time, but since delayed visual maturation may co-exist with ocular or systemic disease, the eventual vision is not necessarily normal. It is noteworthy that the patient who presents with delayed visual maturation in its isolated form is the child with no apparent fixation and following reflexes, and no strabismus. The patient thus appears distinctly different than the infant who presents with poor visual function associated with a bilateral anterior visual pathway disorder in which nystagmus is to be expected and in whom pupillary abnormalities may be present. Delayed visual maturation must be distinguished from those infants who present with poor visual function as a result of visual cortex or associated neurovisual pathway pathology. These patients too may present with poor visual fixation and no nystagmus.

Classification

Uemura *et al.* (1981) present a classification of developmentally delayed visual maturation that includes three categories. This classification was prompted by the observation that many infants with apparent maturation delay were found subsequently to have other significant neurodevelopmental or visual problems. In their original classification, Uemera *et al.* suggested that type I should include patients who exhibit visual maturation delay with no other anomalies; type II should include infants with visual maturation delay who are mentally retarded or who have a seizure disorder; and type III should include children with a primary visual abnormality and a superimposed visual maturation delay. These authors recognized that the simplistic notion that these children simply had a temporary delay in achieving normal visual milestones was often incorrect.

Visual function testing in isolated delayed visual maturation

In these babies general and neurological development is normal (Illingworth 1961), and the only problem is that the baby appears to see less well than expected for his or her age. They have normal ocular examination and no systemic abnormalities.

Thus far, there is a consensus among ophthalmologists that the electroretinogram (ERG) is entirely normal for the adjusted age of the child studied (Hoyt *et al.* 1983; Lambert *et al.* 1989; Tresidder *et al.* 1990). It should be noted that these ERG studies have been standard flash non-focal studies. No attempt to date has been made to study these infants with a focal stimulus or foveal-type ERG.

In contrast to the consensus among ERG studies, visual evoked potentials (VEPs) of these patients have produced variable and conflicting results. Regrettably, none of the VEP studies are entirely free of criticism. Mellor and Fielder (1980) reported that flash VEPs had delayed latencies as well as reduced amplitudes in four children with delayed visual maturation. All of these children were reported to have normal VEPs when tested after achieving apparent normal visual behaviour. Harel *et al.* (1983) describe three infants with delayed visual maturation who had flash VEPs with delayed latencies that became normal by 1 year of age. Fielder *et al.* (1988) reported a large series of children with delayed visual maturation in which 78% had flash VEPs with prolonged latencies, abnormal wave forms and decreased amplitudes. The non-specific stimulus nature of flash VEPs, and the multiple recording artefacts that have been noted in infant visual studies using these techniques, suggest that flash VEP studies are probably not specific enough in their stimulus to be useful in evaluating this group of children.

Pattern VEPs have also been reported in these children. Hoyt *et al.* (1983) reported a series of eight children with delayed visual maturation in which seven had pattern onset/offset VEPs with decreased amplitudes and delayed latencies. The authors unfortunately did not report if these patients were age-matched with normal visually attentive children. Lambert *et al.* (1989) reported the VEP results on nine children with a diagnosis of delayed visual maturation. They reported that there were no abnormalities of amplitude, wave form or latency in these children as compared to an age-matched population. This study unfortunately, because of the unreliability and small amplitude of smaller check sizes in very young infants, utilized a stimulus of 100-minute check size as the standard stimulus: this test of visual function and acuity is relatively coarse. It is possible that had a smaller check size been used in this study, significant abnormalities similar to those reported by Hoyt *et al.* might have occurred.

Tresidder *et al.* (1990) studied 26 infants with delayed visual maturation using a modified forced choice preferential looking apparatus. All infants regardless of the group type showed significant reduction in visual acuity on the initial examination. Visual improvement commenced variably depending on the type of delayed visual maturation.

Clinical course and outcome

Group I: isolated delayed visual maturation

Clinically, the profile of the patient in group I is usually relatively constant. Most patients in this group present by 3–4 months of age, and it is very unusual for improvement to be prolonged beyond 6 months. Quite frequently, the short delay during the referral process is enough to allow for considerable improvement so that the diagnosis in these cases can only be made retrospectively by the history.

Because the measurement of visual function in small children is difficult, and indeed the VEP studies to date conflict in these children, the determination of whether normal vision has been achieved in these infants is largely subjective. However, the eventual outcome should not only be normal for vision but for intellectual and other development.

Several studies have emphasized that children with apparent isolated delayed visual maturation frequently had delays in other spheres of general development upon follow-up examination. Cole *et al.* (1984) reported that several children with delayed visual maturation were slow in learning to speak. Hoyt *et al.* (1983) noted general delays in the motor development of seven of eight children identified with delayed visual maturation. Lambert *et al.* (1989) in a study of nine children noted that four of the children were delayed by 3–5 months in achieving other developmental milestones such as sitting and walking compared with their unaffected siblings. One additional child was hypotonic with marked developmental delay. They concluded that delayed visual maturation may be only one manifestation of global developmental delay in some infants.

Group II: delayed visual maturation with systemic disease or mental retardation

Babies who are very premature, who have severe intercurrent illness early in their life, may present with delay in visual development, but this usually improves in the same way as in group I patients, with residual defects only related to their illness. Most patients in this group have severe mental retardation. It is most frequently seen in children who have infantile spasms, or other seizure disorders in relationship to severe birth asphyxia, hypoglycaemia, hypocalcaemia, tuberous sclerosis, Aicardi's syndrome, and so on. In most cases, these are diagnostic clues to the underlying cause and the neurophysiological studies are more frequently normal, especially the electroencephalogram (EEG). Vision appears to improve with the control of seizures in these children. Children with other causes of mental retardation without seizures, such as hydrocephalus or brain malformations, may also exhibit delayed visual maturation often to a lesser degree. The vision is variable and may be stimulated or excited by sound as well as visual stimulation.

In the group in whom structural central nervous system pathology is associated with delayed visual maturation the long-term prognosis is less good. There are often residual visual defects, or problems with visual perception, or hand–eye co-ordination and the recovery of vision takes considerably longer. This is dramatically demonstrated in the study of Tresidder *et al.* (1990) in which they showed that visual improvement commenced as follows: (i) group I, 7–24 weeks; (ii) group II, 22–78 weeks; and (iii) group III, 13–28 weeks.

Group III: delayed visual maturation with ocular disease

Children with early onset ocular disease associated with nystagmus may have vision that is much worse than would be expected from the primary disease alone. It is a reasonable hypothesis that these children have a form of delayed visual maturation in addition to their organic defect. This is frequently seen in children with albinism, but may also be seen in children with bilateral cataracts, optic nerve hypoplasia, and so on. Children in this group improve to their final level more slowly, and less fully than in group I, but faster and more completely than group II (see above).

Differential diagnoses

The main differential diagnoses for the baby with poor vision, with no apparent nystagmus and no gross ocular or systemic disorder, are delayed visual maturation versus cortical vision impairment. In most cases the child with significant cortical visual impairment will either have a history of significant perinatal hypoxia or other precipitant causes of this disorder, or will present with other associated neurological signs. Occasionally, however, only a magnetic resonance image or computed tomographic scan will be able to discern between these two disorders. Curiously, normal brain myelination does not seem to be affected by early visual loss in most children (Steinlin *et al.* 1992). Nevertheless, in some children with delayed visual maturation a delay in myelination or the visual pathways may be seen on magnetic resonance imaging (Hoyt & Good 1993).

Investigation and management

Delayed visual maturation is an area where the ophthalmologist and paediatrician or paediatric neurologist must work well together (Fielder & Mayer 1991). If the child with suspected delayed visual maturation is developmentally normal, and associated eye or systemic disease has been ruled out by joint consultation, and non-invasive neurophysiological studies are normal or not markedly abnormal, then no further investigations are needed and a good outcome can be expected. These children probably need to be followed rather more carefully than the average patient by their developmental clinician or their general practitioner after their improvement has been observed by the ophthalmologist.

Where the child has eye disease or systemic problems, these should be investigated and managed as appropriate.

References

Beauvieux J. La pseudo-atrophie optique des nouveau-nes. *Ann Oculist* 1926; **163**: 881–921.

Beauvieux M. La cecite apparente chez le nouveau-ne la pseudo-atrophie grise du nerf optique. *Arch Ophthalmol (Paris)* 1947; **7**: 241–9.

Cole GF, Hungerford J, Jones RD. Delayed visual maturation. *Arch Dis Child* 1984; **59**: 107–10.

Fielder AR, Mayer DL. Delayed visual maturation. *Semin Ophthalmol* 1991; **5**: 182–93.

Fielder AR, Russell-Eggitt IR, Dodd KL, Mellor DH. Delayed visual maturation. *Trans Ophthalmol Soc UK* 1988; **104**(6): 653–61.

Harel S, Holtzman M, Feinsod M. Delayed visual maturation. *Arch Dis Child* 1983; **58**: 298–9.

Hoyt CS, Good WV. Visual factors in developmental delay and neurological disorders in infants. In: Simons K, ed. *Early Visual Development: Normal and Abnormal.* New York: Oxford University Press, 1993: 505–12.

Hoyt CS, Jastrzebski G, Marg E. Delayed visual maturation. *Br J Ophthalmol* 1983; **63**: 127–30.

Illingworth RS. Delayed visual maturation. *Arch Dis Child* 1961; **36**: 407–9.

Lambert SR, Kriss A, Taylor D. Delayed visual maturation. *Ophthalmology* 1989; **96**: 524–9.

Mellor DH, Fielder AR. Dissociated visual development: electrodiagnostic studies in infants who are slow to see. *Dev Med Child Neurol* 1980; **22**: 327–35.

Steinlin M, Martin E, Schenker K, Boltshauser E. Myelination of the optic radiation in Leber congenital amaurosis. *Brain Dev* 1992; **14**: 212–15.

Tresidder J, Fielder AR, Nicholson J. Delayed visual maturation: ophthalmic and neurodevelopmental aspects. *Dev Med Child Neurol* 1990; **32**: 872–81.

Uemera Y, Agucci Y, Katsumi O. Visual development delay. *Ophthal Paediatr Genet* 1981; **1**: 4–11.

4: Normal Child Development

Nicholas Cavanagh

Although child development can only be said to have begun from the time of conception, it is clear that there are many factors before conception that will have an important bearing on the outcome. Not only do these include the genetic material, both nuclear and mitochondrial, and the chromosomal configuration of either gamete, but also the immediate environment of the dividing blastocyst. The taking of the family history, the clinical counterpart of the gene probe, is the first step in the elucidation of these factors. The next stage is enquiring about the pregnancy, delivery and neonatal period.

Family history

This should include enquiries about possible consanguinity, and the health of first-degree relatives. Sibling deaths may not be referred to by the parent unless such information is directly (but delicately) sought. Relatives should also be examined when appropriate.

The pregnancy

The answer to a seemingly innocuous question, 'was the pregnancy planned?' may indicate the need for cautious enquiries about attempts to abort, and may also lead on naturally to questions about the mother's health at the time of conception and throughout pregnancy. Whereas the effect of paternal inebriation at the moment of conception remains speculative (how many of us owe our origin to such prevailing conditions?), the deleterious effect of maternally ingested alcohol in moderate or large quantities on the developing fetus is now well recognized. Thus, a drug history should include information about alcohol and tobacco, coffee and tea, in addition to other more readily recognized drugs such as anticonvulsants and hormones, or narcotics and glue-sniffing. The relationship of maternal anaemia, state of nutrition, blood pressure, haemorrhage, intercurrent infection and illness, to fetal growth and development is well known, and such information is often volunteered by the mother, but if not should be asked for directly. Other enquiries about the course of the pregnancy should include the strength of fetal movements, particularly if a neuromuscular condition is suspected, and also if any irradiation was given, especially at an early stage.

Delivery

Since birth injury may be a cause of physical and mental handicap, the following questions are important considerations regarding the delivery: was it at term and, if not, how much pre- or post-term? Was there evidence of fetal distress as shown by meconium staining of the amniotic fluid, irregularities of fetal heart rate on monitoring, intrapartum acidosis, and so on? Was the delivery assisted and, if so, why?

Neonatal period

The state of the infant at birth and within the next few days of life is a summation of much that has happened in the previous 40 weeks of gestation as well as during the delivery. Important questions include the following: did the infant breathe immediately? Was there jaundice requiring specific therapy? Was feeding by breast or bottle and were there any difficulties? Was the baby unduly irritable or quiet? What was the birth weight?

Developmental milestones

It is doubtful whether the answer to questions about stages of development are always reliable. Accuracy of recall is dependent upon a number of factors which include the age of the child (the older the child the more likely the earlier milestones are forgotten), how many siblings there are to confuse with, and whether baby books were kept from which information can be subsequently retrieved. Sometimes no more accurate information can be obtained than whether the development of the child was comparable with the siblings, though most parents are able to remember the age of walking unaided and talking in sentences. The experience of Capute *et al.* (1985) is more hopeful in this respect. He reported a percentage of parents recording motor milestones ranging from 72% for sit up alone to 98% pull to stand in children up to the age of 2 years. The figures in Table 4.1 are derived from that paper.

Whereas the recall of dates and acquisition of skills can be an unreliable basis of developmental assessment, direct observation by the doctor, coupled with information from parents of their child's current ability is likely to produce an accurate record of function. What follows is a practical guide to the normal abilities of children of the following ages: 3 months, 6 months, 1 year, 18 months, 2 years, 3 years, 4 years, 5 years and 7 years. No attempt is made to be fully comprehensive and the information given is intended as a check list which the ophthalmologist may use to decide about the patient. It is presented under the conventional categories of vision and fine movements, hearing and language, posture and gross movements, social and emotional development. These broad headings are useful reminders for the doctor to use in framing questions and channelling observations. The data given here are a composite derived from the author's own experience, the observations of Drs Sheridan (1975) (Table 4.2),

Illingworth (1980), Egan *et al.* (1969) and the revised Denver developmental screening test.

Where recent papers have been published giving precise information about the mean of the age when skills are acquired, these are sometimes quoted, but at all times it should be appreciated that there is considerable normal variation in human development and that care must be taken in interpreting the significance of apparent aberration (see below).

Table 4.2 is one which doctors, who are not themselves developmental specialists but who need to make rapid assessments, may find useful. What follows is a list of skills grouped under the headings used above, with approximate dates when they might be expected to be present. Although the data in this form might appear to be more precise, caution is necessary in interpreting variation from the norm.

Vision and fine movements

Follows with eyes with increasing side-to-side range from birth onwards	
Hand regard	3–5 months
Reaches out	3–4 months
Transfers objects from hand to hand	6–8 months
Pincer grasp between thumb and forefinger	9–10 months
Touches objects with forefinger	9–10 months
Looks for the fallen toy	9–10 months
Builds tower of three bricks	18 months
Copies circle	3 years
Knows colours	3 years
Draws a man with head, trunk, arms and legs	4 years

Hearing and language

Turns to sounds	3–5 months
Single syllable sounds	Up to 6 months
Double syllable sounds	6–8 months
Imitates clapping hands	9–10 months
Waves bye-bye	9–10 months
Many single words with meaning	18 months
Short sentences	2 years
Identifies parts of body	2 years
Asks 'what'	3 years
Asks 'why'	3–4 years

Posture and gross movements

Lifts head when prone	birth onwards
Lifts head when supine	3 months
Rolls from front to back	4 months
Resting on elbows	5 months
Grasps own feet	5 months

Table 4.1 Gross motor milestones which may be recalled by parents of young children. From Capute *et al.* (1985).

Movement	Mean age (months)	Age range (months)
Roll prone to supine	3.7	±1.4
Sit alone	6.4	±1.3
Crawl	7.8	±1.7
Walk	11.5	±1.9

Table 4.2 Normal developmental milestones. Modified from Sheridan (1975).

Age	Vision and fine movements	Hearing and language	Posture and gross movements	Social and emotional development
3 months	Follows adults with eyes Watches own hands before face Fixes still objects briefly	Startled by loud sounds Consoled by comforting sounds Coos	Hands open mostly Lifts head and chest when placed prone	Becomes excited by preparation for happy events, e.g. bath Responds happily to tickle
6 months	Reaches out for small objects he has fixed on Palmar grasp	Uses mostly single syllables, e.g. ah, goo; occasional double sounds, e.g. adah Turns to voices	Grasps own feet Rolls front to back Sits alone very briefly	Takes everything to mouth Beginning to be shy of strangers
1 year	Pincer grasp between forefinger and thumb Looks for toy which has fallen out of sight	Understands several words, e.g. car, spoon Imitates sounds	Has been crawling for several months Beginning to walk holding on or alone	Waves bye-bye Gives on request
18 months	Builds tower with three bricks Enjoys picture books and points	Says 20 or more words	Beginning to run Picks up toys without falling	Drinks well from cup Bowel control Takes off shoes and socks
2 years	Builds tower with six bricks Imitates vertical line Recognizes people in photos	Makes short sentences Can show hands, feet, eyes, etc. on request	Walks up and down Stands alone Can throw a ball	Uses spoon well Bladder control in day Puts on shoes
3 years	Copies a circle Beginning to know colours Cuts with scissors	Knows name, age and sex Asks what, where?	Can stand on one foot Can stand on tip toe	Washes own hands Eats with fork and spoon
4 years	Copies a cross Draws a man with head, trunk and limbs	Asks why? Recounts experiences	Hops	Dresses and undresses and can manage buttons
5 years	Draws a recognizable man and house and copies a square and triangle	Beginning to ask the meaning of abstract words	Can skip on alternate feet	Co-operates with other children and understands the need for rules

Sits alone	6 months	Drinks from cup	9 months
Crawls	8 months	Uses spoon	18 months
Walks alone	1 year		
Stands on one foot	3 years		
Hops	4 years	**Dressing**	
		Helps with dressing	12 months
Social and emotional		Takes off shoes	18 months
		Takes off pants	15–24 months
Smiles	3–8 weeks	Dresses	3–4 years
Shy of strangers	6–12 months	Ties shoe laces	5–7 years

Feeding

Interpreting results

Chews   6 months

There are a number of factors which should be taken into

account when interpreting motor developmental mile-stones, such as racial differences, prematurity, normal variants, and so on.

Racial differences

In general black children achieve motor milestones earlier than white. Capute *et al.* (1985) found this to be true for all motor comparisons except rolling prone to supine, but showed such differences to be small, e.g. less than 1 month difference for milestones prior to walking.

Prematurity

Prematurely born children are generally reported to be delayed in locomotor development. Largo *et al.* (1985) showed that this was the case even when correcting the age for the amount of prematurity and even in neurolo-gically normal children. The differences become more marked with increasing age (hence making it unlikely that the difference is due to inaccurate estimation of prematurity), for example:

- preterm: mean age walking 14.1 months, males;
- term: mean age walking 13.4 months, males;
- preterm: mean age walking 14.4 months, females; and
- term: mean age walking 13.5 months, females.

Although slight sex differences are manifest in the above data and despite the finding of Capute *et al.* (1985) that black/white differences were greater between females than males, comparisons between the sexes in the motor sphere do not show any consistent differences.

Normal variation

For motor milestones it is important to comment on a nor-mal variant, bottom shuffling. Between 8 and 9% of the normal population show this method of early locomotion in preference to crawling and such children walk indepen-dently later than their more conventional colleagues (Rob-son 1970). Forty-eight per cent of idiopathic late walkers were shown by Chaplais and MacFarlane (1984) to be bot-tom shufflers and for there to be a family history of this in half. Apart from mild hypotonia and joint hyperextensi-bility, bottom shufflers are usually normal, though Robson and MacKeith (1971) did point out that one child in eight with spastic diplegia shuffles.

Vision impaired children

The medical literature referring to developmental mile-stones in visually handicapped children is surprisingly limited. Part of the problem is that generalizations cannot be made without reference to the degree of visual impair-ment and sometimes that is difficult to quantitate, particu-larly in a young child.

The single most helpful volume on this topic is *Blindness and Early Childhood Development* (Warren 1984). What follows is a list of highly selective comments and obser-vations which will be helpful to the ophthalmologist.

1 Seventy per cent of congenitally visually handicapped babies have additional major handicaps (Robinson 1977).
2 One-third of 91 babies were found to be hypotonic (Jan *et al.* 1975).
3 In another series of 100 visually impaired children, 68% were at three-quarter level of development or less for their age (Zinkin 1979).
4 Severely visually impaired children's expressive lan-guage tends to develop later than that of sighted children (McConachie & Moore 1994).
5 Developmental set-back in their second or third year of life occurred in 31% of 32 children who were totally blind (Cass *et al.* 1994).

Motor development

Motor development of the congenitally blind child in the first few months of life is not markedly different from that of a sighted child, and adequate maturation of postural milestones is achieved, e.g. independent sitting and standing (Fraiberg 1977). There are, however, qualitative differences, e.g. the blind baby sits in a frozen attitude (Sonksen 1983). Delay becomes manifest in the acquisition of self-initiated mobility, e.g. extension of arms prone, pulling to stand and crawling (achieved late in the first year). The parachute response is delayed by 6 months in blind babies, occurring at 18 months of age.

The blind baby tends to move the legs more than the arms, which may be held flexed at the elbow (Egan 1975). Although the blind baby starts to 'look at' his or her hands by bringing them up to the face at the normal time (16 weeks), reaching out is delayed beyond the 3–4 months norm (Reynell & Zinkin 1975); also, development of the pincer grasp is a year behind normal (Zinkin 1979).

Hearing and language

Babbling is probably the same in sighted and visually impaired children. The evidence is mixed as to whether a 10–20-word vocabulary is acquired at the same stage (Warren 1984), and it may well be that this is because of a difference between mildly and severely visually impaired children, and the difficulty in distinguishing the degree of handicap in young children. The young blind baby is slow to localize sounds by reaching out to touch them, and tends simply to become still to the sound.

Social and emotional development

The blind child smiles at the normal time. However, blind children are very slow to localize their eyes to a part of the body which has been touched. This normally occurs around 7 months and in blind babies it may be 2 years or more before this is done (Sonksen 1983). The social competence of blind children and adolescents is not as strong as normal. Tilman (1967) refers to comparison of sighted and blind children on the various parts of the Wechsler intelligence scale for children (WISC).

What do you do if the child seems abnormal?

The developmental scales above are simply a guide to normal development and as Hall and Baird (1986) indicate, although a below-average performance can be described in terms of age equivalents, i.e. how many months behind, the significance of that delay is uncertain. The best the ophthalmologist can do when a possible delay has been detected is to acknowledge this uncertainty and refer to a paediatrician or to a child psychologist for more formal psychometric assessment when more specific and rigorously standardized tests can be applied.

References

Capute AJ, Shapiro BK, Palmer FB, Ross A, Wachtel RC. Normal gross motor development: the influences of race, sex and socioeconomic status. *Dev Med Child Neurol* 1985; **27**: 635–43.

Cass HD, Sonksen PM, McConachie HR. Developmental setback in severe visual impairment. *Arch Dis Child* 1994; **70**: 192–6.

Chaplais J de Z, MacFarlane JA. A review of 404 late walkers. *Arch Dis Child* 1984; **59**: 512–16.

Egan D. The early development of visually handicapped children. In: Smith V, Keen J, eds. *Visual Handicaps in Children*, Chapter 17, pp 139–153. Clinics in Developmental Medicine No. 73. 1979. Spastics International Medical Publications. London: William Heinemann Medical Books.

Egan DF, Illingworth RS, MacKeith RC. Developmental screening 0–5 years. *Clin Dev Med* 1969; **30**.

Fraiberg S. *Insights from the Blind*. London: Souvenir Press, 1977.

Hall DMB, Baird G. Developmental tests and scales. *Arch Dis Child* 1986; **61**: 213–15.

Illingworth RS. *The Development of the Infant and Young Child, Normal and Abnormal*, 9th edn. Edinburgh: Churchill Livingstone, 1980.

Jan JE, Robinson GC, Scott EP, Kinnis C. Hypotonia in the blind child. *Dev Med Child Neurol* 1975; **17**: 35–40.

Largo RH, Molinari L, Weber M, Comenate Pinto L, Duc C. Early development of locomotion: significance of prematurity, cerebral palsy and sex. *Dev Med Child Neurol* 1985; **27**: 183–91.

McConachie HR, Moore V. Early expressive language of severely visually impaired children. *Dev Med Child Neurol* 1994; **36**: 230–40.

Reynell J, Zinkin P. New perspectives for the developmental assessment of young children with severe visual handicap. *Child Care Health Dev* 1975; **1**: 61–9.

Robinson GC. Causes, ocular disorders, associated handicaps, and incidence and prevalance of blindness in childhood. In: Jan J, Freeman R, Scott E, eds. *Visual Impairment in Children and Adolescents*. New York: Grune & Stratton, 1977: 27–47.

Robson P. Shuffling, hitching, scooting or sliding — some observations in 30 otherwise normal children. *Dev Med Child Neurol* 1970; **12**: 608–17.

Robson P, MacKeith RC. Shufflers with spastic diplegic cerebral palsy: a confusing clinical picture. *Dev Med Child Neurol* 1971; **13**: 651–9.

Sheridan M. *The Developmental Progress of Infants and Young Children*, No. 102. London: HMSO, 1975.

Sonksen P. Vision and early development. In: Taylor D, Wybar K, eds. *Paediatric Ophthalmology*. New York: Marcel Dekker, 1983: 85–95.

Tilman MH. Performance of blind and sighted children on the WISC. *Int J Educ Blind* 1967; **16**: 65–74, 106–12.

Warren DH. *Blindness and Early Childhood Development*, 2nd edn. New York: American Foundation for the Blind, 1984.

Zinkin P. The effect of visual handicap on early development. In: Smith V, Keen J, eds. *Visual Handicap in Children*, Chapter 16; pp. 132–138. Clinics in Developmental Medicine No. 73. International Medical Publications. London: William Heinemann Medical Books.

5: Postnatal Growth of the Eye and Emmetropization

Scott Lambert

The human eye grows rapidly during the first few years of life. While some of this growth is mediated genetically, the visual experience during infancy and childhood also makes a significant contribution to the development of the eye. This is particularly true for the development of the refractive components of the eye.

The premature eye

Premature infants (30–35 gestational weeks) have shorter ocular axial lengths (mean 15.1 ± 0.9 mm), steeper corneas (53.6 ± 2.5 dioptres), and higher lenticular refractive powers (43.5 ± 3.6 dioptres) than full-term infants (Gordon & Donzis 1985). The pupils are miotic and remnants of the tunica vasculosa lentis are frequently present (Kalina 1979). Bilateral symmetrical lens opacities may occur in premature infants. Initially, they consist of vacuoles along the peripheral edges of the posterior Y suture of the lens, but may progress to a dense opacification of the posterior subcapsular area. Their peak incidence occurs 7–10 days after birth. They usually resolve within 1–2 weeks with no residual abnormalities (McCormick 1968).

Vascularization of the retina is completed nasally during the eighth gestational month and temporally during the ninth month. The peripheral retina has a silver–grey appearance in areas in which vascularization is incomplete (Kalina 1979).

The infant eye

By 40 gestational weeks, the mean axial length of the eye increases to 16.8 ± 0.6 mm, the cornea flattens to 51.2 ± 1.1 dioptres, and the lens power decreases to 34.4 ± 2.3 dioptres (Gordon & Donzis 1985). The peripheral retina is fully vascularized and the extrafoveal retina functions at nearly adult levels; however, the fovea is still immature. Neonatal foveolas have both an increased diameter and a lower cone density than adult foveolas. Infants have a rod-free zone or foveola 1000 µm in diameter with a cone density of 18 cones per 100 µm, whereas adults have a rod-free zone with a mean diameter of 650–700 µm and a cone density of 42 cones per 100 µm. This increase in cone density from 36 000 cones/mm² at birth to 108 000 cones/mm² by 4 years of age occurs secondary to the migration of cones centrally. Concurrently, ganglion cells and other components of the inner retina migrate peripherally (Hendrickson 1994). During this same time interval, the length of the cone inner segments increases from 10 to 25 µm and the length of the cone outer segments increases from 3 to 60 µm (Yuodelis & Hendrickson 1986). This compacting process is believed to be partly mediated by Müller cells which span the width of the retina. As the Müller cells are stretched laterally in the inner retina it has been postulated that they squeeze the cone photoreceptors closer together.

The immaturity of the foveal cones during infancy limits visual acuity in at least two ways. First, the lower cone density reduces spatial resolution (Hirsch & Hylton 1984). As the cone density of the foveola increases during the first year of life, there is a comparable improvement in the spatial resolution of the eye (Yuodelis & Hendrickson 1986). Second, the shorter length of the cone outer segments limits the efficiency of the cones in detecting light as well as colour. Although the maturation of the visual cortex and other areas of the visual pathway are important in the enhancement of visual acuity during the first year of life, improvements in acuity thereafter are believed to be mediated by changes in the morphology and packing density of the foveolar cones (Jacobs & Blakemore 1988).

Growth after infancy

The human eye grows rapidly during the first year of life. During the first 6 weeks of life the cornea flattens from a mean of 51 to 44 dioptres (Inagaki 1986), the axial length increases from a mean of 17 mm at birth to 20 mm by 1 year of age, and the power of the lens decreases from 34 dioptres at birth to 28 dioptres by 6 months of age (Gordon & Donzis 1985).

Infants during the first year of life have a mean refractive error of 1.00–1.25 dioptres of hyperopia and a 15–30% incidence of astigmatism exceeding 1.0 dioptre (Ingram *et al.* 1979; Fulton *et al.* 1980). Five per cent of infants between 6 and 9 months of age have greater than 3 dioptres of hyperopia and 0.5% have greater than 3 dioptres of myopia (Atkinson *et al.* 1984). Both the prevalence of astigmatism (Abrahamsson *et al.* 1988) and hyperopia (Mäntyjärvi 1985) decrease with age. By 3 years of age, the incidence of 1 dioptre or more of astigmatism decreases to 8% (Ingram *et al.* 1979).

Emmetropization

Emmetropization refers to the developmental process which co-ordinates the growth of the refractive components of the eye in such a manner as to create a non-Gaussian distribution of refractive errors around emmetropia. Emmetropization is dependent on the visual experience of the infantile eye. Animal studies have shown that inducing a hyperopic or myopic refractive error with external lenses can alter axial elongation. If a myopic refractive error is induced, the eye elongates less whereas if a hyperopic refractive error is induced the eye elongates excessively (Troilo & Wallman 1991; Hung *et al.* 1996). Correcting refractive errors in infants may have a similar effect. Ingram *et al.* (1991) have reported that a higher percentage of children remain hyperopic if the refractive errors are corrected with spectacles during infancy. Aurell and Norrsell (1990) followed longitudinally a cohort of children with a family history of accommodative esotropia. They noted that many children with high hyperopia as infants had a marked shift towards emmetropia during the first 2 years of life. None of these children developed an accommodative esotropia. In contradistinction, a second group retained their hyperopic refractive error and developed an accommodative esotropia when 18–30 months of age. It is unclear why one group of children underwent emmetropization whereas the second group did not since neither group received any treatment prior to the onset of the esotropia.

Visual deprivation during infancy may also interfere with the emmetropization process. Using macaque monkeys, Raviola and Wiesel (1985) have demonstrated that lid closure or corneal opacification during infancy results in axial myopia. The increase in the axial length occurred exclusively in the posterior segment of the eye. Visual deprivation of the nasal or temporal half of the retina in chicks has also been shown to result in asymmetrical growth of the posterior segment of the eye suggesting that the effect can occur regionally within the eye (Wallman *et al.* 1987). This phenomenon appeared to be light-dependent, since myopia does not develop when these animals are reared in the dark (Raviola & Wiesel 1978; Guyton *et al.* 1989). Since myopia develops even after transecting the optic nerve or surgical ablation of the visual cortices, it has been postulated that this process is mediated at the level of the retina. Dopamine is believed to play an important role in regulating this process based on the observations that (i) retinal dopamine levels are reduced in chick and monkey eyes after monocular occlusion, and (ii) axial myopia may be prevented by the topical application of dopamine agonists (Iuvone *et al.* 1989, 1991; Stone *et al.* 1989). As a corollary, the effect of a dopamine agonist on axial elongation may be abolished by the co-administration of a dopamine antagonist (Stone *et al.* 1989).

Other neurotransmitters and growth factors have also been correlated with the development of axial myopia (Stone *et al.* 1988). Many reports have documented axial myopia in children visually deprived during infancy by congenital cataracts (Rabin *et al.* 1981; Johnson *et al.* 1982; von Noorden & Lewis 1987; Rasooly & BenEzra 1988), corneal opacities (Curtin 1985; Gee & Tabbara 1988; Twomey *et al.* 1990), and ptosis (Hoyt *et al.* 1981; von Noorden & Lewis 1987), albeit less dramatically than in experimental animals.

Axial shortening may be produced surgically by removing the crystalline lens during infancy (Wilson *et al.* 1987; Tigges *et al.* 1990; Lambert *et al.* 1996; Kugelberg *et al.* 1996). This phenomenon suggests that factors produced by the crystalline lens may stimulate ocular growth.

Accommodation also may influence the refractive development of infantile eyes. Chronic atropinization during childhood has been reported to reduce the progression of myopia (Kelly *et al.* 1975; Brodstein *et al.* 1984). In addition, a correlation seems to exist between the accommodative demands of near work and the development of myopia (Rosner & Belkin 1987); however, the mechanism whereby excessive accommodation causes myopia is unclear. Interestingly, emmetropization in animals appears to be independent of accommodation since it can occur even after chronic atropinization or ablation of the Edinger–Westphal nucleus (Troilo 1992).

Aberrant growth

Retinal dystrophies are also commonly associated with significant degrees of ametropia. Leber's congenital amaurosis is often associated with high hyperopia (Wagner *et al.* 1985; Lambert *et al.* 1989), whereas retinitis pigmentosa (Sieving & Fishman 1978), blue cone monochromatism and congenital stationary night-blindness (Merin *et al.* 1970) are commonly associated with myopia. Albinos are frequently high myopes or hyperopes or have significant astigmatism (Fonda 1962). Retinopathy of prematurity is also commonly associated with the development of myopia (Kushner 1982; Gordon & Donzis 1986;

Lue *et al.* 1996). Tasman (1979) reported an 8% incidence of 6 dioptres or more of myopia in a series of patients with cicatricial retinopathy of prematurity. Sixty-seven per cent of these patients had a greater axial length in the more myopic eye suggestive of axial myopia. The basis for the development of large refractive errors in these conditions is unknown but again emphasizes the importance of the retina in the refractive development of the human eye.

References

Abrahamsson M, Fabian G, Sjöstrand J. Changes in astigmatism between the ages of 1 and 4 years: a longitudinal study. *Br J Ophthalmol* 1988; **72**: 145–9.

Atkinson J, Braddick OJ, Durden K *et al.* Screening for refractive errors in 6–9 month old infants by photorefraction. *Br J Ophthalmol* 1984; **68**: 105–12.

Aurell E, Norrsell K. A longitudinal study of children with a family history of strabismus: factors determining the incidence of strabismus. *Br J Ophthalmol* 1990; **74**: 589–94.

Brodstein RS, Brodstein DE, Olson RJ *et al.* The treatment of myopia with atropine and bifocals. A long-term prospective study. *Ophthalmology* 1984; **91**: 1373–9.

Curtin BJ. *The Myopias: Basic Science and Clinical Management.* Philadelphia: Harper & Row, 1985.

Fonda G. Characteristics and low-vision corrections in albinism. A report of 161 patients. *Arch Ophthalmol* 1962; **68**: 754–61.

Fulton AB, Dobson V, Salem D *et al.* Cycloplegic refractions in infants and young children. *Am J Ophthalmol* 1980; **90**: 239–47.

Gee KS, Tabbara KF. Increase in ocular axial length in patients with corneal opacification. *Ophthalmology* 1988; **95**: 1276–8.

Gordon RA, Donzis PB. Refractive development of the human eye. *Arch Ophthalmol* 1985; **103**: 785–9.

Gordon RA, Donzis PB. Myopia associated with retinopathy of prematurity. *Ophthalmology* 1986; **93**: 1593–8.

Guyton DL, Greene PR, Scholz RT. Dark-rearing interference with emmetropization in the rhesus monkey. *Invest Ophthalmol Vis Sci* 1989; **30**: 761–4.

Hendrickson AE. Primate foveal development: a microcosm of current questions in neurobiology. *Invest Ophthalmol Vis Sci* 1994; **35**: 3129–33.

Hirsch J, Hylton R. Quality of the primate photoreceptor lattice and limits of spatial vision. *Vision Res* 1984; **24**: 347–55.

Hoyt CS, Stone RD, Fromer C *et al.* Monocular axial myopia associated with neonatal eyelid closure in human infants. *Am J Ophthalmol* 1981; **91**: 197–200.

Hung LF, Crawford MLJ, Smith EJ. Spectacle lenses after eye growth and the refractive status of young monkeys. *Nature Medicine* 1995; **1**: 761–5.

Inagaki Y. The rapid change of corneal curvature in the neonatal period and infancy. *Arch Ophthalmol* 1986; **104**: 1026–7.

Ingram RM, Traynar MJ, Walker C *et al.* Screening for refractive errors at age 1 year: a pilot study. *Br J Ophthalmol* 1979; **63**: 243–50.

Ingram RM, Arnold PE, Dally S, Lucas J. Emmetropisation, squint, and reduced visual acuity after treatment. *Br J Ophthalmol* 1991; **75**: 414–16.

Iuvone PM, Tigges M, Fernandes A *et al.* Dopamine synthesis and metabolism in rhesus monkey retina: development, aging, and the effects of monocular visual deprivation. *Vis Neurosci* 1989; **2**: 465–71.

Iuvone PM, Tigges M, Stone RA *et al.* Effects of apomorphine, a dopamine receptor agonist, on ocular refraction and axial elongation in a primate model of myopia. *Invest Ophthalmol Vis Sci* 1991; **32**: 1674–7.

Jacobs DS, Blakemore C. Factors limiting the postnatal development of visual acuity in the monkey. *Vision Res* 1988; **28**: 947–58.

Johnson CA, Post RB, Chalupa LM *et al.* Monocular deprivation in humans: a study of identical twins. *Invest Ophthalmol Vis Sci* 1982; **23**: 135–8.

Kalina RE. Examination of the premature infant. *Ophthalmology* 1979; **86**: 1690–4.

Kelly TS-B, Chatfield C, Tustin G. Clinical assessment of the arrest of myopia. *Br J Ophthalmol* 1975; **59**: 529–38.

Kugelberg U, Zetterstrom C, Lundgren B, Syren-Nordquist S. Eye growth in the aphakic newborn rabbit. *J Cataract Refract Surg* 1996; **22**: 337–41.

Kushner BJ. Strabismus and amblyopia associated with regressed retinopathy of prematurity. *Arch Ophthalmol* 1982; **100**: 256–61.

Lambert SR, Kriss A, Taylor D *et al.* Follow-up and diagnostic reappraisal of 75 patients with Leber's congenital amaurosis. *Am J Ophthalmol* 1989; **107**: 624–31.

Lambert SR, Fernandes A, Drews-Botsch C, Tigges M. Pseudophakia retards axial elongation in neonatal monkey eyes. *Invest Ophthalmol Vis Sci* 1996; **37**: 451–8.

Lye CL, Hansen RM, Reisner DS *et al.* The course of myopia in children with retinopathy. *Vis Res* 1995; **35**: 1329–35.

McCormick AQ. Transient cataracts in premature infants: a new clinical entity. *Canad J Ophthalmol* 1968; **3**: 202–6.

Mäntyjärvi MI. Changes of refraction in schoolchildren. *Arch Ophthalmol* 1985; **103**: 790–2.

Merin S, Rowe H, Auerbach E *et al.* Syndrome of congenital high myopia with nyctalopia. Report of findings in 25 families. *Am J Ophthalmol* 1970; **70**: 541–7.

Rabin J, Van Sluyters RC, Malach R. Emmetropization: a vision-dependent phenomenon. *Invest Ophthalmol Vis Sci* 1981; **20**: 561–4.

Rasooly R, BenEzra D. Congenital and traumatic cataract. The effect on ocular axial length. *Arch Ophthalmol* 1988; **106**: 1066–8.

Raviola E, Wiesel TN. Effect of dark-rearing on experimental myopia in monkeys. *Invest Ophthalmol Vis Sci* 1978; **17**: 485–8.

Raviola E, Wiesel TN. An animal model of myopia. *N Engl J Med* 1985; **312**: 1609–15.

Rosner M, Belkin M. Intelligence, education, and myopia in males. *Arch Ophthalmol* 1987; **105**: 1508–11.

Sieving PA, Fishman GA. Refractive errors of retinitis pigmentosa patients. *Br J Ophthalmol* 1978; **62**: 163–7.

Stone RA, Laties AM, Raviola E *et al.* Increase in retinal vasoactive intestinal polypeptide after eyelid fusion in primates. *Proc Natl Acad Sci USA* 1988; **85**: 257–60.

Stone RA, Lin T, Laties AM *et al.* Retinal dopamine and form-deprivation myopia. *Proc Natl Acad Sci USA* 1989; **86**: 704–6.

Tasman W. Late complications of retrolental fibroplasia. *Ophthalmology* 1979; **86**: 1724–40.

Tigges M, Tigges J, Fernandes A *et al.* Postnatal axial eye elongation in normal and visually deprived rhesus monkeys. *Invest Ophthalmol Vis Sci* 1990; **31**: 1035–46.

Troilo D. Neonatal eye growth and emmetropisation — a literature review. *Eye* 1992; **6**: 154–60.

Troilo D, Wallman J. The regulation of eye growth and refractive state: an experimental study of emmetropization. *Vision Res* 1991; **31**: 1237–50.

Twomey JM, Gilvarry A, Restori M, Kirkness CM, Moore AT, Holden AL. Ocular enlargement following corneal opacification. *Eye* 1990; **4**: 497–504.

von Noorden GK, Lewis RA. Ocular axial length in unilateral congenital cataracts and blepharoptosis. *Invest Ophthalmol Vis Sci* 1987; **28**: 750–2.

Wagner RS, Caputo AR, Nelson LB *et al*. High hyperopia in Leber's congenital amaurosis. *Arch Ophthalmol* 1985; **103**: 1507–9.

Wallman J, Gottlieb MD, Rajaram V *et al*. Local retinal regions control local eye growth and myopia. *Science* 1987; **237**: 73–7.

Wilson JR, Fernandes A, Chandler CV *et al*. Abnormal development of the axial length of aphakic monkey eyes. *Invest Ophthalmol Vis Sci* 1987; **28**: 2096–9.

Yuodelis C, Hendrickson A. A qualitative and quantitative analysis of the human fovea during development. *Vision Res* 1986; **26**: 847–55.

6: Milestones and Normative Data

H. U. Møller

At birth the infant eye appears to be nearly the same size as the adult eye because the corneal diameter is only 1.7 mm shorter than in the adult; but actually its volume increases almost threefold up to maturity and its weight doubles. Thus the average for the full-term newborn eye is 3.25 cm³ or 3.40 g. The weight of the eyeball increases nearly 40% by the middle of the second year and nearly 70% by the fifth year (Scammon & Armstrong 1925; Wilmer & Scammon 1950).

Many changes occur with maturation and therefore normative data are needed to evaluate clinical observations during childhood. Much of the data is rather old, as the art of anthropometry is out of fashion, but we still rely on these old recordings until they are revised. An extensive textbook *A Biography of the Eye* is published by Weale (1982).

Embryology

The development and growth of an embryo and its eyes is a continuous process; however, there is variability in the rate of growth of the different ocular tissues. Thus the cells which will eventually become the iris are visible as migrated neural crest cells in the seventh week, but they remain dormant until the ciliary muscles are formed in the third month.

Unlike man, Mother Nature does not look at an embryo in terms of stages, weeks of gestation or trimesters; never-

theless the development of the different parts of the eyes are timed according to a meticulously sequenced pattern. Highlighting here a few milestones of embryogenesis may help in the understanding of complex teratogenic syndromes (Fig. 6.1, Table 6.1).

The developing eye comprises more than one germinal layer: (i) neuroectoderm (e.g. the optic sulcus which later becomes the optic vesicle early in the fourth week); (ii) surface ectoderm (e.g. the first sign of the lens which is on day 32); and (iii) migrated neural crest cells which are the stem cells of, among other things, the anterior chamber during the seventh week. The mesodermal embryonic layer contributes only the vascular endothelial cells and extraocular muscles which are visible in the fourth week.

Classical ophthalmological embryology was published by Mann (1928), O'Rahilly (1983) and Torczynski (1989); Barishak (1992) published an extensive and excellent chronological description of eye development. Le Douarin (1982) summarized experiments on neural crest cell migration using chimaeric quail and chick embryos; these provided a basis for understanding the migration defects (neurocristopathies) of anterior segment dysgenesis syndromes. A modern clinical approach to embryology is given by Moore and Persaud (1993) and Larsen (1993).

Intercanthal distance

The distance between the inner canthi and the outer canthi as well as the size of the palpebral fissure are of importance in diagnosing a host of conditions such as craniofacial malformations and fetal alcohol syndrome.

Figure 6.2a shows the linear relationship between gestational age and orbital margin horizontal (OMH) as well as vertical (OMV) diameters. The horizontal and vertical diameters of the orbital margin were determined using a caliper or a metal ruler. Figure 6.2b illustrates the linear relationship between gestational age and conjunctival fornix horizontal (CFH) as well as vertical (CFV) diameters (Isenberg *et al.* 1987). The measurement of the

Table 6.1 Chronological embryology. Modified from Bach and Seefelder (1914), Mann (1928), Hittner (1977), Ozanics and Jacobiec (1982), Torczynski (1989), Barishak (1992), Moore and Persaud (1993) and Larsen (1993).

Development of the eye	The age of the embryo	Development of the eye	The age of the embryo
Optic sulcus, optic primordium	week 3	Vortex veins pierce sclera	month 3
Optic cup	week 4	Eyelids fuse	month 3
Lens placode	week 4	Tarsal plate merges with levator palpebrae	month 3
Retinal disc	week 4	Lacrimal gland	month 3
Embryonic fissure (coloboma)	week 4	Extraocular muscles fuse with sclera	month 3
Primordia, extraocular muscles	week 4	Angle between orbits reduced to 72° due to growth of maxillary processes	month 3
Lens pit invaginates	week 5		
Lens vesicle	week 5	Major retinal constituents present	month 4
Primary vitreous, hyaloid vasculature	week 5	Haller–Zinn arterial circle	month 4
Optic stalk	week 5	Incipient retinal vascularization	month 4
Structures of face and orbit	week 5	Physiological cupping of optic disc	month 4
Angle between orbits reduced to 160° due to growth of maxillary processes	week 5	Anlage of pars plana	month 4
		Arterial circle of iris	month 4
Incipient differentiation of retinal pigment epithelium	week 6	Pupillary membrane replaces anterior tunica vasculosa lentis	month 4
Primordium of sensory retina	week 6	Hyaloid vascular system regresses	month 4
Secondary vitreous fibrils	week 6	Secondary vitreous well developed	month 4
Primary lens fibres	week 6	Tertiary vitreous develops	month 4
First eyelid folds	week 6	Sclera well developed	month 4
Closure of embryonic fissure	week 6	Descemet's membrane	month 4
Retinal pigment epithelium, one cell thick layer of cuboidal cells	week 6	Canal of Schlemm	month 4
First fibrils of secondary vitreous	week 6	Palpebral ligaments	month 4
Primitive corneal epithelium	week 6	Lanugo and sebaceous glands in the caruncle	month 4
First myofibrils of extraocular muscles	week 6	First uncrossed chiasm fibres	month 4
Muscles cone visible	week 6	Differentiation of photoreceptors	month 5
Ciliary ganglion visible	week 6	Rapid growth of retinal vasculature	month 5
Superior anlage of nasolacrimal duct	week 6	Differentiation of cornea	month 5
Inferior anlage of nasolacrimal duct	week 6	Corneal nerves reach the epithelium	month 5
Proliferation and differentiation of future cornea	week 6	Adipose tissue in the orbit	month 5
Sensory retina	week 7	Loss of ganglion cells in the retina	month 5
Choroidal vasculature	week 7	Loss of axons in the optic nerve	month 5
Anterior segment	week 7	Cloquet's canal	month 5
Anterior tunica vasculosa lentis	week 7	Bowman's membrane	month 5
Embryonic fissure completely closed	week 7	Tenon's capsule	month 5
Neural crest cells for corneal endothelium	week 7	Eyelids start to separate	month 5
Neural crest cells for trabecular endothelium	week 7	Scleral spur	month 5
Neural crest cells for corneal stroma	week 7	Dilator muscle of the iris	month 6
Neural crest cells to be future iris stroma	week 7	Vascularization of optic nerve completed	month 6
Anterior chamber between corneal endothelium and lamina irido pupillaris	week 7	Vessels of pupillary membrane start to atrophy	month 6
		Bowman's membrane well defined	month 6
Sclera visible	week 7	Nasolacrimal duct patent	month 6
Circular eyelid fold	week 7	Central fovea starts to thin	month 7
Angle between orbits reduced to 120° due to growth of maxillary processes	week 7	Adult size of avascular zone of fovea	month 7
		Fibrous lamina cibrosa	month 7
Maturation of retinal pigment epithelium	week 8	Myelinization of optic nerve appears from chiasm towards the eye	month 7
Retinal ganglion cells	week 8		
Axons in optic stalk	week 8	Circular muscle of ciliary body	month 7
Bergmeister papilla formed	week 8	Iris completes its pigmentation	month 7
Lacrimal gland	week 8	Pigmentation of choroid	month 7
Optic nerve has 2670 000 axons	week 8	Corneal epithelium 4–5 layers	month 7
Rudimentary chiasm	week 8	Lens diameter 5 mm	month 7
Hyaloid vascular system fully formed	week 8	Iris sphincter	month 8
Y-shaped suture of the lens	week 8	Chamber angle completes formation	month 8
Bergmeister papilla disappears	month 3	Hyaloid system disappears	month 8
Anlage of ciliary processes	month 3	Retinal vessels reach nasal ora serrata	month 8
Iris epithelium	month 3	The length of the muscles cone 25 mm	month 8
Lens completely surrounded by tunica vasculosa lentis	month 3	Retinal vessels reach the periphery	month 9
		Myelination of optic nerve is completed to lamina cibrosa	month 9
Lens comprises embryonal and fetal nucleus	month 3		
Corneal collagen fibrils	month 3	Pupillary membrane disappears	month 9

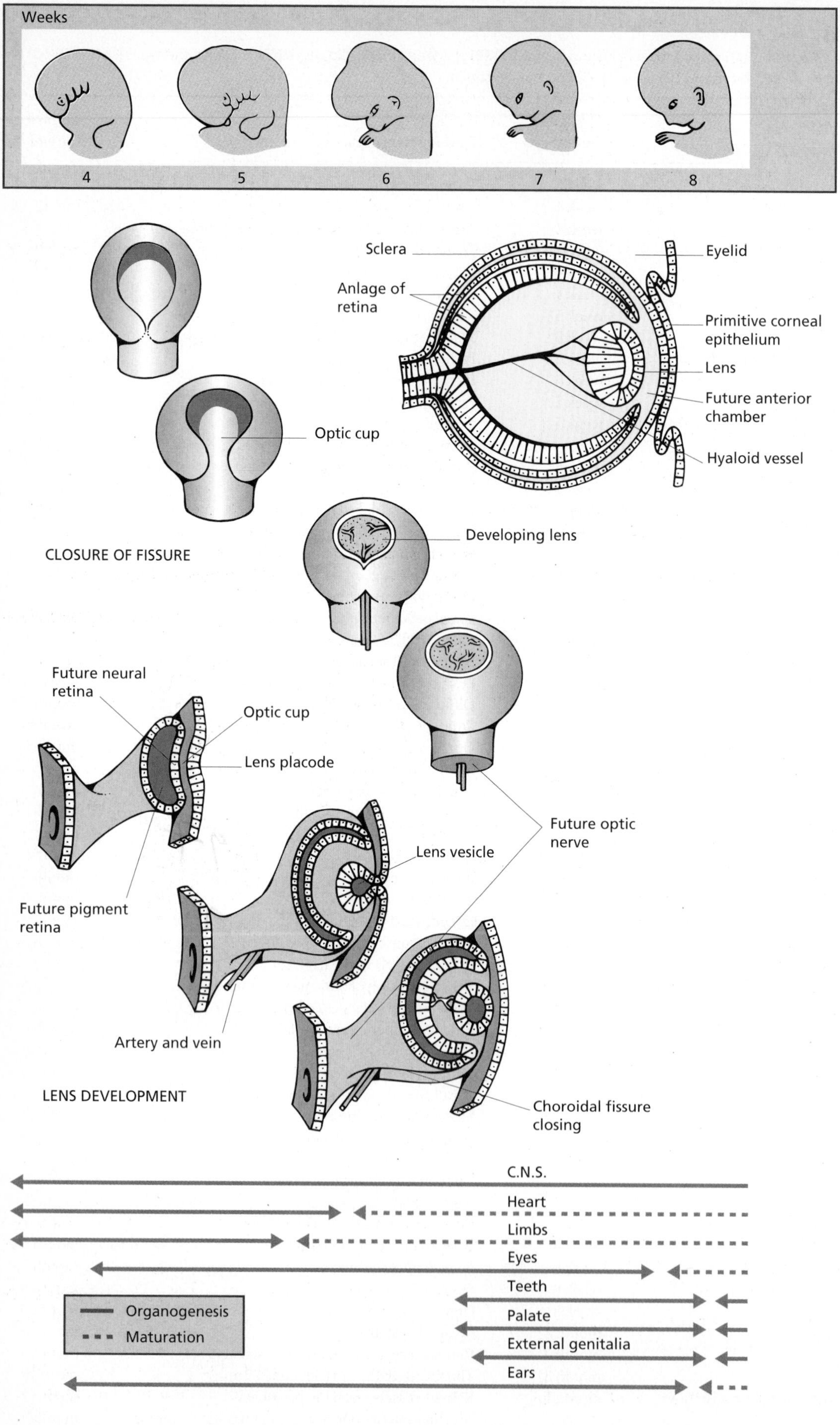

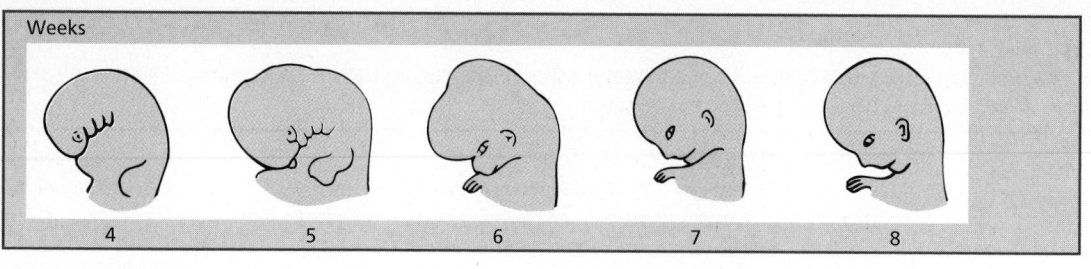

Weeks

4　5　6　7　8

CLOSURE OF FISSURE

Optic cup

Sclera

Anlage of retina

Eyelid

Primitive corneal epithelium

Lens

Future anterior chamber

Hyaloid vessel

Developing lens

Future neural retina

Optic cup

Lens placode

Lens vesicle

Future optic nerve

Future pigment retina

Artery and vein

LENS DEVELOPMENT

Choroidal fissure closing

C.N.S.

Heart

Limbs

Eyes

Teeth

Palate

External genitalia

Ears

—— Organogenesis

- - - Maturation

Fig. 6.1(a) *See caption opposite.*

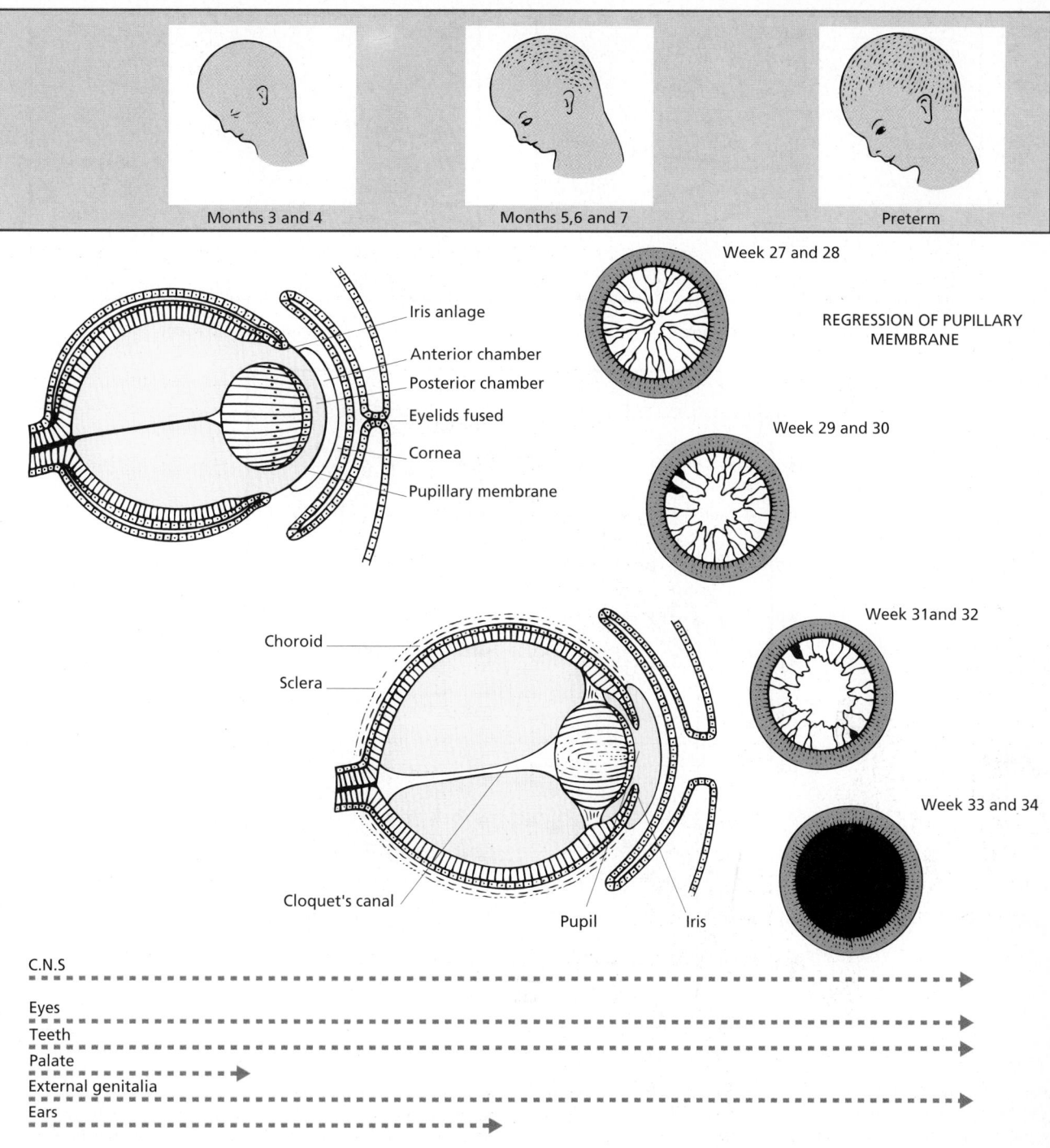

Fig. 6.1 (*above and opposite*) Milestones in ophthalmoembryology. Modified from Bach and Seefelder (1914), Mann (1928), Hittner 1977, Ozanics and Jakobiec (1982), Torczynski (1989), Barishak (1992), Moore and Persaud (1993) and Larsen (1993).

conjunctival fornices was performed using known conformers examining the mobility in millimetres of the conformer.

The palpebral fissures are 15 ± 2 mm at 32 weeks of ges-

tation, 17 ± 2 mm at birth, 24 ± 3 mm at 2 years of age, and 27 ± 3 mm at the age of 14 (data pooled from Jones *et al.* 1978; Thomas *et al.* 1987). Interracial differences may exist: the palpebral fissure is longer in black Americans, with a mean of 30 mm at the age of 3 years (Iosub *et al.* 1985).

Laestadius *et al.* (1969) published extensive data on inner canthal and outer orbital dimensions and found the

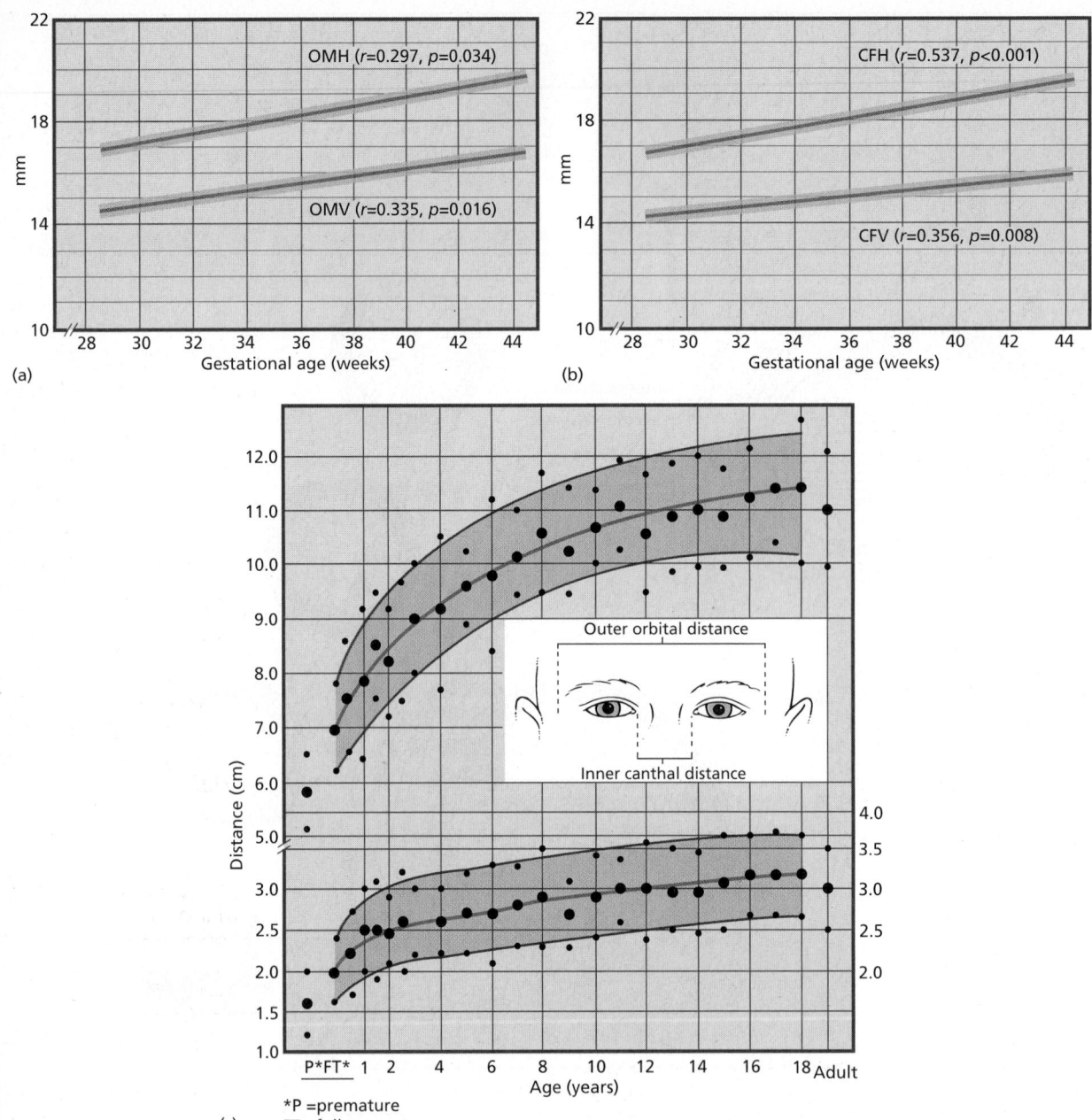

Fig. 6.2 Interocular distance. (a) Linear regression relationship and standard error of the estimate between orbital margin horizontal (OMH) and vertical (OMV) diameters and gestational age. Correlation coefficients with *P* values are indicated. Data from Isenberg *et al*. (1987). Redrawn with permission from the publisher. (b) Linear regression relationship and standard error of the estimate between conjunctival fornix horizontal (CFH) and vertical (CFV) diameters and gestational age. Correlation coefficients with *P* values are indicated. Data from Isenberg *et al*. (1987). Redrawn with permission from the publisher. (c) Graphs of inner canthal and outer orbital distances. The large points represent the mean value for each age group, the smaller points represent 2 SD from the mean. The heavy line approximates the 50th percentile, while the shaded area roughly encompasses the range from the third to the 97th percentile. Data from Laestadius *et al*. (1969). Redrawn with permission from the publisher.

inner canthal distance to be 16 mm and the outer orbital distance to be 59 mm, respectively, in premature infants; 20 ± 4 mm and 69 ± 8 mm in newborn babies; 26 ± 6 and 88 ± 10 mm at the age of 3; and 31 ± 5 mm and 111 ± 12 mm at the age of 14 (Fig. 6.2c).

To simplify matters a universal approach is the canthus index:

$$\text{Canthus Index} = \frac{\text{inner canthus distance} \times 100}{\text{outer canthus distance}}\%$$

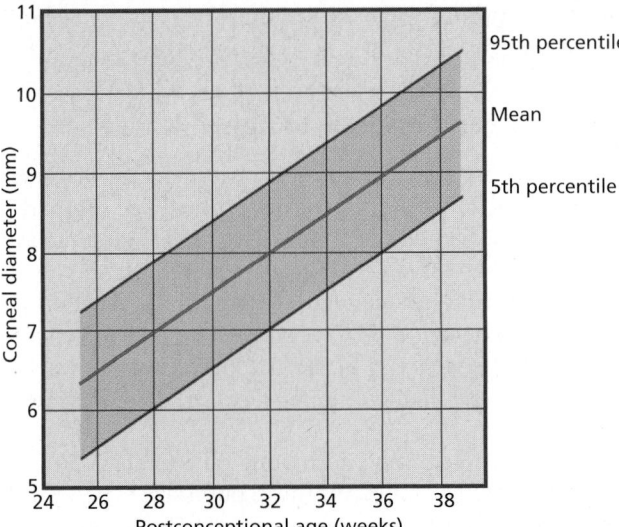

Fig. 6.3 Mean corneal diameter plotted against postconceptional age with 95% prediction limits. Redrawn from Tucker *et al.* (1992). Published with permission from the publisher.

Normative limits, unrelated to age, lie between 28.4 and 38% according to Leiber (1992). Farkas and Munro (1987), however, examined more than 1000 young people between the ages of 6 and 18 years and found conflicting data. A mean for boys and girls at 6 years of age was found at 38.2% (SD 2.1%) and 38.3% (SD 1.8%), respectively, while at the age of 16 years these figures were 37.1% (SD 2.6%) and 36.6% (SD 1.9%).

Cornea

The corneal diameter, measured with corneal templates in premature infants at 25–37 weeks postconceptional age, increases by 0.5 mm every 15 days from 6.2 to 9.0 mm. Figure 6.3 shows the mean corneal diameter plotted against postconceptional age with 95% prediction limits (Tucker *et al.* 1992). Al-Umran and Pandolfi (1992) found values to be about 1 mm higher.

It may be added that the young premature cornea lacks lustre and clarity. Therefore the premature cornea is not a reliable indication of the presence of an abnormality. The narrow anterior chambers, miotic pupils and bluish irides are features of prematurity (Musarella & Morin 1982).

At birth the horizontal and vertical diameters of the cornea for full-term boys were 9.8±0.33 mm and 10.4±0.35 mm and for girls 10.1±0.33 mm and 10.7±0.29 mm (Sorsby & Sheridan 1960).

Scammon and Armstrong (1925) concluded that the last 2 mm of growth in corneal diameter, i.e. approximately 20%, takes place within early infancy and more slowly in early childhood. An adult value of 11.7 mm is reached at the age of 7 years.

Corneal refraction in premature infants is 53.1±1.5 dioptres, in the neonate 48.4±1.7 dioptres, at 1 month 45.9±2.3 dioptres, at 36 months 42.9±1.3 dioptres (Weale 1982).

Central corneal thickness

Abnormal thickness of the central cornea is a possible source of error in applanation tonometry. Central corneal thickness (CCT) in full-term babies is significantly higher, 0.54 mm, than that of children of more than 2 years of age, who have adult readings of 0.52 mm. Results of CCT measured with optical pachometry, as well as corneal curvature and SEM are given for premature and full-term babies in Table 6.2 (Ehlers *et al.* 1976).

CCT was measured by ultrasonic pachometry in 13 babies with gestational ages below 33 weeks (Autzen & Bjørnstrøm 1991); they found a mean of 0.656 mm (SD 0.103 mm) 5 days postnatally, and 0.566 (SD 0.064) at the age of 110 days—a decrease of 12%.

Portellinha and Belfort (1991) looked at 74 full-term neonates, also with ultrasonography, and found CCT 0.573±0.052 mm (range 0.450–0.691 mm). They found peripheral corneal thickness to be 0.650±0.062 mm (range 0.520–0.830 mm). Table 6.3 shows the decrease in thickness during the first few days of life.

Table 6.2 Central corneal thickness (CCT) and curvature (R) in newborns and children. From Ehlers *et al.* (1976).

Age group	No.	CCT (mm ± SEM)	R (mm ± SEM)
Premature newborns	6	0.545 ± 0.014	6.35 ± 0.09
Mature newborns	19	0.541 ± 0.006	7.11 ± 0.07
Children 2–4 years	10	0.520 ± 0.007	7.73 ± 0.09
Children 5–9 years	15	0.520 ± 0.005	7.81 ± 0.09
Children 10–14 years	11	0.520 ± 0.007	8.01 ± 0.05
Adults (own groups and data from literature)		~0.52	~7.8

Table 6.3 Central and peripheral corneal thickness (mm) in newborn babies, time of life in hours. From Portellinha and Belfort (1991).

		Age (hours)		
		0–24	24–48	48–72
Corneal thickness	Central	0.58	0.56	0.54
	Peripheral	0.63	0.63	0.61

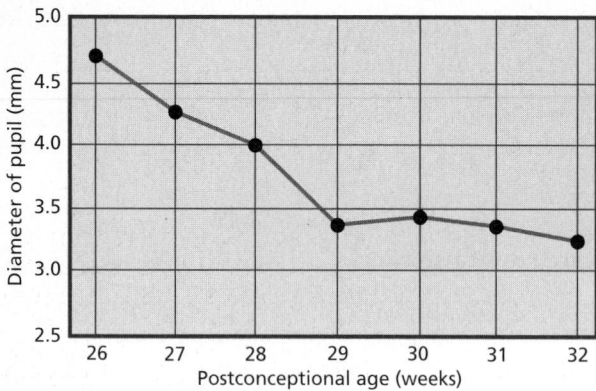

Fig. 6.4 The diameter of the pupil in relative darkness (< 10 ft.-c) in preterm neonates. Data from Isenberg *et al.* 1990. Published with permission from the publisher. © Ophthalmic Publishing Company.

Table 6.4 Values (mm) of the distance from sclerocorneal limbus to the ora serrata in the nasal, temporal, superior and inferior meridians (mean ± SD). From Bonomo (1989).

Nasal meridian	Temporal meridian	Superior meridian	Inferior meridian
3.22	3.33	3.23	3.27
0.30	0.35	0.36	0.37

Remon *et al.* (1992) confirmed these data and the decrease from the values of day 1 by ultrasonic pachometry in full-term newborns. They also studied the peripheral corneal thickness: superior corneal thickness was 0.696 ± 0.055 mm, which was significantly thinner than the inferior corneal thickness (0.744 ± 0.062 mm) and the nasal corneal thickness (0.742 ± 0.058 mm), as well as the temporal corneal thickness (0.748 ± 0.055 mm). The peripheral measurement was taken setting the 1.5-mm probe tip at a tangent to the limbus, i.e. 0.75 mm from the

limbus. They found that adult values are reached at about 3 years of age.

Pupil size and reaction to light

The pupil, in relative darkness, has a mean diameter of 4.7 mm at 26 weeks of postconceptional age compared to a corneal diameter of 7 mm. The pupils subsequently become progressively smaller reaching 3.4 mm at 29 weeks postconceptional age. There is no reaction to light until a mean of 30.6 weeks (±1 week) postconceptional age (Isenberg *et al.* 1990). Figure 6.4 shows the change of pupil diameter in relative darkness in preterm neonates.

Using a photographic technique on 88 babies, Roarty and Keltner (1990) found the mean pupil size to be 3.8 mm (SD ± 0.8 mm) in the newborn period. The incidence of anisocoria of less than 1 mm was 21%. No difference was greater than 1 mm.

Pars plana and ora serrata

Morphological and topographic anatomical studies of 15 fetuses at autopsy (age range 24–40 weeks calculated from the last day of menstruation) have shown the average pars plana to be 1.17 mm in width. Thus the average pars plana is approximately one-third of that found in the adult eye (Bonomo 1989).

The mean value of the distance between the sclerocorneal limbus and the ora serrata was 3.22 mm nasally and 3.33 mm temporally, respectively (Table 6.4). Since there is little growth of the eye between the 30th and 40th weeks of intrauterine life, it could be concluded that the values are close to those in the neonate. Aiello *et al.* (1992) concurred with these estimates finding a mean of 3.06 mm nasally and 3.31 mm temporally soon after birth. Their examinations were based upon 76 paraffin-embedded normal eyes from 1-week to 6-year-old children.

Table 6.5(a) Optic disc parameters in 66 volunteers (values are expressed as means; SDs are listed under the means). From Mansour (1992).

No. of volunteers	Race	Sex	Age	Cycloplegic refraction	Vertical disc diameter (mm)	Horizontal disc diameter (mm)	Cup to disc ratio	Area (mm²)	Neuroretinal rim area (mm²)
16	Black	Female	7.0	+0.8	2.11	1.84	0.32	3.05	2.57
			2.5	1.4	0.21	0.17	0.21	0.54	0.50
14	Black	Male	7.0	+0.5	2.13	1.85	0.40	3.11	2.46
			2.4	0.7	0.19	0.19	0.20	0.56	0.58
18	White	Female	5.2	+1.0	1.88	1.73	0.10	2.57	2.52
			2.4	1.1	0.20	0.17	0.11	0.49	0.48
18	White	Male	6.1	+0.7	1.94	1.79	0.20	2.74	2.54
			2.2	0.7	0.22	0.22	0.18	0.59	0.58

It may be surmised that 76% of the development of the ciliary body has been achieved by the age of 24 months. The pars plana, which occupies 75% of the total length of the ciliary body, follows a similar course.

It is estimated that the external distance from the limbus to the ora serrata is approximately 0.3–0.4 mm more than the corresponding dimension of the ciliary body in the specimens used.

Optic disc parameters

Although one might wish for an objective measurement for optic nerve hypoplasia, this diagnosis is still a subjective one, because it is not only size that is important (see Chapter 50). The optic disc dimensions of 66 children of low refraction error aged 2–10 years were analysed by fundus photography (Mansour 1992). Table 6.5a shows the results, which revealed that vertical disc diameter, the disc area and the cup to disc ratio were significantly larger in black than in white people.

The optic disc dimensions (excluding the meninges) studied at autopsy (Rimmer *et al.* 1993) may produce

Table 6.5(b) Mean vertical and horizontal diameters and area of the optic disc for each age group. From Rimmer *et al.* (1993).

| Age | No. of subjects | Mean diameter (mm) (SD) | | Mean area (mm²) (SD) |
		Vertical	Horizontal	
< 40 weeks gestation	20	1.10 (0.21)	0.93 (0.15)	0.82 (0.26)
Term to 6 months	13	1.37 (0.21)	1.13 (0.19)	1.25 (0.40)
6 months to 2 years	12	1.57 (0.15)	1.40 (0.17)	1.73 (0.32)
2–10 years	17	1.64 (0.20)	1.43 (0.19)	1.87 (0.44)
> 10 years	31	1.73 (0.23)	1.59 (0.21)	2.19 (0.54)

Table 6.5(c) Mean vertical and horizontal diameters and area of the optic nerve for each age group. From Rimmer *et al.* (1993).

| Age | No. of subjects | Mean diameter (mm) (SD) | | Mean area (mm²) (SD) |
		Vertical	Horizontal	
< 40 weeks gestation	20	1.96 (0.36)	1.79 (0.43)	2.85 (1.16)
Term to 6 months	13	2.38 (0.22)	2.23 (0.30)	4.22 (0.87)
6 months to 2 years	12	2.70 (0.33)	2.55 (0.32)	5.47 (1.26)
2–10 years	17	2.84 (0.39)	2.64 (0.27)	5.95 (1.26)
> 10 years	30	3.06 (0.39)	2.85 (0.32)	6.95 (1.62)

Table 6.6(a) Mean and standard deviation of the diameter of the eyeball. From Harayama *et al.* (1981).

| Post-menstrual age (week) | No. of eyes | Diameter of the eyeball (mm) | | |
		Sagittal	Transverse	Vertical
12	18	5.10 ± 0.76	5.48 ± 0.91	4.90 ± 0.89
13	11	5.08 ± 0.93	5.34 ± 1.14	4.98 ± 0.81
14	30	6.14 ± 0.58	6.58 ± 0.66	5.79 ± 0.62
15	20	5.91 ± 0.78	6.37 ± 0.76	5.87 ± 0.88
16	20	6.60 ± 0.65	7.36 ± 0.45	6.55 ± 0.58
17	9	7.12 ± 0.50	7.60 ± 0.41	7.03 ± 0.39
18	20	8.08 ± 0.59	8.70 ± 0.62	7.93 ± 0.67
19	26	8.91 ± 0.97	9.38 ± 0.99	8.67 ± 0.82
20	18	9.36 ± 0.44	9.74 ± 0.41	9.13 ± 0.47
21	71	9.85 ± 0.62	10.34 ± 0.69	9.48 ± 0.61
22	32	10.53 ± 0.77	11.09 ± 0.63	10.23 ± 0.55
23	12	10.89 ± 0.56	11.22 ± 0.62	10.38 ± 0.56
24	28	11.47 ± 0.54	11.99 ± 0.63	11.14 ± 0.59
25	44	11.80 ± 0.53	12.35 ± 0.53	11.33 ± 0.65
26	32	12.65 ± 0.71	13.05 ± 0.52	12.16 ± 0.64
27	14	12.96 ± 0.58	13.22 ± 0.58	12.54 ± 0.58
28	30	13.39 ± 0.99	13.89 ± 0.70	12.85 ± 0.67
29	24	13.82 ± 0.81	14.20 ± 0.66	13.40 ± 0.66
30	6	14.48 ± 0.50	15.18 ± 0.41	14.32 ± 0.60
31	10	14.76 ± 0.69	15.02 ± 0.55	14.17 ± 0.84
32	4	14.70 ± 0.94	14.80 ± 0.57	14.05 ± 0.51
33	4	14.65 ± 0.47	15.23 ± 0.25	14.60 ± 0.39
34	4	15.23 ± 0.34	15.35 ± 0.34	14.30 ± 0.22
35				
36	4	16.08 ± 0.13	16.10 ± 0.14	15.23 ± 0.31
37				
38				
39				
40	10	16.52 ± 1.09	16.96 ± 1.19	15.93 ± 1.59

slightly different results due to fixation shrinkage. Considering this shrinkage (average of 13%) the measurements correlate well with Mansour (1992) (Tables 6.5b and c). Approximately 50% of the growth of the optic disc and nerve occurs by 20 weeks of gestation and 75% by birth. Ninety-five per cent of the growth of the optic disc and nerve occurs before the age of 1 year.

Axial length

In week 9 of fetal life the eye has a sagittal diameter of 1 mm, rapidly increasing to a mean of 5.1 mm by the age of 12 weeks (Harayama *et al.* 1981). Tables 6.6a and b show the relationships between diameter and circumference of the eyeball and gestational age during fetal life.

The total axial length of the premature eye was studied by Tucker *et al.* (1992) in premature babies of 25–37 weeks postconceptional age with A scan ultrasound. The eye increases linearly from 12.6 to 16.2 mm. Figure 6.5

Table 6.6(b) Mean and standard deviation of circumference of the eyeball. From Harayama *et al.* (1981).

Post-menstrual age (week)	Circumference of the eyeball (mm)		
	Transverse	Horizontal meridian	Vertical meridian
12	15.7 ± 2.6	16.3 ± 2.5	15.0 ± 2.5
13	16.5 ± 3.2	16.2 ± 3.3	15.5 ± 2.3
14	18.7 ± 1.9	19.0 ± 2.3	18.0 ± 2.3
15	18.7 ± 2.7	19.0 ± 2.7	18.0 ± 2.7
16	21.4 ± 1.7	21.6 ± 1.5	20.6 ± 1.4
17	23.2 ± 1.2	23.6 ± 1.3	22.6 ± 1.0
18	25.6 ± 2.5	25.8 ± 1.5	24.7 ± 2.1
19	27.5 ± 1.4	27.2 ± 1.6	26.0 ± 1.5
20	29.3 ± 1.4	28.6 ± 1.9	27.8 ± 1.5
21	30.8 ± 2.3	30.8 ± 2.1	29.1 ± 2.1
22	32.8 ± 2.0	32.6 ± 2.3	30.8 ± 2.2
23	33.3 ± 1.0	33.4 ± 1.1	32.2 ± 1.4
24	35.2 ± 1.8	34.9 ± 1.6	33.9 ± 1.5
25	36.4 ± 1.7	36.7 ± 1.7	35.0 ± 1.9
26	38.7 ± 2.1	38.8 ± 2.1	36.9 ± 2.1
27	40.1 ± 1.4	40.2 ± 1.9	38.6 ± 2.1
28	41.9 ± 2.1	41.9 ± 2.2	40.1 ± 2.4
29	42.2 ± 2.1	42.3 ± 2.7	40.7 ± 2.3
30	44.7 ± 1.6	44.1 ± 1.5	42.5 ± 1.5
31	45.1 ± 2.3	44.8 ± 2.3	43.5 ± 2.4
32	44.5 ± 1.8	45.4 ± 2.1	43.4 ± 2.3
33	45.1 ± 0.8	44.4 ± 0.0	43.8 ± 0.8
34	45.0 ± 0.8	45.5 ± 0.7	44.1 ± 0.7
35			
36	47.2 ± 1.6	47.9 ± 0.8	45.8 ± 1.1
37			
38			
39			
40	51.0 ± 3.6	51.5 ± 3.7	48.9 ± 3.0

shows the mean length plotted against postconceptional age.

Ultrasound measurements of the newborn eye (Blomdahl 1979) are as follows:

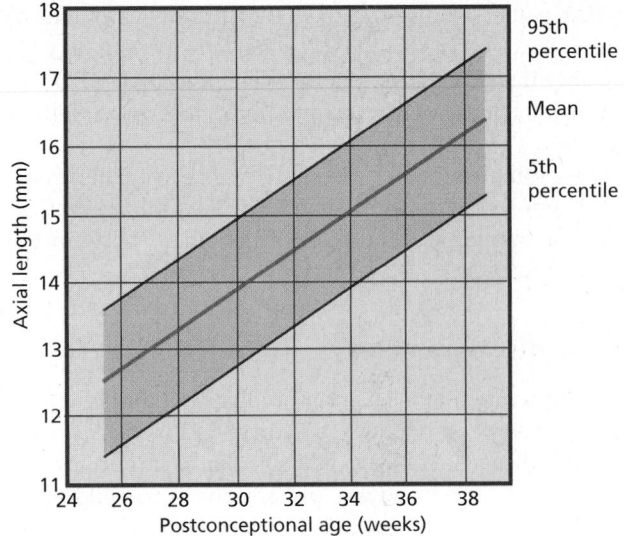

Fig. 6.5 Mean total axial length plotted against postconceptional age with 95% prediction limits. Redrawn from Tucker *et al.* (1992) with permission from the publisher.

1 Average anterior chamber depth (including the cornea) 2.6 mm, ranging from 2.4 to 2.9 mm.
2 Average lens thickness 3.6 mm, ranging from 3.4 to 3.9 mm.
3 Average vitreous length 10.4 mm ranging from 8.9 to 11.2 mm.
4 The total length of the newborn eye is 16.6 mm, range 15.3 to 17.6 mm.

According to an extensive study by Larsen (1971) the postnatal longitudinal growth of the emmetropic eye can be divided into three growth periods. First, there is a rapid postnatal phase with an increase in length of 3.7–3.8 mm during the first 18 months. Second, comes a slower infantile phase from the second to the fifth year of life with an increase in length of 1.1–1.2 mm. Third, a slow juvenile phase begins which lasts until the age of 13 years with an increase of 1.3–1.4 mm. The longitudinal growth is mini-

Table 6.7 Axial length in male series. SD standard deviation, SE standard error. From Larsen (1971).

Length of axis (mm)	Days	Months		Years												
	1–5	6	9	1–2	2–3	3–4	4–5	5–6	6–7	7–8	8–9	9–10	10–11	11–12	12–13	13–14
No. of eyes	86	2	4	36	118	110	100	64	64	70	100	80	56	52	56	24
Mean	16.78	18.21	19.05	20.61	20.79	21.27	21.68	21.85	21.97	22.09	22.33	22.43	22.50	22.70	22.97	23.15
SD	0.51	—	—	0.47	0.61	0.55	0.58	0.59	0.71	0.62	0.51	0.47	0.47	0.82	0.71	0.38
SE	0.055	—	—	0.078	0.056	0.052	0.058	0.074	0.089	0.074	0.051	0.053	0.063	0.114	0.095	0.078

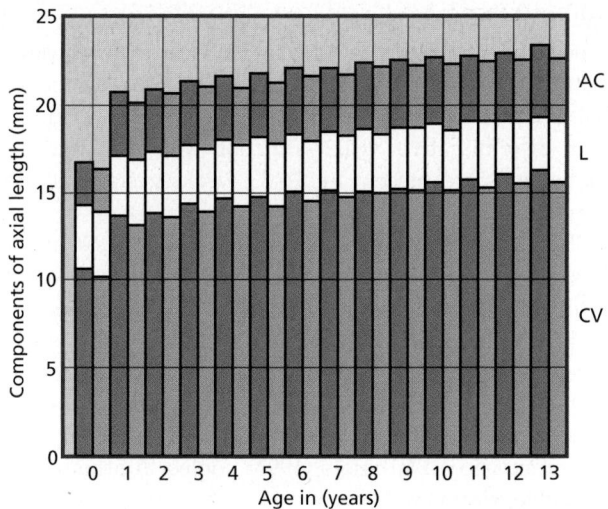

Fig. 6.6 The relationships between the different components of the axis during the growth period. AC, depth of anterior chamber; L, axial thickness of lens; CV, length of vitreous. Redrawn from Larsen (1971) with permission from the publisher ♂ ▣ ♀ ▤ .

Table 6.8(a) Breadth of rectus muscle insertions (mm). From Swan and Wilkins (1984).

Age	No. of specimens	Superior	Medial	Inferior	Lateral
Neonatal	10	7.5	7.6	6.8	6.9
2–3 months	4	7.3	6.8	6.7	7.0
6 months	4	8.9	9.0	8.3	8.4
9 months	4	8.8	8.7	8.3	8.2
20 months	2	10.2	8.9	9.3	7.8
Adult	5	10.8	10.5	9.8	9.2

components of the eye during the growth period (Larsen 1971).

Extraocular muscles and sclera

Most of the enlargement of the eye takes place during the first 6 months of extrauterine life. All diameters increase. The anterior, visible part of the eye in infants, the cornea and the iris, have close to 80% of their adult dimensions at birth. The posterior segment, however, increases more. This has to be taken into consideration in squint surgery of the very young child as the anatomical dimensions make it more difficult to predict the outcome at this age.

mal after this age. Table 6.7 shows the mean of axial length, SD, SE in boys from birth to the age of 14 years. The average values are 0.3–0.4 mm larger in boys than in girls. Figure 6.6 shows the relationship between the different

Table 6.8(b) Millimetres from cornea to rectus muscle insertions. From Swan and Wilkins (1984).

Age	No. of specimens	Superior rectus Nasal End	Superior rectus Temporal End	Medial rectus Sup. End	Medial rectus Inf. End	Inferior rectus Nasal End	Inferior rectus Temporal End	Lateral rectus Sup. End	Lateral rectus Inf. End
Neonatal	10	6.1	7.6	4.7	5.3	6.0	6.6	6.4	5.8
2 months	3	5.5	5.8	5.2	6.0	5.2	6.2	7.8	5.8
3 months	3	6.9	7.5	5.1	5.8	6.6	7.5	7.5	7.0
6 months	4	7.4	8.3	5.8	6.6	7.2	9.0	7.2	7.1
9 months	4	7.2	9.3	6.2	6.9	7.7	8.8	7.5	7.1
20 months	2	7.1	8.7	7.3	7.6	8.5	9.3	8.5	8.5
Adult	5	7.4	10.0	7.8	7.7	8.0	9.2	8.4	8.5

Table 6.8(c) Distance in millimetres of oblique muscle insertions from cornea and optic nerve. From Swan and Wilkins (1984).

Age	No. of specimens	Superior oblique To cornea Ant. edge	Superior oblique To cornea Post. edge	Superior oblique To optic nerve Ant. edge	Superior oblique To optic nerve Post. edge	Inferior oblique To cornea Ant. edge	Inferior oblique To cornea Post. edge	Inferior oblique To optic nerve Ant. edge	Inferior oblique To optic nerve Post. edge
Neonatal	8	9.0	11.6	10.6	5.6	10.2	14.8	8.6	2.2
2–3 months	4	10.3	12.8	10.3	5.6	12.1	16.2	8.2	2.3
6–9 months	8	12.3	14.2	12.0	6.4	13.9	18.0	10.8	3.2
20 months	2	14.2	15.3	12.2	7.8	15.5	19.3	11.7	4.6
Adult	3	14.7	17.7	14.6	8.3	16.2	20.5	14.2	6.6

Tables 6.8a, b and c show the growth of the infant eye, the breadth of rectus muscle insertion, the distance between clear cornea and rectus insertions, as well as the distance of oblique insertions from clear cornea, and from the optic nerve (Swan & Wilkins 1984).

Furthermore, the latter paper describes the thickness of the sclera in 6, 9 and 20 month specimens to be about 0.45 mm, which is similar to that found in adult eyes.

Visual acuity

Most parents appreciate that their newborn baby sees. The neonate stops moving and breathes slowly and regularly when seeing (Warburg 1991). But the image that the brain receives is most probably an unfocused, crude outline to which the infant may not accommodate, and it may even be subcortically mediated via the extrageniculostriate system.

Postnatal maturation of the visual pathways plays an important role in visual development. At birth, the macula is immature. Abramov *et al.* (1982) suggested that vision at birth is extramacular. Hendrickson and Yuodelis (1984) in serially sectioned, normal retinas found that the fovea reaches histological maturity as late as between 15 and 45 months of age. Furthermore, myelination of the optic nerve is not finished until about the age of 2 years (Magoon & Robb 1981).

In an extensive review of visual development Atkinson and Braddick (1981) stated 'The period between 1 and 3 months is a period of radical changes in visual capabilities and behaviour. A rapid rise in acuity, the appearance of the low-frequency cut in contrast sensitivity, the emergence of smooth pursuit eye movements and of symmetrical optokinetic nystagmus, and possibly the establishment of functional binocular vision all occur roughly together'.

In this chapter only a few of the milestones and their experimental background will be included (see Chapter 2).

Lid closure is seen on illumination with a bright light in babies of 25 weeks gestation. The pupillary reflex to light is seen from week 29 to 31 (van Hof-van Duin & Mohn 1984; Isenberg *et al.* 1990). On presenting a red woollen ball at a distance of approximately 17 cm there is evidence that discriminative visual function and tracking eye movements are present by 31–33 weeks gestational age (Dubowitz *et al.* 1980).

The acuity of the newborn infant is close to 6/240 and at 7 weeks of age the infant has eye to face contact. Visual acuity rapidly increases to 6/180–6/90 at 2–3 months. At 6 months visual acuity is between 6/18 and 6/9. The assessment of visual acuity, however, depends on the testing method used; here visual acuities are given as Snellen equivalents which may be a daring interpretation. Table 6.9 summarizes Warburg's (1991) pooled information of visual development.

It is difficult to know at what age adult acuity is normally attained; it is likely that it is approached asymptotically over a number of years (Atkinson & Braddick 1981).

Table 6.10 Mean extent of visual field in degrees (± SEM) in each meridian for the five age groups. From Wilson *et al.* (1991).

Age group	ST	IT	IN	SN
Right eye				
4 years	59.2 (2.1)	84.7 (1.6)	51.4 (2.4)	47.8 (1.8)
5 years	63.4 (2.4)	88.1 (1.9)	52.4 (2.6)	51.7 (1.6)
7 years	66.8 (1.5)	86.0 (2.0)	53.6 (2.0)	58.4 (1.3)
10 years	66.9 (2.3)	86.7 (1.7)	57.9 (1.9)	60.2 (1.3)
Adult	72.6 (2.7)	94.9 (1.4)	54.0 (1.7)	60.2 (2.1)
Left eye				
4 years	66.1 (2.6)	83.8 (2.5)	59.2 (2.9)	49.1 (1.7)
5 years	66.7 (2.8)	83.0 (2.3)	54.8 (2.3)	52.4 (1.9)
7 years	73.7 (1.4)	89.4 (1.7)	51.9 (1.5)	55.9 (1.3)
10 years	71.8 (2.5)	86.7 (1.8)	52.9 (2.1)	55.8 (2.5)
Adult	70.7 (2.5)	93.4 (1.7)	52.4 (2.0)	57.7 (2.1)

S, superior; I, inferior; T, temporal; N, nasal.

Table 6.9 Visual acuity according to different methods, given as Snellen equivalents (pooled information from different sources). Adapted from Warburg (1991).

Technique	Newborn	2 months	4 months	6 months	1 year
Optokinetic nystagmus	20/400	20/400	20/200		20/60
Preferential looking (one study)	20/400	20/200	20/200	20/150	20/50
Preferential looking (other study)	20/800 to 20/1600	20/1200	20/400	20/300	20/100
Visual evoked potential	20/100 to 20/200	20/80	20/80	20/20 to 20/40	20/40

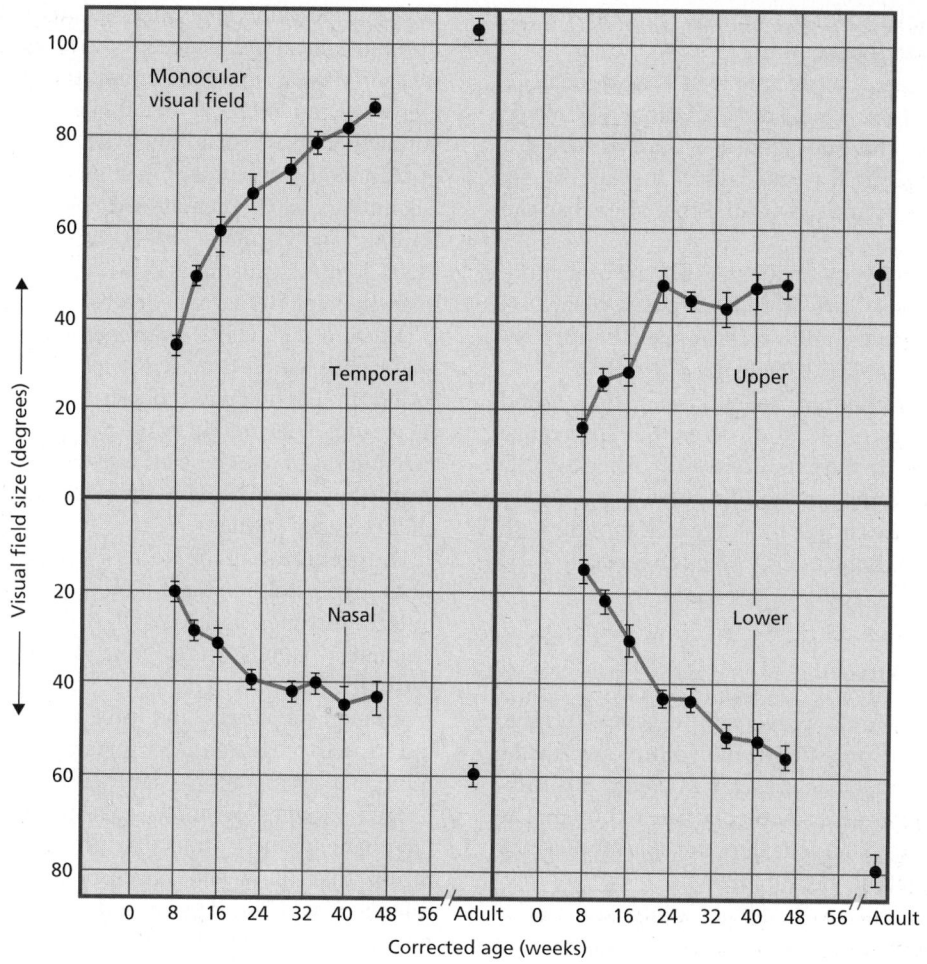

Fig. 6.7 Development of monocular visual field along the horizontal (left) and vertical (right) meridian. Error bars indicate 2 SEM. Redrawn from Mohn and van Hof-van Duin (1986) with permission from the publisher.

Visual field

The visual field of the infant depends on the distance at which the target is presented, whether static or kinetic fields are investigated, and how interesting the targets are, as well as whether a fixation target is present or not. Important milestones seem to be passed between the ages of 2 and 4 months, when the child develops the ability to switch attention to a new object in a controlled way.

The binocular visual field of the infant shows little development between birth and 7 weeks of age. From 2 months onwards there is a rapid expansion of field size until 6–8 months of age. The increase in size of the visual field then continues at a slower rate up to the age of 12 months (Fig. 6.7).

An asymmetry of 13° or more should be considered pathological (Mohn & van Hof-van Duin 1986; J. van Hof-van Duin, personal communication, 1994). The fields were investigated by means of kinetic perimetry using an arc perimeter. Two white balls of 6° diameter served as fixation and peripheral targets. In a similar way Wilson *et al.* (1991) produced normative data for 4–12-year-old children (Table 6.10).

Refraction of the eye, corneal curvature and astigmatism

Slataper (1950) carried out and published the impressive feat of refractions of 35 000 eyes of all ages, but even this was not the end of the story on refractive errors and development. The spectrum of refractive errors is large but the need for normative data when examining any everyday patient is not essential.

There is a large variability among the reported results but most authorities agree that neonatal refractions are distributed in a bell-shaped curve around +2 dioptres.

Later there is a shift towards emmetropia. Hoyt *et al.* (1982) have reviewed the literature.

The normative range for astigmatism is as difficult to quantify as refraction. One study of non-cycloplegic refractions of 1000 children aged 0–6 years revealed a minus cylinder against-the-rule before the age of 4.5 years, and a minus cylinder with-the-rule after that age (Gwiazda 1984).

As would be expected the smaller eyes of the premature and full-term babies have a more curved cornea of 6.35 mm in contrast to the adult measurement of approximately 7.8 mm (see Table 6.2) (Ehlers *et al.* 1976).

In a study of 70 children Asbell *et al.* (1990) found keratometer readings of: 47.59 dioptres (SD 2.10; range 44.08–50.75 dioptres) in the newly born, 45.56 dioptres (SD 2.70; 40.13–52.75 dioptres) in the 12–18-month age group and stabilization of the cornea at the age of 54 months with an average of 42.69 dioptres (SD 1.89; range 40.50–47.50 dioptres).

Intraocular pressure

As in adults, there is no universally accepted normal range for intraocular pressure in the young eye. Awake measurement of intraocular pressure in children is difficult and so a general anaesthetic is often required. The anaesthetic agents used and the depth of anaesthesia may affect the outcome of the measurements.

Despite this, most studies state that the intraocular pressure is lower in children than in adults. Musarella and Morin (1982) measured the intraocular pressure of 37 babies who were 3–11 weeks premature and found mean intraocular pressure values of 18 mmHg (SD 2.3 mmHg; range 13–24 mmHg). They applied a Perkins tonometer on

healthy, topically anaesthetized, relaxed babies under optimal conditions. The face of the tonometer applanator measured 6 mm in diameter and the mean corneal diameter was 8 mm (SD 0.5 mm). Tucker *et al.* (1992) published conflicting results finding, with a hand-held Tonopen applanation tonometer, a mean of 10.3 mmHg (SD 3.5 mmHg) in 70 premature babies aged 25–37 weeks. Radtke and Cohan (1974) found lower values of 11.4 ± 2.4 mmHg using a Perkins tonometer on topically anaesthetized full-term neonates.

Pensiero *et al.* (1992) examined 460 subjects aged 0–16 years with a non-contact Keeler Pulsair tonometer and found in the neonatal phase 9.5 ± 2.3 mmHg rapidly increasing to 14 mmHg at the age of 5 years (Fig. 6.8). Up to 6 months of age these infants were lying down, up to 3 years they were held in their mother's lap, and older children were sitting.

The usefulness of the Keeler Pulsair was confirmed in a study of 53 children aged 6 months to 9 years. Averaged Pulsair readings agreed well with Perkins applanation tonometry values under general anaesthesia (Evans & Wishart 1992).

Among the drugs and procedures known to affect intraocular pressure under general anaesthesia are ketamine, suxamethonium, laryngoscopy and intubation. Large amounts of some anaesthetic agents, such as halothane, reduce intraocular pressure. Dear *et al.* (1987) found that the mean intraocular pressure among 60 infants was 12 mmHg in normal eyes and 22 mmHg in glaucoma after induction on spontaneous ventilation using nitrous oxide and halothane or isoflurane. Using atracurium and controlled ventilation there was a slight increase in intraocular pressure. They recommended measuring the intraocular pressure just after induction well before intubation. This finding was confirmed by Watcha *et al.* (1990) who found constant readings over time in children of different ages after exposure to different concentrations of halothane for 10 minutes before intubation.

An alternative to general anaesthesia with intubation or spontaneous breathing with the problems of a mask could be a laryngeal mask airway, which in a study by Watcha *et al.* (1992) did not increase intraocular pressure.

References

Abramov I, Gordon J, Hendrickson A *et al*. The retina of the newborn human infant. *Science* 1982; **217**: 265–7.

Aiello AL, Tran VT, Rao NA. Postnatal development of the ciliary body and pars plana. *Arch Ophthalmol* 1992; **110**: 802–5.

Al-Umran KU, Pandolfi MF. Corneal diameter in premature infants. *Br J Ophthalmol* 1992; **76**: 292–3.

Asbell PA, Chiang B, Somers ME, Morgan KS. Keratometry in children. *CLAO J* 1990; **16**: 99–102.

Atkinson J, Braddick O. The development of visual function. In: Davis JA *et al.*, eds. *Scientific Foundation of Paediatrics*, 2nd edn. Lon-

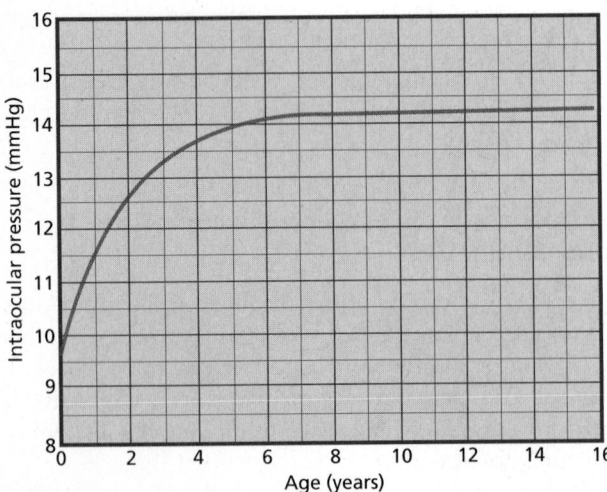

Fig. 6.8 Intraocular pressure by age group. Redrawn from Pensiero *et al.* (1992) with permission from the publisher.

don: Heinemann, 1981: 865–77.

Autzen T, Bjørnstrøm L. Central corneal thickness in premature babies. *Acta Ophthalmol (Copenh)* 1991; **69**: 251–2.

Bach L, Seefelder R. *Atlas zur Entwicklungsgeschichte des menschlichen Auges*. Leipzig and Berlin: Verlag von Wilhelm Engelmann, 1914.

Barishak YR. *Embryology of the Eye and its Adnexae*. Basel, Karger, 1992.

Blomdahl S. Ultrasonic measurements of the eye in the newborn infant. *Acta Ophthalmol (Copenh)* 1979; **57**: 1048–56.

Bonomo PP. Pars plana and ora serrata anatomotopographic study of fetal eyes. *Acta Ophthalmol (Copenh)* 1989; **67**: 145–50.

Dear G de L, Hammerton M, Hatch DJ, Taylor D. Anaesthesia and intra-ocular pressure in young children. *Anaesthesia* 1987; **42**: 259–65.

Dubowitz LMS, Dubowitz V, Verghote AMM. Visual function in the preterm and full-term newborn infant. *Dev Med Child Neurol* 1980; **22**: 465–75.

Ehlers N, Sørensen T, Bramsen T, Poulsen EH. Central corneal thickness in newborns and children. *Acta Ophthalmol (Copenh)* 1976; **54**: 285–90.

Evans K, Wishart PK. Intraocular pressure measurement in children using the Keeler Pulsair tonometer. *Ophthalmic Physiol Opt* 1992; **12**: 287–90.

Farkas LG, Munro IR. Orbital width index. In: Farkas LG, Munro IR, eds. *Anthropometric Facial Proportions in Medicine*. Illinois: Charles C Thomas, 1987, p. 208.

Gwiazda J, Scheiman M, Mohindra I, Held R. Astigmatism in children: changes of axis and amount from birth to 6 years. *Invest Ophthalmol Vis Sci* 1984; **25**: 88–92.

Harayama K, Amemiya T, Nishimura H. Development of the eye ball during fetal life. *J Pediatr Ophthalmol Strabismus* 1981; **18**: 37–40.

Hendrickson AE, Yuodelis C. The morphological development of the human fovea. *Ophthalmology* 1984; **91**: 603–12.

Hittner HM, Hirsch NJ, Rudolph AJ. Assessment of gestational age by examination of the anterior vascular capsule of the lens. *J Pediatr* 1977; **91**: 455–8.

Hoyt CS, Nickel BL, Billson FA. Ophthalmological examination of the infant. *Surv Ophthalmol* 1982; **26**: 177–89.

Iosub S, Fuchs M, Bingol N et al. Palpebral fissure length in black and Hispanic children: correlation with head circumference. *Pediatrics* 1985; **75**: 318–20.

Isenberg SJ, McCarty JW, Rich R. Growth of the conjunctival fornix and orbital margin in term and preterm infants. *Ophthalmology* 1987; **94**: 1276–80.

Isenberg SJ, Molarte A, Vazquez M. The fixed and dilated pupils of premature neonates. *Am J Ophthalmol* 1990; **110**: 168–71.

Jones KL, Hanson JW, Smith DW. Palpebral fissure size in newborn infants. *J Pediatr* 1978; **92**: 787.

Laestadius ND, Aase JM, Smith DW. Normal inner canthal and outer orbital dimensions. *J Pediatr* 1969; **74**: 465–8.

Larsen JS. The sagittal growth of the eye. I–IV. *Acta Ophthalmol (Copenh)* 1971; **49**: 239–62, 427–53, 873–86.

Larsen WJ. *Human Embryology*. Edinburgh: Churchill Livingstone, 1993.

Le Douarin N. *The Neural Crest*. Cambridge: Cambridge University Press, 1982.

Leiber B. Hypertelorismus. HU-Verlag, Mülheim/Ruhr *PAIS* 1992; **11**: 281–5.

Magoon EH, Robb RM. Development of myelin in human optic nerve and tract. A light and electron microscope study. *Arch Ophthalmol* 1981; **99**: 655–9.

Mann I. *The Development of the Human Eye*. Cambridge: Cambridge University Press, 1928.

Mansour AM. Racial variation of the optic disc parameters in children. *Ophthalmic Surg* 1992; **33**: 469–71.

Mohn G, van Hof-van Duin J. Development of the binocular and monocular visual fields of human infants during the first year of life. *Clin Vision Sci* 1986; **1**: 51–64.

Moore KL, Persaud TVN. *The Developing Human*. Philadelphia: WB Saunders, 1993.

Musarella MA, Morin JD. Anterior segment and intraocular pressure measurements of the unanesthetized premature infant. *Metab Pediatr Syst Ophthalmol* 1982; **8**: 53–60.

O'Rahilly R. The timing and sequence of events in the development of the human eye and ear during the embryonic period proper. *Anat Embryol* 1983; **168**: 87–99.

Ozanics V, Jakobiec FA. Prenatal development of the eye and its adnexa. In: Jakobiec FA, ed. *Ocular Anatomy, Embryology and Teratology*. Philadelphia: Harper & Row, 1982.

Pensiero S, Da Pozzo S, Perissutti P, Cavallini GM, Guerra R. Normal intraocular pressure in children. *J Pediatr Ophthalmol Strabismus* 1992; **29**: 79–84.

Portellinha W, Belfort R Jr. Central and peripheral corneal thickness in newborns. *Acta Ophthalmol (Copenh)* 1991; **69**: 247–50.

Radtke ND, Cohan BE. Intraocular pressure measurement in the newborn. *Am J Ophthalmol* 1974; **78**: 501–4.

Remon L, Cristobal JA, Castillo J et al. Central and peripheral corneal thickness in full-term newborns by ultrasonic pachymetry. *Invest Ophthalmol Vis Sci* 1992; **33**: 3080–3.

Rimmer S, Keating C, Chou T et al. Growth of the human optic disc and nerve during gestation, childhood, and early adulthood. *Am J Ophthalmol* 1993; **116**: 748–53.

Roarty JD, Keltner JL. Normal pupil size and anisocoria in newborn infants. *Arch Ophthalmol* 1990; **108**: 94–5.

Scammon RE, Armstrong EL. On the growth of the human eyeball and optic nerve. *J Comp Neurol* 1925; **38**: 165–219.

Slataper FJ. Age norms of refraction and vision. *Arch Ophthalmol* 1950; **43**: 466–81.

Sorsby A, Sheridan M. The eye at birth: measurement of the principal diameters in forty-eight cadavers. *J Anat* 1960; **94**: 192–5.

Swan KC, Wilkins JH. Extraocular muscle surgery in early infancy—anatomical factors. *J Pediatr Ophthalmol Strabismus* 1984; **21**: 44–9.

Thomas IT, Gaitantzis YA, Frias JL. Palpebral fissure length from 29 weeks gestation to 14 years. *J Pediatr* 1987; **111**: 267–8.

Torczynski E. Normal development of the eye and orbit before birth. In: Isenberg SJ, ed. *The Eye in Infancy*. Chicago: Year Book Medical Publishers, 1989: 9–30.

Tucker SM, Enzenauer RW, Levin AV, Morin JD, Hellmann J. Corneal diameter, axial length, and intraocular pressure in premature infants. *Ophthalmology* 1992; **99**: 1296–300.

van Hof-van Duin J, Mohn G. Vision in the preterm infant. In: Prechtl HFR, ed. *Continuity of Neural Functions from Prenatal to Postnatal Life*. Philadelphia: JB Lippincott, 1984: 93–114.

Warburg M. Development of sight. *Ugeskr Laeger* 1991; **153**: 1571–5.

Watcha MF, Chu FC, Stevens JL, Forestner JE. Effects of halothane on intraocular pressure in anesthetized children. *Anesth Analg* 1990; **71**: 181–4.

Watcha MF, White PF, Tychsen L, Stevens JL. Comparative effects of laryngeal mask airway and endotracheal tube insertion on intraocular pressure in children. *Anesth Analg* 1992; **75**: 355–60.

Weale RA. *A Biography of the Eye*. London: HK Lewis, 1982.

Wilmer HA, Scammon RE. Growth of the components of the human eyeball, I and II. *Arch Ophthalmol* 1950; **43**: 599–637.

Wilson M, Quinn G, Dobson V, Breton M. Normative values for visual fields in 4 to 12 year old children using kinetic perimetry. *J Pediatr Ophthalmol Strabismus* 1991; **28**: 151–4.

7: Refraction and Refractive Errors

Hanne Jensen

Evaluation of the optical state of the eye, the refraction, plays an important role in the management of many ophthalmic conditions, and a thorough knowledge of the natural course of refraction with age is important in order to determine what is normal and what is abnormal during childhood.

Postnatal development of the eye

The refraction of the eye depends on four variables and their interaction: (i) corneal power; (ii) anterior chamber depth; (iii) lens power; and (iv) the axial diameter of the globe. The refractive power determines the position of the anterior and posterior focal points of the eye, and the relationship between the power and the axial diameter determines the refractive state of the eye.

The human eye increases in size from birth to adulthood two- to threefold (Raviola & Wiesel 1990), but in some children the development of its components is so precisely regulated, that the image of distant objects can be continuously focused on the photoreceptor layer of the retina.

Children who have refractive errors at birth usually become more emmetropic with increasing age, a process called emmetropization. Clinical conditions such as myopia and hypermetropia probably result from a disturbance in this process. In myopia the posterior focal point lies anterior to the plane of the retinal photoreceptors, whereas in hypermetropia the focal plane lies posterior to the retinal plane.

Hereditary factors are fundamental determinants of the refractive state: the distribution of myopia among races and ethnic groups, its prevalence in families and comparative studies in twins all support hereditary influences in the development of ocular refraction.

Conversely, it is well established that an altered visual input during postnatal eye development may lead to myopia: haemangioma of the lids (Robb 1977), congenital cataract (Johnson *et al.* 1982), corneal scarring (Gee & Tabbara 1988) and ptosis (Hoyt *et al.* 1981) cause myopia in humans; in non-human primates, the use of myopic or hyperopic lenses during development may induce a compensatory refractive error (Hung *et al.* 1995). Animal models of myopia have recently been described by Edwards (1996).

It has also been shown that ocular pathology involving foveal vision, which is not congenital but occurring before the age of 3 years (maculopathies, rod monochromatism), may be accompanied by hypermetropia (Nathan *et al.* 1985). The disruption of central vision in early life is thought to halt the natural emmetropization process, leaving the individual hypermetropic. Failure in emmetropization has also been observed in children, who develop convergent strabismus or amblyopia without strabismus, between 1 and 4 years of age. The deviating eye became anisometropic while the fixating eye became emmetropic (Abrahamsson *et al.* 1992).

If an animal (monkey, cat or chicken) is raised in darkness from birth (regardless of whether the eyelids are sutured) it is likely to remain hypermetropic, whereas raising the animal in a lighted environment with the eyelids sutured or with sight blurred by an optical device is more likely to lead to myopia (Raviola & Wiesel 1978; Yinon & Koslowe 1984; Gottlieb *et al.* 1987). It therefore seems that the refractive error is determined by the genes but influenced by the environment acting through the visual system. For further information see the review by Saunders (1995).

Refractive changes during childhood

Spherical refractive errors

Refractive data from neonates is mainly derived from maternity hospitals, that from schoolchildren is obtained from school vision surveys; preschool children are poorly represented in the available data.

The refractive distribution at birth is characterized by a low degree of hypermetropia and a high standard deviation: Cook and Glasscock (1951) (Fig. 7.1) found among white infants, using atropine cycloplegia and retinoscopy a mean of +2 dioptres hypermetropia (SD 2.75 dioptres), with a range from –7 to +11 dioptres.

Other mean values have been reported: Goldschmidt (1969) found a mean of +0.62 dioptre (SD 2.24 dioptre), and Mohindra and Held (1981) a mean of –0.69 dioptre. These figures demonstrate the consequences of different methods, types of cycloplegics, and especially the age of gestation and maturation.

There is a gradual change with increasing age towards a lower degree of hypermetropia (Sorsby *et al.* 1961; Banks 1980; Edwards 1991). The higher the initial level of

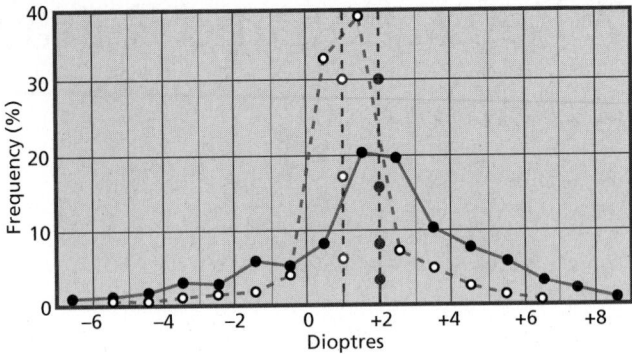

Fig. 7.1 Distribution of refraction in neonates and 10-year-old children. ● Cook and Glasscock (Mean value + 2.0D) neonates. ○ Fledelius (Mean value + 1.0D) 10 year-old children.

ametropia, the more rapidly the refractive error drops during the first year of life (Woodhouse *et al.* 1994). When a child enters school the extreme degrees of both hypermetropia and myopia have disappeared almost completely, and an accumulation of cases around the mean, with a lower SD, characterize the refractive distribution curve (Mohindra & Held 1981; Gwiazda *et al.* 1993). Ten-year-old children have a mean value of +1.0 dioptre (SD 1.61 dioptre) (Fledelius 1976). Figure 7.1 illustrates the increasing degree of leptokurtosis with age.

Children with hypermetropia very frequently become less hypermetropic or even emmetropic, but children who are myopic, or develop myopia during their school years, have greater changes in refraction. Mäntyjärvi (1985a) found an annual change of –0.55 dioptre in myopic children as compared to –0.12 dioptre in those with hypermetropia. Therefore, the refractive distribution curve tends to develop a skew towards the minus direction in the teenage years.

Astigmatism

In astigmatism the optical system of the eye fails to form a point focus of light upon the retina, usually because of toricity of one or more of the eye's refracting surfaces. The front surface of the cornea provides about two-thirds of the refractive power of the eye and most of the eye's astigmatism.

Longitudinal studies show a high prevalence of astigmatism in the first year of life, but this decreases during early infancy (Ingram & Barr 1979a; Fulton *et al.* 1980; Howland & Sayles 1984; Abrahamsson *et al.* 1988). In infancy it is predominantly against-the-rule astigmatism, whilst after the age of 5 years astigmatism with-the-rule is more common (Dobson *et al.* 1984). Infants without astigmatism in the first year of life are unlikely to develop it later (Gwiazda *et al.* 1984).

By the age of 6 years approximately 80% have 0.25 dioptre or less of astigmatism, 12% have 0.25–0.75 dioptre with-the-rule and 5% above 0.75 dioptre with-the-rule astigmatism, while only 3% have astigmatism against-the-rule (Hirsch 1963).

Prediction of refractive errors

At present it is not clear whether an infant who had myopia and later became emmetropic during the preschool years, is the same individual who again becomes myopic at puberty. Establishing this would require longitudinal studies from infancy to adulthood. One longitudinal study of refractive errors in 72 children spanning 9–16 years has recently revealed that infantile refractive errors may be predictive of what occurs with increasing age. After 8 years the refractions manifest during infancy recur in some children. The mean spherical equivalent of the group which showed early negative readings were once again negative, and 42% of those children had become myopic. Only 10% of the children with positive spherical equivalents in infancy had become myopic (Gwiazda *et al.* 1993).

Refractive errors at the age of 5 years are predictive (Hirsch 1964): if the child has any degree of myopia they will remain myopic and the error will probably increase; if the child has hypermetropia in excess of +1.5 dioptre then he or she will very likely remain hypermetropic or possibly even become more hypermetropic. If the child enters school with a refraction between +0.5 and +1.25 dioptre he or she will most likely become emmetropic, and finally if the refraction is between 0 and +0.5 dioptre he or she will very likely be myopic before leaving school.

Assessment of refractive error

Accurate determination of distance refraction requires the suspension of accommodation. The younger the patient the more difficult it is to inhibit accommodative effort.

The most reliable method for relaxing accommodation is the use of a cycloplegic drug. Non-cycloplegic methods for inhibiting accommodation are satisfactory as a patient grows older but there is no definite cut-off age for the use of a cycloplegic. Most children under the age of 15 years are best examined with the aid of a cycloplegic agent, at least once.

Subjective refraction

Subjective refraction can be obtained when the child is old enough to co-operate in a manner similar to that of an adult. Fogging is the most commonly used non-cycloplegic method for relaxing accommodation. Plus lenses are placed in front of the eye to move the posterior focal point of the eye into the vitreous, thus creating a blur at the retinal plane. As any further accommodation will move the posterior focal point even more anteriorly into the vitreous, and thereby increase the blur at the reti-nal plane, the patient will suspend any further accommodative efforts in order to keep the image as clear as possible.

Refraction known from earlier or a retinoscopic measurement can be used as a starting point for subjective refraction. Applying an overcorrection with a +2 dioptre lens should reduce the visual acuity to 0.1 (6/60 or 20/200). If visual acuity is better than this, then more plus lenses are required. Thereafter, the power of the lens is reduced at intervals of 0.25 dioptre (subtracting plus or adding minus) until the best possible vision is obtained. The axes and power of any cylinder can then be refined using a cross cylinder, or an astigmatic fan can be used to detect axis and power of the cylinder.

It is quite difficult to obtain this kind of precision in young children. Although visual acuity can easily be measured in most children at 3 or 4 years of age, asking a child of this age to determine whether the new lens is better or worse than the former is meaningless.

Objective refraction

Objective methods are required for measuring refraction in infants and small children. There are different methods: retinoscopy, autorefraction and photorefraction.

Retinoscopy

Retinoscopy can be performed without cycloplegia by having the child fixate at a distance in order to relax the accommodation, or it can be done dynamically where the child fixates on a near target. Dynamic retinoscopy may be useful as a research tool in order to investigate accommodation in infancy or to evaluate the effectiveness of cycloplegic drugs, but it is rarely used clinically.

Retinoscopy after cycloplegia is useful, and accurate when the technique is mastered — the mean value being within 0.25 dioptre, but it is essential to remember that even trained ophthalmologists can have difficulties. Differences of up to ±0.95 dioptre on the same patient measured by two trained individuals have been reported, the mean figure being 0.1–0.28 dioptre (Hirsch 1956; Zadnik *et al.* 1992) and a 50% probability is found that a trained ophthalmologist would have a difference of 0.40 dioptre or more as a result of lack of precision (Safir *et al.* 1970).

Furthermore, the retinoscopic reflex in young eyes occurs at the vitreous/retinal surface (anterior to the receptors) and produces an objective measurement of refractive error. This is approximately 0.4 dioptre less myopic than the subjective refractive error (Millodot & O'Leary 1978).

Practical aspects

A rack of lenses is often faster (and more portable) than

boxes of individual lenses. It is essential to refract along the visual axis; this necessitates getting the awake child to fix the retinoscopy light or an attractive target near it. In the anaesthetized child a guess must be made at the correct axis to measure: this can be a major source of error and a refraction of a reasonably co-operative awake child is more likely to be accurate than one done under anaesthetic. It should be virtually unnecessary to give an anaesthetic just for the purpose of refraction. In a strabismic eye, the other eye may need to be patched to ensure correct fixation.

In a very unco-operative child the bare minimum information obtained with a +4.00 lens can still be useful; if the retinoscopy without a lens is 'with' the streak or spot you know the child is not significantly myopic and if it is 'against' with a +4.00 lens you know the child is not significantly hypermetropic.

It is worth getting the patient in the best state possible by having a nurse instil the cycloplegic drug and to get the mother to feed the child during the procedure.

The approximate degree of the refractive error can also be estimated from the brightness of the reflex and, in myopia, the distance from the eye that the retinoscope has to be held to find the null point.

Autorefractors

Autorefractors have been in use since the 1970s. The various autorefractors are based on different optical principles (Rassow & Wesemann 1984, 1987), but they have in common that the measurement is performed using infrared, and thus invisible, light. The measurement takes place under standardized conditions, the child being seated in front of the autorefractor fixating the target within the instrument. The test can be done from the age of 3–4 years. The reading is completed in 0.15–1 seconds, depending on the type of autorefractor used. The brief time necessary to obtain a reading appears to be a significant factor in permitting the testing of even young children (Helveston *et al.* 1984).

Despite built-in automatic fogging, autorefractors do not adequately neutralize the patient's accommodative efforts, and the fixation target induces instrument myopia. When the measurements are carried out in cycloplegia, the mean values are within 0 and 0.2 dioptre of the subjectively determined refractive error, and 90% of the values are within ±0.5 dioptre (Rassow & Wesemann 1984, 1987; Grosvenor *et al.* 1985; Ghose *et al.* 1986; Nayak *et al.* 1987; Salvesen & Kohler 1991). The values are comparable to retinoscopy for cylinder axis, power and spherical equivalent when cycloplegia is used.

A new generation of autorefractors has recently been developed: the child can be examined on the parent's knee, sitting about 1 m from the instrument. The test can be performed from the moment the child can sit up and fixate, and both eyes are measured simultaneously. However, reported experience with this type of autorefractor is sparse and only time will show how reliable they are.

Photorefraction

Photorefraction is a photographic technique by which the eye is illuminated by a flash source. The image of the flash is then photographed after it has passed the eye twice on entry and exit. The refractive error can be estimated from the pattern of the image on the camera film (Howland *et al.* 1983).

Two basic photoscreening methods have been developed using either a coaxial light source (on-axis photorefraction) or an eccentric light source (off-axis photorefraction). With the coaxial system three photographs are required per patient: one is focused at the plane of the pupil, the second is defocused by a set dioptric power anteriorly, and the third defocused by an equal amount posteriorly. Spherical and cylindrical errors can be determined by comparing these three photographs (Atkinson & Braddick 1982). Only one photograph is needed for interpretation in the eccentric system. Three reflections are seen: a red fundus reflex, a yellow reflex from the flash source, and a corneal reflex. A yellow crescent is formed in ametropic eyes near the pupil margin, and the size and location of the crescent is dependent on the refractive error. Modifying the eccentric system by having two-flash sources permits estimation of the astigmatic error (Kaakinen *et al.* 1987). The refractive error in both eyes can be calculated from the same photograph, making it easy to detect anisometropia.

Photorefraction is well suited to infants and young children, above the age of 3 months (Atkinson *et al.* 1984; Angi *et al.* 1992; Preslan & Zimmerman 1993). Only brief fixation is needed, the instrument is far away, and the child has little or no fear of the test. The limitation of photorefraction is that it is not accurate enough for the prescription of spectacle correction, and small refractive errors are not detected. The sensitivity of finding children with a refractive error above +3.5 dioptre is about 85% (Hamer *et al.* 1992).

Cycloplegic drugs

Traditionally, atropine has been the standard against which other cycloplegic agents are compared. Since the introduction of the concept of accommodative esotropia by Donders in 1864, refraction under maximal pharmacological cycloplegia has been an essential feature of modern strabismic examination.

In order to obtain a maximum degree of cycloplegia, the usual technique for an atropine retinoscopic examination has been to instil atropine 0.5 or 1% into the conjunctival sac three times a day for 3 days prior to the examination. The recovery of accommodation starts 2–3 days after the last instillation, but 10 days may elapse before full recovery occurs.

Parents have to be aware of both local and universal side-effects, including dryness of the skin and mouth, flushing of the face, irritability, fever and tachycardia. Abdominal distension, arrhythmias, loss of neuromuscular co-ordination, dysarthria, mental aberrations and visual hallucinations have also been observed (Selvin 1987). A 5-ml bottle of 1% atropine contains a potentially lethal dose therefore it is better dispensed in single dose containers (i.e. Minims).

Cyclopentolate and homatropine are shorter acting anticholinergic drugs. The effect of cyclopentolate lasts roughly 24 hours, and it is superior to that of homatropine, having a more rapid onset, a shorter duration, and being more effective. Cyclopentolate only requires 30–60 minutes to reach maximum cycloplegia, making it a convenient drug for office retinoscopic examination.

Two instillations with an interval of 10 minutes has been found to produce maximum cycloplegia in 40% of patients within 15 minutes. Less than 22% of eyes treated with cyclopentolate require 45 minutes or more to reach maximum effect (Milder & Riffenburgh 1953; Gordon & Ehrenberg 1954). Cyclopentolate (Barbee & Smith 1957) has been found to be effective in white subjects with blue and brown eyes, although less potent in children with very pigmented irides, as in black patients.

Parents have to be aware of the dose-related side-effects. Although they are rarely seen, these include signs and symptoms of cerebellar dysfunction, ataxia, dysarthria and visual hallucinations. Cardiopulmonary side-effects have been observed in premature and small infants (Selvin 1987). Cyclopentolate is used in a 1% solution for children over 1 year and 0.5% for infants.

Cyclopentolate has many advantages as compared to atropine, including faster onset, shorter duration, ease of distribution and reduced toxicity. However, it is less effective — especially in the younger age groups. A difference of 0.40 dioptre was found in 1-year-old children, when comparing cyclopentolate to atropine (Ingram & Barr 1979b). Cyclopentolate is also less effective in hypermetropia: atropine uncovers from 0.33 to 0.50 dioptre more hypermetropia than cyclopentolate (Robb & Petersen 1968). In esotropic children less than 5.5 years old 22% of the children had +1 dioptre more hypermetropia disclosed when using atropine than cyclopentolate. Hence, in young patients with esotropia, atropine refraction is essential to reveal the maximum amount of hypermetropia. Almost all of these children had an initial cyclopentolate refraction of +2 dioptre or more (Rosenbaum *et al.* 1981). Conversely, there was no difference between cyclopentolate and atropine, neither in cases of myopia in children <6 years of age (Robb & Petersen 1968), nor in cases with older myopic children (Romano & Shamis 1986).

Recently, tropicamide (1%) has been suggested as an alternative (Mutti *et al.* 1994). It has the shortest duration but is probably the most unreliable. It may give more effective mydriasis in children with deeply pigmented irides. Additional mydriasis can be obtained by using phenylephrine 5% for children and 2.5% for infants. It should not be used for children with cardiovascular disease or on monoamine oxidase inhibitors where it can be fatal.

Recommendations

Determination of refractive error

Cyclopentolate should be used in combination with retinoscopy or an autorefractor. Atropine is sometimes necessary in children with esotropia or those with high degrees of hypermetropia. Atropine given by the parents can be used if the child will not co-operate after having eye drops in the office.

It is important to bring the lens rack forward very slowly and carefully when performing the retinoscopy, because children often become frightened — at times it may be advantageous to use single lenses, even if it is more time-consuming. It is crucial to be sure that the retinoscopy takes places along the optical axis, otherwise false oblique astigmatic refractive errors will occur.

As autorefractors work without visible light many children are not worried by this test, the measurements are obtained rapidly and alignment is automatic. Sometimes the measurements have to be repeated several times, because assessment depends to a great extent on the child's co-operation.

Correction of refractive errors

The main reason for treating refractive errors is to improve visual function. The decision whether to correct a refractive error is seldom a problem in children who can co-operate with visual acuity testing. By no means do all refractive errors require correction. Refractive errors should be corrected according to the needs of the child. It may be desirable to correct a very small error in one child while another may function well without any problems even if a relatively high ametropia is left uncorrected.

Depending on the type of refractive anomaly, prescription of glasses should be considered carefully if the child cannot co-operate. Apart from improving visual acuity, glasses might be needed in order to decrease strabismus, enhance binocular vision, or decrease asthenopic symptoms. Guidelines are provided below.

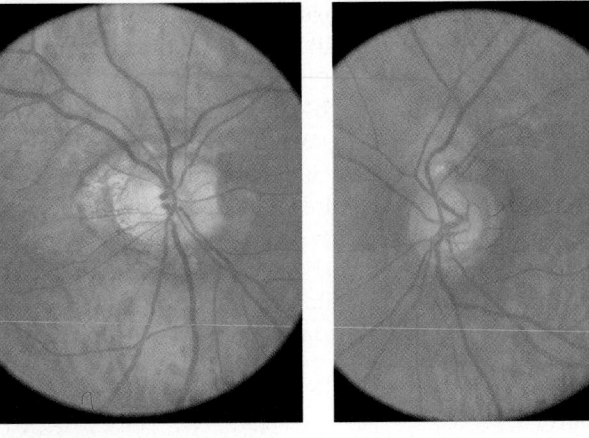
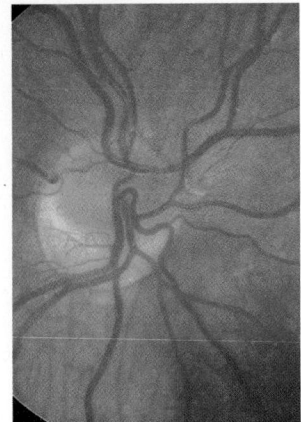
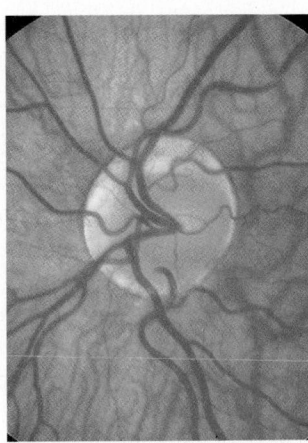

a   b

Fig. 7.2 (a) Peripapillary myopic degeneration; (b) conus defect virtually surrounding the optic discs.

Myopia

Myopia is the most important refractive anomaly with a progressive course in children. There has been increasing interest in this subject within the last few decades due to the hope that arrest of progression or prevention may be possible.

Classification

From both a practical and a theoretical standpoint it is important to distinguish between the various types of myopia. Traditionally, myopia has been divided into low and high myopia — or into simple and pathological myopia — or into congenital, preschool and school myopia, terms based on the degree of myopia, the clinical appearance or the age of onset. However, another classification with three different types of myopia is becoming increasingly accepted (Curtin 1985). It is based on clinical findings and provides a useful description of the various types:

Physiological myopia

Each component of refraction lies upon its normal distribution curve. The postnatal development is normal; the eyes become myopic because of a correlation fault between the total refractive power (cornea and lens) and a normal axial diameter. The fundi of physiologically myopic eyes are therefore normal, and there is no increased morbidity. The onset of this type is common in older children.

Intermediate myopia

This is characterized by an excessive enlargement of the posterior segment of the globe, and distinguished from physiological myopia by clinical changes in the fundus. As the posterior segment enlarges, the eyes show crescent formation at the optic disc (Fig. 7.2), some with supertraction, straightening of the retinal vessels and tessellation of the fundus (Fig. 7.3). The visual function is usually normal, but there is an increase in the incidence of complications: glaucoma, vitreous (Fig. 7.4) and retinal degeneration, and retinal detachment occur in these eyes (Perkins 1979). The onset of this type is most common in younger children. Tilted discs are sometimes seen (Fig. 7.5), and minor degrees may result in pseudopapilloedema (Fig. 7.6).

Pathological myopia

In some children the expansion of the globe becomes worse, and a posterior staphyloma develops. There is peripapillary atrophy, straightening of the retinal vessels and pronounced chorioretinal degeneration, which often

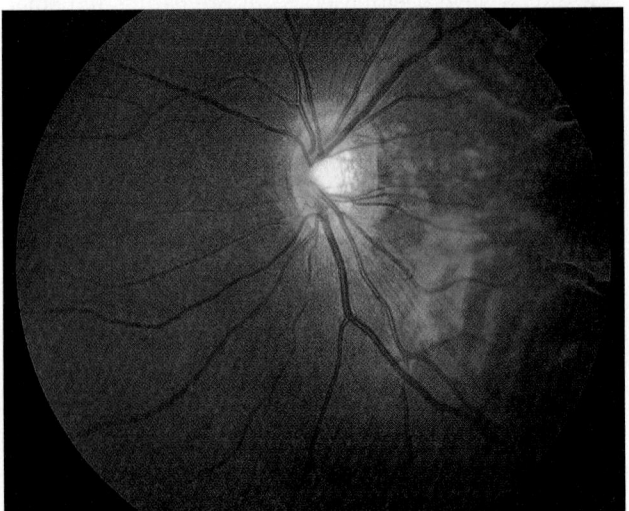

Fig. 7.3 Myopia. The optic disc is vertically oval and has peripapillary degeneration. There is tessellation of the fundus evidenced by the more visible choroidal vascular pattern and the tilting of the optic disc.

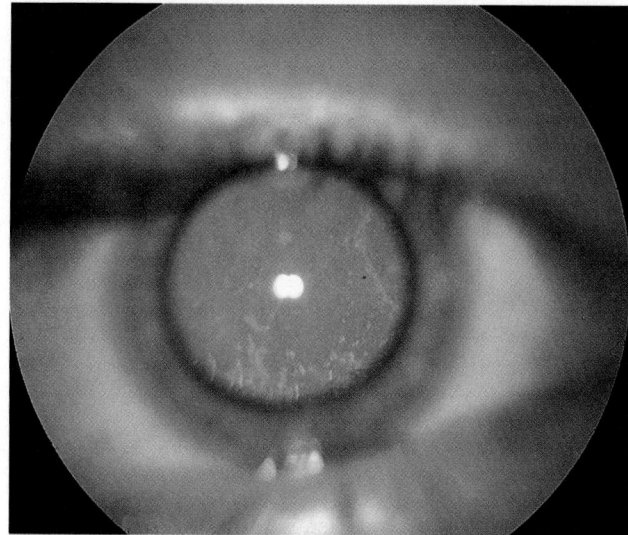

Fig. 7.4 Vitreous floaters in a highly myopic eye with posterior vitreous detachment. The fellow eye had a retinal detachment.

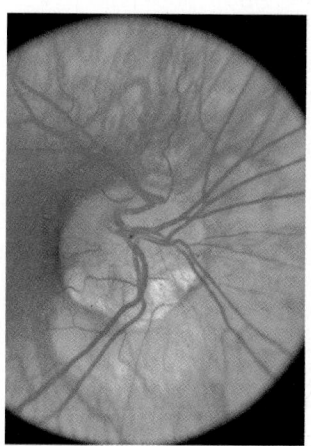
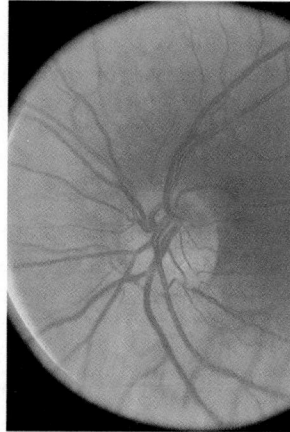

Fig. 7.5 Tilted discs with conus defects. One eye has a staphyloma above the disc and the other below the disc.

About 80% of myopic eyes can be regarded as physiological, a few as pathological and the rest as intermediate. It is highly probable that the many different reports regarding myopia, the aetiology, progression and effects of treatment are the result of comparison of the various types of myopia.

Prevalence

There is a wide variation in the frequency of myopia in

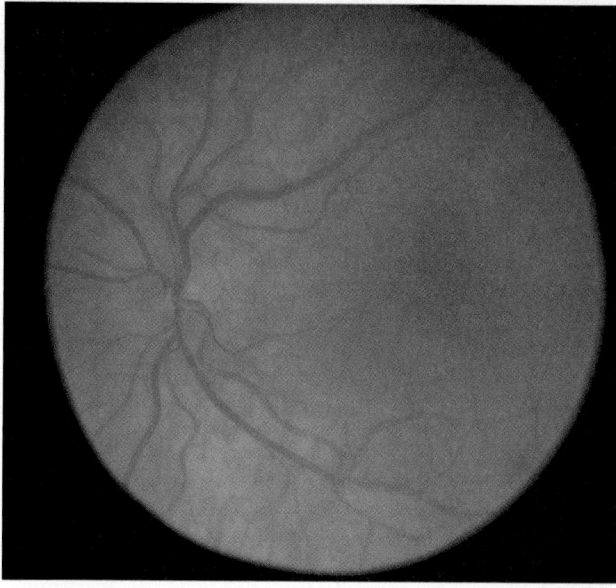

Fig. 7.6 Myopic pseudopapilloedema. This patient has a low degree of myopia and a mildly tilted optic disc with the nasal retina dragged over the optic disc giving a false appearance of mild papilloedema.

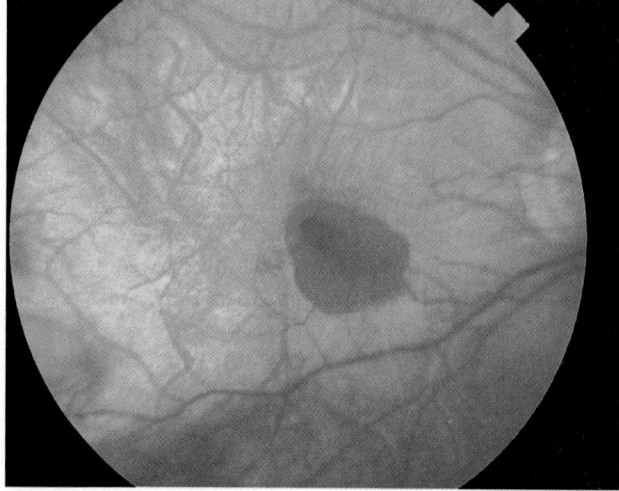

Fig. 7.7 High myopia. There is a small subretinal neovascularization and haemorrhage which obliterate a previously noted lacquer crack.

lead to profound loss of vision. Degeneration of the peripheral retina with local hyperpigmentation, thinning, cystoid and lattice degeneration, schisis and small defects and tears associated with vitreous degeneration (see Fig. 7.4) can induce retinal detachment. Whitish–yellow stripes appear, often multiple which are called lacquer cracks. They are thought to be mechanical breaks in Bruch's membrane and the retinal pigment epithelium. Decrease in visual acuity is especially pronounced when the macula is involved in the atrophic process, and even subretinal neovascularization (Fig. 7.7) can appear. Should these leak, Fuchs' spots can appear — black spots caused by hyperplasia of retinal pigment epithelial cells over the subretinal neovascular membrane (Fig. 7.8). These changes are seldom seen in childhood. Tilted discs are frequent (see Fig. 7.5).

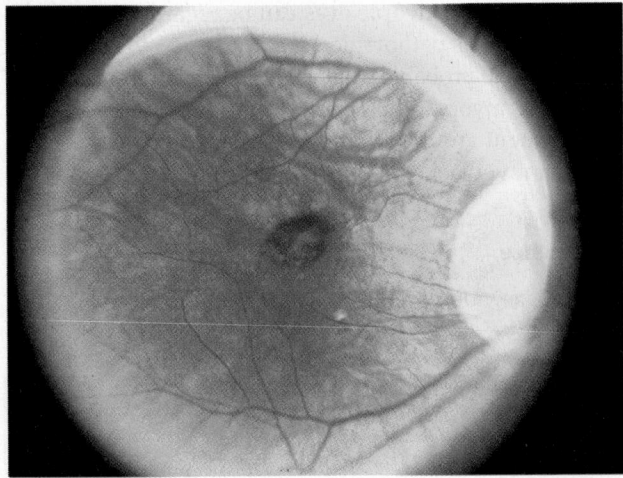

Fig. 7.8 Fuchs' spot.

published reports. This results partly from the methods used, but primarily from the composition of the population. Age, racial and ethnic parameters are the most important.

There are three periods with marked changes in myopia: a sharp reduction in the premature period up to the time of birth, and to a lesser extent from the normal term to 6 months of age. Between 5 and 20 years of age a pronounced rise can be observed.

Premature children have a prevalence of myopia of 30–50%, and this is highest among the most premature (Graham & Gray 1963), especially if they develop retinopathy of prematurity requiring cryotherapy (Kim *et al.* 1992). The prevalence of myopia in normal full-term infants is reported to be between 4 and 6%, but a review of the literature shows large variations, with values of up to 25% (Cook & Glasscock 1951; Goldschmidt 1969). The incidence of myopia is low in the preschool years, and among children just below school age there is a prevalence of 2–3% (Laatikainen & Erkkila 1981; Mohindra & Held 1981).

The incidence shows an increase with age throughout the school years: in 7 year olds, 0.8% become myopic each year, while in 11–13 year olds the incidence has increased to 4% (Mäntyjärvi 1983). Between 20 and 25% of the Caucasian population are myopic after reaching adulthood (Sperduto *et al.* 1983; Pärssinen 1986; Teikari *et al.* 1991).

Eight to ten per cent of healthy offspring can be expected to become near-sighted if both parents are emmetropic. When one parent is myopic it is 23–30%. If both parents are myopic 42–50% of the children become near-sighted (Pärssinen 1986; Gwiazda *et al.* 1993). These figures apply to Western countries. In these areas there has only been a slight increase in the number of myopics over the last generations. Tscherning (1882) investigated con-

scripts and found 8.3% with a degree of myopia above 1.5 dioptre. Goldschmidt (1968) repeated the investigation and found 9.2% had a degree of myopia over 1.5 dioptre. Teasdale *et al.* (1988) found that 10.7% of a comparable group of conscripts were myopic.

Different patterns are seen in other parts of the world. An epidemic increase has taken place among Eskimos; a total of 45% have been classified as myopic (van Rens 1988). This is due to a large percentage of children and youngsters becoming myopic, while the older generation (over 40 years of age) remains emmetropic or hypermetropic. The same tendency is seen in Asia where studies from Taiwan have documented that the prevalence of myopia increases from 4% at 6 years of age to 40% at 12 years and 70% at 15 years of age among children in the cities (Lin *et al.* 1988).

In other places no increase is found in myopia prevalence: among Melanesian school children on the island of Vanuatu only a few had refractive errors and less than 3% were myopic. These children had no electricity in the home, engage very little in reading and had a stress-free existence (Garner *et al.* 1988). Lower degrees of myopia seem to have the same frequency in both sexes, whereas higher degrees of myopia have a higher frequency in females (Curtin 1985).

Aetiology

The aetiology is at present attributed to both hereditary and environmental factors, and myopia is associated with a number of systemic and ocular diseases.

Heredity

The remarkable bilateral symmetry in most myopes and the variations in myopia prevalence among different populations suggest that genetic factors are of great importance. Twin studies have demonstrated a high degree of concordance for refraction in monozygotic compared to dizygotic twins and controls (Sorsby *et al.* 1962; Danning 1981; Chen *et al.* 1985; Teikari *et al.* 1991).

Both autosomal dominant and recessive modes of inheritance have been described in family studies (Edwards & Lewis 1991). The dominant form is often associated with low degrees of myopia (Curtin 1985). Even X-linked pedigrees have been described in families with high degrees of myopia (Gregg & Feinberg 1992).

A common genetic background for low and high myopia is unlikely: myopia is not the product of a single gene. While low myopia is regarded as being polygenic, high myopia is a more heterogeneous group. Some have a monomeric background, some a polymeric and some no genetic background at all (Goldschmidt 1968).

Associated disorders

Myopia is associated with a wide variety of systemic and ocular disorders of a heritable nature and in such cases follows the mode of inheritance of the disease. Chromosomal abnormalities, prenatal and perinatal disorders can be accompanied by myopia, often of an unusually high degree.

Systemic diseases

Among the many systemic disorders accompanied by myopia (Whitmore 1992), the following can be mentioned: Alport's syndrome, Alagille's syndrome, Bassen–Kornzweig syndrome, Ehlers–Danlos syndrome, Fabry's disease, Flynn–Aird syndrome, homocysteinuria, Laurence–Moon–Bardet–Biedl syndrome, Marfan's syndrome and Marshall's syndrome. An overview of the systemic and ocular symptoms, as well as the mode of inheritance is given in Tables 7.1 and 7.2.

Stickler's syndrome is among the most common heritable disorders of connective tissue. Abnormal type II collagen, a key component in cartilage and vitreous, is thought to be responsible, and mutations in the gene encoding for type II collagen on chromosome 12 have been found in families with Stickler's syndrome, as well as in congenital spondyloepiphyseal dysplasia (Hamidi-Toosi & Maumenee 1982; Körkkö *et al.* 1993), and Kniest's syndrome (Winterpacht *et al.* 1993).

Chromosomal abnormalities, among which trisomy 21

Table 7.1 Mode of inheritance and symptoms in systemic disease associated with myopia.

Disorder	Inheritance	Systemic symptoms	Ocular symptoms
Alport's syndrome	AD; AR; X-linked	Deafness; haemorrhagic nephritis	Lenticonus; spherophakia; cataract; retinal detachment
Alagile's syndrome	AD	Intrahepatic cholestatic syndrome	Embryotoxon; cataract; retinal degeneration
Bassen–Kornzweig syndrome	AR	Cerebellar ataxia; sensory neuropathy; dietary fat intolerance	Nyctalopia; nystagmus; pigmentary retinopathy; optic disc pallor
Ehlers–Danlos syndrome	AD	Hyperextensibility of the skin and joints; dislocations	Ectopia of the lens; angioid streaks; posterior staphyloma
Fabry's disease	X-linked	Telangiectasia; peripheral neuropathy; renal disease	Whorl-like corneal deposits; lens opacities; retinal tortuosity
Flynn–Aird syndrome	AD	Dementia; epilepsy; ataxia; deafness; skin atrophy; peripheral neuritis; cystic bone changes	Cataract; pigmentary retinopathy
Homocystinuria	AR	Fair skin and hair spasticity; mental retardation	Dislocation of the lens; cataract; glaucoma; myopia in 90%
Laurence–Moon–Bardet–Biedl syndrome	AR	Short stature; obesity; hypogenitalism; polydactyly; subnormal intelligence; congenital heart disease	Retinitis pigmentosa; ptosis; nystagmus; cataract
Marfan's syndrome	AD	Skeletal changes of long bones; muscular hypoplasia; flat feet; cardiac, pulmonary and renal lesions	Subluxation of the lens; hypoplasia of the iris; cataract; blue sclera; myopia in 83%
Marshall's syndrome	AD	Saddle nose; sensorineural hearing loss	Cataract
Skeletal diseases			
Stickler's syndrome	AD	Arthropathy; cleft palate; micrognathia; flat midface; deafness	Vitreoretinal degeneration; glaucoma; secondary phthisis; cataract; myopia in 83%
Kniest's syndrome	AD	Short stature; flat midface; broad metaphyses; deafness	Vitreoretinal degeneration; high myopia
Congenital spondyloepiphyseal dysplasia	AD	Short stature; cleft palate; deformed tubular bones	Vitreoretinal degeneration

Table 7.2 Mode of inheritance and features in ocular diseases associated with myopia.

Disorder	Inheritance	Features
Albinism ocular	X-linked	Decreased vision; nystagmus; hypopigmentation; hypoplasia of the fundus; high myopia
Choroideraemia	X-linked	Nyctalopia; progressive retinal changes
Coloboma	AD	Decreased vision
Ectopia lentis	AD; AR	Ectopia pupilla; decreased vision; cataract; glaucoma; retinal detachment
Gyrate atrophy	AR	Retinal changes; 90% myopia nyctalopia
Microcornea	AD	High myopia; glaucoma
Myelinated nerve fibres	?	Unilateral/bilateral decreased vision and visual fields; nystagmus; amblyopia
Nyctalopia	X-linked; AR	Reduced vision, colour vision, visual fields; nystagmus; abnormal dark adaptation
Progressive chorioretinal atrophy	AD	Butterfly pattern with loss of choroidal vessels around the optic nerve; nystagmus
Pigment epithelial dystrophy	AD	Nystagmus; choroidal atrophy with pigment clumping
Retinitis pigmentosa	AD; AR; X-linked	Retinal pigmentary deposits; retinal artery attenuation; nyctalopia; decreasing visual fields
Wagner's dystrophy	AD	Retinal artery sheathing; vitreous changes; non-vascular membranes near equator

features and the mode of inheritance is given in Table 7.2. Most of them are rare conditions.

Prenatal and perinatal disorders

The factors governing ocular growth *in utero* are poorly understood. Maternal disease might upset the normal relationship between the refractive components, resulting in myopia either at birth or in early childhood (Gardiner & James 1960). Toxaemia of pregnancy and rubella may give rise to myopia. Low birth weight predisposes to myopia,

is the most well known, are often accompanied by myopia, but it has also been described in combination with trisomy 22, 16 and 17. In patients with trisomy 21 (Down's syndrome) myopia is found in 33%, in addition to blepharitis, pale iris with Brushfield's spots and cataract, which are prominent signs. Systemic signs include mongoloid face, cardiac anomalies, hypogenitalism, mental retardation and obesity.

Ocular diseases

Ocular disorders which are accompanied by myopia include: ocular albinism, choroideraemia, coloboma, ectopia lentis, gyrate atrophy, microcornea, myelinated nerve fibres (Fig. 7.9), nyctalopia, progressive chorioretinal atrophy, pigment epithelial dystrophy, retinitis pigmentosa and Wagner's dystrophy. An overview of ocular

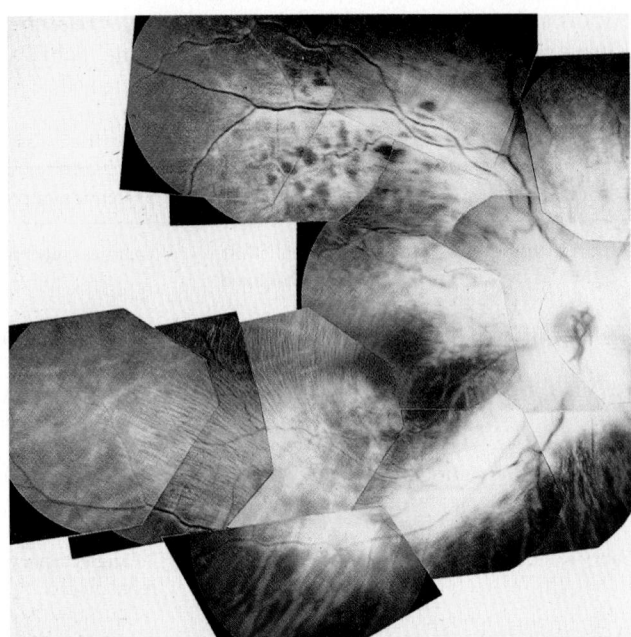

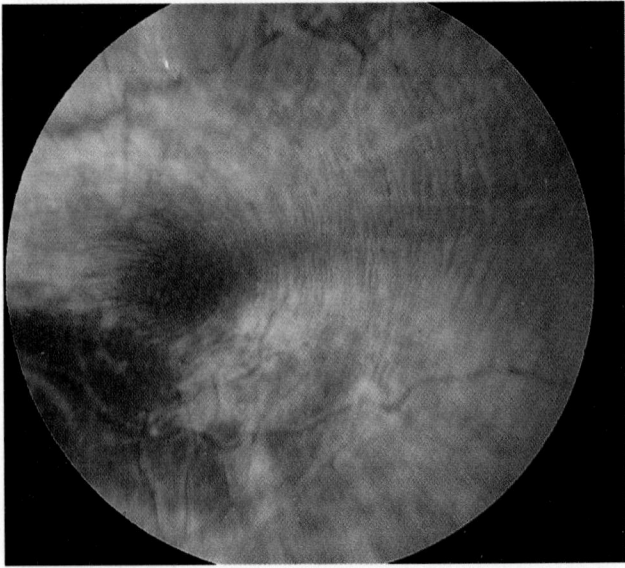

Fig. 7.9 (a) High degree of myopia with myelinated nerve fibres and amblyopia. (b) The anatomy of the median raphe is made outstandingly clear by the visible nerve fibres.

as does prematurity (Page *et al.* 1993). The development of retinopathy of prematurity may cause a permanent myopia, often of a high degree.

Environment (postnatal disorders)

Twin studies also show that environmental factors are important. The classic association of the onset or progression of myopia with schooling naturally leads to the concept of prolonged reading as a cause of this condition.

A recent study of genetically similar samples of teenagers has revealed a statistically significant higher prevalence and degree of myopia in a group of orthodox Jewish male students who differed from the rest in their study habits. Orthodox schooling is characterized by sustained near vision and frequent changes in accommodation (Zylbermann *et al.* 1993).

The mechanism by which prolonged accommodation, convergence or near visual input over long periods of time initiates myopia in humans is unclear. Experimental deprivation myopia in animals suggests that the retinal image (through biochemical or neurochemical mechanisms) may be a factor in the development of myopia. However, mechanical factors, the physical forces on and within the eye from ocular convergence and accommodation, have also been suggested.

Contraction of the extraocular muscles due to convergence has been found to induce increased intraocular pressure (Greene 1980). The contraction of the intraocular muscles during accommodation has been found to elevate the pressure in the posterior chamber (Coleman & Trokel 1969; Young 1975). Thus stress is applied to the scleral wall. Consequently, the axial length may rise, and the subject become myopic.

A decreased scleral resistance, which could be based on inflammation, congestion, optic nerve traction, nutritional deficit or hormonal imbalance rather than stress have been suggested as causes of increased axial diameter. In experimentally lid-sutured highly myopic monkeys, altered fibrillogenesis in the sclera at the fovea was thought to be a key feature in scleral thinning (Funata & Tokoro 1990).

Finally it has been suggested (Avetisov 1979), that the cause of myopia is reduced ability to accommodate in connection with close work. Feeble accommodation can be caused by deficiency of the ciliary muscle or by reduced blood supply to the eye. As a response the axial length increases, and the eye is adapted to near work without the strain of accommodation.

Clinical features

Myopia at birth has usually disappeared by the age of 6 months. The few eyes with pathological myopia are a result of defective development of the posterior segment of the globe. Prematurity has been found to be present in one-third of children with fundus changes.

The near-sighted child will ignore distant objects, while toys and other similar objects are held up close to the eyes for inspection. Some time may pass before the anomaly is discovered, but occasionally, an obvious strabismus will prompt examination. A shift in the visual axis is frequently seen in higher degrees of myopia, so that the angle alpha becomes negative, with the visual axes lying temporal to the pupillary axes, giving rise to an apparent convergent strabismus (Damms *et al.* 1994).

Its clinical course may show wide variations that involve not only the time of onset, but also the nature of the progression (duration, degree and acceleration). The earlier the onset the more likely it is to pursue a more rapidly progressive course (Francois & Goes 1975; Mäntyjärvi 1985b). Progression of myopia usually stops at 16–17 years of age, 1–2 years earlier in girls, but there is a great variability in the time of cessation.

When older, the myopic patient describes blurred distance vision and a need for correcting spectacles. The child has increasing difficulty in reading from the blackboard and has to be seated closer to the teacher. There is a highly quantitative relationship between the degree of refractive error and visual acuity: myopia of −0.5 dioptre corresponds to 0.7 (6/9, 20/30), −1.0 dioptre to 0.3 (6/18, 20/60), and −2.0 dioptre to 0.1 (6/60, 20/200) (Crawford *et al.* 1945).

In order to improve their vision, uncorrected myopics often narrow their eyes to reduce the size of the pupil, thus achieving a sort of pinhole effect. Increased sensitivity to light is a frequent complaint in myopia (Curtin 1985). In close work, convergence and accommodation are combined, but an excess of convergence is required in myopic individuals compared to accommodation, and this can give rise to difficulties. If the accommodation tends to equal the convergence, then ciliary spasm is induced and may increase the myopia, or if convergence is given up, the advantage of binocular vision is abandoned, and a divergent strabismus results.

Asthenopic headache may be seen in people with corrected or uncorrected myopia, caused by peering or by an abnormal convergence/accommodation ratio.

The question is often raised as to whether progression is related to other physical features of the individual. Sorsby *et al.* (1961) found no correlation between the refraction and the changes in components with variations in body growth or such physical traits as the colour of the hair, skin and iris. Neither did spurts in body growth nor the age of menarche have any perceptible effect upon ocular development. However, myopia progression ceases earlier in females than in males, thus indicating some relationship with systemic growth. Also, a tendency towards increased progression rate among those with highest growth rates has been found (Gardiner 1955; Goss *et al.* 1990; Jensen 1991).

Prognosis

No criteria have been found predicting what degree of myopia will develop in the individual child. Age at onset is an important parameter, but variations are pronounced.

Every fourth child with myopia of onset before 10 years of age will have a degree above –6 dioptre, while only 1% of the children with debut after 10 years develop this high degree of myopia (Francois & Goes 1975; Mäntyjärvi 1985b; Jensen 1995).

Treatment and prevention

The spectrum of therapeutic approaches that have been tried is wide — the extreme being heroic surgical approaches designed to stop the progression of myopia. However, no consistent preventive intervention is known.

Non-surgical methods

Training

One of the greatest hopes of all myopic people has been the ability to see clearly without optical aids or surgery. In response to this, William Bates published in 1920 his famous book *The Cure of Imperfect Sight by Treatment without Glasses*. The Bates system had a number of exercises incorporated in the regime, designed to relax the mind and the eye. It has never been confirmed that the refractive error is changed by exercises, but the corrected visual acuity may possibly improve.

Pharmaceutical agents

Cycloplegic agents inducing paralysis of accommodation (atropine, scopolamine), and antiglaucomatous agents reducing the intraocular pressure (pilocarpine, adrenaline, acetazolamide, timolol, labetalol, carteolol) have been used in an attempt at arresting progression.

Assuming that accommodation is an important factor, it is logical to treat progressing myopia with a cycloplegic agent. There have been a large number of studies in this field; reviews of this subject have also been published (Goss 1982; Curtin 1985). Unfortunately, the experimental design of these studies has been less than perfect, and the positive results reported often questionable. Treatment with atropine seems to be the most successful approach (Bedrossian 1979), but there is not yet sufficient documentation to justify the inconvenience and possible dangers of giving atropine to a short-sighted child throughout her or his years at school.

Intraocular pressure is presumed to be a major factor in the normal growth of the eye, as well as in the axial elongation that leads to myopia. The literature on the link between intraocular pressure and progressive myopia was reviewed by Pruett (1988). A prospective study on myopia progression in 9–12-year old children using timolol maleate showed a reduction in intraocular pressure, but no reduction in progression of myopia as compared to a control group (Jensen 1991).

Bifocal lenses

Instead of using medication to avoid elevation of the intraocular pressure when accommodating, bifocal lenses are an easy way to accomplish this. Oakley and Young (1975) published some very encouraging results with almost complete arrest of myopia progression when bifocal lenses were used, but later results have not been as good (Grosvenor *et al.* 1987; Pärssinen *et al.* 1989; Jensen 1991). Goss (1990) found that children with esophoria and astigmatism wearing bifocals had lower mean rates of progression than those wearing single vision lenses.

Prism lenses

Prism lenses can be used to reduce the convergence in order to lower the effect of the extraocular muscles on the globe. It has been impossible to document any effect of this treatment, and these lenses are not prescribed.

Contact lenses ('orthokeratography')

Whether or not hard contact lenses are effective in the control of myopia is a controversial subject. Most of the reported decrease in myopia progression is due to mechanical flattening of the cornea. Grosvenor *et al.* (1989) found that the progression over a 2-year period was 0.5 dioptre less with contact lenses, primarily because of corneal flattening, but also to a minor degree in controlling the axial length. It remains to be established whether this modelling of the cornea and axial length is permanent.

Scleral reinforcing injections

Scleral stabilization is becoming increasingly popular in Russia and at the Helmholtz Institute in Moscow, Avetisov *et al.* (1989) have developed a substance to be injected under Tenon's capsule. The substance polymerizes to form an elastic foam gel, and in 2–3 minutes this composition becomes solid, forming an extra layer on the surface of the sclera. Its slow resorption allows collagen formation and stimulates growth of the connective tissue. This phenomenon is said to improve the strength of the sclera making it stretch less.

Surgical methods

Keratorefractive surgery and eximer laser treatment are not recommended for children, except in some very special cases where standard optical correction cannot be tolerated.

Surgical procedures are used in an attempt to reduce the progression of myopia by reinforcing the sclera. The aim is to avoid ectasia of the posterior pole by implantation of various materials. The long-term results were once questionable, but newer reports from studies in both animals and humans are more promising (Avetisov & Tarutta 1987; Jacob-La Barre *et al.* 1993). The technique has changed and a more simple positioning of foreign bodies in Tenon's space is used. These may be dura mater, fascia lata, tendons or sclera from a donor.

Correction of myopia

The myopic infant can be left uncorrected in infancy. In children with exodeviations full myopic correction may reduce the angle of strabismus. Myopia above –3 dioptres should be corrected and in schoolchildren lower degrees should also be corrected, thus permitting the child to see the blackboard.

It is advisable to give full optical correction, but it has not always been so, there have been advocates of under-correction, even though there is no confirmation regarding the effectiveness of this kind of treatment. The glasses are to be used for distant vision, and as long as it is comfortable, the child should be allowed to read without glasses. It is a very common misunderstanding among parents, that being near-sighted means that the child has to wear the glasses for reading, and not necessarily for distance.

It is sensible to prescribe the weakest glasses that the child can usefully see with, rather than the ones that give them absolutely the best acuity. The child should be discouraged from reading too close and routine follow-up examinations should only be made in non-verbal or retarded children. Children can be relied upon, usually, to tell when their prescription is inadequate and routine appointments usually lead to the prescription of unnecessarily strong lenses.

Hypermetropia (hyperopia)

Hypermetropia is also a common phenomenon. It has not drawn much attention from clinicians, probably because it is perceived as an innocuous condition, a deficiency in optical focusing power. It can be overcome by eyes that have adequate accommodation and can be compensated for by using convex lenses if it causes signs or symptoms that the patient or parent cannot ignore. It does not progress, at least not to an extent that produces concern.

In childhood it does not appear to lead to any significant secondary disorders, although children with high degrees of hypermetropia are at increased risk of developing strabismus and amblyopia (Ingram *et al.* 1986). Bilateral amblyopia has even been described (Abraham 1964), probably due to lack of clear retinal image in early childhood.

Aetiology

It is generally accepted that hypermetropia is of congenital or inherited origin, especially in those with higher degrees of the condition (Teikari *et al.* 1990). The influence of postnatal environmental factors has only been mentioned briefly. It has been suggested, that disruption of central vision early in life halts the natural emmetropization process (Nathan *et al.* 1985).

Hypermetropia is associated with ocular malformations of genetic origin: Leber's congenital amaurosis and Franceschetti's syndrome are among autosomal recessive disorders. Leber's amaurosis is characterized by blindness from early childhood, due to retinal disorders (Babel *et al.* 1989; Lambert *et al.* 1989) and Franceschetti's syndrome is characterized by microphthalmus and makrophakia combined in some cases with tapetoretinal degeneration (Franceschetti & Gernet 1965); usually both have moderate to severe hypermetropia. An early onset type of autosomal dominant retinitis pigmentosa has been found with severe hypermetropia, which is remarkable as patients with retinitis pigmentosa are most often myopic (Lam & Judisch 1991).

Clinical features

The hypermetropic eye is small, not only in its anteroposterior diameter, but in all directions. The cornea is small, the lens is normal and the anterior chamber shallow. Ophthalmoscopically, the fundus may have a characteristic appearance; in high degrees of hypermetropia the retina appears similar to a shot-silk retina (a reflex effect), and the optic disc sometimes resembles optic neuritis (pseudopapillitis or papilloedema) (Fig. 7.10).

The condition is congenital, the vascular reflexes may be accentuated and the vessels may show undue tortuosity and abnormal branchings. If the face is asymmetrical, the most hypermetropic eye is usually found on the smaller side of the face, i.e. that showing the least perfect development. The macula is often situated further from the disc than in the emmetropic eye, and the cornea more decentred, thus the visual axis cuts the cornea at a considerable distance on the inside of the optic axis, hence making a positive angle alpha. This may give rise to an apparent divergent squint, a condition opposite to that found in myopia.

The principal symptoms are headache and blurring of

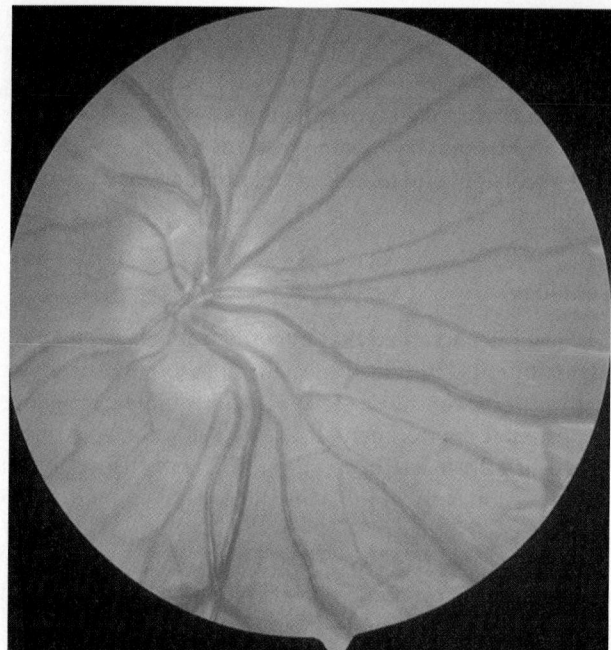

Fig. 7.10 Hypermetropic pseudopapilloedema.

vision during close work. Symptoms may not be present in the first years of life, but may appear with the decline in accommodation during the second decade, or they may appear during times of physical debility or emotional stress. If the available accommodation is inadequate to cope with the degree of hypermetropia, then blurring of vision will also occur for distance vision.

The desire for accommodation in excess of convergence leads to a dissociation of muscle balance and the struggle to maintain binocular vision leads in these circumstances to further strain. Should the fusion faculty be defective, the advantages of binocular vision are abandoned in favour of the more obvious advantage of clear vision, only the better eye is used, and an accommodative convergent squint is provoked.

Occasionally hypermetropic people of moderate or high degree may present with a history of holding a book close to the eyes, a habit more suggestive of myopia. By doing so, the patient achieves enlargement of the retinal image and this compensates for its indistinctness. Hypermetropia is also a factor in infantile esotropia, but in most cases the degree is less than +3.0 dioptres (Robb & Rodier 1986; Nelson *et al.* 1987). The percentage is more skewed in accommodative esotropia: well over 90% are hyperopic, most in excess of +3.0 dioptres (Mazow *et al.* 1984).

Hypermetropia is an important factor in the performance of children at school. The visual characteristics of children with and without satisfactory progress in school have been compared (Rosner & Rosner 1987). Nineteen per cent of the group who had school learning difficulties were myopic; 54% were hypermetropic. The opposite trend was displayed by the group of children who did not have school problems. Fifty-four per cent of that group were myopic and only 16% were hypermetropic.

It has been reported in a study involving 710 elementary schoolchildren that substandard visual analysis skills were observed in 82% of the hypermetropic children, in 38% of the emmetropic children and in only 14% of the myopic children (Rosner & Gruber 1985).

Correction of hypermetropia

The clinical management of hypermetropia varies considerably. Although most agree that compensatory lenses for a 1-year-old child who manifests 1 dioptre of hypermetropia should not be prescribed, opinions differ considerably in respect of higher degrees of hypermetropia.

There is seldom disagreement among practitioners about lens prescription for esotropic children: when the patient is strabismic the refractive error should be fully corrected.

The disagreement appears when there is no strabismus, as some practitioners do not prescribe compensatory lenses, even with high refractive errors. Others take a different point of view, especially when the hypermetropia exceeds 3.0 dioptres, due to the fact that these children are more prone to binocular difficulties. About one-half of the infants with hypermetropia above +3 dioptre have developed amblyopia and/or strabismus by the age of 3.5 years (Ingram *et al.* 1986). Early spectacle correction has been tried, but no evidence found that this improves the outcome with regard to amblyopia and strabismus (Ingram *et al.* 1990).

In conclusion, unrecognized hypermetropia in preschool children may contribute to school learning difficulties, even in children whose cognitive abilities are average or above. The critical degree of hypermetropia below which the hypermetropia may be safely ignored remains to be determined, but until then hypermetropia above +4.0 dioptres probably should be corrected.

Astigmatism

There is a high prevalence of astigmatism in normal infants. It generally diminishes in the first years of life, and between 8 years and adolescence there is virtually no change in mean refractive astigmatism (Hirsch 1963). The change in corneal astigmatism is thought to be a consequence of interaction between changes in the eye axis, lid pressure and ocular rigidity during growth.

Aetiology

Astigmatism may be inherited, and all modes of inheritance—autosomal dominant, autosomal recessive and X-linked — have been reported (Sorsby 1970). Older twin studies demonstrate high correlation coefficients (Wixson 1958) both regarding corneal refractive power and corneal astigmatism, but it is unknown which component is the inherited one. One hypothesis is that it may be low corneal rigidity.

Sorsby *et al.* (1962) found that the correlations between monozygotic twins were higher than those between dizygotic twins in cases of low degrees of astigmatism, while in higher degrees (above 2.25 dioptres) there was no difference. In another study, the amount of astigmatism in monozygotic twins was not statistically significantly different from that of dizygotic twins. This suggests that environmental factors are also of major importance (Teikari & O'Donnell 1989).

This is also confirmed by studies of fetal alcohol syndrome, as it was found that severe corneal astigmatism can be produced by non-hereditary causes (Garber 1984).

Astigmatism has been described together with other conditions such as optic nerve hypoplasia (Zeki 1990) and ptosis (Cadera *et al.* 1992).

Children with low vision have a higher degree of mean astigmatism as compared to normals (Nathan *et al.* 1986), with highest astigmatism in children with albinism, retinitis pigmentosa and idiopathic nystagmus.

Clinical features

Astigmatism may influence the development of amblyopia and possibly also the development of refractive errors. Abrahamsson *et al.* (1990) examined 310 children at 1 year of age and again at 4 years of age. While 280 showed decreasing astigmatism, the 23 with constant or increasing astigmatism were found to be at greater risk for developing amblyopia. Some of this might be meridional amblyopia, which is characterized by reduced acuity even with best optical correction and is presumed to be a form of neural dysfunction.

Astigmatism present at infancy has little effect on visual acuity (Gwiazda *et al.* 1985), but astigmatism presenting between 6 and 24 months is found to correlate with the amblyopia that is detectable later in the child's life (Gwiazda *et al.* 1986). This suggests that there is a connection between optical defects and neural defects: early visual input affects the neural organization of the visual system.

The length of the sensitive period and the minimum amount of astigmatism necessary to produce significant amblyopia are not yet clearly defined. When astigmatism is greater in one eye, then this eye is almost invariably more hypermetropic than its fellow eye. Conversely, it has been found that uncorrected astigmatism in childhood with an unclear retinal focus is likely to be the cause of myopia (Fulton *et al.* 1982).

Correction of astigmatism

As there is a high prevalence of astigmatism in normal infants it is difficult to give dogmatic advice on when to correct it. If the astigmatism does not decrease over the years it should be corrected, especially if it is different in power and axis between the two eyes. The critical period for the development of meridional amblyopia occurs before the end of the child's sixth year, but most probably within the first 2 years. To avoid this condition, it is important to correct the astigmatism as early as possible. Errors of less than 1.5 dioptre can probably be safely ignored.

Older children and adults usually cannot accept the total amount of astigmatism when it is corrected but infants can.

Anisometropia

Anisometropia exists whenever there is a difference between the refractive states of the two eyes. Anisometropia in early infancy is a barrier to the establishment of normal binocular vision. The more ametropic eye may be suppressed and amblyopia may result. Myopic children are anisometropic much more often than those who are hyperopic.

Children with anisometropia often have good visual acuity in one eye and usually straight eyes. These factors, combined with peeking from under the occluder by the child during visual screening may allow monocular reduced visual acuity to go undetected.

The depth of amblyopia has been found to be strongly correlated to the degree of anisometropia (Townshend *et al.* 1993) even though a child with hypermetropic anisometropia is more likely to become amblyopic than a child with myopic anisometropia.

There is evidence that hypermetropic spherical or cylindrical anisometropia greater than 1 dioptre is significantly associated with the later development of amblyopia. Therefore it would seem sensible in infants whose acuity cannot easily be measured to correct any anisometropia of greater than 1.0 dioptre, especially if both eyes are hyperopic. The need for optical correction can be reviewed when the child is old enough to be formally tested.

References

Abraham SV. Bilateral ametropic amblyopia. *J Pediatr Ophthalmol Strabismus* 1964; **1**: 57–61.

Abrahamsson M, Fabian G, Andersson A-K, Sjöstrand J. A longitudinal study of a population-based sample of astigmatic children. *Acta Ophthalmol* (Copenh) 1990; **68**: 428–34.

Abrahamsson M, Fabian G, Sjöstrand J. Changes in astigmatism between the ages of 1 and 4 years: a longitudinal study. *Br J Ophthalmol* 1988; **72**: 145–9.

Abrahamsson M, Fabian G, Sjöstrand J. Refraction changes in children developing convergent or divergent strabismus. *Br J Ophthalmol* 1992; **76**: 723–7.

Angi MR, Pucci V, Forattini F, Formentin PA. Results of photorefractometric screening for amblyogenic defects in children aged 20 months. *Behav Brain Res* 1992; **49**: 91–7.

Atkinson J, Braddick OJ. The use of isotropic photorefraction for vision screening in infants. *Acta Ophthalmol* 1982; (Suppl 157): 36–45.

Atkinson J, Braddick OJ, Durden K *et al*. Screening for refractive errors in 6–9 month old infants by photorefraction. *Br J Ophthalmol* 1984; **68**: 105–12.

Avetisov ES. Unterlagen zur Entstehungstheorie der Myopie. 1. Mitteilung. Die Rolle der Akkommodation in der Entstehung der Myopie. *Klin Monatsbl Augenheilk* 1979; **175**: 735–40.

Avetisov ES, Tarutta EP. Eine neue operation zur Verstärkung der Sklera bei hoher Kurzsichtigkeit und ihre Ergebnisse. *Klin Monatsbl Augenheilk* 1987; **191**: 22–5.

Avetisov ES, Tarutta EP, Smirnova TS *et al*. Immediate and remote results of sclera strengthening injection in the prophylaxis of progressive myopia. In: *Myopia. Proceedings of the International Symposium, Moscow.* 1989, 177–9.

Babel J, Klein D, Roth A. Leber's congenital amaurosis associated with high hyperopia in four sisters. *Ophthal Paediatr Genet* 1989; **10**: 55–61.

Banks M. Infant refraction and accommodation. *Int Ophthalmol Clin* 1980; **20**: 205–32.

Barbee RF, Smith WO. A comparative study of mydriatic and cycloplegic agents. *Am J Ophthalmol* 1957; **44**: 617–22.

Bates W. *The Cure of Imperfect Sight by Treatment without Glasses.* New York: Central Fixation publ. co. 1920.

Bedrossian RH. The effect of atropine on myopia. *Ophthalmology* 1979; **86**: 713–7.

Cadera W, Orton RB, Hakim O. Changes in astigmatism after surgery for congenital ptosis. *J Pediatr Ophthalmol Strabismus* 1992; **29**: 85–8.

Chen CJ, Cohen BH, Diamond EL. Genetic environmental effects on the development of myopia in Chinese twin children. *Ophthal Paediatr Genet* 1985; **6**: 113–9.

Coleman DJ, Trokel S. Direct recorded intraocular pressure variations in a human subject. *Arch Ophthalmol* 1969; **82**: 637–40.

Cook RC, Glasscock RE. Refractive and ocular findings in the newborn. *Am J Ophthalmol* 1951; **34**:1407–13.

Crawford JS, Shagass C, Pashby TJ. Relationship between visual acuity and refractive error in myopia. *Am J Ophthalmol* 1945; **28**: 1220–5.

Curtin BJ. *The Myopias: Basic Science and Clinical Management.* Philadelphia: Harper & Row, 1985.

Damms T, Damms C, Schulz E *et al*. Pseudoesotropie durch Verlagerung der Macula nach nasal bei Patienten mit infantiler hoher Myopie. *Ophthalmologe* 1994; **91**: 77–80.

Danning H. Twin study on myopia. *Chin Med J* 1981; **94**:51–5.

Dobson V, Fulton AB, Sebris SL. Cycloplegic refractions of infants and young children: the axis of astigmatism. *Invest Ophthalmol Vis Sci* 1984; **25**: 83–7.

Edwards M. The refractive status of Hong Kong Chinese infants. *Ophthal Physiol Opt* 1991; **11**: 297–303. •

Edwards MH. Animal models of myopia. *Acta Ophthalmol Scand* 1996; **74**: 213–9.

Edwards M, Lewis WHP. Autosomal recessive inheritance of myopia in Hong Kong Chinese infants. *Ophthal Physiol Opt* 1991; **11**: 227–31.

Fledelius H. Prematurity and the eye. *Acta Ophthalmol* 1976; (Suppl. 128); **54**: 1–243.

Franceschetti A, Gernet H. Diagnostic ultrasonique d'une microphtalmie sans microcornee, avec macrophakie, haute hypermetropie associee a une degenerescence tapeto-retinienne, une disposition glaucomateuse et des anomalies dentaires. *Arch Ophthal* 1965; **25**: 105–16.

Francois J, Goes F. Oculometry of progressive myopia. *Bibl Ophthalmol* 1975; **83**: 277–82.

Fulton AB, Dobson V, Salem D *et al*. Cycloplegic refractions in infants and young children. *Am J Ophthalmol* 1980; **90**: 239–47.

Fulton AB, Hansen RM, Petersen RA. The relation of myopia and astigmatism in developing eyes. *Ophthalmology* 1982; **89**: 298–302.

Funata M. Tokoro T. Scleral change in experimentally myopic monkeys (Graefe's). *Arch Clin Exp Ophthalmol* 1990; **228**: 174–9.

Garber JM. Steep corneal curvature: a fetal alcohol syndrome landmark. *J Am Optometric Assoc* 1984; **55**: 595–8.

Gardiner PA. Physical growth and the progress of myopia. *Lancet* 1955; **ii**: 952–3.

Gardiner PA, James G. Association between maternal disease during pregnancy and myopia in the child. *Br J Ophthalmol* 1960; **44**: 172–8.

Garner LF, Kinnear RF, McKellar M *et al*. Refraction and its components in Melanesian schoolchildren in Vanuatu. *Am J Optom Physiol Opt* 1988; **65**: 182–9.

Gee SS, Tabbara KF. Increase in ocular axial length in patients with corneal opacification. *Ophthalmology* 1988; **95**: 1276–8.

Ghose S, Nayak BK, Singh JP. Critical evaluation of the NR-1000F autorefractometer. *Br J Ophthalmol* 1986; **70**: 221–6.

Goldschmidt E. On the aetiology of myopia. An epidemiological study. *Acta Ophthalmol* 1968; (Suppl. 98); **46**: 1–171.

Goldschmidt E. Refraction in the newborn. *Acta Ophthalmol* 1969; **47**: 570–8.

Gordon DM, Ehrenberg MH. Cyclopentolate hydrochloride: a new mydriatic and cycloplegic agent. *Am J Ophthalmol* 1954; **38**: 831–8.

Goss DA. Attempts to reduce the rate of increase of myopia in young people—a critical literature review. *Am J Optom Physiol Opt* 1982; **59**: 828–41.

Goss DA. Variables related to the rate of childhood myopia progression. *Optom Vis Sci* 1990; **67**: 631–6.

Goss DA, Cox VD, Herrin-Lawson GA *et al*. Refractive error, axial length and height as a function of age in young myope. *Optom Vis Sci* 1990; **67**: 332–8.

Gottlieb MD, Fugate-Wentzek LA, Wallman J. Different visual deprivations produce different ametropias and different eye shapes. *Invest Ophthalmol Vis Sci* 1987; **28**: 1225–35.

Graham MV, Gray OP. Refraction of premature babies eyes. *Br Med J* 1963; **1**: 1452–4.

Greene PR. Mechanical considerations in myopia: relative effects of accommodation, convergence, intraocular pressure and the extraocular muscles. *Am J Optom Physiol Opt* 1980; **57**: 902–14.

Gregg FM, Feinberg EB. X-linked pathologic myopia. *Ann Ophthalmol* 1992; **24**: 310–12.

Grosvenor T, Perrigin DM, Perrigin J. Three-way comparison of retinoscopy, subjective, and Dioptron Nova refractive findings. *Am J Optom Physiol Opt* 1985; **62**: 63–5.

Grosvenor T, Perrigin DM, Perrigin J, Maslovitz B. Houston myopia control study: a randomized clinical trial. Part II. Final report from the patient care team. *Am J Optom Physiol Opt* 1987; **64**: 482–98.

Grosvenor T, Perrigin D, Perrigin J, Quintero S. The use of silicone-acrylate contact lenses for the control of myopia: results after 2 years of lens wear. *Am J Optom Physiol Opt* 1989; **66**: 41–7.

Gwiazda J, Bauer J, Thorn F, Held R. Meridional amblyopia does result from astigmatism in early childhood. *Clin Vision Sci* 1986; **1**: 145–52.

Gwiazda J, Mohindra I, Brill S, Held R. Infant astigmatism and meridional amblyopia. *Vision Res* 1985; **25**: 1269–76.

Gwiazda J, Scheiman M, Mohindra I, Held R. Astigmatism in children: changes in axis and amount from birth to 6 years. *Invest Optom Vis Sci* 1984; **25**: 88–92.

Gwiazda J, Thorn F, Bauer J, Held R. Emmetropization and the progression of manifest refraction in children followed from infancy to puberty. *Clin Vision Sci* 1993; **8**: 337–44.

Hamer RD, Norcia AM, Day SH *et al.* Comparison of on- and off-axis photorefraction with cycloplegic retinoscopy in infants. *J Pediatr Ophthalmol Strabismus* 1992; **29**: 232–9.

Hamidi-Toosi S, Maumenee IH. Vitreoretinal degeneration in spondylepiphyseal dysplasia congenita. *Arch Ophthalmol* 1982; **100**: 1104–7.

Helveston EM, Pachtman MA, Cadera W *et al.* Clinical evaluation of the Nidek AR autorefractor. *J Pediatr Ophthalmol Strabismus* 1984; **21**: 227–30.

Hirsch MJ. Changes in astigmatism during the first 8 years of school — an interim report from the Ojai longitudinal study. *Am J Optom Arch Am Acad Optom* 1963; **40**: 127–32.

Hirsch MJ. Predictability of refraction at age 14 on the basis of testing at age 6—interim report from the Ojai longitudinal study on refraction. *Am J Optom Arch Am Acad Optom* 1964; **41**: 567–73.

Hirsch MJ. The variability of retinoscopic measurements when applied to large groups of children under visual screening conditions. *Am J Optom Arch Am Acad Optom* 1956; **33**: 410–16.

Howland HC, Braddick O, Atkinson J, Howland B. Optics of photorefraction: orthogonal and isotropic methods. *J Opt Soc Am* 1983; **73**: 1701–8.

Howland HC, Sayles N. Photorefractive measurements of astigmatism in infants and young children. *Invest Ophthalmol Vis Sci* 1984; **25**: 93–102.

Hoyt CS, Stone RD, Fromer C. Monocular axial myopia associated with neonatal eyelid closure in human infants. *Am J Ophthalmol* 1981; **91**: 197–200.

Hung L-F, Crawford MLJ, Smith EL. Spectacle lenses alter eye growth and the refractive status of young monkeys. *Nature Medicine* 1995; **1**: 761–5.

Ingram RM, Arnold PE, Dally S, Lucas J. Results of a randomised trial of treating abnormal hypermetropia from the age of 6 months. *Br J Ophthalmol* 1990; **74**: 158–9.

Ingram RM, Barr A. Changes in refraction between the ages of 1 and 3.5 years. *Br J Ophthalmol* 1979a; **63**: 339–42.

Ingram RM, Barr A. Refraction of 1-year-old children after cycloplegia with 1% cyclopentolate: comparison with findings after atropinisation. *Br J Ophthalmol* 1979b; **63**: 348–52.

Ingram RM, Walker C, Wilson JM *et al.* Prediction of amblyopia and squint by means of refraction at age 1 year. *Br J Ophthalmol* 1986; **70**: 12–15.

Jacob-LaBarre JT, Assouline M, Conway MD *et al.* Effects of scleral reinforcement on the elongation of growing cat eyes. *Arch Ophthalmol* 1993; **111**: 979–86.

Jensen H. Myopia progression in young school children. *Acta Ophthalmol* 1991; (Suppl. 200); **69**: 1–79.

Jensen H. Myopia in teenagers. *Acta Ophthalmol Scand* 1995; **73**: 389–93.

Johnson CA, Post RB, Chalupa LM, Lee TJ. Monocular deprivation in humans: a study of identical twins. *Invest Ophthalmol Vis Sci* 1982; **23**: 135–8.

Kaakinen KA, Kaseva HO, Teir HH. Two-flash photorefraction in screening of amblyogenic refractive errors. *Ophthalmology* 1987; **94**: 1036–42.

Kim JY, Kwak SI, Yu YS. Myopia in premature infants at the age of 6 months. *Korean J Ophthalmol* 1992; **6**: 44–9.

Körkkö J, Ritvaniemi P, Haataja L *et al.* Mutation in type II procolla-

gen (COL2A1) that substitutes aspartate for glycine and that causes cataracts and retinal detachment: evidence for molecular heterogeneity in the Wagner syndrome and the Stickler syndrome (arthro-ophthalmopathy). *Am J Hum Genet* 1993; **53**: 55–61.

Laatikainen L, Erkkilä H. Proportion of myopia in visual screening of school children. In: Fledelius HC, Alsbirk PH, Goldschmidt E, eds. *Doc Ophthal Proc*, Series, vol 28. The Hague: Dr W. Junk Publishers, 1981: 1–4.

Lam BL, Judisch GF. Early-onset autosomal dominant retinitis pigmentosa with severe hyperopia. *Am J Ophthalmol* 1991; **111**: 454–6.

Lambert SR, Kriss A, Taylor D *et al.* Follow-up and diagnostic reappraisal of 75 patients with Leber's congenital amaurosis. *Am J Ophthalmol* 1989; **107**: 624–31.

Lin LLK, Chen CH, Hung PT, Ko LS. Nationwide survey of myopia among schoolchildren in Taiwan. *Acta Ophthalmol* 1988; **66** (Suppl. 185): 29–33.

Mäntyjärvi M. Incidence of myopia in a population of Finnish schoolchildren. *Acta Ophthalmol* 1983; **61**: 417–23.

Mäntyjärvi M. Changes of refraction in school children. *Arch Ophthalmol* 1985a; 103: 790–2.

Mäntyjärvi M. Predicting of myopia progression in school children. *J Pediatr Ophthalmol Strabismus* 1985b; **22**: 71–5.

Mazow ML, Kaldis LC, Prager TC, Jenkins PF. Accommodative esotropia. *Am Orthop J* 1984; **34**: 77–82.

Milder B, Riffenburgh RS. An evaluation of cyclogyl (compound 75 GT). *Am J Ophthalmol* 1953; **36**: 1724–6.

Millodot M, O'Leary D. The discrepancy between retinoscopic and subjective measurements: effect of age. *Am J Optom Physiol Opt* 1978; **55**: 309–16.

Mohindra I, Held R. Refraction in humans from birth to five years. In: Fledelius HC, Alsbirk PH, Goldschmidt E, eds. *Doc Ophthal Proc*, Series, vol 28. The Hague: Dr W. Junk Publishers, 1981: 19–27.

Mutti DO, Zadnik K, Egashira S *et al.* The effect of cycloplegia on measurement of the ocular components. *Invest Ophthalmol Vis Sci* 1994; **35**: 515–27.

Nathan J, Kiely PM, Crewther SG, Crewther DP. Astigmatism occurring in association with paediatric eye disease. *Am J Optom Physiol Opt* 1986; **63**: 497–504.

Nathan J, Kiely PM, Crewther SG, Crewther DP. Disease-associated visual image degradation and spherical refractive errors in children. *Am J Optom Physiol Opt* 1985; **62**: 680–8.

Nayak BK, Ghose S, Singh JP. A comparison of cycloplegic and manifest refractions on the NR-1000F (an objective autorefractometer). *Br J Ophthalmol* 1987; **71**: 73–5.

Nelson LB, Wagner RS, Simon JW, Harley RD. Congenital esotropia. *Surv Ophthalmol* 1987; **31**: 363–83.

Oakley KH, Young FA. Bifocal control of myopia. *Am J Optom Physiol Opt* 1975; **52**: 758–64.

Page JM, Schneeweiss S, Whyte HEA, Harvey P. Ocular sequelae in premature infants. *Pediatrics* 1993; **92**: 787–90.

Pärssinen O. *The wearing of spectacles and occurrence of myopia.* Thesis, University of Tampere, 1986; Series A, Vol. 207: 1–158.

Pärssinen O, Hemminki E, Klemetti A. Effect of spectacle use and accommodation on myopic progression: final results of a 3-year randomised clinical trial among school children. *Br J Ophthalmol* 1989; **73**: 547–51.

Perkins ES. Morbidity from myopia. *Sight Saving Rev* 1979; **49**: 11–19.

Preslan MW, Zimmerman E. Photorefraction screening in premature infants. *Ophthalmology* 1993; **100**: 762–8.

Pruett RC. Progressive myopia and intraocular pressure: what is the linkage? A literature review. *Acta Ophthalmol* 1988; (Suppl. 185): 117–27.

Rassow B, Wesemann W. Automatische augenrefractometer. In: Rassow B, ed. *Ophthalmologisch-optische Instrumente. Bucherei des Auge-narztes*, Band 111. Stuttgart: Enke Verlag, 1987: 42–65.

Rassow B, Wesemann W. *Moderne Augenrefractometer. Functionsweise und vergleichende Untersuchungen. Bucherei des Augenarztes*, Band 102. Stuttgart: Enke Verlag, 1984.

Raviola E, Wiesel TN. Effect of dark-rearing on experimental myopia in monkeys. *Invest Ophthalmol Vis Sci* 1978; **17**: 485–8.

Raviola E, Wiesel TN. Neural control of eye growth and experimental myopia in primates. *Ciba Foundation Symp* 1990; **155**: 22.

Robb RM. Refractive errors associated with hemangiomas of the eye-lids and orbit in infancy. *Am J Ophthalmol* 1977; **83**: 52–8.

Robb RM, Petersen RA. Cycloplegic refractions in children. *J Pediatr Ophthalmol* 1968; **5**: 110–14.

Robb RM, Rodier DW. The broad clinical spectrum of early infantile esotropia. *Trans Am Ophthalmol Soc* 1986; **84**: 103–16.

Romano PE, Shamis DJ. Atropine versus cyclopentolate. Cycloplegic refractions in school age myopia. *Am Orthop J* 1986; **36**: 124–6.

Rosenbaum AL, Bateman JB, Bremer DL, Liu PY. Cycloplegic refraction in esotropic children. Cyclopentolate versus atropine. *Ophthalmology* 1981; **88**: 1031–4.

Rosner J, Gruber J. Differences in the perceptual skills development of young myope and hyperopes. *Am J Optom Physiol Opt* 1985; **62**: 501–4.

Rosner J, Rosner J. Comparison of visual characteristics in children with and without learning difficulties. *Am J Optom Physiol Opt* 1987; **64**: 531–3.

Safir A, Hyams L, Philpot J, Jagerman LS. Studies in refraction I. The precision of retinoscopy. *Arch Ophthalmol* 1970; **84**: 49–61.

Salvesen S, Kohler M. Automated refraction. A comparative study of automated refraction with the Nidek AR-1000 autorefractor and retinoscopy. *Acta Ophthalmol* 1991; **69**: 342–6.

Saunders KJ. Early refractive development in humans. *Surv Ophthalmol* 1995; **40**: 207–16.

Selvin BL. Systemic effects of topical ophthalmic medications. In: Lamberts DW, Potter DE, eds. *Clinical Ophthalmic Pharmacology.* Toronto: Little, Brown, 1987: 475–6.

Sorsby A. *Ophthalmic Genetics*, 2nd edn. London: Butterworths, 1970.

Sorsby A, Benjamin B, Sheridan M. Refraction and its component during the growth of the eye from the age of 3. *Medical Research Councils Special Reports*, Series No. 301. HMSO, London: 1961: 1–67.

Sorsby A, Sheridan M, Leary GA. Refraction and its components in twins. *Medical Research Councils Special Reports*, Series No. 303. HMSO, London: 1962: 1–43.

Sperduto RD, Seigel D, Roberts J, Rowland M. Prevalence of myopia in the United States. *Arch Ophthalmol* 1983; **101**: 405–7.

Teasdale TW, Fuchs J, Goldschmidt E. Myopia and its relationship to education, intelligence and height. Preliminary results from an ongoing study of Danish draftees. *Acta Ophthalmol* 1988; **66** (Suppl. 185): 41–3.

Teikari JM, Koskenvuo M, Kaprio J, O'Donnell J. Study of gene-environment effects on development of hyperopia: a study of 191 adult twin pairs from the Finnish Twin Cohort study. *Acta Genet Med Gemello* 1990; **39**: 133–6.

Teikari JM, O'Donnell. Astigmatism in 72 twin pairs. *Cornea* 1989; **8**: 263–6.

Teikari JM, O'Donnell JO, Kaprio J, Koskenvuo M. Impact of heredity in myopia. *Hum Hered* 1991; **41**: 151–6.

Townshend AM, Holmes JM, Evans LS. Depth of anisometropic amblyopia and differences in refraction. *Am J Ophthalmol* 1993; **116**: 431–6.

Tscherning M. *Studier over myopiens ætiologi*. Thesis, Copenhagen: B. Wennstrøms Bogtrykkeri, 1882.

van Rens GHMB. *Ophthalmological Findings among Alaskan Eskimos of the Norton Sound and Bering Straits Region*. Nijmegen: University of Nijmegen, 1988.

Whitmore W. Congenital and developmental myopia. *Eye* 1992; **6**: 361–5.

Winterpacht A, Hilbert M, Schwarze *et al.* Kniest and Stickler dysplasia phenotypes caused by collagen type II gene (COL2A1) defect. *Nature Genet* 1993; **3**: 323–5.

Wixson RJ. The relative effects of heredity and environment upon the refractive errors of identical twins, fraternal twins and like-sex siblings. *Am J Optom Arch Am Acad Optom* 1958; **35**: 346–51.

Woodhouse JM, Saunders KJ, Westall CA. Emmetropisation in human infancy: rate of change is related to initial refractive error. *Invest Ophthalmol Vis Sci* 1994; **35**: 1805.

Yinon U, Koslowe KC. Eyelid closure effects on the refractive error of the eye in dark- and light-reared kittens. *Am J Optom Physiol Opt* 1984; **61**: 271–3.

Young F. The development and control of myopia in human and sub-human primates. *Contacto* 1975; **19**: 16–31.

Zadnik K, Mutti DO, Adams AJ. The repeatability of measurement of the ocular components. *Invest Ophthalmol Vis Sci* 1992; **33**: 2325–33.

Zeki SM. Optic nerve hypoplasia and astigmatism: a new association. *Br J Ophthalmol* 1990; **74**: 297–9.

Zylbermann R, Landau D, Berson D. The influence of study habits on myopia in Jewish teenagers. *J Pediatr Ophthalmol Strabismus* 1993; **30**: 319–22.

Section 2
Management

8: History, Examination and Further Investigation

Susan Day

Taking a history

One initially wonders how detailed a history can be when considering the eyes of infants and children: especially with babies, the vast majority of time seems to be spent sleeping and eating! Many parents do not consciously evaluate how their baby is seeing; yet, when directly questioned about vision, parents often have a very good understanding of how well their baby sees.

The history is of utmost importance in understanding the problem and offering solutions. Although obvious questions about vision will be made, great care must be taken in assessing the child's general health. Perhaps the simplest and most open question to pose is 'Are you, your paediatrician, or doctor, concerned about any aspect of your child's health or development?' Such a question might elicit a response that, for instance, the child has had a special hearing test. As a consequence of this response, one might be alerted to conditions such as retinitis pigmentosa, and Waardenberg's and Alport's syndromes.

Another key question is to ask about the child's general development. Much of a child's motor development within the first year of life is vision-dependent. What appears to be developmental delay may therefore be a clue that not all is right with the child's vision. Similarly, a child who is not growing properly, or who fails to thrive, may have a combination of developmental abnormalities which results in not only endocrine disturbance but also in hypoplasia of the optic nerves or other vision defects.

A query into the prenatal history is also of utmost importance, especially when congenital infections are suspected. Such questions must be carefully phrased because parents may blame themselves unnecessarily for a congenital defect. Nevertheless, the occurrence of maternal rash, fever, use of medications and drug abuse must be reviewed.

A review of medications given to the child and taken by the mother during the pregnancy or while breast feeding must be made. Particularly, use of anticonvulsants may influence a child's apparent visual performance. The possibility of allergies to medications must also be covered. Young children, and particularly those with Down's syndrome, may be sensitive to atropine and other cycloplegic agents.

Once systemic issues have been covered, the baby's vision must be addressed. The most important question to ask the parents is 'How well does your baby see?' Parents and other relatives are keenly perceptive of the baby's vision in an intuitive fashion—they are rarely wrong! Parents often volunteer that they have been concerned about vision for a number of months even though the primary care physician failed to register similar concern. If the child has older siblings, parents also are able to compare the younger child's development to the older child's progress.

Beyond simply intuitive ideas of how good the vision is, the parents should then be questioned about habits which may be directly related to vision or behaviour which implies poor eyesight. A baby with poor vision will often stare at bright lights, have flickering eyelid movements, and may develop nystagmus noticeable to the parents. They may also observe eye-poking or rapid hand waving in front of the eyes by such an infant. This infant may fail to smile or seemingly be disinterested in his or her environment, and hold the head with the chin tucked in when in a sitting position. In contrast, parents of a baby with good sight will volunteer that eye contact is made, or that the baby mimics facial expressions, or that a mobile over the crib fascinates the child. The physician must be cautious in considering behaviour as vision-generated whenever the stimulus also makes a noise, such as a music box playing a lullaby.

Visual behaviour in an older child often centres around the child's playing habits. A child with poor vision may hold the toy within 2–5.5 cm (1–2 inches) of one or both eyes, inspecting the toy in a way that maximizes his or her vision. This child too, may be disinterested in TV, or insist on moving to within inches of the screen where scanning the entire view is not possible without moving the head. Keep in mind, however, that virtually all children do tend to sit more closely to a TV screen than adults, presumably due to (i) their desire to be immersed in the activity on the screen; and (ii) their ability to accommodate more fully and maintain focus at a shorter viewing distance.

Apparent visual difficulty may be present under very specific circumstances, such as in dim illumination or very bright illumination. In the former case, the child may become very irritated when the night light is turned off or have inordinate difficulty in finding his or her way around in dimly lit situations. Conversely, children with poor photopic vision may hate going outside or insist on protection from the sun. An older child must be included in the discussion; valuable information is offered, and rapport is established which leads to better co-operation during the examination.

Children who are born with poor vision are not likely to tell you that their vision is poor. Children who acquire poor vision will usually only volunteer that they are unable to see well if the visual loss is bilateral. Unilateral visual loss, either acute or chronic, is usually not noticed by a young child unless or until the other eye becomes involved.

In summary, the taking of the history is the beginning of a good eye examination in infants and children. Much reliability is placed not only on parental observations, but also on those of other close relatives, as well as the children themselves. A general development and health history, as well as history of medications and allergies, are elementary aspects of history taking. The importance of taking and documenting a family history is described elsewhere (Chapter 10). A detailed history of vision behaviour may give the ophthalmologist an accurate refinement of where to look for pathology.

Finally, the mood set by taking a history helps to establish rapport with the child which makes examination more fun for the child and more rewarding for the doctor.

Clinical examination

Ophthalmologists must keep in mind that the child has already been seen, in all likelihood, by another physician who has raised concern about a potential problem with the eyes. Although great variability exists in the quality of screening examinations by primary care physicians, babies in general will receive an initial examination of the eyes for clarity of the media, evidence of conjunctivitis, and any obvious abnormalities such as a squint or congenital defect of the globe. At the baby clinic within the first 4 months, the ability to 'fix and follow' should be documented with each eye, as well as the assessment of oculomotor alignment and analysis of red reflex. Repeated assessment of vision (both subjectively by the parents and objectively by the physician), alignment and media clarity must be continued on each routine visit within the first 3 years of life. Vision is first routinely quantified by primary care physicians initially between the ages of 3.5 and 7 years.

Once a paediatrician has detected a potential problem, a not insignificant hurdle in the child's care is gaining a prompt appointment. It is absolutely essential that the busy ophthalmologist give specific guidelines to appointment personnel for children as to what represents an urgent problem; leukocoria, for instance, warrants immediate attention to rule out retinoblastoma. A 2-week-old baby with bilateral congenital cataracts represents another urgent matter. Access to the examination is perhaps as important in the practice of paediatric ophthalmology as the examination itself!

The milieu of the examining room is very important. A large examining area is at times almost essential to accommodate the parents, siblings and all the paraphernalia associated with children. As the initial history is being taken from the parents, the patient may be more comfortable in his or her own cradle, or playing quietly with a toy on the floor. Fragile examining equipment or dangerous items such as needles or surgical instruments must be out of reach.

The doctor's image portrayed when the child is initially seen must be carefully considered. Many paediatric ophthalmologists prefer not to wear a traditional white laboratory coat. The child is also less frightened if the doctor is at eye level with the child. Talking directly to the older child (rather than to the parents) initially also focuses the attention appropriately on the patient.

The clinical examination by the ophthalmologist starts

with observation of the child as the history is being taken. How alert is the child? How does the baby react to sudden changes in the environment, such as a change in lighting or noise or someone coming into the room? Does the head appear to be misshapen, enlarged or microcephalic? Are there any signs of external bruising which might suggest non-accidental injury? Does there appear to be any asymmetry between the two eyes? Is fixation steady?

Examination for ptosis, blepharophimosis, the external appearance of the lids and adnexae, and skin lesions must all be made. Early in the visit, an examination of the clarity of the media with a retinoscope provides key information. Examination for factors which lead to amblyopia, including refractive error, strabismus and media opacities can be made with this simple instrument. The retinoscope seems not to bother infants and children as much as ophthalmoscopes which may have brighter lights or which require touching of the child, but an ophthalmoscope with the rheostat turned down can also be used for most purposes, although not for refraction.

Assessment of visual function is a complex task consisting of numerous components including visual acuity, visual fields, colour vision and afferent pupillary function. Visual acuity, or the ability to resolve contrasts, develops over the first year of life and there is plasticity in this system up to the age of 12 years. Methods of visual acuity assessment change as the child grows older.

Fixation and following

In a baby, several techniques of assessing vision on the basis of ocular motor responses are commonly used by paediatric ophthalmologists. Most simply, a baby's ability to fix and follow is noted. Fixation should be steady, and pursuit movements smooth. It must be kept in mind that the ability to follow does not imply any particular Snellen equivalent of visual acuity (Atkinson 1992). Many older children with 20/200–20/400 vision demonstrate a fix and follow response. The fix and follow technique, as well as all of the others mentioned below, should be applied not only binocularly but also monocularly. Occlusion of one eye may result in an unhappy child, and many clinicians rely upon objection to occlusion as an indicator that vision is poor in the unoccluded eye. However, often the occluder itself is enough to upset a child; more subtle occlusion, such as with the examiner's thumb over one eye, may be more successful.

CSM notation

A popular method of notation is the CSM system. The ability of each eye to fixate centrally, steadily, and maintain fixation is documented. Central fixation implies that the patient's fixation is foveal; that is, that the light reflex is in the centre or paracentral area of the pupil. Steady fixa-tion implies that no nystagmoid movements are imposed on the fixing eye which is regarding a static target. Maintained fixation refers to the ability of one eye to maintain fixation when viewing is converted from a monocular to a binocular condition. As an example, a child with a right esotropia is suspected of having an underlying visual problem with the right eye: if the left eye is covered, the right eye takes up fixation which may for the purpose of this illustration be central and steady. Once the occlusion is removed from the left eye, failure of the right eye to move would earn a 'maintained' notation; a shift inward warrants a notation of unmaintained fixation, with implied poor vision in the right eye relative to the left eye.

Quantification of vision

The earliest attempts at visual acuity quantification relied upon an infant's ability to detect stripes on an optokinetic nystagmus drum. The examiner noted the presence or absence of nystagmus by directly observing the baby's eye movements (Gorman *et al.* 1957; Linkz 1973).

Quantification of visual acuity represents a particular challenge in children, due to their communication, developmental and educational skills. This limitation to testing contrasts with the examiner's need to know just how good the vision is—relative to previous examinations, as in the child undergoing occlusion therapy for amblyopia, one eye relative to the other eye, and relative to vision in age-matched controls. (See Chapter 2 for guidelines for visual acuity in different age groups.)

Standard methods of visual acuity testing can rarely be used before the age of 3 years. Near acuity tests, especially with picture optotypes, can often be performed at a young age and should be attempted in co-operative 18–24-month-old children Newer tests which rely upon electrophysiological or behavioural endpoints have been introduced to broaden our knowledge of vision development in infants and children.

Guidelines for the testing of children must adhere to those which we use for adult patients. Whenever possible, distance and near visual acuity measurements must be defined. Testing of each eye separately must be performed, ensuring that complete occlusion of one eye is achieved. Establishment of the specific level of best acuity must be refined by the ophthalmologist with repeated testing of targets around the endpoint. Children may often quit prematurely due simply to lack of interest rather than lack of vision.

Techniques for testing, however, must be artfully refined for children. The examination must be more of a game than a test. Reinforcement and reward for positive responses on the part of the examiner should be somewhat more enthusiastic than with adult patients. Control of parental coaching must be maintained. The testing will only last as long as the child's attention span, and several tries at different times may be necessary. Extraneous competition for the child's attention by active siblings, ringing telephones or unnecessary movement, must be kept at a bare minimum.

Despite the above cautions, proper visual acuity estimates can usually be obtained within a matter of minutes once the examiner's skills for performing them have been adapted to children.

Snellen visual acuity and other optotypes

Quantification of visual acuity depends upon a patient's ability to discriminate differences in contrasting colours (traditionally black and white) and upon the examiner's ability to interpret the patient's response. The standard test is the Snellen visual acuity chart, which relies on letter recognition; the smallest subtended angle is defined by gaps in the letter which give identity clues to the patient.

The Snellen visual acuity chart represents one optotype visual acuity chart. An optotype is any symbol whose identification implies visual acuity, or resolution capability, of a particular subtended angle. The shape of the optotype can vary. Although letters appear on the standard Snellen chart, other examples of optotype acuity charts include the Landolt C rings, number charts, schematic picture, and the E (or illiterate E) charts.

All optotype forms of visual acuity testing are psychophysical tests; i.e. interpretation of the test is a subjective one measured by the patient's ability to communicate this subjective recognition to the examiner.

There are many limitations to optotype testing in paediatric ophthalmology. Although some children are able to recognize a few letters by the age of 4 years, the complexities of Snellen visual acuity testing make it unreliable before the age of 6–8 years. Failure to see a line on the chart must raise the question as to whether the child knows what the letter is.

Many optotype tests have been designed to counter the limitations in letter recognition. The E chart is popularly used not only for the preschool child, but also for illiterate adults as well as people from countries whose alphabet is of non-Roman figures. With children, the E game has basic limitations. First, a child's co-ordination and left–right discrimination may present apparently inaccurate answers. Some examiners will therefore ignore any miss when left is confused with right. Second, the test is inherently repetitious, and the child's attention span may fall short of the examiner's needs.

Picture optotypes may be very helpful in testing 2–5-year-old children, since recognition of pictures of cars, birthday cakes or birds can be adapted into a game format more easily (Fig. 8.1). There are cultural limitations which can impair this test's validity; some children may not recognize a telephone because there is none at home, or

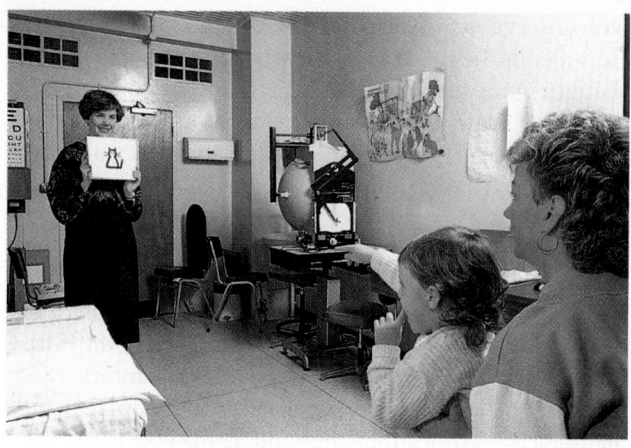

Fig. 8.1 Picture optotypes such as Kay's pictures shown here can be used for acuity measurements but they have cultural limitation due to their being recognition tests.

because the abstracted shape of the telephone on the chart is entirely different from the telephone at home. Another drawback to the picture tests is that the construction of the individual optotypes is less optically accurate than, for instance, the Landolt C ring in which the subtended angle of contrast recognition is very precise. In comparison to the Snellen letter chart, where 26 possible answers are present, the alert child quickly learns that there are usually only five or six possible choices on picture charts.

One adaptation of optotype acuity testing for children is the use of a matching technique. As with the picture chart, the number of possible correct choices is significantly reduced, usually to four or seven possible correct answers. The child need not know the name of a particular optotype but need only pair the examiner's choice of optotype with the patient's available matching optotype which the child holds.

The most popular matching optotypes are the HOTV, Sheridan–Gardner or Sonksen–Silver (Sonksen 1993) charts (Fig. 8.2).

Visual evoked potentials and preferential looking

More recently, researchers have introduced two techniques to define vision development in infant and preverbal children. These two methods — preferential looking (PL or forced PL) (Fulton *et al.* 1981; Jacobson *et al.* 1982; Mayer *et al.* 1982) and visual evoked potentials (VEP) (Sokol 1980; Odom *et al.* 1981) — have aided our understanding of both normal and abnormal visual development. Although still used predominantly in research settings due to time and economic constraints, their impact on clinical ophthalmology is becoming more evident (Ellis *et al.* 1988). Both FPL and VEP provide visual acuity measurements which cannot be directly correlated to Snellen acuity measurements, as their basic principles

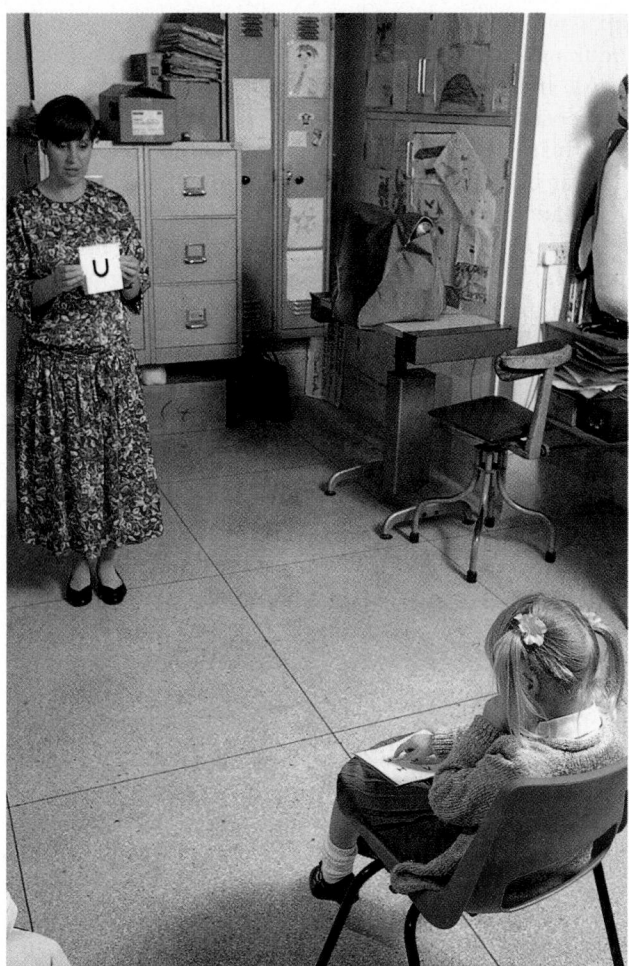

Fig. 8.2 Matching optotypes, such as the Sheridan–Gardner single optotype matching test shown here, cannot be used with children as young as those who can use the picture optotypes but they are nearer to Snellen acuity because recognition is less important.

longer eliciting a response different from the homogeneous targets. The FPL technique has been refined to help eliminate observer bias and to standardize selection of grating size (Teller *et al.* 1974; Held *et al.* 1979). Commercially available FPL cards (McDonald *et al.* 1985; Teller *et al.* 1986) have allowed this technique to enter the clinician's domain.

The FPL technique has been helpful in establishing norms for visual acuity development in infants. Most normal infants reach the ability to resolve 20/20 gratings by the age of 1–3 years (Teller *et al.* 1974; Gwiazda *et al.* 1980; Mayer & Dobson 1978). Abnormal visual development, as occurs with amblyopia, cataract and strabismus, has been assessed with the FPL technique as well (Catalano *et al.* 1987) and correlated when possible with standard Snellen testing (Sokol *et al.* 1983; Birch & Stager 1985; Moskowitz *et al.* 1987) as well as clinical assessment by a paediatric ophthalmologist (Ellis *et al.* 1988). The advantages of the test appear to be a relative ease of administration, a relatively low cost and rapid answers as long as no pathology is present. With any abnormality, however, testing becomes more time-consuming and prone to errors; nystagmus, for instance may require re-orientation of the cards to get the best, and probably the most accurate, acuity (Meiusi *et al.* 1993).

Its use by paediatric ophthalmologists has remained primarily in centres in which ongoing research is present and in which clinicians work in association with infant vision scientists.

VEP represents a second major area of interest in infant vision research. Its recent evolution is in large part a consequence of computer technology. Its value rests upon the occipital cortex's electrical signal in response to a visual stimulation (Sokol 1976; Regan & Spekreijse 1986). The

(behavioural response with FPL and electrophysiological response with VEP) differ from the optotype tests.

Despite the usefulness of these techniques, the clinician should exercise caution in interpreting the results to family and to agencies (for instance as parameters for financial assistance for visual impairment). It is best that grating acuities are not correlated to Snellen optotype acuities.

The FPL technique is based on a child's inherent interest in patterned, as opposed to homogeneous, targets (Fantz *et al.* 1962; Mayer & Dobson 1978). The patient is presented with two targets positioned in a homogeneous background, one of which matches the background, the other of which contains gratings (Fig. 8.3). If the infant responds by turning the eyes or the head towards the striped target as they are simultaneously presented, then this response is interpreted as an ability of the child to see the target. The child is then presented with progressively smaller gratings until the examiner believes the grating targets are no

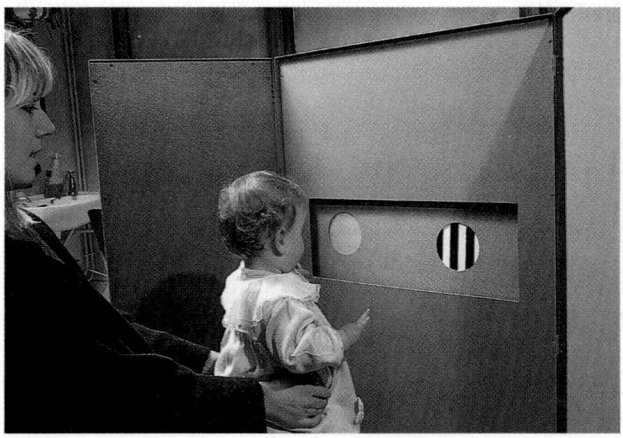

Fig. 8.3 The acuity card procedure. The child sits in front of the screen with as little to distract him or her as possible and cards with varying grating size are placed in the central panel. The child is observed through a minute central peep hole as to whether or not fixation is drawn to the side with the grating.

appearance of the waveform is highly variable as a consequence of different testing circumstances and equipment, and a thorough knowledge of any particular testing situation is required to ensure the validity of the test (Sokol 1976).

In general, two types of stimuli, the unpatterned and the patterned, can evoke visual cortical potentials. The quantification of infant vision is limited to patterned stimuli, which in general are in either bar gratings or in checkerboard form. Focusing of the image is essential in interpreting its results; thus, knowledge and correction of any significant refractive error is essential (Millodot & Riggs 1970).

Two major types of pattern visual evoked responses have been developed for the quantification of infant vision. The pattern reversal technique (Sokol & Dobson 1976) has suggested maturation of 20/20 equivalent grating resolution between the ages of 6 and 12 months. The swept VEP technique, which relies upon extrapolation of the VEP signal generated by a 'sweeping' of grating size from large to small in 10 seconds also suggests this tempo of infant vision development (Norcia & Tyler 1985). The difference in these values compared to FPL data has been thought to be due to the superimposed behavioural requirements placed on the infant with the FPL technique (Allen *et al.* 1987). The VEP has been applied to clinical circumstances in patients with a wide variety of clinical disorders (Sokol 1980; Day *et al.* 1988; Weleber & Palmer 1991; Kriss & Russell-Eggitt 1992). Its current use remains predominantly in the research laboratory and in circumstances in which clinicians and basic scientists closely collaborate, as the VEP remains a time-consuming test in circumstances where there is pathology.

Tests for children with very poor vision

In a child who is obviously poorly sighted, tests must be designed to determine even very low levels of vision. Particularly helpful in the young infant is the spinning or VOR (vestibulo-ocular reflex) test in which the child's fixation reflex is assessed after vestibulo-ocular nystagmus has been induced by spinning, rotating with the child held at arm's length in front of the examiner. With spinning, horizontal nystagmus is induced. After several rotations, the turning is discontinued. The examiner then assesses the baby's eye movements. On cessation of spinning, there are normally only one or two beats of after-nystagmus; in a blind baby, or one with severe cerebellar disease, there will be prolonged after-nystagmus. It is helpful to perform this manoeuvre on normal babies to gain experience in what represents a normal response.

In the most severe cases of poor vision, the examiner simply wishes to know if the child is able to see light at all. A threat response is less helpful in babies than in older individuals because this response may normally not

appear for several months. However, a baby's response by blinking to a bright light or camera flash is easy to obtain.

All these tests, however, rely on the child's motor responses thus, they must be interpreted cautiously bearing this in mind — if he cannot move his eyes he may appear blind until head control improves and he moves his head to the response instead (see Chapter 64).

Other clues that the vision may be poor may be gained by a child's appearance. The presence of nystagmus, eye-poking and a sunken appearance of the eyes all suggest chronically poor vision.

Other visual functions

Visual fields

Visual field testing is often ignored in infants and children since there is a general concept that this test requires sophisticated equipment and an immense amount of co-operation. Although it is true that Goldmann visual field cannot be performed without co-operation, a useful assessment at any age can be made of significant defects such as hemianopias by simple confrontation techniques. The examiner simply faces the child and attracts the child's attention centrally; then a toy or light is introduced silently from the far periphery (Fig. 8.4). A child with normal fields will make a very rapid head movement or saccadic eye movement in the direction of the new stimulus. The child may well become bored with repeated attempts, and the availability of several different toys is helpful. Finger counting or detection of which of the examiner's fingers is wiggling may also be useful in older partially co-operative children (Fig. 8.5). Older children can be tested with more or less conventional techniques (Mutlukan & Damato 1993) (Fig. 8.6). Visual evoked response testing may also reveal significant hemianopias if an array of occipital electrodes is used.

Colour vision

Testing of colour vision also should be attempted. Standard Ishihara colour plates can be used (Fig. 8.7), with adaptation of the usual testing technique so that instead of identification of numbers in the standard way, one can ask a child to trace the area which is coloured with a finger. Ishihara plates test only red–green deficiency but others include blue–yellow testing. The Llantony plates are purely tritan plates (Fig. 8.8). The City University colour vision test (Fig. 8.9) also is adaptable to testing children, since the response does not depend on pattern recognition but rather on the identification of individual dots. The child has to identify which of four different coloured spots is nearer the same colour to a spot around which they are grouped. The HRR plates provide good testing targets for the 3–5 year old, as the geometric targets (circle, Xs and tri-

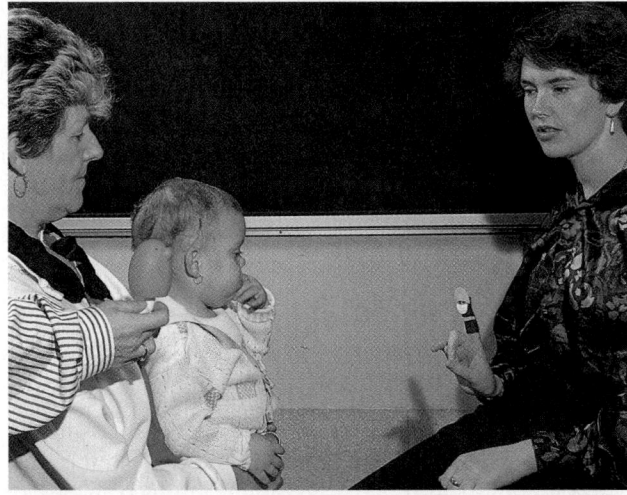

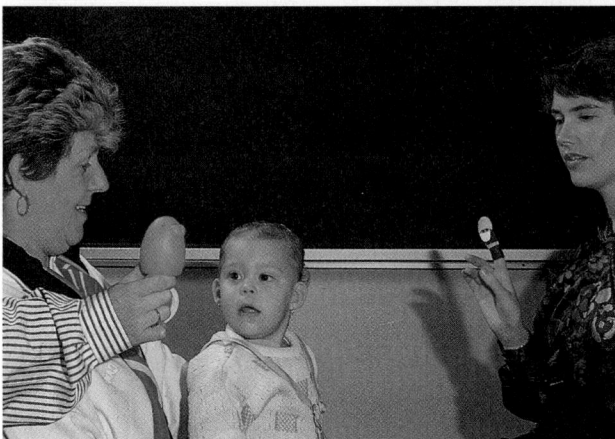

Fig. 8.4 Infant visual field testing. The first tester on the left, attracts the baby's attention (a) whilst the other brings an object in silently from the side to see if the child's attention is drawn to it (b). Although crude, if defects are detected by this method they are likely to be functionally significant in the future.

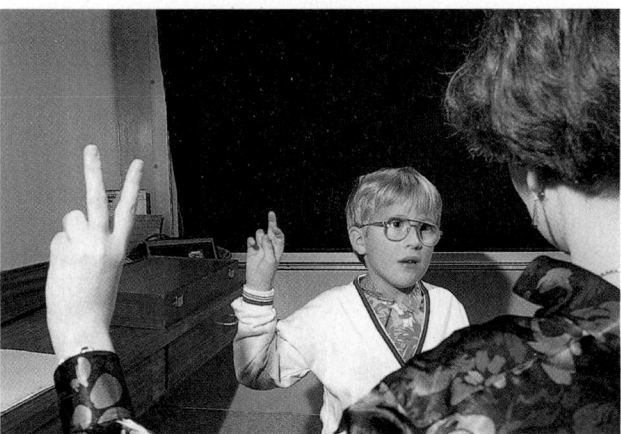

Fig. 8.5 'Finger matching' fields. While the tester watches the fixation, the child tells her when the tester's fingers are wiggling or may watch or count the fingers if able to do so.

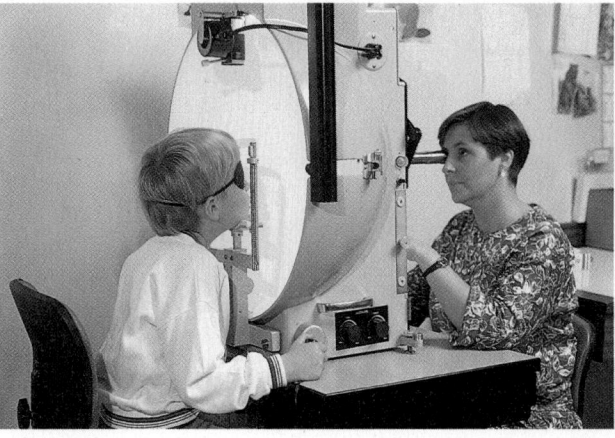

Fig. 8.6 Goldmann visual field testing. Older children, with good attention, can be tested on more sophisticated devices such as the Goldmann field analyser or various forms of automated field analyser.

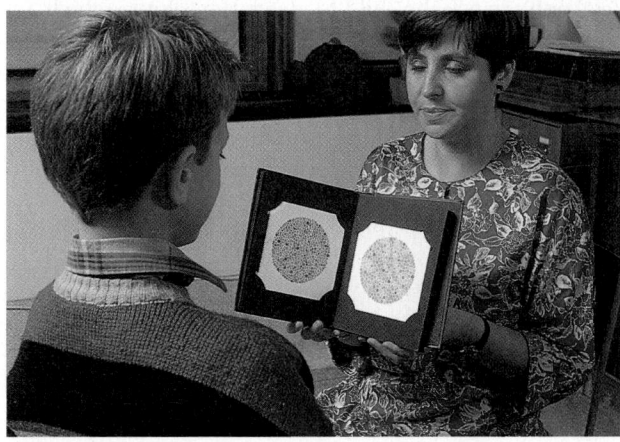

Fig. 8.7 The Ishihara test detects red–green defects only.

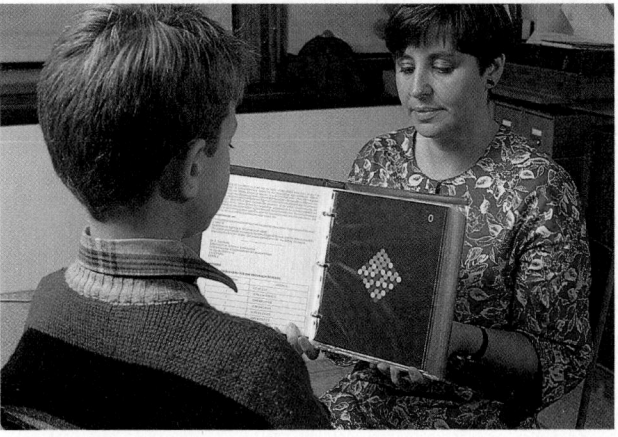

Fig. 8.8 Llantony's tritan plates detect blue–yellow defects.

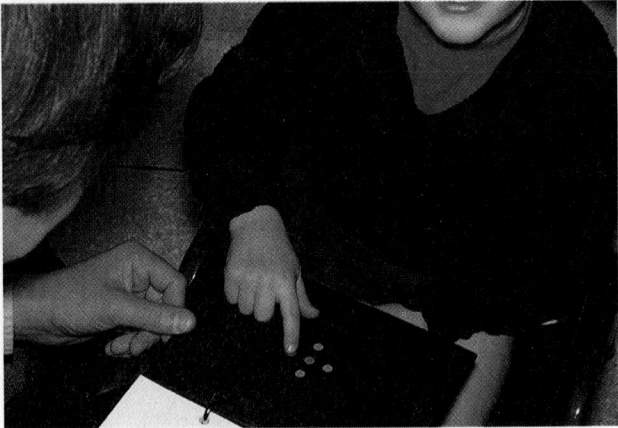

Fig. 8.9 The City University colour test will detect and grade colour defects (see text).

angles) are familiar to them. With tests such as the D-15 test, one can ask the child to match the colours which are more similar to each other. One can also keep a group of different coloured socks and ask the child to pick out the two which match. Colour naming may be useful but should be interpreted with caution because many young children with normal colour vision are rather poor at naming colours.

Pupil inspection

Pupil testing requires interpretation of second cranial nerve function (afferent system) as well as third cranial nerve function (efferent system). Simple inspection of pupil size may reveal anisocoria; unless the size difference exceeds 1 mm and/or there is other evidence of third nerve dysfunction such as ptosis or paralytic exotropia, small differences in pupil size are of no consequence. Typically, the neonatal pupil is small (2–3 mm) and minimally reactive to light. The intrinsic iris muscles, the dilator and the sphincter, develop relatively late embryologically. As a consequence, interpretation of pupil size and reactivity must be modified in the infant less than 3 months old.

In the older child, although pupil size is more easily obtained, the light- and near-pupillary reactions may be difficult to judge. A child's fixation must be controlled at a distance fixation target; otherwise, shifts in fixation may result in either falsely positive or negative interpretation of a relative afferent pupil defect (RAPD). Hippus, or physiological variation in pupil size, also creates difficulty in pupil testing, since this phenomenon is more noticeable in younger individuals. This natural variation in pupil size is particularly noticeable in patients with lightly pigmented irides.

Inevitably, parents are curious about the colour of their child's eyes. 'Can you tell what colour they will be?' and

'When will the eyes turn the final colour?' are foremost in young parents' minds. The evolution of iris pigmentation tends to be complete by 9–12 months; in many circumstances, eye colour can be predicted much earlier on the basis of the colour of the parents' eyes as well as the relative degree of pigmentation of the neonate's eyes. Conditions which result in lightening of the eyes with age are rare; thus it is fairly safe to provide this information to parents.

Tests of binocular vision

Binocularity carries a vast overlap into the field of strabismus where maintenance or improvement of this function influences the management of the child with strabismus. Several clinical tests have become traditional means of assessing binocularity.

Stereopsis

Stereopsis is a binocular function in which a perception of depth is created by either nasal or temporal disparity in the projection of similar retinal images, one from each eye, to the brain. It is not synonymous with 'depth perception' which contains many monocular clues. Although stereopsis implies excellent visual acuity in each eye, poor stereopsis can occur in patients with excellent monocular acuity as well as diminished acuity in one or both eyes (Donzis *et al.* 1983). Although some screening programmes have advocated stereopsis tests as helpful in young children it must be remembered that visual acuity and stereopsis are two different functions.

In clinical practice, the Titmus fly and Randot stereopsis test remains the most commonly used form of assessment (Fig. 8.10). A child wearing polarized lenses is asked to point to apparently elevated figures in a book with two

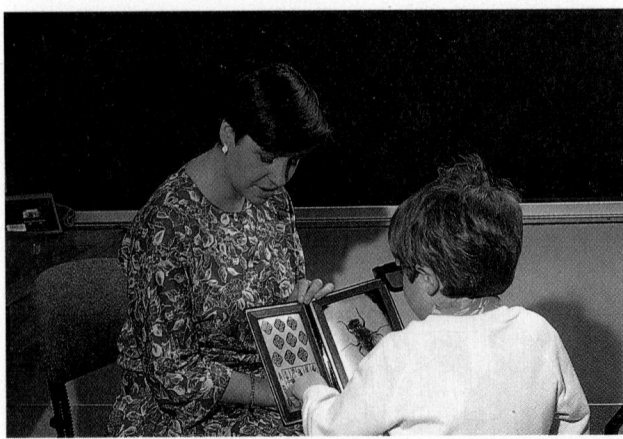

Fig. 8.10 The Titmus stereoacuity test requires the use of polaroid glasses with the plane of polarization at right angles to each other in the spectacles.

superimposed, slightly displaced images creating a three-dimensional effect. The test is therefore a psychophysical one, and the less refined targets can in fact be seen using monocular clues. Other tests use red–green goggles to create disparate images (Fig. 8.11). Co-operation is required, and in general a failed response is regarded as unreliable in children less than 5 years old. Other stereopsis tests may be used for younger children, in which they point to figures that are elevated or depressed by their position in special plastic cards, such as the Lang or Frisby tests (Fig. 8.12) in which no special lenses or glasses are required.

In recent years, research has expanded in the field of stereopsis, again largely as a consequence of computer technology. One avenue of study has been to explore stere-

opsis development, which appears to be most impressive between 3 and 7 months of age (Teller & Movshon 1986). A second area has explored different forms of testing, especially the random dot stereogram (Julesz 1986). Clinicians have compared the various forms of commercially available stereopsis tests and raised their potential use as screening tests for vision since excellent visual acuity is required in each eye for good stereopsis (Donzis *et al.* 1983). Researchers also have begun to study young infant stereopsis and the effects of esotropia on stereopsis in an effort to better define the most appropriate time for surgery in children with infantile esotropia (Mohindra *et al.* 1985).

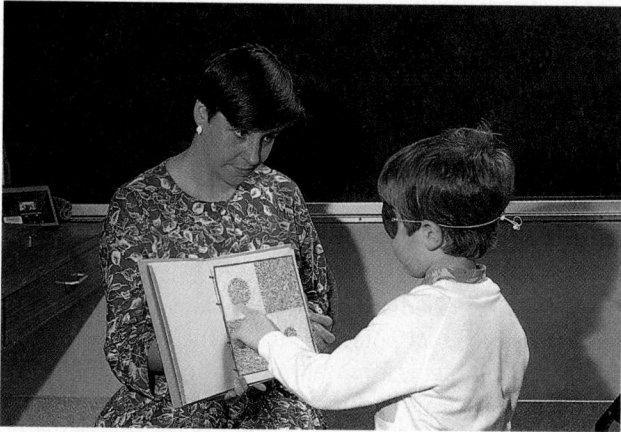

Fig. 8.11 Other stereoacuity tests use a red–green system for creating the disparity between the eyes which allows the child to see shapes on the test card. This child is viewing the demonstration plate.

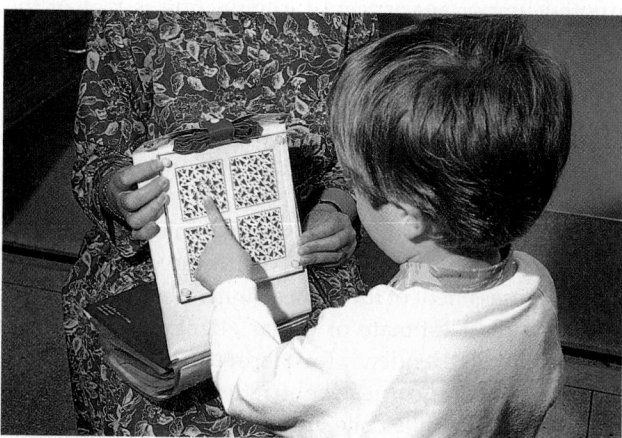

Fig. 8.12 The Frisby test does not require glasses; instead the figures in a central panel of one of the test squares are printed on the other side of the perspex sheets so that the child can only see it if he or she has binocular depth perception. In this picture this is demonstrated by the flash gun's shadow cast by the test figure to which the child points. The thickness of the perspex varies; the thicker plates give greater disparity and therefore are easier to see.

Fusion

The binocular function of fusion includes both sensory and motor fusion. In the former, the visual cortex receives and unifies two images, one from each eye, similar in size and shape. Sensory fusion infers that corresponding retinal points are present in the two eyes which project to one site within the cortex. When fusion is not present, then the abnormal binocular sensory states of diplopia, confusion, or suppression are present (see Chapter 2).

Sensory fusion is most commonly tested with the Worth four-dot test. The child is instructed to wear a pair of glasses in which a red filter is over one eye and a green filter over the other eye. An illuminated target consisting of one red dot, two green dots, and one white dot is held at near (33 cm) and at distance (6 m) and the child is asked the number and colour of the dots. When fusion is present, four dots are seen, with the white dot changing colours due to retinal rivalry. When diplopia is present, five dots are seen. Suppression results in the child seeing two or three dots, depending on which eye is suppressed. This test is performed at distance and near to assess for central (with the distance testing) and peripheral (with the near testing) fusion as a consequence of the subtended angle covered by the dots at varied distances. Although the Worth four-dot test is widely used to assess preoperative fusional status in children with strabismus its reliability has been criticized on the basis of the artificiality of an environment interrupted by red and green filters.

Motor fusion refers to vergence movements — either convergence or divergence — evident when an apparent image is 'moved' on the retina, such as holding a prism in front of one eye. Although there is a natural limit to normal fusional amplitudes (von Noorden 1985) the ability of a patient to make this vergence movement implies excellent binocular function since the impetus for the motor response is unification of the images.

Retinal correspondence

With orthophoria, binocular vision develops as a consequence of normal retinal correspondence, or a point-to-point coupling of retinal receptor information in the two eyes which is projected to a single cortical region. With early onset malalignment, or strabismus, this coupling is altered, resulting in abnormal input to the visual cortex, or anomalous retinal correspondence. The retinal receptor fields are in a sense reordered such that under binocular circumstances, there is a shift in the coupling of the projected images from the two eyes that achieves an alteration in binocularity. Tests for normal and anomalous retinal correspondence (ARC) rely upon a subjective interpretation by the patient of two groups of tests. The 'after image' test stimulates the fovea of each eye viewing under monocular conditions. A bright flash with a central gap is horizontally viewed first by one eye; this eye is then occluded and the fellow eye views a vertically oriented flash. With both eyes closed, the patient then is asked to describe the orientation of these two relative positions as a cross with one gap (normal correspondence) or as a cross in which the gaps are shifted. The alignment of the eyes must be known as well, since a similar description in an esotropic patient would imply abnormal retinal correspondence, or an apparent reordering of object perception which allows for the basic deviation.

The second form of testing for ARC involves simultaneous viewing of an object which is thus projected onto one foveal and one extrafoveal retinal locus in the patient with strabismus. Since one goal of sensory testing is to create as little interruption to the natural environment as is possible (or, in strabismus jargon, to try to maintain fusion), the Bagolini lenses (Fig. 8.13) have gained popularity in this group of testing. The surfaces of plano lenses are 'scratched' in a way that a pinpoint source of light is displayed through the lens in a linear fashion. The orientation of the striations is projected so that the striations in one eye are perpendicular to the fellow eye. The patient's interpretation of the direction of the striation as well as the point source of light will then allow the examiner to judge

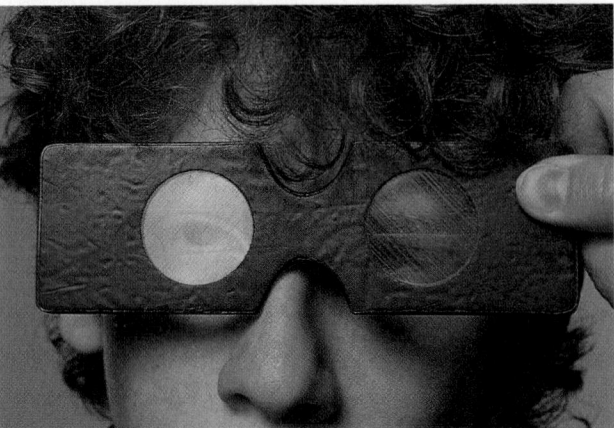

Fig. 8.13 Bagolini's striated glasses. The striations can be clearly seen in the glass in front of the patient's left eye (see text).

normal and anomalous retinal correspondence as well as the type of ocular deviation when the patient's alignment and fixation are also known.

A second test in which the patient views one target through dissimilar circumstances for the two eyes is the red glass, or diplopia test. A white light is viewed by the patient with a red filter over one eye. A vertical prism will allow separation of the red and white. Interpretation of the patient's responses must be correlated with the patient's alignment at a similar testing distance. The patient responds by assessing the relative position of the red and white lights. By comparing to the alignment of the eye, the examiner can then define whether normal or abnormal retinal correspondence is present.

Contrast sensitivity

Contrast sensitivity testing has proved helpful in patients with subtle visual loss, especially in conditions such as visual pathway gliomas, optic neuritis and glaucoma. Its value has been that its testing may be abnormal when other standard tests such as visual acuity, colour vision and visual field testing have been normal (Zimmern *et al.* 1979; Regan *et al.* 1980; Stamper *et al.* 1982).

Although contrast sensitivity testing is not routinely performed by paediatric ophthalmologists, researchers have considered its potential role in the management of paediatric problems such as monitoring of amblyopia. Contrast sensitivity function appears to develop rapidly during the first few months of life (Norcia *et al.* 1987).

Eye movements and strabismus

Another important aspect of examination is that of the ocular motor system; strabismus is an extremely common referral diagnosis in children. One must constantly keep in mind the interplay between strabismus and amblyopia. Thus, the examination of the motor system is a reflection of both eye movements and visual function, both monocular and binocular.

As with visual acuity assessment, oculomotor assessment varies in its completeness with the child's age. In infancy, assessment of the corneal light reflex (Hirschberg) is the simplest estimate of ocular alignment. One must keep in mind the tendency for children to have a nasal displacement of the corneal light reflex or 'positive angle kappa'. Additionally, one must be aware that despite apparently straight eyes as judged by corneal light reflex testing, a small tropia may be present with more sophisticated cover test techniques. Nevertheless, corneal light reflex testing is a very important technique to master as a screening technique for strabismus.

In the Krimsky test a prism bar is used to equalize the position of the light reflex in the two eyes—it is particular-

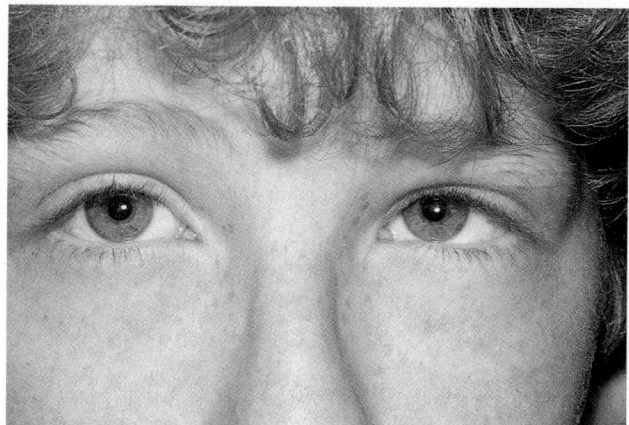
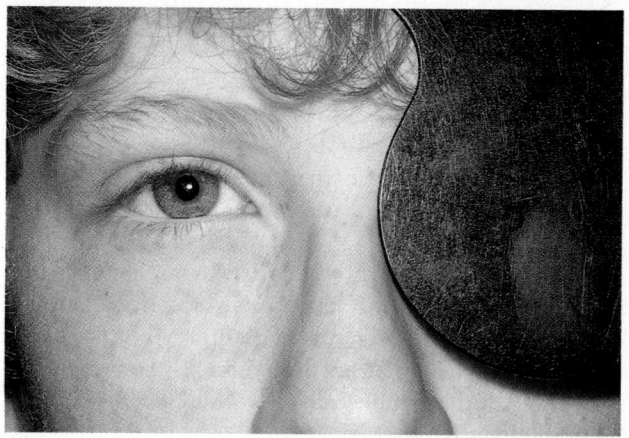
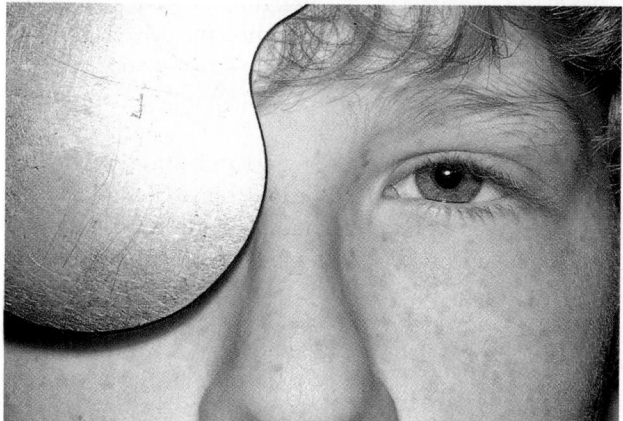

Fig. 8.14 The cover test. (a) The asymmetrical light reflexes in the pupils can be seen. (b) No shift of the right eye on left eye cover. (c) On the right eye being covered the left eye moves out to take up fixation. Meticulous control over fixation must be maintained (see text).

ly useful in non-fixing eyes because it does not need the eye to shift to take up fixation to indicate the magnitude of the deviation.

There are several useful tips about testing for the corneal light reflex: (i) when the corneal light reflex is checked at near, the light source itself must also be held at near, at the same distance as the observer; and (ii) the child should fix not on the light source but preferably on a small, accommodative, target, such as a small picture. With this type of stimulus, an accommodative component of the strabismus can more easily be elicited.

Confirmation of strabismus is made with the alternate cover test and the cover–uncover test (Fig. 8.14). Both of these tests are difficult to perform on the younger child, since control of fixation is mandatory and often children tend to refixate randomly. Also, children tend to object to the presence of a large plastic occluder. The examiner's thumb may be used as an occluder as long as one is careful to hold the thumb close enough so as to truly prevent fixation with the occluded eye.

When a small angle strabismus is present which cannot be detected on traditional cover techniques, the 4 dioptre base-out prism test (Jampolsky 1964) may reveal information about the patient's alignment and sensory status (Fig. 8.15). With controlled distance fixation, the prism is introduced over one eye, and the examiner assesses for a

fixation shift. The test is then repeated with the prism held over the fellow eye. If there is a difference between the two eyes a refixation movement is made with the prism over one eye only. The complete ocular motility examination, however, must be far more comprehensive. Measurement of the deviation at near, definition of phoric versus tropic deviations, measurements in the nine positions of gaze, and head tilt measurements are indicated in patients with strabismus (see Chapters 65–67).

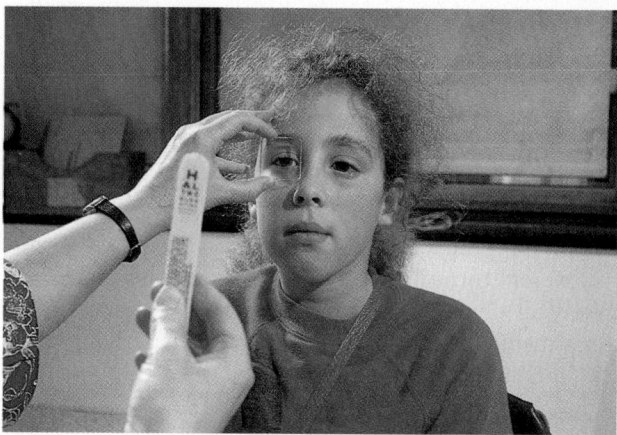

Fig. 8.15 The 4 dioptre base-out prism test. Holding fixation with a target appropriate to the age of the child is vital (see text).

Although measurement of the deviation in the primary position is the most important part of the strabismus examination, assessment of versions is an essential element as well. Limitations of versions may be suggested by an abnormal head posture. Assessment of versions is essential in the detection of incomitant squints and cranial nerve palsies. A and V patterns are detected by testing versions.

Strabismus may be subtly hidden by an abnormal or preferred head position. Other ocular causes of abnormal head positions are nystagmus with null-point, refractive error (usually astigmatism or myopia), a homonymous hemianopia or torticollis caused by muscular, skeletal or neuro-otological defect.

In some circumstances, attention must be given to supranuclear eye movement function including saccades and pursuits, especially when one suspects oculomotor apraxia, progressive external ophthalmoplegia and other neurological conditions.

In general, the oculomotor examination gives information about the function of cranial nerves III, IV and VI, as well as the supranuclear control of eye movements. One additional assessment of cranial nerve III is pupillary shape, size and response to light as well as accommodation.

Slit-lamp examination

Slit-lamp examination is one vital test which is often overlooked in young children. Examination of the young infant is made easier by the simple measure of raising the slit lamp to a comfortable height for the parent to hold the baby in a prone position, steadying the chin with one hand and supporting the body with that arm. The second arm steadies the head posteriorly. The mother is instructed to bring the baby in this prone position up towards the slit lamp until the baby's forehead rests against the forehead strap (Fig. 8.16). Alternatively, hand-held slit lamps may be of particular benefit in other situations, such as inpatient consultations or in the operating room.

Slit-lamp examination is particularly important in infants with nystagmus, as patients with albinism may clearly show iris transillumination defects on retroillumination.

Other specific indications for slit-lamp examination include determination of the level of media opacity, examination for foreign bodies and corneal abrasions, determination of corneal abnormalities such as breaks in Descemet's membrane from congenital glaucoma, and assessment of the conjunctiva to identify underlying causes of inflammation.

Refraction

See Chapter 7.

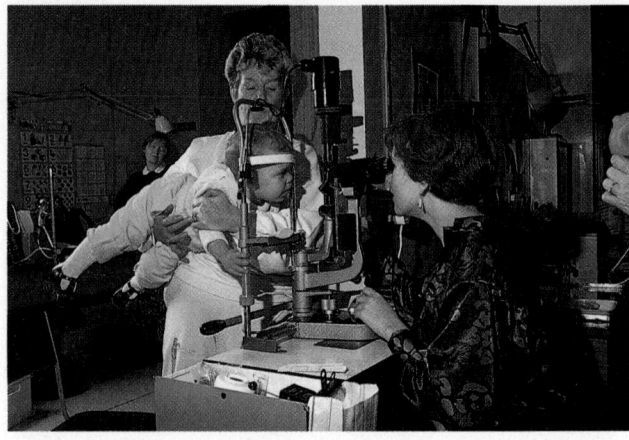

Fig. 8.16 Slit-lamp examination can be performed at almost any age in nearly all children but requires a firm but gentle person to hold the child so that the forehead touches the strap.

Photorefraction

New screening devices based on photographic refraction techniques are offered for screening the preverbal child. Using several optical principles (Howland & Howland 1974; Kaakinen 1979) these devices are primarily designed to detect refractive error photographically. In addition to detecting refractive error (Atkinson *et al.* 1987), other amblyogenic factors such as cataract and strabismus have been documented with this technique in infants and preverbal children (Day & Norcia 1986).

As more systems become available, the clinician must answer several questions prior to endorsing a particular system. Has the system been validated for the intended age of usage? As a corollary, what age will be screened? Each system has a refractive error for which it is most sensitive. The domain of refractive error which is potentially problematic will be different for the 6-month infant, the 3-year-old child and the school aged child. Who will interpret the results? How carefully will parameters such as pupil size be respected? To what extent will the interpreter be trained?

Finally, one must realize that there are few scientific data available to address the clinical issues which will potentially be raised by this technique, such as the need to prescribe glasses in a straight-eyed hyperopic infant (see Chapter 7).

Fundoscopy

Fundoscopy in infants and children represents a particular challenge, not only due to limited co-operation, but also due to the different appearance of the fundus in very young children compared to adults. Adequate mydriasis is essential and is best obtained by supplementing the cycloplegic agent (cyclopentolate 0.5 or 1%) with a mydriatic agent such as either tropicamide (Mydriacyl 0.5 or 1%)

or phenylephrine 2.5%, especially in an infant with brown irides (Bolt *et al.* 1992). Both indirect and direct ophthalmoscopy should be performed if possible. The first instrument to be used should be the indirect ophthalmoscope, as a quick overview of the fundus can lead one to pay particular attention to areas with the direct ophthalmoscope. Although the +20 dioptre lens is frequently used, the +28 to +30 lens can provide a wider field and the +14 lens can provide further details of structures such as the optic nerve. With the tiny infant, it is best to ensure that the baby is quiet and content during the indirect examination. Often this can be achieved by feeding the baby. The baby can be cradled in the parent's arms or lying on the parent's lap, whichever makes the baby most comfortable. Usually the lids can be held with the examiner's fingers. It is best to line the lens up first and, once in place, quickly bring the ophthalmoscope light into view. Several quick glimpses seem to allow greater co-operation than one attempted prolonged look. As soon as the baby begins to squeeze the lids, the Bell's phenomenon will occur, and the examiner is thwarted!

In the older child, the fundus examination itself can become a game. One technique would be to suggest that by looking in the eyes, the examiner is able to determine what the child has eaten for breakfast (a guess is made based on the current best selling cereal or local favourite!). Another trick is to suggest that there is a particular animal that can be seen, describing the features of the animal until the child is able to identify what the animal is. It is sometimes helpful to demonstrate on either the parents or older siblings what the examination is like, and then the child may ask for his or her own turn or understand that fundoscopy is not painful.

With children of all ages, it is best to have the room lights dimmed to improve the image of the fundus, but the room should not be completely darkened, as some children may be afraid.

In examining with the direct ophthalmoscope, specific anatomical features must be sought. Examination of the fovea is often easy, as the child will look at the light. If one can get the child's attention away from the light by asking the child to look at a distance fixation target, then control of the area of examination is easier to obtain. Some children will tolerate the red-free light more easily.

The premature baby

Examination of the premature infant requires special preparation, since the eye evaluation is most commonly in the setting of an intensive care nursery. Co-ordination of the examination must be made with the neonatologists and charge nurses, as these infants often require other tests or special care throughout the day. A telephone call 30–60 minutes in advance of the examination should be made to ensure adequate mydriasis for the examination.

One must use low doses of dilating agents due to the systemic absorption of the medication. A combination drop, such as Cyclomydril (0.2% cyclopentolate, 0.1% phenylephrine) is best used as one drop to each eye, repeated once in 5–10 minutes. Alternatively, one drop of cyclopentolate 0.5% and phenylephrine 2.5% should ensure adequate mydriasis. *Never* allow phenylephrine 10% to be used, as its systemic absorption may result in severe hypertensive crises or death in the premature baby. Equipment must be brought for the examination as well, including an indirect ophthalmoscope, +20 or +30 lens, lid speculum, scleral indentation device and topical anaesthesia.

The examination itself is often performed in the large intensive care nursery room which is brightly lit and hectic. It is necessary to keep in mind the precarious state of health of these infants. At all times during the eye examination, a nurse should be assisting as minor positioning changes can quickly compromise airways or other important lines. The examination may require a lid speculum and scleral indentor since the peripheral retina must be assessed thoroughly due to concerns about retinopathy of prematurity. If pupil dilation is poor, look carefully for synechiae formation, which may be a clue that significant retinopathy of prematurity is present.

One must keep in mind other features besides retinal status in the premature infant as the examination continues. Slight haziness of the cornea and vitreous haze, in the premature infant, may obscure examination but may be entirely normal.

Additional portable equipment, such as hand-held slit lamps and the Perkins applanation tonometers, may be invaluable in the premature infant. Concern about congenital glaucoma, metabolic or infectious disorders, and other particular reasons for ophthalmological consultation should be known prior to arrival in the neonatal unit. Retinoscopy may also be highly desirable in the older premature infant still dependent on life-support systems since high refractive errors may be present. Retinoscopy bars (hand-held racks of lenses) can be obtained to aid in this part of the examination.

The treatment of retinopathy of prematurity has remained controversial (Sira *et al.* 1988). A multicentre prospective trial has demonstrated the efficacy of treating these patients with cryotherapy in certain stages of disease (Cryotherapy for Retinopathy of Prematurity Cooperative Group 1988). Thus, the compulsion for examination of premature infants has gained even greater significance (see Chapter 43).

Examination under sedation

Rarely, a standard examination is insufficient to provide all the information which is necessary in making the appropriate medical decisions. An oral form of sedation such as chloral hydrate may be considered in such circumstances when general anaesthesia is to be avoided. When chloral hydrate sedation is to be performed, great care must be given that support staff trained in the management of sedated infants and children is available, or the sedation should not be carried out. It should not be carried out without appropriate resuscitation equipment being available. Sedated examinations must be used especially judiciously in infants less than 6 months old and in infants who have neurological abnormalities. An oral dose between 50 and 100 mg/kg of chloral hydrate will usually provide adequate sedation. Patients must be healthy, and their cardiovascular as well as pulmonary status must be ascertained prior to sedation. The infant should have no food or drink for approximately 4 hours beforehand. When chloral hydrate sedation is used, the child must be isolated in a quiet dimly lit room. Adequate sedation will usually allow checking of intraocular pressure, use of a portable slit lamp, use of lid speculum and fundus photography. If any manipulation is to be performed, such as removal of nasolacrimal stents or removal of sutures which will require pulling, chloral hydrate sedation is often not sufficient. Chloral hydrate sedation is most commonly indicated in children who have congenital glaucoma and require repeated follow-up, in children who have unexplained visual loss who cannot co-operate well enough on a routine examination, and in severely retarded children who are unable to co-operate with an examination. Ketamine is a useful alternative, although its use does require the presence of an anaesthetist which in itself implies the use of hospital facilities.

Ketamine has gained popularity as an agent for oculinum administration to young children (Magoon 1988); its hallucinogenic potential must be recognized and included in informed consent.

Examination under anaesthetic

Occasionally, an examination under anaesthesia (EUA) is warranted. The indications include: (i) inability to sedate sufficiently with a safe dose of chloral hydrate; (ii) the need for manipulation such as stent removal or suture removal; (iii) re-examination of a child with congenital glaucoma who may require further glaucoma surgery immediately after the examination; and (iv) examination of children with suspected retinoblastoma who will subsequently undergo enucleation.

Additionally, children with known retinoblastoma who require follow-up bone marrow aspirations and lumbar punctures may be co-ordinated under one anaesthetic to allow follow-up ophthalmoscopy in addition to the other testing.

Finally, EUA may be warranted when detailed electroretinography studies, fluorescein angiography, and combined procedures with other paediatric subspecialities are needed. In most infants, neurophysiological studies do not require anaesthesia. When an EUA is scheduled, all possible data must be obtained during this golden opportunity. These measurements include corneal diameters, gonioscopy, tonometry, slit-lamp examination, cycloplegic retinoscopy, and microscopic examination of the anterior and posterior segment of the eye with special contact lenses when indicated. The consequences of an EUA often require proceeding immediately to surgery such as goniotomy, lensectomy, biopsy or enucleation. Thus, proper counselling of the parents of these possible procedures must be performed prior to the EUA, so that a subsequent anaesthetic can be avoided. If an EUA is planned, it is appropriate to check if the child requires other elective surgery such as hernia repair, cleft palate repair or even venesection, as simultaneous procedures or sequential procedures may be performed with proper co-ordination.

Other examination and diagnostic testing of infants and children warrants particular co-ordination, including electrophysiology, ultrasonography, photography and radiology.

The measurement of intraocular pressure in suspected congenital glaucoma is critical to its management. Ketamine sedation, although not universally accepted by anaesthetists, is in widespread use as an agent for producing narcosis. Standard techniques of anaesthesia can be used (Dear *et al.* 1987) providing the pressure is measured before or at least 10 minutes after intubation.

Neurophysiological studies

See Chapter 9.

Ultrasound

Ultrasonography has particular applications to infants and children. In general, the A- and B-scan ultrasound can be performed on infants and children and has been used to detail the development of the eye (Larsen 1971a, b). With skilled examiners, sedation is rarely required in order to answer specific questions in a baby with opaque media, where details of the vitreous cavity and posterior pole are sought. This is particularly helpful in an infant with a corneal opacity or a cataract when the normality of the posterior segment must be ensured before surgery. Ultrasonography is also helpful before vitrectomy (Restori & McLeod 1977) in cases of ocular trauma in which retinal detachments or retained foreign bodies are suspected. Real-time studies, in which the movements of the intraocular contents can be observed, are particularly helpful (McLeod & Restori 1977). Care must be taken in cases where a ruptured globe is suspected, however, as inadvertent pressure on the globe may result in further damage to the eye. In cases of retinoblastoma, intralesional calcification may be demonstrable by ultrasonography.

The use of A-scan ultrasound is helpful to determine axial length. Although this may be of help to an infant who is having an intraocular lens or is being fitted with a contact lens, axial lengths may also be of interest in following a child who has high ametropia, and in which the retinoscopic or refractive error appears to have other factors than axial length (Belkin *et al.* 1973). The power of an intraocular lens may also be determined by B-scans, in the unco-operative child. Orbital ultrasound (Restori & Wright 1977) is helpful in some cases, especially if real-time studies are carried out.

Photography

Photography in infants and children can be of particular value, providing documentation to assess changes or to demonstrate pathology to patients, other physicians or for medicolegal purposes. Photographs of the lens or fundus are especially helpful to the parents when the pathology is not obvious to them as they look at their child. Photography may also be helpful in demonstrating pre- and postoperative differences, such as in children with strabismus or ptosis. Children are often most easily photographed with a portable fundus camera since the special positioning of the patient, necessary with formal fundus photography, is difficult. When a child is to receive sedation or a general anaesthetic, it is wise to co-ordinate this with the ophthalmic photographer so that the photographs can be taken at the time of the EUA (Johns 1983; Reeves 1985).

Radiology

Radiology plays a particularly important role in the examination of a child with ocular trauma, suspected non-accidental injury, orbital tumours, intraretinal masses and disorders of the optic nerve and brain (Lloyd *et al.* 1991). Additionally, such studies may be valuable in the assessment of suspected phakomatoses. Computed tomography (CT) and magnetic resonance imaging (MRI) scans have in large part replaced plain X-rays of the orbits and skull (Lloyd *et al.* 1991). The merits of the CT scan include details of the orbit, oculomotor nerves and muscles, as well as concurrent study of the central nervous system. Calcification of intracranial masses, in particular retinoblastoma, can be well demonstrated with the CT scan. Newer MRI techniques may be less valuable in retinoblastoma cases, since calcification is not so well detected with this technique. Nevertheless, MRI may be helpful in determining preoperatively whether optic nerve extension is present since bone artefact is reduced (Schulman *et al.* 1986).

MRI is very valuable in assessing posterior fossa abnormalities, suspected demyelinating processes and in identifying parachiasmal structures. Plain X-rays of the orbits may still have special indications in identifying histiocytosis, defects in association with dermoids, and in fibrous dysplasia and other bony defects. Blow-out or skull fractures may also be better demonstrated by plain X-rays or tomograms of the orbits and skull.

A child who is sedated for a CT scan can easily be assessed for fundus examination if dilating drops have been used and the ophthalmologist co-ordinates an appropriate time for examination with the radiology staff.

Summary

The examination of the infant and child entails the same components as that of the adult ophthalmological examination. The techniques, however, differ due to the different disease processes, differing degrees of co-operation, and the child's personality. Ancillary testing, although not routine, can usually be performed in children as long as the indications for the tests are weighed against their inherent risks. It is of foremost importance that the examination of a child be systematic and complete. It can in fact be great fun if the physician develops the skills necessary to play with children while completing a detailed examination.

References

Allen D, Bennett P, Banks M. Effects of luminance on FPL and VEP acuity in human infants. *Invest Ophthalmol Vis Sci* 1987; **28**(Suppl.): 5.

Atkinson J. Early visual development: differential functioning of parvocellular and magnocellulr pathways. *Eye* 1992; **6**: 129–35.

Atkinson J, Braddick O, Wattam-Bell J *et al.* Photorefractive screening of effects of refractive correction. *Invest Ophthalmol Vis Sci* 1987; **28**: 399.

Belkin M, Ticho U, Susal A, Levinson A. Ultrasonography in the refraction of aphakic infants. *Br J Ophthalmol* 1973; **57**: 845–8.

Birch E, Stager D. Monocular acuity and stereopsis in infantile esotropia. *Invest Ophthalmol Vis Sci* 1985; **26**: 1624–30.

Bolt B, Benz B, Koerner F, Bossi E. A mydriatic eye-drop combination without systemic effects for premature infants: a prospective double-blind study. *J Pediatr Ophthalmol Strabismus* 1992; **29**: 157–62.

Catalano R, Simon J, Jenkins P, Kandel G. Preferential looking as a guide for amblyopia therapy in monocular infantile cataracts. *J Pediatr Ophthalmol Strabismus* 1987; **24**: 56–63.

Cryotherapy for Retinopathy of Prematurity Cooperative Group (CRPCG). Multi-centre trial of cryotherapy for retinopathy of prematurity. *Arch Ophthalmol* 1988; **106**: 471–9.

Day S, Norcia A. Photographic detection of amblyogenic factors. *Ophthalmology* 1986; **93**: 25–8.

Day S, Orel-Bixter D, Norcia A. Abnormal grating acuity in infants with esotropia. *Invest Ophthalmol Vis Sci* 1988; **29**: 327–92.

Dear G De L, Hammerton M, Hatch DJ, Taylor D. Anaesthesia and intraocular pressure in young children. *Anaesthesia* 1987; **42**: 259–65.

Donzis P, Rapazzo J, Burde R, Gordon M. Effect of binocular variations of Snellen's visual acuity on Titmus stereoacuity. *Arch Ophthalmol* 1983; **101**: 930–2.

Ellis G, Hartmann E, Love A, May J, Morgan K. Teller acuity cards versus clinical judgement in the diagnosis of amblyopia with strabismus. *Ophthalmology* 1988; **95**: 788–91.

Fantz RL, Ordy JM, Udele MS. Maturation of pattern vision in infants during the first 6 months. *J Comp Physiol Psychol* 1962; **55**: 907–17.

Fulton AB, Hanson RM, Manning KA. Measuring visual acuity in infants. *Surv Ophthalmol* 1981; **25**: 325–32.

Gorman JJ, Cogan DG, Gellis SS. An apparatus for grading the visual acuity of infants on the basis of optokinetic nystagmus. *Pediatrics* 1957; **19**: 1088–92.

Gwiazda J, Brill S, Mohindra I, Held R. Preferential looking estimates of visual acuity in infants from 2 to 58 weeks of age. *Am J Optom Physiol Opt* 1980; **57**: 428–32.

Held R, Gwiazda J, Brill S *et al*. Infant visual acuity is underestimated because near threshold gratings are not preferentially fixated. *Vision Res* 1979; **19**: 1377–9.

Howland H, Howland B. Photorefraction: a technique for study of refractive state at a distance. *J Optom Soc Am* 1974; **64**: 240–9.

Jacobson SG, Mohindra I, Held R. Visual acuity of infants with ocular diseases. *Am J Ophthalmol* 1982; **93**: 198–209.

Jampolsky A. The prism test for strabismus screening. *J Pediatr Ophthalmol Strabismus* 1964; **1**: 30–3.

Johns M. Fluorescein angiography in the young child. In: Wybar K, Taylor D, eds. *Pediatric Ophthalmology Current Aspects*. New York: Dekker, 1983: 77–81.

Julesz B. Stereoscopic vision. *Vision Res* 1986; **26**: 1601–12.

Kaakinen K. A simple method for screening of children with strabismus, anisometropia or ametropia by simultaneous photography of the corneal and the fundus reflexes. *Acta Ophthalmol (Copenh)* 1979; **57**: 161–71.

Kriss A, Russell-Eggitt I. Electrophysiological assessment of visual pathway function in infants. *Eye* 1992; **6**: 145–53.

Larsen JS. The sagittal growth of the eye I. Ultrasonic measurement of the depth of the anterior chamber from birth to puberty. *Acta Ophthalmol (Copenh)* 1971a; **49**: 239–62.

Larsen JS. The sagittal growth of the eye II. Ultrasonic measurement of the axial diameter of the lens and the anterior segment from birth to puberty. *Acta Ophthalmol (Copenh)* 1971b; **49**: 427–52.

Linkz A. Visual acuity in the newborn with notes on some objective methods to determine visual acuity. *Documenta Ophthalmol* 1973; **34**: 259–70.

Lloyd IC, Demaerel P, Kendall BE, Taylor D. MRI and CT in pediatric ophthalmology: a guide to their use. *Semin Ophthalmol* 1991; **6**: 169–81.

McDonald M, Dobson V, Sebris S *et al*. The acuity card procedure: a rapid test of infant acuity. *Invest Ophthalmol Vis Sci* 1985; **26**: 1158–62.

McLeod D, Restori M. Real-time B-scanning of the vitreous. *Trans Ophthal Soc UK* 1977; **97**: 547–51.

Magoon EH. The use of oculinum in children. *Ophthalmology* 1988; **95**(Suppl.): 142.

Mayer D, Dobson V. Visual acuity development in infants and young children, as assessed by apparent preferential looking. *Vision Res* 1978; **18**: 1469.

Mayer DL, Fulton AB, Hansen RM. Preferential looking obtained with a staircase procedure in pediatric patients. *Invest Ophthalmol Vis Sci* 1982; **23**: 538–43.

Meiusi R, Lavoie J, Summers CG. The effect of grating orientation on resolution acuity in patients with nystagmus. *J Pediatr Ophthalmol Strabismus* 1993; **30**: 259–326.

Millodot M, Riggs LA. Refraction determined electrophysiologically:

responses to alternation of visual contours. *Arch Ophthalmol* 1970; **84**: 272–8.

Mohindra I, Zwaan J, Held R *et al*. Development of acuity and stereopsis in infants with esotropia. *Ophthalmology* 1985; **92**: 691–7.

Moskowitz A, Sokol S, Hansen V. Rapid assessment of visual function in pediatric patients using pattern VEPs and acuity cards. *Clin Vis Sci* 1987; **2**: 11–20.

Mutlukan E, Damato B. Computerised perimetry with moving and steady fixation in children. *Eye* 1993: **7**: 554–61.

Norcia A, Tyler C. Spatial frequency sweep VEP: visual acuity during the first year of life. *Vision Res* 1985; **25**: 1399–408.

Norcia A, Tyler C, Hamer R. Development of contrast sensitivity in human infants. *Invest Ophthalmol Vis Sci* 1987; **28**(Suppl.): 5.

Odom JV, Hoyt CS, Marg E. Effect of natural deprivation and unilateral eye patching, on visual acuity of infants and children; evoked potential measurements. *Arch Ophthalmol* 1991; **99**: 1412–16.

Reeves C. *Paediatric ophthalmic photography*. FBIPP thesis. Institute of Child Health, London, 1985.

Regan D, Spekreijse H. Evoked potentials in vision research 1961–86. *Vision Res* 1986; **26**: 1461–80.

Regan D, Whitlock J, Murray T, Beverly K. Orientation-specific losses of contrast sensitivity in multiple sclerosis. *Invest Ophthalmol Vis Sci* 1980; **19**: 324–8.

Restori M, McLeod D. Ultrasound in pre-vitrectomy assessment. *Trans Ophthalmol Soc UK* 1977; **97**: 232–4.

Restori M, Wright J. C-scan ultrasonography in orbital diagnosis. *Br J Ophthalmol* 1977; **61**: 735–40.

Schulman J, Peyman G, Mafee M *et al*. The use of magnetic resonance imaging in the evaluation of retinoblastoma. *J Pediatr Ophthalmol Strabismus* 1986; **23**: 144–7.

Sira I, Nissenkorn I, Kremer I. Retinopathy of prematurity. *Surv Ophthalmol* 1988; **33**: 1–16.

Sokol S. Pattern visual evoked potentials: their use in pediatric ophthalmology. *Int Ophthalmol Clin* 1980; **20**: 251–68.

Sokol S. Visually evoked potentials: theory, technique and clinical applications. *Surv Ophthalmol* 1976; **21**: 18–44.

Sokol S, Dobson V. Pattern reversal visually evoked potentials in infants. *Invest Ophthalmol Vis Sci* 1976; **15**: 58–62.

Sokol S, Hansen V, Moskowitz A, Greenfield P, Towle V. Evoked potentials and preferential looking estimates of visual acuity in pediatric patients. *Ophthalmology* 1983; **90**: 552–62.

Sonksen P. The assessment of vision in the preschool child. *Arch Dis Child* 1993; **68**: 513–16.

Stamper R, Hsu-Winges C, Sopher M. Arden contrast sensitivity in glaucoma. *Arch Ophthalmol* 1982; **100**: 947–52.

Teller D, McDonald M, Preston K *et al*. Assessment of visual acuity in infants and children: the acuity card procedure. *Dev Med Child Neurol* 1986; **28**: 779–89.

Teller DY, Morse R, Borton R, Regal D. Visual acuity for vertical and diagonal gratings in human infants. *Vision Res* 1974; **14**: 1433–9.

Teller D, Movshon A. Visual development. *Vision Res* 1986; **26**: 1483–521.

von Noorden GK. *Burian–von Noorden's Binocular Vision and Ocular Motility: Theory and Management of Strabismus*, 3rd edn. St Louis: CV Mosby, 1985: 205.

Weleber RG, Palmer EA. Electrophysiological evaluation of children with visual impairment. *Semin Ophthalmol* 1991; **6**: 161–8.

Zimmern R, Campbell F, Wilkinson I. Subtle disturbances of vision after optic neuritis elicited by studying contrast sensitivity. *J Neurol Neurosurg Psychiatry* 1979; **42**: 407–12.

9: Visual Electrophysiology

Tony Kriss and Dorothy Thompson

Visual electrodiagnostic studies offer objective methods of assessing sensory visual pathway function which will complement, and often supplement, clinical examination. They are not hazardous; can be used for serial monitoring; are relatively swift to perform; give immediate access to results; and are not dependent on eye movement or a verbal response from the subject (e.g. as is preferential looking or visual field testing). Electrodiagnostic tests are particularly useful in appraising visual pathway function in preverbal children, and do not normally require sedation or anaesthesia (Fulton *et al.* 1989; Harden *et al.* 1989; Apkarian & Spekreijse 1990; Sokol 1990b; Kriss & Russell-Eggitt 1992; Taylor & McCulloch 1992).

A set of tests is available which will provide information about processing at different pathway levels: retinal function is gauged by the electroretinogram (ERG) and the electro-oculogram (EOG), and postretinal pathway integrity can be assessed by the visual evoked potential (VEP).

The results of ERG, EOG and VEP testing, used in combination, can indicate the following:

1 The location and possible nature of the dysfunction along the visual pathway (indicating a disturbance of optic nerve, chiasmal or postchiasmal/cortical function).

2 The involvement of particular retinal cell types (rod and cone receptors, bipolar/Muller cells, pigment epithelium).

3 The involvement of a particular subpopulation of visual fibres or processing by a visual subsystem (e.g. macular/paramacular, magnocellular/parvocellular, binocular, motion or colour submodalities).

4 A non-organic aetiology, in a context where this is a possibility and normal responses are obtained (see Chapter 56).

The concurrent recording of ERG and VEP can complement other forms of testing which provide information about biochemical activity or anatomical structure. For example, an abnormal ERG may signal the necessity for metabolic screening, and an abnormal VEP can indicate the need for imaging studies. Computed tomography (CT) and magnetic resonance imaging (MRI) scans are more costly and more hazardous in young children, but they show the position and size of structural lesions with precision. However, although magnetic imaging techniques offer exquisite visualization of anatomy, they do not give such detailed information for appraising visual pathway function, compared with electrophysiology. At

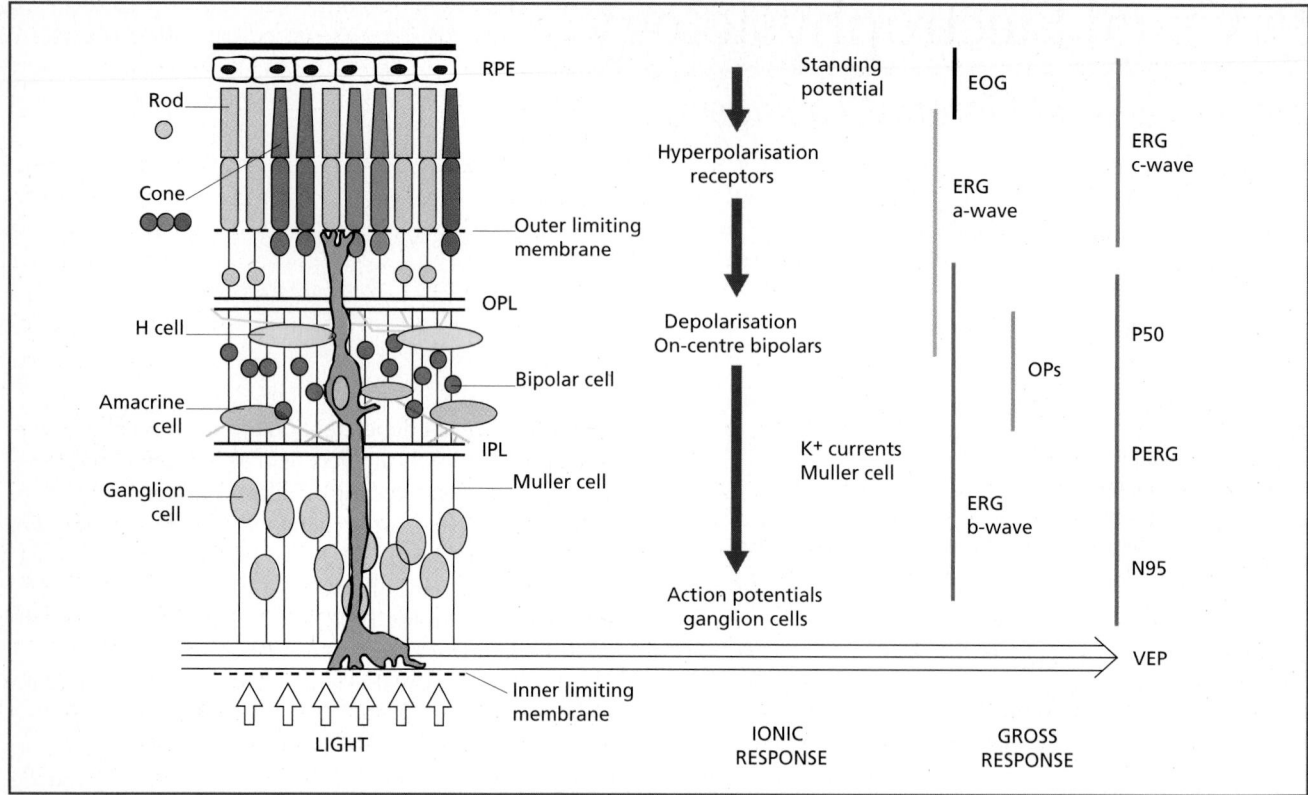

Fig. 9.1 Schematic diagram of retinal anatomy showing main cell types and their relationship to the generation of the ERG, EOG and VEP.

present, sedation and anaesthesia are overwhelming confounding factors for functional MRI testing.

Visual electrophysiological testing in children demands attention to technique. Stimulating and recording conditions have to be closely controlled to avoid the numerous physiological, physical and technical factors which alter responses and lead to possible misinterpretation (Kriss 1993a, 1994).

Although some have questioned the usefulness of evoked potentials, dwelling on their misuse and overuse (Griner & Glaser 1982; Hoyt 1984; Chiappa & Young 1985), others have clearly demonstrated their wide-ranging usefulness, and have emphasized the caveat that evoked potentials have the status of a useful clinical sign (Chiappa 1990; Halliday 1993).

Physiology

Electroretinography

The flash ERG represents bioelectric activity arising in the outer and middle retinal layers. It is the algebraic summation of retinal potentials which have different polarity, amplitude and latency. The bright flash ERG from a dark-adapted eye has three major components, the a-, b- and c-waves, plus oscillatory potentials which are a series of wavelets between the a- and b-waves (see Fig. 9.3).

The a-wave is the first major negative component, and reflects the hyperpolarization of retinal photoreceptors by incident light (Falk 1991). On-centre bipolar cells are depolarized by photoreceptor activation—the potassium ions released in the depolarization are transported through Muller cells — and the spread of ionic current associated with this process produces the corneal positive b-wave (Newman & Frishman 1991). The current flow associated with the initial movement of potassium ions into the receptors leads to ionic flow into the distal parts of Muller cells, with depletion of the amount of potassium present between the receptors and the retinal pigment epithelium (RPE). The ionic imbalance across the apical membrane of the RPE results in a positivity which interacts with a smaller negativity produced by distal parts of Muller cells, and the net result is the positive c-wave, identifiable (but not invariably so) after the b-wave (Griff 1991).

Oscillatory potentials represent radial currents in the retina, which are probably generated by bipolar and/or interplexiform cells (Wachtmeister & Dowling 1978; Heynen *et al.* 1985; Karowski & Kawasaki 1991) (Fig. 9.1). Assessment of a- and b-waves has a more general clinical application in ophthalmology. Measuring oscillatory potentials can be useful, but mainly in relation to retinal vascular disturbance associated with diabetes (Bresnick 1991), and to inner retinal dysfunction occuring in certain forms of night-blindness (Speros & Price 1981; Miyake 1991).

Electro-oculography

The RPE has several functions.

1 The phagocytosis of outer segment discs shed by rods and cones.

2 Absorption of light scattered within the eye.

3 The synthesis of the interreceptor matrix and transport of retinal binding proteins.

The difference in ionic activity at the apices of RPE cells, abutting the photoreceptors and their basal ends, results in a standing potential across the RPE. This potential measures about 6 mV at the corneal apex (Berson 1992). A physiological differential amplifier connected to recording electrodes at the outer canthi will pick up a relatively large potential change when the eyes move horizontally— this is the EOG. Ionic activity in the RPE greatly increases under photopic conditions, and decreases under scotopic conditions. The fluctuations in ionic concentrations associated with the state of adaptation of the eye are reflected as changes in the size of the EOG (Kolder 1991; Marmor & Zrenner 1993). Non-photic increases in the EOG potential can also occur in response to induced hyperosmolarity with mannitol, and by acetazolamide, and possibly sodium bicarbonate (Marmor 1991), although the clinical value of these chemically produced procedures is yet to be firmly established.

Visual evoked potentials

The VEP is recorded over the occipital scalp. It is elicited using bright flashes or patterned stimuli. The latter are most usually black and white checks or stripes, which are made to either alternate (pattern reversal) or to appear and disappear from a uniform field of equivalent overall luminance (pattern onset/offset). Flash stimulation is used mainly where visual acuity is poor, and it is not possible to elicit pattern VEPs. However, the flash VEP can have a complex waveform with considerable interindividual variability compared with all types of pattern VEP (e.g. see Fig. 9.4), and consequently its application for routine clinical assessment is more limited. The VEP to pattern reversal has a simple triphasic waveform with a predominant major positive component (called P100). P100 appears to be a reflection of cortical activation initiated by the arrival of an afferent volley from the retinogeniculate pathway. The volley initially causes depolarization in lamina 4c of the striate cortex V1 (Schroeder *et al.* 1991; Givre *et al.* 1994). Recordings in monkeys demonstrate that pattern reversal stimulation activates the same structures as diffuse flash stimulation, but is additionally accompanied by more prominent activity at supra- and infra-granular layers of striate cortex. Other specialized visual areas are also activated, in particular V4 in the macaque. V4 is found to contribute to the later components of the flash VEP (Givre *et al.* 1994).

Experimental studies in the monkey and cat indicate that the parvocellular (P) and magnocellular (M) projections are two important parallel processing streams involved in transferring visual information within the retinogeniculocortico pathway. In the monkey, and probably also in humans, as many as 30 visually specialized cortical areas have been identified (Fellman & Van Essen 1991). Areas V1–V5, in particular, have been well studied (Zeki 1993). It is clear that P- and M-cell projections retain a considerable, though not complete, degree of segregation in their projections to these areas. Stimuli can be designed to activate a particular processing stream optimally (Tolhurst 1973; Livingstone & Hubel 1988; Merigan 1991) and, combined with topographic mapping, have been used to elicit VEPs from certain visual subsystems (e.g. Drasdo *et al.* 1993). The P-system may be preferentially stimulated using isoluminant chromatic patterns, or high contrast, high spatial frequency patterns presented at a low temporal rate (e.g. Thompson & Drasdo 1992). Conversely, low contrast, low spatial frequency stimuli presented at high temporal rates, will preferentially tap the M-system; and stimuli moving with velocities less than 4 degrees/second appear to elicit VEPs optimally from cortical areas concerned with motion processing (e.g. Markwardt *et al.* 1988). However, in practice there is a substantial degree of functional overlap between the M- and P- systems and it remains to be proved that incorporating these more sophisticated stimuli into a clincial protocol will improve the sensitivity and specificity of visual electrodiagnostic testing (Norcia *et al.* 1991; Kubova & Kuba 1992).

Random-dot correlograms and stereograms have been successfully applied to study the development of binocular function (Braddick *et al.* 1980; Skarf *et al.* 1993).

Paradoxical lateralization of pattern reversal visual evoked potentials

Paradoxical lateralization is important when interpreting VEPs to activation of one occipital hemisphere only, as occurs in half-field stimulation in controls or when testing patients with hemianopia. The P100 of the pattern reversal VEP is predominantly lateralized over the occipital scalp ipsilateral to the field stimulating the activated hemisphere (Fig. 9.2) (Barrett *et al.* 1976). The ipsilateral N80–P100–N145 complex represents macular pathway activity predominantly, whereas the P75–N105–P150 complex recorded over the contralateral scalp reflects mainly activation of paramacular areas of the visual field (Halliday *et al.* 1979). Patients with well-circumscribed

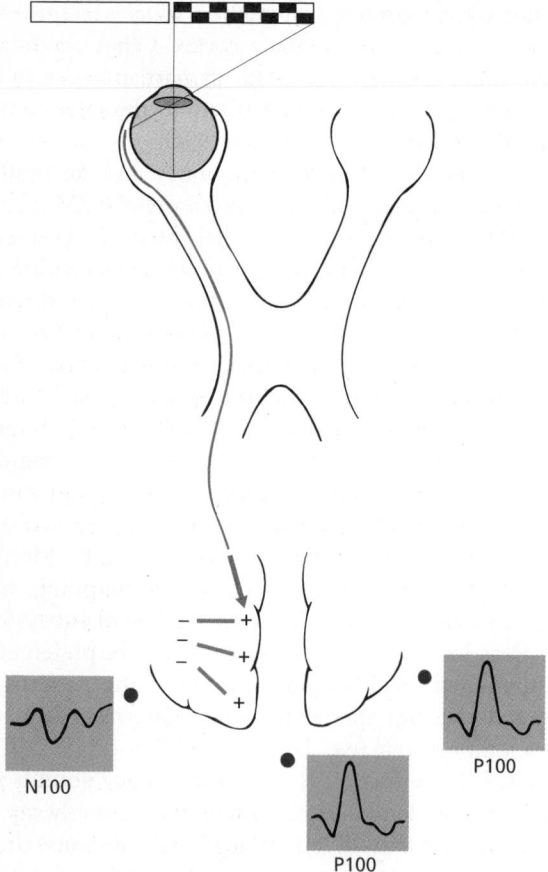

Fig. 9.2 Paradoxical lateralization of pattern VEPs to half-field stimulation. The afferent volley activates cortical generators which have dipole-like properties. Electrodes at the midline and over the hemisphere ipsilateral to the stimulated half-field are well placed to pick up P100 activity produced by the visual cortex of the activated hemisphere.

central scotomas will produce full-field pattern reversal VEPs from paramacular areas, which are characterized by negative peaks best seen on either side of the occipital midline (see Halliday *et al.* 1979 and Kriss *et al.* 1982 for examples).

Methodology

Several international professional bodies have published recommendations for recording the ERG (Marmor *et al.* 1989; Marmor & Zrenner 1995), VEP (American EEG Society 1994), and EOG (Marmor & Zrenner 1993). These guidelines are mostly applicable to co-operative subjects, though some recognize that strict adherence to the advocated standards will be difficult when dealing with young children, and suggestions are made relating to these circumstances.

The International Society for Clinical Electrophysiology of Vision (ISCEV) standards strongly endorse the use of a contact lens electrode with speculum to record the ERG,

for both adults and children. Contact lens electrodes indisputably give the largest retinal responses, and in our view, use of the ISCEV technique in young children is advantageous when detecting small magnitude ERG changes near the laboratory limits of normality. They are also useful for accurately monitoring disease progression or small changes due to therapeutic intervention. However, our electrophysiological recording experience in paediatrics has led us to conclude that the ISCEV approach is unnecessarily demanding for screening purposes as, with proper control of recording variables and signal averaging, skin ERGs can provide good quality data from which reliable diagnosis can be made (Kriss & Russell-Eggitt 1992; Kriss *et al.* 1992a). Other workers have similarly reported that skin ERGs can be successfully used for clinical purposes (Papakostopoulos 1982; France 1984; Coupland & Janaky 1989; Harden *et al.* 1989; Brecelj & Stirn-Kranjc 1992; Ikeda 1993). Two important disadvantages of contact lens ERG recording are the requirement for young children to be sedated, anaesthetized or physically restrained for a protracted period, and the risk of corneal abrasion (Vey *et al.* 1979).

Skin ERG recording is easier to perform, and it can be simultaneously combined with VEP recording, without anaesthesia or sedation (as this degrades the VEP). Combined ERG/VEP recording is more informative in identifying the level of visual pathway dysfunction, especially with infants in whom the cause for poor vision has not been established. We have performed around 8000 recordings in children with a wide variety of eye and brain conditions, and find the combined skin ERG/VEP technique is very effective in helping to establish a diagnosis. It can distinguish reliably between rod and cone dysfunction, when appropriate stimulus techniques are used; and, with pattern stimulation, can be used to estimate the quality of vision (Lambert *et al.* 1989a; Kriss & Russell-Eggitt 1992; Kriss *et al.* 1992a). In children with nystagmus, EOG eye movement assessment at the same hospital visit complements electrophysiological findings, and is useful in characterising the nature of the nystagmus (see Chapters 63 and 64).

Electroretinography recording

Corneal electroretinography

ISCEV recommends that electroretinography should include the following methodological points: (i) the use of a contact lens electrode with speculum; (ii) pupil dilation; (iii) full-field (ganzfeld) stimulation; and (iv) at least 20 minutes of dark adaptation (Marmor & Zrenner 1995). Recording of five standard responses is advocated (Fig. 9.3) for the following.

1 A maximal mixed cone–rod response elicited from a dark-adapted eye by a bright white flash (the 'standard'

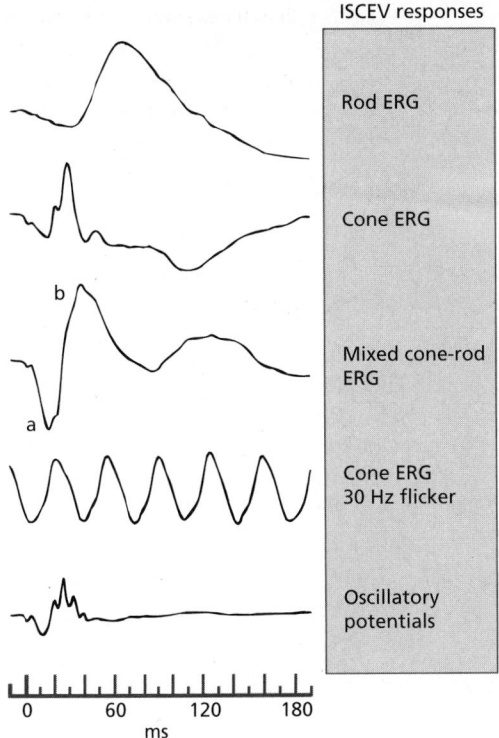

ISCEV responses

Rod ERG

Cone ERG

Mixed cone-rod ERG

Cone ERG 30 Hz flicker

Oscillatory potentials

b

a

0   60   120   180
ms

Fig. 9.3 The five standard ERGs recorded with a contact lens electrode. The ISCEV guidelines recommend recording ERGs to a dim white light (rod-mediated) and a bright white light (mixed cone- and rod-mediated) following dark adaptation for at least 20 minutes. Cone-mediated ERGs are recorded under photopic conditions, both to single flash and to 30 Hz flicker. Amplifier filter settings of the order of 100–300 Hz are used to record oscillatory potentials, which arise mainly from inner retinal layers. Note the figure is illustrative and the display gain for the various responses is different. The negative a-wave from the photoreceptors and positive b-wave from inner retinal layers are shown for a mixed rod cone ERG.

flash strength measures 1.5–3.0 cd/m² at the surface of a ganzfeld bowl in a maximum time of 5 milliseconds).

2 A rod response elicited from a dark-adapted eye by a dim white flash (2.5 log units less than the standard flash).

3 Oscillatory potentials obtained from a dark-adapted eye to a standard flash.

4 A cone-mediated response elicited from the light-adapted eye by a single standard flash.

5 Cone-mediated 30/second light flicker.

The latest guidelines indicate that most children can be studied without sedation, though they may be restrained if necessary (Marmor & Zrenner 1995). They also state that where restraint is difficult, a sedative such as chloral hydrate may be used. The ERG is changed little by light anaesthesia (Wongpichedchai *et al.* 1992), though it is stressed that full anaesthesia may modify ERGs. Use of a contact lens electrode designed for children together with a speculum is advised, with the caveat that care should be used to minimize corneal and psychological trauma, though it is not made clear how this can be achieved.

Advice is given that the infant ERG needs to be interpreted with caution due to maturational variability. Repeat recordings in a given session are advised to ensure reproducibility, and it is advocated that the largest, most normal looking, response should be chosen for measurement. Test findings should indicate the degree of co-operation and medications used (Marmor & Zrenner 1995).

A large variety of electrodes are available for recording corneal ERGs. Many are non-contact lens types which rest on or hook over the lower eyelid, and thus are better for recording pattern ERGs since they do not interfere with the optics of the visual axis. However, it is important to have normative data for each electrode used, as there are significant differences in the size of ERG when comparing electrode types. In our experience, the Burian–Allen unipolar contact lens electrode consistently gives the largest flash ERG compared with non-contact lens electrodes; the size of the scotopic b-wave recorded for the same condition from some other electrodes relative to that recorded from the Burian–Allen (471 µV) is as follows:

- Jet 89%,
- C-glide 77%,
- gold foil 56%,
- DTL thread 46%, and
- lower lid skin electrode 12% (Esakowitz *et al.* 1993).

Several authors have described their techniques for recording corneal ERGs in young children. Some prefer not to sedate and will restrain as necessary (Marmor 1976; Fulton *et al.* 1989; Fishman & Sokol 1990), others will sedate routinely, commonly with chloral hydrate (Weleber & Palmer 1991).

The neonatal ERG is markedly attenuated, being from about 20 to 50% the size of that found in adults. It can be detected in premature infants from about 34 weeks gestational age. ERG responses mature rapidly over the first 3 months following birth, and more slowly thereafter, so that by 12 months of age the amplitude of the infant ERG is approximately within 10% of that of the adult (Horsten & Winkleman 1962; Fulton & Hansen 1985; Macetier *et al.* 1988; Grose *et al.* 1989).

Skin electroretinography

Disorders affecting rod and/or cone function can be detected reliably with skin ERGs in young children when signal averaging and suitable stimulus conditions are employed (Lambert *et al.* 1989a, b; Kriss & Russell-Eggitt 1992; Kriss *et al.* 1992a). The skin ERG electrode is best placed centrally, 1 cm below the margin of the lower eyelid; a midfrontal common reference location (Fz) is adequate for both ERG and VEP recordings. There are moderate changes in ERG amplitude when the eye is in maintained left or right lateral gaze, or downward gaze. In cases of constant heterotropia, it is advisable to displace the active electrode so that it sits directly under the centre

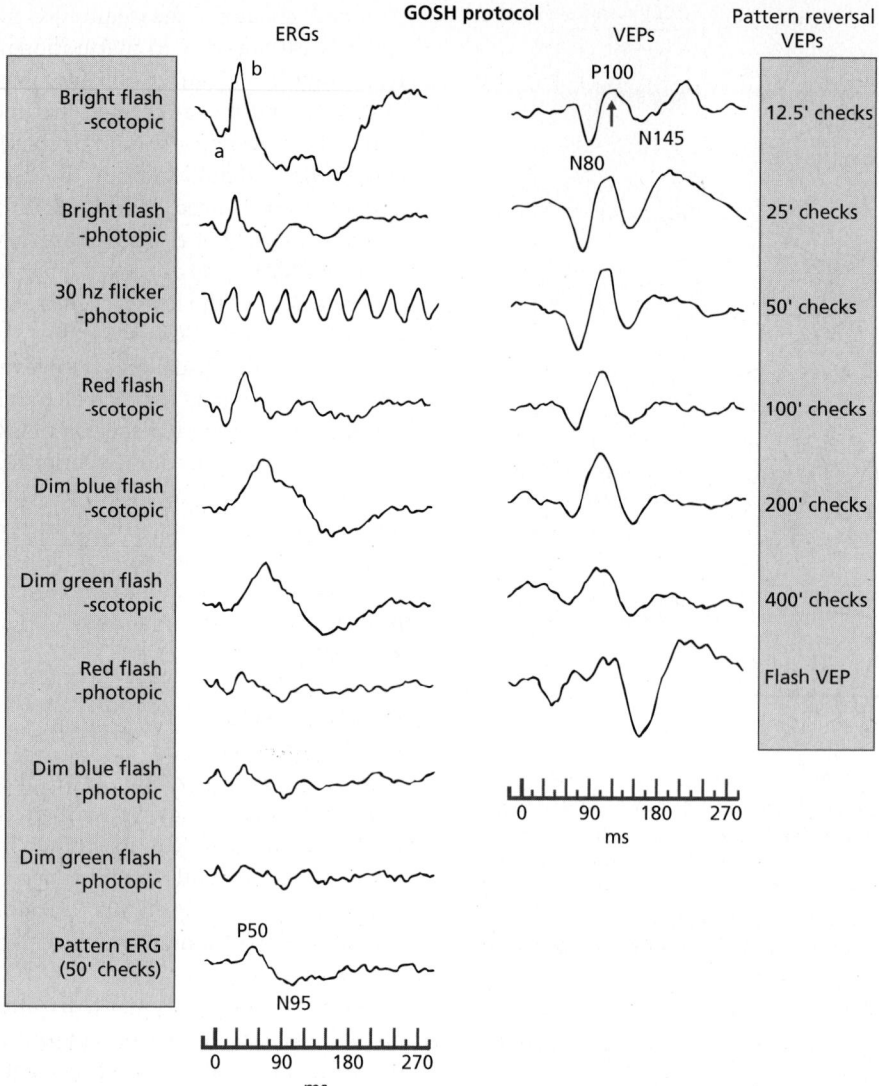

Fig. 9.4 Great Ormond Street Hospital (GOSH) protocol for combined skin ERG and VEP averaged recording. ERGs to bright white flash (mixed cone–rod), dim blue and green flash (both rod-mediated), and red flash (predominantly cone-mediated), are recorded under scotopic conditions. Photopic ERGs to white flash and 30 Hz flicker are also recorded (cone-mediated). Cone-mediated responses are recorded to red, dim blue and green flashes delivered under photopic conditions; these are smaller and earlier as the longer latency and larger amplitude activity associated with rods is not generated. The pattern reversal ERG has a similar waveform as it stimulates the predominantly cone-rich macular region. The pattern reversal VEP is characterized by its main positive component (P100), and the preceding negativity (N80). N80 and P100 are best defined for stimulation with checks between 25′ and 50′. The flash VEP usually has a more complex waveform compared with the pattern VEP. Note that the figure is illustrative; the display gain of cone-mediated responses is increased with respect to the other responses.

of the pupil. The ERG can be markedly attenuated, or even inverted, when the eye is held consistently in upward gaze during averaging. This can occur during sleep or in some patients who have an exaggerated Bell's phenomenon. In this instance repositioning of the active electrode to the upper eyelid or brow is recommended (Kriss 1994).

It is essential to have scotopic conditions to elicit rod-mediated activity. A moderately bright flash (Grass PS22 photic stimulator: intensity 4, 3.7×10^5 cd) delivered under scotopic conditions will elicit a mixed cone–rod ERG which, on average, has an a–b amplitude of 25 μV in subjects over 6 months of age without retinal disease. In infants of 1 month of age the b-wave is broad and less than half the amplitude of that of the adult (mean a–b amplitude = 10.5 μV) (Kriss *et al.* 1992a). The latency of the b-wave indicates the relative contribution of rods and cones to the averaged signal. Under scotopic conditions, the mixed cone–rod response has a b-wave latency of 39 milliseconds (we usually record the flash ERG after recording pattern VEPs for 10–15 minutes in the dark) (Fig. 9.4). A red flash (peak transmission from 670 nm) will elicit a predominantly cone-mediated ERG with a mean b-wave latency of 40.4 ms (2.5 SD upper limit of normal = 46.9 milliseconds), and dim blue (peak transmission 450 nm) will elicit a predominantly rod-mediated response (Grass intensity 1, 1.6×10^4 cd) with a–b-wave mean latency of 61.7 milliseconds (2.5 SD upper limit of normal = 84.0 milliseconds). Both ERGs to red flash and dim blue flash have mean amplitudes of approximately 13 μV (Kriss *et al.* 1992a).

The pupil size is not usually a significant confounding factor if physiological dilation is normal and testing is carried out under fully darkened conditions. We find that using a hand-held Grass lamp in front of the eyes and presenting a bright flash (intensity setting 4) under fully darkened laboratory conditions, that the a–b-wave amplitude for the mixed cone–rod ERG is similar (i.e. <15% difference) when responses recorded under pharmacologically dilated conditions are compared with responses under normal pupil conditions. If the pupils are constricted to less than 3 mm, from any cause, then this may lead to significant attenuation of the ERG (Kriss 1994).

Visual evoked potential recording

VEP testing has an established place in assessing postretinal visual function (Halliday 1993). Flash stimulation is most commonly used in children as it is relatively easy to perform, with either a hand-held lamp, or LED goggles (Taylor & McCulloch 1992). However, it is being increasingly recognized that pattern testing can be successfully accomplished in children, with the advantage that pattern VEPs will not only give more accurate information regarding the level at which dysfunction is occurring, but also provide information about the level of acuity (Sokol 1978; Apkarian *et al.* 1986; Kriss & Russell-Eggitt 1992). Monocular stimulation and a transoccipital VEP recording are essential procedures for helping to localize postretinal visual pathway dysfunction (Halliday 1993). Field defects are most accurately detected when each half-field is independently tested with pattern reversal stimulation (Blumhardt *et al.* 1982). However, half-field testing is not usually possible in infants, though a reliable indication of postchiasmal dysfunction can be obtained when there is a marked occipital VEP asymmetry with activity of opposite polarity on either side of the scalp (Lambert *et al.* 1990; Jacobs *et al.* 1993; Patel *et al.* 1993).

When recording VEPs, it is best to adopt a common reference montage with at least three occipital electrodes. We place active electrodes midoccipitally (0z, 10–20 system of electrode placement (Jasper 1958); about 3 cm above the inion) and half way between 0z and the mastoid process behind the ear (4–5 cm laterally, depending on head size).

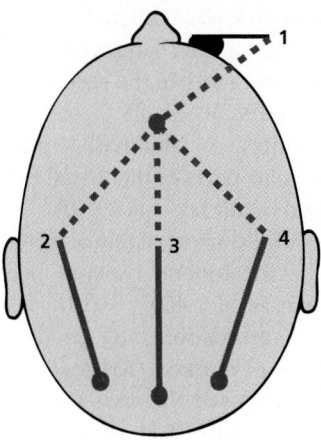

Fig. 9.5 Montage for skin ERG/VEP recording. Occipital VEP electrodes are placed at 0z (about 3 cm above the inion), and halfway between 0z and the mastoid (4–5 cm laterally, depending on head size). The ERG electrode is placed centrally, 1 cm below the rim of the lower eyelid. All active electrodes are referred to a common midfrontal reference at Fz.

All three occipital electrodes are referred to a common midfrontal reference (Fz, 10–20 system) of electrode placement (Fig. 9.5). A monopolar derivation in which 'active' occipital electrodes are referred to a common 'indifferent' reference well away from the occipital area is preferable to a bipolar derivation, in which occipital electrodes have separate references nearby, usually on the same side of the scalp (e.g. an occipital to parietal derivation) (see Kriss 1993 for fuller discussion).

During pattern stimulation, the patients' visual performance has to be carefully monitored as constant fixation near the left or right edges of the screen, droopy eyelids and poor concentration may give VEP changes which can be easily misinterpreted as clinically significant. We use closed-circuit television (with zoom, and pan and tilt facilities) to focus in on the eyes. Averaging is manually halted when fixation is inadequate. A child's attention is directed towards the stimulus pattern by alternating the checkerboard with cartoons, or playing the sound track of a nursery rhyme video while averaging responses. Alternatively, noisy toys such as rattles are erratically moved along the upper part of the screen. The retinotopic map projects the lower part of the visual field on the occipital cortex underlying electrodes placed near 0z (the upper field is mainly represented on the undersurface of the occipital lobe). Thus, VEPs recorded at the scalp have a predominant contribution from the lower half-field, so it is best to stimulate this half-field preferentially by attracting the child's attention to the top part of the screen.

We prefer pattern reversal to pattern onset stimulation for routine clinical testing for the following reasons.
1 The reversal VEP waveform or component structure

does not change markedly with maturation: pattern onset VEPs show morphological changes during childhood and attain the adult form early in the second decade (DeVries Khoe & Spekreijse 1982)

2 VEP components associated with stimulation of macular and paramacular parts of the visual field can be more readily identified (Halliday *et al.* 1979).

3 The reversal VEP shows reliable occipital lateralization in association with lesions causing hemianopic field defects (Blumhardt *et al.* 1982).

Pattern onset stimulation may produce larger VEPs when nystagmus is marked (Kriss *et al.* 1989). Several stimulus modes are used to assess for albinism, because infant flash VEPs (and ERGs) give the clearest changes (Russell-Eggitt *et al.* 1990; Apkarian 1994), whereas pattern onset stimulation tends to be the better stimulus mode for demonstrating the albino crossed asymmetry in older children and adults (Apkarian *et al.* 1984).

Flash and pattern VEPs can be used to give a useful qualitative assessment of vision. We test using 12.5', 25', 50', 100', 200' and 400' check sizes and provide routinely a qualitative, but clinically very useful, feedback about the level of infant vision based on our empirical experience. Thus, when pattern VEPs to 12.5' and 25' checks are detectable visual acuity is deemed to be 'good'; when not evident to smaller checks but detectable to 50' checks and larger it is reported as 'moderate'; when elicited to the largest 200' and 400' checks only, it is reported as 'poor'; and 'rudimentary' if detectable to flash stimulation only.

The flash VEP of preterm infants between 24 and 27 weeks gestational age has a simplified waveform characterized by negativity peaking around 250–300 milliseconds. The positivity characteristic of the adult VEP emerges at about 32–35 weeks of age and has a latency of 190–230 milliseconds. The latency of the main positivity progressively decreases to within 10 milliseconds of adult values by about 4 months after a full-term birth. It is claimed that the VEP matures at a faster rate in preterm infants compared with full-term subjects (Barnet *et al.* 1980; Mushin *et al.* 1984; Kurzberg & Vaughan 1985; Taylor *et al.* 1987).

Grose *et al.* (1989) were able to elicit pattern reversal VEPs reliably in premature infants using 2 degree checks displayed on a small TV. It is generally agreed that latencies of pattern reversal VEPs to small checks (<20') reach mature (adult) levels at a slower rate than those to larger checks (Moscowitz & Sokol 1983; Harding *et al.* 1989).

Combined electroretinography and visual evoked potential recording

In our laboratory (Fig. 9.6) ERGs and VEPs are recorded simultaneously and the amplifier and averager settings are selected to optimize recordings from infants (i.e. to reduce the effects of myogenic and electrode movement

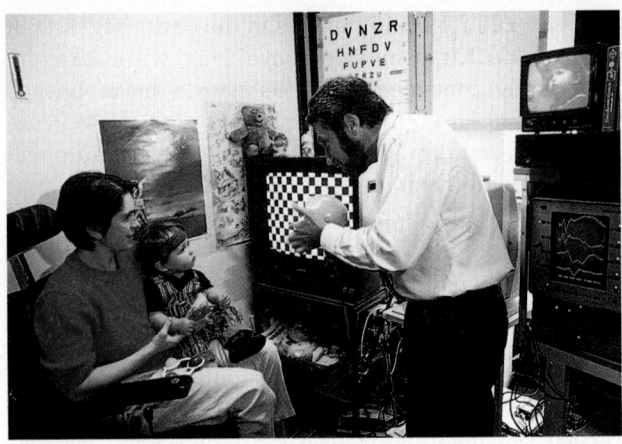

Fig. 9.6 Laboratory set-up. A young child sits on a carer's lap at 1 m from the large TV display. Fixation is monitored using closed-circuit television and, when inadequate, averaging is halted. The laboratory is fully blacked out. A hand-held lamp is used to present white and colour flashes at 3/second under scotopic conditions, and white flashes at 3 and 30/second under photopic conditions. Averaged responses are stored and processed using a computer.

artefacts). The amplifier band pass is set at 3–125 Hz and the stimulus is presented three times a second, with signal sampling carried out over 300 milliseconds (15 milliseconds pre-stimulus and 285 milliseconds post-stimulus) in infants over 6 weeks of age. During the first 6 weeks of life the latency of the pattern reversal VEP P100 component is usually in the range of 150–250 milliseconds (Kriss & Russell-Eggitt 1992), and better defined responses are obtained by reducing the frequency of stimulation to 1 per second and increasing the averaging period to 500 milliseconds. Between 64 and 128 repetitions are averaged for each test condition.

Parents cuddle their child while the electrodes are attached, and during the recording. They also help by encouraging the child to fix on the test stimuli. Pattern testing is routinely performed first in a fully darkened room, and typically this takes about 10–15 minutes. Flash testing is then performed, first under fully darkened conditions, and then photopically. On average, the whole recording session lasts 35 minutes.

Electro-oculography

The EOG is recorded routinely by positioning skin electrodes adjacent to the inner and outer canthi of the eye. A potential difference (the EOG) is recorded between the two electrodes when the eye makes a saccade. The amplitude of the EOG depends upon the size of the saccade, and also on the state of light adaptation of the eye To control the size of the saccade in routine testing, patients are instructed to fix alternately illuminated lights positioned a known distance apart (usually 20–30 degrees), and placed either in a ganzfeld or in a large flat back-illuminated screen. Under fully darkened conditions, the EOG size progressively diminishes to a minimum after about 8 minutes — the 'dark trough'. Testing continues usually for a total of 12–15 minutes in the dark. The eye is then exposed to bright photopic conditions and the EOG increases in amplitude, to reach a maximum after 8–10 minutes — the 'light rise'. The ratio of the light maximum to the dark minimum EOG amplitude (light rise/dark trough), is called the Arden index (Arden & Kelsey 1962). Values greater than about 1.8, depending on test conditions and subject variables, are considered to be normal (see Fig. 9.8 which shows normal and abnormal EOGs).

Considerable attention is required to make saccades accurately at 1–2 minute intervals for the total of 30 minutes necessary for routine EOG testing. The EOG procedure is unlikely to be successfully completed by children aged 6 years or less. Other techniques have been proposed for the younger child, for example, utilizing the vestibulo-ocular reflex. The child holds his fixation on a target while sitting on a chair which rotates the child's body by a fixed amount. Alternatively, a rocking chair is used to produce a sinusoidal turn of 22 degrees, which in turn gives 30–50 degrees of vestibulo-ocular reflex (Fulton *et al.* 1989).

The EOG is a mass response reflecting interaction of photoreceptor membranes and the pigment epithelium. It has an essential role in helping to diagnose Best's disease, which is electrodiagnostically characterized by a markedly reduced Arden ratio (near 1.0) in association with normal ERG (both to flash and pattern stimulation). An abnormal EOG is also seen in retinitis pigmentosa, advanced Stargardt's disease and myopic chorioretinal degeneration, though in distinction to Best's disease, in these conditions there are also ERG abnormalities. In achromatopsia, it has been reported that the EOG scotopic phase is reduced and the latency of the light peak is delayed (Thaler *et al.* 1986). The circadian rhythm can influence the EOG, and this should be taken into account in longitudinal studies of disease progression (Anderson & Purple 1980).

Clinical applications

The following sections give a wide-ranging overview and thus topics are covered somewhat tersely (for greater detail see Davson 1990; Fishman & Sokol 1990; Heckenlively & Arden 1991; Hart 1992; Halliday 1993).

Pre-retinal disorders

When pre-retinal eye conditions prevent adequate visualization of the fundus; combined flash ERG and VEP recording can provide valuable information about retinal and postretinal function. A very bright flash is likely to penetrate all but the most dense corneal and lenticular opacities, and will stimulate the retina effectively. Thus, retinal function can be assessed in corneal opacities, cataract, anterior segment dysgenesis and in cryptophthalmos. ERGs are occasionally larger than normal due to light scatter by a cataract (Galloway 1988), but are mostly attenuated when the opacification is dense. In cryptophthalmos, the use of a bright flash can be used to indicate the functional status of the retina and the postretinal pathway (Hing *et al.* 1990).

Congenital cataracts are often associated with microphthalmia or other ocular abnormalities: the presence of a normal flash ERG and a well-preserved flash VEP, together with ocular ultrasound assessment, can indicate the visual outcome after surgery (Thompson & Harding 1978; Vrjland & Van Lith 1983). Postoperatively, pattern VEPs are more useful as they may indicate the extent of any amblyopia (Beller *et al.* 1981; Odom & Green 1984; Kriss *et al.* 1994; McCulloch & Skarf 1994). We find that, where cataracts appear to be mild in young children (e.g. lamellar or dot cataracts), pattern VEPs are detectable, and can be used to monitor changes in acuity associated with progressive opacification.

When there is intraocular haemorrhage, the presence of an ERG and VEP following bright flash stimulation can be a useful indicator of the eventual visual outcome (Fuller & Hutton 1982; Hutton & Fuller 1984). However, several authors warn that in the acute stage visual responses may not be recordable but can appear within a few weeks of the onset of intraocular bleeding (Babel *et al.* 1977; Crews *et al.* 1978; Mandelbaum *et al.* 1980).

In foveal hypoplasia (e.g. as occurs in aniridia and albinism, or coloboma), the mixed cone–rod ERG is normal but the VEP to flash and pattern reversal VEP are markedly attenuated and degraded. VEPs can provide a useful indication of visual quality when it is not clear from ophthalmoscopy to what extent coloboma is affecting macular vision in infants (Apkarian & Spekreijse 1990).

Retinal disorders

Rod and cone dysfunction

Leber's amaurosis is an autosomal recessive condition with severe rod and cone dysfunction which is evident from birth. The flash ERG is usually not detectable and this finding is an essential part of establishing the diagnosis. Recording the flash VEP concurrently can be valuable as it may indicate those infants who are likely to have rudimentary vision. Lambert *et al.* (1989c) found that of 43 older children and adults with Leber's amaurosis, 19 had an attenuated flash VEP, and none had a detectable bright flash ERG. All 19 patients with flash VEPs had only rudimentary vision; in only one of these patients could a very degraded pattern reversal VEP to very large checks be recorded.

Predominantly rod dysfunction

Many retinal conditions appear to affect one set of photoreceptors initially, but in the course of time it becomes evident that there is both rod and cone involvement with variable emphasis. Rod–cone degenerations or dystrophies (e.g. retinitis pigmentosa in its various forms) will demonstrate more severe degradation of rod-mediated activity as compared with cone-mediated activity, and vice versa for the cone–rod degenerations (e.g. progressive cone deterioration and maculopathies). We have followed traditional lines in order to simplify presentation and have grouped conditions according to the initial predominance in the involvement of rods and cones, the presence or otherwise of retinal pigmentation, and the tendency or otherwise for progressive deterioration.

Rod dysfunction associated with pigmentary retinopathy

Isolated pigmentary retinopathy. Retinitis pigmentosa is the most common monogenic cause of inherited blindness. When fully established, it is characterized by severe night-blindness, very reduced or non-detectable rod-mediated ERG, and subnormal EOG. ERG changes are apparent early, commonly before the characteristic bone spicule retinal pigmentation. Retinitis pigmentosa is genetically heterogeneous and transmitted by autosomal recessive, autosomal dominant or X-linked recessive inheritance modes. Autosomal dominant forms tend to be the mildest and have a later onset; subnormal cone- and rod-mediated ERGs are often recordable in these cases (Moore *et al.* 1993). Autosomal recessive and X-linked recessive forms are usually severe and progress rapidly, leading to severe visual loss by the second decade. Fishman *et al.* (1988) reported that 71% of X-linked cases show no detectable ERG. In early retinitis pigmentosa, b-waves of rod- and cone-mediated flicker ERGs tend to be delayed (Berson 1992). Children of over 6 years with a hereditary risk of retinitis pigmentosa and who have b-waves of normal amplitude and latency for both cone- and rod-mediated activity, are not likely to develop the disease (Berson 1992). ERGs, and the fundal reflex, can be abnormal in a high proportion (80–90%) of X-linked and heterozygote carriers (Berson *et al.* 1979; Fishman *et al.* 1986).

The pattern ERG is normal or near normal when central vision is well preserved (Arden *et al.* 1984). VEPs both to flash and pattern stimulation are usually of normal size and latency in the early stages of retinitis pigmentosa (Lennerstrand 1982; Papathanasopoulos & Papakostopoulos 1994). However, in later stages, when macular vision is poor, the VEP will be attenuated and frequently moderately delayed also.

Pigmentary retinopathy associated with inborn errors of metabolism and systemic disease. The article by Poll The *et al.* 1992 offers a useful review of this aspect (see also Chapter 44).

Gyrate atophy. The ERG is generally reduced depending upon the extent of retinal involvement (Berson *et al.* 1979), and the EOG is subnormal (Kaiser-Kupfer *et al.* 1985). However, the pattern VEP is normal, at least in childhood and early adulthood, when macular function is well preserved (Fig. 9.7).

Abetalipoproteinaemia. The ERG can be subnormal in childhood when fundal examination is normal (Lamy *et al.* 1963). The EOG is abnormal when retinal pigmentation is observed. Vitamins A and E, by injection or orally, effectively stabilize symptoms and electrophysiological changes (Runge *et al.* 1986b; Fagan & Taylor 1987).

Peroxisomal disorders. See Folz and Trobe (1991) for fuller descriptions.

Zellweger's syndrome. Flash ERGs and VEPs are very attenuated or absent in keeping with widespread photoreceptor and ganglion cell degeneration (Cohen *et al.* 1983; Garner *et al.* 1982; Stanesu & Evrard 1989).

Infantile Refsum's disease. The flash ERG is usually subnormal or undetectable (Weleber & Kennaway 1990), and flash VEPs are very degraded. Arrest of the retinopathy, as monitored by the ERG, has been reported following dietary restriction of phytanic acid and phytol (Gouras *et al.* 1971; Claridge *et al.* 1992).

Infantile adrenoleucodystrophy. There is rod and cone degeneration, cerebral demyelination with eventual complete demyelination of the visual system (Cohen *et al.* 1983; Wilson 1990). Flash ERGs and VEPs are undetectable from an early stage in this infantile condition in contrast to the X-linked childhood form which does not affect the retina (Battaglia *et al.* 1981).

Bardet–Biedl syndrome. The ERG is markedly reduced or unrecordable from an early stage (Fig. 9.8). Flash and pattern VEPs are usually present but are smaller and later compared with matched age controls (Lavy *et al.* 1995). The course of central and peripheral field deterioration varies considerably between individuals (Fulton *et al.* 1993).

Joubert's syndrome. This condition is primarily characterized by cerebellar vermis hypoplasia, and very attenuated or undetectable rod-mediated ERGs, though it is not clear from the literature if the retinal abnormality is an invariable feature. Macular function is usually good in

Gyrate atrophy (KC)

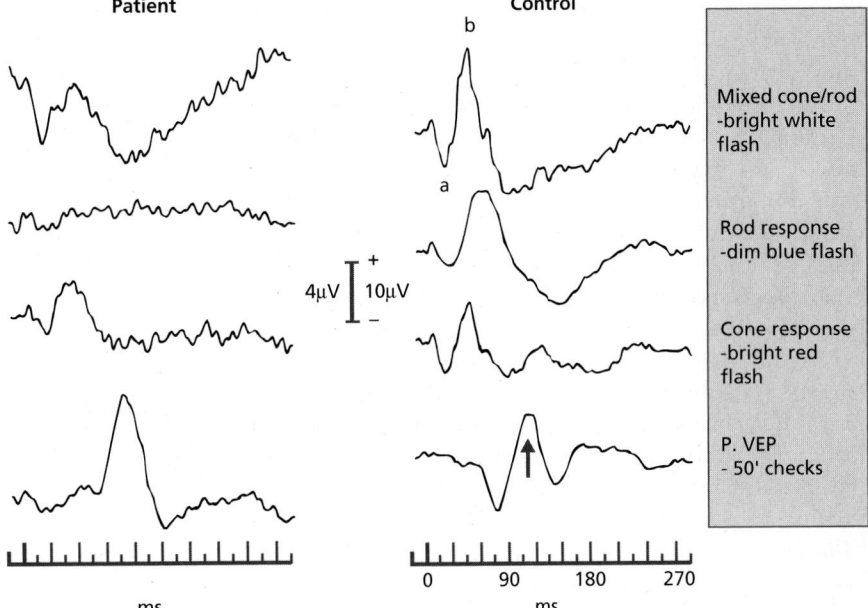

Fig. 9.7 Flash ERGs and pattern VEPs from a patient with gyrate atrophy, pigmentary retinopathy (left side) and a control subject (right side). Note the difference in display gain. The patient has abnormal ERGs (rod-mediated are more abnormal than cone-mediated). However, macular function as reflected by the pattern VEP is essentially normal.

Bardet-Biedl syndrome KM

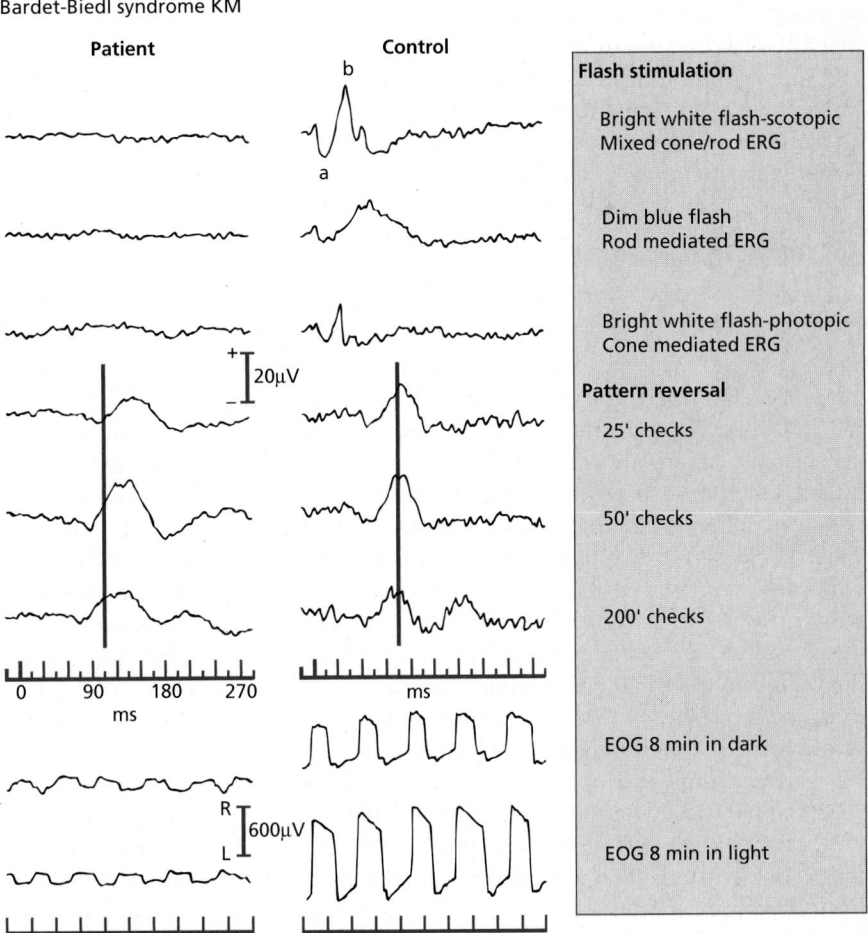

Fig. 9.8 Flash ERGs, pattern VEPs and EOG from a patient with pigmentary retinopathy associated with Bardet–Biedl syndrome (left) and a control subject (right). No ERGs are detectable from the patient indicating marked extramacular dysfunction. Pattern VEPs are of normal size but significantly delayed, suggesting mild macular dysfunction. The EOG potential is markedly attenuated with no enlargement following light adaptation, pointing to a severe abnormality of the pigment epithelium also.

childhood, and VEPs to both flash and pattern reversal stimulation are well preserved (Lambert *et al.* 1989b).

Mucopolysaccharidoses and neurolipidoses. Hurler's (mucopolysaccharidosis type l-H), Sanfilippo's (mucopolysaccharidosis type III), Scheie's (mucopolysaccharidosis type I-S) and Hunter's syndromes are all associated with pigmentary retinopathy. ERGs can show a wide spectrum of abnormality, varying from small near normal abnormality to undetectable responses. ERGs are usually normal in Morquio's and Maroteaux–Lamy types of mucopolysaccharidosis. Many of the mucopolysaccharidoses are associated with corneal clouding and optic nerve neuropathy. Flash VEPs can give a useful indication of postretinal function in these situations. Neurolipidosis type IV may have a retinal degeneration with an abnormal ERG, and all forms have abnormal VEPs at later stages of the disease (see also Chapter 57).

Mitochondrial disease. This encompasses a wide range of syndromes with no common phenotype. The diagnosis is made biochemically and/or by identifying abnormal mitochondria on electron microscopy studies in striated muscle or other tissue (Lestienne & Bataille 1994). Ophthalmic abnormalities, especially ophthalmoplegia, are frequent. Atypical pigmentary retinopathy and subnormal ERGs have been reported in Kearne–Sayers syndrome and mitochondrial myopathy (Mullie *et al.* 1985; Lang & Maumenee 1988). Optic atrophy occurs in Leigh's disease and Leber's optic atrophy, and in both conditions the VEP is markedly attenuated (Halliday 1993; Taylor 1993).

Rod pathway dysfunction without pigmentary retinopathy

Congenital stationary night-blindness. This is a non-progressive disorder, predominantly affecting the rod pathways (Fig. 9.9). The main sign is an elevation of dark adaptation threshold, and many patients have nystagmus in childhood. Congenital stationary night-blindness occurs most commonly with high myopia and has an X-linked inheritance pattern: rarely, it has an autosomal recessive inheritance. Both forms produce a 'negative ERG' ('Schubert–Bornschein' type) characterized by a well-preserved a-wave, and attenuated or undetectable b-wave on scotopic testing with bright flash. They show no abnormalities on fundal reflectometry, suggesting that there are no abnormalities in either the amount or the dynamic properties of rhodopsin (Ripps 1982). It may be due to inadequacies in synaptic transmission, most probably between rods and optic nerve bipolar cells (Ripps 1982; Carr 1991; Sieving 1993; Fitzgerald *et al.* 1994).

Miyake (Miyake *et al.* 1986; Ruether *et al.* 1993) has further classified congenital stationary night-blindness into the following categories.

1 'Complete' congenital stationary night-blindness. No

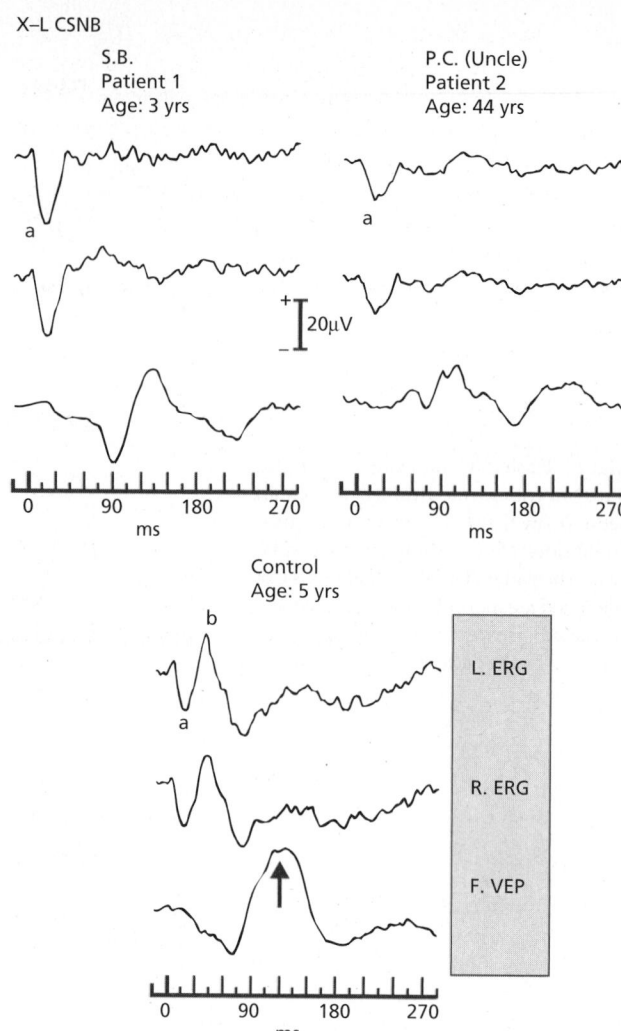

Fig. 9.9 Mixed cone–rod ERGs and VEPs from a young 3-year-old boy and his maternal uncle, both of whom have X-linked congenital stationary night-blindness (upper traces), and those of a 5-year-old control (lower traces). Note both patients have a negative ERG, with clearly discernible a-wave.

rod function is detectable on dark adapatation and negative ERG to bright flash tested under scotopic conditions. Cone responses are well preserved or show mild amplitude or latency changes only (Hill *et al.* 1974; Lachapelle *et al.* 1983).

2 'Incomplete' congenital stationary night-blindness. Subnormal rod function demonstrable by dark adaptation and ERG. Negative ERG to bright flash tested under scotopic conditions. Cone responses well preserved and usually enhance following 15 minutes of light adaptation. Recordable oscillatory potentials (OPs).

Patients with complete congenital stationary night-blindness tend to have pattern VEPs with normal or near normal, latency, though amplitudes are often marginally smaller than average (Kriss & Russell-Eggitt 1992). Asymptomatic carriers of X-linked congenital stationary night-blindness can show attenuation of OPs (Miyake 1991).

Autosomal dominant congenital stationary night-blindness (Nougaret or Riggs type) is associated with an attenuated ERG, involving attenuation of both a- and b-waves. The rod dark adaptation curve in these patients has a slower course than normal.

Oguchi's disease is a rare autosomal recessive condition; most documented cases are from Japan. Patients have night-blindness and a negative ERG. The fundus has an unusual yellow, phosphorescent discoloration, but after dark adaptation for several hours it regains normal colouring (Mizuo–Nakamura phenomenon), and the ERG b-wave is normal for the first few flashes. Photopic ERGs, and the EOG are normal, and the basis of the condition is thought to be postreceptoral (Carr 1991).

Fundus albipunctatus is an autosomal recessive condition in which there is night-blindness and abnormally prolonged dark adaptation. The fundus is spotted throughout with yellow–white dots. The ERG and EOG come within the normal range only after dark adaptation for several hours. This condition has been ascribed to abnormally slowed regeneration of visual pigment (Carr 1991).

Predominantly cone dysfunction

Patients with cone dysfunction have decreased acuity, abnormal colour vision, abnormal photopic and flicker ERGs with relatively well-preserved rod-mediated ERGs. The fundal picture of patients with cone dysfunction varies: young patients with achromatopsia may show only subtle ophthalmoscopic changes in which the fovea is poorly discernible, whereas patients with a variety of maculopathies may have abnormal perimacular pigmentation, often giving the fundus a 'bull's eye' appearance.

Alstrom's syndrome

In Alstrom's syndrome there is a rapid initial loss of cone function in infancy and a more slowly progressive degeneration of rod function. Tremblay *et al.* (1993) described an infant with a reduced cone-mediated ERG at 6 months, which by 1 year was unrecordable. The rod-mediated ERG was normal during the early stages, but deteriorated rapidly and was not detectable by 5 years of age. They suggest this electrophysiological picture is pathognomic of Alstrom's syndrome.

Rod monochromatism (congenital cone dysfunction or achromatopsia)

The photopic ERG, the response to 30 Hz flicker, and the ERG to red flash, are all usually absent. A few patients have evidence of rudimentary colour vision and produce very attenuated, degraded cone-mediated ERGs (Fig. 9.10).

Children with rod monochromatism usually have nystagmus which contributes to degradation of the pattern reversal VEPs for check sizes smaller than 100′ (Lambert *et al.* 1989d). Some rod monochromats have delayed VEPs to both flash and large check pattern reversal stimulation (Halliday & Kriss 1993).

Blue cone monochromatism

This is a rare X-linked condition in which only the sparse blue cones are preserved (Farley & Heckenlively 1991). It is better detected by psychophysical than by ERG testing (Berson 1992), since blue cone ERGs are very small (b-wave amplitude $< 15 \mu V$ with contact lens electrode) and require very bright flashes to be discerned. Although Berson's test distinguishes X-linked blue cone monochromats from achromatopsia, it does not discriminate from X-linked progressive cone dystrophies (Pinckers 1992).

In both rod and blue cone monochromatism, cone-mediated ERGs to red flash and white flash under photopic conditions are grossly attenuated. Since the VEP (both to flash and pattern stimulation) is predominantly cone-mediated, it is very attenuated and delayed (Ikeda 1993; Kriss 1993b).

Dyschromatopsia

Patients with a mild colour vision deficit or dyschromatopsia (incomplete colour defect) have deficiency of one of the cone systems (most commonly either red or green). The pattern VEP is usually detectable and of normal latency when black and white checks are used (Regan 1989). Detection of a VEP abnormality in patients with minor red–green defects relies on using properly balanced isoluminant stimuli (Regan & Spekreijse 1974; Regan 1975, 1989).

Maculopathies

In these patients, the scotopic ERG is normal and the photopic ERG to white light is also within normal limits, but the latter becomes subnormal in later stages, when macular changes are more apparent. Red flicker and pattern reversal ERGs and VEPs, which preferentially stimulate macular cones, are also likely to give abnormalities in patients with maculopathies (Babel *et al.* 1977).

Best's disease. An exception to other maculopathies is Best's disease (vitelliform macular dystrophy), as pattern and flash ERGs and VEPs are usually normal in the early stages, though typically the EOG is markedly subnormal. Best's disease carriers also have abnormal EOGs (Deutman 1969), and normal ERG and VEPs. The EOG ratio

Rod monochromatism (SI)

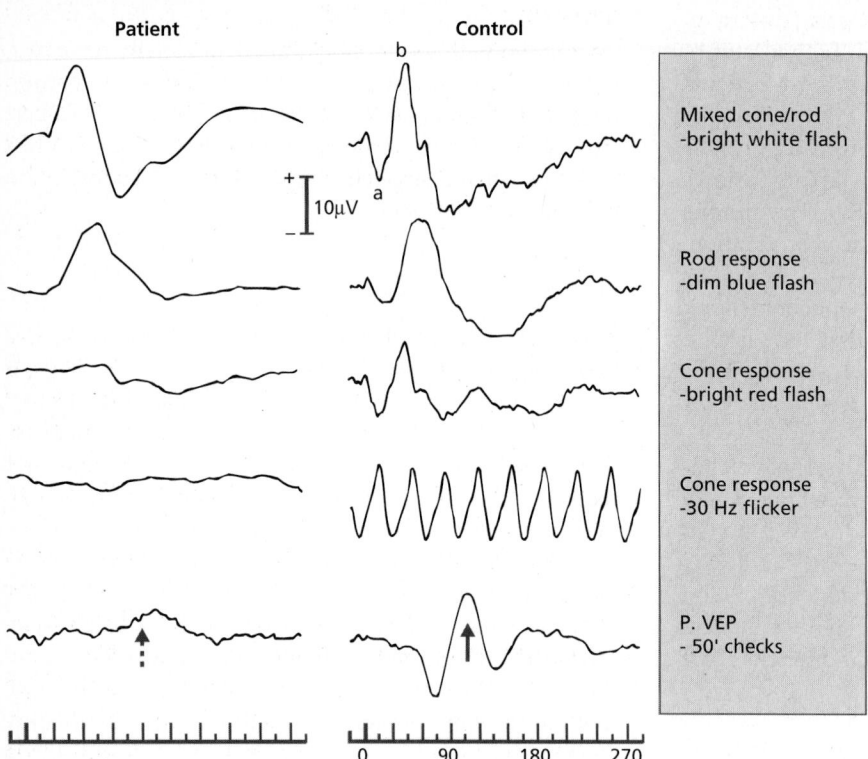

Patient	Control	
		Mixed cone/rod -bright white flash
		Rod response -dim blue flash
		Cone response -bright red flash
		Cone response -30 Hz flicker
		P. VEP - 50' checks

10μV

0   90   180   270
ms

Fig. 9.10 Flash ERGs and VEPs from a young patient with rod monochromatism (left) and a control subject (right). She produces well-preserved rod-mediated ERGs to bright and dim white flashes, but no discernible cone-mediated ERGs to red flashes at 3 or 30/second flicker. Her pattern VEPs to 50' checks (and larger check sizes) were broad and delayed (⁑).

does not correlate well with the appearance or severity of the macular lesions (Wajima *et al*. 1993).

Juvenile macular degeneration (Stargardt's disease). The scotopic ERG, and EOG are normal but the photopic b-wave amplitude may be decreased in the early stages (Noble & Carr 1979; Aaberg 1986), as are cone-mediated ERGs to red flash (Ikeda 1993). The scotopic ERG becomes abnormal as retinal changes progress to the flavimaculatus appearance. The EOG is commonly normal, except in a few severely affected cases (Lennerstrand 1982). In the early stages, P100 of the pattern VEP is often marginally delayed and attenuated, and in advanced disease the pattern VEP is frequently not detectable (Stadtler 1984).

Benign pigment epithelial macular defects ('benign concentric macular dystrophy' or 'annular macular dystrophy') tend to show mildly attenuated photopic and scotopic ERGs.

The pattern ERG elicited by checkerboard or grating reversal can be a sensitive indicator of macular function (Sokol 1972; Lawill 1974; Arden *et al*. 1984; Hull *et al*. 1992). The pattern ERG is of small amplitude (around 5μV in controls), even when recorded with a corneal electrode, with steady fixation and minimal blinking. It has two components: a positive peak at 50 milliseconds (P50), and a negative peak at 95 milliseconds (N95) (see Fig. 9.4),

these probably represent the activity of outer and inner retinal elements respectively (Holder 1987). The P50 component is reduced in maculopathies, and the N95 reduced where ganglion cell activity is compromised (e.g. Holder 1987). Recording the pattern ERG with a corneal electrode is difficult in children less than 6 years old. We record the pattern ERG from skin electrodes, and find interocular comparisons of P50 useful when only one eye is affected. However, use of N95 is more limited as it is poorly represented in skin ERG recordings, and it is also often contaminated by periorbital myogenic activity.

Vitreoretinal disorders

X-linked retinoschisis

In the early stages, the ERG characteristically shows a well-preserved a-wave but markedly reduced b-wave. The EOG is usually normal. The VEP, both to flash and to pattern stimulation, tends to be attenuated and delayed (Harris & Yeung 1976; Hirose *et al*. 1977; Papakostopoulos *et al*. 1989).

Hirose *et al*. (1977) found that VEPs of retinoschisis patients to a focal 4.5° stimulus were delayed by more than 50 milliseconds compared with controls. Papakostopoulos *et al*. (1989) reported that pattern reversal VEPs were delayed by more than 4SD above the mean values of controls. Both X-linked retinoschisis and congenital stationary night-blindness give negative ERGs to bright flash, but pattern VEPs are of increased latency in retinoschisis (Papakostopoulos *et al.* 1989). Some cases have a golden fundus reflex and a Mizuo–Nakamura phenomenon (de-Jong *et al.* 1991).

Goldmanm–Favre disease

Visual electrophysiological changes in autosomal recessive Goldmanm–Favre disease are usually very marked with highly attenuated or undetectable ERGs (Fishman *et al.* 1976; Nasr *et al.* 1990), subnormal EOG and poor flash VEPs.

Wagner's disease and erosive vitreoretinopathy. Wagner's disease and erosive vitreoretinopathy are allelic autosomal dominant diseases that share some similarities with, but appear genetically distinct from, COL2A1-associated Stickler's syndrome (Brown *et al.* 1995). Both disorders have associated retinal pigment epithelial changes, poor night vision, visual field defects and abnormal ERG findings, which are not found in families with COL2A1-associated Stickler's syndrome. In addition, rhegmatogeneous retinal detachments are uncommon in Wagner's disease, but occur in approximately 50% of patients with either erosive vitreoretinopathy or Stickler's syndrome. Myopia is common in Wagner's disease and the ERG is usually of subnormal size (Hirose *et al.* 1973).

Stickler's disease. Stickler's disease is also a dominantly inherited connective tissue disorder and has several associated characteristic musculoskeletal features. About two-thirds of affected families demonstrate linkage to the gene encoding type II procollagen (COL2A1) (Snead *et al.* 1994). Affected members tend to have progressive myopia and are prone to retinal detachment. The ERG relates to the degree of fundal involvement and may be normal or abnormal, the latter if there is evidence for retinal degeneration and detachment (Fishman & Sokol 1990).

Toxic conditions

Chloroquine. When the changes are apparent at the macula only and the ERG is normal or near normal then chloroquine toxicity should be suspected. The ERG is markedly attenuated in advanced disease.

Quinine. High doses can affect the outer retinal layer leading to attenuation of both a- and b-waves. The ERG can show partial recovery when the drug is withdrawn.

Indomethacin. Abnormal scotopic ERG a- and b-wave amplitudes may occur with prolonged use (Burns 1968).

Vincristine and vinblastine. These can lead to b-wave attenuation (Ripps *et al.* 1989) and an abnormal VEP may occur if there is optic neuropathy.

Desferoxamine. The ERG can show subtle changes in b-wave sensitivity, i.e. when assessing changes in b-wave amplitude with alterations in flash intensity (Niemeyer 1991).

Optic nerve disorders

Established optic nerve demyelination associated with good to moderate vision, usually will give a VEP which is delayed (in the order of 20–40 milliseconds) but with a well-preserved waveform. During the acute stage of optic neuritis when acuity is poor, the pattern VEP is likely not to be detectable (Halliday *et al.* 1973).

In compressive and ischaemic abnormalities, and in many degenerative conditions causing optic atrophy, the pattern VEP will be attenuated and only mildly delayed (in the order of 10–20 milliseconds) (Halliday 1993).

Ethambutol-induced optic neuropathy is associated with reduced pattern VEP amplitude and mildly increased latency, but this may be reversible (Yiannikas *et al.* 1983; Harding *et al.* 1984).

Monocular VEP stimulation has to be performed in order to help define whether a disease process is affecting the optic nerve, chiasm or posterior hemisphere. Testing half-fields improves the sensitivity (Brecelj 1994; Halliday 1993), but usually this is only satisfactorily achievable in older children and adults.

The combined ERG/VEP approach will distinguish between retinal and postretinal problems—thus a normal mixed cone–rod ERG and reduced VEP (flash or pattern) strongly suggests dysfunction beyond the eye, for example optic nerve hypoplasia, optic atrophy associated with inflammatory, compressive, vascular or neurometabolic disease (Halliday & Kriss 1993).

Infant patients with uncomplicated delayed visual maturation, have normal flash ERGs and VEPs from the outset, compared with age-matched controls (Lambert *et al.* 1989a).

Hysterical (or functional) visual loss

Hysterical or functional visual loss is associated with normal flash and pattern VEP findings. It is particularly important to monitor fixation performance carefully and not to use small check sizes (< 15′) only, as voluntary changes in accommodation by patients may lead to apparently significant VEP changes, whereas larger check sizes are far more resistant to such manoeuvres (see Halliday 1993 and Sokol 1990b for further discussion).

Optic nerve hypoplasia

The combined ERG/VEP picture of cases with severe optic nerve dysplasia (Fig. 9.11) shows a normal or larger than normal ERG, and a variably attenuated VEP (Kriss *et al.* 1994) sometimes with a moderate increase in latency (Apkarian & Spekreijse 1990). There is discrepancy between studies concerning the ERG in optic nerve hypoplasia. Some studies claim the ERG to be of small amplitude and increased latency (Cibis & Fitzgerald 1994; Janaky *et al.* 1994), while others describe super-normal ERGs, and ascribe this effect to a reduction in inhibitory feedback or gain control, analogous to that reported following optic nerve section (Francois & DeRouck 1976; Sprague & Wilson 1981; Kriss & Russell-Eggitt 1992).

Optic nerve compression

Infantile osteopetrosis

Infantile osteopetrosis is distinguished by increased bone density and mass, and by its characteristic 'bone-within-bone' radiological appearance. The autosomal recessive form is evident from infancy and is more severe than the adult onset, autosomal dominant form. It is due to poor osteoclast function which leads to excessive deposition of bone and narrowing of cranial foramina (Gerritson *et al.* 1994). The ERG has been reported to be attenuated (Keith 1968; Hoyt & Billson 1979), but in our series, the majority

(92%, 12 of 13 patients) had normal ERGs (Kriss & Thompson 1995). It is generally found that in most cases the VEP is abnormal. In our series, 77% of cases had delayed (on average 14 milliseconds above laboratory norms), and attenuated flash VEPs. The VEP provides an early sign of anterior visual pathway compression and provides a better functional evaluation of visual pathway compromise than neuroimaging or ophthalmoscopy (Kriss & Thompson 1995).

Optic nerve glioma

Optic nerve glioma is most commonly associated with attenuation, broadening and mild delay of the pattern VEP from the affected eye. The flash VEP is usually more robust to waveform changes than the pattern VEP. In the series studied by Groswasser *et al.* (1985), the main positivity of the pattern VEP from the affected eye was delayed (in the order of 20 milliseconds) and attenuated (5–12 µV) compared with the fellow eye. Pattern VEPs are more valuable than flash VEPs when testing the fellow eye. In 20% of cases the occipital asymmetry of the pattern VEP distribution (not evident for flash stimulation) indicated posterior spread of the glioma to involve the temporal field fibres crossing at the chiasm. Spontaneous improvement in optic nerve function can occur occasionally (Groswasser *et al.* 1985). Jabbari *et al.* (1985) have stressed the value of pattern VEPs in identifying patients with neurofibromatosis who also have optic nerve glioma.

Optic neuritis

In a follow-up study of 39 cases of childhood optic neuritis (mean follow-up 8.8 years), only 20% had developed multiple sclerosis (Kriss *et al.* 1988). Pattern VEPs in 45% of those 20 patients recorded had significantly delayed VEPs at follow-up 9.3 years after the onset of the attack which occurred at a mean age of 9.4 years (Halliday *et al.* 1986). In 64% of the eyes which showed significant delays, pattern VEP latencies were increased by 15–35 milliseconds. In contrast to childhood optic neuritis, 90% of adult optic neuritis cases maintain delays in their pattern VEPs (Halliday 1993).

Hereditary optic atrophy and cerebellar ataxias

Pattern VEPs are usually attenuated, degraded and sometimes mildly delayed, in all forms of hereditary optic atrophy, though there may be differences between conditions as to which VEP components are affected.

In Leber's optic neuropathy, pattern VEPs are markedly attenuated in the active stage of the disease, and tend to remain attenuated and degraded even when acuity improves (Dorfman *et al.* 1977; Carroll & Mastaglia 1979; Halliday 1993).

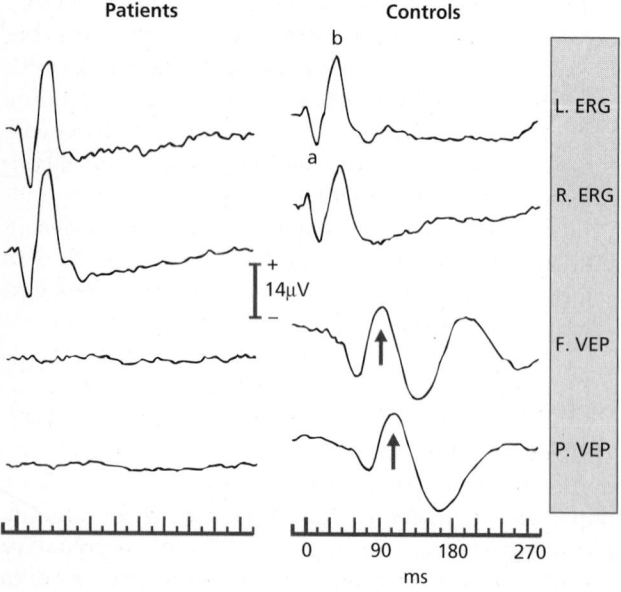

Optic nerve hypoplasia
Group average of 6

Patients   Controls

L. ERG
R. ERG
F. VEP
P. VEP

14 µV

0   90   180   270
ms

Fig. 9.11 Mixed cone–rod ERGs, and VEPs to flash and pattern reversal—a group average of six patients with severe optic nerve hypoplasia. Note patients have large well-preserved ERGs but no detectable VEPs.

In dominant optic atrophy, many patients may show 'W' or bifid morphology, both in their pattern and flash VEPs (Harding & Crews 1982; Halliday 1993). For pattern VEPs, this W waveform can be ascribed to macular VEP attenuation ('scotomatous' changes) with consequent predominance of paramacular VEP components (Halliday *et al.* 1979). Those without scotomatous VEP features may have attenuated and mildly delayed responses.

Some cerebellar ataxias have a pigmentary retinopathy, not necessarily with optic atrophy. In Friedreich's ataxia there is mild axonal degeneration and pattern VEPs are mildly attenuated and marginally delayed (Carroll *et al.* 1980).

Reports of pattern VEPs in olivopontocerebellar atrophy are somewhat variable; some authors describe delayed and attenuated responses in about 50% (Nuwer *et al.* 1983; Sridhan 1983; Cosi *et al.* 1984), others find pattern VEPs to be normal (Bird & Crill 1981; Chokroverty *et al.* 1985).

Vitamin deficiency

Vitamin B_{12} deficiency can lead to patchy demyelination of the visual pathway and spinal cord, particulary the papillomacular bundle and spinal posterior columns (Agamanolis *et al.* 1976). Abnormal pattern VEPs occur in patients with pernicious anaemia, subacute combined degeneration and tobacco–alcohol amblyopia (Troncoso *et al.* 1979; Fine & Hallett 1980; Krumholz *et al.* 1981; Kriss *et al.* 1982); all show partial improvement in pattern VEPs following vitamin B_{12} administration.

Vitamin E deficiency over a long period can be associated with spinocerebellar degeneration, neuromuscular weakness, ophthalmoplegia and pigmentary retinopathy. In cystic fibrosis and abetalipoproteinaemia there is fat malabsorption leading to vitamin E deficiency. ERG and pattern VEP abnormalities (attenuation and increased latency) have been reported in humans (Willison *et al.* 1985; Runge *et al.* 1986b; Fagan & Taylor 1987) and rats (Goss-Sampson *et al.* 1991).

Chiasmal abnormalities

Electrophysiological detection of chiasmal anomalies is optimally accomplished by left and right half-field testing of each eye (Halliday 1993; Brecelj 1994). Pattern VEP half-field testing is difficult to perform in young children because of poor fixation but it is possible to detect an occipital asymmetry reliably on monocular full-field testing, which reverses in distribution when the other eye is tested. This change in occipital distribution is called 'crossed asymmetry' (Halliday 1993) and is an important VEP indicator of a chiasmal defect. The VEP asymmetry is of greatest significance when there is activity of opposite polarity on either side of the occipital midline. Binocular VEP testing is not helpful in identifying chiasmal abnormalities as there will be cancellation of activity recorded at lateral electrodes due to algebraic summation of activity with opposite polarity.

Crossed asymmetry anomalies can be of two opposite forms: (i) compromise of fibres crossing at the chiasm due to compression and achiasmia; and (ii) excessive decussation of fibres at the chiasm.

Compromise of fibres crossing at the chiasm, and achiasmia

Chiasmal glioma. As described above, when optic nerve glioma spreads backwards, it frequently affects visual fibres from the fellow eye crossing at the chiasm. The pattern VEP provides a useful indication of the degree of visual pathway involvement, as responses from the affected eye are usually markedly attenuated and degraded. Those from the fellow eye can demonstrate an occipital asymmetry indicating compromise of temporal field fibres crossing at the chiasm. Gliomas intrinsically located within the chiasm have a more deleterious effect, and VEPs are generally very degraded and markedly attenuated (Kupersmith *et al.* 1981; Groswasser *et al.* 1985).

Craniopharyngioma (Fig. 9.12). In our experience, children treated for craniopharyngioma have pattern VEPs which, on average, are 8 milliseconds later, and about one-third the size of age-matched controls (Lavy *et al.* 1995). About 20% of young patients with craniopharyngioma have a pattern VEP crossed asymmetry, with poor temporal field responses from each eye. In 44%, VEPs to both pattern and flash are very attenuated and degraded or undetectable. Ten per cent have an uncrossed asymmetry indicating unilateral postchiasmal compression; whilst in 2% VEPs from one eye only are degraded and attenuated indicating optic nerve compression. In a further 24%, pattern VEPs are within normal latency and amplitude limits. There was good agreement between field loss indicated by pattern VEPs and Goldmann visual field studies, except in a small minority of patients who had peripheral field loss confined to the upper quadrants, in whom the pattern VEPs were deemed normal. Others have similarly emphasized the value of pattern VEPs in detecting and monitoring chiasmal compression due to craniopharyngioma or pituitary tumours (Holder 1978; Flanagan & Harding 1987; Halliday 1993; Brecelj 1994).

Achiasmia. In achiasmia, the chiasm fails to develop (see Chapter 52). The pattern onset VEP was reported to demonstrate a crossed asymmetry for the first positive component (C1) in two patients with isolated achiasmia (Apkarian *et al.* 1994). We have detected achiasma in an infant with midline brain abnormalities using flash VEPs. The chiasmal abnormality was detected with MRI only

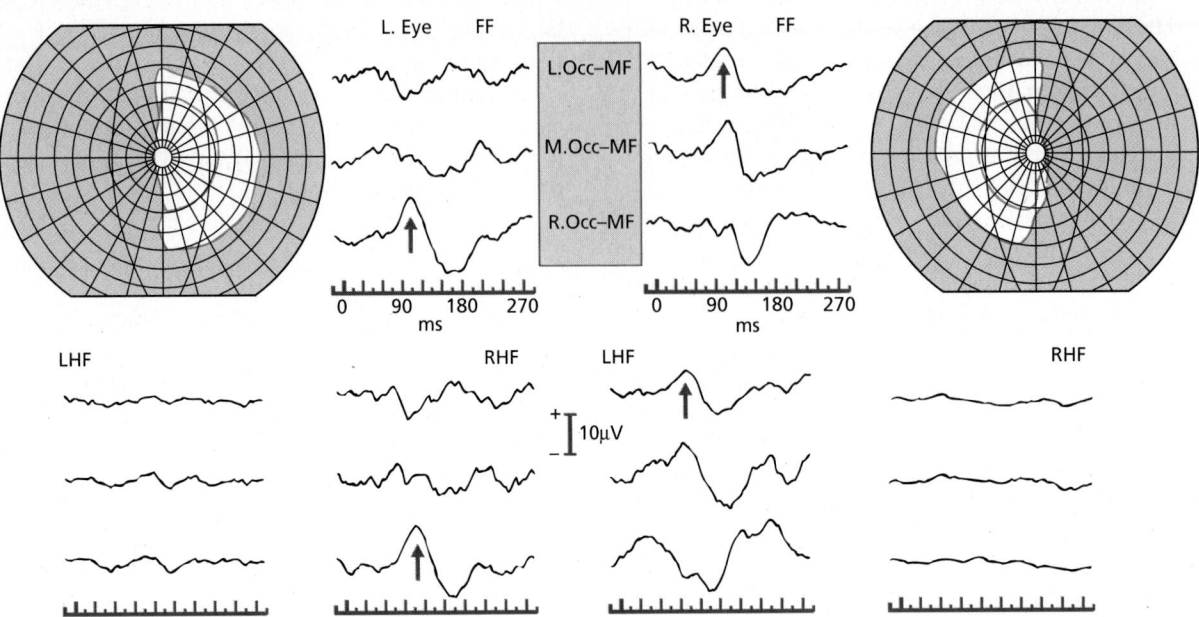

Fig. 9.12 Pattern VEPs of patient with a bitemporal hemianopia who had been operated on for removal of a craniopharyngioma. Note the opposite occipital distribution when comparing full-field (FF) stimulation of each eye (crossed asymmetry), and the preserved nasal field responses on half-field stimulation (HF); P100 (arrow) is on the side of scalp ipsilateral to the preserved half-field.

after a re-review of images following the abnormal flash VEP findings (see Fig. 52.6) (Leitch *et al*. 1996).

Excessive decussation of fibres at the chiasm

This occurs uniquely in albinism. The pattern of crossed asymmetry in albinism is opposite to chiasmal compression or achiasmia (Figs 9.12, 9.13). In infancy, the albino crossed asymmetry is best shown with flash stimulation. Large amplitude ERGs also occur (Kriss *et al*. 1990; Russell-Eggitt *et al*. 1990). When albinos have nystagmus it is best to use large check sizes for pattern VEPs as smaller check sizes are not reliable. In older children and adult albinos, the crossed asymmetry is most conspicuous when using pattern onset stimulation (Creel *et al*. 1979, 1981; Apkarian 1994). A minority of albinos have near normal acuity and no nystagmus, but they also show a crossed asymmetry for pattern onset and pattern reversal VEPs (Kriss *et al*. 1992b).

Postchiasmal dysfunction

Generalized

Hypoxic, infective, most neurodegenerative conditions and hydrocephalus commonly cause widespread dys-

function of the postchiasmal visual pathway. Flash and pattern VEPs are usually attenuated and degraded but latencies are normal or near normal. Although there are case reports of a few individuals who appear cortically blind yet have normal flash VEPs (Bodis-Wollner 1977; Celesia *et al*. 1980), in studies reporting on a large series of young children in acute onset cortical blindness, the presence of a flash VEP was a useful indicator of visual prognosis, regardless of aetiology (Taylor & McCulloch 1991). Well-preserved flash VEPs predict good recovery, whereas patients with abnormal flash VEPs are likely to remain behaviourally blind (Regan *et al*. 1982; Regan 1989; Taylor & McCulloch 1991; Taylor *et al*. 1992).

Perinatal hypoxia

The visual cortex is susceptible to hypoxic damage (Pryds & Greisen 1990). In perinatal hypoxia, the flash VEP can give an indication of visual function and eventual outcome during the acute stage (Whyte *et al*. 1986; Taylor *et al*. 1992). In milder cases of cerebral palsy, pattern VEPs are attenuated and recordable to the larger check sizes (>100') only, and in many severe cases with rudimentary vision the flash VEPs have an atypical morphology and distribution with positivity at 80 milliseconds, which has maximal amplitude 3–5 cm lateral to the midocciput.

Hydrocephalus

A common electrodiagnostic picture associated with hydrocephalus is normal flash ERGs and attenuated, degraded and delayed VEPs to both flash and pattern

Achiasmic

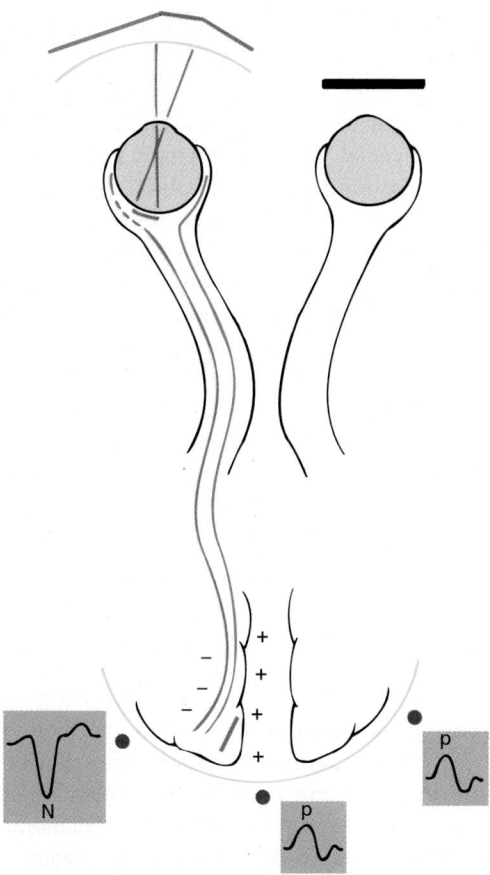

Albino

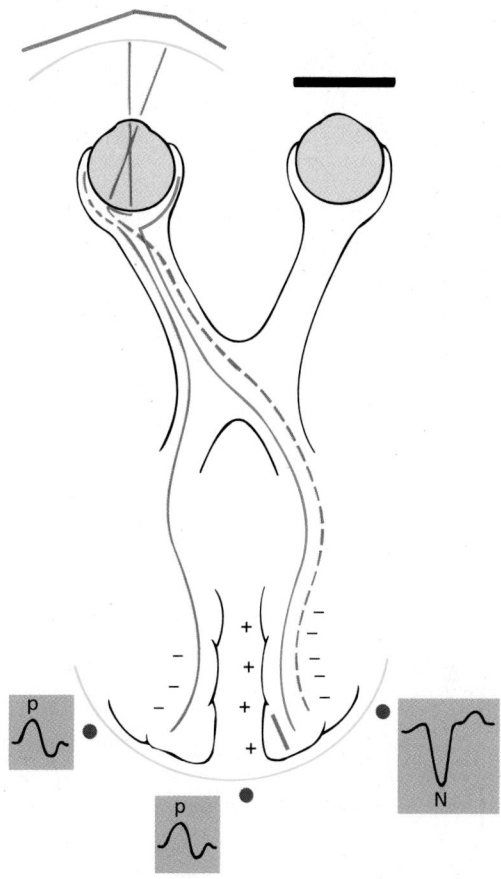

Fig. 9.13 Schematic comparing the visual pathway and VEP distribution in albino and achiasmic patients for flash stimulation of the left eye. Stimulation of the right eye produces the mirror image distribution for either condition. In the achiasmic subject, all the visual fibres from the left eye project to the left occipital cortex, and at 80–100 milliseconds, a positivity is recorded over the right scalp and a negativity over the left. In contrast, most of the fibres from one eye cross at the chiasm in albinism, and the VEP distribution is the opposite, with a positivity recorded over the left scalp, and a negativity over the right.

stimulation. Often this picture is evident before optic atrophy is evident on fundoscopy. VEP latency shows a close relationship with intracranial pressure and parallels improvements after shunting, and deterioration with shunt blockage (Sklar *et al.* 1979; York *et al.* 1981; Watanabe *et al.* 1984; Alani 1985). The flash VEP may a better indicator of hydrocephalic effects in infants than in older children (George & Taylor 1987).

Neurodegenerative conditions

Batten's disease (neuronal ceroid lipofuscinosis) (see Chapter 57, and Baker *et al.* 1995 for more extensive electrophysiological review). All childhood onset forms of Batten's disease are associated with retinal degeneration and visual failure. The photopic ERG is very attenuated or abolished (Harden & Pampiglione 1982).

In the infantile and juvenile forms of Batten's disease,

the VEP is not detectable when the disease is well established. In the late infantile form the flash VEP is reported to be markedly enlarged (12–20 times larger than normal) even though the flash ERG is usually not detectable (Harden & Pampiglione 1982). The occipital response may not be a true VEP as each flash elicits what appears to be 'epileptic' activity (analogous to a myoclonic response following somatosensory stimulation) with different morphology and distribution to a normal VEP (Fig. 9.14).

Tay–Sachs disease. The ERG is usually normal throughout the course of the disease. The flash VEP is poorly defined during the early stages, and not detectable in the later stages: this distinguishes Tay–Sachs electrophysiologically from Batten's disease.

Metachromatic leucodystrophy and adrenoleucodystrophy. In these conditions, the flash ERG is normal, but the VEP

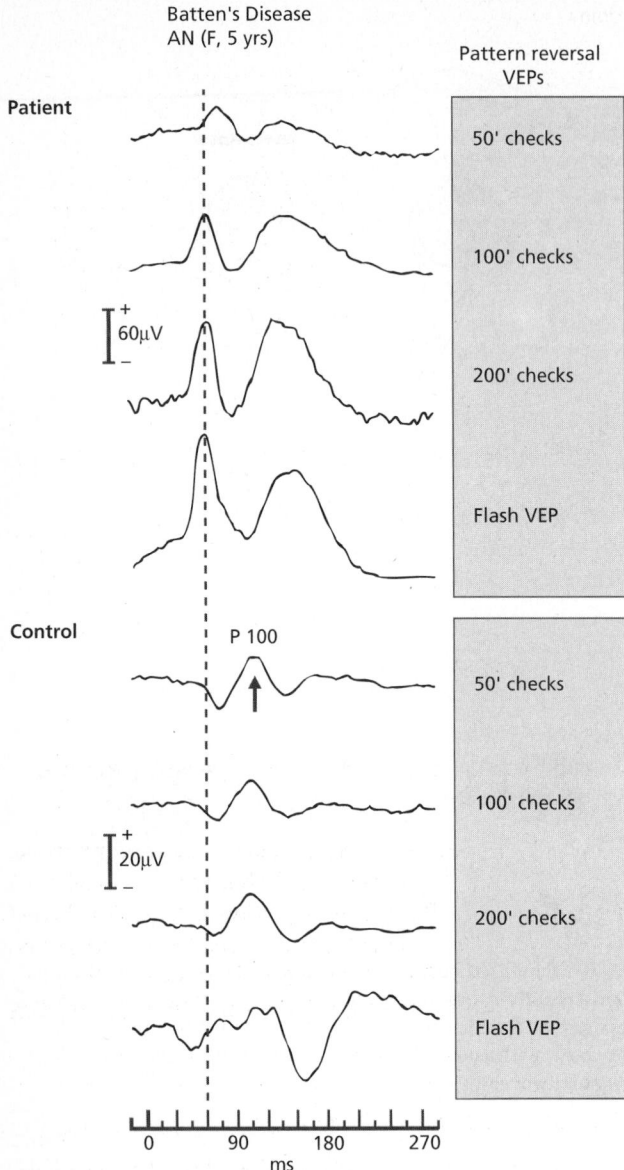

Batten's Disease
AN (F, 5 yrs)

Pattern reversal
VEPs

Patient

50' checks

100' checks

60µV

200' checks

Flash VEP

Control   P 100

50' checks

20µV

100' checks

200' checks

Flash VEP

0   90   180   270
ms

Fig. 9.14 Pattern reversal and flash VEPs in a patient with Late Infantile Batten's disease (upper traces), and a healthy subject of similar age (lower traces). Note the different morphology, and much larger size, of the patient's VEPs compared with the normal control. In patients, the VEPs tend to get larger as the luminance contribution increases with larger checks; in contrast, the control gives a VEP with better defined components to the smaller checks.

findings are somewhat variable: in some patients they are normal, in others they are poorly formed and delayed, or absent.

Pelizaus–Merzbacher disease. This is associated with poor central myelination, and patients have markedly delayed VEPs (Apkarian *et al.* 1993; Hodes *et al.* 1993; Wang *et al.* 1995).

Unilateral posterior hemisphere dysfunction

In young children, both pattern and flash VEPs show a conspicuous occipital asymmetry when there is dysfunction in one hemisphere, most commonly due to space-occupying or vascular lesions (Fig. 9.15). The P100 of the pattern reversal VEP, and the main positivity of the flash VEP (also around 100 milliseconds), is seen over the midline, and over the dysfunctional hemisphere, and a negativity with peak latency of about 100 milliseconds is often recorded over the opposite hemisphere. This asymmetry is evident for binocular stimulation, and is virtually the same for independent stimulation of each eye (hence it is called 'uncrossed asymmetry'). The distribution may appear paradoxical (see Fig. 9.2) because electrodes over the abnormal hemisphere pick up activity produced by the normal hemisphere (Barrett *et al.* 1976; Blumhardt *et al.* 1982). VEPs can demonstrate hemisphere dysfunction in young children where clinical signs are not obvious (Lambert *et al.* 1990; Jacobs *et al.* 1993; Patel *et al.* 1993).

Visual electrophysiology and ophthalmogenetics

Electrophysiology helps to distinguish between phenotypes of certain retinal disorders (Apkarian 1994), and to define clinical conditions for molecular genetic studies. For example, some patients with Duchenne's or De Becker's muscular dystrophy have negative scotopic ERGs without clinical evidence of retinal dysfunction, e.g nyctalopia as found in X-linked congenital stationary night-blindness, or retinal folding found in retinoschisis. The ERG findings in Duchenne's muscular dystrophy can be distinguished from congenital stationary night-blindness by use of prolonged on/off flashes delivered under photopic conditions (Fitzgerald *et al.* 1994). In Duchenne's muscular dystrophy there is preservation of 'on' function, in contrast to congenital stationary night-blindness in which it is abnormal. Duchenne's muscular dystrophy has been mapped to deletions in the Xp21 region, an area associated with the dystrophin gene. The ERG changes relate to the position and extent of the mutation or deletion (De Becker *et al.* 1994; Sigesmund *et al.* 1994). Milder ERG abnormalities tend to be associated with deletion at the 5' or proximal end of the gene.

Autosomal dominant retinitis pigmentosa has been mapped to chromosome 7p in a large English family which showed variable expression reflected both in the ERG and psychophysical differences between individuals (Kim *et al.* 1995).

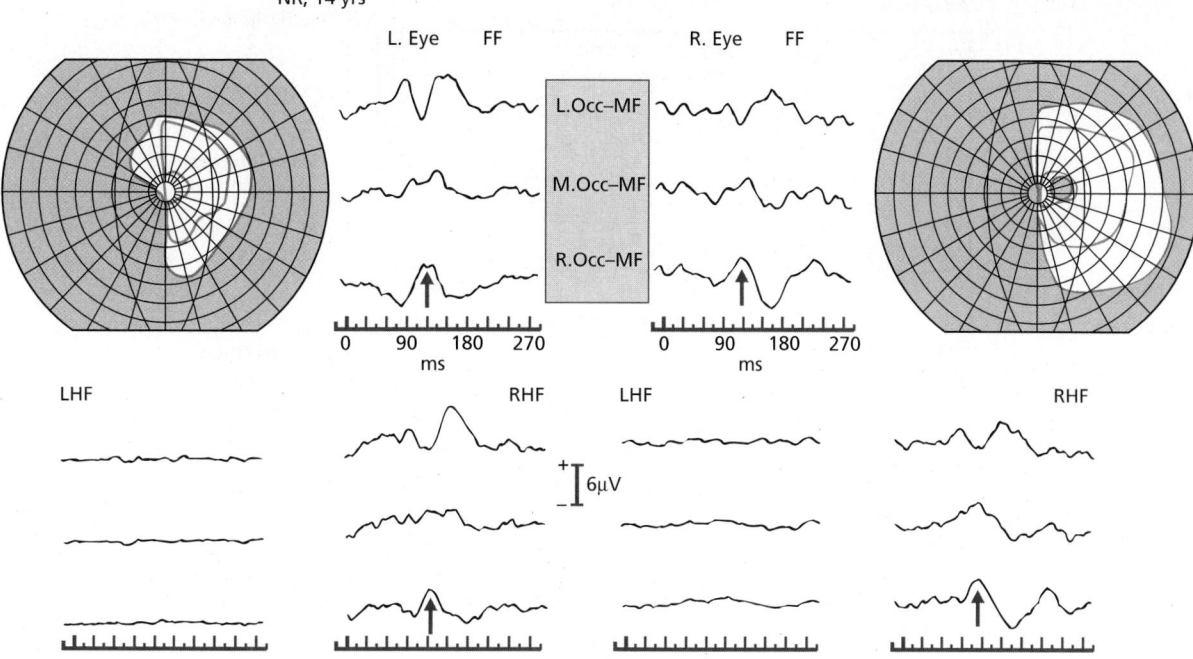

Fig. 9.15 Pattern VEPs of patient with a left homonymous hemianopia who had been operated on for removal of a craniopharyngioma. The occipital distribution for full-field (FF) stimulation of each eye is the same (uncrossed asymmetry): the right half-field (RHF) produces a well-preserved response, for either eye (lowermost traces).

Investigating the child with nystagmus

Nystagmus in infancy is likely to be a sign of poor vision due to retinal, optic nerve or chiasmal abnormalities or of brain-stem and/or cerebellar dysfunction. The majority of patients with congenital nystagmus have retinal or optic nerve disease (Gelbart & Hoyt 1988; Cibis & Fitzgerald 1994). Nystagmus is rarely seen in postchiasmal disorders even with poor vision. Combined ERG/VEP recording helps greatly in establishing a diagnosis: Leber's amaurosis, achromatopsia, X-linked congenital stationary night-blindness will have abnormal ERGs, whereas albinism, osteopetrosis, optic nerve hypoplasia, glioma and craniopharyngioma have normal ERGs, but abnormal monocular VEPs. In infancy, all these conditions may present with nystagmus as the only conspicuous clinical sign.

If both ERGs and VEPs are normal, the nystagmus is likely to be either associated with brain-stem or cerebellar disease, or is idiopathic. Eye movement studies are useful for characterizing the nystagmus waveform (see Chapter 63; Yee 1990) and combined electrophysiological and eye movement recording can help in deciding which cases require neuroimaging.

Estimating acuity with pattern visual evoked potentials

Pattern VEPs can be used to estimate visual acuity: this is particularly useful in preverbal children, or those with expressive or motor communication difficulties. When using pattern VEP acuity, interest is concentrated on the smallest test element size that can be consistently detected. Any refractive error must be corrected during pattern VEP recording.

Transient visual evoked potentials

Transient VEPs, to pattern reversal or pattern onset stimulation, can give a quantitative assessment of vision (Marg *et al.* 1976; Sokol 1978; Spekreijse 1978; Odom & Green 1984; Apkarian *et al.* 1986; Orel-Bixler *et al.* 1989; McCulloch & Skarf 1994). The amplitude of the transient pattern reversal VEP varies with spatial frequency, demonstrating an inverted U-shaped tuning curve. The peak of the tuning curve is broadly associated with the size of the stimulus field. Stimulus fields used for clinical work are greater than 10 degrees; these sizes of stimulus field, and patterns with element sizes of 10–20 minutes, give the largest pattern VEPs from 5 to 6 years of age and onwards (Wenzel & Brandl 1984).

The morphology of the transient pattern onset VEP alters as element size becomes smaller and preferentially stimulates the foveal occipital representation (Spekreijse 1978). The adult pattern onset VEP has a positive (C1) to negative (C2) to positive (C3) waveform. The negative C2

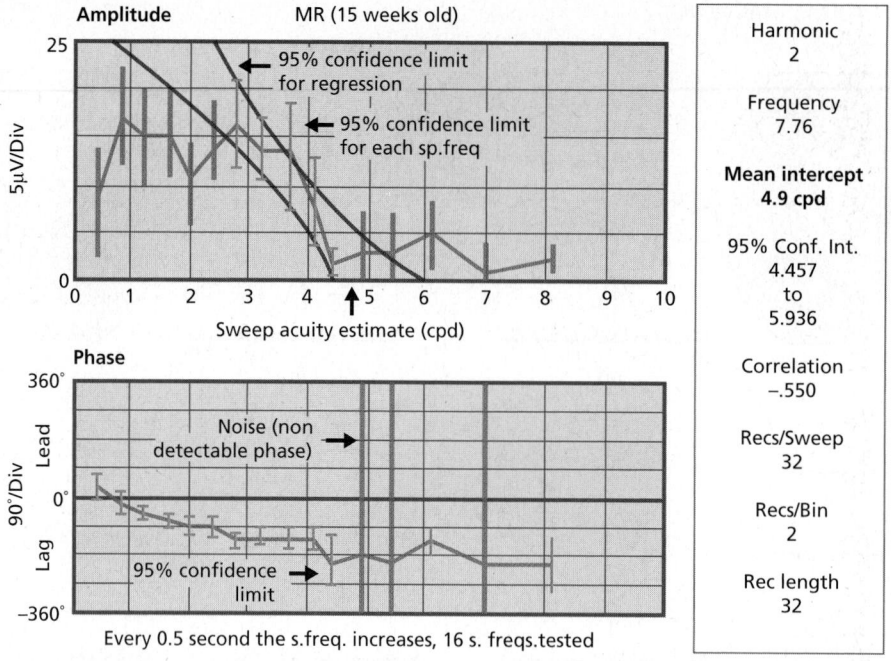

Fig. 9.16 Sweep VEP. Rapid rates of stimulation are used to elicit a quasi-sinusoidal VEP which is characterized by its amplitude and phase. A range of spatial frequencies are presented. There is a trend for VEP amplitude to decrease with increasing spatial frequency. The regression is computed and the VEP acuity estimate is where the regression line intersects the x-axis.

peak has particular sensitivity to contour, and correlates well with acuity; however, this component is not usually evident until around 8 years of age (DeVries Khoe & Spekreijse 1982). Latencies of all onset components reach adult levels at puberty. In distinction to that of the adult, the infantile and juvenile pattern onset VEP is characterized by a single positive peak (C1) and changes in this component have been used successfully to estimate acuity in young children (Apkarian & Spekreijse 1990).

The near threshold pattern VEP amplitude is proportional to stimulus contrast (Campbell & Maffei 1970), although near the acuity limit log contrast sensitivity is also linearly related to spatial frequency (Campbell & Gubisch 1966). Thus, near the acuity limit VEP amplitude falls off linearly with spatial frequency. The extrapolation of the high spatial frequency limb of the spatial tuning function to zero amplitude (or the noise level) produces an intercept which correlates with the subjective visual resolution.

Extrapolation has been used to derive acuity estimates from transient pattern reversal and pattern onset VEPs (DeVries Khoe & Spekreijse 1982; Orel-Bixler & Norcia 1987), and flashed pattern stimuli (Harter *et al.* 1977). A direct estimate of threshold can be obtained by recording

the VEP to successively smaller patterns until a response is no longer reliably distinguished from background activity (Marg *et al.* 1976; McCulloch & Skarf 1994). A young child's interest in the test stimulus often wanes as threshold is approached, and this leads to difficulties in determining the acuity endpoint due to noise from intrusive electroencephalogram (EEG) and electromyogram (EMG) activity.

Sweep visual evoked potentials

Recording independent responses to a range of pattern sizes to estimate acuity using the transient VEP can be a lengthy procedure and difficult to implement satisfactorily in children. 'Sweep techniques' test a range of spatial frequencies very rapidly and determine VEP thresholds as an estimate of visual acuity (Regan 1973, 1977; Tyler *et al.* 1979; Seiple *et al.* 1984). The sweep technique has been used to study visual development (Fig. 9.16) (Norcia *et al.* 1985a, b).

Sweep techniques elicit steady-state VEPs and progressively change spatial frequency. The change can be continuous or sampled, each spatial frequency presented for a discrete interval of time (commonly 5–10 seconds) (Seiple & Holopigian 1989). The 'optimal' temporal frequency giving the largest VEPs increases with maturation (Moscowitz & Sokol 1980), and is around 8 reversals/second in adults, and about 4 reversals/second in young infants less than 3 months old.

Discrete Fourier transform is a mathematical technique for examining the relative power of different frequencies deduced as contributing to the make-up of the quasi-sinusoidal VEP. Analysis is often confined to the second harmonic component as this mainly represents the response to each pattern reversal. The fundamental refers to a full to-and-fro cycle of activity, e.g. the change from a white stimulus element to black, and then back to white, and this is described by the rate of pattern reversal expressed in hertz. Thus 8 Hz is equivalent to 16 reversals/second; however, a response is expected for every reversal, thus the second harmonic frequency 2 F = 16 is a measure of this activity.

We compute a linear regression on the descending limb of the second harmonic amplitude versus spatial frequency plot—the sweep acuity is taken as the threshold point, where the extrapolation meets the x-axis, i.e. zero amplitude (Fig. 9.16). We present eight or 16 spatial frequencies during an 8-second period, depending on the resolution required and the level of co-operation of the subject. The responses to each spatial frequency are averaged and confidence limits are displayed to allow estimation of variability and statistical validity of the sweep run. Response phase is expected to lag as the pattern size presented progressively becomes smaller. A sudden change in phase, or marked increase in the phase confidence limit, gives an additional indication of unreliability in distinguishing the response from background noise.

There is a degree of interindividual and age-related variability in the spatial tuning function of the sweep VEP: it may monotonically decrease with increasing spatial frequency, or may have two or even three maximal peaks. A double peak is not uncommon in older infants and adults (Tyler *et al.* 1978; Strasburger *et al.* 1988). Pattern onset/offset stimulation gives larger amplitude responses than reversal to equivalent pattern sizes and has a simpler tuning function. However, the phase change with spatial frequency (which is a useful indicator of signal reliability with pattern reversal stimulation) is not present for onset/offset stimulation (Strasburger *et al.* 1990).

A wide range of spatial frequencies should be used to give a more accurate estimation of the threshold using linear regression. There is a need to replicate and average spatial sweeps to even out intertrial variability. It is important to maintain a child's attention on the stimulus for the duration of the spatial frequency sweep (Norcia & Tyler 1985a, b; Regan 1980, 1989). The temporal rate of pattern presentation must be age appropriate. Children with good optotype acuity have higher sweep acuity at lower temporal frequencies, and those with poor optotype acuity tend to have better sweep acuity at higher temporal rates (Gottlob *et al.* 1990).

An assessment of acuity can also be made by determining the VEP contrast sensitivity threshold to a reversing sinusoidal grating over a range of spatial frequencies (Seiple *et al.* 1984; Allen *et al.* 1986; Norcia *et al.* 1989; Spileers *et al.* 1992). There is good correlation between subjective perceptual judgements and pattern VEP amplitude estimates of contrast threshold (Campbell & Maffei 1970; Allen *et al.* 1986).

Relationship between pattern reversal visual evoked potentials and behavioural acuity

Transient VEP estimates of acuity indicate that adult levels are reached between 6 and 10 months of age (Marg *et al.* 1976; Sokol 1978; De Vries Khoe & Spekreijse 1982). Sweep VEP estimates indicate acuities of about 4.5 cycles per degree (cpd) in the first month of life, and increasing to the adult level of 20 cpd by 8 months of age (Norcia & Tyler 1985b; Allen *et al.* 1992). During the first year of life, sweep VEP acuity is higher and has a slower developmental course compared with transient VEPs. Methodological factors are also important: scoring criteria, the method of extrapolating to zero amplitude, and noise estimation have all been highlighted (Orel-Bixler & Norcia 1987). Intertrial acuities within 0.5 octave of each other can be obtained with the sweep VEP technique, and within 1–2 octaves with the transient VEP, providing it is ensured that there is close sampling near threshold.

In infancy, VEP estimates are most often compared with forced choice preferential looking acuity. VEP estimates exceed forced choice looking acuity in the first year of life but they converge later (Orel-Bixler *et al.* 1989; Sokol *et al.* 1992; Thompson *et al.* 1993). The differences between electrophysiological and behavioural acuity assessments may be accounted for by central field for VEPs versus smaller peripheral field for forced choice preferential looking, and/or by static stimulus versus changing stimulus involving motion for pattern reversal VEPs. There is good agreement of interocular acuity estimates between the two methods. We have found pattern VEPs particularly sensitive in monitoring the effects of occlusion in infants operated on for unilateral cataracts. Although the lensectomized eye shows significant improvements in acuity, we find the fellow (patched) eye shows smaller transient pattern VEPs and reduced recognition acuity using a logarithmic Minimum Angle of Resolution (log MAR) chart, compared with untreated unilateral cataract patients and healthy controls (Thompson *et al.* 1996).

References

Aaberg TB. Stargardt's disease and fundus flavimaculatus: evaluation of morphological progression and intrafamilial coexistence. *Trans Am Ophthalmol Soc* 1986; **84**: 453–87.

Agamanolis DP, Chester EM, Victor M, Kark JA, Hines JD, Harris JW. Neuropathology of experimental vitamin B_{12} deficiency in monkeys. *Neurology* 1976; **26**: 905–14.

Alani SM. Pattern reversal visual evoked potentials in patients with hydrocephalus. *J Neurosurg* 1985; **62**: 234–7.

Allen D, Banks MS, Norcia AM. Does chromatic sensitivity develop more slowly than luminance sensitivity? *Vision Res* 1993; **33**: 2553–62.

Allen D, Bennett PJ, Banks MS. The effects of luminance on FPL and VEP acuity in human infants. *Vis Res* 1992; **32**: 2005–12.

Allen D, Norcia AM, Tyler CW. A comparative study of electrophysiological and psychophysical measurement of the contrast sensitivity function in humans. *Am J Optom Physiol Opt* 1986; **63**: 442–9.

American Electroencephalographic Society. Clinical evoked potential guidelines. *J Clin Neurophysiol* 1994; **11**: 40–73.

Anderson ML, Purple RL. Circadian rhythms and variability of the clinical electro-oculogram. *Invest Ophthalmol Vis Sci* 1980; **19**: 278–88.

Apkarian P. Electrodiagnosis in paediatric ophthalmogenetics. *Int J Psychophysiol* 1994; **16**: 229–43.

Apkarian P, Bour L, Barth PG. A unique achiasmatic anomaly detected in non-albinos with misrouted retinal–fugal projections. *Eur J Neurosci* 1994; **6**: 501–7.

Apkarian P, Koetsveld-Baart JC, Barth PG. Visual evoked potential characteristics and early diagnosis of Pelizaeus–Merzbacher disease. *Arch Neurol* 1993; **50**: 981–5.

Apkarian P, Reits D, Spekreijse H. Component specificity in albino VEP asymmetry: maturation of the visual pathway anomaly. *Exp Brain Res* 1984; **53**: 285–94.

Apkarian P, Spekreijse H. The use of the electroretinogram and visual evoked potentials in ophthalmogenetics. In: Desmedt JE, ed. *Visual Evoked Potentials*. Amsterdam: Elsevier, 1990: 169–223.

Apkarian P, Van Veenendal W, Spekreijse H. Measurement of visual acuity in infants and young children by visual evoked potentials. *Doc Ophthalmol Proc Ser* 1986; **45**: 168–89.

Arden GB, Carter RM, MacFarlan A. Pattern and ganzfeld electroretinograms in macular disease. *Br J Ophthalmol* 1984; **68**: 878–84.

Arden GB, Kelsey JB. Changes produced by light in the standing potential of the human eye. *J Physiol* 1962; **61**: 189–204.

Babel J, Stangos N, Korol S, Spiritus M. *Ocular Electrophysiology: a Clinical and Experimental Study of Electroretinogram, Electro-oculogram and Visual Evoked Response*. Stuttgart: Georg Thieme, 1977.

Baker RS, Schmeisser ET, Epstein AD. Visual system electrodiagnosis in neurologic disease in childhood. *Pediatr Neurol* 1995; **12**: 99–110.

Barnet AB, Friedman SL, Weiss IP, Ohlrich ES, Shanks B, Lodge A. VEP development in infancy and early childhood. A longitudinal study. *Electroencephalog Clin Neurophysiol* 1980; **49**:476–89.

Barrett G, Blumhardt L, Halliday AM, Halliday E, Kriss A. A paradox in the lateralisation of the visual evoked response. *Nature* 1976; **261**: 253–5.

Battaglia A, Harden A, Pampiglione G, Walsh PJ. Adrenoleucodystrophy: neurophysiological aspects. *J Neurol Neurosurg Psychiatr* 1981; **44**: 781–5.

Beller R, Hoyt CS, Marg E, Odom JV. Good visual function after neonatal surgery for congenital monocular cataracts. *Am J Ophthalmol*, 1981; **91**: 559–65.

Berson EL. Electrical phenomena in the retina. In: Hart WH, ed. *Adler's Physiology of the Eye Clinical Application*. St. Louis: Mosby Year Book, 1992: 641–707.

Berson EL, Rosen JB, Siminoff EA. Electroretinographic testing as an aid in detection of X chromosome linked retinitis pigmentosa. *Am J Ophthalmol* 1979; **87**: 460–8.

Berson EL, Schmidt SY, Shih VE. Ocular and biochemical abnormalities in gyrate atrophy of the choroid and retina. *Ophthalmology* 1978; **85**: 1018–27.

Bird TD, Crill WE. Pattern-evoked potentials in the hereditary ataxias and spinal degenerations. *Ann Neurol* 1981; **9**: 243–50.

Blumhardt LD, Barratt G, Kriss A, Halliday AM. The pattern-evoked potential in lesions of the posterior visual pathways. *Ann NY Acad Sci* 1982; **388**: 264–89.

Bodis-Wollner I, Atkin A, Raab E, Wolkstein M. Visual association cortex and vision in man: pattern evoked potentials in a blind boy. *Science* 1977; **198**: 629–31.

Braddick O, Atkinson J, Julesz B, Kropfl W, Bodis-Wollner I, Raab E. Cortical binocularity in infants. *Nature* 1980; **288**: 363–5.

Brecelj J. Electrodiagnostics of chiasmal compressive lesions. *Int J Psychophysiol* 1994; **16**: 263–72.

Brecelj J, Stirn-Kranjc B. Electrophysiologic evaluation of the visual pathway in children. *Doc.Ophthalmol* 1992; **79**: 313–23.

Bresnick GH. Diabetic retinopathy. In: Heckenlively JR, Arden GB, eds. *Principles and Practice of Clinical Electrophysiology of Vision*. St Louis: CV Mosby, 1991: 619–35.

Brown DM, Graemiger RA, Hergersberg M *et al*. Genetic linkage of Wagner disease and erosive vitreoretinopathy to chromosome 5q13–14. *Arch Ophthalmol* 1995; **113**: 671–5.

Burns CA. Indomethacin, reduced retinal sensitivity and corneal deposits. *Am J Ophthalmol* 1968; **66**: 825–35.

Campbell FW, Gubisch RW. Optical quality of the human eye. *J Physiol* 1966; **186**: 558–78.

Campbell FW, Maffei L. Electrophysiological evidence for the existence of orientation and size detectors in the human visual system. *J Physiol* 1970; **207**: 635–52.

Carr RE. Congenital stationary night blindness In: Heckenlively JR, Arden GB, eds. *Principles and Practice of Clinical Electrophysiology of Vision*. St Louis: CV Mosby, 1991: 713–20.

Carroll WM, Kriss A, Baraitser M, Barrett G, Halliday AM. The incidence and nature of visual pathway involvement in Friedreich's ataxia: a clinical and visual evoked potential study of 22 patients. *Brain* 1980; **103**: 413–34.

Carroll WM, Mastaglia FL. Leber's optic neuropathy: a clinical and visual evoked potential study of affected and asymptomatic members of a six generation family. *Brain* 1979; **102**: 559–80.

Celesia GG, Archer CR, Kurroiwa Y, Goldfader PR. Visual function of the extrageniculate–calcarine system in man. *Arch Neurol* 1980; **37**: 704–6.

Chiappa K. *Evoked Potentials in Clinical Medicine* 2nd edn. New York: Raven Press, 1990.

Chiappa KH, Young RR. Evoked potentials: overused, underused and misused. *Arch Neurol* 1985; **42**: 76–7.

Chokroverty S, Duvoisin RC, Sachdeo R, Sage J, Lepore F, Nicklas W. Neurophysiologic study of olivopontocerebellar atrophy with or without glutamate dehydrogenase deficiency. *Neurology* 1985; **35**: 652–9.

Cibis GW, Fitzgerald KM. Optic nerve hypoplasia in association with brain anomalies and an abnormal ERG. *Doc Ophthalmol* 1994; **86**: 11–22.

Claridge KG, Gibberd FB, Sidney MC. Refsum disease: the presentation and ophthalmic aspects of Refsum disease in a series of 23 patients. *Eye* 1992; **6**: 371–5.

Cohen SMZ, Brown FR, Martyn L *et al*. Ocular histopathologic and biochemical studies of the cerebrohepatorenal syndrome (Zellweger's syndrome) and its relationship to neonatal adrenoleucodystrophy. *Am J Ophthalmol* 1983; **96**: 488–501.

Cosi V, Piccolo G, Callieco R. Evoked potential studies in Friedreich's ataxia and olivopontocerebellar atrophy. *Ital J Neurol Sci* 1984; **4**(Suppl.): 172–81.

Coupland SG, Janaky M. ERG electrode in pediatric patients: comparison of DTL fiber, PVA-gel, and non-corneal skin electrodes. *Doc Ophthalmol* 1989; **71**: 427–33.

Creel D. Luminance-onset, pattern onset and pattern reversal evoked potentials in human albinos demonstrating visual system anomalies. *J Biomed Eng* 1979; **1**: 100–4.

Creel D, Spekreijse H, Reits DT. Evoked potentials in albinos: efficacy of pattern stimuli in detecting misrouted optic fibers. *Electroencephalogr Clin Neurophysiol* 1981; **52**: 595–603.

Crews SJ, Thompson CRS, Harding GFA. The ERG and VEP in patients with severe eye injury. *Doc Ophthalmol Proc* 1978: **15**: 203–9.

Davson H. *Physiology of the Eye*. Oxford: Pergamon Press, 1990.

De Becker I, Riddell DC, Dooley JM, Tremblay F. Correlation between electroretinogram findings and molecular analysis in the Duchenne muscular dystrophy phenotype. *Br J Ophthalmol* 1994; **78**: 719–22.

de Jong PT, Zrenner E; van Meel GJ, Keunen JE, van Norren D. Mizuo phenomenon in X-linked retinoschisis. Pathogenesis of the Mizuo phenomenon. *Arch Ophthalmol* 1991; **109**: 1104–8.

Deutman AF. Electro-oculogram in families with vitelliform dystrophy of the fovea: detection of the carrier state. *Arch Ophthalmol* 1969; **81**: 305–16.

De Vries Khoe LH, Spekreijse H. Maturation of luminance and pattern EPs in man. *Doc Ophthalmol Proc* 1982; **31**: 461–75.

Dorfman LJ, Nikoskelainen E, Rosenthal AR, Sogg RL. Visual evoked potentials in Leber's optic neuropathy. *Ann Neurol* 1977; **1**: 565–8.

Drasdo N, Edwards L, Thompson DA. Models of the visual cortex based on visual evoked potentials. In: Gulyas B, Ottoson D, Roland PE, eds. *Functional Organisation of the Human Visual Cortex*, Wenner Gren International Series, Vol. 61. Oxford: Pergamon Press, 1993: 255–70.

Esakowitz L, Kriss A, Shawkat F. A comparison of flash electroretinograms recorded from Burian–Allen, JET, C-glide, gold foil, DTL and skin electrodes. *Eye* 1993; **7**: 169–71.

Fagan ER, Taylor MJ. Longitudinal multimodal evoked potential studies in abetalipoproteinaemia. *Canad J Neurol Sci* 1987; **14**: 617–21.

Falk G. Retinal physiology. In: Heckenlively JR, Arden GB, eds. *Principles and Practice of Clinical Electrophysiology of Vision*. St Louis: CV Mosby, 1991: 69–84.

Farley MK, Heckenlively JR. Blue cone monochromatism. In: Heckenlively JR, Arden GB, eds. *Principles and Practice of Clinical Electrophysiology of Vision*. St Louis: CV Mosby, 1991: 753–5.

Fellman DJ, Van Essen D. Distributed hierarchical processing in the primate visual cortex. *Cerebral Cortex* 1991; **1**: 1–47.

Fine EJ, Hallett M. Neurophysiological study of subacute combined degeneration. *J Neurol Sci* 1980; **45**: 331–6.

Fishman GA, Farber MD, Derlacki DJ. X-linked retinitis pigmentosa: profile of clinical findings. *Arch Ophthalmol* 1988; **106**: 369–75.

Fishman GA, Jampol LM, Goldberg MF. Diagnostic features of the Favre–Goldman syndrome. *Br J Ophthalmol* 1976; **60**: 345–55.

Fishman GA, Sokol S. *Electrophysiological Testing*. San Francisco: American Academy of Ophthalmology Monograph, 1990.

Fishman GA, Weinburg AB, McMahon TT. X-linked recessive retinitis pigmentosa: clinical characteristics of carriers. *Arch Ophthalmol* 1986; **104**: 1329–35.

Fitzgerald KM, Cibis GW, Giambrone SA, Harris DJ. Retinal signal transmission in Duchenne muscular dystrophy: evidence for dysfunction in the photoreceptor depolarising bipolar cell pathway. *J Clin Invest* 1994; **93**: 2425–30.

Flanagan JG, Harding GFA. Multi-channel visual evoked potentials in early compressive lesions of the optic chiasm. *Doc Ophthalmol* 1987; **69**: 271–82.

Folz SJ, Trobe JD. The peroxisome and the eye. *Surv Ophthalmol* 1991; **35**: 353–68.

France TD Electrophysiologic testing and its specific application in unsedated children. *Trans Am Ophthalmol Soc* 1984; **82**: 383–445.

Francois J, DeRouck A. Electroretinographic study of the hypoplasia of the optic nerve. *Ophthalmologica* 1976; **172**: 308–30.

Fuller DG, Hutton WL. *Presurgical Evaluation of Eyes with Opaque Media*. New York: Grune & Stratton, 1982.

Fulton AB, Hansen RM. Electroretinography: application to clinical studies of infants. *J Pediatr Ophthalmol Strabismus* 1985; **22**: 251–5.

Fulton AB, Hansen RM, Glynn RJ. Natural course of visual functions in the Bardet–Biedel syndrome. *Arch Ophthalmol* 1993; **111**: 1500–6.

Fulton AB, Hartmann EE, Hansen RM. Electrophysiological testing techniques for children. *Documenta Ophthalmol* 1989; **71**: 341–54.

Galloway NR. Electrophysiological testing of eyes with opaque media. *Eye* 1988; **2**: 615–24.

Garner A, Fielder AR, Primavesi R, Steven A. Tapetoretinal degeneration in the cerebro-hepato-renal (Zellweger) syndrome. *Br J Ophthalmol* 1982; **66**: 422–31.

Gelbart SS, Hoyt CS. Congenital nystagmus: a clinical perspective in infancy. *Graefe's Arch Clin Exp Ophthalmol* 1988; **266**: 178–80.

George SR, Taylor MJ. VEPs and SEPs in hydrocephalic infants before and after shunting. *Clin Neurol Neurosurg* 1987; (Suppl. 1): 96.

Gerritson EJA, Vossen JM, van Loo IGH *et al.* Autosomal recessive osteopetrosis: variability of findings at diagnosis and during the natural course. *Pediatrics* 1994; **93**: 247–53.

Givre SJ, Schroeder CE, Arezzo JC. Contribution of extrastriate area V4 to the surface recorded flash VEP in the awake macaque. *Vision Res* 1994; **34**: 415–28.

Goss-Sampson MA, Muller DPR, Kriss A. Abnormalities of the electroretinogram and visual evoked potentials in vitamin E deficient rats. *Exp Eye Res* 1991; **53**: 623–7.

Gottlob I, Fendick MG, Guo S, Zubcov AA, Odom JV, Reinecke RR. Visual acuity measurement by swept spatial frequency visual-evoked cortical potentials (VECPs): clinical application in children with various disorders. *J Pediatr Ophthalmol Strabismus* 1990; **27**: 40–7.

Gouras P, Carr RE, Gunkel RD. Retinitis pigmentosa in abetalipoproteinemia: effects of vitamin A. *Invest Ophthalmol Vis Sci* 1971: **10**: 784–93.

Griff ER. Electroretinographic components arising in the distal retina. In: Heckenlively JR, Arden GB, eds. *Principles and Practice of Clinical Electrophysiology of Vision*. St Louis: CV Mosby, 1991: 91–8.

Griner PF, Glase RJ. Misuse of laboratory tests and diagnostic procedures. *N Engl J Med* 1982; **307**: 1336–9.

Grose J, Harding GFA, Wilton AY, Bissenden JG. The maturation of the pattern reversal VEP and flash ERG in pre-term infants. *Clin Vis Sci* 1989; **4**: 239–46.

Groswasser Z, Kriss A, Halliday AM, McDonald WI. Pattern- and flash-evoked potentials in the assessment and management of optic nerve gliomas. *J Neurol Neurosurg Psychiatr* 1985; **48**: 1125–34.

Halliday AM. *Evoked Potentials in Clinical Testing*, 2nd edn. Edinburgh: Churchill Livingstone, 1993.

Halliday AM, Barrett G, Blumhardt LD, Kriss A. The macular and paramacular components of the pattern evoked response. In: Lehmann D, Callaway E, eds. *Human Evoked Potentials: Applications and Problems*. New York: Plenum Press, 1979: 135–51.

Halliday AM, Kriss A. The visual evoked potential and electroretinogram in the investigation of diseases of the eye. In: Halliday AM, ed. *Evoked Potentials in Clinical Testing*, 2nd edn. Edinburgh: Churchill Livingstone, 1993: 141–94.

Halliday AM, Kriss A, Cuendent F, Francis D, McDonald WI, Taylor D. Childhood optic neuritis: a study of pattern and flash evoked potentials. In: Gallai V, ed. *Maturation of the CNS and Evoked Potentials*. Amsterdam: Elsevier, 1986: 41–50.

Halliday AM, McDonald WI, Mushin J. Delayed pattern-evoked responses in optic neuritis in relation to visual acuity. *Trans Ophthalmol Soc UK* 1973; **93**: 315–24.

Harden A, Adams GG, Taylor D. The electroretinogram. *Arch Dis*

Child 1989; **64**: 1080–7.

Harden A, Pampiglione G. Neurophysiological approach to disorders of vision. *Lancet* 1970; **i**: 805–9.

Harden A, Pampiglione G. Neurophysiological studies (EEG/ERG/VEP/SEP) in 88 children with so-called neuronal ceroid lipofuscinosis. In: Armstrong D, Koppang N, Rider JA, eds. *Ceroid Lipofuscinosis (Batten's disease)*. Amsterdam: Elsevier, 1982: 61–70.

Harding GFA, Crews SJ. The VER in hereditary optic atrophy of the dominant type. In: Mauguiere F, Courjon F, eds. *The Clinical Applications of Evoked Potentials in Neurology*. New York: Raven Press, 1982: 21–30.

Harding GFA, Grose J ,Wilton A, Bissenden JG. The pattern reversal VEP in short gestation infants. *Electroencephalogr Clin Neurophysiol* 1989; **74** : 76–80.

Harding GFA, Williams DE, Innes JA. The visual evoked potentials and psychophysics during ethambutol therapy. In: Nodar RH, Barber C, eds. *Evoked Potentials*, Vol. II. Boston: Butterworth, 1984: 339–44.

Harris GS, Yeung J. Maculopathy of sex-linked juvenile retinoschisis. *Canad J Ophthalmol* 1976; **11**: 1–10.

Hart WM, ed. *Adler's Physiology of the Eye, Clinical Application*. St Louis: CV Mosby Year Book, 1992.

Harter MR, Deaton FK, Odom JV. Maturation of evoked potentials and visual preference in 6–45 day old babies: effects of check size, visual acuity and refractive error. *Electroencephalogr Clin Neurophysiol* 1977; **42**: 595–607.

Heckenlively JR, Arden GB. *Principles and Practice of Clinical Electrophysiology of Vision*. St Louis: CV Mosby Year Book, 1991.

Heynen H, Wachtmeister L, van Norren D. Origin of the oscillatory potentials in the primate retina. *Vision Res* 1985; **25**: 1365–74.

Hill DA, Arbel KF, Berson EL. Cone electroretinograms in congenital nyctalopia with myopia. *Am J Ophthalmol* 1974; **78**: 127–36.

Hing S, Wilson-Holt N, Kriss A, Flueler U, Taylor DSI. Complete cryptophthalmos: a case report with normal flash VEP and ERG. *Pediatr Opthalmol Strabismus* 1990; **27**: 133–5.

Hirose T, Lee KY, Schepens C. Wagner's hereditary vitreoretinal degeneration and retinal detachment. *Arch Ophthalmol* 1973; **89**: 176–85.

Hirose T, Wolf E, Hara A. Electrophysiological and psychophysical studies in congenital retinoschisis X-linked recessive inheritance. *Documenta Ophthal Proc* 1977; **13**: 173–84.

Hodes ME, Pratt VM, Dlouhy SR. Genetics of Pelizaeus–Merzbacher disease. *Dev Neurosci* 1993; **15**: 383–94.

Holder G. The significance of abnormal pattern electroretinograms in anterior pathway dysfunction. *Br J Ophthalmol* 1987; **71**: 166–71.

Holder GE. The effects of chiasmal compression on the pattern visual evoked potential. *Electroencephalogr Clin Neurophysiol* 1978; **45**: 278–80.

Horsten GPM, Winkleman JE. Electrical activity of the retina in relation to histological differentiation in infants born prematurely and at full term. *Vision Res* 1962; **2**: 269–76.

Hoyt CS. The clinical usefulness of the visual evoked response. *J Pediatr Ophthalmol Strabismus* 1984; **21**: 231–4.

Hoyt CS, Billson FA. Visual loss in osteopetrosis. *Am J Dis Child* 1979; **133**: 955–8.

Hull BM, Thompson DA. A review of the clinical applications of the pattern electroretinogram. *Ophthalmic Physiol Opt* 1989; **9**: 143–52.

Hutton WL, Fuller DG. Factors influencing final visual results in severely injured eyes. *Am J Ophthalmol* 1984; **97**: 715–22.

Ikeda H. Electrodiagnosis of the primary afferent visual system. Past, present and future. *Zdrv Vestn* 1993; (Suppl. 1): 57–66.

Jabbari B, Maitland CG, Morris LM, Morales J, Gunderson CH. The value of visual evoked potential as a screening test in neurofibromatosis. *Arch Neurol* 1985; **42**: 1072–4.

Jacobs M, Shawkat F, Harris CH, Kriss A, Taylor D. Eye movement and electrophysiological findings in an infant with hemispheric pathology. *Dev Med Child Neurol* 1993; **35**: 431–5.

Janaky M, Deak A, Pelle Z, Benedek G. Electrophysiologic alterations in patients with optic nerve hypoplasia. *Documenta Ophthalmol* 1994; **86**: 247–57.

Jasper HH. Report of the committee on methods of clinical examinations in electroencephalography. *Electroenceph Clin Neurophysiol* 1958; **10**: 370–5.

Kaiser-Kupfer MI, Ludwig IH, de Monasterio FM *et al.* Gyrate atrophy of the choroid and retina: early findings. *Ophthalmology* 1985; **92**: 394–410.

Karwoski C, Kawasaki K. Oscillatory potentials. In: Heckenlively JR, Arden GB, eds. *Principles and Practice of Clinical Electrophysiology of Vision*. St Louis: CV Mosby Year Book, 1991: 125–8.

Keith CG. Retinal atrophy in osteopetrosis. *Arch Ophthalmol* 1968; **79**: 234–41.

Kim RY, Fitzke FW, Moore AT *et al.* Autosomal dominant retinitis pigmentosa mapping to chromosome 7p exhibits variable expression. *Br Ophthalmol* 1995; **79**: 23–7.

Kolder HE. Electro-oculography. In: Heckenlively JR, Arden GB, eds. *Principles and Practice of Clinical Electrophysiology of Vision*. St Louis: CV Mosby Year Book, 1991: 301–14.

Kolodny EH. Dysmyelinating and demyelinating conditions in infancy. *Curr Opin Neurol Neurosurg* 1993; **6**: 379–86.

Kriss A. Recording technique. In: Halliday AM, ed. *Evoked Potentials in Clinical Testing*, 2nd edn. Edinburgh: Churchill Livingstone, 1993a: 1–56.

Kriss A. Skin ERGs their effectiveness when recording from young children and comparision with ERGs recorded using various types of corneal electrode. *Int J Psychophysiol* 1994; **16**: 137–46.

Kriss A. Visual electrophysiological testing of young children. *Zdrav Vestn* 1993b; **62**(Suppl 1): 85–90.

Kriss A, Carroll WM, Blumhardt LD, Halliday AM. Pattern and flash evoked potential changes in toxic (nutritional) optic neuropathy. In: Courjon J, Maugiere F, Revol M, eds. *Clinical Applications of Evoked Potentials in Neurology*, Vol. 32. *Advances in Neurology*. New York: Raven Press, 1982: 11–19.

Kriss A, Francis D, Cluendet F *et al.* Recovery after optic neuritis in childhood. *J Neurol Neurosurg Psychiatr* 1988; **51**: 1253–8.

Kriss A, Gresty M, Shawkat F, Taylor D. Effects of induced nystagmus on pattern and flash VEPs. *Ophthalmol Physiol Optics* 1989; **9**: 103–9.

Kriss A, Jeffrey B, Taylor D. The electroretinogram in infants and young children. *J Clin Neurophysiol* 1992a; **9**: 373–93.

Kriss A, Russell-Eggitt I. Electrophysiological assessment of visual pathway function in infants. *Eye* 1992; **6**: 145–53.

Kriss A, Russell-Eggitt I, Harris CM, Lloyd IC, Taylor DSI. Aspects of albinism. *Ophthalmol Paediatr Genet* 1992b; **13**: 89–100.

Kriss A, Russell-Eggitt I, Taylor DSI. Childhood albinism. Visual electrophysiological features. *Ophthalmol Paediatr Genet* 1990; **11**: 185–92.

Kriss A, Thompson DA. Value of ERG and VEP tesing in infantile osteopetrosis. *Inv Ophthalmol Vis Sci* 1995; **36**(Suppl.): 4.

Kriss A, Thompson DA, Lloyd IC, Jeffrey B, Russell-Eggitt I, Taylor D. Pattern VEP findings in young children treated for unilateral congenital cataract . In: Cottlier E, ed. *Congenital Cataracts*. Austin: RG Landes, 1994: 79–88.

Krumholtz A, Weiss HD, Goldstein PJ, Harris KC. Evoked responses in vitamin B_{12} deficiency. *Ann Neurol* 1981; **9**: 407–9.

Kubova Z, Kuba M. Clinical application of motion-onset potentials. *Documenta Ophthalmol* 1992; **81**: 209–18.

Kuppersmith MJ, Siegel IM, Carr RE, Ransohoff J, Flamm E, Shakin E. Visual evoked potentials in chiasmal gliomas in four adults. *Arch Neurol* 1981; **38**: 362–6.

Kurtzberg D, Vaughan HG. Electrophysiologic assessment of auditory and visual function in the newborn. *Clin Perinatol* 1985; **12**: 277–99.

Lachapelle P, Little JM, Polomeno RC. The photopic electroretinogram in congenital stationary night blindness with myopia. *Invest Ophthalmol Vis Sci* 1983; **24**: 442–50.

Lambert SR, Kriss A, Taylor D. Delayed visual maturation: a longitudinal clinical and electrophysiological assessment. *Ophthalmol* 1989a; **96**: 534–29.

Lambert SR, Kriss A, Taylor D. Detection of isolated occipital lobe anomalies during early childhood. *Dev Med Ch Neurol* 1990; **32**: 451–5.

Lambert SR, Kriss A, Taylor DSI. Joubert syndrome. *Arch Ophthalmology* 1989b; **107**: 709–13.

Lambert SR, Kriss A, Taylor D, Coffey R, Pembrey M. Follow-up and diagnostic re-appraisal of 75 patients with Leber's congenital amaurosis. *Am J Ophthalmol* 1989c; **107**: 624–31.

Lambert SR, Taylor DSI, Kriss A. The infant with nystagmus, normal appearing fundi but an abnormal ERG. *Surv Ophthalmol* 1989d; **34**: 176–86.

Lamy M, Frezal J, Polonovski J *et al*. Congenital absence of beta-lipoproteins. *Pediatrics* 1963; **31**: 277–89.

Lang GE, Maumenee IH. Retinal dystrophies associated with storage diseases. In: Newsome DA, ed. *Retinal Dystrophies and Degenerations*. New York: Raven Press, 1988: 319–40.

Lavy T, Harris CM, Shawkat F, Thompson D, Kriss A. An ERG, VEP and eye movement assessment of children with Bardet–Biedel syndrome In: Lennerstrand G, ed. *Update on Strabismus and Pediatric Ophthalmology*. Boca Raton: CRC Press, 1995: 549–52.

Lawill T. The bar pattern electroretinogram for clinical evaluation of the central retina. *Am J Ophthalmol* 1974; **78**: 121–6.

Leitch J, Thompson DA, Harris C, Shawkat F, Kriss A. Achiasmia in a case of midline craniofacial cleft with see-saw nystagmus. *Brit J Ophthalmol* 1997 (in press).

Lennerstrand G. Delayed visual evoked cortical potentials in retinal disease. *Acta Ophthalmol (Copenh)* 1982; **60**: 497–504.

Lestienne P, Bataille N. Mitochondrial DNA alterations and genetic diseases: a review. *Biomed Pharmacother* 1994; **48**: 199–214.

Livingstone MS, Hubel DH. Segregation of form, colour, movement and depth: anatomy, physiology and perception. *Science* 1988; **240**: 740–50.

Mactier H, Dexter JD, Hewett JE, Latham CB, Woodruff CW. The electroretinogram in preterm infants. *J Pediatr* 1988; **113**: 607–12.

Mandelbaum S, Cleary PE, Ruan SJ, Ogden TE. Bright flash electroretinography and vitreous hemorrhage. *Arch Ophthalmol* 1980; **98**: 1823–8.

Marg E, Freeman DN, Peltzman P, Goldstein PJ. Visual acuity development in human infants: evoked potential measurements. *Invest Ophthalmol Vis Sci* 1976; **15**: 150–3.

Markwardt F, Gopfert E, Muller R. Influence of velocity, temporal frequency and initial phase position of grating patterns on the motion VEP. *Biomed Biochem Acta* 1988; **47**: 753–60.

Marmor MF. Clinical electrophysiology of the retinal pigment epithelium. *Documenta Ophthalmol* 1991; **76**: 301–14.

Marmor MF. Corneal electroretinograms in children without sedation. *J Pediatr Ophthalmol* 1976; **13**: 112–16.

Marmor MF, Arden GB, Nilsson SE, Zrenner E. Standard for clinical electroretinography. *Arch Ophthalmol* 1989; **107**: 816–19.

Marmor MF, Zrenner E. Standard for clinical electroretinography (1994 update). *Documenta Ophthalmol* 1995; **89**: 199–210.

Marmor MF, Zrenner E. Standard for clinical electro-oculography. International Society of Clinical Electrophysiology of Vision. *Arch Ophthalmol* 1993; **111**: 601–4.

McCulloch DL, Skarf B. Pattern reversal visual evoked potentials following early treatment of unilateral congenital cataract. *Arch Ophthalmol* 1994; **112**: 510–18.

Merigan WH. P and M pathway specialisation in the macaque. In: Valberg A, Lee BB, eds. *From Pigments to Perception Advances in Understanding Visual Processes*. NATO ASI Series No. 203. Plenum Press: 117–25.

Miyake Y. Carrier state of congenital stationary night blindness. In: Heckenlively JR, Arden GB, eds. *Principles and Practice of Clinical Electrophysiology of Vision*. St. Louis: Mosby Year Book, 1991: 711–12.

Miyake Y, Yagasaki K, Horiguchi M, Kawase Y, Kanda T. Congenital stationary night blindness with a negative electroretinogram: a new classification. *Arch Ophthalmol* 1986; **104**: 1013–20.

Moore AT, Fitzke F, Jay M *et al*. Autosomal dominant retinitis pigmentosa with apparent incomplete penetrance: a clinical, electrophysiological, psychophysical, and molecular genetic study. *Br J Ophthalmol* 1993; **77**: 473–9.

Moskowitz A, Sokol S. Developmental changes in the visual system as reflected by the latency of the pattern reversal VEP. *Electroencephalogr Clin Neurophysiol* 1983; **56**: 1–15.

Moskowitz A, Sokol S. Spatial and temporal interaction of pattern-evoked cortical potentials in human infants. *Vision Res* 1980; **20**: 699–707.

Mullie MA, Harding AE, Petty RKP, Ikeda H, Morgan-Hughes JA, Sanders MD. The retinal manifestations of mitochondrial myopathy: a study of 22 cases. *Arch Ophthalmol* 1985; **103**: 1825–30.

Musarella MA, Anson-Cartwright C, McDowell C *et al*. Physical mapping at a potential X-linked retinitis pigmentosa locus (RP3) by pulsed field gel electrophoresis. *Genomics* 1991; **11**: 263–72.

Mushin J, Hogg CR, Dubowitz LMS, Skouteli H, Arden GB. Visual evoked responses to light emitting diode (LED) photostimulation in newborn infants. *Electroencephalogr Clin Neurophysiol* 1984; **58**: 317–20.

Nasr YG, Cherfan GM, Michels RG, Wilkinson CP. Goldmann–Favre maculopathy. *Retina* 1990; **10**: 178–80.

Newman EA, Frishman L. The b-wave. In: Heckenlively JR, Arden GB, eds. *Principles and Practice of Clinical Electrophysiology of Vision*. St Louis: CV Mosby, 1991: 101–11.

Niemeyer G. Pharmacological effects in retinal electrophysiology. In: Heckenlively JR, Arden GB, eds. *Principles and Practice of Clinical Electrophysiology of Vision*. St Louis: CV Mosby, 1991: 151–62.

Nobel KG, Carr RE. Stargardt's disease and fundus flavimaculatus. *Arch Ophthalmol* 1979; **97**: 1281–5.

Norcia AM, Garcia H, Humphry R, Holmes A, Hamer ARD, Orel-Bixler D. Anomalous motion VEPs in infants and in infantile esotropia. *Invest Ophthalmol Vis Sci* 1991; **32**: 436–9.

Norcia AM, Tyler CW. Infant VEP acuity measurements: analysis of individual differences and measurement error. *Electroencephalogr Clin Neurophysiol* 1985a; **61**: 359–69.

Norcia AM, Tyler CW. Spatial frequency sweep VEP: visual acuity during the first year of life. *Vision Res* 1985b; **25**: 1399–408.

Norcia AM, Tyler CW, Hamer RD, Weseman W. Measurement of spatial contrast sensitivity with the swept contrast VEP. *Vision Res* 1989; **29**: 627–37.

Nuwer MR, Perlman SL, Packwood JW, Kark RAP. Evoked potential abnormalities in the various inherited ataxias. *Ann Neurol* 1983; **13**: 20–7.

Odom JV, Green M. Visual evoked potential (VEP) acuity: testability in a clinical pediatric population. *Acta Ophthalmol* 1984; **62**: 993–8.

Orel-Bixler D, Haegerstrom-Portnoy G, Hall A. Visual assessment of the multiply handicapped patient. *Optom Vis Sci* 1989; **66**: 530–6.

Orel-Bixler DA, Norcia AM. Differential growth for steady state pattern reversal and transient onset–offset VEPs. *Clin Vis Sci* 1987; **2**: 1–10.

Papakostopoulos D. Clinical electrophysiology of the human visual system. In: Chiarenza GA, Papakostopoulos D, eds. *Clinical Applications of Cerebral Evoked Potentials in Pediatric Medicine*. Amsterdam: Excerpta Medica, 1982: 3–40.

Papakostopoulos D, Dean Hart JC, Papathanasopoulos P, Vougioucas A, Harney B. The pattern VEP and flicker following electroretinogram and EEG in cone and rod dystrophies. *Electroencephogr Clin Neurophysiol* 1987; **67**: 45P–51P.

Papakostopoulos D, Doran RM, Ragge NK, Dean Hart JC. Electroretinography and pattern reversal evoked potentials in retinoschisis. *Electroencephalogr Clin Neurophysiol* 1989; **72**: 40.

Papathanasopoulos PG, Papakostopoulos D. Pattern reversal visual evoked potentials in retinitis pigmentosa. *Int J Psychophysiol* 1994; **16**: 245–50.

Patel CK, Taylor D, Russell-Eggitt I, Kriss A, Demaeral P. Congenital third nerve palsy associated with mid-trimester amniocentesis. *Br J Ophthalmol* 1993; **77**: 530–3.

Pinckers A. Berson test for blue cone monochromatism. *Int Ophthalmol* 1992; **16**: 185–6.

Poll The BT, Billettee de Villemeur T, Abitol M, Dufier JL, Saudubray JM. Metabolic pigmentary retinopathies; diagnosis and therapeutic attempts. *Eur J Pediatr* 1992 **151**: 2–11.

Pryds O, Greisen G. Preservation of single flash visual evoked potentials at very low cerebral oxygen delivery in preterm infants. *Pediatr Neurol* 1990; **6**: 151–8.

Regan D. Colour coding of pattern responses in man investigated by evoked potential feedback and direct plot techniques. *Vision Res* 1975; **15**: 175–83.

Regan D. *Human Brain Electrophysiology*. Amsterdam: Elsevier, 1989.

Regan D. Rapid methods for refracting the eye and for assessing visual acuity in amblyopia, using steady-state visual evoked potentials. In: Desmedt JE, ed. *Visual Evoked Potentials in Man: New Developments*. Oxford: Clarendon Press, 1977: 418–26.

Regan D. Rapid objective refraction using evoked brain potentials. *Invest Ophthalmol* 1973; **12**: 669–79.

Regan D. Speedy evoked potential methods for assessing vision in normal and amblyopic eyes: pros and cons. *Vision Res* 1980; **20**: 265–70.

Regan D, Regal D, Tibbles JAR. Evoked potentials during recovery from blindness recorded serially from an infant and his normally sighted twin. *Electroencephalogr Clin Neurophysiol* 1982; **54**: 465–8.

Regan D, Spekreijse H. Evoked potential indications of colour blindness. *Vision Res* 1974; **14**: 89–95.

Ripps H. Night blindness revisited: from man to molecules. Proctor lecture. *Invest Ophthalmol Vis Sci* 1982; **23**: 588–609.

Ripps H, Mahaffy L, Siegel IM, Niemeyer G. Vincristine-induced changes in the retina of isolated arterially perfused cat eye. *Exp Eye Res* 1989; **48**: 771–90.

Ruether K, Apfelstedt-Sylla E, Zrenner E. Clinical findings in patients with congenital stationary night blindness of the Schubert–Bornschein type. *Geriatr J Ophthalmol* 1993; **2**: 429–35.

Runge P, Calver D, Marshall J, Taylor D. Histopathology of mitochondrial cytopathy and the Laurence–Moon–Biedl syndrome. *Br J Ophthalmol* 1986a; **70**: 782–96.

Runge P, Muller DPR, McAllister J *et al.* Oral vitamin E can prevent the retinopathy of abetalipoproteinaemia. *Br J Ophthalmol* 1986b; **70**: 166–73.

Russell-Eggitt I, Kriss A, Taylor D. Albinism in childhood: a flash VEP and ERG study. *Br J Ophthalmol* 1990; **74**: 136–40.

Schroeder CE, Tenke CE, Givre SJ, Arezzo JC, Vaughan HG Jr. Striate cortical contribution to the surface recorded pattern reversal VEP in the alert monkey. *Vision Res* 1991; **31** (7–8): 1143–57 (also published erratum *Vision Res* 1991 **31** (11): 1).

Seiple W, Holopigian K. An examination of VEP response phase. *Electroencephalogr Clin Neurophysiol* 1989; **73**: 520–31.

Seiple WH, Kupersmith MJ, Nelson JJ, Carr RE. The assessment of evoked potential contrast thresholds using real time retrieval. *Invest Ophthalmol Vis Sci* 1984; **25**: 627–31.

Sieving PA. Photopic ON. OFF-pathway abnormalities in retinal dystrophies. *Trans Am Ophthalmol Soc* 1993; **91**: 701–73.

Sigesmund DA, Weleber RG, Pillers DM *et al.* Characterisation of the ocular phenotype of Duchenne and Becker muscular dystrophy *Ophthalmology* 1994; **101**: 856–65.

Skarf B, Eizenmann M, Katz LM, Bachynski B, Klein R. A new VEP system for studying binocular single vision in human infants. *J Pediatr Ophthalmol Strabismus* 1993; **30**: 237–42.

Sklar FH, Ehle AL, Clarke WK. Visual evoked potentials: a non-invasive technique to monitor patients with shunted hydrocephalus. *Neurosurgery* 1979; **4**: 529–34.

Snead MP, Payne SJ, Barton DE *et al.* Stickler syndrome: correlation between vitreoretinal phenotypes and linkage to COL 2A1. *Eye* 1994; **8**: 609–14.

Sokol S. An electrodiagnostic test of macular degeneration. *Arch Ophthalmol* 1972; **88**: 619–24.

Sokol S. Maturation of visual function studied by visual evoked potentials. In: Desmedt JE, ed. *Visual Evoked Potentials*. Amsterdam: Elsevier, 1990a: 35–44.

Sokol S. Measurement of infant visual acuity from pattern reversal evoked potentials. *Vision Res* 1978; **18**: 33–9.

Sokol S. The visually evoked cortical potential in optic nerve and visual pathway disorders. In: Fishman GA, Sokol S, eds. *Electrophysiological Testing in Disorders of the Retina, Optic Nerve, and Visual Pathway*. San Francisco: American Academy of Ophthalmology, 1990b: 105–42.

Sokol S, Moskowitz A, McCormack G. Infant VEP and preferential looking acuity measured with phase alternating gratings. *Invest Ophthalmol Vis Sci* 1992; **33**: 3156–61.

Spekreijse H. Maturation of contrast EPs and development of visual resolution. *Arch Ital Biol* 1978; **116**: 358–69.

Speros P, Price J. Oscillatory potentials: history, techniques, and potential use in the evaluation of disturbances of retinal circulation. *Surv Ophthalmol* 1981; **25**: 237–52.

Spileers W, Maes H, Van Hulle M, Missotten L, Orban GA. Contrast modulated steady state evoked potentials (CMSS VEPS) measuring static and dynamic contrast sensitivity. *Clin Vis Res* 1992; **7**: 93–106.

Sprague JB, Wilson WB. Electrophysiological findings in bilateral optic nerve hypoplasia. *Arch Ophthalmol* 1981; **99**: 1028–9.

Sridharan R. Visual evoked potentials in spinocerebellar degenerations. *Clin Neurol Neurosurg* 1983; **85**: 235–43.

Stadtler G. Electrophysiological results in several types of macular dystrophy. *Dev Ophthalmol* 1984; **9**: 204–12.

Stanesu-Segal B, Evrard P. Zellweger syndrome, retinal involvement. *Metab Pediatr Syst Ophthalmol* 1989; **12**: 96–9.

Strasburger H, Scheider W, Rentschler I. Amplitude and phase characteristics of the steady state visual evoked potential. *Applied Optics* 1988; **27**: 1069–87.

Taylor MJ. Evoked potentials in paediatrics. In: Halliday AM, ed. *Evoked Potentials in Clinical Testing*. Edinburgh: Churchill Livingstone, 1993: 489–521.

Taylor MJ, Menzies R, MacMillan LJ, Whyte HE. VEPs in normal full-term and premature neonates: longitudinal versus cross-sectional data. *Electroencephalogr Clin Neurophysiol* 1987; **68**: 20–7.

Taylor MJ, McCulloch DL. The prognostic value of VEPs in young children with acute onset cortical blindness. *Pediatr Neurol* 1991; **7**: 86–90.

Taylor MJ, McCulloch DL. Visual evoked potentials in infants and children. *J Clin Neurophysiol* 1992; **9**: 357–72.

Taylor MJ, Murphy WJ, Whyte HE. Prognostic reliability of SEPs and VEPs in asphyxiated term infants. *Dev Med Child Neurol* 1992; **34**: 507–15.

Thaler A, Lessel MR, Heilig P. Light induced oscillations of the standing potential in achromatopisa. *Doc Ophthalmol* 1986; **63**: 333–6.

Thompson CRS, Harding GFA. The visual evoked potential in patients with cataracts. *Doc Ophthalml Proc* 1978; **15**: 193–201.

Thompson DA, Drasdo N. Temporal patterns and the topography of the visual evoked potential. In: *Noninvasive Assessment of the Visual System*, Vol. 1, Technical Digest series. (Optical Society of America) 1992; **1**: 150–3.

Thompson DA, Lloyd IC, Dowler J *et al.* The development of spatial resolution measured by swept VEP and forced choice preferential looking techniques. *Inv Ophthalmol Vis Sci* 1993; **34**(Suppl.): 1354.

Thompson DA, Moller H, Russell-Eggitt RE, Kriss A. Visual acuity in unilateral cataract. *Br J Ophthalmol* 1996; **80**: 1–5.

Tolhurst DJ. Separate channels for the analysis of the shape and movement of a moving visual stimulus. *J Physiol* 1973; **231**: 385–402.

Tremblay F, LaRoche RG, Shea SE, Ludman MD. Longitudinal study of the early electroretinographic changes in Alstrom's syndrome. *Am J Ophthalmol* 1993; **115**: 657–65.

Troncoso J, Mancall EL, Schatz NJ. Visual evoked responses in pernicious anemia. *Arch Neurol* 1979; **36**: 168–9.

Tyler CW, Apkarian P, Levi DM, Nakayama K. Rapid assessment of visual function: an electronic sweep technique for the pattern VEP. *Invest Ophthalmol Vis Sci* 1979; **18**: 703–13.

Tyler CW, Apkarian P, Nakayama K. Multiple spatial frequency tuning of electrical responses from human visual cortex. *Expl Brain Res* 1978; **33**: 535–50.

Vey EK, Wlodzimierz MK, Danowski TS. Electroretinographic testing in diabetics: a comparision study of the Burian–Allen and Henkes corneal electrodes. *Doc Ophthalmol* 1979; **48**: 337–44.

Vjijland HR, Van Lith GH. Cataract, pattern stimulation and visually evoked potentials. *Doc Ophthalmol* 1983; **55**: 107–12.

Wachtmeister L, Dowling J. The oscillatory potentials of the mud-

puppy retina. *Invest Ophthalmol Vis Sci* 1978; **17**: 1176–88.

Wang PJ, Young C, Liu HM, Chang YC, Shen YZ. Neurophysiologic studies and MRI in Pelizaeus–Merzbacher disease: comparison of classic and connatal forms. *Pediatr Neurol* 1995; **12**(1): 47–53.

Watanabe K, Yamaday H, Hara K, Miyazaki S, Nakamura S. Neurophysiological evaluation of newborns with congenital hydrocephalus. *Clin Electroencephalogr* 1984; **15**: 22–31.

Wattam-Bell J. Development of motion specific cortical responses in infancy. *Vision Res* 1991; **31**: 287–97.

Weiss AH, Biersdorff WR. Visual sensory disorders in congenital nystagmus. *Ophthalmology* 1989; **96**: 517–23.

Weleber RG, Kennaway NG. Clinical trial of vitamin B6 for gyrate atrophy of the choroid and retina. *Ophthalmology* 1981; **88**: 316–24.

Weleber RG, Kennaway NG. Infantile Refsum's disease. In: Gold DH, Weingeist TA, eds. *The Eye in Systemic Disease*. Philadelphia: JP Lippincott, 1990: 409–11.

Weleber RG, Palmer EA. Electrophysiologic evaluation of children with visual impairment. *Semin Ophthalmol* 1991; **6**: 161–8.

Wenzel D, Brandl U. Maturation of evoked potentials elicited by checkerboard reversal. *Dev Ophthalmol* 1984; **9**: 87–93.

Whyte HE, Taylor ME, Menzies R, Chin K, Macmillan LJ. Prognostic utility of visual evoked potentials in term asphyxiated neonates. *Pediatr Neurol* 1986; **2**: 220–3.

Willison HJ, Muller DPR, Matthews S *et al.* A study of the relationship between neurological function and serum vitamin E concentrations in patients with cystic fibrosis. *J Neurol Neurosurg Psychiatr* 1985; **48**: 1097–102.

Wilson WB. Peroxisomal disorders In: Gold DH, Weingeist TA, eds. *The Eye in Systemic Disease*. Philadelphia: JB Lippincott, 1990: 402–6.

Wongpichedchai S, Hansen RM, Koka B, Gudas VM, Fulton AB. Effects of halothane on children's electroretinograms. *Ophthalmology* 1992; **99**: 1309–12.

Yee RD. Evaluating nystagmus in young children. *Arch Ophthalmol* 1990; **108**: 793.

Yiannikas C, Walsh JC, McCleod JG. Visual evoked potentials in the detection of subclinical optic toxic effects secondary to ethambutol. *Arch Neurol* 1983; **40**: 645–8.

York DH, Pulliam MW, Rosenfeld JG, Watts C. Relationship between visual evoked potentials and intracranial pressure. *J Neurosurg* 1981; **55**: 909–16.

Zeki SA. *Vision of the Brain*. Oxford: Blackwell Scientific Publications, 1993.

10: Ophthalmic Genetics

Michael Baraitser and Elizabeth Thompson

There are a number of indications for formal genetic counselling. These include a family history of eye problems, the birth of a child with a malformation of the eye, or with a progressive disease leading to visual impairment. Not only will the parents want to discuss the possibility that the handicap could be genetically determined but also whether there is a way of preventing it during a subsequent pregnancy. This might be handled by the ophthalmologist or at the genetic clinic or perhaps by a combination of the two at separate or combined clinics. It should be noted that the word counselling is a misnomer as few parents would expect 'counsel', i.e. advice, but would want to receive all the available information so that they can come to a meaningful decision, given their individual circumstances.

An approach to counselling

There are two essential requirements before counselling. One is an accurate three-generation family history — something which can usually be achieved even in a busy ophthalmic clinic (this will include questions about consanguinity); and the other is an accurate diagnosis.

The diagnosis will often necessitate an input from other disciplines and most geneticists will study the available information at a preclinical meeting. This meeting also allows the geneticist to search the literature before seeing the patient. In the absence of a specific diagnosis, a category diagnosis, i.e. an anterior chamber defect or colobomatous microphthalmia, is useful. These latter two diagnoses do not describe single entities but at least the geneticist can draw on empirical data to counsel approximate risks. It should be noted that empirical data must be carefully assessed. For instance anophthalmia seems to be a recessive disorder in the Middle East, but experience in the UK is different and it could be that only one-half of the cases seen are recessive. A recurrence risk of 12% (i.e. one-half of 25%) would be appropriate in Europe, after the birth of a single case to unrelated parents.

Counselling in recessively inherited disease

A condition is thought to be recessively inherited for a number of reasons. It might be frequently seen and studies have shown a segregation ratio close to that expected in autosomal recessive inheritance. Such is the case with albinism. Alternatively, in rare recessives a single case report of a sibship in the literature affecting both sexes might be sufficient to suggest recessive inheritance. There will probably not be enough information to exclude dominant inheritance with reduced expression or even dominant inheritance with gonadal mosaicism (i.e. a parent carries the gene only in the gonad and is therefore clinically unaffected). But on balance whatever the precise mechanism, the practical conclusion can be drawn that recurrence risks are high and a recessive risk would be appropriate. In other words a balance has to be drawn between the various possibilities. Occasionally, a suggestion of a genetic disorder, possibly recessively inherited, might be arrived at in a girl with a multitude of problems one of which includes a pigmentary retinopathy. The last-named sign might strongly suggest a recessive metabolic process even if no diagnosis is forthcoming.

Whereas in recessive inheritance the carrier parents will mostly be found to be normal, confusion might arise because occasionally a parent manifests a minor degree of the condition. For instance in oculocutaneous albinism a carrier parent might show translucency of the iris, and some people who are carriers have slightly lighter skin and hair colour, but in general, carriers do not show signs. If the condition is such that carriers can be detected then it would be expected that both parents would be found to have the changes. The fact that oculocutaneous albinism might be heterogeneous (tyrosinase-positive or tyrosinase-negative) does not make any difference as all the subgroups seem to be recessively inherited. That the genes are at separate loci might, however, affect counselling if there were DNA markers for a specific type of albinism. Prenatal prediction would apply only to that specific category and indeed tyrosinase-positive albinism has been mapped to chromosome 15q, and tyrosinase-negative albinism to chromosome 11q14–21.

Many different loci for albinism would also affect the counselling of two albinos who wanted to marry and have children. The prediction would be that all their children would be affected if albinism was always the result of homozygosity at a single locus. If different loci were involved, then all the children would have normal pigmentation of the skin, hair and iris.

Genetic counselling in autosomal recessive conditions is usually straightforward. The risk of recurrence in subsequent children of the same parents is one in four or 25%; this is known as a high-risk category, as are all risks greater that one in 10, but counselling is non-directive and parents will choose whether the risk is acceptable or not. It is clear that in albinism, the ocular complications are not necessarily severe and some parents are happy to accept the risk. What is needed, given this variability, is that parents should be furnished with information about the proportion of children who will have mild, moderate or severe handicap. In order to understand the risks in general, it is always helpful for parents to know the background risk that any couple run every time they have a child. This figure is in the vicinity of one in 50, i.e. about 2% of children are born with a major malformation. From this perspective, a 1–2% risk should be regarded as a reasonable risk. Despite a general acceptance that a one in four risk is high, no couple should be made to feel guilty for taking that risk. Counselling remains essentially information-giving. Risks should be numerically expressed in the form of odds which should always be put into perspective. Directive counselling should seldom be given and is rarely asked for.

The biggest problem for parents is how to cope with high risks of serious conditions. Leber's amaurosis is a good example. It is often difficult for parents whose first child is diagnosed as having this serious autosomal recessive condition to contemplate another pregnancy especially in the absence of prenatal diagnosis. Only artificial insemination by donor (AID) or ovum transplantation are ways around the problem, but the first option is not acceptable to many people and the latter option is not readily available at present. The decision whether to accept the risk will also depend on the family structure. If parents already have two other normal children, then they might not want to enlarge the family. The most agonizing choice is for those parents where the affected child is the first in the family. They might be reluctant to accept the genetic implications by suggesting that it 'cannot be genetic because there is no family history', but unfortunately there is often no family history in those conditions which are inherited as an autosomal recessive. In the face of unpleasant information which the parents will receive, the counsellor will often seek to balance the gloomy news by pointing out that neither their normal nor their affected children are likely to have affected children themselves unless they marry a close relation, or a visually handicapped person with exactly the same diagnosis, i.e. one who carries the same gene. It is also at times difficult for parents who must be carriers not to feel responsible for the child's handicap; it should therefore be pointed out that on average, everyone in the population is a carrier for at least one potentially harmful recessive gene which in a single 'dose' is harmless. The realization that often results from this explanation is that somehow the parents had been unlucky enough to have chosen from the population at large a partner who is another gene carrier for a rare condition, e.g. Leber's amaurosis. This may provoke a situation where one partner says to the other with some regret, that they had clearly made a wrong choice of partners and the counsellor should be aware of the tensions that could arise from each statement that is made.

Genetic counselling must always be dynamic and flexible so that misconceptions or an overemphasis on blame or bad luck must be countered and put into perspective. An interview might take longer than anticipated and ample time should be allowed.

The risks to the offspring of the parents' siblings or the affected child's siblings are likely to be small, even allowing for there being a 50% chance that a parent's sibling is a carrier and a two-thirds chance that a normal sibling of an affected child is a carrier. The probability that they would marry another carrier is small, unless they marry a cousin, and cautious reassurance is mostly all that is necessary. A figure quantifying the risk is usually possible to derive. For instance, given that the population frequency for Leber's amaurosis is one in 40 000 then the carrier frequency in the population is only about one in 100. The chance therefore of a parent's sibling having an affected child is one in two multiplied by one in a 100 multiplied by one in four ($1/2 \times 1/100 \times 1/4$). This gives an overall risk of one in 800, which is acceptable to most people.

Counselling in dominantly inherited disease

This follows one of three sequences. If there is a family history of a rare condition stretching over at least two generations and there has been male to male transmission thereby excluding X-linked inheritance, counselling of risks to offspring of those who are affected is simple. The risk is one in two or 50% (a high risk) and if the condition is serious and no prenatal diagnosis is available, then a significant number of people decide that the risk is unacceptable. AID should be discussed if the gene carrier is male. At present, ovum donation is a less practical consideration.

The second common situation is where the condition is known to be dominant, but there is no family history, i.e. a child has uncomplicated aniridia with normal chromosomes and the parents have normal irides. Given that the condition is usually totally penetrant, then it would be reasonable to reassure the parents that the affected child may have the condition as a fresh mutation. This concept will nearly always need an explanation and by far the easiest is to indicate that each child inherits half of its genes from each parent and in order to do so, DNA has to replicate itself by a process of copying. It is a mis-copy of one of the genes that leads to a fresh mutation. It is comforting for parents to be told that there is nothing wrong with their genes *per se*, but the fault lies in the innate difficulty of accurately copying many thousands of genes. Even in those situations where the evidence seems to suggest that we are dealing with a fresh mutation, recurrence risks are small but never nil. Indeed experienced genetic counsellors seldom are able to quote risks of less than 1%. The reason is that an unaffected parent could be a gonadal mosaic, i.e. have the mutation only in an ovum or testis and then proceed to have another affected child despite being unaffected themselves. This is the reason why parents of normal stature have on rare occasions produced two affected children with achondroplasia, a dominantly inherited condition.

It should also be noted that in some dominantly inherited conditions, where for instance a pigmentary retinopathy has been transmitted for many generations, the parents usually have a good understanding of the burden of the condition and it would be inappropriate for the counsellor to comment in a directive way. Parents will always decide whether or not they could cope although they might want to know whether a particular condition could be more or less severe than their own experience of it.

The third counselling problem in dominantly inherited conditions concerns variable expression and penetrance. For instance in dominant optic atrophy, it could appear on taking a pedigree that certain members seem to transmit the condition without being affected themselves. However, if they are examined by an experienced ophthalmologist, then pale optic discs will in all probability be found. No parent should therefore be reassured that recurrence risks are small in any condition known to be dominantly inherited with variable expression until they themselves have been examined.

Counselling in X-linked disorders

It might be that a simple appraisal of the pedigree will be sufficient to recognize an X-linked condition. If a mother has an affected son and an affected brother but is herself unaffected, or if an affected father produces both normal male and female children but his grandsons through his daughters have the same condition, then this is good evidence for X-linkage. It is more difficult in those situations where a woman has two affected sons as this could be either autosomal recessive or X-linked. If a diagnosis has been made, i.e. of ocular albinism which is mostly X-linked but might occasionally be inherited as an autosomal recessive condition, then on balance, counselling should proceed as if the inheritance pattern were X-linked but a small autosomal recessive risk should be added to the calculation. However, if both males have an unidentifiable but similar condition, then it becomes impossible from the pedigree to distinguish between an X-linked and an autosomal recessive mode of transmission.

When a single male is born with a known X-linked condition, the relevant counselling problem is to know whether the mother is a carrier. The affected male could arise in two ways; either as a fresh mutation or because the mother is a carrier. Even an absence of a family history does not preclude the possibility that the mother is a carrier as she might be a fresh mutation herself or the mutation could have arisen in her own mother. Some female carriers of an X-linked condition show minimal manifestations which should always be looked for. For instance, carriers for Lowe's syndrome might show lens opacities and despite some overlap with the normal population, there are those situations where a slit-lamp examination of the mother might give a clear-cut result, or at least a high probability that the mother is a carrier. If there is no way of carrier detection, as is the case in Norrie's disease, then there are theoretical reasons for assuming that in X-linked conditions which are so handicapping that boys seldom reproduce, at least two-thirds of mothers are carriers. This presumes equal mutation rates in sperm and ova (which unfortunately is not always the case). In this situation, the risk of having an affected child is half of two-thirds, i.e. one-third, which is unfortunately an uncomfortably high risk.

More recently carrier detection using DNA markers has become possible (see below).

Mitochondrial inheritance

The zygote receives virtually all its cytoplasmic DNA from maternal mitochondria, which in humans are the only source of extranuclear DNA. Each mitochondrion contains a number of DNA molecules which encode the RNA and protein needed by the mitochondrion.

Some diseases, most notably Leber's optic neuropathy (see Chapter 51) and mitochondrial cytopathy (see Chapter 44), are now known (not inevitably in the case of some of the mitochondrial cytopathies) to result from mutations in mitochondrial DNA. They have virtually exclusively maternal transmission as opposed to transmission through affected males via carrier daughters, to grandsons as in X-linked disease. A carrier female could theoretically produce a high proportion of affected offspring but it is a difficult counselling situation even if you detect the mitochondrial mutation in a female, as it is not possible to know the proportion of mitochondria with the mutation that she has, or will transmit in her ova, making predictions about the clinical situation very difficult (she might pass some mutations on and yet insufficient in number to cause disease)!

Chromosomal disorders

All children with multiple malformations should have their chromosomes checked. If an abnormality is found, i.e. a deletion or an unbalanced translocation, both parents should have their karyotypes examined. If the parental results are normal then the recurrence risks are small (1–2%). The figure is never zero as one or both parents could be a mosaic for the abnormality that cannot be detected in the blood chromosomes. If a parent is a translocation carrier the risk depends on how the translocation was ascertained. If through an abnormality in a child the recurrence is 20%, if through a family history of a chromosomal problem, i.e. before the birth of an abnormal child, it is 10%.

Counselling when no diagnosis is possible

Problems in genetic counselling arise where there is no precise diagnosis. For instance, a girl with normal chromosomes who is mentally retarded presents with congenital blindness due to a retinal coloboma. Experience suggests that the majority of these cases seem to be sporadic although rare recessives have been reported. Parents should be given the complete facts, but be told that recurrence risks are still likely to be small in view of the fact that the vast majority of reported cases have been single events. A risk of 2–3% might be appropriate in this situation and parents should understand that this is a small risk but that there is no way totally to exclude the unusual possibility of a recurrence due to an undiagnosable unique recessive.

It becomes even more difficult when the affected person is a single male without a specific diagnosis as there is the added problem of X-linked inheritance. Experienced dysmorphologists used to looking at congenital malformations and having experience in the diagnosis of rare syndromes will argue that if he or she cannot make a diagnosis, then at least a large proportion of genetic diseases have been excluded. Recurrence risks are therefore reduced to an empirical figure of between 3 and 5% depending on the specific combination of defects. The careful counsellor will also make use of one of the dysmorphology databases (for instance the London Dysmorphology Database; Winter & Baraitser 1995) which can be easily used in the office on a microcomputer in order to scan the available world literature to make sure that the specific combination has not been described in a possibly obscure paper.

Prenatal diagnosis can occasionally be achieved by high-resolution ultrasonography. Measurements of the globe in microphthalmia or anophthalmos should be considered, and in these conditions the test could be offered early in a subsequent pregnancy.

Clinical application of DNA technology

DNA analysis can be used to provide information for carrier detection, and presymptomatic and prenatal diagnosis of an increasing number of genetic disorders. This is accomplished by detection of the actual mutation causing the disease or of DNA markers that are linked to the disease gene locus.

In a genetic linkage study, DNA of relevant family members is analysed to track the inheritance of a particular disease gene. One example of this involves use of restriction enzymes which recognize specific DNA sequences and cut the DNA at these sites. Normal variation (polymorphisms) in the presence or absence of cutting sites gives rise to differently sized fragments which can be separated by electrophoresis. Such restriction fragment length polymorphisms (RFLPs) can be detected by radioactively or biotin-labelled DNA probes, in a process called Southern blotting (Emery 1988; Weatherall 1991). RFLPs are inherited in a simple mendelian fashion and, when close to the particular disease gene (closely linked), can be used to determine whether an individual has inherited the disease gene, without knowing anything about the disease gene itself. If the marker is not closely linked to the disease gene, then there is a high risk that the two loci will become separated at meiosis (during recombination) resulting in a false prediction.

Early prenatal diagnosis by chorionic villus sampling (CVS) around 11 weeks of pregnancy can be offered if the fetus is at risk of a genetic disorder for which reliable DNA markers are available or if the mutation itself is detectable. It is always preferable for the family to have genetic counselling before a pregnancy, so that the preliminary gene tracking can be done. Occasionally, for various reasons, the gene cannot be tracked in a particular family and a prenatal test is not possible. In addition, the accuracy and limitations of the test, the risks of the procedure and decisions regarding termination of the pregnancy all need to be fully discussed. Currently, the risk of miscarriage from CVS is about 2%. The analysis of DNA from the CVS sample takes at least 2 weeks, but the use of polymerase chain reaction (PCR), a method for amplifying minute quantities of DNA, means that the results can be available in a few days in some cases.

Two genetic disorders of the eye, Norrie's disease and retinoblastoma, are discussed in order to highlight the principles for the uses and limitations of DNA technology for families.

Norrie's disease

This X-linked disorder is characterized by early vascular proliferation (pseudoglioma) in both retinas, atrophic irides, corneal clouding and cataracts, progressing to shrinkage of the globes (phthisis bulbi). About two-thirds of cases are moderately or severely mentally retarded (Warburg 1966) and about one-third develop progressive sensorineural deafness. Other abnormalities may be present including odd behaviour patterns, seizures, microcephaly, poor muscle bulk and perhaps a characteristic facial appearance with a narrow nasal bridge, hypotelorism, flattened nasal area, thin upper lips and large ears (Donnai *et al.* 1988). The diagnosis is usually made on the ocular findings but can be difficult in isolated cases. Rarely, a female heterozygote manifests symptoms (Chen Z-Y *et al.* 1993c; Woodruff *et al.* 1993).

About two-thirds of mothers of an isolated affected male are carriers, and 50% of the sons of a known carrier will be affected. Until recently, no method of detection of carriers or prenatal diagnosis was available, and families were counselled on the basis of Bayesian calculation of risks which depends upon the number of unaffected male relatives.

Linkage studies

Gal *et al.* (1985b) reported close linkage of Norrie's disease and the polymorphic X chromosome locus DXS7 defined by the DNA probe L1.28, which localized the Norrie's disease gene to the short arm of the X chromosome at band 11.3, i.e. at Xp11.3. This linkage was confirmed (Bleeker-Wagemakers *et al.* 1985; Gal *et al.* 1985a; Kivlin *et al.* 1987) and can be used to provide carrier detection and prenatal diagnosis in suitable families.

For example, in Fig. 10.1 using probe L1.28 to detect DNA polymorphisms, it can be seen that the two X chromosome RFLPs of the mother (an obligate carrier) can be distinguished and can be called A and B. Her affected sons both inherited allele A, so that, in this family, the disease gene is 'tracking' with allele A. The daughter, at 50% risk of being a carrier on pedigree grounds, has inherited the A allele from the father and the B from the mother. Thus she

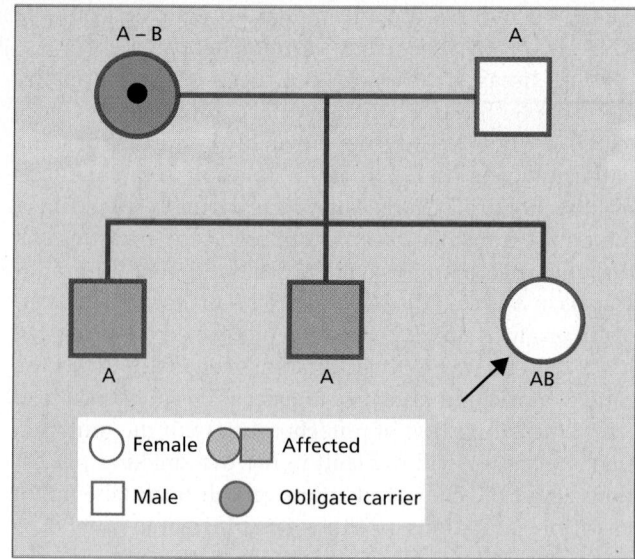

Fig. 10.1 Norrie's disease. The probe L1.28 reveals RFLPs with the enzyme *Eco*RI. The RFLPs have been designated A and B. The mother (a carrier) has alleles A and B; the affected sons inherited allele A. The maternal allele A is tracking with the Norrie's disease gene. The daughter inherited allele A from father and B from mother, so is predicted not to be a carrier.

is predicted not to be a carrier, barring the risk of recombination, estimated at about 5%, and so her risk of having an affected son is 2.5% (half her risk). The mother herself could be offered a prenatal test; if a male fetus inherited the maternal A or B allele, he would be at 95 or 5% risk, respectively.

This example highlights three important points in linkage studies. First, the mother must be heterozygous for the DNA markers, that is, her two alleles must be distinguishable, in order to be able to be offered a prenatal test. This is called being 'informative' for the test. If the mother were homozygous, i.e. AA or BB, then her two alleles could not be distinguished and a prenatal test would be impossible. However, as new markers are identified, it becomes increasingly likely that a given female will become informative for the test. The second point is that the risk of a wrong prediction due to recombination must be explained to the woman and her partner. Some couples would not be prepared to take this risk and would opt for fetal sexing and termination of a male fetus. The degree of risk that a woman is prepared to take often reflects her experience of the disease; a woman who has two affected brothers may be prepared to take less risk than her cousin who has never lived with an affected boy. Third, in the example shown in Fig. 10.1 the accuracy of the prediction that the daughter is unlikely to be a carrier is based on the assumption of correct paternity. If her true father in fact had allele B, then the prediction would be that the girl is

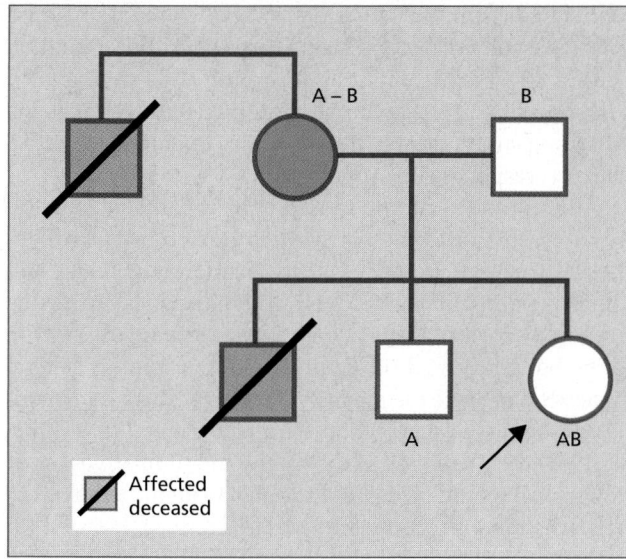

Fig. 10.2 Norrie's disease. Although the affected brother has died, it can be seen that the normal brother inherited the maternal A allele. Barring recombination, the maternal B allele must be tracking with the disease in this family and so the daughter would be predicted not to be a carrier.

likely to be a carrier. Thus a DNA test for paternity should be carried out where a result is dependent on correct paternity.

A factor which can limit the availability of a test based on linkage is family structure. For example, if the affected boys had died, it would be impossible to 'track' the gene and know which RFLP was travelling with the disease gene in this family. For this reason, it is important to store a DNA sample from an affected individual, particularly if they are likely to die. Note, however, that all may not be lost if an affected individual has died without a DNA sample being stored. In Fig. 10.2 the healthy brother gives information about the normal allele and so it could be predicted that his sister is not a carrier. Even if the healthy brother were not available and the daughter's own risk could not be altered by DNA analysis, she could be offered a 'prenatal exclusion' test in pregnancy. If a male fetus inherited the allele B, which she inherited from her normal father, the fetus would be at very low risk and would be excluded as being affected. An example of this was reported by Gal *et al.* (1988). If the male fetus inherited the A allele which the woman got from her mother, he would be at essentially the same risk as his mother of being a carrier and the woman could opt for termination of pregnancy.

Submicroscopic deletions

In several families (de la Chapelle *et al.* 1985; Gal *et al.* 1985a; Donnai *et al.* 1988; Zhu *et al.* 1989) a submicroscopic deletion of the Norrie's disease gene locus was detected:

the DNA probe L1.28 did not hybridize to the patient's DNA. In families in which a deletion is found, females at risk of being carriers can be offered a virtually 100% accurate prenatal test because the mutation itself is being detected. In a male fetus, the presence of an L1.28 allele indicates that the deletion and therefore the disease is absent; if there is no L1.28 allele then the baby has a deletion and would be affected. Such a prenatal test was reported by de la Chapelle *et al.* (1985). Deletion detection can sometimes be used to see if at-risk females are carriers (de la Chapelle *et al.* 1985; Donnai *et al.* 1988). In sporadic cases whose diagnosis is in doubt, identification of a deletion confirms the diagnosis.

Norrie's disease gene

The gene for Norrie's disease was isolated by positional cloning (Berger *et al.* 1992a; Chen *et al.* 1992). Eleven different point mutations in the gene were identified in 12 patients (Berger *et al.* 1992b). As the diagnosis of Norrie's disease is often difficult, the ability to test for specific mutations will help clarify the diagnosis of Norrie's disease, and will allow accurate carrier detection and prenatal diagnosis.

Genotype–phenotype correlations

It is interesting to note that the monoamine oxidase genes MAOA and MAOB are close to the Norrie's disease gene locus though distinct from it (Sims *et al.* 1989) but some males with Norrie's disease have a submicroscopic deletion which includes the MAOA and MAOB loci (Sims *et al.* 1989; Collins *et al.* 1992) which probably accounts for the behavioural problems in these patients and in some female carriers. In other words, these individuals have a contiguous gene syndrome, involving two or more adjacent genes. Other patients with Norrie's disease, however, have non-ocular manifestations, but they have discrete mutations within the Norrie gene only. It has been noted that there is no particular correlation of the phenotype with genotype with regard to the extent of disruption within the Norrie gene itself. For example, a patient with a deletion encompassing the whole Norrie gene had ocular symptoms only, whilst others with a variety of mutations in the Norrie gene, such as point mutations, had a severe phenotype with mental retardation and deafness (Berger *et al.* 1992b). Some patients have myoclonic epilepsy and growth retardation, but these were not seen in association with point mutations (Berger *et al.* 1992b).

The Norrie's disease protein (NDP) may be involved in the pathway that regulates neural cell differentiation and proliferation (Chen *et al.* 1993b). Meitinger *et al.* (1993) reported that the NDP has a tertiary structure similar to that of an emerging family of growth factors with implications for the physiological role of the NDP.

Recently, a family with an X-linked form of familial exudative vitreoretinopathy (FEVR) was reported with a mutation in the Norrie gene (Chen *et al.* 1993a). The two disorders are similar but distinct clinically. In FEVR, there is failure of peripheral retinal vascularization resulting in fibrovascular proliferation in the affected area, with a variety of consequences, ranging from peripheral vitreous opacities to a total fibrovascular mass. Most cases are autosomal dominantly inherited with a less common X-linked form. This study suggests that Norrie's diesase and X-linked FEVR result from mutations in the same gene. The authors suggest that other X-linked eye diseases should be similarly investigated, e.g. X-linked primary retinal dysplasia.

Retinoblastoma

Retinoblastoma (Rb), the most common ophthalmic malignancy in childhood, occurs in about one in 20 000 live births (Vogel 1979). The tumour develops in infancy and rarely occurs after 6 years. The majority of cases are sporadic, that is, they have no family history of Rb; about 25% in the UK have a positive family history (Jay *et al.* 1988). In most cases (60%) the disease affects only one eye; in the minority it is bilateral (Vogel 1979). In the familial form, the predisposition is inherited in an autosomal dominant fashion, with a penetrance of about 90% (Vogel 1979). Familial cases are more likely to be bilateral and to have an earlier onset (at or before 15 months) than sporadic cases, which are more likely to be unilateral, and to begin between 2 and 3 years. Familial cases can be unilateral, but bilateral or multifocal cases are always considered to be hereditary, especially if they present in the early months of life. Hereditary cases may have either inherited the predisposing mutation from a parent or it may have arisen as a fresh germinal mutation. In the former, there is a subsequent risk to siblings and offspring but in the latter there is a risk only to the offspring of the affected individual. In a truly sporadic case, there is no risk to siblings or offspring. Germ-line mutations are thought to underlie all sporadic bilateral cases and about 10–15% of sporadic unilateral cases (Vogel 1979; Murphree & Benedict 1984).

A mechanism to explain tumour formation in Rb was proposed in 1971 by Knudson who suggested that two independent mutation events are required to trigger tumour development (the 'two-hit' hypothesis). The first mutational event could be inherited from a parent or could arise as a fresh mutation in gametogenesis, while the second occurred in immature retinal cells. Patients with unilateral non-hereditary Rb had two new mutations in a retinal cell, which explained why their tumour developed later and was unifocal.

Genetic counselling is straightforward in familial Rb — an affected individual's offspring has a 45% risk of developing Rb (assuming 90% penetrance). A sporadic bilateral case is assumed to represent a new germ-line mutation with a 45% risk to offspring. Empiric data are used for risks to a sibling of a sporadic bilateral case (6%) and to the offspring and siblings of a sporadic unilateral case (5.5 and 1%, respectively) (Vogel 1979).

Although surgical and radiotherapy treatment are highly successful, outcome is greatly improved by early diagnosis. Current practice is to examine siblings and offspring at regular (often 3 monthly) intervals during the high-risk period. Satisfactory ocular examinations can only be performed in young children under general anaesthesia. Since the majority of cases have sporadic unilateral disease and most of these are non-hereditary (Jay *et al.* 1988) the likelihood is that many infant relatives are at low risk. It would be useful to be able to identify the risk to relatives more precisely and perhaps reduce the need for screening. Individuals who carry a heritable mutation also have a greatly increased risk of developing independent second primary cancers later in life — 14% in the series of Abramson *et al.* (1984), most frequently osteosarcoma. Patients with a family history of Rb and those with bilateral sporadic Rb are at risk of this, but so are 10–15% of sporadic unilateral cases (who carry a germ-line mutation) and it would be useful to be able to identify and then screen the latter group. Finally, many families request prenatal diagnosis.

Much progress has been made in recent years towards these goals. The gene for Rb lies on chromosome 13, at band 14 of the long arm, i.e. at 13q14. About 5% of patients with Rb have a constitutional chromosome deletion which includes band 13q14 (Yunis & Ramsay 1978; Cowell *et al.* 1986; Jay *et al.* 1988). Deletions at the same site have been found in Rb tumour cells (Balaban *et al.* 1982). The gene for esterase D (ESD), an enzyme ubiquitous in human tissues whose biological function is unknown, was also localized to chromosome 13q14 (Sparkes *et al.* 1980). The enzyme shows electrophoretic variants, and using these, Sparkes *et al.* (1983) showed that the ESD and Rb loci are closely linked. Using DNA polymorphisms, it has been shown by comparing the somatic cells with tumour cells in patients that the normal allele at the Rb locus is lost, that is, the mutation which predisposes to the cancer is a 'loss of function' mutation (Benedict *et al.* 1983; Cavanee *et al.* 1983; Dryja *et al.* 1984). In other words, the normal gene acts as a suppressor of tumour formation (Huang *et al.* 1988). In keeping with this, the RB1 gene product has the properties of a cell cycle regulatory element (Buchkovich *et al.* 1989; Chen *et al.* 1989; De Caprio *et al.* 1989).

To develop the tumour, both alleles at the Rb locus must be lost. One abnormal allele may be inherited from a parent or may arise during gametogenesis; the individual is then predisposed to develop the tumour, but this would not occur until, by various mechanisms, the normal allele was lost in the retina. In a true sporadic case, a mutation of both alleles occurs by chance in the same retinoblast. Thus there is now evidence to support Knudson's two-hit hypothesis and to suggest that the mutational events involve 'loss of function' alleles. Rb is a prototype of a group of human cancers apparently caused by recessive 'loss of function' mutations at distinct genetic loci. Other examples are aniridia, Wilms' tumour, familial renal cell carcinoma, neuroblastoma and small cell carcinoma of the lung (Murphree & Benedict 1984). This recessive mechanism may seem paradoxical, given the dominant inheritance of Rb, but it is explained by a dominantly inherited predisposition, with only a few cells undergoing the second mutation (Buchanan & Cavanee 1987). The retinoblastoma gene (RB1) has been cloned (Friend *et al.* 1986) and a number of DNA polymorphisms close to and within the locus have been identified. At the present time, it is possible to offer prenatal or presymptomatic screening to many families by a variety of means. The following procedure is recommended for genetic counselling for Rb families.

Family history and examination

Occasionally, Rb may regress spontaneously and so it is important to examine first-degree relatives for the presence of a scar, calcification or other evidence of a regressed tumour (Carlson & Desnick 1979; Onadim *et al.* 1991). Obviously, if one were found in a parent of an affected child, the case would be considered familial.

Chromosome analysis of peripheral lymphocytes

About 5% of cases of Rb have a constitutional deletion of chromosome 13q14 which is detectable cytogenetically. Large deletions are associated with congenital anomalies and mental retardation, but these features may be mild or absent if the deletions are small (Benedict *et al.* 1983); these patients have a heritable form of Rb and cytogenetic detection of the deletion can be used for prenatal and presymptomatic screening, with virtually 100% accuracy.

DNA studies

Linkage studies using DNA polymorphisms. This is now rarely needed but could still play a role when a mutation cannot be detected. In families with more than one affected family member, presymptomatic and prenatal testing is usually done by linkage studies using RFLPs. The DNA markers used may be very close to the Rb gene (linked markers) but inaccurate predictions can result from recombination at meiosis. The reliability can be improved by using more markers, especially flanking markers which lie outside and flank the Rb gene (Cavanee *et al.* 1986; Greger *et al.* 1988). Intragenic markers which

lie within the Rb gene give very reliable results, since the marker is in the gene itself and is unlikely to become separated from the mutation at meiosis (Mitchell *et al.* 1988; Wiggs *et al.* 1988; Goddard *et al.* 1990). If flanking and intragenic markers are used, the accuracy is even greater (Scheffer *et al.* 1989). Using intragenic RFLPs, Onadim *et al.* (1990) found that 90% of 55 families were informative for prenatal screening and it is expected that this figure will rise as new probes are developed. It has been suggested that infants shown not to have inherited the high-risk allele need not undergo repeated ophthalmological screening examinations (Onadim *et al.* 1992) and if this advice is to be followed, the accuracy of prenatal and predictive tests is of vital importance. An example using intragenic DNA markers is shown in Fig. 10.3.

Direct mutation analysis. If the mutation itself is detectable, then this provides a virtually 100% accurate predictive test for other members of the family in familial Rb (Horsthemke *et al.* 1987). The other advantage of direct mutation analysis is that isolated cases may be distinguishable as hereditary or non-hereditary, which is important in genetic counselling (Yandell *et al.* 1989). Take, for example, a patient with a unilateral Rb and no family history of Rb. If the mutation in the Rb gene were identified in the tumour cells but not in peripheral lymphocytes, then the patient has a truly sporadic Rb, with no increased risk to other family members and a low risk to the child of second primary Rb-related tumours. If the child did have the mutation in lymphocytes, then the child has a high offspring risk and the parents can be offered a test. If neither parent carries the mutation in peripheral lymphocytes, then the risk to their other offspring is low (but not zero, as occasionally, a parent carries the mutation in the gonad, but not in the somatic cells).

Sporadic cases. If direct mutation analysis were not available, as described above, linkage studies using DNA RFLPs could be used to exclude the predisposition to Rb in siblings of a case with no family history, without knowing whether or not the case is heritable. For example, if the sibling shared no Rb gene marker in common with the affected child, then the sibling would be at very low risk of developing the tumour and frequent examinations under anaesthetic could perhaps be avoided (Fig. 10.4).

A variety of other manoeuvres can be used to help individual cases. For example, a sporadic case with bilateral tumours (which must be heritable) has a deletion in the tumour but not in peripheral lymphocytes. This implies that the 'second hit' was the deletion. The 'first hit' or germ-line mutation must be in the other allele of the Rb gene. This information could be used for a prenatal test for the patient in future.

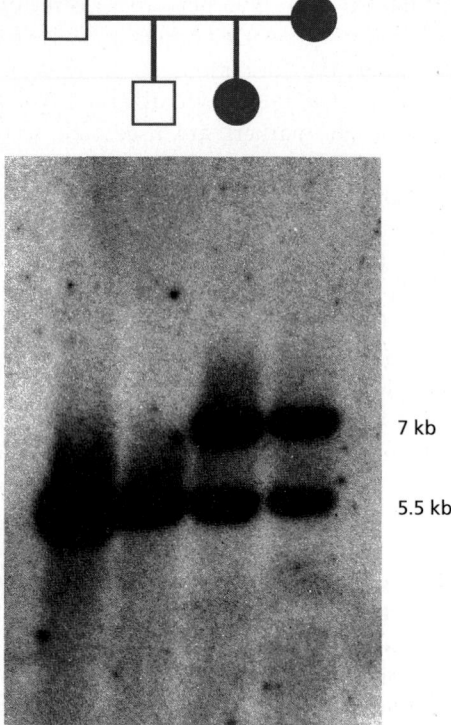

Fig. 10.3 Predictive tests using intragenic DNA polymorphisms. The family has been studied with probe p88PR0.6 using the restriction enzyme *Xba*1 which reveals a 2 allele polymorphism. The smaller lower band is 5.5 kb (kilobases) in length and the upper band is 7 kb. The affected daughter inherited the 7 kb band from her affected mother. In this family, the retinoblastoma predisposing gene is tracking with the 7 kb band. The father is homozygous for the 5.5 kb band. The son inherited a 5.5 kb band from father and from mother and so is predicted not to be at risk of retinoblastoma. (Father's band looks larger than son's because there is more DNA in the track.) (Photograph by courtesy of Dr. C. Mitchell.)

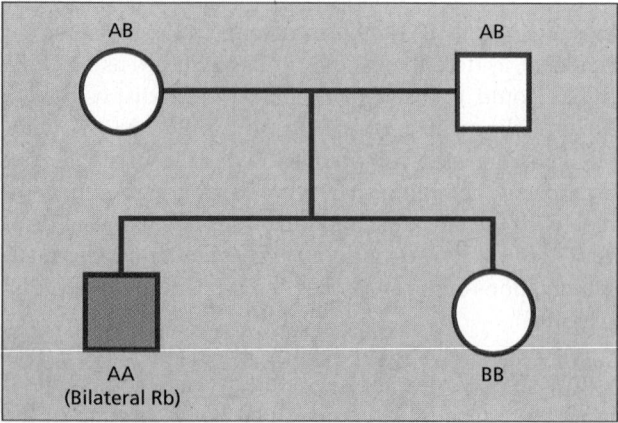

Fig. 10.4 Sporadic retinoblastoma: use of intragenic DNA polymorphisms in a sporadic case to exclude risk to siblings. Since the sibling of the affected boy has no alleles in common with her brother, it is unlikely that she carries the predisposition to Rb, even if one parent has the predisposing gene but has not manifested Rb.

Since molecular analysis of tumour DNA is often useful, it is important to arrange storage of DNA from all Rb tumours and national registers can help co-ordinate the arrangements (Jay *et al.* 1988). If tumour DNA is not stored, it may be possible to isolate DNA from a histopathological specimen from the tumour (Onadim & Cowell 1991).

References

Abramson DH, Ellsworth RM, Kitchin TD, Tung G. Second nonocular tumour in retinoblastoma survivors. *Ophthalmology* 1984; **91**: 1351–5.

Balaban G, Gilbert F, Nichols W, Meadows AT, Shields J. Abnormalities of chromosome 13 in retinoblastomas from individuals with normal constitutional karyotypes. *Cancer Genet Cytogenet* 1982; **6**: 213–21.

Benedict WF, Murphee AL, Banerjee A, Spina CA, Sparkes MC, Sparkes RS. Patients with 13 chromosome deletion: evidence that the retinoblastoma gene is a recessive cancer gene. *Science* 1983; **219**: 973–5.

Berger W, Meindl A, van de Pol TJR *et al.* Isolation of a candidate gene for Norrie disease by positional cloning. *Nature Genet* 1992a; **1**: 199–203.

Berger W, van de Pol D, Warburg M *et al.* Mutations in the candidate gene for Norrie disease. *Hum Molec Genet* 1992b; **1**: 461–5.

Bleeker-Wagemakers LM, Friedrich U, Gal A, Wienker TF, Warburg M, Ropers H-H. Close linkage between Norrie disease, a cloned DNA sequence from the proximal short arm, and the centromere of the X chromosome. *Hum Genet* 1985; **71**: 211–14.

Buchanan JA, Cavanee WK. Review article. Genetic markers for assessment of retinoblastoma predisposition. *Dis Markers* 1987; **5**: 141–52.

Buchkovich K, Duffy LA, Harlow E. The retinoblastoma protein is phosphorylated during specific phases of the cell cycle. *Cell* 1989; **58**: 1097–105.

Carlson EA, Desnick RJ. Mutational mosaicism and genetic counselling in retinoblastoma. *Am J Med Genet* 1979; **4**: 365–81.

Cavanee WK, Dryja TP, Phillips RA *et al.* Expression of recessive alleles by chromosomal mechanisms in retinoblastoma. *Nature* 1983; **305**: 779–84.

Cavanee WK, Murphree AL, Shull MM *et al.* Prediction of familial predisposition to retinoblastoma. *N Engl J Med* 1986; **314**: 1201–7.

Chen P-L, Scully P, Shew J-Y, Wang JYJ, Lee WH. Phosphorylation of the retinoblastoma gene product is modulated during the cell cycle and cellular differentiation. *Cell* 1989; **58**: 1193–8.

Chen Z-Y, Battinelli EM, Fielder A *et al.* A mutation in the Norrie disease gene (NDP) associated with X-linked familial exudative vitreoretinopathy. *Nature Genet* 1993a; **5**: 180–3.

Chen Z-Y, Battinelli EM, Hendriks RW *et al.* Norrie disease gene: characterization of deletions and possible function. *Genomics* 1993b; **16**: 533–5.

Chen Z-Y, Battinelli EM, Woodruff G, Young I, Breakefield XO, Craig IW. Characterization of a mutation within the NDP gene in a family with a manifesting female carrier. *Hum Molec Genet* 1993c; **2**: 1727–9.

Chen Z-Y, Hendriks RW, Jobling MA *et al.* Isolation and characterization of a candidate gene for Norrie disease. *Nature Genet* 1992; **1**: 204–8.

Collins FA, Murphy DL, Reiss AL *et al.* Clinical, biochemical, and neuropsychiatric evaluation of a patient with a contiguous gene syndrome due to a microdeletion Xp11.3 including the Norrie disease gene locus and monoamine oxidase (MAOA and MAOB) genes. *Am J Med Genet* 1992; **42**: 127–34.

Cowell JK, Rutland P, Jay M, Hungerford J. Deletions of the esterase D locus from a survey of 200 retinoblastoma patients. *Hum Genet* 1986; **72**: 164–7.

de la Chapelle A, Sankila EM, Lindlof M, Aula P, Norio R. Norrie disease caused by a gene deletion allowing carrier detection and prenatal diagnosis. *Clin Genet* 1985; **28**: 317–20.

DeCaprio JA, Ludlow JW, Lynch D *et al.* The product of the retinoblastoma susceptibility gene has properties of a cell cycle regulatory element. *Cell* 1989; **58**: 1085–95.

Donnai D, Mountford RC, Read AP. Norrie disease resulting from a gene deletion: clinical features and DNA studies. *J Med Genet* 1988; **25**: 73–8.

Dryja TP, Cavanee W, White R *et al.* Homozygosity of chromosome 13 in retinoblastoma. *N Engl J Med* 1984; **310**: 550–3.

Emery AEH. *An Introduction to Recombinant DNA.* Chichester: John Wiley, 1988.

Friend SH, Bernards R, Rogelj S *et al.* A human DNA segment with properties of the gene that predisposes to retinoblastoma and osteosarcoma. *Nature* 1986; **323**: 643–6.

Gal A, Bleeker-Wagemakers L, Wienker TF, Warburg M, Ropers HH. Localisation of the gene for Norrie's disease by linkage to the DXS7 locus HGM8. *Cytogenet Cell Genet* 1985a; **40**: 633.

Gal A, Stolzenberger C, Weinker TF *et al.* Norrie's disease: close linkage with genetic markers from the proximal short arm of the X chromosome. *Clin Genet* 1985b; **27**: 282–3.

Gal A, Uhlhaas S, Glaser D, Grimm T. Prenatal exclusion of Norrie disease with flanking DNA markers. *Am J Med Genet* 1988; **31**: 449–53.

Goddard AD, Phillips RA, Greger V *et al.* Use of the RB1 cDNA as a diagnostic probe in retinoblastoma families. *Clin Genet* 1990; **37**: 117–26.

Greger V, Kerst S, Messmer E, Hopping W, Passarge E, Horsthemke B. Application of linkage analysis to genetic counselling in families with hereditary retinoblastoma. *J Med Genet* 1988; **25**: 217–21.

Horsthemke B, Barnet HJ, Gregor V, Passarge E, Hopping W. Early diagnosis in hereditary retinoblastoma by detection of molecular deletions at gene locus. *Lancet* 1987; **1**: 511–12.

Huang H-J, Yee J-K, Shew J-Y *et al.* Suppression of the neoplastic phenotype by replacement of the Rb gene in human cancer cells. *Science* 1988; **242**: 1563–6.

Jay M, Cowell J, Hungerford J. Register of retinoblastoma: preliminary results. *Eye* 1988; **2**: 102–5.

Kivlin JD, Sanborn GE, Wright E, Cannon L, Carey J. Further linkage data on Norrie disease. *Am J Med Genet* 1987; **26**: 733–6.

Knudson AG. Mutation and cancer: a statistical study of retinoblastoma. *Proc Natl Acad Sci USA* 1971; **68**: 820–3.

Meitinger T, Meindl A, Bork P *et al.* Molecular modelling of the Norrie disease protein predicts a cystine knot growth factor tertiary structure. *Nature Genet* 1993; **5**: 376–80.

Mitchell C, Nicolaides K, Kingston J, Hungerford J, Jay M, Cowell J.

Prenatal exclusion of hereditary retinoblastoma. *Lancet* 1988; **i**: 826.

Murphree AL, Benedict WF. Retinoblastoma: clues to human oncogenesis. *Science* 1984; **223**: 1028–33.

Onadim Z, Cowell JK. Application of PCR amplification of DNA from paraffin-embedded tissue sections to linkage analysis in familial retinoblastoma. *J Med Genet* 1991; **28**: 312–16.

Onadim Z, Hungerford J, Cowell JK. Follow-up of retinoblastoma patients having prenatal and perinatal predictions for mutant gene carrier status using intragenic probes from the RB1 gene. *Br J Cancer* 1992; **65**: 711–16.

Onadim Z, Hykin PG, Hungerford JL, Cowell JK. Genetic counselling in retinoblastoma: importance of ocular fundus examination of first-degree relatives and linkage analysis. *Br J Ophthalmol* 1991; **75**: 147–50.

Onadim ZO, Mitchell CD, Rutland PC *et al.* Application of intragenic DNA probes in prenatal screening for retinoblastoma gene carriers in the United Kingdom. *Arch Dis Child* 1990; **65**: 651–6.

Scheffer H, te Meerman GJ, Kruize YCM *et al.* Linkage analysis of families with hereditary retinoblastoma: non-penetrance of mutation, revealed by combined use of markers within and flanking the RB1 gene. *Am J Hum Genet* 1989; **45**: 252–60.

Sims KB, Ozelius L, Corey T *et al.* Norrie disease gene is distinct from the monoamine oxidase genes. *Am J Hum Genet* 1989; **45**: 424–34.

Sparkes RS, Murphree AL, Lingua RW *et al.* Gene for hereditary retinoblastoma assigned to human chromosome 13 by linkage to esterase-D. *Science* 1983; **219**: 971–3.

Sparkes RS, Sparkes MC, Wilson MG *et al.* Regional assignment of genes for human esterase D and retinoblastoma to chromosome band 13q14. *Science* 1980; **208**: 1042–4.

Vogel F. Genetics of retinoblastoma. *Hum Genet* 1979; **52**: 1–54.

Warburg M. Norrie's disease, a congenital progressive oculo-acoustico-cerebral degeneration. *Acta Ophthalmol Kbh* 1966; **89**(Suppl.): 1–147.

Weatherall DJ. *The New Genetics and Clinical Practice*, 3rd edn. Oxford: Oxford University Press, 1991.

Wiggs J, Nordenskjold M, Yandell D *et al.* Prediction of the risk of hereditary retinoblastoma, using DNA polymorphisms within the retinoblastoma gene. *New Engl J Med* 1988; **318**: 151–7.

Winter RM, Baraitser M. The London Dysmorphology Database: A computerized database for the diagnosis of rare dysmorphic syndromes. New York: Oxford University Press, 1995.

Woodruff G, Newbury-Ecob R, Plaha DS, Young ID. Manifesting heterozygosity in Norrie's disease? *Br J Ophthalmol* 1993; **77**: 813–14.

Yandell DW, Campbell TA, Dayton SH *et al.* Oncogenic point mutations in the human retinoblastoma gene: their application to genetic counselling. *N Engl J Med* 1989; **321**: 1689–95.

Yunis JJ, Ramsay N. Retinoblastoma and sub-band deletion of chromosome 13. *Am J Dis Child* 1978; **132**: 161–3.

Zhu D, Antonarakis SE, Schmeckpeper BJ, Diergaarde PJ, Greb AE, Maumenee IH. Microdeletion in the X chromosome and prenatal diagnosis in a family with Norrie disease. *Am J Med Genet* 1989; **33**: 485–8.

11: The Paediatric Ophthalmology Genome

R. Jane Leitch

This chapter lists conditions where the genetic locus is known or suspected. The order of the list follows the chapters in outline so that some conditions with more than one major ocular feature appear in more than one section. Not all minor ocular features have been represented with multiple entries, and since the genome literature is expanding very rapidly, this section cannot be all-encompassing; in some instances review articles are cited, especially where the literature on that subject is large. There are a few entries in brackets; these are conditions where their position on the genome is of particular interest in relation to another condition, e.g. the proximity of a gene abnormality resulting in meningioma is at a similar locus to neurofibromatosis type 2. References are indicated by superior numbers.

Myopia

1p	Ehlers–Danlos (6)[73]
3p24.25	Marfan's syndrome[69]
8q22–23	Cohen's syndrome[34]
10q26	Gyrate atrophy (B_6 responsive and B_6 unresponsive)[3]
12q13.11–13.2	Stickler's syndrome[2]
12q13	Spondoepiphyseal dysplasia tarda[5]
12q13	Kniest's dysplasia[2]
12q22–qter	Noonan's syndrome[36]
15q11	Prader–Willi syndrome/Angelman[5]
15q15–21	Marfan's syndrome/dominant ectopia lentis[5]
16p13.3	Rubinstein–Tabi syndrome[5]
17p12	Smith–Magenis syndrome[24]
17	Marfan atypical[5]
21q22.3	Homocystinuria[1]
Xq28	Bornholm eye disease[5]

18 External eye diseases

11q12–13	Atopy[27]

20 Disorders of the eye as a whole

2q21–31	Bilateral microphthalmia and cataract[56]
3q26	De Lange syndrome[90]
14q22–23	Anophthalmia and pituitary abnormalities[35]
Xp22.3	MIDAS[39]
Xp22.31	Microphthalmia and linear skin defects (Goltz)[64]
Xq27–28	Anophthalmia[5]

21 Lids

2p12/2p14	Baraitser/Winter iris coloboma and ptosis[91]
3p	3p syndrome[80]
3q22–23	Blepharophimosis epicanthus inversus and ptosis[1,11]
7q21–22	Ectrodactyly ectodermal dysplasia and clefting[78]
7q32	Smith–Lemli–Optiz syndrome (ptosis)[75]
9q22.3–31	Naevoid basal cell carcinoma syndrome[45]
14q11.2–13	Oculopharyngeal muscular dystrophy[25]
19p13.2–13.1	Familial hypercholesterolaemia[1]

22 Conjunctiva and subconjunctival tissue

1p	Naevoid basal cell carcinoma syndrome[5]
1q21	Gaucher type 2[94]
1q41–42	Xeroderma pigmentosum[5]
2q21	Xeroderma pigmentosum (group B)[61]

3p15–21	Epidermolysis bullosa dystrophica[79]
5	Xeroderma pigmentosa[59]
8q24	Epidermolysis bullosa ogna type[1]
8	Xeroderma pigmentosa (group A)[60]
9q34.1	Xeroderma pigmentosum[58]
10q21–22	Gaucher's disease variant form[1]
11q22–23	Ataxia telangiectasia[5]
13q	Xeroderma pigmentosum[1]
15q23–25	Tyrosinaemia type 1[1]
15	Xeroderma pigmentosum (group F)[1]
16q13.3–13.2	Xeroderma pigmentosum[57]
16q22.1–24	Tyrosinaemia type 2[1]
17q	Epidermolysis bullosa simplex[2]
19q13.2–13.3	Xeroderma pigmentosum[5]
Xq21.33–22	Fabry's disease[5]
Xq28	Dyskeratosis congenita[1]

23 Developmental anomalies of the anterior segment

4q25–27	Rieger's syndrome[5]
4q25	Autosomal dominant iris hypoplasia[148]
4q28–31	Anterior segment mesenchymal dysgenesis[5]
11p13	PAX 6 aniridia and Peters' anomaly[5]

24 Corneal abnormalities in childhood

1p	Ehlers–Danlos (6)[73]
3p15–21	Epidermolysis bullosa dystrophica[79]
3p14.2–21	Mucopolysaccharidosis 4B (Morquio)[1]
4p16.3	Mucopolysaccharidosis 1 (Hurler)[96,106]
4p16.3	Mucopolysaccharidosis 1S (Scheie)[96,106]
4q21–23	Mucolipidosis 3[1]
5q11–13	Mucopolysaccharidosis 6 (Maroteaux–Lamy)[5]
7q21	Osteogenesis imperfecta types 1–3[98]
9q34	Amyloidosis[1]
9q31–34	Riley–Day syndrome[38]
11q23–qter	Amyloidosis[1]
13q14–21	Wilson's disease[1,8]
15q23–25	Tyrosinaemia type 1[1]
16q22.1–24	Tyrosinaemia type 2[1]
17q21.3–22.05	Osteogenesis imperfecta[5]
20p12.1–11.3	Alagille's syndrome[5]

20p11	Amyloidosis type 6[5]
22pter–q11	Hurler–Scheie mucopolysaccharidosis[5]
Xpter–22.32	Ichthyosis X-linked[1]
Xp22.2–22.1	Corneal dermoids[63]
Xp22–21	Megalocornea[5]
Xq12–13	Anhidrotic ectodermal dysplasia[5]
Xq21.33–22	Fabry's disease[5]
Xq28.1	Hunter's syndrome[5]

25 Corneal dystrophies

5q31	Lattice corneal dystrophy type 1[30]
5q31	Granular dystrophy[30]
5q31	Avellino (autosomal dominant corneal dystrophy)[30]

26 Lacrimal system

7q21–22	Ectrodactyly ectodermal dysplasia and clefting[78]

28 Neurofibromatosis

17q11	Von Recklinghausen neurofibromatosis type 1[143]
(17q11–12	Watson's syndrome[2])
22q11.21–11.23	Neurofibromatosis type 2[136,137]
(22q12.3–qter	Meningioma[1])

29, 30 Orbital tumours

1p31–32	Neuroblastoma[22,120]
2q35–37	Rhabdomyosarcoma (alveolar)[92]
11p15.5	Rhabdomyosarcoma[92]
11q	Neuroblastoma[120]
14q32–qter	Neuroblastoma[120]

34 Craniofacial abnormalities

3p21	Greig craniopolysyndactyly
5q32–33	Treacher–Collins syndrome[1]
5qter	Craniosynostosis type 2[111]
7p21	Saethre–Chotzen[9]
7p13	Greig craniosyndactyly[66]
7p11.2–14	Craniosynostosis syndrome 2
8p	Pfeiffer's syndrome[7]
8q22	Cleidocranial dysostosis[1]
10q25–26	Crouzon's craniofacial dysostosis[7]
10q25–26	Jackson–Weiss syndrome[7]
10q25–26	Pfeiffer syndrome[145,146]
10q25–26	Apert syndrome[147]
15q15	Craniosynostosis[132]
22 (trisomy)	Goldenhar[40]
Xq13	Aarskog's syndrome[84]

38 Uveal tract

1q43	Chediak–Higashi syndrome[5]
2pter–p25.1	Coloboma of iris[1,5]
2p12/2p14	Baraitser/Winter iris coloboma and ptosis[91]
2q37.3	Waardenburg's syndrome[5]
3p12–14	Waardenburg's syndrome type 2[81]
4q28–31	Sclerotylisis[2]
4q33–qter	Williams' syndrome[97]
6q13–15	Recessive ocular albinism[115]
6	Williams–Beurren syndrome[114]
7q11	Williams' syndrome[76]
9q34	Nail–patella syndrome[1]
11p13	PAX 6 aniridia and Peters' anomaly[5]
11q14–21	Oculocutaneous albinism (types 1A, 1B and 1C)[5]
13	Williams' syndrome[102,103,104]
15p11–q13	Oculocutaneous albinism[72,131]
19q13.4–qter	Facial dysmorphism coloboma and heart defects[3]
22q11	Cat's eye syndrome[5]
Xp22.3–22.2	Ocular albinism[3]
Xq26.3–27.1	Albinism and deafness[5]

39 Lens

1p21–22	Zellweger type 2[100,101] Dislocated lens
1q21–25	Cataract zonular pulverulent
1q2	Cataract zonular pulverulent[119]
1	Cataract, Coppock[5]
2p25	Cataract anterior polar[5]
2q21–31	Bilateral microphthalmia and cataract[56]
2q31	Ehlers–Danlos (4)[5] Dislocated lens
2q33–35	Cataract, Coppock-like[1]
3p24.25	Marfan's syndrome[69] Dislocated lens
3p22–23	Pseudo-Zellweger[2] Cataract
5q15.2	Cri du chat[139] Cataract
6q16.1–16.3	Diabetes mellitus, juvenile[5]cataract
7q11.23	Zellweger's syndrome[74] Cataract
7q32	Smith–Lemli–Optiz syndrome[75] Cataract
8p11.2–21.1	Werner's syndrome[105] Cataract
8q21	Zellweger[99] Cataract
9p13	Galactosaemia[2] Cataract
9q34	Nail–patella syndrome[1,58]
10q11.21	Cockayne's syndrome[125] Cataract
11q12–13	Atopy[27] Cataract
11q23	Ataxia microcephaly and cataract[126]
12q22–24.1	Phenylketonuria[5] Cataract
13q14–21	Wilson's disease[1,8] Cataract
14q24	Anterior polar cataract[5]

15q15–21	Marfan's syndrome/dominant ectopia lentis[5]
16p13.3	Rubinstein–Tabi syndrome[5] Cataract
16q16.3	Autosomal dominant congenital cataract and microphthalmia[153]
16q	Familial posterior polar[5] Cataract
16q22.1–23.1	Cataract Marmar type[1]
17q11–12	Cataract congenital zonular with sutural opacities[154]
17q21–22 17q24	Galactokinase deficiency Cataract
17q24	Caerulean cataract[6]
17	Marfan atypical[5] Dislocated lens
19p13.2–q12	Mannosidosis[1] Cataract
19q13.3	Myotonic dystrophy[5] Cataract
19q	Cataract with high serum ferritin Autosomal dominant[151]
21q22.3	Homocystinuria[1] Dislocated lens
22q11	Velocardiofacial syndrome[138] Cataract
Xp	Cataract with microcornea and microphthalmos[5]
Xp22	Chondrodysplasia punctata[1] Cataract
Xp21.1–22.3	Nance–Horan syndrome[5] Cataract
Xq24–26	Lowe's syndrome[5] Cataract
Xq28	G-6-PD[5] Cataract
Xq28	Happle's syndrome[55] Cataract

40 Childhood glaucoma

1q21–23	Open angle glaucoma[140]
3p24.25	Marfan's syndrome[69]
3p14.2–21	Mucopolysaccharidosis 4B[1]
5q11–13	Mucopolysaccharidosis 6 (Maroteaux–Lamy)[5]
11q	Congenital glaucoma[1]
15q15–21	Marfan's syndrome/dominant ectopia lentis[5]
16p13.3	Rubinstein–Tabi syndrome[5]
22pter–q11	Hurler–Scheie mucopolysaccharidosis[5]
Xq24–26	Lowe's syndrome[5]

41 Vitreous (and retinal dysplasia)

11q13.5–22	Autosomal dominant exudative vitreoretinopathy[3]
12q13.11–13.2	Stickler's syndrome[5]
12q13	Spondoepiphyseal dysplasia tarda[5]
Xp11.3–11.4	Norrie's disease[3]
Xp11/Xq28	Incontinentia pigmenti[5]
Xq21.3	Familial exudative vitreoretinopathy[3]

42 Retinoblastoma

13q14.1–14.2	Retinoblastoma and osteosarcoma in survivors[3]

44 Inherited retinal dystrophies

1p21–22	Zellweger type 2[100,101]
1q32	Usher type 2[3]
1q32	Retinitis pigmentosa[50]
1q31–32.1	Autosomal recessive retinitis pigmentosa (RP12)[155]
1q42–qter	Choroideraemia like[47]
2p24	Hypobetalipoproteinaemia[1]
2p24	Abetalipoproteinaemia[1]
2q	Oguchi's disease[26]
2	Familial juvenile nephrophthisis associated with ARRP (Senior–Loken syndrome)[51]
3p14.2–21	Mucopolysaccharidosis 4B[1]
3q21–24	Retinitis pigmentosa 4 (autosomal dominant)[3]
3q21–23	Retinitis pigmentosa 5 (autosomal recessive)[82]
3q21–25	Usher's syndrome type 3 (USH3)[12]
4p16.3	Autosomal dominant stationary night-blindness[65]
4p16.3	Mucopolysaccharidosis 1 (Hurler)[96,106]
4p16.3	Mucopolysaccharidosis 1S (Scheie)[96,106]
4p16.3	Retinitis pigmentosa (cGMP phosphodiesterase)[144]
4q21–23	Mucolipidosis 2[2]
5q11–13	Mucopolysaccharidosis 6 (Maroteaux–Lamy)[5]
5q13	Gangliosidosis 2 (Sandhoff disease)[5]
6p21.3–21.1	Autosomal recessive retinitis pigmentosa (RP14)[158]
6pcen–p21.1	Retinitis pigmentosa 7 (peripherin-related slow)[3]
6q25–26	Autosomal dominant cone dystrophy[3]
7p	Autosomal dominant retinitis pigmentosa (RP9)[3]
7q11.23	Zellweger's syndrome[74]
7q	Retinitis pigmentosa (RP10)[52,53]
8p11–q21	Retinitis pigmentosa (RP1)[3,122]
8q21	Zellweger[99]
10q11.21	Cockayne's syndrome[125]
10q23–24	Deficiency of retinol-binding protein[1]
10q26	Gyrate atrophy (B_6 responsive and B_6 unresponsive)[3]
11p15.2–14	Usher's syndrome type 1C[3]
11q21	Bardet–Biedl[62]
11q13.5	Usher's syndrome type 1B[3]
12q14	Mucopolysaccharidosis D (Sanfillipo)[67]
14q32.1–32.3	Usher's syndrome type 1[3]
14	Rod monochromacy[130]
15q11	Angleman's syndrome[5]
16q11	Batten's disease[1]
16q13–22	Bardet–Biedl[3]
16q24	Mucopolysaccharidosis (4A)[95]
17p13.1	Autosomal dominant retinitis pigmentosa[135]
17p12.1	Recoverin gene[49]
17	Niemann–Pick disease[5]
17	Usher's type 1[46]
17p	Leber's congenital amaurosis[149]
17q	Cone–rod dystrophy[3]
17q	Autosomal dominant retinitis pigmentosa[150]
18q21.1	Cone–rod dystrophy[54]
19q13.1–13.2	Cone–rod dystrophy[3]
19q13.3	Myotonic dystrophy[5]
19q13.4	Autosomal dominant retinitis pigmentosa (RP8)[3]
19q13.4	Autosomal dominant retinitis pigmentosa (RP11)[156]
20p12.1–11.3	Alagille's syndrome[5]
22pter–q11	Hurler–Scheie mucopolysaccharidosis[5]
22q13–qter	Sorsby retinal dystrophy[10]
Xp21.1	Retinitis pigmentosa RP3[3]
Xp21.3–21.2	Retinitis pigmentosa 6 (X-linked recessive)[77]
Xp21–11.1	Progressive cone dystrophy[3,47]
(Xp21	Duchenne muscular dystrophy[14])
Xp11	Ocular albinism 2[3]
Xp11.23	Retinitis pigmentosa RP2[47]
Xp11.23	Aland Island eye disease[13]
Xp11.3	CSNB (Congenital Stationary Night Blindness)[5]
(Xp11.3–11.4	Norrie's disease[3])
Xp	Gyrate atrophy[83]
Xp21	Oregon eye disease[68]
Xp22.1–q21.31	Choroideraemia[3]
Xp22.13–22.11	Retinitis pigmentosa (RP15)[157]
Xq22	Pelizaeus–Merzbacher[2]
Xq28.1	Hunter's syndrome[5]
Xq28	Adrenoleucodystrophy[5]
Xq28	Cone degeneration[3]

45 Inherited macular dystrophies

1p	Stargardt/flavimaculatus[3] fundus
3p12–21.1	Autosomal dominant cerebellar

ataxia and pigmentary macular dystrophy[16,17]
6pcen–p21.1   Vitelliform macular dystrophy[109]
6pcen–21.1   Butterfly macular dystrophy[110]
6q11–15   Stargardt/fundus flavimaculatus[3]
6q16.1–16.3   North Carolina macular dystrophy[3]
7p15–21   Dominant cystoid macular oedema[37]
8q24   Macular dystrophy, atypical vitelliform[3]
11q13.1–13.5   Best's disease (vitelliform dystrophy)[3]
13q34   Stargardt macular dystrophy[3]
16p   Macular dystrophy (atypical vitelliform)[5]
Xp22.3–21.1   Retinoschisis[3]

46 Congenital and vascular abnormalities of the retina

3p25–26   Von Hippel–Lindau[71]
9q3   Rendu–Osler–Weber telangiectasia[21]
9q33–34   Tuberous sclerosis[5]
9q33–34   Rendu–Osler–Weber telangiectasia[20]
11q22–23   Tuberous sclerosis 2[5]
12q23   Tuberous sclerosis 3[1]
12q   Rendu–Osler–Weber telangiectasia[19]
16p13.4   Tuberous sclerosis type 4[5]
Xp11/Xq28   Incontinentia pigmenti[5]
Xq21.33–22   Fabry's disease[5]

47 Retinal detachment in childhood

1p36.3–36.2   Ehlers–Danlos (6)[73]
3p24.25   Marfan's syndrome[69]
12q13.11–13.2   Stickler's syndrome[2,5]
12q13   Spondoepiphyseal dysplasia tarda[5]
15q15–21   Marfan's syndrome/dominant ectopia lentis[5]
17   Marfan atypical[5]

48 Flecked retina syndromes

1p   Stargardt's/fundus flavimaculatus[3]
2p24   Abetalipoproteinaemia[1]
2q36–q37   Oxalosis type 1[5]
6pcen–p21.1   Retinitis punctata albescens[3]

49 Miscellaneous retinal disorders

1p36.3–36.2   Ehlers–Danlos (6)[73]

2p16–21   Autosomal dominant Radial Drusen[88]
2p24   Abetalipoproteinaemia[1]
5q22–23   Familial poliposis coli (CHRPE: Congenital Hypertrophy of the Retinal Pigment Epithelium)[1]
6q16.1–16.3   Diabetes mellitus, juvenile[5]
7q22–qter   Tritan colour blindness[3]
11p15.5   Sickle cell anaemia[5]
11p15   Beta-thalassaemia[1]
Xq28   Colour blindness[3]

50 Optic nerve—congenital abnormalities

2p   Optic atrophy[5]
3q21–24   Dominant optic atrophy[89]
10q24–25   PAX 2 (optic nerve colobomas)[18]
13   Trisomy 13 Patau's syndrome[87]
Xp22.31   Goltz's syndrome[64]
Xp22.3   Kalmann's syndrome[33]
Xp22   Aicardi's syndrome[5]

51 Optic neuropathies

1q21   Gaucher type 2[94]
3p21.33   GM1 gangliosidosis[141]
3p14.2–21   Mucopolysaccharidosis 4B[1]
4p   Wolfram's syndrome[31]
4q21–q23   Mucolipidosis 3[1]
5q11–q13   Mucopolysaccharidosis 6 (Maroteaux–Lamy)[5]
6q16.1–16.3   Diabetes mellitus, juvenile[5]
9q13–21   Friedreich ataxia[124]
10q21–22   Metachromatic leucodystrophy (two genes)[1]
10q21–22   Gaucher's disease variant form[1]
11p15.4–15.1   Niemann–Pick disease[1]
14q21–24.3   Krabbe's disease[1]
15q22–25.1   Tay–Sachs disease[70]
15q22–25.1   GM2 gangliosidosis juvenile[1]
16q24   Mucopolysaccharidosis (4A)[95]
17p11.2–12   Charcot–Marie–Tooth 1A[121]
17q21.3–22.05   Krabbe's disease[5]
20q   Galactosialidosis[2]
22pter–q11   Hurler–Scheie mucopolysaccharidosis[5]
22q13.31–qter   Metachromatic leucodystrophy[1]
Xq12–13   Menke's syndrome[5]
Xp13.1   Charcot–Marie–Tooth
Xq28   Adrenoleucodystrophy[5]

52 Chiasmal defects

14q22–23   Anophthalmia and pituitary abnormalities[35]

53 Hydrocephalus

Xp26	Dandy–Walker malformation[142]
Xq28	Hydrocephalus[86]

54 Brain problems

2p21	Holoprosencephaly 2
3p24	Holoprosencephaly
7q36–qter	Holoprosencephaly[117]
10q11–21	Holoprosencephaly
13q	Holoprosencephaly[128,129]
17p13.3	Miller–Dicker lissencephaly[5]
18 (ring)	Holoprosencephaly[133]
21q22.3	Holoprosencephaly[118]

57 Neurometabolic disease

1p34.1–36.1	Fucosidosis[93]
1p36.1–34	Hypophosphatasia[1]
1p21	Glycogen storage disease type 2[113]
1p21–22	Zellweger type 2[100,101]
1p13	Maple syrup urine disease[44]
1q21	Gaucher type 2[94]
2p24	Hyperlipoproteinaemia[5]
3p22–23	Pseudo-Zellweger[2]
3p21.33	GM1 gangliosidosis[141]
3p14.2–21	Mucopolysaccharidosis 4B (Morquio)[1]
3q24	Maple syrup urine disease[44]
4p16.3	Mucopolysaccharidosis 1 (Hurler)[96,106]
4p16.3	Mucopolysaccharidosis 1S (Scheie)[96,106]
4p15	Phenylketonuria (dihydropteridine reductase deficiency)[1]
4q21–23	Mucolipidosis 2[2]
4q21–23	Mucolipidosis 3[1]
5q11–13	Mucopolysaccharidosis 6 (Maroteaux–Lamy)[5]
5q13	Gangliosidosis 2 (Sandhoff disease)[5]
6p21–22	Maple syrup urine disease[43]
7q11.23	Zellweger's syndrome[74]
8p22	Hyperlipoproteinaemia 1[1]
8q21	Zellweger[99]
10q21–22	Metachromatic leucodystrophy (two genes)[1]
10q21–22	Gaucher's disease variant form[1]
10q24–25	Wolman's disease[1]
11p15.4–15.1	Niemann–Pick disease[1]
14q21–24.3	Krabbe's disease[1]
12q14	Mucopolysaccharidosis D (Sanfillipo)[67]
12q22–24.1	Phenylketonuria[5]

14q32.1	Glycogen storage disease type 4
15q22–25.1	Tay–Sachs disease[70]
15q22–25.1	GM2 gangliosidosis juvenile[1]
16q11	Batten's disease[1]
16q22.1–24	Tyrosinaemia type 2[1]
16q24	Mucopolysaccharidosis (4A)[95]
17q21.3–22.05	Krabbe's disease[5]
17	Niemann–Pick disease[5]
19p13.2–q12	Mannosidosis[1]
19q13.1	Hyperlipoproteinaemia type 1B[1]
19q13.1	Hyperlipoproteinaemia type III[1]
19q13	Maple syrup urine disease[42]
20q	Galactosialidosis[2]
22pter–q11	Hurler–Scheie mucopolysaccharidosis[5]
22q13.31–qter	Metachromatic leucodystrophy[1]
Xq12–13	Menkes syndrome[5]
Xq28.1	Hunter's syndrome[5]
Xq28	Adrenoleucodystrophy[5]

60 Leukaemia

1p31–32	Leukaemia/lymphoma T cell[1]
2q33–35	Leukaemia/lymphoma T cell[1]
8q24.1	Burkitt's lymphoma[108]
9p23	Acute lymphoblastic leukaemia[1]
9q22	Leukaemia 2 acute lymphoblastic[1]
9q34	Acute T-cell leukaemia[1]
10q23–24	Acute T-cell leukaemia [1]
11q13.3	T-cell leukaemia/lymphoma[5]
12 (trisomy)	Chronic lymphatic leukaemia[108]
13q14	Chronic lymphatic leukaemia[108]
14q32.1	B-cell leukaemia/lymphoma[1]
21q22	Acute myeloid leukaemia[1]

61 Phakomatoses

3p25–26	Von Hippel–Lindau[71]
9q33–34	Tuberous sclerosis[5]
11q22–23	Tuberous sclerosis 2[5]
12q23	Tuberous sclerosis 3[1]
16p13.4	Tuberous sclerosis type 4[5]

64 Other eye movement disorders

1p31	Maple syrup urine disease[44]
3q24	Maple syrup urine disease[44]
3p12–21.1	Autosomal dominant cerebellar ataxia and pigmentary macular dystrophy[16,17]
6p23–2	Spinocerebellar ataxia (type 1)[28]
6p21–22	Maple syrup urine disease[43]
9q13–21	Friedreich's ataxia[124]
11q22–23	Ataxia telangiectasia[5]
11q23	Ataxia microcephaly and cataract[126]

13q14–21	Wilson's disease[1,8]
19q13	Maple syrup urine disease[42]
20q13–11	Creutzfeld–Jakob disease[1]
20	Seizures, benign neonatal[1]
21q22.3	Epilepsy, progressive myoclonus[1]

66 Incomitant strabismus and cranial nerve palsies

12cen	Congenital fibrosis of the extraocular muscles[29]
13q12–13	Mobius syndrome[127]
19q13.3	Myotonic dystrophy[5]

Miscellaneous

1p13	Hypothyroidism[1]
1q21.3–p23	Charcot–Marie–Tooth type 1B[125]
1q32	Protein S deficiency[107]
2q14	Protein C deficiency[1]
2q33–35	Amyotrophic lateral sclerosis[32]
3cen–3q11	Protein S deficiency[1]
4q31–32	Gilles de la Tourette's syndrome[5]
8q24	Hypothyroidism[123]
10q11.21	Multiple endocrine neoplasia II[1]
10q21.1	Multiple endocrine neoplasia IIB[1]
11p15.4–pter	Beckwith–Wiedemann syndrome[41]
11q23	Hypertriglyceridaemia[1]
16q22.1	Fish eye disease[5]
17p12	Smith–Magenis syndrome[24]
19	Green/blue eye colour[5]
20q13	Severe combined immunodeficiency[1]
22q11	Di George syndrome[23]
22q11	Velocardiofacial syndrome[138]
22q11	Ewing's sarcoma[1]
Xp22	Deafness and cortical blindness[15]

References

1 McKusick VA, Amberger JS. The morbid anatomy of the human genome: chromosomal location of mutations causing disease. *J Med Genet* 1993; **30**: 1–26.

2 Wilkie AOM, Amberger JS, McKusick VA. A gene map of congenital malformations. *J Med Genet* 1994; **31**: 507–17.

3 Rosenfeid PJ, McKusik VA, Amberger JS, Dryja T. Recent advances in the gene map of inherited eye disorders: primary hereditary diseases of the retina, choroid and vitreous. *J Med Genet* 1994; **31**: 903–15.

4 Tommerup N. Mendelian cytogenetics. Chromosome rearrangements associated with mendelian disorders. *J Med Genet* 1993; **30**: 713–27.

5 Klintworth GK. Genetically determined disorders affecting the eye. In: Garner A, Klintworth GK, eds. *The Pathobiology of Ocular Disease: a Dynamic Approach*. New York: Marcel Dekker, 1994, pp. 811–38.

6 Armitage MM, Kilvin JD, Ferrell A. Progressive early onset

cataract gene maps to human chromosome 17q24. *Nat Genet* 1995; **9**: 37–40.

7 Mulvihill JJ. Craniofacial syndromes: no such thing as a single gene disease. *Nat Genet* 1995; **9**: 101–2.

8 Thomas GR, Forbes JR, Roberts EA, Walsh JM, Cox DW. The Wilson disease gene: spectrum of mutations and their consequences. *Nat Genet* 1995; **9**: 210–17.

9 Wilkie AO, Yang SP, Summers D, Poole MD, Reardon W, Winter RM. Saethre–Chotzen syndrome associated with balanced translocations involving 7p21: three further families. *J Med Genet* 1995; **32**: 174–80.

10 Weber BHF, Vogt G, Wolz W *et al.* Sorsby's fundus dystrophy is genetically linked to chromosome 22q13–qter. *Nat Genet* 1994; **7**: 158–61.

11 Warburg M, Bugge M, Brondu–Nielsen K. Cytogenetic findings indicate heterogeneity in patients with blepharophimosis, epicanthus inversus and developmental delay. *J Med Genet* 1995; **32**: 19-24.

12 SanKila E, Pakarinen L, Kaarlainen *et al.* Assignment of Usher syndrome type 3 (USH 3) gene to chromosome 3q. *Hum Mol Genet* 1995; **4**: 93–8.

13 Glass IA, Good P, Coleman MP *et al.* Genetic mapping of a cone and rod dysfunction (Aland Island eye disease) to the proximal short arm of the human X chromosome. *J Med Genet* 1993; **30**: 1044–50.

14 Jensen H, Warburg M, Sjo O *et al.* Duchenne muscular dystrophy: negative electroretinograms and normal dark adaptation. Reappraisal of assignment of X-linked incomplete congenital stationary night blindness. *J Med Genet* 1995; **32**: 348–51.

15 Tranebjaerg L, Schwartz C, Eriksen H *et al.* A new X-linked recessive deafness syndrome with blindness, dystonia, fractures, and mental deficiency is linked to Xq22. *J Med Genet* 1995; **32**: 257–63.

16 Benomar A, Krols L, Stevanin G *et al.* The gene for autosomal dominant cerebellar ataxia with pigmentary macular dystrophy maps to chromosome 3p12–p21.1. *Nat Genet* 1995; **10**: 84–8.

17 Gouw LG, Kaplan CD, Haines JH *et al.* Retinal degeneration characterizes a spinocerebellar ataxia mapping to chromosome 3p. *Nat Genet* 1995; **10**: 89–93.

18 Sanyanusin P, Schimmenti LA, McNoe *et al.* Mutation of the PAX2 gene in a family with optic nerve colobomas, renal anomalies and vesicoureteral reflux. *Nat Genet* 1995; **9**: 358–63.

19 Vincent P, Planchu H, Faure S *et al.* A third locus for hereditary haemorrhagic telangiectasia maps to chromosome 12q. *Hum Mol Genet* 1995; **4**: 945–9.

20 McDonald MT, Papenberg KA, Ghosh S *et al.* A disease locus for hereditary haemorrhagic telangiectasia maps to chromosome 9q33–34. *Nat Genet* 1994; **6**: 197–204.

21 Shovlin CL, Hughes JMB, Tuddenham EGD *et al.* A gene for hereditary haemorrhagic telangiectasia maps to chromosome 9q3. *Nat Genet* 1994; **6**: 205–9.

22 Caron H, Peter M, van Sluis P *et al.* Evidence for two tumour suppressor loci on chromosomal bands 1p35–36 involved in neuroblastoma: one probably imprinted, another associated with N-*myc* amplification. *Hum Mol Genet* 1995; **4**: 535–9.

23 Driscoll DA, Budarf ML, Emanuel BS. A genetic aetiology for Di George syndrome. Consistent deletions and microdeletions of 22q11. *Am J Hum Genet* 1992; **50**: 924–33.

24 Zhao Z, Lee C, Jiralerspong S *et al.* The gene for a human microfibril-associated glycoprotein is commonly deleted in Smith–Magenis syndrome patients. *Hum Mol Genet* 1995; **4**: 589–97.

25 Brais B, Xie Y, Sanson M *et al.* The oculopharyngeal muscular

dystrophy locus maps to the region of the cardiac a and b myosin heavy chain genes on chromosome 14q11.2–q13. *Hum Mol Genet* 1995; **4**: 429–34.

26 Maw MA, John S, Jablonka S *et al*. Oguchi disease suggestion to markers on chromosome 2q. *J Med Genet* 1995; **32**: 396–8.

27 Sandford AJ, Shirakawa T, Moffat MF *et al*. Localisation of atopy and the b subunit of high-affinity IgE receptor (FceRI) on chromosome 11q. *Lancet* 1993; **341**: 332–4.

28 Banfi S, Servadio A, Chung MY *et al*. Identification and characterisation of the gene causing type 1 spinocerebellar ataxia. *Nat Genet* 1994; **7**: 513–20.

29 Engle EC, Kunkel LM, Specht A *et al*. Mapping a gene for congenital fibrosis of the extraocular muscles to the centromeric region of chromosome 12. *Nat Genet* 1994; **7**: 69–73.

30 Stone E, Mathers WD, Rosenwasser GOD *et al*. Three autosomal dominant corneal dystrophies map to chromosome 5q. *Nat Genet* 1994; **6**: 47–51.

31 Polymeropoulous MH, Gorman Swift R, Swift M. Linkage of the gene for Wolfram syndrome to markers on the short arm of chromosome 4. *Nat Genet* 1994; **8**: 95–7.

32 Hentati A, Bejaoui K, Pericak-Vance MA *et al*. Linkage of recessive familial amyotrophic lateral sclerosis to chromosome 2q33–q35. *Nat Genet* 1994; **7**: 425–8.

33 Ballabio A, Sebastio G, Corrozzo R *et al*. Deletions of the steroid sulphatase gene in classical X-linked icthyosis associated with Kallman syndrome. *Hum Genet* 1987; **77**: 338–41.

34 Tahvanainen E, Norio R, Karila E *et al*. Cohen syndrome gene assigned to the long arm of chromosome 8 by linkage analysis. *Nat Genet* 1994; **7**: 201–4.

35 Bennet CP, Betts DR, Seller MJ. Deletion 14q(q22q23) associated with anophthalmia, absent pituitary and other abnormalities. *J Med Genet* 1991; **28**: 280–1.

36 Jamieson CR, van de Burgt I, Brady AF *et al*. Mapping a gene for Noonan syndrome to the long arm of chromosome 12. *Nat Genet* 1994; **8**: 357–60.

37 Kremer H, Pinckers A, van dem Helm B *et al*. Localisation of the gene for dominant cystoid macular dystrophy on chromosome 7p. *Hum Mol Genet* 1994; **3**: 299–302.

38 Blumenfeld A, Slaugenhaupt SA, Axelrod FB *et al*. Localisation of the gene for familial dysautonomia on chromosome 9 and definition of DNA markers for genetic diagnosis. *Nat Genet* 1993; **4**: 160–4.

39 Happle R, Daniels O, Koopman RJ. MIDAS syndrome (microphthalmia, dermal aplasia and sclerocornea): an X-linked phenotype distinct from Goltz syndrome. *Am J Med Genet* 1993; **47**: 710–13.

40 Korbrynski L, Chitayat D, Zahed L *et al*. Trisomy 22 and facioauriculovertebral (Goldenhar) sequence. *Am J Med Genet* 1993; **46**: 68–71.

41 Weksberg R, Teshima I, Williams BR *et al*. Molecular characterisation of cytogenetic alterations associated with the Beckwith–Wiedemann syndrome (BWS) phenotype refines the localisation and suggests the gene for BWS is imprinted. *Hum Mol Genet* 1993; **2**: 549–56.

42 Zhang B, Zhao Y, Harris RA *et al*. Molecular defects in the E1 alpha subunit of branched chain alpha ketoacid dehydrogenase complex that cause maple syrup urine disease. *Mol Biol Med* 1991; **8**: 39–47.

43 Zneimer SM, Lau KS, Eddy RL *et al*. Regional assignment of two genes of the human branched-chain alpha-ketoacid dehydrogenase complex: the E1 beta gene (BCKDHB) to chromosome 6p21–22 and the E2 gene (DBT) to chromosome 1p31. *Genomics* 1991; **10**: 740–7.

44 Chuang DT, Fisher CW, Lau KS *et al*. Maple syrup urine disease: domain structure, mutations and exon skipping in the dihydrolipoyl transacylase (E2) component of the branched-chain alpha-ketoacid dehydrogenase complex. *Mol Biol Med* 1991; **8**: 49–63.

45 Goldstein AM, Stewart C, Bale AE *et al*. Localisation of the gene for the nevoid basal cell carcinoma syndrome. *Am J Hum Genet* 1994; **54**: 765–73.

46 Cotran Pr, Bruns GA, Berson EL *et al*. Genetic analysis of patients with retinitis pigmentosa using a cloned DNA probe for the human gamma subunit of cyclic GMP phosphodiesterase. *Exp Eye Res* 1991; **53**: 557–64.

47 Teague PW, Aldred MA, Jay M *et al*. Heterogeneity analysis in 40 X-linked retinitis pigmentosa families. *Am J Hum Genet* 1994; **55**: 105–11.

48 von Bokhoven H, von Genderen C, Molloy CM *et al*. Mapping of the choroideraemia-like (CHML) gene at 1q42–qter and mutation analysis in patients with Usher syndrome type II. *Genomics* 1994; **19**: 385–7.

49 Wiechmann AF, Akots G, Hammarback JA *et al*. Genetic and physical mapping of human recoverin: a gene expressed in retinal photoreceptors. *Invest Ophthalmol Vis Sci* 1994; **35**: 325–31.

50 Sparkes RS, Lee RH, Shinohara T *et al*. Assignment of the phosducin (PDC) gene to human chromosome 1q25–1q32.1 by somatic cell hybridisation and *in situ* hybridisation. *Genomics* 1993; **18**: 426–8.

51 Hildebrant F, Singh-Sawhney I, Schnieders B *et al*. Mapping of a gene for familial juvenile nephronophthisis: refining the map and defining flanking markers on chromosome 2. APN study group. *Am J Hum Genet* 1993; **53**: 1256–61.

52 Jordan SA, Farrar GJ, Kenna P *et al*. Localisation of an autosomal dominant retinitis pigmentosa gene to chromosome 7q (comment). *Nat Genet* 1993; **4**: 54–8.

53 Inglehearn CF, Carter SA, Keen TJ *et al*. A new locus for dominant retinitis pigmentosa on chromosome 7p. *Nat Genet* 1993; **4**: 51–3.

54 Warburg M, Sjo O, Tranebjaerg L *et al*. Deletion mapping of a retinal cone–rod dystrophy: assignment to 11q21.1. *Am J Med Genet* 1991; **39**: 288–93.

55 Traupe H, Muller D, Atherton D *et al*. Exclusion mapping of the X-linked dominant chondroplasia punctata–icthyosis–cataract–short stature (Happle) syndrome: possible involvement of an unstable premutation. *Hum Genet* 1992; **89**: 659–65.

56 Weaver RG, Rao N, Thomas IT *et al*. De novo inv (2) (p21q31) associated with isolated bilateral microphthalmia and cataracts. *Am J Med Genet* 1991; **40**: 509–12.

57 Liu P, Siciliano J, White B *et al*. Regional mapping of human DNA excision repair gene ERCC4 to chromosome 16p13.13–p13.2. *Mutagenesis* 1993; **8**: 199–205.

58 Ozelius LJ, Kwiatkowski DJ, Schuback DE *et al*. A genetic linkage map of human chromosome 9q. *Genomics* 1992; **14**: 715–20.

59 Kaur GP, Athwal RS. Complementation of DNA repair defect in xeroderma pigmentosum cells of group C by the transfer of human chromosome 5. *Somat Cell Mol Genet* 1993; **19**: 83–93.

60 Mori T, Rinaldy TL, Thwal RS *et al*. A xeroderma pigmentosum complementation group A related gene: confirmation using monoclonal antibodies against the cyclobutane dimer and (6–4) photoproduct. *Mutat Res* 1993; **293**: 143–50.

61 Weeda G, Wiegant J, van der Ploeg M *et al*. Localisation of the xeroderma pigmentosum group b correcting gene ERCC3 to human chromosome 2q21. *Genomics* 1991; **10**: 1035–40.

62 Leppert M, Baird L, Anderson KL *et al*. Bardet–Biedl syndrome is linked to DNA markers on chromosome 11q and is genetically

heterogeneous. *Nat Genet* 1994; **7**: 108–12.

63 Igbal MA, Chitayat D, Hahm SYE *et al*. Linkage of gene for corneal dermoids with the DXS43 (Xp22.2–22.1) locus. *Am J Hum Genet* 1987; **41**: A171.

64 Friedman PA, Rao PW, Teplin SW *et al*. Provisional deletion mapping of the focal dermal hypoplasia (FDH) gene to Xp22.31. *Am J Hum Genet* 1988; **43**: A50.

65 Gal A, Orth N, Baehr W *et al*. Heterogeneous mis-sense mutation in the rod cGMP phosphodiesterase b-subunit gene in autosomal dominant stationary night blindness. *Nat Genet* 1994; **7**: 64–8.

66 Brueton L, Huson SM, Winter RM *et al*. Chromosomal localisation of a developmental gene in man: direct DNA analysis determines that Greig cephalopolysyndactyly maps to 7p13. *Am J Med Genet* 1988; **31**: 799–804.

67 Robertson DA, Callen DF, Baker EG *et al*. Chromosomal localisation of the gene for human glucosamine-6-sulphatase 10 12q14. *Hum Genet* 1988; **79**: 175–8.

68 Pillers DA, Seltzer W, Powell B *et al*. Negative configuration electroretinogram Oregon eye disease: consistent phenotype Xp21 deletion syndrome. *Arch Ophthalmol* 1993; **111**: 1558–72.

69 Collod G. A second locus for Marfan syndrome maps to chromosome 3p24.2–25. *Nat Genet* 1994; **8**: 264–8.

70 Nakai H, Byers MG, Shows TB. Mapping HEXA to 15q23–q24. *Cytogenet Cell Genet* 1987; **46**: 667.

71 Vance JM, Small K, Stajich H *et al*. Linkage studies in Von Hippel–Lindau disease. *Cytogenet Cell Genet* 1989; **51**: 1097.

72 Durham-Pierre D, Gardner JM, Nakatsu Y *et al*. African origin of an intragenic deletion of the human P gene in tyrosinase positive oculocutaneous albinism. *Nat Genet* 1994; **7**: 176–9.

73 Hautala T, Byers MG, Eddy RC *et al*. Cloning of human lysyl hydroxylase: Complete DNA derived amino acid sequence and assignment of the gene (PLOD) to chromosome 1p36.3–p36.2. *Genomics* 1992; **13**: 62–9.

74 Saulos MJ, Moser AB, Drwinga H *et al*. Analysis of peroxisomes in lymphoblasts; Zwellweger syndrome and a patient with a deletion in chromosome 7. *Paediatr Res* 1993; **33**: 441–4.

75 Wallace M, Zori RT, Alley T. Smith–Lemli–Optiz syndrome in a female with *de novo* balanced translocation involving 7q32: probable disruption of an SLOS gene. *Am J Med Genet* 1994; **50**: 368–74.

76 Morris CA, Loker J, Ensig G *et al*. Supravalvular aortic stenosis co-segregates with a familial 6;7 translocation that disrupts the elastin gene. *Am J Med Genet* 1993; **46**: 737–44.

77 Musarella M, Anson-Cartwright L, Leal SM *et al*. Multipoint linkage analysis and heterogeneity testing in 20 X-linked retinitis pigmentosa families. *Genomics* 1990; **8**: 286–96.

78 Akita S, Kuratomi H, Abe K *et al*. EC syndrome in a girl with paracentric inversion 7(q22.1q36.3). *Clin Dysmorphol* 1993; **2**: 627.

79 Uitto J, Chung-Honet LC, Christiano AM. Molecular biology and pathology of type VII collagen. *Exp Dermatol* 1992; **1**: 2–11.

80 Phipps ME, Latif F, Prowse A *et al*. Molecular genetic analysis of the 3p syndrome. *Hum Mol Genet* 1994; **3**: 903–8.

81 Hughes A, Newton V, Liu X *et al*. A gene for Waardenburg syndrome type 2 maps close to the human chromosome of the microphthalmia gene chromosome 3p12-p14.1. *Nat Genet* 1994; **7**: 509–12.

82 Kumavamanickaral G, Maw M, Dento M *et al*. Missense rhodopsin mutation in a family with recessive RP. *Nat Genet* 1994; **8**: 10–11.

83 Akaki Y, Hotta Y, Mashima Y *et al*. A deletion in the ornithine aminotransferase gene in gyrate atrophy. *J Biol Chem* 1992; **267**: 12950–4.

84 Porteous ME, Curtis A, Lindsay S *et al*. The gene for Aarskog syndrome located between DXS255 and DXS566 (Xp11.2–Xq13). *Genomics* 1992; **14**: 298–301.

85 Bergoffen J, Scherer SS, Wang S *et al*. Connection mutations in X-linked CMT disease. *Science* 1993; **262**: 2039–42.

86 Lyonnet S, Pelet A, Reyer G *et al*. The gene for X-linked hydrocephalus maps to Xq28 distal to DXS52. *Genomics* 1992; **14**: 508–10.

87 Koole FD, Velzebber CM, van der Harten JJ. Ocular anomalies in the Patau syndrome (chromosome 13 trisomy syndrome). *Ophthalmol Paediatr Genet* 1990; **11**: 15–21.

88 Heon E, Piguet B, Munier F *et al*. Linkage of Autosomal Dominant radial drusen (malattia leventinesse) to chromosone 2p16–21. *Arch Ophthalmol* 1996; **114**: 193–8.

89 Eiberg H, Kjer B, Kjer P *et al*. Dominant optic atrophy (OPA1) mapped to chromosome 3q region 1. Linkage analysis. *Hum Mol Genet* 1994; **3**: 977–80.

90 Holder SE, Grimsley LM, Palmer RW *et al*. Partial trisomy of 3q causing mild Cornelia de Lange phenotype. *J Med Genet* 1994; **31**: 150–2.

91 Pallotta R. Iris coloboma ptosis hypertelorism and mental retardation a new syndrome possibly localised on chromosome 2. *J Med Genet* 1991; **28**: 342–4.

92 Barr FG, Galilli N, Holick J *et al*. Rearrangement of the PAX3 paired box gene in the paediatric solid tumour alveolar rhabdomyosarcoma. *Nat Genet* 1993; **3**: 113–17.

93 Williamson M, Cragg H, Grent J *et al*. A 5′ splice site mutation in fucosidosis. *J Med Genet* 1993; **30**: 218–23.

94 Glenn D, Gelbart T, Beutler E. Tight linkage of pyruvate kinase (PKLR) and glucocerebrosidase (GBA) genes. *Hum Genet* 1994; **93**: 635–8.

95 Masuno M, Tomatsu S, Nakashima Y *et al*. Mucopolysaccharidosis IVA: assignment of the human *N*-acetylgalactosamine 6 sulfate sulfatase (GALNS) gene to chromosome 16q24. *Genomics* 1993; **16**: 777–8.

96 Scott HS, Ashton LJ, Eyre HJ *et al*. Chromosomal localisation of the human alpha L-iduronidase gene (1DUA) to 4p16.3. *Am J Hum Genet* 1990; **47**: 802–7.

97 Tupler R, Maraschio P, Gerardo A *et al*. A complex chromosome rearrangement with 10 break points: tentative assignment of the locus for Williams syndrome to 4q33–q35.1. *J Med Genet* 1992; **29**: 253–5.

98 Byers PH, Steiner RD. Osteogenesis imperfecta. *Ann Rev Med* 1992; **43**: 269–82.

99 Masuno M, Scimozawa N, Suzuki Y *et al*. Assignment of the human peroxisome assembly factor 1 gene (PXMP3) responsible for Zellweger syndrome to chromosome 8q21.1 by fluorescence *in situ* hybridization. *Genomics* 1994; **20**: 141–2.

100 Gartner J, Valle D. The 70 kDa peroxisomal membrane protein: an ATP binding cassette transporter protein involved in peroxisome biogenesis. *Semin Cell Biol* 1993; **4**: 45–52.

101 Gartner J, Moser H, Valle D. Mutations in the 70 K peroxisomal membrane protein gene in Zellweger syndrome. *Nat Genet* 1992; **1**: 16–23.

102 Gosch A, Paukau R. Chromosome abnormalities in the Williams–Beuren syndrome. *J Med Genet* 1993; **30**: 886.

103 Colley A, Thakker Y, Ward H *et al*. Unbalanced 13:18 translocation and Williams syndrome. *J Med Genet* 1992; **29**: 63–5.

104 Menko FH, Stouthart PJ. Williams syndrome and chromosome 18 (letter). *J Med Genet* 1992; **29**: 679–80.

105 Yu CE, Oshima J, Goddard KA *et al*. Linkage disequilibrium and haplotype studies of chromosome 8p11.1–21.1 markers and Werner syndrome. *Am J Hum Genet* 1994; **55**: 356–64.

106 Riess O, Winkelmann B, Epplen JT. Toward the complete genomic map and molecular pathology of human chromosome 4. *Hum Genet* 1994; **94**: 1–18.

107 Dahlback B. Protein S and C4b binding protein: components involved in the regulation of the C protein anticoagulant system. *Thromb Haemostat* 1991; **66**: 49–61.

108 Juliusson G, Gahrton G. Cytogenetics in CLL and related disorders. *Bailliéres Clin Haematol* 1993; **6**: 821–48.

109 Wells J, Wroblewski J, Keen J *et al*. Mutations in the human retinal degeneration slow RDS gene can cause either retinitis pigmentosa or macular dystrophy. *Nat Genet* 1993; **3**: 213–18.

110 Nichols BE, Sheffield VC, Vandenburgh K *et al*. Butterfly shaped pigment dystrophy of the fovea caused by a point mutation in codon 167 of the RDS gene. *Nat Genet* 1993; **3**: 202–7.

111 Muller U, Warman MI, Mulliken JB *et al*. Assignment of a gene locus involved in craniosynostosis to chromosome 5qter. *Hum Mol Genet* 1993; **2**: 119–22.

112 Clark BJ, Lowther GW, Lee WR. Congenital ocular defects associated with an abnormality of human chromosome 1 trisomy 1q32–qter. *J Paediatr Ophthalmol Strabismus* 1994; **31**: 41–5.

113 Yang Feng TL, Zheng K, Yu J *et al*. Assignment of the human glycogen debrancher gene to chromosome 1p21. *Genomics* 1992; **13**: 931–4.

114 Pankau R, Gosch A, Simeoni E *et al*. Williams–Beuren syndrome in monozygotic twins with variable expression. *Am J Med Genet* 1993; **47**: 475–7.

115 Rose NC, Menacker SJ, Schnur RE *et al*. Ocular albinism in a male with del (6)(q 13–q15): candidate region for autosomal recessive ocular albinism. *Am J Med Genet* 1992; **42**: 700–5.

116 Kajiwara K, Sandberg MA, Berson EL *et al*. A null mutation in the human peripherin/RDS gene in a family with autosomal dominant retinitis punctata albescens. *Nat Genet* 1993; **3**: 208–12.

117 Muenke M, Gurrien F, Bay C *et al*. Linkage of a human brain malformation familial holoprosencephaly to chromosome 7 and evidence for genetic heterogeneity. *Proc Natl Acad Sci USA* 1994; **91**: 102–6.

118 Estabrooks LL, Rao KW, Donahue RP *et al*. Holoprosencephaly in an infant with a minute deletion of chromosome 21(q22.3). *Am J Med Genet* 1990; **36**: 306–9.

119 Cook PJ, Hamerton JL. Report of the committee on the genetic constitution of chromosome 1. *Cytogenet Cell Genet* 1979; **25**: 9–20.

120 Tonini GP. Neuroblastoma: the result of multistep transformation? *Stem Cells* 1993; **11**: 276–82.

121 Lebo RV, Martelli L, Su Y *et al*. Prenatal diagnosis of Charcot–Marie–Tooth disease type 1A by multicolour *in situ* hybridisation. *Am J Med Genet* 1993; **47**: 441–50.

122 Blanton SH, Heckenlively JR, Cottingham AW. Linkage mapping of autosomal dominant RP (RP1) to pericentric region of chromosome 8. *Genomics* 1991; **11**: 857–69.

123 Leiri T. Thyroglobulin Tg gene and familial Tg defect. *Nippon Rinsho* 1994; **52**: 869–74.

124 Fujita R, Hanauer A, Vincent A *et al* Physical mapping of two loci (D955 and D9515) tightly linked to Friedreich ataxia locus (FRDA) and identification of nearby CpG islands by pulse field electrophoresis. *Genomics* 1991; **10**: 915–20.

125 Fryns JP, Bukke J, Verdu P. Apparent late onset Cockayne syndrome and interstitial deletion of the long arm of chromosome 10. *Am J Med Genet* 1991; **40**: 343–4.

126 Ziv Y, Frydman M, Lange E. Ataxia telangiectasia: linkage analysis in highly inbred Arab and Druze families and differentiation from an ataxia microcephaly syndrome. *Hum Genet* 1992; **88**: 619–26.

127 Slee JJ, Smart RD, Viljoeu DL. Deletion of chromosome 13 in Moebius syndrome. *J Med Genet* 1991; **28**: 413–18.

128 Sellor MJ, Chitty LS, Dunbar H. Pseudotrisomy 13 and autosomal recessive holoprosencephaly. *J Med Genet* 1993; **30**: 970–1.

129 Verloes A, Ayme S, Gambarelli D *et al*. Holoprosencephaly–polydactyly (pseudotrisomy 13) syndrome: a syndrome with features of hydrocephalus and Smith–Lemli–Optiz syndrome. A collaborative multicentre study. *J Med Genet* 1991; **28**: 297–303.

130 Pentao L, Lewis RA, Ledbetter DH *et al*. Maternal uniparental isodisomy of chromosome 14: association with autosomal recessive rod monochromacy. *Am J Hum Genet* 1992; **50**: 690–9.

131 Lee ST, Nicholls RD, Bundey S *et al*. Mutation of the P gene in oculocutaneous albinism, ocular albinism and Prader–Willi syndrome and albinism. *N Engl J Med* 1994; **330**: 529–34.

132 Fukushima Y, Wakui K, Nishida T *et al*. Craniosynostosis in an infant with an interstitial deletion of 15q [46XYdel (15) (q15q22.1)]. *Am J Med Genet* 1990; **36**: 209–13.

133 Tavin E, Stecker E, Marion R. Nasal pyriform aperture stenosis and the holoprosencephaly spectrum. *Int J Paediatr Otorhinolaryngol* 1994; **28**: 199–204.

134 Van Essen AJ, Schoots CJ, van Lingen RA *et al*. Isochrome 18q in a girl with holoprosencephaly, Di George anomaly and streak ovaries. *Am J Med Genet* 1993; **47**: 85–8.

135 Greenberg J, Goliath R, Beighton P *et al*. A new locus for autosomal dominant retinitis pigmentosa on the short arm of chromosome 17. *Hum Mol Genet* 1994; **3**: 915–18.

136 Rouleau GA, Merel P, Lutchman M *et al*. Alteration in a new gene encoding a putative membrane organising protein cause for neurofibromatosis type 2. *Nature* 1993; **363**: 515–21.

137 Ruttledge MH, Xie YG, Han FY *et al*. Physical mapping of the NF2/meningioma region on human chromosome 22q12. *Genomics* 1994; **19**: 52–9.

138 Mitnick RJ, Bello JA, Shprintzen RJ. Brain anomalies in velocardio-facial syndrome. *Am J Med Genet* 1994; **54**: 100–6.

139 Church DM, Bengtsson U, Nielsen KV *et al*. Molecular definition of deletions of different segments of distal 5p that result in distinct phenotypic features. *Am J Hum Genet* 1995; **56**: 1162–72.

140 Lichter PR. Genetic clues to glaucoma's secrets. The L Edward Jackson Memorial Lecture. Part 2. *Am J Ophthalmol* 1994; **117**: 706–27.

141 Takano T, Yamanouchi Y. Assignment of human beta galactosidase A gene to 3p21.33 by fluorescence *in situ* hybridization. *Hum Genet* 1993; **92**: 403–4.

142 Cowles T, Furman P, Wilkins I. Prenatal diagnosis of Dandy Walker malformation in a family displaying X-linked inheritance. *Prenat Diagn* 1993; **13**: 87–91.

143 Ragge NK. Clinical and genetic patterns of neurofibromatosis 1 and 2. *Br J Ophthalmol* 1993; **77**: 662–72.

144 McLaughlin ME, Sandberg MA, Berson EL *et al*. Recessive mutations in the gene encoding the beta-subunit of rod phosphodiesterase in patients with retinitis pigmentosa. *Nat Genet* 1993; **4**: 130–4.

145 Rutland P, Pulleyn LJ, Reardon W *et al*. Identical mutations in the FGFR2 gene cause both Pfeiffer and Crouzon syndrome phenotypes. *Nat Genet* 1995; **9**: 173–6.

146 Lajeunie E, Ma HW, Bonaventure J *et al*. FGFR2 mutations in Pfeiffer syndrome. *Nat Genet* 1995; **9**: 108.

147 Wilkie AOM, Slaney SF, Oldridge M *et al*. Apert's syndrome results from localised mutations of FGFR2 and is allelic with Crouzon syndrome. *Nat Genet* 1995; **9**: 165–72.

148 Heon E, Sheth BP, Kalenak JW *et al*. Linkage of autosomal dominant iris hypoplasia to the region of the Rieger syndrome locus

(4q25). *Hum Mol Genet* 1995; **4**: 1435–9.

149 Camuzat A, Dollfus H, Rozet JM *et al.* A gene for Leber's congenital amaurosis maps to chromosome 17p. *Hum Mol Genet* 1995; **4**: 1447–52.

150 Bardien S, Ebenezer N, Greenberg J *et al.* An eighth locus for autosomal dominant retinitis pigmentosa is linked to chromosome 17q. *Hum Mol Genet* 1995; **4**: 1459–62.

151 Bonneau D, Winter-Fuseau I, Loiseau MN *et al.* Bilateral cataract and high serum ferritin: a new dominant genetic disorder. *J Med Genet* 1995; **32**: 778–9.

152 Van Camp G, Van Thienen MN, Handig I *et al.* Chromosome 13q deletion with Waardenburg syndrome: further evidence for a gene involved in neural crest function on 13q. *J Med Genet* 1995; **32**: 531–6.

153 Yokayama Y, Narahara K, Tsuji K *et al.* Autosomal dominant congenital cataract and microphthalmia associated with familial t(2; 16) translocation. *Hum Genet* 1992; **90**: 177–8.

154 Padma T, Ayyagari R, Murty JS *et al.* Autosomal dominant zonular cataract with sutural opacities localised to chromosome 17q11–12. *Am J Hum Genet* 1995; **57**: 840–5.

155 Vansoest S, Vandenborn LI, Gal A *et al.* Assignment of a gene for autosomal recessive retinitis pigmentosa (RP 12) to chromosome 1q31–q32.1 in an inbred and genetically heterogeneous disease population. *Genomics* 1994; **22**: 499–504.

156 al-Maghtheh M, Inglehearn C, Keen T *et al.* The identification of a sixth locus for autosomal dominant retinitis pigmentosa on chromosome 19. *Hum Mol Genet* 1994; **3**: 351–4.

157 McGuire RE, Sullivan LS, Blanton SH *et al.* X-linked dominant cone-rod degeneration: linkage mapping of a new locus for retinitis pigmentosa (RP 15) to Xp22.13–p22.11. *Am J Hum Genet* 1995; **57**: 87–94.

158 Knowles J, Shugart Y, Banerjee P *et al.* Identification of a locus, distinct from RDS-peripherin, for autosomal recessive retinitis pigmentosa on chromosome 6p. *Hum Mol Genet* 1994; **3**: 1401–3.

12: The Visually Handicapped Baby and the Family

David Taylor

Although it is preferable to work with, or refer to, a paediatrician or another professional with a special interest in the development of visually handicapped or multiply handicapped children, the ophthalmologist and general paediatrician must learn to understand the needs of the visually impaired baby and his family. By understanding the whole family's needs their shock and pain of having a child with special needs will be eased, and the baby himself will be helped to best overcome his handicap (Sonksen & Stiff 1991).

The blind child

Effect of visual handicap on the baby

The absence or blunting of sight from birth has effects that stretch far beyond the simple loss of vision (Cass *et al.* 1994) because vision is necessary in the development of other primary senses and perceptions and also for normal social integration. Early in the baby's life, as any parent knows, there is a deep bond that forms aided by visual communication—the mother knows that her baby is not just pointing both his eyes at her but actually communicating and their relationship builds on that early interaction. The poverty of facial expression of a blind child may be a problem to the parents unless it is explained that they only show extremes of facial expressions, that the smile may be rather fixed and that their face becomes passive when they are concentrating on speech.

The meaning of things touched such as other parts of the child's body, other people or objects, is enhanced by the use of vision. In a sighted child, the full meaning of an object that is explored by touch may be gained, and a visual memory of that object is developed; because a blind baby lacks this visual memory his tactile exploration is less rewarding.

Sight is partly necessary for the learning of speech; the baby mimics the parent's lip movements. Also, by using his hearing to modify the sounds he makes, speech is formed. Sightless babies do not turn their head towards a source of sound nearly as accurately, as quickly or as persistently as sighted babies and there are other secondary motor problems (Cass *et al.* 1994).

The blind baby is very late in appreciating the disposition of the world around him in three dimensions. Sounds, touch and other communication reach him as though from anywhere and it is a long time before he builds up a 'map' or frame of reference that is similar to that of a sighted person. The concept of permanence of the surroundings, and perspective are difficult to grasp—perspective in particular is almost impossible for a blind person to understand. Descriptions of brightness and colour are meaningless and names of colours with second meanings (such as blue, yellow, purple) probably mean less as well!

The social interaction of a blind child with other blind or with sighted children is more difficult; their lack of mobility, sometimes odd appearance and delay in other areas of development makes them poor companions for sighted children. Even as toddlers, the blind have greater difficulties in socializing and interacting in their play groups and in infant school. This pattern is set in early life and persists, although at some stage many children over-react against it, and go through a precocious stage that lasts a variable period. Later they often lack drive, initiative and independence, and tend to prefer their own company or that of close relatives.

Blind babies who do not have appropriate help in the early years, especially if they have additional handicaps, are at risk of developing a form of autism the effects of which are life long and may be devastating.

There is little doubt that advice and help can enable many parents to help their child to lead a more fulfilling life. Their intellectual and developmental achievements and potential need to be assessed using special scales for visually handicapped children (Reynell & Zinkin 1979).

The older visually handicapped children

The advantage of referring a visually handicapped child to an expert in child development is that they can get specific help and preventive advice, so that it is best to refer them routinely and as early as possible. Every ophthalmologist and paediatrician involved in the case of visually handicapped children should read about the subject — a book such as that by Scott *et al.* (1985) provides insight into the problems and practical advice on how to help. It is helpful if the advice given is consistent and even offered before a problem arises, so the ophthalmologist and general paediatrician should be conversant with the main problems that confront blind babies. It is important that a strong, early relationship builds up between the doctor, the parents and the children and that it is based on mutual trust and respect.

The advice given has to be tailored to each child's needs, so that, for example, specific advice regarding schooling in the later years is not usually the province of the primary doctor but of the educators, agencies and local authorities working in concert. Particularly in cases of multiple handicap, doctors will be required to give advice about not only the child's visual capabilities but also how these problems interact with the other handicaps.

Mannerisms and stereotyped behaviour

Blind children develop a wide variety of mannerisms; eye-poking or rubbing, body rocking, head banging, light seeking or sun staring, making repetitive noise, and even, in severe cases usually associated with mental retardation, self mutilation. There is no clear cause for these abnormal forms of behaviour but it may be related to the way in which they are handled in early life. Early intervention by encouraging the parents to handle the baby frequently and to keep him occupied for much of his waking hours may help. Once the mannerisms have become established it is very difficult to stop them. Most doctors involved with visually handicapped children do not recommend psychiatric treatment by aversive therapy, preferring to encourage the parents to intervene when the child is employing the mannerism and substitute it for another one with less risk and that is less socially odd; for instance to exchange eye-rubbing for thumb-sucking.

Self image, self esteem and cosmetic problems

Cosmetic problems, such as an ugly appearance of the eyes, a squint or roving eye movements need to be considered early because of their potential to alter the way other people may react to the baby. Older children, where reasonably possible, should be reassured that they look nice as this will all help with their confidence and self esteem which is easily shaken and often only rises to levels that would be considered low in sighted people.

Psychological and psychiatric problems

Psychiatric problems are more common in blind children, and especially those with multiple handicaps. Many of these problems, including the autistic behaviour of some blind children, may be prevented by appropriate early management. However, once established these may require expert help. Behaviour disorders, personality abnormalities and manipulative behaviour are all frequent and require patience and understanding together with pre-emptive counselling as a way of prevention by appropriate handling. Interestingly, clinical depression is probably no more frequent in blind than sighted children.

Sport and mobility

One of the major difficulties in social interaction and the building of self esteem is the immobility of blind children and their inability to take part in games and sport like sighted children. It is only very rarely that blind or partially sighted children need to be excluded from sport and activity on the grounds that it might endanger their eyes, so the main reasons why they don't take part are visual. Water sports, even sailing, skiing, walking, running, pottery, wood-carving, sculpture, tandem bicycle riding, bungee jumping, gymnastics, and many other activities can be enjoyed by blind children. However, from very early on the parents need to be encouraged to let their child take part in the rough and tumble of nursery games and to stifle their natural desire to overprotect the child.

The degree to which a visually handicapped child is mobile depends on several factors: intelligence, the amount of vision that he has, how well and how early he was encouraged to be mobile, the type of visual defect, when he became blind and above all his drive and personality. Mobility is essential to achieve independence and it usually requires a very high degree of commitment to training by the child, his parents and the agencies.

The parents and other family members

Impact of the diagnosis on the parents

Most parents react positively to the diagnosis of blindness in their child but others may react in a negative and even destructive way (Hunt & Wilh 1983). However, even those who have an outwardly calm demeanour will later admit that the realization of the extent of the visual handicap and its awesome implications on their and their children's lives brought with it the most difficult time in their lives.

Parents may react with a mixture of anger, resentment, terror and aggression in varying mixtures which may be destructive and against the best interests of their child. These reactions start early and until they are overcome they only make things worse for the child; they are all made worse by the lack of a cure, the absence of a diagnosis, the making of a diagnosis that is later changed, and the great uncertainty about the future.

The uncertainty is compounded by a changing handicap, uncertainty about the medical diagnosis and prognosis, a failure by the parents to grasp the full impact of the diagnosis and much deeper worries about the educational implications (will it take him away from home?), genetic worries, and rarely discussed but none the less important concerns about the cause (is it a throwback, was it anything that the parents did?).

Early and positive intervention and good consistent advice can help prevent all of these worries.

When and how to talk to the parents

Every doctor will acquire his or her own way of doing this very rewarding but difficult job but it is generally best to save the definitive discussion until the diagnosis is established, if this is not immediately apparent. A preliminary discussion will be necessary until the diagnosis is established to keep the parents informed of the plan of investigation and how much is known so far.

Repeated interviews are very helpful, as even the most intelligent parents (or their doctor!) can remember only a few items from each interview. It is essential to give them plenty of time for questions and to leave an open invitation to come back at any time. Encouraging parents to write down their questions is a helpful invitation but it is surprisingly rarely taken up. A booklet on how parents can best help their child is most helpful (Sonksen & Stiff 1991).

The way in which the parents' questions are answered is vital. A friendly, simple approach using simple diagrams and no jargon, will help the parents to understand the defect and its impact on the life of their baby, and on the rest of the family. It is essential to be honest about how much or how little you know; it is just as important to most parents to know the limits of your knowledge about their child's problem as it is to know how much you know.

The role of the first adviser is by far the most difficult. Very few non-ophthalmologists understand how difficult it is to be the first adviser in the chain of visual handicap experts that the parents of a blind child will meet. The first ophthalmologist is often blamed by the parents and their later advisers, sometimes with justification, because he or she has been too blunt, too indirect, too evasive, too insensitive, and so on; perhaps the later adviser should try being the first!

The meaning of visual handicap to a family

The terms 'blindness', 'partial sight', 'visual handicap' and 'blunted sight' all have different meanings to different people. Statutory definitions usually involve the ability of the child to be educated by sighted or non-sighted means, or in older people involve employment. A child may be blind from the educational point of view but able to behave almost normally until the time comes for him to read and write. It is vital to define for the parents what you mean by any of these terms; for instance to define that blindness does not necessarily mean to be stone blind and that a child may be able to do many things whilst still being registered blind. The most common mistake is to be too pessimistic, which makes things more difficult for the parents. Be accurate as far as you can and build up the value of the residual vision. Even ability to perceive light only is better than no perception of light. Use all the diagnostic aids at your disposal but rely most on clinical judgement as this still provides the best guide. It is probably not an exaggeration to say that the parents should not be told that the child is stone blind unless he is anophthalmic!

Other children in the family can be profoundly affected by the blind sibling and show reactions of anger, jealousy because of the attention the child gets, hysterical conversion symptoms, attention-seeking behaviour difficulties, and embarrassment because of the appearance of the child. There is no one way to handle these problems, but pre-emptive advice to the parents on not overprotecting the blind baby (or the sibling), being fair in their attentions, especially early in the life of the handicapped baby, and being equal in their rewards and punishment, all help to make the other sibling feel at least equal. The sighted older sibling can be given special responsibilities for the blind baby and often reacts positively to this. It is important to let the children sort out their own interpersonal problems and for the parents to interfere as little as possible.

The second opinion

It is better if the doctor suggests getting a second opinion to the parents. It is more confidence building for the parents if the suggestion comes from the doctor but if the parents or their other advisers suggest it first it is only sensible for the doctor to co-operate whole-heartedly with the suggestion. When the first specialist suggests a second opinion he can usually influence to whom the child is referred to make sure that the best opinion is obtained.

Positive ways of helping

Early and positive intervention

The diagnosis of a severe visual handicap need not be accompanied by negative advice as the parents are often aware of what a blind child cannot do and they need positive advice to help them to help their child (they need to know what he can do). This is not just a way of 'keeping them occupied' but appropriate advice and early stimulation (Hyvärinen 1983; Sonksen *et al.* 1991) can help the baby to make the best of his life.

Starting the advice early (early intervention) is helpful not only to the baby but it can help the parents in the early days to live with the awful shock of the discovery of blindness in their child (Sonksen & Stiff 1991).

One of the most common reactions of the parents is to feel overawed by their baby's problems and to have a rather stand-offish attitude to the child, they treat him like porcelain. It is good to show them that he is like any other baby and can enjoy all the cuddling, playing and the gentle rough and tumble that sighted children get.

Any residual vision, however little, should be encouraged by stimuli appropriate to the visual defect. These include the use of lights, mirrors, brightly coloured and broad patterned toys, and especially toys that have interesting and different textures and preferably ones which make a noise.

Helping the child to learn to explore things with his hands can be started from birth. The parents can be encouraged to hold their baby close to them and to hold his hands to their faces to explore them.

The more auditory–tactile stimuli that the blind baby gets the better he will learn to understand and react to new stimuli later.

Physiotherapy

Home physiotherapy and posture-improving exercises are advised by some experts who rightly note that the odd posture and mannerisms of blind children may contribute to their difficulties in communication with others.

Consistent advice, where possible from the same doctor or other adviser, is very much to be encouraged; inconsistency leads to loss of confidence and failure to take any advice. Unfortunately not many state medical systems make this possible.

Other family members

Other children in the family need to be remembered. It is very easy for them to be overlooked by the parents in their desire to do their best for the blind child; they can often be encouraged to help the baby with visual stimulation and just general play, with mutual benefit.

The parents of a blind child are often so involved with the immediate problems that it is very easy for them to overlook the needs of their own parents. The baby's grandparents are often less able to accept his problem than the parents but they can be given help by the parents who should be encouraged to involve the grandparents in any discussion and in getting them to help with the day-to-day life of the baby; not least in baby-sitting while the parents get out by themselves.

The burdens (and the joys) should be shared between all the members of the family. Often the doctor can be helpful in identifying the 'expert' parent or grandparent; one who takes on all the tasks, reads and knows all about blindness, and tends to exclude other members.

When there is no treatment

Three-quarters of child blindness is totally untreatable. The parents often expect that treatment will be available somewhere or sometime; we are so bombarded with news reports of medical breakthroughs that many people believe that most conditions are treatable.

A frank discussion, emphasizing that although no formal cure is possible there is still a lot that can be done for the child, and that no cure is available anywhere else (if this is true) will help the parents to accept the situation and look forward positively. In this respect it is often best to broach the subject of eye transplant to the parents and to tell them why no such operation is possible or is likely to be possible in the future. Many parents think that a transplant (of one of their eyes) might help the baby but some are too shy to bring up the question themselves.

Support measures

Most support measures are the province of the blind

agency workers, the community or others local to the family home but it is important for all to be aware of the possibility of helping the parents and the rest of the family by simple means.

It may be possible to arrange help with baby-sitting, either for evenings or parts of weekends so that the parents can be together and go to do things such as shopping, meeting the bank manager, visiting friends, and so on, whilst being confident that the child is safe and happy. Longer term child care, short-term fostering, or even admission to hospital, nursing home or children's home for short periods may enable parents to go on holiday together or accompany each other on business trips or visit a partner who is working away from home.

When the day-to-day management of the child is a major stress factor in a family it may be possible to reduce the burden, and increase the family's positive attitude towards the child by arranging for the child to board at a school or home during the week, coming home at the weekends.

Blindness agency workers may have access to a toy library of suitable toys for visually handicapped children. These workers become very expert at understanding and helping parents and perform a valuable service in the broader management of the child; by intervention, advice and counselling.

Specific problems for the family

Lack of bonding

The lack of mutual visual communication, together with the shock of the diagnosis and many other factors, can give rise to an incomplete bonding or even a source of rejection or distancing in the parents. These feelings probably reflect on the child and affect him too. It is best prevented by early intervention and encouraging bodily contact and game playing.

Guilty feelings

Many parents feel a sense of guilt that they have brought a handicapped child into the world; this is most especially so if the cause is thought to be genetic, due to prenatal infection or drug ingestion or postnatal injury. The effect of these feelings can be all-consuming with harmful effects on both parents, the baby and the rest of the family: many are irrational but many are founded on lack of understanding of the condition and its cause, so the best remedy is in the fullest explanation and early intervention.

Family stress

Whilst the birth of a blind baby can result in a deeper and stronger relationship between the parents and other members of the family it very frequently results in enormous stresses within the family. The parents may argue, start to drink alcohol heavily or behave aggressively towards each other or their children, and the marriage may break up especially if there were pre-existing problems. The ophthalmologist is usually in no position to help here; it is usually the paediatrician, health worker or blindness agency worker who is in closer contact and who may be able to help in small but positive ways.

Parents who reject help

Sometimes the reaction of the parents is very strongly against what is seen as the conventional medical wisdom especially if the doctors are seen as failing to provide a cure. They may fail to recognize the handicap and are determined to treat their child as normal until he 'gets better' or they reject any help or counselling. This is quite a common problem and will vary in degree, and it can be handled in various ways but it is unlikely to be resolved by forcing or bullying the parents who, providing the physical and mental welfare of the child is being looked after, are usually well within their rights. Usually the best approach is to maintain contact and there are often small problems that the parents can be helped with that may gradually establish a useful relationship again between the parents and the doctor. Again prevention by early and positive advice is the best cure.

Genetic counselling

Unless the cause of the child's blindness is clearly non-genetic, such as in cases of proven (not suspected) congenital infection, the parents should be encouraged to have genetic counselling. Even if the condition is not obviously hereditary, or if the diagnosis is not known there is usually a lot that the geneticist can do to help the parents either in diagnosis by association of ocular and non-ocular conditions, by giving empirical recurrence risks or by newer forms of genetic and chromosomal investigation. Advice is also helpful for older children and young adults who may be concerned about their chances of passing on the defect. Around one-half of blind children have an hereditary condition.

Parents' groups

In many parts of the world parents meet in self-help groups. These may be disease orientated, i.e. rubella or retinitis pigmentosa, or handicap based, i.e. deaf–blind or partially sighted, and the parents meet for discussion of mutual problems, or act as local or nationwide pressure groups. Some of the disease-orientated groups have charity status and raise money for research. Some parents derive great comfort and help from these groups but initially it is often best to arrange for a meeting with one parent, on the understanding that the 'new' parent of a blind baby realizes that no two cases are the same. It is often very reassuring to the new parent to hear how the older child is getting on and managing; often much better than the new parent would have guessed.

Multiple handicaps

Further handicaps do not just add to the visual handicap, they multiply it. One of the biggest problems that face the parent is that numerous experts become involved. It is therefore most important that there is only one conductor to the medical orchestra (usually it is best if this is a paediatrician with a special interest in handicap) and that he or she works in close co-operation with, and preferably geographically close to, the specialists. Multidisciplinary teams are one way of getting around this problem although they may be a relatively inefficient use of specialists' time. If the care can be confined within one hospital and the number of visits curtailed there is an enormous saving to the parents of time, money and stress.

Visual problems are frequent in children with developmental delay and there is a high incidence of other defects in children with poor vision. Vigilance for both is necessary to give the child his best chance in life.

Mental retardation is defined by the World Health Organization as 'incomplete or insufficient general development of mental capacities'. There are many other definitions.

In the UK the term educationally subnormal (ESN) is used, with moderate (M) or severe (S) subclassifications. ESN(M) children have IQs between 50 and 69, and ESN(S) children have IQs below 50; those below 30 usually being designated profound ESN(S).

In assessing the ability of visually handicapped children special tests are necessary to reduce the effect of the visual handicap on the child's performance (Reynell & Zinkin 1979).

Chromosomal abnormalities (e.g. Down's syndrome), genetic conditions (e.g. the phakomatoses), 'acquired' causes such as congenital infection, antepartum haemorrhage or toxaemia and intrauterine growth retardation, or prenatal toxic effects (such as drugs and alcohol), are all important prenatal causes. Perinatal anoxia is probably a major cause of cerebral palsy and many affected children are also mentally retarded. Postnatal damage is a less frequent cause of mental retardation in most developed countries. Nonetheless malnutrition, deprived social conditions as well as meningitis, hydrocephalus, hypoglycaemia, encephalitis, and trauma (including non-accidental injury) all play their role. One form of epilepsy in infancy is the so-called infantile spasm which is characteristically a generalized seizure with spasm in flexion.

Many children who have infantile spasms appear to be blind as their EEG is grossly abnormal and they are constantly fitting. Most of these children turn out to be substantially mentally retarded even when the spasms are controlled. They may have structural brain disease, e.g. tuberose sclerosis or Aicardi's syndrome (in which infantile spasms, agenesis of the corpus collosum, ectopic grey matter and characteristic retinal defects are associated in girls). Neurometabolic disease such as phenylketonuria, Tay–Sachs, or Batten's disease are unusual associations of epilepsy with blindness and congenital infections are uncommon but significantly preventable causes.

The apparently poor vision in these children appears to improve as the fits are controlled and mental development occurs.

Cerebral palsy is a common cause of disability in childhood. It is a motor defect due to non-progressive brain damage in infancy or early childhood. It may be characterized by spasticity, rigidity, athetosis, ataxia or occasionally tremor, or it may be mixed. Various forms occur such as hemiplegia, or double hemiplegia (tetraplegia), diplegia (bilateral but legs more affected than arms) or athetoid (with involuntary movements). From the ophthalmologist's point of view the two most common problems in cerebral palsy are optic atrophy and squint. Optic atrophy is common in children with perinatal anoxia as the cause of their cerebral palsy and its effects are often multiplied by the presence of widespread cerebral damage. Early diagnosis is important so as to institute early intervention. Squints in children with cerebral palsy should be treated in the same way as normal children. There is often a temptation to think it is kind to spare a child with cerebral palsy surgery just for cosmetic reasons. The cosmetic indication is even more important in a child with cerebral palsy, who already has a good enough reason for strangers reacting oddly with him, and in any case some of these children with squints may develop useful binocular vision if treated appropriately. Caution should be exercised with surgery as they often make a more substantial response than usual to standard amounts of surgery and consecutive squints are frequent.

Education

Playgroups

Preschool contact with other blind and with sighted children is helpful in improving the blind child's confidence and inquisitiveness. Many ordinary playgroups will accept visually handicapped babies and young children and in some areas there are playgroups attached to schools for older visually handicapped children.

Preschool training

It is important to start thinking about education long before the child actually needs to go to school. The availability of special education and extra help with education in a normal school varies enormously from country to country and in different areas within each country. The visual defect needs to be registered so that the education authorities are aware of the further needs of the child and of the needs for special education within a community. The earlier these needs are known the easier it is to arrange for appropriate education. Registration may be delayed, or the categorization left uncertain if the vision of the child is changing but in general it is still best for the child's handicap to be registered and his needs recognized for the future.

There is a very strong trend towards integration of children into local schools, either in the normal classroom for those with minimal defect or into a local special school for visual handicap, the type of education offered depending on the visual abilities of the child and the presence of any other handicap. Many normal schools have visual handicap units within them, offering specialized extra help in teaching together with special facilities for the partially sighted such as closed circuit TV reading aids.

Special boarding schools are usually available for older children and may have the advantage of special facilities and a more independent environment.

The agency responsible for placement varies from country to country but ultimately it is the parent who has to decide on the best of the alternatives on offer. The school which has the right atmosphere and facilities for the child's combination of defects is often difficult to find near to the parental home and there has to be a major commitment to travelling throughout the child's education. The parents will need to visit all the schools available and to hold discussions with the staff before they can be sure of their choice—and time will show a proportion of parents that theirs was not the right choice!

Boarding schools

Although integration into the sighted community is the aim, in many countries there can be little doubt that there is still a role for boarding or weekly boarding schools for certain categories of children.

The young and some older multiply handicapped children may fare better in a more ordered environment, and the families of such children may benefit from a rest from their child's demands during the week in cases where weekly boarding is possible.

The older child may benefit from the special facilities available, from the training of the staff, and from contact with other children in the same predicament.

Bibliography for parents (see also Chapter P30)

Carson S, Arthbertson D, Forbes C. *Off to a Good Start! A Rescue Manual for Parents of Young Blind and Visually Impaired Children*. Newton, Massachusetts, Massachusetts International Institute for the Visually Impaired. (This book is largely for those in Massachusetts, USA, but with ideas for others.)

Heart to Heart. Parents of Blind and Partially Sighted Children Talk about their Feelings. Blind Children's Center, 412 Marathan Street, PO Box 29159, Los Angeles, California 9002, USA.

Scott EP, Jan JE, Freeman RD. *Can't Your Child See?*, 2nd edn. Pro-Ed 5341. Industrial Oaks Boulevard, Austin, Texas 78735, USA, 1985.

Sonksen P, Stiff B. *Show Me What My Friends Can See. A Developmental Guide for Parents of Babies with Severely Impaired Sight and their Professional Advisers*. Institute of Child Health, London WC1N 1EH, UK, 1991.

References

Cass HD, Sonksen PM, McConachie HR. Developmental setback in severe visual impairment. *Arch Dis Child* 1994; **70**: 192–6.

Fraiberg S. *Insights from the Blind: Comparative Studies of Blind and Sighted Infants*. New York: Basic Books, 1977.

Hunt H, Wilh DM. The visually handicapped child. In: Wybar KC, Taylor DSI, eds. *Paediatric Ophthalmology — Current Aspects*. New York: Marcel Dekker, 1983: 85–141.

Hyvärinen L. Early stimulation of visually impaired infants. *Ophth Paed Genet* 1983; **2**: 129–33.

Jan JE, Freeman RD, Scott EP. *Visual Impairment in Children and Adolescents*. New York: Grune & Stratton, 1977.

Reynell J, Zinkin P. Developmental aids for young visually handicapped children. *Child Care Health Dev* 1979; **1**: 61–9.

Sonksen PM, Petrie A, Drew KJ. Promotion of visual development in severely visually impaired babies; evaluation of a developmentally based programme. *Dev Med Child Neurol* 1991; **33**: 320–50.

Section 3
Infectious, Allergic and External Eye Disorders

13: Ocular Manifestations of Intrauterine Infections

Scott Lambert

While most maternal infections during pregnancy do not affect the developing fetus, there are several notable exceptions including the TORCH infections (i.e. toxoplasmosis, syphilis, rubella, cytomegalovirus (CMV), and herpes simplex), human immunodeficiency virus (HIV) and varicella. While certain of these infections have decreased in prevalence with the introduction of vaccinations and antibiotics, the incidence of others, such as neonatal HIV infections, have increased exponentially during recent years.

Neonates may be infected either by haematogenous spread, an ascending infection from the maternal genitourinary tract, or during the delivery process. Primary rubella and varicella infections impart life-long immunity, virtually eliminating any risk of an intrauterine infection during subsequent pregnancies, while other infections such as CMV and toxoplasmosis may recur (Embil *et al.* 1970; Knech *et al.* 1971; Stagno *et al.* 1977). Maternal syphilis infection may result in significant intrauterine disease, regardless of whether it is a primary, secondary or latent infection. Similarly, women with HIV infections have a high incidence of affected offspring even if the infection is long standing or asymptomatic.

Intrauterine infections may injure the fetus by disturbing embryogenesis, damaging vital organs, or as an ongoing infection into postnatal life. Rubella infections primarily damage the fetus by interfering with embryogenesis and as a consequence rarely result in serious malformations after the first trimester. Varicella and CMV infections damage the fetus by causing necrosis of vital organs and may result in severe abnormalities even if contracted during the second and, rarely, the third trimesters of gestation. Intrauterine HIV and syphilis infections continue to damage neonates postnatally and as part of an ongoing infection.

Intrauterine infections are difficult to distinguish on clinical grounds alone. Laboratory confirmation may sometimes be obtained by culturing the responsible pathogen; cultures from neonates with intrauterine CMV, rubella and herpes simplex infections are frequently positive. Other infections, such as varicella and toxoplasmosis, are difficult to culture after intrauterine infections and usually require serological confirmation of the diagnosis. An elevated titre of immunoglobulin M (IgM) antibodies in a neonate suggests an intrauterine infection since maternal IgM antibodies are too large to cross the blood–placental barrier. An elevated titre of IgG antibodies is less specific since maternal IgG antibodies cross the blood–placental barrier; however, a higher IgG antibody titre in a neonate than the mother is suggestive of an intrauterine infection.

Rubella

In 1941, Greg reported congenital cataracts in 78 children following a rubella epidemic in Australia. Most had pearly white central opacities with a clear peripheral zone. In 68 instances, the mothers had had symptomatic rubella infections while pregnant with the affected children. In addition, many of these children had microphthalmos, growth retardation, and congenital heart defects. The congenital rubella syndrome has since been expanded to include sensorineural hearing loss, mental retardation, hepatosplenomegaly, thrombocytopenic purpura, microcephaly, osteopathy, lymphadenopathy, diabetes, abnormal dermaglyphics, a retinal pigmentary disturbance, glaucoma and keratitis (Alfano 1966; Wolff 1972). Computed tomography (CT) may show low density areas and flecks of calcification of the white matter, and calcification in the basal ganglia (Ishikawa *et al.* 1982).

The prevalence of these abnormalities correlates closely with the gestational stage during which the rubella infection occurs. Intrauterine infections during the first 3 months of pregnancy result in a 50% incidence of the rubella embryopathy (Hanshaw *et al.* 1985), whereas

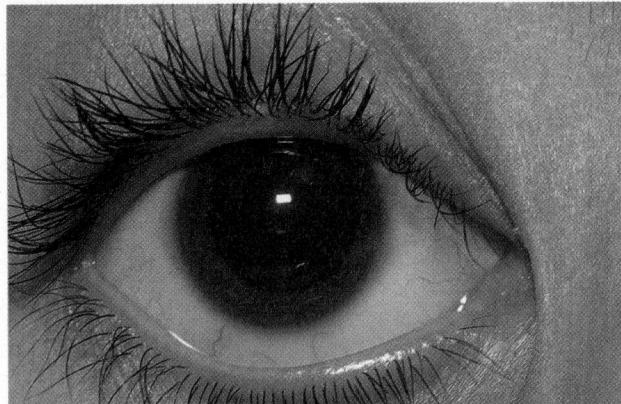

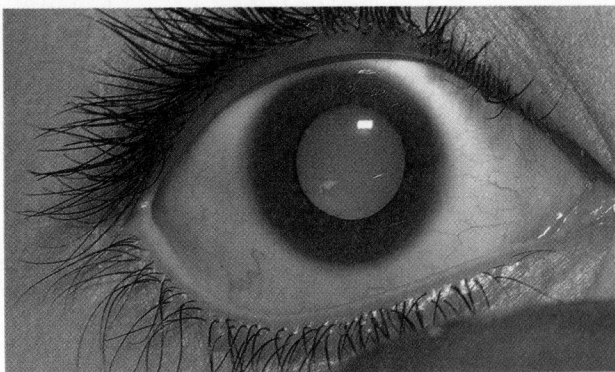

Fig. 13.1 Unilateral congenital rubella cataract. Twenty-five per cent have a unilateral cataract associated with microphthalmos. They are usually 'shaggy' and central but may be complete.

infections after the fourth gestational month rarely result in the full rubella syndrome (Manson *et al.* 1960).

Cataracts (Fig. 13.1) are present in 20–30% of children with the congenital rubella syndrome (Hertzberg 1968; Givens *et al.* 1993). They are bilateral 75% of the time (Fig. 13.1) and conform closely to Greg's original description. The rubella virus has been cultured from the catarac-

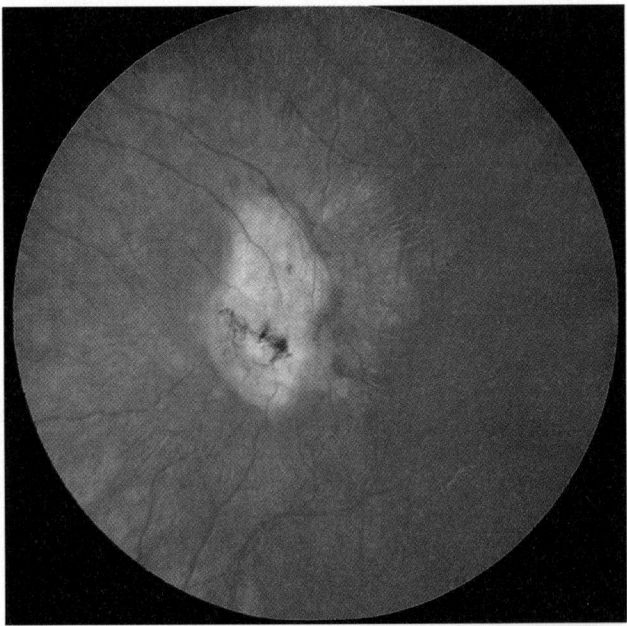

a

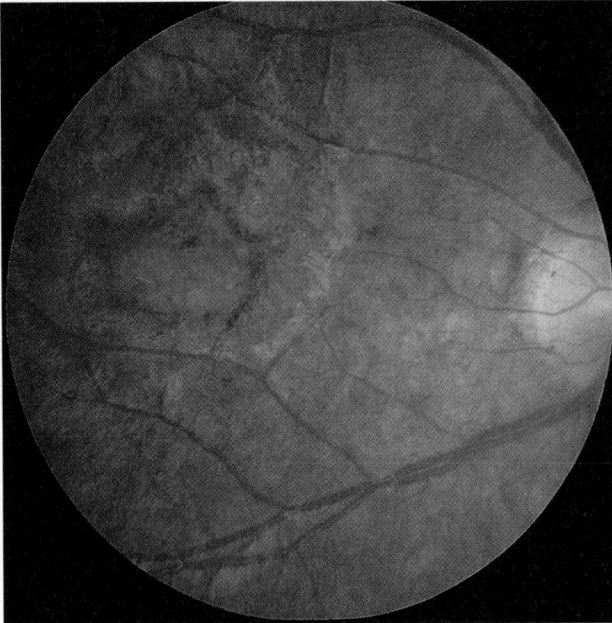

Fig. 13.2 Congenital rubella retinopathy. There are diffuse retinal pigment epithelial changes most marked at the posterior pole. The acuity is 6/12.

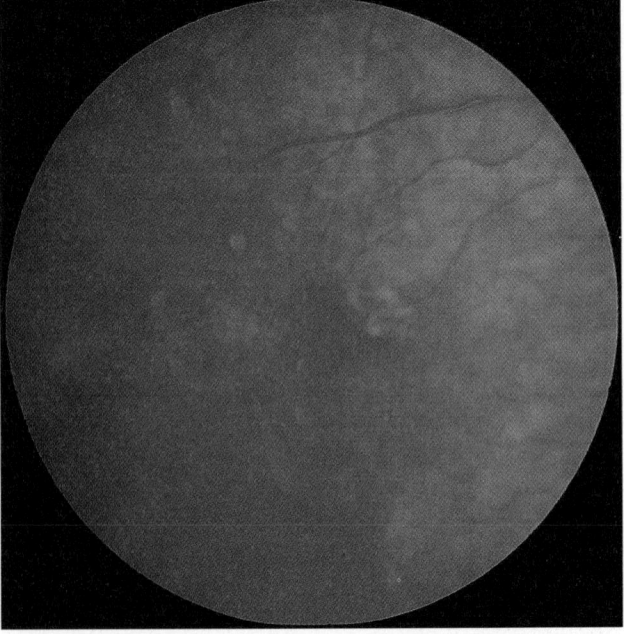

b

Fig. 13.3 (a) Left eye showing disciform scarring in congenital rubella. The patient aged 9 years has an acuity (secondary to subretinal neovascularization in this eye) of 5/60. (b) Same patient. The right eye has a mild retinal pigment epithelial disturbance and 6/6 acuity.

tous lenses of children with the congenital rubella syndrome up to 4 years of age and is probably responsible for the intense inflammatory response that may occur after cataract surgery (Cotlier *et al*. 1966).

The most common ocular abnormality of the congenital rubella syndrome is a pigmentary retinopathy (Fig. 13.2) (Marks 1946). It is usually bilateral and is present in 40% of affected patients. The retinopathy is characterized by mottled pigmentary changes throughout the fundi which are most marked in the posterior pole (Fig. 13.2). Although progression of the pigmentary changes may occur, the vision typically remains 6/12 or better (Hertzberg 1968; Collis & Cohen 1970). Rarely subretinal neovascularization may occur with a precipitous fall in the visual acuity (Fig. 13.3). The electro-oculogram and electroretinogram are usually normal, indicating that the function of the retinal pigment epithelium and retina are not affected by the pigment mottling (Krill 1967). A disturbance of iris pigmentation is also common (Fig. 13.4) and may be associated with glaucoma (Brooks & Gillies 1994).

The corneas of infants with the rubella syndrome may be hazy, secondary either to a keratitis (Fig. 13.5) or less commonly to an elevation of the intraocular pressure. The keratitis typically clears in weeks or a few months. Glaucoma is found most frequently in eyes with iris hypoplasia and microphthalmos (Wolff 1972; Brooks & Gillies 1994). It occurs in approximately 10% of children with the congenital rubella syndrome (Sears 1967). Severe anterior segment damage may result from the combination of keratitis, glaucoma and cataract (Fig. 13.6).

The development of an attenuated rubella virus vaccine and its subsequent widespread usage beginning in 1969

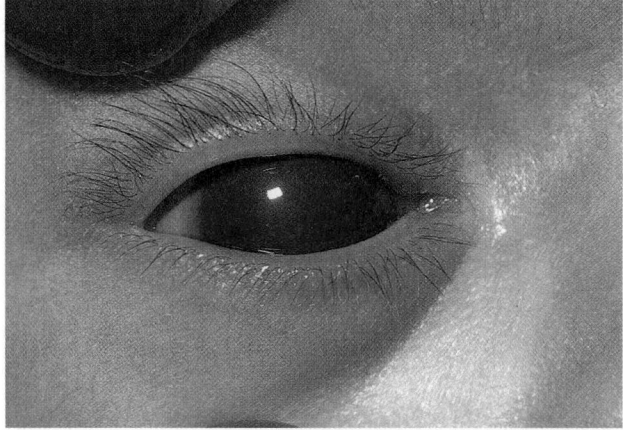
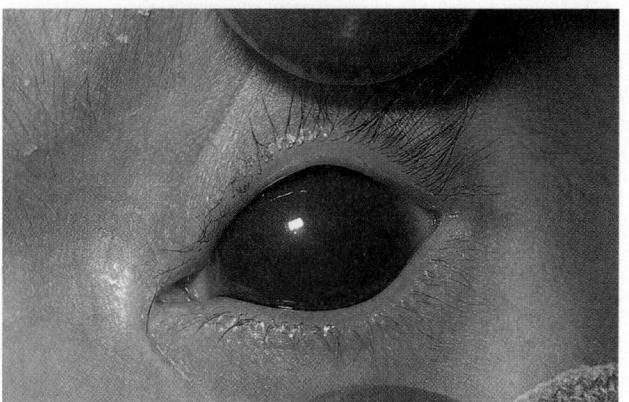
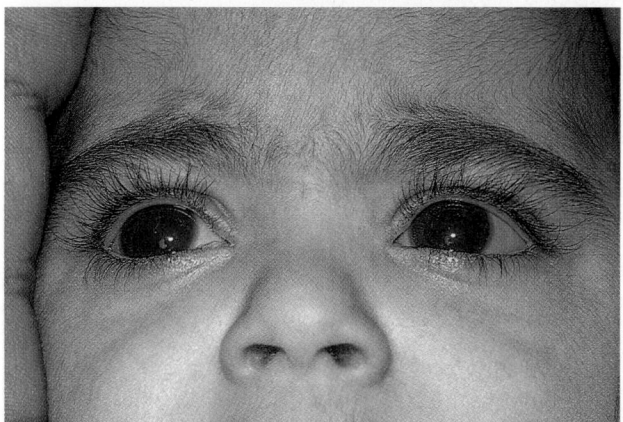

Fig. 13.5 (a) Neonate with congenital rubella with hazy large appearing corneas. The intraocular pressure was normal. (b) Same patient aged 3 years. The intraocular pressure has not been raised at any of the subsequent examinations. The corneas had cleared by 3 months of age.

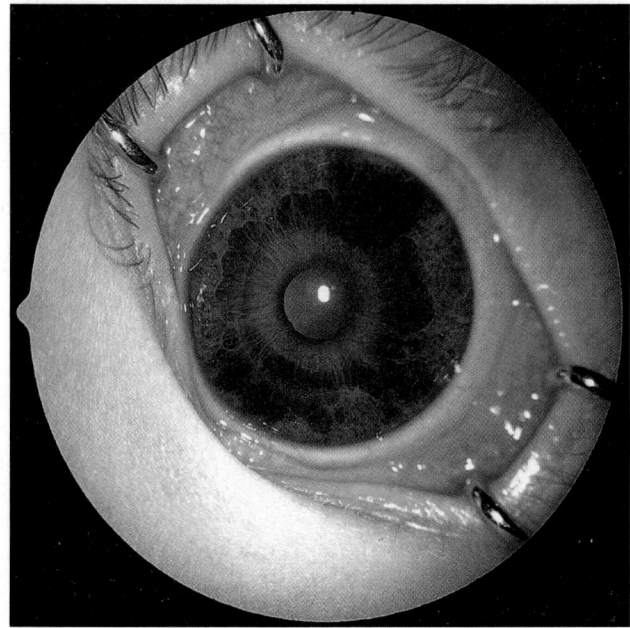

Fig. 13.4 Congenital rubella. Iris pigment disturbance.

has dramatically decreased the incidence of the congenital rubella syndrome (Meyer *et al*. 1966; Krugman 1969). Whereas 30 000 children were estimated to have been born with the congenital rubella syndrome during the rubella epidemic of 1964 in the USA, the condition is now rare there.

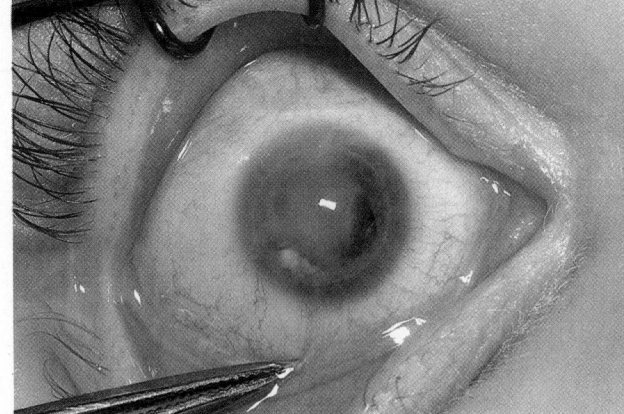

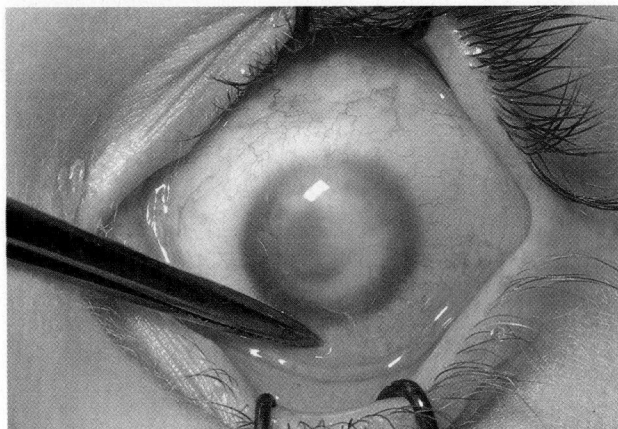

Fig. 13.6 (a, b) Congenital rubella with microphthalmos, cataract, iris damage, glaucoma, and corneal scarring. The right eye (a) had had a partially successful graft and had navigation vision.

Toxoplasmosis

Intrauterine toxoplasmosis was first recognized as a cause of chorioretinitis and intracranial calcification in 1939 (Wolf *et al.* 1939). Chorioretinitis is the most frequently recognized feature of the congenital toxoplasmosis syndrome (Figs 13.7–13.9). Other common findings include intracranial calcification (Fig. 13.10), seizures, hydrocephalus, microcephaly, hepatosplenomegaly, jaundice,

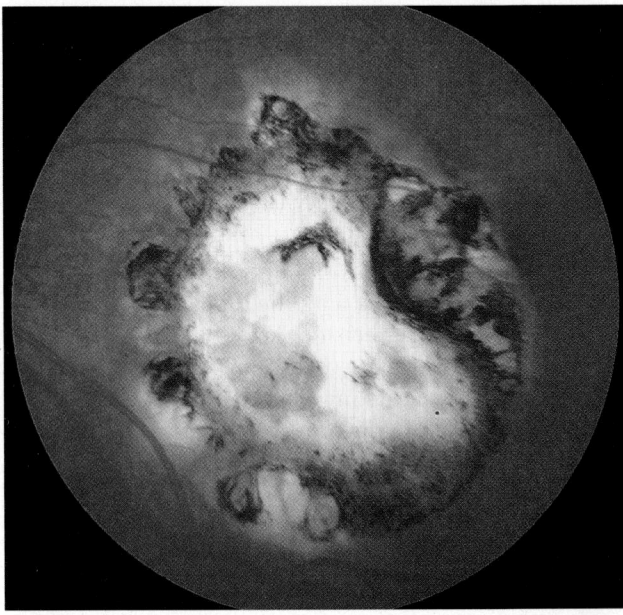

Fig. 13.8 Raised toxoplasmosis macular scar.

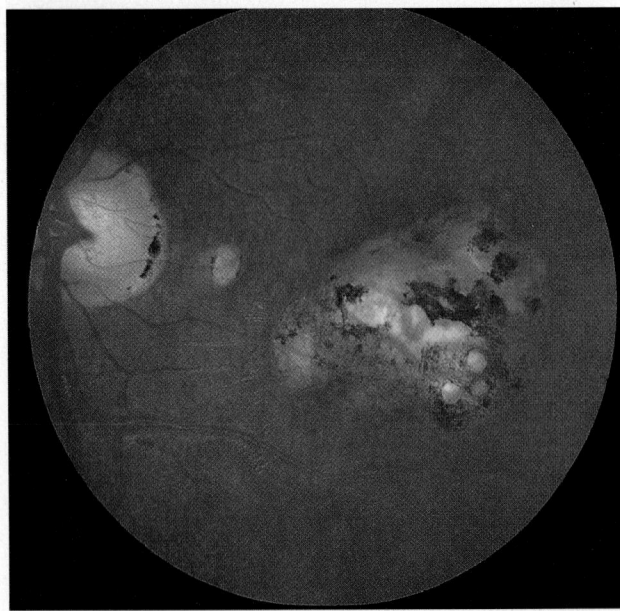

Fig. 13.7 Toxoplasmosis macular retinal pigment epithelial disturbance.

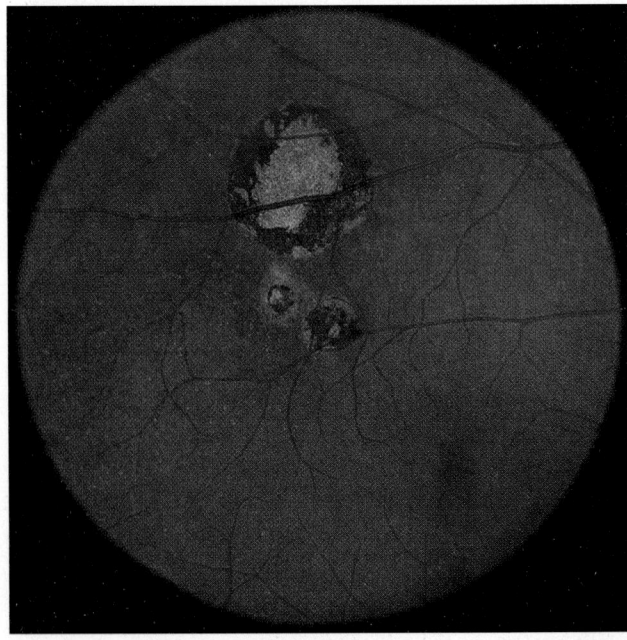

Fig. 13.9 Paramacular toxplasmosis scar.

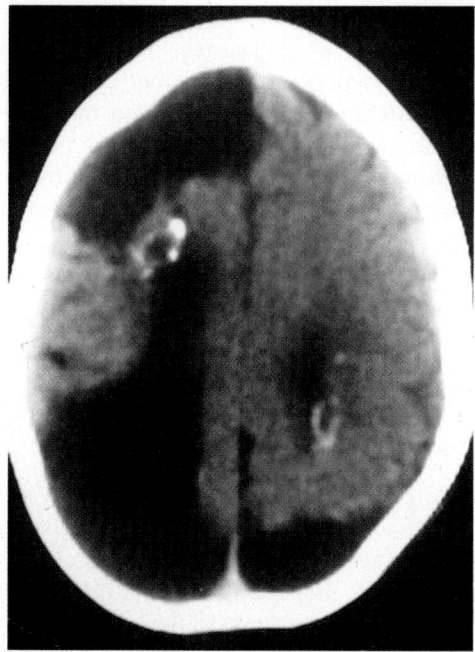

Fig. 13.10 Congenital toxoplasmosis, intracranial calcification, cerebral necrosis.

anaemia and fever (Eichenwald 1957). In the USA, it has been estimated to have an incidence ranging from one in 1000 live births to one in 10 000 live births (Remington & Desmonts 1990). Only 10–15% of the offspring of women who become infected with toxoplasmosis during the first trimester demonstrate serological evidence of intrauterine disease. However, these children typically have the most severe manifestations of the syndrome. A higher percentage of fetuses infected during the later stages of gestation are seropositive for toxoplasmosis, but usually have minimal if any abnormalities (Desmonts & Couvreur 1974). However, it is now recognized that some of these infants who are apparently normal on initial examination develop chorioretinitis, blindness, hydrocephalus, mental retardation and deafness later in childhood (Wilson *et al.* 1980; Koppe *et al.* 1986).

Toxoplasmosis is acquired from eating undercooked meat or exposure to cat faeces. Marked regional differences occur in the prevalence of seropositivity to toxoplasmosis presumably due to differing dietary and living customs. For example, 84% of pregnant women in Paris are seropositive to toxoplasmosis (Desmonts & Couvreur 1974) versus only 22% of pregnant women in London (Ruoss & Bourne 1972). Women of childbearing years emigrating from an area of low immunity to a region of high immunity are at the greatest risk of contracting toxoplasmosis.

Ocular manifestations of congenital toxoplasmosis include chorioretinitis (see Figs 13.7–13.9), microphthalmos, cataracts, panuveitis and optic atrophy. The chorioretinal scarring is usually heavily pigmented and associated with areas of chorioretinal atrophy (Noble & Carr 1982). A large prospective study demonstrated a 30% incidence of chorioretinal scarring in infants with congenital toxoplasmosis (Guerina *et al.* 1994); in severe disease, it may approach 100% (Meenken *et al.* 1995). The chorioretinal scarring is usually bilateral and frequently involves the macula. Toxoplasmosis acquired after birth only rarely results in chorioretinitis (Asbell *et al.* 1982; Nussenblatt & Belfort 1994).

All neonates with serological evidence of an intrauterine toxoplasmosis infection, whether or not they have signs of active infection, should be treated with systemic antibiotics. McAuley *et al.* (1994) recommended a 1-year course of pyrimethamine and sulfadiazine with the concurrent administration of folinic acid to reduce the haemotoxicity of pyrimethamine. They noted a dramatic reduction in the incidence of adverse neurological sequelae in children treated with this drug regimen; however, 80% of these children still developed chorioretinitis. In Massachusetts and New Hampshire, all children are screened serologically for congenital toxoplasmosis at birth in an attempt to treat all infected infants (Guerina *et al.* 1994). Others have argued that there are disadvantages to screening and that this is not cost-effective (Peckham & Logan 1993).

Women seronegative to toxoplasmosis should not eat undercooked meat and should minimize their exposure to cats during pregnancy. Fruits and vegetables, which might be contaminated with toxoplasmosis oocytes, should be washed carefully before being eaten. If a pregnant woman is found to have a primary toxoplasmosis infection, treatment with spiramycin may mitigate the severity of the disease in her offspring (Daffos *et al.* 1988).

Cytomegalovirus

A congenital CMV infection is the most common intrauterine infection recurring in 0.4–2.3% of all newborns (Stagno *et al.* 1986). Most children with congenital CMV infections develop normally, but 10–20% have congenital abnormalities (Hanshaw 1971; Pass *et al.* 1980).

Intrauterine CMV infections damage the fetus as a consequence of tissue necrosis rather than interfering with organogenesis. Infections early in gestation are probably more embryopathic, although it is often difficult to determine the gestational age at which the infection occurred since 95% of primary CMV infections are asymptomatic (Stagno *et al.* 1986). Primary CMV infections are much more embryopathic than recurrent infections (Fowler *et al.* 1992). Abnormalities associated with congenital CMV infections include jaundice, hepatosplenomegaly, microcephaly, psychomotor retardation, cerebral calcifications (Fig. 13.11), a petechial rash, optic atrophy and chorioretinitis (Weller 1971).

Ocular manifestations of congenital CMV are not com-

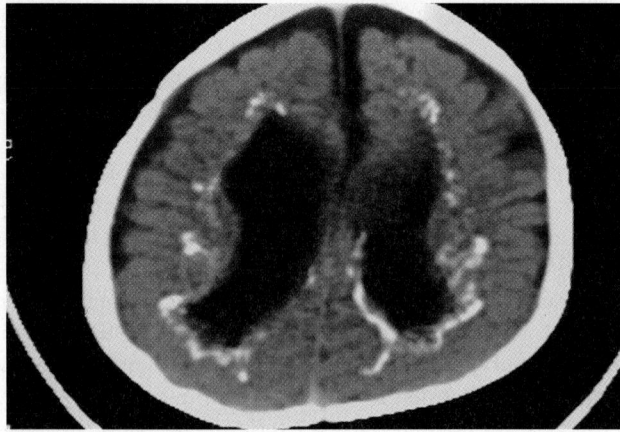

Fig. 13.11 Congenital CMV infection with periventricular calcification, hydrocephalus and cerebral atrophy shown on this CT scan.

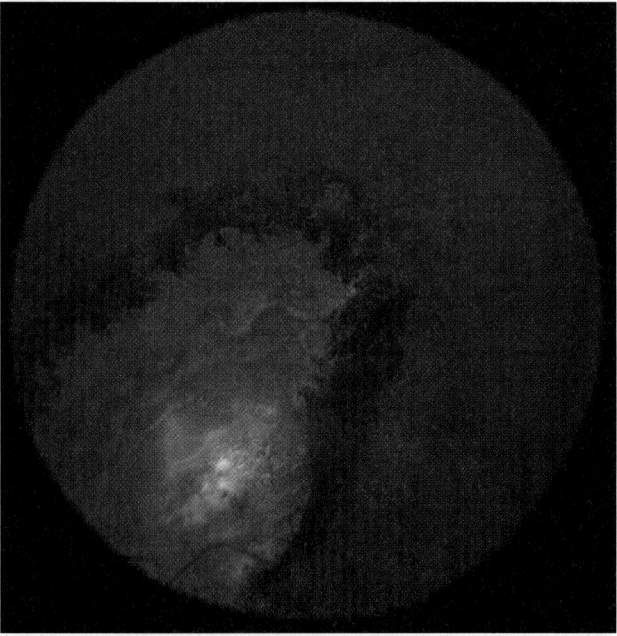

Fig. 13.12 Chorioretinal lesion in a child with proven CMV infection.

mon, but include chorioretinitis (Fig. 13.12), microphthalmos, cataracts, keratitis (Fig. 13.13) and optic atrophy (Tarrkanen *et al.* 1972). Congenital CMV infections result in chorioretinal scarring in 6% of infants after a primary maternal CMV infection and 2% of infants after a recurrent maternal CMV infection (Fowler *et al.* 1992). Congenital CMV chorioretinal scars are usually less heavily pigmented than those associated with congenital toxoplasmosis.

The diagnosis of congenital CMV should be suspected in neonates with hepatosplenomegaly, jaundice, petechiae or thrombocytopenia, cerebral calcification, chorioretinitis

and microcephaly. The diagnosis should be confirmed by viral isolation and serological tests since these findings occur in association with many other congenital infections. The virus can usually be cultured from the urine, stool and throat of congenitally infected neonates for many months. CMV-specific IgM antibody titres are also usually elevated. Most maternal CMV infections are believed to be acquired from younger children in a family rather than from casual contacts in the community since it is probably necessary to have intimate contact with a person excreting CMV in order to acquire the infection (Divorsky *et al.* 1983; Pass *et al.* 1987).

Herpes simplex

Herpes simplex infections most commonly occur in neonates delivered to mothers with active genital herpes simplex infections. The risk of neonates becoming infected is much higher after primary genital herpes infection than from recurrent infections (Nahmias *et al.* 1971; Prober *et al.* 1987). While most infants are infected during parturition, a small percentage are infected secondary to an infection ascending into the uterus after premature rupture of the amniotic membranes (Fig. 13.14) or postnatal innoculation. The herpes simplex type 2 strain is responsible for most neonatal infections.

Neonatal herpes simplex infections are often first detected as a cutaneous vesicular eruption. In 50% of infants, this then progresses to a systemic infection. Systemic involvement may result in hepatitis, pneumonia, disseminated intravascular coagulation or encephalitis. Seventy per cent of neonates with disseminated infections have involvement of both the viscera and the central nervous system.

Ocular involvement most commonly consists of blepharoconjunctivitis with vesicles on the eyelids or a keratitis with epithelial dendrites (Nahimas & Hagler 1972).

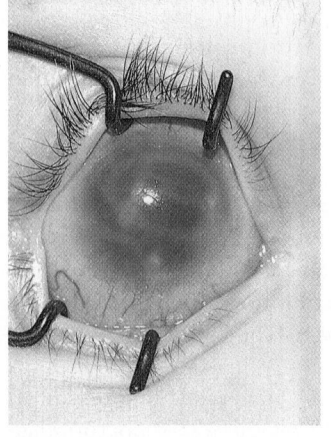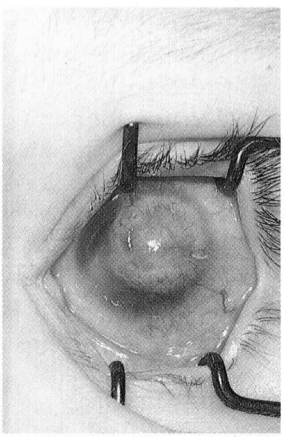

Fig. 13.13 Congenital CMV with bilateral keratopathy and glaucoma.

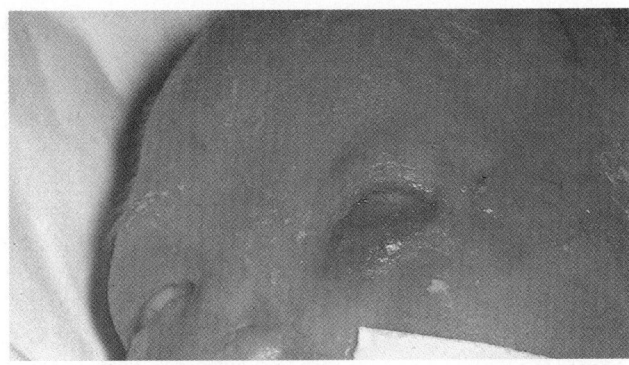

Fig. 13.14 Prenatal herpes simplex infection, facial and corneal scarring.

Chorioretinitis with an accompanying vitritis and optic atrophy may also occur, particularly in infants with central nervous system involvement (Azazi *et al.* 1990). The chorioretinitis typically involves the peripheral retina and results in well-circumscribed hyperpigmented scars. A recrudescence of the herpes virus in these scars later in life can result in acute retinal necrosis (Thompson *et al.* 1994). On rare occasions a fulminant retinitis may develop during infancy which involves the entire retina. Cataracts may also form secondary to the accompanying uveitis. In addition, cortical visual impairment is a common sequela after herpes simplex encephalitis.

A disseminated neonatal herpes simplex infection is associated with a 70% mortality rate. In addition, a high percentage of children surviving herpes simplex encephalitis are neurologically handicapped (Whitley *et al.* 1980). Because of the risk of dissemination, all neonates less than 1 month of age with a herpes simplex infection, even if it is initially limited to cutaneous or ocular involvement, should be treated with systemic acyclovir. Herpetic keratitis should be treated with either acyclovir ointment or triflurothymidine solution topically. Herpes simplex blepharoconjunctivitis should also be treated with topical antiviral therapy as prophylaxis against the development of keratitis.

The diagnosis of a herpes simplex infection should be considered in infants with progressive icterus, fever, hepatosplenomegaly and cutaneous vesicular lesions. The isolation of herpes simplex from fresh vesicles or from corneal scrapings confirms the diagnosis. The presence of multinucleated giant cells on scraping from vesicles or from the cornea is suggestive of a herpes simplex infection, but is not diagnostic since they may occur with several other viral infections.

Syphilis

Congenital syphilis only occurs in fetuses exposed to *Treponema pallidum* after the 16th gestational week. Virtually all of the offspring of women with primary syphilis acquired after the 16th gestational week have congenital syphilis, whereas the incidence decreases to 90% with secondary syphilis and 30% with latent syphilis. Syphilis infections acquired at an earlier gestational age frequently result in fetal death.

Congenital syphilis is associated with early manifestations occurring during infancy secondary to an active infection or late manifestations occurring later in childhood secondary to ongoing inflammation or a hypersensitivity reaction. Early manifestations include skeletal abnormalities, rhinitis, a maculopapular rash, fissures around the lips, nares and anus, hepatosplenomegaly, anaemia and uveitis. Late manifestations include sensorineural hearing loss, bone changes, dental abnormalities and interstitial keratitis (Fiumara & Lessell 1983). The finding of interstitial keratitis, deafness and malformed incisors is known as Hutchinson's triad.

Ocular manifestations of congenital syphilis include chorioretinitis (Fig. 13.15), interstitial keratitis, anterior uveitis and optic atrophy. Interstitial keratitis occurs in 10–40% of children with untreated congenital syphilis. It most commonly occurs in individuals of 5–20 years of age. It is characterized by either sectorial or diffuse corneal oedema infiltrated by interstitial vessels. Visual loss occurs secondary to corneal scarring and residual ghost vessels. It is bilateral in 80% of affected children and usually accompanied by an iridocyclitis and iris atrophy. It occurs secondary to a hypersensitivity reaction and responds to topical corticosteroids. The chorioretinitis

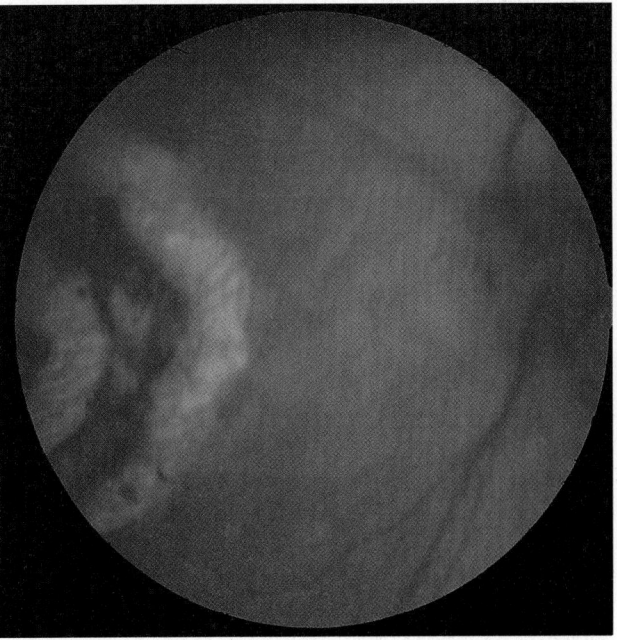

Fig. 13.15 Macular chorioretinitis in a baby with proven congenital syphilis; it was bilateral. Other serological studies were normal.

occurring with congenital syphilis most commonly results in peripheral areas of pigment mottling, but in severe cases may result in extensive pigmentary changes resembling retinitis pigmentosa. This form of syphilitic chorioretinitis is sometimes referred to as pseudoretinitis pigmentosa.

Congenital syphilis predominantly occurs in the offspring of young, unmarried women with poor antenatal care. Improved antenatal care, community surveillance of known cases of syphilis, and follow-up after treatment could prevent many cases of congenital syphilis (Mascola *et al.* 1984).

The diagnosis of congenital syphilis may be difficult to establish in neonates since few have symptoms of the disease and serological tests may initially be negative (Dorfman & Glaser 1990). A quantitative rapid plasma reagin (RPR) or venereal disease reference laboratory (VDRL) result higher in an infant than the mother is highly suggestive of congenital disease.

Occasionally dark-field microscopy or a direct fluorescent antibody test of a scraping from a fresh lesion will reveal *Treponema pallidum*. *T. pallidum* is very sensitive to penicillin. A 10–14-day course of intravenous penicillin is usually adequate to treat congenital syphilis; however, a more protracted course of treatment is occasionally necessary (Ryan *et al.* 1972). Serologies should be repeated after a course of penicillin to ensure that the treatment was adequate.

Varicella

In 1947, a child was reported with multiple birth defects following an intrauterine varicella infection (Laforet & Lynch 1947). The abnormalities included a hypotrophic limb, a low birth weight for gestational age, seizures, cortical atrophy and cicatricial skin lesions (DeNicola & Hanshaw 1979). Subsequent reports have confirmed these findings and expanded the congenital varicella syndrome to include chorioretinitis (Charles *et al.* 1977), cataracts (Cotlier 1978), microphthalmos, Horner's syndrome (Savage *et al.* 1973) and neuropathic bladder (Borzyskowski *et al.* 1981). Unlike the rubella syndrome, which occurs almost exclusively after first trimester infections, the congenital varicella syndrome frequently occurs after second, and even third trimester infections. Several prospective studies have shown that the risk of the varicella embryopathy developing after a maternal varicella infection during the first trimester is about 2% (Paryani & Arvin 1986; Pastuszak *et al.* 1994). In some instances, the congenital varicella syndrome may be overlooked since the clinical findings may be subtle and non-specific. Attempts to culture the varicella virus from congenitally infected neonates have been unsuccessful.

Chorioretinitis (Fig. 13.16) is probably the most common ocular manifestation of the syndrome. It closely

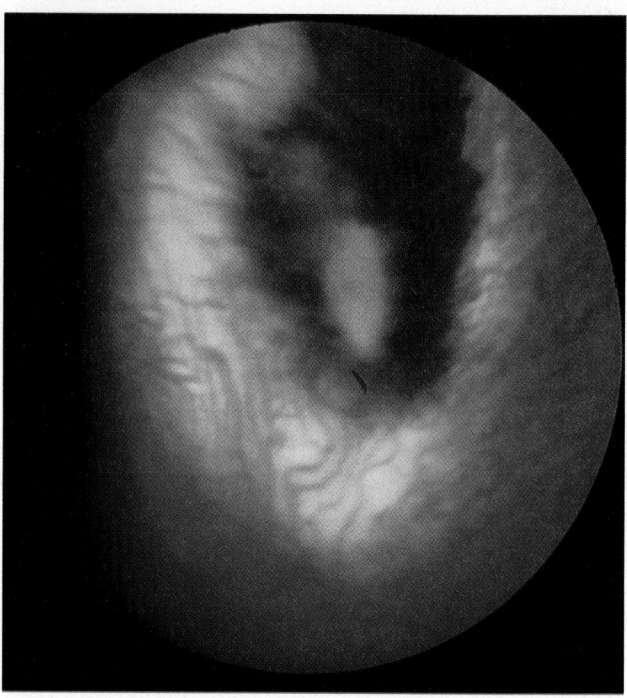

Fig. 13.16 Chorioretinal scar in a child with congenital varicella syndrome.

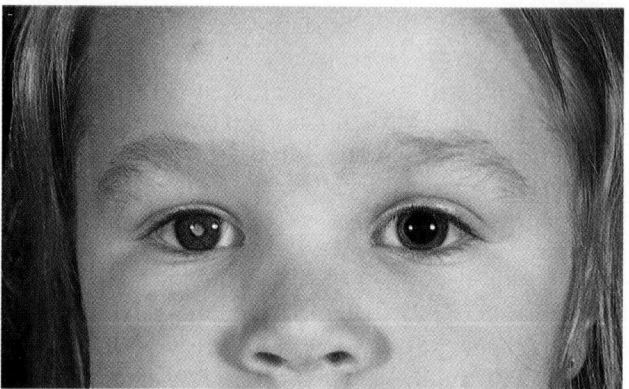

Fig. 13.17 Congenital varicella. Congenital cataracts and microphthalmos.

resembles the chorioretinitis of toxoplasmosis with either single (see Fig. 13.13) or multiple deeply pigmented chorioretinal scars and atrophy (Lambert *et al.* 1989). It may be unilateral or bilateral. In some instances the chorioretinal scarring may be so severe as to result in tractional retinal detachments.

Mature cataracts in microphthalmic eyes (Fig. 13.17) may also occur with the congenital varicella syndrome (Cotlier 1978; Lambert *et al.* 1989). The associated chorioretinal disease often limits the visual potential of these eyes even if the cataracts are extracted.

A unilateral Horner's syndrome (Fig. 13.18) also occasionally occurs with the congenital varicella syndrome (Savage *et al.* 1973; Lambert *et al.* 1989). Congenital herpes

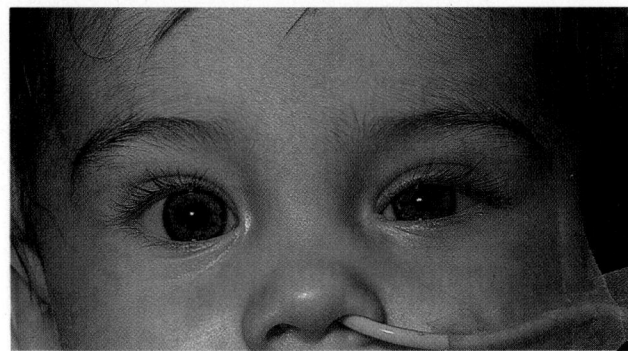

Fig. 13.18 Left Horner's syndrome in the congenital varicella syndrome (Lambert *et al.* 1989).

zoster ophthalmicus has been described (Singh & Gibson 1993).

Varicella infections usually occur during childhood and confer life-long immunity. However, 5–16% of women of child-bearing years are seronegative to varicella (Gershon *et al.* 1976). An estimated 0.7 cases of primary varicella infections occur per 1000 pregnancies (Myers 1974). Severe infection during pregnancy has led to pneumonitis and even death (Paryani & Arvin 1986).

Although the risks to the fetus of acquiring the congenital varicella syndrome are small, because the associated malformations may be so severe it has been recommended that pregnant women exposed to varicella who are seronegative should promptly receive an injection of zoster immunoglobulin (DeNicola & Hanshaw 1979). While this does not prevent an infection from developing, it may attenuate the severity of the infection (McIntosh & Isaacs 1993).

References

Alfano JE. Ocular aspects of the maternal rubella syndrome. *Trans Am Acad Ophthalmol Otolaryng* 1966; **70**: 235–66.

Asbell PA, Bermund SH, Hofeldt AJ. Presumed toxoplasmic retinochoroiditis in four siblings. *Am J Ophthalmol* 1982; **94**: 456–63.

Azazi M. El, Malm G, Forsgren M. Late ophthalmologic manifestations of neonatal herpes simplex virus infection. *Am J Ophthalmol* 1990; **109**: 1–7.

Borzyskowski M, Harris RF, Jones RWA. The congenital varicella syndrome. *Eur J Pediatr* 1981; **137**: 335–8.

Brooks AMV, Gillies WE. Congenital rubella syndrome (letter). *Br J Ophthalmol* 1994; **78**: 77–8.

Charles NC, Bennet TW, Margolis S. Ocular pathology of the congenital varicella syndrome. *Arch Ophthalmol* 1977; **95**: 2034–7.

Collis WJ, Cohen DN. Rubella retinopathy. A progressive disorder. *Arch Ophthalmol* 1970; **84**: 33–5.

Cotlier E. Congenital varicella cataract. *Am J Ophthalmol* 1978; **86**: 627–9.

Cotlier E, Fox J, Smith M. Rubella virus in the cataractous lens of congenital rubella syndrome. *Am J Ophthalmol* 1966; **62**: 233–6.

Daffos F, Forestier F, Capella-Pavlovsky M *et al.* Prenatal management of 746 pregnancies at risk for congenital toxoplasmosis.

N Engl J Med 1988; **318**: 271–5.

DeNicola LK, Hanshaw JB. Congenital and neonatal varicella. *J Pediatr* 1979: **94**: 175–6.

Dennehy PJ, Warman R, Flynn JT, Scott GB, Mastrucci MT. Ocular manifestations in pediatric patients with acquired immunodeficiency syndrome. *Arch Ophthalmol* 1989; **107**: 978–82.

Desmonts G, Couvreur J. Congenital toxoplasmosis: a prospective study of 378 pregnancies. *N Engl J Med* 1974; **290(2)**: 1110–16.

Divorsky ME, Welch K, Cassady, Stagno S. Occupational risk for primary cytomegalovirus infections among pediatric health-care workers. *N Engl J Med* 1983; **309**: 950–3.

Dorfman DH, Glaser JH. Congenital syphilis presenting in infants after the newborn period. *N Engl J Med* 1990; **323**: 1299–302.

Eichenwald HF. Congenital toxoplasmosis. A study of 150 cases. *Am J Dis Child* 1957; **94**: 411–12.

Embil JA, Ozene RL, Haldone EV. Congenital CMV infection in two siblings from consecutive pregnancies. *J Pediatr* 1970; **77**: 417–21.

Fiumara NJ, Lessell S. The stigmata of late congenital syphilis: an analysis of 100 patients. *Sex Trans Dis* 1983; **10**: 126–9.

Fowler KB, Stagno S, Pass RF *et al.* The outcome of congenital cytomegalovirus infection in relation to maternal antibody status. *N Engl J Med* 1992; **326**: 663–703.

Gershon AA, Raker R, Steinberg S *et al.* Antibody to varicella zoster virus in parturient women and their offspring during the first year of life. *Pediatrics* 1976; **58**: 692–6.

Givens KT, Lee DA, Jones T, Ilstrup DM. Congenital rubella syndrome: ophthalmic manifestations and associated systemic disorders. *Br J Ophthalmol* 1993; **77**: 358–63.

Greg NM. Congenital cataract following German measles in the mother. *Trans Ophthalmol Soc Austr* 1941; **3**: 35–44.

Guerina NG, Hsu HW, Meissner HC *et al.* Neonatal serologic screening and early treatment for congenital *Toxoplasma gondii* infection. *N Engl J Med* 1994; **330**: 1858–63.

Hanshaw JB. Congenital cytomegalovirus infections. A 15-year perspective. *J Infect Dis* 1971; **123**: 555–61.

Hanshaw JB, Dudyen JA, Marshall CUL. *Viral Diseases of the Fetus and Newborn*, 2nd edn. London: WB Saunders, 1985: 13–91.

Hertzberg R. Twenty-five year follow-up of ocular defects in congenital rubella. *Am J Ophthalmol* 1968; **66**: 269–71.

Ishikawa A, Murayama T, Sakuma N *et al.* Computed tomography in congenital rubella syndrome. *Arch Neurol* 1982; **39**: 420–1.

Knech V, Kojajev Z, Jung M. Congenital CMV in siblings from consecutive pregnancies. *Helv Pediatr Acta* 1971; **26**: 355–62.

Koppe JG, Loewer-Sieger DH, Roever-Bonnet H. Results of 20-year follow-up of congenital toxoplasmosis. *Lancet* 1986; **i**: 254–6.

Krill AE. The retinal disease of rubella. *Arch Ophthalmol* 1967; **77**: 445–9.

Krugman S. International Conference on Rubella Immunization. *Am J Dis Child* 1969; **118**: 1–410.

Laforet EG, Lynch CL. Multiple congenital defects following maternal varicella. Report of a case. *N Engl J Med* 1947; **236**: 534–7.

Lambert SR, Taylor D, Kriss A, Holzel H, Heard S. The ocular manifestations of the congenital varicella syndrome. *Arch Ophthalmol* 1989; **107**: 52–6.

McAuley J, Boyer KM, Patel D *et al.* Early and longitudinal evaluations of treated infants and children and untreated historical patients with congenital toxoplasmosis: the Chicago Collaborative Treatment Trial. *Clin Infect Dis* 1994; **18**: 38–72.

McIntosh D, Isaacs D. Varicella zoster virus infection in pregnancy. *Arch Dis Child* 1993; **68**: 1–20.

Manson MM, Logan WPD, Loy RM. *Rubella and Other Virus Infections in Pregnancy*. Reports on Public Health and Medical Subjects, No. 101. London: Ministry of Health, 1960.

Marks EO. Pigmentary abnormality in children congenitally deaf following maternal German measles. *Trans Ophthalmol Soc Austr* 1946; **6**: 122–5.

Mascola L, Pelosi R, Bloutt JH *et al.* Congenital syphilis: why is it still occurring? *J Am Med Assoc* 1984; **252**: 1719–22.

Meenken C, Assies J, van Nieuwenhuizen O *et al.* Long-term ocular and neurological involvement in severe congenital toxoplasmosis. *Br J Ophthalmol* 1995; **79**: 581–4.

Meyer HM, Parkman PD, Panos TC. Attenuated rubella virus II. Production of an experimental live-virus vaccine and clinical trial. *N Engl J Med* 1966; **275**: 575–80.

Myers JD. Congenital varicella in term infants. Risk reconsidered. *J Infect Dis* 1974; **129**: 215–20.

Nahmias AJ, Hagler AJ. Ocular manifestations of herpes simplex in the newborn. *Int Ophthalmol Clin* 1972; **12**: 191–213.

Nahmias AJ, Josey WE, Naib SM. Neonatal risk associated with maternal genital herpes simplex virus infection. *Am J Obstet Gynecol* 1971; **110**: 825–36.

Noble K, Carr R. Disorders of the fundus: *Toxoplasma* retinochoroiditis. *Ophthalmology* 1982; **89**: 1289–91.

Nussenblatt RB, Belfort R Jr. Ocular toxoplasmosis: an old disease revisited. *J Am Med Assoc* 1994; **271**: 304–7.

Paryani SLG, Arvin AM. Intrauterine infection with varicella zoster virus after maternal varicella. *N Engl J Med* 1986; **314**: 1542–5.

Pass RF, Little A, Stagno S *et al.* Young children as a probable source of maternal and congenital cytomegalovirus infection. *N Engl J Med* 1987; **316**: 1366–70.

Pass RF, Stagno S, Myers GJ, Alford CA. Outcome of symptomatic congenital cytomegalovirus infection: results of long-term longitudinal follow-up. *Pediatrics* 1980; **66**: 758–62.

Pastuszak AL, Levy M, Schick B *et al.* Outcome after maternal varicella infection in the first 20 weeks of pregnancy. *N Engl J Med* 1994; **330**: 901–5.

Peckham C, Logan S. Screening for toxoplasmosis during pregnancy. *Arch Dis Child* 1993; **68**: 3–50.

Prober CG, Sullender WLM, Yasukawa LL. Low risk of herpes simplex virus infections in neonates exposed to the virus at the time of vaginal delivery to mothers with recurrent genital herpes simplex virus infections. *N Engl J Med* 1987; **316**: 240–4.

Remington JS, Desmonts G. Toxoplasmosis. In: Remington JS, Klein JO, eds. *Infectious Diseases of the Fetus and Newborn Infants*, 3rd edn. Philadelphia: WB Saunders, 1990: 89–195.

Rouss CF, Bourne GL. Toxoplasmosis in pregnancy. *J Obstet Gynaecol Br Commonw* 1972; **779**: 1115–18.

Ryan SJ, Hardy PH, Hardy JM *et al.* Persistence of a virulent *Treponema pallidum* despite penicillin therapy in congenital syphilis. *Am J Ophthalmol* 1972; **73**: 258–61.

Savage MO, Moosa A, Gordon RR. Maternal varicella infection as a cause of fetal malformations. *Lancet* 1973; **i**: 352–4.

Sears ML. Congenital glaucoma in neonatal rubella. *Br J Ophthalmol* 1967; **51**: 744–8.

Singh J, Gibson J. A case of presumed congenital herpes zoster ophthalmicus. *Br J Ophthalmol* 1993; **77**: 459–61.

Stagno S, Pass RF, Coud G *et al.* Primary cytomegalovirus infection in pregnancy: incidence, transmission to foetus, and clinical outcome. *J Am Med Assoc* 1986; **256**: 1904–8.

Stagno S, Reynolds DW, Hurry E. Congenital CMV infection: occurrence in immune population. *N Engl J Med* 1977; **296**: 1254–8.

Tarkkanen A, Merenmias L, Holmstron T. Ocular involvement in congenital cytomegalic inclusion disease. *J Pediatr Ophthalmol* 1972; **9**: 82–6.

Thompson WS, Culbertson WW, Smiddy WE *et al.* Acute retinal necrosis caused by reactivation of herpes simplex virus type 2. *Am J Ophthalmol* 1994; **118**: 205–11.

Weller TH. The cytomegaloviruses: ubiquitous agents with protean clinical manifestations. *N Engl J Med* 1971; **285**: 203–14.

Whitley RJ, Nahmias AJ, Visentine AM *et al.* The natural history of herpes simplex virus infection of mother and newborn. *Pediatrics* 1980; **66**: 489–94.

Wilson CB, Remington JS, Stagno S, Reynolds DW. Development of adverse sequelae in children born with subclinical congenital *Toxoplasma* infection. *Pediatrics* 1980; **66**: 767–74.

Wolf A, Cowen D, Paige BH. Toxoplasmosis encephalomyelitis. III. A new case of granulomatous encephalomyelitis due to a protozoan. *Am J Pathol* 1939; **15**: 657–94.

Wolff SM. The ocular manifestations of congenital rubella. *Trans Am Ophthalmol Soc* 1972; **70**: 577–614.

14: AIDS and the Child's Eye

R. Jane Leitch

Epidemiology

Human immunodeficiency virus (HIV) infection in children is increasing in incidence; the incidence in the adult male population has plateaued but the incidence in females is still rising. The majority of the affected females are within the reproductive age group and acquire their infection via intravenous drug abuse or, increasingly, via heterosexual transmission: as a direct result vertical transmission of HIV to offspring is rapidly increasing in incidence (Frenkel & Sunanda 1994). An increasing incidence is also being seen in the adolescent population particularly among females (Lindegren *et al.* 1994). The suggested reason, in addition to intravenous drug abuse, is heterosexual contact with older men. In the USA HIV is the seventh leading cause of death in children 1–4 years of age (Rogers & Jaffe 1994) and the sixth leading cause of death in the age group 15–24 years (Lindegren *et al.* 1994).

Transmission

There are three main modes for children to become infected with HIV.

Maternal

There are three modes of maternal transmission.
1 Prenatal—transplacental.

2 Perinatal—at birth.
3 Postnatal—via breast milk.
Infants of infected mothers become infected themselves in 15–40% of cases. Thomas *et al.* (1994) have attempted to highlight maternal predictors for transmission and recommend that women who have evidence of HIV-related immunosuppression manifested by a low CD4+ count (which reflects T-helper cells) with or without a relatively elevated CD8+ count (which reflects T-suppressor cells) should be advised of an increased risk of transmission. However, transmission can be seen without evidence of immunosuppression in the mother. Other factors that may influence transmission are a protective effect from caesarean section, the length of time between rupture of membranes and delivery, and the influence of concurrent infections, for example syphilis.

Connor *et al.* (1994) have shown a reduction in the maternal transmission of HIV with zidovudine treatment (transmission rate was 8.3% in treated group compared to 25.5% in the placebo group). Treatment was given to the mother during pregnancy (after organogenesis was complete), during labour and to the infant for the first 6 weeks of life. This finding raises many ethical questions about the compulsory testing of pregnant mothers and newborns (Bayer 1994).

Infected blood products

The screening of all blood products has reduced this cause of HIV infection; however, some new cases are still presenting as a result of this mode of transmission. Goedent *et al.* (1989) in their study of haemophiliacs at risk of developing acquired immunodeficiency syndrome (AIDS) showed that children and adolescents had the lowest risk (13.3%), followed by young adults aged 18–34 years (26.8%) and adults over 34 years of age (43.7%).

Adolescents

HIV infection in the adolescent population tends to reflect that seen in the adult population. However, the incidence in this group is increasing rapidly in both males and females and although over-represented in some ethnic groups it is represented in all socioeconomic groups (Lindegren *et al.* 1994). This has implications as to where HIV education needs to be directed. Knowledge of the risk of HIV infection alone is not sufficient to change the behaviour of people and more practical advice in communication skills may be beneficial.

HIV in the neonate

Children born to HIV-positive mothers are infected themselves in up to 40% of cases (Blanche *et al.* 1989; Connor *et al.* 1994). The confirmation of a congenital infection is not easy because of the free transfer of maternal antibodies across the placenta after the 27th week of gestation. Positive serology in the newborn does not necessarily confirm the diagnosis and one of the following three assays must be positive (Frenkel & Sunanda 1994).
1 HIV viral culture.
2 HIV p24 antigen (specific antigen of HIV that implies infection) in the infant serum.
3 HIV viral-specified DNA detected in the infant's lymphocytes by polymerase chain reaction (PCR) only.

Neonates tend to fall into two groups: (i) those patients who are sick from opportunistic and other bacterial infections from an early age (a few weeks to months) and suffer a fulminant course; and (ii) those patients who may survive to the age of 10 or 12 years (Frenkel & Sunanda 1994). Mofenson *et al.* (1994) show that intravenous immunoglobulin can reduce the number of bacterial infections and hospital admissions of HIV-positive children and that this treatment benefit may continue for several years. Current reports (Frenkel & Sunanda 1994; Mofenson *et al.* 1994) indicate that early diagnosis and treatment aimed both at the HIV infection and opportunistic infections can increase the lifespan of some affected children.

Ocular manifestations

The involvement of the ocular structures in HIV can be observed in the ocular adnexae, the external eye, anterior segment, retina and choroid.

In adults up to 50% of patients with AIDS (Holland *et al.* 1983, 1987; Palestine *et al.* 1984; Dhillon 1994) have ocular pathology: the incidence in children appears to be much lower. The routine eye examination of all affected children appears unwarranted but in those children where there is extensive systemic or central nervous system opportunistic infection, for example with cytomegalovirus (CMV) or *Toxoplasma*, then ocular examination would be indicated (Dennehy *et al.* 1989).

The most frequently encountered problems in HIV are seen in the retina, and these include the following.

1 HIV retinopathy.
2 CMV retinitis.
3 Toxoplasmosis.
4 Chronic progressive retinal necrosis.

HIV retinopathy

This is usually asymptomatic and characterized by cotton-wool spots, retinal haemorrhages and other microvascular abnormalities (Figs 14.1, 14.2). These changes may be seen to resolve over a few weeks. If the changes are pronounced and there is a lot of retinal haemorrhage care should be taken to differentiate from CMV retinitis (Holland *et al.* 1983; de Smet & Nussenbatt 1991).

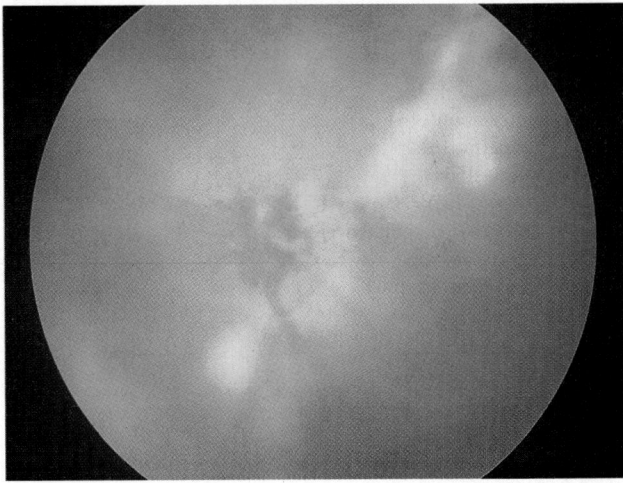

Fig. 14.1 CMV retinitis in a child with maternally transmitted HIV, showing extensive haemorrhages and exudates, the so-called 'scrambled egg and tomato ketchup' appearance.

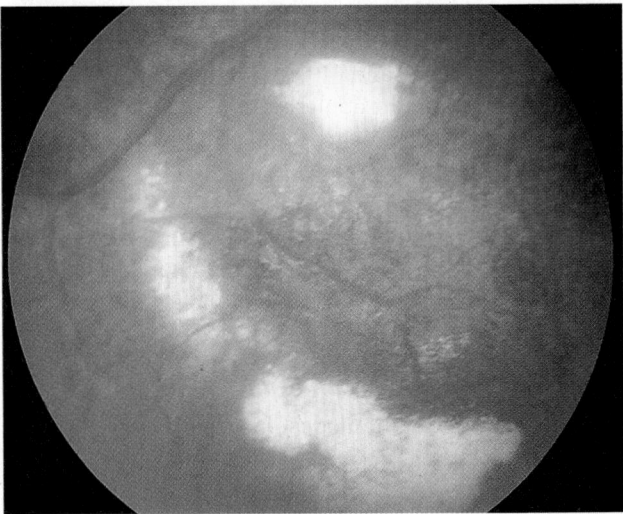

Fig. 14.2 Chronic CMV retinitis, showing extensive subretinal exudates and retinal vascular changes.

CMV retinitis

Up to 45% of patients with AIDS can be affected with CMV retinitis and it is associated with severe immunodeficiency (Holland *et al.* 1983, 1987; Palestine *et al.* 1984; Salvador *et al.* 1993). If untreated, the infection can become bilateral in 80% of cases (de Smet & Nussenbatt 1991). CMV retinitis in children tends to occur in patients with central nervous system or multisystem involvement and is rarely seen in isolation. As in adults, the appearance of CMV retinitis is an indicator of advanced disease and limited life-expectancy (Dennehy *et al.* 1989; Peters *et al.* 1995). Early changes are asymptomatic but as the disease progresses symptoms of floaters, loss of visual field and blurred vision are appreciated. The initial lesion can resemble a cotton-wool spot with an active edge that may be associated with haemorrhage. As the infection spreads through the retina the primary lesion will expand in size and satellite lesions occur.

With treatment the affected areas of retina become atrophic with a sharp demarcation line between healthy and affected retina. Retinal tears with retinal detachment can occur in up to 50% of cases by 1 year. Surgery has been undertaken in some of these cases (Holland 1991; Chuang & Davis 1992). The therapeutic agents available are only virostatic and consequently maintenance therapy is required once the retinitis is under control. Ganciclovir is the treatment of choice in CMV retinitis with 80% of patients showing a response. However, a neutropenia can be induced in up to 40% and concurrent administration of zidovudine may not be possible. Foscarnet may be preferred if neutropenia is a problem. Intravenous access and the introduction of a long line is required for the administration of these drugs and patients and their families have to be taught the appropriate care. Parents of affected children may refuse to accept treatment with an indwelling long line and in these cases high-dose oral acyclovir has been used (Peters *et al.* 1995). Intravitreal ganciclovir and foscarnet have been used in adults who would not tolerate systemic treatment (Akula *et al.* 1994; Dhillon 1994; Diaz-Llopis *et al.* 1994). It is also important to try to boost the CD4+ count as this will improve patient response to the infection (Kozal & Merrigan 1994).

In a clinicopathological report of Bylsma *et al.* (1995) peripapillary CMV retinitis was seen as a predictor of central nervous system infection (75% of cases). However, histological examination of the peripapillary lesions showed involvement of all layers of the retina without penetration into the papilla or the peripapillary nerve fibre layer and only two of 47 cases examined showed a papillitis. From the literature, ocular involvement with CMV is not uncommon in advanced disease in adults and may occur in the absence of an encephalitis, although the incidence of a concurrent encephalitis is greater in those patients with peripapillary involvement. In children, particularly in cases of vertical transmission of HIV, retinitis appears more commonly in association with profound systemic infection with or without an encephalitis. This difference in clinical pattern remains unexplained.

Toxoplasmosis

Toxoplasmosis although not frequently reported in HIV (Bottoni *et al.* 1990) usually presents as a necrotizing retinochoroiditis associated with vasculitis, papillitis and vitritis. Toxoplasmosis in a patient who is not HIV positive is generally thought of as a reactivation of congenital disease. However, in some cases of HIV the retinochoroiditis occurs as part of a multisystem infection, for example in the presence of *Toxoplasma* encephalitis. *Toxoplasma* responds well to treatment with sulphadiazine and pyrimethamine with folinic acid supplements but in these patients a maintenance regime may be required in addition to a standard treatment programme to prevent relapse.

Chronic progressive retinal necrosis

This represents a similar clinical picture to bilateral acute retinal necrosis (BARN) but it evolves much more slowly. The retina appears pale and swollen in the midperiphery and the lesions extend to become confluent. The infective agent is thought to be herpes zoster and a clinical response is seen to acyclovir (Forster *et al.* 1990).

Adnexal and external eye disease

Kaposi's sarcoma can occur as a violaceous subconjunctival mass that may be solitary or multiple. Treatment tends to be conservative or by radiotherapy. The incidence of Kaposi's sarcoma is much less in adolescents and young adults and increases with age. It is associated with chronic CMV infection in individuals who are not HIV infected. In HIV-positive individuals it can run a fulminant course (Holland *et al.* 1983).

Neonates infected with HIV can suffer an increase in bacterial infections with recurrent attacks of bacterial conjunctivitis and orbital cellulitis (Dennehy *et al.* 1989). Lesions of molluscum contagiosum can occur and be much more extensive than normally seen (Dennehy *et al.* 1989). If herpes simplex virus 1 infection occurs the initial infection may be severe and additional treatment may need to be continued to prevent recurrence.

Keratoconjunctivitis sicca has been described in young male patients with HIV at an increased frequency to their unaffected counterparts. It appears that they respond to lubricant treatment (Lucca *et al.* 1990).

Other manifestations

Abnormalities of ocular movement, particularly the saccadic system, have been demonstrated in HIV-infected individuals (Merrill *et al.* 1991). These abnormalities can be demonstrated in both asymptomatic patients and those patients with AIDS both with and without dementia.

Contrast sensitivity has also been shown to be reduced in HIV-positive individuals prior to the appearance of any retinopathy or evidence of retinal infection (Mutlukan *et al.* 1992).

References

Akula SK, Ma PE, Peyman GA *et al.* Treatment of cytomegalovirus retinitis with intravitreal injection of liposome encapsulated gancyclovir in a patient with AIDS. *Br J Ophthalmol* 1994; **78**: 677–80

Bayer R. Ethical challenges posed by zidovudine treatment to reduce vertical transmission of HIV. *New Engl J Med* 1994; **331**: 1123–5.

Blanche S, Ronzioux C, Guilard Moscato ML *et al.* A prospective study of infants born to women seropositive for human immunodeficiency virus type 1. *New Engl J Med* 1989; **320**: 1643–8.

Bottoni F, Gonella P, Autelitano A, Orzalesi N. Diffuse necrotising retinochoroiditis in a child with AIDS and toxoplasmic encephalitis. *Graefe's Arch Clin Exp Ophthalmol* 1990; **228**: 36–9.

Bylsma SS, Achim CL, Wiley CA *et al.* The predictive value of cytomegalovirus retinitis for cytomegalovirus encephalitis in acquired immunodeficiency syndrome. *Arch Ophthalmol* 1995; **11**: 89–95.

Chuang EL, Davis JL. Management of retinal detachment associated with CMV retinitis in AIDS patients. *Eye* 1992; **6**: 28–34.

Connor EM, Sperling RS, Geber R *et al.* Reduction of maternal infant transmission of human immunodeficiency virus type 1 with zidovudine treatment. *New Engl J Med* 1994; **331**: 1173–80.

de Smet, Nussenbatt R. Ocular manifestations in AIDS. *JAMA* 1991; **266**: 3019–22.

Dennehy P, Warman R, Flynn JT *et al.* Ocular manifestations in pediatric patients with acquired immunodeficiency syndrome. *Arch Ophthalmol* 1989; **107**: 978–82.

Dhillon B. The management of cytomegalovirus retinitis in AIDS. *Br J Ophthalmol* 1994; **78**: 66–9.

Diaz Lopez M, Espana E, Munoz G *et al.* High dose intravitreal foscarnet in the treatment of cytomegalovirus retinitis in AIDS. *Br J Ophthalmol* 1994; **78**: 677–80.

Forster DJ, Dugel PU, Frangeigh GT *et al.* Rapidly progressive outer retinal necrosis in the acquired immunodeficiency syndrome. *Am J Ophthalmol* 1990; **104**: 341–8.

Frenkel LD, Sunanda G. Perinatal HIV infection and AIDS. *Clin Perinatol* 1994; **21**: 95–107.

Goedent J, Kessler LM, Aledort LM *et al.* A prospective study of human immunodeficiency virus type 1 infection and the development of AIDS in subjects with hemophilia. *New Engl J Med* 1989; **321**: 1141–8.

Holland GN. The management of retinal detachments in patients with acquired immunodeficiency syndrome (editorial). *Arch Ophthalmol* 1991; **109**: 791–3.

Holland GN, Pepose JS, Pettit TH, Gotleib MS, Yee RD, Foos RY. Acquired immune deficiency syndrome: ocular manifestations. *Ophthalmology* 1983; **90**: 859–71.

Holland GN, Sidikaro Y, Kreiger AF *et al.* Treatment of cytomegalovirus retinopathy with gancyclovir. *Ophthalmol* 1987; **94**: 815–23.

Kozal MJ, Merrigan TC. Therapy of HIV-1 infection. *Curr Opinion Infect Dis* 1994; **7**: 72–81.

Lindegren ML, Hanson C, Miller K, Byers R, Onorato I. Epidemiology of human immunodeficiency virus infection in adolescents in the United States. *Paediatr Infect Dis J* 1994; **13**: 525–35.

Lucca JA, Farris RL, Bielory L, Caputo A. Keratoconjunctivitis sicca in male patients infected with human immunodeficiency virus type 1. *Ophthalmology* 1990; **97**: 1008–10.

Merrill PT, Paige GD, Abrams RA *et al.* Ocular motor abnormalities in human immunodeficiency virus infection. *Ann Neurol* 1991; **30**: 130–8.

Mofenson L, Maye J, Karelitz J *et al.* Crossover of placebo patients to intravenous immunoglobulin confirms efficacy for prophylaxis of bacterial infections and reduction of hospitalisation in human immunodeficiency virus infected children. *Paediatr Infect Dis J* 1994; **13**: 477–84.

Mutlukan E, Dhillon B, Aspinal P, Cullen JF. Low contrast visual acuity changes in human immunodeficiency virus (HIV) infection. *Eye* 1992; **6**: 39–42.

Palestine AG, Rodrigues M, Machou AM *et al.* Ophthalmic involvement in acquired immunodeficiency syndrome. *Ophthalmology* 1984; **91**: 1092–9.

Peters MJ, Moller HU, Russell-Eggitt I, Novelli V. Cytomegalovirus retinitis in AIDS. *Arch Dis Child* 1995; **72**: 54–5.

Rogers MF, Jaffe HW. Reducing the risk of maternal–infant transmission of HIV: a door is opened. *N Engl J Med* 1994; **331**: 1222–3.

Salvador F, Blanco R, Colin A, Galon A, Gil-Gibernau J. Cytomegalovirus retinitis in pediatric acquired immunodeficiency syndrome: report of two cases. *J Pediatr Ophthalmol Strabismus* 1993; **30**:159–62.

Thomas PA, Weedon J, Krasinski K *et al.* Maternal predictors of perinatal human immunodeficiency virus transmission. *Paediatr Infect Dis J* 1994; **13**: 489–95.

15: Conjunctivitis of the Newborn

Scott Lambert

Conjunctivitis of the newborn is the term used by the World Health Organization to describe conjunctivitis during the neonatal period (Chandler 1989). Previously it was referred to as ophthalmia neonatorum. It was originally described in 1750 (Quellmalz 1750) and is one of the most common infections occurring during the first month of life (Sandstrom *et al.* 1984; Foster and Krause 1995). Its incidence has been reported to be as high as 7–19% of all newborns (Pierce *et al.* 1982; Fransen *et al.* 1986; Laga *et al.* 1988; Dannevig *et al.* 1992).

The period of time after birth until the onset of neonatal conjunctivitis is quite variable and may be helpful in suggesting the causative agent. Conjunctivitis during the first few days of life commonly occurs as a toxic effect of topically administered silver nitrate at the time of birth. Gonococcal conjunctivitis usually develops during the first week of life. Chlamydial conjunctivitis may also develop during the first week of life, but is frequently delayed in its onset until the second week of life or later (Dannevig *et al.* 1992). Prophylactic treatment with erythromycin may prolong the interval until chlamydial conjunctivitis is detected. Bell *et al.* (1987) reported that chlamydial conjunctivitis was not detected in infants who had received erythromycin prophylaxis until 9–45 days after birth, whereas infants who received silver nitrate prophylaxis presented with chlamydial conjunctivitis 6–26 days after birth. Conjunctivitis caused by other bacterial pathogens may occur at any time during the first month of life.

The pathogens responsible for neonatal conjunctivitis vary between different geographical areas due to differences in the prevalence of maternal infections and the use of prophylactic antibiotics or silver nitrate. In a large hospital in Nairobi, Kenya where 6% of all pregnant women had cervical gonococcal cervicitis, 3% of all newborns had gonococcal conjunctivitis (Laga *et al.* 1986). In contrast, gonococcal conjunctivitis is rare in neonates in the USA, with a prevalence as low as 0.4% (Rothenberg 1979). *Chlamydia trachomatis* is a more common cause of neonatal conjunctivitis in most industrialized countries than *Neisseria gonococcus* (Rapoza *et al.* 1986; Dannevig *et al.* 1992) where women are routinely cultured for *Neisseria gonorrhoeae* during pregnancy.

Laboratory studies

Because of the difficulty in distinguishing between the various types of neonatal conjunctivitis by clinical characteristics alone, laboratory studies are paramount in establishing the correct diagnosis and selecting the best treatment. A Gram stain should be performed on a conjunctival scraping from the palpebral conjunctiva of all infants with conjunctivitis (Winceslaus *et al.* 1987). If Gram-negative diplococci are present in polymorphonuclear leucocytes, the child should be treated for presumed gonococcal conjunctivitis. Sandstrom *et al.* (1984) reported that while the identification of Gram-negative coccobacilli on a Gram stain of the conjunctiva correlated with the isolation of *Haemophilus* species, the presence of Gram-positive cocci did not correlate with positive cultures *of Staphylococcus aureus*, enterococci or *Streptococcus pneumoniae*. White blood cells are also present more frequently on the Gram stain of infants with conjunctivitis than controls (Sandstrom *et al.* 1984).

McCoy cell culture has been the standard for diagnosing *Chlamydia* conjunctivitis in the past. While the specificity of this technique is 100%, the sensitivity varies between 65 and 85% and several days are needed before the culture results are available. Polymerase chain reaction (PCR) analysis achieves a comparable specificity, with a higher sensitivity (Talley *et al.* 1992). Talley *et al.* (1994) compared PCR tests with McCoy cell cultures and found that only two of seven (28%) patients with positive PCR analyses had positive McCoy cell cultures suggesting a much higher sensitivity for PCR analysis. They also emphasized the fact that the diagnosis could be established more quickly with the PCR analysis which allowed treatment to be initiated earlier.

A Giemsa stain may also be helpful in identifying intracytoplasmic inclusion bodies in infants with chlamydial conjunctivitis. Unlike adults with chlamydial conjunctivitis, intracytoplasmic inclusion bodies may be seen in 60–80% of all infants with chlamydial conjunctivitis.

Gonococcal conjunctivitis

Gonococcal conjunctivitis in newborns is still common in developing countries, but is rare in the most industrialized countries (Laga *et al.* 1986). However, because of its propensity to produce a severe keratitis, a gonococcal infection should be excluded in all children with neonatal conjunctivitis by Gram staining and culturing a conjunctival scraping. *Neisseria gonorrhoeae* isolates are resistant to penicillin in many urban areas in the USA and many other parts of the world (50–60% in certain areas of Africa) (Laga *et al.* 1986). For this reason, infants with gonococcal conjunctivitis should be treated with a third-generation cephalosporin for 7 days in areas where penicillinase-producing strains of *N. gonorrhoeae* are endemic (1% or more of isolates) (Lepage *et al.* 1988). Irrigation of the eyes with saline at least hourly until the accompanying ocular discharge is eliminated is also recommended. Newborn infants whose mothers are known to have a gonococcal infection at the time of delivery should receive a single dose of ceftriaxone (25–50 mg/kg) soon after birth, in addition to ocular prophylaxis. A concurrent infection with *Chlamydia trachomatis* should be considered in neonates who do not respond to this therapy.

Chlamydial conjunctivitis

Chlamydia trachomatis is one of the most commonly isolated pathogens in infants with neonatal conjunctivitis in industrialized countries, with a prevalence of three to four per 1000 live births (Schachter 1978; Pierce *et al.* 1982). It usually begins as a unilateral process but often becomes bilateral (Fig. 15.1). Because chlamydial conjunctivitis may also be associated with a neonatal pneumonitis, it is important that the correct diagnosis be promptly established (Schachter *et al.* 1975; Beem & Saxon 1977; Harrison *et al.* 1978). The pneumonitis generally develops during the first 6 weeks of life and is associated with a nasal discharge, cough and tachypnoea. The recommended treatment for infants with chlamydial conjunctivitis is a 4-day course of oral erythromycin syrup (50 mg/kg per day) in four divided doses (Peter 1991). Oral erythromycin not only treats chlamydial pneumonitis and eradicates nasopharyngeal carriage *of Chlamydia,* but it is also more effective than topical erythromycin in preventing a

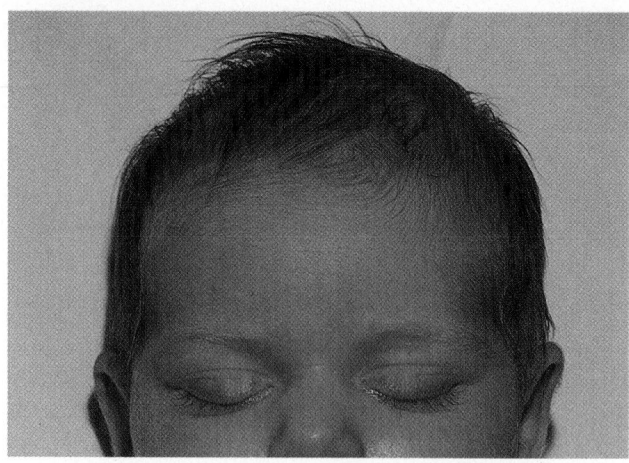

Fig. 15.1 Mild neonatal chlamydial conjunctivitis. The lids are slightly swollen and there is a discharge.

relapse of chlamydial conjunctivitis (Patamasucon *et al.* 1982). However, chlamydial conjunctivitis may recur even after a course of oral erythromycin, possibly due to poor compliance with antibiotic therapy, an inadequate dose of antibiotics or a reinfection (Rees *et al.* 1981). A second course of oral erythromycin should be given when a recurrence occurs. Adjuvant therapy with topical erythromycin or tetracycline may also be beneficial. In addition, parents of infected children should be treated with oral tetracycline or erythromycin for 2 weeks. If possible, pregnant women with chlamydial cervicitis should be treated before delivery of their child with oral erythromycin. Untreated chlamydial conjunctivitis usually resolves spontaneously after 8–12 months but may result in the formation of a micropannus and scarring of the tarsal conjunctiva (Mordhorst & Dawson 1971). In addition, children with untreated chlamydial conjunctivitis are at increased risk of developing a pneumonitis or otitis (Beem & Saxon 1977; Harrison *et al.* 1978).

Non-gonococcal, non-chlamydial conjunctivitis

The most common pathogen isolated from neonates with conjunctivitis in most studies is *Staphylococcus aureus* (Dannevig *et al.* 1992; Zanoni *et al.* 1992). Other Gram-positive organisms including *Staphylococcus epidermitis, Streptococcus viridans* and *Streptococcus pneumoniae* can also frequently be cultured from newborns with conjunctivitis. Gram-negative organisms such as enterococcus, *Escherichia coli, Serratia* and *Pseudomonas* account for a smaller percentage of cases (Rapoza *et al.* 1986; Sandstrom 1987). Conjunctival cultures are negative in up to 25% of children with neonatal conjunctivitis. Broad-spectrum antibiotics should be administered to infants with severe conjunctivitis until culture results have identified the pathogen and its antibiotic sensitivity. Infants with mild to moderate conjunctivitis may be treated with lid hygiene alone until a microbe has been isolated. Lid hygiene alone may be sufficient for infants with negative conjunctival cultures (Sandstrom 1987).

Congenital dacrostenosis

A congenital nasolacrimal duct obstruction is also frequently associated with neonatal conjunctivitis. Dacrostenosis should be suspected in children with unilateral conjunctivitis and epiphora who have a reflux of mucopurulent material from the lacrimal punctae after massaging the lacrimal sac. Dacrocystitis in infants with congenital dacrostenosis is usually caused by *Haemophilus* species and *S. pneumoniae* (Sandstrom *et al.* 1984). Congenital dacrostenosis should be treated initially with topical antibiotics and massaging of the lacrimal sac to increase the hydrostatic pressure in the lacrimal sac (Crigler 1923). If the dacrostenosis fails to resolve spontaneously by 6–12 months of age, the nasolacrimal system should be probed (Kushner 1982). A dacryocystocoele is an enlargement of the lacrimal sac secondary to a distal and proximal obstruction of the nasolacrimal system. While mucinous material may be expressed from the lacrimal sac by massaging a dacryocystocoele, the lacrimal sac rapidly fills again, presumably due to the ball-valve effect of the proximal obstruction. Infants with dacryocystocoeles should be probed soon after birth before dacryocystitis develops (Katowitz & Welsh 1987; Pollard 1991).

Viral conjunctivitis

Viral conjunctivitis occurs infrequently in neonates. Herpes simplex conjunctivitis usually occurs in neonates exposed to a maternal herpes infection at the time of birth. Vesicles may be present on the eyelids or on other parts of the body. Herpetic keratitis may also develop. The diagnosis can be confirmed by culturing the fluid in a vesicle. Neonates with a suspected herpes simplex infection should be treated with systemic acyclovir to reduce the risk of a disseminated infection developing.

Prophylaxis

Crede (1881), introduced 2% silver nitrate as a prophylactic treatment for conjunctivitis in newborns in Leipzig in 1881. The widespread use of silver nitrate prophylaxis was subsequently associated with a dramatic decline in the incidence of gonococcal conjunctivitis in newborns throughout Europe and the USA (Barsam 1966; Forbes & Forbes 1971). Topical erythromycin and tetracycline are also now used for ocular prophylaxis in newborns. All are considered to be quite effective in preventing gonococcal conjunctivitis (Laga *et al.* 1988; Peter 1991); but less effective as a prophylactic treatment for chlamydial conjunctivitis (Bell *et al.* 1987; Laga *et al.* 1988; Hammerschlag *et al.* 1989). Bell *et al.* (1993) randomized 630 infants to silver nitrate, erythromycin or no prophylaxis. Mild conjunctivitis developed in 17% of the infants. While the incidence of conjunctivitis was slightly lower in the children receiving silver nitrate and erythromycin prophylaxis, the effect was modest and the conjunctivitis was caused in most cases by micro-organisms of low virulence which were believed to be acquired postnatally. These findings suggest that most cases of neonatal conjunctivitis are caused by postnatally acquired pathogens. This helps to explain why the incidence of conjunctivitis in newborns is similar between infants born by caesarean and vaginal delivery.

Povidone-iodine (Isenberg *et al.* 1994) is under evaluation and looks promising (Isenberg *et al.* 1995) as it may be more effective, less costly and less toxic than silver nitrate or erythromycin.

References

Barsam PC. Specific prophylaxis of gonorrheal ophthalmia neonatorum: a review. *N Engl J Med* 1966; **274**: 731–4.

Beem MO, Saxon EM. Respiratory tract colonization and a distinctive pneumonia syndrome in infants with *Chlamydia trachomatis*. *N Engl J Med* 1977; **296**; 306–10.

Bell TA, Grayson JT, Krohn MA *et al.* Randomized trial of silver nitrate, erythromycin, and no eye prophylaxis for the prevention of conjunctivitis among newborns not at risk for gonococcal ophthalmitis. *Pediatrics* 1993; **92**: 755–60.

Bell TA, Sandstrom KI, Gravett MG *et al.* Comparison of ophthalmic silver nitrate solution and erythromycin ointment for prevention of natally acquired *Chlamydia trachomatis*. *Sex Trans Dis* 1987; **14**: 195–200.

Chandler JW. Controversies in ocular prophylaxis of newborns. *Arch Ophthalmol* 1989; **107**: 814–15.

Crede CSF. Reports from the obstetrical clinic in Leipzig: prevention of eye inflammation in the newborn. *Arch Gynaekol* 1881; **17**: 50–3.

Crigler LW. The treatment of congenital dacrocystitis. *JAMA* 1923; **81**: 23–4.

Dannevig L, Straume B, Melby K. Ophthalmia neonatorum in northern Norway II. Microbiology with emphasis on *Chlamydia trachomatis*. *Acta Ophthalmol* 1992; **70**: 19–25.

Forbes GB, Forbes GM. Silver nitrate and the eyes of the newborn: Crede's contribution to preventive medicine. *Am J Dis Child* 1971; **121**: 1–3.

Foster A, Krause V. Ophthalmia neonatorum in developing countries (editorial). *N Engl J Med* 1995; (Mar 2):600–2.

Fransen L, Nsanze H, Klauss V *et al.* Ophthalmia neonatorum in Nairobi, Kenya: the roles of *Neisseria gonorrhoeae* and *Chlamydia trachomatis*. *J Infect Dis* 1986; **153**: 862–9.

Hammerschlag MR, Cummings C, Roblin PM *et al.* Efficacy of neonatal ocular prophylaxis for the prevention of chlamydial and gonococcal conjunctivitis. *N Engl J Med* 1989; **320**:769–72.

Harrison HR, Phil D, English MG *et al. Chlamydia trachomatis* infant pneumonitis. Comparison with matched controls and other infant pneumonitis. *N Engl J Med* 1978; **298**: 702–8.

Isenberg SJ, Apt L, Wood M. A controlled trial of Povidone-iodine as prophylaxis against ophthalmia neonatorum. *N Engl J Med* 1995; March 2: 562–6.

Isenberg S, Apt L, Yoshimori R, Leake R, Rick R. Povidone-iodine for ophthalmia neonatorum prophylaxis. *Am J Ophthalmol* 1994; **118**: 701–6.

Katowitz IA, Welsh MG. Timing of initial probing and irrigation in congenital nasolacrimal duct obstruction. *Ophthalmology* 1987; **94**: 698–705.

Kushner BJ. Congenital nasolacrimal system obstruction. *Arch Ophthalmol* 1982; **100**: 597–600.

Laga M, Naamara W, Brunham RC *et al*. Single-dose therapy of gonococcal ophthalmia neonatorum with ceftriaxone. *N Engl J Med* 1986; **315**: 1382–5.

Laga M, Plummer FA, Piot P *et al*. Prophylaxis of gonococcal and chlamydial ophthalmia neonatorum. *N Engl J Med* 1988; **318**: 653–7.

Lepage P, Bogaerts J, Kestelyn P *et al*. Single-dose cefotaxime intramuscularly cures gonococcal ophthalmia neonatorum. *Br J Ophthalmol* 1988; **72**: 518–20.

Mordhorst CH, Dawson C. Sequelae of neonatal inclusion conjunctivitis and associated diseases in parents. *Am J Ophthalmol* 1971; **71**: 861–7.

Patamasucon P, Rettig PJ, Faust KL *et al*. Oral versus topical erythomycin therapies for chlamydial conjunctivitis. *Am J Dis Child* 1982; **136**: 817–21.

Peter G. *Red Book: Report of the Committee on Infectious Diseases*, 20th edn. Elk Grove, Illinois: American Academy of Pediatrics, 1991.

Pierce JM, Ward ME, Seal DV. Ophthalmia neonatorum in the 1980s: incidence, aetiology and treatment. *Br J Ophthalmol* 1982; **66**: 728–31.

Pollard ZF. Treatment of acute dacryocystitis in neonates. *J Pediatr Ophthalmol Strabismus* 1991; **28**: 341–3.

Quellmalz ST. *De Caecitate Infantum Fluoris Albi Materni Ejusque Virulentae Pedissqua*. Lipsiae. 1750.

Rapoza PA, Quinn TC, Kiessling LA *et al*. Assessment of neonatal conjunctivitis with a direct immunofluorescent monoclonal antibody stain for *Chlamydia*. *JAMA* 1986; **255**: 3369–73.

Rees E, Tait A, Hobson D *et al*. Persistence of chlamydial infection after treatment for neonatal conjunctivitis. *Arch Dis Child* 1981; **56**: 193–8.

Rothenberg R. Ophthalmia neonatorum due to *Neisseria gonorrhoea*: prevention and treatment. *Sex Trans Dis* 1979; **6**: 187–91.

Sandstrom I. Treatment of neonatal conjunctivitis. *Arch Ophthalmol* 1987; **105**: 925–8.

Sandstrom KI, Bell TA, Chandler JW *et al*. Microbial causes of neonatal conjunctivitis. *J Pediatr* 1984; **5**: 706–11.

Schachter J. Chlamydial infections. *N Engl J Med* 1978; **298**: 540–9.

Schachter J, Lun L, Gooding CA *et al*. Pneumonitis following inclusion blennorrhea. *J Paediatr* 1975; **87**: 779–80.

Talley AR, Garcia-Ferrer KF, Laycock KA *et al*. Comparative diagnosis of neonatal chlamydial conjunctivitis by polymerase chain reaction and McCoy cell culture. *Am J Ophthalmol* 1994; **117**: 50–7.

Talley AR, Garcia-Ferrer F, Laycock KA *et al*. The use of polymerase chain reaction for the detection of chlamydial keratoconjunctivitis. *Am J Ophthalmol* 1992; **114**: 685–92.

Winceslaus J, Goh BT, Dunlop EM *et al*. Diagnosis of ophthalmia neonatorum. *Br Med J* 1987; **295**: 1377–9.

Zanoni D, Isenberg SJ, Apt L. A comparison of silver nitrate with erythromycin for prophylaxis against ophthalmia neonatorum. *Clin Pediatr* 1992; **31**: 295.

16: Preseptal and Orbital Cellulitis

Anthony Moore and Donal Brosnahan

Periorbital infections, particularly sinusitis, may cause infection or a severe inflammatory reaction of the orbital tissues leading to preseptal or orbital cellulitis. The proximity of the paranasal sinuses to the orbital walls, and the interconnection between the venous system of the orbit and the face allow infection to spread from the sinuses to the orbit either directly or via the blood stream. The orbital venous system is devoid of valves and two-way communication is permitted with the venous system of the nose, face and pterygoid fossa. The superior and inferior ophthalmic veins which drain the orbit empty into the cavernous sinus, hence orbital and facial infections may lead to the serious complication of cavernous sinus thrombosis.

Certain anatomical structures help to limit the direct spread of infection. The orbital periosteum acts as a barrier to spread from infected sinuses, but may become stripped from the orbital wall by a collection of pus which forms a subperiosteal abscess. The orbital septum limits the spread of infection from the preseptal space to the orbit.

Orbital infections and their complications can be classified into five types (Chandler *et al.* 1970) (Table 16.1). Combining both clinical and CT findings permits more accurate staging (Eustis *et al.* 1986).

Preseptal cellulitis

Aetiology

Preseptal cellulitis occurs when the infection is anterior to the orbital septum. It is much more common than orbital cellulitis and may have a variety of causes including eyelid trauma, extraocular infections and upper respiratory tract infections (Barkin & Todd 1978; Weiss *et al.* 1983). Children with this condition can be divided into three main groups (Jones 1982). The first group includes those who have developed periorbital oedema from an associated lid infection such as impetigo, herpes simplex or varicella, or have a local cause for the oedema such as infected chalazion, or dacrocystitis (Fig. 16.1). Second, suppurative cellulitis may develop from lid trauma (Fig. 16.2), in which case the causative organism is usually *Staphylococcus aureus* or a beta-haemolytic streptococcus. Third, in preseptal cellulitis associated with an upper respiratory tract infection (Fig. 16.3), *Haemophilus influenzae* and *Streptococcus aureus* are the usual organisms involved (Smith 1978; Weiss 1983). In this last group of children there is often an associated sinusitis (Barkin & Todd 1978; Weiss *et al.* 1983).

Molarte (1989) in a review of 30 patients under 1 year of age all of whom had periorbital cellulitis, noted that the most frequent predisposing condition in neonates was a ruptured dacryocoele. However, in older infants upper respiratory tract infection was most prevalent. *Streptococcus pneumoniae* and *Staphylococcus aureus* were associated with cellulitis in the neonatal period and *Haemophilus influenzae* in later infancy.

Clinical manifestations

The usual clinical presentation is unilateral orbital oedema in a child with recent lid trauma or upper respiratory tract infection. Bilateral involvement is rare (Barkin & Todd 1978). In contrast with orbital cellulitis vision is usually normal and there is no proptosis and/or limitation of ocular motility. The child is often generally unwell and febrile and full blood count will usually show a leucocyto-

Table 16.1 Classification of orbital infections. Modified from Chandler *et al.* (1970).

Preseptal cellulitis
Orbital cellulitis
Subperiosteal abscess
Orbital abscess
Cavernous sinus thrombosis

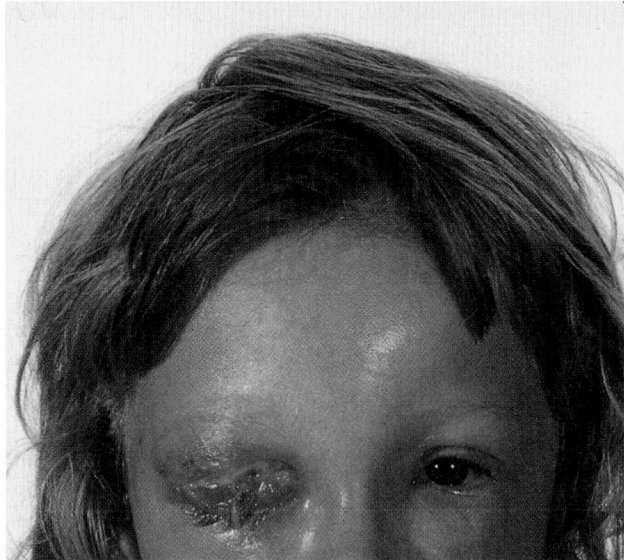

Fig. 16.1 Preseptal cellulitis caused by spread from a stye in a patient with leukaemia.

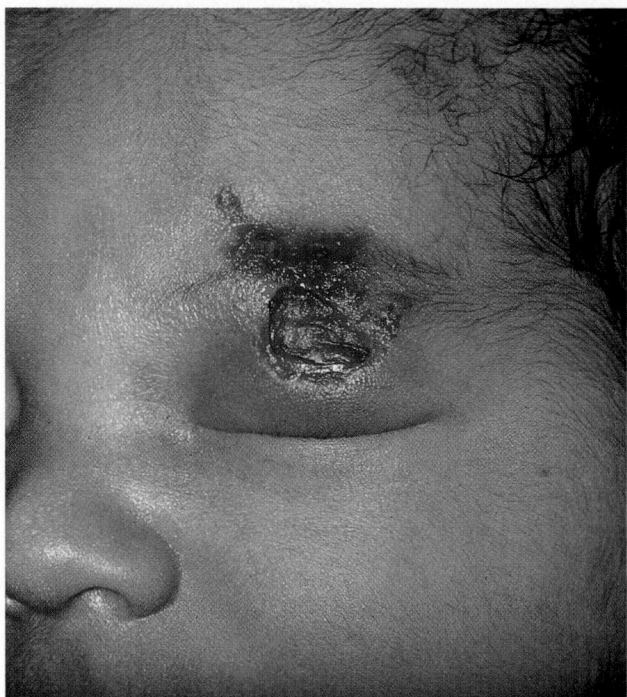

Fig. 16.2 Preseptal cellulitis caused by infection of a necrotic ulcer caused by a forceps injury (Dr S. Day's patient).

sis. Local causes for the lid swelling such as chalazion or dacryocystitis are easily excluded on clinical examination. In the neonate it is important to exclude inclusion conjunctivitis and osteomyelitis of the maxilla (Cavenagh 1960), and Caffey's disease (infantile cortical hyperostosis).

The clinical picture may vary with different organisms involved. In staphylococcal infections there is a purulent discharge, whilst *Haemophilus* infection leads to a nonpurulent cellulitis with a characteristic blueish-purple discoloration of the eyelid. This may be accompanied by irritability, raised temperature and otitis media. In streptococcal infection there is usually a sharply demarcated red area of induration (Jones 1983), heat and marked tenderness.

Preseptal cellulitis may be complicated by meningitis particularly if the infection is due to *Haemophilus influenzae* type b (Ciarallo & Rowe 1993).

Management

Children with a local cause for the periorbital oedema, such as dacryocystitis, need specific treatment for the underlying condition and rarely need further investigation. In suppurative cellulitis following lid trauma it is

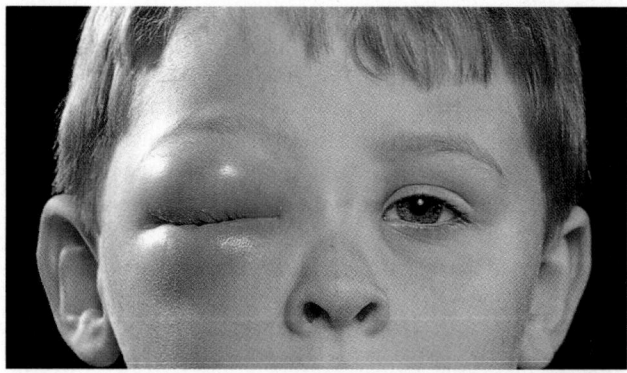

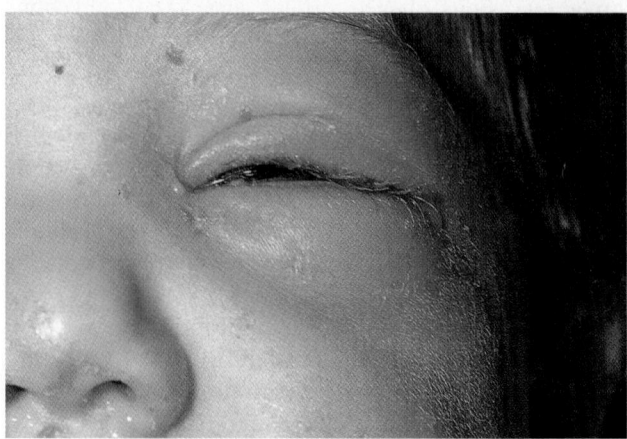

Fig. 16.3 (a) Preseptal cellulitis associated with sinusitis in an otherwise healthy child. (b) Preseptal cellulitis due to *Haemophilus influenzae* in a 6-month-old infant.

sufficient to culture the wound discharge as there is rarely any bacteraemia and blood cultures are usually negative (Weiss *et al.* 1983). Parenteral antibiotics are administered and tetanus prophylaxis provided, if appropriate. In children who develop preseptal cellulitis following an upper respiratory tract infection, cultures should be taken from the nose, throat, conjunctiva and from any aspirates of the periorbital oedema.

In one study blood cultures were positive in 27% of patients (Molarte *et al.* 1989) and they are indicated if there is fever or systemic upset. Sinus X-rays are usually performed, although they may be difficult to interpret in children under the age of 2 years due to the lack of development of the sinuses (Weiss *et al.* 1983). Lumbar puncture may be required to rule out meningitis, particularly if the infecting organism is thought to be *Haemophilus influenzae*. A computed tomography (CT) scan (Fig. 16.4) to exclude orbital involvement is indicated when marked lid swelling prevents an adequate examination of the globe (Goldberg *et al.* 1978).

Older children with a suppurative cellulitis following lid trauma who are not generally unwell, can be managed

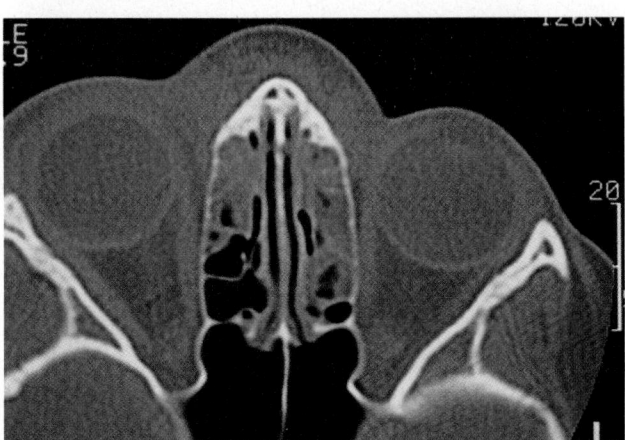

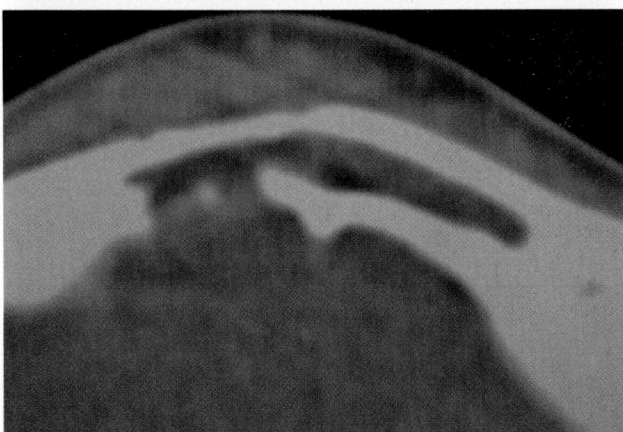

Fig. 16.4 (a, b) CT scans of a 13-year-old child with an anomalous frontal sinus. The initial cellulitis responded to low doses of antibiotics which were then stopped. One month later she developed osteomyelitis, meningitis and frontal lobe oedema.

as an outpatient using oral antibiotics. The most likely infecting organisms are *Staphylococcus aureus* or *Streptococcus pyogenes* and should respond to a penicillinase-resistant penicillin such as nafcillin or oxacillin, 150–200 mg/kg per day administered in divided doses at 6-hourly intervals (Table 16.2). If the skin has been penetrated by organic material or following animal bites penicillin G should be added to cover anaerobic organisms.

In the absence of trauma or predisposing skin lesion, *Haemophilus influenzae* and *Streptococcus pneumoniae* infections predominate. A second-generation cephalosporin such as cefuroxime 100–150 mg/kg per day should be administered intravenously in divided doses at 8-hourly intervals. An alternative combination is ampicillin 50–100 mg/kg per day and chloramphenicol 75–100 mg/kg per day in divided doses, though ampicillin-resistant strains of *Haemophilus influenzae* are frequently encountered (Lerman *et al.* 1980; Noel *et al.* 1990). Antibiotics should be administered intravenously initially and regimens may need to be modified on the basis of culture and sensitivity.

In young children and infants overall management is best undertaken by a paediatrician and/or an infectious diseases specialist in consultation with the ophthalmologist and ENT surgeon.

Surgical treatment is seldom necessary; about 10% of children will require surgical drainage of a lid abscess or paranasal sinus (Weiss *et al.* 1983).

Orbital cellulitis

Orbital cellulitis is an uncommon but important condition which may give rise to a variety of serious systemic and ocular complications (Table 16.3). In the pre-antibiotic era one-fifth of patients died from septic intracranial complications and one-third of the survivors had visual loss in the affected eye (Duke-Elder & MacFaul 1974). This poor outlook has been dramatically altered by the introduction of effective antibiotics but prompt diagnosis and vigorous treatment are essential if such complications are to be avoided.

Aetiology

In contrast to preseptal cellulitis, orbital cellulitis is more frequent in children older than 5 years, and in over 90% of cases occurs secondary to sinusitis (Watters *et al.* 1976; Weiss *et al.* 1983) especially of the ethmoid. When it does occur in infants it is usually due to infection with type b *Haemophilus influenzae* (Londer & Nelson 1974). Other less common causes are penetrating orbital trauma, especially when there is a retained foreign body, dental infections (Flood *et al.* 1982), extraocular muscle and retinal surgery (Von Noorden 1972) and haematogenous spread during a systemic infectious illness.

Table 16.2 Initial antibiotic treatment of preseptal and orbital cellulitis.

Preseptal cellulitis	*Associated with trauma/suppurative* Oxacillin or nafcillin 150–200 mg/kg per day in divided doses (p.o. *or* i.v.) *Associated with upper respiratory tract infection* Cefuroxime 100–150 mg/kg per day *or* ampicillin 50–100 mg/kg per day *and* chloramphenicol 75–100 mg/kg per day (i.v. in divided doses)
Orbital cellulitis	Ceftazidime 100–150 mg/kg per day *or* ceftoxamine 100–150 mg/kg per day *or* ceftriaxone 100–150 mg/kg per day (i.v. in divided doses) and oxacillin or nafcillin 150–200 mg/kg per day (in divided doses)

The exact dose will vary with age and severity of infection.

The common bacterial pathogens are *Staphylococcus aureus*, *Streptococcus pyogenes*, *Streptococcus pneumoniae* and *Haemophilus influenzae*. Other Gram-negative organisms such as *Escherichia coli* and anaerobic bacteria which may form gas within the orbit (Sevel *et al.* 1973), may occasionally be implicated. Atypical mycobacteria have also been reported to cause orbital cellulitis in young children (Levine 1969). Fungal infections are rare but should be excluded when orbital cellulitis occurs in an immunosuppressed or diabetic child (Schwartz *et al.* 1977).

Clinical manifestations

The usual presentation is with a painful red eye and increasing lid oedema in a child who has had a recent upper respiratory tract infection. The child is usually pyrexial and generally unwell. There is usually conjunctival chemosis and injection, axial proptosis and limitation of eye movements (Fig. 16.5). Visual loss when it occurs is usually due to an associated optic neuritis but may also be caused by exposure keratitis or even a retinal vascular occlusion (Jarrett & Gutman 1969; Sherry 1973; Schramm *et al.* 1978) (Fig. 16.6).

The acute onset, pain, fever and systemic illness help to differentiate orbital cellulitis from other causes of unilateral proptosis. Occasionally, orbital cellulitis may cause proptosis and limitation of ocular motility without marked inflammatory signs and may be confused clinically with a rapidly growing orbital tumour or inflammatory pseudotumour. In such cases the distinction is made on plain films and CT scan of the orbit. Rarely a necrotic retinoblastoma (Rozanksy 1964; Shields *et al.* 1991) (Fig. 16.7) or Coats' disease (Judisch 1980) may cause severe panophthalmitis and orbital inflammation which can be confused with orbital cellulitis. Orbital myositis

may also mimic orbital cellulitis (Takahashi 1983; Moorman & Elston 1995).

In young infants under 3 months of age osteomyelitis of the superior maxilla (Cavenagh 1960), which gives a similar clinical picture, should be excluded.

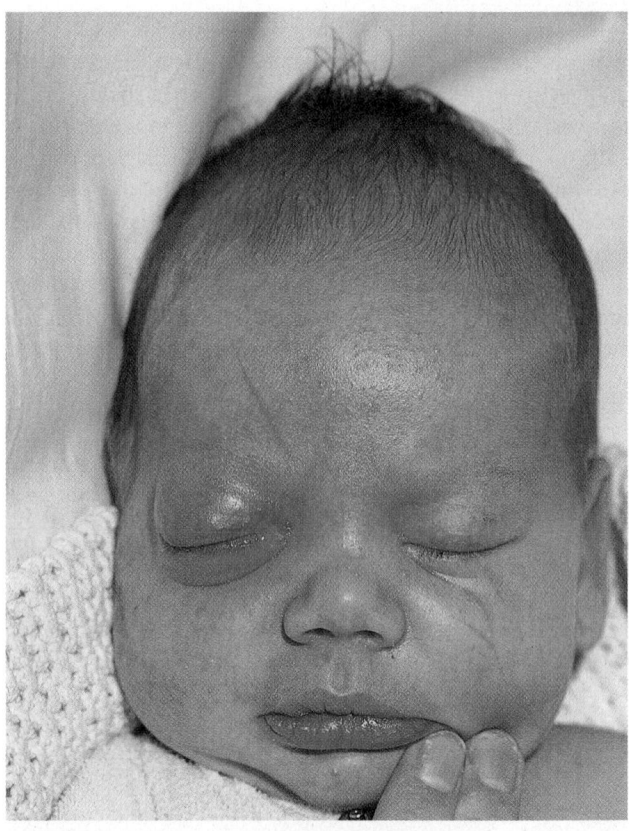

Fig. 16.5 Orbital cellulitis.

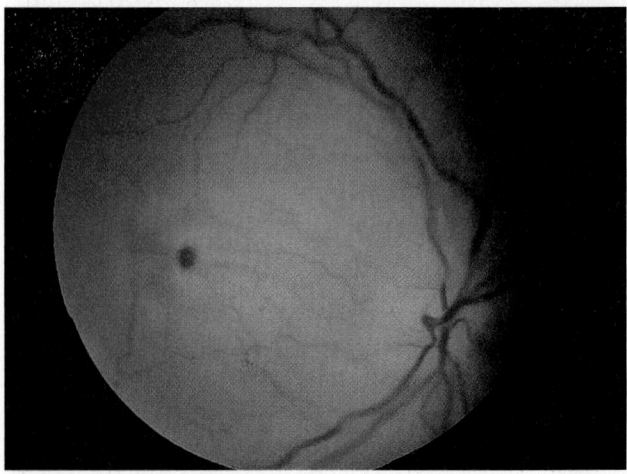

Fig. 16.6 Central retinal artery occlusion in orbital cellulitis (Dr S. Day's patient).

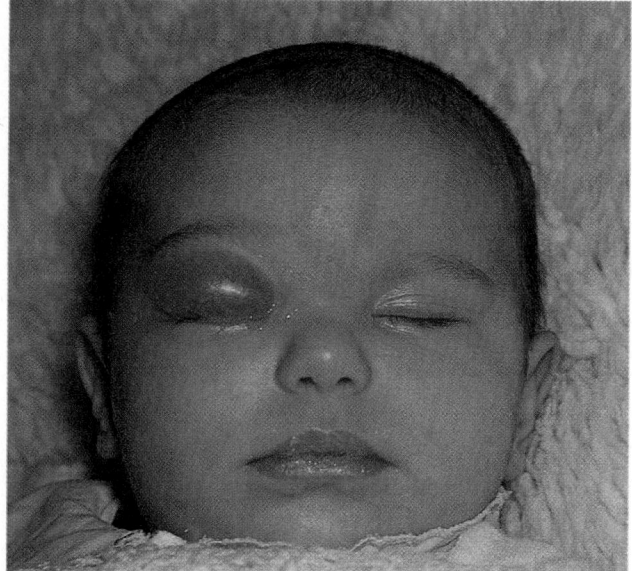

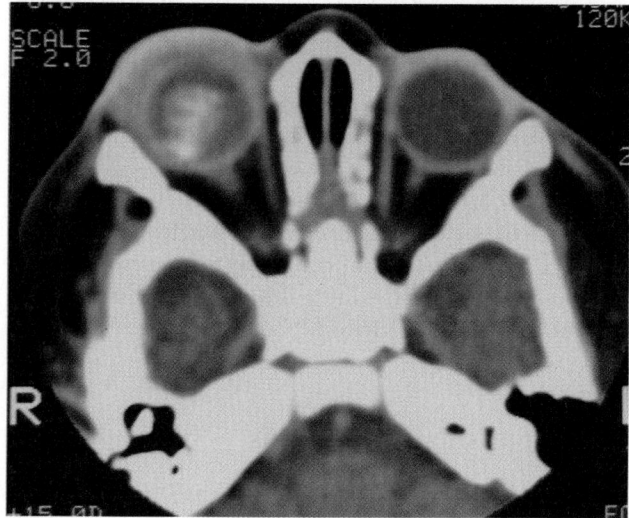

Fig. 16.7 (a) This 9-month-old child presented with a severe unilateral orbital oedema. She was unwell but apyrexial. (b) CT scan shows bilateral retinoblastoma; large and calcified on the right, small on the left. She was treated with systemic steroids which abolished the orbital oedema, the right eye was enucleated and the left given local treatment. She is alive and well 7 years later with a left visual acuity of 6/5.

Management

Children with orbital cellulitis should be admitted to hospital immediately for investigation and treatment. Initial investigations should include blood cultures and cultures from nose, throat and conjunctivae. These are often negative, but a positive result is helpful in planning antibiotic treatment. Sinus X-rays and a dental examination should be performed and an ENT consultation obtained. In the absence of any local cause for the orbital cellulitis a careful search should be made for any septic focus elsewhere in

the body. If there are signs of meningism lumbar puncture is indicated. As in preseptal cellulitis close liaison between paediatrician, ENT surgeon and ophthalmologist is required for optimal treatment.

It is preferable to obtain a CT scan in all cases of orbital cellulitis as CT scan has been shown to detect subperiosteal and orbital abscesses which are not apparent clinically or on plain films (Goldberg *et al.* 1978; Schramm *et al.* 1978). Orbital ultrasound may also detect orbital abscess but is less reliable (Schramm *et al.* 1978; Krohel *et al.* 1980).

The initial treatment of orbital cellulitis in infants should be with high-dose intravenous third-generation cephalosporin such as ceftoxamine 100–150 mg/kg per day, ceftazidime 100–150 mg/kg per day or ceftriaxone 100–150 mg/kg per day combined with a penicillinase-resistant penicillin (Table 16.2). In older children sinusitis is frequently caused by mixed aerobic and anaerobic organisms so clindamycin 10 mg/kg per day may be substituted for penicillinase-resistant penicillin. An alternative regimen is the combination of penicillinase-resistant penicillin with chloramphenicol. The initial regime may be modified in the light of later culture results. Nasal decongestants such as ephedrine may be helpful in promoting intranasal drainage of infected sinuses. About 60% of children will be cured by antibiotics alone but the remainder will require surgical drainage of an infected sinus or orbital abscess (Weiss *et al.* 1983). With prompt treatment complications are fortunately rare.

Subperiosteal and orbital abscess

The incidence of subperiosteal and orbital abscess complicating orbital cellulitis varies in different series but is probably about 10% (Hornblass *et al.* 1984). The vast majority of such cases have associated sinus infection. In the first decade of life infection most frequently arises from the maxillary or ethmoidal sinus (Harris 1983). In subperiosteal abscess, a purulent infection within a sinus breaks through the thin orbital bony wall (lamina papyracea) and lies beneath the periosteum which is stripped from the bone. Orbital abscess occurs either when a subperiosteal abscess breaches the periorbita or

Table 16.3 Complications of orbital cellulitis.

Optic neuritis
Optic atrophy
Exposure keratitis
Central retinal artery occlusion (Jarrett & Gutman 1969)
Retinal and choroidal ischaemia (Sherry 1973)
Subperiosteal and orbital abscess (Schramm *et al.* 1978; Krohel *et al.* 1980)
Cavernous sinus thrombosis (Clune 1963)
Meningitis (Weiss *et al.* 1983)
Brain abscess
Septicaemia (Krohel *et al.* 1980)

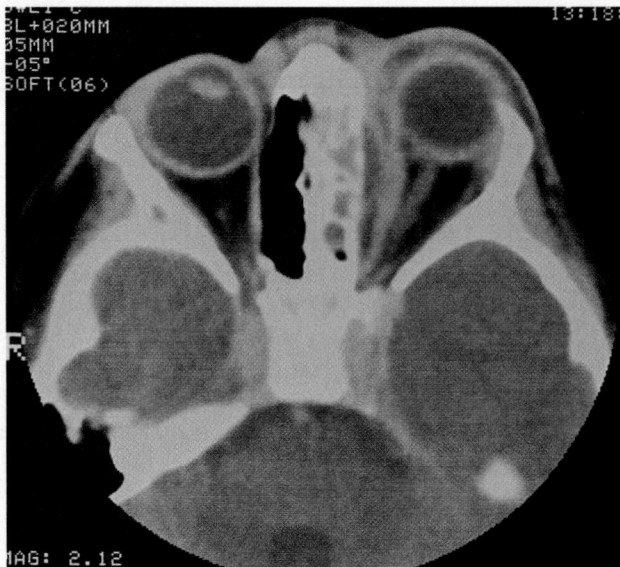

Fig. 16.8 CT scan showing left ethmoidal sinusitis and subperiosteal abscess.

when a collection of pus forms within the orbit in a child with orbital cellulitis. The usual causative organism is *Staphylococcus* but *Streptococcus, Haemophilus influenzae* and anaerobic organisms may also be responsible. Unless there is non-axial proptosis or a palpable fluctuant swelling at the orbital rim, it is difficult to distinguish orbital abscess from uncomplicated orbital cellulitis clinically. It should be suspected whenever there is marked systemic toxicity and severe orbital signs, or when orbital cellulitis is slow to respond to adequate doses of intravenous antibiotics. The presence of subperiosteal abscess may be indicated by lateral displacement of the globe away from the infected sinus, impaired adduction and resiliency on retropulsion (Harris 1983). Initial CT (Fig. 16.8) scanning of all new cases of orbital cellulitis will allow early detection of orbital and subperiosteal abscess, and serial orbital ultrasound may be used to follow the course of the abscess once treatment has been started.

While there is general agreement that orbital abscess should be drained the management of subperiosteal abscess is more controversial. A number of authors have reported resolution of subperiosteal abscess treated medically (Rubin & Zito 1994; Catalano & Smoot 1990; Noel *et al.* 1990). Harris (1994) in a review of 37 patients with subperiosteal abscess secondary to sinusitis noted that resolution occurred in 83% of patients under 9 years of age who were treated medically or who had negative cultures on drainage. In contrast only 25% of those aged between 9 and 14 years cleared without drainage or had negative cultures on drainage. The remaining group aged 15 years and over were refractory to medical therapy alone. These findings are attributed to differences in the bacterial flora found in the different groups, with single aerobic organisms cultured from younger patients and mixed aerobic and anaerobic infections from the older groups. Thus it would seem reasonable to treat medically initially if vision is normal, the subperiosteal abscess is of moderate size, in the absence of intracranial extension and if the child is under 9 years of age (Harris 1994).

Osteomyelitis of the superior maxilla

This condition, which usually presents in the first few months of life with fever, general malaise and marked periorbital oedema, may be confused with orbital cellulitis, or subperiosteal abscess (Cavenagh 1960). There may be conjunctival chemosis, mild proptosis and early central abscess formation in the superior maxilla with pointing at the inner or outer canthus. The diagnosis should be suspected if there is pus in the nostril and oedema of the alveolus and palate on the affected side. A fistula may be present in the area of the first deciduous molar.

Staphylococcus aureus is the usual infecting organism but the mode of infection is uncertain; it may result from haematogenous spread to the dental sac of the first deciduous molar, which has a rich blood supply, or may develop secondary to mastitis in the mother.

Treatment is with high-dose intravenous antibiotics chosen on the basis of culture and sensitivity and surgical drainage of the abscess preferably via the nose. Cavenagh (1960) has reviewed the literature on this condition and reported a series of 24 infants she has personally treated with excellent results.

Cavernous sinus thrombosis

Since the introduction of antibiotics this dreaded complication of orbital cellulitis has become rare. In the pre-antibiotic era the mortality rate was almost 100% (Grove 1936). Antibiotics have reduced the mortality of this complication of orbital cellulitis to 25% (Clune 1963). In its early stages cavernous sinus thrombosis may be difficult to distinguish clinically from orbital cellulitis. In the former there is more severe pain and a marked systemic illness, proptosis develops rapidly and there may be third, fourth and sixth cranial nerve palsies compared with the purely mechanical limitation seen in orbital cellulitis. Hyperalgesia in the distribution of the fifth cranial nerve is common. The presence of retinal venous dilatation and optic disc swelling, especially if bilateral, is very suggestive of cavernous sinus thrombosis. In the later stages, bilateral involvement in cavernous sinus thrombosis makes the clinical distinction from orbital cellulitis easier. Diagnosis can be confirmed by performing digital orbital venography and CT scan. Cavernous sinus thrombosis is most frequently associated with *Staphylococcus aureus* infection (Southwick *et al.* 1986).

The management of cavernous sinus thrombosis is best undertaken by a paediatric neurologist or neurosurgeon and involves treatment with high-dose intravenous antibiotics, anticoagulants and systemic steroids in selected cases.

Fungal orbital cellulitis

Fungal orbital cellulitis is rare in childhood but fungi of the class zygomycetes (formerly known as phycomycetes), may cause orbital infection in children who are acidotic, diabetic or immunosuppressed.

This class contains two orders, Mucorales and Entomophthorales. *Mucor*, *Rhizopus* and *Absidia*, which have been isolated in fungal orbital cellulitis, are members of the class Mucorales hence the term mucormycosis.

Orbital zygomycosis

In adults this infection is seen mainly in diabetics in ketoacidosis but may occur in mild diabetes (Schwartz *et al.* 1977) and in patients who are immunosuppressed. The main predisposing condition in childhood is metabolic acidosis associated with gastroenteritis (Hale 1971) although less commonly it may occur in children who are diabetic or immunosuppressed (Schwartz *et al.* 1977). Fungal orbital cellulitis has been described in otherwise healthy children (Blodi *et al.* 1969; Whitehurst & Liston 1981). Untreated, it is rapidly fatal so that prompt diagnosis is essential.

The condition begins with colonization of the sinuses by spores followed by direct or haematogenous spread to the orbit. Orbital involvement is heralded by periorbital pain, marked lid oedema, conjunctival chemosis and proptosis. Later spread to the orbital apex will result in third, fourth and sixth cranial nerve palsies and optic neuropathy. Central retinal artery occlusion may occur. Sinus X-rays will normally show ethmoid or maxillary sinusitis. Zygomycetes have a tendency to invade arteries causing thrombosis and subsequent ischaemic necrosis; involvement of the facial arteries causes gangrene of the nose, palate and facial tissues. Once spread to the cavernous sinus and intracranial vessels has occurred, the prognosis is very poor.

Orbital fungal infection should therefore be suspected in any diabetic, acidotic or immunosuppressed child who develops a rapidly progressive orbital cellulitis, especially if accompanied by necrosis of the skin or nasal mucosa. To confirm the diagnosis, scrapings from infected tissues should be cultured and Gram and Giemsa stained. Larger tissue biopsies should be fixed in 10% formalin and processed for histological examination. These fungi have an affinity for haematoxylin and are therefore easily recognized in haematoxylin and eosin sections. Histological examination of biopsy specimens reveals invasion of vascular structures and thrombosis. A positive culture result should be interpreted with caution as zygomycetes are common contaminants in most microbiology laboratories.

The management of this condition consists of specific antifungal therapy, correction of the underlying metabolic or immunological abnormality and surgical debridement of necrotic tissues. The specific treatment of choice is amphotericin B, which should be given intravenously and may also be used locally to irrigate infected sinuses. It is nephrotoxic so renal function should be carefully monitored. Any metabolic abnormality should be corrected and immunosuppressive drugs, especially steroids, should be withdrawn if possible. Surgical debridement of necrotic tissues should be performed when the patient's general condition allows.

References

Barkin, RM, Todd JK, Amer J. Periorbital cellulitis in children. *Paediatrics* 1978; **62**: 390–2.

Blodi FC, Hannah FT, Wadsworth JAC. Lethal orbitocerebral phycomycosis in otherwise healthy children. *Am J Ophthalmol* 1969; **67**: 698–704.

Catalano RA, Smoot CN. Subperiosteal masses in children with orbital cellulitis: time for reevaluation? *J Pediatr Ophthalmol Strabismus* 1990; **27**: 141–2.

Cavenagh F. Osteomyelitis of the superior maxilla in infants. *Br Med J* 1960; **1**: 468–72.

Chandler JR, Langenbrunner DJ, Stevens ER. The pathogenesis of orbital complications of acute sinusitis. *Laryngoscope* 1970; **80**: 1414–28.

Ciarallo LR, Rowe PC. Lumbar puncture in children with periorbital and orbital cellulitis. *J Pediatr* 1993; **122**: 355–9.

Clune JP. Septic thrombosis within the cavernous sinus. *Am J Ophthalmol* 1963; **56**: 33–9.

Duke-Elder S, MacFaul PA. In: Duke Elder S, ed. *Ocular Adnexae: Lacrimal Orbital and Para-orbital Diseases. System of Ophthalmology*, Vol. XIII, Part 2. St Louis: CV Mosby, 1974: 859–89.

Eustis HS, Armstrong DC, Buncic JR, Morin JD. Staging of orbital cellulitis in children: computerized tomography and treatment guidelines. *J Pediatr Ophthalmol Strabismus* 1986; **23**: 246–51.

Flood TP, Braude LS, Jampol LM, Herzog S. Computed tomography in the management of orbital infections associated with dental disease. *Br J Ophthalmol* 1982; **66**: 26–74.

Goldberg F, Berne AS, Oski FA. Differentiation of orbital cellulitis from preseptal cellulitis by computed tomography. *Paediatrics* 1978; **62**: 1000–9.

Grove WE. Septic and aseptic types of thrombosis of the cavernous sinus. *Arch Otolaryngol* 1936; **24**: 29–50.

Hale LM. Orbito-cerebral phycomycosis. *Arch Ophthalmol* 1971; **86**: 39–43.

Harris GJ. Subperiosteal abscess of the orbit. *Arch Ophthalmol* 1983; **101**: 751–7.

Harris GJ. Subperiosteal abscess of the orbit. *Ophthalmology* 1994; **101**: 585–95.

Hornblass A, Herschorn BJ, Stern K, Grimes C. Orbital abscess. *Surv Ophthalmol* 1984; **29**: 169–78.

Jarrett W, Gutman F. Ocular complications of infection in the paranasal sinuses. *Arch Ophthalmol* 1969; **81**: 683–8.

Jones DB. Discussion on paper by Weiss *et al*. Bacterial periorbital cellulitis and orbital cellulitis in childhood. *Ophthalmology* 1983; **90**: 201–3.

Jones DB. Microbial pre-septal and orbital cellulitis. In: Duane TD, Jaeger AJ, eds. *Clinical Ophthalmology*, Vol. 4. London: Harper & Row, 1982: 1–19.

Judisch F. Orbital cellulitis secondary to Coats' disease. *Arch Ophthalmol* 1980; **98**: 2004–6.

Krohel GB, Krauss HR, Christensen RE, Minckler D. Orbital abscess. *Arch Ophthalmol* 1980; **98**: 274–6.

Lerman SJ, Brunken JM, Bollinger M. Prevalence of ampicillin-resistant strains of *Haemophilus influenzae* causing systemic infection. *Antimicrobiol Agents Chemother* 1980; **18**: 474–5.

Levine RA. Infection of the orbit by an atypical mycobacterium. *Arch Ophthalmol* 1969; **82**: 608–10.

Londer L, Nelson DL. Orbital cellulitis due to *Haemophilus influenzae*. *Arch Ophthalmol* 1974; **91**: 89–98.

Molarte AB, Isenberg SJ. Periorbital cellulitis in infancy. *J Pediatr Ophthalmol Strabismus* 1989; **26**: 232–4.

Moorman CM, Elston JS. Acute orbital cellulitis. *Eye* 1995; **9**: 96–101.

Noel LP, Clarke WN, MacDonald N. Clinical management of orbital cellulitis in children. *Canad J Ophthalmol* 1990; **25**: 11–16.

Rozansky NM. A necrotic retinoblastoma simulating panophthalmitis. *Surv Ophthalmol* 1964; **9**: 381–3.

Rubin SE, Zito J. Orbital sub-periosteal abscess responding to medical therapy. *J Pediatr Ophthalmol Strabismus* 1994; **31**: 325–6.

Schramm VL, Myers EN, Kennerdell J. Orbital complications of acute sinusitis. Evaluation management and outcome. *Otolaryngology* 1978; **86**: 221–30.

Schwartz JN, Donnelly EH, Klintworth GK. Ocular and orbital phycomycosis. *Surv Ophthalmol* 1977; **22**: 3–28.

Sevel D, Tobias B, Sellars SL *et al*. Gas in the orbit associated with orbital cellulitis and paranasal sinusitis. *Br J Ophthalmol* 1973; **57**: 133–7.

Sherry T. Acute infarction of the choroid and retina. *Br J Ophthalmol* 1973; **57**: 133–7.

Shields JA, Shields CL, Suvarnamani C, Schroeder RP, DePotter P. Retinoblastoma manifesting as orbital cellulitis. *Am J Ophthalmol* 1991; **112**: 442–9.

Smith TF, O'Day D, Wright PF. Clinical implications of preseptal (periorbital) cellulitis in childhood. *Pediatrics* 1978; **62**: 1006–9.

Southwick FS, Richardson EP, Swartz MN. Septic thrombosis of the dural sinuses. *Medicine* 1986; **65**: 82–106.

Takahashi T. Orbital myositis simulating infectious cellulitis. *Jpn J Ophthalmol* 1983; **27**: 626–30.

Von Noorden GK. Orbital cellulitis following extraocular muscle surgery. *Am J Ophthalmol* 1972; **74**: 627–9.

Watters E, Waller H, Hiles D, Michaels RH. Acute orbital cellulitis. *Arch Ophthalmol* 1976; **94**: 785–8.

Weiss A, Friendly D, Eglin K, Chang M, Cold B. Bacterial periorbital and orbital cellulitis in childhood. *Ophthalmology* 1983; **90**: 195–203.

Whitehurst FO, Liston TE. Orbital aspergillosis: Report of a case in a child. *J Pediatr Ophthalmol Strabismus* 1981; **18**: 50–4.

17: Endophthalmitis

Donal Brosnahan and Anthony Moore

Intraocular infections may be caused by bacteria, fungi or parasites; organisms may enter the eye directly (exogenous endophthalmitis) or may be blood-borne from a distant source of infection (endogenous endophthalmitis). Many authors now make a distinction between acute and chronic postoperative endophthalmitis as different infecting organisms are responsible and different therapeutic approaches indicated (Mandelbaum & Meisler 1993; Speaker & Menikoff 1993). Bacterial infections will be considered separately from fungal and parasitic endophthalmitis.

Bacterial endophthalmitis

Bacterial endophthalmitis is rare in childhood but prompt recognition and early treatment are essential if blindness and destruction of the globe is to be avoided. The true incidence of endophthalmitis following paediatric intraocular surgery is unknown but has been estimated to be 0.45% in a study by Good *et al.* (1990) and 0.071% by Wheeler *et al.* (1992). A high index of suspicion is necessary to diagnose this rare condition early and a systematic approach to diagnosis and management should be followed for optimum results.

Exogenous bacterial endophthalmitis

Aetiology

Pathogenic bacteria may enter the eye by a variety of routes; direct infection may occur during intraocular surgery or follow penetrating trauma or inadvertent perforation of the globe during extraocular surgical procedures such as strabismus and retinal surgery (McMeel *et al.* 1978; Salamon *et al.* 1982). Endophthalmitis may also develop secondary to an infected glaucoma drainage bleb, suppurative keratitis (Fig. 17.1) or even orbital cellulitis.

In adults most bacterial infections develop following intraocular surgery but this complication is fortunately rare (for example the incidence of postoperative endophthalmitis following cataract surgery is about 0.1%) (Javitt *et al.* 1991; Kattan *et al.* 1991). The patient is the usual source of infection although contaminated instruments or irrigating solutions (McCray *et al.* 1986) or less commonly the surgeon may be the cause. Bacteria which colonize the eyelids and conjunctiva may contaminate intraocular lenses as they are being placed within the eye (Vafidis *et al.* 1984). There is a higher incidence of endophthalmitis following intracapsular cataract extraction or when there has been a tear of the posterior capsule in the course of extracapsular cataract extraction. It would seem that integrity of the posterior capsule limits spread of pathogens to the vitreous. This may be relevant to paediatric cataract extraction where posterior capsulotomy is frequently performed either at the time of surgery or subsequently. Neuteboom & De Vries-Knoppert (1988) reported endophthalmitis following neodymium–yttrium aluminium garnet (Nd–YAG) laser capsulotomy, a procedure which is increasingly being used to manage posterior capsular opacification in the paediatric population. Removal of sutures postoperatively may initiate endophthalmitis allowing pathogens to enter the eye along suture tracks (Gelender 1982). Both Good (1990) and Wheeler *et al.* (1992) noted a strong association between blockage of the nasolacrimal duct, upper respiratory tract infection and

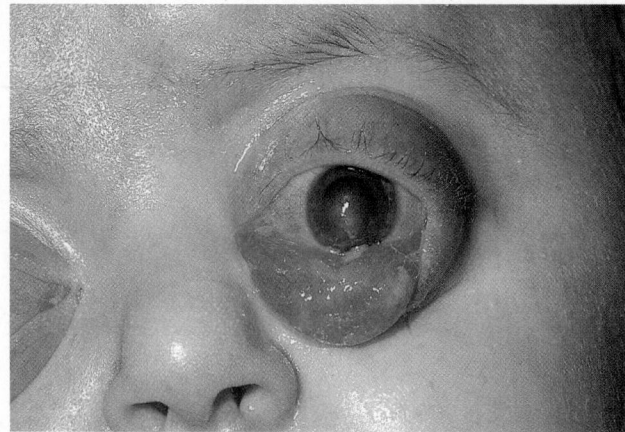

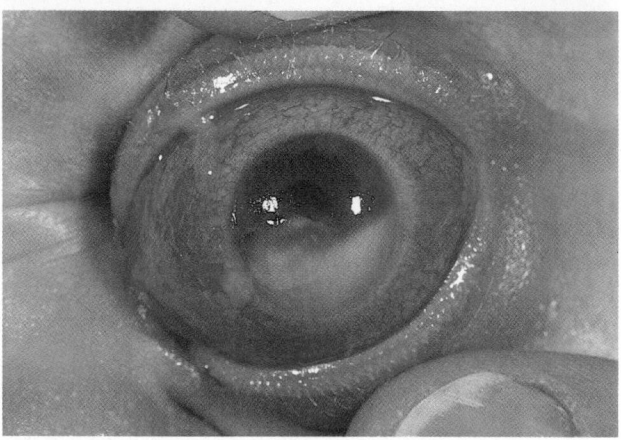

Fig. 17.1 (a) Exposure keratitis with conjunctival chemosis in a child with subluxation of the globe caused by shallow orbits in Crouzon's disease. (b) Same patient with endophthalmitis and hypopyon following exposure keratitis. Although the eye was saved by prompt antibiotic treatment the acuity 5 years later was very poor due to amblyopia. Occlusion of the other eye was made difficult by craniofacial deformity.

endophthalmitis. In children, in whom intraocular surgery is rarely performed, trauma is a more important predisposing factor (Weinstein *et al.* 1979).

Pathogenic organisms

Acute bacterial endophthalmitis most frequently results from infection with *Staphylococcus epidermidis*, which forms part of the normal flora of the eyelids, conjunctiva and face; until recently these organisms were considered to be only moderately pathogenic. The term acute is generally used to describe infection which occurs within days or weeks of intraocular surgery, while chronic has been reserved for those cases where infection occurs more than 1 month following surgery. *Staphylococcus epidermidis* accounts for approximately 38% of cases and *Staphylococcus aureus* for a further 10–20% of culture-positive cases (Shrader *et al.* 1990; Hughes & Hill 1994). Gram-negative

organisms such as *Pseudomonas aeruginosa*, *Proteus* species and *Haemophilus influenzae* have been cultured in about 16% of cases (Driebe *et al.* 1986). Most studies of the bacteriology of endophthalmitis have been concerned with the adult population but in Weinstein's study of children with endophthalmitis the results were very similar with 75% of culture-positive cases being caused by Gram-positive organisms (Weinstein *et al.* 1979). Both Wheeler *et al.* (1992) and Good *et al.* (1990) reporting on a paediatric population identified *Staphylococcus epidermidis*, *Streptococcus pneumoniae* and *Staphylococcus aureus* as the most frequent infective agents. Endophthalmitis associated with filtering blebs is most likely to result from *Staphylococcus aureus*, streptococcal species or *Haemophilus influenzae* rather than *Staphylococcus epidermidis* (Mandelbaum *et al.* 1985). A single organism is usually responsible though in post-traumatic endophthalmitis mixed infections are common.

Propionibacterium acnes is the organism most frequently identified in chronic endophthalmitis though staphylococci and streptococci have also been found. This opportunistic pathogen, which has previously been associated with infection of prosthetic heart valves and shunts, is a Gram-positive anaerobe forming part of the normal flora of the conjunctiva and skin. In chronic endophthalmitis, inflammation may develop gradually or suddenly some time after an uneventful immediate postoperative period.

Clinical presentation

The clinical presentation of bacterial endophthalmitis depends on the route of infection and the virulence of the organism. Acute postoperative endophthalmitis typically presents 1–3 days after surgery with pain and blurring of vision. There is usually lid swelling, conjunctival injection and chemosis, a severe uveitis, hypopyon and vitreous haze. With less virulent organisms such as *Staphylococcus epidermidis* the onset of symptoms and signs may be delayed for several weeks after surgery.

Chronic endophthalmitis may run a more indolent course with exacerbations and remissions. Intraocular inflammation is less severe though hypopyon and vitreous haze may occur. The presence of creamy white plaques on the posterior capsule or the intraocular lens is suggestive of *Propionibacterium acnes* infection (Mandlebaum & Meisler 1993). In endophthalmitis following penetrating trauma there is a persistent severe uveitis and vitreous haze often with infiltration of the wound edges. Retinal periphlebitis may be an early sign of bacterial endophthalmitis in those cases in which a fundus examination is possible. Endophthalmitis should always be suspected after intraocular surgery or traumatic perforation whenever the degree of inflammation is greater than expected. Serial examinations should be performed if

Table 17.1 Causes of hypopyon in childhood.

Endophthalmitis
Severe uveitis
Retinoblastoma
Leukaemia
Lymphoma
Neuroblastoma
Langerhans' cell histiocytosis

there is any doubt as early diagnosis and treatment offer the best hope of good visual outcome.

The main differential diagnoses are from fungal endophthalmitis and severe uveitis. Rarely retinoblastoma or metastatic tumour may present with uveitis and hypopyon (Table 17.1).

Bacteriological investigation

Culture specimens from aqueous, vitreous and any other obviously infected site should always be taken before starting therapy. Children with suspected endophthalmitis often need a general anaesthetic to allow a thorough examination and bacteriological specimens to be taken. The microbiologist should be informed so that fresh culture media are available in the operating room and that immediate Gram and Giemsa stains can be performed.

We recommend the protocol suggested by Forster *et al.* (1980). Aqueous and vitreous specimens are plated out on blood agar, chocolate agar and thioglycollate broth and incubated at 37°C for bacterial isolation; further specimens are incubated at 25°C on Sabouraud's medium and blood agar for fungal growth. In addition, both aqueous and vitreous should be placed on glass slides and stained with Gram and Giemsa stains. Culture for up to 2 weeks is required to allow growth of anaerobes such as *Propionibacterium acnes*. *Propionibacterium acnes* may be sequestered in folds of posterior capsule and removal of capsular remnants may be helpful in achieving a diagnosis and may have an additional therapeutic effect. Electron microscopy may provide important diagnostic information and should be performed if available.

Both aqueous and vitreous specimens are obtained either by aspiration or using an automated suction cutter. Use of a suction cutter is probably a safer alternative in that retinal traction is minimized. In infants the pars plana is poorly developed and an anterior approach may be more appropriate if lensectomy and anterior vitrectomy have been performed. Once all specimens have been taken, intravitreal and subconjunctival antibiotic injections can be given during the same anaesthetic.

Management

There are few published reports on the management of endophthalmitis in childhood and as it seems that similar organisms are responsible for childhood and adult infections, antimicrobial therapy should be guided by experience in treating adult endophthalmitis (Forster *et al.* 1980; Olson *et al.* 1983; Ramsey *et al.* 1982; Doft 1991; Speaker & Menikoff 1993). Young children present special problems in management and frequent sedation or general anaesthetics may need to be given to allow the progress of treatment to be monitored and subconjunctival injections to be given. Before starting treatment, the Gram and Giemsa stains of aqueous and vitreous should be reviewed; if there is no evidence of fungal infection treatment should be started with broad-spectrum antibiotics (Gram stain results are not sufficiently reliable to allow specific antibacterial treatment to be given at this stage). Intravitreal ceftazidime or amikacin or gentamicin and vancomycin are given as detailed in Table 17.2. There are reports suggesting retinal toxicity related to use of intravitreal aminoglycosides (Campochiaro & Conway 1991), ceftazidime is proposed as a suitable alternative. In addition subconjunctival ceftazidime and vancomycin together with intravenous ceftazidime and vancomycin should offer effective cover until Gram stain and culture are available. Topical antibiotics such as gentamicin and cefuroxime provide broad-spectrum cover while atropine ensures cycloplegia. If aminoglycosides are used intravenously blood levels must be monitored and dosage altered accordingly. Special care should be taken in preparing the intravitreal antibiotics because of the risk of retinal toxicity if higher doses are inadvertently given (Jeglum *et al.* 1981). Antibiotic therapy is reviewed in the light of culture and sensitivity results. Once a causative organism has been isolated and there is improvement on specific antibacterial therapy local and systemic steroids should

Table 17.2 Initial treatment* of bacterial endophthalmitis.

Intravitreal
gentamicin 0.1 mg (in 0.1 ml water)
or amikacin 0.4 mg (0.1 ml water)
or ceftazidime 2.25 mg (0.1 ml water)
and vancomycin 1.0 mg (0.1 ml water)

Subconjunctival
vancomycin 25 mg
ceftazidime 100 mg

Systemic
ceftazidime 100–150 mg/kg per day, i.v. 8-hourly
vancomycin 44 mg/kg per day, i.v. 8-hourly

Topical
atropine 1% b.d. (0.5% b.d. in infants)
gentamicin 1.5% hourly
cefuroxime 5%

*Review therapy when culture results available. Dosage may need to be adjusted for children under 1 year of age.

be given to reduce intraocular inflammation. (Steroids are, however, contraindicated if a co-existent fungal infection is suspected.)

The role of vitrectomy in the early management of bacterial endophthalmitis is not established. Although it offers the theoretical advantage of allowing removal of bacterial toxins from the eye and facilitating the spread of intraocular antibiotics it is technically difficult in infected eyes and complications such as retinal detachment may occur (Olson *et al.* 1983); in children especially, the lens may have to be sacrificed to allow a complete vitrectomy to be performed. Patients who already have very poor vision may be the most likely to benefit (Endophthalmitis Vitrectomy Study Group 1995).

In cases where medical treatment is not successful in controlling the infection and vision is lost, evisceration should be performed.

Prevention

In postoperative endophthalmitis the patient is the usual source of infection; children with extraocular infection such as blepharitis or conjunctivitis or with impaired nasolacrimal drainage should have ocular surgery deferred until these conditions are remedied. Surgery should also be deferred in the presence of upper respiratory tract infection.

We routinely use topical chloramphenicol for 24 hours preoperatively and give a subconjunctival injection of gentamicin or a cephalosporin at the end of intraocular surgery. Preoperative application of topical povidone-iodine 5% solution to the conjunctival sac and the lid margins has been shown to decrease the incidence of endophthalmitis (Speaker & Menikoff 1991). In addition, meticulous attention should be paid to a sterile non-touch operative technique.

In penetrating trauma it is important to remove any intraocular foreign body or devitalized tissue and to commence local and systemic antimicrobial therapy immediately after wound repair. Topical povidone-iodine 5% solution should not be applied in the presence of globe perforation.

Aphakic infants wearing contact lenses are at risk of developing suppurative keratitis and endophthalmitis; the parents should be warned to remove the contact lens immediately and seek advice if there is conjunctival injection, corneal haze, purulent discharge, photophobia or pain.

Endogenous bacterial endophthalmitis

Metastatic endophthalmitis results from haematogenous spread of infection from a distant focus of infection such as meningitis (Hedges *et al.* 1956; Jenson & Naidof 1973), bacterial endocarditis, skin infections, abdominal sepsis and otitis media (Gammel & Allansmith 1974). Diabetes mellitus, heart disease and gastrointestinal disorders are significant risk factors. Bilateral involvement is reported to occur in 14–50% of cases (Gammel & Allensmith 1974; Okada *et al.* 1994). *Staphylococcus aureus* was identified in 25% of patients though various species of *Streptococcus* were the largest group accounting for 32% of cases in one study (Okada *et al.* 1994). In earlier studies meningococci and pneumococci (Figs 17.2, 17.3) were the organisms most commonly isolated.

The usual presentation is with insidious onset of blurred vision, often bilaterally (Jensen & Naidoff 1973), and photophobia. Initially the clinical picture may be confused with a chronic uveitis (Gammel & Allansmith 1974) and the diagnosis delayed until there are signs of a severe vitritis or hypopyon. The presence of significant vitreous inflammation and posterior segment changes such as vasculitis and localized choroidal or retinal infiltration suggests an infective aetiology.

Metastatic endophthalmitis should be managed in the same way as postoperative infection. Aqueous and vitreous specimens should be obtained for culture before starting treatment with appropriate intravitreal and intravenous antibiotics. Blood cultures are indicated and may prove positive in up to 72% of cases (Okada *et al.* 1994). The role of therapeutic vitrectomy remains unclear and must be evaluated on a case-by-case basis. In children who are too sick to undergo a general anaesthetic, antibiotic therapy can be guided by the results of blood culture.

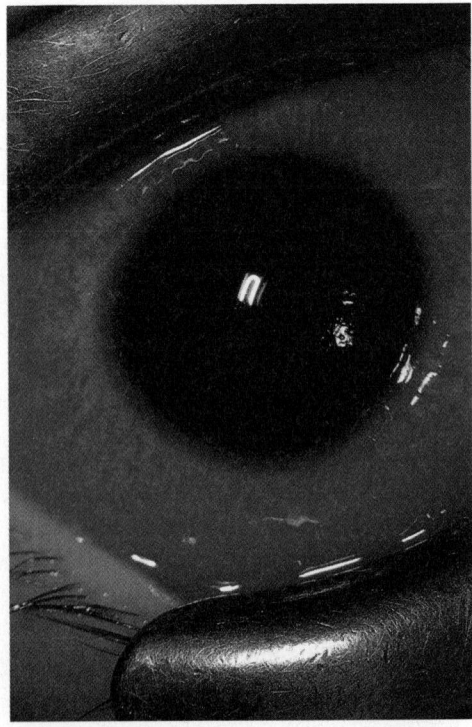

Fig. 17.2 Panophthalmitis in meningococcal septicaemia. Fifty per cent of such cases are bilateral.

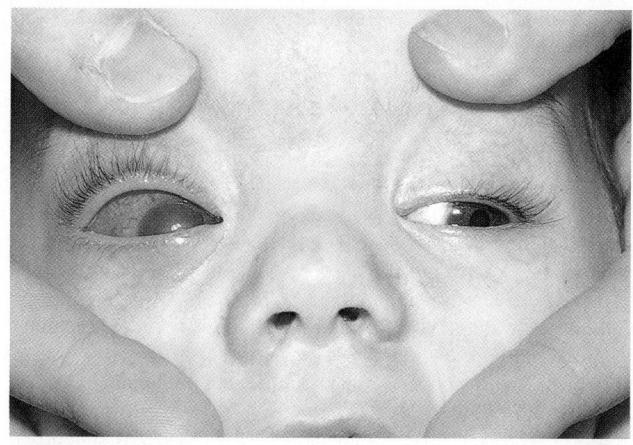

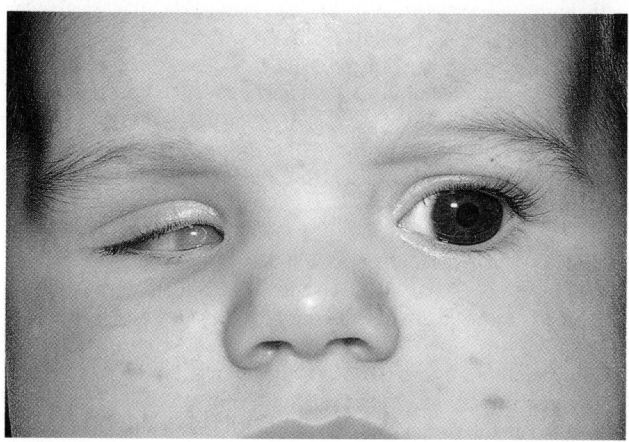

Fig. 17.3 Meningococcal endophthalmitis (a) leading to phthisis bulbi (b).

Visual outcome is often disappointing, which may reflect delay in diagnosis and institution of effective treatment in this rare condition. Eye symptoms in the presence of bacteraemia should raise suspicions of metastatic endophthalmitis.

Fungal endophthalmitis

Fungal endophthalmitis is fortunately rare in childhood and is usually seen as a complication of fungal septicaemia in sick children with compromised immunity. Rarely fungal infection may complicate penetrating trauma especially when there is retained foreign material (Meyer & Hood 1977).

Endogenous fungal endophthalmitis

Candida albicans is the organism most commonly implicated in endogenous fungal endophthalmitis although other fungal pathogens are occasionally responsible. It usually develops in sick children with *Candida* septicaemia; risk factors include immunosuppression, intravenous feeding (Parke *et al.* 1982), haemodialysis (Parke *et al.* 1982), prematurity (Baley *et al.* 1981) and broad-spectrum antibiotic

use (Baley *et al.* 1981). The prevalence of *Candida* endophthalmitis has been estimated to be between 28 and 45% in patients with candidal septicaemia (Brooks 1989; Bross *et al.* 1989) although postmortem studies (Edwards *et al.* 1974) have shown histopathological evidence of intraocular infection in 85% of cases. However, Donahue *et al.* (1994) in a large prospective study detected *Candida* chorioretinitis in 9.3% of patients with positive blood cultures yet found no cases of *Candida* endophthalmitis. These findings are attributed to stricter diagnostic criteria and also a possible effect of earlier treatment.

The typical appearance of intraocular *Candida* infection is of discrete fluffy white chorioretinal lesions sometimes with an associated retinal haemorrhage. Rarely *Candida* endophthalmitis may present as cataract (Clinch *et al.* 1989).

There is usually overlying vitreous inflammation, and as the condition evolves the retinal lesions enlarge and white 'snowballs' may appear in the vitreous (Edwards *et al.* 1974). In most cases, when the ocular lesions are small and *Candida* has been isolated from blood cultures treatment can be started without the need for culture of aqueous and vitreous. Diagnostic vitrectomy is indicated when the diagnosis is in doubt or when there is a large vitreous abscess. Amphotericin B remains the treatment of choice; renal and hepatic function must be closely monitored. Initial dosage is 250 µg/kg infused over 6 hours once daily increasing gradually to 1 mg/kg over a number of days. Low birth weight babies are particularly prone to renal complications and a maximum dose of 0.5 mg/kg per day has been recommended (Baley *et al.* 1984). Blood levels need to be monitored regularly. Flucytosine may be added but should not be used on its own as resistance quickly develops. The overall management of these children should be undertaken by a paediatrician with a special interest in infectious disease.

Exogenous fungal endophthalmitis

This may rarely complicate penetrating trauma in children, especially if there is a retained wooden foreign body. Symptoms and signs of intraocular infection may develop weeks or months after the injury following which there is a slow progression, with uveitis, vitritis and later hypopyon and vitreous abscess.

In suspected fungal endophthalmitis aqueous and vitreous specimens should be aspirated and cultured as for bacterial endophthalmitis. Gram and Giemsa stains will often show fungal hyphae and allow a prompt diagnosis to be made. If fungi are seen on microscopic examination amphotericin B (5 µg) is injected intravitreally and broad-spectrum antifungal treatment given locally and systemically. Steroids should not be used. The detailed treatment of fungal endophthalmitis has been reviewed by Jones (1978) and Smolin *et al.* (1984).

Parasitic endophthalmitis

Toxocara

See Chapter 38.

Toxoplasmosis

See Chapter 13.

Immune-mediated ophthalmitis

Mahdi *et al.* (1988) proposed an immune-mediated mechanism for endophthalmitis in a 7-month-old patient with meningococcal septicaemia whose panophthalmitis failed to respond to systemic antibiotic therapy but which responded to topical steroids and mydriatics.

References

Baley J, Annable WL, Kliegmann RM. *Candida* endophthalmitis in the premature infant. *J Pediatr* 1981; **98**: 458–61.

Baley L, Kliegman RM, Fanaroff AA. Disseminated fungal infection in very low birth weight infants: therapeutic toxicity. *Pediatrics* 1984; **73**: 153–7.

Brooks RG. Prospective study of *Candida* endophthalmitis in hospitalized patients with candidemia. *Arch Intern Med* 1989; **149**; 2226–8.

Bross J, Talbot GH, Maislin G *et al.* Risk factors for nosocomial candidemia: a case control study in adults without leukemia. *Am J Med* 1989; **87**: 614–20.

Campochiaro PA, Conway BP. Aminoglycoside toxicity: a survey of retinal specialists: implications for intraocular use. *Arch Ophthalmol* 1991; **109**: 946–50.

Clinch TE, Duker JS, Eagle RC *et al.* Infantile endogenous *Candida* endophthalmitis presenting as a cataract. *Surv Ophthalmol* 1989; **34**:107–12.

Doft BH. The endophthalmitis vitrectomy study. *Arch Ophthalmol* 1991; **109**: 487–8.

Donahue SP, Greven CM, Zuravleff JJ *et al.* Intraocular candidiasis in patients with candidemia. *Ophthalmology* 1994; **101**: 1302–9.

Driebe WT, Mandelbaum S, Forster RK *et al.* Pseudophakic endophthalmitis. *Ophthalmology* 1986; **93**: 442–8.

Edwards JE. Severe candidal infections, clinical perspectives, immune defense mechanisms and current concepts of therapy. *Ann Intern Med* 1978; **89**: 91–106.

Edwards JE, Foos R, Montgomerie J, Gaze L. Ocular manifestations of *Candida* septicaemia. Review of 76 cases of haematogenous *Candida* endophthalmitis. *Medicine* 1974; **53**: 47–55.

Endophthalmitis Vitrectomy Study Group. Results of the Endophthalmitis Vitrectomy Study: a randomized trial of immediate vitrectomy and of intravenous antibiotic for the treatment of postoperative bacterial endophthalmitis. *Arch Ophthalmol* 1995; **113**: 1479–96.

Forster RK, Abbot RL, Gelender H. Management of infectious endophthalmitis. *Ophthalmology* 1980; **87**: 313–19.

Gammel J, Allansmith M. Metastatic staphylococcal endophthalmitis presenting as chronic iridocyclitis. *Am J Ophthalmol* 1974; **77**: 454–8.

Gelender H. Bacterial endophthalmitis following cutting of sutures after cataract surgery. *Am J Ophthalmol* 1982; **94**: 528–33.

Good WV, Hing S, Irvine AR, Hoyt CS, Taylor DSI. Postoperative endophthalmitis in children following cataract surgery. *J Pediatr Ophthalmol Strabismus* 1990; **27**: 283–5.

Hedges TR, McAllister R, Coriell LL *et al.* Metastatic endophthalmitis as a complication of meningococcic meningitis. *Arch Ophthalmol* 1956; **55**: 513–15.

Hughes DS, Hill RJ. Infectious endophthalmitis after cataract surgery. *Br J Ophthalmol* 1994; **78**: 227–32.

Javitt JC, Vitale S, Canner JK *et al.* National outcomes of cataract extraction. *Arch Ophthalmol* 1991; **109**:1085–9.

Jeglum EL, Rosenberg SB, Benson WE. Preparation of intravitreal drug doses. *Ophthalmic Surg* 1981; **12**: 355–9.

Jensen AD, Naidoff MA. Bilateral meningococcal endophthalmitis. *Arch Ophthalmol* 1973; **90**: 396–8.

Jones DB. Therapy of post surgical fungal endophthalmitis. *Ophthalmology* 1978; **85**: 357–70.

Kattan HM, Flynn HW, Pflugfelder SC *et al.* Nosocomial endophthalmitis survey: current incidence of infection after intraocular surgery. *Ophthalmology* 1991; **98**: 227–38.

McCray E, Rampell N, Solomon SL *et al.* Outbreak of *Candida parapsilosis* endophthalmitis after cataract extraction and intraocular lens implantation. *J Clin Microbiol* 1986; **24**: 625–8.

McMeel JW, Naegele DF, Badrinath SS, Murphy PL. Acute and subacute infections following scleral buckling operations. *Ophthalmology* 1978; **85**: 341–9.

Mahdi G, Tulton M, Evans-Jones G. Ophthalmitis in meningococcal disease. *Arch Dis Child* 1988; **63**: 550–1.

Mandelbaum S, Forster RK, Gelender H *et al.* Late onset endophthalmitis associated with filtering blebs. *Ophthalmology* 1985; **92**: 946–72.

Mandelbaum S, Meisler DM. Postoperative chronic microbial endophthalmitis. *Int Ophthalmol Clin* 1993; **33**: 71–9.

Meyer R, Hood I. Fungus implantation with wooden intraocular foreign bodies. *Ann Ophthalmol* 1977; **9**: 271–8.

Neuteboom GHG, De Vries-Knoppert WAEJ. Endophthalmitis after Nd : YAG laser capsulotomy. *Doc Ophthalmol* 1988; **70**: 175–8.

Okada AA, Johnson RP, Liles WC *et al.* Endogenous bacterial endophthalmitis. *Ophthalmology* 1994; **101**: 832–8.

Olson JC, Flynn HW, Forster RK, Clubertson WW. Results in the treatment of post operative endophthalmitis. *Ophthalmology* 1983; **90**: 692–9.

Parke D, Jones D, Gentry L. Endogenous endophthalmitis among patients with candidemia. *Ophthalmology* 1982; **89**: 789–96.

Ramsey JJ, Newsom DL, Sexton DJ, Harms WK. Endophthalmitis current approaches. *Ophthalmology* 1982; **89**: 1055–65.

Salamon S, Friberg T, Lukenberg M. Endophthalmitis after strabismus surgery. *Am J Ophthalmol* 1982; **93**: 39–41.

Shrader SK, Band JD, Lauter CB *et al.* The clinical spectrum of endophthalmitis: incidence, predisposing factors, and features influencing outcome. *J Infect Dis* 1990; **162** :115–20.

Smolin G, Tabbara K, Whitaker J. *Infectious Diseases of the Eye.* Baltimore: Williams & Wilkins, 1984: 161–71.

Speaker MG, Menikoff JA. Postoperative endophthalmitis: pathogenesis, prophylaxis, and management. *Int Ophthalmol Clin* 1993; **33**: 51–70.

Speaker MG, Menikoff JA. Prophylaxis of endophthalmitis with topical povidone-iodine. *Ophthalmology* 1991; **1**: 1769–75.

Vafidis GC, March RJ, Stacey AR. Bacterial contamination of intraocular lens surgery. *Br J Ophthalmol* 1984; **68**: 520–3.

Weinstein GS, Mondino BJ, Weinberg RJ, Biglan AW. Endophthalmitis in a pediatric population. *Ann Ophthalmol* 1979; **11**: 935–43.

Wheeler DT, Stager DR, Weakley DR. Endophthalmitis following pediatric intraocular surgery for congenital cataracts and congenital glaucoma. *J Pediatr Ophthalmol Strabismus* 1992; **29**: 139–41.

18: External Eye Diseases

David Taylor

Infections of the external eye

Epidemiology

Corneal disease is the most common cause of blindness in many parts of the world today (Foster 1988; Foster & Gilbert 1992; Gilbert *et al.* 1993). In pre-antibiotic days infective keratitis was the major cause of child blindness and that situation still applies to the developing world especially in areas where there is chronic malnutrition, endemic trachoma and unhygienic living conditions.

In developed countries external eye infections comprise one of the most common referrals to casualty clinics (Chiapella & Rosenthal 1985), and keratitis is a small but significant cause of blindness especially amongst children whose health is already compromised.

The normal flora of the conjunctiva is different to that of adults, with children having fewer anaerobic bacteria and more *Streptococcus* species (Singer *et al.* 1988).

The 'soil and the seed'

Normally the eye has a very strong resistance to the damaging effects of even the most virulent of micro-organisms. That resistance is based on a number of factors.

1 A normal volume tear production, and the ability to produce more when needed.

2 Normal tear constituents, including lysozyme and other antibacterial substances, immunoglobulins, cells and interferon.

3 A stable tear film that covers the whole cornea evenly and does not break down between blinks.

4 Normal tear spreading by blinking.
5 Corneal sensation and the ability to detect and react to corneal foreign bodies.
6 An intact epithelium with properties of resistance to penetration by micro-organisms, rapid repair and a continual turnover of cells.

Should there be a breakdown in any one of those mechanisms the cornea and the eye itself are at threat from infection. In the developed world German measles (rubella) gives rise to a keratoconjunctivitis with photophobia, grittiness and redness of the eyes that lasts a few days, clearing without residua. In the malnourished child, low in vitamin A, it results in a liquefactive keratitis and blindness. The soil is as important as the seed. Other common examples are the severity of herpes simplex keratitis in leukaemic children, the severity of fungal ulcers on the immunosuppressed, the devastating rapidity of deterioration of corneal ulcers in children with a combination of fifth and seventh nerve palsy, and the almost exclusive occurrence of *Candida* keratitis in the immunocompromised, i.e. in mucocutaneous candidiasis (Wagman *et al.* 1987).

Symptoms and signs

The classic symptom of conjunctivitis is discharge giving rise to an eye that is stuck in the morning and has a greenish or yellowish discharge during the day. The eye is also red from blood vessel dilatation and haemorrhages may occur from endothelial damage and dilatation. Swelling of the conjunctiva is due to oedema and to follicles — nests of lymphoid tissue within the conjunctiva which quickly swell during infections and in response to other antigenic stimuli; they have blood vessels around their margins whereas the papillae seen in chronic conjunctivitis are solid blocks of cellular aggregations around a central vascular core. Acute conjunctivitis causes the eye to feel hot and sometimes to itch a little. Vision is unaffected except by the strands of mucous floating around which can be blinked away to clear the vision.

The history of the conjunctivitis — chronological and symptomatic — is vital to the diagnosis (Jackson 1993). Itching suggests allergy, purulent discharge, a bacterial infection, an associated pharyngitis, a virus conjunctivitis, eczema, vernal catarrh, and so on.

Keratitis results in discomfort (except in anaesthetic eyes) and a foreign-body sensation or grittiness; fresh ulcers may be frankly painful. The vision is unaffected until the corneal transparency is impaired, especially in the axial area. Eyes with keratitis almost invariably have a degree of conjunctivitis. Examination with magnification, preferably the slit lamp, is mandatory and fluorescein is helpful, painless and safe in demonstrating breaks in corneal and conjunctival epithelium.

Laboratory diagnosis

Although there is no necessity for culture of the discharge in every case seen in a general ophthalmic practice, the ophthalmologist must have access to good microbiology services if the correct diagnosis is to be made and the best treatment instituted. Collaboration with a microbiologist colleague is the way in which most ophthalmologists achieve their goal. The pace of change in antibiotic therapy and microbiological diagnosis is so great that few ophthalmologists have adequate expertise in this area.

Culture is important in severe cases, in chronic or recurrent infections and follicular and atypical reactions (Jackson 1993). In keratitis, the ulcer that fails to respond to antibiotics may need to have all treatment stopped for 48 hours before reculturing. Scrapings are useful for culture and direct examination for fungi and bacteria when stained. Viral isolation is important in the neonate and also in suspected herpes simplex keratitis.

Acute catarrhal conjunctivitis

Acute conjunctivitis without specific features in childhood results from infection with a vast array of organisms; probably the most common are the influenza virus, infectious mononucleosis, and with exanthemas such as measles. For conjunctivitis in neonates see Chapter 15.

Gigliotti *et al.* (1981) identified an organism in 72% of children with acute conjunctivitis. *Haemophilus influenzae* accounted for 42% of those, adenovirus for 20% and *Streptococcus pneumoniae* for 12%. *Haemophilus influenzae* was found to be more common in the winter, adenovirus in the late summer. If the children had pharyngitis then adenovirus was the most common organism. It was interesting that *Moraxella* and *Chlamydia* were not isolated in the group of children up to 18 years of age. *Moraxella* species usually cause a subacute conjunctivitis. Weiss *et al.* (1993), looking at 95 children with acute conjunctivitis and 91 controls found 76 cases of bacterial infection (*Haemophilus influenzae*, *Streptococcus pneumoniae*, *Moraxella catarrhalis*). *Staphylococcus aureus*, *Corynebacterium* and alpha-haemolytic streptococci were the most common commensals in the controls. Viral conjunctivitis was less common in this series.

In hyperacute conjunctivitis it is most important to culture and exclude *Neisseria* species and other causes of membranous conjunctivitis.

Acute follicular keratoconjunctivitis

Acute follicular conjunctivitis is usually bilateral, affecting the eye within a few days. There is usually a history of contact with someone with similar symptoms. After the first few days the conjunctival follicles are enlarged and 'juicy' and there is often a systemic upset.

Epidemic keratoconjunctivitis

Epidemic keratoconjunctivitis is often caused by adenovirus type 8, 19 and 37 but other adenoviruses have been implicated. It is highly infectious. The incubation period is between 2 days and 2 weeks and the follicular conjunctivitis which mostly affects the lower fornix is associated with a keratitis with multiple small, round, raised, white epithelial and subepithelial lesions which cause considerable discomfort and photophobia. The symptoms may last some weeks and small white stromal lesions, which represent an immune reaction, may remain for months. A systemic illness occurs in nearly half the patients (Darougar *et al.* 1983). The disease spreads rapidly and is notorious for infecting patients and staff in an ophthalmology department.

Persistent lacrimation may be caused by a multifocal nasolacrimal duct and canalicular obstruction which may require probing, corticosteroid irrigation and intubation if dacryocystorhinostomy is to be avoided (Hyde & Berger 1988).

Treatment is not usually helpful but dilute steroids may improve the symptoms and chloramphenicol may be used to prevent secondary bacterial infection.

Pharyngoconjunctival fever

Pharyngoconjunctival fever is highly infectious and is usually due to adenovirus type 3 or other subtypes. The patient has a fever, pharyngitis and a keratoconjunctivitis similar to epidemic keratoconjunctivitis. No treatment alters the course of the disease which lasts up to 2 weeks.

Herpes simplex keratoconjunctivitis

Darougar *et al.* (1985) studied primary herpes virus infections in 108 patients: 69% were over 15 years and 7% were under the age of 5 years. Upper respiratory tract infections were found in 35% and other systemic disturbance including fever, malaise and aching in 31%. Symptoms included redness, watering, discharge, itching lids and a pre-auricular adenopathy. The major signs were lid vesicles and ulcers, papillary conjunctivitis mainly in the upper lid conjunctiva and follicles in the lower lid conjunctiva. Punctate epithelial keratitis was common but dendritic ulcers occurred in 15% and disciform keratitis in 2%. Seven per cent of patients presented with a keratoconjunctivitis without any clinical clues as to the diagnosis and a chronic blepharoconjunctivitis developed in 15% of patients.

The conjunctivitis may be severe with a pseudomembrane obscuring the conjunctiva but it is self-limiting in most patients. Special precautions need to be taken for the immunocompromised patient who should be treated with topical antiviral agents in conjunction with an infectious diseases specialist.

One of the most interesting things about the ubiquitous herpes simplex virus is why in some individuals the normally amicable relationship between the virus and host is disturbed (Monnickendam 1988). Most infected patients resolve spontaneously (Simon *et al.* 1986), only the minority developing keratitis. Recurrence of the infection is common (Darougar *et al.* 1989).

Treatment of superficial or dendritic keratitis is with antivirals such as idoxuridine, trifluorothymidine or acyclovir. Herpetic stromal keratitis is usually treated with topical steroids (Wilhelmus *et al.* 1994), often in diluted form, and topical antivirals; systemic antivirals are probably not effective (Barron *et al.* 1994), but may be indicated in immunocompromised children.

Haemorrhagic keratoconjunctivitis

This occurs in epidemics and is due to various picornavirus types (enterovirus type 70). The epithelial keratitis is painful and the presence of multiple subconjunctival haemorrhages and the short duration (often only a few days) are characteristic. Coxsackie virus type A24 has also been implicated (Yin-Murphy *et al.* 1993).

Chlamydia infections and trachoma

Chlamydia trachomatis strains cause neonatal inclusion conjunctivitis and *Chlamydia* strains cause acute trachoma and trachoma inclusion conjunctivitis (oculogenital disease). The oculogenital types are not common in sexually inactive persons but acute trachoma occurs in children and young adults as a more or less subacute bilateral keratoconjunctivitis which is characterized by follicles prominent on the upper tarsal plate and a marginal keratitis. Pannus, limbal follicles and pitted scarring at the upper limbus (Herbert's pits) are most characteristic. The changes which make it such a prominent cause of blindness relate to subconjunctival scarring with consequent dry eyes, entropion and trichiasis. The clinical picture and progression vary with the health of the population in which trachoma is endemic and the area of the world in which it is found. Treatment is with tetracycline ointment for 2 months and systemic erythromycin.

Acute conjunctivitis with other systemic diseases

Acute conjunctivitis may occur in acute exanthemas such as varicella, with Lyme borreliosis, influenza and Epstein–Barr virus infection. In Parinaud's oculoglandular syndrome there is a unilateral acute or subacute conjunctivitis with ipsilateral pre-auricular or submandibular lymphadenopathy. The cat-scratch disease

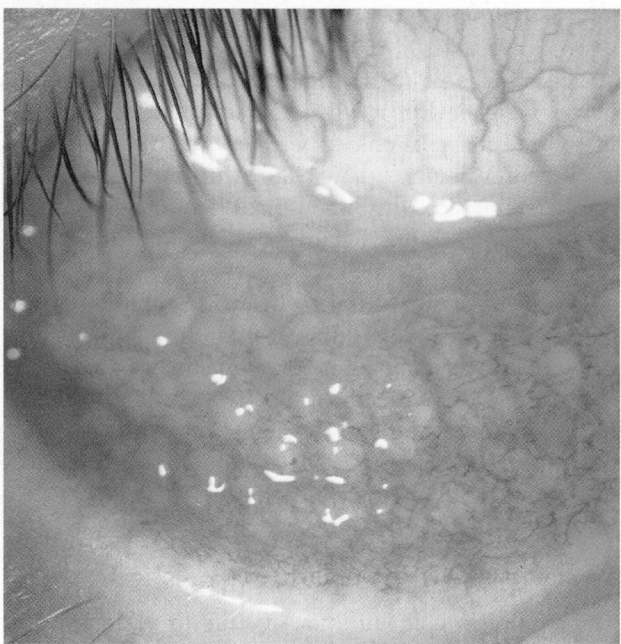

Fig. 18.1 Acute follicular conjunctivitis in a child with multiple molluscum contagiosum lesions.

bacillus is a major cause (Wear *et al.* 1985). Sweet's syndrome of fever, arthritis and nodular or pseudovesicular peripheral and facial rash may present as conjunctivitis (Cohen 1993).

Other micro-organisms

Molluscum contagiosum infections (Fig. 18.1), mononucleosis, psittacosis and occasionally bacteria and fungi may cause a follicular conjunctivitis.

Membranous conjunctivitis

Membranous conjunctivitis is a severe, sight-threatening conjunctivitis that may also be part of a systemic infection. The eye is very red, the lids swollen and the conjunctiva is covered by a variably sized fibrin plaque. The underlying conjunctiva bleeds when the plaque is removed, the membrane may involve the cornea. Pseudomembranous conjunctivitis is less severe and represents a fibrin coagulum on the surface of the conjunctiva. It occurs in Stevens–Johnson syndrome and toxic epidermal necrolysis, herpes simplex and herpes zoster.

Causes include *Corynebacterium diphtheriae*, *Streptococcus pyogenes*, *Staphylococcus aureus*, *Neisseria* species, *Shigella*, *Salmonella* and *Escherichia coli* and it occurs in neonatal inclusion conjunctivitis.

The diagnosis must be made early and appropriate treatment instituted.

Subacute and chronic follicular conjunctivitis

Normal childhood folliculosis

It is normal in childhood to have prominent follicles especially in the fornices, in the lower lid and without much evidence of inflammation. It seems to be analogous to the normal lymphoid hyperplasia that occurs in tonsils, lymph nodes and so on.

Moraxella conjunctivitis

The bacterium *Moraxella lacunata* causes 'external angular conjunctivitis' — so called because it tends to affect the external angle most particularly with bulbar injection and involvement of the lids. It is a subacute infection which may give rise to marginal infiltrates.

Other micro-organisms

Molluscum contagiosum and some bacterial or fungal conjunctivitides, especially if partially treated, may give rise to a chronic follicular conjunctivitis. The clue to the diagnosis is the finding of or a history of the pearly lid lesions — this may be difficult as they may be small and away from the lid. They should be curetted. Occasionally they are large (Al-Hazza & Hidayat 1993).

Tuberculous conjunctivitis is rarely seen in recent decades (Helm 1993) but may be seen again with increasing frequency as the disease spreads, especially in vulnerable populations. Primary conjunctival tuberculosis is usually unilateral, affecting the upper palpebral conjunctiva, and is associated with ulceration and a regional lymphadenopathy. It may be associated with a stromal and ulcerative keratitis (Aclimandos & Kerr Muir 1992).

Pulmonary tuberculosis is not necessarily associated. Phlyctenular disease is also associated with tuberculosis.

Drugs

Various drugs including idoxuridine, eserine and adrenaline can cause a subacute or chronic follicular conjunctivitis (Wilson 1979). It is sometimes known as conjunctivitis medicamentosa.

Rosacea keratoconjunctivitis

Acne rosacea is rare in prepubescent children but it may occur giving meibomitis and subepithelial marginal infiltrates (Erzurum *et al.* 1993).

Blepharoconjunctivitis

Chronic conjunctivitis with seborrhoeic blepharitis and

chronic meibomitis gives disproportionately severe symptoms of irritation and burning compared with the relatively mild findings of conjunctival hyperaemia and lid disease. Treatment is directed at the lid disease (see Chapter 21).

Keratitis

The most common forms of keratitis are those associated with acute virus infections but these are almost invariably self-limiting except in sick children. Herpes simplex keratitis forms a small but important group of children with chronic disease who may lose vision as a result of the disease and amblyopia combined.

Bacterial keratitis

Microbial keratitis in healthy children is a small cause of blindness (Coster *et al.* 1981), but one in which predisposing factors are vitally important (Ormerod *et al.* 1986); these include contact lens wear (Erie *et al.* 1993), overwhelming systemic infections, immunodeficiency, orbital malignancies, exposure, trauma or dry eye (Cruz *et al.* 1993; Clinch *et al.* 1994).

Pseudomonas species (Fig. 18.2) (Ormerod *et al.* 1986; Cruz *et al.* 1993) and *Streptococcus viridans* (Seal *et al.* 1982) are the most common bacteria isolated in early life. Mixed infections are common (Jones 1981; Cruz *et al.* 1993). Older children are most commonly infected with *Streptococcus pneumoniae* (Okumoto & Smolin 1974) and males are most frequently affected (Klein 1981; Ormerod *et al.* 1986). Beta-haemolytic streptococci, *Staphylococcus*, *Haemophilus* species, *Moraxella* species, coliforms and *Shigella* (Schmiedt & Cimma 1983) are less frequent pathogens.

Prevention

Prevention of microbial keratitis is important: paediatricians need to understand the relevance of corneal exposure, trichiasis and dry eyes and orbital neoplasms may require special attention due to the combination of exposure, dryness, immunodeficiency, radiation keratitis, and corneotoxicity of chemotherapeutic drugs (Ormerod *et al.* 1986). Correct and careful nursing techniques may prevent many severe nosocomial corneal infections in children in intensive care units (Hilton *et al.* 1983).

Treatment

Treatment relies on skilled paediatric management and nursing so that frequently repeated eye drops can be instilled and subconjunctival doses of antibiotics given using oral or intravenous sedation or anaesthesia if neces-

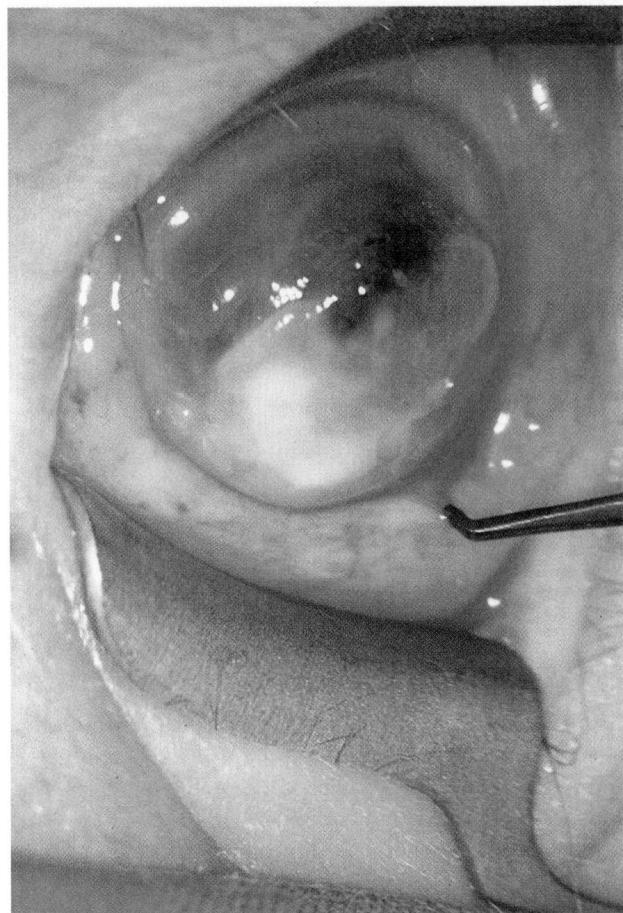

Fig. 18.2 *Pseudomonas* keratitis in a neonate with no known predisposing factors.

sary. Delivering the treatment is the most difficult part of the management but delivering the right treatment is also vital and usually requires collaboration with the microbiology team. Culture of the discharge and scraping is the most important prelude to treatment, which should not be withheld awaiting the culture and antibiotic sensitivity results, but started immediately. Chloramphenicol remains the most effective topical treatment and tetracycline is also useful (Seal *et al.* 1982). Gentamicin is the most effective against *Pseudomonas* species (Dart & Seal 1988). Hourly drops are usually best given in a form without preservative because irritation by most preservatives can cause slow healing.

Intravenous antibiotics based on the sensitivity of the cultured organism should be given in the immunocompromised or septicaemic child.

Later treatment such as tectonic grafts, debridement, conjunctival flap and penetrating keratoplasty may have their place but the visual prognosis is often poor due to the scarring from the disease and amblyopia in younger children.

Specific features of various forms of bacterial keratitis

Pseudomonas

Pseudomonas aeruginosa ulcers most frequently affect young children and contact-lens wearers. It is a virulent organism that is mobile and produces collagenase which gives rise to a rapidly spreading liquefactive ulcer with hypopyon. Gentamicin remains the most frequently used antibiotic against *Pseudomonas*, and most other Gram-negative bacteria, but medical adjunctive therapy (i.e. cycloplegics, steroids and protease inhibitors) and surgical treatment may help in some cases (Dart & Seal 1988).

Moraxella

Moraxella species are diplococci which give rise to external angular keratitis and indolent corneal ulcers that are oval in shape with undermined edges.

Staphylococcus

Staphylococcal ulcers tend to be limited or with satellite lesions and rather round in shape. *Staphylococcus aureus* is more virulent and causes central hypopyon ulcers. *Staphylococcus epidermidis*, though much more common, only causes infection when the corneal resistance is compromised; the ulcers are superficial and indolent.

Streptococcus

Streptococcus pneumoniae is a common organism that may invade corneas compromised by disease or contact lens wear and in children with chronic dacryocystitis. The ulcers may be very rapid in onset and spread, with an undermined edge, and hypopyon and perforation are frequent. *Streptococcus pyogenes* usually causes marginal ulcers in an eye with blepharoconjunctivitis or dacryocystitis.

Streptococcus viridans is the usual cause of infectious crystalline keratopathy. The majority of hosts have had corneal surgery, trauma, herpes simplex or *Acanthamoeba* keratitis. The characteristic appearance is of a white, feathery crystalline deposit in the anterior stroma without much inflammation. Previous steroid treatment is frequent. The diagnosis is usually made by microscopy of corneal donor buttons but culture of a corneal scrape or swab may be possible (Watson *et al.* 1988).

Gonococci

Gonococcal keratitis leads to a very rapidly spreading ulcer, especially dangerous in the neonate. Perforation occurs rapidly if untreated. Meningococci give rise to similar ulcers.

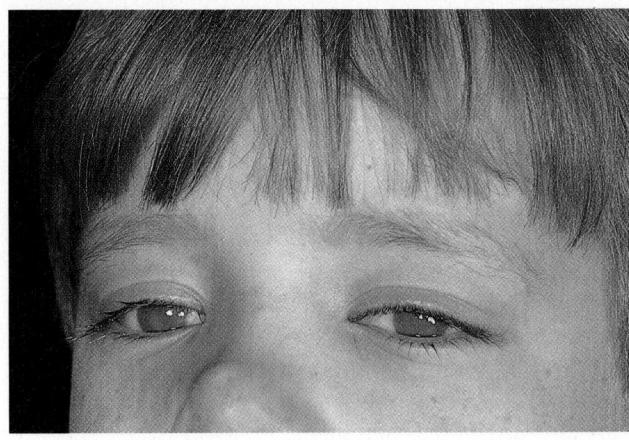

Fig. 18.3 Interstitial keratitis of unknown cause.

Enterobacteria

Escherichia coli, *Aerobacter*, *Proteus* and *Klebsiella* species usually affect debilitated children.

Interstitial keratitis

Interstitial keratitis is a non-ulcerative stromal keratitis with vascularization which affects a variable proportion of the cornea.

Classically interstitial keratitis was caused by congenital syphilis early in the course of the disease, more frequently in girls. Pain, photophobia and limbal vascular engorgement occur, and the cornea becomes cloudy, usually diffusely and bilaterally (Fig. 18.3); a uveitis accompanies the corneal changes. Heavy vascularization extends from the limbus giving the orangey–red 'salmon patch'. Clearing proceeds from the periphery leaving a central hazy cornea and ghost vessels.

Diagnosis depends on clinical suspicion of the disease and the finding of a positive fluorescent treponemal antibody absorption (FTA-ABS) test. Treatment consists of treating the underlying disease and topical steroids. Syphilitic interstitial keratitis may represent an allergic mechanism.

Interstitial keratitis also occurs with onchocerciasis, leprosy and tuberculosis, all of which give rise to localized disease. Viral interstitial keratitis is usually discoid. Causes include mumps, measles, herpes simplex and trypanosomiasis: a sclerosing form of interstitial keratitis occurs in onchocerciasis.

Cogan's syndrome

See Chapter 24.

Nummular keratitis

Nummular keratitis is a localized form of keratitis often

with multiple round, anterior stromal corneal lesions with minimal conjunctivitis. The coin-shaped lesions may be faceted but not ulcerated. They are mostly caused by viruses including adenovirus, herpes simplex, varicella-zoster (Wilhelmus *et al.* 1991) and Epstein–Barr virus (Nummular Keratitis) (Palay *et al.* 1993). It also occurs with sarcoid (Lennarson & Barney 1995), onchocerciasis and tuberculosis. The lesions often respond to topical steroids, which must be used with care when herpes simplex is a possibility.

Viral keratitis

Epithelial lesions occur in herpes simplex, commonly punctate lesions; dendrites occur less frequently in acute cases with skin lesions. Dendrites are more common than geographical or disciform lesions in more chronic cases, and they carry a much better visual prognosis (Beigi *et al.* 1994). Dendrites also occur in herpes zoster. Many acute virus conjunctivitides, lid papillomas, verrucae and molluscum contagiosum may also cause a punctate keratitis.

Round subepithelial opacities (Fig. 18.4) occur in epidemic keratoconjunctivitis, Epstein–Barr virus infection, infectious mononucleosis, trachoma and inclusion conjunctivitis.

Deep non-suppurative ('disciform') keratitis occurs with herpes simplex and rarely with the Epstein–Barr and varicella-zoster infection. In herpes simplex infectious disciform keratitis appears as a grey vascularized stromal opacity with corneal anaesthesia and a uveitis: it has been described following neonatal herpes simplex infection (Hammond & Harden 1994). Varicella, mumps and cytomegalovirus also cause a stromal keratitis.

Fungal keratitis

Fungi are unusual causes of keratitis and occur in children predisposed by severe systemic disease (Wagman *et al.* 1987), trauma with dirty wounds (Hirst *et al.* 1979), topical and systemic steroid (Ralph *et al.* 1976). Prior administration of steroids remains a significant problem in weakening resistance to the infection and although they may have a role in the treatment of some infective keratitis when combined with antibiotics, they should be withheld where possible.

The most common causative organisms are Actinomycetaceae (*Actinomyces*) and *Candida*. *Candida* produces marginal infiltration or elevated multiple chronic white anterior stromal and epithelial defects (see Fig. 18.5) with later penetration of the stroma, liquefaction and endophthalmitis. *Nocardia* are aerobic and produce penetrating single corneal ulcers with a slow onset but later they may have a severe keratitis, with hypopyon that may be resistant to antibiotic treatment and may require debridement and a conjunctival flap (Hirst *et al.* 1979).

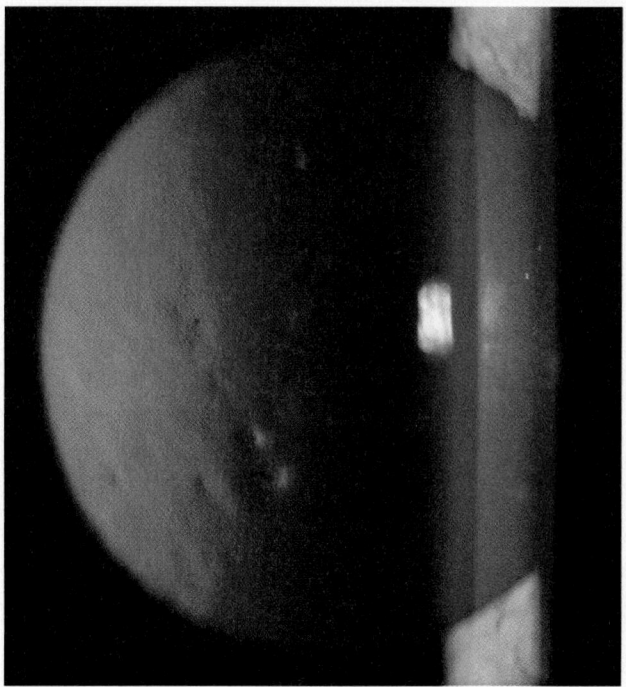

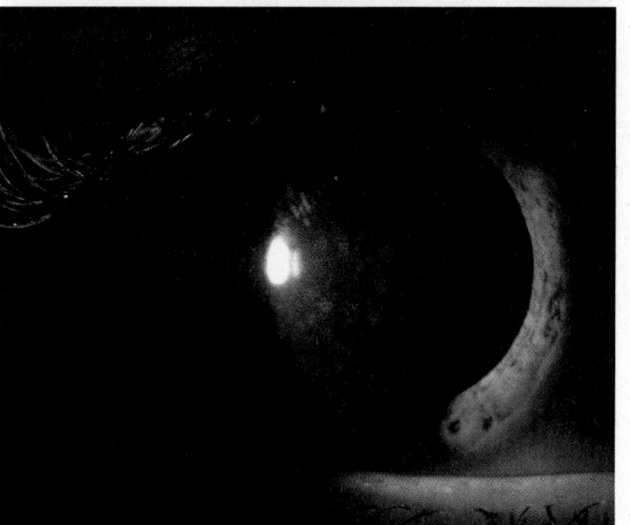

Fig. 18.4 Epidemic keratoconjunctivitis. The round slightly raised epithelial lesions can be seen on (a) retroillumination, and (b) direct illumination.

Small satellite lesions around the main ulcer occur and coalesce with each other. They may respond to treatment with sulphonamides and co-trimoxazole.

Filamentous fungi such as *Fusarium* species, *Mucor*, *Penicillium* and *Aspergillus* also cause keratitis in dirty wounds and in compromised hosts.

Protozoal keratitis

Acanthamoeba species are ubiquitous protozoa that exist in soil and water. *Acanthamoeba* keratitis occurs in people

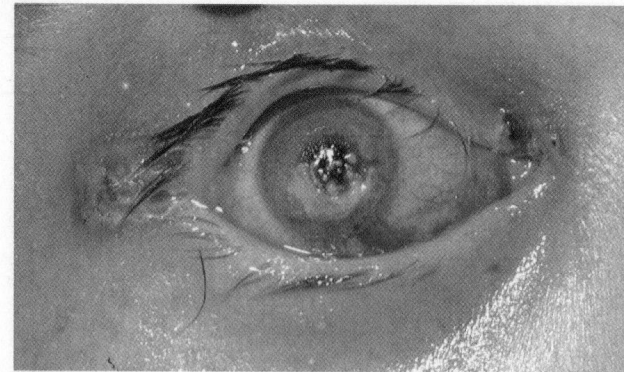

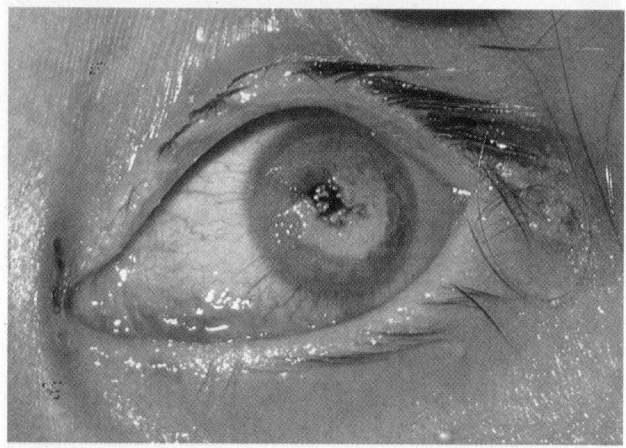

Fig. 18.5 (a, b) Bilateral *Candida* keratitis in a severely immunocompromised child.

exposed to the organism by swimming in brackish and standing water, in chlorinated swimming pools or hot tubs and by using contact lenses that are inadequately sterilized (Palmer & Hindiuk 1993). Even disposable lenses are not immune (Bacon *et al.* 1993).

The ulcers are chronic and indolent, but are associated with few inflammatory signs. Infection often follows minor trauma, exposure to soil, standing water, and so on, and pain is a prominent symptom. The lesions are stromal infiltrates, often ring-shaped with variable anterior uveitis (Mannis *et al.* 1986). Diagnosis is made by Giemsa stain or fluorescent antibody techniques from corneal scrapes or keratoplasty buttons (Epstein *et al.* 1986).

It may be that the use of corticosteroids should only be instituted with caution because of the occurrence of an additional bacterial keratitis, i.e. with *Streptococcus viridans* causing infectious crystalline keratopathy (Ficker 1988), or *Pseudomonas* (Davis *et al.* 1987).

Treatment with 0.1% propamidine isesthionate, 0.15% dibromopropamidine, neomycin or miconazole has been successful (Wright *et al.* 1985), but the infection is often resistant to treatment and results in stromal keratitis which may require keratoplasty, often with recurrence in the graft. A progressive sclerokeratitis may occur (Dougherty *et al.* 1994).

Heat sterilizing of contact lenses is important in prevention, together with the once only use of contact lens solution or sterilizing solutions that are discarded weekly (Ficker 1988). Contact lens cases should also be sterilized regularly.

Non-infective external eye disease

Phlyctenular disease

Phlyctenular conjunctivitis occurs in all parts of the world, often in undernourished children. There is a single localized inflammatory lesion with a white centre that is raised and later ulcerates. The lesions are usually transient, lasting up to 2 weeks before disappearing without trace, only to reappear elsewhere. There are few symptoms. The cornea may be involved with a marginal infiltrate and an ulcer that is painful. Most cases are associated with staphylococcal lid disease by some form of immunological mechanism. No direct infective agent has been proved but it seems to be associated with systemic infections including tuberculosis, fungal and worm infections.

Ligneous conjunctivitis

Ligneous conjunctivitis is a disorder of children which presents with redness and watering, sometimes following acute conjunctivitis. There are thickened nodular masses composed of amorphous fibrous hyalinized material.

It has been reported in siblings (Bateman *et al.* 1986) and following strabismus surgery (Bierly *et al.* 1994). An autosomal recessive inheritance is suggested. Infective causes have never been proven. Other mucous membranes may be involved.

Treatment has included excision, steroids, cromoglycate and antifibrin agents with varying success. Excision by itself is followed by rapid recurrence (Hidayat & Riddle 1987). Spontaneous resolution occurs and cases in Hidayat and Riddle's series of 17 had the disease for between 4 months and 44 years.

Chronic papillary conjunctivitis

Papillae form as a chronic response to a variety of stimulants. They are characterized by the presence of loops of vessels surrounded by variable cellular aggregations so that the papillae measure from 0.5 to 5 mm. The cells are inflammatory and later there is organization of the whole mosaic-like mass which is best seen on the tarsal plates of the upper lids.

Chronic atopic conjunctivitis and keratoconjunctivitis

The prime symptom of this condition is itching (Friedlaender 1993), with redness, burning, watering and stickiness also being present. It is usually seen in older children and can be very troublesome but on examination there are often very few signs — usually limited to the finding of numerous small pale tarsal papillae. It may be seasonal or perennial. There is often a personal or family history of atopy and conjunctival swabs show eosinophils in the mucous discharge. The serum immunoglobulin E (IgE) levels are raised. Although many cases are, like the eczema from which many of them suffer, self-limited, some go on to form a troublesome chronic keratoconjunctivitis (Jay 1981) and some develop keratoconus possibly related to eye-rubbing. Plaque formation occurs (Tuft *et al.* 1991) and subepithelial fibrosis with symblepharon or a keratopathy may cause a serious visual defect (Foster & Calonge 1990). The co-existence of herpes simplex keratitis and staphylococcal blepharitis can make management very difficult.

Treatment is best kept to the minimum required for the symptoms. Decongestants, antihistamine drops and systemic antihistamines may be useful (Abelson & Schaefer 1993) and many patients feel better with simple lubricants. Sodium cromoglycate is often helpful but needs to be used prophylactically if there is a seasonal element, and started well before the onset of symptoms. Steroids are best avoided, only being used in short courses under strict supervision.

Physical and chemical irritants

Ecothiopate, phenylephrine, antiviral agents, atropine (Wilson 1979), skin irritants, eye drop preservatives, oily vehicles and atmospheric and industrial chemicals may give rise to a chronic papillary conjunctivitis. Physical irritants include contact lenses, artificial eyes, eye sutures and 'teddy bear fibres' (Ferry 1994). Lacrimal concretions with fungal infection may also cause a similar picture.

In some countries corneal ulcers may be caused by the use of traditional eye medicines by non-medically trained healers: these ulcers tend to be peripheral in the cornea (Lewallen & Courtright 1995).

Acute conjunctivitis or keratoconjunctivitis in a contact lens wearer is most frequently due to trauma or over wear but certain 'soft' contact lenses and artificial eyes are associated with a giant papillary conjunctivitis almost identical to vernal disease. It starts after months or years of successful wear and develops gradually. It seems to be related to mechanical disturbance of the conjunctival epithelium. A painful red eye in a contact lens wearer should always be treated as an infection; infection by a variety of organisms including *Pseudomonas*, fungi and *Acanthamoeba* are more frequent in contact lens wearers.

Vernal disease

Vernal disease is a chronic conjunctivitis with an onset in childhood that is more frequent in boys than girls. It is seasonally exacerbated and occurs in all parts of the world although its incidence and manifestations vary greatly from area to area.

The onset is rarely before 4 years and many patients have a personal or family history of atopy (Frankland & Easty 1971) and there is often other evidence of hypersensitivity including high IgE levels in blood and tears and an eosinophilia.

Pollen-specific IgE and IgG have been found in tears and blood (Ballow & Mendelson 1980; Ballow *et al.* 1983) indicating that various forms of immune reaction may be involved.

The main symptom is itching with redness, watering and lid swelling; a mucus discharge is usual. The itching is invariable and matches the severity of the disease. There are two forms, palpebral and limbal with a mixed form.

The palpebral form is characterized by a generally more severe course with characteristic flat-topped giant papillae (Fig. 18.6) in the upper tarsal conjunctiva which are red at first, become whiter with ageing and in remission (Fig. 18.7). The papillae may be mucus laden and become very hypertrophic and when actively inflamed they may be indirectly associated with keratopathy but probably do not cause it.

Limbal vernal disease (Fig. 18.8) starts as a swelling and opacification at the limbus, often nodular. The nodules are papillae with a central vascular tuft; they may become cystic or have white deposits in them known as Trantas' spots. The cornea becomes vascularized in the

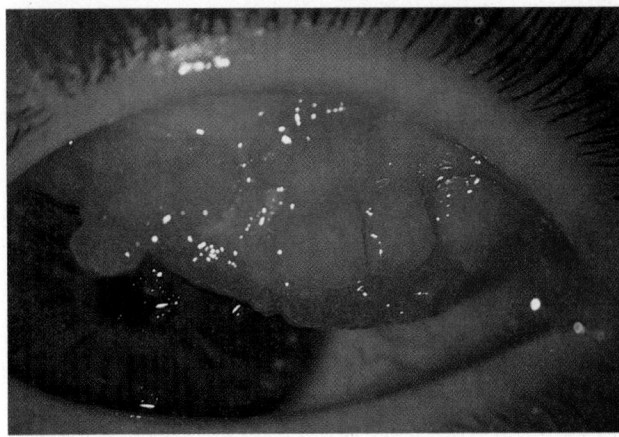

Fig. 18.6 Giant papillae in active vernal disease.

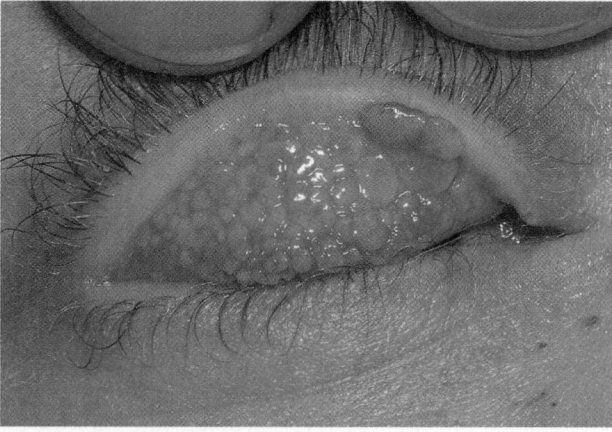

Fig. 18.7 Large papillae and residual giant papillae in treated chronic vernal disease.

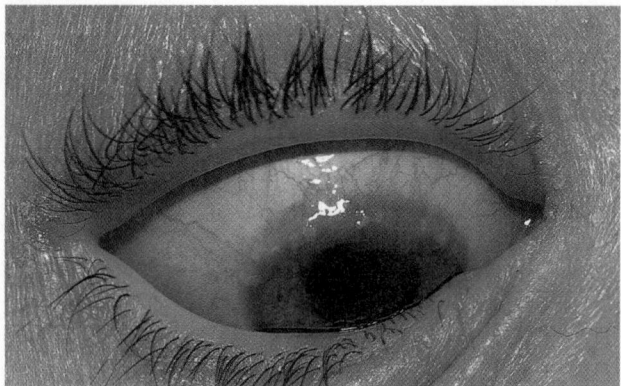

Fig. 18.8 Limbal vernal disease showing Trantas' spots.

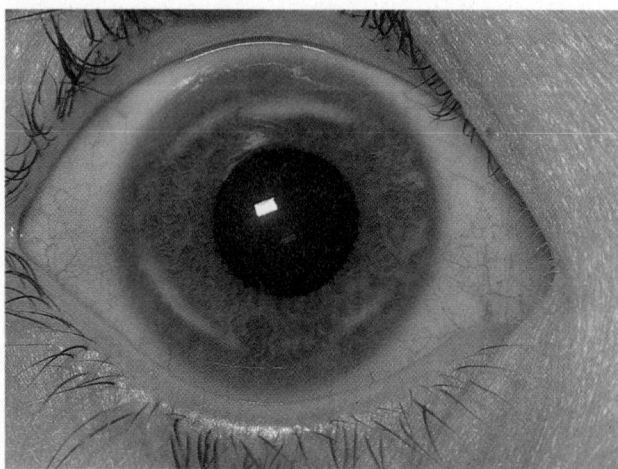

Fig. 18.9 Arcus lipoides in long-standing vernal disease, currently in remission.

affected area of the limbus and arcus-like changes occur (Fig. 18.9). Limbal vernal disease is more frequent in females, black people and Asians and atopic disease is less frequently associated compared with the palpebral form (Tuft *et al.* 1989).

Vernal keratopathy usually starts in the upper third of the cornea as punctate epithelial opacities which coalesce and extend to form a fluorescein-staining area which may form a 'macro-erosion' (Buckley 1981). These erosions are very indolent with a slightly raised margin and a base which becomes filled with mucus, fibrin and cellular debris known as vernal plaque. Subepithelial scarring and arcus lipoides ('pseudo-gerontotoxon') occur related to the affected areas.

Treatment has been greatly aided by two drugs. The first, soluble steroids, can be used with great effect in acute and severe disease, usually being started in high doses and rapidly tailed off, but chronic usage is often necessary. Therein lies the greatest problem because up to 10% may be susceptible to steroid-induced glaucoma. Since these children often pose great difficulty in examination, if tonometry is not possible they may require periodic anaesthetics in order to be sure that glaucoma has not supervened. The practice of prescribing acetazolamide routinely with steroids to 'prevent' glaucoma may not be justified in view of the side-effects of acetazolamide and the low risk of an anaesthetic. The second drug is disodium cromoglycate, which seems to lack side-effects and to be at least moderately effective (Foster 1988). The drops sting especially in an already inflamed eye and they may take some time to become effective; it is often best to start them before an exacerbation if it is predictable or to cover the start of their use by increasing the steroid dose. Some cases can be controlled by disodium cromoglycate alone. Lodoxamide is an equivalent, newer, drug which is also an effective treatment (Santos *et al.* 1994).

Vernal keratitis usually responds to the medical treatment outlined above. There is no benefit to the cornea from removing the lid papillae, however large and vicious looking, but corneal plaque may simply be excised (Buckley 1981). Simple measures such as avoidance of contact with allergies, cold compresses, the use of filtered air conditioning, and goggles are important (Abelson & Schaefer 1993).

Seasonal allergic (hay fever) conjunctivitis

These children have recurrent, often seasonal red eyes and running nose in response to a variety of more or less well-defined allergens, the most common being pollen, moulds, horse dander and cat fur. The onset is rapid with itching and pale, baggy swelling of the lids and conjunctiva. They water and become red with time with mucoid discharge. There may be a personal or family history of atopy.

Treatment may be by desensitization, topical (rarely systemic) steroids, or antihistamines by drop or systemically. In principal treatment is usually started with antihistamines or decongestants being used depending on response.

Perennial allergic conjunctivitis

This is a similar condition to the seasonal variant but it is present all year round with seasonal exacerbations. A family history of atopy may be obtained.

Staphylococcal hypersensitivity

A form of hypersensitivity to staphylococcal exotoxins is used to explain a variety of external eye diseases including some forms of blepharoconjunctivitis, meibomitis, and acute keratitis as in toxic epidermal necrolysis.

Avitaminosis

See Chapter 22.

Biotinidase deficiency

In biotinidase deficiency (Fig. 18.10), hypotonia, seizures, alopecia, skin rashes (pinpoint maculopapular lesions), ataxia and optic atrophy may be associated with a chronic conjunctivitis (Wolf & Heard 1991).

Episcleritis

Episcleritis occurs in self-limiting attacks lasting up to a month and recurring after an interval of some months. The eye becomes red in a circumscribed area deep to the conjunctiva (Fig. 18.11) which may be swollen ('nodular') and irritable. No cause is found in children but in adults there is a definite association with gout. Treatment with a short course of topical steroids usually shortens the attack and oral non-steroidal anti-inflammatory agents may help.

Laryngo-onychocutaneous syndrome (LOGIC syndrome) (Shabbir *et al.* 1986)

This devastating condition which comprises laryngeal and ocular granulation tissue in Punjabi Muslim children is probably autosomal recessively inherited (Ainsworth *et al.* 1992). In the first year of life relentlessly progressive (Fig. 18.12) conjunctival, laryngeal, nailbed, oral and oesophageal granulitides appear that are resistant to all forms of treatment (Ainsworth *et al.* 1991). It may be a form of junctional epidermolysis bullosa (Phillips *et al.* 1994).

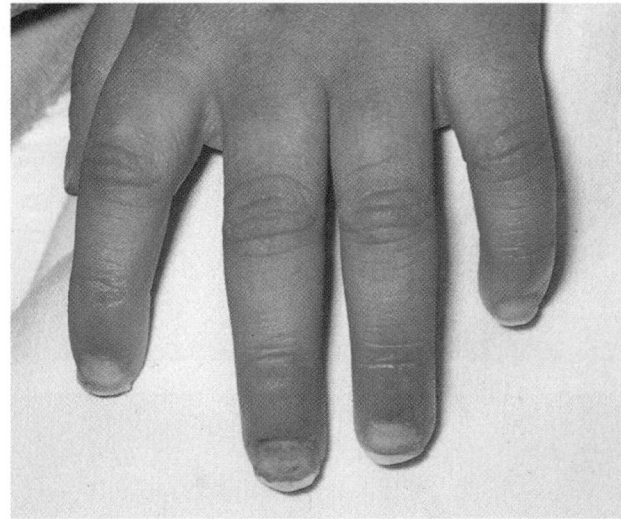

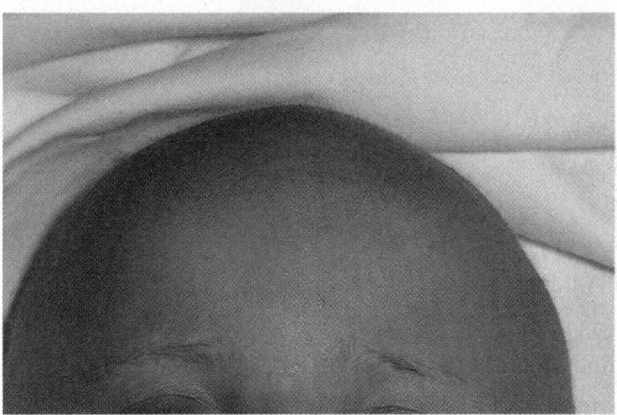

Fig. 18.10 Biotinidase deficiency. Patients with this condition may present with a chronic conjunctivitis, skin and nail abnormalities and alopecia. Seizures, hypotonia, ataxia and optic atrophy may be found.

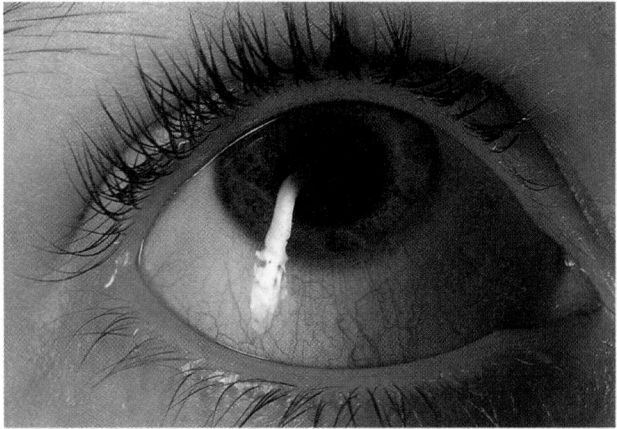

Fig. 18.11 Episcleritis.

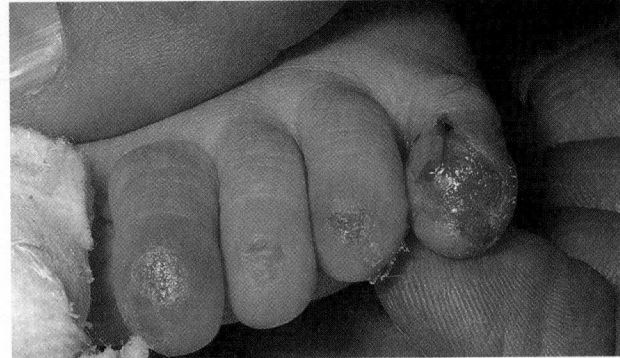

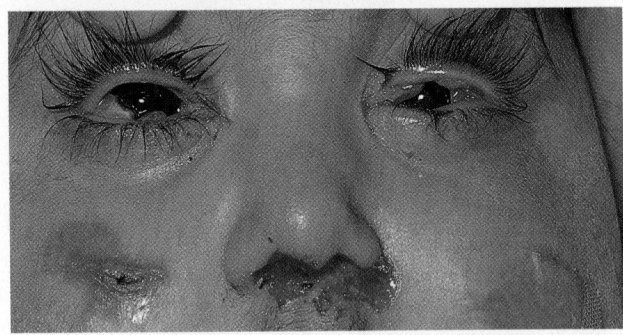

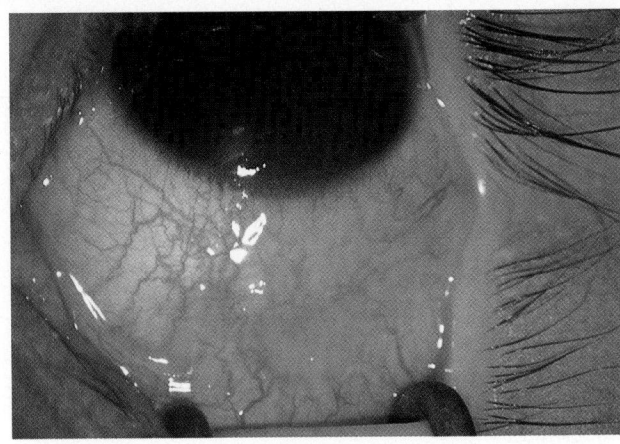

Fig. 18.12 Shabbir's syndrome. The laryngo-onychocutaneous syndrome comprises laryngeal, nailbed (a), oral and oesophageal lesions. In (b) a conjunctival granuloma with a necrotic slough can be seen, and in (c) there is bilateral conjunctival and nasal mucosal involvement.

Ophthalmia nodosa

Caterpillar or other insect hairs, both barbed and unbarbed (Arora *et al.* 1994), can cause a prolonged inflammatory nodular conjunctivitis; keratitis, iridocyclitis and even endophthalmitis have been recorded.

Lyme disease

In stage 1 up to 11% of patients with Lyme borreliosis have conjunctivitis, in stage 2, VII and other cranial nerve palsies occur (Winterkorn 1990; Zaidman 1993) (see Chapter 38).

References

Abelson M, Schaefer K. Conjunctivitis of allergic origin: immunologic mechanisms and current approaches to therapy. *Surv Ophthalmol* 1993; **38**: 115–32.

Aclimandos WA, Kerr-Muir M. Tuberculous keratoconjunctivitis. *Br J Ophthalmol* 1992; **76**: 175–6.

Ainsworth JR, Shabbir G, Spender AF, Cockburn F. Multisystem disorder of Punjabi children exhibiting spontaneous dermal and submycosal granulation tissue formation: LOGIC syndrome. *Clin Dysmorphol* 1992; **1**: 3–14.

Ainsworth J, Spencer A, Dudgeon J, Geddes N, Lee W. Laryngeal and ocular granulation tissue formation in two Punjabi children: LOGIC syndrome. *Eye* 1991; **5**: 717–22.

Al-Hazza S, Hidayat A. Molluscum contagiosum of the eyelid and infra-orbital margin—a clinicopathologic study with light and electron microscopic observations. *J Pediatr Ophthalmol Strabismus* 1993; **30**: 58–9.

Arora R, Gupta AK, Chaturvedi KU, Bhatnagar A. Ophthalmia nodosa: due to unbarbed hairs. *J Pediatr Ophthalmol Strabismus* 1994; **31**: 104–6.

Bacon A, Frazer D, Dart J, Matheson M, Ficker L, Wright P. A review of 72 consecutive cases of acanthamoeba keratitis, 1984–1992. *Eye* 1993; **7**: 719–25.

Ballow M, Danshik PC, Mendelson L, Rapacz P, Sparks K. IgG-specific antibodies to rye grass and ragweed pollen antigens in the tear secretions of patients with vernal conjunctivitis. *Am J Ophthalmol* 1983; **95**: 161–8.

Ballow M, Mendelson L. Specific immunoglobulin E antibodies in tear secretions of patients with vernal conjunctivitis. *J Allergy Clin Immunol* 1980; **66**: 112–18.

Barron B, Gee L, Hauck W *et al.* Herpetic eye disease study: a controlled trial of oral acyclovir for herpes simplex stromal keratitis. *Ophthalmology* 1994; **101**: 1871–82.

Bateman JB, Isenberg SJ, Pettit TH, Simons KB. Ligneous conjunctivitis: an autosomal recessive disorder. *J Pediatr Ophthalmol Strabismus* 1986; **23**: 137–40.

Beigi B, Algawi K, Foley-Nolan A, O'Keefe M. Herpes simplex keratitis in children. *Br J Ophthalmol* 1994; **78**: 458–60.

Bierly JR, Blandford DL, Weeks JA, Baker RS. Ligneous conjunctivitis as a complication following strabismus surgery. *J Pediatr Ophthalmol Strabismus* 1994; **31**: 99–103.

Buckley RJ. Vernal keratopathy and its management. *Trans Ophthalmol Soc UK* 1981; **101**: 234–8.

Chiapella AP, Rosenthal AJR. One year in an eye casualty clinic. *Br J Ophthalmol* 1985; **69**: 865–70.

Clinch T, Dalmon F, Robinson M, Cohen E, Barron B, Liabson P. Microbial keratitis in children. *Am J Ophthalmol* 1994; **117**: 65–71.

Cohen P. Sweet's syndrome presenting as conjunctivitis. *Arch Ophthalmol* 1993; **111**: 587–8.

Coster DJ, Wilhelmus K, Jones BR. Suppurative keratitis in London. In: Trevor-Roper PD, ed. *The Cornea in Health and Disease*. London: Academic Press, 1981: 395–8.

Cruz D, Sabir S, Capo H, Alfonso E. Microbial keratitis in childhood. *Ophthalmology* 1993; **100**: 192–6.

Darougar S, Grey RHB, Thaker U, McSwiggan DA. Clinical and epidemiological features of adenovirus keratoconjunctivitis in London. *Br J Ophthalmol* 1983; **67**: 1–7.

Darougar S, Monnickendam MA, Woodland RM. Management and prevention of ocular viral and chlamydial infections. *Crit Rev Microbiol* 1989; **16**: 369–418.

Darougar S, Wishart MS, Viswalingham ND. Epidemiological and clinical features of primary herpes simplex virus ocular infection. *Br J Ophthalmol* 1985; **69**: 2–6.

Dart JK, Seal DV. Pathogenesis and therapy of *Pseudomonas aeruginosa* keratitis. *Eye* 1988; **2**(Suppl.): 546–57.

Davis RM, Schroeder RJP, Rowsey JJ, Jensen HG, Tripathi R. *Acanthamoeba* keratitis and infectious crystalline keratopathy. *Arch Ophthalmol* 1987; **105**: 1524–7.

Dougherty PJ, Binder PS, Mondino BJ, Glasgow BJ. *Acanthamoeba* sclerokeratitis. *Am J Ophthalmol* 1994; **117**: 475–9.

Epstein RJ, Wilson LA, Visvesvara GS, Plourde EG. Rapid diagnosis of acanthamoeba keratitis from corneal scraping using indirect fluorescent antibody staining. *Arch Ophthalmol* 1986; **104**: 1318–21.

Erie J, Nevitt M, Hodge D, Ballard D. Incidence of ulcerative keratitis in a defined population from 1950 to 1988. *Arch Ophthalmol* 1993; **111**: 1665–71.

Erzurum S, Feder R, Greenwald M. Acne rosacea with keratitis in childhood. *Arch Ophthalmol* 1993; **111**: 228–30.

Ferry A. Synthetic fiber granuloma: 'teddy bear' granuloma of the conjunctiva. *Arch Ophthalmol* 1994; **112**: 1339–41.

Ficker L. *Acanthamoeba* keratitis. The quest for a better prognosis. *Eye* 1988; **2**(Suppl.): 537–45.

Foster A. Childhood blindness. *Eye* 1988; **2**(Suppl.): 527–36.

Foster A, Gilbert C. Epidemiology of childhood blindness. *Eye* 1992; **6**: 173–6.

Foster CS and the Cromolyn Sodium Collaborative Study Group. Evaluation of topical cromolyn sodium in the treatment of vernal keratoconjunctivitis. *Ophthalmology* 1988; **95**: 19–202.

Foster CS, Calonge M. Atopic keratoconjunctivitis. *Ophthalmology* 1990; **97**: 992–1000.

Frankland AW, Easty DL. Vernal keratoconjunctivitis, an atopic disease. *Trans Ophthalmol Soc UK* 1971; **91**: 479–82.

Friedlaender M. Conjunctivitis of allergic origin: clinical presentation and differential diagnosis. *Surv Ophthalmol* 1993; **38**: 105–14.

Gigliotti F, Williams WT, Hayden FG, Hendley JO. Etiology of acute conjunctivitis in children. *J Pediatr* 1981; **98**: 531–6.

Gilbert C, Canovas R, Hagan M, Rao S, Foster A. Causes of childhood blindness: results from West Africa, South India and Chile. *Eye* 1993; **7**: 184–8.

Hammond C, Harden A. Progressive corneal vascularisation as a previously unreported complication of neonatal herpes simplex infection. *Br J Ophthalmol* 1994; **78**: P654.

Helm CJ. Ocular tuberculosis. *Surv Ophthalmol* 1993; **38**: 229–56.

Hidayat AA, Riddle PJ. Ligneous conjunctivitis. *Ophthalmology* 1987; **94**: 949–59.

Hilton E, Uliss A, Samuels S, Adams AA, Leser, ML, Lowy FD. Nosocomial bacterial eye infections in intensive care units. *Lancet* 1983; **i**: 1318–20.

Hirst LW, Harrison, GK, Merz WG, Stark WJ. Nocardia asteroides keratitis. *Br J Ophthalmol* 1979; **63**: 449–54.

Hyde KJ, Berger ST. Epidemic keratoconjunctivitis and lacrimal excretory system obstruction. *Ophthalmology* 1988; **95**: 1447–9.

Jackson WB. Differentiating conjunctivitis of diverse origins. *Surv Ophthalmol* 1993; **38**: 91–104.

Jay JL. Clinical features and diagnosis of adult atopic keratoconjunctivitis and the effect of treatment with sodium cromoglycate. *Br J Ophthalmol* 1981; **65**: 335–40.

Jones DB. Polymicrobial keratitis. *Trans Am Ophthalmol Soc* 1981; **79**: 153–67.

Klein JO. The epidemiology of pneumococcal disease in infants and children. *Rev Infect Dis* 1981; **3**: 246–53.

Lennarson P, Barney NP. Interstitial keratitis as presenting ophthalmic sign of sarcoidosis in a child. *J Pediatr Ophthalmol Strabismus* 1995; **32**: 194–6.

Lewallen S, Courtright P. Peripheral corneal ulcers associated with use of African traditional eye medicines. *Br J Ophthalmol* 1995; **79**: 343–6.

Mannis MJ, Tamaru R, Roth AM *et al*. Acanthamoeba sclerokeratitis: determining diagnostic criteria. *Arch Ophthalmol* 1986; **104**: 1313–17.

Monnickendam MA. Herpes simplex ophthalmia. *Eye* 1988; **2**(Suppl.): S56–69.

Okumoto M, Smolin G. Pneumococcal infections of the eye. *Am J Ophthalmol* 1974; **77**: 346–52.

Ormerod LD, Murphree AL, Gomez DS, Schanzlin DJ, Smith RE. Microbial keratitis in children. *Ophthalmology* 1986; **93**: 449–55.

Palay D, Litoff D, Krachmer J. Stromal keratitis associated with Epstein–Barr virus infection in a young child. *Arch Ophthalmol* 1993; **111**: 1323–4.

Palmer ML, Hindiuk RA. Contact lens-related infectious keratitis. *Int Ophthalmol Clin* 1993; **33**: 23–49.

Phillips R, Atherton D, Gibbs M, Strobel S, Lake B. Laryngo-onychocutaneous syndrome: an inherited epithelial defect. *Arch Dis Child* 1994; **70**: 319–26.

Ralph RA, Lemp MA, Liss G. Nocardia keratitis: a case report. *Br J Ophthalmol* 1976; **60**: 104–6.

Santos CI, Huang AJ, Abelson MB, Foster CS, Friedlaender M, McCulley JP. Efficacy of iodoxamide 0.1% ophthalmic solution in resolving corneal epitheliopathy associated with vernal keratoconjunctivitis. *Am J Ophthalmol* 1994; **117**: 488–97.

Schmiedt R, Cimma R. *Shigella* corneal ulceration. *Clin Pediatr* 1983; **24**: 460–1.

Seal DV, Barrett SP, McGill JI. Aetiology and treatment of acute bacterial infection of the external eye. *Br J Ophthalmol* 1982; **66**: 357–60.

Shabbir G, Hassan M, Kazim A. Laryngo-onycho-cutaneous syndrome. *Biomedica* 1986; **2**: 15–25.

Simon JW, Lango F, Smith RS. Spontaneous resolution of herpes simplex blepharoconjunctivitis in children. *Am J Ophthalmol* 1986; **102**: 598–600.

Singer TR, Isenberg SJ, Apt L. Conjunctival anaerobic and aerobic bacterial flora in paediatric versus adult subjects. *Br J Ophthalmol* 1988; **72**: 448–52.

Tuft SJ, Dart JK, Kemery M. Limbal vernal keratoconjunctivitis: clinical characteristics and immunoglobulin E expression compared with palpebral vernal. *Eye* 1989; **3**: 420–8.

Tuft SJ, Kemeny DM, Dart JK, Buckley RJ. Clinical features of atopic keratoconjunctivitis. *Ophthalmology* 1991; **98**: 150–8.

Wagman RD, Kazdan JJ, Kooh SW, Fraser D. Keratitis associated with the multiple endocrine deficiency, autoimmune disease, and candidiasis syndrome. *Am J Ophthalmol* 1987; **103**: 569–75.

Watson AP, Tullo AB, Kerr-Muir MG, Ridgway ACA, Lucas DR. Arborescent bacterial keratopathy (infectious crystalline keratopathy). *Eye* 1988; **2**(Suppl.): 517–22.

Wear DJ, Malaty RH, Zimmerman LE, Hadfield TL, Margileth AM.

Cat scratch disease bacilli in the conjunctiva of patients with Parinaud's oculoglandular syndrome. *Ophthalmology* 1985; **92**: 1282–7.

Weiss A, Brinser JH, Nazar-Stewart V. Acute conjunctivitis in childhood. *J Paediatr* 1993; **122**: 10–14.

Wilhelmus K, Gee L, Hauck W *et al.* Herpetic Eye Disease Study: a controlled trial of topical corticosteroids for herpes simplex stromal keratitis. *Ophthalmology* 1994; **101**: 1883–96.

Wilhelmus K, Hamill M, Jones D. Varicella disciform stromal keratitis. *Am J Ophthalmol* 1991; **111**: 575–81.

Wilson FM. Adverse external ocular effects of topical ophthalmic medications. *Surv Ophthalmol* 1979; **24**: 57–88.

Winterkorn J. Lyme disease: neurologic and ophthalmic manifestations. *Surv Ophthalmol* 1990; **35**: 191–205.

Wolff B, Heard G. Biotinidase deficiency. *Adv Pediatr* 1991; **38**: 1–21.

Wright P, Warhurst D, Jones BR. *Acanthamoeba* keratitis successfully treated medically. *Br J Ophthalmol* 1985; **69**: 778–82.

Yin-Murphy M, Goh K, Phoon M, Yao J, Ishak B. A recent epidemic of acute hemorrhagic conjunctivitis. *Am J Ophthalmol* 1993; **116**: 212–17.

Zaidman GW. The ocular manifestations of Lyme disease. *Int Ophthalmol Clin* 1993; **33**: 9–22.

19: Erythema Multiforme (Stevens–Johnson Syndrome)

Anthony Moore

Erythema multiforme is an acute systemic disorder with variable skin and mucous membrane involvement. In its mildest form it is characterized by a localized or generalized skin eruption often with typical 'target' or 'iris' lesions. In the more severe form, often termed the Stevens–Johnson syndrome (Stevens & Johnson 1922), there is an extensive bullous form of erythema multiforme with involvement of mucous membranes and conjunctiva. Toxic epidermal necrolysis is a closely related disorder in which there is epidermal necrosis and shedding of skin (Lyell 1956; Kaufman 1994). Toxic epidermal necrolysis shares many of the same precipitating factors as Stevens–Johnson syndrome, has some overlap in its clinical features and may represent the severe end of a disease spectrum which includes erythema multiforme and Stevens–Johnson syndrome (Roujeau 1994).

Aetiology

Although the exact aetiology is unknown, the disorder is thought to be due to an acute hypersensitivity reaction and may follow bacterial, protozoal, fungal, viral (particularly herpes simplex) or mycoplasmal infection, or be related to food or drug sensitivity (Gottschalk & Stone 1976; Hurwitz 1981). In many cases the cause is unknown. Histological and immunohistochemical studies suggest that the skin and mucous membrane abnormalities are caused by an immune complex-mediated vasculitis (Kazmierowski & Wuepper 1978; Wuepper *et al.* 1980; Foster *et al.* 1988; Mondino 1990). In children most cases probably follow infection. Although the acute disorder is self-limiting it can produce serious long-term ocular abnormalities (Wright & Collin 1983; Mondino 1990). Recurrent disease of the skin, eyes and mucous membranes may occur in a minority of patients (Bean & Quezada 1983; Foster *et al.* 1988).

Clinical features

The clinical features are extremely variable; in some cases there is a mild self-limiting skin rash with no mucous membrane involvement, whereas in others there is widespread skin and mucous membrane disease. Conjunctival involvement is similarly variable and tends to parallel the severity of the skin involvement. The acute phase of the disease lasts from 2 to 6 weeks.

In most cases the onset of the skin eruption is preceded by a prodromal period with mild fever, malaise and joint and muscle pains. The skin lesions are symmetrical, and may involve any part of the surface including palms and soles of the feet. The appearance is variable and includes patchy erythema, bullae or the typical target lesions (Hurwitz 1981; Wilkins *et al.* 1992; Feldman 1993). Oral lesions are common and are seen as swelling and blistering of the lips and erosions of the oral mucosa and tongue. Conjunctival involvement varies from mild injection to severe disease with membrane formation and symblepharon.

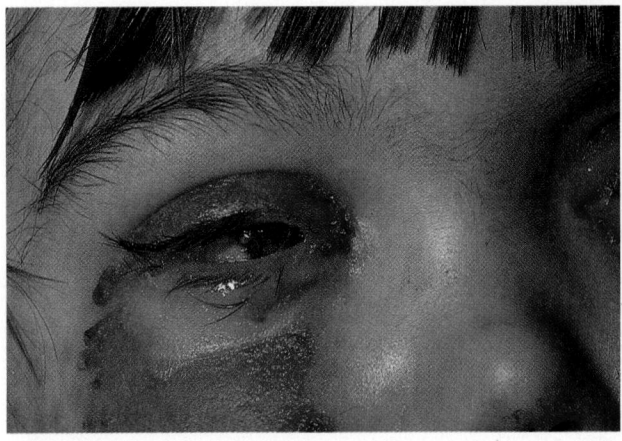

Fig. 19.1 Stevens–Johnson syndrome; early stage with acute keratoconjunctivitis and skin lesions.

199

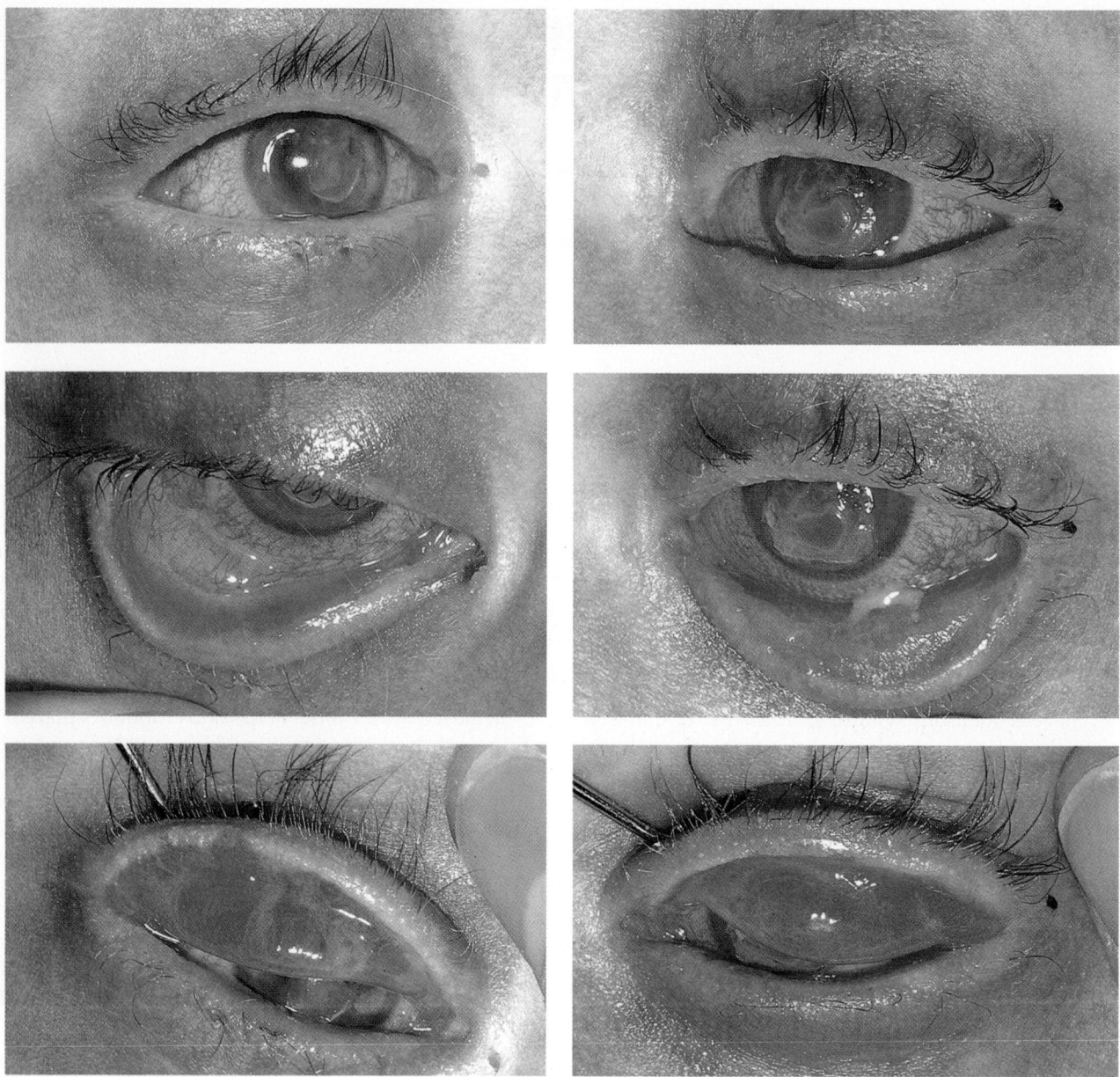

Fig. 19.2 Stevens–Johnson syndrome; bilateral desquamative conjunctivitis with areas of necrosis. There is a severe keratitis which resulted in chronic scarring worsened by the later occurrence of a dry eye.

The most severe involvement occurs in Stevens–Johnson syndrome. In this variant there is usually a prodromal period of general malaise, fever, gastrointestinal upset and arthralgia followed by acute onset of an extensive bullous skin eruption with severe involvement of ocular, oral, anal and genital mucosa with later scarring.

Ocular involvement

In the acute phase (Fig. 19.1) there is usually a mucopuru-lent conjunctivitis with a marked papillary reaction of the subtarsal conjunctiva. In more severe cases there may be infarction of the conjunctiva (Fig. 19.2) with membrane formation, and adhesions may form between the lid and bulbar conjunctiva (Howard 1963; Arstikaitis 1973; Wright & Collin 1983; Mondino 1990). Vesicles and less common-ly conjunctival cysts (Goodglick *et al.* 1992) may develop on the bulbar or palpebral conjunctiva. Desai *et al.* (1992) have reported an unusal complication of an orbital cyst developing in a 10-year-old girl with Stevens–Johnson syndrome.

Although the initial conjunctival changes are self-limit-ing, secondary bacterial infection, late scarring and sec-ondary epithelial changes may give rise to serious ocular problems. Lid margin deformities, punctal occlusion,

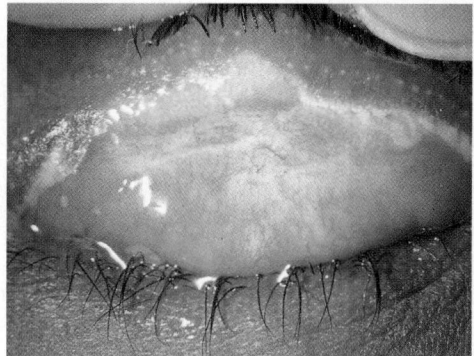 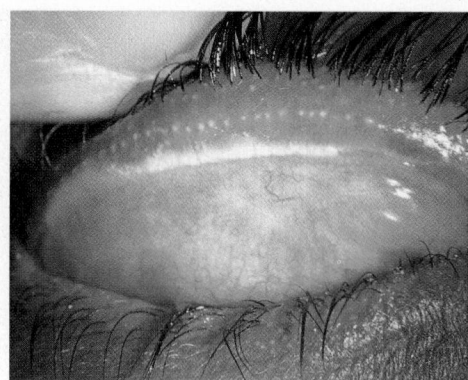

Fig. 19.3 Stevens–Johnson syndrome; late stage with subconjunctival scarring and squamous metaplasia of the lid margins.

metaplastic lashes, and trichiasis are common, and conjunctivalization of the lid has been described (Navon & Rubin 1994). Keratinization of the tarsal conjunctiva (Fig. 19.3) may lead to chronic irritation (Wright & Collin 1983). Some patients develop a dry-eye syndrome due to loss of goblet cells and obliteration of the lacrimal and meibomian gland orifices by extensive mucosal scarring. Corneal changes such as punctate epithelial keratitis, and neovascularization may be seen and are usually secondary to conjunctival and lid margin abnormalities. The combination of tear film and lid margin abnormalities may predispose to recurrent corneal epithelial breakdown, corneal infection, ulceration and subsequent scarring. Patients with severe skin disease usually have equally severe conjunctival disease (Fig. 19.4).

Management

Most children with the Stevens–Johnson syndrome require hospital admission and systemic steroids are often prescribed to control the widespread vasculitis (Rasmussen 1976; Mondino 1990; Wilkins *et al.* 1992). The acute eye management includes frequent topical steroids (without preservatives), and less frequent topical antibiotics to prevent any secondary infection. Topical cycloplegics are helpful if there is evidence of uveitis or pain from ciliary spasm. The nursing management is vital because these miserable sick children are almost always reluctant to accept the treatment that is so vital. If adhesions start to form between the bulbar conjunctiva and lid these may be separated with a glass rod ('rodding') or divided with scissors under local anaesthesia. This may need to be carried out daily to prevent permanent adhesions. The acute conjunctival changes settle within a few weeks but the late complications may present long-term problems in management. Dry eyes may require frequent treatment with artificial tear drops and a simple ointment lubricant at night. Squamous metaplasia and keratinization of the conjunctiva may respond to topical retinoid therapy (Kaz

Soong *et al.* 1988). Trichiasis is best treated with cryotherapy although if there is a true cicatricial entropion a lid everting procedure such as a Trabut's operation may be necessary (Wright & Collin 1983). If there is extensive scarring and shortening of the tarsus a mucous membrane graft may be required in addition. Cicatricial ectropion may require treatment with skin grafting. Penetrating keratoplasty has a poor prognosis in Stevens–Johnson syn-

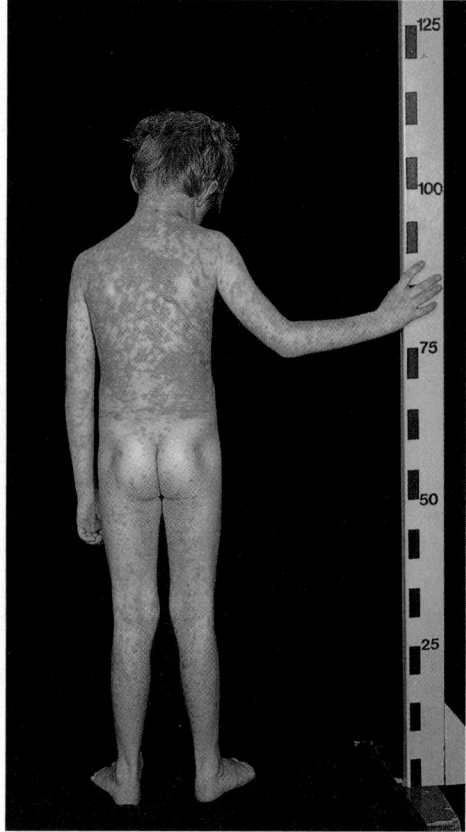

Fig. 19.4 Stevens–Johnson syndrome; same patient as in Fig. 19.2. There is extensive scarring and pigmentation of the skin.

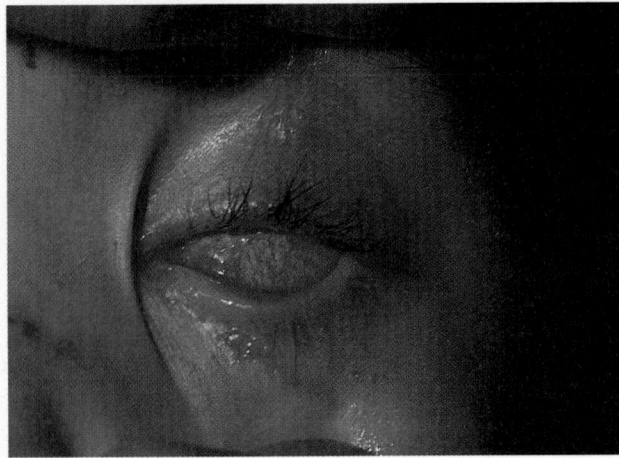

Fig. 19.5 Toxic epidermal necrolysis with conjunctivitis in a 3-year-old girl.

drome due to the poor tear film and lid abnormalities. If there is bilateral severe corneal scarring keratoprosthesis may need to be considered but the results are still disappointing in the long term (Kozarsky *et al.* 1987).

Children with Stevens–Johnson syndrome should be followed carefully in the eye department and any lid margin deformity or trichiasis corrected early to prevent permanent corneal damage.

Toxic epidermal necrolysis

There is considerable overlap between this disorder and Stevens–Johnson syndrome (Kaufman 1994; Roujeau 1994). Toxic epidermal necrolysis is usually drug-induced and starts with a painful eruption of the skin which initially involves the face and upper trunk and then extends rapidly to involve the rest of the cutaneous surface. The face, trunk and proximal part of the limbs are predominantly affected. The skin is initially erythematous but subsequently there is detachment of large areas of necrotic epidermis with exudation of fluid from the exposed dermis (Wilkins *et al.* 1992; Roujeau 1994). The epidermis may separate when gently stroked (the Nikolsky sign). Typical target lesions may be present at the border of the necrotic lesions. Mucous membrane and conjunctival involvement is very common (Fig. 19.5) and the ophthalmological features and management are similar to those described in Stevens–Johnson syndrome (Bennet *et al.* 1977).

References

Arstikaitis MS. Ocular aftermath of Stevens–Johnson syndrome: review of 33 cases. *Arch Ophthalomol* 1973; **90**: 376–9.

Bean SF, Quezada RK. Recurrent oral erythema multiforme. Clinical experience with 11 patients. *J Am Med Assoc* 1983; **249**: 281–2.

Bennet TO, Sugar J, Sahgal S. Ocular manifestations of toxic epidermal necrolysis associated with allopurinol use. *Arch Ophthalmol* 1977; **95**: 1362–4.

Desai VN, Shields CL, Shields JA. Orbital cyst in a patient with Stevens–Johnson syndrome. *Cornea* 1992; **11**: 592–4.

Feldman SR. Bullous dermatoses associated with systemic disease. *Dermatol Clin* 1993; **11**: 597–609.

Foster CS, Fong LP, Azar D, Kenyon KR. Episodic conjunctival inflammation after Stevens–Johnson syndrome. *Ophthalmology* 1988; **95**: 453–62.

Goodglick TA, Wolfley D, Cavanagh HD, Zimmerman L. Ciliated respiratory-like epithelium forming cystic conjunctival lesions in a patient with Stevens–Johnson syndrome. *Ophthalmic Surg* 1992; **23**: 557–9.

Gottschalk HR, Stone OJ. Stevens–Johnson syndrome from ophthalmic sulphonamide. *Arch Dermatol* 1976; **112**: 513–14.

Howard GM. The Stevens–Johnson syndrome. Ocular prognosis and treatment. *Am J Ophthalmol* 1963; **55**: 893–900.

Hurwitz S. Hypersensitivity syndromes. In: Hurwitz S, ed. *Clinical Pediatric Dermatology*. London: WB Saunders, 1981: 392–4.

Kaufman DW. Epidemiological approaches to the study of toxic epidermal necrolysis. *J Invest Dermatol* 1994; **102**: 31S–33S.

Kaz Soong H, Martin NF, Wagener MD. Topical retinoid therapy for squamous metaplasia of various ocular surface disorders. *Ophthalmology* 1988; **95**: 1442–6.

Kazmierowski JA, Wuepper KD. Erythema multiforme: immune complex vasculitis of the superficial cutaneous microvasculature. *J Invest Dermatol* 1978; **71**: 366–9.

Kozarsky AM, Snight SH, Waring GO III. Clinical results of keratoprosthesis placed through the eyelid. *Ophthalmology* 1987; **84**: 904–11.

Lyell A. Toxic epidermal necrolysis: an eruption resembling scalded skin. *Br J Dermatol* 1956; **68**: 355–61.

Mondino BJ. Cicatricial pemphigoid and erythema multiforme. *Ophthalmology* 1990; **97**: 939–52.

Navon SE, Rubin PAD. Ectopic conjunctivalisation in Stevens–Johnson syndrome. *Br J Ophthalmol* 1994; **78**: 727–8.

Rasmussen JE. Erythema multiforme in children—response to treatment with systemic steroids. *Br J Dermatol* 1976; **95**: 181–5.

Roujeau J-C. Epidemiology of toxic epidermal necrolysis: the spectrum of Stevens–Johnson syndrome and toxic epidermal necrolysis: a clinical classification. *J Invest Dermatol* 1994; **102**: 28S–30S.

Stevens AM, Johnson FC. A new eruptive fever associated with stomatitis and ophthalmia: a report of two cases in children. *Am J Dis Child* 1922; **24**: 526–33.

Wilkins J, Morrison L, White CR. Oculocutaneous manifestations of erythema multiforme/Stevens–Johnson syndrome/toxic epidermal necrolysis spectrum. *Dermatol Clin* 1992; **10**: 571–81.

Wuepper KD, Watson PA, Kazmerowski JA. Immune complexes in erythema multiforme and the Stevens–Johnson syndrome. *J Invest Dermatol* 1980; **74**: 368–71.

Wright P, Collin JRO. Ocular complications of erythema multiforme and their management. *Trans Ophthalmol Soc UK* 1983; **103**: 338–41.

Section 4
Systematic Paediatric Ophthalmology

20: Disorders of the Eye as a Whole

David Taylor and Susan Day

Influence of the eye on the development of the orbit

Although the absence of a developing eye in itself does not affect the initial development of a bony orbit (Mann 1937), the growth of the orbit is highly influenced by the presence or absence of an eye. At birth, the normal eye occupies a higher percentage of the orbital volume; growth of the orbital volume increases dramatically during the first year of life (Peyton 1940).

How does absence of an eye, either congenitally or surgically at an early age, influence the growth of the bony orbit? Although orbital volume cannot be assessed with X-rays, the horizontal and vertical measurement of the orbital rim can be taken easily. Kennedy (1965) has shown that these parameters are reduced by 15% in adults who had anophthalmos or had the eye removed within the first year of life. He has also shown that in humans, cats and rabbits this retardation of orbital growth is approximately halved when an orbital implant is used and that the severity of the overall reduction in volume diminishes if the insult occurs at a later date. Orbital growth appears to be complete by the age of 15 years, so that subsequent enucleation will not result in any appreciable size difference.

Determination of the influence of an eye on orbital volume cannot be detected radiologically, but measurements of skulls have shown a 60% reduction in volume (Kennedy 1973).

Orbital growth may be secondarily influenced by radiotherapy (Guyuron *et al.* 1983). This consideration as well as intracranial radiotherapeutic effects becomes important clinically in the management of children with retinoblastoma, rhabdomyosarcoma, and other radiosensitive neoplasms involving the orbit (Starceski *et al.* 1987).

Anophthalmos

Anophthalmos is the term used when the eye is non-existent as a true eye or more commonly a tiny cystic remnant of the eye is present, when the term 'clinical anophthalmos' (Fig. 20.1) may be used: this term emphasizes that there is a spectrum between anophthalmos and microphthalmos.

Variable abnormalities of the orbit occur and orbital growth is retarded to some extent (Pfeiffer 1945; Kennedy 1965). Extraocular muscles may be absent, and optic foramen size decreased (Pico & Townsend 1979). The conjunctival sac may be very small in size, and its growth may be stimulated with insertion of a prosthesis within the first few years of life; these prostheses require periodic enlargement.

Anophthalmos represents either a complete failure of budding of the optic vesicle or early arrest of its development. To differentiate between anophthalmos and extreme microphthalmos, the examiner can touch the lids to feel for any movements representing rudimentary extraocular muscle function. Computed tomography (CT) or magnetic resonance imaging (MRI) scans may demonstrate buried residual soft tissue mass in cases of extreme microphthalmos, but histological sectioning alone can clarify the presence of neural ectoderm derived cells or microphthalmos, or their absence in true anophthalmos (Pearce *et al.* 1974; Brownstein *et al.* 1977; Sassani & Yanoff 1977; Brunquell *et al.* 1984; Guyer & Green 1984; Pe'er & BenEzra 1986). Functional assessment, using electrophysiology (see Chapter 9) may demonstrate rudimentary function in cases thought to be anophthalmic on

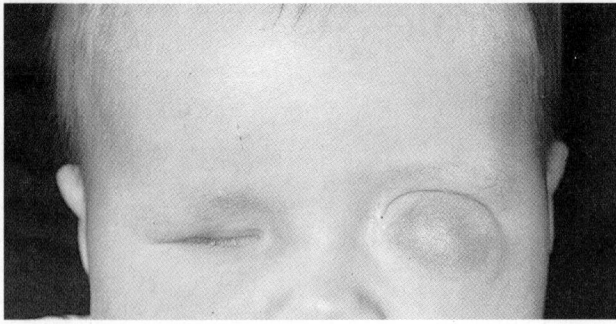

Fig. 20.1 Right clinical anophthalmos. Left microphthalmos with cyst. The baby had presented at birth with a clinically anophthalmic right eye and extreme colobomatous microphthalmos in the left eye. A blue swelling was initially thought to be vascular but it transilluminated and was found to be a cyst associated with microphthalmos.

clinical examination. Unilateral anophthalmos is often associated with anomalies of the other eye (O'Keefe *et al.* 1987).

Many underlying causes have been proposed for anophthalmos: these merge almost imperceptibly with the causes of microphthalmos (see below). Its bilaterality and severity implies an early generalized teratogenic event. Many are sporadic (Warburg 1981a) although case reports involving siblings do exist (Zeiter 1963). Chromosomal abnormalities (Zimmerman & Font 1966; Warburg 1981b; Glaser *et al.* 1994; McLeod *et al.* 1994) include many syndromes in which extreme microphthalmos is one of many congenital defects. A family in which both parents had PAX6-related cataracts and aniridia had a child with total anophthalmos, microcephaly, agenesis of the corpus callosum and choanal atresia (Glaser *et al.* 1994). Prenatal parvovirus infections (Burton & Caul 1988; Hartwig *et al.* 1989), X-rays, chemical agents such as LSD (Bogdanoff *et al.* 1972) and other environmental agents (Gilbert 1993) may all play a role in the anophthalmos–microphthalmos spectrum of disorders (Guyer & Green 1984). Some families have shown a dominant gene for coloboma with variable expression with extreme microphthalmos at one end of the spectrum and coloboma, sometimes quite trivial colobomatous defects, at the other.

The ophthalmologist's management of anophthalmos is twofold:

1 To stimulate growth of the adnexal structures and orbit (Kennedy 1973; Soll 1982) (see Chapter 27). Orbital expansion can be achieved by the use of serially larger prostheses, and hydrophilic or inflatable expanders (Tucker *et al.* 1995).

2 To provide support for the parents of such a child. When bilateral, blindness is inevitable and networking with the appropriate agencies will provide great support. A search for possible causes in conjunction with a primary care physician may help ease guilt. Genetic counselling

will aid the parents in understanding risks of future children being involved. When unilateral, emphasis must be placed on the integrity of the fellow eye if this is the case, and on the relatively normal life that can be expected in a monocular child. Safety glasses may be considered at an early age to protect the good eye.

Microphthalmos

The spectrum of anophthalmos merges with microphthalmos. The net volume of a microphthalmic eye is reduced. Often, clinical suspicion is created on the basis of cornea size. Although microphthalmos is usually associated with a small cornea, there may be microphthalmos with a normal cornea (Bateman 1984) and microcornea without microphthalmos (Judisch *et al.* 1979). Ultrasonographic determination of an axial length less than 21 mm in an adult or 19 mm in a 1-year-old child substantiates a diagnosis of microphthalmos (François & Goes 1977; Weiss *et al.* 1989a, b). This represents 2 SD below normal.

Bilateral microphthalmos is a relatively rare condition (Heimonen *et al.* 1977) but it accounted for approximately 10% of blind children in one study (Fujiki *et al.* 1989).

The defect of vision depends on whether it is bilateral and on the severity of the microphthalmos, specifically the horizontal corneal diameter, the presence of cataract and coloboma (Elder 1994).

Microphthalmos may be designated as simple (without other ocular disease) or complex (associated with cataract, retinal or vitreous disease, or more complex malformations) (Weiss *et al.* 1989a, b). It can be further divided into colobomatous (Fig. 20.2) and non-colobomatous categories (Bateman 1984; Warburg 1993) on the basis of associated uveal abnormalities. The association between eye growth and closure of the fetal fissure are linked and important since closure of the cleft is completed early in development (Mann 1964).

Microphthalmos probably represents a non-specific growth failure in response to a very wide variety of prenatal insults. Many causal associations of microphthalmos have been suggested, and possible causes must be kept in mind while considering the child's overall health. Bateman (1984) and others have carefully identified and classified microphthalmos according to heredity, environmental causes, chromosomal aberration and unknown causes which have additional systemic abnormalities (Lindsay *et al.* 1994).

Isolated microphthalmos

Idiopathic microphthalmos

Some eyes that are otherwise healthy may be below 2 SD in size. Vision is variably affected, depending on the degree to which the eye is microphthalmic. There may be

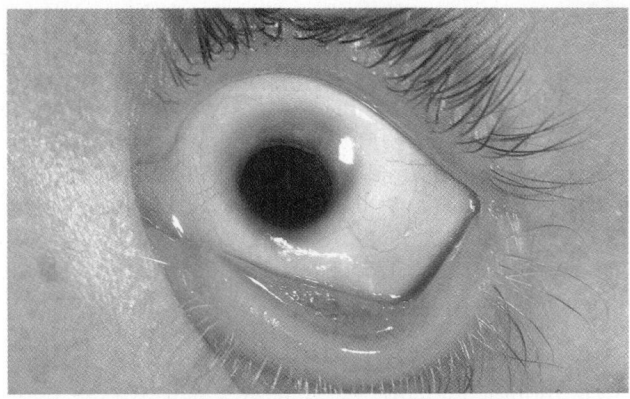

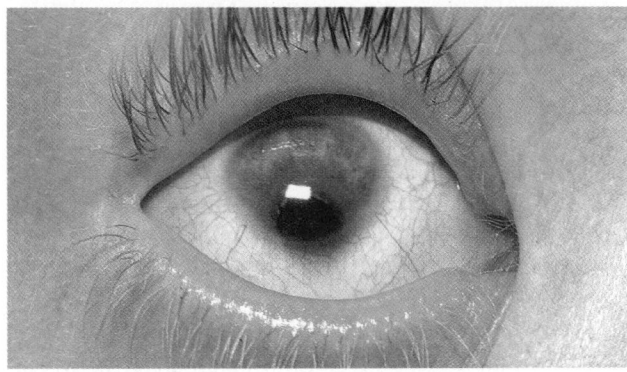

Fig. 20.2 Colobomatous microphthalmos. Both eyes are generally small with an inferior coloboma in the fundus. Although vision was limited to an acuity of 2/60 in each eye, the patient had a useful field and navigated without problems.

no obvious inheritance pattern, but care is needed in genetic counselling because of the possibility of new mutations and recessive inheritance

Inherited isolated microphthalmos

These are inherited as follows.
1 Autosomal dominant (Figs 20.3, 20.4) (Russell-Eggitt *et al.* 1985).
2 Autosomal recessive (Kohn *et al.* 1988).
3 X-linked recessive (Graham *et al.* 1991).
Graham *et al.*'s seven males from three generations also had mental retardation; the gene was localized to Xq27–28.

Microphthalmos with ocular abnormalities

Microphthalmos is a non-specific response to a wide variety of influences; therefore it occurs with many severe eye diseases, including the following.
1 Anterior segment malformations, i.e. Peters' anomaly, Rieger's anomaly, and so on (Siber 1984; Shields *et al.* 1985; Ghose *et al.* 1991; DePaepe *et al.* 1993).
2 Cataract (see Chapter 39). Yokoyama *et al.* (1992) described a family with a translocation defect t(2;16), the

breakpoint was at 16p13.3 (Witkop-Oostenrijk 1956; Capella *et al.* 1963).
3 Persistent hyperplastic vitreous (see Chapter 39) (Haddad *et al.* 1978). Traboulsi and Parks (1990) described this in the autosomal dominant oculodentodigital syndrome.
4 Retinal diseases:
 • retinopathy of prematurity (see Chapter 43);
 • retinal dysplasia, i.e. Norrie's disease HARD+/-E syndrome (see Chapter 41), the osteoporosis–pseudoglioma syndrome (De Paepe *et al.* 1993);
 • retinal folds (Young *et al.* 1987);
 • retinal degeneration and glaucoma (Herrmann 1958; Franceschetti & Gernet 1965).
5 Aniridia. Edwards *et al.* (1984) described a family of three generations with aniridia, anophthalmos, and microcephaly.
6 Coloboma (see Chapter 50). Coloboma is the most common association of microphthalmos (Pagon *et al.* 1981; Schachenmann *et al.* 1965; Schinzel *et al.* 1981; Traboulsi *et al.* 1988) and is found in many of the microphthalmos syndromes below.

Microphthalmos with systemic disease

1 MIDAS, or the Temple–al Gazali, syndrome. The microphthalmos, dermal aplasia and sclerocornea (MIDAS) syndrome (Fig. 20.5) is the result of a deletion of Xp22.2–pter; patients have linear, irregular areas of skin aplasia especially of the head and neck, microphthalmos with variable sclerocornea and usually normal intelli-

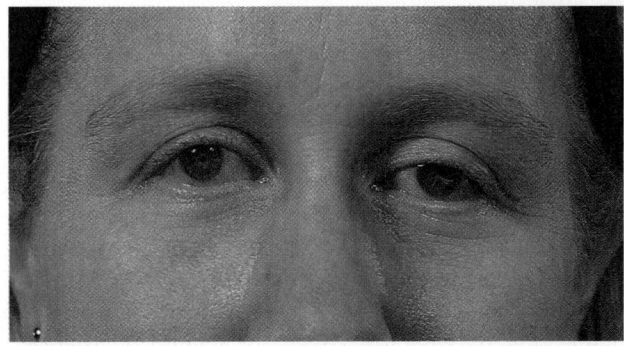

Fig. 20.3 Bilateral non-colobomatous microphthalmos in an adult.

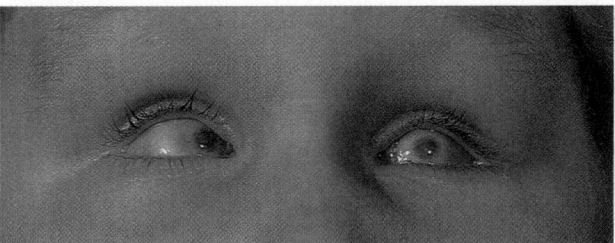

Fig. 20.4 Child of the patient in Fig. 20.3 was born with bilateral marked microphthalmos.

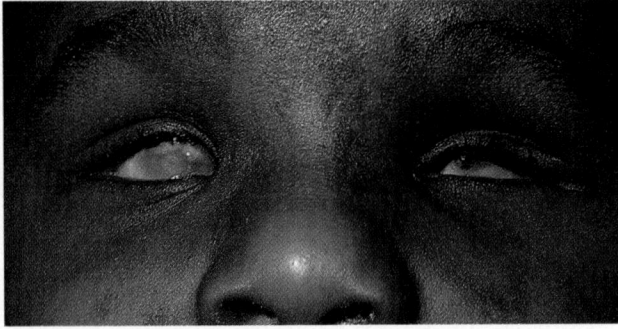

Fig. 20.5 The Temple–al-Gazali (MIDAS) syndrome showing extreme microphthalmos and characteristic skin lesions.

gence (al Gazali 1990; Temple *et al.* 1990b; McLeod *et al.* 1994). They are female or at least have two X chromosomes (Lindsay *et al.* 1994).

2 Chromosomal syndromes. Chromosomal disorders are often associated with colobomatous microphthalmos (see Chapter 50). Warburg and Friedrich (1987) have reviewed the association of coloboma or microphthalmos with mental retardation and found that chromosomal aberrations were common.

3 Mental retardation. Many patients with microphthalmos-associated syndromes are mentally retarded. Isolated mental retardation may also occur: Wilkes and Stephenson (1983) described it as an autosomal recessive disorder; Graham *et al.* (1991) as an X-linked trait.

4 Macrosomia/cleft palate (Teebi *et al.* 1989).

5 Facial defects:
- with midline brain defects (Fig. 20.6a) (Temple *et al.* 1990a);
- in the branchio-oculofacial syndrome: broad nose with large lateral pillars, branchial sinuses and orbital cysts (Fielding and Fryer 1992; McCool & Weaver 1994);
- in frontal facionasal dysplasia (White *et al.* 1991; Reardon *et al.* 1994);
- other clefting syndromes (Fig. 20.6b).

6 Delleman syndrome. Skin tags, punched-out lesions of the skin on ears and elsewhere, mental retardation, hydrocephalus, brain malformations and orbital cysts (DeCock & Merizian 1992).

7 Ectodermal dysplasia (Wallis & Beighton 1992).

8 Blepharophimosis, ptosis, epicanthus inversus. Fujita *et al.* (1992) described a boy with a chromosomal deletion (3)(q12 q32).

9 Microcephaly, urogenital anomalies (Siber 1984).

10 Growth retardation, microcephaly, brachycephaly, oligophrenia syndrome (GOMBO syndrome) (Verloes *et al.* 1989).

11 Dental anomalies. The oculodentodigital syndrome (Traboulsi & Parks 1990). Enamel hypoplasia, spasticity, glaucoma (Franceschetti & Gernet 1965).

12 Fetal infections: rubella, varicella, influenza, and toxoplasmosis.

13 Fetal toxins: vitamin A, alcohol, warfarin, thalidomide, hyperthermia (Milunsky *et al.* 1992).

14 Microphthalmos with syndactyly, oligodactyly and other limb defects and mental retardation: 'Waardenburg's recessive anophthalmia syndrome' (Richieri-Costa 1983; Traboulsi *et al.* 1984).

15 Cross syndrome. This autosomal recessive syndrome associates microphthalmos with corneal opacities and albinism and severe mental retardation (Lerone *et al.* 1992).

The ophthalmologist faced with a new patient with microphthalmos must carefully address several questions:

1 What is the level of visual function?

2 What is the refractive error; if it is asymmetrical is amblyopia present in addition?

3 Are any colobomas present?

4 Is there evidence of glaucoma or uveal effusion?

Additionally, the ophthalmologist in conjunction with the primary care physician must answer these critical questions:

1 Are there any contributing factors to its presence such as congenital infection, chromosomal abnormality or environmental factors?

2 Is there a risk of involvement in future children?

3 Are there life-threatening associations (such as cardiac defect) or factors which may alter parental expectations of the child (such as mental retardation or deafness)?

Ophthalmic intervention *per se* is limited to prescribing glasses to offset amblyogenic refractive errors, arranging

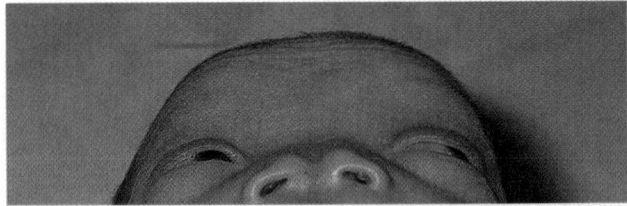

a

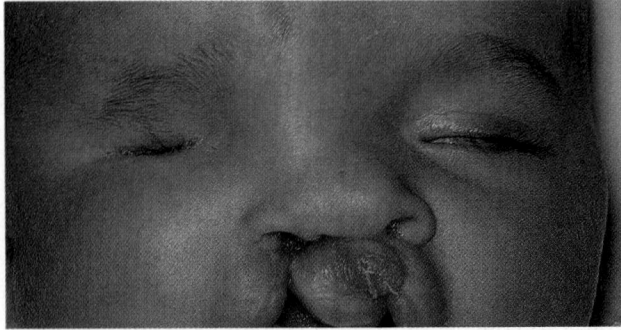

b

Fig. 20.6 (a) Bilateral microphthalmos with a midline defect. Note the bifid nose. (b) Right clinical anophthalmos, left microphthalmos in a child with bilateral cleft lip and palate.

for assessment of low vision, supervising the ocularist's role in fitting cosmetic shells or contact lenses in non-seeing eyes, and diagnosing and treating glaucoma. Microphthalmic eyes with corneal opacities may rarely be successfully treated by corneal grafting (Feldman *et al.* 1987).

Microphthalmos with orbital cyst

One unusual form of microphthalmos can present with progressive swelling from birth (see Fig. 20.1). The eye often cannot be seen, and the uninitiated ophthalmologist often initially fears a rapidly growing neoplasm. This condition is a colobomatous microphthalmos where cyst formation occurs on the course of the optic nerve, often with free communication with the intraocular contents (Dollfus *et al.* 1968; Makley & Battles 1969; Helveston *et al.* 1970; Waring *et al.* 1976; Leatherbarrow *et al.* 1990; Pasquale *et al.* 1991). Presentation may be as a massive orbital mass distending the lids and hiding the eye or as proptosis in which a microphthalmic eye is visible. Ultrasonography (Fisher 1978) and CT or MRI scanning (Weiss *et al.* 1985) aid in its diagnosis. Although management is usually conservative, extremely large cysts may be handled either with repeated aspiration (Weiss *et al.* 1985) or surgical removal of the cyst (Makley & Battles 1969; Waring *et al.* 1976). Because of the communication of the cyst with the eye, the removal of the cyst may necessarily deflate the microphthalmic eye which may need to be removed. Microphthalmos may occur in the Delleman syndrome (Pasquale *et al.* 1991; DeCock & Merizian 1992), and may be inherited as an autosomal trait (Porges *et al.* 1992). The relationship between microphthalmos and congenital cystic eye (Pasquale *et al.* 1991) is not clear (see also Chapter 35).

Cryptophthalmos

The cryptophthalmos syndrome (Walton *et al.* 1990) describes the concurrence of microphthalmos with a varying degree of skin covering the eyeball and lids being variably attached to the cornea.

Francois (1969) described three subgroups:
1 Complete cryptophthalmos (Fig. 20.7). The lids are replaced by a layer of skin without lashes or glands, and the skin is fused with the microphthalmic eye without a conjunctival sac. Normal electrophysiological responses have been recorded in this form of cryptophthalmos (Hing *et al.* 1990).
2 Incomplete cryptophthalmos. The lids are colobomatous (often medially), or rudimentary and there is a small conjunctival sac. The exposed cornea is often opaque.
3 Abortive form. In this form the upper lid is partly fused with the upper cornea and conjunctiva (Fig. 20.8) and may

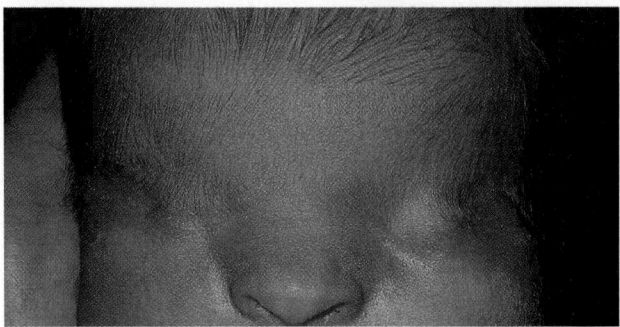

Fig. 20.7 Complete cryptophthalmos. Note the characteristic abnormality of the hair extending to the brow and the abnormality of the nose.

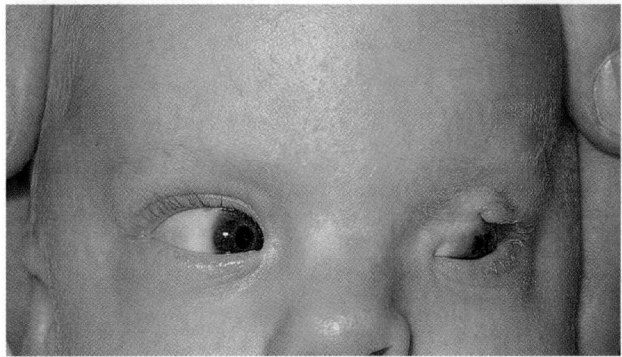

Fig. 20.8 Partial cryptophthalmos of the left eye. The eye is small and the cornea is opaque. There is a colobomatous upper lid and a characteristic 'lick' of hair from the temple to the brow with a unilateral nose abnormality.

be colobomatous (Walton *et al.* 1990). The globe is often small.

The systemic associations include nose deformities, cleft lip and palate, syndactyly, abnormal genitalia, renal agenesis, mental retardation, and many others (François 1969; Ide & Wollschlaeger 1969; Brazier *et al.* 1986; Thomas *et al.* 1986; Walton *et al.* 1990). Surgical treatment is often unsatisfactory and mainly indicated to protect an eye at risk from further deterioration of corneal clarity (see also Chapter 21).

Nanophthalmos

Nanophthalmos (Figs 20.9–20.12) is a rare disease characterized by a small eye, high hypermetropia, a weak but thick sclera with abnormal collagen (Stewart *et al.* 1991), and a tendency to angle closure glaucoma (O'Grady 1971; Calhoun 1975) and uveal effusion (Brockhurst 1974). There is an increased fibronectin level in nanophthalmic sclera and cells (Yue *et al.* 1988). Fibronectin is a glycoprotein involved with cellular adhesion and healing.

Any surgery, but especially intraocular surgery and

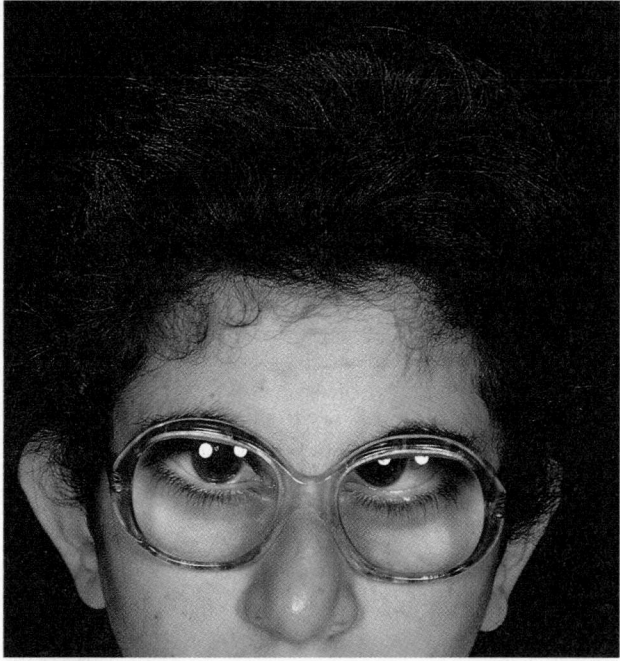

Fig. 20.9 Nanophthalmos showing the high hypermetropia. The phakic correction was +10.0 right, +11.0 left.

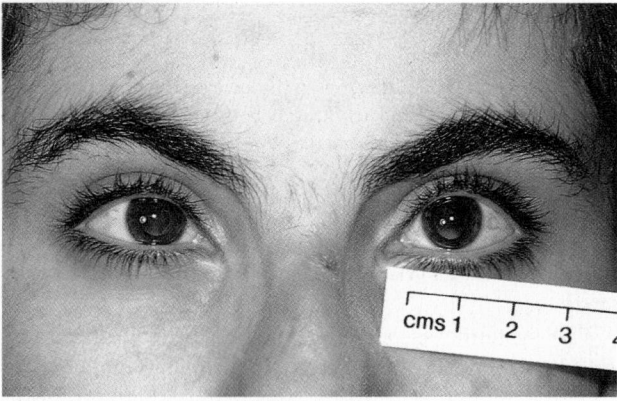

Fig. 20.10 Nanophthalmos showing small eyes and abnormal reflex.

even laser trabeculoplasty (Good & Stern 1988; Brockhurst 1990; Jin & Anderson 1990) may be complicated by severe uveal effusion and should be avoided where possible. Vortex vein decompression may reduce the incidence of uveal effusion (Brockhurst 1990). Some cases may be autosomal recessive. MacKay *et al.* (1987) described a consanguineous family with seven affected offspring, with a pigmentary retinopathy, cystic macular degeneration, high hypermetropia, nanophthalmos and angle closure glaucoma.

Cyclopia and synophthalmos

Complete (cyclopic) or partial (synophthalmos) fusion of

the two eyes is a very rare birth defect. The brain also fails to develop two hemispheres (Llorca 1955), and the orbit has gross deformities. The defects are incompatible with life except in very rare circumstances (Panum 1878).

These conditions result from inadequate embryonic neural tissue anteriorly, with subsequent maldevelopment of midline mesodermal structures (Torczynski *et al.* 1977). Because of the close parallel of eye and central nervous system embryological development, the brain is almost always malformed as well (Leech & Shuman 1986), the telencephalon fails to divide, and a large dorsal cyst develops (Mettler 1947). Midline structures such as the corpus callosum, septum pellucidum, and olfactory lobes are often not present (Jellinger *et al.* 1981; Kuchle *et al.* 1991) and anomalies may extend to the mesencephalic region with thalamic abnormalities.

The orbits are markedly affected as a consequence of

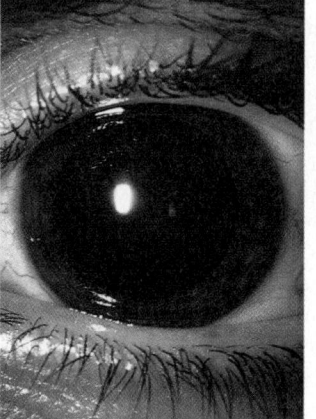
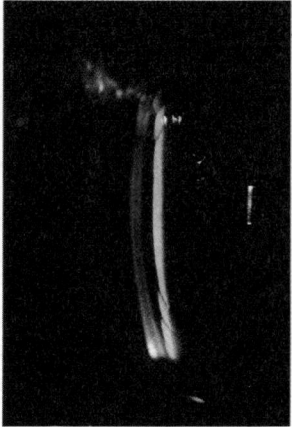

Fig. 20.11 Nanophthalmos showing the shallow anterior chamber. The eyes are prone to angle closure glaucoma.

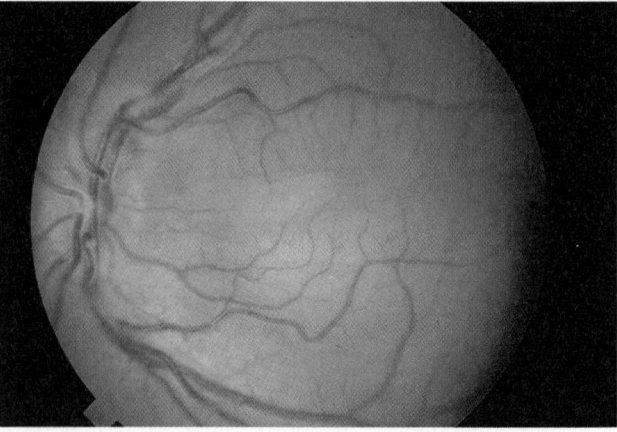

Fig. 20.12 Nanophthalmos showing the crowded optic disc and prominent yellow foveal pigment with a fold between the fovea and the macula. Nanophthalmic eyes are very prone to choroidal effusions in response to intraocular surgery.

the abnormal development of midline mesodermal structures. The normal nasal cavity is replaced by the 'pseudo-orbit' (Duke-Elder 1964), and the bones show multiple malformations, especially in midline structures. The defects additionally involve the skull, with absence of the sella turcica and clinoids.

The eyes are more commonly partly fused than completely fused. One optic nerve is present, and no chiasm is recognizable. Structures are best developed laterally, such as the muscles innervated by cranial nerves IV and VI in comparison to those innervated by cranial nerve III (Gartner 1947). Other intraocular abnormalities may exist such as persistent hyperplastic primary vitreous, cataract, coloboma and microcornea (Spencer 1985).

Chromosomal aberrations are commonly present (Batts *et al.* 1972; Fujimoto *et al.* 1973; Howard 1977; Kuchle *et al.* 1991). Familial occurrences and association with consanguineous marriages have also been noted (Howard 1977).

Other aetiological considerations include maternal health (Stabile *et al.* 1985) and toxic factors. Evidence for this is based on a high incidence in animals who grazed on an alkaloid-containing substance (Bryden *et al.* 1971).

The importance of cyclopia and synophthalmos is primarily one of academic embryological interest; the overwhelming systemic abnormalities place management of this condition in the hands of perinatologists and geneticists.

Diplophthalmos

Stefani *et al.* (1991) reported the presence of a double eye unilaterally with associated head and neck abnormalities.

References

al Gazali LI, Mueller RF, Caine A, Antonion A, McCartney A, Fitchett M, Dennis NR. Two 46,XX,t(X;Y) females with linear skin defects and congenital microphthalmia: a new syndrome of Xp 22.3. *J Med Genet* 1990; **27**: 59–63.

Bateman JB. Microphthalmos. *Int Ophthalmol Clin* 1984; **24**: 87–107.

Batts JA, Punnett HH, Valdes-Dapena M, Coles JW, Green WR. A case of cyclopia. *Am J Obstet Gynecol* 1972; **112**: 657–61.

Bogdanoff B, Rorke LB, Yanoff M, Warren WS. Brain and eye abnormalities: possible sequelae to prenatal use of multiple drugs including LSD. *Am J Dis Child* 1972; **123**: 145–8.

Brazier DJ, Hardman-Lea SJ, Collin JRO. Cryptophthalmos: surgical treatment of the congenital symblepharon variant. *Br J Ophthalmol* 1986; **70**: 391–5.

Brockhurst R. Cataract surgery in nanophthalmic eyes. *Arch Ophthalmol* 1990; **108**: 965–8.

Brockhurst RJ. Nanophthalmos with uveal effusion: a new clinical entity. *Trans Am Ophthalmol Soc* 1974; **72**: 371–403.

Brownstein S, Bright M, Kirkharn TH, Carpenter S. Anophthalmos. Report of two cases. *Can J Ophthalmol* 1977; **12**: 143–6.

Brunquell PJ, Papale JH, Horton JC *et al.* Sex-linked hereditary bilat-

eral anophthalmos, pathologic and radiologic correlation. *Arch Ophthalmol* 1984; **102**: 108–13.

Bryden MM, Evans HE, Keeler RF. Cyclopia in sheep caused by plant teratogens. *J Anat* 1971; **110**: 507.

Burton PA, Caul EO. Fetal cell tropism of human parvovirus B19. *Lancet* 1988; **ii**: 767.

Calhoun FP. The management of glaucoma in nanophthalmos. *Trans Am Ophthalmol Soc* 1975; **73**: 97–122.

Capella JA, Kaufman HE, Lill FJ, Cooper G. Hereditary cataracts and microphthalmia. *Am J Ophthalmol* 1963; **56**: 454–8.

De Cock R, Merizian A. Delleman syndrome: a case report and review. *Br J Ophthalmol* 1992; **76**: 115–16.

De Paepe A, Leroy J, Nuytinck L *et al.* Osteoporosis–pseudoglioma syndrome. *Am J Med Genet* 1993; **45**: 30–7.

Dollfus MA, Marx P, Langlois J, Clement JC, Forthomme J. Congenital cystic eyeball. *Am J Ophthalmol* 1968; **66**: 504–9.

Duke-Elder S. Anomalies in the size of the eye. In: *Normal and Abnormal Development. System of Ophthalmology*, Vol. III, Part 2. London: Kimpton, 1964: 429–51, 488–90.

Edwards J, Lampert R, Hammer M, Young S. Ocular defects and dysmorphic features in three generations. *J Clin Dysmorphol* 1984; **2**: 8–12.

Elder MJ. Aetiology of severe visual impairment and blindness in microphthalmos. *Br J Ophthalmol* 1994; **78**: 332–4.

Feldman ST, Frucht-Pery J, Brown SI. Corneal transplantation in microphthalmic eyes. *Am J Ophthalmol* 1987; **104**: 164–7.

Fielding DW, Fryer AL. Recurrence of orbital cysts in the branchio-oculo facial syndrome. *J Med Genet* 1992; **29**: 430–1.

Fisher YL. Microphthalmos with ocular communicating cyst — ultrasonic diagnosis. *Ophthalmology* 1978; **85**: 1208–11.

Franceschetti A, Gernet H. Diagnostic ultrasonique d'une microphthalmic sans microscornee, avec macrophakie haute hypermetropie associee avec une degeneresence tapeto retinienne, une disposition glaucomateuse et des anomalies dentaires. *Arch Ophthal (Paris)* 1965; **25**: 105–16.

Francois J. Syndrome malformatif avec cryptophtalmie. *Acta Genet Med Gemellol (Roma)* 1969; **18**: 18–50.

Francois J, Goes F. Ultrasonographic study of 1010 emmetropic eyes. *Ophthalmologica* 1977; **175**: 321–7.

Fujiki K, Nakajima A, Yasuda N *et al.* Genetic analysis of microphthalmos. *Ophthal Paediatr Genet* 1989; **1**: 139–49.

Fujimoto A, Ebbin AJ, Towner JW, Wilson MG. Trisomy 13 in two infants with cyclops. *J Med Genet* 1973; **10**: 294–6.

Fujita H, Meng J, Kawamura M *et al.* Boy with a chromosome deletion (3)(q12q23) and blepharophimosis syndrome. *Am J Med Genet* 1992; **44**: 434–6.

Gartner S. Cyclopia. *Arch Ophthalmol* 1947; **37**: 220–31.

Ghose S, Singh N, Kaur D, Verma I. Microphthalmos and anterior segment dysgenesis in a family. *Ophthal Paediatr Genet* 1991; **12**: 177–82.

Gilbert R. 'Clusters' of anophthalmia in Britain. *Br Med J* 1993; **307**: 340–1.

Glaser T, Jepeal L, Edwards J, Young S, Favor J, Maas I. PAX6 gene dosage effect in a family with congenital cataracts, aniridia, anophthalmia, and central nervous system defects. *Nature Genet* 1994; **7**: 463–71.

Good WV, Stern WH. Recurrent nanophthalmic uveal effusion syndrome following laser trabeculoplasty. *Am J Ophthalmol* 1988; **106**: 234–5.

Graham CA, Redmond RM, Nevin L. X-linked clinical anophthalmos: localisation of the gene to Xq27-Xq28. *Ophthal Paediatr Genet* 1991; **12**: 43–8.

Guyer DR, Green WR. Bilateral extreme microphthalmos. *Ophthal*

Paediatr Genet 1984; **4**: 81–90.

Guyuron B, Dagys AP, Munro IR, Ross RB. Effect of irradiation on facial growth: a 7- to 25-year follow-up. *Ann Plast Surg* 1983; **11**: 493–7.

Haddad R, Font RL, Resser F. Persistent hyperplastic primary vitreous: a clinicopathological study of 62 cases and review of the literature. *Surv Ophthalmol* 1978; **23**: 123–43.

Hall BD. Choanal atresia and associated multiple anomalies. *J Pediatr* 1979; **95**: 395–8.

Hartwig NG, Vermeij-Keers C, Van Elsacker-Niele AMW, Fleuren CJ. Embryonic malformations in a case of intrauterine Parvovirus B19 infection. *Teratology* 1989; **39**: 295–302.

Heinonen OP, Shapiro S, Slone D. *Birth Defects and Drugs in Pregnancy*. Massachusetts: Publishing Sciences Group, 1977.

Helveston EM, Malone E, Lashmet MH. Congenital cystic eye. *Arch Ophthalmol* 1970; **84**: 622–4.

Hermann P. Le syndrome: microphthalmie-retinite pigmentaine-glaucome. *Arch Ophthal (Paris)* 1958; **18**: 17–24.

Hing S, Wilson-Holt N, Kriss A, Flueler U, Taylor D. Complete cryptophthalmos: case report with normal flash VEP and ERG. *J Pediatr Ophthalmol Strabismus* 1990; **27**: 133–6.

Howard RO. Chromosomal abnormalities associated with cyclopia and synophthalmia. *Trans Am Ophthalmol Soc* 1977; **75**: 505–38.

Ide CH, Wollschlaeger PB. Multiple congenital abnormalities associated with cryptophthalmia. *Arch Ophthalmol* 1969; **81**: 640–4.

Jellinger K, Gross H, Kaltenback E, Grisold W. Holoprosencephaly and agenesis of the corpus callosum: frequency of associated malformations. *Acta Neuropathol (Berlin)* 1981; **55**: 1–10.

Jin J, Anderson D. Laser and unsutured sclerotomy in nanophthalmos. *Am J Ophthalmol* 1990; **109**: 575–81.

Judisch GF, Martin-Casals A, Hanson JW, Olin WH. Oculodentodigital dysplasia. Four new reports and a literature review. *Arch Ophthalmol* 1979; **97**: 878–84.

Kennedy RE. The effect of early enucleation on the orbit in animals and humans. *Am J Ophthalmol* 1965; **60**: 277–306.

Kennedy RE. Growth retardation and volume determination of the anophthalmic orbit. *Am J Ophthalmol* 1973; **76**: 294–302.

Kohn G, Shawwa ER. Isolated 'clinical anophthalmia' in an extremely affected Arab kindred. *Clin Genet* 1988; **33**: 321–4.

Kuchle M, Kraus J, Rummelt C, Naumann GOM. Synophthalmia and holoprosencephaly in chromosome 18p deletion defect. *Arch Ophthalmol* 1991; **109**: 136–8.

Leatherbarrow B, Kwartz J, Noble J. Microphthalmos with cyst in monozygous twins. *J Pediatr Ophthalmol Strabismus* 1990; **27**: 294–9.

Leech RW, Shuman RM. Holoprosencephaly and related midline cerebral anomalies: a review. *J Child Neurol* 1986; **1**: 3–18.

Lerone M, Persagno A, Taccone A *et al*. Oculocerebral syndrome with hypopigmentation. *Clin Genet* 1992; **41**: 87–9.

Lindsay EA, Gutto A, Ferrero GB *et al*. Microphthalmia with linear skin defects (MLS) syndrome. *Am J Med Genet* 1994; **49**: 229–34.

Llorca FO. Le cerveau et l'oeil de deux embryons humains cyclopes de 37 et 45 jours. *Acta Anat (Basel)* 1955; **23**: 379–85.

McCool M, Weaver DD. Branchio-oculo-facial syndrome: broadening the spectrum. *Am J Med Genet* 1994; **49**:414–21.

McLeod S, Sugar J, Elejalde B, Eng A, Lebel R. Gazali–Temple syndrome. *Arch Ophthalmol* 1994; **112**: 851–2.

MacKay CJ, Shek MS, Carr RE, Yanuzzi LA, Gouras P. Retinal degeneration with nanophthalmos, cystic macular degeneration, and angle closure glaucoma. A new recessive syndrome. *Arch Ophthalmol* 1987; **105**: 366–71.

Makley TA, Battles M. Microphthalmos with cyst. Report of two cases in the same family. *Surv Ophthalmol* 1969; **13**: 200–6.

Mann I. *Developmental Abnormalities of the Eye*. Cambridge: Cambridge University Press, 1937: 46–64.

Mann I. *The Development of the Human Eye*, 3rd edn. London: British Medical Association, 1964: 277.

Mettler FA. Congenital malformation of the brain. Critical review. *J Neuropathol Exp Neurol* 1947; **6**: 98–110.

Milunsky A, Ulcickas M, Rothman AJ *et al*. Maternal heat exposure and neural tube defects. *J Am Med Assoc* 1992; **268**: 882–5.

O'Grady RB. Nanophthalmos. *Am J Ophthalmol* 1971; **71**: 1251–3.

O'Keefe M, Webb M, Pashby RC, Wagman RD. Clinical anophthalmos. *Br J Ophthalmol* 1987; **71**: 635–8.

Pagon RA, Graham JM, Zonana J, Young S-L. Coloboma, congenital heart disease, and choanal atresia with multiple anomalies: CHARGE association. *J Pediatr* 1981; **99**: 223–7.

Panum PL. Beitrage zur Kenntniss der physiologischen Bedeutung der argebornen Missbildungen. *Virch Arch Pathol Anat* 1878; **72**: 289–324.

Pasquale LR, Romayananda N, Kubacki J, Johnson MH, Chan GH. Congenital cystic eye with multiple ocular and intracranial anomalies. *Arch Ophthalmol* 1991; **109**: 985–7.

Pearce WG, Nigam S, Rootman J. Primary anophthalmos histological and genetic features. *Can J Ophthalmol* 1974; **9**: 141–5.

Pe'er J, BenEzra D. Heterotopic smooth muscle in the choroid of two patients with cryptophthalmos. *Arch Ophthalmol* 1986; **104**: 1665–70.

Peyton WT. A topographic study of the orbit and bulbus oculi during a part of the growth period. *Anat Rec* 1940; **76**: 343–55.

Pfeiffer RL. The effect of enucleation on the orbit. *Trans Am Acad Ophthalmol Otolaryngol* 1945; **49**: 236–9.

Pico G, Townsend W. Congenital and developmental anomalies of the orbit. In: Jones IS, Jakobiec FA, eds. *Diseases of the Orbit*. Hagerstow: Harper & Row, 1979: 123–33.

Porges Y, Gersoni-Baruch R, Leibu R, Zanis S, Shapira I, Miller B. Hereditary microphthalmia with colobomatous cyst. *Am J Ophthalmol* 1992; **114**: 30–4.

Reardon W, Winter RM, Taylor D, Baraitser M. Frontofacionasal dysplasia: a new case and review of the phenotype. *Clin Dysmorph* 1994; **3**: 70–4.

Richiem-Costa A, Gallop TR, Otto P. Autosomal recessive anophthalmia with multiple congenital abnormalities — type Waardenburg. *Am J Med Genet* 1983; **14**: 607–15.

Russell-Eggitt I, Fielder A, Levene M. Microphthalmos in a family. *Ophthal Paediatr Genet* 1985; **6**: 121–8.

Sassani JW, Yanoff M. Anophthalmos in an infant with multiple congenital anomalies. *Am J Ophthalmol* 1977; **83**: 43–8.

Schachenmann G, Schmid W, Fraccaro M, Mannini A, Tiepolo L, Perona GP, Sartori E. Chromosomes in coloboma and anal atresia. *Lancet* 1965; **ii**: 290.

Schinzel A, Schmid W, Fraccaro M *et al*. The cat-eye syndrome: dicentric small marker chromosome probably derived from a 22 (tetrasomy 22 pter-qt1) associated with a characteristic phenotype: report of 11 patients and delineation of the clinical picture. *Hum Genet* 1981; **57**: 148–58.

Sheilds MB, Buckley E, Klintworth GK, Thresher R. Axenfeld–Rieger syndrome; a spectrum of developmental disorders. *Surv Ophthalmol* 1985; **29**: 387–409.

Siber M. X-linked recessive microcephaly microphthalmia with corneal opacities, spastic quadriplegia, hypospadius and cryptorchidism. *Clin Genet* 1984; **26**: 453–6.

Soll DB. The anophthalmic socket. *Ophthalmology* 1982; **89**: 407–23.

Spencer WH. Abnormalities of scleral thickness and congenital anomalies. In: Spencer WH, ed. *Ophthalmic Pathology. An Atlas and Textbook*, 3rd edn. Philadelphia: WB Saunders, 1985: 394–5.

Stabile M, Bianco A, Iannuzzi S, Buonocore MC, Ventruto V. A case of suspected keratogenic holoprosencephaly. *J Med Genet* 1985; **22**: 147–9.

Starceski PJ, Lee PA, Blatt J, Finegold D, Brown D. Comparable effects of l800- and 2400-rad (18- and 24-cGy) cranial irradiation on height and weight in children treated for acute lymphocytic leukemia. *Am J Dis Child* 1987; **141**: 550–2.

Stefani FH, Hausmann N, Lund OE. Unilateral diplophthalmos. *Am J Ophthalmol* 1991; **112**: 581–6.

Stewart DH, Streeten BW, Brockhurst RJ, Anderson DR, Hirose T, Gass JD. Abnormal scleral collagen in nanophthalmos: an ultra-structural study. *Arch Ophthalmol* 1991; **109**: 1017–19.

Teebi AS, Al Saleh Q, Hassoon M *et al*. Macrosomia microphthalmia with or without cleft palate and early infant death: a new autoso-mal recessive syndrome. *Clin Genet* 1989; **36**: 174–7.

Temple IK, Brunner H, Jones B *et al*. Midline facial defects with ocular colobomata. *Am J Med Genet* 1990a; **37**: 23–7.

Temple IK, Hurst JA, Hing S, Butler L, Baraitser M. *De novo* deletion of Xp22.2pter in a female with linear skin lesions of the face and neck, microphthalmia and anterior chamber eye anomalies. *J Med Genet* 1990b; **27**: 56–8.

Thomas IT, Frias JL, Felix V, Sanchez de Lear L, Hernandez RA, Jones MC. Isolated and syndromic cryptophthalmos. *Am J Med Genet* 1986; **25**: 85–98.

Torczynski E, Jacobiec FA, Johnston MC, Font RL, Madewell JA. Syn-ophthalmia and cyclopia: a histopathologic, radiographic, and organogenetic analysis. *Documenta Ophthalmol* 1977; **94**: 311–28.

Traboulsi EI, Lenz W, Gonzales-Ramas M, Siegel J, Macrae WG, Maumenee IH. The Lenz microphthalmia syndrome. *Am J Ophthal-mol* 1988; **105**: 40–5.

Traboulsi EI, Nasr A, Fahd S *et al*. Waardenberg's recessive anoph-thalmia syndrome. *Ophthal Paediatr Genet* 1984; **4**: 3–18.

Traboulsi EI, Parks MM. Glaucoma in oculo-dento-osseous dyspla-sia. *Am J Ophthalmol* 1990; **109**: 310–13.

Tucker SM, Sapp N, Collin R. Orbital expansion of the congenitally anophthalmic socket. *Br J Ophthalmol* 1995; **79**: 667–71.

Verloes A, Delfortrie J, Lambott C. GOMBO syndrome of growth retardation, ocular abnormalities, microcephaly, brachydactyly and digephrenia: a possible 'new' recessively inherited syndrome. *Am J Med Genet* 1989; **32**: 13–18.

Yokoyama Y, Narahara K, Tsuji K *et al*. Autosomal dominant congeni-tal cataract and cataract associated with a familial translocation +(2;16). *Hum Genet* 1992; **90**: 177–8.

Wallis CE, Beighton P. Ectodermal dysplasia with blindness in sibs on the island of Rodrigues. *J Med Genet* 1992; **29**: 323–5.

Walton WT, Enzenauer RW, Cornell FM. Abortive cryptophthalmos: a case report and a review of cryptophthalmos. *J Pediatr Ophthalmol Strabismus* 1990; **27**: 129–33.

Warburg M. Classification of microphthalmos and coloboma. *J Med Genet* 1993; **30**: 664–9.

Warburg M. Genetics of microphthalmos. *Int Ophthalmol* 1981a; **4**: 45–65.

Warburg M. Diagnostic precision in microphthalmos and coloboma of heterogenous origin. *Ophthal Paediatr Genet* 1981b; **1**: 37–42.

Warburg M, Friedrich U. Coloboma and microphthalmos in chromo-somal aberrations. Chromosomal aberrations and neural crest cell developmental field. *Ophthal Paediatr Genet* 1987; **8**: 105–18.

Waring GO, Roth AM, Rodrigues MM. Clinicopathologic correlation of microphthalmos with cyst. *Am J Ophthalmol* 1976; **82**: 714–21.

Weiss AH, Kausseff BG, Ros EA, Longbottom J. Complex microph-thalmos. *Arch Ophthalmol* 1989a; **107**: 1619–24.

Weiss AH, Kausseff BG, Ros EA, Longbottom J. Simple microph-thalmos. *Arch Ophthalmol* 1989b; **107**: 1625–30.

Weiss A, Martinez C, Greenwald M. Microphthalmos with cyst: clini-cal presentations and computed tomographic findings. *J Pediatr Ophthalmol Strabismus* 1985; **22**: 6–12.

White E, Figueroa R, Flannery DB. Frontofacionasal dysplasia. *Am J Med Genet* 1991; **40**: 338–40.

Wilkes G, Stephenson R. Microphthalmia, microcornea and mental retardation: an autosomal recessive disorder. *Proc Or Genet Center* 1983; **2**: 14–19.

Witkop-Oostenrijk GA. Microphthalmia, microcornea and congeni-tal cataract. *Ned Tijdschr Geneeskd* 1956; **100**: 2910–13.

Young I, Fielder A, Simpson K. Microcephaly, microphthalmos and retinal folds: report of a family. *J Med Genet* 1987; **24**: 172–84.

Yue BYJT, Kurosawa A, Duvall J, Goldberg MF, Tso MOM, Sugar J. Nanophthalmic sclera. Fibronectin studies. *Ophthalmology* 1988; **95**: 56–60.

Zeiter HJ. Congenital microphthalmos. A pedigree of four affected siblings and an additional report of 44 sporadic cases. *Am J Oph-thalmol* 1963; **55**: 910–22.

Zimmerman LE, Font RL. Congenital malformations of the eye. Some recent advances in knowledge of the pathogenesis and histopatho-logical characteristics. *J Am Med Assoc* 1966; **196**: 684–92.

21: Lids

David Reynolds and Richard Collin

Embryology and anatomy

During the first month of embryonic development, the optic vesicle is covered by a thin layer of surface ectoderm. During the second month, active cellular proliferation of the adjacent mesoderm results in the formation of a circular fold of mesoderm lined on both sides by ectoderm. This fold constitutes the rudiments of the eyelid which gradually elongates over the eye. The mesodermal portion of the upper lid arises from the frontal nasal process, the lower lid from the maxillary process. The covering layer of ectoderm becomes skin on the outside and the conjunctiva on the inside. Tarsal plate, connective and muscular tissues of the eyelids are derived from the mesodermal core.

The process of fusion of the eyelids by an epithelial seal begins at the two extremities at 8 weeks and is soon complete. The eyelids remain adherent until the end of the fifth to the seventh month. Separation begins from the nasal side, and is usually completed during the sixth or seventh month of development. Very rarely, this process is incomplete at birth in a full-term infant. The specialized structures in the lids develop between 8 weeks and 7 months and by term the lid is fully developed with functioning muscles, lashes and meibomian glands (Sevel 1988).

The eyelids have several characteristic folds. The most conspicuous is a well-demarcated skin crease 3–4 mm above the lid margin which flattens out on depression and becomes deeply recessed when the upper lid is elevated. It divides each lid into an orbital and tarsal portion. The orbital portion lies between the margin of the orbit and the crease, and the tarsal portion lies in direct relationship to the globe. The palpebral fissure—the opening between the upper and lower lids—is the entrance into the conjunctival sac bounded by the margins of the eyelids. This aperture forms an asymmetrical ellipse that is approximately 22–30 mm long and 12–15 mm high when the lids are open (Feingold & Bossert 1974).

When the eyelids are opened in a newborn infant, the upper eyelid may rise well above the cornea while the lower eyelid crosses the inferior margin of the cornea. However, by adulthood the upper eyelid covers the upper 1–2 mm of the cornea while the lower lid lies slightly below its inferior margin (Feingold & Bossert 1974).

The principle muscle involved in opening the upper lid and in maintaining normal lid position is the levator palpebrae superioris. Muller's muscle and the frontalis muscle play an accessory role.

The levator palpebrae superioris arises as a short tendon blended with the underlying origin of the superior rectus from the undersurface of the lesser wing of the sphenoid bone. Its flat muscle belly passes forward below the orbital roof and just superior to the superior rectus muscle until it is about 1 cm behind the orbital septum where it ends in a membranous expansion or aponeurosis. The aponeurosis of the levator spreads out in a fan-shaped manner across the length of the eyelid, inserting primarily into the septum that separates the bundles of the orbicularis oculae muscle in the lower half of the eyelid. Some of the fibres of the aponeurosis also attach to the anterior surface of the tarsal plate. The lateral and medial extensions of the aponeurosis are referred to as its horns. The lateral horn is attached to the orbital tubercle and to the upper aspect of the lateral palpebral ligament. The medial horn is attached to the medial palpebral ligament. The levator palpebrae superioris is innervated by branches from the superior division of the oculomotor nerve.

Muller's muscle is composed of a thin band of smooth muscle fibres about 10 mm in width that arise on the inferior surface of the levator palpebrae superioris. The muscle courses anteriorly directly between the levator aponeurosis and the conjunctiva of the upper eyelid to insert into the superior margin of the tarsus. Branches of the ocular sympathetic pathway innervate the fibres of Muller's muscle.

The eyelid is indirectly elevated by attachment of the frontalis muscle into the superior orbital portions of the orbicularis oculae muscle. The frontalis muscle is innervated by the temporal branch of the facial nerve. A tarsal plate composed of dense connective tissue is found in both the upper and lower eyelids. The upper lid tarsal plate has a marginal length of 29 mm and is 10–12 mm wide. The lower lid tarsal plate is about 4 mm wide.

Congenital eyelid abnormalities

Cryptophthalmos

Cryptophthalmos is a rare condition in which there are marked abnormalities in eyelid development. Several subtypes exist (see Chapter 20). In complete cryptophthalmos, the epithelium that is normally differentiated into cornea and conjunctiva becomes part of the skin that passes continuously from the forehead to the cheek. The eyebrow is usually absent and the globe microphthalmic. In the incomplete form, a rudimentary lid and conjunctival sac is present. Finally, abortive (or symblepharon) cryptophthalmos presents with a normal lower lid and an absent or abnormal upper lid, the forehead skin passing directly to and fusing with the superior cornea (Fig. 21.1). Cryptophthalmos may be an isolated finding or present as part of Fraser's syndrome. Multiple abnormalities may be seen in association including syndactyly and abnormal genitalia (Gupta & Saxena 1963; Sullivan *et al.* 1992).

Ophthalmic management is directed towards protecting the globe and promoting visual development where possible. The reconstructive efforts must be based on the individual deformities. When visual potential exists, or ophthalmic exposure is problematic, surgery should be performed as soon as practicable. Where no visual potential exists and exposure is controlled, surgery should be delayed to allow for the relaxation of tissues which occur as the infant matures (Brazier *et al.* 1986; Sullivan *et al.* 1992).

Coloboma

A congenital eyelid coloboma is a clefting defect which

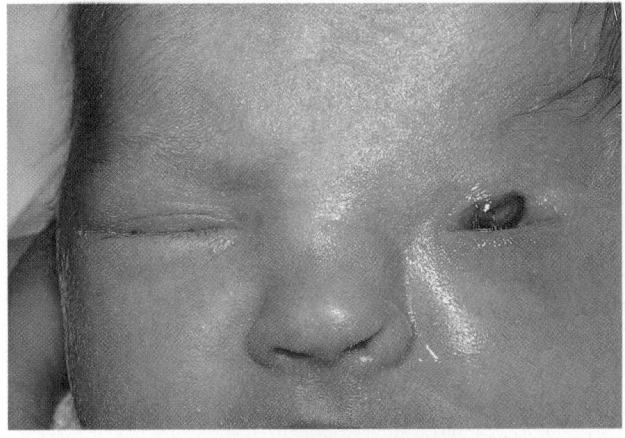

Fig. 21.1 Cryptophthalmos (Fraser's) syndrome. This child with a unilateral form has a fused eye and lid. The upper lid is also defective. The nares are notched on the left. Other features include partial syndactyly, ear anomalies and anomalous genitalia (Gupta & Saxena 1963).

affects primarily the lid margin. It may occur as an isolated anomaly or in association with other clefting abnormalities or first arch syndromes. Eyelid colobomas may be found in all areas of the eyelids but are most commonly found in the nasal half of the upper lid (Roper-Hall 1969). More than one lid may be involved in the same patient, or there may be multiple colobomas in the same lid (Fig. 21.2). The eye itself may be normal or show any degree of abnormalities such as corneal opacities, iris and retinal colobomas extending to microphthalmos and anophthalmos. There may be associated bands which can limit ocular motility and strabismus is common (Collin 1986). Dermoids and dermolipomas are common and are seen in association with external ear abnormalities in Goldenhar's and first arch syndromes.

There may be failure of the eyelid folds to form and fuse which if it is minor leads to a localized eyelid coloboma and if it is major leads to cryptophthalmos. Facial clefts may be caused by a failure of fusion or by pressure from amniotic bands. First arch syndromes may be due to haemorrhages in the developing vascular system or failure of cellular migration. Heredity does not usually play a significant role in the aetiology of most lid colobomas (Smith & Cherubini 1970). An exception is the lower lid coloboma associated with mandibulofacial dysostosis (Treacher–Collins syndrome) which appears to be an autosomal dominant trait of varying penetrance and expressivity.

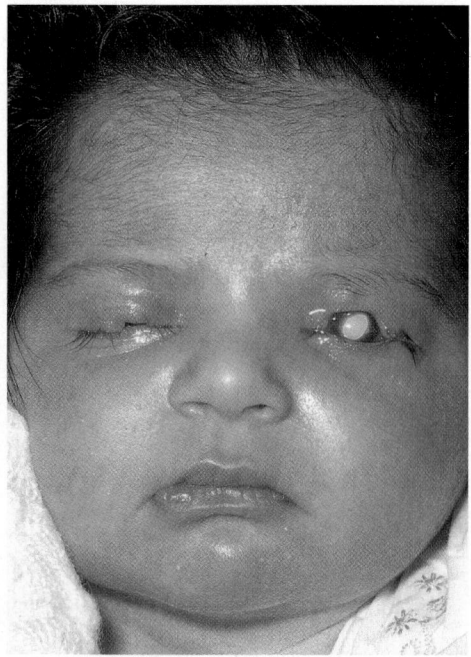

Fig. 21.2 Bilateral lid colobomas in a patient with Goldenhar's syndrome. Since birth this child had corneal exposure on the left from a large lid coloboma which has given rise to drying of the cornea, corneal ulceration and ultimately scarring.

A full ocular examination should be carried out to exclude ocular abnormalities and a forced duction test should be performed on all children with an eyelid coloboma because of the risk of underlying bands. This should be carried out as soon as possible and usually requires an examination under anaesthesia. If the coloboma is small it can often be closed directly at the same time. If a more complicated repair is required this can often wait until early childhood when the tissues are a little larger and the repair simpler, provided any ocular exposure can be controlled with lubricants. If corneal exposure cannot be controlled the eyelid reconstruction must proceed urgently. If any bands limiting ocular motility are detected they must be excised as early as possible attempting to avoid secondary strabismus (Collin 1986).

Ablepharon

Congenital absence of the eyelids has been reported in several settings. The association with ichthyosis was reported by Chaurasia and Goswani (1971). In the Neu–Laxova syndrome, ablepharon is associated with intrauterine growth retardation, syndactyly, swollen 'collodion' skin, microcephaly and severe developmental brain defects (Shapiro *et al.* 1992): survival is limited. In the ablepharon–macrostomia syndrome, patients have congenitally absent or rudimentary eyelids (McCarthy & West 1977), a hypoplastic nose, ambiguous genitalia (Hornblass & Reiffler 1985), an absent zygoma (Jackson 1988) and macrostomia. Some cases have mental retardation and the presence of a hairy forehead (Cenarino *et al.* 1988) suggests that some cases may actually be examples of the cryptophthalmos syndrome (see Chapter 20). Surgical management is challenging, the priority being to preserve the cornea by early postnatal treatment with lubricants and early lid reconstruction (Price *et al.* 1991).

Ankyloblepharon

In ankyloblepharon the eyelid margins are partially or completely fused together. The horizontal palpebral aperture is reduced. The condition must be differentiated from blepharophimosis in which the palpebral aperture is also reduced and there is telecanthus but the eyelid margins are normal. This abnormality may be inherited as an autosomal dominant trait, and may occur in association with ectodermal defects such as cleft lip and palate (Ehlers & Jensen 1970; Hay & Wells 1976; Akkerman & Stern 1979).

Ankyloblepharon filiforme adnatum is a similar condition in which one or more skin tags join the two lids centrally, with a normal horizontal palpebral fissure. They are usually isolated but have been described with systemic abnormalities including meningomyelocoele and hydrocephalus (Kazarian & Goldstein 1977), ectodermal defects

(Weiss *et al.* 1992) or in trisomy 18 (Clarke & Patterson 1985; Weiss *et al.* 1992; Bacal *et al.* 1993). Recently, Scott *et al.* (1994) described a patient with co-existing anterior chamber dysgenesis. The tags may be surgically excised. The recognition of this uncommon condition necessitates careful systemic evaluation to detect associated abnormalities.

Euryblepharon

Euryblepharon is a condition of generalized enlargement of the palpebral aperture, usually greatest in the lateral aspect (Keipert 1975). There is localized outward and downward displacement of the lateral canthus, with a downward displacement of the lower lid. This may superficially mimic the appearance of congenital ectropion. It may occur as an isolated anomaly, inherited as an autosomal dominant trait, or may be associated with Down's syndrome (Markowitz *et al.* 1994) or with craniofacial dysostoses. Correction using lateral canthal tightening, tarsorraphy and skin grafting has been described.

Ectropion

Congenital ectropion refers to an outward rotation of the eyelid margin present at birth. The condition may occur in either the upper or lower lids and rarely occurs as an isolated anomaly. Reported associations of congenital or acquired ectropion include the blepharophimosis syndrome, Down's syndrome (Sellar *et al.* 1992), mandibulofacial or other facial dysostoses, skin disorders, i.e. lamellar ichthyosis (Oestreicher & Nelson 1990), microphthalmos, buphthalmos and orbital cysts (Fig. 21.3).

Therapy may be initially conservative using lubrication. Surgical intervention is indicated for exposure keratitis or cosmesis. The procedure should address the underlying deficiency and may include skin grafting, horizontal shortening or tarsorraphy (Callahan 1973; Morris & Collin 1986; Miller *et al.* 1988; Oestreicher & Nelson 1990).

Eversion

Congenital eversion of the lids is an acute ectropion. It can occur intermittently in neonates when the child cries. It is caused by spasm of the orbicularis muscle and usually corrects itself spontaneously. If it becomes established the conjunctiva becomes chemotic and may obscure the globe. This condition, which has been reported in association with Down's syndrome (Fig. 21.4), black babies and difficult deliveries, should be treated initially by pressure patching or repositioning of the lids and taping (Kronish & Lingua 1991). More severe cases have been treated by intermarginal sutures, inverting sutures, tarsorraphy, hor-

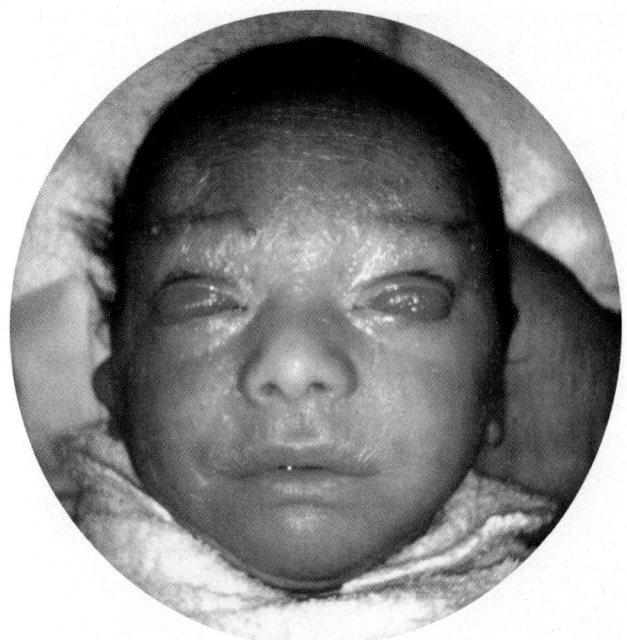

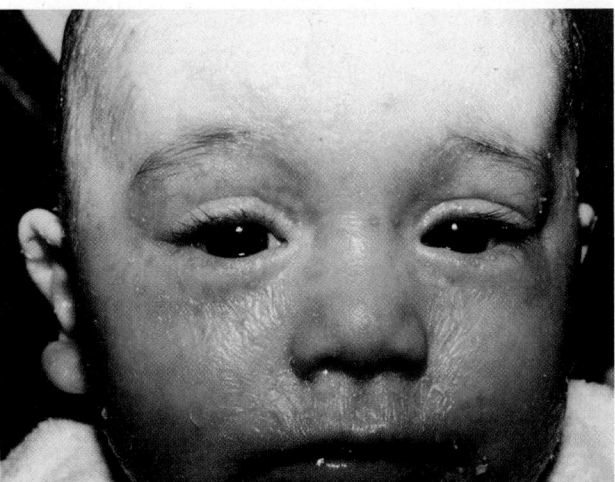

Fig. 21.3 (a) Bilateral ectropion in a patient with severe congenital ichthyosis. (b) Same patient after bilateral lid suture. Dr Geoffrey Hipwell's patient.

izontal shortening procedures or by the insertion of a skin graft (Bentsi-Enchill 1981; Moanie *et al.* 1982; Raab & Saphir 1985; Alvarez *et al.* 1988; Miller *et al.* 1988).

Epitarsus

Primary epitarsus is an apron-like fold of conjunctiva attached to the inner surface of the upper lid. It occurs secondary to conjunctivitis, amniotic bands or as a congenital anomaly (Khurana *et al.* 1986).

Epiblepharon

Epiblepharon is a condition characterized by the presence

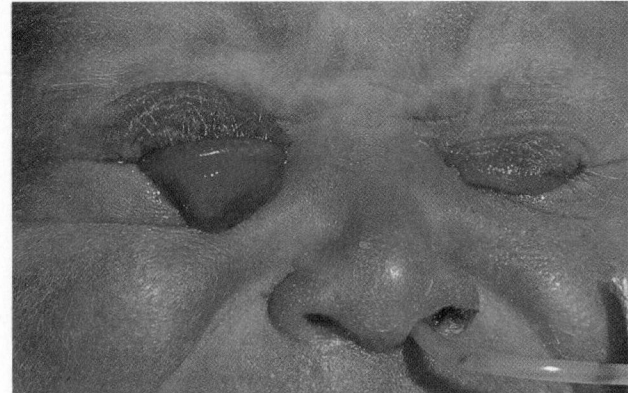

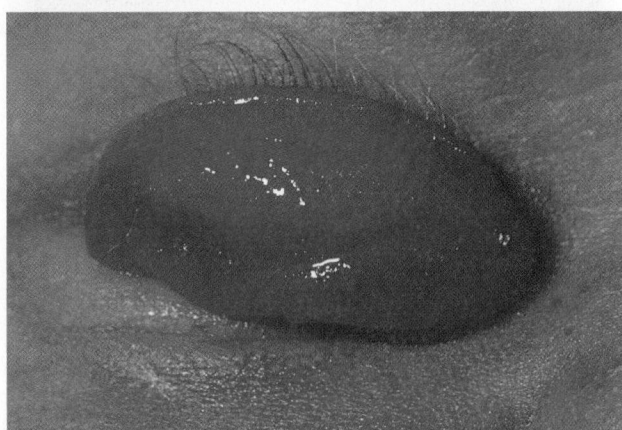

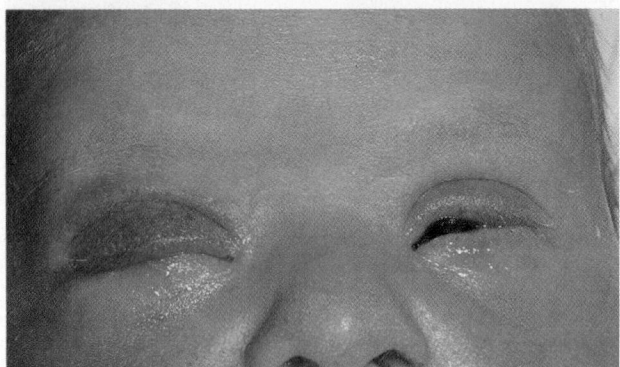

Fig. 21.4 (a) This neonate with Down's syndrome developed lid eversion when crying that rapidly became permanently present. The birth history was unremarkable. (b) The lid eversion was maintained by the very marked chemosis. (c) After taping the lids for 4 days the swelling resolved leaving bruising, indicating that haemorrhage may play a causative role.

of a horizontal fold of skin across either the upper or lower eyelid which forces the lashes against the cornea (Fig. 21.5). There is often a familial tendency towards this condition. It occurs more frequently in chubby-cheeked and in Oriental infants. Epiblepharon usually corrects itself within the first 2 years of life as a result of differential growth of the facial bones. It is seldom associated with keratitis.

Surgical intervention is therefore rarely indicated except when foreign-body symptoms, photophobia or corneal compromise persist despite conservative treatment (i.e. lubrication). Surgery may consist simply of lid bracing sutures or a subciliary excision of an ellipse of skin and orbicularis muscle (Hayasaka *et al.* 1989; O'Donnell & Collin 1994).

Entropion

Congenital entropion refers to turning inward of the lid margin, with associated malposition of the tarsal plate. It usually involves the lower lid, although involvement of the upper lid has been documented (Fig. 21.6). Congenital entropion must be distinguished from epiblepharon, where a skinfold causes a secondary turning of the lower lid eyelashes. Entropion may be secondary to microphthalmos and enophthalmos, resulting from lack of support of the posterior border of the eyelid. The aetiology of primary congenital entropion is controversial. Hypertro-

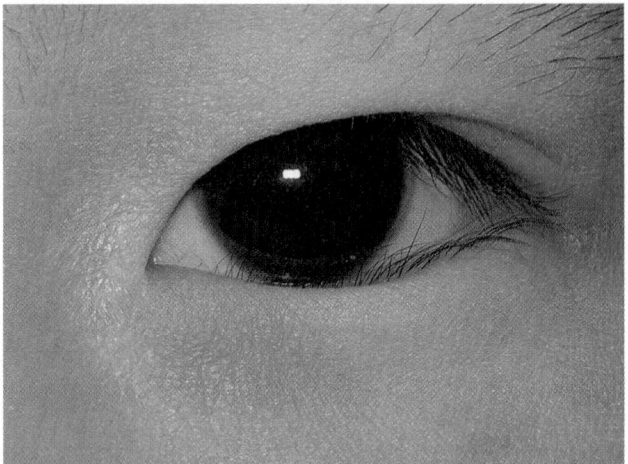

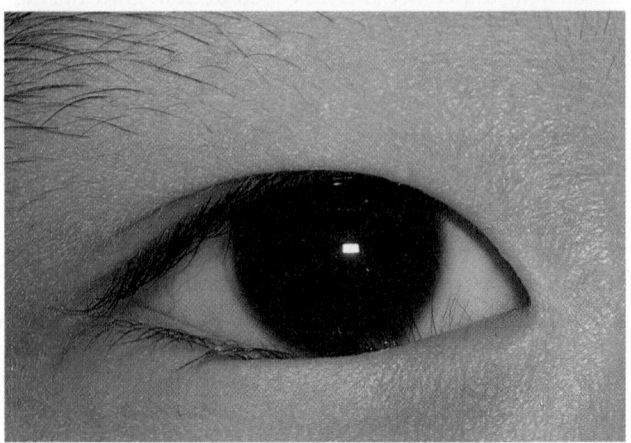

Fig. 21.5 Epiblepharon. In this child the lower lid lashes have turned in from birth, but the cornea has remained undamaged. Spontaneous improvement usually occurs.

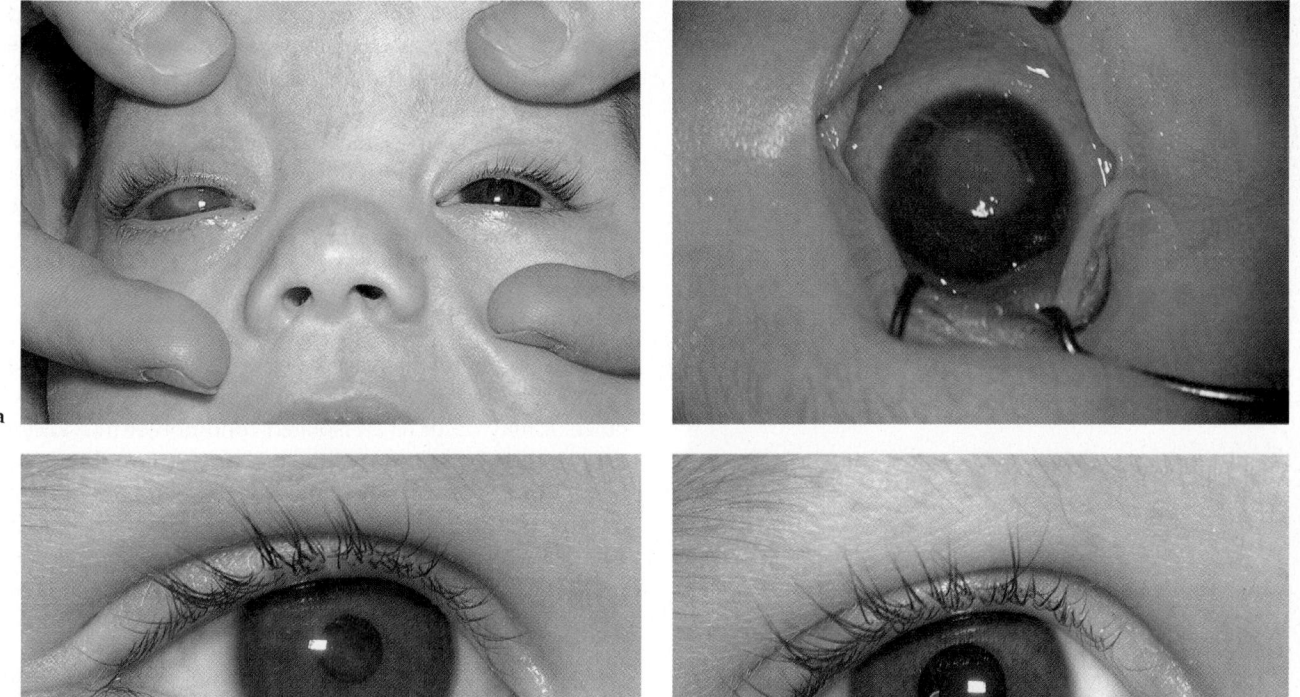

Fig. 21.6 (a) Congenital entropion. Shortly after birth this child's eye was found to be swollen. During examination under anaesthetic right upper lid entropion was found. (b) A corneal abrasion caused by the entropion. (c) After taping the lids, the entropion resolved and (d) ultimately there was only minimal subepithelial opacity.

phy of the marginal portion of the orbicularis muscle and disinsertion of the lower lid retractors have been considered responsible factors according to various authors (Tse *et al.* 1983; Bartley *et al.* 1991; Jordan 1993). Entropion occurs in association with Larsen's syndrome: multiple large joint dislocations, flattened facies, cleft palate and, sometimes, mental retardation (Eiferman *et al.* 1993).

Congenital entropion, as opposed to congenital epiblepharon, often requires prompt surgical intervention to prevent corneal scarring and infection (Young *et al.* 1996). Surgical procedures are usually directed towards myocutaneous resection and plication or reattachment of the lower lid retractors to the inferior tarsal border. A trial of simpler treatment may be worthwile (Fig. 21.7).

Tarsal kink

Congenital horizontal kinking of the tarsus causes secondary upper lid entropion which can be corrected by repositioning of the anterior lamella of the eyelid with a simple upper lid entropion correction (Bosniak *et al.* 1985; Price & Collin 1987). Lid suture with mechanical flattening of the kink may be successful (Fig. 21.8).

Distichiasis

Distichiasis refers to a congenital abnormality in which a second row of lashes exits from the mouths of the meibomian gland orifices (White 1975). It may occur as an isolated anomaly, or be inherited as an autosomal dominant trait. It may be associated with chronic lymphoedema of the lower extremities or the Fall–Kertesz syndrome (Anderson & Harvey 1981; Temple & Collin 1994). Other features include a webbed neck, cardiac defects, vertebral anomalies, extradural spinal cysts and bifid uvula (Kolin *et al.* 1991). It is inherited as an autosomal dominant trait.

Jalili (1989) described an autosomal recessive condition with a cone–rod dystrophy, hairy face and eyebrows, synophrys, coarse scalp hair and distichiasis.

In the Setleis forceps marks syndrome (Frederick & Robb 1992), there are scar-like skin defects on the forehead and temple, absent lashes, distichiasis, a fleshy nose and thick lips.

The Tuomaala–Haapanen syndrome (Tuomaala & Haapanen 1968) consists of mental retardation, myopia,

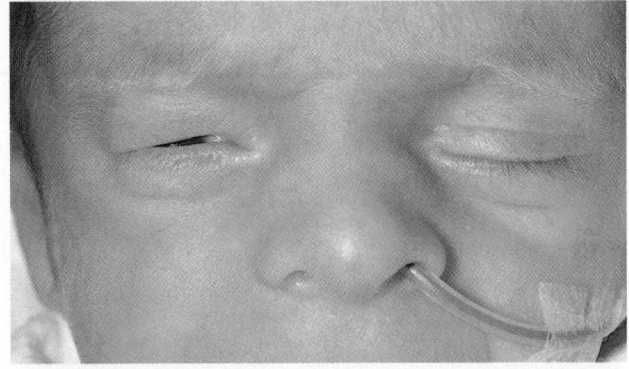

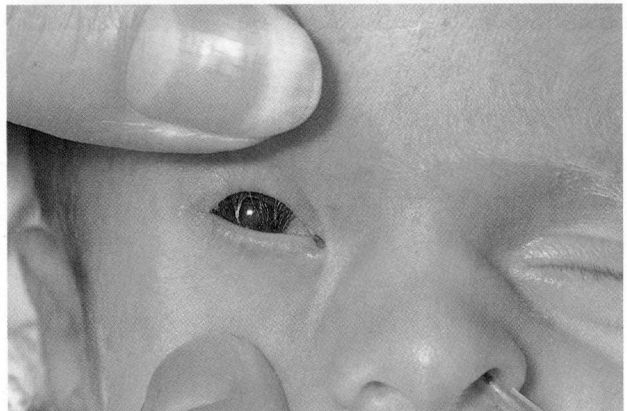

Fig. 21.7 (a) Congenital entropion. This child presented with irritability and an abnormality of the right lids which were slightly swollen. (b) Same child with the lid everted showing the lashes inturned and abrading the cornea without damage at this stage. It was treated with simple lid suture and resolved without complication.

cataracts, short stature, hypogonadism, hypopigmentation and distichiasis.

Distichiasis occurs in association with the Cornelia de Lange syndrome.

Pseudodistichiasis occurs in chronic lid disease with metaplasia, in the Stevens–Johnson syndrome or with ectodermal dysplasia (Howard & Wilson 1993).

If patients are symptomatic or show signs of significant corneal staining, treatment is indicated. Epilation, electrolysis, cryotherapy, lid splitting with cryotherapy to the posterior lamella, and excision of individual follicles (Wolfley 1987; O'Donnell & Collin 1993) have all been used. The decision regarding the appropriate procedure depends on the extent of involvement.

Epicanthus

Epicanthal folds are folds of skin which extend from the upper eyelid towards the medial canthus (Fig. 21.9). They can be subdivided by the area where they occur such as preseptal, pretarsal or orbital. If they extend from the lower lid they are known as inverse epicanthal folds (epi-

canthus inversus). They are common in Asian races and may occur as an isolated anomaly or in association with other conditions, such as the blepharophimosis syndrome (Mustarde 1963, 1971). The folds represent lines of relative skin shortage which can be broken up and lengthened with various Z-plasty techniques (Anderson & Nowinski 1989). The epicanthus may give rise to a false appearance of strabismus (pseudosquint) (Fig. 21.10).

Telecanthus

Telecanthus is an increased width between the medial canthi (Fig. 21.11). There is a normal interpupillary distance. It may occur as an isolated condition or in association with other abnormalities such as epicanthus and blepharophimosis. It is usually due to an abnormality of the soft tissues in the medial canthal region. If there is an overgrowth of bone with an increase in the interorbital width the condition is referred to as hypertelorism. The

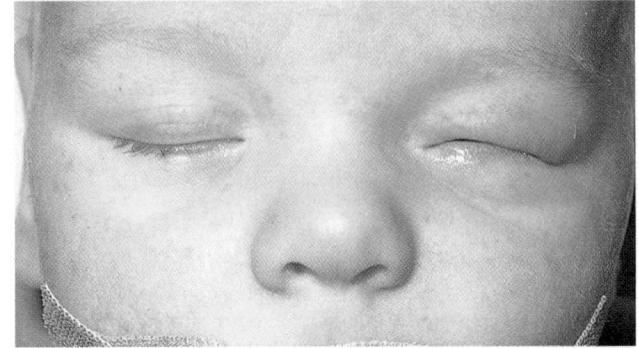

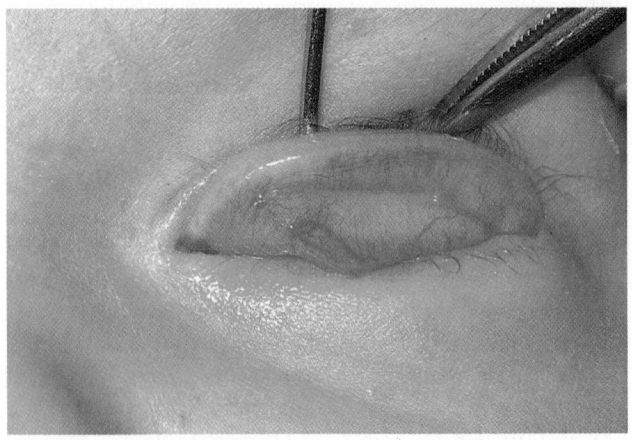

Fig. 21.8 (a) Horizontal tarsal kink. This child presented with a swollen and sore left eye with blepharospasm. (b) On eversion of the lid the horizontal kink in the tarsus can be seen. It runs the whole length of the tarsal plate which is bent to 90%. It was treated by forced eversion using a strabismus hook to straighten the tarsus by force while the margin of the lid was held. This was followed by a week of lid suture and the condition resolved following that treatment but there was severe corneal scarring and the eye was blind.

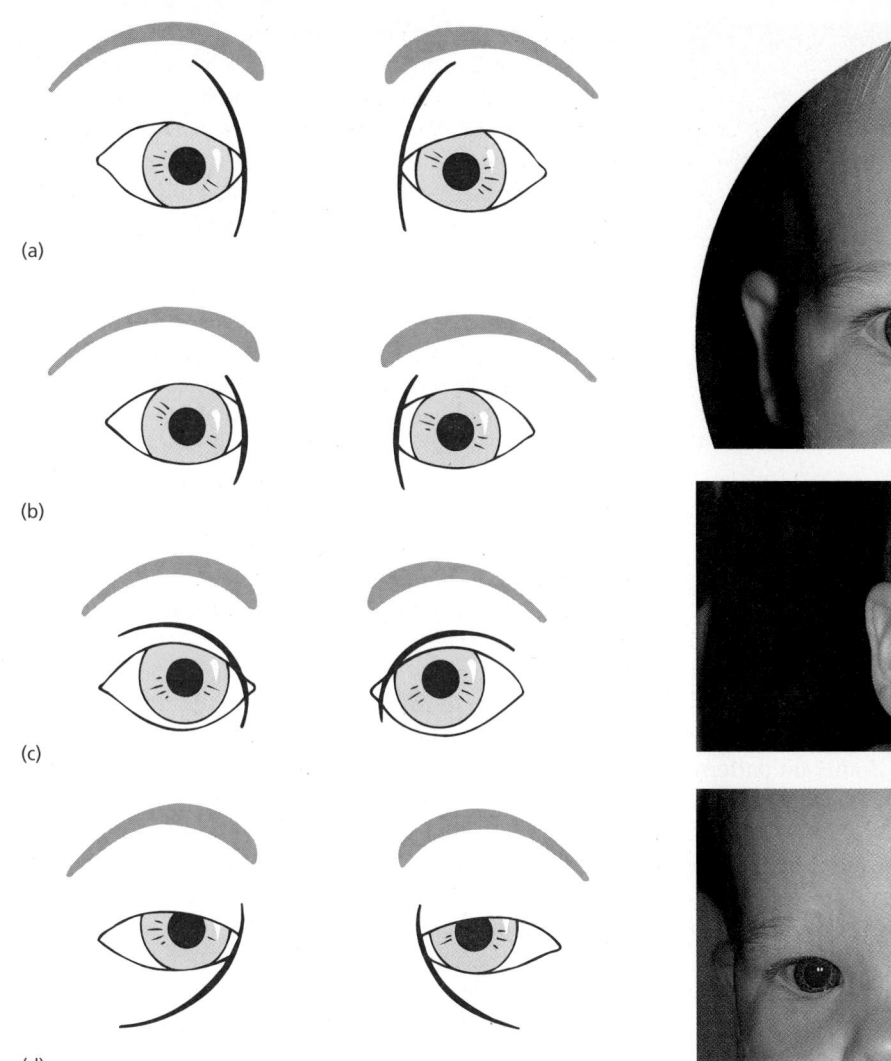

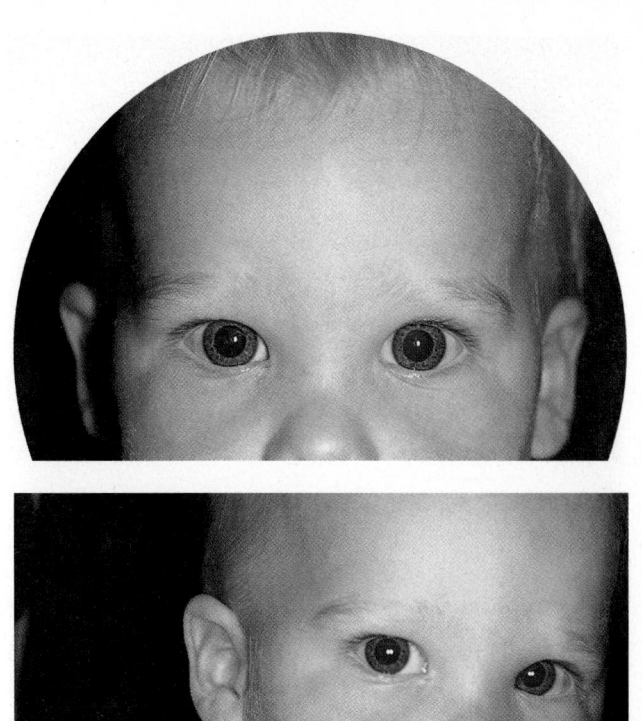

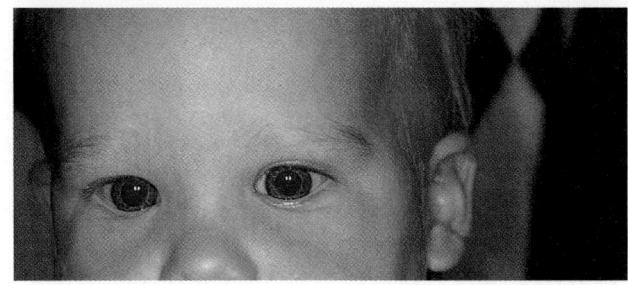

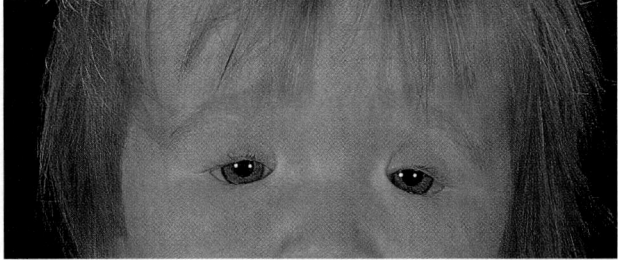

Fig. 21.9 Clinical forms of epicanthus. (a) superciliaris; (b) palpebralis (most frequent); (c) tarsalis ('Asian' epicanthus); (d) inversus (blepharophimosis and ptosis frequent).

Fig. 21.10 (a) Epicanthus in the straight-ahead position. This child can be seen to have a broad base to his nose and mild epicanthus. In the straight-ahead position his eyes appear straight. (b) On looking right or left the adducting eye appears to be convergent giving rise to a pseudosquint.

Fig. 21.11 Telecanthus in a patient with ptosis. Telecanthus and epicanthus inversus.

normal intercanthal distance is 20 ± 2 mm (1 SD) at birth increasing to 26 ± 1.5 mm by 2 years of age. The normal interpupillary distance is 39 ± 3 mm at birth increasing to 48 ± 2 mm by 2 years of age (Feingold & Bossert 1974) (see Chapter 6).

Telecanthus can usually be improved by shortening the medial canthal tendons and soft tissues without involving a significant reduction of bone (McCord 1980). If a transnasal wire is required, it is essential to have preoperative radiological evidence of the height of the cribriform plate to avoid the risk of damage to the intracranial structures. The correction of hypertelorism requires the mobilization of the orbital rims and the reduction of the ethmoidal bones which involves craniofacial surgery. In many instances, since perfection cannot be obtained surgically, surgery for the only functional element, the ptosis, may be the preferred option.

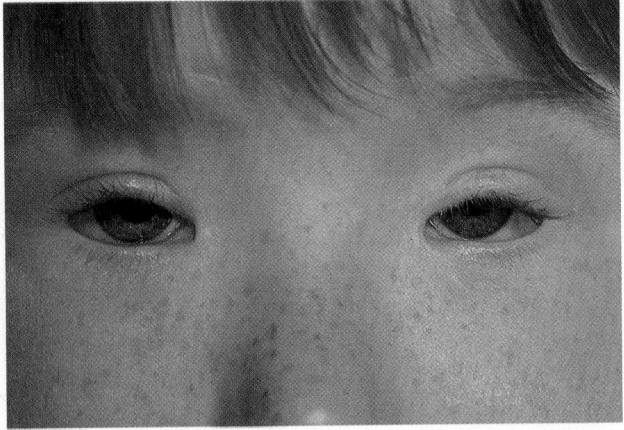

Fig. 21.12 Blepharophimosis. The patient has the blepharophimosis syndrome with blepharophimosis, ptosis (treated) and telecanthus.

Blepharophimosis

Blepharophimosis literally means small eyelids. In the blepharophimosis syndrome, the horizontal palpebral aperture is reduced and this is associated with ptosis, telecanthus (Fig. 21.12) and epicanthus inversus. Though the condition is inherited in an autosomal dominant pattern, 50% of cases occur without a family history. The gene locus may be at 3q22.3–23 (Jewett *et al.* 1993). Some females with the condition are relatively infertile (Jones & Collin 1984). Strabismus may occur and amblyopia as high as 56.4% occurred in one large series (Beaconsfield *et al.* 1991).

The ophthalmologist's participation is directed towards promoting visual development and improving cosmesis. Patients should be evaluated for the presence of refractive errors, amblyopia and strabismus. Resting lid position will determine the urgency of ptosis correction. If a markedly ptotic lid obstructs the visual axis and contributes to the development of amblyopia, lid elevation should proceed promptly. Surgical intervention for ptosis correction usually involves a frontalis sling procedure, as levator function is often poor. Medial canthal reconstruction of the telecanthus and epicanthus inversus may be achieved by shortening the medial canthal tendons and by various flap techniques (Mustarde 1963; Anderson & Nowinski 1989).

Lid retraction in infancy

Occasionally infants may present with a history of one or both eyelids appearing to be retracted. Upper lid retraction is considered to exist when the resting position of the lid is above the superior limbus. For lower lid retraction the affected lower lid rests below the inferior limbus. There is often significant asymmetry between the two sides. There are several conditions which can give rise to this appearance.

1 Physiological, in the newborn.

2 Congenital idiopathic lid retraction (Collin 1990). There are patients in whom one eyelid, usually the upper, is retracted. Several anatomical variants may be responsible for this such as an increase in the number and size of the levator muscle fibres and a thickened or shortened levator aponeurosis or orbital septum. No definite aetiology has been established.

3 A false appearance of lid retraction may be given by ipsilateral proptosis, contralateral ptosis when the child is trying to elevate the ptosed lid, and with inferior rectus fibrosis, double elevator palsy, Brown's syndrome or orbital pathology which restrict upward movement of the eye.

4 Bilateral lid elevation with an upgaze palsy is the classic 'setting sun' sign in hydrocephalus of any cause and also in dorsal midbrain disease.

5 Lid retraction, unilateral or bilateral, may occur with the Marcus Gunn jaw-winking phenomenon. Sometimes there is no ptosis—the lid just elevates.

6 Neonatal Graves' disease (Shields *et al.* 1988).

7 A sequel to third nerve palsy with aberrant regeneration (Stout & Borchert 1993).

8 Myasthenic patients may have transient lid retraction particularly after looking down for a period.

9 Lid lag is a defective relaxation of the lids which occurs in hyperthyroidism, myopathic disease, a congenitally short levator tendon (Zak 1984) or occasionally in myasthenia gravis.

10 Seventh nerve palsy.

11 Levator fibrosis (Stout & Borchert 1993).

12 Vertical nystagmus.

Treatment necessarily depends upon the aetiology. For primary congenital eyelid retraction, initial management should consist of observation and lubrication. Indications for surgical intervention include corneal exposure and cosmesis. Corneal exposure, when not responsive to lubrication, will require early surgery. Cosmetic surgery may be delayed into early childhood. Upper lid retraction is generally corrected by a lid lowering procedure such as levator recession or Z-myotomy. Lower lid retraction may be corrected by retractor recession, usually in combination with a spacer graft (Collin 1990).

Ptosis

This section aims to provide the ophthalmologist with a guide to the differential diagnoses of a child with ptosis and an outline of the subsequent management.

Ptosis is usually classified as congenital or acquired but many conditions, such as third nerve palsies and Horner's syndrome, may be either. The essential differentiation is between a simple congenital dystrophy of the levator muscle and other causes of ptosis. If the levator is dystrophic, it will not relax properly and there will be some

Table 21.1 Classification of ptosis.

Congenital ptosis
Dystrophic
  simple congenital ptosis
  no superior rectus weakness (Mustarde 1963)
  with superior rectus weakness
  with the blepharophimosis syndrome
Non-dystrophic
  aponeurotic defects
  neurogenic, mechanical

Acquired
Aponeurotic defects
  blepharochalasis, trauma, oedema, etc.
Neurogenic
  third nerve palsy and associated syndromes
  Horner's syndrome
Myogenic
  progressive external opthalmoplegia
  ocular myopathies
  myasthenia gravis
Mechanical
  lid tumours
  cicatricial conditions
  lacerations, etc.

Pseudoptosis
Hypotropia
Enophthalmos
Excess skin, etc.

lid lag on downgaze; whereas if the levator muscle is not dystrophic, the ptotic eyelid will remain ptotic in all positions of gaze.

The following classification emphasizes this differentiation and covers most of the causes of ptosis. Traumatic ptosis is not included as a separate entity since the ptosis can be due to nerve, muscle or aponeurotic damage and is therefore included under the headings below (Table 21.1).

Classification

Congenital ptosis

Dystrophic ptosis

Simple congenital ptosis is by far the most common type of ptosis in childhood. It is due to a dystrophy of the levator palpebrae superioris muscle. The number of healthy-looking levator muscle fibres which can be found on histology is directly related to the degree of levator function (Berke & Wadsworth 1955). Lid lag on downgaze and the extent of the skin crease are also usually related to the levator function. In view of the close embryological development of the levator and superior rectus muscles, it is not surprising that a ptosis may be associated with a superior rectus weakness (Figs 21.13, 21.14). There is no well-

defined pattern of heredity, and it is not known why an isolated unilateral dystrophy of the levator muscle should be relatively common.

The blepharophimosis syndrome is inherited as an autosomal dominant trait, although fresh mutations are common. There is a bilateral, usually severe, dystrophy of the levator muscle, with a phimotic palpebral aperture, telecanthus and epicanthus inversus. Other features may include a lateral ectropion of the outer third of the lower lid, maxillary hypoplasia and external ear abnormalities (see also Congenital eyelid abnormalities above).

Non-dystrophic ptosis

Aponeurotic defects may occur anywhere in the aponeurosis. They are associated with good levator function and no lid lag on downgaze. The most common sites are at the origin or insertion of the aponeurosis. If a defect occurs at the origin and the terminal aponeurosis is normal, the child will have a ptosis with good levator function and a normal skin crease. If the defect occurs at the insertion of the aponeurosis, as commonly occurs with trauma, the ptosis will be associated with a high skin crease.

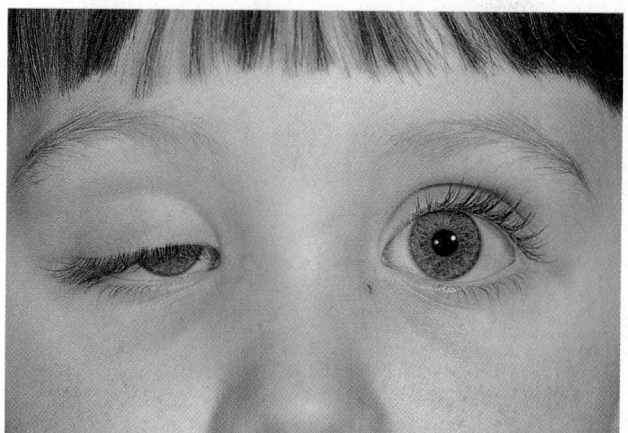

a

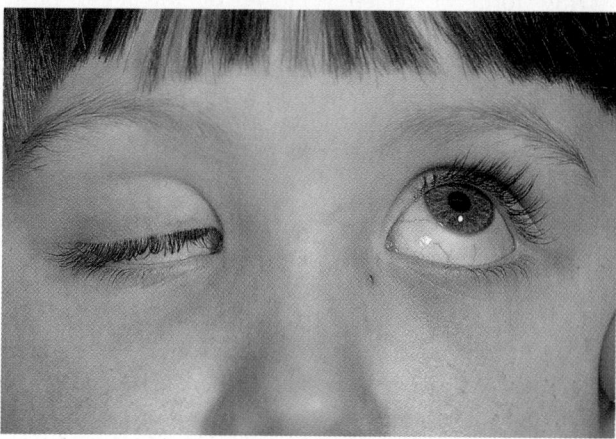

b

Fig. 21.13 (a, b) Unilateral simple congenital ptosis with mildly defective superior rectus action on the right (b).

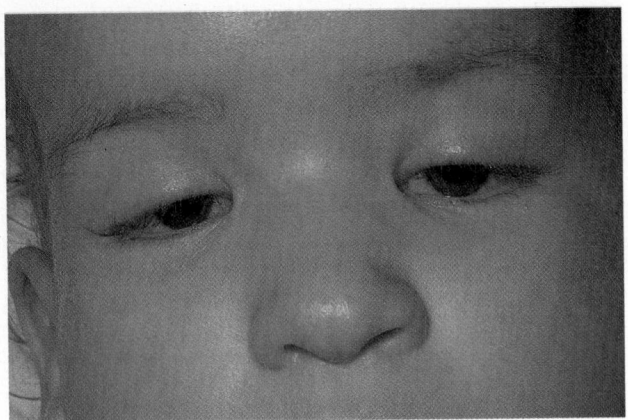

Fig. 21.14 Bilateral severe simple congenital ptosis.

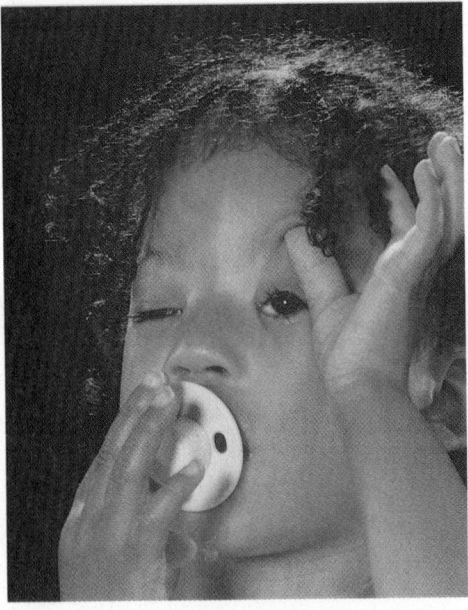

Fig. 21.15 This girl with bilateral ptosis adapts to the condition by lifting her lid anytime that she wants to see more clearly.

Any form of bilateral ptosis, or unilateral ptosis when the non-ptotic eye is patched, will lead to adaptive strategies to secure a clear visual axis. These include lid lifting (Fig. 21.15) or a chin-up head position (Fig. 21.16).

Acquired ptosis

Aponeurotic defects. These may be congenital or acquired due to trauma or to any cause of eyelid oedema. Blepharochalasis is an idiopathic form of eyelid oedema which may start in the first decade of life but more often begins between 10 and 20 years of age. Intermittent attacks of eyelid oedema occur which may be unilateral or bilateral usually affecting the upper eyelids (Curter *et al.* 1985). The frequency and duration of attacks do not seem to follow any predictable pattern. The aetiology of this syndrome is unknown. Each succeeding attack leaves

some residual damage to the tissues. Excessive fine wrinkled skin, atrophy of subcutaneous tissues and fat, ptosis due to aponeurotic weakness, herniated orbital fat, lacrimal gland prolapse, pseudoepicanthic folds, entropion and ectropion may occur. Treatment of the acute attack is supportive, e.g. cool compresses. Steroids and antihistamines have not been shown to be effective. In the quiescent phase, surgical correction may consist of a combination of levator aponeurosis reinsertion, blepharoplasty, lateral canthoplasty and dermis fat graft in atrophic cases (Collin 1979, 1991; Bergin *et al.* 1988; Jordan 1990).

Neurogenic defects. A third nerve palsy may be either congenital or acquired. The many causes and appropriate investigations are not detailed here. There is a ptosis and the eye is abducted by the lateral rectus and intorted by the superior oblique muscle. There may be associated neurological defects (Balkan & Hoyt 1984). The pupil is usually large with loss of accommodation if the parasympathetic supply is involved. Recognition of the condition in its complete form is easy, but in partial form the diagnosis may be missed and investigation delayed (see Chapter 66).

Aberrant third nerve regeneration may occur after a congenital or acquired oculomotor palsy. The nucleus and its connections may be abnormal or nerve fibres may regenerate misdirectedly across the site of an injury and supply the levator muscle. In traumatic cases the damage is usually central to the orbital apex before the superior and inferior divisions of the nerve separate. Eyelid movements are abnormal and the ptotic eyelid may elevate when the patient attempts to adduct, depress or elevate the eye, depending on whether the nerve supply to the

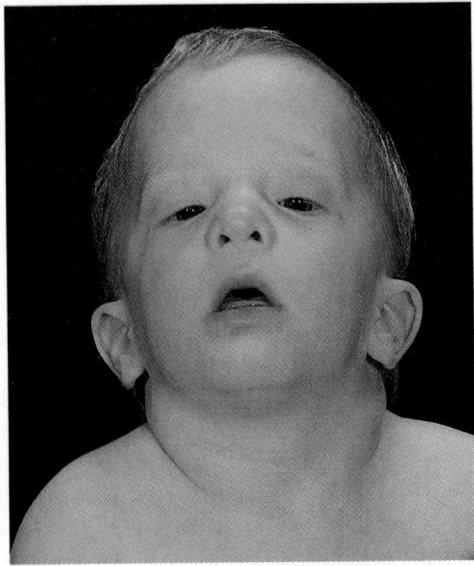

Fig. 21.16 Bilateral congenital ptosis with abnormal head posture. The abnormal head posture is an adaptive mechanism to allow binocular vision.

medial, inferior or superior rectus is misdirected (see Chapter 66).

Cyclic oculomotor palsy is a rare condition in which the third nerve palsy is interrupted intermittently by involuntary activity in the nerve (Fells & Collin 1979). In the paretic phase there is a ptosis and the eye is abducted with a large pupil. In the spastic phase the eyelid elevates, the pupil becomes miosed and the eye may adduct. The periodicity of the cycle and severity of its phases varies considerably in different patients, the paretic phase usually lasting 1–2 minutes and the spastic phase up to 30 seconds. Parents usually detect the anomaly of the eye within the first few months of life and before the age of 2 years. It is thought that an injury occurring by this age to some of the intracranial third nerve fibres causes the partial third nerve palsy. Retrograde degeneration occurs, which secondarily affects part of the oculomotor nucleus before normal supranuclear connections have formed. Some of the injured nuclear cells recover and regenerating fibres sprout diffusely across the scar to join normal efferent fibres. These injured neurones have abnormal connections both centrally and peripherally and produce the cyclic spasms by summation of subthreshold stimuli which are constantly arriving at the oculomotor nucleus. The normal nuclear cells that avoided injury still produce normal oculomotor movements, while the relative proportions of damaged and undamaged neurones determine the inverse relationship between cyclical and physiological movements. It is important to recognize this condition and prevent unnecessary neurological investigation, since nothing is found unless it is associated with other signs (see Chapter 66).

Marcus Gunn's jaw–winking syndrome is due to an abnormal synkinesis between the levator and usually the lateral pterygoid muscle. The affected eyelid is usually ptotic but elevates when the jaw is opened and deviated to the contralateral side (Figs 21.17, 21.18). A medial pterygoid synkinesis in which the affected eyelid elevates when the jaw is clenched or protruded occurs less commonly. The voluntary levator excursion is always decreased and frequently there is a weakness of the superior rectus muscle. The condition is almost always congenital, sporadic and unilateral, but acquired and familial cases may occur. There is normally a synkinesis between the lateral pterygoid and the levator muscles. It is mediated by proprioceptive fibres from the pterygoid muscles which travel in the motor root of the trigeminal nerve. Their cell bodies lie in the mesencephalic nucleus, which has synaptic connections with the motor nucleus of the fifth nerve and the oculomotor nucleus. The normal lateral pterygoid synkinesis is exaggerated in Marcus Gunn's syndrome, possibly as a result of a small brainstem lesion such as a haemorrhage, which reduces central inhibition of the reflex (Sano 1959). Other synkinetic eye movements can occasionally be associated (Hamed *et al.* 1990).

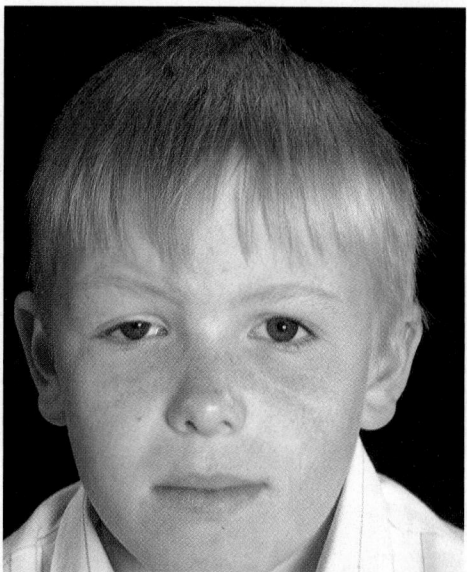

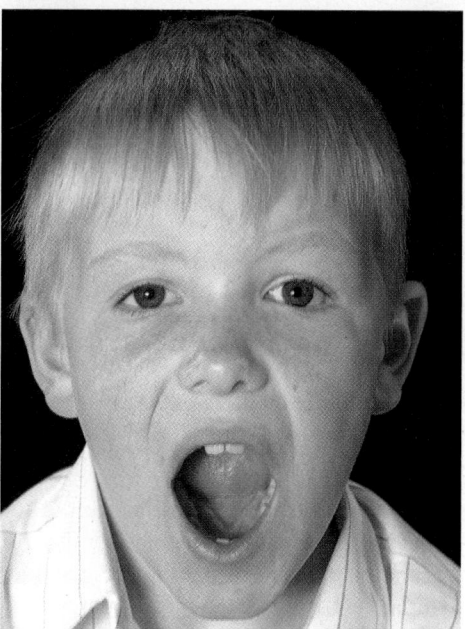

Fig. 21.17 (a) Right ptosis (Marcus Gunn). (b) With jaw open the right upper lid rises.

Horner's syndrome comprises ptosis, miosis and sometimes anhidrosis on the affected side of the face and neck. If the lesion is congenital, iris pigmentation may be defective. There is about 2 mm of ptosis, which is probably accounted for mainly by the denervation of Muller's muscle. The apparent ptosis may be increased by some elevation of the lower lid due to denervation of the smooth muscle of the lower lid retractors. This also provides the impression of the enophthalmos, which in humans is more apparent than real. The syndrome is due to an interruption of the sympathetic supply anywhere along its course through the brainstem and cervical spinal cord, via the thoracic outlet to the superior cervical ganglion and

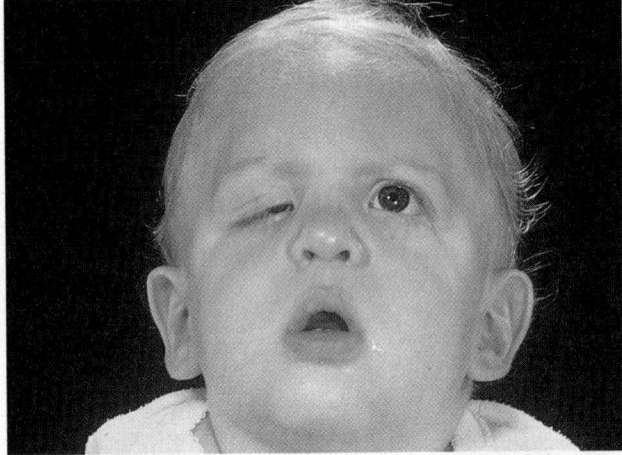

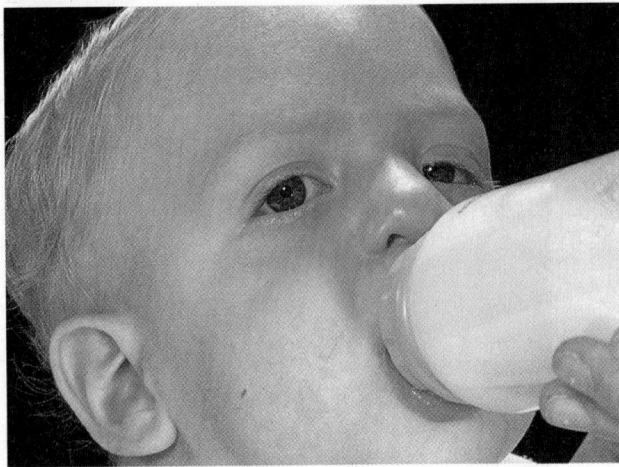

Fig. 21.18 Marcus Gunn ptosis showing marked right ptosis which completely elevates on jaw movement; in this instance during feeding

thence with the carotid arteries to the orbit. The clinical diagnosis of Horner's syndrome can be confirmed by taking the patient into a dark room and noting an increase in the anisocoria, the uninvolved pupil dilates very much more than the pupil with Horner's syndrome. Four per cent cocaine drops similarly increase the inequality in pupil size, the uninvolved pupil dilating more readily. One per cent hydroxyamphetamine (Paredrine) differentiates between a lesion proximal or distal to the superior cervical ganglion. The drops only dilate the pupil if the postganglionic fibres are intact. Preganglionic lesions usually require further investigation, as the course of the sympathetic nerve fibres prior to the superior cervical ganglion is discrete. The nerve fibres can be interrupted in children by such lesions as cervical vertebral fractures, brainstem, cervical cord and mediastinal tumours, apical tuberculosis and enlarged cervical lymph glands. After the superior cervical ganglion the course of the sympathetic nerve supply is less discrete and postganglionic lesions probably require investigation only if there are other indications (see Chapter 59).

Myogenic ptosis

Progressive external ophthalmoplegia may present in childhood with ptosis, which may initially be unilateral but becomes bilateral. There is an associated slowly progressive palsy of all the extraocular muscles, which usually limits elevation first but progresses until the eyes are practically immobile (Fig. 21.19). The pupil and accommodation are not involved. It may occur sporadically, but a familial incidence is common and it is frequently inherited as a dominant characteristic. Histology, electron microscopy and electromyography suggest that it is a muscular dystrophy. Characteristic ragged red fibres may be seen on muscle biopsy stained with a modified trichrome method. It is probably due to a generalized mitochondrial abnormality and may progress to involve the orbicularis, facial pharyngeal and skeletal muscles, especially of the neck and shoulders. A pigmentary retinopathy and cardiomyopathy may occur and there is an increased anaesthetic risk of malignant hyperthermia.

Myasthenia gravis is a chronic disease characterized by an abnormal fatiguability of striated muscles. It may be confined indefinitely to a single group of muscles or may become generalized. Ten per cent of cases occur in children before puberty and it may occur transitorily in newborns of myasthenic mothers. A familial incidence is recognized although there is no clear hereditary pattern. Many cases are associated with hyperplasia of the thymus or a thymic tumour. The cause is an autoimmune defect in the acetylcholine mechanism at the neuromuscular junction, to which the ocular muscles are particularly sensitive. Ptosis, which may be unilateral and variable, but is usually worse at the end to the day, is often the presenting symptom. Diplopia commonly occurs and the child may present with an unusual squint. The orbicularis oculi is usually also weak.

Clinically, fatiguability may cause an increase in the ptosis after repeated up- and downgaze. The abnormality of neuromuscular control may be demonstrated by an overshoot to the eyelid on upgaze, and the horizontal eye

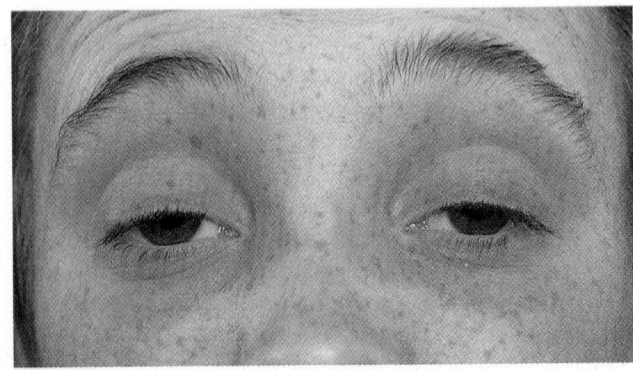

Fig. 21.19 Bilateral ptosis and brow elevation in chronic external ophthalmoplegia.

movements may show hypometric saccades. Myasthenia can sometimes be confirmed pharmacologically; it must be said, however, that unless pre- and post-test parameters (such as a Hess chart or orthoptic measurements) are taken the test is often equivocal except in cases that are clinically obvious. In an adult-sized child, 2 mg of Tensilon (edrophonium chloride) is given intravenously as a test dose followed by 8 mg given rapidly. This may produce quick relief of the ptosis. If the child is under 10 kg in weight, the dose is reduced or Prostigmin (neostigmine) can be given by intramuscular injection 20 minutes after an intramuscular injection of atropine. The test must only be carried out in circumstances where proper resuscitation facilities are available, appropriate to the age of the child.

Mechanical ptosis

Mechanical ptosis may be caused by anything increasing the weight of the eyelid, such as neurofibroma, haemangioma or meibomian cyst; by scar tissue limiting eyelid movement, such as after surgery, chemical burns and so on; or by trauma (including birth trauma, Fig. 21.20) interfering with the action of the levator muscle.

Pseudoptosis

A pseudoptosis is any condition in which the eyelid margin is at the normal level but the eyelid appears ptotic. If the eye is hypotropic, there may be such an apparent ptosis which disappears when the eye takes up fixation. In enophthalmic conditions such as microphthalmos or with anophthalmos, the apparent ptosis can be corrected by restoring the orbital volume. Excess skin from a resolving haemangioma may overhang the lid margin and be another cause of pseudoptosis.

Management

History

The essential questions, such as length of history, associated signs and symptoms, variability, family history and so on, are obvious from the preceding account of the causes of ptosis. With a simple congenital ptosis there is often a history that the condition seemed to improve initially after birth then became static.

Examination

A full eye examination should be performed, with particular attention to the position of the lid on downgaze, the extraocular muscle movements, any squint (Anderson & Baumgartner 1980a, b), the facial appearance, evidence of jaw–winking, aberrant movements of the lid, the pupil,

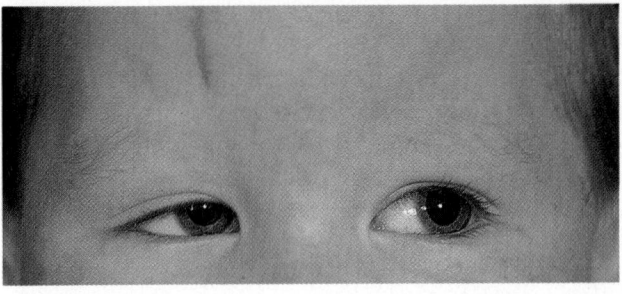

Fig. 21.20 Right ptosis associated with forceps injury at birth.

variability in the signs, pseudoepicanthic folds and so on. Associated abnormalities, such as astigmatism with haemangiomas or pigmentary retinopathy with progressive external ophthalmoplegia may be found. Further investigations may be indicated depending on the findings (e.g. with third nerve palsies) (Collin 1988).

The degree of ptosis should be assessed both by comparing the vertical interpalpebral aperture measurements on both sides and by assessing the height of the lid above the corneal reflex from a spot source of light. This obviates inaccuracies from malposition of the lower eyelid. The levator function should be measured by pressing over the brow to prevent any frontalis action and then measuring the excursion of the lid between full up- and downgaze. The position of the skin crease on both sides and the presence or absence of Bell's phenomenon should be noted.

Treatment

This depends on the diagnosis and physical findings. Surgical correction is urgent only if there is a risk of amblyopia because the eyelid is occluding the pupil in infancy. This is rare but does occur (Harrad *et al.* 1988). Even in the setting of severe unilateral ptosis, a chin-up head posture may be adopted in an attempt to maintain binocular fusion (McCulloch & Wright 1993). Hence, ptosis surgery usually can be delayed until the child is old enough for an accurate assessment of the levator function, which usually occurs about the age of 4 years. However, if there is any suggestion of the eyelid being close to the visual axis, the child must be kept under appropriate medical supervision, and occlusion instituted whenever necessary. With a simple congenital ptosis the levator function and degree of ptosis govern the choice of operation.

In mild congenital ptosis, if there is about 2 mm of ptosis with good levator function of 10 mm or more, a Fasanella Servat procedure is very effective. The upper border of the tarsal plate with the lower part of the Muller's muscle and its overlying conjunctiva are clamped and excised and the wound edges are held together by a continuous suture of 6–0 collagen or nylon. The levator aponeurosis is not involved in this surgery.

In moderate congenital ptosis, a greater degree of ptosis with a levator function between 4 and 10 mm can usually be corrected with a levator resection graded according to the amount of levator function and degree of ptosis. Either an anterior or a posterior approach to the levator can give satisfactory results. The posterior approach has the advantage that the resected levator muscle is held by pull-out sutures which are tied in the skin crease. These can be removed in the early postoperative period and the eyelid lowered if an overcorrection occurs. The anterior approach is suitable for a maximum levator resection, as it gives a slightly better exposure of the levator muscle and allows the creation of an enhanced lid fold. The disadvantage of a large levator resection is that it increases the lid lag on downgaze. If there is a weakness of the superior rectus muscle, a larger levator resection is required for any given degree of ptosis and levator function.

In severe congenital ptosis, if there is less than 4 mm of levator function, two basic techniques have been advocated. First, the eyelid can be suspended from the brow and elevated by the frontalis muscle. If it is necessary to elevate an eyelid urgently to prevent amblyopia, this can be done with a unilateral procedure using a non-autogenous material (Downes & Collin 1989). Non-autogenous materials may slip, become infected, extrude or lead to granuloma formation. If the operation does not have to be done to prevent amblyopia, it is better to wait until the child's leg is large enough to take autogenous fascia lata (usually by the age of 3–4 years). A unilateral sling may produce an unacceptable degree of asymmetry if the contralateral levator muscle is working normally. It is therefore reasonable to consider correcting a severe unilateral ptosis by first weakening or excising the normal levator muscle and then lifting both eyelids symmetrically with a bilateral brow suspension procedure (Fig. 21.21).

An alternative to the brow suspension procedure in a patient with poor levator function is to excise the aponeurosis anterior to Whitnall's ligament and suture the ligament to the tarsus, possibly combining this with a partial tarsectomy (Holds *et al.* 1993). Whitnall's ligament is attached to the orbital roof in the region of the trochlea and lacrimal fossa and therefore acts as an 'internal sling'. This may elevate the eyelid satisfactorily in the primary position but may cause unacceptable unilateral lagophthalmos.

Finally, a maximal levator resection may be performed. In this technique, the levator muscle is dissected free of all attachments, including Whitnall's, and resected such that the lid rests at the superior limbus intraoperatively. Mauriello *et al.* (1986) reported no persistent exposure-related problems in their series, but if the levator muscle is very dystrophic it may stretch in time with a recurrence of the ptosis.

Specific conditions

In the blepharophimosis syndrome levator function is usually poor and bilateral autogenous fascia lata brow suspensions are required. If the levator function is good, bilateral levator resections can be performed instead. The epicanthus inversus is usually best treated with a medial canthoplasty about 6 months before the lids are lifted.

In Marcus Gunn's syndrome, if the jaw–winking element is unobtrusive, the ptosis alone can be corrected based on the levator function. If the jaw–winking is severe, it can be abolished by cutting the levator muscle. The ptosis must then be corrected with a brow suspension procedure. The logical treatment is perhaps to excise both levator muscles and correct the ptosis with a bilateral autogenous fascia lata brow suspension in the interest of symmetry (Beard 1965). Some cases may become less marked with time and it may therefore be justifiable to delay surgery until the child is old enough to help in the decision-making.

With third nerve lesions the eye should be straightened first with horizontal muscle surgery, supplemented if necessary by transplanting the superior oblique muscle from the trochlea and suturing it adjacent to the medial rectus muscle insertion to hold the eye just in adduction. The correction of the ptosis depends as usual on the levator function. If a brow suspension procedure is required, it may be reasonable to consider unilateral surgery as the result is not going to be symmetrical because of the ocular position. If Bell's phenomenon is defective, there is a risk of exposure keratitis and ptosis surgery should be more conservative.

The same remarks apply to the correction of aberrant third nerve regeneration syndromes and cyclic oculomotor palsy, both of which may require excision of the levator muscle and brow suspension procedure.

Horner's syndrome usually does well with a Fasanella Servat procedure.

Myasthenics should rarely be operated on. Appropriate medication, and ptosis prop contact lenses usually offer a better solution, but conservative surgery may sometimes be justified.

Progressive external ophthalmoplegia is similar but autogenous fascia lata brow suspensions may be successful if the slings are left loose enough to allow the lids to be closed on the operating table. When the patient raises his eyebrows the ptosis will be improved without causing lagophthalmos and corneal exposure. There is, however, always the risk of exposure problems as the ocular movements become more limited and the orbicularis muscle becomes weaker. This may necessitate cutting the fascial bands to allow complete eyelid closure and then using ptosis props which will be tolerated if the orbicularis muscle is sufficiently weak.

Aponeurotic defects occurring congenitally, traumatically, or in blepharochalasis should be repaired.

A hypotropia should be corrected before embarking on ptosis surgery. If it is due to mechanical restriction, this

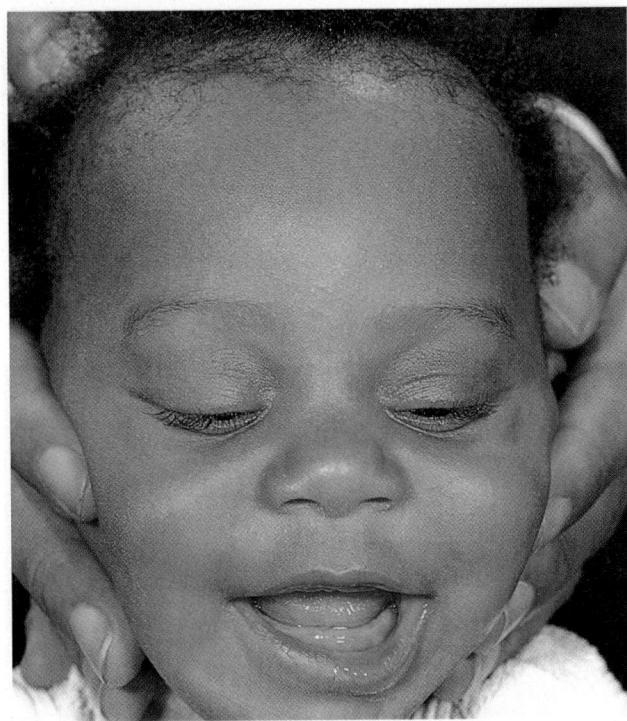

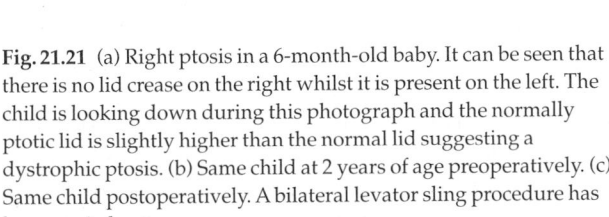

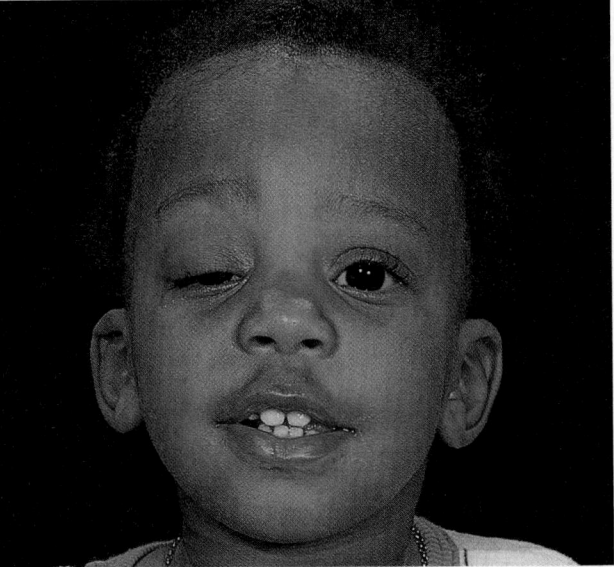

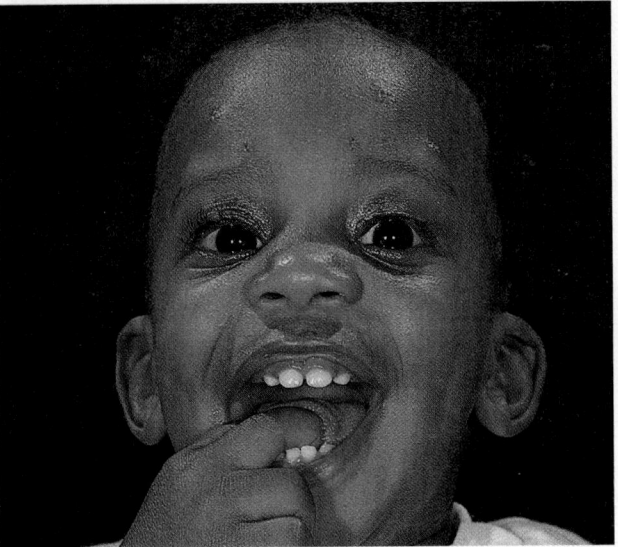

Fig. 21.21 (a) Right ptosis in a 6-month-old baby. It can be seen that there is no lid crease on the right whilst it is present on the left. The child is looking down during this photograph and the normally ptotic lid is slightly higher than the normal lid suggesting a dystrophic ptosis. (b) Same child at 2 years of age preoperatively. (c) Same child postoperatively. A bilateral levator sling procedure has been carried out.

should be relieved. A superior rectus muscle resection may increase the ptosis. If the medial and lateral rectus muscles are disinserted and reattached close to the insertion of the superior rectus, the eye may be elevated. If a forced duction test shows inferior rectus restriction, the inferior rectus muscle must be recessed. Any residual ptosis can then be corrected with a subsequent ptosis operation.

In the ocular fibrosis syndrome, a brow suspension with careful postoperative management to prevent exposure may give good results.

Lid tumours

Haemangioma

Capillary haemangiomas are usually noticed soon after birth as a reddish discolouration of the eyelid skin which rapidly develops into an enlarging mass. The size of the tumour can distort the globe leading to astigmatism and it can affect the eyelid position causing simultaneous ptosis and deprivation amblyopia. Growth is variable but often occurs maximally in the first 2 years of life and then slows down progressing to involution which is usually complete by 8 years of age (Fig. 21.22). Various treatments have been tried to limit the growth of these tumours and to hasten the involution such as radiotherapy, carbon dioxide snow and sclerosing agents. These often created more problems than they solved. Systemic or intra- and perilesional injections often work well (Kushner 1982; Boyd & Collin 1991) but adrenal suppression and growth retardation can be induced by such therapy. Local steroid injections are probably safer than systemic steroids. One regimen is to give 4 mg Triamcinolone (Decadron) subcu-

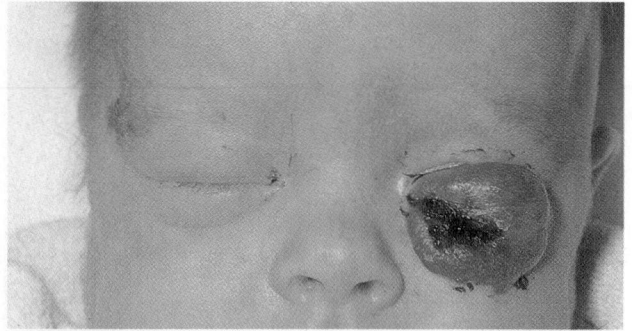

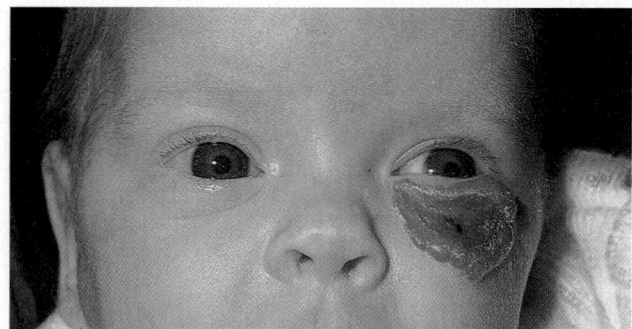

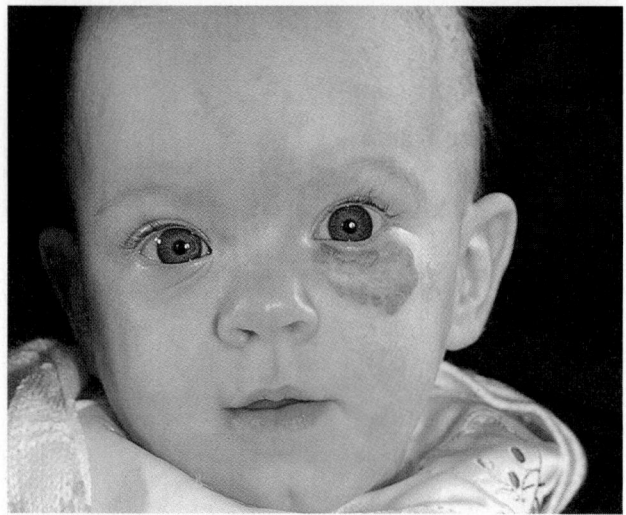

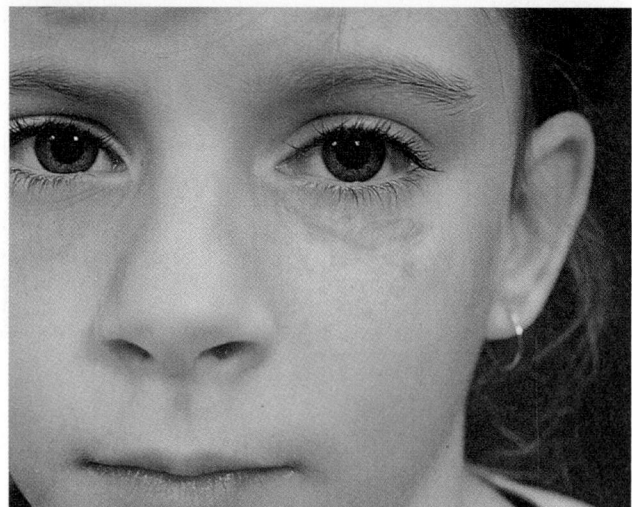

Fig. 21.22 (a) Lower lid haemangioma. This presented as a rapidly increasing mass in the left lower lid which occluded the eye by the age of 6 weeks. It was treated with three separate injections of depot steroid and resolved leaving minimal skin changes (b–d).

taneously around the lesion and 40 mg of Depo-Medrone deep into the lesion, taking care that the chalky deposits do not become immediately subcutaneous as they may remain visible permanently. If there is a dramatic response or no change after 2 or 3 weeks, there is little point in repeating the injections. If there is some response, the injections can be repeated at monthly intervals. After a total of three rounds of injections, it is wise to observe the child before considering a further course of treatment. A child should be kept under refractive and orthoptic supervision with occlusion of the uninvolved eye as required (Robb 1977). Involution has usually occurred by the age of 8 years and surgery may be required at this stage for such sequelae as excess discoloured skin, lash ptosis, entropion, ptosis, tumour bulk, contour deformity and skin crease distortion.

Naevi

Melanocytic naevi are flat lesions and usually small, becoming larger and darker with age. Divided naevi (Fig. 21.23) are a form of congenital melanocytic naevus which involves the upper and lower lids (McDonnell & Mayou 1988).

Dermoid cysts

Dermoid cysts may occur in the lids, but these are usually primary tumours of the orbit and orbital margin and involve the lid secondarily (see Chapter 35).

Molluscum contagiosum and warts

Molluscum contagiosum and warts of viral origin also frequently occur on the eyelids; they may rarely obtain large size (Al-Hazzaa & Hidyat 1993) (Fig. 21.24) and 'kiss' lesions may occur on upper and lower lids (Fig. 21.25). They may be associated with a follicular conjunctivitis (Fig. 21.26). Molluscum lesions may require curettage and diathermy of their core.

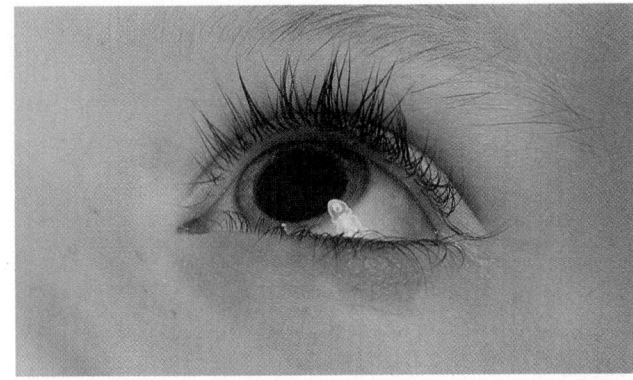

a

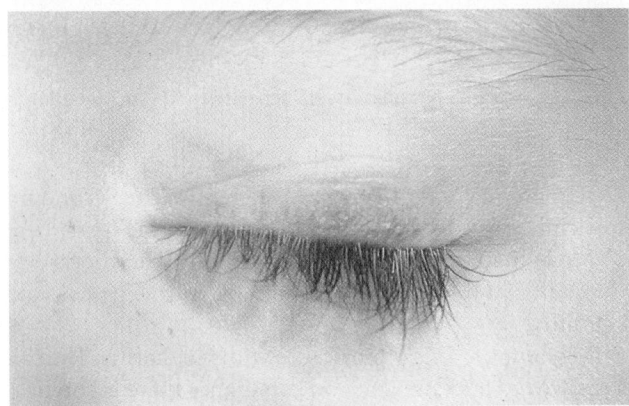

b

Fig. 21.23 (a, b) Divided naevus.

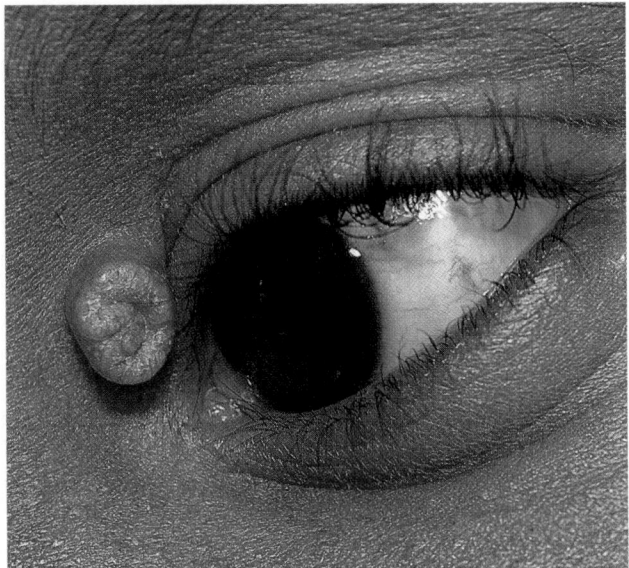

Fig. 21.24 Large molluscum contagiosum lesion. Dr S. Day's patient.

Juvenile xanthogranuloma

Juvenile xanthogranulomatous lesions occasionally occur in the lids (Mansour *et al.* 1985; Kavalec & Harvey 1993) (see Chapter 33).

Complex choristoma

These are rare lid tumours; a 2-year-old child with an aggregate of lashes in the upper lid, associated with an ectopic lacrimal gland which produced tears has been described (Gordon *et al.* 1991).

Calcifying epithelioma of Malherbe (pilomatrixoma)

These are small, hard, benign nodules of the lid or brow (Ni *et al.* 1982; Shields *et al.* 1995).

Carney's complex

This constitutes the association of multiple systemic myxomas (heart and elsewhere), schwannomas and facial lentigines. Lid lentigines are common and a lid myxoma has been described in a young man who had an asympto-

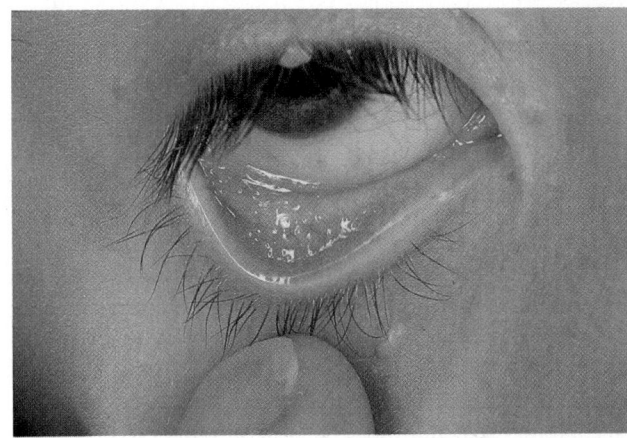

Fig. 21.25 Molluscum contagiosum showing multiple lesions and a follicular conjunctivitis.

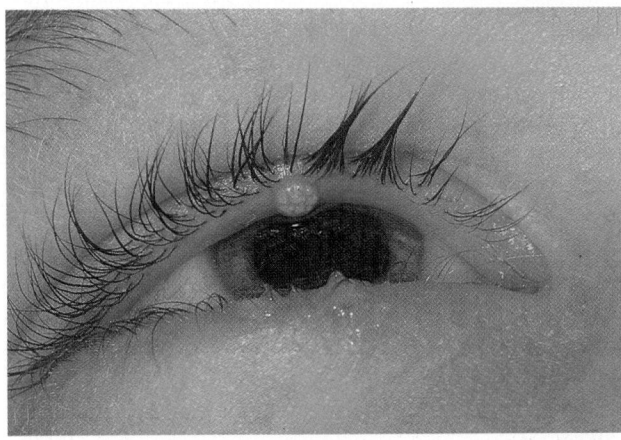

Fig. 21.26 Molluscum contagiosum showing 'kiss' lesions on upper and lower lid.

matic cardiac myxoma (Kennedy *et al.* 1991; Mansell *et al.* 1991). The condition is inherited in an autosomal dominant manner.

Lid hamartoma

These may be associated with Cowden's disease (Bardenstein *et al.* 1988). They have multiple facial and lid trichilemmomas, and carcinomas of the breast and thyroid. It is inherited as an autosomal dominant trait.

Rhabdomyosarcoma

These may occasionally start in the lid.

Meibomian gland diseases

Bron *et al.* (1991) described the functions of the meibomian glands as:
1 reduce tear evaporation;
2 enhance tear stability;
3 prevent tear spillover at the lid margin;
4 prevent tear contamination by sebum; and
5 sealing the apposed lid margins during sleep.

Chalazia (meibomian cysts)

A chalazion is a lipogranuloma of the meibomian gland that results from obstruction of the gland duct and is usually located in the midportion of the tarsus, away from the lid border; sometimes they may occur well away from the lid margin (Gonnering 1988). It may occur on the lid margin if the opening of the duct is involved. A secondary infection of the surrounding tissues may develop with swelling of the entire lid. Chalazia can cause pressure on the globe thereby altering the refractive error. Small chalazia may resolve spontaneously. If they are large, however, or secondarily infected, treatment is usually required. This involves the use of warm compresses with topical antibiotic therapy. Incision of the conjunctival wall of the lesion and curettage is sometimes necessary, although this is avoided whenever possible in young children since it usually necessitates a general anaesthetic. Chronic meibomitis and blepharitis, which may predispose to recurrent chalazia, should be treated by lid cleaning together with antibiotic/hydrocortisone ointment for a circumscribed period before resorting to incision and curettage. Chronic chalazia should be treated with suspicion as rhabdomyosarcoma may present in this guise.

Other diseases of the meibomian glands include the following.
1 Absent or deficient glands. (i) Primary — congenital, ectodermal dysplasia (see Chapter 24), ichthyosis (see Chapter 24). (ii) Secondary to lid disease.

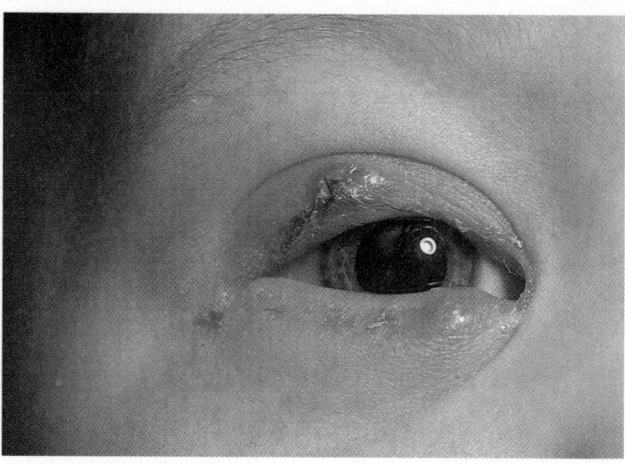

Fig. 21.27 Acute blepharitis with lid ulceration and stye formation.

2 Replacement. (i) Primary distichiasis. (ii) Secondary distichiasis due to metaplasia.
3 Meibomian seborrhoea — associated with seborrhoeic dermatitis and acne rosacea. The meibum is greasy and solidified.
4 Meibomitis. This often occurs with blepharitis. The orifices are red and swollen and sometimes there is soreness with associated lid oedema. Treatment is similar to blepharitis.

Acute blepharitis

Acute blepharitis (Fig. 21.27) presents with ulceration of the lid margins and is usually caused by *Staphylococcus aureus*, other organisms and viruses, including *Moraxella* species, herpes simplex, and various fungi in immunosuppressed patients. Staphylococcal and *Moraxella* blepharitis usually respond well to antibiotic cream and lid toilet. Fungi or herpes simplex usually respond to appropriate chemotherapy.

Chronic blepharitis

Chronic blepharitis is much more common than the acute form. It presents as irritable eyelids that are red, scaly and sometimes rather swollen (Fig. 21.28). The anterior lid margin is usually most affected but occasionally the posterior lid margin is more red and swollen when the meibomian glands are affected (chronic meibomitis). Infection plays a role with *Staphylococcus aureus*, *Propionibacterium acnes* or coagulase-negative staphylococcal species being important (Dougherty & McCully 1984). The role of yeasts like *Pityrosporum ovale* is uncertain but it seems clearer that the mite *Demodex folliculorum* plays a role, perhaps as a vector for bacteria and yeasts.

Most cases of chronic blepharitis have a seborrhoeic element with greasy, scaly lids associated in some cases

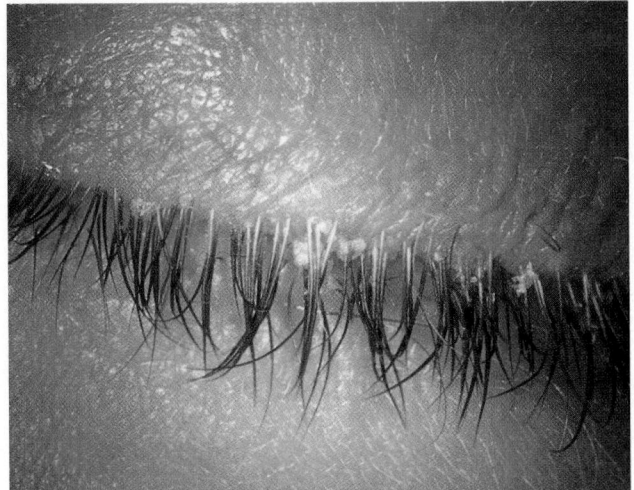

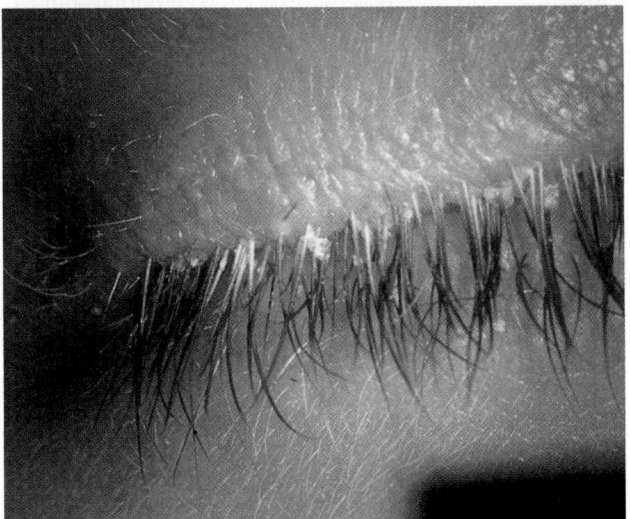

Fig. 21.28 Chronic blepharitis associated with chronic *Staphylococcus* infection.

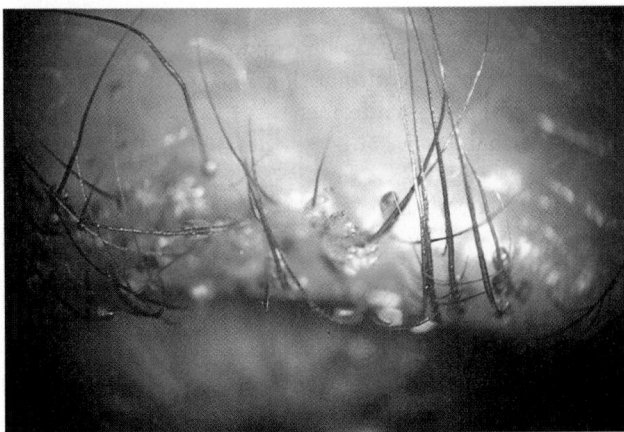

Fig. 21.29 Lid lice.

with seborrhoeic dermatitis of the scalp (dandruff) or elsewhere.

Treatment is by regular lid cleaning, with particular attention to the lid margins. Expression of greasy meibomian secretion by firm pressure may also help the symptoms of burning and irritation. This simple treatment should be carried out long after the symptoms have improved. Recurrent or severe cases, which may be associated with keratoconjunctivitis, may be treated in addition by a short course of a steroid–antibiotic combination ointment.

Lid lice

Lice, *Phthirus palpebrarum* or *P. pubis*, may be found on slit-lamp examination of the lash bases (Fig. 21.29) or their eggs ('nits') may be found attached to the lashes.

Trichiasis

Trichiasis is an acquired condition of the eyelash roots in which the cilia are misdirected, usually backward, causing corneal and conjunctival irritation. It differs from entropion in that the lid margin itself is in a normal position, but because of fibrosis or cicatrization, the ciliae are misplaced. Historically, the most common cause of this condition has been trachoma. In most developed countries, however, more common causes of trichiasis include the Stevens–Johnson syndrome, severe burns and pemphigus.

The treatment of trichiasis depends on the number of abnormal lashes. One or few lashes can be treated with electrolysis or surgery either to excise the lash roots or to resect the affected portion to the eyelid margin. More numerous lashes are best treated with cryotherapy but all the lashes in the treated area are liable to be destroyed and it may cause depigmentation. In black patients it can sometimes be combined with a lid splitting technique as described for distichiasis.

Eyebrows

Synophrys

Eyebrows which join medially (synophrys) have numerous associations.

1 Cornelia de Lange syndrome is the association of mental retardation, hirsutism, growth retardation, flared nostrils and synophrys (Levin *et al.* 1990; Jackson *et al.* 1993).

2 The Jalili retinal dystrophy–hypertrichosis syndrome (Jalili 1984).

3 Waardenburg's syndrome. This autosomal dominant syndrome includes a white forlock, deafness, iris heterochromia, dystopia canthorum and poliosis. In type 1,

234   *Chapter 21*

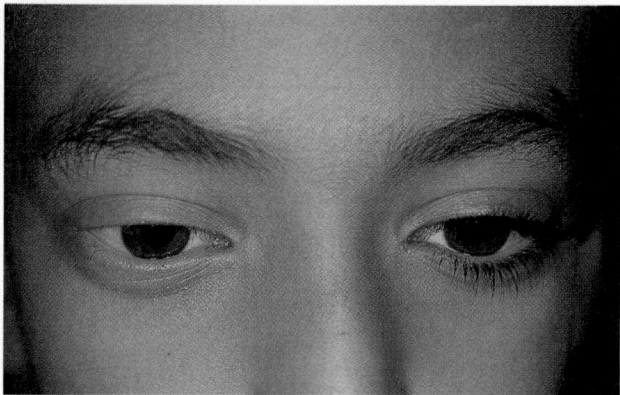

Fig. 21.30 Trichotillomania. The lashes have been plucked. A few remaining broken lashes can be seen in the upper lid.

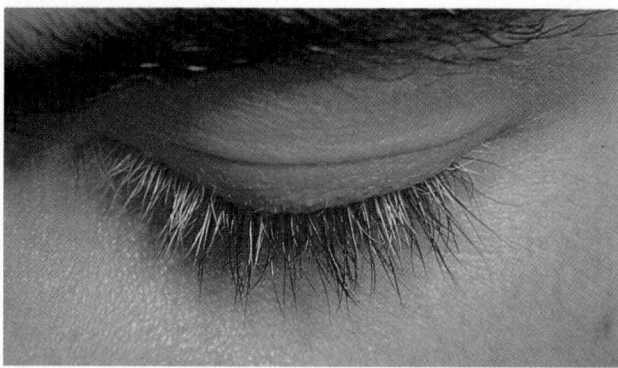

Fig. 21.31 Poliosis in a patient with a Waardenburg's syndrome. The poliosis can be clearly seen against the normally dark lashes.

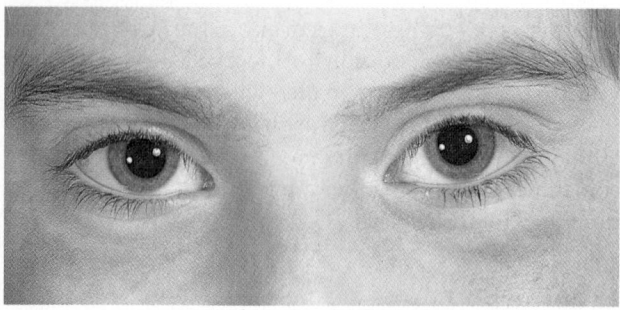

Fig. 21.32 Poliosis in a patient with vitiligo. The poliosis is subtle because of the patient's relatively normal lashes. Preserved skin pigment can be seen on the malar regions.

dystopia canthorum and deafness are most prominent. The gene locus is at 2q37 (Asher *et al.* 1991). In type 2, there is no dystopia and the gene locus is at 3p12-14 (see Chapter 38).
4 Some mucopolysaccharidoses.
5 The Temtamy–Sinbawy syndrome (Temtamy & Sinbawy 1991) includes symptoms of cataract, generalized hypertrichosis and mental retardation; it is an autosomal recessive trait.

6 Other rare syndromes (Winter & Baraitser 1995).

Sparse or absent eyebrows or eyelashes

These occur in the following.
1 Ablepharon–macrostomia syndrome
2 Alopecia unversalis.
3 Trichotillomania — eyelash or eyebrow pulling as a manifestation of psychological stress (Fig. 21.30).
4 Ectodermal dysplasia.
5 Dyskeratosis congenita.
6 Trichomegaly syndrome.
7 Many forms of ichthyosis.
8 Progeria.
9 The cardiofaciocutaneous syndrome (Young *et al.* 1993) — the association of cardiac defects, macrocephaly, growth retardation, hypertelorism and hypoplasia of the supraorbital ridge.
10 Hallerman–Streiff–Francois syndrome (see Chapter 39).
11 Killian–Pallister syndrome.
12 Parry–Romberg syndrome.
13 Rothmund–Thompson syndrome.
14 Woolly hair syndrome (Taylor 1990).

Eyebrow infection

The eyebrows can be affected by many of the afflictions of the eyelids. They are especially prone to abscesses around the eyebrow follicles in eyebrow pluckers and in herpes zoster (Marsh & Cooper 1993). Herpes zoster occasionally occurs in children, and quite frequently in children who are immunosuppressed.

White brows or lashes (poliosis)

1 Albinism. In ocular albinism, the lashes may be pigmented.
2 Vogt–Koyangi–Harada syndrome.
3 Waardenburg's syndrome (Fig. 21.31).
4 Parry–Romberg syndrome.
5 Ectodermal dysplasia.
6 Vitiligo (Fig. 21.32).
7 As an isolated event.

References

Akkerman CHI, Stern LM. Ankyloblepharon filiforme adnatum. *Br J Ophthalmol* 1979; **63**: 129–31.
Al-Hazzia S, Hidayat A. Molluscum contagiosum of the eye lid. *J Pediatr Ophthalmol Strabismus* 1993; **30**: 58–9.
Alvarez EV, Wakakura M, Alvarez E. Surgical management of persistent congenital eversion of the upper eyelids. *Ann Ophthalmol* 1988; **20**: 353–7.
Anderson L, Baumgartner A. Amblyopia in ptosis. *Arch Ophthalmol* 1980a; **98**: 1068–9.

Anderson L, Baumgartner A. Stabismus in ptosis. *Arch Ophthalmol* 1980b; **98**: 1062–7.

Anderson RL, Harvey JT. Lid splitting in posterior lamellar cryosurgery for congenital and acquired distichiasis. *Arch Ophthalmol* 1981; **99**: 631–41.

Anderson RL, Nowinski TS. The five-flap technique for blepharophimosis. *Arch Ophthalmol* 1989; **107**: 448–52.

Asher JH Jr, Morrel R, Friedman TB. Waardenburg syndrome. *Am J Hum Genet* 1991; **48**: 43–52.

Bacal DA, Nelson LB, Zackai EH *et al.* Ankyloblepharon filiforme adnatum in trisomy 18. *J Pediatr Ophthalmol Strabismus* 1993; **30**: 337–9.

Balkan R, Hoyt CS. Associated neurologic abnormalities in congenital third nerve palsies. *Am J Ophthalmol* 1984; **97**: 315–19.

Bardenstein DS, McLean IW, Nerney J, Boatwright RS. Cowden's disease. *Ophthalmology* 1988; **95**: 1038–42.

Bartley GB, Nerad JA, Kersten RC, Maguire LJ. Congenital entropion with intact lower eyelid retractor insertion. *Am J Ophthalmol* 1991; **112**: 437–41.

Beard C. A new treatment for severe unilateral ptosis and for ptosis with jaw–winking. *Am J Ophthalmol* 1965; **59**: 252–7.

Beaconsfield M, Walker JW, Collin JRO. Visual development in blepharophimosis syndrome. *Br J Ophthal* 1991; **75**: 746–8.

Bentsi-Enchill KO. Congenital total eversion of the upper eyelids. *Br J Ophthalmol* 1981; **65**: 209–13.

Bergin DJ, McCord CD, Berger T, Friedberg H, Waterhouse W. Blepharochalasis. *Br J Ophthalmol* 1988; **72**: 863–7.

Berke RN, Wadsworth JAC. Histology of levator muscle in congenital and acquired ptosis. *Arch Ophthalmol* 1955; **53**: 413–16.

Berry C, Cree J, Mann T. Aarskog's syndrome. *Arch Dis Child* 1980; **55**: 706–11.

Bosniak, Hornblass A, Smith B. Re-examining the tarsal kink syndrome: consideration of its etiology and treatment. *Ophthalmic Surg* 1985; **16**: 437–40.

Boyd MJ, Collin JRO. Capillary haemangiomas: an approach to their management. *Br J Ophthalmol* 1991; **75**: 298–300.

Brazier DJ, Hardman-Lea SJ, Collin JR. Cryptophthalmos: surgical treatment of the congenital symblepharon variant. *Br J Ophthalmol* 1986; **70**: 391–5.

Bron AJ, Benjamin L, Snibson GR. Meibomian gland disease. *Eye* 1991; **5**: 395–411.

Calahan AC. Surgical correction of blepharophimosis syndromes. *Trans Am Acad Ophthalmol Otolaryngol* 1973; **77**: 687–95.

Caplan LR. Ptosis. *J Neurol Neurosurg Psychiatry* 1974; **34**: 1–7.

Cenarino EJ, Pinheiro M, Freire-Maia N, Meira-Silva MC. Ablepharon–macrostomia syndrome. *Am J Med Genet* 1988; **31**: 299–304.

Chaurasia BD, Goswani HK. Congenitally malformed female infant with hairy pinnae. *Clin Genet* 1971; **2**: 111–14.

Clarke DI, Patterson A. Ankyloblepharon filiforme adnatum in trisomy 18 (Edward's syndrome). *Br J Ophthalmol* 1985; **69**: 471–3.

Collin JRO, Beard C, Stern WH, Schoengarth D. Blepharochalasis. *Br J Ophthalmol* 1979; **63**: 542.

Collin JRO. Blepharochalasis: a review of 30 cases. *Ophthalmol Plastic Reconstr Surg* 1991; **7**: 153–7.

Collin JRO. Congenital upper lid coloboma. *Austral New Zeal J Ophthalmol* 1986; **14**: 313–17.

Collin JRO. New concepts in the management of ptosis. *Eye* 1988; **2**: 185–9.

Collin JRO, Castronovo S, Allen L. Congenital eyelid retraction. *Br J Ophthalmol* 1990; **9**: 542–4.

Curter PL, Tenzel RR, Kewalczyk AP. Blepharochalasis syndrome. *Am J Ophthalmol* 1985; **99**: 424–8.

Dougherty JM, McCully JP. Comparative bacteriology of chronic blepharitis. *Br J Ophthalmol* 1984; **68**: 524–9.

Downes RN, Collin JR. The Mersilene mesh sling—a new concept in ptosis surgery. *Br J Opthalmol* 1989; **73**: 498–501.

Ehlers N, Jensen IK. Ankyloblepharon filiforme congenitum: associated with harelip and cleft palate. *Acta Ophthalmol* 1970; **48**: 465–7.

Eiferman R, Lane L, Law M. Larsen's syndrome. *Am J Ophthalmol* 1993; **15**: 395–6.

Feingold M, Bossert WH. Normal values for selected physical parameters: an aid to syndrome delineation. *Birth Defects* 1974; **10**: 13.

Frederick D, Robb R. Setleis syndrome. *J Pediatr Ophthalmol Strabismus* 1992; **29**: 127–9.

Fells P, Collin JRO. Cyclic oculomotor palsy. *Trans Ophthal Soc UK* 1979; **99**: 192.

Gonnering RS. Extratarsal chalazia. *Br J Ophthalmol* 1988; **72**: 202–4.

Gordon A, Patrinely J, Krupp J, Font R. Complex choristoma of the eyelid containing ectopic cilia and lacrimal gland. *Ophthalmology* 1991; **98**: 1547–50.

Gupta SP, Saxena RC. Cryptophthalmos. *Br J Ophthalmol* 1963; **46**: 629–31.

Hamed LM, Dennehy PJ, Lingua RW. Synergistic divergence and jaw–winking phenomenon. *J Pediatr Ophthalmol Strabismus* 1990; **27**: 88–91.

Harrad RA, Graham CM, Collin JR. Amblyopia and strabismus in congenital ptosis. *Eye* 1988; **2**: 625–7.

Hay RJ, Wells RS. The syndrome of ankyloblepharon, ectodermal defects and cleft lip and palate: an autosomal dominant condition. *Br J Dermatol* 1976; **94**: 277–89.

Hayasaka S, Noda S, Setogawa T. Epiblepharon with inverted eyelashes in Japanese children. II. Surgical repairs. *Br J Ophthalmol* 1989; **73**: 28–130.

Holds JB, McLeish WM, Anderson RL. Whitnall's sling with superior tarsectomy for the correction of severe unilateral blepharoptosis. *Arch Ophthalmol* 1993; **111**: 1285–91.

Hornblass A, Reiffler DM. Ablepharon macrostomia syndrome. *Am J Ophthalmol* 1985; **99**: 552–6.

Howard G, Wilson M. Pseudodistichiasis as a manifestation of anhidrotic ectodermal dysplasia. *J Pediatr Ophthalmol Strabismus* 1993; **30**: 204–5.

Jackson IT. Macrostomia syndrome. *Br J Plastic Surg* 1988; **41**: 410–16.

Jackson L, Kline AD, Barr MA *et al.* De Lang syndrome. *Am J Educ Genet* 1993; **47**: 940–6.

Jalili IK. Congenital amaurosis associated with congenital hypertrichosis. *J Med Genet* 1989; **26**: 504–10.

Jewett T, Kao N, Weaver RS, Stewart W, Thomas IT, Pettenati MV. Blepharophimosis ptosis and epicanthus inversion syndrome. *Am J Med Genet* 1993; **47**: 1147–50.

Jones CA, Collin JRO. Blepharophimosis and its association with female infertility. *Br J Ophthalmol* 1984; **68**: 533–4.

Jordan R. Blepharochalasis syndrome. *Arch Ophthalmol* 1990; **108**: 1633.

Jordan R. The lower lid retractors in congenital entropion and epiblepharon. *Ophthalmic Surg* 1993; **24**: 494–6.

Kavalec C, Harvey J. Xanthoma disseminatum. *Arch Ophthalmol* 1993; **111**: 1428–9.

Kazarian El, Goldstein P. Ankyloblepharon filiforme adnatum with hydrocephalus, meningomyelocele and imperforate anus. *Am J Ophthalmol* 1977; **84**: 355–7.

Keipert JA. Euryblepharon. *Br J Ophthalmol* 1975; **59**: 57–8.

Kennedy R, Flanagan J, Eagle R, Carney J. Carney's complex. *Am J Ophthalmol* 1991; **111**: 699–703.

Khurana A, Ahluwalia B, Mehtani V. Primary epitarsus: a case report. *Br J Ophthalmol* 1986; **70**: 931–2.

Kolin T, Johns K, Wadlington W, Butter M, Sunalp M, Wright K. Dystichiasis. *Arch Ophthalmol* 1991; **109**: 980–1.

Kronish J, Lingua R. Pressure patch treatment for congenital upper eyelid eversion. *Arch Ophthalmol* 1991; **109**: 767–8.

Kushner BJ. Intralesional corticosteroid injection for infantile adnexal hemangioma. *Am J Ophthalmol* 1982; **93**: 496–506.

Levin AV, Feidman DJ, Hebart B, Jackson LG. Cornelia de Lang syndrome. *J Pediatr Ophthalmol Strabismus* 1990; **27**: 94–102.

McCarthy GT, West CM. Ablepharon macrostomia syndrome. *Div Med Child Neurol* 1977; **19**: 659–63.

McCord CD. The correction of telecanthus and epicanthal folds. *Ophthalmic Surg* 1980; **11**: 446–56.

McCulloch DL, Wright KW. Unilateral congenital ptosis: compensatory head posturing and amblyopia. *Ophthal Plastic Reconstr Surg* 1993; **9**: 196–200.

McDonnell PJ, Mayou BJ. Congenital divided naevus of the eyelids. *Br J Ophthalmol* 1988; **72**: 198–202.

Mansell PI, Higgs E, Reckless JPD. Carney's complex. *J Roy Soc Med* 1991; **84**: 496–7.

Mansour AM, Traboulsi E, Frangieh G. Multiple recurrences of juvenile xanthogranuloma of the eyelid. *J Pediatr Ophthalmol Strabismus* 1985; **22**: 156–7.

Markowitz G, Hsandler L, Katowitz J. Congenital euryblepharon and nasolacrimal anomalies in a patient with Down syndrome. *J Pediatr Ophthalmol Strabismus* 1994; **31**: 330–1.

Marsh R, Cooper M. Ophthalmic herpes zoster. *Eye* 1993; **7**: 350–70.

Mauriello JA, Wagner RS, Caputo AR. Treatment of congenital ptosis by maximal levator resection. *Ophthalmology* 1986; **93**: 466–8.

Miller R, Martin F, Allen H. A case of congenital ectropion in Down's syndrome. *Austral N Zeal J Ophthalmol* 1988; **16**: 119–25.

Moainei R, Kopelowitz N, Rosenfeld W, Jhaderi R. Congenital eversion of the eyelids. *J Pediatr Ophthalmol Strabismus* 1982; **19**: 326–7.

Morris RJ, Collin JRO. Functional lid surgery in Down's syndrome. *Br J Ophthalmol* 1986; **73**: 494–7.

Mustarde JC. Epicanthal folds and the problem of telecanthus. *Trans Ophthalmol Soc UK* 1963; **83**: 397–411.

Mustarde JC. *Plastic Surgery in Infancy and Childhood*. London: Longman, 1971: 251–60.

Ni C, Kimball GP, Craft JL *et al*. Calcifying epithelioma of Malherbe. *Int Ophthalmol Clin* 1982; **22**: 63–86.

Noda S, Hayasaka S, Setogawa T. Epiblepharon with inverted lashes in Japanese children I. Incidence and symptoms. *Br J Ophthalmol* 1989; **73**: 126–7.

O'Donnell BA, Collin JRO. Congenital lower eyelid deformity with trichiasis, epiblepharon and entropion. *Austral N Zeal J Ophthalmol* 1994; **22**: 33–7.

O'Donnell BA, Collin JRO. Distichiasis: management with cryotherapy to the posterior lamella. *Br J Ophthalmol* 1993; **77**: 289–92.

Oestreicher JH, Nelson CC. Lamellar ichthyosis and congenital ectropion. *Arch Ophthalmol* 1990; **108**: 1772–3.

Price NC, Collin JR. Congenital horizontal tarsal kink: a simple surgical correction. *Br J Ophthalmol* 1987; **71**: 204–7.

Price NC, Pugh R, Farndon P, Willshaw H. Ablepharon macrostomia syndrome. *Br J Ophthalmol* 1991; **75**: 317–320.

Raab EL, Saphir RL. Congenital eyelid eversion with orbicularis spasm. *J Pediatr Ophthalmol Strabismus* 1985; **22**: 125–8.

Robb RM. Refractive errors associated with hemangiomas of the eyelids in infancy. *Am J Ophthalmol* 1977; **83**: 52–8.

Roper-Hall MJ. Congenital colobomata of the lids. *Trans Ophthalmol Soc UK* 1969; **88**: 556–7.

Sano K. Trigemino-oculomotor synkinesis. *Neurolgia* 1959; **I**: 29–51.

Scott MH, Richard JM, Farris BK. Ankyloblepharon filiforme adnatum associated with infantile glaucoma and tridogonoidysgenesis. *J Pediatr Ophthalmol Strabismus* 1994; **31**: 93–5.

Sellar PW, Bryars JH, Archer DB. Congenital ectropion in child with Down's syndrome. *J. Pediatr Ophthalmol* 1992; **29**: 64–7.

Sevel D. A reappraisal of the development of the eyelids. *Eye* 1988; **2**: 123–9.

Shapiro I, Borochowitz Z, Deganis S *et al*. Neu–Laxova syndrome. *Am J Med Genet* 1992; **43**: 602–5.

Shields JA, Shields CL, Eagle RC, Mulvey L. Pilomatrixoma of the eyelid. *J Pediatr Ophthalmol Strabismus* 1995; **32**: 260–1.

Shields LC, Nelson LB, Carpenter GC, Shields JA. Neonatal Grave's disease. *Br J Ophthalmol* 1988; **72**: 424–8.

Smith B, Chrubini T. *Oculoplastic Surgery*. St Louis: CV Mosby, 1970: 9–12, 18–20.

Stout A, Borchert M. Etiology of eyelid retraction in children. *J Pediatr Ophthalmol Strabismus* 1993; **30**: 96–9.

Sullivan TJ, Clarke MP, Rootman DS, Pashby RC. Eyelid and fornix reconstruction in bilateral abortive cryptophthalmos (Fraser syndrome). *Austral N Zeal J. Ophthalmol* 1992; **20**: 51–6.

Taylor AEM. Hereditary woolly hair with ocular involvement. *Br J Dermatol* 1990; **123**: 523–5.

Temple IK, Collin JRO. Distichiasis-lymphoedema syndrome: a family report. *Clin Dysmorph* 1994; **3**: 139–42.

Temtamy SA, Synbawy AHH. Cataract, hypertrichosis, and mental retardation (CAHMR): a new autosomal recessive syndrome. *Am J Med Genet* 1991; **41**: 432–3.

Tse DP, Anderson RL, Fratkin JD. Aponeurosis disinsertion in congenital entropion. *Arch Ophthalmol* 1983; **101**: 436–40.

Tuomaala P, Haapanen L. Three siblings with similar anomalies of the eyes, bone, and skin. *Acta Ophthalmol* 1968; **46**: 365–71.

Weiss AH, Riscile G, Kousseff BG. Ankyloblepharon filiforme adnatum. *Am J Med Genet* 1992; **42**: 369–73.

White JH. Correction of distichiasis by tarsal resection and mucous membrane grafting. *Am J Ophthalmol* 1975; **80**: 507–8.

Winter RM, Baraitser M. The London Dysmorphology Database: A computerised database for the diagnosis of rare dysmorphic syndromes. New York, Oxford University Press, 1995.

Wolfley D. Excision of individual follicles for the management of congenital distichiasis and localised trichiasis. *J Pediatr Ophthalmol Strabismus* 1987; **24**: 22–6.

Young LLH, Lambert SR, Chapman J, Stulting RD. Congenital entropion and congenital corneal ulcer. *Am J Ophthalmol* 1996; **121**: 329–31.

Young T, Ziylan S, Schaffer D. Cardiofaciocutaneous syndrome. *J Pediatr Ophthalmol Strabismus* 1993; **30**: 48–52.

Zak TA. Congenital primary upper eyelid entropion. *J Pediatr Ophthalmol Strabismus* 1984; **21**: 69–73.

22: Conjunctiva and Subconjunctival Tissue

David Taylor

Structure, function and embryology

The conjunctiva is derived from a band of mesenchyme around the limbus which also forms the sclera, episclera, and Tenon's capsule. In childhood the conjunctiva is thicker than in old age and the epithelial cells are more square in shape and they are more numerous than in mid-life. In childhood Tenon's capsule is thick and the blood vessels are fewer, less tortuous, smaller and less prominent than they are in old age. As every strabismus surgeon knows, the conjunctiva of a child is a much tougher tissue than the underlying Tenon's 'capsule': it holds sutures well. The subconjunctival tissues do not develop the fatty infiltrates that occur especially in the exposed areas in an adult, this being one of the factors behind the 'bright eyes' of youth. The conjunctiva contains goblet cells which produce mucus, vital to the normal structure of the tear layer and therefore vital to the protection of the eye. The growth of the conjunctival fornix, orbital margin, and palpebral fissure correlates with weight and gestational age of term and premature neonates (Isenberg *et al.* 1987).

Vascular abnormalities

Haemangioma and lymphohaemangioma

Usually occurring predominantly as a haemangioma composed only of blood vessels, these are usually associated with lid and orbital haemangiomas (Fig. 22.1) and sometimes with intracranial haemangiomas but these may be isolated. They appear as bright red masses (Fig. 22.2) which blanch on pressure and which not infrequently haemorrhage spontaneously or with trivial trauma (Fig. 22.3). Treatment may be difficult because removal is often but not always (Sujatha *et al.* 1994) followed by recurrence. Radiotherapy may play some role in their treatment.

Lymphohaemangiomas (Fig. 22.4) are usually more widespread, with the whole of one side of the face being affected and the abnormality appearing in other parts of the face, in the nose causing nose bleeds or on the palate causing bleeding when eating. Lymphohaemangiomas are less prone to the cessation of growth which many of the haemangiomas show by the time the child is a few years of age, but nonetheless some do show resolution and therefore surgery should be restricted only to those cases where relentless growth has occurred, where the cosmetic appearance is extremely poor, or where there

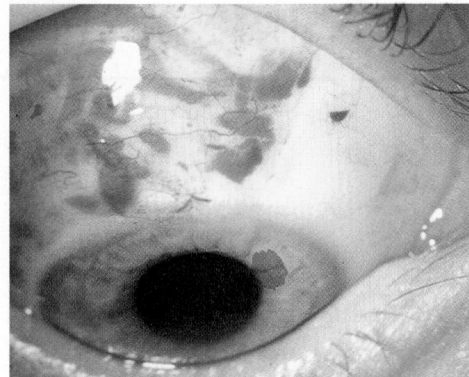

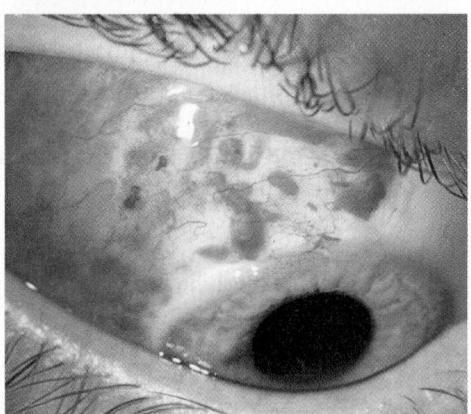

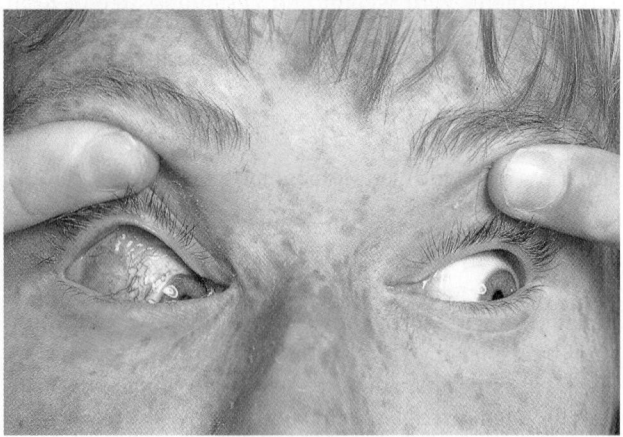

Fig. 22.1 Conjunctival haemangioma. (a) As a baby this 17-year-old girl had an orbital and lid haemangioma. The subconjunctival vascular abnormality had bled repeatedly and did not respond to surgical excision of the subconjunctival vessels. (b) The conjunctival haemangiomas became devascularized with low-dose radiotherapy (same patient).

appears to be no cessation of growth. Clinically they may be distinguished by the appearance of clear fluid-filled cystic areas amongst the blood-filled haemangioma tissue.

Sturge–Weber syndrome

Naevus flammeus, the flat form of facial haemangioma,

may sometimes be associated with congenital glaucoma, intracranial calcification and fits, when it is known as the Sturge–Weber syndrome. The conjunctiva may be involved (Fig. 22.5) showing only a faint blush on the normal whiteness of the conjunctiva or it may be more extensive. It may be limited to sectors of the conjunctiva and may cause difficulty because of bleeding at the time of surgery for glaucoma associated with Sturge–Weber syndrome (Chapter 40). The vessels consist of a very fine network of capillary-sized vessels.

Klippel–Trenaunay–Weber syndrome

This syndrome (Klippel & Trenaunay 1900; Weber 1907),

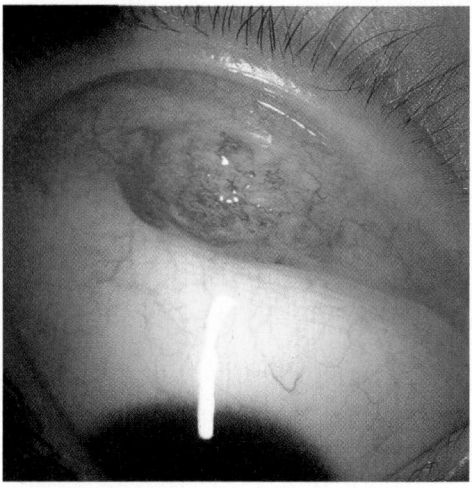

Fig. 22.2 An isolated conjunctival haemangioma in a 2-year-old child that disappeared by the age of 6 years.

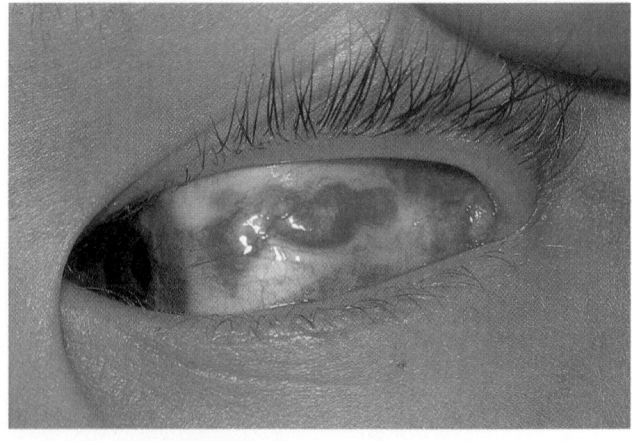

Fig. 22.3 Subconjunctival haemangioma in an otherwise normal child. Although it had regressed spontaneously from being quite large at birth, it was prone to repeated subconjunctival haemorrhages. On this occasion the haemorrhage is contained within the subconjunctival tissue but can be seen to be spreading anteriorly.

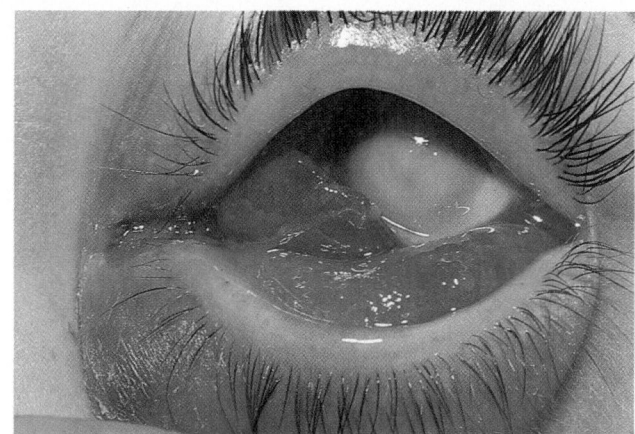

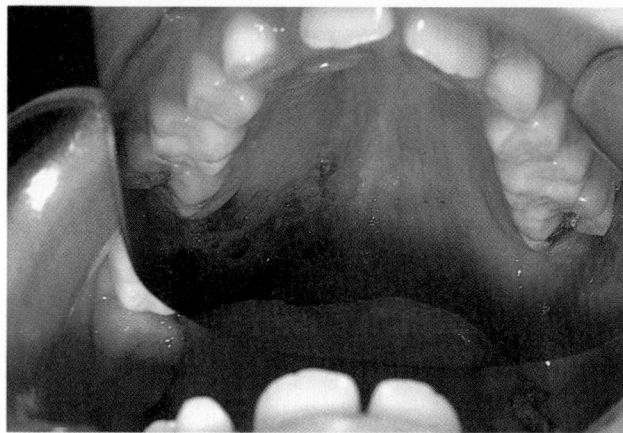

Fig. 22.4 (a) This 2-year-old child had an anomalous left eye from birth; at 18 months of age the lids became swollen due to a lymphohaemangioma which also involved the orbit and maxilla. (b) Palatal clear and blood-filled cysts typical of lymphohaemangioma (same patient).

which consists of a widespread vascular anomaly causing limb hypertrophy and bluish vascular anomalies of the skin, may also have conjunctival angiomas (Stewart & Farmer 1990).

Orbital, cerebral and ocular vascular malformations

A variety of intracranial abnormalities may be associated with orbital and conjunctival varices. The best known of the ocular abnormalities is in the Wyburn–Mason syndrome, in which huge racemose angiomatous malformation of the retina, sometimes with remarkably well-preserved vision, is associated with intracranial, orbital, and sometimes conjunctival vascular malformations (Theron *et al.* 1974).

A variety of other ocular and adnexal abnormalities occur including small optic nerves and eye muscle enlargement (O'Connor & Smith 1978; Good & Hoyt 1989), orbital varix (Rathburn *et al.* 1970), retinal varicosity

(Limaye *et al.* 1979) and glaucoma (Hudelo 1929). Most cases do not have ocular involvement. Intracranial tumours with Klippel–Trenaunay–Weber syndrome have also occasionally been described (Djinjian *et al.* 1977; Howitz *et al.* 1979) and it may be associated with oculodermal melanocytosis (Teekhasaenee 1990) (see Chapter 37).

Ataxia telangiectasia (Louis–Bar syndrome)

This disease is autosomal recessively inherited and usually presents with a cerebellar ataxia after a normal early development. Limb and truncal ataxia occurs in the first decade and is slowly progressive. Later dysarthria and other movement disorders including extrapyramidal disorders are seen. Usually the child becomes severely handicapped by 12 years of age. Mental retardation is frequent, as is dementia, and growth retardation occurs especially in those who have recurrent infections. These infections are due to an immunological defect with reduced synthesis of immunoglobulin A (IgA), IgM and, to a certain extent, IgG. They are also susceptible to a variety of neoplasms and abnormal carbohydrate metabolism (McFarlan & Strober 1972). The characteristic ocular feature is the presence of extremely tortuous and telangiectatic conjunctival vessels which usually occur in the exposed areas (Fig. 22.6). Sometimes they may be quite gross, but they are usually subtle. The bulbar conjunctiva is affected first (Harley *et al.* 1967) and the lesions consist of a postcapillary venular link with vessels of non-uniform calibre with slow flow of red blood cells (Kulikov 1974). Later, telangiectases develop on exposed areas of skin, especially the ears.

Another characteristic finding is an eye movement defect consisting of nystagmus and a form of saccade palsy or oculomotor apraxia (Smith & Cogan 1959; Baloh *et al.* 1978) (see Chapter 64).

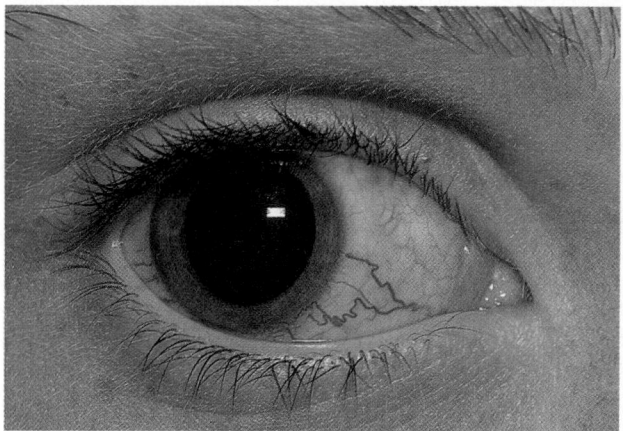

Fig. 22.5 Sturge–Weber syndrome. Conjunctival capillary haemangioma with dilated larger vessels associated with glaucoma.

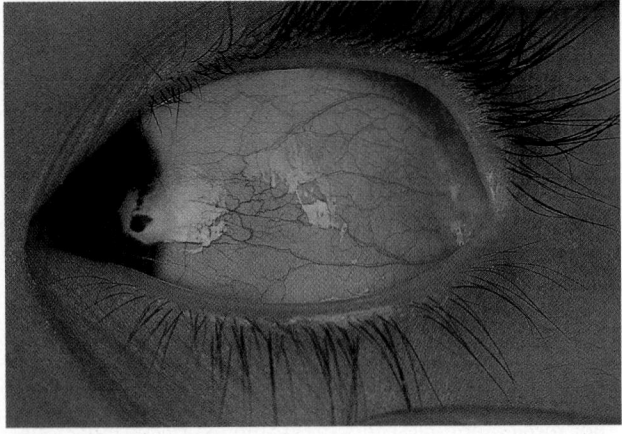

Fig. 22.6 Ataxia telangiectasia. There is a group of telangiectatic and tortuous vessels in the exposed area of the conjunctiva especially temporally.

Rendu–Osler–Weber disease

Brant *et al.* (1989) found conjunctival telangiectases in seven of 20 patients with Rendu–Osler–Weber syndrome; two also had a retinal vascular malformation.

Carotid cavernous fistula

Children who develop a red eye following head trauma by a few days, but occasionally some weeks, should be suspected of having a carotid cavernous fistula. Although relatively rare in childhood it is sometimes severe and may be associated with raised intraocular pressure (see Chapter 62).

Sickle cell disease

Although not symptomatic, the conjunctiva is a useful site for observing the vascular changes by slit-lamp microscopy. Comma-shaped conjunctiva capillaries and slow flow may be seen.

Hyperviscosity

In blood hyperviscosity states the conjunctiva appears suffused, the capillaries dilated and tortuous with slow flow seen on slit-lamp microscopy.

Conjunctival haemorrhage

Most frequently this occurs after minor trauma and it occurs when there has been a rise in central venous pressure such as after a seizure, immediately after birth or any activity involving valsalva type manoeuvres. The haemorrhages usually improve spontaneously within 2 weeks and do not require treatment.

Spontaneous conjunctival haemorrhages are not infrequent in childhood and are the subject of some mythology as to causation, but they are generally not known to be associated with any serious abnormality. Sometimes they occur repeatedly in one area and slit-lamp examination may reveal an anomalous vessel which occasionally needs treatment by cautery to prevent recurrence.

Subconjunctival haemorrhages occur in thrombocytopenic states, for instance in leukaemia. Various forms of conjunctivitis may be associated with subconjunctival haemorrhage (see Chapter 18).

Fabry's disease

Small conjunctival aneurysms occur in Fabry's disease.

Conjunctival lymphangiectasia

Conjunctival lymphangiectasia may be associated with generalized lymphoedema (Milroy–Meige disease). It has been described with Turner's syndrome (Perry & Cossari 1986) and dilated subconjunctival lymph vessels may be seen adjacent to plexiform neuromas (Fig. 22.7).

Linear scleroderma (morphoea en coup de sabre)

A perilimbal dilated vascular network is a not uncommon finding in morphoea en coup de sabre (Taylor & Talbot 1985) (Fig. 22.8). Morphoea appears as a linear groove in the scalp or forehead skin and may spread to the lids, orbit and eye. Uveitis is not infrequent (Fig. 22.9), and ipsilateral glaucoma may occur (Perrot *et al.* 1977).

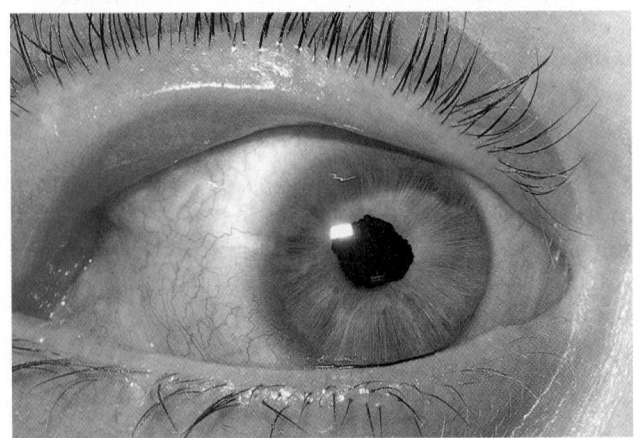

Fig. 22.7 Neurofibromatosis with orbital plexiform neuroma adjacent to which there are dilated lymph vessels; note the ectropion pupillae.

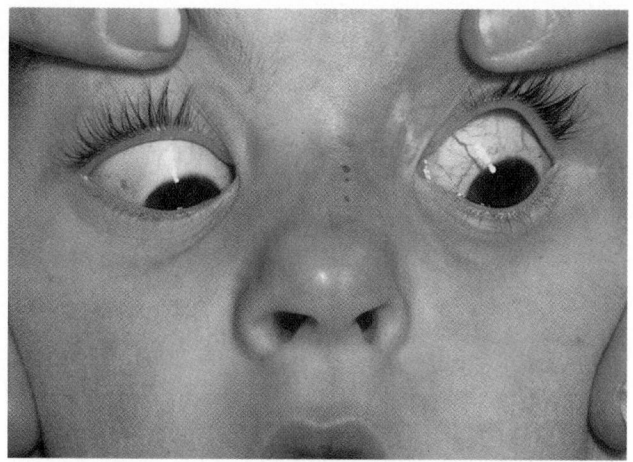

Fig. 22.8 Morphoea en coup de sabre. This child had a left frontal linear scleroderma which can be seen to affect the side of the nose, together with conjunctival telangiectasia, uveitis and glaucoma.

Pigmented lesions

Oculodermal melanosis (naevus of Ota) and ocular melanosis

Pigmentation of the conjunctiva and subconjunctival tissue may be known as ocular melanosis; when the ipsilateral skin and mucous membrane are involved the condition is known as oculodermal melanocytosis (Fig. 22.10) or naevus of Ota.

Ocular melanosis (Fig. 22.11) shows as a variable slatey blue scleral, conjunctival and subconjunctival pigmentation associated with skin and mucous membrane hyperpigmentation usually on the same side (Charlin 1973). Ipsilateral iris hyperpigmentation occurs due to diffuse iris naevus (Ticho *et al.* 1989). It is usually noticed in the first year or two of life but sometimes does not present until later. It may get worse initially and then again later at puberty. There is an increased risk in this condition of the child later developing uveal or other (Unal *et al.* 1992) malignant melanomas (Jay 1965a; Yamamoto 1969; Singh *et al.* 1988). Although more frequent in black and oriental people, malignant change may be less frequent than in white people (Gonder *et al.* 1982; Nik *et al.* 1982; Dutton *et al.* 1984). The incidence of malignant change is not known but is probably not high. Intracranial vascular malformations may also be associated (Orr *et al.* 1978; Massey *et al.* 1979).

Teekhasaenee *et al.* (1990) examined 194 patients with oculodermal melanocytosis; 60% had skin and eye involvement, 6% had only eye involvement and 34% only skin involvement. Ten per cent had raised intraocular pressure with or without glaucomatous changes. Familial occurrence was unusual in this series but has been described before (Dutton *et al.* 1984).

Children with this condition should be reviewed periodically because of a risk of pigmentary glaucoma and the risk of melanoma (Roldan *et al.* 1987).

Oculodermal melanocytosis may be associated with neurofibromatosis and the Klippel–Trenaunay–Weber syndrome (Teekhasaenee 1990).

Naevi

These do not usually beome obvious until after the first few years of life (Jay 1965b) often after 10 years or even later. They are composed of melanocytic naevus cells sometimes located only within the epithelial layer of the conjunctiva, when they are known as junctional naevi. When subepithelial and epithelial naevus cells are present

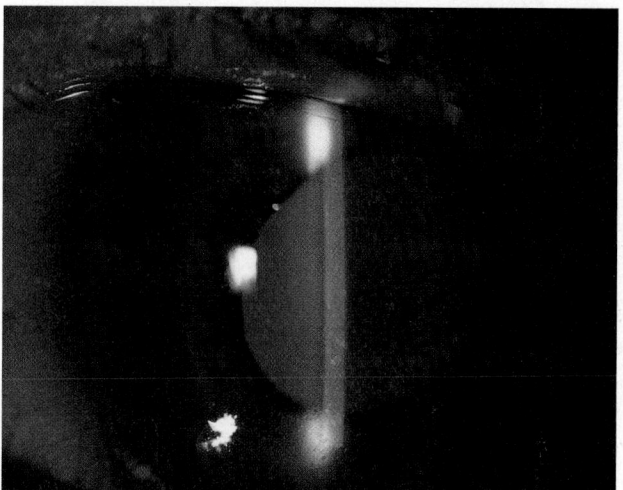

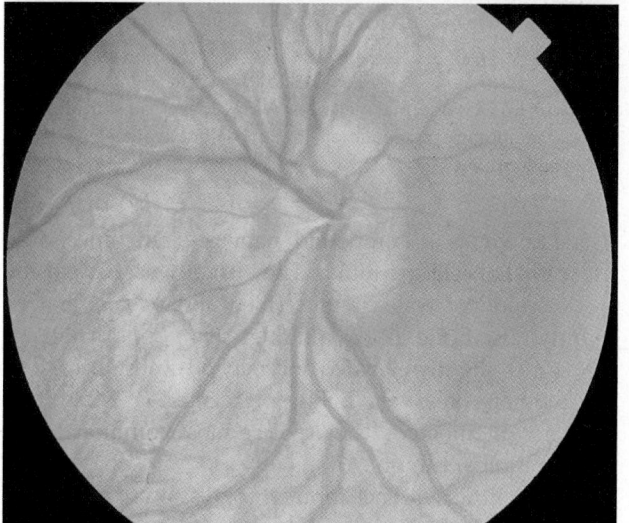

Fig. 22.9 Morphoea en coup de sabre. (a) On the same side as the linear scleroderma there was a uveitis with keratic precipitates. (b) Hypotony with disc oedema.

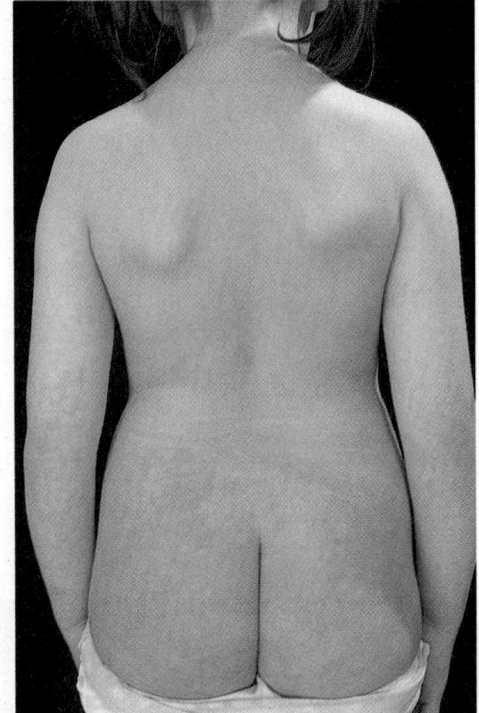

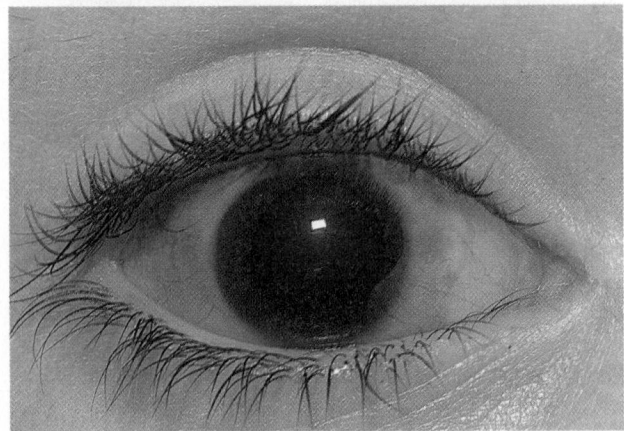

Fig. 22.10 (a) Oculodermal melanosis with widespread skin and mucous membrane pigmentation. (b) Subconjunctival melanosis (same patient).

it is known as a compound naevus. Sometimes only subepithelial cells are found. They usually occur near the limbus and are well circumscribed and usually flat or slightly raised (Fig. 22.12), although compound naevi are sometimes slightly elevated and may be cystic. Occasionally they are only very lightly pigmented (Fig. 22.13) or even non-pigmented. They are the most common childhood epibulbar tumour.

There is little evidence for the progression of naevi into melanomas. Melanomas of the conjunctiva are extremely rare in childhood but when they occur they are characterized by being somewhat more raised, vascular and fleshy than naevi (Fig. 22.14), with histological differences, and

they should carry a more guarded prognosis (McDonnell *et al.* 1989a).

Gaucher's disease

Pingueculae and conjunctival pigmentation occur in the chronic forms of Gaucher's disease (see Chapter 57).

Alkaptonuria

Episcleral and conjunctival pigmentation occur in the area

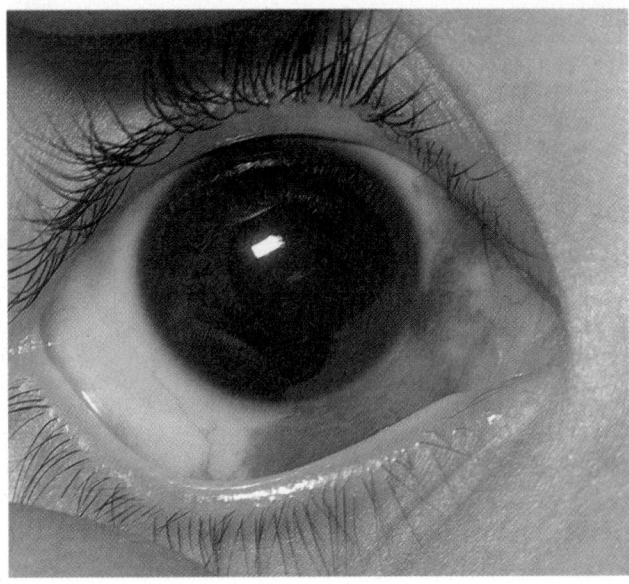

Fig. 22.11 Ocular melanosis. Congenital slate-blue episcleral pigmentation.

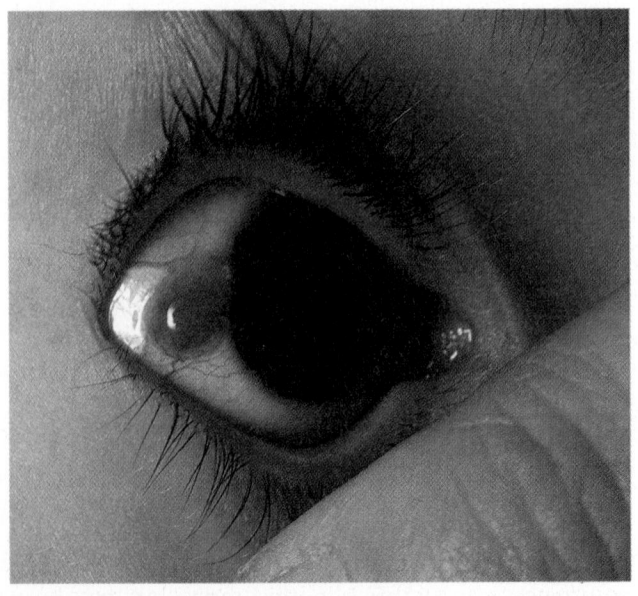

Fig. 22.12 Raised pigmented limbal naevus.

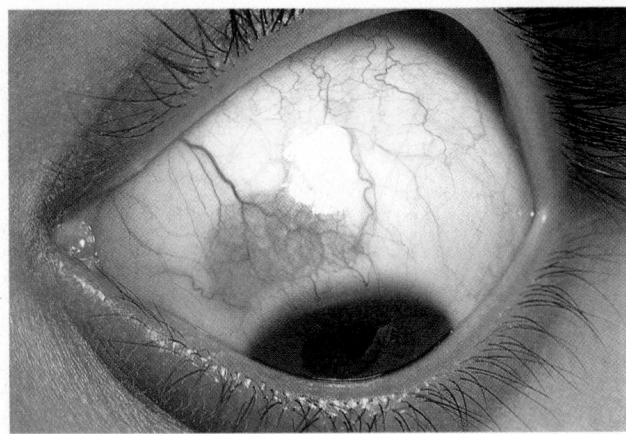

Fig. 22.13 Lightly pigmented cystic compound naevus of the conjunctiva in a 14-year-old patient.

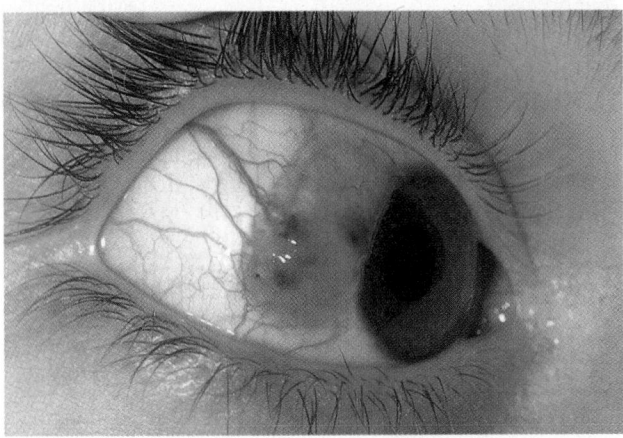

Fig. 22.14 A raised vascular fleshy naevus that may be a melanoma.

of the horizontal rectus muscle insertions. These children, whose urine turns black on standing, have bone disease with arthritis and valvular and atherosclerotic heart disease.

Kartagener's syndrome

In this recessively inherited syndrome children may be born with dextrocardia and they develop bronchiectasis, bronchitis and respiratory tract infections. They are sometimes myopic and may develop glaucoma. They characteristically have marked conjunctival melanosis and hypertrophy of the plica semilunaris (Segal *et al.* 1963).

Peutz–Jeghers syndrome

This is an autosomal dominantly inherited syndrome with polyposis of the gastrointestinal tract, especially the small bowel. The polyps may bleed and may become malignant.

Freckles are seen around the orifices, on the lids and conjunctiva; scleral and corneal pigmented spots have been described. Gass and Glatzer (1991) described an adult who presented with pigmented freckles of the lips and penis, thought to be due to Peutz–Jeghers syndrome, but who actually had malignant bilateral diffuse uveal melanocytic proliferation.

Tumours and infiltrates

The most common epibulbar tumours are naevi, dermoids, inclusion cysts and papillomas (Cunha *et al.* 1987).

Epibulbar dermoids

These are choristomas which contain a combination of fat, hair follicles and sebaceous glands. They may occur at the limbus or even on the cornea alone. Corneal and limbal dermoids appear as yellowish white, usually rounded elevations sometimes with pigmentation and hair at the apex (Figs 22.15, 22.16) and sometimes associated with intraocular abnormalities (Fig. 22.17). The more posterior dermoids, known as dermolipomas, may be associated with a larger amount of fatty tissue without hairs and they extend posteriorly for some considerable distance and cannot safely be removed as a whole. They may be closely related to eye muscles and surgeons need to limit their ambitions to the safely achievable (Fry & Leone 1994).

Either type of dermoid may be associated with Goldenhar's syndrome (Fig. 22.18) in which often bilateral epibulbar dermoids occur with a lid coloboma and with pre-auricular skin tags or appendages; a variety of first branchial arch abnormalities; and occasionally a neurotrophic or neuroparalytic keratitis (Romano 1978) (see

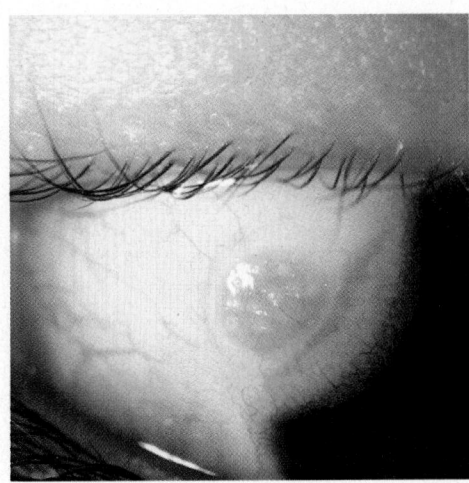

Fig. 22.15 A hairy limbal dermoid.

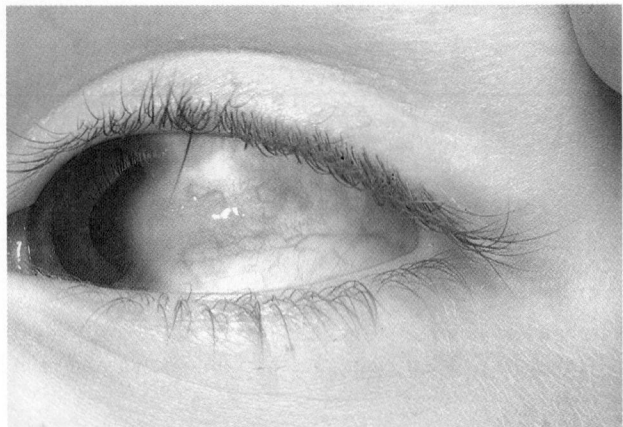

Fig. 22.16 A limbal dermoid encroaching on the cornea and extending back to the temporal fornix.

Chapter 24). Other systemic associations are the linear naevus sebaceous syndrome (Fuerstein–Mimms), and encephalocraniocutaneous lipomatosis (Kodsi *et al.* 1994), in which ipsilateral ocular, cutaneous, and intracranial choristomas and hamartomas occur.

Epibulbar osseous choristomas are flatter, bony and

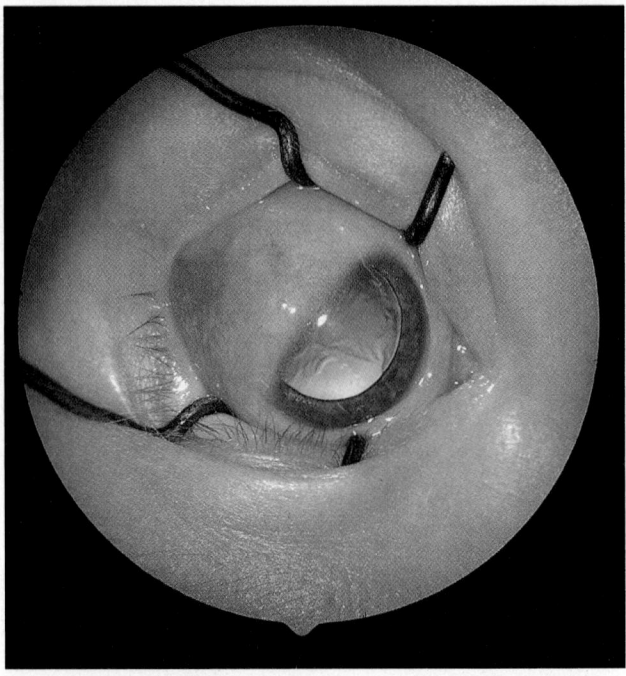

Fig. 22.17 A limbal epibulbar dermoid encroaching on the lateral third of the cornea. Although removed, leaving minimal scarring, the eye had profound amblyopia due to astigmatism.

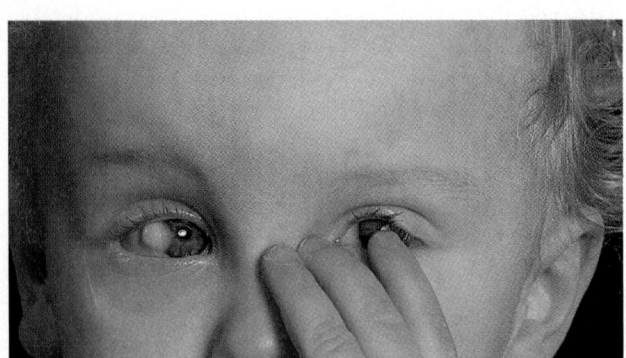

a

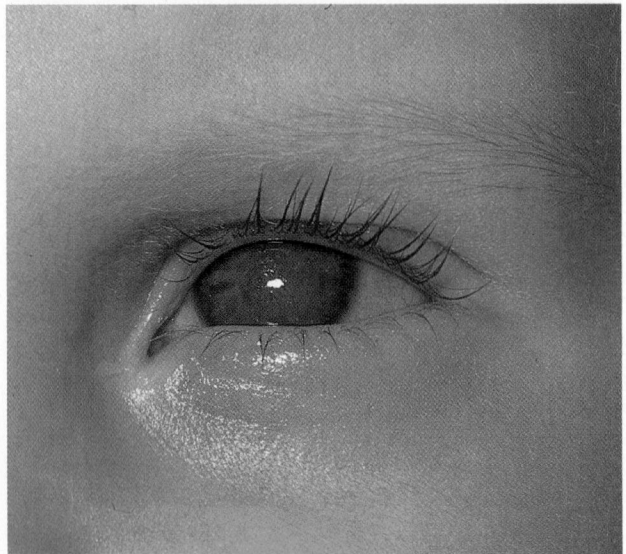

b

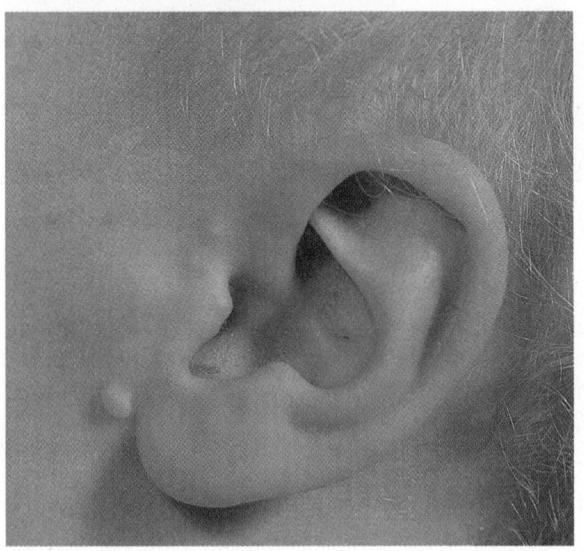

c

Fig. 22.18 (a) Right limbal dermoid in a child with Goldenhar's syndrome. He also had corneal anaesthesia affecting particularly the left eye and can be seen scratching the cornea at the time when the picture was taken. (b) Corneal scarring and vascularization resulting from chronic traumatization of the anaesthetic, left eye. (c) Pre-auricular skin tags in the same patient with Goldenhar's syndrome.

fatty abnormalities (Fig. 22.19) which may overlie ectopic lacrimal gland in the temporal or superotemporal region under the conjunctiva (Hered & Hiles 1987; Pokorny *et al.* 1987).

Proteus syndrome

The proteus syndrome (Fig. 22.20) is characterized by a warty overgrowth of the sole of the foot, craniofacial anomalies, intradermal naevi, variable mental retardation, epibulbar hamartomas (Burke *et al.* 1988) and lid hamartomas (Lessner & Margo 1991).

Most dermoids can be simply excised for cosmetic reasons; when the cornea is involved a lamellar keratectomy has to be carried out and the results are often only moderately good with an improvement in that the elevated mass

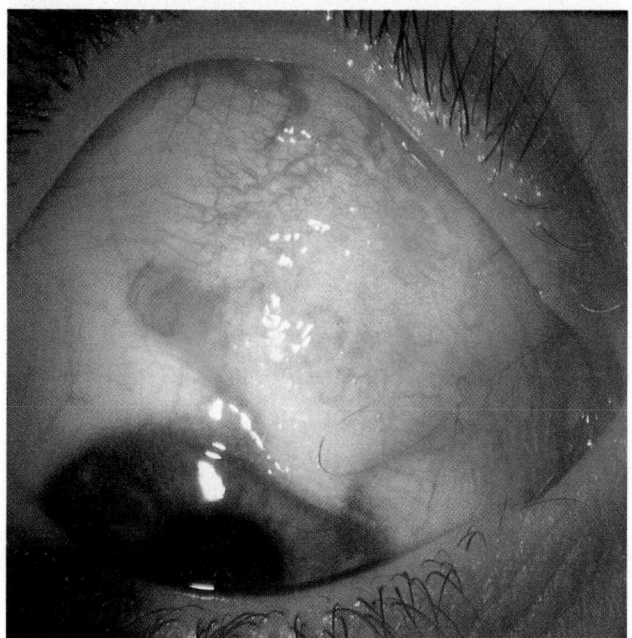

Fig. 22.19 Epibulbar osseous choristoma overlying ectopic lacrimal gland.

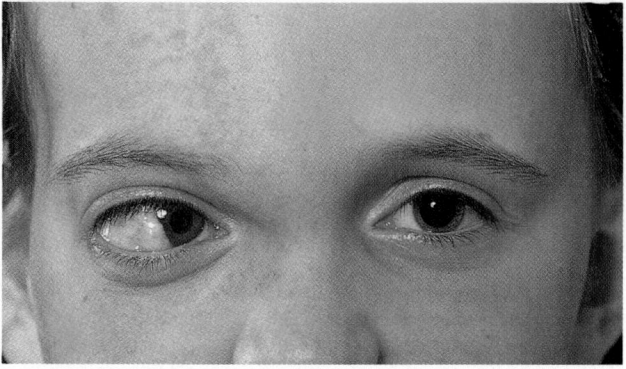

Fig. 22.20 Proteus syndrome showing an epibulbar hamartoma.

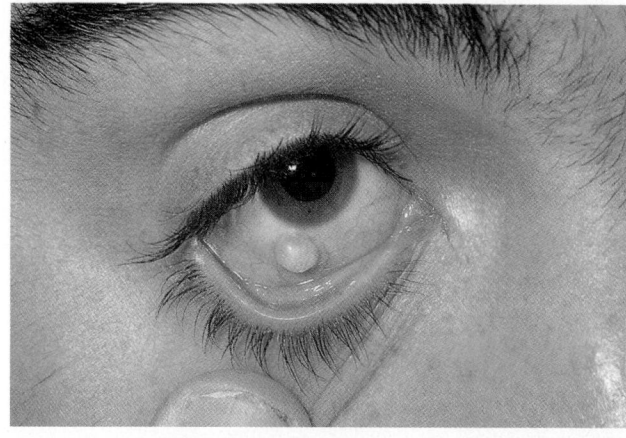

Fig. 22.21 Clear cyst of the conjunctiva in a teenager with no history of trauma or surgery.

is removed, but the remaining cornea is sometimes opalescent or may even become opaque. Freehand corneal lamellar grafting may improve the appearance in refractory cases but the results are sometimes not very satisfactory.

Clear cysts

Occasionally small, clear fluid-filled cysts (Fig. 22.21) appear in the conjunctiva in older children. These are of no significance and usually disappear spontaneously; if they cause symptoms they can be simply excised. They may be post-traumatic or surgical.

Secondary tumours

The conjunctiva may be invaded by other tumours including rhabdomyosarcoma (Fig. 22.22) and retinoblastoma; rarely retinoblastoma may present as a conjunctival or subconjunctival swelling. Histiocytosis-X occasionally involves the conjunctiva as does juvenile xanthogranuloma. Conjunctival infiltrates occur in childhood leukaemia and neurofibromas, usually associated with a plexiform neuroma of the orbit, may present with a whitish or clear cystic knotted mass in the subconjunctival tissue. A Burkitt's lymphoma has been presented with a subconjunctival mass (Weisenthal *et al.* 1995).

Xeroderma pigmentosa

This is a rare autosomal recessive disease of infancy and childhood in which the skin is excessively sensitive to light resulting in pigmentation, telangiectasis, keratosis, and the development of basal cell and squamous cell carcinomas, malignant melanomas (Vivian *et al.* 1993; Goyal *et al.* 1994), and a variety of other tumours. These may include squamous cell carcinomas of the conjunctiva

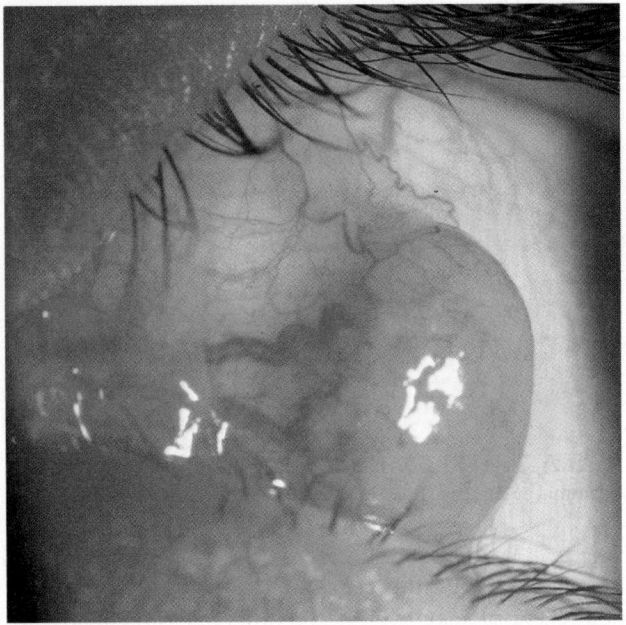

Fig. 22.22 Rhabdomyosarcoma presenting as a subconjunctival nodule.

(Fig. 22.23) (Bellows *et al.* 1974; Vivian *et al.* 1993). The syndrome is sometimes associated with progressive neurological abnormalities including deafness, ataxia, mental retardation and cerebellar atrophy, when it is known as the De Sanctis–Cacchione syndrome (Handa *et al.* 1978; Kraemer *et al.* 1987).

Patients with xeroderma pigmentosa have a defect in DNA repair (Arlett 1986) and their tissues are vulnerable to ultraviolet light exposure. In addition to covering the skin and the use of sunscreens the eyes should be protected by the use of 100% ultraviolet barrier spectacles with sidearms. Frequent slit-lamp examinations for conjunctival and lid tumours are mandatory.

It is genetically complex with several genes involved; the most common in white people is in group C (XP-C) which encodes a protein that complements the repair deficiency of XP-C cells; there are six distinct mutations in XP-C (Li *et al.* 1993).

Benign hereditary epithelial dyskeratosis

This dominantly inherited condition consists of the presence of elevated whitish plaques of hyperkeratotic and vascular tissue in the exposed areas of the conjunctiva and it may be associated with dyskeratosis of the buccal mucosa (Yanoff 1968). It is rare and has been described in a small group of North American patients.

Papilloma

Conjunctival papillomas are not uncommon in childhood. They present as elevated, sometimes pedunculated lesions that are usually white or yellowish, but may be quite heavily pigmented or pink in colour (Fig. 22.24). On lamp examination they can be seen to consist of translucent 'flesh' with small red spots which represent the vessels in the core of the papillomatous tissue. They may be multiple and may occur in more than one member of the family. In young children they are usually associated with a virus infection and they often disappear spontaneously (Wilson & Ostler 1974), but if they do not disappear after a few months or if they are causing considerable trouble

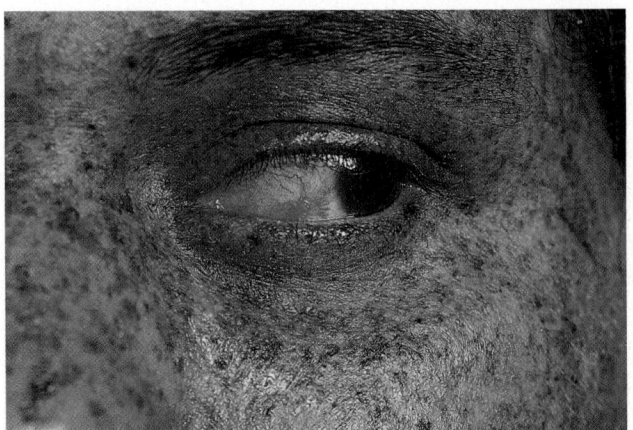

a

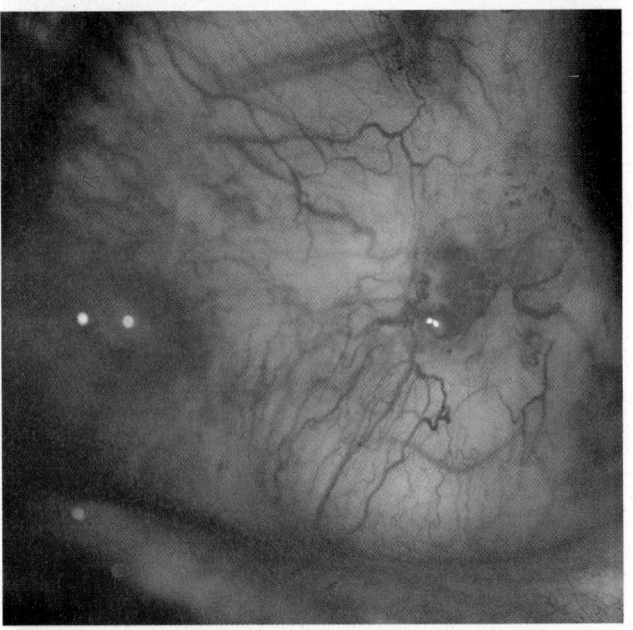

b

Fig. 22.23 (a) Xeroderma pigmentosa. The widespread skin pigmentation can be seen in this girl of Indian origin. (b) The conjunctiva was affected by multifocal recurrent squamous cell carcinomas.

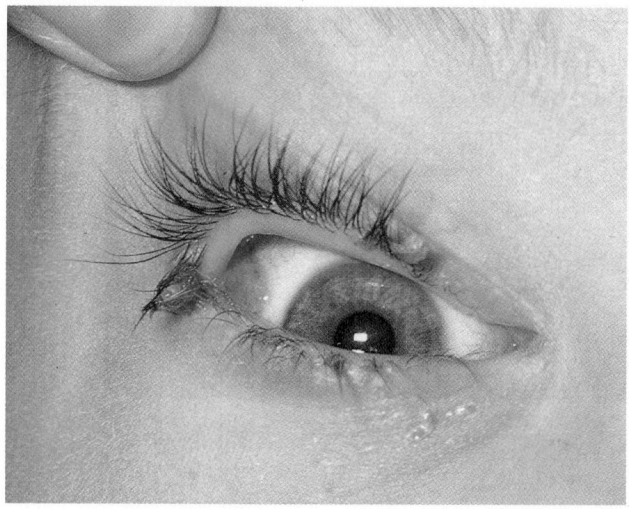

Fig. 22.24 Conjunctival papilloma of the temporal bulbar conjunctiva associated with lid papillomas.

cryotherapy, surgical excision or diathermy may be indicated.

Neurofibromas

These are benign, raised, solid, grey–white or pinkish nodules often near the limbus but they may occur at any site. They occur mostly in patients with neurofibromatosis type 1 (NF1), occasionally with multiple endocrine neoplasia type IIb (when they are usually on the lid conjunctiva) and in NF2 (Kalina *et al.* 1991).

Sarcoidosis

The conjunctiva was once thought to be frequently involved in sarcoidosis and it was not infrequent for 'blind' biopsies of the conjunctiva to be carried out in order to diagnose sarcoidosis. The histological diagnosis must be carefully considered because meibomian 'cysts' have a similar appearance. Conjunctival biopsy is indicated in suspected sarcoidosis (Hoover *et al.* 1986) especially if a discrete elevated lesion is seen. Conjunctival sarcoidosis does not usually cause any symptoms and in itself requires no treatment.

Avitaminosis

Malnutrition is one of the most common causes of blindness in the world today. Although it warrants deeper study only the conjunctival aspects will be referred to here.

Xerophthalmia, the term applied to the external eye manifestations of blinding malnutrition, usually occurs in the setting of a more widespread protein/calorie malnu-

trition and is often associated with infection (Brown *et al.* 1979). Following a period of night-blindness, which is often the first symptom but only discovered on direct questioning, a dry appearance or dullness of the eyes appears with the conjunctiva appearing wrinkled (Fig. 22.25), reddened, dull and sometimes pigmented. Bitot's spots are flaky, elevated patches usually in exposed areas of the conjunctiva and most significant if present on both sides of the cornea (Sommer *et al.* 1980). Most of these cases are associated with vitamin A deficiency as well as a more generalized malnutrition, and infection of the conjunctiva and cornea, already weakened by dryness and vitamin A deficiency, plays a major role. Keratomalacia, an acute liquefactive keratitis, may ensue rapidly, often related to exacerbations of the state of general nutrition; the cornea may perforate, and endophthalmitis may occur or a leucoma adherens and cataract may be found later when the cornea clears. In any country, there may be marked regional variations due to differences in local nutritional status (Rahi *et al.* 1995).

Xanthogranulomas

These present as fleshy raised nodules, usually at the limbus, sometimes with a yellowish orange colour. Simple excision is often effective but recurrences may be treated

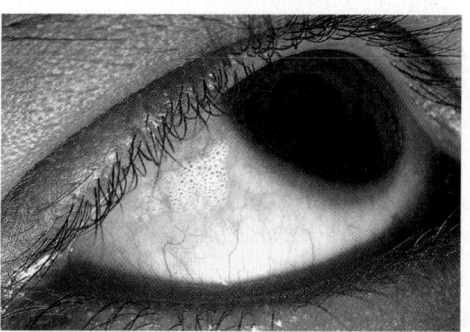

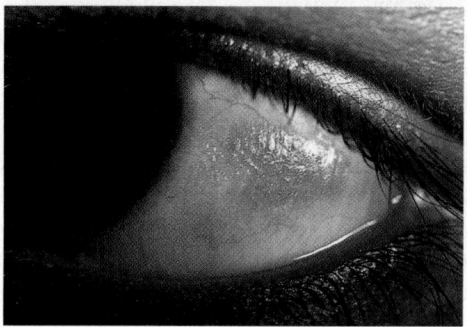

Fig. 22.25 Xerophthalmia: (a) right eye, (b) left eye. Bitot's spots are flaky elevated patches in the exposed areas of the conjunctiva. As in this case, they are often pigmented. Photographs by kind permission of Mr Michael Eckstein.

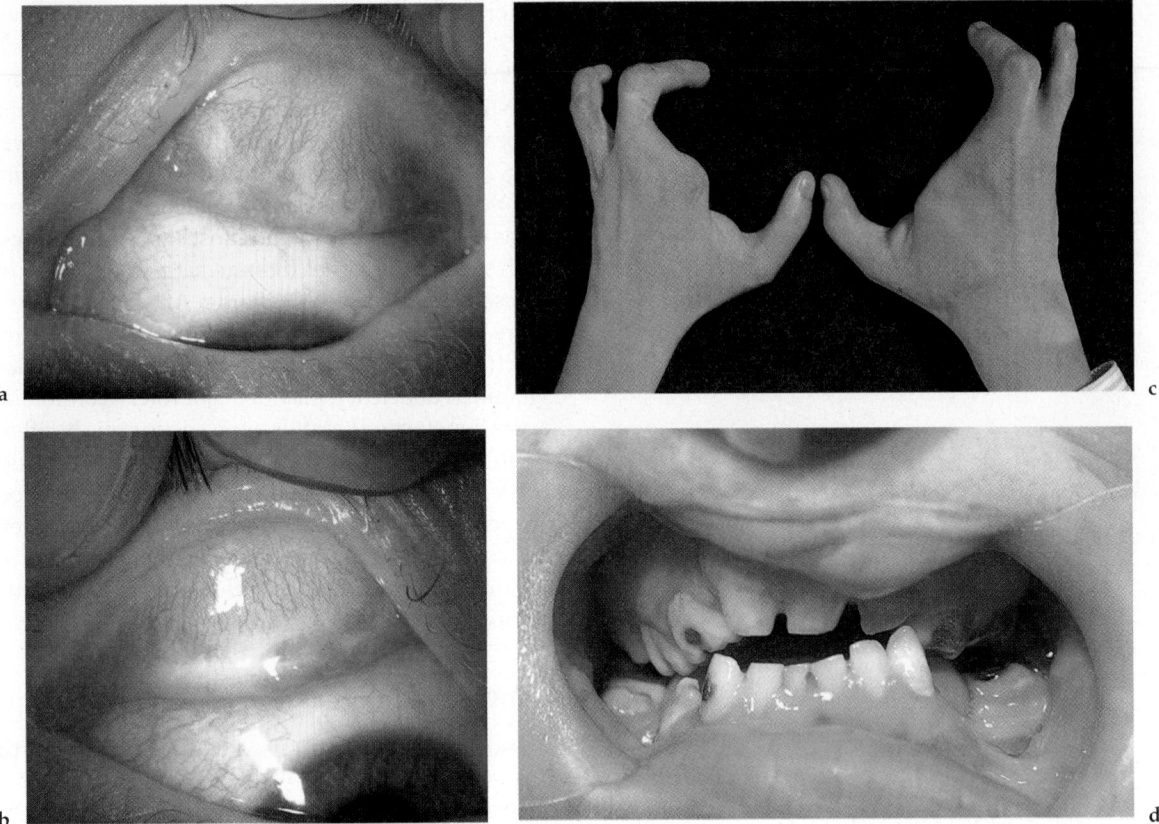

Fig. 22.26 EEC syndrome. (a, b) This child had conjunctival thinning especially affecting the tarsal plates. (c) Marked ectrodactyly. (d) Dental abnormalities.

with beta-irradiation (750 cGy) or keratectomy with lamellar graft (Collum *et al.* 1991).

Pingueculum and pterygium

Pingueculae and pterygia are rare in childhood but can occur occasionally in children who come from hot and dry countries. It is unusual for them to give rise to substantial problems in childhood. Conversely, pseudopterygia are not uncommon following inflammatory corneal disease or excision of a corneal lesion, for instance, an epibulbar dermoid. If cosmetically unsightly they may be excised with a wide conjunctival margin and a superficial keratectomy but occasionally a mucous membrane graft may be required.

Conjunctival thinning

Conjunctival thinning occurs in Dego's disease, the scalded baby syndrome, epidermolysis bullosa (Iwamoto *et al.* 1991) and in ectodermal dysplasia.

Dego's disease is a rare, multiple organ system disease characterized by a papular eruption, on the trunk and extremities, with atrophic white-centred lesions surrounded by a telangiectatic border. A variety of ocular manifestations may occur including an abnormal retinal vascular pattern (Lee *et al.* 1984), ophthalmoplegia, papilloedema and optic atrophy, together with atrophic telangiectatic conjunctival lesions.

In ectodermal dysplasia there is conjunctival and corneal thinning which may lead to spontaneous perforation. The ectrodactyly, ectodermal dysplasia, clefting (EEC) syndrome (Fig. 22.26) is an autosomal dominant syndrome with variable expression which has prominent eye complications (Wilson *et al.* 1973; McNab *et al.* 1989).

In dystrophic epidermolysis bullosa eye changes are common including symblepharon, broadening of the limbus, corneal opacities (Fig. 22.27) and recurrent erosions (McDonnell & Spalton 1988; McDonnell *et al.* 1989b).

Conjunctival thickening

Conjunctival thickening occurs in conjunctival scarring, pemphigus, and the Richner–Hanhart syndrome. In the Richner–Hanhart syndrome, also known as tyrosinaemia type 2, there are hyperkeratotic lesions of the palm, soles

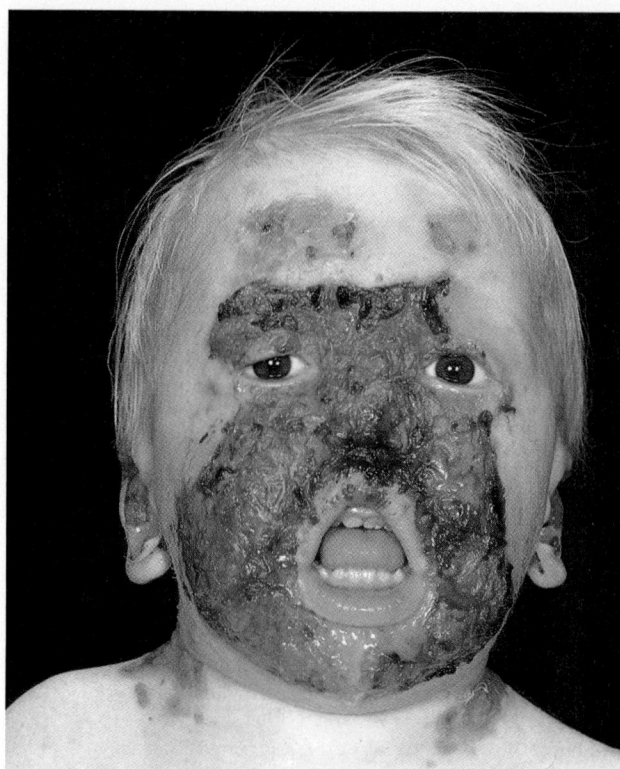

Fig. 22.27 Dystrophic epidermolysis bullosa. Most of the facial skin had debrided but the conjunctiva and corneal epithelium were only mildly affected in this case.

(see Fig. 24.32) and elbows and occasionally mental retardation. It is associated with an increase in serum and urine tyrosine. It is transmitted as an autosomal recessive trait. Children with this condition are photophobic and have watering eyes with thickened conjunctiva and hypertrophy of the tarsal conjunctiva. There are epithelial and subepithelial opacities of the cornea and corneal ulceration which appear dendritic at times. The lesions on the cornea tend to heal spontaneously but may take some time. When they first appear they are dendritiform and they are often bilateral. The corneal lesions may be treated with corticosteroids; with an appropriate diet (Michalski *et al.* 1988) the lesions rapidly improve (see Chapter 24).

Conjunctival scarring

Conjunctival scarring occurs in a wide variety of conditions (see Bernauer *et al.* 1993 for an excellent review) some of which affect children:

1 Burns:
  (a) thermal;
  (b) chemical; and
  (c) ionizing radiation.
2 Traumatic, including squint surgery and surgery to remove dermoids, etc.
3 Infection:
  (a) trachoma; and
  (b) severe and prolonged bacterial and viral infections and membranous conjunctivitis.
4 Avitaminosis.
5 Inflammatory disease:
  (a) Stevens–Johnson syndrome and erythema multiforme (see Chapter 19);
  (b) Richner–Hanhart syndrome;
  (c) chronic vernal conjunctivitis;
  (d) toxic epidermal necrolysis;
  (e) epidermolysis bullosa; and
  (f) linear IgA disease.
6 Dry eye.
7 Ectodermal dysplasia.
8 Epidermolysis bullosa (Iwamoto *et al.* 1991).
9 Drugs
  (a) systemic; and
  (b) topical (lower fornix).

References

Arlett CF. Human DNA repair defects. *J Inherit Metab Dis* 1986; **9** (Suppl.): 69–84.

Baloh RW, Yee RD, Boder E. Eye movements in ataxia telangiectasia. *Neurology* 1978; **28**: 1099–104.

Bellows RA, Lahour M, Lepreau FJ, Albert DM. Ocular manifestations of xeroderma pigmentosa in a black family. *Arch Ophthalmol* 1974; **92**: 113–19.

Bernauer W, Broadway D, Wright P. Chronic progressive conjunctival cicatrisation. *Eye* 1993; **7**: 371–8.

Brown KH, Gaffar A, Alamgir SM. Xerophthalmia, protein–calorie malnutrition and infections in children. *J Pediatr* 1979; **95**: 651–6.

Brant AM, Schachat AP, White RI. Ocular manifestations in hereditary hemorrhagic telangiectasia (Rendu–Osler–Weber disease). *Am J Ophthalmol* 1989; **107**: 642–7.

Burke JP, Bowell R, O'Doherty N. Proteus syndrome: ocular complications. *J Pediatr Ophthalmol Strabismus* 1988; **25**: 99–104.

Charlin C. Oculo-dermo-mucous melanosis. Naevus of ota. *Arch Ophthalmol (Paris)* 1973; **33**: 19–28.

Collum LMT, Power WJ, Mullaney J, Farrell M. Limbal xanthogranuloma. *J Pediatr Ophthalmol Strabismus* 1991; **280**: 157–60.

Cunha RP, Cunha MC, Shields JA. Epibulbar tumours in children: a survey of 282 biopsies. *J Pediatr Ophthalmol Strabismus* 1987; **24**: 249–55.

Djindjian M, Djindjian R, Hurth M, Rey A, Houdact R. Angiomes médullaires et syndrome de Klippel–Trénaunay–Weber. *Dev Neurol* 1977; **133**: 609–19.

Dutton JJ, Anderson RL, Schelper RL, Purcell JJ, Tse DT. Orbital malignant melanoma and oculodermal melanocytosis: report of two cases and review of the literature. *Ophthalmology* 1984; **91**: 497–507.

Fry C, Leone C. Safe management of dermolipomas. *Arch Ophthalmol* 1994; **112**: 1114–16.

Gass JDM, Glatzer RJ. Acquired pigmentation simulating Peutz–Jeghers syndrome: initial manifestation of diffuse uveal melanocytic proliferation. *Br J Ophthalmol* 1991; **75**: 693–5.

Gonder JR, Shields JA, Albert DM, Augsburger JJ, Lavin PT. Uveal malignant melanoma associated with ocular and oculodermal melanocytosis. *Ophthalmology* 1982; **89**: 853–60.

Good WV, Hoyt CS. Optic nerve shadow enlargement in the Klippel–Trenaunay–Weber syndrome. *J Pediatr Ophthalmol Strabismus* 1989; **26**: 288–90.

Goyal J, Rao V, Srinivasan R, Agarawal K. Oculocutaneous manifestations in xeroderma pigmentosa. *Br J Ophthalmol* 1994; **78**: 295–7.

Handa J, Nakano Y, Akiguchi I. Cranial computed tomography findings in xeroderma pigmentosum with neurologic manifestations (De Sanctis–Cacchione syndrome). *J Comp Assoc Tomogr* 1978; **2**: 456–9.

Harley RD, Baird HW, Craven J. Ataxia telangiectasia. *Arch Ophthalmol (Chic)* 1967; **77**: 582–92.

Hered RW, Hiles DA. Epibulbar osseous choristoma and ectopic lacrimal gland underlying a dermolipoma. *J Pediatr Ophthalmol Strabismus* 1987; **24**: 255–9.

Hoover DL, Khan JA, Giangiacomo J. Review. Pediatric ocular sarcoidosis. *Surv Ophthalmol* 1986; **30**: 215–29.

Howitz P, Howitz J, Gjerris F. A variant of the Klippel–Trenaunay–Weber syndrome with temporal lobe astrocytoma. *Acta Paediatr Scand* 1979; **68**: 116–21.

Hudelo A. Glaucome et naevus faciale. *Ann Occul* 1929; **166**: 889–902.

Isenberg SJ, McCarty JW, Rich R. Growth of the conjunctival fornix and orbital margin in term and premature infants. *Ophthalmology* 1987; **94**: 1276–81.

Iwamoto M, Haik BG, Iwamoto T, Harrison W, Carter M. The ultrastructural defect in conjunctiva from a case of recessive dystrophic epidermolysis bullosa. *Arch Ophthalmol* 1991; **109**: 1382–6.

Jay B. Malignant melanoma of the orbit in a case of oculodermal melanosis (naevus of ota). *Br J Ophthalmol* 1965a; **49**: 359–63.

Jay B. Naevi and melanomata of the conjunctiva. *Br J Ophthalmol* 1965b; **49**: 169–83.

Kalina P, Bartley G, Campbell, Buettner H. Isolated neurofibromas of the conjunctiva. *Am J Ophthalmol* 1991; **111**: 694–9.

Klippel M, Trénaunay P. Du naevus variqueux osteohypertrophique. *Arch Gen Med (Paris)* 1900; **3**: 641.

Kodsi S, Bloom K, Egbert J, Holland E, Cameron J. Ocular and systemic manifestations of encephalocraniocutaneous lipomatosis. *Am J Ophthalmol* 1994; **118**: 77–82.

Kraemer KH, Rapini RP, Beran M. Xeroderma pigmentosum: cutaneous, ocular and neurologic abnormalities in 830 published cases. *Arch Dermatol* 1987; **123**: 241–50.

Kulikov W. Changes in the microvascular bed of the eye conjunctiva in ataxia-telangiectasis (syndrome of Louis–Bar). *Arch Patologi (Moscow)* 1974; **36**: 311–18.

Lee DA, Su D, Liesegang TJ. Systemic ophthalmology. Ophthalmic changes of Dego's disease (malignant atrophic papulosis). *Ophthalmology* 1984; **91**: 295–9.

Lessner A, Margo CE. Eyelid tumours in the proteus syndrome. *Am J Ophthalmol* 1991; **111**: 521–2.

Li L, Bales ES, Peterson CA, Legerski RJ. Characterisation of molecular defects in xeroderma pigmentosum group C. *Nature Genet* 1993; **5**: 413–17.

Limaye SR, Doyle HA, Tang RA. Retinal varicosity in Klippel–Trenaunay–Weber syndrome. *J Pediatr Ophthalmol Strabismus* 1979; **16**: 371–3.

McDonnell JM, Carpenter JD, Jacobs P, Wan L, Gilmore JE. Conjunctival melanocytic lesions in children. *Ophthalmology* 1989a; **96**: 986–93.

McDonnell PJ, Schofield OMV, Spalton DJ, Mayou BJ, Eady RAJ. The eye in dystrophic epidermolysis bullosa. *Eye* 1989b; **3**: 79–84.

McDonnell PJ, Spalton DJ. The ocular signs and complications of epidermolysis bullosa. *J. Roy. Soc Med* 1988; **81**: 576–8.

McFarlan DE, Strober W. Ataxia telangiectasia. *Medicine* 1972; **51**: 281–314.

McNab A, Potts MJ, Welham RAN. The EEC syndrome and its ocular manifestations. *Br J Ophthalmol* 1989; **73**: 261–5.

Massey EW, Brannon WL, Morland M. Naevus of Ota and intracranial arteriovenous malformation. *Neurology* 1979; **29**: 1625–7.

Michalski A, Leonard JV, Taylor DSI. The eye in inherited metabolic disease. *J Roy Soc Med* 1988; **81**: 286–90.

Nik NA, Glew WB, Zimmerman LE. Malignant melanoma of the choroid in the nevus of Ota of a black patient. *Arch Ophthalmol* 1982; **100**: 1641–3.

O'Connor PS, Smith JL. Optic nerve variant in the Klippel–Trenaunay–Weber syndrome. *Ann Ophthalmol (Chic)* 1978; **10**: 131–4.

Orr LS, Osher RH, Savino PJ. The syndrome of facial nevi, anomalous cerebral venous return, and hydrocephalus. *Ann Neurol* 1978; **3**: 316–18.

Perrot H, Durand L, Thivolet J, Millon M, Ortonne JP. Sclerodermie en coup de sabre et glaucome chronique homolateral. *Ann Dermatol Venereol* 1977; **104**: 381–6.

Perry HD, Cossari AJ. Chronic lymphangiectasis in Turner's syndrome. *Br J Ophthalmol* 1986; **70**: 396–9.

Pokorny KS, Hyman BM, Jakobiec FA, Perry HD, Caputo AR, Iwamoto T. Epibulbar choristomas containing lacrimal tissue: clinical distinction from dermoids and histologic evidence of an origin from the palpebral lobe. *J Am Acad Ophthalmol* 1987; **94**: 1249–58.

Rahi JS, Stripathi S, Gilbert CE, Foster A. Childhood blindness due to vitamin A deficiency in India: regional variations. *Arch Dis Child* 1995; **72**: 330–3.

Rathbun JE, Hoyt WF, Beard C. Surgical management of orbitofrontal varix in Klippel–Trenaunay–Weber syndrome. *Am J Ophthalmol* 1970; **70**: 109–12.

Roldan M, Llanes F, Negrete O, Valverde F. Malignant melanoma of the choroid associated with melanosis oculi in a child. *Am J Ophthalmol* 1987; **104**: 662–3.

Romano P. Neuroparalytic keratitis in Goldenhar's syndrome. *Am J Ophthalmol* 1978; **85**: 111–13.

Segal P, Kikela M, Mrzyglod S, Keromska-Zbierska I. Kartagener's syndrome with familial eye changes. *Am J Ophthalmol* 1963; **55**: 1043–9.

Singh M, Kaur B, Annwar NM. Malignant melanoma of the choroid is a naevus of ota. *Br J Ophthalmol* 1988; **72**: 131–4.

Smith JL, Cogan DG. Ataxia telangiectasia. *Arch Ophthalmol (Chic)* 1959; **62**: 364–9.

Sommer A, Emran N, Tjakrasudjatma S. Clinical characteristics of vitamin A responsive and non-responsive Bitot's spots. *Am J Ophthalmol* 1980; **90**: 160–71.

Stewart G, Farmer G. Sturge–Weber and Klippel–Trenaunay syndrome with absence of inferior vena cava. *Arch Dis Child* 1990; **65**: 546–8.

Sujatha S, Sampath R, Bonshek R, Tullo A. Conjunctival haemangiopericytoma. *Br J Ophthalmol* 1994; **78**: 497–9.

Taylor P, Talbot EM. Perilimbal vascular anomaly associated with ipsilateral en coup de sabre morphoea. *Br J Ophthalmol* 1985; **69**: 60–2.

Teekhasaenee C, Riteh R, Rutnin U, Leelawongs N. Ocular findings in oculodermal melanocytosis. *Arch Ophthalmol* 1990; **108**: 1114–21.

Theron J, Newton TH, Hoyt WF. Unilateral retino-cephalic vascular malformations. *Neuroradiology* 1974; **7**: 185–96.

Ticho BH, Tso MO, Kishi S. Diffuse iris nevus in oculodermal melanocytosis: a light and electron microscopic study. *J Pediatr Ophthalmol Strabismus* 1989; **26**: 244–51.

Unal M, Gunalp I, Deery A, Durak I, Erekul S, Bulay O. Malignant melanoma of the optic nerve head in a case of oculodermal melanocystosis. *Br J Ophthalmol* 1992; **76**: 313–15.

Vivian A, Ellison D, McGill J. Ocular melanosis in xeroderma pigmentosum. *Br J Ophthalmol* 1993; **77**: 597–8.

Weber FP. Angioma formation in connection with hypertrophy of the limbus and hemihypertrophy. *Br J Dermatol* 1907; **19**: 231–2.

Weisenthal R, Streeten B, Dubonsky S, Hutchison R, Pecora J. Burkitt lymphoma presenting as a conjunctival mass. *Ophthalmology* 1995; **102**: 129–34.

Wilson FM, Grayson M, Pieroni D. Corneal changes in ectodermal dysplasia. *Am J Ophthalmol* 1973; **75**: 17–27.

Wilson FM, Ostler HB. Conjunctival papillomas in siblings. *Am J Ophthalmol* 1974; **77**: 103–10.

Yamamoto T. Malignant melanoma of the choroid in the nevus of ota. *Ophthalmologica* 1969; **159**: 1–10.

Yanoff M. Hereditary benign intra epithelial dyskeratosis. *Arch Ophthalmol* 1968; **79**: 291–5.

23: Developmental Abnormalities of the Anterior Segment

John Elston

The prenatal development of the cornea, trabecular meshwork and iris takes place in a co-ordinated, integrated fashion (Mann 1957a). Different structures in the anterior segment are subject to common influences, so that developmental abnormalities of one component are often accompanied by abnormalities of others. Clinically, these disorders are therefore usually bilateral, but often asymmetrical, and present as abnormal corneal size, corneal opacity, glaucoma and iris abnormalities, or combinations of these.

Embryology

By the sixth week of intrauterine life, the surface ectoderm has been restored after the separation of the lens vesicle, and therefore constitutes the future anterior epithelium of the cornea. Mesenchymal tissue accumulates between the surface ectoderm and the anterior lens capsule (O'Rahilly 1975). There is evidence that the mesenchymal differentiation and cell division is determined by neural crest cells (Kupfer & Kaiser-Kupfer 1979). These are cells derived from the dorsal margin of the neural tube and therefore of neuroectodermal origin. They are pluripotent, and have an important role in the migration and terminal induction of tissues in many sites (Beauchamp & Knepper 1984). For example, the development of cartilage, bone, meninges, peripheral nerve, Schwann cells and the neuroendocrine system is dependent on neural crest cells (Tripathi & Tripathi 1989). The mesenchyme involved in anterior segment development shows three distinct phases of increased activity from the sixth week onwards.

The first phase (primary mesenchymal development) involves cell multiplication and migration deep to the surface ectoderm (Kenyon 1975; O'Rahilly 1975). A solid disc of tissue, two cells thick by the eighth week, is formed and will become the corneal endothelium (Wulle 1972). The central corneal endothelial cell density diminishes rapidly from the 16th week onwards as the cornea grows, creating a monolayer of cells by the 18th week. The evidence suggests that there is little endothelial cell division after the second trimester (Murphy *et al.* 1984b). Descemet's membrane is secreted by the endothelial cells and from the eighth week onwards they show evidence of high metabolic activity, with plentiful endoplasmic reticulum, mitochondria, Golgi bodies and nucleoli and the deposition of a basement membrane (Wulle 1972). The membrane is regularly thickened by the addition of further lamellae, approximately 30 being present at term. The lamellae are bound by short cross-linking bridges (Murphy *et al.* 1984a). The prenatally developed striated Descemet's membrane is 3.0 μm thick. Postnatally it is thickened by the addition of amorphous material. Schwalbe's ring marks the posterior limit of Descemet's membrane and is developmentally part of the trabecular meshwork (see below). Histological examination for the presence of striations in Descemet's membrane in developmental abnormalities of the anterior segment can therefore indicate whether there has been a primary or secondary failure of endothelial cell function.

The second phase of mesenchymal activity results in the migration and multiplication of cells between the developing Descemet's membrane and the surface ectoderm; these cells become keratocytes, and produce the corneal stroma (Mann 1957b). The third phase of cell migration is accompanied by blood vessels and occurs superficial to the lens, thereby creating the anterior chamber between itself and the first phase tissue. Until the 28th week this chamber is lined by a continuous sheet of mesothelium (O'Rahilly 1975).

The trabecular meshwork develops from a circumferential mass of mesenchyme situated at the periphery of the developing cornea, adjacent to the sclera. The anterior border of the mesenchyme develops into Schwalbe's ring; posterior to this, the trabeculae are formed. The neural crest origin of the trabecular meshwork has been demonstrated by the presence of neuronal-specific enolase (NSE) in these cells (Tripathi & Tripathi 1989). The angle between the developing cornea and iris progressively extends further posteriorly during intrauterine life. The developing canal of Schlemm, initially posterior to the anterior chamber and separated from it by a layer of mesenchyme, thereby comes to lie superficial to the trabecular meshwork. Similarly, the extension of the anterior chamber angle posteriorly means that Schwalbe's ring becomes separated from the iris stroma (Hansson & Jerndal 1971).

The process of intrauterine anterior chamber angle extension was originally ascribed to tissue atrophy or resorption. In 1955, a new hypothesis, based on examinations of fetal eyes and measurement of the relative positions of the angle, ciliary body and corneoscleral junction, was put forward (Allen *et al.* 1955). It was suggested that the angle extended by cleavage of tissue, the splitting force being the relatively high rate of growth and increase in curvature of the cornea. Failure of proper cleavage of the angle could result in the various types of anterior segment and angle maldevelopment, for this reason called 'anterior segment cleavage syndromes' (Allen *et al.* 1955; Reese & Ellsworth 1966; Waring *et al.* 1975).

Subsequent histological studies have provided no support for the theory of tissue cleavage, which is probably an artefact related to the postfixation detachment of the ciliary body from the overlying sclera (Kupfer 1969; Kupfer & Ross 1971). The angle appears to form by a process of differential growth, altering micro-anatomical relations, and the term anterior segment cleavage syndrome should therefore be abandoned. Because abnormal migration or defective terminal induction is responsible for many anterior segment developmental anomalies, the generic term neural crestopathy (or neurocristopathy) is more appropriate.

The discontinuity in the monolayer of polyhedral endothelial cells lining the trabecular meshwork that develops around the 28th week is reflected in an increase in outflow facility (Kupfer & Ross 1971). Again, the process involved is probably differential cell growth.

At full-term birth, the cornea is less than 10 mm in horizontal and vertical diameter (9.3 mm; Murphy *et al.* 1984b), and Descemet's membrane is 3.0 μm thick. The cornea continues to grow relatively quickly in infancy, reaching adult size (11.7 mm diameter) by 24 months, during which period the endothelial cell density also falls relatively rapidly since cell division is minimal (Speedwell *et al.* 1988). The outflow facility through the trabecular meshwork has usually reached postnatal values by the 32nd week of intrauterine life (Kupfer & Ross 1971).

Patterns of anterior segment maldevelopment

Anterior segment dysgenesis may affect the cornea, (including the limbus) the trabecular meshwork or the iris. Combinations of abnormalities and involvement of other intraocular structures such as the lens are common. Recognizable patterns of clinical presentation, physical signs, natural history and systemic associations are seen, but there is considerable overlap. Anterior segment maldevelopment may be genetically determined with or without systemic features. Heterogeneity is an important aspect of these conditions and the family of an affected individual must be examined systemically and on the slit lamp before genetic advice can be given (Holmstrom *et al.* 1991).

Ocular embryogenesis is also susceptible to toxic insult and anterior segment anomalies are amongst the characteristic features of the fetal alcohol syndrome (see below) (Chan *et al.* 1991).

Although the embryological basis of the subdivision of anterior segment maldevelopment given below is limited, it has clinical merit.

Primary corneal abnormalities

Whole cornea

Megalocornea

If the cornea is adult size at birth, or 13 mm diameter by 2 years, and provided buphthalmos has been excluded, and preferably if endothelial cell density and corneal thickness are normal, 'simple' megalocornea is diagnosed (Fig. 23.1). Most commonly this is an X-linked disorder, although autosomal recessive and dominant inheritance has been described (Duke-Elder 1964). The corneal diameter ranges between 13 and 18 mm and intraocular pressure

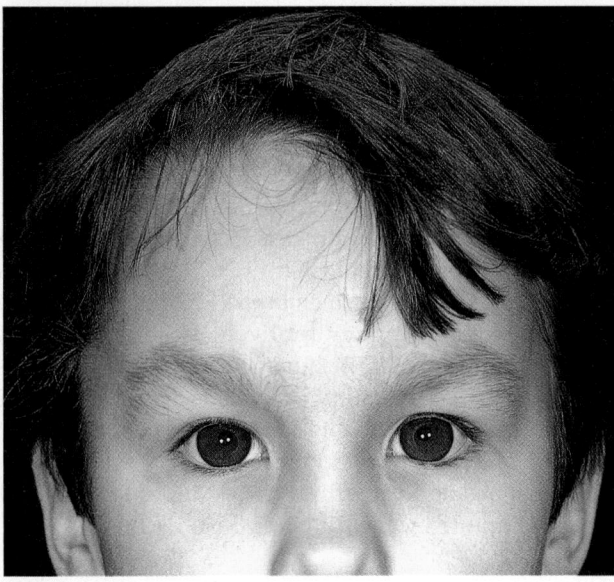

Fig. 23.1 Megalocornea. Corrected acuities were normal.

is normal. Unlike buphthalmos, the radius of curvature of the cornea is increased. The condition is non-progressive, bilateral, symmetrical and congenital. The corneal thickness is normal, as is endothelial cell density, indicating a process of total corneal hypertrophy (Skuta *et al.* 1983).

Other ocular features are arcus juvenilis, mosaic corneal dystrophy, pigment dispersion, cataract (usually developing in early adult life) and lens dislocation. Biometry shows that the axial length is normal or slightly increased, the anterior chamber is deep, the lens is normal, and the posterior segment is short (Meire 1994). Visual development is usually normal with the refraction showing emmetropia or low myopia with astigmatism (Kraft *et al.* 1984; Meire & Delleman 1994).

A gene locus has been identified on the X chromosome in the region Xq12–q26 (Mackey *et al.* 1991). No clinical abnormality has been identified in female carriers.

Systemic associations

Systemic associations of X-linked megalocornea include:
1 Ichthyosis and poikiloderma congenitale.
2 Aarskog's syndrome. Megalocornea is a feature of Aarskog's syndrome (faciodigital–genital syndrome). This is an X-linked recessive disorder characterized by short stature, hypertelorism, an antimongoloid slant, saddle deformity of the scrotum and syndactly. All cases described have corneas between 12 and 13 mm in diameter (Kirkham *et al.* 1975). The gene locus for Aarskog's syndrome is close to that for X-linked megalocornea.
3 Marfan's syndrome (Ramsey *et al.* 1973).
4 Megalocornea–mental retardation (MMR or Neuhauser) syndrome. This associates megalocornea

with mental retardation, short stature, ataxia, and seizures (Neuhauser *et al.* 1975; Santolaya *et al.* 1992; Gibbs *et al.* 1994).
5 Others (Meire 1994) including Kniest's syndrome and non-ketotic hyperglycinaemia.

Ocular associations (Meire 1994)

1 Ectopia lentis et pupillae. In this autosomal recessive condition, posterior displacement of the lens–iris diaphragm is combined with severe axial myopia, cataract, iris transillumination, persistent pupillary membrane, retinal detachment and, sometimes, megalocornea. Visual development is poor (Goldberg 1988).
2 Congenital miosis.
3 Rieger's anomaly.
4 Albinism.
5 Weill–Marchesani syndrome (Soriano & Psilas 1970).
6 Crouzon's syndrome (Gorlin 1990a).
7 Marshall–Smith syndrome — increased axial length, failure to thrive, mental retardation, dysmorphia (Gorlin 1990b).
8 SHORT syndrome — short stature, hyperextensible joints, ocular depression, Rieger's anomaly and teething delay (Lipson *et al.* 1989).

Microcornea

In simple microphthalmos the axial length of the eye is greater than 2 SD below the mean; the corneal diameter is normal. The condition is due to reduced growth of the posterior segment (Weiss *et al.* 1989a). Nanophthalmos is simple microphthalmos plus microcornea (see Chapter 20). Simple microphthalmos and nanophthalmos may be unilateral or bilateral.

In complex microphthalmos, as well as having a reduced axial length, the globe is malformed (Fig. 23.2) and microcornea is common (Weiss *et al.* 1989b). The cornea may be opaque or vascularized. Other associations are anterior segment dysgenesis, cataract (or absent lens), coloboma (with or without cyst), persistent hyperplastic primary vitreous (PHPV), retinal dysplasia and ipsilateral facial malformation. If bilateral, complex microphthalmos is often associated with systemic malformations especially of the central nervous system (e.g. holoprosencephaly, hydrocephalus) and cardiovascular system (patent ductus arteriosus and other structural defects) (Foxman & Cameron 1984).

Complex microphthalmos with microcornea and cyst may be seen in the 13q deletion syndrome, ring deletion of chromosome 18 and Edward's syndrome (trisomy 18) (Guterman *et al.* 1990; Porges *et al.* 1992). The cyst may be present in the neonate or develop in infancy or childhood. Microphthalmos with cyst may also occur as an autosomal recessive trait.

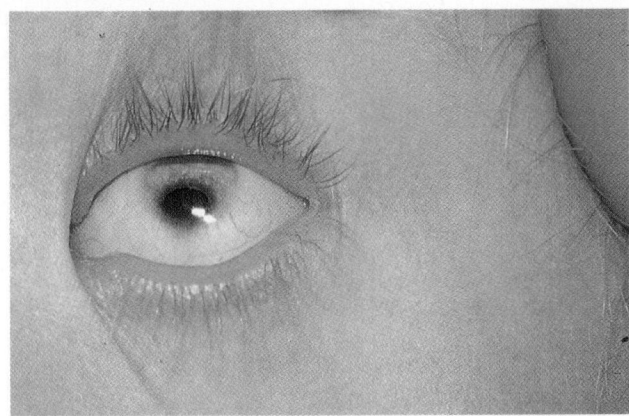

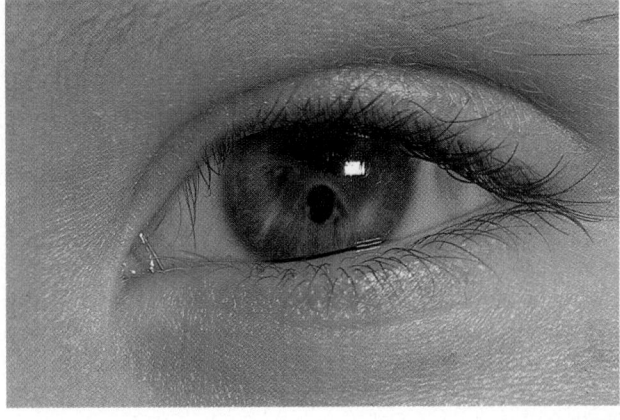

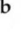

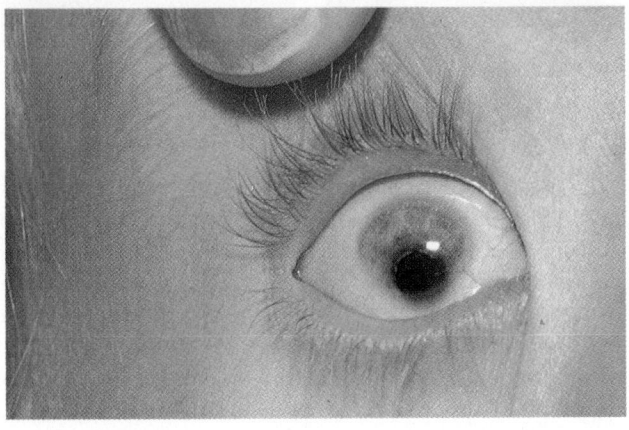

a

b

Cornea plana

Cornea plana is an abnormality of curvature of the cornea, which is relatively flattened. It may be found as a component of microphthalmos, coloboma or sclerocornea, and is not an isolated condition.

Congenital corneal clouding

Diffuse corneal clouding may be a feature of the fetal alcohol syndrome (Edward *et al.* 1993). It is due to primary endothelial cell failure *in utero* and associated with an absent or poorly formed anterior banded zone of Descemet's membrane. There is corneal stromal oedema and thickening or loss of Bowman's membrane. Corneal grafting is the only possible treatment. Other ocular features include microphthalmos, optic nerve hypoplasia, strabismus, short palpebral fissures, epicanthus and ptosis (Jones *et al.* 1973; Chan *et al.* 1991; Spour *et al.* 1993). The differential diagnosis of congenital corneal opacification is as follows.
1 Congenital glaucoma.
2 Birth trauma (endothelial and Descemet's membrane damage, usually by forceps).
3 Developmental defects—Peters' anomaly.
4 Congenital corneal dystrophy.
5 Fetal alcohol syndrome.

Fig. 23.2 (a) Colobomatous microphthalmos, microcornea and cornea plana. (b) Microcornea with iris abnormalities, congenital idiopathic microcoria (see Chapter 38).

6 Corneal dermoid.
7 Intrauterine infection (rubella, cytomegalovirus, syphilis).
8 Severe neonatal conjunctivitis.

Agenesis of Bowman's layer

Congenital absence of Bowman's layer of the cornea has been documented histopathologically as a component of Peters' anomaly, sclerocornea and osteogenesis imperfecta type II (Kasner *et al.* 1993).

Peripheral

Choristoma

A choristoma is a congenital overgrowth of normal tissue in an abnormal location. A dermoid choristoma consists of collagen connective tissue with an epithelium giving a white solid mass. A lipodermoid choristoma has fatty tissue and dermis connective tissue. Epibulbar dermoids may be conjunctival, scleral, limbal or corneal. As an isolated abnormality they may be sporadic or genetically determined. In the ring dermoid syndrome there are bilateral 360° dermoids with corneal, limbal, scleral and conjunctival components. The condition is autosomal dominant and corneal astigmatism with amblyopia and strabismus is common (Mattos *et al.* 1980). X-linked corneal dermoid may present as a diffuse congenital bilateral corneal opacity (Topilow *et al.* 1981). Corneal dermoid also occurs in various syndromes (see Chapter 24).

Sclerocornea

Sclerocornea is congenital, bilateral, often asymmetrical, predominantly peripheral corneal opacification with vascularization. It may be isolated, or more usually, associated with abnormal corneal size (microcornea) or curvature (cornea plana). With time a relatively clear midcorneal zone may develop (Figs 23.3, 23.4). Other associations are raised intraocular pressure due to an associated angle dysgenesis, strabismus in asymmetrical cases, and nystagmus if the central cornea becomes opaque (Goldstein & Cogan 1962; Elliott *et al.* 1985).

Rarely, there are systemic abnormalities, e.g. mental retardation, and abnormal facies. Sclerocornea has also

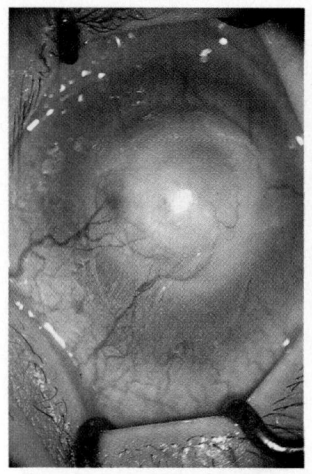
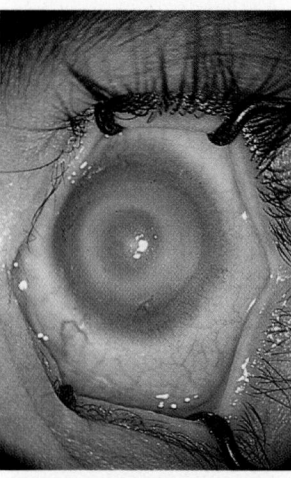

Fig. 23.4 Sclerocornea. With time a relatively clear zone may develop between the opaque centre and the periphery.

been described in a number of unrelated conditions involving multiple congenital abnormalities. It may be autosomal dominant (Elliott *et al.* 1985) or sporadic. Segregation analysis suggests autosomal recessive inheritance in some cases (Block 1965). Minor sclerocornea is common in dysgenesis of other anterior segment structures. Histology shows variable collagen fibre diameters, vascularization and a poorly developed or absent Descemet's membrane (Howard & Abrahams 1971).

Management

Glaucoma should be excluded, at an examination under anaesthetic (EUA), which is usually necessary to make the diagnosis. If present, it should be treated medically if possible. An accurate refraction and appropriate correction will also be required. Repeated EUAs may be necessary. The inheritance should be established where possible and the parents offered genetic counselling.

Central

Peters' anomaly

This consists of a congenital central corneal opacity: 80% of cases are bilateral, and the peripheral cornea is usually clear although scleralization of the limbus is common. There may be an associated cataract. Peters' anomaly is a morphological finding and not a distinct entity.

1 Peters' anomaly may be isolated (Fig. 23.5).

2 Peters' anomaly may be accompanied by other ocular malformations (Figs 23.6, 23.7). Over half of the cases have glaucoma, and other ocular associations include microcornea, microphthalmos, cornea plana, coloboma, cataract, and mesenchymal dysgenesis of the iris (Kenyon

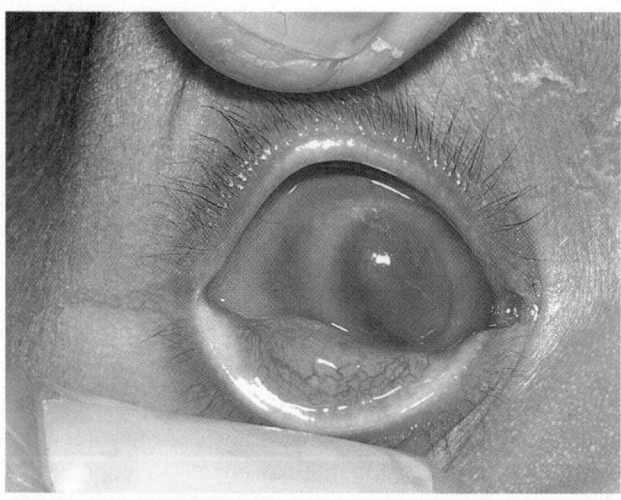

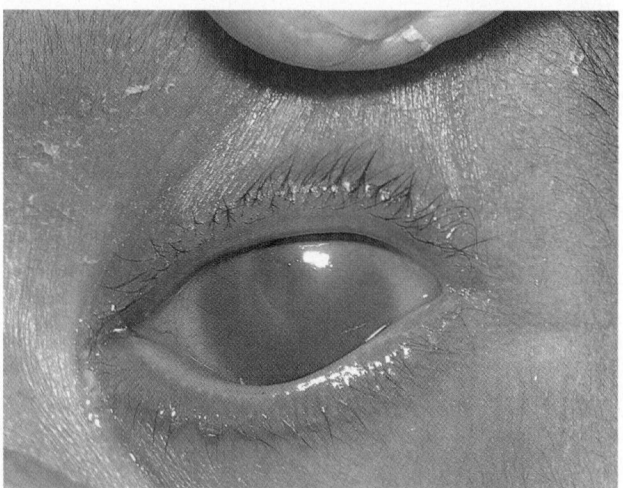

Fig. 23.3 Sclerocornea.

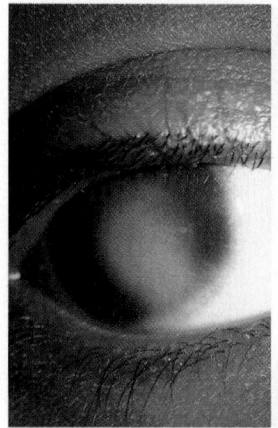
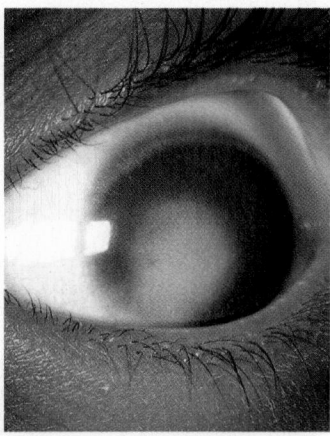

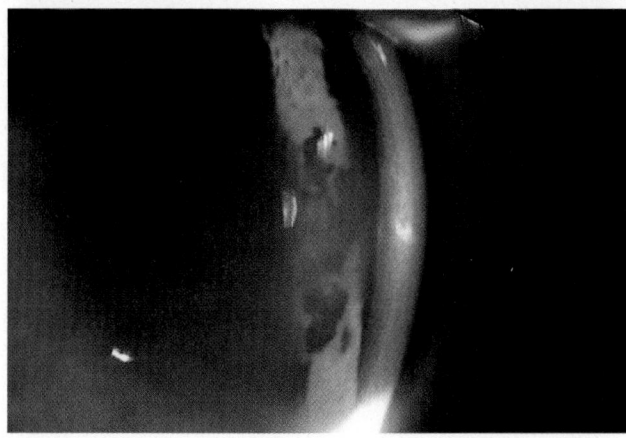

Fig. 23.5 (a) Bilateral Peters' anomaly with peripheral scleralization of the cornea. (b) Left eye in the same patient 5 years later showing clearing of the cornea with underlying iridocorneal adhesion.

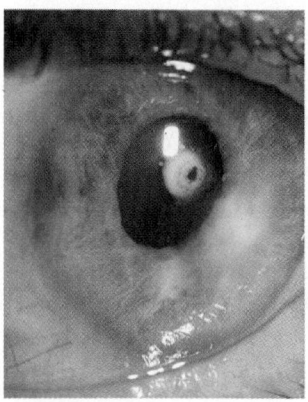
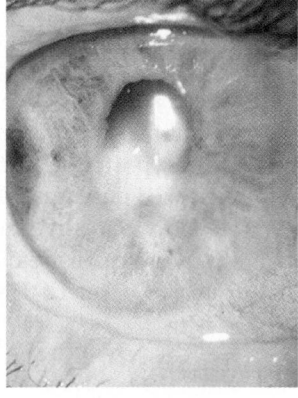

Fig. 23.6 Peters' anomaly with cataract underlying the corneal opacity. The iris defect to the left of both pictures is surgical.

1975). Congenital perforation of the cornea has also been described (Fig. 23.8) (Heckenlively & Kielar 1979).

3 Peters' anomaly may be accompanied by systemic features. Sporadic cases may have other features including developmental delay, congenital heart disease, midline central nervous system defects and genitourinary malformations (Traboulsi & Maumenee 1992).

4 Peters' anomaly may be a component of a syndrome (Kirlin *et al*. 1986).

Peters' plus syndrome

Peters' plus syndrome consists of the ocular anomaly with short stature, cleft lip and/or palate, abnormal ears and developmental delay (Van Schooneveld *et al*. 1984). In two-thirds of cases, the Peters' anomaly is bilateral (Traboulsi & Maumenee 1992). Cardiac anomalies (Kresca & Goldberg 1978; Chen & D'Sousa 1988), and multiple congenital contractures (arthrogryposis) may be associated with Peters' anomaly as well as chorioretinal coloboma (Sullivan *et al*. 1992). Children with Warburg's syndrome (mental retardation, hydrocephalus, agyria, microphthalmos and congenital retinal detachment) can also have Peters' anomaly (Myles *et al*. 1992).

Peters' anomaly in the fetal alcohol syndrome is due to a direct toxic effect of ethyl alcohol or a metabolite on the development of the corneal endothelium. Peters' anomaly has also been described in association with the ring 21 chromosomal abnormality (Cibis *et al*. 1985) and partial deletion of the long arm of chromosome 11 (Bateman *et al*. 1984). Families with anterior segment malformations, including Peters' anomaly, may have mutations of the PAX6 homeobox gene (Hanson *et al*. 1994).

The histopathological hallmark of Peters' anomaly is absence of the central corneal endothelium and Descemet's membrane. Immunohistochemical studies show abnormal corneal stromal lamellae with an enhanced fibronectin-staining reaction. Fibronectin is an extracellular glycoprotein that maintains cell morphology, regulates cell spread and has a role in cell differentiation in the embryo. Its persistence postnatally reflects the abnormal corneal development (Lee *et al*. 1989). The lens is normal ultrastructurally, but may be adherent to the central corneal opacity. The endothelial defect is the primary abnormality (with secondary failure of secretion of Descemet's membrane), but it can be the result of several different pathogenetic mechanisms. These include primary dysgenesis and secondary disruption, e.g. in rubella embryopathy (Stone *et al*. 1976). Secondary keratolenticular contact from a variety of causes *in utero* may produce the clinical and histopathological features of Peters' anomaly (Townsend *et al*. 1974). An associated PHPV has been described in one case (Myles *et al*. 1992).

Management

An EUA and microscopy will usually be required to establish the diagnosis, to exclude glaucoma, and document other ocular features. Paediatric referral to determine systemic involvement is sensible. If the condition is predominantly unilateral, with normal pressure and no

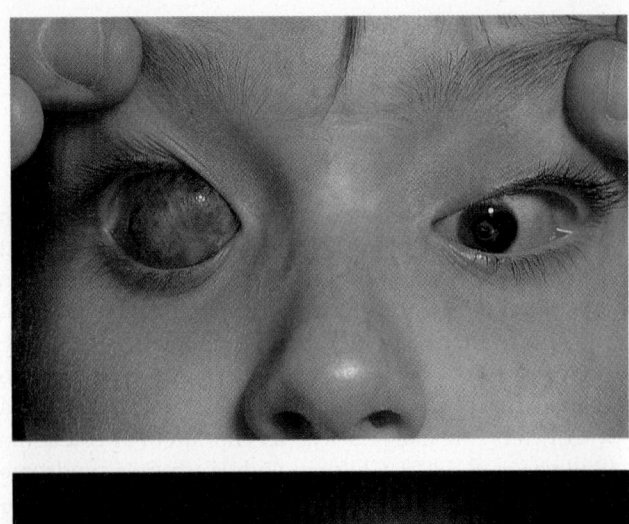

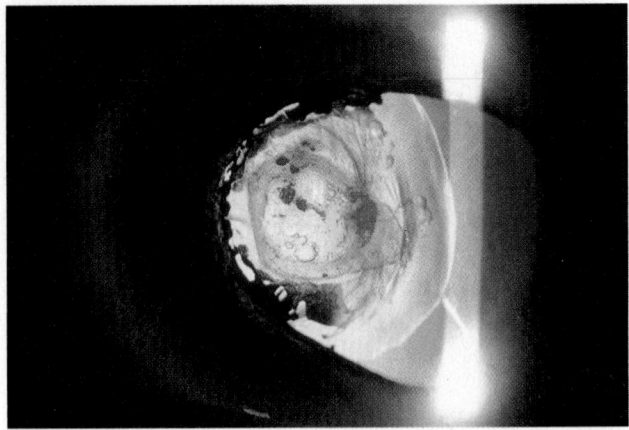

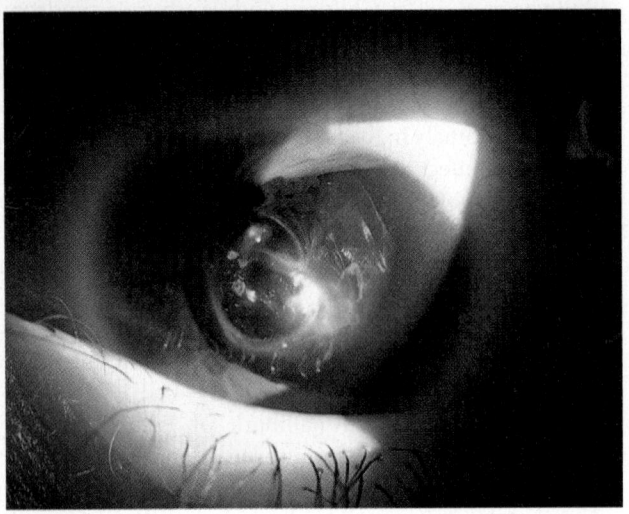

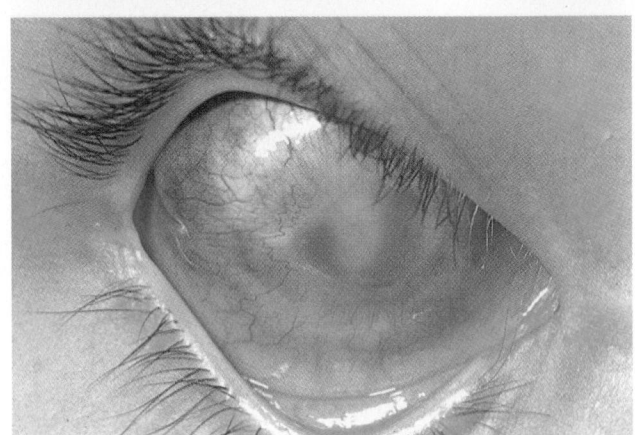

Fig. 23.7 (a) Bilateral Peters' anomaly with intractable glaucoma in the right eye requiring enucleation. (b, c) The left eye also had glaucoma which was controlled by a single trabeculectomy. The eye is phakic, with lens–cornea adhesion and extensive iris hypoplasia. (d) Right eye showing intractable buphthalmos. A more cosmetically satisfactory appearance was achieved by enucleation.

axial corneal opacity in the less involved eye, no treatment will be required. Intraocular pressure should be measured regularly, and treated if raised. If pressure control with drops fails, cyclodestructive treatment or surgery, usually trabeculectomy, is performed (see Chapter 40).

For dense bilateral corneal opacities, surgical treatment may be offered. Ultrasound will exclude keratolenticular contact and retinal detachment (Townsend *et al.* 1974). An 'open sky' lensectomy, anterior vitrectomy, and corneal graft will usually be required, although rarely only the corneal graft is necessary. The prognosis should be extremely guarded (Waring & Laibson 1977; Stultins *et al.* 1984). Despite occasional good results (Cameron 1993) the prognosis is so poor that grafts for unilateral cases are not usually recommended.

Posterior keratoconus

In posterior keratoconus the anterior corneal curvature is normal, but there is a circumscribed area of stromal thinning on the posterior surface, usually axial, associated with increased curvature. The condition is bilateral, congenital, non-progressive, and very rare (Wolter & Haney 1963). Familial cases are described associated with short stature and a thick neck (Haney & Falls 1961).

Management

These children have myopic astigmatism which should be treated with the appropriate spectacle correction.

Primary angle abnormalities

Schwalbe's ring, developmentally part of the angle, marks the posterior limit of Descemet's membrane. The anterior border is visible as a narrow grey–white line on the inner surface of the cornea, known as posterior embryotoxon.

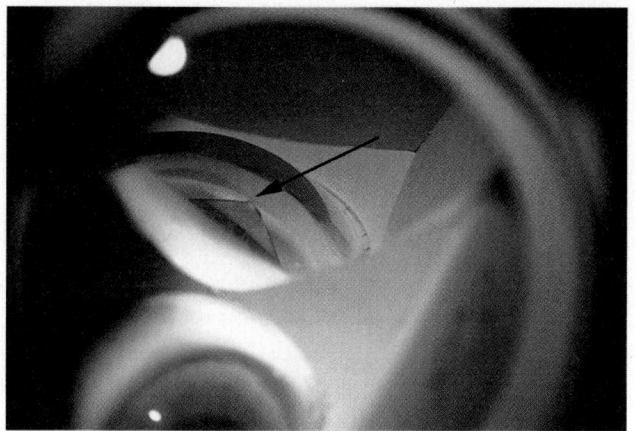

Fig. 23.8 Peters' anomaly showing a small anterior extension of the lens which is attached to the posterior part of the cornea (arrow) at which site there is an opacity. The lens and cornea may be fused in some cases.

Posterior embryotoxon

Posterior embryotoxon is a common variant of normality, and may be visible in up to 32% of eyes (Forsius *et al.* 1964). It is more prominent temporally than nasally, and as an isolated finding has no pathological significance. Developmental abnormalities of the anterior segment are, however, frequently accompanied by posterior embryotoxon (Forsius & Eriksson 1964).

Alagille's syndrome (see Chapter 44)

Posterior embryotoxon is a major feature of Alagille's syndrome (Wells *et al.* 1993): in this condition (Fig. 23.9), congenital intrahepatic bile duct hypoplasia leads to jaundice. There are associated skeletal (vertebral arch malformation) and cardiovascular defects (pulmonary stenosis in 85%) with deep-set eyes, hypertelorism and a pointed chin. A pigmentary retinopathy due to vitamin A and E deficiency develops and all affected individuals must receive vitamin supplementation (Johnson 1990).

Axenfeld's anomaly

Axenfeld's anomaly consists of posterior embryotoxon with, in addition, bridges of iris tissue crossing the angle to Schwalbe's ring (iridogoniodysgenesis) (Figs 23.10, 23.11). It indicates significant angle dysgenesis, and is associated with glaucoma in 50% of patients (Waring *et al.* 1975). It may occur sporadically, or show autosomal dominant inheritance, sometimes associated with cataract (Hodes *et al.* 1993). The glaucoma may be manifest at birth as buphthalmos, or develop in later life, so that regular monitoring of the intraocular pressure is mandatory. Autosomal dominant inherited Axenfeld's anomaly has been noted in one pedigree with pigment dispersion syn-

drome and presenile hypermature cataracts (Hodes *et al.* 1993). Other ocular features may include a pupil–iris–lens membrane (Cibis *et al.* 1986).

Congenital glaucoma

Primary congenital glaucoma (buphthalmos) is a form of angle dysgenesis due to a failure of development of the normal discontinuity of cells lining the angle (Kupfer & Ross 1971; Kupfer & Kaiser-Kupfer 1979).

Secondary congenital glaucoma is seen in eyes with additional developmental abnormalities, for example of the iris (e.g. Rieger's anomaly, or aniridia), or in conditions such as neurofibromatosis type 1 (NF1) and rubella embryopathy where the angle may be developmentally or functionally defective (see Chapter 40).

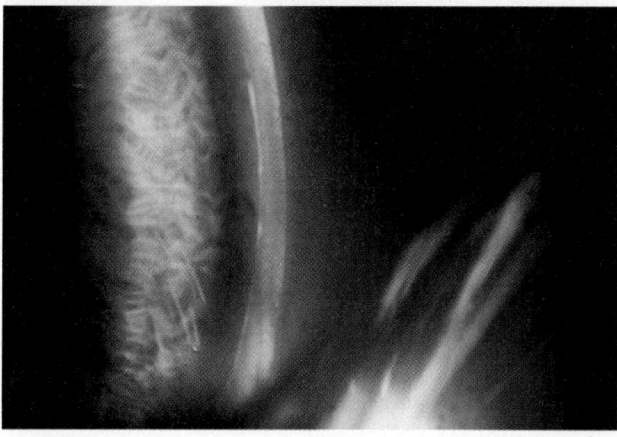

Fig. 23.9 Posterior embryotoxon. This common anomaly can be seen in the slit beam.

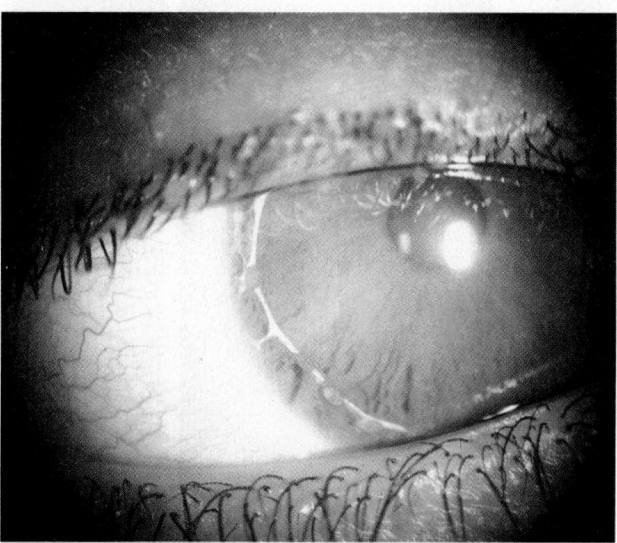

Fig. 23.10 Axenfeld's anomaly. Marked posterior embryotoxon to which is attached strands of iris.

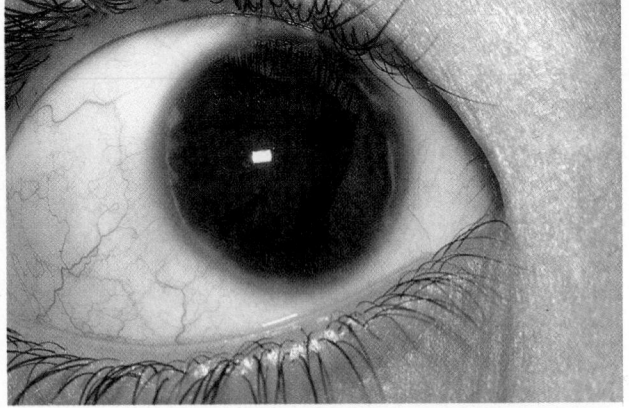

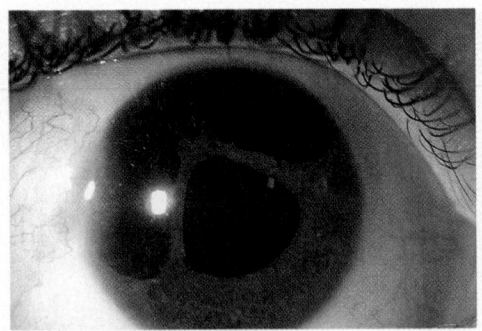

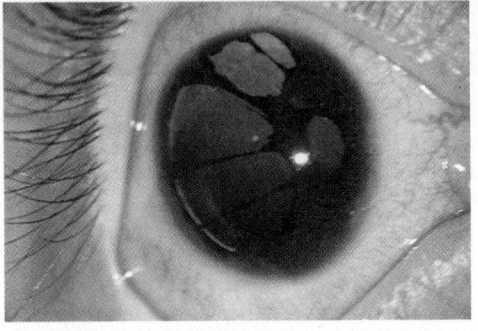

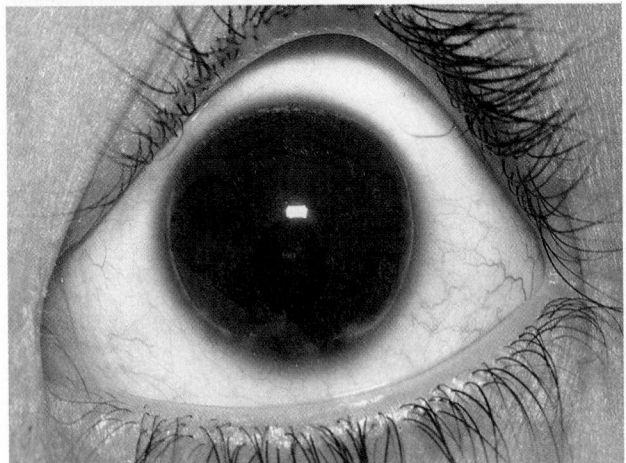

Fig. 23.13 (a) Rieger's anomaly showing iris hypoplasia and polycoria. (b) Rieger's anomaly in retroillumination showing corectopia and polycoria.

Fig. 23.11 Rieger's anomaly with posterior embryotoxon with iris adhesions, polycoria and glaucoma.

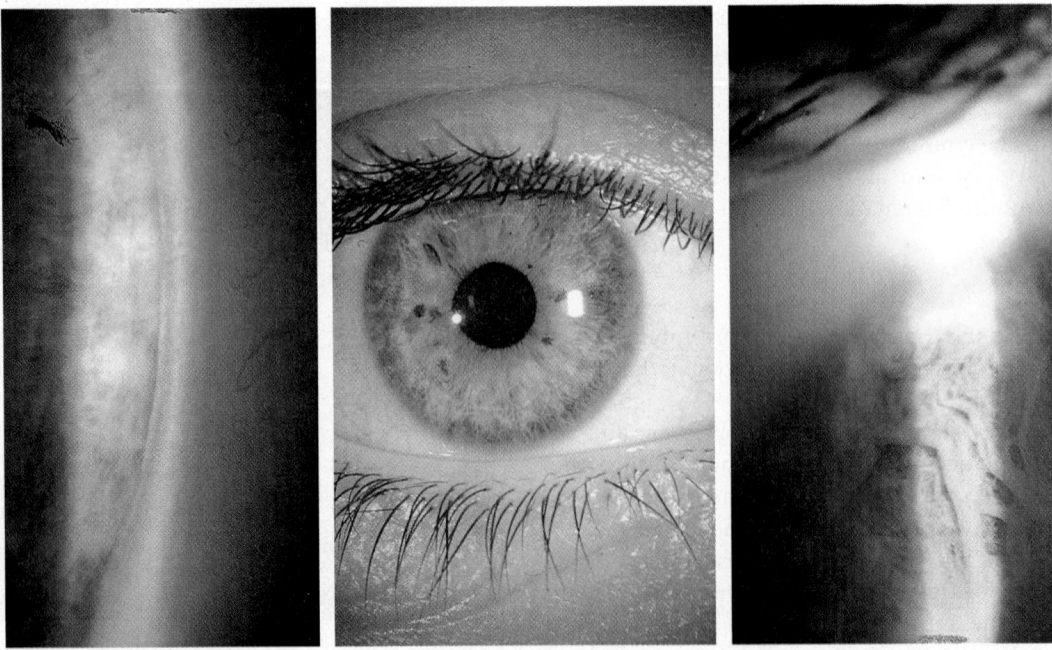

Fig. 23.12 Rieger's anomaly with focal iris hypoplasia.

Primary iris abnormalities

Rieger's anomaly

Rieger's anomaly consists of hypoplasia of the anterior iris stroma, which gives the iris a flat featureless appearance, accompanied by iridotrabecular bridges to Schwalbe's line, and posterior embryotoxon (Fig. 23.11, 23.12). The iris hypoplasia may be full thickness and the pupil may have an abnormal shape, size or position, or rarely, there may be more than one pupil (Fig. 23.13).

Ectropion uveae is common (Henkind *et al.* 1965; Dowling *et al.* 1985) and coloboma of the iris has been described (Pearce & Kerr 1965). Other ocular features include high myopia and retinal detachment which may be bilateral or due to a giant retinal tear (Spallone 1989). Glaucoma occurs in 60% of cases, but its occurrence and severity do not correspond to the extent of the iris changes (Henkind *et al.* 1965).

Other developmental abnormalities such as sclerocornea (Figs 23.14, 23.15) may be seen in Rieger's anomaly. In addition there are consistent corneal endothelial abnor-

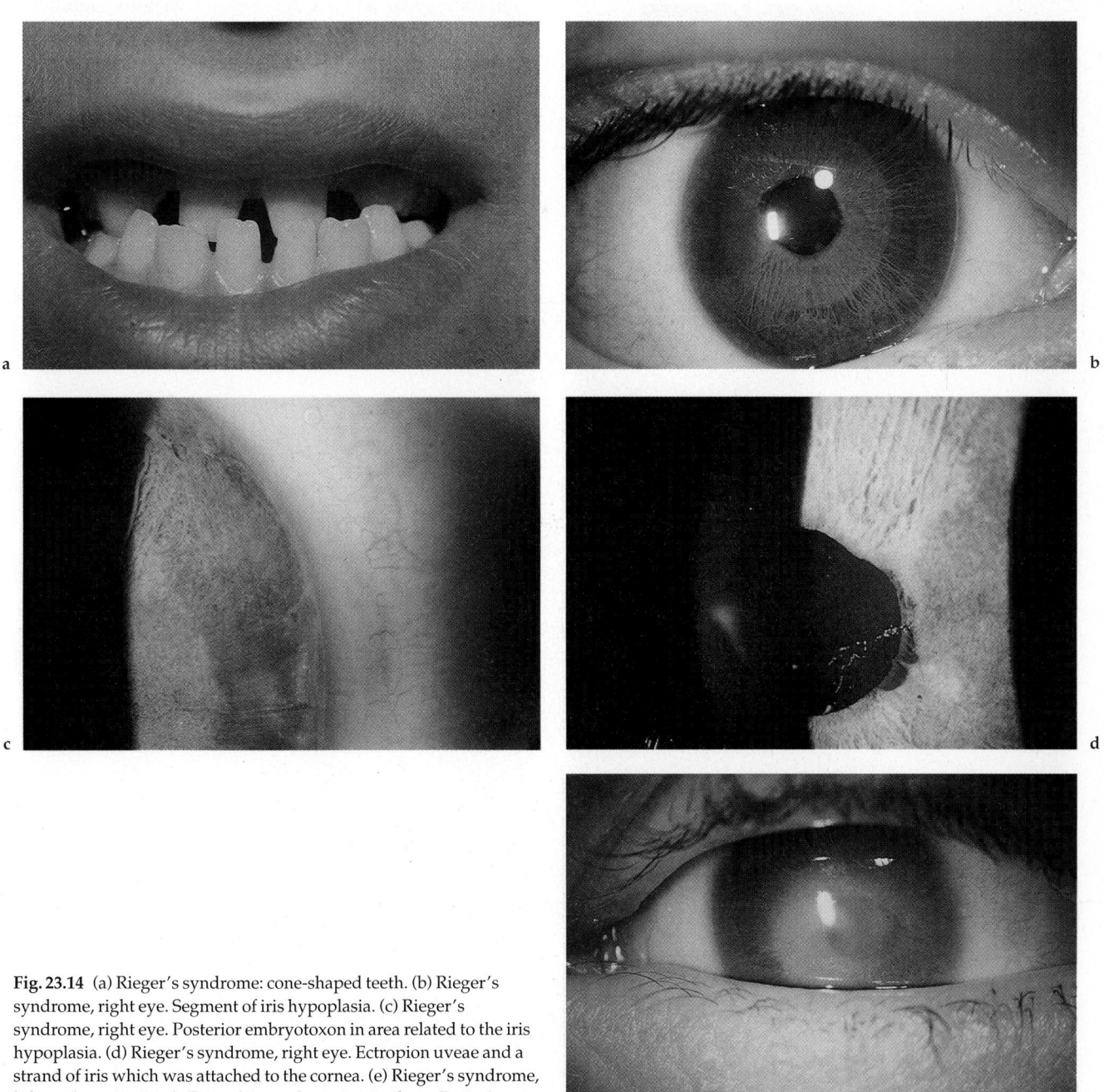

Fig. 23.14 (a) Rieger's syndrome: cone-shaped teeth. (b) Rieger's syndrome, right eye. Segment of iris hypoplasia. (c) Rieger's syndrome, right eye. Posterior embryotoxon in area related to the iris hypoplasia. (d) Rieger's syndrome, right eye. Ectropion uveae and a strand of iris which was attached to the cornea. (e) Rieger's syndrome, left eye (same patient). Central corneal opacity similar to Peters' anomaly.

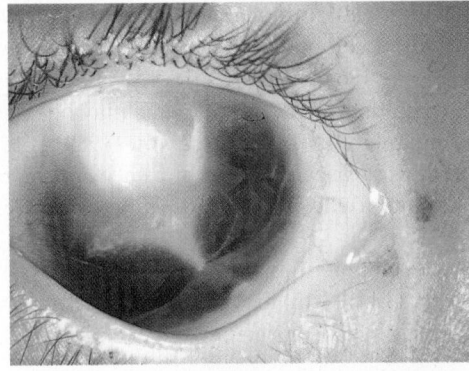

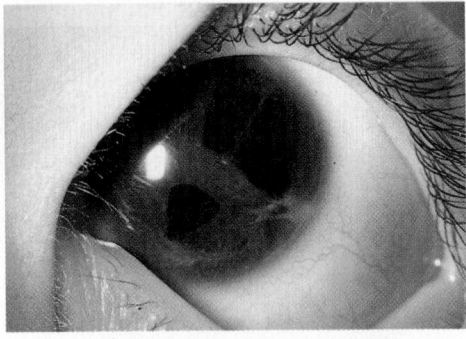

Fig. 23.15 Rieger's syndrome. Brother of patient in Fig. 23.14 with features of Rieger's and Peters' syndromes.

malities. Large, heterogeneous cells, visible on specular microscopy indicate that both the first and third phase of mesenchymal activity in anterior segment development is defective (Hittner *et al.* 1982).

Corneal opacities are common but are usually small and peripheral, at the level of Descemet's membrane. Rarely, however, Rieger's anomaly may present as a central corneal opacity (Hittner *et al.* 1982). Posterior keratoconus has also been described as an association (Mullaney 1968).

Lens changes are another consistent finding; they consist of small localized cortical opacities (Hittner *et al.* 1982) or epicapsular stars (Henkind *et al.* 1965; Chisholm & Chudley 1983) and are not usually visually significant. Other ocular associations include optic disc anomalies (e.g. tilting, myelination) and high myopia (Tabbara *et al.* 1973).

Rieger's anomaly may be inherited as an autosomal dominant characteristic with variable expressivity; some 30% of cases appear to be either sporadic or new mutations (Henkind *et al.* 1965).

Rieger's syndrome

Rieger's syndrome consists of the eye anomaly with somatic features. Most prominent are the facial abnormal-

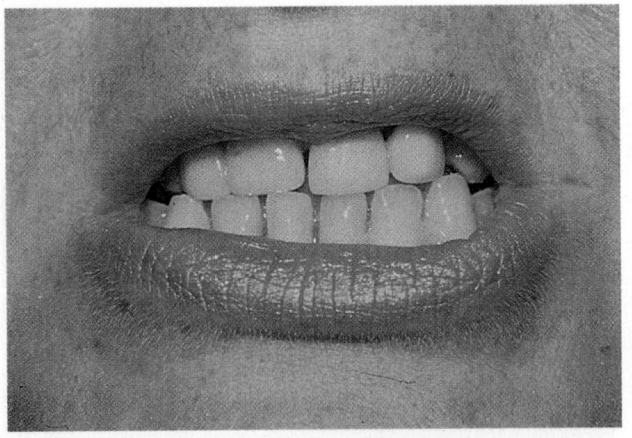

a

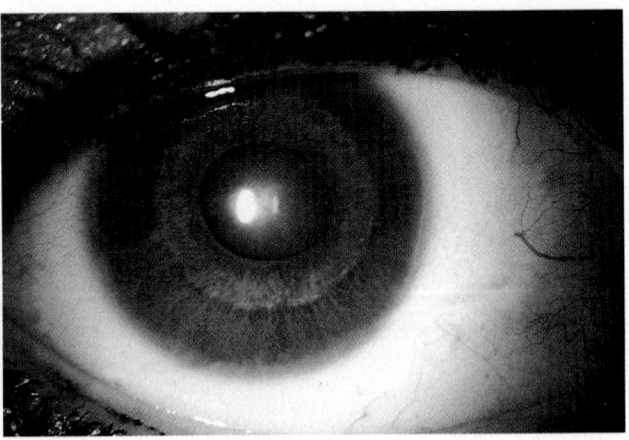

b

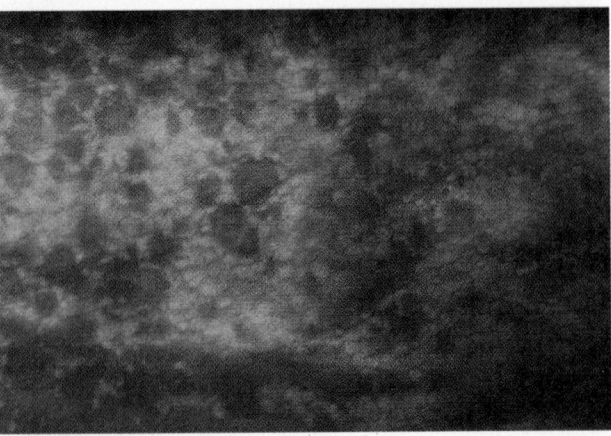

c

Fig. 23.16 (a) Rieger's syndrome. Mother of patients in Figs 23.14 and 23.15 with capped teeth. (b) Iris hypoplasia (same patient). (c) Corneal endothelium. Endothelial photographs by courtesy of Mr J. Dart.

ities; maxillary hypoplasia and short philtrum (Figs 23.14, 23.16), and dental abnormalities (Figs 23.17, 23.18) which affect both primary and secondary dentition, and consist of small, widely spaced cone-shaped teeth, or even partial anodontia (Wesley *et al.* 1978). Other features of Rieger's syndrome are umbilical and inguinal hernias and hypospadias. Isolated growth hormone deficiency is recognized as an inconstant feature (Sadeghi-Nejad & Sencot 1974; Heinemann *et al.* 1979). All the involved tissues are derived in part from neural crest cells or developed *in utero* under the influence of these cells. For this reason, other systemic features such as cardiac valvular disease (e.g. aortic stenosis, Tsai & Crajewski 1994) may be found, as may abnormalities of gonadal development (Steinsapir *et al.* 1990).

Abnormalities of chromosome 6 have been described (Tabbara *et al.* 1973; Heinemann *et al.* 1979) as has deletion of chromosome 13 (Stathacopoulos *et al.* 1987) and 4q25–27 deletion (Vaux *et al.* 1992). Linkage to the epidermal growth factor suggests 4q as the locus (Murray *et al.* 1992).

Rieger's syndrome is an autosomal dominant condition; some members of a pedigree may have the somatic manifestations without ocular signs (Chisholm & Chudley 1983). Identical twins have been described with characteristic dental abnormalities, only one of whom had eye involvement, which was unilateral (Geyer *et al.* 1994). Glaucoma occurs in 25–50% of affected individuals.

Other syndromes with anterior segment maldevelopment

1 Michels' syndrome. Affected individuals have cleft lip and palate, epicanthus, telecanthus, ptosis, subnormal intelligence, telangiectatic conjunctival vessels, peripheral corneal opacities, and iridocorneal adhesions (Michels *et al.* 1978; De La Paz *et al.* 1991). It is probably autosomal recessive.

2 Oculodentodigital dysplasia. In this autosomal dominant syndrome, microphthalmos, iris hypoplasia, persistent pupillary membranes, and an abnormal angle are associated with a small nose, hypoplastic alae, narrow and short palpebral fissures, telecanthus, epicanthus, sparse eyebrows, dental enamel hypoplasia, and camptodactyly or syndactyly of the ulnar two or three digits (Dudgeon & Chisholm 1974; Judisch *et al.* 1979; Traboulsi & Parks 1990).

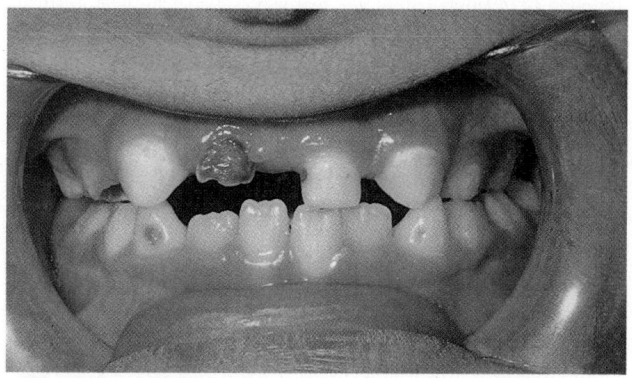

Fig. 23.17 Rieger's anomaly showing the dental abnormalities, widely spaced conical teeth and partial anodontia. There is also caries.

Management

Cases may present as buphthalmos, corneal opacity, or abnormal appearing irises or eyes. The diagnosis may require an examination under anaesthetic. Somatic features should be sought and the relatives will need examination on the slit lamp as a prelude to genetic counselling.

Glaucoma should be treated if possible medically, since it may resolve spontaneously. If uncontrolled, a trabeculectomy may be required (see Chapter 40).

Life-long monitoring of intraocular pressure is required, since the intraocular pressure may become elevated in later life. Genetic counselling should be offered to the parents of affected children.

Other primary iris developmental abnormalities

Another primary iris developmental abnormality consists of the association of dysgenesis of the angle with a persistent pupillary membrane attached to the lens (Cibis *et al.* 1986).

References

Allen L, Burian HM, Braley AE. A new concept of the development of the anterior chamber angle. *Arch Ophthalmol* 1955; **53**: 783–98.
Bateman JB, Maumenee IH, Sparkes RS. Peters' anomaly associated

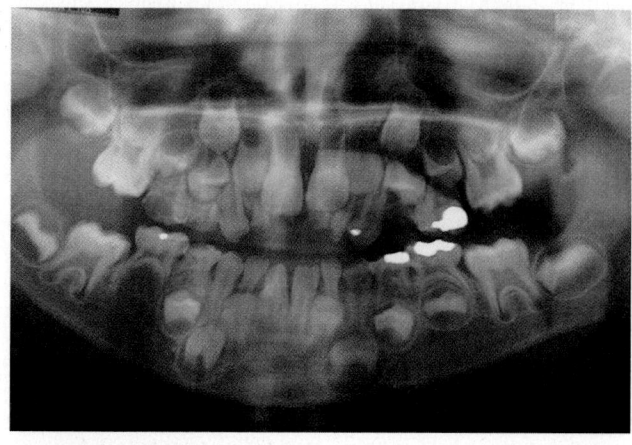

Fig. 23.18 Rieger's anomaly. Dental X-ray.

with partial deletion of the long arm of chromosome 11. *Am J Ophthalmol* 1984; **97**: 11–15.

Beauchamp GR, Knepper PA. Role of the neural crest in anterior segment development and disease. *J Pediatr Ophthalmol Strabismus* 1984; **21**: 209–14.

Block N. Les differents types de sclerocornee, leurs modes d'heredite et les malformations congenitales concomitantes. *J Genet Hum* 1965; **14**: 133–72.

Cameron J. Good visual result following early penetrating keratoplasty for Peters' anomaly. *J Pediatr Ophthalmol Strabismus* 1993; **30**: 109–112.

Chan T, Bowell R, O'Keefe M, Lanagan B. Ocular manifestations in fetal alcohol syndrome. *Br J Ophthalmol* 1991; **75**: 524–6.

Chen S-C, D'Sousa IV. Familial tetralogy of Fallot and glaucoma. *Am J Med Genet* 1988; **37**: 40–1.

Chisholm IA, Chudley AE. Autosomal dominant iridogoniodysgenesis with associated somatic anomalies: four generation family with Rieger's syndrome. *Br J Ophthalmol* 1983; **67**: 529–34.

Cibis GW, Waeltermann J, Harris DJ. Peters' anomaly in association with ring 21 chromosomal abnormality. *Am J Ophthalmol* 1985; **100**: 733–4.

Cibis GW, Waeltermann JM, Hurst E, Tripathi RC, Richardson W. Congenital pupillary–iris–lens membrane with goniodysgenesis. *Ophthalmology* 1986; **93**: 847–53.

De La Paz M, Lewis RA, Patrinely JR, Merin L, Greenberg F. A sibship with unusual anomalies of the eye and skeleton (Michels' syndrome). *Am J Ophthalmol* 1991; **112**: 572–80.

Dowling JL, Albert DM, Nelson LB, Walton DS. Primary glaucoma associated with iridotrabecular dysgenesis and ectropion uveae. *Ophthalmology* 1985; **92**: 912–21.

Dudgeon J, Chisholm JA. Oculo-dento-digital dysplasia. *Trans Ophthal Soc UK* 1974; **94**: 203–10.

Duke-Elder S. *System of Ophthalmology*, Vol. III, Part 2. London: Henry Kimpton, 1964: 498–505.

Edward DP, Li J, Sawaguchi S, Sugar J, Yue BYJT, Tso MOM. Diffuse corneal clouding in siblings with fetal alcohol syndrome. *Am J Ophthalmol* 1993; **150**: 484–93.

Elliott JH, Feman SS, O'Day DM, Garber N. Hereditary sclerocornea. *Arch Ophthalmol* 1985; **103**: 676–9.

Forsius H. Eriksson A. Embryotoxon corneae posterius in a family with slit pupil and in cases with other anomalies of the iris. *Acta Ophthalmol* 1964; **42**: 68–77.

Forsius H, Eriksson A, Fellman J. Embryotoxon corneae posterius in an isolated population. *Acta Ophthalmol* 1964; **42**: 42–9.

Foxman S, Cameron JT. The clinical implications of bilateral microphthalmos with cyst. *Am J Ophthalmol* 1984; **97**: 632–8.

Geyer O, Loewenstein A, Garty BZ, Lazar M. Different manifestations of Rieger's syndrome in monozygotic twins. *J Pediatr Ophthalmol Strabismus* 1994; **31**: 57–8.

Gibbs M, Wilkie A, Winter R, Taylor D, Baraitser M. Megalocornea developmental retardation and dysmorphic features: two further patients. *Clin Dysmorphol* 1994; **3**: 132–8.

Goldberg MF. Clinical manifestations of ectopia lentis et pupillae in 16 patients. *Ophthalmology* 1988; **95**: 1080–7.

Goldstein JE, Cogan DG. Sclerocornea and associated congenital anomalies. *Arch Ophthalmol* 1962; **67**: 760–8.

Gorlin RJ, Cohen MM, Levin LS. Syndromes with Craniosynostosis, part II. *Syndromes of the Head and Neck*. New York: Oxford University Press, 1990a: 524–6.

Gorlin RJ, Cohen MM, Levin LS. Syndromes with Craniosynostosis, part I. *Syndromes of the Head and Neck*. New York: Oxford University Press, 1990b: 340–2.

Guterman C, Abboude E, Mets MB. Microphthalmos with cyst and

Edward's syndrome. *Am J Ophthalmol* 1990; **109**: 228–30.

Haney WP, Falls HF. The occurrence of congenital keratoconus posticus circumscriptus. *Am J Ophthalmol* 1961; **52**: 53–5.

Hanson I, Fletcher J, Jordan T *et al.* Mutations at the PAX6 locus are found in heterogenous anterior segment malformations including Peters' anomaly. *Nature Genet* 1994; **6**: 168–73 .

Hansson HA, Jerndal T. Scanning electron microscopic studies on the development of the iridocorneal angle in human eyes. *Invest Ophthalmol* 1971; **10**: 252–65.

Heckenlively J, Kielar R. Congenital perforated cornea in Peters' anomaly. *Am J Ophthalmol* 1979; **88**: 63–5 .

Heinemann M-H, Breg R, Cotlier E. Rieger's syndrome with pericentric inversion of chromosome 6. *Br J Ophthalmol* 1979; **63**: 40–4.

Henkind P, Siegel IM, Carr RE. Mesodermal dysgenesis of the anterior segment: Rieger's anomaly. *Arch Ophthalmol* 1965; **73**: 810–17.

Hittner HM, Kretzer FL, Antoszyk JM, Ferrell RE, Mehta RS. Variable expressivity of autosomal dominant anterior segment mesenchymal dysgenesis in six generations. *Am J Ophthalmol* 1982; **93**: 57–70.

Hodes BL, Noecker RJ, Prendeville KJ. Autosomal dominant inheritance of iridogoniodysgenesis and cataract. *Ophthalmology* 1993; **100**: 168–72.

Holmstrom GE, Reardon WP, Baraitser M, Elston JS, Taylor DS. Heterogeneity in dominant anterior segment malformations. *Br J Ophthalmol* 1991; **75**: 591–7.

Howard RO, Abrahams IW. Sclerocornea. *Am J Ophthalmol* 1971; **71**: 1254–60.

Johnson BL. Ocular pathologic features of arteriohepatic dysplasia (Alagille's syndrome). *Am J Ophthalmol* 1990; **110**: 504–12.

Jones KL, Smith DW, Ulleland CN, Streissguth AP. Pattern of malformation in off-spring of chronic alcoholic mothers. *Lancet* 1973; **i**: 1267–71.

Judisch GF, Martin-Casals A, Hansar JW, Olin WH. Oculodentodigital dysplasia: four new reports and a literature review. *Arch Ophthalmol* 1979; **97**: 878–84.

Kasner L, Meitz H, Green WR. Agenesis of Bowman's layer. *Cornea* 1993; **12**: 163–70.

Kenyon KR. Mesenchymal dysgenesis in Peters' anomaly, sclerocornea and congenital endothelial dystrophy. *Exp Eye Res* 1975; **21**: 125–42.

Kirkham TH, Milot J, Berman P. Ophthalmic manifestations of Aarskog (facial-digital-genital) syndrome. *Am J Ophthalmol* 1975; **79**: 441–5.

Kirlin JD, Fineman RM, Crandall AS, Obon RJ. Peters' anomaly as a consequence of genetic and non-genetic syndromes. *Arch Ophthalmol* 1986; **104**: 61–4.

Kraft SP, Judisch GF, Grayson DM. Megalocornea: a clinical and echographic study of an autosomal dominant pedigree. *J Pediatr Ophthalmol Strabismus* 1984; **21**: 190–4.

Kresca LJ, Goldberg MF. Peters' anomaly: dominant inheritance in one pedigree, and dextrocardia in another. *J Pediatr Ophthalmol Strabismus* 1978; **15**: 141–6.

Kupfer C. A note on the development of the anterior chamber angle. *Invest Ophthalmol* 1969; **8**: 69–74.

Kupfer C, Kaiser-Kupfer MF. Observations on the development of the anterior chamber angle with reference to the pathogenesis of congenital glaucomas. *Am J Ophthalmol* 1979; **88**: 424–6.

Kupfer C, Ross K. The development of outflow facility in human eyes. *Invest Ophthalmol* 1971; **10**: 513–17.

Lee CF, Yue BYJT, Robin J, Sawagoochi S, Sugar J. Immunohistochemical studies of Peters' anomaly. *Ophthalmology* 1989; **96**: 958–64.

Lipson AH, Cowell C, Gorlin RJ. The SHORT syndrome: further delineation and natural history. *J Med Genet* 1989; **26**: 473–5.

Mackey DA, Buttery RG, Wise GM, Denton MJ. Description of X-linked megalocornea with identification of the gene locus. *Arch Ophthalmol* 1991; **109**: 829–33.

Mann I. The iris. In *Developmental Abnormalities of the Eye*. London: British Medical Association, 1957a: 224.

Mann I. The cornea. In *Developmental Abnormalities of the Eye*. London: British Medical Association, 1957b; 342–64.

Mattos J, Contreras F, O'Donnell FE. A new syndrome of autosomal dominantly inherited bilateral annular limbal dermoids with corneal and conjunctival extension. *Arch Ophthalmol* 1980; **98**: 1069–71.

Meire FM. Megalocornea: clinical and genetic aspects. *Doc Ophthalmol* 1994; **87**: 1–121.

Meire FM, Delleman JW. Biometry in X-linked megalocornea: pathognomonic findings. *Br J Ophthalmol* 1994; **78**: 781–5.

Michels VV, Hittner HM, Beaudet AL. A clefting syndrome with ocular anterior chamber defect and lid anomalies. *J Pediatr* 1978; **93**: 444.

Mullaney J. The anterior chamber cleavage syndrome. *Trans Ophthalmol Soc UK* 1968; **88**: 757–66.

Murphy C, Alvarado J, Juster R. Prenatal and postnatal growth of human Descemet's membrane. *Invest Ophthalmol Vis Sci* 1984a; **25**: 1402–15.

Murphy C, Alvarado J, Juster R, Maglio M. Prenatal and postnatal cellularity of the human corneal endothelium. *Invest Ophthalmol Vis Sci* 1984b; **25**: 312–22.

Murray JC, Bennett SR, Kwitek AE *et al*. Linkage of Rieger syndrome to the region of the epidermal growth factor gene on chromosome 4. *Nature Genet* 1992; **2**: 46–9.

Myles WM, Flanders ME, Chitayat D, Brownstein S. Peters' anomaly —a clinicopathologic study. *J Paediatr Ophthalmol Strabismus* 1992; **29**: 374–81.

Neuhauser G, Kaveggia, France TD, Opitz JM. Syndrome of mental retardation, seizures, hypotonic cerebral palsy and megalocorneas recessively inherited. *Z Kinderheikd* 1975; **120**: 1–18.

O'Rahilly R. The prenatal development of the human eye. *Exp Eye Res* 1975; **21**: 93–112.

Pearce WG, Kerr CB. Inherited variation in Rieger's malformation. *Br J Ophthalmol* 1965; **49**: 503–37.

Porges Y, Gershoni-Baruch R, Leibu R *et al*. Hereditary microphthalmia with colobomatous cyst. *Am J Ophthalmol* 1992; **114**: 30–4.

Ramsey MS, Fine BS, Shields JA, Yanoff M. The Marfan syndrome. A histological study of ocular findings. *Am J Ophthalmol* 1973; **76**: 102–16.

Reese AB, Ellsworth RM. The anterior chamber cleavage syndrome. *Arch Ophthalmol* 1966; **75**: 307–18.

Sadeghi-Nejad A, Sencot B. Autosomal dominant transmission of isolated growth hormone deficiency in iris–dental dysplasia (Rieger's syndrome). *J Pediatr* 1974; **85**: 644–8.

Santolaya J, Grijalbo A, Delgado A, Eidozain G. Additional case of Nehauser megalocornea and mental retardation syndrome with congenital hypotonia. *Am J Med Genet* 1992; **43**: 609–11.

Skuta GL, Sugar J, Ericson ES. Corneal endothelial cell measurements in megalocornea. *Arch Ophthalmol* 1983; **101**: 51–3.

Soriano H, Psilas K. Syndrome e marchesani associe a une a megalocornee et a une atrophie de l'iris; etude echographique. *Ophthalmologica (Basel)* 1970; **161**: 269–73.

Spallone A. Retinal detachment in Axenfeld–Rieger syndrome. *Br J Ophthalmol* 1989; **73**: 559–62.

Speedwell L, Novakovic P, Sherrard GS, Taylor DSI. The infant corneal endothelium. *Arch Ophthalmol* 1988; **106**: 771–5.

Spour H-L, Willms J, Steinhousen HC. Prenatal alcohol exposure and long-term developmental consequences. *Lancet* 1993; **341**: 907–10.

Stathacopoulos RA, Bateman JB, Sparkes RS, Hepler RS. Rieger's syndrome and chromosome 13 deletion. *J Pediatr Ophthalmol Strabismus* 1987; **24**: 198–203.

Steinsapir KD, Lehman E, Ernest JRT, Tripathi RC. Systemic neurocristopathy associated with Rieger's syndrome. *Am J Ophthalmol* 1990; **110**: 437–8.

Stone DL, Kenyon KR, Green R, Ryan SJ. Congenital central corneal leukoma, (Peters' anomaly). *Am J Ophthalmol* 1976; **81**: 74–193.

Sullivan TJ, Clarke MP, Heathcote JG, Hunter WS, Routeman DS, Morin JD. Multiple congenital contractures (arthrogryposis) in association with Peters' anomaly and chorioretinal colobomata. *J Pediatr Ophthalmol Strabismus* 1992; **29**: 370–3.

Stultins RD, Sumers KD, Cavanagh HD, Waring GO, Gammon JA. Penetrating keratoplasty in children. *Ophthalmology* 1984; **91**: 1222–30.

Tabbara KF, Knouri FP, Derkaloustian VM. Rieger's syndrome with chromosome anomaly. *Can J Ophthalmol* 1973; **8**: 488–91.

Topilow HW, Cykiert RC, Goldman K, Palmer E, Henkind P. Bilateral corneal dermis-like choristomas. *Arch Ophthalmol* 1981; **99**: 1387–91.

Townsend WM, Font RL, Zimmerman LE. Congenital corneal leukomas. *Am J Ophthalmol* 1974; **77**: 192–206.

Traboulsi BI, Maumenee IH. Peters' anomaly and associated congenital malformations. *Arch Ophthalmol* 1992; **110**: 1739–42.

Traboulsi EI, Parks MM. Glaucoma in oculo-dento-osseous dysplasia. *Am J Ophthalmol* 1990; **109**: 310–13.

Tripathi BJ, Tripathi RC. Neural crest origin of human trabecular meshwork and its implications for the pathogenesis of glaucoma. *Am J Ophthalmol* 1989; **107**: 583–90.

Tsai JC, Crajewski AL. Cardiovascular disease and Axenfeld–Rieger syndrome. *Am J Ophthalmol* 1994; **118**: 255–6.

Van Schooneveld MJ, Delleman JW *et al*. Peters' plus: a new syndrome. *Ophthal Paediatr Genet* 1984; **4**: 141–6.

Vaux C, Sheffield L, Keith CG, Voullaire L. Evidence that Rieger's syndrome maps to 4q25 or 4q27. *J Med Genet* 1992; **29**: 256–8.

Waring GO, Laibson PR. Keratoplasty in infants and children. *Trans Am Acad Ophthalmol Otolaryngol* 1977; **83**: 283–96.

Waring GO, Rodrigues MM, Laibson PR. Anterior chamber cleavage syndrome: a stepladder classification. *Surv Ophthalmol* 1975; **20**: 3–27.

Weiss AH, Kousseff BG, Ross EA, Longbottom J. Complex microphthalmos. *Arch Ophthalmol* 1989a; **107**: 1619–24.

Weiss AH, Kousseff BG, Ross EA, Longbottom J. Simple microphthalmos. *Arch Ophthalmol* 1989b; **107**: 1625–30.

Wells K, Pulida J, Judisch G, Ussoinig K, Fisher T, La Breque D. Ophthalmic features of Alagille syndrome (arteriohepatic dysplasia). *J Pediatr Ophthalmol Strabismus* 1993; **30**: 130–5.

Wesley RK, Baker JD, Golnick AL. Rieger's syndrome. *J Pediatr Ophthalmol Strabismus* 1978; **15**: 67–70.

Wolter JR, Haney WP. Histopathology of keratoconus posticus circumscriptus. *Arch Ophthalmol* 1963; **69**: 357–62.

Wulle KG. Electron microscopy of the fetal development of the corneal endothelium and Descemet's membrane of the human eye. *Invest Ophthalmol* 1972; **11**: 897–904.

24: Corneal Abnormalities in Childhood

William V. Good and Creig S. Hoyt

Corneal disease is still the most common cause of blindness in the world today. It is not surgery but the combination of better nutrition, public and private health measures, and antibiotics that have made corneal disease an unusual cause of blindness in the Western world. Nonetheless corneal diseases are a small but significant cause of disability from visual defect, glare or pain and corneal abnormalities may form important clues to the nature of systemic diseases.

Trisomy 18 and trisomy 8 mosaic

In trisomy 18, the eyelid may be abnormal, and the eye frequently is colobomatous. The cornea may be diffusely opaque at birth. Discrete corneal opacities caused by breakdown of the corneal epithelium occasionally occur.

In trisomy 8 mosaic syndrome geographical corneal opacities (Fig. 24.1) are characteristic (Frangoulis & Taylor 1983; Stark *et al.* 1987). These opacities have been histologically studied and consist of richly vascularized fibrous tissue in the superficial layers of the cornea (Stark *et al.* 1987).

Dermoids (choristomas)

Choristomas are benign congenital overgrowths of abnormally located tissue; in the eye they consist of masses of skin, hair follicles (Figs 24.2–24.4), hair and sebaceous glands. They may be multiple (Fig. 24.5). These masses were originally destined to become skin but were displaced onto the eye.

Single-tissue choristomas contain ectopic tissues of mesenchymal or ectodermal origin (Mansour *et al.* 1989), i.e. dermis, lacrimal gland, fat, respiratory epithelium (Young *et al.* 1990), brain, nerve, bone, teeth, and so on. Complex choristomas contain two or more tissues of mesenchymal or ectodermal origin.

A dermoid (or lipodermoid) is a congenital, solid mass of dermis-like and pilosebaceous material covered with keratinized, often hairy squamous epithelium. They are usually found at the corneoscleral junction, in the inferotemporal quadrant, but they may be much more widespread and overlie a microphthalmic (Murata *et al.* 1991) or staphylomatous (Bernuy *et al.* 1981) eye. Dermoids can involve the entire thickness of the cornea (Oakman *et al.* 1993) and sclera. They reduce vision by blocking light (if they occur across the cornea) or by distorting the contour of the cornea giving astigmatism and amblyopia; they may sometimes cover the cornea (Fig. 24.6).

Dermolipomas are similar to dermoids but have a large amount of fat and few or no pilosebaceous apparati. Some are inherited in an autosomal dominant fashion, though X-linked recessive inheritance has also been described (Topilow *et al.* 1981). Dermoids and dermolipomas also occur in Goldenhar's syndrome (Mansour *et al.* 1985),

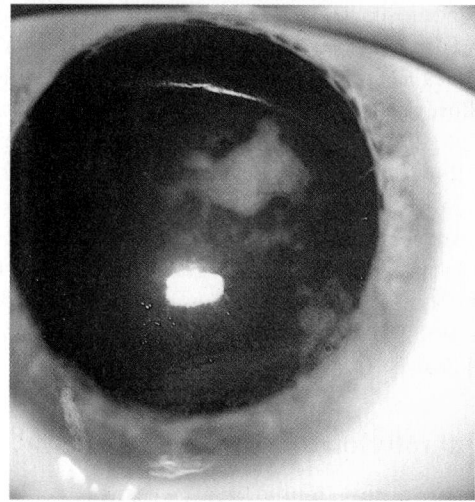

Fig. 24.1 Trisomy 8 mosaic syndrome with characteristic geographical corneal opacity.

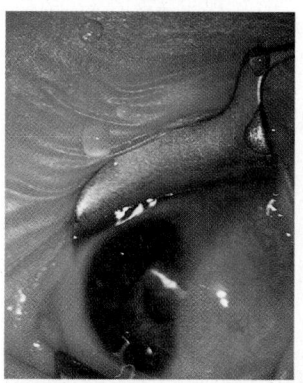 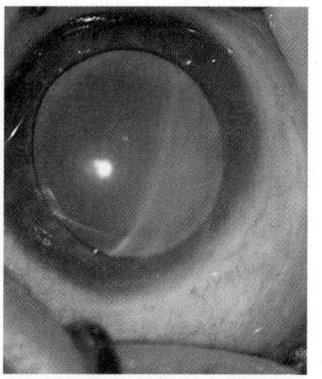

a   b

Fig. 24.2 (a) Limbal dermoid which covered half of the cornea and extended posteriorly in the fornix. (b) Same patient, 1 year following lamellar keratectomy which was carried out at 2 months of age. Although the cosmetic appearance was satisfactory and remained so for 5 years after this photograph the eye was deeply amblyopic due to high astigmatism and the corneal opacity.

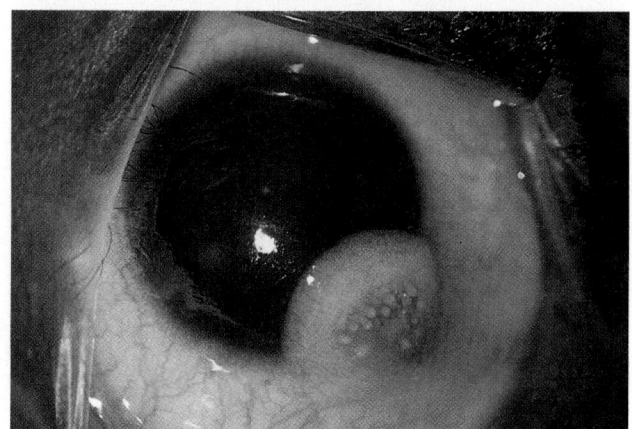

Fig. 24.3 Hairy limbal dermoid.

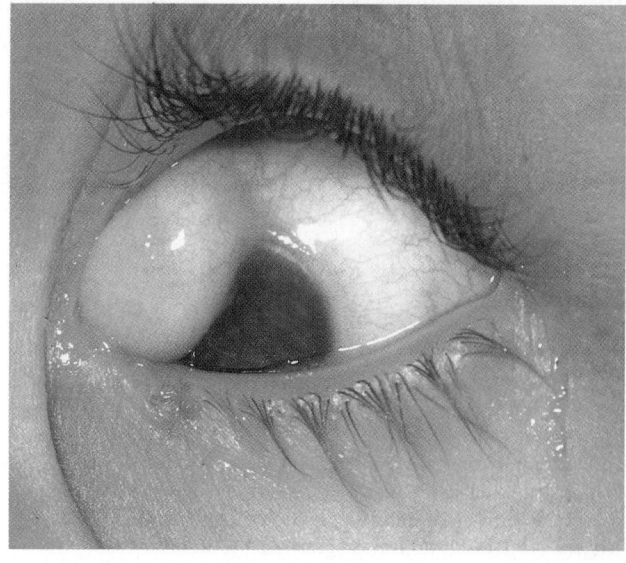

Fig. 24.4 Large bulky hairy superior limbal dermoid.

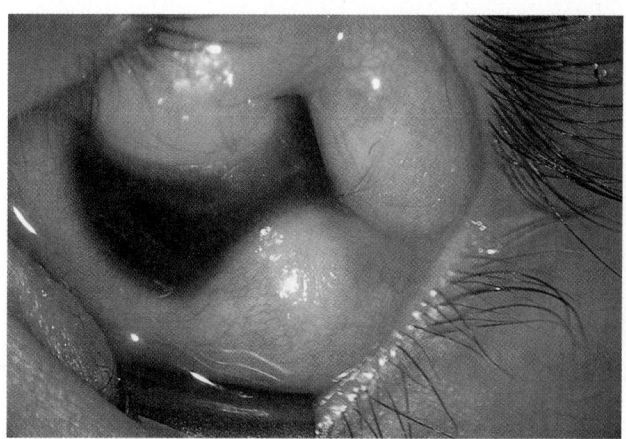

Fig. 24.5 Multiple corneal dermoids in a patient with Goldenhar's syndrome.

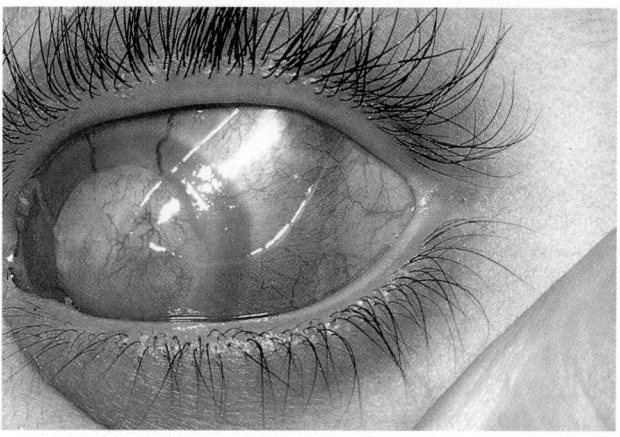

Fig. 24.6 Dermis-like choristoma overlying an anomalous eye that has become buphthalmic.

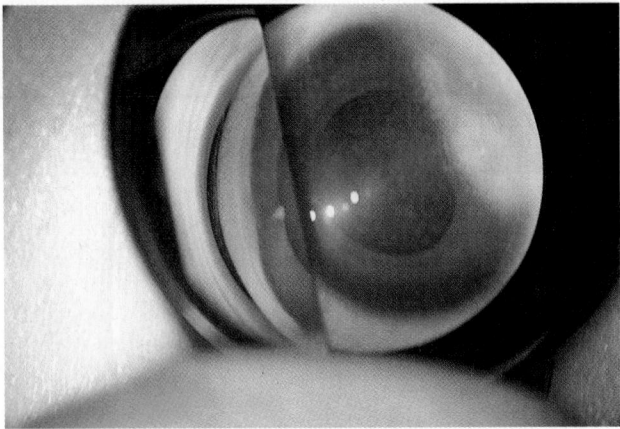

Fig. 24.7 Limbal dermoid: gonioscopic view. Through the gonioscope it can just be seen that the dermoid involves the inner part of the cornea indicating that caution should be taken during surgery. A full thickness corneal graft may be the only way to treat this sort of problem and may not be indicated unless the cosmetic appearance is extreme.

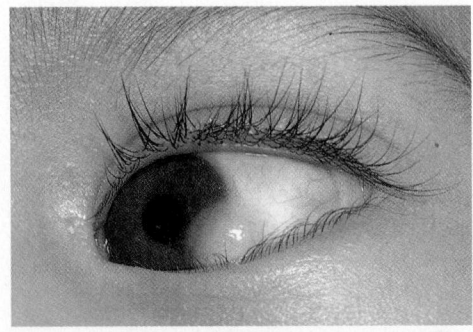

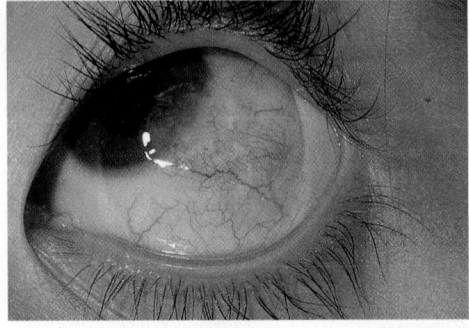

Fig. 24.8 (a) Limbal dermoid. The indication for surgery was the cosmetic appearance. It can be seen that the dermoid is raised and pale coloured. (b) Same case as in (a) after lamellar keratectomy. Although there is still some residual corneal opacity the lesion is now flat and cosmetically acceptable.

encephalocraniocutaneous lipomatosis (Kodsi *et al.* 1994), congenital generalized fibromatosis (Vangsted & Limpaphayom 1983), and the linear naevus sebaceous syndrome of Fuerstein and Mimms (Mansour *et al.* 1986).

Treatment is usually necessary on cosmetic grounds alone but must be preceded by a full ocular examination including gonioscopy to assess the extent of the mass (Fig. 24.7). Lamellar keratectomy is sufficient in most cases and improves the appearance by not only removing the white–yellow appearance and any hairs but also the elevation (Fig. 24.8); many cases re-opacify but the appearance is often adequate postoperatively and freehand lamellar grafting is not usually required. Full thickness dermoids may be treated by excision and corneal (not scleral) grafting (Fig. 24.9) but the prognosis is guarded. Enucleation is occasionally the best option for widespread dermoids, but is best left for as long as possible to allow for orbital growth.

Corneal staphyloma

In congenital corneal staphyloma the cornea is enlarged, ectatic and opaque (Figs 24.10, 24.11); the Descemet's membrane is missing (Schanzlin *et al.* 1983). The posterior segment of the eye is usually normal (Leff *et al.* 1986), but glaucoma occurs and may cause buphthalmos. Corneal metaplasia is a similar condition; both this, sclerocornea and staphyloma may be caused by a neural crest cell migration defect. Intraocular defects sometimes co-exist (Klauss & Riedel 1983) and the cornea may become opaque and keratinized with time.

Amniotic bands

Amniotic bands may be associated with congenital

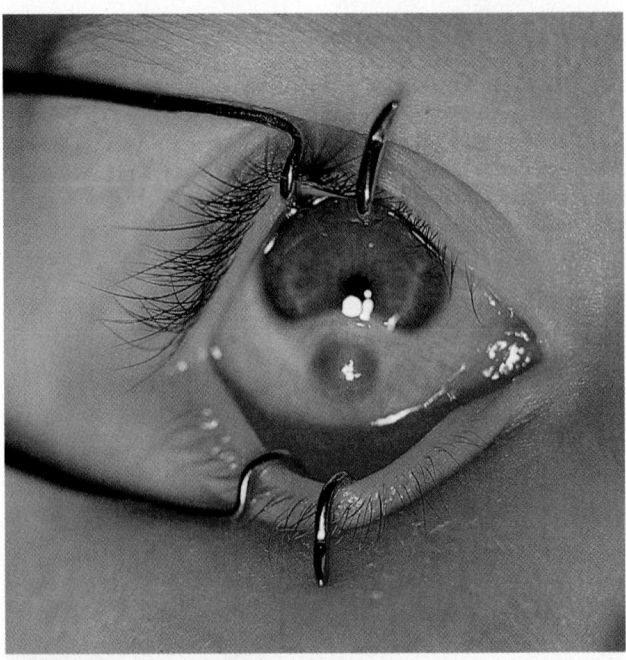

Fig. 24.9 Limbal ectasia following scleral graft for a full thickness limbal dermoid. This has been repeated on three occasions, but the graft repeatedly dissolved and the area became ectatic. It was successfully treated with a corneal graft which lasted permanently.

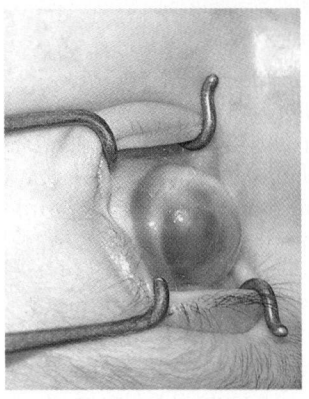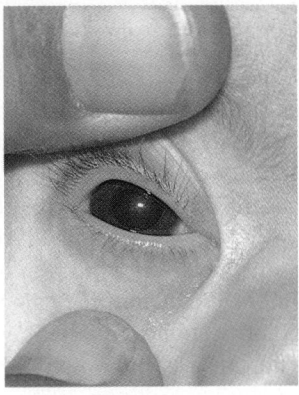

Fig. 24.10 Congenital corneal staphyloma of the right eye. The left eye was normal.

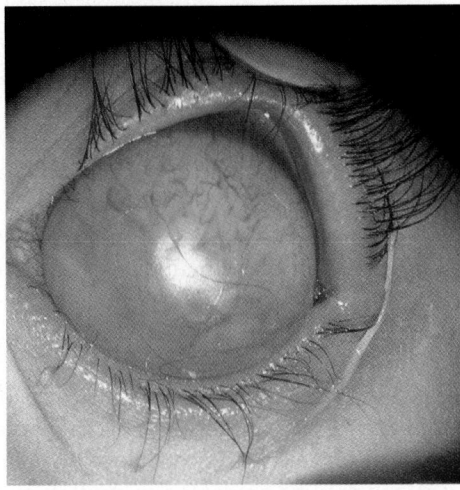

Fig. 24.11 Corneal staphyloma that has become keratinized and the cornea thickened.

corneal leucomas (Miller *et al.* 1987) or with exposure keratitis from lid defects (Ben-Ezra *et al.* 1982).

Treatment of the congenitally opaque cornea

Treatment for these conditions is often hopeless, so unilateral cases are usually treated as cosmetic problems and the eye is covered with a cosmetic shell or contact lens. The eye is enucleated if painful or excessively large or ugly. Bilateral cases are best left alone if there is any possibility of an increase in corneal clarity with time (as in many developmental anomalies of the cornea), and if there is likely to be useful vision for at least navigation in one eye. If the infant is blind corneal grafting is indicated, with occasional good results (Zaidman *et al.* 1982; Hwang & Hwang 1991). Although surgical valour is more appealing than conservatism, the high rate of failure in complex cases especially when compared to adults (Mackenson *et al.* 1977; Knobel & Demeler 1978; Brown & Salamon 1983;

Cowden 1990), the possibility of spontaneous improvement, and secondary complications in failures leads most experienced surgeons to prefer conservatism in all but the most hopeless bilateral cases.

Grafting is probably best performed either early in infancy when the baby can be examined more easily on the slit lamp or later in childhood when he or she is more co-operative. Grafts in infants are often followed by myopia (Gloor *et al.* 1992), especially if infant graft material is used; this may be used to advantage in aphakic cases.

Keratitis

Allergic

See Chapter 18.

Infection

See Chapter 18.

Exposure keratitis

Exposure keratitis is a disorder of the ocular surface due to failure to maintain adequate lubrication and protection for the corneal epithelium, which results in its breakdown. The cornea will lose its lustre, and this may be followed by punctate loss of corneal epithelium. Larger areas of epithelial loss are followed by thinning of the corneal stroma. In severe cases, corneal perforation can occur. Usually these cases are associated with a bacterial infection which occurs because of the loss of protection afforded by the normal spread of tears.

Eyelid abnormalities may cause exposure keratitis (Miller *et al.* 1987). An ectropion, for example, can result in poor eyelid apposition; the cornea, then, is relatively unprotected. Disorders of the lacrimal gland (e.g. tumours, congenital malfunctions, central nervous system disease, radiation necrosis) (Fig. 24.12) result in poor lubrication of the corneal surface. Exophthalmos from orbit disease results in poor lid closure. Seventh nerve palsies affect closure of the eyelids. Fifth nerve palsies also result in keratitis and combined fifth and seventh cranial nerve palsies cause the most serious problems especially if the eye is also dry (Fig. 24.13). Sensory innervation of the cornea may play an important role in maintaining its integrity (Schimmelpfennig & Beurman 1979). Blinking is also influenced by sensory input.

Non-accidental injury

A spectrum of corneal injuries can occur in child abuse. The corneal epithelium may be abraded, producing a characteristic stain when fluorescein is placed on the eye.

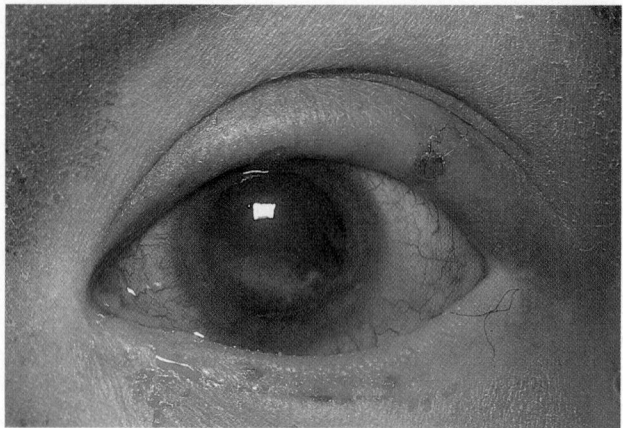

Fig. 24.12 Keratitis resulting from a combination of exposure, drying and the direct effects of irradiation for orbital rhabdomyosarcoma.

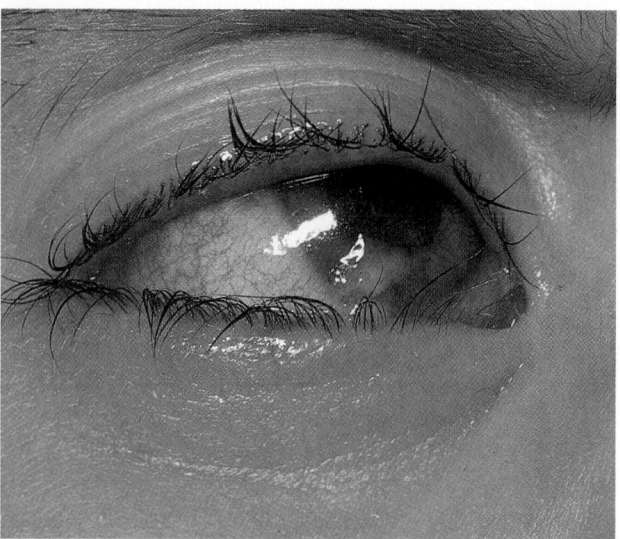

Fig. 24.13 Dry and exposed eye giving rise to keratitis in a patient with seventh nerve palsy associated with the CHARGE association.

Deeper injuries are produced when the object striking the eye is sharp. Corneal perforation with flattening of the anterior chamber occurs rarely. The presence of lid ecchymoses accompanying the corneal injury should arouse suspicion of abuse. A careful history and physical examination should be conducted, searching for other unexplained injuries. Forceps injuries cause ruptures of Descemet's membrane usually in a vertical direction and are associated with high astigmatism in the axis of the ruptures, myopia and deep amblyopia (Angell *et al.* 1981). Chemical injuries, sometimes repeated, may be due to non-accidental injury by the parents (Fig. 24.14) (Taylor & Bentovim 1976) (see Chapter 62).

Cogan's syndrome

Cogan's syndrome consists of interstitial keratitis and audiovestibular disease (Cogan 1945). The cornea shows bilateral patchy stromal infiltrates, with vascularization and uveitis. Eventually, vascularization of the cornea occurs. The eighth nerve impairment may precede or follow corneal involvement. An association of this syndrome with polyarteritis nodosa has been described (Gilbert & Talbot 1969), and there are many case reports of this and other systemic associations (Bicknell & Holland 1978). The cause is unknown although immunological factors (Cogan & Sullivan 1975), viral agents (Darougar *et al.* 1978) and vasculitis (Podder *et al.* 1994) have been implicated.

Vitamin A deficiency and measles

Deficiency of vitamin A damages the cornea. The surface loses its normal lustre, even though the eye is not always excessively dry. The tears show abnormal electrophoretic responses to measles infection, especially in malnourished children (Kogbe & Listet 1987). Corneal vascularization, keratinization, and oedema can occur. When vitamin deficiency is accompanied by malnourishment and protein deficiency, an acute liquefactive necrosis of the cornea can occur (Fig. 24.15).

This is particularly marked when associated with measles infection, herpes simplex or the use of traditional eye medicines (Foster & Sommer 1987). If diagnosed early, some of these problems are reversible with vitamin A replacement and may be prevented by dietary measures,

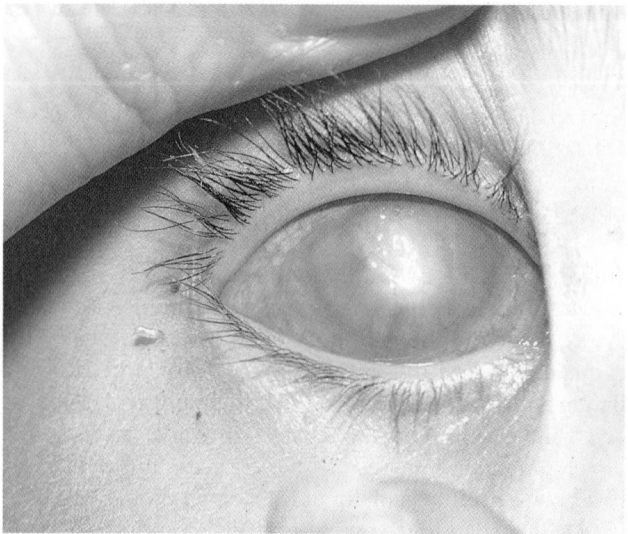

Fig. 24.14 Non-accidental chemical injury to the cornea. This child suddenly developed a profoundly severe keratitis in one eye on the day that his mother's boyfriend left home. Although never proven the situation was highly suggestive.

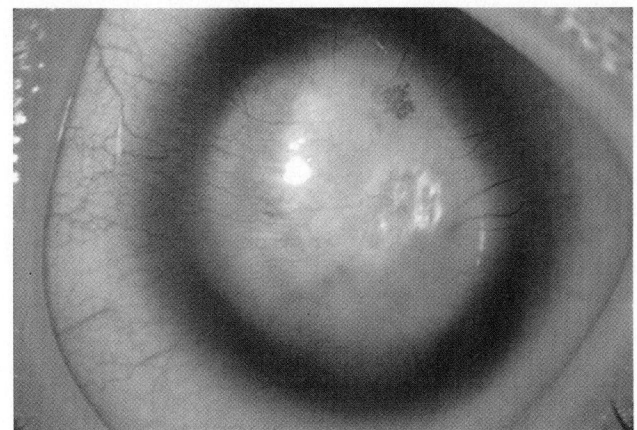

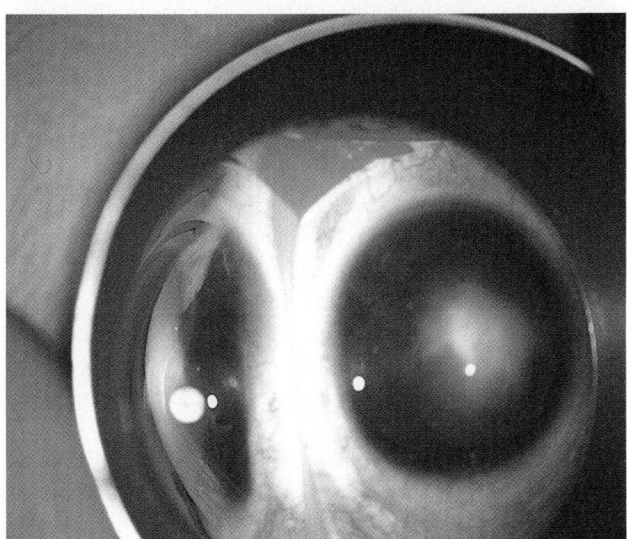

Fig. 24.15 (a) Keratomalacia showing the large axial scar. (b) Gonioscopic view showing the iris attached to the posterior surface of the cornea—leucoma adherans.

vitamin A replacement and measles vaccination (Monnickendam & Darougar 1987). Higher doses of vitamin A are necessary when the child has worms or diarrhoea (Gujral *et al.* 1993). The Bitot spot (Fig. 22.25) is a triangular foamy appearing lesion that occurs over the conjunctiva in vitamin A deficiency; its presence on the temporal side of the eye suggests active deficiency (Sommer 1978). Vitamin A deficiency also causes night-blindness.

Ectodermal dysplasia

Ectodermal dysplasia is a very rare (1 : 100 000 live births), usually X-linked or autosomal recessive condition, with abnormal eccrine glands, whispy or absent hair, and abnormal teeth or nails. Innumerable syndromes make up the ectodermal dysplasia group, the two main groups being the hidrotic and the anhidrotic (or hypohidrotic)

forms. General management poses numerous problems (Masse & Perusse 1994).

Occasionally, corneal changes occur (Wilson *et al.* 1973). Epithelial corneal cysts and opacities (Fig. 24.16) that are best seen with a slit lamp develop. Pannus, the abnormal growth of superficial blood vessels onto the cornea, occurs. A dry-eye state may result from deficient tear production. A more severe keratopathy with severe visual consequences (Fig. 24.17) occurs in some cases. This may be due to the combination of the underlying dysplasia, tear film abnormalities and infection (Mawhorter *et al.* 1985). If the tear film is adequate, grafting may help (Mader & Stulting 1990).

Epidermolysis bullosa

Severe corneal abnormalities are surprisingly infrequent in epidermolysis bullosa, but changes include limbal

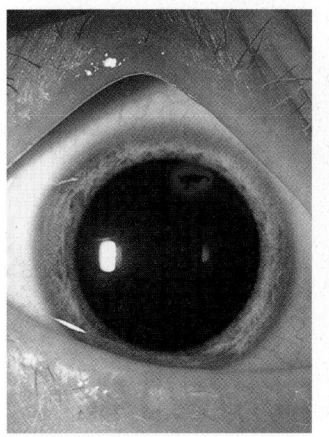
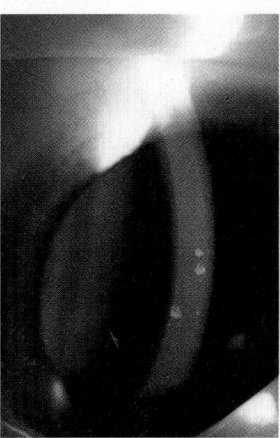

Fig. 24.16 Ectodermal dysplasia with small superficial corneal opacities.

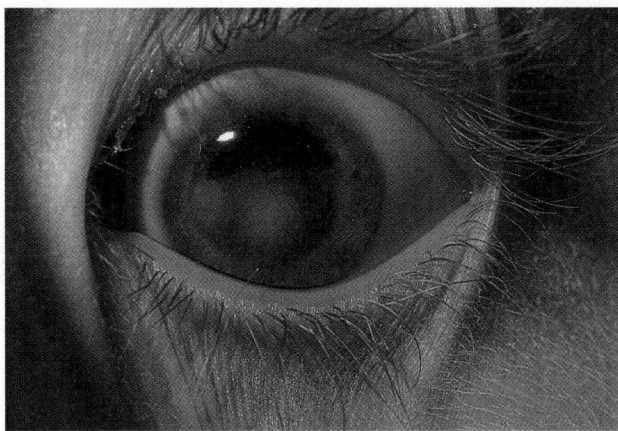

Fig. 24.17 Ectodermal dysplasia with an axial keratopathy which resulted in poor vision.

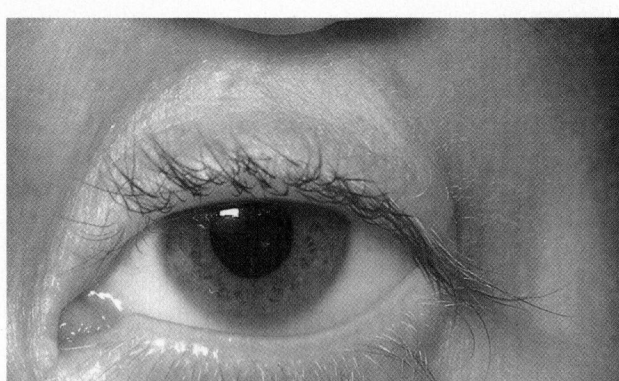

Fig. 24.18 Epidermolysis bullosa showing expanded limbus and peripheral pannus.

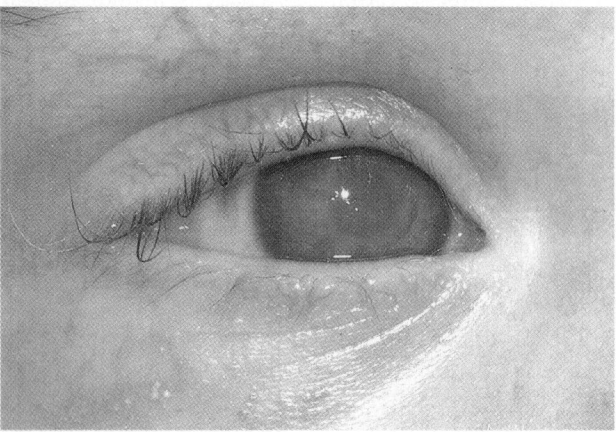

Fig. 24.19 Epidermolysis bullosa. Although many cases of epidermolysis bullosa do not have corneal changes, some, like this patient, develop acute epithelial erosions as a result of minor trauma, which if repeated result in permanent corneal opacity.

broadening (Fig. 24.18), corneal reticular opacities at the level of Bowman's capsule and symblepharon (McDonnell & Spalton 1988). Symblepharon is more frequent in dystrophic epidermolysis bullosa (Lin *et al.* 1994). Although the lesions are usually small and anterior (Aurora *et al.* 1975) they may develop widespread corneal epithelial erosions (Fig. 24.19) and abrasions (Lin *et al.* 1994). In dystrophic epidermolysis bullosa, there are absent anchoring fibrils at the conjunctival dermoepidermal junction (Iwamoto *et al.* 1991) and abnormal attachment complexes between the corneal epithelium and its basement membrane (Adamis *et al.* 1993); these may be due to mutations in genes encoding type VII collagen (Epstein 1992).

Ichthyosis

The ichthyosiform dermatoses are a group of disorders characterized by scaling. 'Harlequin baby' and 'collodian baby' (Orth *et al.* 1974) are extreme congenital forms which may have congenital ectropion. They frequently succumb to skin infections in the neonatal period. Ichthyosis vulgaris is the most common form, inherited as an autosomal dominant trait, with scaling of the extensor surfaces and back. No eye problems occur.

X-linked ichthyosis is congenital and occurs in one in 6000 men (Kerr & Wells 1965; Wells & Kerr 1966). Afflicted individuals note scaling of the scalp, face and neck, abdomen and limbs; palms and soles are spared. Corneal nerves may be thickened and band keratopathy occurs as an isolated abnormality (Jay *et al.* 1968). Superficial corneal lesions, which stain with fluorescein, occur; they are usually transient but recur and eventually cause superficial scarring (Fig. 24.20). The scarring and superficial lesions may be caused by eyelid abnormalities, or may occur independently of eyelid problems. Macsai and Doshi (1994) found abnormalities of the corneal epithelial basement membrane in a patient with X-linked ichthyosis and steroid sulphatase deficiency, and hypothesized that this was the result of increased production of proteins by the basal layer of the corneal epithelium.

Posterior corneal opacities are also known to occur. These opacities are small and located in deep corneal stroma or Descemet's membrane. Seldom do corneal lesions diminish visual acuity (Jay *et al.* 1968; Sever *et al.* 1968).

Lamellar ichthyosis (Katowitz *et al.* 1974) and ichthyosis linearis circumflexa are severe autosomal recessive disorders that give rise to ectropion and keratoconjunctivitis mainly due to exposure. Epidermolytic hyperkeratosis and erythrokeratoderma variabilis are two autosomal dominant varieties. Ichthyosis also occurs in the Sjögren–Larssen syndrome (see Chapter 48), Netherton's syndrome (ichthyosis, sparse hair, eyebrows and eyelashes, and atopic diathesis), Refsum's disease (see Chapter 57), chondrodysplasia punctata (Conradi's disease and rhizomelic dwarfism), IBIDS syndrome (ichthyosis, brittle hair, impaired intelligence, decreased fertility and short stature; see Chapter 39), and the KID syndrome of

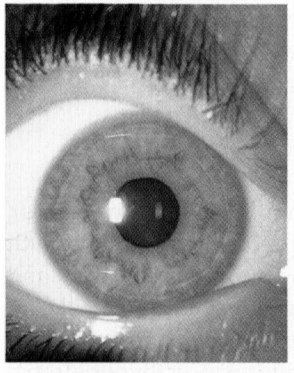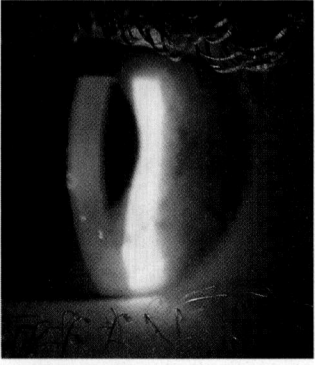

Fig. 24.20 Ichthyosis with superficial corneal lesions.

ichthyosis, deafness and keratitis (Tuppurainen *et al.* 1988; Langer *et al.* 1990; McGrae 1990a, b).

Corneal anaesthesia and hypoaesthesia

Defective corneal sensation may give rise to a keratitis that is chronic, recurrent and often severe. Although termed neurotropic, implying that the lack of some nerve factor is important, it is most likely that the main aetiological factors are drying, reduced blinking and repeated trivial trauma. Defective corneal sensation may arise from any cause of fifth nerve damage. As in adults, it occurs with trauma, herpes zoster ophthalmicus, developmental or acquired brain stem lesions, and tumours, in particular cerebellopontine angle or pontine tumours. It may occur with herpes simplex keratitis, or after carbon disulphide

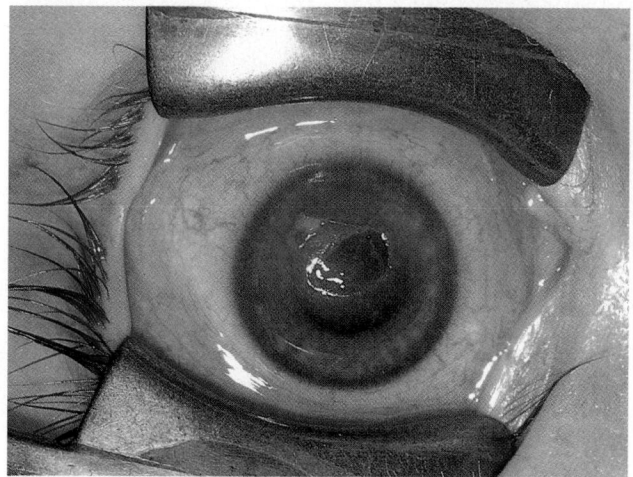

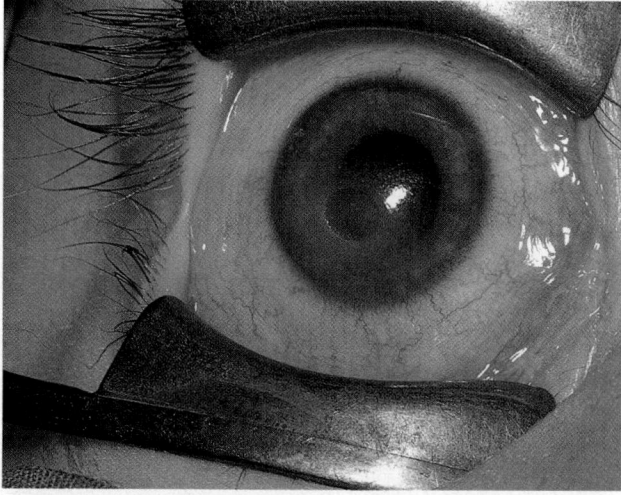

Fig. 24.21 Riley–Day syndrome. This child had a combination of anaesthetic corneas and dry eyes that had been treated for several months by topical wetting agents without success. He responded well to a bilateral tarsorrhaphy and lubricant ointment. Later, punctal occlusion allowed enough wetting of his eyes to allow the tarsorraphies to be undone.

(McDonald 1938) or hydrogen sulphide (Sjogren 1939) poisoning.

In addition, corneal hypoaesthesia has been described together with leprosy (Shields *et al.* 1974), Goldenhar's syndrome (Mohandesson & Romano 1978) and other oculofacial syndromes (Bowen 1971). It occurred in a family of Navajo Indians with an acromutilating neuropathy (Appenzeller *et al.* 1976; Shorey & Lobo 1990) and it can be found in a subclinical form in Adie's pupil (Purcell *et al.* 1977), and in some corneal dystrophies (Birndorff & Ginsberg 1972; Purcell *et al.* 1977). It is common in the Riley–Day syndrome (Fig. 24.21). It has been described in the MURCS association — Mullerian duct aplasia/hypoplasia, renal agenesis or ectopy, and cervico-thoracic somite dysplasia. Patients with this syndrome have absent uterus and upper vagina, renal ectopy or agenesis, short stature, and cervicothoracic vertebral defects (Esakowitz & Yates 1988).

It may be unilateral (Hennis & Saunders 1989), familial (Keys *et al.* 1990), and occasionally associated with fifth nerve motor involvement (Heath & Long 1993). A proportion of these children have other neurological disorders. An interesting feature in some is an element of self-mutilation which can be difficult to treat—elbow splinting being the most satisfactory method (Trope *et al.* 1985).

Corneal hypoaesthesia occurs as an isolated abnormality (Fig. 24.22), or with an associated trigeminal (usually first division) hypoaesthesia. Because it is unusual it is often diagnosed late. When it is severe it may give rise to blinding keratitis. Lawford (1907) and MacNab (1907) described some early cases in the Ophthalmological Society of the UK, and J.F. Cunningham, cited by Lawford (1907) had seen a case in which a horse hair with a bending strain of 1200 mg was used to test corneal sensation. The child was not aware of being touched on either cornea, superior palpebral conjunctiva, or upper part of the bulbar conjunctiva; there was some sensation in the inferior conjunctiva demonstrated by this precursor of the Cochet and Bonnet aesthesiometer indicating that the second division of the trigeminal nerve was intact.

The Cochet and Bonnet aesthesiometer is a patent device in which a 'synthetic hair' can have its length varied to decrease the pressure on the tip as it is lengthened; it may be used to detect small areas of corneal hypoaesthesis. Most clinical cases in which there is a neurotrophic keratitis are profoundly anaesthetic — even to the extent that these patients do not mind having their conjunctiva picked up with forceps!

Although in many cases the corneal anaesthesia is part of a more widespread anaesthesia (Ford & Wilkins 1938; Appenzeller *et al.* 1976; Manfredi *et al.* 1981) it is most often confined to the cornea (Hewson 1963; Anseth 1968; Carpel 1978). It may be unilateral (Shenk 1958; Stewart *et al.* 1972). Familial cases have been recorded (Purcell & Krachmer 1979).

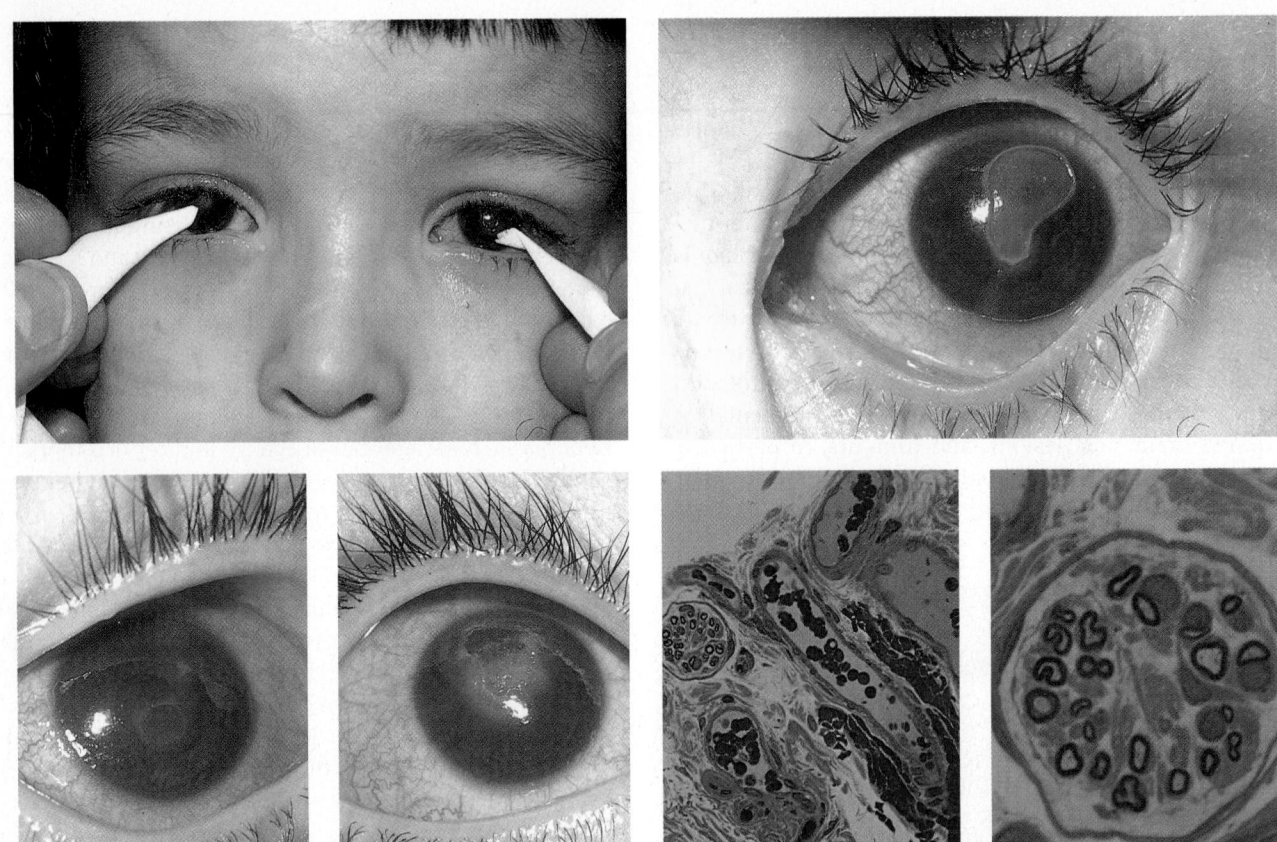

Fig. 24.22 (a) Profound corneal anaesthesia which allows the eye to be touched and for keratitis to occur without pain. (b) In this child acute episodes of erosion due to direct trauma resulted in corneal scarring. (c) Repeated corneal ulceration and keratitis gave rise to bilateral scarring. (d) Histology of the conjunctival nerves was normal. This child himself was of normal intellect and had no systemic abnormalities. The anaesthesia was confined to the cornea in the first division of the fifth nerve (a–d same patient).

Children with neurotrophic keratitis are rarely diagnosed when they first present. It is the recurrent nature of the disease, and to a certain extent their relative lack of symptoms, that draws the ophthalmologist's attention to the real cause. They have several attacks of redness, watering and sometimes discharging eye. Pain may be present from an associated uveitis. Sometimes the presence of scars on the forehead gives the clue to trigeminal anaesthesia. Care should be taken over the diagnosis remembering that in almost any severe keratitis the corneal sensation may be reduced. As a general rule, unless combined with lagophthalmos or a dry eye, the corneal anaesthesia has to be profound to assure the diagnosis. The child is usually insensitive to any corneal stimulus, therefore care needs to be taken to avoid causing an abrasion. Repeated trauma may cause hypertrophic corneal scars (Fig. 24.23).

Cases with lagophthalmos or defective tears (most anaesthetic corneas are associated with reduced reflex tearing because an afferent of the tearing reflex is missing) are much more severe. This combination is seen in the Riley–Day syndrome, leprosy and some brain stem lesions.

Treatment in small children is very difficult but it improves with age; it may require dedicated parents to

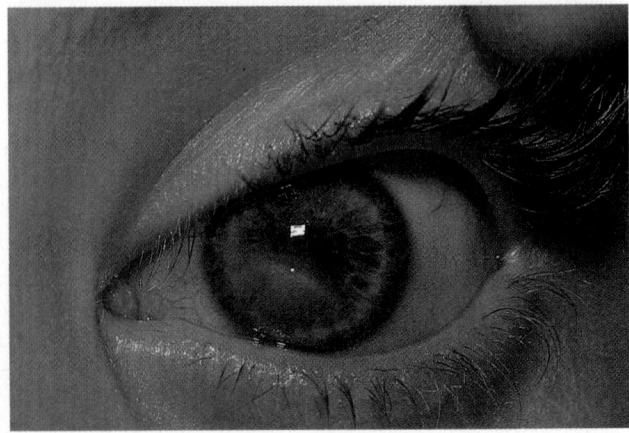

Fig. 24.23 Chronic trauma in corneal anaesthesia may give rise to a hypertrophic scar.

avoid blindness. There are a variety of regimes, but the following regimes have been successful in most cases.

Treatment in infancy

Acute cases are treated with frequent antibiotic drops (without preservative) and ointment with temporary taping of the eye. Frequent use of lubricant drops in mild cases is sufficient, but once keratitis has occurred more than once, the child has to have the exposed area of the cornea reduced. Taping or glueing the lids or using protective bubble shields or spectacles is good as a temporary measure, but an early tarsorrhaphy has been the most effective measure in the long term. An outer half or third tarsorrhaphy is used, remembering that it is easier to undo than to increase the procedure. Simple eye ointment (containing no antibiotic) is used at night, or day and night in severe cases. This can blur vision and may cause amblyopia in young children so should be used sparingly. Rubbing the eye may be a problem in infants and young children, especially if they are developmentally delayed: elbow splinting may be the only solution here.

Treatment in childhood

Children can usually be treated with simple ointment and antibiotics in the acute phase but more severe cases require a tarsorrhaphy which is better done early than late.

Corneal trauma

A condition mistaken for trauma is spontaneous corneal perforation in premature infants (Bachynsky *et al.* 1986) (see Chapter 62).

Keratoconus

Keratoconus is a condition causing usually bilateral, central thinning of the cornea. It usually starts in adolescence and may progress rapidly or stabilize; the younger the presentation, and occurrence in black people, are poor prognostic factors (Tuft *et al.* 1994). The cause is unknown, but an association with atopic skin disease has led to the speculation that, amongst other factors, eye-rubbing may play a role (Spencer & Fisher 1959). Keratoconus is occasionally familial, it may occur with atopy (Rahi *et al.* 1977), floppy lids (Donnenfeld *et al.* 1991), Down's syndrome, increased maternal age (Woodward 1981), Marfan's syndrome, retinal dystrophies, congenital cone/rod dystrophy, aniridia, Ehlers–Danlos syndrome, and congenital rubella (Boger *et al.* 1981). Posterior polymorphous dystrophy (PPMD) is a condition characterized by vesicular lesions of the posterior cornea, and epithelialization of corneal endothelium. Keratoconus may occasionally occur in PPMD (Driver *et al.* 1994).

First symptoms are usually related to visual impairment. Corneal thinning leads to increasing amounts of astigmatism (Fig. 24.24). Ultimately, contact lens use becomes necessary to compensate for irregular corneal curvature because spectacle correction is inadequate.

When Descemet's membrane is stretched beyond its breaking point, it may rupture. This condition is called acute hydrops (Fig. 24.25). The symptoms of hydrops are blurred vision, caused by corneal oedema, and pain. Hydrops resolves in several months, leaving variable corneal scarring; treatment is usually conservative, as

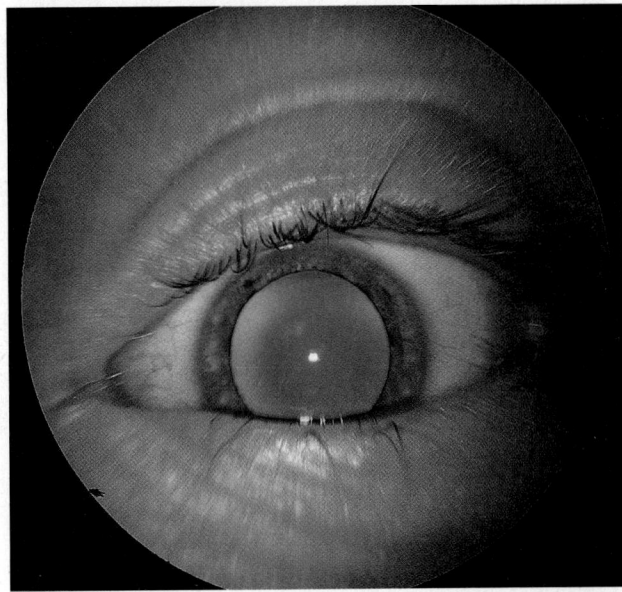

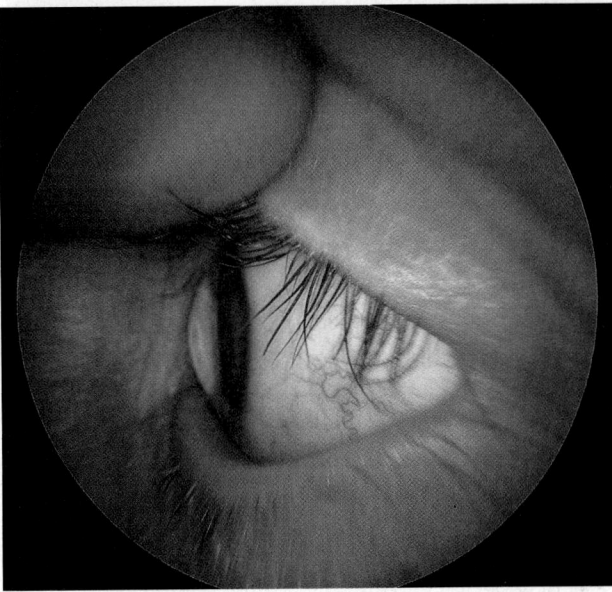

Fig. 24.24 (a) Keratoconus. The retinoscopy reflex in keratoconus is abnormal with no clear end point. (b) Keratoconus. Side view showing the conical cornea and the outward bowing of the lower lid (Munsen's sign).

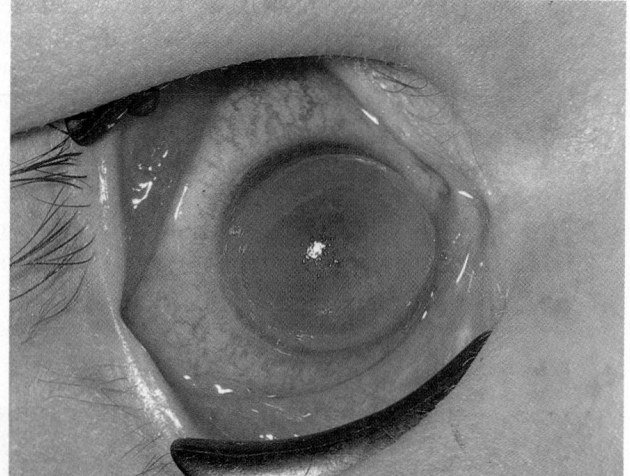

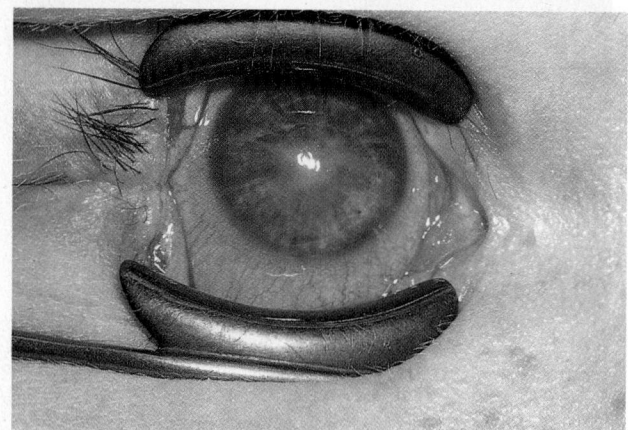

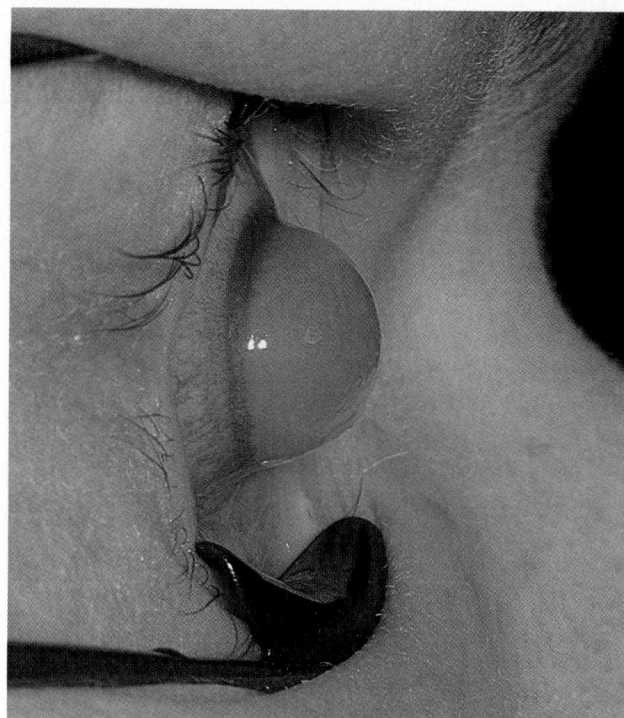

Fig. 24.25 (a) Acute hydrops in a child with Down's syndrome and keratoconus. (b) Same patient. Side view showing extreme keratoglobus. (c) After using elbow restraints to stop her rubbing her eyes, bilateral tarsorrhaphies and padding of the eye, the keratoglobus resolved and became asymptomatic but vision was reduced by axial scarring.

padding and bandaging the eye are successful even in severe cases, although where neovascularization occurs, early grafting may be indicated (Rowson *et al.* 1992).

Most cases of keratoconus can be managed conservatively, with contact lenses (Smiddy *et al.* 1988). Occasionally, corneal transplant is indicated, but even then, continued hard contact lens wear may be necessary after surgery to obtain good vision.

Keratoglobus

In keratoconus, the stromal thinning occurs in the centre of the cornea; in keratoglobus, which may occur in families with keratoconus, the thinning is in the mid-periphery. The result is that the cornea takes on a globular rather than conical appearance (Fig. 24.26). This can often be appreciated by standing over the patient's head and looking down on the protruding cornea. Keratoglobus may be associated with blue sclerae (Hyams *et al.* 1969), joint hyperextensibility, deafness and mottled teeth (Biglan *et al.* 1977). The collagen defect in these patients may give rise to perforation of the eye after minimal trauma.

Acute keratoglobus is a form of hydrops, as in keratoconus; it occurs in Down's syndrome and the Rubinstein–Taybi syndrome (Nelson & Talbot 1989).

Metabolic diseases and the cornea

Metabolic diseases, by abnormal accumulation of enzymatic byproducts, can stain the cornea. Systemic medications, like chloroquine and amiodarone, form deposits in the cornea. Sometimes the cornea is secondarily altered by ocular disease (band keratopathy). Occasionally, the degree of accumulation is enough to degrade vision. Some toxic diseases can be diagnosed by the pattern of corneal involvement.

The corneal epithelium may be stained by toxins. Chloroquine diphosphate and hydroxychloroquine sulphate are used to treat malaria and systemic lupus erythematosis. These compounds stain the corneal epithelium and form whorl-like opacities. Amiodarone (Fig. 24.27), Fabry's disease and mucolipidois type IV (Fig. 24.28) also induce a vortex pattern of corneal epithelium staining (Wilson *et al.* 1980). Indomethacin can cause fine opacities in the corneal epithelium. A vortex-

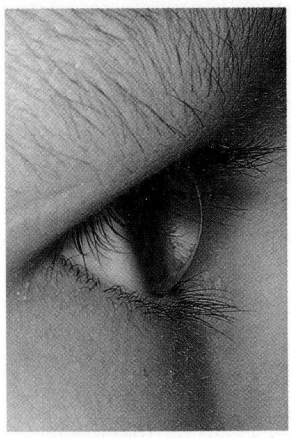
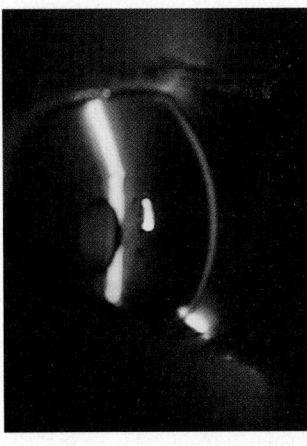

Fig. 24.26 X-linked keratoglobus. On the left it is possible to see into the iridocorneal angle by looking laterally at the eye without using a gonioscope.

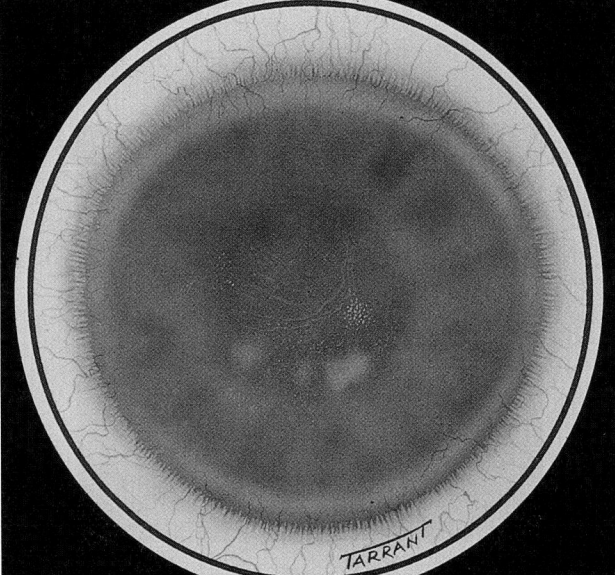

Fig. 24.27 Amiodarone keratopathy. It is unusual for these patients to have a significant visual defect. The most common abnormality is a mild whorl-like opacity as seen in the centre of this painting.

like pattern is sometimes seen in corneal oedema (Fig. 24.29).

Wilson's disease is an inherited disorder of copper metabolism. Low levels of the copper-transporting protein, ceruloplasmin, accompany low serum, and high tissue levels of copper. The gene, which is similar to the Menkes gene (Bull *et al.* 1993; Tanzi *et al.* 1993), is at 13q14.3 (Petrukhin *et al.* 1993).

Wilson's disease usually presents in the second decade of life. Four organ systems are involved. Central nervous system involvement leads to basal ganglia degeneration with tremor, choreoathetosis, and neuropsychiatric changes. Renal tubular staining causes aminoaciduria.

The liver is affected by nodular cirrhosis. The cornea often develops staining of the peripheral Descemet's membrane, most marked in the 12 and 6 o'clock positions (Kayser–Fleischer ring). The stain, which is due to copper deposition, is brown–green and is best seen at the slit lamp (Fig. 24.30). Gonioscopy may be necessary for visualization in some cases. The ring is not absolutely pathognomonic of Wilson's disease; other causes of liver failure, carotenaemia, and multiple myeloma may lead to a similar ring (Fleming *et al.* 1977).

In Wilson's disease, a rare but characteristic abnormality is the 'sunflower' subcapsular cataract. Penicillamine is the drug of choice, but trientene and zinc may be safe and effective; liver transplant may be necessary (Yarze *et al.* 1992).

Acrodermatitis enteropathica is associated with radial, subepithelial lines in the superior portion of the cornea (Matta *et al.* 1975). The lines are whorl-like and pass from the corneoscleral junction towards the centre of the cornea. Keratomalacia may be associated (Feldberg *et al.* 1981). This rare dermatitis is characterized by an asymmetrical rash that begins in infancy. The nails are dystrophic. A gastrointestinal disturbance causes diarrhoea

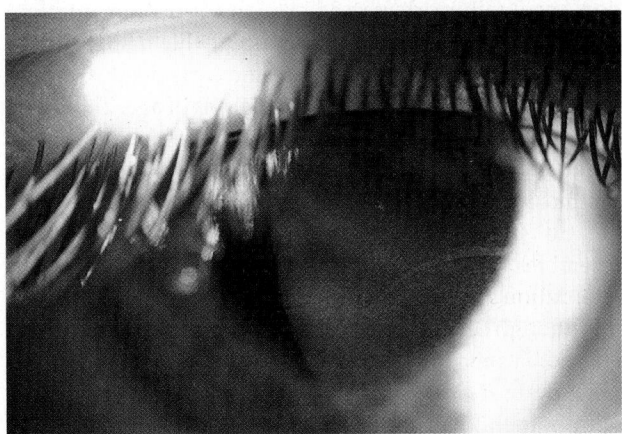

Fig. 24.28 Corneal verticillata in mucolipidosis type IV.

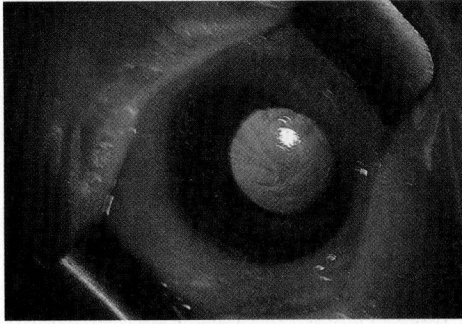

Fig. 24.29 A verticillata-like appearance in a patient with corneal oedema from congenital glaucoma.

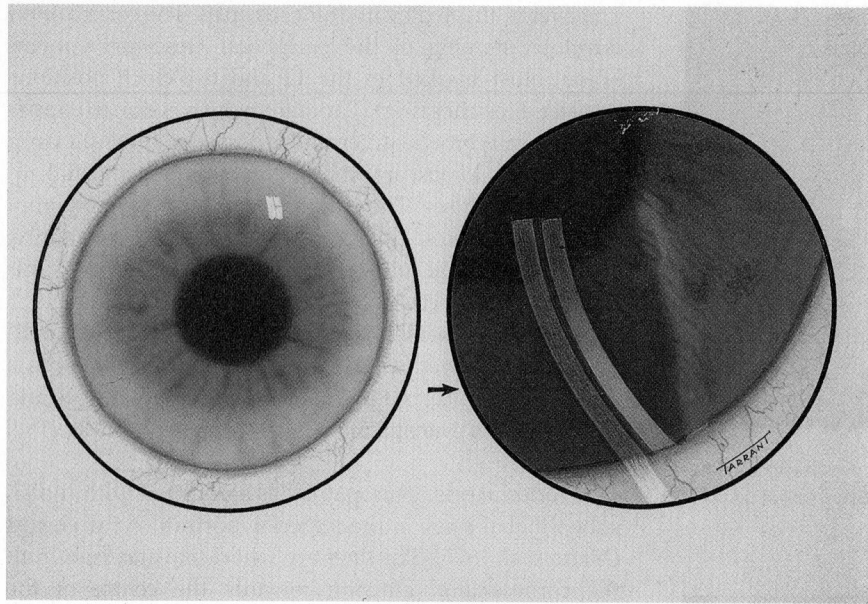

Fig. 24.30 Wilson's disease. The brown deposits are most prominent in the 6 and 12 o'clock positions and consist of deposition of brown–green copper-containing substance in the peripheral parts of Descemet's membrane. Gonioscopy may be necessary for visualization.

and poor growth; it is treated successfully with zinc dietary supplements.

In cystinosis, a defect in lysosomal transport leads to accumulation of cystine in lysosomes. Growth retardation, renal failure, decreased skin and hair pigmentation, and corneal crystalline deposits occur (Fig. 24.31). Infantile cystinosis causes renal failure and early death. Corneal crystals are detected as early as 2 months of age. They start anteriorly, progressing posteriorly (Melles *et al.* 1987). A pigmentary retinopathy also develops. An adult form of cystinosis (non-nephronopathic) causes corneal deposits but no systemic manifestations. The adolescent form resembles the infantile form, with the absence of growth retardation and skin hypopigmentation.

Although corneal crystals in cystinosis are mainly in the anterior stroma, they occur in all tissues and the cornea is thick (Katz *et al.* 1989). They seldom reduce visual acuity, but photophobia is frequent (Katz *et al.* 1987c, 1990). The glare disability may be profound. Patients may also have an abnormal contrast sensitivity (Katz *et al.* 1987a) and reduced corneal sensitivity (Katz *et al.* 1987b). A superficial punctate keratopathy (Richler *et al.* 1991), and recurrent erosions (Elder & Astin 1994) occur. The crystals have different morphologies depending on the site (Frazier & Wong 1968) and can be studied by specular microscopy (Dale *et al.* 1981). Cysteamine treatment has been shown to have beneficial effects (Kaiser-Kupfer *et al.* 1987, 1990; Bradbury *et al.* 1991; Jones *et al.* 1991; Graf *et al.* 1992). Corneal grafts may remain clear at least in the medium term (Kaiser-Kupfer *et al.* 1986). Glaucoma may occur due to crystal accumulation in intraocular tissues (Wan *et al.* 1986).

Photic sneezes have been described in cystinosis (Katz *et al.* 1990); they may also be autosomal dominantly inher-

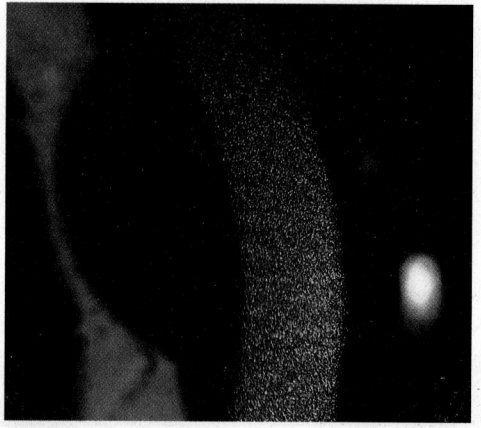

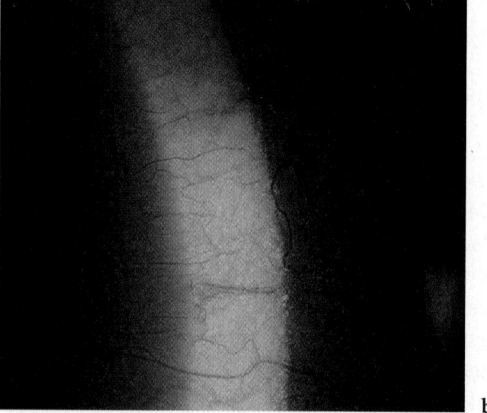

Fig. 24.31 (a) Cystinosis. Corneal crystals can be seen by slit-lamp microscopy. The children are often blonde, fair-skinned and very photophobic. (b) Cystinosis. Crystal deposition occurs in many tissues throughout the body, including the conjunctiva which can be seen here on slit-lamp biomicroscopy.

ited (Peroutka & Peroutka 1984). Photic sneezes have been given the catchy name ACHOO syndrome (autosomal dominant compelling helio-ophthalmic outburst syndrome) (Collie *et al.* 1978).

Corneal crystals

Crystalline corneal deposits or crystal-like deposits occur in the following conditions:

1 Cystinosis.

2 Crystalline corneal dystrophy (Schnyder's dystrophy):

(a) this may present in infancy;

(b) there are anterior central corneal ring-like aggregations of stromal crystals that may be yellowish and hard; they are composed of cholesterol (Rodriguez *et al.* 1987; Brooks *et al.* 1988);

(c) they are usually asymptomatic, it does not affect the epithelium;

(d) it may be autosomal dominant (Rodriguez *et al.* 1987);

(e) it may be accompanied by an arcus lipoides and white limbus girdle;

(f) there are not usually systemic associations (Lisch *et al.* 1986).

3 Lecithin cholesterol acyltransferase (LCAT) deficiency disease.

4 Uric acid crystals (brownish coloured).

5 Granular dystrophy and Bietti's marginal dystrophy (Wilson *et al.* 1989).

6 Multiple myeloma (Knapp *et al.* 1987). In the monoclonal gammopathies, crystals are rare (Bourne *et al.* 1989).

7 Calcium deposition.

8 Dieffenbachian plant keratoconjunctivitis (Ellis *et al.* 1973).

9 A syndrome of corneal crystals, myopathy and nephropathy (Arnold *et al.* 1987).

10 Tyrosinaemia type II—the Richner–Hanhart syndrome (see Chapter 22):

(a) plaque-like pseudodendritic lesions with crystalline edges occur. They are intra- and subepithelial, raised, and bilateral, and conjunctival; thickening also occurs;

(b) children usually present with photophobia and watering eyes (Heidemann *et al.* 1989);

(c) ulceration occurs;

(d) steroid treatment may help corneal lesions;

(e) a low tyrosine, low phenylalanine diet may rapidly abolish the symptoms (Bienfang *et al.* 1976; Grayson 1983; Michalski *et al.* 1988; Heidemann *et al.* 1989) and prevent recurrence;

(f) mental and physical retardation may be present;

(g) the skin lesions occur particularly on the pressure areas (Fig. 24.32) of the palms and soles (Paige *et al.* 1992);

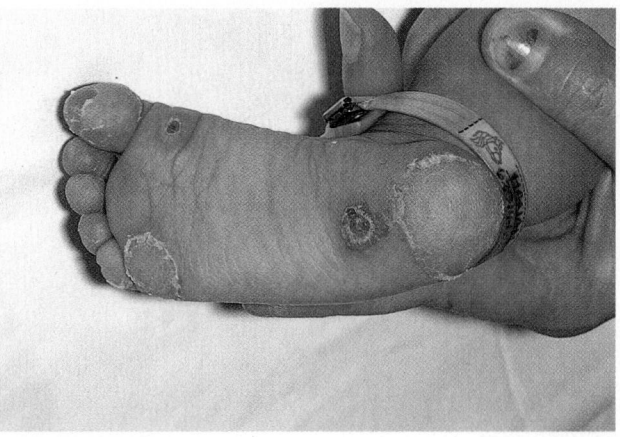

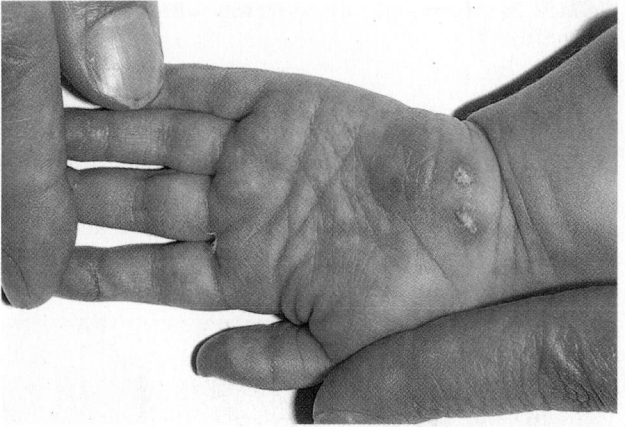

Fig. 24.32 (a) Tyrosinaemia type II. Skin lesions on pressure points of the sole. (b) Tyrosinaemia type II. Skin lesions on the pressure points of the palms.

(h) significant intrafamilial phenotypic variation occurs (Chitayat *et al.* 1992).

Band keratopathy

Band keratopathy is the result of ocular inflammation or systemic disease. The band occurs in the region between the eyelids (interpalpebral region), usually with a clear region between the band and the corneoscleral limbus. Bowman's membrane is infiltrated with calcium. Eventually, Bowman's membrane will be destroyed. The deposits of calcium take on a 'Swiss-cheese' appearance, which helps distinguish this condition from simple corneal calcific degeneration. This latter condition is the end-product of phthisis bulbi or a necrotic ocular tumour and may involve all corneal layers.

Any condition causing systemic hypercalcaemia can cause band keratopathy. Thus, sarcoidosis, parathyroid disease, and multiple myeloma, are occasionally associated with a band. Chronic ocular inflammation also causes band keratopathy. This is most characteristic in Still's disease (juvenile chronic arthritis) in its pauci-

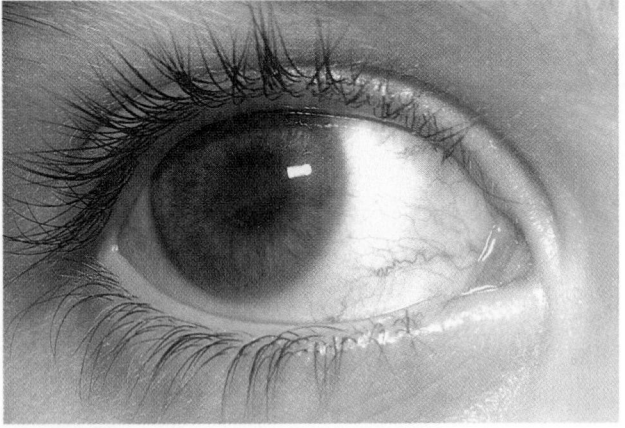

Fig. 24.33 Band keratopathy in a patient with Still's disease (see Chapter 38)

articular form (Fig. 24.33). Prolonged corneal oedema and glaucoma rarely lead to band formation. Toxic mercury vapours or eye drops and gout are uncommonly associated with band keratopathy. Gouty band kerotopathy differs from other causes by being brown. Band

keratopathy may occur with some forms of ichthyosis (Jay *et al.* 1968).

Lecithin cholesterol acyltransferase deficiency

LCAT deficiency is a rare autosomal recessive condition that causes a central corneal haze in homozygotes; at least two mutations in the LCAT gene are associated with fish-eye disease (Klein 1992). Premature arcus senilus develops in heterozygotes (Vrabec *et al.* 1988). LCAT esterifies free cholesterol for use in the synthesis of cell membranes. Its absence causes proteinuria, renal failure, anaemia, and hyperlipidaemia.

Corneal arcus

Arcus lipoides is due to a deposition of a variety of phospholipids, low density lipoproteins and triglycerides in the stroma of the peripheral cornea. Unlike xanthomas, corneal arcus is not invariably associated with hyperlipidaemia, but when corneal arcus appears in youth it is highly suggestive of raised plasma low density lipoproteins (Fig. 24.34). Arcus is not correlated with plasma high

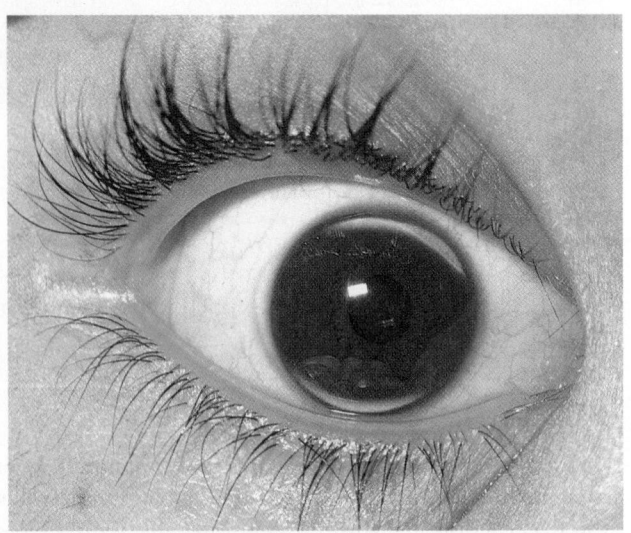

a

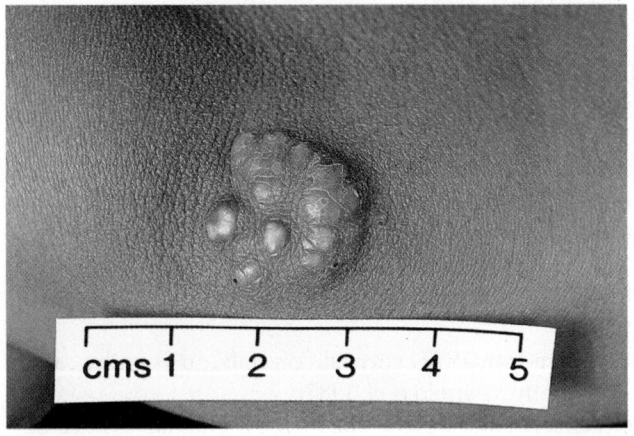

b

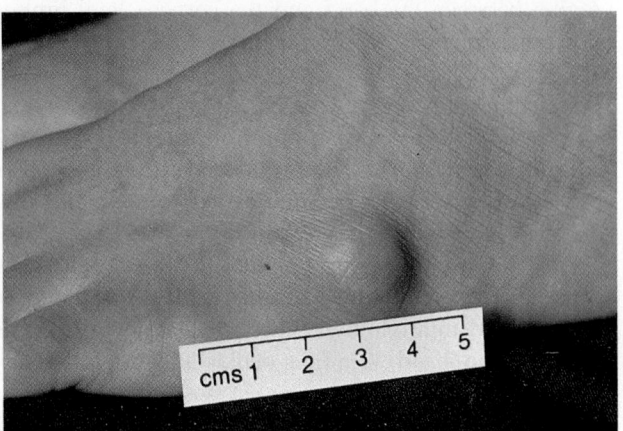

c

Fig. 24.34 (a) Corneal arcus in a patient with hyperlipidaemia. (b) Skin xanthoma in hypercholesterolaemia. (c) Tendon xanthoma in the same patient.

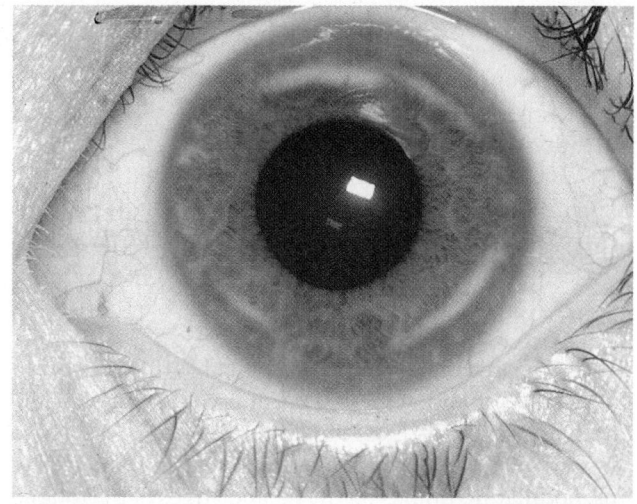

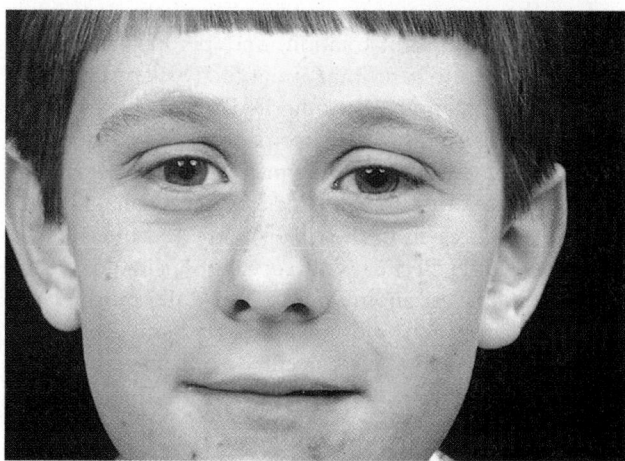

Fig. 24.35 Corneal arcus remaining in a child who had had severe vernal catarrah.

density lipoprotein or very low density lipoprotein. Arcus appears in youth in familial hypercholesterolaemia (Fredrickson's type II) and in familial hyperlipoproteinaemia (type III).

Arcus lipoides may also occur in children adjacent to areas of corneal disease including vernal keratopathy (Fig. 24.35), herpes simplex, and limbal dermoid.

Disorders of high density lipoprotein metabolism tend to cause diffuse corneal clouding; these include LCAT disease, Tangier's disease, fish-eye disease, and apoprotein A1 absence; occasionally however, an arcus-like peripheral condensation occurs.

Primary lipoidal degeneration of the cornea is an arcus that occurs in a healthy cornea in a person with normal plasma lipids.

White or cloudy cornea at birth

The white cornea at birth poses an important differential diagnosis. The first consideration is that the newborn suf- fers congenital glaucoma. The corneal diameter will be large (due to expansion of the globe from increased pressure). Ruptures in Descemet's membrane that are limbus parallel may be present. Intraocular pressure is elevated. The optic nerves will show increased cupping. Urgent intervention in the form of surgery is usually indicated if vision is to be preserved.

In most countries the most common cause of a congenitally opaque cornea is a developmental abnormality of the anterior segment (see Chapter 23). The next possibility is a forceps injury. Forceps marks may be visible on the lids or cheek. A linear, usually vertical, rupture of Descemet's membrane will be present. This causes corneal oedema. Oedema always resolves, leaving varying degrees of astigmatism. Late corneal decompensation is possible.

Certain metabolic conditions are in the differential diagnosis. Cystinosis rarely causes a cloudy cornea at birth. Mucopolysaccharidoses, occasionally present as congenital cloudy cornea, and rare conditions such as acromesomelic dysplasia (Clarke *et al.* 1994) may have congenital scarring.

Congenital hereditary corneal dystrophy usually presents in the first months of life (Kirkness *et al.* 1987) (see Chapter 25). A rare Bowman's layer dysgenesis may cause congenital corneal clouding (Apple *et al.* 1984).

Infection of the cornea will also cause it to turn white. Rubella keratitis should be considered. Neonatal infection with *Gonococcus* is also in the differential diagnosis.

Blue sclerae

Hereditary conditions that cause a defect in the mesodermal structures will produce a blue appearing sclera. The characteristic blue discoloration is probably related to thinning of the sclera. In a study by Chan *et al.* (1982), a defect in the fine structure of collagen fibrils was the morphological abnormality that explained blue sclera. Blue sclera is a consistent finding in osteogenesis imperfecta. This condition is associated with brittle bones and a conductive hearing loss (Van der Hoeve & Kleyn 1918). Six types of osteogenesis imperfecta have been described; four of these are autosomal dominantly inherited and two are recessive. Autosomal recessive osteogenesis imperfecta is characterized by early infant death or severe growth retardation.

Blue sclera also occurs in the Ehlers–Danlos syndrome. The Ehlers–Danlos syndrome is a heterogeneous group of disorders with characteristics such as fragile skin and hypermobile joints. At least 10 types have been described, all of which may show blue sclera. Type 6 is caused by hydroxylysine deficiency (Pinnel *et al.* 1972). Ocular findings in Ehlers–Danlos include spontaneous corneal rupture (Cameron 1993), keratoglobus (Biglan *et al.* 1977), cornea plana, peripheral sclerocornea, and microcornea.

Rarely, blue sclera occurs in the Hallermann–Streiff syndrome, Marfan's syndrome and in association with brittle corneas (Stein *et al.* 1968; Zlotogora *et al.* 1990) or ectodermal dysplasia (Wilson *et al.* 1973). In infancy many normal children have blueish corneas and some myopic children also have the same appearance.

Hyphaema and corneal blood staining

Blood staining of the cornea is an important and devastating complication of hyphaema. Generally, duration of hyphaema, degree of elevation of intraocular pressure, the integrity of the corneal endothelium and the occurrence of secondary haemorrhages are the factors associated with staining. The doctor should observe the patient with hyphaema at least daily, administering non-aspirin-containing analgesics and acetazolamide if the intraocular pressure is raised, and, when staining of the cornea is suspected, an anterior chamber lavage may be recommended; the efficacy of antifibrinolytic drugs is not established (Kraft *et al.* 1987). Corneal blood staining may occur within 3 days if the intraocular pressure is high.

The incidence in one series (Agapitos *et al.* 1987) was 17 per 100000 paediatric population per year. Rebleeds occurred in 7.6% but did not correlate with age, the use of cycloplegics or steroids. Ninety-one per cent of this series achieved acuity of 20/30 or better. Amblyopia occurred in the two children who required cataract extraction of the 316 in the series.

Corneal nerves

Corneal nerves are visible in the periphery of the cornea in normal people but they may be more visible in certain conditions (Menscher 1974), including the following.
1 Dystrophies: Fuchs' corneal dystrophy, keratoconus.

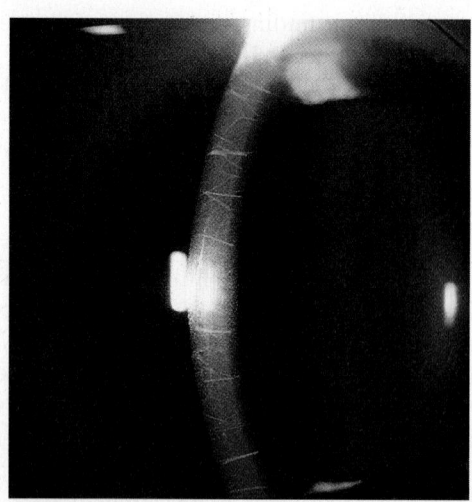

Fig. 24.36 Multiple endocrine neoplasia type IIb. Thickened corneal nerves can be seen crossing even the axial area of the cornea.

2 Buphthalmos.
3 Inflammatory disease: leprosy; after corneal grafts; corneal trauma.
4 Refsum's disease.
5 Ichthyosis.
6 Multiple endocrine neoplasia (MEN) type IIb.
7 Neurofibromatosis (described but may have been cases of MEN type IIb).

Multiple endocrine neoplasia

There are three main syndromes in which tumours occur in a variety of endocrine organs at a young age. For the ophthalmologist the most prominent of these is MEN type IIb. Patients show a marfanoid habitus, full and fleshy lips, nodular neuromas on the tip and edges of the tongue and on the margins of the eyelids (Wortham & Nguyen 1990). Pes cavus, constipation, and peroneal muscular atrophy are due to neuroma formation (Dyck *et al.* 1979). It is autosomal dominantly inherited. Prominent corneal nerves within an otherwise normal cornea (Spector *et al.* 1981) are an important diagnostic feature (Fig. 24.36). They are a mixture of myelinated and unmyelinated fibres and are also present in the ciliary body and iris (Riley & Robertson 1981). Because of a very high incidence of thyroid medullary carcinoma in MEN type IIb, prophylactic thyroidectomy may be recommended in childhood. Phaeochromocytoma also occurs. Somewhat enlarged corneal nerves may occur in MEN type Ia (Kinoshita *et al.* 1991).

References

Adamis AP, Schein OD, Kenyon KR. Anterior corneal disease of epidermolysis bullosa simplex. *Arch Ophthalmol* 1993; **111**: 499–502.

Agapitos PJ, Noel L-P, Clarke WN. Traumatic hyphema in children. *Ophthalmology* 1987; **94**: 1238–42.

Angell LK, Robb RM, Benson FG. Visual prognosis in patients with ruptures in Descemet's membrane due to forceps injuries. *Arch Ophthalmol* 1981; **99**: 2137–9.

Anseth A. Congenital bilateral corneal anaesthesia. *Acta Ophthalmol* 1968; **46**: 909–11.

Appenzeller O, Kornfield M, Snyder R. Acromutilating paralyzing neuropathy with corneal ulceration in Navajo children. *Arch Neurol* 1976; **33**: 733–8.

Apple DJ, Olson RJ, Jones GR *et al.* Congenital corneal opacification secondary to Bowman's layer dysgenesis. *Am J Ophthalmol* 1984; **98**: 320–8.

Arnold RW, Stickler G, Bourne W *et al.* Corneal crystals, myopathy and nephropathy: a new syndrome? *J Pediatr Ophthalmol Strabismus* 1987; **24**: 151–5.

Aurora AL, Madhaven M, Rao S. Ocular changes in epidermolysis bullosa letalis. *Am J Ophthalmol* 1975; **79**: 464–70.

Bachynski BN, Andreu R, Flynn JR. Spontaneous corneal perforation and extrusion of intraocular contents in premature infants. *J Pediatr Ophthalmol Strabismus* 1986; **23**: 25–8.

Beinfang D, Kuwabara T, Pueschel S. The Richner–Hanhart syndrome: report of a case with associated tyrosinemia. *Arch Ophthal-*

mol 1976; **94**: 1133–7.

BenEzra D, Frucht Y, Paez JH *et al*. Amniotic band syndrome and strabismus. *J Pediatr Ophthalmol Strabismus* 1982; **19**: 33–6.

Bernuy A, Contreras F, Maumenee AE, O'Donnell FE. Bilateral, congenital, dermis-like choristomas overlying corneal staphylomas. *Arch Ophthalmol* 1981; **99**: 1995–8.

Bicknell JM, Holland JV. Neurologic manifestations of Cogan syndrome. *Neurology* 1978; **28**: 218–33.

Biglan AW, Brown SI, Johnson BL. Keratoglobus and blue sclerae. *Am J Ophthalmol* 1977; **83**: 225–33.

Birndorff LA, Ginsberg SP. Hereditary fleck dystrophy associated with decreased corneal sensitivity. *Am J Ophthalmol* 1972; **73**: 670–2.

Boger WP, Petersen RA, Robb RM. Keratoconus and acute hydrops in mentally retarded patients with congenital rubella syndrome. *Am J Ophthalmol* 1981; **91**: 231–3.

Bourne WM, Kyle RA, Brubaker RF, Greipp PR. Incidence of corneal crystals in the monoclonal gammopathies. *Am J Ophthalmol* 1989; **107**: 192–3.

Bowen DI, Collum LM, Rees DO. Clinical aspects of oculo-auriculovertebral dysplasia. *Br J Ophthalmol* 1971; **55**: 145–54.

Bradbury JA, Danjoux J-P, Voller J *et al*. A randomised placebo-controlled trial of topical cysteamine therapy in patients with nephropathic cystinosis. *Eye* 1991; **5**: 755–60.

Brooks AM, Grant G, Gillies WE. Determination of the nature of corneal crystals by specular microscopy. *Ophthalmology* 1988; **95**: 448–52.

Brown SI, Salamon SM. Wound healing of grafts in congenitally opaque infant corneas. *Am J Ophthalmol* 1983; **95**: 641–4.

Bull PC, Thomas GR, Rommens JM, Forbes J *et al*. The Wilson disease gene is a putative copper transporting P-type ATPase similar to the Menkes gene. *Nature Genet* 1993; **5**: 327–37.

Cameron JA. Corneal abnormalities in Ehlers–Danlos syndrome type VI. *Cornea* 1993; **12**: 54–9.

Carpel EF. Congenital corneal anesthesia. *Am J Ophthalmol* 1978; **85**: 357–9.

Chan CC, Green WR, de la Cruz ZC, Hillis A. Ocular findings in osteogenesis imperfecta. *Arch Ophthalmol* 1982; **100**: 1458–63.

Chitayat D, Balbul A, Hani V, Mamer OA, Clow C, Scriver CR. Hereditary tyrosinaemia type II in a consanguinous Ashkenazy Jewish family: intrafamilial variation in phenotype; absence of phenotype effects on the fetus. *J Inherit Metab Dis* 1992; **15**: 198–203.

Clarke WN, Munro S, Brownstein S, Agapitos P, Hughes–Benzie R. Ocular findings in acromesomelic dysplasia. *Am J Ophthalmol* 1994; **118**: 797–804.

Cogan DG. Syndrome of non–syphilitic interstitial keratitis and vestibular auditory symptoms. *Arch Ophthalmol* 1945; **33**: 144–9.

Cogan DG, Sullivan WR. Immunologic study of non-syphilitic interstitial keratitis with vestibuloauditory symptoms. *Am J Ophthalmol* 1975; **80**: 491–5.

Collie WR, Pagon RA, Hall JG, Shokeir MHK. ACHOO syndrome (autosomal dominant compelling helio–ophthalmic outburst syndrome). *Birth Defects* 1978; **14**: 361–3.

Cowden JW. Penetrating keratoplasty in infants and children. *Ophthalmology* 1990; **97**: 324–8.

Dale RT, Rao GN, Aquavella JV, Metz HS. Adolescent cystinosis: a clinical and specular microscopic study of an unusual sibship. *Br J Ophthalmol* 1981; **65**: 828–32.

Darougar S, John AC, Viswalingam M, Cornell L, Jones BR. Isolation of *Chlamydia psittaci* from a patient with interstitial keratitis and uveitis associated with otological and cardiovascular lesions. *Br J Ophthalmol* 1978; **62**: 709–13.

Donnenfeld E, Perry H, Gibralter R, Ingraham H, Udell I. Keratoconus associated with floppy eyelid syndrome. *Ophthalmology*

1991; **98**: 1674–8.

Driver PJ, Reed JW, Davis RH. Familial cases of keratoconus associated with posterior polymorphous dystrophy. *Am J Ophthalmol* 1994; **118**: 256–7.

Dyck PJ, Carney JA, Sizemore GW, Okazaki H, Brimijoin WS, Lambert EH. Multiple endocrine neoplasia type 2b: phenotype recognition, neurological features and their pathological basis. *Ann Neurol* 1979; **6**: 302–14.

Elder MJ, Astin CL. Recurrent corneal erosion in cystinosis. *J Pediatr Ophthalmol Strabismus* 1994; **31**: 270–1.

Ellis W, Barfort P, Mastman GJ. Keratoconjunctivitis with corneal crystals caused by the dieffenbachian plant. *Am J Ophthalmol* 1973; **76**: 143–7.

Epstein EH. Molecular genetics of epidermolysis bullosa. *Science* 1992; **256**: 799–804.

Esakowitz L, Yates JR. Congenital corneal anaesthesia and the MURCs association: a case report. *Br J Ophthalmol* 1988; **72**: 236–9.

Feldberg R, Yassur Y, Ben-Sira I, Versamo I *et al*. Keratomalacia in acrodermatitis enteropathica. *Metab Pediatr Ophthalmol* 1981; **5**: 207–11.

Fleming CR, Dickson ER, Wahner HW, Hollenhorst RW, McCall JT. Pigmented rings in non-Wilsonian liver disease. *Ann Intern Med* 1977; **86**: 285–8.

Ford FR, Wilkins L. Congenital universal insensitiveness to pain. *Bull Johns Hopkins Hosp* 1938; **62**: 448–66.

Foster A, Sommer A. Corneal ulceration, measles and childhood blindness in Tanzania. *Br J Ophthalmol* 1987; **71**: 331–43.

Frangoulis M, Taylor D. Corneal opacities — a diagnostic feature of the trisomy 8 mosaic syndrome. *Br J Ophthalmol* 1983; **67**: 619–22.

Frazier PD, Wong VG. Cystinosis. Histologic and crystallographic examination of crystals in eye tissues. *Arch Ophthalmol* 1968; **80**: 87–91.

Gilbert WS, Talbot FJ. Cogan's syndrome. Signs of periarteritis nodosa and cerebral venous sinus thrombosis. *Arch Ophthalmol* 1969; **82**: 633–6.

Gloor P, Keech RV, Krachmer JH. Factors associated with high postoperative myopia after penetrating keratoplasties in infants. *Ophthalmology* 1992; **99**: 775–9.

Graf M, Grote A, Wagner F. Cysteamin–Augentropfen zur Behandlung kornealer Zystineinlagerungen bei infantiler Zystinose. *Klin Mbl Augenheilk* 1992; **201**: 48–50.

Grayson M. *Diseases of the Cornea*. St Louis: CV Mosby, 1983: 222–6.

Gujral S, Abbi R, Golpaldas T. Xerophthalmia, vitamin A supplementation and morbidity in children. *J Trop Pediatr* 1993; **39**: 89–92.

Heath JD, Long G. Neurotropic keratitis presenting in infancy with involvement of the motor component of the trigeminal nerve. *Br J Ophthalmol* 1993; **77**: 679–80.

Heidemann DG, Dunn SP, Bawle EV, Shepherd JM. Early diagnosis of tyrosinemia type II. *Am J Ophthalmol* 1989; **107**: 559–60.

Hennis HL, Saunders RA. Unilateral corneal anesthesia. *Am J Ophthalmol* 1989; **108**: 331–2.

Hewson GE. Congenital trigeminal anaesthesia. *Br J Ophthalmol* 1963; **47**: 308–11.

Hwang DG, Hwang PH. Pediatric penetrating keratoplasty. *Semin Ophthalmol* 1991; **6**: 212–18.

Hyams SW, Kar H, Neumann E. Blue sclerae and keratoglobus. Ocular signs of a systemic connective tissue disorder. *Br J Ophthalmol* 1969; **53**: 53–8.

Iwamoto M, Haik BG, Iwamoto T, Harrison W, Carter M. The ultrastructural defect in conjunctiva from a case of recessive dystrophic epidermolysis bullosa. *Arch Ophthalmol* 1991; **109**: 1382–6.

Jay B, Blach RK, Wells RS. Ocular manifestations of ichthyosis. *Br J Ophthalmol* 1968; **52**: 217–26.

Jones NP, Postlethwaite RJ, Noble JL. Clearance of corneal crystals in nephropathic cystinosis by topical cysteamine 0.5%. *Br J Ophthalmol* 1991; **75**: 311–2.

Kaiser-Kupfer MI, Caruso RC, Minkler DS, Gahl WA. Long-term ocular manifestations in nephropathic cystinosis. *Arch Ophthalmol* 1986; **104**: 706–11.

Kaiser-Kupfer MI, Fujikawa L, Kuwabara T, Jain S, Gahl WA. Removal of corneal crystals by topical cysteamine in nephropathic cystinosis. *N Engl J Med* 1987; **316**: 775–9.

Kaiser-Kupfer MI, Gazzo MA, Datiles MB, Caruso RC, Kueche EM, Gahl WA. A randomized placebo-controlled trial of cysteamine eye drops in nephropathic cystinosis. *Arch Ophthalmol* 1990; **108**: 689–93.

Katowitz JA, Yolles EA, Yanoff M. Ichthyosis congenita. *Arch Ophthalmol* 1974; **91**: 208–10.

Katz B, Melles RB, Schneider JA. Contrast sensitivity function in nephropathic cystinosis. *Arch Ophthalmol* 1987a; **105**: 1667–70.

Katz B, Melles RB, Schneider JA. Corneal sensitivity in nephropathic cystinosis. *Am J Ophthalmol* 1987b; **104**: 413–16.

Katz B, Melles RB, Schneider JA. Glare disability in nephropathic cystinosis. *Arch Ophthalmol* 1987c; **105**: 1670–1.

Katz B, Melles RB, Schneider JA, Rao NA. Corneal thickness in nephropathic cystinosis. *Br J Ophthalmol* 1989; **73**:665–9.

Katz B, Melles RB, Swenson MR, Schneider JA. Photic sneeze reflex in nephropathic cystinosis. *Br J Ophthalmol* 1990; **74**: 706–8.

Kerr CB, Wells RS. Sex-linked ichthyosis. *Am Hum Genet* 1965; **29**: 33.

Kinoshita S, Tanaka F, Ohashi Y, Ikeda M, Takai S. Incidence of prominent corneal nerves in multiple endocrine neoplasia type 2a. *Am J Ophthalmol* 1991; **111**: 307–11.

Keys C, Sugar J, Mafee M. Familial trigeminal anesthesia. *Arch Ophthalmol* 1990; **108**: 1720–3.

Kirkness CM, McCartney A, Rice NS *et al*. Congenital hereditary corneal oedema of Maumenee: its clinical features, management and pathology. *Br J Ophthalmol* 1987; **71**: 130–44.

Klauss V, Reidel K. Bilateral and unilateral mesodermal corneal metaplasia. *Br J Ophthalmol* 1983; **67**: 320–3.

Klein HG, Lohse P, Pritchard PH, Bojanovski D, Schmidt H, Brewer HB Jr. Two different allelic mutations in lecithin–cholesterol acyltransferase gene associated with fish-eye syndrome. Lecithin–cholesterol acyltransferase (Thr123—Ile) and lecithin–cholesterol acyltransferase (Thr347—Met). *J Clin Invest* 1992; **89**: 499–506.

Knapp AJ, Gartner S, Henkind P. Multiple myeloma and its ocular manifestations. *Surv Ophthalmol* 1987; **31**: 343–51.

Knobel H, Demeler U. Keratoplastik bei kindern und jugendlichen. *Ophthalmologica (Basel)* 1978; **177**: 146–51.

Kodsi SR, Bloom KE, Egbert JE, Holland EJ, Cameron JD. Ocular and systemic manifestations of encephalocraniocutaneous lipomatosis. *Am J Ophthalmol* 1994; **118**: 77–82.

Kogbe O, Listet S. Tear electrophoretic changes in Nigerian children after measles. *Br J Ophthalmol* 1987; **71**: 326–30.

Kraft SP, Christianson MD, Crawford JS, Wagman RD, Antoszyk JH. Traumatic hyphema in children. Treatment with epsilon–aminocaproic acid. *Ophthalmology* 1987; **94**: 1232–7.

Langer K, Konrad K, Wolff K. Keratitis, ichthyosis and deafness (KID) syndrome: report of three cases and a review of the literature. *Br J Dermatol* 1990; **122**: 689–97.

Lawford JB. Bilateral (?congenital) anaesthesia of conjunctiva and cornea; neuroparalytic keratitis. *Trans Ophthalmol Soc UK* 1907; **27**: 80–4.

Leff SR, Shields JA, Augsburger JJ, Sakowski AD Jr, Blair CJ. Congenital corneal staphyloma: clinical, radiological and pathological correlation. *Br J Ophthalmol* 1986; **70**: 427–30.

Lin A, Murphy F, Brodie S, Carter D. Review of ophthalmic findings

in 204 patients with epidermolysis bullosa. *Am J Ophthalmol* 1994; **118**: 384–90.

Lisch W, Weidle EG, Lisch C *et al*. Schnyder's dystrophy. Progression and metabolism. *Ophthalmol Pediatr Genet* 1986; **7**: 45–56.

McDonald R. Carbon disulfide poisoning. *Arch Ophthalmol* 1938; **20**: 839.

McDonnell PJ, Spalton DJ. The ocular signs and complications of epidermolysis bullosa. *J Roy Soc Med* 1988; **81**: 576–8.

McGrae J. Keratitis, ichthyosis and deafness (KID) syndrome. *Int J Dermatol* 1990a; **29**: 88–93.

McGrae J. Keratitis, ichthyosis and deafness syndrome with adult onset of keratitis component. *Int J Dermatol* 1990b; **29**: 145–6.

Mackensen G, Sundmachen R, Trauzettel S. Keratoplasty in childhood. *Klin Monatsbl Augenheilk* 1977; **171**: 199–209.

MacNab A. Opacity of the cornea in three members of one family. *Trans Ophthalmol Soc UK* 1907; **27**: 81–2.

Macsai MS, Doshi H. Clinical pathologic correlation of superficial corneal opacities in X-linked ichthyosis. *Am J Ophthalmol* 1994; **118**: 477–84.

Mader TH, Stulting RD. Penetrating keratoplasty in ectodermal dysplasia. *Am J Ophthalmol* 1990; **110**: 319–20.

Manfredi M, Bini G, Cruccu G, Accornero N, Berardelli A, Medolago L. Congenital absence of pain. *Arch Neurol* 1981; **38**: 507–11.

Mansour AM, Barber JC, Reinecke RD, Wang FM. Ocular choristomas. *Surv Ophthalmol* 1989; **33**: 339–58.

Mansour AM, Laibson P, Reinecke R, Henkind P, Nikati M. Bilateral total corneal and conjunctival choristomas associated with epidermal nevus. *Arch Ophthalmol* 1986; **104**: 245–8.

Mansour AM, Wang F, Henkind P, Goldberg R, Shprintzein R. Ocular findings in facio-auriculovertebral sequence (Goldenhar–Gerlin syndrome). *Am J Ophthalmol* 1985; **100**: 555–9.

Masse J-F, Perusse R. Ectodermal dysplasia. *Arch Dis Child* 1994; **71**: 1–20.

Matta CS, Felker GV, Ide CH. Eye manifestations in acrodermatitis enteropathica. *Arch Ophthalmol* 1975; **93**: 140–2.

Mawhorter LG, Ruttum MS, Koenig SR. Keratopathy in a family with the ectrodactyly ectodermal dysplasia clefting syndrome. *Ophthalmology* 1985; **92**: 1427–31.

Melles RB, Schneider JA, Ras NA, Katz B. Spatial and temporal sequence of corneal crystal deposition in nephropathic cystinosis. *Am J Ophthalmol* 1987; **104**: 598–604.

Mensher JH. Corneal nerves. *Surv Ophthalmol* 1974; **19**: 1–18.

Michalski A, Leonard JV, Taylor DS. The eye and inherited metabolic disease. *J Roy Soc Med* 1988; **82**: 286–90.

Miller MT, Deutsch TA, Cronin C, Keys CL. Amniotic bands as a cause of ocular anomalies. *Am J Ophthalmol* 1987; **104**: 270–9.

Mohandessan MM, Romano PE. Neuroparalytic keratitis in Goldenhar–Gorlin syndrome. *Am J Ophthalmol* 1978; **85**: 111–13.

Monnickendam M, Darougar S. Editorial: postmeasles blindness. *Br J Ophthalmol* 1987; **71**: 325.

Murata T, Ishibashi T, Ohnishi Y, Inomata H. Corneal choristoma with microphthalmos. *Arch Ophthalmol* 1991; **109**: 1130–3.

Nelson ME, Talbot JF. Keratoglobus in the Rubenstein–Taybi syndrome. *Br J Ophthalmol* 1989; **73**: 385–7.

Oakman J, Lambert S, Grossniklaus H. Corneal dermoid: case report and review of classification. *J Pediatr Ophthalmol Strabismus* 1993; **30**: 388–91.

Orth DH, Fretzin DF, Abramson V. Collodian baby with transient bilateral upper lid ectropion. Review of ocular manifestations in ichthyosis. *Arch Ophthalmol* 1974; **91**: 206–7.

Paige D, Clayton P, Bowron A, Harper J. Richner–Hanhart syndrome (oculocutaneous tyrosinaemia, tyrosinaemia type II). *J Roy Soc Med* 1992; **85**: 759–60.

Peroutka SJ, Peroutka LA. Autosomal dominant transmission of the 'photic sneeze reflex'. *N Engl J Med* 1984; **310**: 599–600.

Petrukhin K, Fischer S, Pirastu M *et al.* Mapping, cloning and genetic characterization of the region containing the Wilson disease gene. *Nature Genet* 1993; **5**: 338–43.

Pinnel SR, Krane SM, Kenzora JE, Glimcher MJ. A heritable disorder of connective tissue: hydroxylysine-deficient collagen disease. *N Engl J Med* 1972; **286**: 1013–20.

Podder S, Shepherd R. Cogan's syndrome: a rare systemic vasculitis. *Arch Dis Child* 1994; **71**: 163–4.

Purcell JJ, Krachmer JH. Familial corneal hyperesthesia. *Arch Ophthalmol* 1979; **97**: 872–4.

Purcell JJ, Krachmer JH, Thompson HS. Corneal sensation in Adie's pupil. *Am J Ophthalmol* 1977; **84**: 496–500.

Rahi A, Davies P, Ruben M, Lobascher D, Menon J. Keratoconus and coexisting atopic disease. *Br J Ophthalmol* 1977; **61**: 761–4.

Richler M, Milot J, Quigley M, O Regan S. Ocular manifestations of nephrotic cystinosis. The French-Canadian experience in a genetically homogeneous population. *Arch Ophthalmol* 1991; **109**: 359–62.

Riley FC, Robertson DM. Ocular histopathology in multiple endocrine neoplasia type 2b. *Am J Ophthalmol* 1981; **91**: 57–64.

Rodrigues MM, Kruth HS, Krachmer JH, Willis R. Unesterified cholesterol in Schnyder's corneal crystalline dystrophy. *Am J Ophthalmol* 1987; **104**: 157–63.

Rowson N, Dart J, Buckley R. Corneal neovascularisation in acute hydrops. *Eye* 1992; **6**: 404–6.

Schanzlin DJ, Robin JB, Erickson G, Lingra R, Minckler D, Pickford M. Histopathologic and ultrastructural analysis of congenital corneal staphyloma. *Am J Ophthalmol* 1983; **95**: 506–14.

Schimmelpfennig B, Beurman RW. Evidence for neurotropism in the cornea (abstract). *Invest Ophthalmol Vis Sci* 1979; **18**: 125.

Sever RJ, Frost P, Weinstein G. Eye changes in ichthyosis. *J Am Med Assoc* 1968; **206**: 2283–6.

Shenk Van H. Hornhautbefunde bei idiopathischer anasthesie der-hornhaut. *Klin Monatsbl Augenheilkd* 1958; **133**: 506–18.

Shields JA, Waring GO, Monte LG. Ocular findings in leprosy. *Am J Ophthalmol* 1974; **77**: 880–90.

Shorey P, Lobo G. Congenital corneal anesthesia: problems in diagnosis. *J Pediatr Ophthalmol Strabismus* 1990; **27**: 143–8.

Sjogren H. A contribution to our knowledge of the ocular changes induced by sulphuretted hydrogen. *Acta Ophthalmol* 1939; **17**: 166–71.

Smiddy WE, Hamburg TR, Kracher GP, Stark WJ. Keratoconus: contact lens or keratoplasty? *Ophthalmology* 1988; **95**: 487–92.

Sommer A. Renewed interest in the ancient scourge xerophthalmia (editorial). *Am J Ophthalmol* 1978; **86**: 284–5.

Spector B, Klintworth GK, Wells SA. Histologic study of the ocular lesions in multiple endocrine neoplasia syndrome type IIb. *Am J Ophthalmol* 1981; **91**: 204–15.

Spencer WH, Fisher JJ. The association of keratoconus with atopic dermatitis. *Am J Ophthalmol* 1959; **47**: 332–4.

Stark DJ, Gilmore D, Vance J, Pearn J. A corneal abnormality associated with trisomy 8 mosaicism syndrome. *Br J Ophthalmol* 1987; **71**: 29–31.

Stein R, Lazar M, Adam A. Brittle cornea. A familial trait associated with blue sclera. *Am J Ophthalmol* 1968; **66**: 67–9.

Stewart HL, Wind CA, Kaufman HE. Unilateral congenital corneal anesthesia. *Am J Ophthalmol* 1972; **74**: 334–5.

Tanzi R, Pertrukhin K, Chernov I *et al.* The Wilson disease gene is a copper transporting ATPase with homology to the Menkes disease gene. *Nature Genet* 1993; **5**: 344–50.

Taylor D, Bentovim A. Recurrent nonaccidentally inflicted chemical eye injuries to siblings. *J Pediatr Ophthalmol Strabismus* 1976; **13**: 238–42.

Topilow HW, Cykiert RC, Goldman K, Palme E, Henkind P. Bilateral corneal dermis-like choristoma: an X-chromosome-linked disorder. *Arch Ophthalmol* 1981; **99**: 1387–91.

Trope GE, Jay JL, Dudgeon J, Woodruff G. Self-inflicted corneal injuries in children with congenital anaesthesia. *Br J Ophthalmol* 1985; **69**: 551–4.

Tuft S, Moodaley L, Gregory W, Davison C, Buckley R. Prognostic factors for the progression of keratoconus. *Ophthalmology* 1994; **101**: 439–47.

Tuppurainen K, Fraki J, Karjalainen S, Paljarri L, Suhonen R, Ryynanen M. The KID syndrome in Finland. *Acta Ophthalmol* 1988; **66**: 692–8.

Van der Hoeve J, Kleyn JE. Blaue sclera, knochenbruchigkeit und schwerhorigkeit. *Albrecht Von Graefe Arch Klin Exp Ophthalmol* 1918; **95**: 81–93.

Vangsted P, Limpaphayom P. Dermoid of the cornea in association with congenital generalized fibromatosis. A case report. *Acta Ophthalmol* 1983; **61**: 927–33.

Vrabec MB, Shapiro MB, Koller E, Wiebe DA, Henricks J, Albers JJ. Ophthalmic observations in lecithin cholesterol acyltransferase deficiency. *Arch Ophthalmol* 1988; **106**: 225–9.

Wan WL, Minckler DS, Rao NA. Pupillary block glaucoma associated with childhood cystinosis. *Am J Ophthalmol* 1986; **101**: 700–5.

Wells RS, Kerr CB. Clinical features of autosomal dominance in sex-linked ichthyosis in an English population. *Br Med J* 1966; **1**: 947.

Wilson DJ, Weleber RG, Klein M, Welch RB, Green WR. Bietti's crystalline dystrophy: a clinicopathologic correlative study. *Arch Ophthalmol* 1989; **107**: 213–21.

Wilson FM, Grayson M, Pieroni D. Corneal changes in ectodermal dysplasia: case report, histopathology and differential diagnosis. *Am J Ophthalmol* 1973; **75**: 17–27.

Wilson FM, Schmitt TE, Grayson M. Amiodarone induced corneal verticillata. *Ann Ophthalmol* 1980; **12**: 657–60.

Woodward EG. Keratoconus: maternal age and social class. *Br J Ophthalmol* 1981; **65**: 104–7.

Wortham E, Nguyen C-X. Multiple endocrine neoplasia. *Arch Ophthalmol* 1990; **108**: 1338.

Yarze JC, Martin P, Munoz SJ, Friedman LS. Wilson's disease: current status. *Am J Med* 1992; **92**: 643–54.

Young TL, Buchi E, Kaufman L, Sugar J, Tso M. Respiratory epithelium in a cystic choristoma of the limbus. *Arch Ophthalmol* 1990; **108**: 1736–9.

Zaidman GW, Johnson B, Brown SI. Corneal transplantation in an infant with corneal dermoid. *Am J Ophthalmol* 1982; **93**: 78–83.

Zlotogara J, BenEzra D, Cohen T, Cohen E. Syndrome of brittle cornea, blue sclera and joint hyperextensibility. *Am J Med Genet* 1990; **36**: 269–72.

25: Corneal Dystrophies

H. U. Møller

Corneal dystrophies are mendelian inherited conditions which exhibit bilateral and usually symmetrical changes. No two reviews on corneal dystrophies comprise the same entities: some such as 'cornea guttata' are assumed to be corneal dystrophies by some review authors, but not by others. Some rare diseases are excluded by some authors as not being essential.

Furthermore, the prevalence and the importance of the different conditions vary. The founder effect has in some countries given rise to large pedigrees and subsequent publications of cases, which may be almost non-existent elsewhere.

This chapter focuses on dystrophies proven to be the most common at the European Cornea Conference, held in 1992, and highlights the clinical presentation in the young patient when it differs from the adult appearance.

Definition and classification

The term dystrophy is derived from the Greek words *dys* (meaning wrong or difficult) and *trophe* (nourishment). Warburg and Møller (1989) suggested the following definition of dystrophy as 'The process and consequences of hereditary progressive affections of specific cells in one or more tissues that initially show a normal function'. This definition would comprise most diseases traditionally named corneal dystrophies, with or without systemic manifestations.

The classical subdivision of corneal dystrophies according to the layer of their main involvement, e.g. stromal dystrophies, has historical interest but little practical importance; often the classification antedates the slit lamp. Most corneal dystrophies have had an eponym attached to the descriptive name.

Dystrophies should be distinguished from corneal degenerations (Friedlaender & Smolin 1979), which are secondary, non-genetic processes resulting from ageing or previous corneal inflammation. 'Cornea guttata, Fuchs' endothelial dystrophy' as seen in an adult cataract clinic rarely shows a mendelian inheritance pattern. Thus it is an example of a disease of old age, often called a dystrophy but probably best described as a degeneration.

Mutation rate

As the mutation rates for many of the corneal dystrophies are probably very low, it is important to be cautious when diagnosing apparently sporadic cases and a family history and examination of parents are mandatory. Phenocopies do exist although they may be rare in children; paraproteinaemic crystalline keratopathy is an example of a disease mimicking granular dystrophy (Møller *et al.* 1993).

Map, dot and fingerprint dystrophy; Cogan's microcystic basement membrane dystrophy

This entity (Cogan *et al.* 1964) may not be a true dystrophy. It can be autosomal dominant (Laibson & Krachmer 1975), but many patients present with no family history. Furthermore, the typical map, dot and fingerprint changes may be the result of trauma or corneal surgery (Nelson *et al.* 1985) and may be present in one eye only. On the slit lamp, refractile geographical changes, dots (Fig. 25.1) or fingerprint-type lines just beneath the epithelium are seen on retroillumination. The findings are sharply demarcated and the rest of the cornea is healthy (Fig. 25.2). The slit-lamp appearance changes with time. These changes repre-

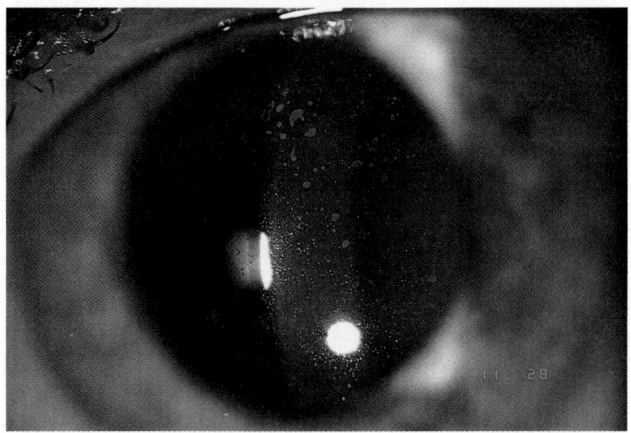

Fig. 25.1 Map, dot and fingerprint dystrophy in an adult.

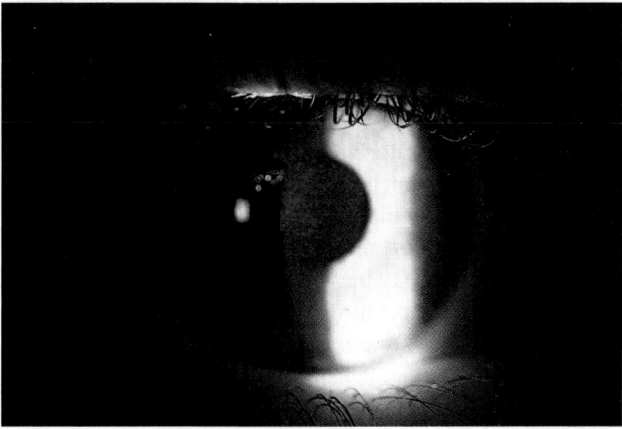

Fig. 25.2 Unknown superficial dystrophy, probably map, dot and fingerprint type. There was no family history and both parents were normal on slit-lamp examination. Dr Wittebol-Post's patient.

sent alterations in the epithelial basement membrane and may give rise to intraepithelial cysts (Ehlers & Møller 1988) which are often discovered on routine examination. If symptomatic, the patient experiences painful, recurrent erosions (see below): careful slit-lamp examination in a non-symptomatic phase will often reveal microcystic changes. This disease has no systemic manifestations and vision is rarely affected.

Recurrent erosions

Recurrent erosions present in childhood as a result of underlying corneal disease or previous trauma (Hope-Ross *et al.* 1994). There is often associated meibomian gland dysfunction. Affected children usually have recurrent attacks of severe foreign-body pain in one or both eyes, often starting when they wake in the morning. The pain lasts 1–5 hours, sometimes longer, and is accompanied by redness and watering.

Treatment is aimed at preventing the recurrent epithelial erosions by prescribing hypertonic ointment at night. Patching, pupil dilatation, analgesics, and ocular lubricants are the mainstay of acute treatment of the erosions. Epithelial debridement and soft contact lens use may all help in more severe cases. Excimer laser treatment may prove effective.

Juvenile epithelial dystrophy; Meesmann–Wilke dystrophy

This condition (Meesmann & Wilke 1939), has a varied expression (Thiel & Behnke 1968). Although often asymptomatic it may present in early childhood with symptoms of ocular irritation and photophobia due to recurrent erosions. The typical patient has a huge number of tiny epithelial vesicles (Fig. 25.3). In the young child, small areas may be spared. It is rare; the best documented pedigree is from northern Germany (Behnke & Thiel 1965). Treatment may be with soft contact lenses, corneal abrasion or excimer laser treatment, the indication being a decrease in visual acuity caused by basement membrane changes. Recurrence will follow soon, however.

Vision is rarely severely affected in childhood and the patients are otherwise healthy.

Reis–Bücklers dystrophy

The old literature on this condition (Bücklers 1949) is rather confusing. Møller (1991) reviewed it and suggested that these patients have a variety of granular corneal dystrophy, whereas Wittebol-Post *et al.* (1989) believed that they have a well-described entity identical to the 'corneal dystrophy of Waardenburg and Jonkers', and the 'honeycomb dystrophy of Thiel and Behnke'. It has been linked to 5q (Small *et al.* 1996), as has granular dystrophy. It is an autosomal dominant disease presenting in infancy

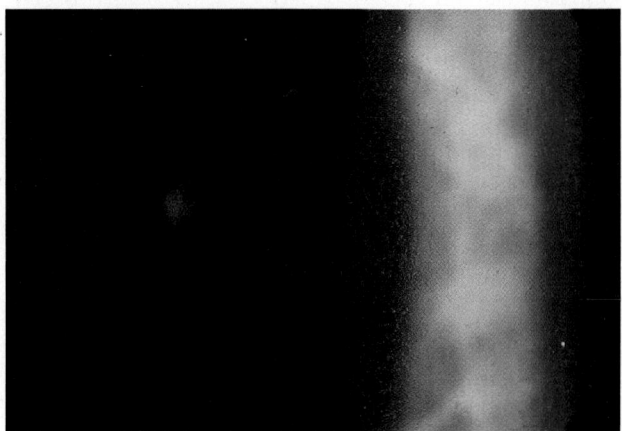

Fig. 25.3 Meesmann–Wilke dystrophy showing multiple epithelial vesicles. Dr Wittebol-Post's patient.

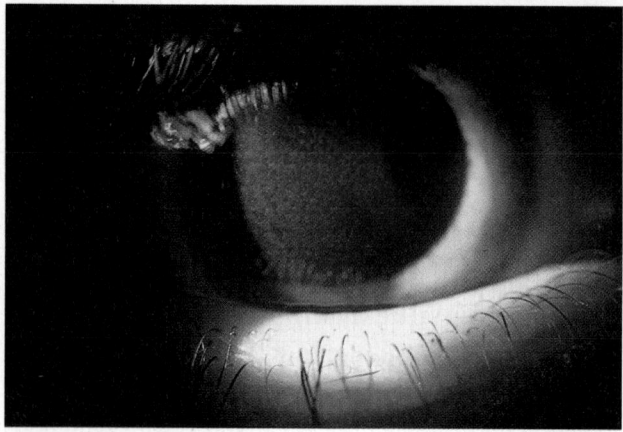

Fig. 25.4 Reis–Bücklers dystrophy showing the irregular corneal surface with subepithelial opacities. Dr Wittebol-Post's patient.

or early childhood with recurrent attacks of photophobia, pain, redness and watering which last days or weeks. Treatment of the acute attacks is similar to that of the recurrent erosions (see above).

The corneal surface is irregular with microscopic subepithelial protrusions (Fig. 25.4) caused by accumulation of abnormal material at the level of Bowman's membrane. Eventually the opacities become more numerous and opaque with a honeycomb appearance, worse in the mid-peripheral zone. Corneal sensation is reduced. Vision is impaired by infiltration of Bowman's layer and its replacement by scar tissue in the mid-twenties (Rice *et al.* 1968) at which time it becomes less symptomatic. Vision is affected in early adulthood and keratoplasty is often required; this may be followed by recurrence in the graft (Olson & Kaufmann 1978).

Granular dystrophy; Groenouw type I

Granular dystrophy (Groenouw 1890) is an autosomal dominant dystrophy. It is distinguished by discrete granular-appearing corneal opacities in an otherwise clear cornea. The opacities are white in direct illumination, and transparent, like a crack in glass, by retroillumination. In the child of 5 years of age or so, these may be brownish and superficial to Bowman's membrane and present in a verticillata configuration (Fig. 25.5). The granules increase in number and size and progress into the stroma during early adulthood. There is always a 2 mm clear, limbal zone. One striking feature is that unlike most dominant disorders the expressivity is constant in all generations (Møller 1991); some families have several hundred granules in one cornea, whereas in other families (with a later onset) members have between 50 and 100 granules. Granular dystrophy has been linked to chromosome 5q (Eiberg *et al.* 1994; Stone *et al.* 1994).

Grafting is rarely required until the fifth or sixth decade when visual acuity may drop below 6/12; recurrence in the graft is the rule. It has no extra ocular signs or symptoms. Superficial keratectomy, or lamellar keratoplasty alone may be successful if the deposits are limited to the superficial cornea (Sajjadi & Javadi 1992; Lyons *et al.* 1994).

A so-called superficial, unusual variety with a very severe clinical outcome in young children has been described. They have an almost white central cornea before the age of 10 years. These patients are homozygous for the dominant gene (Møller & Ridgway 1990; Diaper 1994).

Lattice dystrophy; Haab–Biber–Dimer dystrophy

Lattice dystrophy (Biber 1890) is also an autosomal dominant condition. The deposition of amyloid in the child cornea is recognized by three distinct slit-lamp observations (Dubord & Krachmer 1982).
1 Tiny non-refractile, whitish spots, round or ovoid (Fig. 25.6a).
2 A diffuse axial, anterior stromal haze.
3 White, anterior, stromal dots as well as (in the somewhat older patient) filamentary lines which are refractile (Fig. 25.6b) on indirect illumination.

The deposition may be symmetrical or asymmetrical in both eyes. The intervening stroma becomes increasingly hazy in the adult. The appearance of the lattice lines giving rise to the name of the condition will only become evident in adulthood. Lattice dystrophy has been linked to chromosome 5q (Stone *et al.* 1994), i.e. to the very same area as granular dystrophy. It is likely that granular, lattice, Reis-Bücklers and Avellino dystrophy are different mutations within the same gene (Folberg *et al.* 1994). Avellino dystrophy has features of both lattice and granular dystrophy (Rosenwasser *et al.* 1993; Lucorelli & Adamis 1994).

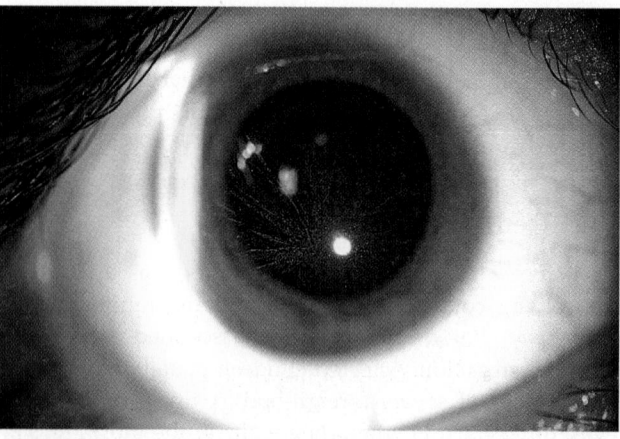

Fig. 25.5 Granular dystrophy showing a verticillata-like configuration of the corneal opacities.

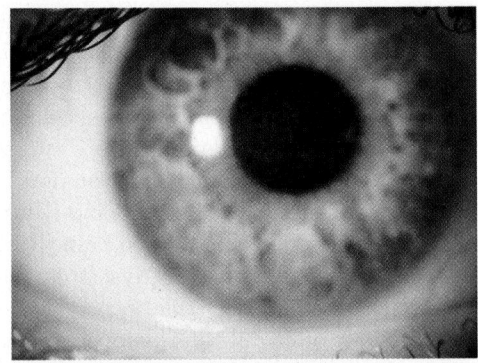

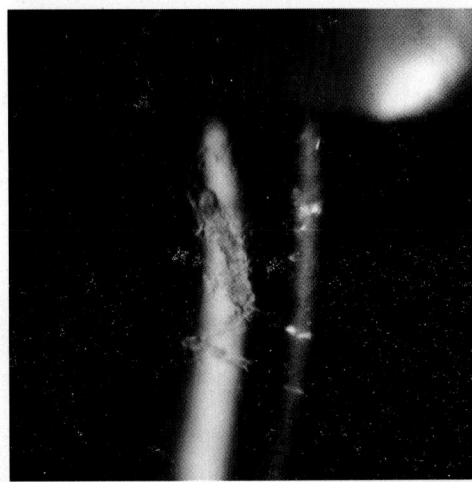

Fig. 25.6 (a) Lattice dystrophy. Early changes showing non-refractile round spots. Mr A.E.A. Ridgway's patient. (b) Later changes showing filamentary lines.

Many patients experience recurrent erosions and corneal grafting may be necessary in early adult life due to visual impairment. Recurrence in the graft is often troublesome. Subtypes exist (Meretoja 1972) and are associated with systemic amyloidosis with progressive cranial and peripheral nerve palsies.

Macular dystrophy; Groenouw type II

Not many ophthalmologists will have the opportunity to diagnose macular dystrophy (Groenouw 1890) in a very young child. The very first subtle findings are discrete, nebulous, whitish opacities in the centre of the cornea which itself is very thin (Malbran 1972). However, over the years it increases in thickness and the corneal stroma becomes increasingly hazy (Fig. 25.7) between the opacities with an irregular surface. Deposits of glycosaminoglycan cause the opacification. As it is inherited as a recessive trait, consanguinity is frequent. The high prevalence of macular dystrophy in Iceland is an example of the founder effect in a particular geographical area (Jonasson *et al.* 1989). Macular dystrophy has been linked to chromosome 16 (Vance *et al.* 1996).

Visual deterioration is symmetrical and inevitable, but patients do not usually require corneal grafting until late in the second or third decade. Patients experience no systemic symptoms, but there is immunohistochemical evidence of heterogeneity (Yang *et al.* 1988).

Central crystalline Schnyder's dystrophy

This autosomal dominant corneal dystrophy (Schnyder 1929; Weiss 1992) can be diagnosed in children and may have a variable expression. The central anterior cornea has a slowly progressing (Ingraham 1993), disc-like central opacification with or without polychromatic crystals. It may be visible from a few years of age. In their twenties patients develop an arcus lipoides and a diffuse stromal haze. Vision is variably affected and keratoplasty may be necessary in the adult. The crystals comprise cholesterol and other lipids (Rodrigues *et al.* 1990).

Dermochondral dystrophy

This is a rare central anterior dystrophy with confluent opacities, anterior cortical cataract, skin nodules and limb deformities (Bierley *et al.* 1992).

Posterior polymorphous dystrophy

This is also an autosomal dominant dystrophy (Schlichting 1941) which may be seen in the very young (Levy *et al.* 1996). It is asymmetrical and slowly progressive. Slit-lamp appearances show small, round, discrete, transparent, vesicular lesions surrounded by a ring of opacity deep in the cornea at the level of Descemet's membrane (Fig. 25.8). The opacities are best seen on retroillumination. Geographical and band varieties exist as well.

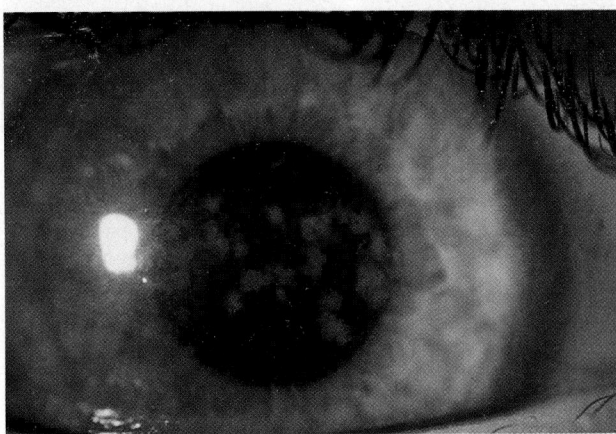

Fig. 25.7 Macular dystrophy in a 13-year-old girl. Typical macular corneal opacities. What cannot be seen in a picture is the opaque ground substance between opacities and the thin cornea.

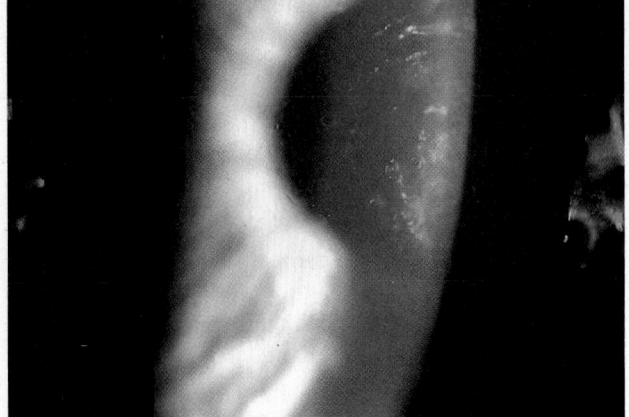

a

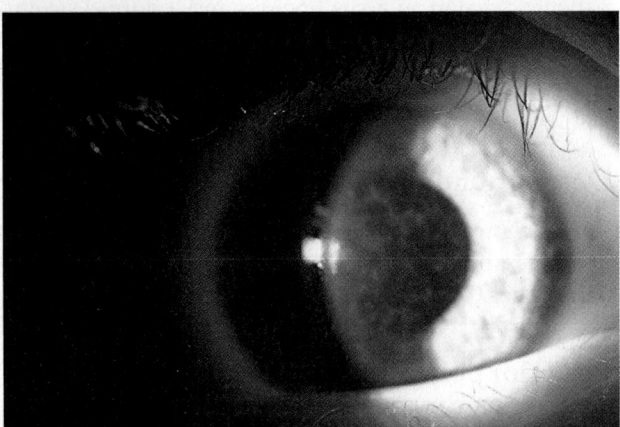

b

c

Fig. 25.8 (a) Posterior polymorphous dystrophy showing deep transparent vesicular lesions. (b) Posterior polymorphous dystrophy. Direct illumination showing geographical opacities. (c) Posterior polymorphous dystrophy. Slit-lamp picture showing deep posterior stromal-endothelial ring-like opacities.

There is controversy over whether or not posterior polymorphous dystrophy is an isolated corneal condition, and what its relationship is with anterior chamber cleavage abnormalities and how they overlap. Posterior polymorphous dystrophy may have some features of anterior chamber cleavage disorders, such as a pro-

minent Schwalbe's line and iridocorneal adhesions, glaucoma and corectopia according to Krachmer's description in 1985. Laganowski *et al.* (1991) distinguished the corneal affections in iridocorneal endothelial syndrome from posterior polymorphous dystrophy by means of specular microscopy. Ultrastructural studies show a mosaic of better preserved and dystrophic endothelial cells and Descemet's membrane (Sekundo *et al.* 1994). Posterior polymorphous dystrophy has been linked to chromosome 20 (Héon *et al.* 1995).

The symptoms are often mild and vision unaffected and most patients do not require corneal grafting (McCartney & Kirkness 1988).

Congenital hereditary endothelial dystrophy

This important but rare corneal disease was clearly described by Maumenee (1960). Strictly speaking it may

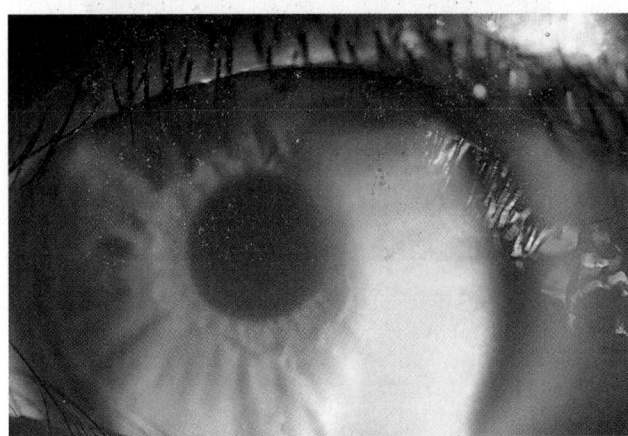

a

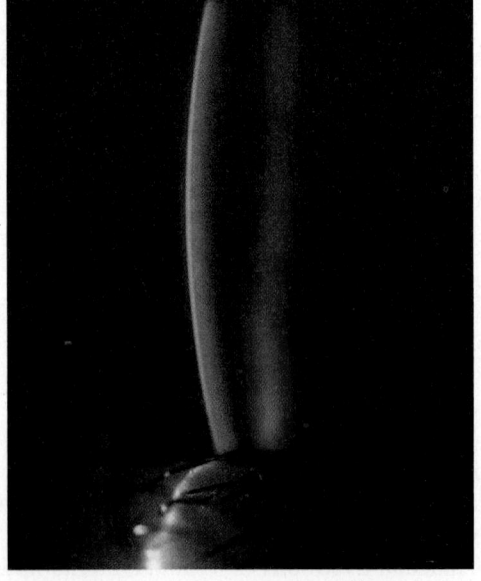

b

Fig. 25.9 (a) Congenital hereditary endothelial dystrophy showing opaque cornea. (b) Congenital hereditary endothelial dystrophy showing opaque and thickened cornea on slit-lamp illumination.

not be a true dystrophy as it is congenital but usually it is included among the dystrophies. Autosomal dominant as well as recessive inheritance patterns seem to exist. It has been described in association with nail hypoplasia (Stirling *et al.* 1994).

Usually the presentation is at birth with a variable diffuse avascular haziness, ground-glass, bluish-white opacity of the cornea (Fig. 25.9). The cornea is thicker than normal. The opacification may clear in the first few weeks of life. It may also, however, progress. It is suggested that congenital hereditary endothelial dystrophy patients should be observed rather than operated on in early life. If grafting proves necessary it carries a relatively good prognosis (Kirkness *et al.* 1987). Differentiation from congenital glaucoma is important but often very difficult.

References

Behnke H, Thiel H-J. Über die hereditäre Epitheldystrophie der Hornhaut (Typ Meesmann–Wilke) in Schleswig–Holstein. *Klin Monatsbl Augenheilk* 1965; **147**: 662–72.

Biber H. *Ueber einige seltenere Hornhauterkrankungen*. Dissertation, Zürich, 1890.

Bierly J, George S, Volpicelli M. Dermochondral corneal dystrophy (of Francois). *Br J Ophthalmol* 1992; **76**: 760–1.

Bücklers M. Ueber eine weitere familiäre Hornhautdystrophie (Reis). *Klin Monatsbl Augenheilkd* 1949; **114**: 386–400.

Cogan DG, Donaldson DD, Kuwabara T, Marshall D. Microcystic dystrophy of the corneal epithelium. *Trans Am Ophthalmol Soc* 1964; **62**: 213–25.

Diaper CJM. Severe granular dystrophy: a pedigree with presumed homozygotes. *Eye* 1994; **8**: 448–52.

Dubord PJ, Krachmer JH. Diagnosis of early lattice corneal dystrophy. *Arch Ophthalmol* 1982; **100**: 788–90.

Ehlers N, Møller HU. Pathology and pathomechanisms of epithelial microcystic and basement membrane abnormalities of the cornea. *Acta Ophthalmol (Copenh)* 1988; **66**: 318–26.

Eiberg H, Møller HU, Berendt I, Mohr J. Assignment of granular corneal dystrophy Groenouw type I (CDGG1) to chromosome 5q. *Eur J Hum Genet* 1994; **2**: 132–8.

Folberg R, Stone E, Sheffield V, Mathers W. The relationship between granular, lattice type 1, and Avellino corneal dystrophies. A histopathologic study. *Arch Ophthalmol* 1994; **112**: 1080–5.

Friedlaender MH, Smolin G. Corneal degenerations. *Ann Ophthalmol* 1979; **11**: 1485–95.

Groenouw A. Knötchenförmige Hornhauttrübungen (Noduli corneae). *Archiv Augenheilkd* 1890; **21**: 281–9.

Héon E, Mathers WD, Alward WLM *et al.* Linkage of posterior polymorphous dystrophy to 20q11. *Hum Mol Genet* 1995; **4**: 485–8.

Hope-Ross MW, Chell PB, Kerrick GN, McDonnell P. Recurrent erosion: clinical features. *Eye* 1994; **8**: 373–7.

Ingraham H, Perry H, Donnenfeld E, Donaldson D. Progressive Schnyder's corneal dystrophy. *Ophthalmology* 1993; **100**: 1824–7.

Jonasson F, Johannsson H, Garner A, Rice NSC. Macular corneal dystrophy in Iceland. *Eye* 1989; **3**: 446–54.

Kirkness CM, McCartney AC, Rice NSC, Garner A, Steele ADMcG. Congenital hereditary corneal oedema of Maumenee: its clinical features, management and pathology. *Br J Ophthalmol* 1987; **71**: 130–44.

Krachmer JH. Posterior polymorphous corneal dystrophy. *Trans Am Ophthalmol Soc* 1985; **83**: 413–75.

Laganowski HC, Sherrard ES, Kerr-Muir MG, Buckley RJ. Distinguishing features of the iridocorneal endothelial syndrome and posterior polymorphous dystrophy: value of endothelial specular microscopy. *Br J Ophthalmol* 1991; **75**: 212–16.

Laibson PR, Krachmer JH. Familial occurrence of dot (microcystic), map, fingerprint dystrophy of the cornea. *Invest Ophthalmol* 1975; **14**: 397–9.

Levy GL, Moss J, Noble BA, McCartney ACE. Early-onset posterior polymorphous dystrophy. *Arch Ophthalmol* 1996; **114**: 1265–68.

Lucorelli M, Adamis A. Avellino corneal dystrophy. *Arch Ophthalmol* 1994; **112**: 418–19.

Lyons C, McCartney ACE, Kirkness CM, Ficker LA, Steele AD, Rice N. Granular corneal dystrophy. *Ophthalmology* 1994; **101**: 1812–17.

McCartney ACE, Kirkness CM. Comparison between posterior polymorphous dystrophy of the cornea and congenital hereditary endothelial dystrophy of the cornea. *Eye* 1988; **2**: 63–71.

Malbran ES. Corneal dystrophies: a clinical, pathological and surgical approach. *Am J Ophthalmol* 1972; **74**: 771–809.

Maumenee AE. Congenital hereditary corneal dystrophy. *Am J Ophthalmol* 1960; **50**: 1114–24.

Meesmann A, Wilke F. Klinische und anatomische Untersuchungen über eine bisher unbekannte, dominant vererbte Epitheldystrophie der Hornhaut. *Klin Monatsbl Augenheilkd* 1939; **103**: 361–91.

Meretoja J. Comparative histopathological and clinical findings in eyes with lattice corneal dystrophy of two different types. *Ophthalmologica* 1972; **165**: 15–37.

Møller HU. Granular corneal dystrophy Groenouw type I. *Acta Ophthalmol (Copenh)* 1991; **69** (Suppl. 198): 1–40.

Møller HU, Ehlers N, Bojsen-Møller M, Ridgway AEA. Differential diagnosis between granular corneal dystrophy Groenouw type I and paraproteinemic crystalline keratopathy. *Acta Ophthalmol (Copenh)* 1993; **71**: 552–5.

Møller HU, Ridgway AEA. Granular corneal dystrophy Groenouw type I. A report of a probable homozygous patient. *Acta Ophthalmol (Copenh)* 1990; **68**: 97–101.

Nelson JD, Williams P, Lindstrom RL, Doughman DJ. Map fingerprint dot changes in the corneal epithelial basement membrane following radial keratotomy. *Ophthalmology* 1985; **92**: 199–205.

Olson RJ, Kaufmann HE. Recurrence of Reis–Bücklers' corneal dystrophy in a graft. *Am J Ophthalmol* 1978; **85**: 349–51.

Rice NSC, Ashton N, Jay B, Blach RK. Reis–Bücklers' dystrophy. *Br J Ophthalmol* 1968; **52**: 577–603.

Rodrigues MM, Kruth HS, Krachmer JH, Vrabec MP, Blanchette-Mackie J. Cholesterol localization in ultra thin frozen sections in Schnyder's corneal crystalline dystrophy. *Am J Ophthalmol* 1990; **110**: 513–18.

Rosenwasser G, Sucheski B, Rosa N *et al.* Phenotypic variation in combined granular lattice (Avellino) corneal dystrophy. *Arch Ophthalmol* 1993; **111**: 1546–52.

Sajjadi SH, Javadi M. Superficial juvenile granular dystrophy. *Ophthalmology* 1992; **99**: 95–102.

Schlichting H. Blasen- und dellenförmige Endotheldystrophie der Hornhaut. *Klin Monatsbl Augenheilkd* 1941; **107**: 425–35.

Schnyder WF. Mitteilung über einen neuen Typus von familiärer Hornhauterkrankung. *Schweiz Med Wochenschr* 1929; **59**: 559–71.

Sekundo W, Lee W, Kirkness C, Aitken D, Fleck B. An ultrastructural investigation of an early manifestation of the posterior polymorphous dystrophy of the cornea. *Ophthalmology* 1994; **101**: 1422–31.

Small KW, Mullen L, Barletta J *et al.* Mapping of Reis–Bücklers corneal dystrophy to chromosome 5q. *Am J Ophthalmol* 1996; **121**: 384–90.

Stone E, Mathers W, Rosenwasser G *et al.* Three autosomal dominant corneal dystrophies map to chromosome 5q. *Nature Genet* 1994; **6**: 47–51.

Stirling R, Pitts J, Galloway N, Robson K, Newbury-Ecob R. Congenital hereditary endothelial dystrophy associated with nail hypoplasia. *Br J Ophthalmol* 1994; **78**: 77–8.

Thiel HJ, Behnke H. Über die Variationsbreite der hereditären Hornhautepitheldystrophie Typ Meesmann–Wilke. *Ophthalmologica* 1968; **155**: 81–6.

Vance JM, Jonasson F, Lennon F. *et al*. Linkage of a gene for macular corneal dystrophy to chromosome 16. *Am J Hum Genet* 1996; **58**: 757–62.

Warburg M, Møller HU. Dystrophy. A revised definition. *J Med Genet* 1989; **26**: 769–71.

Weiss JS. Schnyder's dystrophy of the cornea. A Swede–Finn connection. *Cornea* 1992; **11**: 93–101.

Wittebol-Post D, van Schooneveld MJ, Pels E. The corneal dystrophy of Waardenburg and Jonkers. *Ophthal Paediatr Genet* 1989; **10**: 249–55.

Yang CJ, SundarRaj N, Thonar EJ-MA, Klintworth GK. Immunohistochemical evidence of heterogeneity in macular corneal dystrophy. *Am J Ophthalmol* 1988; **106**: 65-71.

26: Lacrimal System

Susan Day

The lacrimal system consists of a secretory portion, lacrimal and accessory lacrimal glands, meibomian glands, and goblet cells; and an excretory portion, punctae, canaliculus, lacrimal sac, and nasolacrimal duct. Its function is to produce and remove tears. Tears themselves serve in multiple ways to protect the eyes, including lubrication, provision of oxygen, and an antibacterial role; when the tears drain away, irritating substances as well as cellular debris are similarly removed (Lemp & Blackman 1983; Werb 1983). Epiphora represents one of the most common indications for referral in a paediatric ophthalmology practice. Other rare conditions in infants and children warrant a thorough knowledge of its pathology.

Lacrimal gland

Anatomy

The lacrimal gland occupies the lacrimal gland fossa in the superotemporal aspect of the orbit. It is divided into the orbital and palpebral lobes by the levator aponeurosis. The palpebral lobe can normally be directly prolapsed into the superotemporal cul-de-sac and with abnormal enlargement of the lacrimal gland, direct visualization or direct biopsy of the lacrimal gland can usually be made.

Embryology

The lacrimal gland commences differentiation from the nasal cells by the conjunctiva at 40–45 days of gestation. By the fifth month, lobules are relatively well formed. The lacrimal gland continues to grow up to 3–4 years of age after birth. Reflex tearing, however, begins in infants anywhere from a few weeks to several months (Duke-Elder & Cook 1963; Sevel 1981). The accessory lacrimal glands have common origins but remain within the lids rather than migrating with the remainder of the lacrimal gland precursors.

Congenital abnormalities

Congenital absence of the lacrimal gland is rare, but has been documented neuroradiologically (Uleckas *et al.* 1994). This is usually associated with conditions in which congenital absence of at least part of the conjunctiva is present, such as anophthalmos, cryptophthalmos (including Fraser's syndrome), and the lacrimo-auriculodentodigital (LADD) syndrome (Thompson *et al.* 1985; Heinz *et al.* 1993).

Anomalous lacrimal ductules surface on the skin, medial or lateral to the lacrimal gland (Blanksma & Pol 1980; Cogen *et al.* 1994); they may be best treated by careful dissection and excision.

Alacrima

Congenital alacrima or hyposecretion of tears is relatively common; the lacrimal gland may be present despite the absence of tears (Uleckas *et al.* 1994). Because tear production, especially reflex tear production, is often small until 6 months after birth, investigation of these patients is not usually indicated unless other systemic disorders seem apparent (Riley *et al.* 1949; Riley 1952; Riley & Moore 1966; Thompson *et al.* 1985; Heinz *et al.* 1993). Patrick (1974) has shown that neonates do produce tears and suspected that the apparent absence of tearing was accounted for by an efficient tear pump created by the lids and lacrimal system. Children with familial dysautonomia, or Riley–Day syndrome, can develop severe keratopathy as a consequence of the dry eyes and corneal hypoaesthesia (Goldberg *et al.* 1968) (see Chapter P8).

Other congenital abnormalities include ectopic lacrimal gland tissue in which tissue is embryologically misplaced deeper in the orbit. Since no drainage system exists, an apparent enlarging orbital mass may develop (Green & Zimmerman 1967; Jacobs *et al.* 1977). Neoplasms have been reported in association with ectopic tissue; thus its diagnosis is significant (Mindlin *et al.* 1977; Mueller & Borit 1979).

Since the embryology of the lacrimal gland is closely linked to that of the conjunctival epithelium, the common position of some forms of dermoid cysts superotemporally can be understood. Dermoid cysts must be distinguished from dacryops, or ectasia of the lacrimal gland ducts, in certain circumstances (Rush & Leone 1981; Brownstein *et al.* 1984).

Fistulae are probably the same as anomalous ductules (see above); they may be present in the region of the lateral canthus (Duke-Elder & Cook 1963; Blanksma & Pol 1980; Welham *et al.* 1992) and pre-auricular region (Mukherji & Mukhopadhay 1972).

Crocodile tears (Chorobski 1951), in which tearing is elicited by chewing or sucking, occur as a consequence of congenital aberrant innervation between the fifth cranial nerve (innervating the lacrimal gland) and the gustatory fibres of the seventh cranial nerve. This has been found in instances of aberrant innervation including the Marcus Gunn jaw–winking phenomenon and Duane's syndrome (Ramsey & Taylor 1980).

Dacryoadenitis

This may occur either unilaterally or more typically bilaterally in children. Often the child is systemically ill. Mumps may result in lacrimal gland as well as parotid gland swelling (Riffenburgh 1961). Other causes include mononucleosis, herpes zoster, histoplasmosis and gonococcal infection (Duke-Elder & MacFaul 1974). The diagnosis of dacryoadenitis is aided by assessment of the 'S-sign' in which there is a drooping of the lateral aspect of the upper lid. Direct inspection of the palpebral lobe of the gland may confirm evidence of inflammation. Computed tomography (CT) scans can confirm the presence of enlargement but also help in ruling out lacrimal or other orbital masses if signs and symptoms of dacryoadenitis do not resolve.

Lacrimal gland infarct

This occurs rarely in children with sickle cell disease. The rapid onset can mimic and must be differentiated from orbital cellulitis, but its treatment consists of reversal of the sickle cell crisis. A bone scan may be particularly helpful in defining the lacrimal infarct.

Lacrimal gland tumour and pseudotumour

With the exception of a dermoid involving the lacrimal gland, tumours are extremely rare in childhood (Duke-Elder & Cook 1963). Pseudotumour is rare in childhood but may affect the lacrimal gland in young people (Chavis *et al.* 1978; Mottow & Jakobiec 1978). Malignant epithelial tumours including mixed cell, adenocystic and other carcinomas (Dagher *et al.* 1980) are also rare but recorded in childhood (Wright *et al.* 1979; Wright 1982).

Lacrimal duct cyst

These appear to be rare in childhood (Smith & Rootman 1986) but occur as translucent swellings under the conjunctiva or swelling of the lacrimal gland.

Lacrimal gland prolapse

Lacrimal gland prolapse, usually bilateral, may appear clinically as subconjunctival masses in the outer part of the upper fornix; it is uncommon before puberty, and is more frequent in black people. It usually requires neuroimaging and other studies to exclude underlying diseases such as sarcoidosis, tumours or leukaemia; most cases are of unknown cause.

Lacrimal drainage system

Embryology

The development of the lacrimal drainage system includes an epithelial lined ectodermal component as well as mesodermal components. The ectodermal precursors of the canaliculi and ducts are in place at the 28–30 mm stage of the embryo. Growth continues with gradual formation of a lumen, and patency is established to the lids. The most distal region of the nasolacrimal duct remains non-patent, consisting of mesodermal components of the nasolacrimal duct and the mucosa of the inferior nasal meatus.

At birth, a substantial number of infants still do not have patency of this terminal region. Murube-del-Castillo (1983) probed 181 full-term infants and found bilateral patency in 131, unilateral patency in 46, and bilateral blockage in four, concluding a 15% non-patency of 362 passages. Other anatomical studies have revealed between 35 and 73% non-patency in full-term infants (Schwarz 1935; Cassady 1952). The bones related to the lacrimal excretory passage are incompletely developed at birth; chondrification and ossification commence 6 weeks after birth and may cause significant difficulty with probing by 18 months.

Congenital abnormalities

Congenital punctal and canalicular abnormalities

These abnormalities, including imperforate punctae and absent punctae, can involve both the upper and lower punctae. If the punctae are absent, the associated canaliculi are often absent (Lyons *et al.* 1993). A thin grey membrane is often present and additional punctae or slit-like fistulae may be present. Non-patency of the punctae may be suspected when epiphora is present in the absence of any significant discharge, since stagnation within the nasolacrimal sac is not present.

Treatment

Isolated absence of the upper punctum requires no treatment, but absence of the lower or both upper and lower punctum may require treatment only if there are significant symptoms. Initially, a simple puncturing of a membrane using magnification, combined with syringing and probing, may be sufficient for cases where the obstruction is purely punctal, but more widespread obstruction requires microdissection or retrograde cannulation with intubation for at least 6 weeks postoperatively. If that fails a conjunctivodacryocystal rhinostomy with Lester Jones tubes (Lyons *et al.* 1993) is the only, albeit usually unsatisfactory, treatment.

Fistula of the nasolacrimal system

Fistulas may occur due to false passage formation after incision of a lacrimal sac abscess but more frequently they are bilateral developmental abnormalities, perhaps aberrant canaliculi (Welham *et al.* 1992). They are usually asymptomatic unless there is an associated nasolacrimal duct obstruction when they may leak tears or pus. Typically they appear just below the medial canthus (Fig. 26.1); they can be multiple. If they cause symptoms they can be excised after careful delineation of the canaliculi with or without a dacryocystorhinostomy (DCR) (Welham *et al.* 1992).

Congenital dacryocystocoele (amniotocoele, mucocoele, lacrimal sac cyst)

An unusual presentation of non-patent nasolacrimal system(s) (Mansour *et al.* 1991) may occur in the neonate

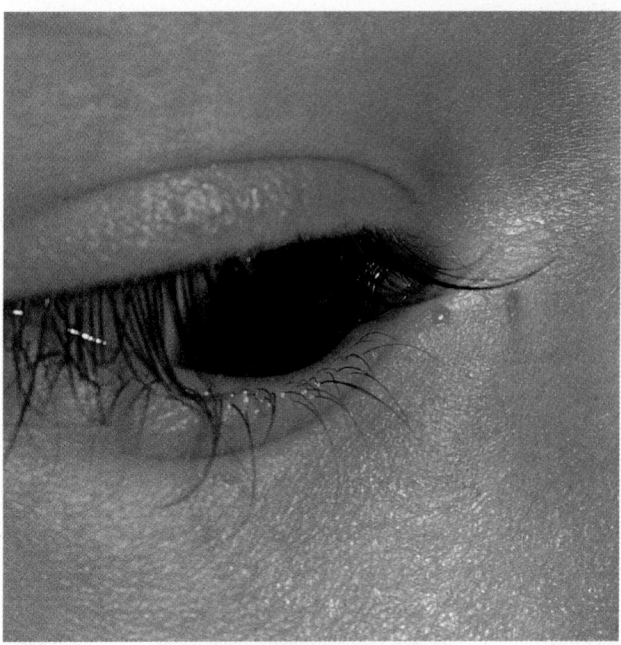

Fig. 26.1 Congenital fistula of the nasolacrimal system. The fistula can be seen as a tiny mark below the medial canthus.

when fluid has become trapped within the nasolacrimal sac and distends it. Various terms have been suggested for this condition; 'amniotocoele' has been used since, in part, the fluid within the sac was derived from amniotic fluid (Levy 1979), and 'mucocoele' to coincide with the appearance of the fluid obtained from the mass (Jackson & Lambert 1963; Scott *et al.* 1979). 'Dacryocystocoele' has been suggested (Harris & DiClementi 1982) as an attempt to describe the condition anatomically without implying the specific content of the swelling.

The baby has a bluish appearing mass (see Fig. 26.5), often 10–12 mm in diameter, in the region of the nasolacrimal sac. Appropriate management of the swelling has included prevention of secondary dacryocystitis, conservative massage (Levy 1979; Harris & DiClementi 1982) to probing within a few days (Scott *et al.* 1979). Rarely, this condition has resulted in respiratory compromise through obstruction (Edmond & Keech 1991; Grin *et al.* 1991), warranting prompt management by the ophthalmologist. Although meningocoele must be considered in the differential diagnosis, the appearance is so classic that further investigation is unnecessary unless the condition is not resolved within a week or unless clinical findings progress. One helpful differentiating feature is the presence of pulsations with a meningocoele on palpation. They must also be differentiated from midline nasal dermoids (Whelehan & Rose 1995).

Many can be expressed via the punctum, a proportion resolve spontaneously, others may require probing (Mansour *et al.* 1991).

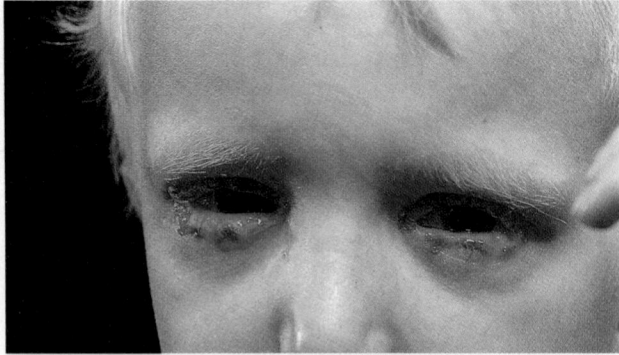

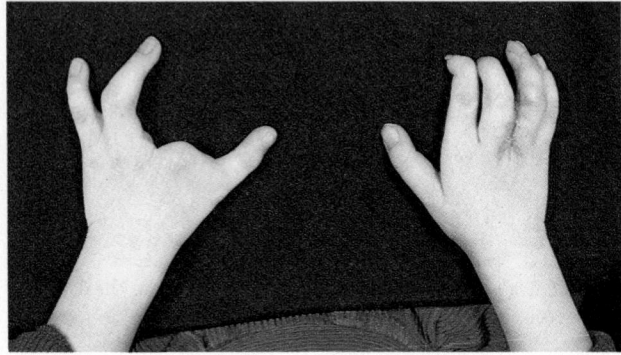

Fig. 26.2 EEC syndrome with a nasolacrimal duct obstruction. The bottom picture shows the 'lobster claw' deformity of the hands (see also p. 248).

Congenital nasolacrimal duct obstruction

This is frequent (MacEwan & Young 1991) and involves failure of the lacrimal system to establish patency to the nasal mucosa. It is usually an isolated defect but may be associated with the EEC syndrome (ectrodactyly, ectodermal dysplasia, clefting) (Fig. 26.2) or with craniofacial abnormalities such as the branchio-oculofacial syndrome (Lin *et al.* 1991; Fielding & Fryer 1992), craniometaphyseal or craniodiaphyseal dysplasia, Down's syndrome (Markowitz *et al.* 1994), LADD syndrome (Heinz *et al.* 1993), and the CHARGE association (Bowling & Chandna 1994) (see Chapter 50). The infant characteristically develops epiphora at 2–6 weeks; recurrent conjunctivitis, discharge, or dacryocystitis may also be associated. The condition is bilateral in approximately one-third of children (Crawford & Pashby 1984). The symptoms may be aggravated by wind or dust, but photophobia is absent.

Diagnosis can be supported by applying gentle pressure to express discharge through the punctae. Alternatively, agents such as fluorescein can be instilled and assessment made of its disappearance (MacEwen 1991), or within the oropharynx with the cobalt blue light—not easy in an infant! The fluorescein disappearance test is performed as follows.

1 Instil 1 drop of 1% fluorescein into the conjunctival sac.
2 Inspect at 2 and 5 minutes.
3 Grade the amount of fluorescein left between 0 and

3 (0 = no fluorescein left, 3 = no fluorescein disappeared). Normally, at 5 minutes the score should be between 0 and 1.

The management of the infant with nasolacrimal duct obstruction depends largely on the age of the infant and severity of symptoms. In general, primary care physicians assume this responsibility until the child is 6 months old unless the symptoms are particularly prominent or the parents are particularly worried. Many paediatricians will instruct the parents to massage the nasolacrimal sac region in an effort to hasten resolution (Kushner 1982). The most appropriate motion for this manoeuvre is to initially milk any discharge from the sac by gently stroking in an upward motion. Once cleaned, the nasolacrimal system should be firmly massaged with downward pressure. This technique forces any remaining fluid to press against the (presumably) remaining thin mucous membrane between the nasolacrimal duct and the nose. The number of strokes should be between three and five and repeated frequently throughout the day. The strokes should be firm, and done with an index finger with a well-trimmed nail! It may be helpful to recommend that every nappy change would be an appropriate time to perform this manoeuvre, before the nappy is changed.

The use of topical antibiotics in infants with epiphora is rather widespread amongst primary care physicians. This author's practice is to reserve antibiotics until there is evidence of conjunctivitis or pus enough to demand frequent cleaning of the discharge.

On the first visit, a complete ophthalmological assessment is indicated. Assessment of the patency or non-patency of the system can be made with fluorescein (MacEwen 1991). Congenital glaucoma must be excluded as an underlying cause for the epiphora, especially when there is no discharge. Diagrams should be drawn for the parents so that they can understand the proposed treatment. Topical antibiotics, usually sulfacetamide, can be prescribed if evidence of infection is present. Proper massage technique should be encouraged.

The decision to proceed with nasolacrimal probing is based primarily on the natural history (Fig. 26.3) of the condition (Paul & Shepherd 1994), severity, age, parental concern, and is tempered by the general health and the standard practice within the community. Most nasolacrimal probings are performed between 9 and 12 months of age. By waiting until this age, a chance of allowing spontaneous resolution is given (Kushner 1982; MacEwen & Young 1991). There is, however, nothing sacred about any particular age, and if the symptoms warrant it, or if there is a family history of dacryocystitis among siblings, probing in the first few months or even weeks of life may be appropriate.

The choice of venue for probing, either office or hospital, depends in large part on the training of the ophthalmologist, but is also influenced by medical economics and

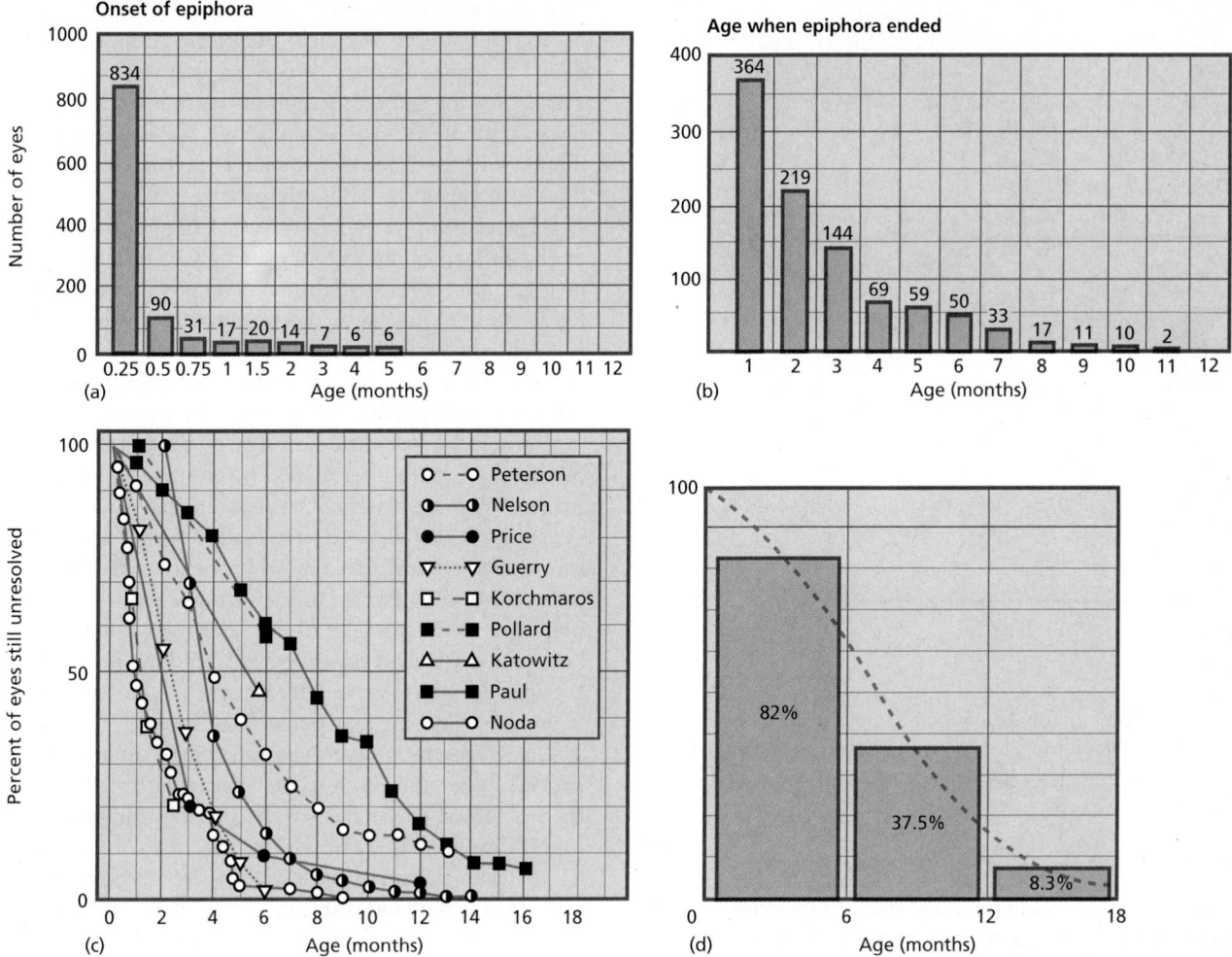

Fig. 26.3 (a) Age of onset of epiphora. In 95%, the epiphora presented during the first month of life. From MacEwen & Young (1991). (b) Spontaneous resolution. Each column represents the number of eyes that showed resolution of symptoms during that month of life. From MacEwan & Young (1991). (c) The rate of spontaneous resolution of nasolacrimal duct obstruction expressed as a percentage still unresolved at a given age in months. From Paul and Shepherd (1994). (d) Proportion of original cohort still symptomatic at various age ranges. From Paul and Shepherd (1994) with permission.

parental requests. The office-based probing procedure avoids a general anaesthetic and the expense of a hospital stay, and many parents will choose this option. The hospital-based probing procedure, in a controlled environment, undoubtedly involves less anxiety for the ophthalmologist. With current medical economics, a hospital-based procedure may cost 50–100 times as much as an office-based procedure. Probing under chloral hydrate sedation cannot be performed since manipulation is required. An office-based procedure requires a flat surface with overhead illumination, a restraint (or 'papoose') board, sterile nasolacrimal probing set, standard topical anaesthetic drops, applicators, and steady hands (earplugs for the ophthalmologist are optional!).

Some ophthalmologists prefer that the parents be with their baby: others will ask them to wait elsewhere. A detailed discussion of the procedure will be necessary if they are to observe, especially emphasizing that the procedure (i) is entirely outside of the globe itself; (ii) during the actual probing, the instrument will be rotated such that it appears almost like an acupuncture needle; and (iii) the major side-effect is a bloody nose or regurgitation of blood into the conjunctival sac. When the parents ask if the procedure hurts, it should be explained that there will be discomfort, but much of the crying is a consequence of being restrained in a foreign setting. The trauma to the baby is probably analogous to the discomfort when an intravenous line is placed in a baby. Virtually all parents report that their baby sleeps afterwards, presumably from being stressed by the procedure. Very few say their child acts differently; the worst reaction registered by parents has been that the baby experiences anxiety over being placed in a supine position for a day or two. Parents rarely say that, if given the choice again, they would prefer hospital-

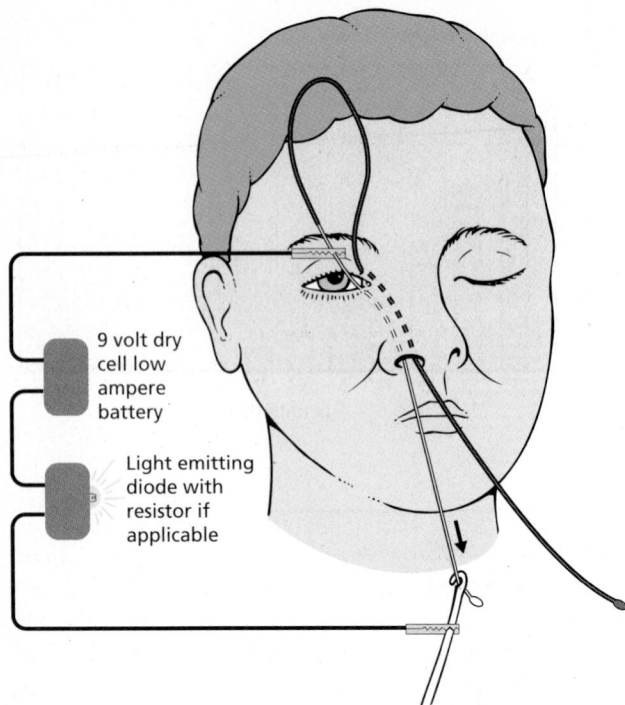

9 volt dry
cell low
ampere
battery

Light emitting
diode with
resistor if
applicable

Fig. 26.4 Silicone tube intubation of the nasolacrimal system can be facilitated by location of the Crawford's probe under the turbinate by the use of a low amperage electrical circuit.

ization, but some feel that as the risk of anaesthetic is negligible the psychological trauma is unwarranted.

Hospital-based probing is undoubtedly a more controlled procedure and is in many ways simpler for the physician since the child is under anaesthesia and the familiar operating room milieu is present. The same instrumentation is required, and the same steps are taken with the exception of instillation of anaesthetic drops and holding an applicator moistened with 4% xylocaine over the punctum. One initially dilates the superior or inferior punctum; a small gauge probe is then introduced at the superior punctum, perpendicular to the lid margin, for a short distance (approximately 1 mm). The probe is then rotated and advanced to follow the canalicular system in a horizontal and then inferoposterior direction. The probe should pass without much force so that false passages are not created. At the distal extreme, a resistance will be felt from the mucous membrane. A slight pop can be felt as this is broken with the probe. The feeling is similar to popping a balloon with a blunt needle. The 000 probe is removed and a larger gauge 00 or 0 probe inserted to provide further dilation. The now-patent system should be irrigated with 1 ml of balanced salt solution.

Probing of the opposite side, if indicated, may be performed at the same time if the baby has tolerated the procedure well. Probing should not be performed if there is

evidence of acute dacryocystitis.

Postoperatively, a topical antibiotic drop four times daily for a few days may be used as well as a nasal decongestant for the same time period (such as 0.25 or 0.125% phenylephrine or 0.5% ephedrine); do not use this in infants with cardiac disease or for prolonged periods of time, as it may induce hypertension.

The success of office-based procedures approaches 80% on the initial probing. Patency can usually be judged within days after the procedure. Most physicians prefer a repeat simple probing to tube placement unless the child is older or symptoms are severe.

If the turbinates are large, with boggy mucosa and a very tight ostium, they may be gently infractured. Tube insertion must be considered if two failed probings have occurred (Aggarwal *et al.* 1993), or in cases of trauma involving the nasolacrimal system. They may also be used in conjunction with dacryocystorhinostomy. Silicone tubes are used in which a metal probe is wedged or glued onto each end. Crawford tubes include a probe with a bulbous enlargement at the tip; Guibor tubes have a larger bore probe attached on either end. Under general anaesthesia, the superior and inferior systems are probed and irrigated to ensure that patency is present. The inferior system is then probed with one end of the tubing until the probe reaches the nasal cavity. Retrieval of the probe is then obtained either with a special hook-shaped instrument (Crawford 1977) or with a straight clamp. Although direct visualization of the metal probe can be attempted with appropriate nasal speculae, the young child's anatomy with large inferior turbinates often makes this difficult. A good coaxial light, a nasal endoscope and cocaine paste are also very useful.

The contact of the hook with the probe can be difficult to feel and is improved by connecting the probe and the hook to different levels of an electrical circuit (low amperage) in which there is a light bulb and when contact is made, it lights up (Fig. 26.4). A good coaxial headlight, and suitable nasal speculae, and other nose instruments, such as a nasendoscope, make the task much easier, but even the experienced must be humble, and be prepared to call for their ENT colleague if necessary!

One gains skill in prompt location of the probe by visualizing the angle formed between the inserted probe and the retrieving instrument. In comparison to adults, the probe is far more anteriorly located. Once the inferior system has its portion of tubing in place, the superior system is then canalized, leaving a loop of tubing which extends from superior to inferior punctum and two metal probes coming out of the nose. The loose ends are then securely tied to each other with multiple (six to eight) squared knots and the tubing then cut 1 cm from the knot. Future retrieval of the knotted end can be ensured by securing a 4.0 silk suture around the knot and cutting its end long. A single square knot in the silicone tubing (Ratliff & Meyer

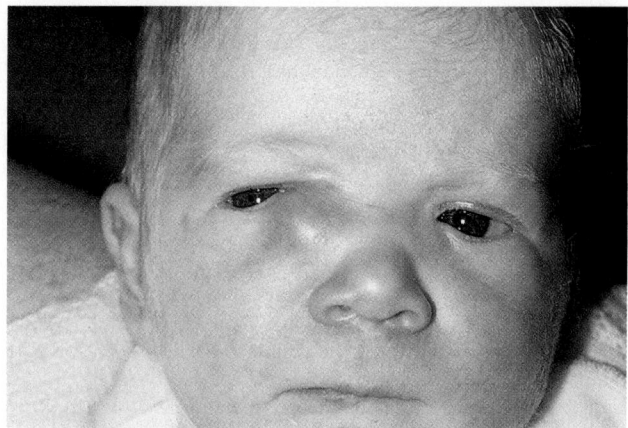

Fig. 26.5 Congenital dacryocystocele.

1994), an absorbable suture (Hunter 1995), or looping a single tube via both upper canaliculi over the nose (Arnold 1995) may make later removal more easy.

Tubes are usually left in place for 3–6 months so that patency may be established (Crawford & Pashby 1984). Removal in the young child usually requires a general anaesthetic unless the portion of tubing or silk suture can easily be seen in the nasal cavity. The loop is bisected, and tubing is then pulled through the nose.

Rarely, a dacryocystorhinostomy (DCR) must be performed in children. Indications include recurrent epiphora despite prior silicone intubation, inability to establish patency with simple probings and intubation, and trauma (Billson *et al.* 1978) involving the nasolacrimal sac. Although ophthalmologists have traditionally avoided its use in children, success is comparable to adult DCRs when particular attention is given to paediatric anatomy (Nowinski *et al.* 1985).

Children with cranial or facial anomalies, whether congenital or acquired, may be treated much as other children, although great care needs to be taken over identification of the anatomy (Hicks *et al.* 1994).

Acquired nasolacrimal duct obstruction

Acquired nasolacrimal duct obstruction may be caused by diseases of the nose, or paranasal sinuses, especially chronic allergic rhinitis. Rarely, acquired obstruction may herald a tumour (Baron *et al.* 1993), or bone disease such as fibrous dysplasia, craniometaphyseal or craniodiaphyseal dysplasia. Although DCR may be appropriate in some cases (McHugh *et al.* 1994), many would consider the high recurrence rate too high, and opt for dacryocystectomy, which stops the discharge and leaves surprisingly little watering. The use of dyed tissue adhesive to make the sac more visible makes this an easy technique (Rowson *et al.* 1994).

Acute dacryocystitis

Acute dacryocystitis (Fig. 26.6) frequently accompanies non-patent nasolacrimal systems since a stagnant system is present. Congenital acute dacryocystitis is very rare; the swelling usually represents a dacryocystocoele. Infantile acute dacryocystitis (Pollard 1991) requires systemic antibiotics, in much the same way as preseptal cellulitis. Rarely, an acute involvement may be associated with more generalized illness such as infectious mononucleosis (Atkinson *et al.* 1990). Prompt treatment is mandatory or a retrobulbar abscess may occur (Weiss & Leib 1993). Cultures should be taken if discharge can be expressed through the punctum. Probing should not be performed, since false passages can lead to orbital cellulitis and fistulae. Similarly, incision should preferably not be made in the acute phase since fistularization can occur even though much of the inflammation takes place around rather than in the lacrimal sac. If a fluctuant mass remains after resolution of the acute phase, evacuation can be performed with a 19-gauge needle into the lower pole of the sac, reducing the chances of fistularization, and placing the potential fistula track in the region where a DCR incision would be performed anyway. Once all signs of infection have been resolved, probing to establish patency should be performed.

Chronic dacryocystitis

Chronic dacryocystitis is more common than the acute form. The nasolacrimal sac is enlarged (Fig. 26.7) but the

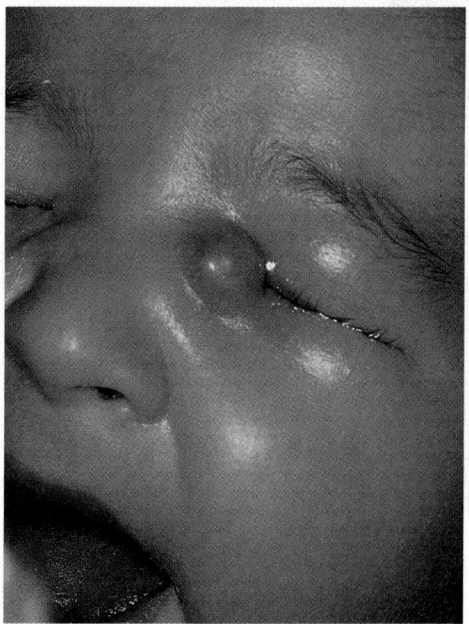

Fig. 26.6 Acute dacryocystitis. Mr R. Welham's patient.

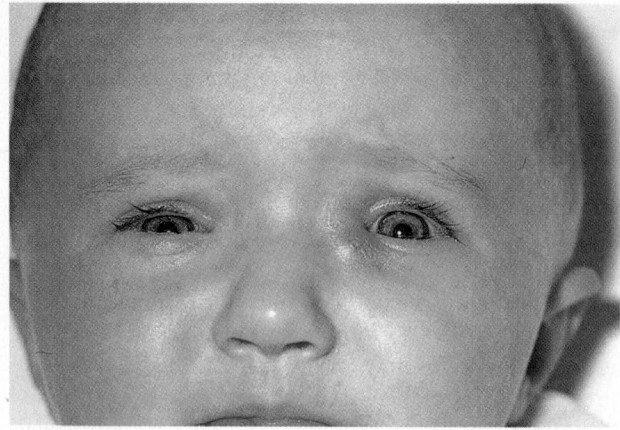

Fig. 26.7 Chronic recurrent dacryocystitis associated with nasolacrimal duct obstruction.

child is comfortable. Rarely, purulent discharge can be obtained. These patients require establishment of patency with probing after attempted irrigation. If a spontaneous fistula has occurred, probing should be hastened to encourage the fistula to close spontaneously.

Canaliculitis

Canaliculitis in children is uncommon. Treatment involves cultures and antibiotics. Probing in the active phase is to be avoided.

HIV

Although it is highly unlikely that tears were the transmitting vector, it is sensible for the ophthalmologist to wash their hands between cases and to be particularly cautious when examining a baby with HIV (Fujikawa *et al.* 1986). One might also take special precautions such as gloving in procedures such as the examination of a neonate that is failing to thrive.

References

Aggarwal R, Misson G, Donaldson I, Willshaw H. The role of naso-lacrimal intubation in the management of childhood epiphora. *Eye* 1993; **7**: 760–2.

Arnold RW. Bilateral monocanalicular silicone loop: predictable home removal of nasolacrimal stents. *J Pediatr Ophthalmol Strabismus* 1995; **32**: 200–1.

Atkinson P, Ansons A, Patterson A. Infectious mononucleosis presenting as bilateral acute dacryocystitis. *Br J Ophthalmol* 1990; **74**: 750–1.

Baron E, Kersten R, Kulevin D. Rhabdomyosarcoma manifesting as acquired nasolacrimal duct obstruction. *Am J Ophthalmol* 1993; **115**: 239–42.

Billson FA, Taylor HR, Hoyt CS. Trauma to the lacrimal system in children. *Am J Ophthalmol* 1978; **86**: 828–33.

Blanksma LJ, Pol BAE. Congenital fistulae of the lacrimal gland. *Br J Ophthalmol* 1980; **64**: 515–17.

Bowling B, Chandna A. Superior lacrimal canalicular atresia and nasolacrimal duct obstruction in the CHARGE association. *J Pediatr Ophthalmol Strabismus* 1994; **31**: 336–7.

Brownstein S, Belin MW, Krohel GB, Smith RS, Condon G, Codere F. Orbital dacryops. *Ophthalmology* 1984; **91**: 1424–9.

Cassady JV. Developmental anatomy of the nasolacrimal duct. *Arch Ophthalmol* 1952; **47**: 141–58.

Chavis RM, Garner A, Wright JE. Inflammatory orbital pseudotumour. *Arch Ophthalmol* 1978; **96**: 1817–22.

Chorobski J. Syndrome of crocodile tears. *Arch Neurol Psychiatr* 1951; **65**: 299–318.

Cogen M, Lewis A, Kelly A. Anomalous lacrimal ductule: case report and review. *J Pediatr Ophthalmol Strabismus* 1994; **31**: 327–9.

Crawford JA. Intubation of obstructions in the lacrimal system. *Can J Ophthalmol* 1977; **12**: 289–93.

Crawford JA, Pashby RC. Lacrimal system disorders. *Int Ophthalmol Clin* 1984; **24**: 39–53.

Dagher G, Anderson RL, Ossoinig KC, Baker JD. Adenoid cystic carcinoma of the lacrimal gland in a child. *Arch Ophthalmol* 1980; **98**: 1098–100.

Duke-Elder S, Cook C. The lacrimal gland. In: Duke-Elder S, ed. *System of Ophthalmology*, Vol. III, Part 1. London: Kimpton, 1963: 239–41.

Duke-Elder S, MacFaul PA. The ocular adnexa. In: Duke-Elder S, ed. *System of Ophthalmology*, Vol. VIII, Part 1. St Louis: CV Mosby, 1974: 605–10.

Edmond JC, Keech RV. Congenital nasolacrimal sac mucocele associated with respiratory distress. *J Pediatr Ophthalmol Strabismus* 1991; **28**: 287–9.

Fielding DW, Fryer AE. Recurrence of orbital cysts in the branchio-oculofacial syndrome. *J Med Genet* 1992; **29**: 430–1.

Fujikawa L, Salahuddin S, Ablashi D *et al.* HTLV III in the tears of AIDS patients. *Ophthalmology* 1986; **93**: 1471–81.

Goldberg MF, Payne JW, Brunt PW. Ophthalmologic studies of familial dysautonomia; the Riley–Day syndrome. *Arch Ophthalmol* 1968; **80**: 732–46.

Green WR, Zimmerman LE. Ectopic lacrimal gland tissue: report of eight cases with orbital involvement. *Arch Ophthalmol* 1967; **78**: 318–27.

Grin TR, Mertz JS, Stass-Isern M. Congenital nasolacrimal duct cysts in dacryocystocele. *Ophthalmology* 1991; **98**: 1238–42.

Guerry D, Kendig EL. Congenital impatency of the nasolacrimal duct. *Arch Ophthalmol* 1948; **39**: 193–204.

Harris GJ, DiClementi D. Congenital dacryocystocele. *Arch Ophthalmol* 1982; **100**: 1763–5.

Heinz G, Bateman J, Barrett D, Thargarel M, Crandall B. Ocular manifestations ot the lacrimo-auriculo-dento-digital syndrome. *Am J Ophthalmol* 1993; **115**: 243–8.

Hicks C, Pitts J, Rose G. Lacrimal surgery in patients with congenital cranial or facial anomalies. *Eye* 1994; **8**: 583–91.

Hunter LR. Crawford tubes (without suture) secured with absorbable suture. *J Pediatr Ophthalmol Strabismus* 1995; **32**: 197–9.

Jackson H, Lambert TD. Congenital mucocele of the lacrimal sac. *Br J Ophthalmol* 1963; **47**: 690–1.

Jacobs L, Sirkin S, Kinkel W. Ectopic lacrimal gland in the orbit identified by computerized axial transverse tomography. *Ann Ophthalmol* 1977; **9**: 591–3.

Katowitz JA, Welsh MG. Timing of initial probing and irrigation in congenital nasolacrimal duct obstruction. *Ophthalmology* 1987; **94**: 698–705.

Korchmaros I, Szalay E. Cannula-probing combined with nasal procedure for dacryocystitis neonatorum. *Acta Ophthalmol (Copenh)*

1978; **56**: 357–62.

Kushner B. Congenital nasolacrimal system obstruction. *Arch Ophthalmol* 1982; **100**: 597–600.

Lemp M, Blackman H. Physiology of tears. In: Milder B, Weil B, eds. *The Lacrimal System*. Connecticut: Appleton-Century-Crofts, 1983: 49–62.

Levy NS. Conservative management of congenital amniotocele of the nasolacrimal sac. *J Pediatr Ophthalmol Strabismus* 1979; **16**: 254–6.

Lin AE, Lasken HW, Jaffe R, Biglan A. The branchio-oculo-facial syndrome. *Cleft Palate Craniofacial J* 1991; **28**: 96–102.

Lyons C, Rosser P, Welham R. The management of punctal agenesis. *Ophthalmology* 1993; **100**: 1851–5.

MacEwen CJ. The fluorescein disappearance test (FDT): an evaluation of its use in infants. *J Pediatr Ophthalmol Strabismus* 1991; **28**: 302–5.

MacEwen CJ, Young JD. Epiphora during the first year of life. *Eye* 1991; **5**: 596–600.

Mansour A, Cheng K, Mumma J *et al.* Congenital dacryocele: a collaborative review. *Ophthalmology* 1991; **98**: 1744–51.

Markowitz G, Handler L, Katowitz J. Congenital euryblepharon and nasolacrimal anomalies in a patient with Down syndrome. *J Pediatr Ophthalmol Strabismus* 1994; **31**: 330–1.

McHugh D, Rose G, Garner A. Nasolacrimal obstruction and facial bone histopathology in craniodiaphyseal dysplasia. *Br J Ophthalmol* 1994; **78**: 501–3.

Mindlin A, Lamberts D, Barsky D. Mixed lacrimal gland tumors arising from ectopic lacrimal gland tissue in the orbit. *J Pediatr Ophthalmol* 1977; **14**: 44–6.

Mottow LS, Jakobiec FA. Idiopathic inflammatory orbital pseudotumour in childhood I. Clinical characteristics. *Arch Ophthalmol* 1978; **96**: 1410–17.

Mueller EC, Borit A. Aberrant lacrimal gland and pleomorphic adenoma within the muscle cone. *Ann Ophthalmol* 1979; **11**: 661–3.

Mukherji R, Mukhopadhay SD. Congenital bilateral lacrimal and pre-auricular fistulas. *Am J Ophthalmol* 1972; **73**: 595–6.

Murube-del-Castillo J. Development of the lacrimal apparatus. In: Milden B, Weil B, eds. *The Lacrimal System*. Connecticut: Appleton-Century-Crofts, 1983: 9–22.

Nelson LB, Calhoun JH, Menduke H. Medical management of congenital nasolacrimal duct obstruction. *Ophthalmology* 1985; **92**: 1187–90.

Noda S, Hayasaka S, Setogawa T. Congenital nasolacrimal duct obstruction in Japanese infants: its incidence and treatment with massage. *J Pediatr Ophthalmol Strabismus* 1991; **28**: 20–2.

Nowinski TS, Flanagan JC, Mauriello J. Pediatric dacryocystorhinostomy. *Arch Ophthalmol* 1985; **103**: 1226–8.

Patrick RK. Lacrimal secretions in full-term and premature babies. *Trans Ophthalmol Soc UK* 1974; **94**: 283–310.

Paul TO. Medical management of congenital nasolacrimal duct obstruction. *J Pediatr Ophthalmol Strabismus* 1985; **22**: 68–70.

Paul TO, Shepherd R. Congenital nasolacrimal duct obstruction: natural history and the timing of optimal intervention. *J Pediatr Ophthalmol Strabismus* 1994; **31**; 362–7.

Peterson RA, Robb RM. The natural course of congenital obstruction of the nasolacrimal duct. *J Pediatr Ophthalmol Strabismus* 1978; **15**: 246–50.

Pollard Z. Treatment of acute dacryocystitis in neonates. *J Pediatr Ophthalmol Strabismus* 1991; **28**: 341–3.

Pollard ZF. Tear duct obstruction in babies. *J Med Assoc Georgia* 1978; **68**: 464–6.

Price HW. Dacryostenosis. *J Pediatr* 1947; **30**: 302–5.

Ramsay J, Taylor D. Congenital crocodile tears: a key to the aetiology of Duane's syndrome. *Br J Ophthalmol* 1980; **64**: 518–22.

Ratliff C, Meyer D. Silicone intubation without intranasal fixation for treatment of congenital nasolacrimal duct obstruction. *Am J Ophthalmol* 1994; **118**: 781–5.

Riffenburgh RS. Ocular manifestations of mumps. *Arch Ophthalmol* 1961; **66**: 739–43.

Riley CM. Familial autonomic dysfunction. *J Am Med Assoc* 1952; **149**: 1532–5.

Riley CM, Day RL, Greeley D, Langford WS. Central autonomic dysfunction with defective lacrimation: I. Report of five cases. *Pediatrics* 1949; **3**: 468–78.

Riley CM, Moore RH. Familial dysautonomia differentiated from related disorders. *Pediatrics* 1966; **37**: 435–46.

Rowson N, Kent D, Taylor D. The use of fibrin adhesive as an aid to dacryocystectomy. *Orbit* 1994; **13**: 81–3.

Rush JA, Leone CR Jr. Ectopic lacrimal gland cyst of the orbit. *Am J Ophthalmol* 1981; **92**: 198–201.

Schwarz M. Congenital atresia of the nasolacrimal canal. *Arch Ophthalmol* 1935; **13**: 301–2.

Scott WE, Fabre JA, Ossoinig KC. Congenital mucocele of the lacrimal sac. *Arch Ophthalmol* 1979; **97**: 1656–8.

Sevel D. Development and congenital abnormalities of the nasolacrimal apparatus. *J Pediatr Ophthalmol Strabismus* 1981; **18**: 13–19.

Smith S, Rootman J. Clinical pathological review lacrimal ductal cysts. Presentation and management. *Surv Ophthalmol* 1986; **30**: 245–51.

Thompson E, Pembury M, Graham JM. Phenotypic variation in the LADD syndrome. *J Med Genet* 1985; **22**: 382–5.

Uleckas JK, Garel L, Milot J, Mathieu-Millaire F. Orbital CT scan in congenital alacrima. *J Pediatr Ophthalmol Strabismus* 1994; **31**: 114–17.

Weiss G, Leib M. Congenital dacryocystitis and retrobulbar abscess. *J Paediatr Ophthalmol Strabismus* 1993; **30**: 217–72.

Whelehan I, Rose GE. Midline nasal dermoids presenting like discharging lacrimal sac mucocoeles. *Eye* 1995; **9**: 479–84.

Welham R, Bates A, Stasior G. Congenital lacrimal fistula. *Eye* 1992; **6**: 211–14.

Werb A. The anatomy of the lacrimal system. In: Milder B, Weil B, eds. *The Lacrimal System*. Connecticut: Appleton-Century-Crofts, 1983: 23–32.

Wright JE. Factors affecting the survival of patients with lacrimal gland tumours. *Can J Ophthalmol* 1982; **17**: 3–9.

Wright JE, William B, Krohel GB. Clinical presentation and management of lacrimal gland tumours. *Br J Ophthalmol* 1979; **63**: 600–6.

27: Orbital Disease in Children

Christopher Lyons and Jack Rootman

Abnormalities of the orbit in childhood may result from developmental anomalies, or may be acquired from orbital disease.

Developmental abnormalities may be confined to the orbit or be part of a more widespread craniofacial malformation. The orbit may be smaller than normal or may be shallow, resulting in proptosis. The relationship between the two orbits may be disturbed: in hypertelorism the orbits are widely separated; conversely, in hypotelorism, they are set close together. Part of the orbital walls may be deficient at birth allowing prolapse of intracranial tissue into the orbit, a cause of pulsating exophthalmos. Normally, the orbits continue to develop throughout childhood but congenital absence of the globe, enucleation or radiotherapy may result in failure of the orbit to grow normally on the affected side.

Children with acquired orbital disease most commonly present with signs and symptoms of a mass within the orbit. The term 'mass effect' encompasses these signs and includes proptosis which may be axial or non-axial, as well as the soft tissue signs which may accompany the presence of an orbital mass. Occasionally, the mass itself is seen or palpated by the parents. Other presenting symptoms and signs include reduced vision, restriction of ocular movements, pain and inflammation. Occasionally, enophthalmos may be a presenting sign, for instance following orbital trauma resulting in a blow-out fracture.

The relative frequencies of the conditions causing proptosis in childhood have varied considerably in previous series (Porterfield 1962; MacCarty & Brown 1964; Youseffi 1969; Templeton 1971; Eldrup-Jorgensen & Fledelius 1975; Crawford 1983; Shields *et al.* 1986; Kodsi *et al.* 1994) depending, in part, on the source of the material. Series from eye hospitals (Youseffi 1969) are different from those from neurosurgical (MacCarty & Brown 1964) or paediatric units (Crawford 1983). Geographical factors are also important. For example, the major causes of proptosis in African children (Templeton 1971) are different from those seen in Europe and North America. Series which have relied solely on histopathological examination of biopsy specimens (Porterfield 1962; Eldrup-Jorgensen & Fledelius 1975; Shields *et al.* 1986; Kodsi *et al.* 1994) reflect the incidence of lesions which are encountered surgically. However, biopsy-based studies do not represent the many conditions which can be diagnosed and treated without biopsy or surgery, such as capillary haemangioma, or those in which biopsy may be more conveniently obtained at another site of involvement, such as neuroblastoma or histiocytosis. In that sense, they are not helpful in formulating the differential diagnosis of a child with proptosis.

Orbital disease and age

The reviews discussed above have stressed the major differences between childhood and adult orbital disease. However, even within the 'childhood' years, defined here as ages up to and including 16 years, there are trends in the incidence of the causative disorders which, when understood, can usefully contribute to the diagnostic process.

We have reviewed the clinical data of the 320 children seen by the orbital service in Vancouver since 1976 (Table 27.1). This period postdates the introduction of the computed tomography (CT) scan, a watershed in the non-invasive investigation of orbital disease. It is clear from Figure 27.1 that structural abnormalities (including cysts) and neoplasia account for the great majority of children presenting with orbital disease. This is quite different from the adult pattern of orbital disease, in which over 50% of presentations are due to inflammatory causes and structural abnormalities account for less than 20% of cases (Rootman 1988). The distribution of orbital disease

Table 27.1 Orbital disease in children—multiseries data comparison.

	Rootman 1993		Bullock *et al.* 1989		Crawford 1983		All series	
	No.	%	No.	%	No.	%	Total	%
Neoplasia								
Optic nerve glioma	16	5.6	5	3.6	17	3.0	38	3.9
Meningioma	3	1.0	2	1.4			5	0.5
Other neurogenic tumour	1	0.3					1	0.1
PNS tumours	11	3.8	9	6.4	14	2.5	34	3.4
Lymphocytic	2	0.7	1	0.7	23	4.1	26	2.6
Other lymphocytic	4	1.4	4	2.9			8	0.8
Histiocytic	5	1.7	1	0.7	20	3.6	26	2.6
Vascular	55	19.1	19	13.6	18	3.2	92	9.3
Secondary/metastatic	4	1.4	4	2.9	21	3.8	29	2.9
Mesenchymal								
rhabdomyosarcoma	6	2.1	3	2.1	11	2.0	20	2.0
fibrous	1	0.3	3	2.1	1	0.2	5	0.5
histiocytic	3	1.0	2	1.4			5	0.5
bone	5	1.7	1	0.7	6	1.1	12	1.2
neoplasia	7	2.4	2	1.4	1	0.2	10	1.0
other	2	0.7					2	0.2
Unknown neoplasia			1	0.7	3	0.5	4	0.4
Lacrimal (adenoid cystic)	2	0.7					2	0.2
Teratoma					1	0.2	1	0.1
Structural								
Cystic	51	17.7	59	42.1	6	1.1	116	11.8
Bone anomalies	8	2.8			50	8.9	58	5.9
Ectopia	6	2.1	11	7.9			17	1.7
Other—acquired	2	0.7					2	0.2
Inflammatory								
Infectious diseases	17	5.9			232	41.5	249	25.2
NSOIS	14	4.9	6	4.3	5	0.9	25	2.5
Other—inflammatory	6	2.1	3	2.1			9	0.9
Thyroid orbitopathy	36	12.5			107	19.1	143	14.5
Vascular	16	5.6	4	2.9	10	1.8	30	3.0
Atrophy/degeneration	3	1.0					3	0.3
Unknown	2	0.7			13	2.3	15	1.5
Total	288	100.0	140	100.0	559	100.0	987	100.0

NSOIS, non-specific orbital inflammatory syndrome; PNS, peripheral nervous system.

in children aged over 11 years largely conforms to the adult pattern (Fig. 27.2).

Surprisingly, only a small proportion of the neoplasia can be considered malignant, which concurs with previously published series (Crawford 1983; Shields *et al.* 1986; Bullock *et al.* 1989). Under 2 years of age (Fig. 27.3), the major causes of proptosis are capillary haemangioma and lymphangioma, inclusion and dermoid cysts, and structural abnormalities. Figure 27.3, in which the distribution of the major diagnostic groups is shown by age at presentation, shows that whilst some lesions are distributed evenly throughout childhood (lymphangioma, varices and arteriovenous malformations), others tend to occur within a specific age range. Six patients with rhabdomyosarcoma were seen, whose ages ranged from 4 to 11 years. The five patients with histiocytosis-X ranged in age from 5 to 9 years. Capillary haemangiomas did not present after the age of 7 years. Inflammatory conditions con-

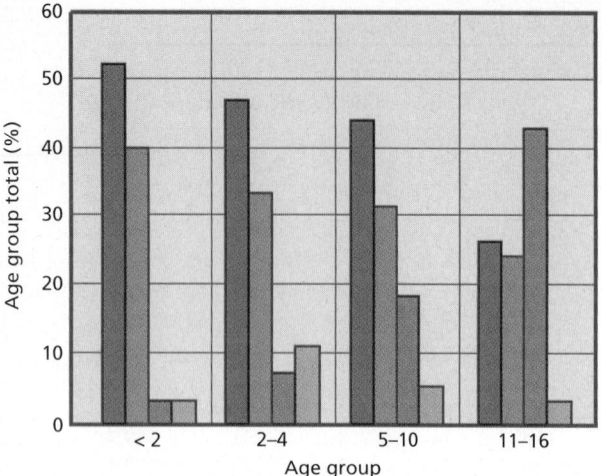

Fig. 27.1 Distribution of orbital disease by age group in patients less than 17 years of age. ▪ Neoplastic; ▪ structural; ▪ inflammatory; ▫ vascular.

tributed increasingly to numbers after the age of 5 years, especially orbital cellulitis, non-specific orbital inflammatory syndromes (6 years and over) and thyroid orbitopathy (10 years and over). The small numbers involved do not allow hard and fast rules to be stated since, for example, histiocytosis is well known to occur in infancy and early childhood, but this series may provide clinicians with a framework for the working diagnosis of a child with mass effect. It is also noteworthy that there were two cases of lacrimal gland carcinoma and two of Wegener's granuloma in this series, a reminder that, although rare, these potentially lethal conditions do occur in children.

Clinical assessment

When assessing a child with orbital disease, a careful history, examination and differential diagnosis in the context of the child's age are essential before investigations can be planned.

History

The age of onset, laterality (unilateral or bilateral) and the tempo of onset are important clues to the underlying diagnosis. As with adult orbital disease, the duration is often difficult to determine accurately. A review of old photographs may be helpful to identify the time of onset of an orbital problem.

Bilateral proptosis in early infancy is often due to orbital shallowing in craniofacial malformations. This can occasionally be unilateral, as in plagiocephaly. Usually, however, unilateral proptosis is due to the globe being displaced forward by a mass within the orbit.

Benign tumours such as optic nerve glioma or dermoid cyst grow slowly. Rapidly increasing proptosis suggests a metastatic deposit or rapidly growing tumour such as rhabdomyosarcoma. Rapid tumour growth may be associated with necrosis, resulting in periorbital ecchymosis. The presence of bilateral ecchymosis is suggestive of orbital deposits in neuroblastoma.

A catastrophic onset (within hours) implies a bleed within an (often unsuspected) pre-existing lesion such as a lymphangioma. Occasionally, the onset of orbital cellulitis may also be very sudden. Here, it is usually accompanied by pain, local inflammation and limitation of ocular motility in a child who is generally ill and febrile. The presence of clinically detectable orbital and periorbital inflammatory symptoms and signs in childhood is overwhelmingly associated with either infection or non-specific orbital inflammatory disease. Although inflammation is part of the classical description of rhabdomyosarcoma, this sign was absent in all six patients with this diagnosis treated by the orbital service at this centre over the last 18 years.

Most round-cell tumours in childhood, including rhabdomyosarcoma, granulocytic sarcoma (chloroma) and Ewing's sarcoma, present as a mass developing over weeks in a subacute manner except neuroblastoma, which can present with onset of proptosis over days.

An increase in proptosis with crying or straining is sug-

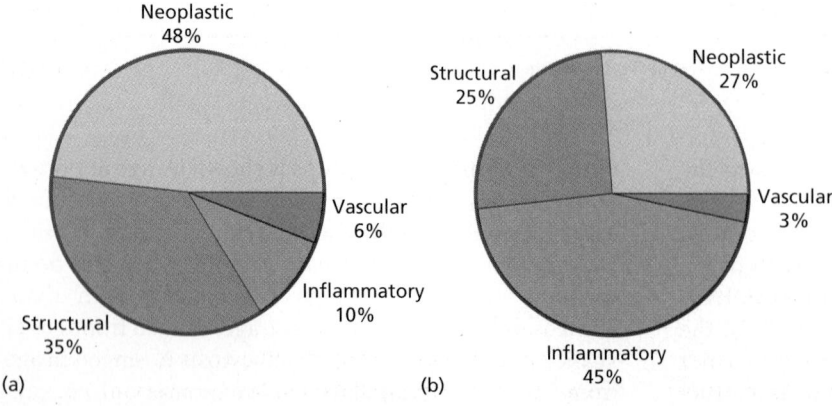

Fig. 27.2 (a) Distribution of orbital disease in patients less than 11 years of age. (b) Distribution of orbital disease in patients 11–17 years.

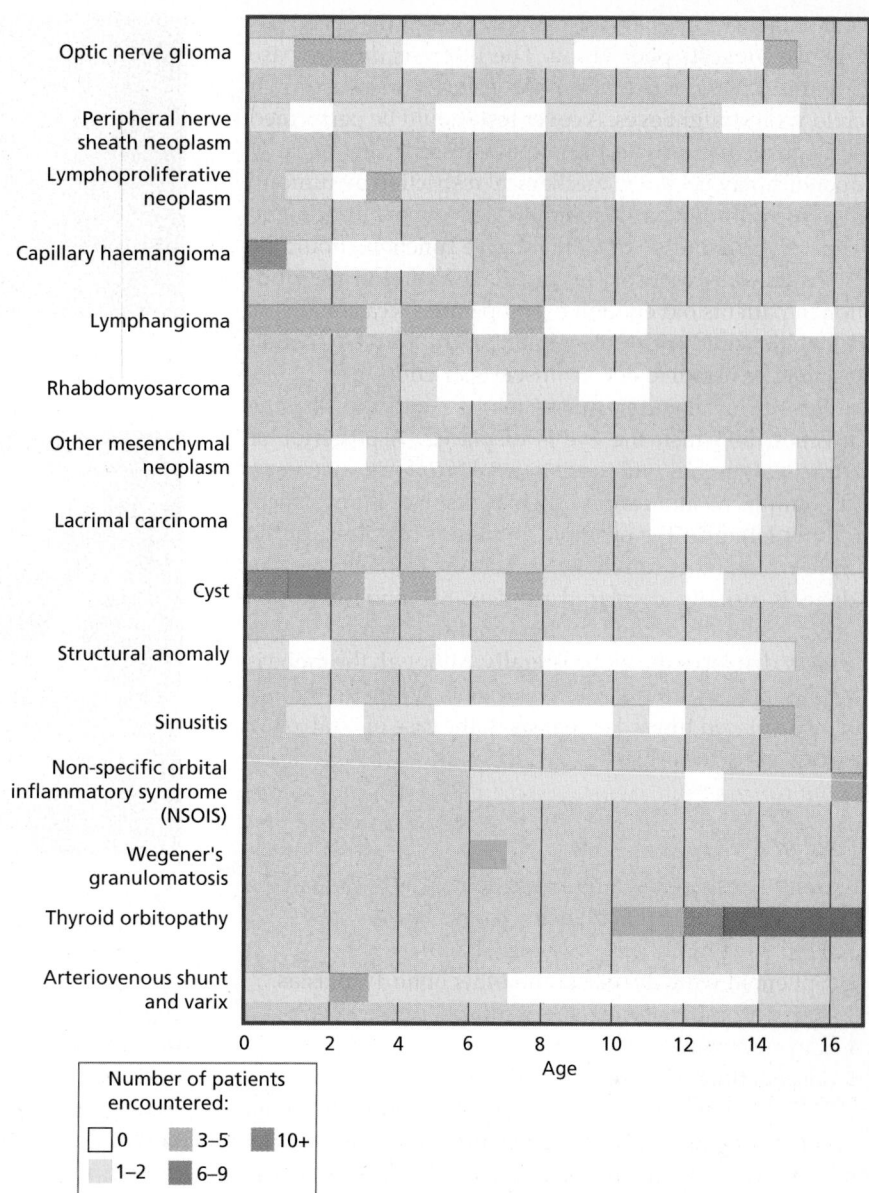

Fig. 27.3 Age distribution of common orbital diseases.

gestive of capillary haemangioma, lymphangioma, varices or absence of the sphenoid wing (as in neurofibromatosis type 1, NF1). This sign is useful in the neonate, where crying is almost invariably elicited by a thorough examination. When very obvious, its presence helps to exclude malignancy as a cause of the proptosis.

Pulsating exophthalmos may be associated with congenital defects of the orbital wall (as seen in NF1) or encephalocoele. Occasionally, large capillary haemangiomas may pulsate due to their rich arterial blood supply, as may high-flow arteriovenous shunts. The latter are rare in childhood.

Skin discoloration may offer a clue to the underlying aetiology. Red is suggestive of the arterial supply of capil-

lary haemangioma which, when superficial to the septum, almost invariably involves the overlying skin. When deep, these may have a blueish or purple hue. Venous lesions, such as varices or lymphangiomas, appear blue or purple, as do some cystic lesions such as lacrimal or conjunctival cysts. The brownish cutaneous discoloration of haemosiderin is usually caused by previous bleeds into a lymphangioma or, rarely, by neuroblastoma. Both of these may present with spontaneous ecchymosis.

Examination

Children with proptosis must have a visual acuity assessment. In infants, this may be limited to observing the fixation of the two eyes; resentment to cover of the contralateral eye suggests poor vision. The 10-prism dioptre base down test may be useful if poor vision is suspected in a child with straight eyes. A cover test should be performed and ocular ductions and versions assessed. Limitation of ductions may be due to mechanical restriction by tumour, muscle infiltration, inflammation, oedema or entrapment. Third, fourth and sixth cranial nerve function should be tested, as well as sensory testing in the Vi and Vii distribution in patients old enough to co-operate. Occasionally, as in an older child with a blow-out fracture, a forced duction test may be useful to detect muscle restriction.

The site of an orbital mass may be indicated by the direction in which the eye is displaced. A posterior or intraconal tumour will result in axial proptosis, whereas a tumour placed more anteriorly may displace the eye vertically or laterally. For example, in fibrous dysplasia of the orbit, which most commonly affects the frontal bone, the globe is usually displaced downwards and forwards. Orbital cellulitis secondary to ethmoidal sinus infection usually displaces the globe laterally. Although the globe is displaced away from most mass lesions, it can occasionally be displaced towards them, as in the case of cicatrizing metastasis to the orbit.

Enophthalmos

Enophthalmos, or a relative recession of the eyeball in the orbit, may occur in the following cases.
1 Following radiotherapy (Fig. 27.4).
2 Sphenoid wing dysplasia and other bone dysplasias.
3 Parry–Romberg syndrome or morphoea (Fig. 27.5).
4 Developmental tumours (Fig. 27.6).
5 Orbital floor blow-out fracture.

The position of the globe should be recorded using an exophthalmometer with a transparent ruler to measure the amount of vertical and horizontal displacement. The eyelid position should be recorded; retraction or lag may

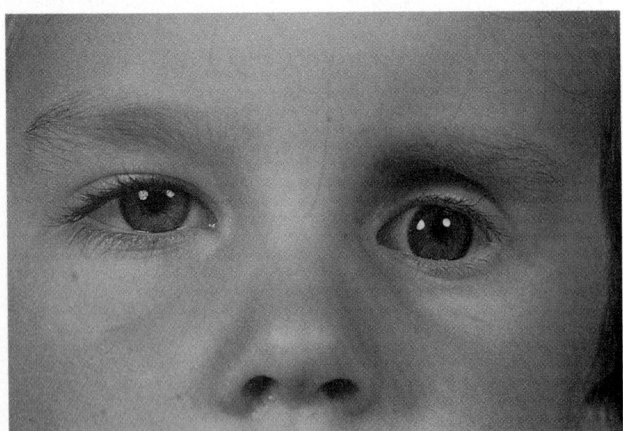

Fig. 27.4 Left enophthalmos following radiotherapy for retinoblastoma. Dr Jack Rootman's patient.

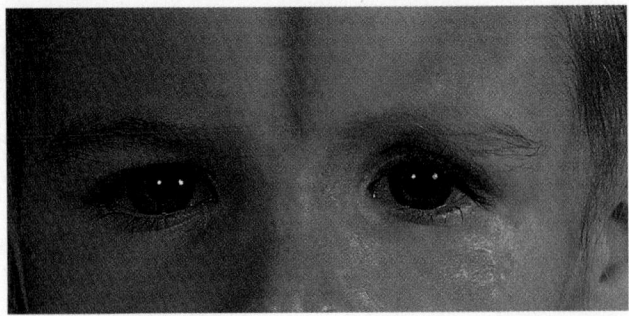

Fig. 27.5 Enophthalmos with morphoea en coup de sabre.

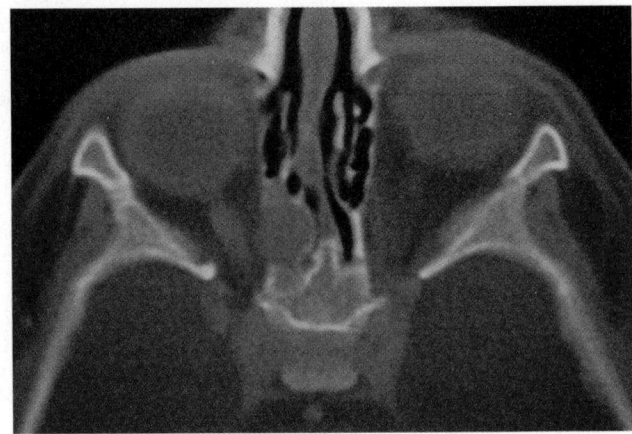

Fig. 27.6 Acquired enophthalmos caused by an astroglial tumour involving the paranasal sinuses.

suggest thyroid orbitopathy, but may also be indicative of tethering by tumour such as Langerhans' cell histiocytosis.

Slit-lamp examination may show dilated venous channels in the conjunctiva of patients with varices. Lymphangioma may be associated with visible conjunctival lymphangiectasis or cysts, which occasionally contain a meniscus of blood. The presence of Lisch nodules on the iris is one of the earliest diagnostic signs of NF1. Their identification might suggest plexiform neurofibroma or sphenoid wing dysplasia as causes of proptosis. Optic nerve glioma is thought to run a relatively benign course in the presence of NF1 and identification of Lisch nodules in an affected patient may suggest a relatively good visual prognosis, but a poorer prognosis for survival due to the risk of developing other central nervous system tumours. Juvenile cataract is increasingly realized as an early marker for NF2 and its identification may suggest meningioma or schwannoma as a cause of orbital mass effect, possibly prompting audiological assessment for the presence of vestibular schwannomas.

The presence of an afferent pupillary defect indicates optic neuropathy which may be due to extrinsic compression, as in fibrous dysplasia involving the optic canal, or to intrinsic disease, as in glioma. In the co-operative child, the use of neutral density filters allows accurate comparison of the affected nerve with its fellow. In this situation, field testing might reveal the central scotoma of optic neuropathy; chiasmal involvement, for example by glioma, may show bitemporal field loss. In the older age group, colour vision may be assessed using subjective red desaturation or an Ishihara chart, to confirm the presence of a subtle optic neuropathy.

Cycloplegic refraction is important to detect the presence of astigmatism due to distortion of the globe by an orbital mass. Retrobulbar lesions tend to result in a hyperopic shift whilst lesions at or anterior to the equator produce astigmatism. Left untreated, these changes are important causes of amblyopia (Bogan *et al.* 1987). Occasionally, myopia may mimic proptosis. This is particularly so when unilateral. Long-term occlusion of an eye, as in uncorrected unilateral ptosis due to capillary haemangioma, results in ipsilateral axial myopia.

Optic disc swelling or atrophy may be present in patients with optic nerve compression or glioma. Choroidal folds may be evident if the mass is close behind the globe. Opticociliary shunt vessels, classically associated with meningioma, are also commonly seen with optic nerve glioma.

Palpation of the orbit reveals the consistency of a localized mass. Capillary haemangiomas feel firm and spongy, and their contents cannot be expelled by palpation, whereas orbital varices are easily drained of blood, even with gentle pressure. Dermoids should be carefully examined for mobility and the presence of a tail extending into the posterior orbit or temporalis fossa. A posterior extension or extension through the lateral wall of the orbit is more likely to be present in dermoids which are situated inside the orbital rim than in those directly overlying the rim.

Although the orbit does not have true lymphatics, the pre-auricular and submandibular lymph nodes should be palpated to exclude enlargement from metastasis, as in rhabdomyosarcoma involving the eyelids, or infection, as in orbital cellulitis.

The evaluation of children with orbital disease should include systemic examination, since this may give useful clues to the diagnosis. Café-au-lait spots may suggest a diagnosis of neurofibromatosis, and skin pigmentation may also be seen in fibrous dysplasia. Characteristic skin lesions may also be present in Langerhans' cell histiocytosis and juvenile xanthogranuloma. Capillary haemangioma of the orbit is often associated with cutaneous capillary haemangiomas elsewhere. In suspected metastatic disease there may be other involved sites such as an abdominal mass in neuroblastoma or skin, scalp or bony lesions in Langerhans' cell histiocytosis. Thyroid orbitopathy may be accompanied by systemic signs of hyperthyroidism suggestive of this diagnosis.

Opinions from other specialists, particularly general paediatricians and ENT surgeons, may help to determine the cause of unexplained proptosis in a child.

Investigations

Investigation of children with proptosis should be guided by the history and clinical findings and tailored to each individual case. In some cases, like craniofacial abnormalities, the abnormalities fit a clear pattern and further investigations are not warranted. In others further tests will be necessary to confirm the suspected diagnosis or to assess the degree of orbital involvement. When other systems are involved, such as extension of tumour into the brain or sinuses or systemic involvement in malignancy, investigation of the child should, from the outset, be planned with the other specialists who may become involved in the child's care.

Radiology

Plain X-rays

Although CT scan is the initial radiological investigation in most patients with orbital disease, plain X-rays are still useful in certain circumstances. These include the assessment of orbital bony trauma, the localization of a radio-opaque orbital foreign body, assessment of systemic disease (such as absence of the sphenoid wing in neurofibromatosis) and morphometric studies when planning craniofacial surgery.

Sinus X-rays in suspected sinus disease with orbital cellulitis should be interpreted with care, since sinus anatomy is very variable under the age of 10 years. Although the finding of bony distortion on the affected side suggests a long-standing or slow-growing process in adults, this sign is unreliable in children, where it may be seen with rapidly enlarging lesions (see Fig. 32.4).

The principal merits of plain X-rays are the ubiquity of the equipment, low cost and the fact that sedation is rarely required. Although the dose of radiation delivered in a CT scan of the orbit is higher than that used in a plain X-ray, the diagnostic yield per unit of radiation exposure is much greater with CT (Weiss *et al.* 1984).

Computed tomography and magnetic resonance imaging

Diagnostic imaging of orbital structures was revolutionized by the development of CT in the early 1970s (Ambrose *et al.* 1974; Gawler *et al.* 1974). Optimal imaging requires 2–3 mm slice thickness and both direct coronal and axial images. CT will provide information about intracranial as well as orbital structures (Lloyd 1977). This technique yields more information on bony detail if soft tissue and 'bone window' settings are specifically requested. The differential diagnostic yield is increased by the use of contrast in selected cases (Moseley & Sanders 1982), since vascular, inflammatory and some malignancies are enhanced after its injection. Sedation is usually necessary under the age of 5 years. Other disadvantages include the relatively high dose of radiation delivered to the eye and the fact that only coronal or axial images can be obtained directly. Other images can be created by reformatting the information acquired in different planes, although this process often results in loss of definition.

Magnetic resonance imaging (MRI) provides higher resolution without exposure to ionizing radiation. This is particularly important if repeat imaging is necessary, for example a child with NF1 and optic nerve glioma who is being followed up regularly. Any desired plane can be chosen at the time of the examination, e.g. directly along the optic nerve. Orbital views may be obtained with a 0.5–1.5 tesla field, and surface coils may be used to increase the surface to noise ratio. Contrast enhancement can be obtained for similar indications to those outlined above for CT, using agents such as Gadolinium. These result in T1 shortening. Because fat has a bright signal on T1-weighted images, fat saturation techniques must be used to maximize the conspicuity of contrast enhancement in the orbit. Multiple image sequences can provide characteristic signal patterns, such as the fluid/fluid levels typical of slow-flow vascular malformations. Identification and dating of blood within haemorrhagic lesions such as lymphangiomas, presence or absence of flow within mass lesions and contrast enhancement of the optic nerve in optic neuritis are further strengths of this technique in the orbit.

Disadvantages include the time taken to image an orbit, which is in the order of 30–45 minutes (compared with CT which takes 15 minutes), the contraindications of the technique in patients with ferromagnetic foreign bodies, including aneurysm clips, and the necessity to sedate most patients aged 7 years or less because of the noise and duration of the procedure. A more specific problem of MRI for orbital work is its relative inability to image bone and calcification (Leib & Kates 1988), which is particularly important when differentiating glioma from meningioma in the orbit.

The texts by Newton and Bilaniuk (1990) and Bilaniuk and Farber (1992) are useful for readers seeking further information on imaging of the orbit in childhood.

Surgery

The surgical approach for access to the child's orbit differs markedly from that taken in adult orbital disease. This is due to the relative shallowness of the orbit in childhood. Lateral orbitotomy, in which the lateral orbital wall is removed, is unnecessary in most cases since the lesions can usually be reached via the relatively atraumatic anterior approach.

References

Ambrose JAE, Lloyd GAS, Wright JE. A preliminary evaluation of fine matrix computerized axial tomography (EMI scan) in the diagnosis of orbital space-occupying lesions. *Br J Radiol* 1974; **47**: 747–51.

Bilaniuk LT, Farber M. Imaging of developmental anomalies of the eye and orbit. *Am J Neuroradiol* 1992; **13**: 793–803.

Bogan S, Simon JW, Krohel GB, Nelson LB. Astigmatism associated with adnexal masses in infancy. *Arch Ophthalmol* 1987; **105**: 1368–70.

Bullock JD, Goldberg SH, Rakes SM. Orbital tumors in children. *Ophthal Plastic Reconstr Surg* 1989; **5**: 13–16.

Crawford JS. In: Crawford JS, Morin JD, eds. Diseases of the Orbit. In: *The Eye in Childhood*. New York: Grune & Stratton, 1983: 361–94.

Eldrup-Jorgensen P, Fledelius H. Orbital tumours in infancy: an analysis of Danish cases from 1943–1962. *Acta Ophthalmol* 1975; **53**: 887–93.

Gawler J, Sanders MD, Bull JWD, de Boulay G, Marshall J. Computer-assisted tomography in orbital disease. *Br J Ophthalmol* 1974; **58**: 571–87.

Leib ML, Kates MR. Orbital computer-assisted tomography. In: Lessel S, Van Dalen JTW, eds. *Current Neuro-ophthalmology*, Vol. 1. Chicago: Year Book Medical Publishers, 1988. Chapter 20.

Lloyd GAS. The impact of CT scanning and ultrasonography on orbital diagnosis. *Clin Radiol* 1977; **28**: 583.

MacCarty CS, Brown DN. Orbital tumours in children. *Clin Neurosurg* 1964; **11**: 76–84.

Moseley IF, Sanders MD. *Computerized Tomography in Neuro-ophthalmology*. London: Chapman & Hall, 1982.

Newton TH, Bilaniuk LT, eds. *Radiology of the Eye and Orbit. Modern Neuroradiology*, Vol 4. New York: Raven Press, 1990.

Porterfield JF. Orbital tumours in children: a report on 214 cases. *Int Ophthalmol Clin* 1962; **2**: 319–26.

Rootman J. *Diseases of the Orbit: A Multidisciplinary Approach*. Philadelphia: JB Lippincott, 1988, Chapter 8.

Shields JA, Bakewell B, Augsburger JJ, Donso L, Bernardino V. Space-occupying orbital masses in children. A review of 250 consecutive biopsies. *Ophthalmology* 1986; **93**: 379–84.

Templeton AC. Orbital tumours in African children. *Br J Ophthalmol* 1971; **55**: 254–61.

Weiss RA, Haik BG, Smith ME. Introduction to diagnostic imaging techniques in ophthalmology. *Int Ophthalmol Clin* 1986; **26**: 1–24.

Youseffi B. Orbital tumours in children: a clinical study of 62 cases. *J Pediatr Ophthalmol Strabismus* 1969; **6**: 177–81.

28: The Neurofibromatoses

Christopher Lyons

The term 'neurofibromatosis' originally described a condition which is now known to be a group of genetically distinct neurocristopathies. Although they have a number of similar features, their clinically significant manifestations are, to a large extent, different. The overlap which gave rise to the common name is principally seen in their common cutaneous manifestations which include cutaneous neurofibromas, café-au-lait patches and plexiform neurofibromas. Affected patients also have a propensity to develop hamartomas. Central nervous system tumours are common in all groups, and there also appears to be some overlap in their type. Nevertheless, it is useful to consider these diseases as separate entities. The most common are neurofibromatosis types 1 and 2 (NF1 and NF2), although up to seven distinct entities have been identified by some workers (Riccardi 1992). Each name describes a specific disease entity whose range of manifestations can, to a large extent, be predicted. Each disease requires different screening and follow-up protocols. The numeric suffix is therefore useful and the global term 'neurofibromatosis' should be abandoned.

Neurofibromatosis type 1

This disease, described by von Recklinghausen in 1882 and eponymous thereafter, has also been called peripheral neurofibromatosis in contrast to the central form which is now known as NF2. The National Institutes of Health (NIH) diagnostic criteria are listed in Table 28.1. These are by no means the only findings in NF1 and many others are described below.

Genetic aspects

NF1 is a progressive disease whose final manifestations are extremely variable. With time, however, existing lesions tend to enlarge gradually and new lesions develop. The parents of a newly diagnosed child will wish to know the likely severity of their NF1 manifestations and their potential effects on life, sight and cosmesis. They will also enquire about the likelihood of further children being affected. Careful counselling is important to allay the fears of gross physical deformity which folklore has often incorrectly attributed to this diagnosis.

NF1 is probably the most common single gene disorder affecting the nervous system, occurring in approximately one in 3000 people. It is autosomal dominantly inherited. Although it has 100% penetrance, its expressivity is highly variable from generation to generation. Moreover, there is a high spontaneous mutation rate, possibly related to the very large size of the gene, which is situated in the pericentromeric region of the long arm of chromosome 17. The absence of a family history therefore does not preclude the diagnosis of NF1.

The exact mechanism for the appearance of benign stigmata in NF1 has not been elucidated but it is known that the NF1 gene codes for a cytoplasmic protein called neurofibromin, which has a role in the regulation of growth and differentiation of a variety of cell types. It is thought that part of this protein catalyses the inactivation of a proto-oncogene (*p21ras*). Since its active form stimulates cell growth and its inactive form inhibits it, a defective neurofibromin from a mutation in the NF1 gene would result in uncontrolled cell growth and multiple tumour

309

Table 28.1 Diagnostic criteria for NF1.

The diagnostic criteria are met if two or more of the following are found

1 Six or more *café-au-lait* macules over 5 mm in greatest diameter in prepubertal individuals and over 15 mm in greatest diameter in postpubertal individuals

2 Two or more neurofibromas of any type *or* one plexiform neurofibroma

3 Freckling in the axillary or inguinal regions

4 Optic glioma

5 Two or more Lisch nodules (iris hamartomas)

6 A distinctive osseous lesion such as sphenoid dysplasia or thinning of long bone cortex, with or without pseudoarthrosis

7 A first-degree relative (parent, sibling or offspring) with NF1 by the above criteria

---

formation. The genetic mechanism through which NF1 mutations give rise to malignant tumours may be similar to that of retinoblastoma formation (Knudson 1971), which results from the deletion of both copies of a tumour-suppressor gene. The first 'hit' is the germ-line mutation of one copy of the gene and the second hit corresponds to a spontaneous mutation within a specific cell, allowing tumour development due to loss of the *p21ras* pathway. Loss of both alleles of the NF1 gene has been identified in neurofibrosarcoma (Legius *et al.* 1992) and bone marrow cells of children with myeloid leukaemia (Shannon *et al.* 1994).

Clinical presentation

The NIH diagnostic criteria for NF1 (see Table 28.1) include the ocular finding of Lisch nodules and orbital findings of plexiform neurofibroma, sphenoid wing dysplasia and optic nerve glioma.

Lisch nodules

These dome-shaped, discrete lesions may occur anywhere on the anterior surface of the iris, including the angle where they may only be seen with a gonioscope. They are usually orange–brown, the colour of burnt sienna (Fig. 28.1), appearing darker than blue irides but paler than brown irides (Fig. 28.2). Most are round, evenly distributed on the iris and bilateral. Their size varies from a pinpoint to involvement of a segment of iris. They are usually bilateral. Histologically, they are melanocytic hamartomas. They may be confluent.

In NF1, they are present in one-third of 2.5 year olds, half of 5 year olds, three-quarters of 15 year olds and almost all adults over 30 (Ragge *et al.* 1993). Lubs *et al.* (1991) found them in 100% of the 65 patients with NF1 aged 21 or above whom they examined with a slit lamp. Although patients with NF2 have been reported to have iris nodules (Charles *et al.* 1989; Garretto *et al.* 1989), true Lisch nodules are overwhelmingly more common in NF1. They occur earlier than neurofibromas in children (Lubs *et*

al. 1991) and are therefore a useful marker for NF1. Since their recognition can trigger the early detection of central nervous system tumours and contribute to genetic counselling of other family members, it is important for ophthalmologists to recognize them, and be able to distinguish them from iris naevi.

Anterior segment and uvea

Because the differentiation of NF1 from the other types of

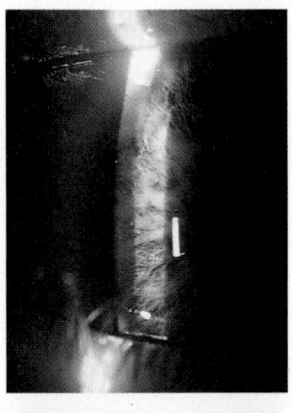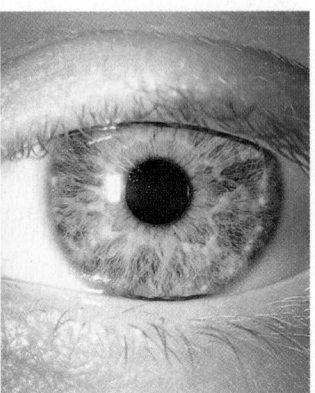

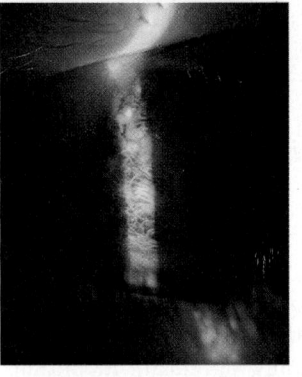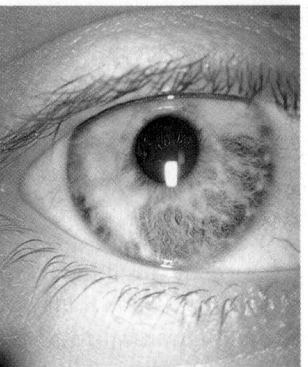

a

b

Fig. 28.1 (a) Multiple Lisch nodules in neurofibromatosis. (b) Right eye with confluent Lisch nodule (same patient).

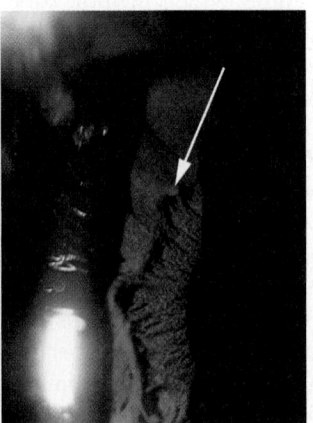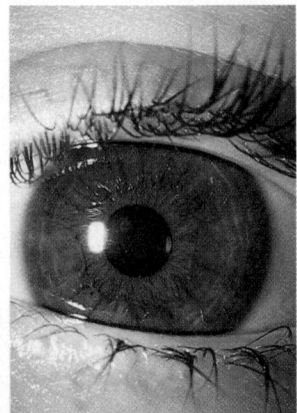

Fig. 28.2 Very small Lisch nodule, but of diagnostic importance in neurofibromatosis. In brown irides Lisch nodules appear light brown (arrow).

neurofibroma is fairly recent, our understanding of the ocular and other findings in any particular neurofibroma type is still evolving.

Prominent nerves have been reported in the cornea, although this finding is rare. They are more commonly seen in the multiple endocrine neoplasia (MEN) syndrome (Knox *et al.* 1969), another neurocristopathy which is now known to be genetically distinct from NF1. Neurofibromas may occur in the perilimbal conjunctiva (Insler *et al.* 1985). Buphthalmos from congenital glaucoma is well recognized in NF1 (Grant & Walton 1968; Castillo *et al.* 1988; Tripathi & Tripathi 1989), particularly in association with a plexiform neurofibroma involving the ipsilateral upper lid. It is virtually always unilateral. Grant and Walton (1968) suggested the major cause was involvement of the angle by neurofibroma, although other causes such as angle obstruction by neurofibromatous thickening of the ciliary body and failure of differentiation of the angle structures have been invoked. Brownstein and Little (1983) also reported synechial angle closure and endothelialization of the iris in one case of congenital glaucoma with NF1. Congenital ectropion uveae (Fig. 28.3), iris heterochromia, angle abnormalities and posterior embryotoxon may predispose to later onset glaucoma. Cataract is not a notable feature of NF1.

Pigmentary hamartomas may also involve the posterior uveal tract. Huson *et al.* (1987) found choroidal naevi in 35% of their patients with NF1. Rarely, the whole uveal tract may be involved by diffuse thickening which can give rise to glaucoma (Kurosawa & Kurosawa 1982; Brownstein & Little 1983). Malignant melanoma may arise

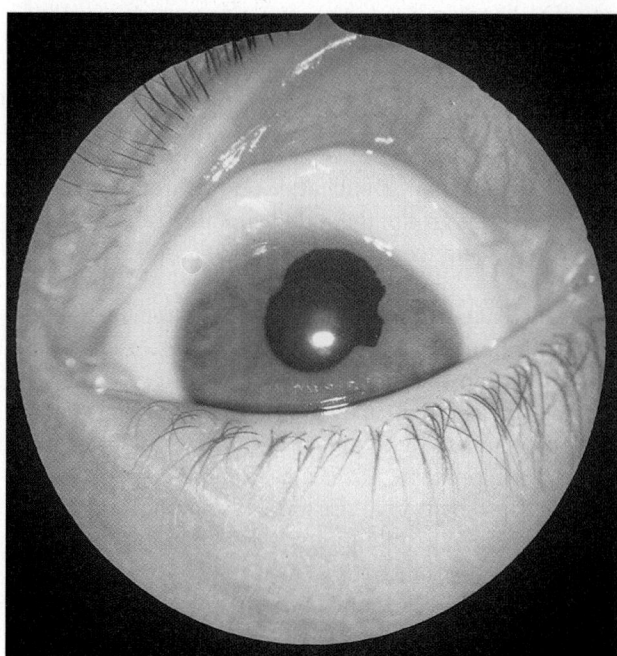

Fig. 28.3 Ectropion uveae, another iris abnormality occurring in NF1. Dr Andrew McCormick's patient.

within these pigmentary hamartomas, as in one of our patients with NF1 in whom a contralateral optic nerve glioma was also present.

Retina and optic disc

Retinal manifestations are rare in NF1. They may include astrocytic hamartomas, like those found in tuberous sclerosis but are occasionally much more extensive (Destro *et al.* 1991). Combined hamartoma of the retina and pigment epithelium has also been described in NF1. Retinal detachment may complicate these lesions. Retinal haemangiomas with exudation may require treatment with laser photocoagulation (Destro *et al.* 1991). Central retinal vein obstruction by optic nerve glioma can give rise to clinical findings of central retinal vein occlusion or venous stasis retinopathy, and rubeosis has been described in this context (Buchanan & Hoyt 1982). Retinal arterial vascular occlusive disease with low flow retinopathy and retinal ischaemia has recently been described in a 4-year-old boy with NF1 and no evidence of glioma on computed tomography (CT) scan (Moadel *et al.* 1994). Gliomas limited to the optic disc may occur (Malbrel *et al.* 1986) although some of the cases reported as having optic disc glioma with von Recklinghausen's disease may actually have had NF2 (Dossetor *et al.* 1989). Pallor of the optic disc may suggest optic nerve or chiasmal glioma. Optic disc swelling may be due to optic nerve glioma (Fig. 28.4), or may be secondary to increased cerebrospinal fluid pressure from tumour or congenital anomalies such as aqueductal stenosis.

Skin, lids and orbits

Café-au-lait spots are hyperpigmented macular lesions which are usually present at birth, and will all have appeared by the age of 1 year (Riccardi 1992). They tend to enlarge at puberty. They are particularly common on the trunk but are absent from the scalp and eyebrows as well as the palms and soles. Histologically, there is melanocytic hyperplasia with increased pigmentation in the basal layer of epidermis. The presence of six 1 cm café-au-lait spots after the age of 1 year is one of the diagnostic criteria for NF1 (NIH 1988).

Neurofibromas

The term 'neuroma' should perhaps be replaced by the correct histopathological terms (Fig. 28.5). These masses arising from peripheral nerves are usually neurofibromas in NF1 and usually schwannomas in NF2 (Evans *et al.* 1992) although some overlap is possible. The 'acoustic neuromas' of NF2 are actually vestibular schwannomas.

Four types of neurofibromas are recognized (Riccardi 1992). First, the discrete cutaneous neurofibroma occurs in

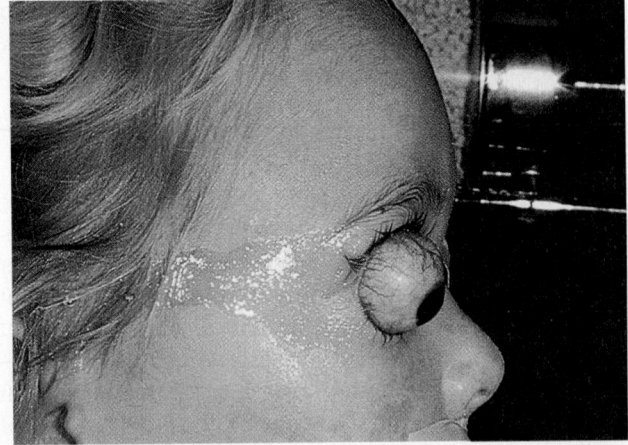

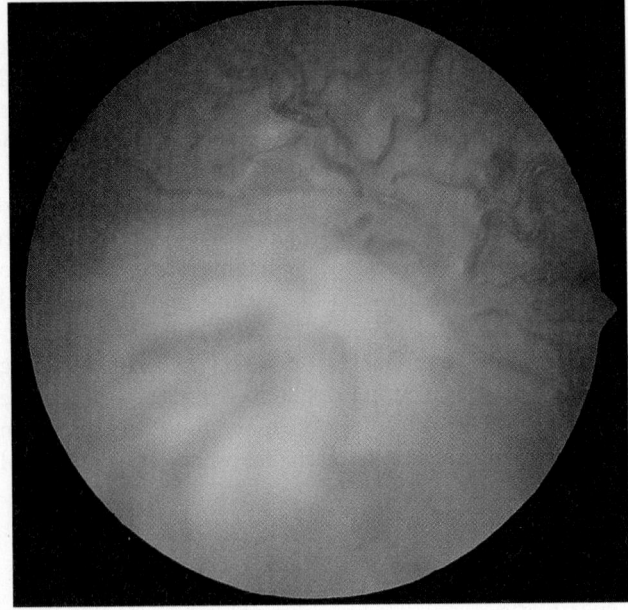

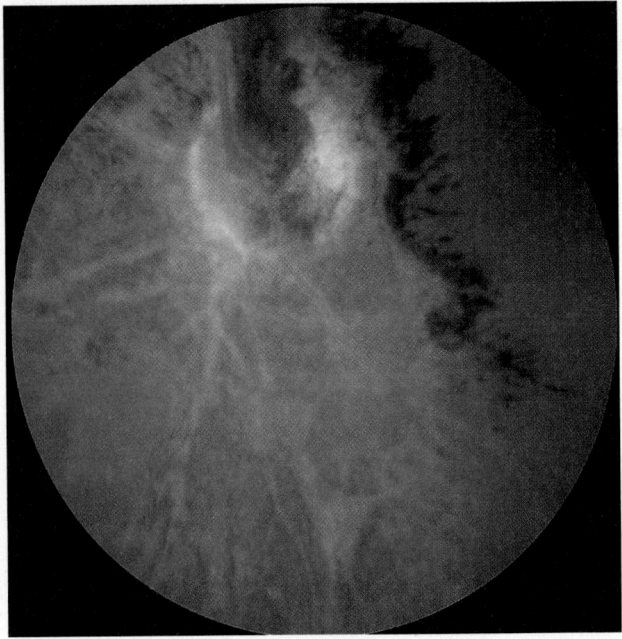

Fig. 28.4 (a) Subluxated globe in optic nerve glioma. (b) Tumour and optic disc oedema (same patient). (c) Fundus of a patient with optic nerve glioma. The tumour had been excised 4 years previously with excision of the central vessels and ciliary vessels. There are extensive areas of healthy choroid and retina anteriorly presumably supplied by the anterior ciliary circulation. By preservation of the posterior ciliary vessels this complication can be avoided.

the epidermis and dermis, moves with the skin and may be blueish-tinged. Second, in contrast, subcutaneous neurofibromas are deep to the dermis. Skin moves over them, they feel firm and rounded and tend to occur along the course of peripheral nerves. Third, nodular plexiform neurofibromas interdigitate with normal tissues in a localized manner. Fourth, diffuse plexiform neurofibromas infiltrate widely and deeply into surrounding tissues. Classically, they feel like a 'bag of worms' when palpated (Figs 28.6, 28.7). They are always congenital but may only manifest clinically later in life. They may be associated with ipsilateral congenital dysplasia of the greater wing of the sphenoid although this can also occur without this tumour (Riccardi 1992). Although the overlying skin is often deeply pigmented, this is not a true café-au-lait spot.

The presence and growth pattern of neurofibromas is age-related; in infancy and early childhood, diffuse plexiform neurofibromas are most active and give rise to

cosmetic and visual problems within the orbit. Manifestations of cutaneous or subcutaneous neurofibromas are rare in this age group; these develop and grow fastest at puberty, the late teens (see Fig. 28.6c), and during pregnancy.

The medial portion of the upper lid is often the first site for a neurofibroma to develop, giving rise to the classically described sinusoid lid margin or a diffusely swollen appearance. Its growth may cause a mechanical ptosis and distort the globe. Amblyopia may result from this or from induced astigmatism. Orbital involvement by plexiform neurofibromas may give rise to early complications as the tumour tends to grow rapidly in the first 3 years of life. Growth may be directed backwards, eroding the orbital walls into the middle cranial fossa, producing enophthalmos or exophthalmos which may be pulsatile (Fig. 28.8). It is not clear whether the sphenoid defect is dysplastic or secondary to the plexiform neurofibroma. They may also grow forwards onto the face (Savino *et al.* 1977; Scully *et al.*

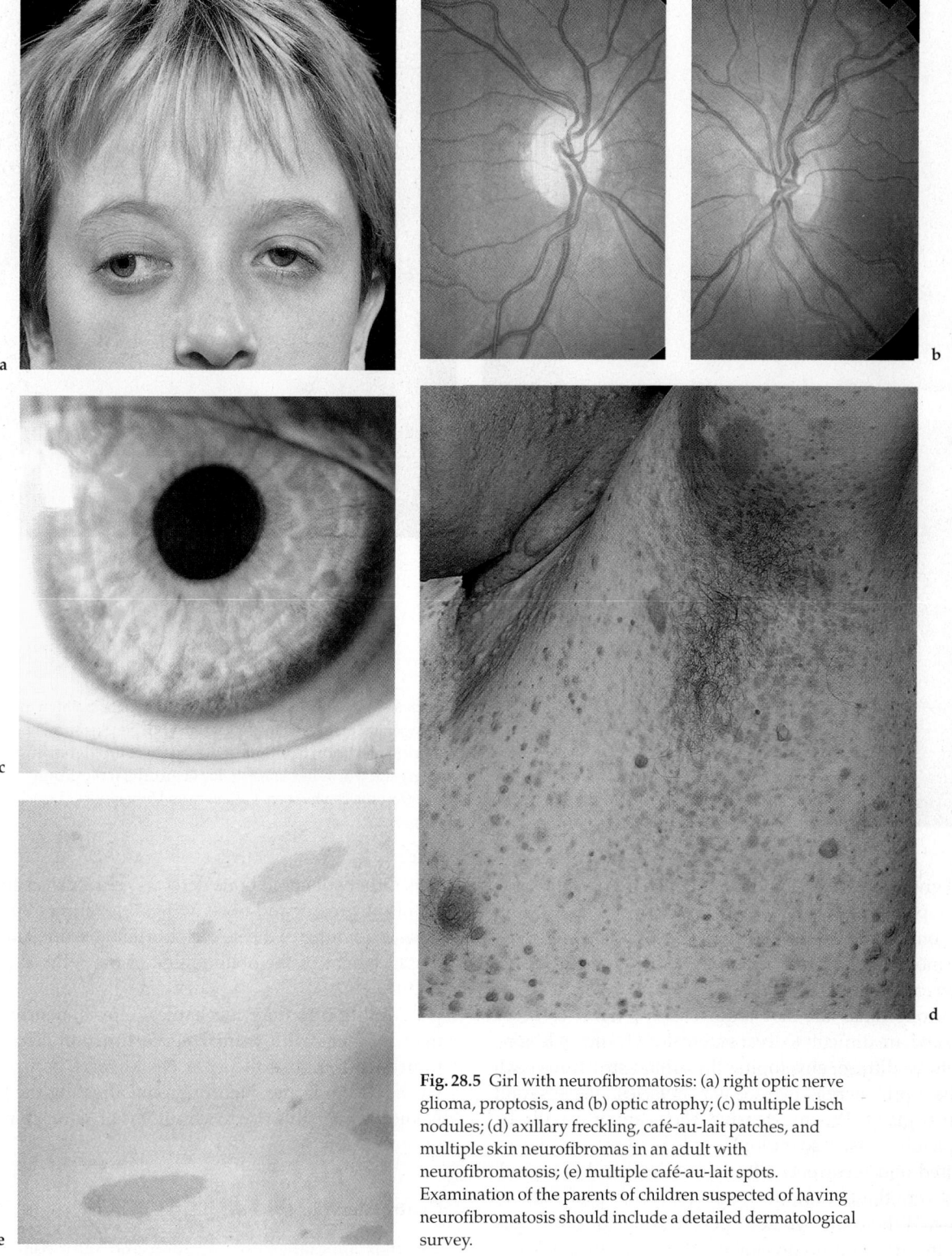

Fig. 28.5 Girl with neurofibromatosis: (a) right optic nerve glioma, proptosis, and (b) optic atrophy; (c) multiple Lisch nodules; (d) axillary freckling, café-au-lait patches, and multiple skin neurofibromas in an adult with neurofibromatosis; (e) multiple café-au-lait spots. Examination of the parents of children suspected of having neurofibromatosis should include a detailed dermatological survey.

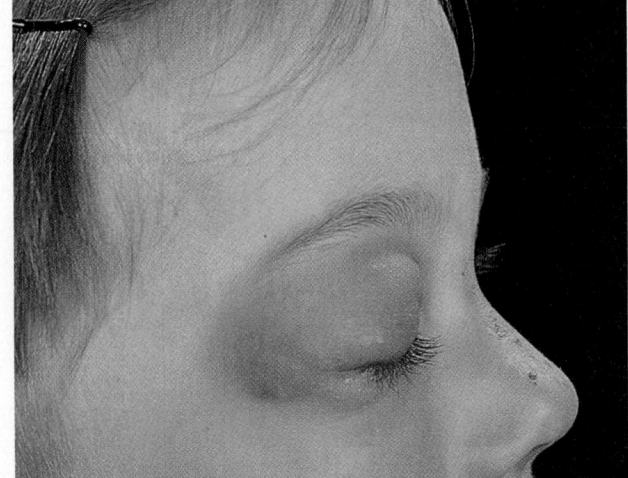

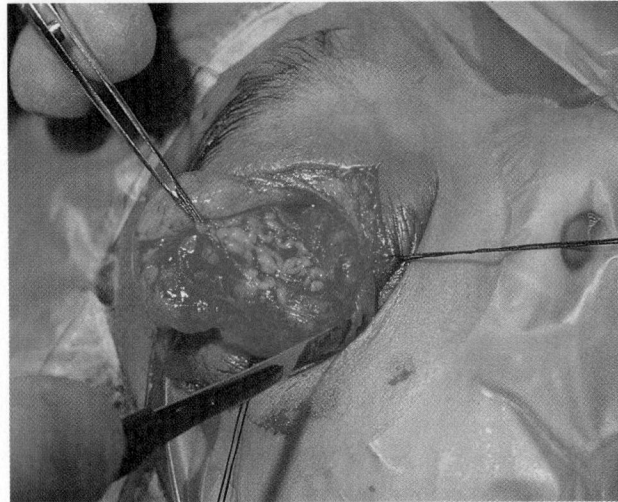

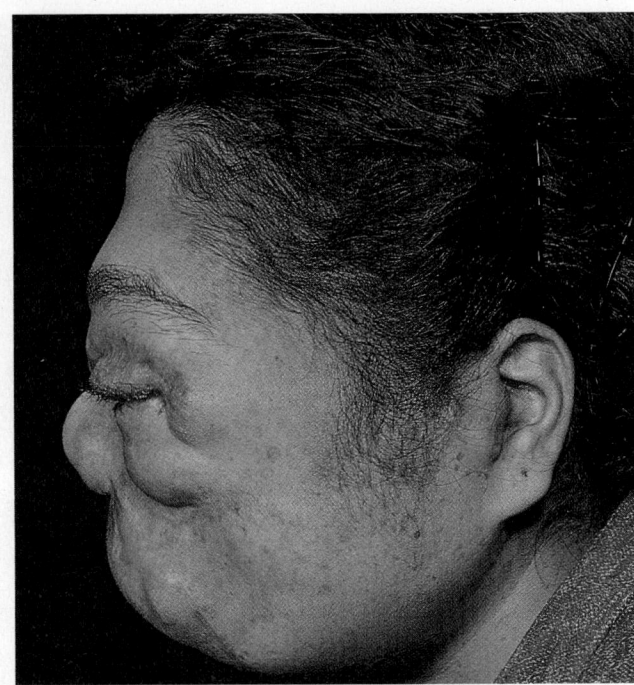

Fig. 28.6 (a) Plexiform neuroma of the lid. There is a high incidence of congenital glaucoma in association with lid plexiform neuromas. (b) Large plexiform neuroma of the face in neurofibromatosis. (c) At surgery the worm-like consistency of an orbital plexiform neurofibroma can be seen. Patient from University of British Columbia.

1984) giving rise to disfigurement which may require surgical repair. Plexiform neurofibroma appears on CT scan as a non-encapsulated, poorly defined, infiltrating mass with moderate contrast enhancement (Reed *et al.* 1986; Linder *et al.* 1987).

Neurofibromas are not radiosensitive (Font & Ferry 1972) and are difficult to treat surgically. Plexiform lesions tend to be diffuse, enveloping the orbital structures such as the optic nerve, extraocular muscles, vessels and lacrimal gland. When extensive, they cannot usually be completely excised, so multiple subtotal resections may be required and recurrence after partial removal is typical. Moreover, these tumours tend to bleed profusely at surgery. Where an eye sees poorly (due to amblyopia resulting from lid involvement or to optic atrophy) and the cosmetic defect is considerable, exenteration with orbital bone grafting is a possibility (Hoyt & Billson 1977; Jackson *et al.* 1983). Lid neurofibroma can be reduced by plastic surgical procedures (Tenzel *et al.* 1977).

In some cases orbital enlargement is not associated with an intraorbital mass and is due instead to bony malforma-

tion. Other sphenoid bone defects occur, such as hypoplasia of the greater and lesser wings, elevation of the lower wing, widening of the superior orbital fissure, and lateral displacement of the oblique line of the orbit (Binet *et al.* 1969).

In addition to their mechanical effects, neurofibromas may interfere with cranial nerve function. Thus, third, fourth, fifth and sixth nerve palsies may occur, as may Horner's syndrome. Neurofibroma affecting the trigeminal nerve may give rise to symptoms of aching pain in the orbital region.

Central nervous system

Vascular anomalies are common and may contribute to the seizures, problems with co-ordination, learning disabilities and mental retardation which are more common with NF1 than in unaffected patients. Hydrocephalus may occur as a complication of congenital or tumoral aqueductal stenosis (Riviello *et al.* 1988; Chapman 1989). It may present with headache, dorsal midbrain syndrome, and

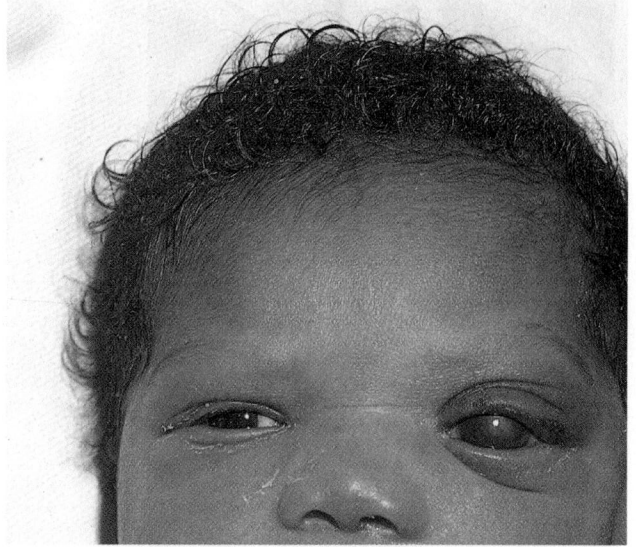

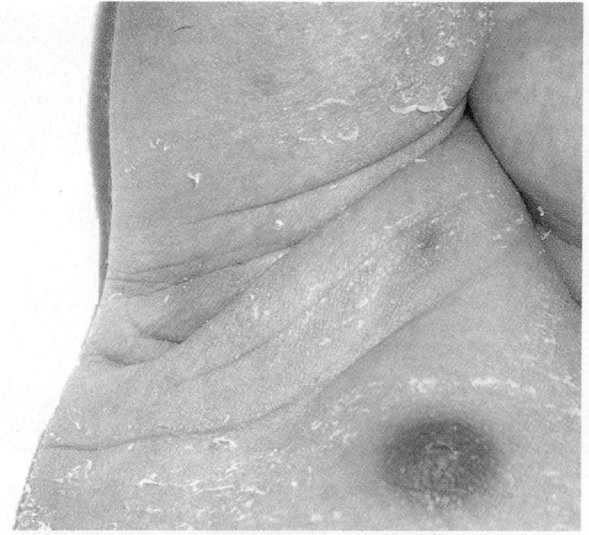

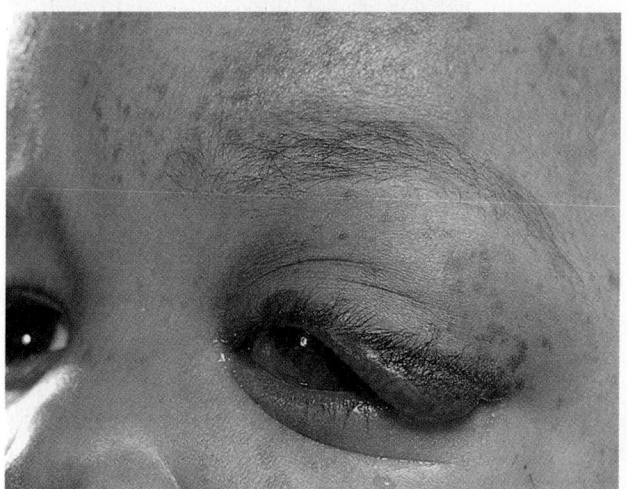

Fig. 28.7 (a) Neonate with enlarged glaucomatous eye and thickened pigmented lid. (b) Same patient showing axillary freckling suggesting NF1. (c) Same patient 2 years later showing S-shaped lid with plexiform neuroma. The glaucoma failed to respond to treatment.

should be remembered as a cause of sixth nerve palsy in NF1. Arachnoid cysts arising from the meninges are a common incidental finding in NF1. These rarely produce clinical features of space-occupying lesions.

The incidence of strabismus is said to be higher than in the general population (Riccardi 1992). Strabismus may be the presenting sign of optic nerve glioma.

Optic nerve and chiasmal glioma with and without NF1 is considered in the section on neurogenic tumours.

Other systems

Tumours of the spinal cord, sympathetic nerves and adrenals may be encountered in patients with neurofibromatosis. The patient may first present with malignant hypertension from phaeochromocytoma. There may be multiple neurofibromas of the gastrointestinal tract and various osseous abnormalities including abnormal vertebrae, scoliosis, pseudoarthrosis of long bones and subperiosteal changes.

However, it is the other central nervous system tumours associated with NF1 which are of greatest importance in reducing the life-expectancy of these patients.

Neurofibromatosis type 2

NF2, formerly known as central neurofibromatosis, is characterized by the development of vestibular schwannomas (acoustic neuromas). Other features include meningiomas, spinal nerve root schwannomas and presenile lens opacities. The severe disease features of NF2 are limited to the central nervous system, in contrast to NF1 where any system may be affected.

Genetics

This autosomal dominantly transmitted defect is about 10 times rarer than NF1, since it is found only in one in 37 000 of the population. Like NF1 the gene has almost complete penetrance and there is considerable inter-

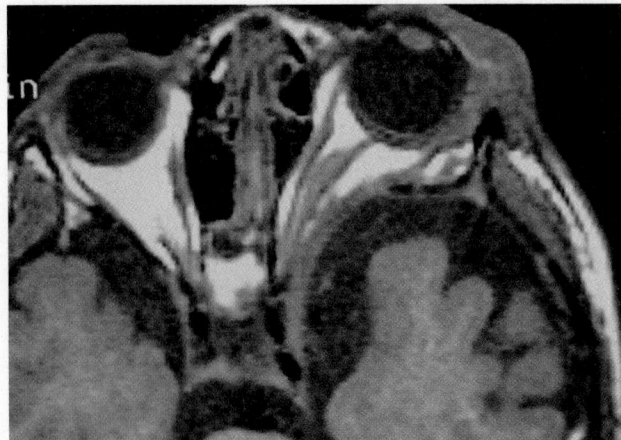

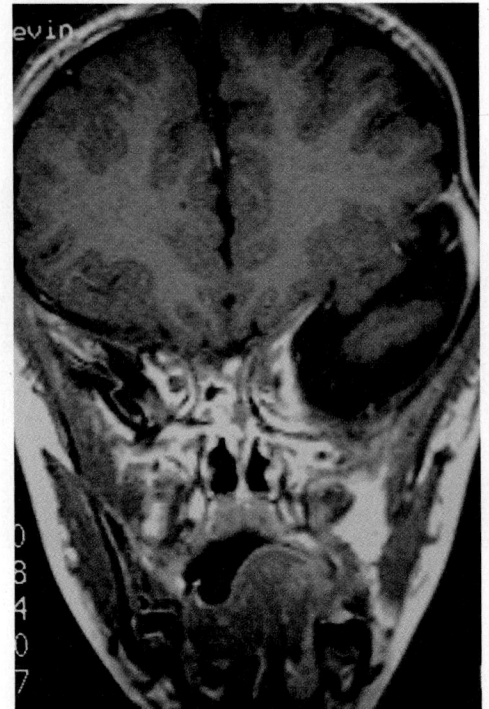

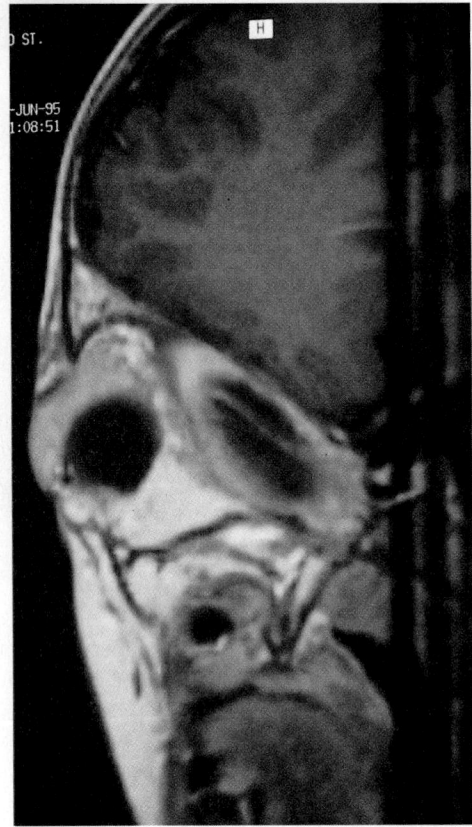

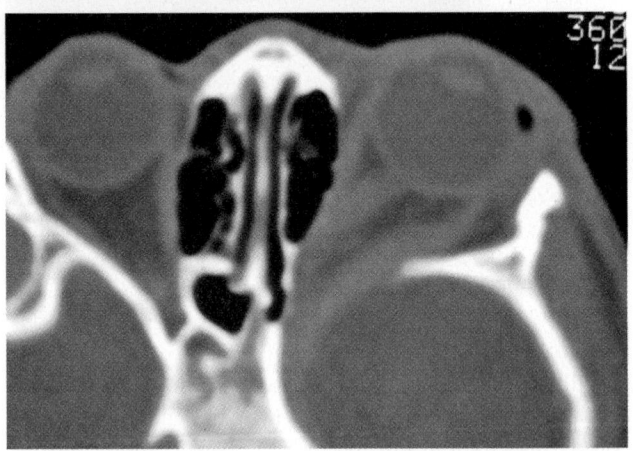

Fig. 28.8 (a–c) NF1. MRI scan shows plexiform neuroma in lid, sphenoid dysplasia with temporal lobe herniation giving pulsating proptosis. (d) CT scan showing bony sphenoid defect (same patient).

individual variation in the phenotypic manifestations of NF2, but unlike NF1 the phenotype of NF2 seems to 'breed true' within affected families. A negative family history does not preclude the diagnosis of NF2 since at least half of patients with NF2 have a new mutation (Riccardi 1992). A maternal effect has been suggested, with earlier onset of clinical manifestations among patients born to a mother with NF2 than those whose father was affected (Kanter *et al.* 1980). It seems that virtually all gene carriers develop tumours of the central nervous system with significant morbidity and mortality (Evans *et al.* 1992).

NF2 has only recently been defined as genetically distinct from NF1. Linkage studies have shown that the gene for NF2 is situated on chromosome 22, coding for a membrane organizing protein called Merlin or (less enchantingly) Schwannomin (Rouleau *et al.* 1993; Trofatter *et al.* 1993). This protein is thought to connect the cytoskeleton to its plasma membrane. The gene implicated in NF2 also probably has a tumour-suppressor role since it has been found to be altered in meningiomas, schwannomas (Bolger *et al.* 1985; Sainz *et al.* 1994) and several human malignancies (Bianchi *et al.* 1994).

Systemic findings

Patients with NF2 often have a few café-au-lait spots, and cutaneous lesions which are usually schwannomas. There are usually less than six café-au-lait spots, often on the trunk, and axillary and groin freckling is absent. Deep plexiform neurofibromas rarely occur and were not found in 120 patients reviewed by Evans *et al.* (1992).

The hallmark of NF2 is the presence of bilateral vestibular schwannomas ('acoustic neuromas') which may only be evident on CT scan. Gadolinium-enhanced magnetic resonance imaging (MRI) is the modality of choice for imaging schwannomas in NF2. It is thought that the gene for NF2 can produce either bilateral vestibular schwannomas if there is a germ-line mutation or unilateral schwannomas if the mutation is somatic. The origin of the trigeminal nerve is another frequent intracranial site for schwannomas (Riccardi 1992), and they have been noted on multiple cranial nerves in affected patients (Tonsgard & Oesterle 1993). The NIH criteria necessary to reach a diagnosis of NF2 are shown in Table 28.2.

In Kanter *et al.*'s (1980) study, the most common presenting symptom was bilateral hearing loss (50%), followed by unilateral hearing loss (21%), usually presenting in the mid-teens to twenties. Vestibular problems (10%), tinnitus (9%), and other presentations including headache, visual symptoms, facial nerve paresis (10%) accounted for most of the remainder.

Whereas patients with NF1 tend to develop neural or astrocytic tumours (astrocytomas, optic nerve 'gliomas'), the nervous system tumours of NF2 typically involve neural coverings or linings (meningiomas, optic nerve sheath meningiomas, schwannomas, ependymomas) (Ragge 1993). Astrocytomas are rare in the brain in NF2, especially involving the optic pathways, but are relatively common in the spinal cord. Although usually of low histological grade, they may have serious sequelae if they occur in the brainstem or spinal cord. Spinal cord meningiomas are also commonly seen, with a predilection for the exit point of foramina, perhaps due

to the stretching of the nerves which occurs at these sites (Riccardi 1992).

Ocular findings

Bouzas *et al.* (1993b) reviewed 54 patients with NF2 and found decreased vision (20/40 or worse) in 18, five bilaterally. Nineteen per cent of the affected eyes had vision of 20/100 or worse. Visual loss is particularly significant in NF2 since progressive bilateral hearing loss is so common in this condition: in this series of 54 patients, whose mean age was 36 years, 26 patients had bilateral profound hearing loss, and nine others had profound hearing loss in one ear and moderate hearing loss in the other. Only eight patients had normal hearing.

Anterior segment

As in NF1, it is becoming obvious that the ocular changes of NF2 are early markers of the disease which may be of diagnostic importance. In particular, 55 to 87% of affected patients have presenile central posterior subcapsular lens opacities (Kaiser-Kupfer *et al.* 1989; Kaye *et al.* 1992; Bouzas *et al.* 1993a). Cataracts (Fig. 28.9) were present in 44 of the 54 patients reviewed by Bouzas *et al.* (1993b) but they only interfered significantly with vision in seven of these, and produced symptomatic glare in a further six. Evans *et al.* (1992) reported that 16 (18%) of their 90 patients had cataracts in the paediatric period, congenital in five. Cataracts presented before any other feature in 11 of 97 patients. Lens opacities may therefore serve as a sensitive marker for predisposition to develop bilateral vestibular schwannomas since they often precede the development of these tumours. The types of cataract that are most suggestive of NF2 are plaque-like posterior subcapsular or capsular cataract and cortical cataract with onset under the age of 30 years (Ragge *et al.* 1995). Juvenile onset peripheral cortical lens opacities have also been described in NF2 (Kaye *et al.* 1992; Bouzas *et al.* 1993a; Landau *et al.* 1993). Corneal hypoaesthesia from trigeminal nerve schwannoma, and decreased tear production, reduced blinking and lagophthalmos from facial nerve palsy may adversely affect the outcome of cataract extraction in patients requiring surgery. These causes resulted in corneal opacification and visual impairment (20/40 or less) in six of the 54 patients reviewed by Bouzas *et al.* (1993b).

Lisch nodules are rare but have been reported in NF2 (Charles *et al.* 1989; Garretto *et al.* 1989; Kaye *et al.* 1992).

Several patients with NF2 and childhood third nerve palsies (Fig. 28.10) have been reported (Kaye *et al.* 1992; Mautner *et al.* 1993; Ragge *et al.* 1993). Tonsgard & Oesterle (1993) reported a patient with epiretinal membrane noted at the age of 4 years, who developed an ipsilateral third nerve palsy when aged 10 years and whose vestibular

Table 28.2 Diagnostic criteria for NF2 (NIH 1988).

NF2 may be diagnosed when one of the following is present
1 Bilateral eighth nerve masses seen by appropriate imaging techniques (e.g. CT scan or MRI). Preferably MRI with gadolinium (Mulvihill *et al.* 1990)
2 A parent, sibling or child with NF2 and either unilateral eighth nerve mass or any two of the following
  (a) neurofibroma
  (b) meningioma
  (c) glioma
  (d) schwannoma
  (e) juvenile posterior subcapsular lens opacity

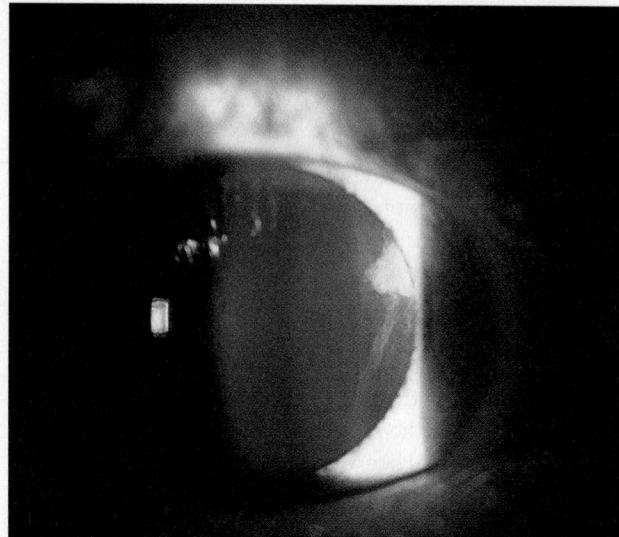

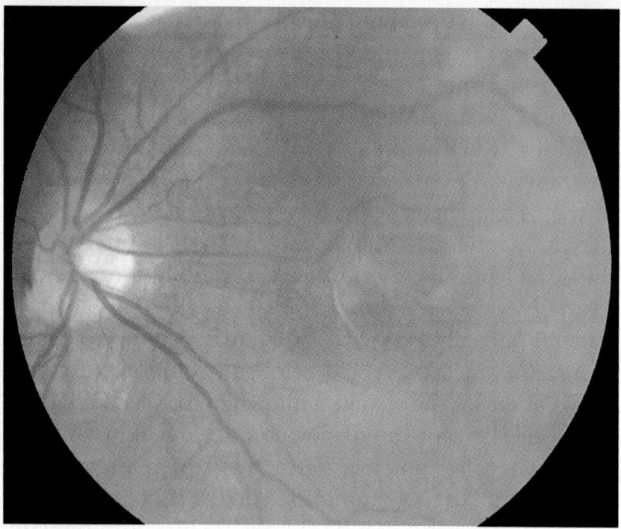

Fig. 28.9 NF2. (a) Cataract in a patient with NF2. (b) Epiretinal membrane in the same patient. There is a preretinal membrane which is causing kinking of the arteriole running above the macula.

schwannomas were identified after symptomatic hearing loss at the age of 17 years. We have seen one patient with congenital third nerve palsy and NF2 whose other eye was blind due to combined hamartoma of the retina and pigment epithelium (see Fig. 28.10). Fourth and sixth nerve involvement has also been described in NF2 (Landau *et al.* 1993; Tonsgard & Oesterle 1993).

Posterior segment

Combined retinal and pigment epithelial hamartomas (CRPEH) have been reported in NF2 (Landau *et al.* 1990; Sivalingam *et al.* 1991). They were present in two of the 54 patients with NF2 reported by Bouzas *et al.* (1992). They may be bilateral (Good *et al.* 1991) and familial (Bouzas *et al.* 1992). They typically occur at the posterior pole and

their characteristic appearance is shown in Fig. 28.10. The severity of the abnormality ranges from mild, with a visual acuity of 20/80 (Sivalingam *et al.* 1991), to severe, as in Landau *et al.*'s (1990) patient whose acuity was 'finger-counting' and the case we present here who did not take up fixation with the affected eye. There may be co-existing epiretinal membranes (Schachat *et al.* 1984).

Epiretinal membranes may occur alone in NF2, usually affecting the posterior pole. They may represent an abortive form of CRPEH. They were reported in seven of the nine patients with NF2 studied by Kaye *et al.* (1992) and in four of six patients by Landau and Yasargil (1993). The severity of these membranes ranged from cellophane maculopathy (two eyes) to macular pucker (three eyes) with visual acuities ranging from 20/20 to 20/200, respectively. Histologically, intraretinal glial proliferation is seen, with an overlying membrane consisting of astrocytic glial fibrillary acidic protein (GFAP)-staining cells (Kaye *et al.* 1992). It is interesting that uncontrolled glial proliferation, a process which is widely implicated in the other central nervous system manifestations of NF2, should be seen in the retina.

Other rare fundus abnormalities have been described in NF2, including astrocytic hamartomas (Kaye *et al.* 1992; Landau & Yasargil 1993) and optic disc gliomas (Stallard 1938; Dossetor *et al.* 1989; Landau & Yasargil 1993).

Optic nerve sheath meningiomas, which may be bilateral, can also cause visual loss in NF2. These may easily be missed on MRI unless fat suppression techniques are used.

Progress

The progression of vestibular schwannoma (acoustic neuroma) is unpredictable but is more rapid with NF2 than without, and appears to be hastened by pregnancy. The use of oestrogens is contraindicated in NF2 (Riccardi 1992). Others have questioned the effect of pregnancy on the progression of NF2-related tumours (Evans *et al.* 1992). The mere presence of a vestibular schwannoma on MRI scan is not an indication for its removal, since many of these tumours remain unchanged for years (Mulvihill *et al.* 1990).

Unfortunately, patients with NF2 often present to ophthalmologists with facial nerve paresis after vestibular schwannoma excision. The incidence of this complication is higher for larger tumours, but is reduced by the use of the operating microscope and intraoperative physiological monitoring of facial nerve function. Recent series, possibly reflecting a trend towards earlier surgery, suggest that anatomical preservation of the facial nerve is possible in up to 97% of cases, with good function in three-quarters of these (Kartush & Lundy 1992). Unfortunately, hearing preservation after vestibular schwannoma excision is only possible in a minority of patients. Small preoperative tumour size is a favourable prognostic factor, but hear-

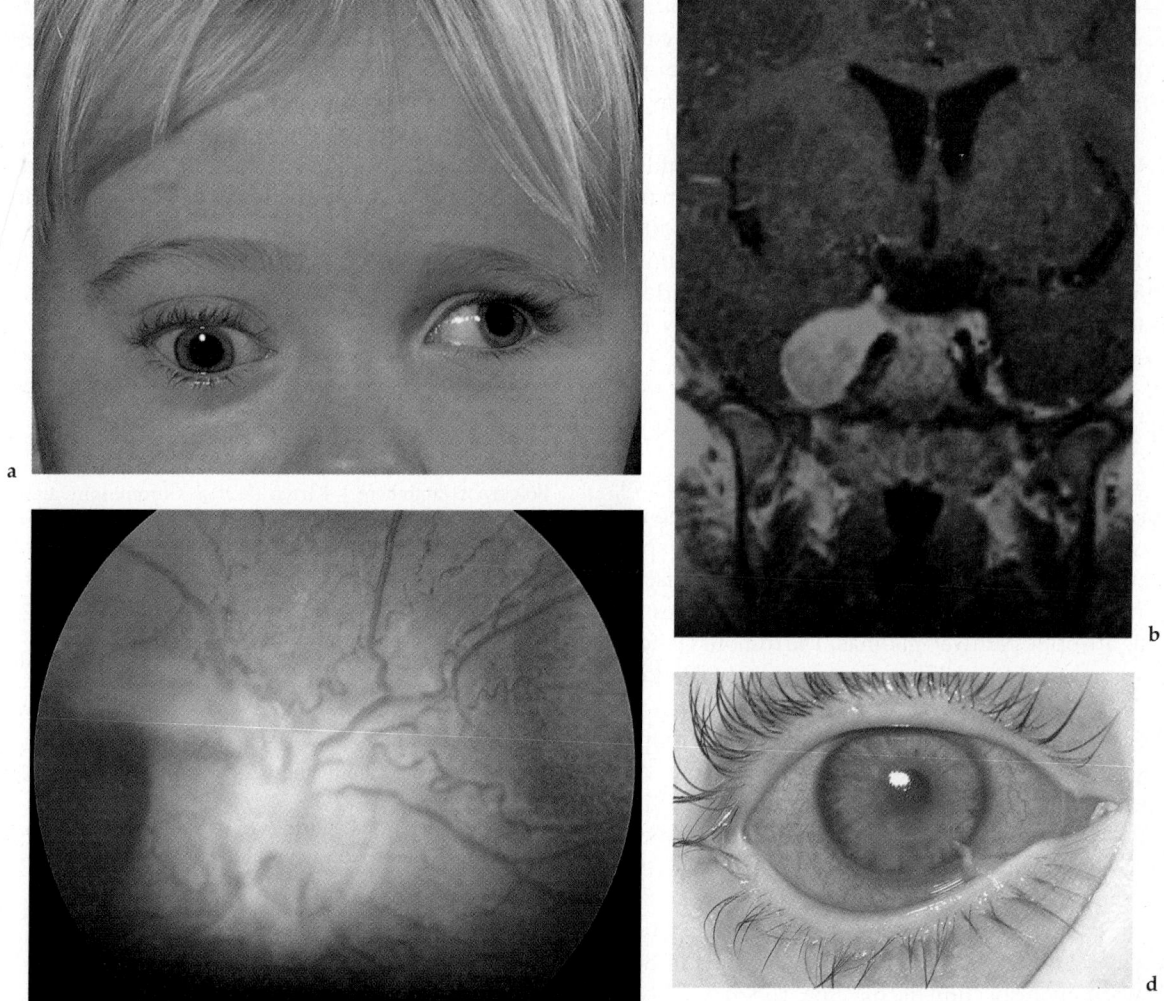

Fig. 28.10 NF2. This 2-year-old boy with NF2 presented with a long-standing head tilt. There is a partial right third and sixth nerve palsy (a). He fixes with the right eye as the acuity in the left eye is poor due to a combined hamartoma of the retina and retinal pigment epithelium (c). An enhancing lesion, probably a meningioma, fills the cavernous sinus and floor of the middle cranial fossa (b). Bilateral vestibular schwannomas were also demonstrated on MRI. Corneal anaesthesia developed on the right side with corneal ulceration due to repeated trauma to the right eye (d).

ing preservation is less likely for bilateral tumours (Shelton 1992). The 'gamma knife' or highly collimated radiotherapy, is currently under evaluation for the non-invasive treatment of vestibular schwannoma.

Since morbidity from the excision of vestibular schwannoma increases with tumour size, early diagnosis and surgery may be advantageous. Early evaluation of the offspring of parents with NF2 for vestibular schwannoma is essential. Nine children who had either one parent with NF2 or skin or spinal tumours suggestive of NF2 were studied by Mautner *et al.* (1993). Vestibular schwannomas were identified in seven of these by MRI scanning with gadolinium. Six of these, whose age ranged from 9 to 16 years, had no clinical signs or symptoms. Slit-lamp examination revealed posterior subcapsular cataracts in four of these, two of whom were 10 years old. In retrospect, the first signs of NF2 were present in infancy in four of the nine children, and by age 5 years in six of the nine. Although NF2 is generally considered a disease of teenage and adulthood, it is becoming evident that this gene defect gives rise to manifestations occurring much earlier in life. Evans *et al.* (1992) have suggested ophthalmological screening with a slit-lamp examination is indicated in early childhood, and screening for vestibular schwannoma with annual brainstem evoked responses should start in the early teens. A genetic screening test for at-risk relatives will help to determine whether the germ-line mutation is present or not (Merel *et al.* 1995).

Paediatric ophthalmologists should remain alert to the possibility of NF2 and initiate investigations such as hearing tests and gadolinium-enhanced MRI scans of the cerebellopontine angle and vestibular nerves in patients with characteristic ocular findings. These include combined hamartomas of the retina and pigment epithelium, apparently idiopathic juvenile posterior subcapsular cataracts and, possibly, unexplained third nerve palsy in a child. Moreover, a child who has too few café-au-lait spots and neurofibroma-like cutaneous lesions to meet the criteria for a diagnosis of NF1 may actually have NF2.

Affected patients and their at-risk relatives should be warned of the risks associated with this diagnosis. In particular, drowning or near-drowning due to loss of direction under water, occurred in eight of 73 patients studied by Kanter *et al.* (1980) and two others died in accidents related to insidious hearing loss such as being hit by cars or trains.

Other forms of neurofibromatosis

NF3 is a mixed form of neurofibromatosis in which features of both NF1 and NF2 are present. Palmar neurofibromas are characteristic lesions. Café-au-lait spots occur but are few in number. Intracranial, spinal or paraspinal tumours occur commonly. Lisch nodules are absent, as are optic pathway gliomas. The tumours tend to behave aggressively and life prognosis is poor (Riccardi 1992).

NF4 or variant neurofibromatosis designates a group of patients whose phenotypic features do not fit into any other group of neurofibromatosis. This is really a 'sorting' category, devised to prevent these patients from masking the relative uniformity found in other groups for investigational purposes.

NF5 is segmental. Café-au-lait spots, freckling, and other signs of NF1 are restricted to one side or quadrant of the body, strictly respecting the midline. The possibility of this form of neurofibromatosis being due to a somatic mutation is called into question by Weleber and Zonana's (1983) report of Lisch nodules and the report of NF1 in the offspring of an affected patient (Boltshauser *et al.* 1989).

NF6 and NF7 describe 'café-au-lait spots only' and 'late onset' neurofibromatosis, respectively.

Conclusion

There has been a revolution in our understanding of the group of neurocristopathies previously referred to under the generic term of neurofibromatosis.

The ophthalmologist may have a pivotal role in making the diagnosis of NF1, by correctly identifying Lisch nodules, orbital plexiform neurofibromas, characteristic sphenoid wing defects, and optic nerve gliomas. In NF2 also, it is becoming clear that ocular findings such as juvenile posterior subcapsular cataract, idiopathic epiretinal membrane and combined hamartoma of the retina and pigment epithelium are important in making a presymptomatic diagnosis.

In both cases, ocular findings may precede other, sometimes sight- or even life-threatening manifestations of NF1

or NF2. It is therefore essential for paediatric ophthalmologists to be aware of their ocular features, and refer early and appropriately for audiological, neuroradiological or other relevant investigations.

As our understanding improves, and gene probes become freely available for diagnostic testing and genetic counselling, we will be better able to define the phenotype of each gene defect.

References

Bianchi AB, Hara T, Ramesh V *et al.* Mutations in transcript isoforms of the neurofibromatosis 2 gene in multiple human tumour types. *Nature Genet* 1994; **6**: 185–92.

Binet E, Keiffer SA, Martin SH, Peterson HO. Orbital dysplasia in neurofibromatosis. *Radiology* 1969; **93**: 829–33.

Bolger GB, Stamberg J, Kirsch IR *et al.* Chromosome translocation t(14;22) and oncogene (*c-cis*) variant in a pedigree with familial meningioma. *New Engl J Med* 1985; **312**: 564–7.

Boltshauser E, Stocker H, Machler M. Neurofibromatosis type 1 in a child of a parent with segmental neurofibromatosis (NF5). *Neurofibromatosis* 1989; **2**: 244–5.

Bouzas EA, Parry DM, Eldridge R, Kaiser-Kupfer MI. Familial occurrence of combined pigment epithelial and retinal hamartomas associated with neurofibromatosis 2. *Retina* 1992; **12**: 103–7.

Bouzas EA, Freidlin V, Parry DM, Eldridge R, Kaiser-Kupfer MI. Lens opacities in neurofibromatosis 2: further significant correlations. *Br J Ophthalmol* 1993a; **77**: 354–7.

Bouzas EA, Parry DM, Eldridge R, Kaiser-Kupfer MI. Visual impairment in patients with neurofibromatosis 2. *Neurology* 1993b; **43**: 622–3.

Brownstein S, Little JM. Ocular neurofibromatosis. *Ophthalmology* 1983; **90**: 1595–9.

Buchanan TAS, Hoyt WF. Optic nerve glioma and neovascular glaucoma: report of a case. *Br J Ophthalmol* 1982; **66**: 96–8.

Castillo M, Quencer RM, Glaser J, Altman N. Congenital glaucoma and buphthalmos in a child with neurofibromatosis. *J Clin Neuroophthalmol* 1988; **8**: 69–71.

Chapman PH. Von Recklinghausen's neurofibromatosis and aqueduct stenosis. *Neurosurgery* 1989; **25**: 318.

Charles SJ, Moore AT, Yates JRW, Ferguson-Smith MA. Lisch nodules in neurofibromatosis type 2. Case report. *Arch Ophthalmol* 1989; **107**: 1571–2.

Destro M, D'Amico DJ, Gragoudas ES *et al.* Retinal manifestations of neurofibromatosis. Diagnosis and management. *Arch Ophthalmol* 1991; **109**: 662–6.

Dossetor FR, Landau K, Hoyt WF. Optic disk glioma in neurofibromatosis type 2. *Am J Ophthalmol* 1989; **108**: 602–3.

Evans DG, Huson SM, Donnai D *et al.* A genetic study of type 2 neurofibromatosis in the UK. II. Guidelines for genetic counselling. *J Med Genet* 1992; **29**: 847–52.

Font RL, Ferry AP. Phakomatoses. *Int Ophthalmol Clin* 1972; **12**: 1–50.

Garretto NS, Ameriso S, Molina HA *et al.* Type 2 neurofibromatosis with Lisch nodules. *Neurofibromatosis* 1989; **2**: 315–21.

Good WV, Brodsky MC, Edwards MS, Hoyt WF. Bilateral retinal hamartomas in neurofibromatosis type 2. *Br J Ophthalmol* 1991; **75**: 190.

Grant WM, Walton DS. Distinctive gonioscopic findings in glaucoma due to neurofibromatosis. *Arch Ophthalmol* 1968; **79**: 127–34.

Hoyt CS, Billson FA. Buphthalmos in neurofibromatosis: is it an expression of regional giantism? *J Pediatr Ophthalmol Strabismus* 1977; **14**: 228–34.

Huson S, Jones D, Beck L. Ophthalmic manifestations of neurofibromatosis. *Br J Ophthalmol* 1987; **71**: 235–9.

Insler MS, Helm C, Napoli S. Conjunctival hamartoma in neurofibromatosis. *Am J Ophthalmol* 1985; **99**: 731–3.

Jackson IT, Laws ER, Martin RD. The surgical management of orbital neurofibromatosis. *Plastic Reconstr Surg* 1983; **71**: 751–8.

Kaiser-Kupfer MI, Freidlin V, Datiles MB *et al.* The association of posterior capsular lens opacities with bilateral acoustic neuromas in patients with neurofibromatosis type 2. *Arch Ophthalmol* 1989; **107**: 541–4.

Kanter WR, Eldridge R, Fabricant R *et al.* Central neurofibromatosis with bilateral acoustic neuroma: genetic, clinical and biochemical distinctions from peripheral neurofibromatosis. *Neurology* 1980; **30**: 851–9.

Kartush JM, Lundy LB. Facial nerve outcome in acoustic neuroma surgery. *Otolaryngol Clin N Am* 1992; **25**: 623–47.

Kaye L, Rothner A, Beauchamp G, Meyer S, Estes M. Ocular findings associated with neurofibromatosis type 2. *Ophthalmology* 1992; **99**: 1424–9.

Knox DL, Payne JW, Hartmann WH. Thickened corneal nerves and eyelids as signs of neurofibromatosis and medullary thyroid carcinoma. In: *Progress in Neuro-ophthalmology*, No. 176. Amsterdam: Exerpta Medica, 1969: 262–6.

Knudson AG Jr. Mutation and cancer: statistical study of retinoblastoma. *Proc Natl Acad Sci USA* 1971; **68**: 820–3.

Kurosawa A, Kurosawa H. Ovoid bodies in choroidal neurofibromatosis. *Arch Ophthalmol* 1982; **100**:1939–41.

Landau K, Dossetor FM, Hoyt WF, Muci-Mendoza R. Retinal hamartoma in neurofibromatosis 2. *Arch Ophthalmol* 1990; **108**: 328–9.

Landau K, Yasargil GM. Ocular fundus in neurofibromatosis type 2. *Br J Ophthalmol* 1993; **77**: 646–9.

Legius E, Marchuk DA, Hall BK *et al.* NF1-related locus on chromosome 15. *Genomics* 1992; **13**: 1316–18.

Linder B, Campos M, Schafer M. CT and MRI of orbital anomalies in neurofibromatosis and selected craniofacial anomalies. *Radiol Clin N Am* 1987; **25**: 787–802.

Lubs ML, Bauer MS, Formas ME, Djokic B. Lisch nodules in neurofibromatosis type 1. *New Engl J Med* 1991; **324**: 1264–6.

Malbrel C, Hecart JF, Malbrel G *et al.* Gliome de la papille. *Bull Soc Ophtalmol France* 1986; **86**: 289–91.

Mautner VF, Tatagiba M, Guthoff R *et al.* Neurofibromatosis 2 in the pediatric age group. *Neurosurgery* 1993; **33**: 92–6.

Merel P, Khe HX, Sanson M *et al.* Screening for germ-line mutations in the NF2 gene. *Genes, Chromosomes and Cancer* 1995; **12**: 117–27.

Moadel K, Yannuzzi LA, Ho AC, Ursekar A. Retinal vascular occlusive disease in a child with neurofibromatosis (letter). *Arch Ophthalmol* 1994; **112**: 1021–3.

Mulvihill JJ, Parry DM, Sherman JL *et al.* NIH Conference. Neurofibromatosis 1 (Recklinghausen disease) and neurofibromatosis 2 (bilateral acoustic neurofibromatosis). An update. *Ann Intern Med* 1990; **113**: 39–52.

NIH. National Institutes of Health consensus development conference statement: neurofibromatosis. *Neurofibromatosis* 1988; **1**: 172–8.

Ragge NK. Clinical and genetic patterns of neurofibromatosis 1 and 2. *Br J Ophthalmol* 1993; **77**: 662–72.

Ragge NK, Baser ME, Klein J *et al.* Ocular abnormalities in neurofibromatosis. *Am J Ophthalmol* 1995; **120**: 534–41.

Ragge NK, Falk R, Cohen WE, Murphree AL. Images of Lisch nodules across the spectrum. *Eye* 1993; **7**: 95–101.

Reed D, Robertson WD, Rootman J, Douglas G. Plexiform neurofibromatosis of the orbit. CT evaluation. *Am J Neuroradiol* 1986; **7**: 259–63.

Riccardi VM. *Neurofibromatosis: Phenotype, Natural History, and Pathogenesis*, 2nd edn. Baltimore: Johns Hopkins University Press, 1992.

Riviello JJ, Marks HG, Lee MS, Mandell GA. Aqueductal stenosis in neurofibromatosis. *Neurology* 1988; **1**: 312–17.

Rouleau GA, Merel P, Lutchman M *et al.* Alteration in a new gene encoding a putative membrane-organizing protein causes neurofibromatosis type 2. *Nature* 1993; **363**: 515–21.

Sainz J, Huynh DP, Figueroa K *et al.* Mutations of the neurofibromatosis type 2 gene and lack of the gene product in vestibular schwannomas. *Hum Mol Genet* 1994; **6**: 885–91.

Savino PJ, Glaser JS, Luxenburg MN. Pulsating enophthalmos and choroidal hamartomas: two rare stigmata of neurofibromatosis. *Br J Ophthalmol* 1977; **61**: 483–8.

Schachat AP, Shields JA, Fine SL *et al.* Combined hamartomas of the retina and retinal pigment epithelium. *Ophthalmology* 1984; **91**: 1609–15.

Scully RE, Mark EJ, McNeely BU. Case records of the Massachusetts General Hospital. Weekly clinicopathological exercises. Case 34-1984. *N Engl J Med* 1984; **311**: 520–7.

Shannon KM, O'Connell P, Martin GA *et al.* Loss of the normal NF1 allele from the bone marrow of children with type 1 neurofibromatosis and malignant myeloid disorders. *New Engl J Med* 1994; **330**: 597–601.

Shelton C. Hearing preservation in acoustic tumor surgery. *Otolaryngol Clin N Am* 1992; **25**: 609–21.

Sivalingam A, Augsburger J, Perilongo G *et al.* Combined hamartoma of the retina and retinal pigment epithelium in a patient with neurofibromatosis type 2. *J Pediatr Ophthalmol Strabismus* 1991; **28**: 320–2.

Stallard HB. A case of intra-ocular neuroma (von Recklinghausen's disease) of the left optic nerve head. *Br J Ophthalmol* 1938; **21**: 11.

Tenzel RR, Boynton JR, Miller GR, Buffam FV. Surgical treatment of eyelid neurofibromas. *Arch Ophthalmol* 1977; **95**: 479–83.

Tonsgard JH, Oesterle CS. The ophthalmologic presentation of NF2 in childhood. *J Pediatr Ophthalmol Strabismus* 1993; **30**: 327–30.

Tripathi BJ, Tripathi RC. Neural crest origin of human trabecular meshwork and its implications for the pathogenesis of glaucoma. *Am J Ophthalmol* 1989; **107**: 583–90.

Trofatter JA, MacCollin MM, Rutter JL *et al.* A novel moesin-, ezrin-, radixin-like gene is a candidate for the neurofibromatosis 2 tumor suppressor. *Cell* 1993; **72**: 791–800.

von Recklinghausen FD. *Ueber die multiplen Fibrome der Haut und ihre Beziehung zu den multiplen Neuromen. Festschrift zur Feier des 25 Jährigen Bestchens des Pathologischen Instituts zu Berlin.* Berlin: Herrn Rudolf Virchow Dargebracht, 1882.

Weleber RG, Zonana J. Iris hamartomas (Lisch nodules) in a case of segmental neurofibromatosis. *Am J Ophthalmol* 1983; **96**: 740–3.

29: Neurogenic Tumours

Christopher Lyons and Jack Rootman

Optic nerve tumours

Glioma

Gliomas (astrocytomas) are the most common intracranial tumours in neurofibromatosis type 1 (NF1), occurring most frequently in the anterior visual pathways, brainstem and posterior fossa (Lewis *et al.* 1984). They rarely affect the brain in NF2 but are found in the spinal cord. Conversely, Riccardi (1992) has questioned whether meningiomas and schwannomas are part of the NF1 phenotype, and suggested that these tumours are more typical of NF2.

Anterior pathway gliomas

The overall prevalence has been estimated at 19% of patients with NF1 (Listernick *et al.* 1994), and 10–15% in the absence of visual symptoms (Lewis *et al.* 1984; Listernick *et al.* 1994). Depending on the series, between 10 and 70% of patients with anterior pathway glioma have been said to have NF1 (Miller 1988). Glioma shows no particular predilection for any part of the anterior visual pathway and may arise in one or both optic nerves, the chiasm or the chiasm and one or both nerves. Bilateral optic nerve glioma is one of the diagnostic criteria of NF1. Patients with anterior pathway gliomas should be examined for signs of neurofibromatosis in the eye (Lisch nodules, glaucoma, fundus lesions), orbit (neurofibromas, sphenoid defects), and skin (café-au-lait spots, neurofibromas). Family members should also be examined.

Does the presence of NF1 affect the mode of presentation, behaviour, visual prognosis and life prognosis of patients with optic pathway gliomas? This question has been a source of heated debate for some time. The true answer is still masked by the lack of reference to this point in much of the glioma literature. Some argue that the vast majority of these tumours have an excellent visual prognosis, and the number which behave aggressively is so small that it is difficult to make a statement about relative prognosis with and without NF1 (Miller 1988). Nevertheless, there is a strong clinical impression (Rootman 1988; Wright *et al.* 1989; Listernick *et al.* 1994; Janss *et al.* 1995) that glioma occurring in the presence of NF1 has different characteristics at presentation, different radiological findings, a better visual prognosis, but that survival is poorer due to the development of other central nervous system tumours. Where possible, the differences between these will be highlighted and the practical management of glioma in each context will be discussed.

The management of optic nerve and chiasmal glioma is fundamentally different and it is important to distinguish optic nerve glioma, where the chiasm is not involved from chiasmal glioma, where the optic nerves may be involved.

Optic nerve glioma

Presentation. The reported age of presentation has ranged from birth to 79 years but most series suggest between 4 and 12 years to be most common, with an overall mean from several large combined series of 8.8 years (Dutton 1994). The vast majority have presented by 20 years of age. Females are more often affected than males. Optic nerve glioma is occasionally bilateral, especially in patients with neurofibromatosis (Eggers *et al.* 1976), but florid outward signs of NF1 such as orbital plexiform neurofibromas are no more common in patients with a glioma than in other patients with NF1 (Listernick *et al.* 1994). Indeed, they may be absent, further confusing the debate on the relative prognosis of glioma with NF1.

The presenting signs depend on the site of the tumour;

gliomas involving the intraorbital portion of the nerve commonly present with axial proptosis (Wright *et al.* 1980) (Fig. 29.1). This may be quite sudden in onset or recognition and is occasionally rapidly progressive. The eye is painless and uninflamed unless there is corneal exposure or neovascular glaucoma (Buchanan & Hoyt 1982). Limitation of elevation was present in almost half of Wright *et al.*'s (1980) 31 patients. Strabismus associated with unilateral visual loss may be the presenting feature (Hoyt & Baghdassarian 1969). The older patient may complain of visual loss. Colour vision deficits with central field defects (Wright *et al.* 1980) may be identified. Other visual field abnormalities may occur, such as altitudinal hemianopias, depending on the relationship of the tumour to the nerve and its blood supply. In patients with unilateral or asymmetrical optic nerve involvement, there is usually an afferent pupillary defect on the side which is most affected.

Poor vision, disc swelling or more commonly pallor, may be noted at a routine examination of an asymptomatic patient. Opticociliary shunt vessels may be found and involvement of the disc by tumour is occasionally seen. However, many series have shown these tumours to be silent in as many as 10% of patients with NF1 (Lewis *et al.* 1984). In the absence of visual symptoms, optic nerve glioma is rarely identified by fundus examination alone. Listernick *et al.* (1989) have suggested that routine neuroimaging is of value at the time of presentation with NF1 in order to detect asymptomatic glioma. It could be argued, however, that this would rarely, if ever, alter the patient's management.

Patients with the stigmata of NF1 often present with relatively good visual acuity which may fluctuate at follow-up, with spontaneous improvement. Bilaterality (Fig. 29.2) and multifocal optic nerve/chiasmatic involvement is relatively common. Patients without NF1 tend to present with an isolated localized lesion, and poor visual acuity on the affected side. The major features of glioma with and without NF1 are described in Table 29.1.

Radiographic features. In patients with a suggestive history, the radiographic appearances of optic nerve glioma are so characteristic that biopsy is not needed to make a diagnosis. Indeed, biopsy was shown frequently to be misleading in optic nerve glioma since reactive changes in the arachnoid can mimic meningioma (Wright *et al.* 1980). Furthermore, biopsy may permanently disable the patient visually. Although optic canal enlargement on plain X-ray suggests a diagnosis of glioma, this modality has largely been abandoned since it yields insufficient information for diagnostic and management purposes. Computed tomography (CT) scanning reveals a smooth fusiform optic nerve enlargement with variable contrast enhancement. The optic nerve is commonly kinked in the immediate retrobulbar zone, due to its elongation (Imes & Hoyt 1991) and the soft nature of the tumour, a finding which helps to

Table 29.1 Characteristics of optic nerve glioma with and without NF1.

	NF1	No NF1
Associated features	*Café-au-lait* spots; Lisch nodules; other tumours (see text)	None
Presentation	Asymptomatic; routine examination finding; visual loss	Visual loss; strabismus; proptosis
Tumour distribution	Multifocal, diffuse bilateral	Discrete, unilateral
Progression	Stable–slow progression Fluctuating vision	Stable–slow progression; occasionally rapid
Histology	Arachnoid gliomatosis; perineural gliomatous and mucinous accumulation	Obliteration of perineural space by expanding optic nerve
Radiographic findings	Fusiform optic nerve enlargement; high signal intensity of perineural arachnoid gliomatosis on T2-weighted MRI; kinking of intraorbital nerve	Fusiform optic nerve enlargement; loss of perineural space
Visual prognosis	Good	Poor
Life-expectancy	Reduced	Normal

differentiate glioma from the much less common and more aggressive childhood optic nerve sheath meningioma (Jakobiec *et al.* 1984). Nevertheless, these two entities are easily confused radiologically (Rootman 1988; Wright *et al.* 1989). Calcification rarely occurs in glioma, whereas it is a typical feature of meningioma. There is smooth enlargement of the optic canal when this area is involved.

Magnetic resonance imaging (MRI) (Fig. 29.3) is the modality of choice for evaluation and follow-up of anterior pathway gliomas since this has superior definition in distinguishing involved from uninvolved tissue (especially T2 weighting), axial views along the nerve can easily be acquired, and there is no exposure to radiation. In Wright *et al.*'s (1989) series, two of 31 patients with optic nerve glioma were found to have chiasmal involvement on MRI which had been unsuspected clinically and had not been detected by visual evoked potentials (VEP) and CT scan. The optic nerve gliomas found in NF1 are thought to differ histopathologically from others: arachnoid gliomatosis with mucinous accumulation in the perineural subarachnoid space is a characteristic feature whereas obliteration of the subarachnoid space with replacement of the nerve is typical of gliomas in the absence of NF1 (Stern *et al.*

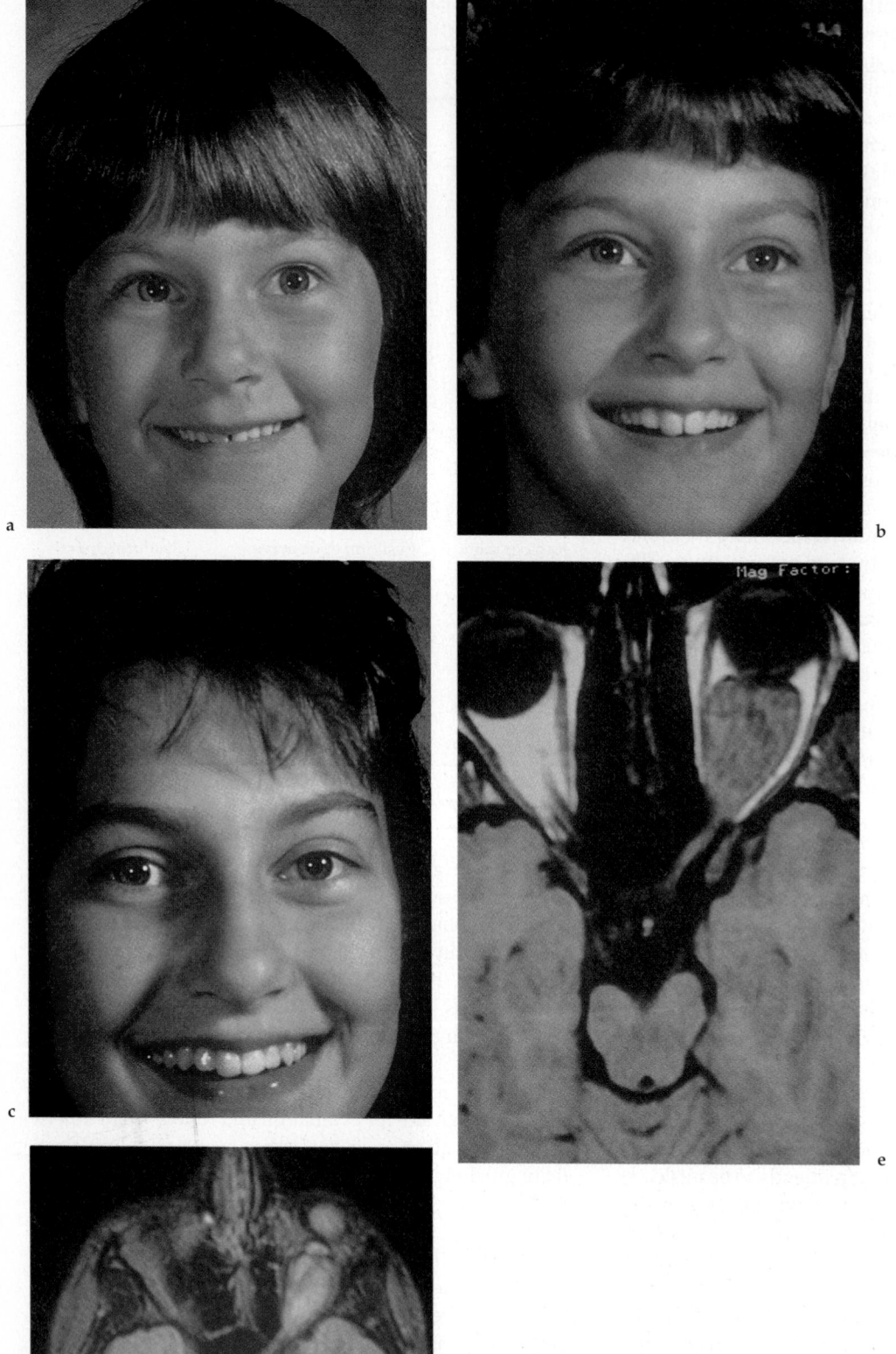

Fig. 29.1 This patient with no stigmas of NF1 was followed up from 8 to 22 years of age (a–c) with deterioration of her visual acuity from 20/80 to 20/200 and increasing proptosis of the left eye. The chiasm appeared to be free of tumour (d, e). Patient from the University of British Columbia.

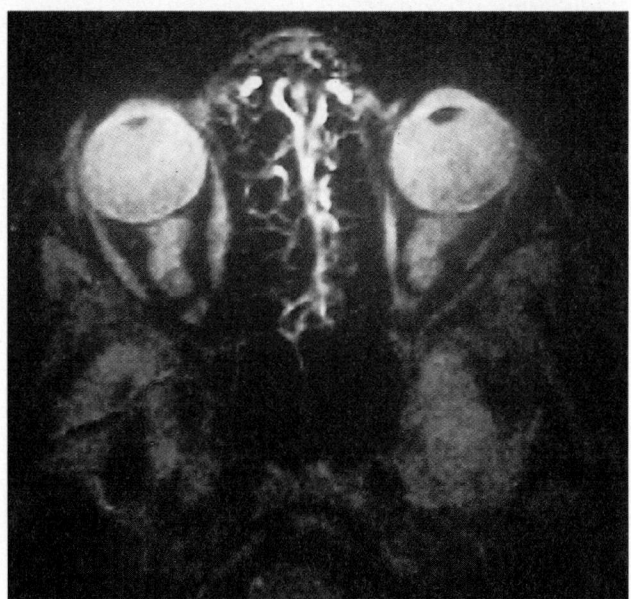

Fig. 29.2 Bilateral optic nerve glioma in a patient with NF1 who had been followed with no change in vision or neuroimaging for many years.

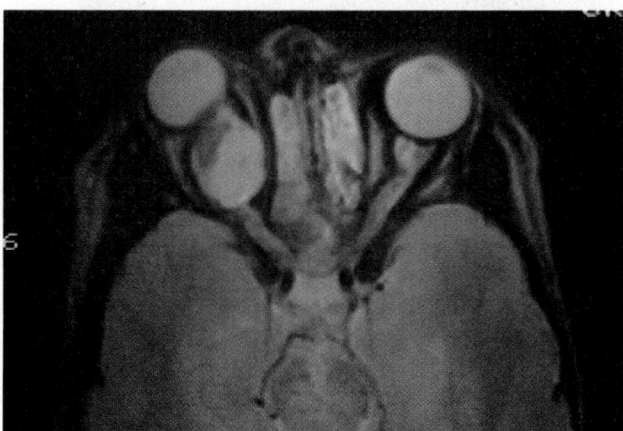

a

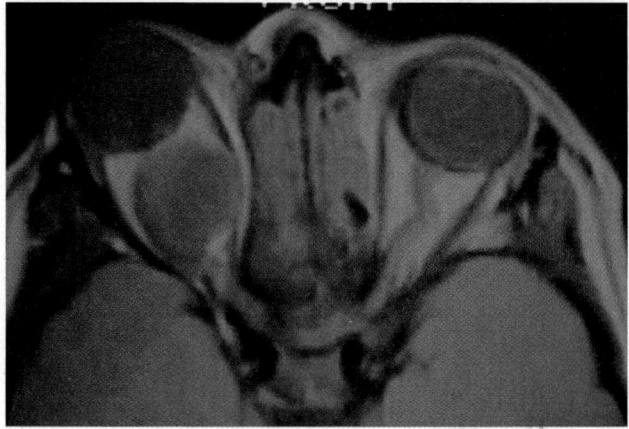

b

Fig. 29.3 (a, b) Optic nerve glioma with cystic area anteriorly.

1980). T2-weighted images of NF1 gliomas show an area of high signal intensity (corresponding to the mucinous element) surrounding a central core of lower signal intensity (the intraneural tumour) (Seiff *et al.* 1987; Imes & Hoyt 1991; Brodsky 1993).

Biological behaviour and management. Optic nerve gliomas are low grade pilocytic astrocytomas. Their behaviour parallels the behaviour of these tumours elsewhere in the central nervous system. The vast majority have little potential for growth and their management is therefore conservative wherever possible. Static findings or slow growth are usually documented at annual or 6-monthly follow-up. Fluctuation of visual acuity is known to occur, and improvement of vision is well documented (Hoyt & Baghdassarian 1969; Frohman *et al.* 1985; Miller 1988; Wright *et al.* 1989). However, rare cases run a more aggressive course (Miller 1988; Wright *et al.* 1989). Enlargement, which can be rapid and substantial, takes place by a combination of glial proliferation, mucoid degeneration and meningeal hyperplasia (Spencer 1972; Wright *et al.* 1980). The difficulty is in identifying which patient is going to progress. Disc oedema (as opposed to atrophy), restriction of movement and the absence of neurofibromatosis were identified as risk factors for rapid progression by Wright *et al.* (1989).

There is no doubt that the prognosis for survival is excellent after excision of optic nerve gliomas (Miller 1988). The question which has been widely debated over the past 25 years and is still unresolved is: which patient needs to undergo this surgery? Until a large prospective study is done on carefully, genetically classified patients comparing conservative management versus the option of surgery or radiotherapy, the answer will have to be based on retrospective data.

Our practical approach to glioma management is this: in our view, a child with a unilateral optic nerve glioma, good vision and no evidence of chiasmal involvement on MRI scan or contralateral VEP studies should be followed up regularly with VEP and MRI studies. Intervention is then based on evidence of prechiasmal progression and/or proptosis. Patients with NF1 are more likely to have stable findings and an indolent course, diffuse or multifocal involvement of their visual pathways and to have chiasmal involvement. They also tend to have good preservation of visual function, and fluctuation of vision is well known to occur. The emphasis of management in this group is therefore conservative. Visual deterioration without fluctuation may be an indication for treatment with low-dose chemotherapy, as advocated by Packer *et al.* (1983) or radiotherapy (Howrich & Bloom 1985) which may halt or even reverse the decline (Taveras *et al.* 1956; Miller 1988). If the tumour is associated with visual obscurations due to mucoid accumulation within the nerve sheath, nerve sheath decompression can be considered.

Patients without evidence of NF1 tend to present with worse visual acuity and localized involvement of the optic nerve. These gliomas also behave in a very benign way with slow or no progression at annual assessment. However, tumours situated anterior to the chiasm showing progression and threatening to involve this structure, or evidence of steady enlargement on sequential MRIs with disfiguring proptosis or globe luxation as well as poor vision are indications for surgical excision. This is performed through a lateral orbitotomy if the tumour is restricted to the intraorbital portion of the nerve, or a temporofrontal panoramic orbitotomy if extension beyond the orbit is noted. The affected nerve is divided posterior to the tumour, with frozen section control to ensure complete removal. In cases where there is intracranial extension, the nerve is divided just anterior to the chiasm. The globe is usually spared after tumour excision, even if the central retinal and posterior ciliary arteries appear to be involved. Dissection of the posterior ciliary vessels prior to resection of the nerve prevents postoperative ocular ischaemia (Rootman *et al.* 1995), which was previously reported to be a common complication after glioma excision (Wright *et al.* 1989). Obviously, vision is sacrificed in the ipsilateral eye. Orbitotomy has minimal effect on the subsequent growth of the facial and orbital bones.

It is important to stress that excision is only indicated in the absence of chiasmal involvement by tumour. However, accurate assessment of this remains problematic even with the most modern techniques. Clinicians who believe gliomas to be congenital lesions which behave like hamartomas (Hoyt & Baghdassarian 1969) argue that these tumours do not truly 'grow' into previously uninvolved neural tissue, but rather that pre-existing and hitherto subclinical involvement manifests itself with time. If this was the case, chiasmal involvement would not be prevented by excision of the affected optic nerve. Borit and Richardson (1982) reported histological and postmortem studies following optic nerve glioma excision showing multicentric involvement of the visual pathways by glioma. Nevertheless, Wright *et al.* (1989) reported no evidence of recurrent chiasmal disease in all six patients in whom the proximal end of the excised optic nerve was histologically free of tumour, with a mean follow-up of 6.5 years. It is not clear whether these patients had NF1 or not. Enlargement of glioma proximal to the cut end of the optic nerve is well recorded.

The next generation of MRI scanners may help to define chiasmal involvement more accurately.

Chiasmal glioma (see also Chapter 52)

Presentation. Glioma affecting predominantly the chiasm is more common than optic nerve glioma (Moseley & Sanders 1982; Rush *et al.* 1982). Unlike optic nerve glioma, which is more common in girls, there is no sex predilec-

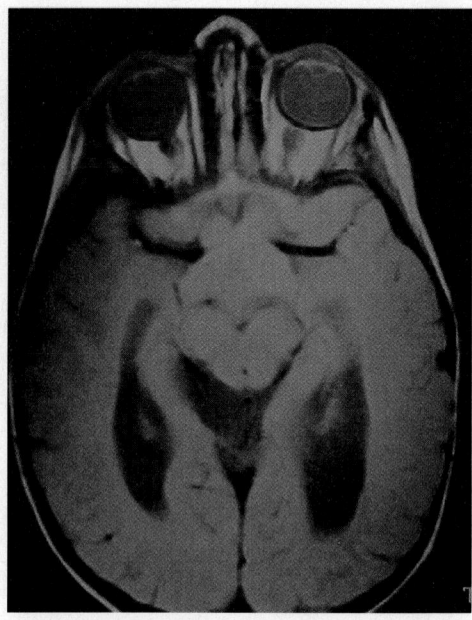

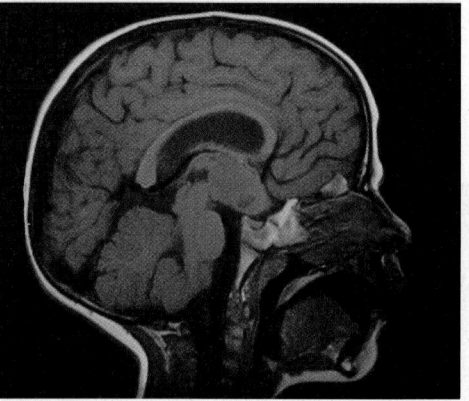

Fig. 29.4 (a, b) Chiasmal and hypothalamic glioma with thickened intracranial optic nerves.

tion. They are seen in a slightly older age group than children with optic nerve glioma (Rush *et al.* 1982). The usual presentation to the ophthalmologist is with bilateral visual loss (Fig. 29.4, 29.5), although chiasmal glioma may be discovered during investigation of hydrocephalus or endocrine dysfunction (Hoyt & Baghdassarian 1969) or in a hitherto asymptomatic patient by neuroimaging studies (Listernick *et al.* 1994). The history is usually of slowly deteriorating vision, but sudden visual loss mimicking optic neuritis may occur as a result of haemorrhage within the tumour, a complication Maitland *et al.* (1982) called 'chiasmal apoplexy'.

Strabismus is an occasional presenting sign. Unilateral or asymmetrical (dissociated) nystagmus caused by chiasmal glioma may mimic spasmus nutans (Farmer & Hoyt 1984). Neuroradiological studies are therefore indicated in any child with asymmetrical nystagmus, particularly in the presence of optic atrophy, poor feeding or hydro-

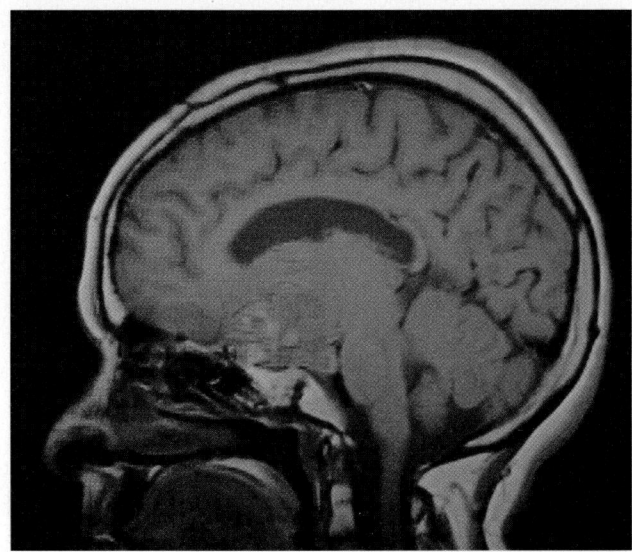

Fig. 29.5 Large, vascular, chiasmal and hypothalamic glioma.

cephalus since this is suggestive of chiasmal glioma with or without posterior extension (Lavery *et al.* 1984).

Proptosis is an unusual presenting sign (Fig. 29.6), although tumour often extends forwards into one or both optic nerves and occasionally into the orbit. The tumour can also extend into the optic tracts and the visual field findings are therefore variable (Glaser *et al.* 1971), but bitemporal loss is common (Rush *et al.* 1982). The discs may be normal, but are more likely to be atrophic or, more rarely, swollen (Rush *et al.* 1982).

Extension of the lesion into the hypothalamus produces various endocrine abnormalities. Precocious puberty was reported in seven of 18 children with chiasmal glioma, with ages ranging from 4.8 to 5.9 years (Listernick *et al.* 1994). Reduced growth and sexual maturation, diabetes insipidus and obesity may also occur. In some cases, there may be extreme wasting, reduced development and often vertical or rotary nystagmus, an association known as Russell's diencephalic syndrome (Russell 1951; Moseley & Sanders 1982).

Radiologically, chiasmal glioma is seen as a suprasellar mass which may be accompanied by a diagnostic contiguous enlargement of the optic nerve or tract (Fletcher *et al.* 1986). Minor degrees of chiasmal enlargement are relatively difficult to detect with CT. MRI is better for studying the chiasm, intracranial optic nerves and optic tract (Holman *et al.* 1985; Haik *et al.* 1987; Savino 1987).

The diagnosis can be made on the basis of neuroimaging studies and tissue diagnosis is rarely necessary for lesions which appear intrinsic to the chiasm.

Biological behaviour and management. Several long-term studies have documented stability in the majority of chiasmal gliomas (Hoyt & Baghdassarian 1969; Glaser *et al.* 1971; Imes & Hoyt 1986). Surgery may be of benefit in gliomas in which a significant exophytic component is compressing the chiasm or either optic nerve (Venes *et al.* 1984). Surgery on the chiasm carries an appreciable risk of hypothalamic syndrome and sudden death. Moreover, surgical removal of intrinsic chiasmal glioma is not possible without sacrificing vision bilaterally. The management options are observation, radiotherapy and, possibly, chemotherapy. The management plans suggested by Packer *et al.* (1983) and reinforced by Kennerdell and Garrity (1988) seem logical.

In view of remaining uncertainty about the natural history of chiasmal glioma, no treatment is given if the tumour is confined to the chiasm at the time of diagnosis. These patients are reviewed regularly with clinical evaluation of acuity, fields and regular MRI.

There is no single accepted indication for treatment of chiasmal glioma. If there is involvement of the hypothalamus or third ventricle or gross enlargement of the optic tract, treatment by radiotherapy is advised. Whilst the effectiveness of radiotherapy for chiasmal glioma is still in doubt (Rush *et al.* 1982; Imes & Hoyt 1986), some authors consider that disease control in up to 50% of patients is possible (Packer *et al.* 1983; Howrich & Bloom 1985). Radiotherapy therefore appears the best treatment option available, especially when visual loss has been rapid and recent. However, radiotherapy can have numerous adverse effects on the developing brain, including mental and growth retardation, psychiatric problems and the induction of second tumours. Chemotherapy may delay radiation and its unwanted side-effects, but 60% of children eventually relapse (Janss *et al.* 1995). Endocrine abnormalities associated with chiasmal glioma require assessment and treatment. Hydrocephalus may require ventricular shunting.

Screening for anterior visual pathway gliomas. The National Institutes of Health (NIH) conference on neurofibromatosis stated that tests such as CT, MRI and VEPs are unlikely to be of value in asymptomatic patients with NF1. Annual ophthalmological follow-up was recommended for patients with NF1 and those with gliomas of the optic pathways documented to have stable findings. Many would now argue that baseline imaging of the optic pathways is indicated for all patients with NF1 (Riccardi 1992; Listernick *et al.* 1994). VEPs may provide a low cost and safe alternative to the general anaesthetic which is necessary for MRI of children under the age of 6 years. Jabbari *et al.* (1985) found abnormal pattern reversal VEPs in eight of 30 asymptomatic patients with NF1 whose ocular examination, including visual fields, was normal. In seven, there was increased latency. Of the eight, seven had CT scans. Six of these showed ipsilateral optic nerve enlargement suggestive of optic nerve glioma.

Groswasser *et al.* (1985) recorded VEPs in 25 patients with optic nerve glioma. The mean age in their study

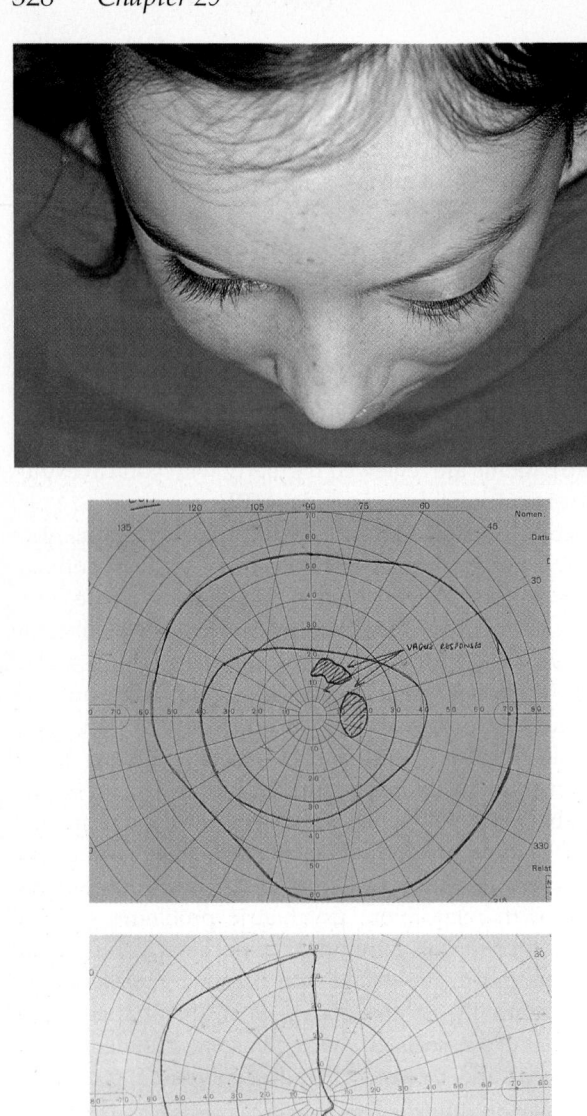

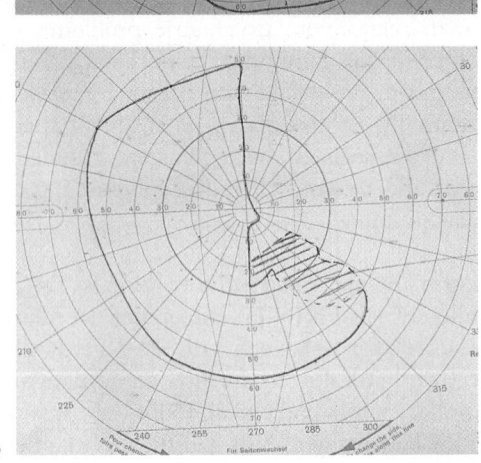

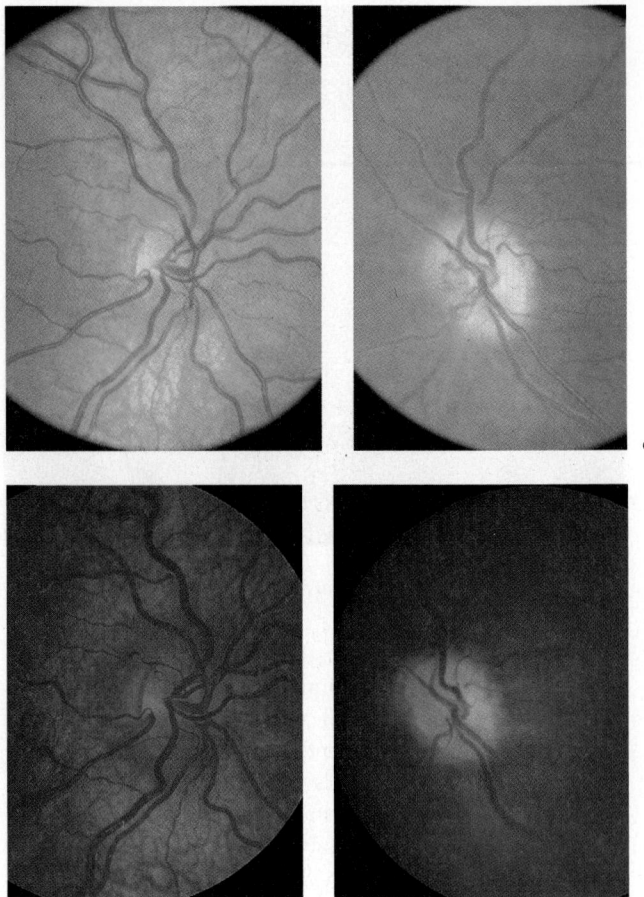

Fig. 29.6 (a) Chiasmal and left optic nerve glioma with left proptosis.
(b) Right visual field on 13 November 1974 (top). Right visual field
(bottom) on 14 April 1976 showing temporal field defect from
increased chiasmal involvement (same patient in a–c). A clear-cut
temporal field loss is unusual in chiasmal glioma because there are
frequently associated tract and optic nerve lesions.
(c) In November 1974 her left eye had very poor vision. There was
optic atrophy, the disc was swollen and there were shunt vessels
visible. The right eye shows mild band atrophy.
(d) In April 1976 the left optic nerve was completely atrophic and
the eye is blind. The shunt vessels have disappeared. The right eye
has papilloedema due to raised intracranial pressure and this
demonstrates clearly the bilobed nature of the papilloedema
associated with a temporal field defect ('twin peaks' papilloedema).

group was 11.3 years (range 2–29 years). They reported
delay and reduction in amplitude from eyes with optic
nerve gliomas in which there was moderate visual impairment. In severe visual impairment, the pattern reversal
VEP was unrecordable, but flash VEP showed an increase
in latency. They also described *de novo* involvement and
subsequent deterioration of the contralateral temporal
hemifield VEP in a patient with clinically unsuspected
progressive chiasmal involvement from optic nerve
glioma with, later, spontaneous improvement.

More recently (and worryingly) Rossi *et al.* (1994)
reported normal pattern reversal VEPs in six children

with optic nerve gliomas documented with MRI, probably
confirming the latter as the best diagnostic modality available today. North *et al.* (1994), however, reported a sensitivity of 90% for detecting optic gliomas, with an increase
to 100% when hemifield stimulation was used. The specificity was 60%, suggesting that there were a lot of false positive results. Perhaps the use of MRI could be limited
to those children with NF1 whose VEPs are found to
be abnormal using pattern reversal and hemifield
techniques.

Malignant gliomas of the anterior visual pathway
which behave aggressively, also known as glioblastoma

multiforme, are recognized in adults (Hoyt *et al.* 1973; Spoor *et al.* 1980) and may occasionally occur in children (Moseley & Sanders 1982; Rush *et al.* 1982).

Meningiomas

Meningiomas are very rare in childhood, but become slightly more common in the teenage years. They result from proliferation of meningothelial cap cells of the arachnoid and may arise in association with NF1 or NF2. They may occur within the sheath of the optic nerve or from the dura of the sphenoid bone, affecting the sphenoid wing and/or parasellar region. The site of origin determines the pattern of presentation: tumours arising from the lateral third of the greater wing of the sphenoid present with mass effect and relative visual preservation whereas those situated at the inner third tend to present with earlier visual loss with or without cranial nerve palsies. Optic nerve sheath tumours, particularly when intracanalicular, present with early visual loss and relatively little mass effect.

Optic nerve sheath meningiomas

Clinical presentation of optic nerve sheath meningioma is with visual loss; proptosis is less common as a presenting sign, especially with posteriorly situated orbital lesions (Dutton 1992). A tendency to grow through the dura makes extraocular muscle involvement relatively frequent (Jakobiec & Jones 1983). Diplopia may be a feature, due to splinting of the optic nerve by the tumour. Compression of the optic nerve results in an optic neuropathy. Duction-induced obscurations may occur at first, followed by visual loss as the tumour enlarges. An afferent pupillary defect may be present as well as disc swelling or pallor and opticociliary shunt vessels. Although the latter may also occur with optic nerve gliomas, their presence is more suggestive of meningioma (Jakobiec & Jones 1983).

Investigation

CT offers certain advantages over MRI for intraorbital optic nerve imaging, since the latter may fail to highlight calcification within the lesion, and optic nerve sheath enlargement may be missed unless specific fat-suppression techniques are used. Nevertheless, if facilities are available, MRI with fat saturation and gadolinium enhancement is the modality of choice for defining the extent of the tumour (Lindblom *et al.* 1992) since it better demonstrates intracanalicular and intracranial extension. On CT scans (Fig. 29.7a), meningioma usually causes a tubular enlargement of the optic nerve, sometimes with calcification causing a tram-line appearance (Jakobiec *et al.* 1984) or excrescent growth through the dura (Rothfus *et al.* 1984). The nerve can usually be identified as a radiolu-

cent region within the tumour on axial and coronal scans (Jakobiec *et al.* 1984; Rothfus *et al.* 1984). Since these tumours may be quite vascular, enhancement with intravenous contrast, and tumour blush on angiography are common features, unlike glioma where they are rare (Moseley & Sanders 1982). Furthermore, kinking of the nerve, a common feature in glioma, is not seen. Dutton and Anderson (1985) have drawn attention to the radiological similarity of the perineural variant of non-specific orbital inflammation and optic nerve sheath meningioma. MRI (see Fig. 29.7b) may clearly delineate the difference between the nerve and the tumour.

Biopsy may not be helpful in differentiating meningioma from glioma, due to the presence of meningeal hyperplasia in the latter which appears similar to meningioma (Anonymous 1979). It should be possible to distinguish these two entities on clinical and radiological grounds (Jakobiec *et al.* 1984; Rothfus *et al.* 1984).

Treatment

The main choice lies between observation and surgical excision, although radiotherapy may also be considered (Kennerdell & Garrity 1988). Tumour involving the anterior two-thirds of the intraorbital nerve can be excised via a lateral orbitotomy. If the tumour extends to the posterior orbit or intracranially, a combined orbital–neurosurgical approach is required via a panoramic orbitotomy. The eye will be blind but cosmetically satisfactory (Rootman 1988; Wolter 1988). The clinical course of optic nerve sheath meningioma is reported to be more aggressive in children than adults so surgical treatment may be favoured (Jakobiec *et al.* 1984). Conversely, these lesions have no metastatic potential and may grow slowly, so observation to establish the pattern of growth in individual cases appears a reasonable option.

Extraoptic meningioma

This type of meningioma is slightly more common in childhood than optic nerve tumours, with a tendency to occur during the teenage years. The sites of ophthalmic relevance are the sphenoid wing, suprasellar area and olfactory groove. The ophthalmic features reflect the position of the tumour, since those situated medially present with visual loss, cranial nerve palsies and symptoms and signs of venous obstruction at the orbital apex, whilst those arising laterally cause mass effect, and swelling in the temporalis fossa. Very rarely, meningiomas can arise at extradural sites in children (Johnson *et al.* 1993).

The best diagnostic modality for these is CT scan which demonstrates the hyperostosis underlying the tumour. The lesion is of homogeneously increased density, and enhances evenly after contrast injection. Fine calcification may be present in psammomatous tumours.

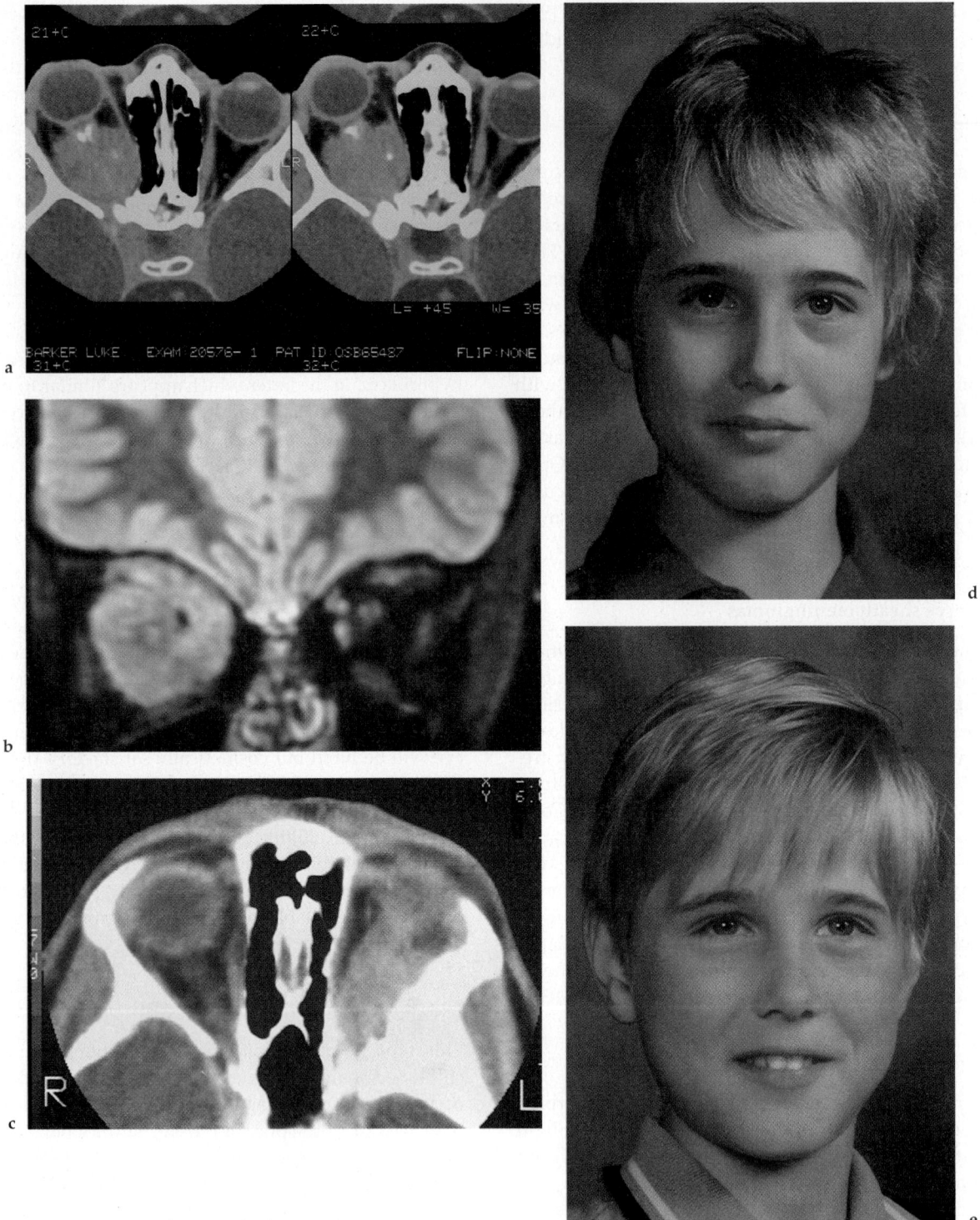

Fig. 29.7 (a) Optic nerve meningioma in a 5-year-old boy. CT scan showing calcification around the optic nerve and orbital expansion on the right. (b) MRI of same patient showing the clear differentiation between the peripheral tumour and the axial optic nerve. The calcium is not demonstrated. (c) Sphenoid wing meningioma in a 9-year-old boy: CT scan showing marked hyperostosis on the left. (d) Sphenoid wing meningioma (same patient) aged 9 years, showing lid swelling and proptosis. (e) Sphenoid wing meningioma: same patient aged 12 years after resection and radiotherapy. Patient from the University of British Columbia.

Since tumour growth is slow, observation is warranted in most cases. The course tends to be more aggressive in childhood. Excision is indicated for cosmesis or visual loss, but encasement of orbital structures or bone invasion may preclude complete clearance. Debulking may be sufficient to improve cosmesis and decompress the orbital apex, with improvement of optic neuropathy. Encouraging results have been reported with radical excision followed by radiotherapy to any residual tumour (Maroon *et al.* 1994).

Rare optic nerve tumours in childhood

Leukaemic infiltration of the optic nerve traditionally has a grave systemic prognosis although with combined radiotherapy and chemotherapy the prognosis is greatly improved when the infiltration is prelaminar, the optic disc has a fluffy appearance with oedema and haemorrhage without marked visual loss. Retrolaminar involvement results in moderate disc swelling but profound visual loss (Kincaid & Green 1983; Rosenthal 1983).

Tumours of the optic disc such as melanocytoma, angiomatous malformations, or glial hamartoma (as seen in tuberous sclerosis) may involve the very anterior parts of the optic nerve. Ganglioma, ganglioglioma (Bergin *et al.* 1988), inflammatory lesions, aneurysms, histiocytosis, sarcomas, and other rare entities have also been described (Eggers *et al.* 1976; Brown & Shields 1985). Medulloepithelioma is a tumour which arises from the medullary epithelium of the optic vesicle, and is much more commonly found in the ciliary body. It can affect the optic nerve head and may extend into the substance of the optic nerve. Both benign and malignant forms have been described. Margo and Kincaid (1988) found a vascular malformation in the retrolaminar portion of two eyes removed for suspicion of retinoblastoma, one eye had a neuroblastic tumour and the other a form of retina dysplasia.

The importance of many of these rare optic nerve tumours is in the differential diagnosis of the much more common optic nerve glioma, for which biopsy is rarely performed.

Schwannoma

Schwannomas (formerly known as neurilemmomas or neurinomas) are tumours which arise from the Schwann cells of peripheral nerve sheath (Fig. 29.8). They are rare in childhood, generally occurring in middle-aged patients. They are more common in NF1 and NF2. The sensory nerves are much more frequently affected, but schwannomas of the ocular motor nerves are well recognized, particularly the third nerve.

The tumour is composed of proliferating Schwann cells, without significant admixture of axons and endoneural cells, in a collagenous matrix (Harkin & Reed 1969) and is

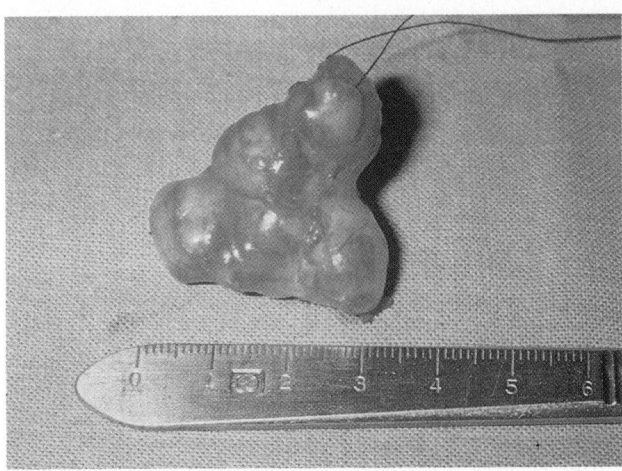

Fig. 29.8 A lobulated orbital schwannoma after surgical excision. Patient from the University of British Columbia.

circumscribed by a fibrous capsule. Two cellular patterns, which may occur in the same tumour, are recognized. The Antoni A pattern consists of compactly arranged spindle cells with long oval nuclei, frequently orientated with their long axes parallel. The Antoni B type pattern consists of Schwann cells with twisted and elongated shapes widely separated by a featureless collagen matrix.

Transformation into a malignant Schwann cell tumour is exceedingly rare in childhood but Miller (1988) described a 6-week-old infant with increasing proptosis from birth and NF1 stigmata who was affected bilaterally.

Orbital schwannoma generally presents with proptosis. Since the trigeminal nerve is often involved, facial paraesthesia may be a feature. Diplopia may result from third nerve involvement or compression by a tumour in the trigeminal ganglion. Progression tends to be slow and sometimes intermittent over a period of years. Schwannoma may also occur in the eyelid (Reese 1976). Orbital schwannomas tend to be localized and can be excised or their contents can be evacuated without undue difficulty (Reese 1976; Nicholson & Green 1981; Rootman 1988).

References

Anonymous. Primary optic nerve meningioma (editorial). *Br J Ophthalmol* 1979; **63**: 595.

Bergin DJ, Johnson TE, Spencer WH, McCord CD. Ganglioglioma of the optic nerve. *Am J Ophthalmol* 1988; **105**: 146–50.

Borit A, Richardson EF. The biological and clinical behaviour of pilocytic astrocytomas of the optic pathways. *Brain* 1982; **105**: 161–88.

Brodsky MC. The 'pseudo-CSF' signal of orbital optic glioma on magnetic resonance imaging: a signature of neurofibromatosis. *Surv Ophthalmol* 1993; **38**: 213–18.

Brown GC, Shields JA. Tumours of the optic nerve head. *Surv Ophthalmol* 1985; **29**: 239–64.

Buchanan TAS, Hoyt WF. Optic nerve glioma and neovascular glaucoma: report of a case. *Br J Ophthalmol* 1982; **66**: 96–8.

Dutton JJ. Gliomas of the anterior visual pathway. *Surv Ophthalmol* 1994; **38**: 427–52.

Dutton JJ. Optic nerve sheath meningiomas. *Surv Ophthalmol* 1992; **37**: 167–83.

Dutton JJ, Anderson RL. Idiopathic inflammatory perioptic neuritis simulating optic nerve sheath meningioma. *Am J Ophthalmol* 1985; **100**: 424–30.

Eggers H, Jakobiec FA, Jones IS. Tumours of the optic nerve. *Documenta Ophthalmol* 1976; **41**: 43–128.

Farmer J, Hoyt CS. Monocular nystagmus in infancy and early childhood. *Am J Ophthalmol* 1984; **98**: 504–9.

Fletcher WA, Imes RK, Hoyt WF. Chiasmal gliomas: appearance and long-term changes demonstrated by computerized tomography. *J Neurosurg* 1986; **65**: 154–9.

Frohman LP, Epstein F, Kupersmith MJ. Atypical visual prognosis with an optic nerve glioma. *J Clin Neuro-ophthalmol* 1985; **5**: 90–4.

Glaser JS, Hoyt WF, Corbett J. Visual morbidity with chiasmal glioma. Long-term studies of visual fields in untreated and irradiated cases. *Arch Ophthalmol* 1971; **85**: 3–12.

Groswasser Z, Kriss A, Halliday AM, McDonald WI. Pattern- and flash-evoked potentials in the assessment and management of optic nerve gliomas. *J Neurol Neurosurg Psychiatry* 1985; **48**: 1125–34.

Haik B, Saint Louis L, Bierly J et al. Magnetic resonance imaging in the evaluation of optic nerve gliomas. *Ophthalmology* 1987; **94**: 709–18.

Harkin J, Reed R. Tumours of the peripheral nervous system. In: *Atlas of Tumour Pathology*, 2nd Series, Fascicle 3. Washington: Armed Forces Institute of Pathology, 1969.

Holman RE, Grimson BS, Drayer BP et al. Magnetic resonance imaging of optic gliomas. *Am J Ophthalmol* 1985; **100**: 596–601.

Howrich A, Bloom HJG. Optic gliomas: radiation therapy and prognosis. *Int J Radiat Oncol Biol Phys* 1985; **11**: 1067–79.

Hoyt WF, Baghdassarian SA. Optic glioma of childhood. Natural history and rationale for conservative management. *Br J Ophthalmol* 1969; **53**: 793–8.

Hoyt WF, Meshel LG, Lessell S et al. Malignant optic glioma of adulthood. *Brain* 1973; **96**: 121–32.

Imes RK, Hoyt WF. Childhood chiasmal gliomas: update on the fate of patients in the 1969 San Francisco study. *Br J Ophthalmol* 1986; **70**: 179–82.

Imes RK, Hoyt WF. Magnetic resonance imaging signs of optic nerve glioma in neurofibromatosis 1. *Am J Ophthalmol* 1991; **111**: 729–34.

Jabbari B, Maitland CG, Morris LM et al. The value of visual evoked potential as a screening test in neurofibromatosis. *Arch Neurol* 1985; **42**: 1072–4.

Jakobiec FA, Depot MJ, Kennerdell J et al. Combined clinical and computed tomographic diagnosis of orbital glioma and meningioma. *Ophthalmology* 1984; **91**: 137–55.

Jakobiec FA, Jones IS. Neurogenic tumours. In: Duane T, ed. *Clinical Ophthalmology*, Vol. 2. Hagerstown: Harper & Row, 1983: 1–16.

Janss AJ, Grundy R, Canan A et al. Optic pathway and hypothalamic/chiasmatic gliomas in children younger than age 5 years with a 6-year follow-up. *Cancer* 1995; **75**: 1051–9.

Johnson TE, Weatherhead RG, Nasr AM, Siqueira EB. Ectopic (extradural) meningioma of the orbit: a report of two cases in children. *J Pediatr Ophthalmol Strabismus* 1993; **30**: 43–7.

Kennerdell JS, Garrity JA. Tumours of the optic nerve. In: Lessell S, Van Dalen JTW, eds. *Current Neuro-ophthalmology*, Vol. 1. Chicago: Year Book Medical Publishers, 1988: 25–32.

Kincaid MC, Green WR. Ocular and orbital involvement in leukemia. *Surv Ophthalmol* 1983; **15**: 123–6.

Lavery MA, O'Neill JF, Chu FE, Martyn LJ. Acquired nystagmus in early childhood: a presenting sign of intracranial tumour. *Ophthalmology* 1984; **91**: 425–34.

Lewis RA, Gerson LP, Axelson KA et al. Von Recklinghausen neurofibromatosis II: incidence of optic glioma. *Ophthalmology* 1984; **91**: 929–35.

Lindblom B, Truwit C, Hoyt WF. Optic nerve sheath meningioma. Definition of intraorbital, intracanalicular and intracranial components with magnetic resonance imaging. *Ophthalmology* 1992; **99**: 560–6.

Listernick R, Charrow J, Greenwald MJ, Esterly NB. Optic gliomas in children with neurofibromatosis type 1. *J Pediatr* 1989; **114**: 788–92.

Listernick R, Charrow J, Greenwald M, Mets M. Natural history of optic pathway tumors in children with neurofibromatosis type 1: a longitudinal study. *J Pediatr* 1994; **125**: 63–6.

Maitland CG, Abiko S, Hoyt WF et al. Chiasmal apoplexy: report of four cases. *J Neurosurg* 1982; **56**: 118–22.

Margo CE, Kincaid MC. Angiomatous malformation of the retrolaminar optic nerve. *J Pediatr Ophthalmol Strabismus* 1988; **25**: 37–40.

Maroon JC, Kennerdell JS, Vidovich DV et al. Recurrent sphenoorbital meningioma. *J Neurosurg* 1994; **80**: 202–8.

Miller NR, ed. *Walsh and Hoyt's Clinical Neuro-ophthalmology*, 4th edn. Baltimore: Williams & Wilkins, 1988: 1559.

Moseley IF, Sanders MD. *Computerised Tomography in Neuro-ophthalmology*. London: Chapman & Hall, 1982.

Nicholson DH, Green WR. *Pediatric Ocular Tumours*. New York: Masson, 1981.

North K, Cochineas C, Tang E, Fagan E. Optic gliomas in neurofibromatosis type 1: role of visual evoked potentials. *Pediatr Neurol* 1994; **10**: 117–23.

Packer RJ, Savino PJ, Bilaniuk LT et al. Chiasmatic gliomas of childhood. A reappraisal of natural history and effectiveness of cranial irradiation. *Child's Brain* 1983; **10**: 393–403.

Reese AB. *Tumours of the Eye*, 3rd edn. Hagerstown: Harper & Row, 1976: 156–65.

Riccardi VM. *Neurofibromatosis: Phenotype, Natural History, and Pathogenesis*, 2nd edn. Baltimore: Johns Hopkins University Press, 1992.

Rootman J. *Diseases of the Orbit: A Multidisciplinary Approach*. Philadelphia: JB Lippincott, 1988, Chapter 12.

Rootman J, Kao SCS, Graeb D. Multidisciplinary approaches to complicated vascular lesions of the orbit. *Ophthalmology* 1992; **99**: 1440–6.

Rootman J, Stewart B, Goldberg RA. *Surgery of the Orbit*. New York: Raven Press, 1995.

Rosenthal AR. Ocular manifestations of leukemia: a review. *Ophthalmology* 1983; **90**: 899–905.

Rossi LN, Pastorino G, Scotti G et al. Early diagnosis of optic glioma in children with neurofibromatosis type 1. *Child's Nervous System* 1994; **10**: 426–9.

Rothfus WE, Curtin MD, Slamovits TL, Kennerdell JS. Optic nerve/sheath enlargement. *Radiology* 1984; **150**: 409–15.

Rush JA, Younge BR, Campbell RJ, MacCarthy CS. Optic glioma: long-term follow-up of 85 histopathologically verified cases. *Ophthalmology* 1982; **89**: 1213–19.

Russell A. A diencephalic syndrome of emaciation in infancy and childhood. *Arch Dis Child* 1951; **26**: 274.

Savino PJ. The present role of magnetic resonance imaging in neuro-ophthalmology. *Canad J Ophthalmol* 1987; **22**: 4–12.

Seiff SR, Brodsky MC, MacDonald G et al. Orbital optic glioma in neurofibromatosis. *Arch Ophthalmol* 1987; **105**: 1689–93.

Spencer WH. Primary neoplasms of the optic nerve and its sheaths. *Trans Am Ophthalmol Soc* 1972; **70**: 490–505.

Spoor TC, Kennerdell JS, Martinez AJ, Zoras D. Malignant gliomas of the optic pathways. *Am J Ophthalmol* 1980; **89**: 284–92.

Stern J, Jakobiec FA, Housepian EM. The architecture of optic nerve gliomas with and without neurofibromatosis. *Arch Ophthalmol* 1980; **98**: 505–11.

Taveras JM, Mount LA, Wood EH. The value of radiation therapy in the management of glioma of the optic nerves and chiasm. *Radiology* 1956; **66**: 518–28.

Venes JL, Latack J, Kandt RS. Postoperative regression opticochiasmic astrocytoma: a case for expectant therapy. *Neurosurgery* 1984;

15: 421–3.

Wolter JR. Ten years without orbital optic nerve: late clinical results after removal of retrobulbar gliomas with preservation of blind eyes. *J Pediatr Ophthalmol Strabismus* 1988; **25**: 55–60.

Wright JE, McDonald WI, Call NB. Management of optic nerve gliomas. *Br J Ophthalmol* 1980; **64**: 545–52.

Wright JE, McNab AA, McDonald WI. Optic nerve glioma and the management of optic nerve tumours in the young. *Br J Ophthalmol* 1989; **73**: 967–74.

30: Rhabdomyosarcoma

Christopher Lyons and Jack Rootman

Primary orbital malignant lesions are an exceedingly rare cause of proptosis in children, but rhabdomyosarcoma is the most common of these. In the combined clinical series presented (see Table 27.1), it accounted for 2% of all children presenting with orbital problems. In Shields' (1986) biopsy-based series, it accounted for 4% of paediatric orbital space-occupying lesions.

It is a tumour of primitive connective tissue or mesenchyme, which has the capacity to differentiate towards striated muscle. Interestingly, the tumours seen in children are not usually situated in extraocular muscles but in orbital connective tissue. The prognosis for affected children has vastly improved over the past 25 years as treatment has evolved from radical surgery to biopsy, radiotherapy and chemotherapy (Haik *et al.* 1986).

Epidemiology and genetics

The great majority of rhabdomyosarcomas present before the age of 10 years, with an overall mean age at onset of 7–8 years (Knowles *et al.* 1983). They may occasionally occur as early as the first year of life and have even been reported in the newborn (Jones *et al.* 1965; Himmel & Siegel 1967). Rarely, they may present in adulthood; the oldest recorded case was 78 years old (Kassel *et al.* 1965). The tumours found in older patients are usually of pleomorphic type, arising within the extraocular muscles. Overall, males are more likely to be affected than females by a ratio of 5:3 (Knowles *et al.* 1976).

Familial cases have been reported. In particular, Li and Fraumeni (1969) and Li *et al.* (1988) described families with a positive history of malignancy, in which pairs of offspring of young mothers with carcinoma developed rhabdomyosarcoma. This association, the Li–Fraumeni syndrome, is now known to be related to mutations of the *p53* gene, a tumour-suppressor gene situated on the short arm of chromosome 17. Rhabdomyosarcoma has also been reported to be more common in patients with neurofibromatosis 1 (Riccardi 1992), another gene defect situated on chromosome 17 (long arm).

As in the case of other malignancies, rhabdomyosarcoma is associated with an increased prevalence of congenital malformations. These were present in one-third of the 115 children and adolescents with rhabdomyosarcoma reviewed at autopsy by Ruymann *et al.* (1988). The malformations most commonly involved the genitourinary, gastrointestinal and central nervous systems.

There are no constitutional chromosome translocations in patients with rhabdomyosarcoma, although in alveolar rhabdomyosarcoma, a t(2:13)(q35:q14) translocation is found in tumour cells (Cowell 1994). Other translocations have been described, with the same breakpoint in chromosome 2. This corresponds with breakage of the *PAX3* gene (Barr *et al.* 1993), a homeobox gene concerned with control of transcription of important developmental genes. A different translocation has also been identified in alveolar rhabdomyosarcoma; the consistent breakpoint here is at 13q14, and this possibly causes tumours in younger children (Douglass *et al.* 1991).

Clinical features

The most common presenting feature is proptosis (Figs 30.1–30.3) which may appear suddenly and progress over a few days or weeks (Frayer & Enterline 1959; Jones *et al.* 1965) often with eyelid erythema and oedema, as well as increasing ophthalmoplegia. The lid signs may occasionally precede the proptosis (Lederman & Wybar 1976). The absence of local heat, pyrexia and general malaise may help to distinguish this entity from orbital cellulitis.

Other presentations include ptosis or a palpable lid mass (Fig. 30.4) occurring at onset of the proptosis or shortly after (Knowles *et al.* 1983). Forty-eight per cent of the 58 patients in one series (Abramson *et al.* 1979) present-

gopalatine fossa or nasal cavity may occur. The latter may give rise to nasal stuffiness or nosebleeds. Rarely, it arises within the cranial cavity, only giving rise to proptosis when orbital involvement occurs (Shuangshoti & Phonprasert 1976). Although there are no lymphatics within the orbit, involvement of the eyelids may be complicated by spread to the cervical or pre-auricular lymph nodes, especially in alveolar rhabdomyosarcoma. Blood-borne spread to the lungs or bones may occasionally occur (Knowles *et al.* 1983). Congenital presentation may occur (Fig. 30.7).

Diagnosis

Rhabdomyosarcoma is one of the causes of rapidly progressive proptosis in childhood. As discussed above, it is rare under the age of 4 years. In this age group, haeman-

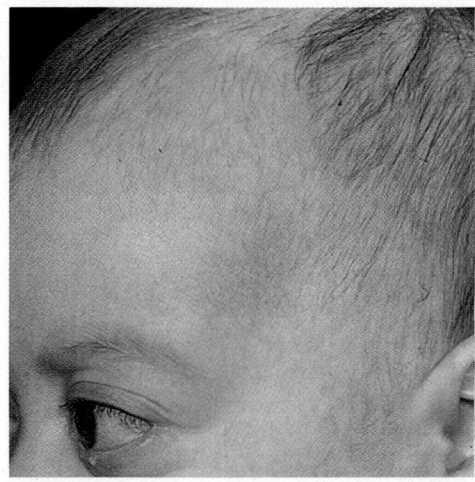

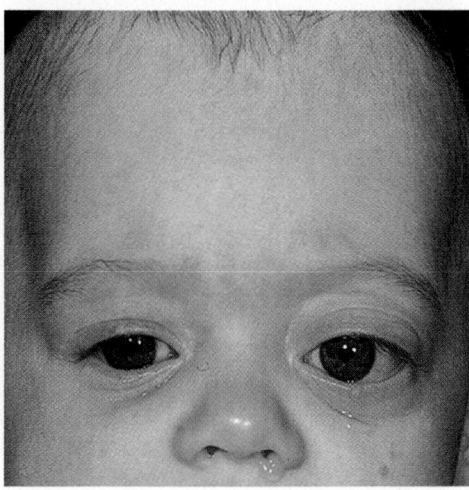

Fig. 30.1 Rhabdomyosarcoma. This 3-month-old boy had a 2-week history of left proptosis.

ed in this way. The lid lump may occasionally be mistaken for a chalazion and erroneously treated as such. It is therefore important to consider rhabdomyosarcoma in the differential diagnosis of any childhood lid lump or unexplained ptosis. Rarely, rhabdomyosarcoma can present as grape-like subconjunctival nodules (botryoid variant), or periorbital swellings (Fig. 30.5).

The location of the tumour affects the direction of displacement of the globe. In the review of 62 patients by Jones *et al.* (1965), half of the tumours were retrobulbar and one-quarter were situated superiorly. Twelve per cent were inferior, 6% nasal and 6% temporal. Although commonly retrobulbar, visual symptoms are unusual (Frayer & Enterline 1959). Rhabdomyosarcomas in the lids or cheeks may easily be mistaken for haemangiomas (Fig. 30.6).

Rhabdomyosarcoma spreads early by rapid local invasion. The tumour is usually confined to the orbit at the time of diagnosis, but later extension into the anterior or middle cranial fossa (parameningeal spread), ptery-

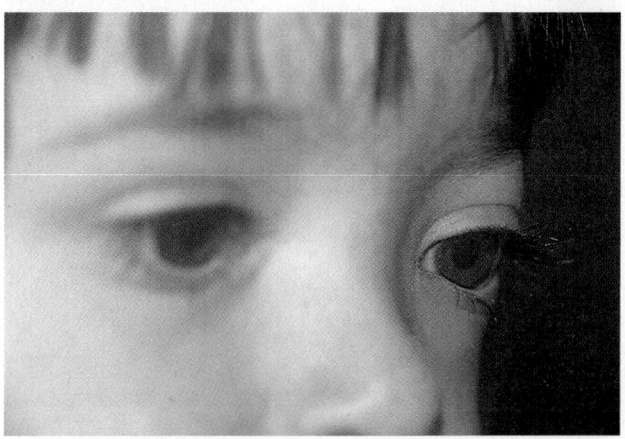

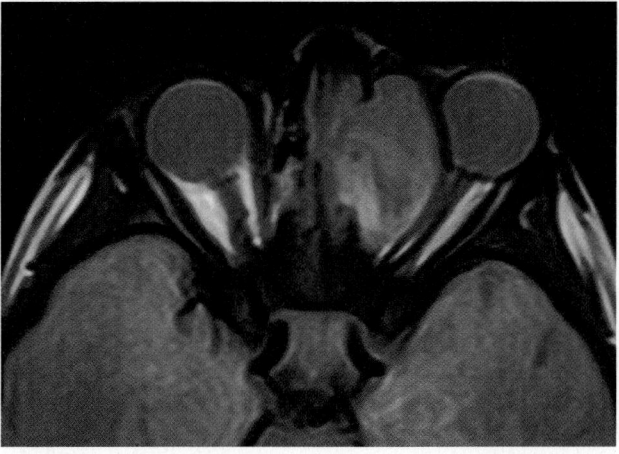

Fig. 30.2 (a) This 20-month-old girl had a 3-week history of left proptosis, nasal discharge and nosebleeds. There is 7 mm of proptosis of the left eye with 5 mm lateral globe displacement. (b) On MRI, an ethmoidal mass had eroded through the medial orbital wall and displaced the orbital contents anteriorly and laterally. The mass has also obstructed the nasal cavity. Intranasal biopsy demonstrated rhabdomyosarcoma of alveolar type. Patient from the University of British Columbia.

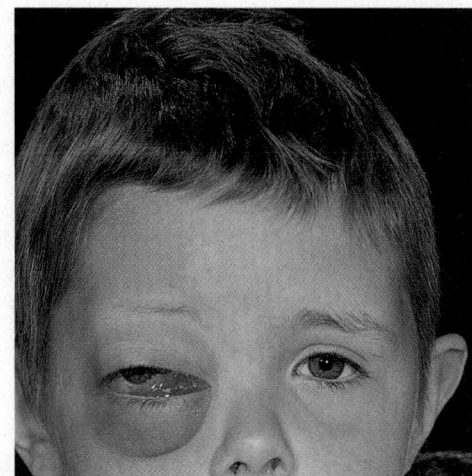

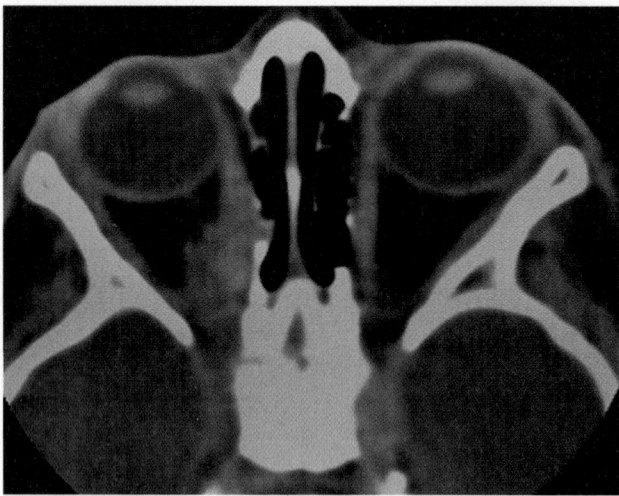

Computed tomography (CT) scanning or magnetic resonance imaging (MRI) are the best investigation in this context. CT typically shows a non-enhancing poorly defined mass of homogeneous tissue density. There may be low density areas within the tumour. Bone windows on CT are important to determine whether there is invasion of the orbital walls, a sign associated with a poorer prognosis.

CT or MRI will delineate the tumour in order to plan the best approach for biopsy. If these modalities are not available, plain orbital X-ray may show increased soft tissue density in the orbit or evidence of bone erosion by the tumour, and orbital ultrasound may contribute to the imaging of anteriorly situated tumours.

Since tumour seeding along the biopsy tract is well rec-

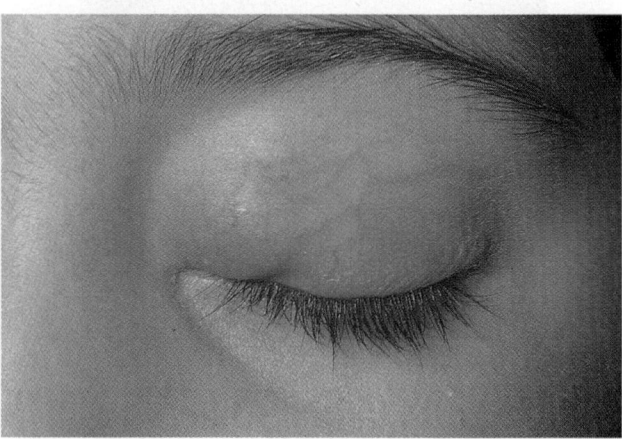

Fig. 30.4 A localized swelling in this 8-year-old girl's left upper lid was clinically diagnosed as a chalazion. Pathological examination was not requested at the time of incision and curettage. The mass recurred and a biopsy confirmed the diagnosis of rhabdomyosarcoma which was treated with radio- and chemotherapy. Patient from the University of British Columbia.

Fig. 30.3 (a) Rhabdomyosarcoma. This 6-year-old girl had tumour involving the medial wall of the orbit with chronic proptosis. (b) Rhabdomyosarcoma. CT scan showing involvement of the left medial rectus and medial wall of the orbit. Transethmoidal biopsy was performed. Intramuscular rhabdomyosarcoma is unusual in childhood.

gioma, lymphangioma, orbital cellulitis, metastatic neuroblastoma, leukaemia or granulocytic sarcoma are more likely to cause this clinical picture. Rarely, retinoblastoma which has spread into the orbit may present in this way. It is also very rare above the age of 10 years, where orbital cellulitis, inflamed dermoid cyst, secondary tumour, non-specific orbital inflammation and sudden haemorrhage into a pre-existing lymphangioma are predominant causes of rapidly increasing proptosis. Nevertheless rhabdomyosarcoma can present outside the typical age group and early identification and treatment of this tumour can be life-saving. Since its diagnosis is based on histopathological examination of tissue, the clinician dealing with rapidly progressive proptosis in childhood should keep a high index of suspicion for this tumour, proceeding to biopsy where indicated.

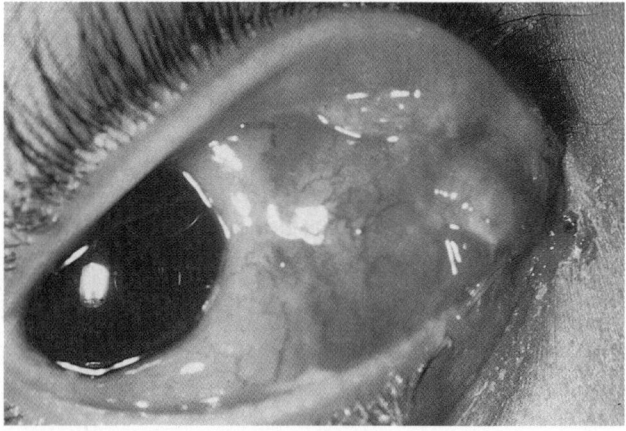

Fig. 30.5 This 8-year-old boy presented with a 5-week history of 'red eye'. Examination revealed the grape-like configuration of botryoid rhabdomyosarcoma. Patient from the University of British Columbia.

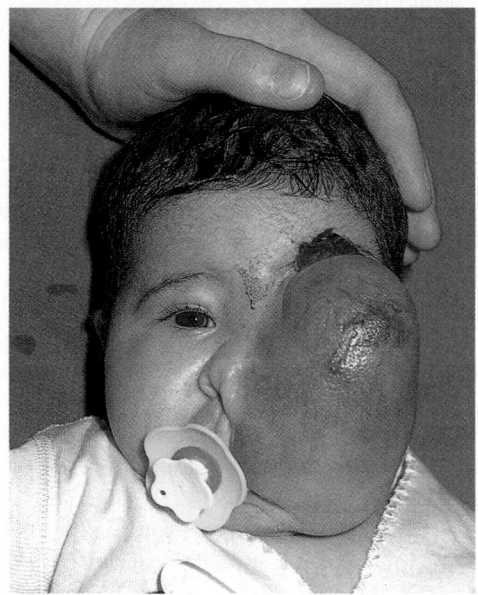

Fig. 30.6 Rhabdomyosarcoma. This 15-month-old child had a tumour which had previously been treated as a haemangioma—it involved only the soft tissues of the face.

ognized (Jones *et al.* 1965), the most direct approach should be taken to obtain a biopsy and the transcranial route should be avoided. Knowles *et al.* (1983) have stressed the importance of taking a large biopsy for accurate histopathological diagnosis. The largest amount of tumour that can be safely removed is taken at surgery; it is completely excised if the surgeon feels that this will not result in permanent functional or cosmetic sequelae. The tumour may be debulked with the aid of CUSA, an ultrasonic suction device similar in principle to a phacoemulsifier which is often used by neurosurgeons. Since irradiation and chemotherapy are started almost immediately following surgery, the incision should be closed with particular care.

Pathology

Rhabdomyosarcoma originates in undifferentiated mesenchyme which is either prospective muscle or capable of differentiation into muscle (Harry 1975; Knowles *et al.* 1983). Orbital rhabdomyosarcomas are classified on the basis of their histopathological features into embryonal, alveolar or pleomorphic types (Hogan & Zimmerman

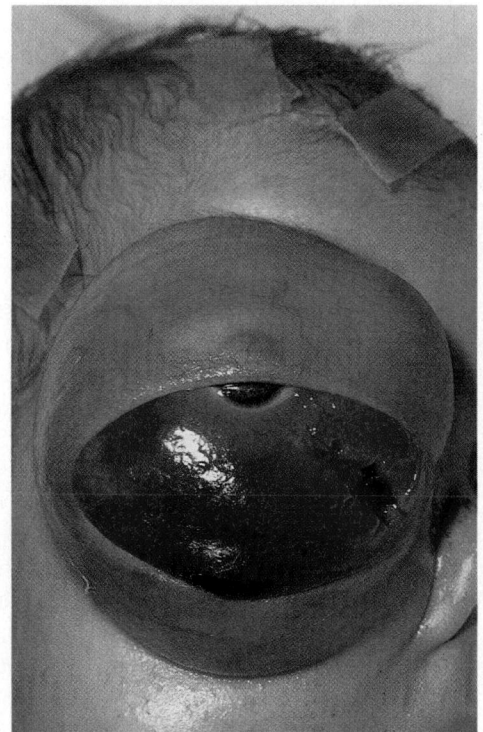

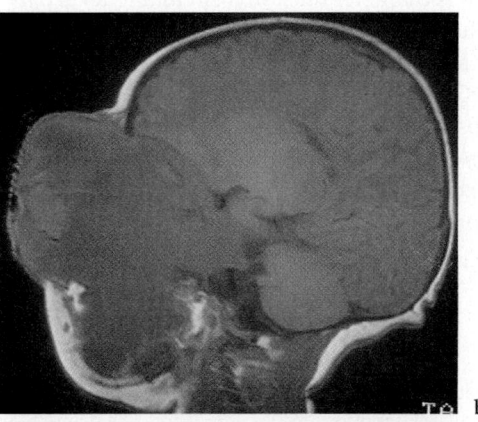

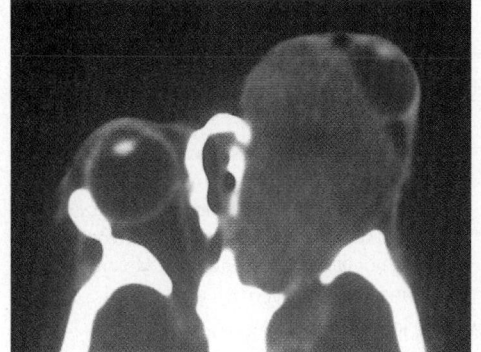

Fig. 30.7 (a) Congenital rhabdomyosarcoma. This child was born with a massive orbital tumour and proptosis. The eye itself was of normal size and the lids can be seen to be stretched by the huge tumour. (b) Same patient. MRI scan showing extensive extraorbital maxillary and intracranial involvement. (c) Same patient. CT scan showing bony destruction, intracranial involvement and the gross distortion of the globe. The main differential diagnosis is with orbital teratoma.

1962; Porterfield & Zimmerman 1962; Yanoff & Fine 1976). Embryonal tumours are the most common in the orbit (Ashton & Morgan 1965), accounting for roughly two-thirds of childhood rhabdomyosarcomas. The alveolar type, which has the worst prognosis (Knowles *et al.* 1983), and is often situated in the inferior orbit or nasopharynx, is the next most common in childhood. Pleomorphic rhabdomyosarcomas are the rarest, accounting for only 1% of rhabdomyosarcomas. They occur in teenagers and adults, arising from differentiated muscle. These have the best prognosis (Porterfield & Zimmerman 1962; Charles 1979).

The histopathological features of the various types overlap and diagnosis by light microscopy alone may be difficult. The pathological differential diagnosis is highlighted in Table 30.1. In particular, cross-striations, which are a helpful light microscopic feature, are only seen in about 50% of the common embryonal rhabdomyosarcomas, and about 30% of alveolar tumours. Nevertheless, other light microscopic features such as abundant eosinophilic cytoplasm and vacuolated web-like cytoplasm may be used to characterize rhabdomyoblasts. Electron microscopy is extremely useful in confirming the diagnosis, since identification of myofilamentary differentiation can be diagnostic (Ghafoor & Dudgeon 1985). The presence of 150 Å diameter thick myosin filaments is particularly significant. Immunohistochemical stains (e.g. for desmin, actin and myoglobin) may also be contributory (Kahn *et al.* 1983; Garrido & Arra 1986).

Rhabdomyosarcoma has been classified into three groups by Palmer *et al.* (1982, 1983): anaplastic, monomorphous and mixed. The latter are the most common and have the best prognosis.

Table 30.1 Pathological differential diagnosis of poorly differentiated small cell tumours.

Tissue of origin	Differential diagnosis
Epithelial or presumed epithelial	Undifferentiated carcinoma; oat cell carcinoma; rhabdoid tumour
Mesenchymal rhabdomyosarcoma	Embryonal Ewing's sarcoma; small cell osteosarcoma; mesenchymal chondrosarcoma; thoracopulmonary small cell tumour; undifferentiated sarcoma; synovial sarcoma; epithelial sarcoma; mesotheliomas
Neural or presumed neural crest	Neuroblastoma; retinoblastoma; glioblastoma; medulloblastoma; melanoma; alveolar soft part sarcoma
Lymphoreticular sarcoma	Lymphoma; leukaemia: granulocytic; plasmacytoma

Management

Historical aspects

Orbital rhabdomyosarcoma was treated by surgery alone until the mid-1960s (Jones *et al.* 1965). Frayer and Enterline (1959) reported recurrence requiring orbital exenteration in all five patients treated by local tumour resection in a series of 12 patients. Exenteration remained the treatment of choice, the best published results being those of Jones *et al.* (1965) with 32% 3-year and 29% 5-year survival. Even extensive and mutilating surgery was therefore associated with a poor prognosis.

In 1968 Cassady *et al.* (1968) reported five patients treated by surgery and primary radiotherapy rather than radical surgery. All five patients were alive at follow-up varying from 15 months to 5 years. During the succeeding years there followed reports of improved survival with radiotherapy and benefits of adjuvant chemotherapy (Heyn *et al.* 1974; Abramson *et al.* 1979; Weichselbaum *et al.* 1980).

It is now widely recognized that excellent survival rates can be achieved with biopsy, followed by different combinations of radiotherapy and chemotherapy depending on the extent of the disease (Knowles *et al.* 1983; Wybar 1983; Ellsworth 1987). Currently, the 5-year survival is 71% if tumours arising in all sites of the body are considered together (Maurer *et al.* 1993). Orbital tumours have a better prognosis (Rodary *et al.* 1988; Maurer *et al.* 1993), possibly because of their earlier symptomatic presentation and the orbit's poorly developed lymphatic system. The 5-year survival for these is in the order of 93%.

Treatment

Once the diagnosis has been confirmed histopathologically, the patient's tumour is staged. In conjunction with the surgeon's opinion regarding the amount of residual tumour and the clinical findings on cranial nerve examination, the CT or MRI scans are reviewed for evidence of local spread. The patient should also be worked up for metastases, with a chest X-ray, full blood count, renal and liver function tests, bone marrow aspiration for cytology and bone scan. The cerebrospinal fluid should be examined for cytology if there is any suggestion of meningeal spread.

There are several different methods of staging rhabdomyosarcoma. The Intergroup Rhabdomyosarcoma Study system (Wharam *et al.* 1987) is presented in Table 30.2. Fortunately, most orbital tumours are identified at stages I or II. The Intergroup Rhabdomyosarcoma Studies I and II (IRS I and II) were large prospective studies in which patients were randomized to treatment groups which differed according to the stage of their disease (see Table 30.2). The IRS I study recruited 686 patients from

Table 30.2 Staging of rhabdomyosarcoma (Intergroup Rhabdomyosarcoma Study).

Group		Survival (%)
Group I	Localized disease, completely resected	91
Group II	Regional disease, with or without lymph node involvement, grossly resected	86
Group III	Incomplete resection or biopsy with gross residual disease	35
Group IV	Distant metastases (lung, bone marrow, brain, distant muscle and nodes)	32

1972 to 1978 and the results were published in 1988 (Maurer *et al.* 1988). The IRS II study recruited 999 patients from 1978 to 1984. This was published in 1993 (Maurer *et al.* 1993).

Although radiotherapy alone can be expected to control orbital disease in 90% of cases (Ellsworth 1987), this modality was abandoned for patients in whom a localized tumour had been completely resected (group I) after IRS I showed it did not improve survival compared to chemotherapy alone using vincristine and dactinomycin. IRS II showed that the addition of cyclophosphamide to this regimen did not increase 5-year survival significantly.

Patients in groups II, III and IV received radiation to the orbit and surrounding bony tissues; 4500–5000 cGy were administered in divided doses over 4–5 weeks. Distant metastases were also treated by radiotherapy. Treatment of the orbit with the eyelids open helps to preserve accessory lacrimal tissue and reduces the incidence of dry eye post-treatment (Sagerman 1993).

Patients with evidence of intracranial spread also underwent radiotherapy to the whole cranium and primary tumour. In addition, intrathecal chemotherapy was given with methotrexate, hydrocortisone and cytosine arabinoside. Adoption of this regimen of central nervous system prophylaxis was associated with an increase in survival rate from 45 to 67% in this group of patients.

Patients with gross evidence of residual tumour and distant metastases (groups III and IV) received repetitive pulses of vincristine, dactinomycin and cyclophosphamide with irradiation. The addition of adriamycin to this regimen did not improve survival significantly in the most recent Intergroup Rhabdomyosarcoma Study.

The vast majority of recurrences occur within 3 years of the original presentation but prolonged follow-up is indicated as late recurrence is an occasional problem (Chestler *et al.* 1988).

The clinical stage of the disease was the most important determinant of survival in both IRS I and II. Considering stage I patients, the only characteristic consistently related to survival was histology. Patients with alveolar tumours had the poorest survival (Crist *et al.* 1990).

Complications of treatment

Although much effort has been devoted to avoiding mutilating surgery in rhabdomyosarcoma, Abramson *et al.* (1979) reported that in one-third of 58 treated orbits, the eye eventually had to be enucleated due to treatment-related morbidity. Heyn *et al.* (1986) reviewed the complications of treatment by radiotherapy and chemotherapy in 50 patients from IRS I; they found cataract to be a virtually universal contributor to the visual loss which was recorded in 90% of patients after treatment. Other ocular sequelae included keratoconjunctivitis (Figs 30.8, 30.9), dry eye and radiation retinopathy. Facial asymmetry from bony hypoplasia was present in many cases and its severity was found to be inversely related to the age of the patient at the time of treatment. Enophthalmos, lacrimal

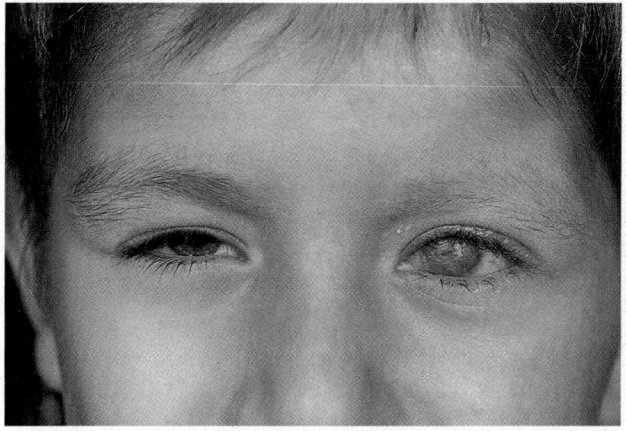

Fig. 30.8 Rhabdomyosarcoma. Radiation keratitis and dry eye.

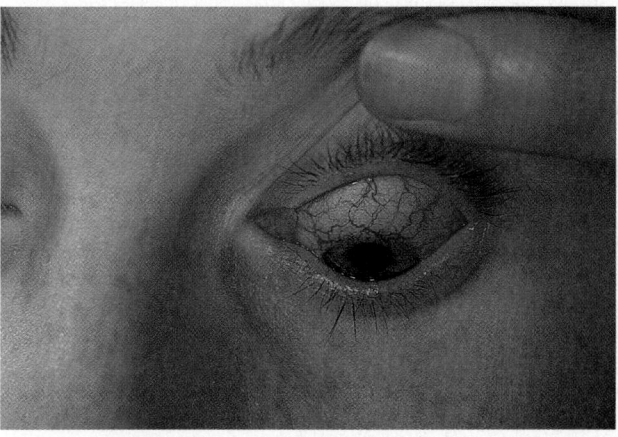

Fig. 30.9 Rhabdomyosarcoma. Radiation-induced conjunctival vascular changes.

duct stenosis, dry eye and even dental defects occurred. Growth reduction from incidental irradiation of the pituitary gland was present in almost two-thirds of the patients. However, only four eyes of the 50 patients in this series had to be enucleated. It is likely that the avoidance of radiotherapy and of prolonged treatment with cyclophosphamide for stage I disease, as recommended by the IRS, will result in a reduction in the ocular morbidity associated with treatment.

Heyn *et al.* (1993) reviewed the incidence of secondary malignant neoplasms in 1770 patients treated on IRS I and II. They found 22 cases; the most common secondary neoplasm was osteogenic sarcoma, followed in frequency by acute non-lymphoblastic leukaemia. The affected patients were more likely to have been treated with alkylating agents and radiotherapy. Most patients had neurofibromatosis or a family history suggestive of the Li–Fraumeni syndrome (see above).

Conclusion

Rhabdomyosarcoma is the most common orbital tumour of childhood. Its onset is typically rapid with features which may mimic inflammatory orbital disease. Its diagnosis and assessment has been helped by the availability of CT and MRI scans but still ultimately depends on histopathological examination of biopsy tissue. The prognosis of patients with orbital rhabdomyosarcoma has dramatically improved with newer treatment modalities. The next challenge, as in other areas of ocular oncology, is to reduce the ocular morbidity associated with treatment so that useful vision may be retained.

References

Abramson DH, Ellsworth RM, Tretter P *et al.* The treatment of orbital rhabdomyosarcoma with irradiation and chemotherapy. *Ophthalmology* 1979; **86**: 1330–5.

Ashton N, Morgan G. Embryonal sarcoma and embryonal rhabdomyosarcoma of the orbit. *J Clin Pathol* 1965; **18**: 644–714.

Barr FG, Galili N, Holick J, Biegel JA *et al.* Rearrangement of the PAX3 paired box gene in the paediatric solid tumour alveolar rhabdomyosarcoma. *Nature Genet* 1993; **3**: 113–17.

Cassady JR, Sagerman RH, Tretter P, Ellsworth RM. Radiation therapy for rhabdomyosarcoma. *Radiology* 1968; **91**: 116–20.

Charles NC. Pathology and incidence of orbital disorders: an overview. In: Hornblass A, ed. *Tumours of the Ocular Adnexa and Orbit*. St Louis: CV Mosby, 1979: 190–3.

Chestler RJ, Dortzbach RK, Kronisch JW. Late recurrence in primary orbital rhabdomyosarcoma (letter). *Am J Ophthalmol* 1988; **106**: 92–3.

Cowell JK. Genetics of paediatric solid tumours. *Br Med Bull* 1994; **50**: 600–23.

Crist WM, Garnsey L, Beltangady MS *et al.* Prognosis in children with rhabdomyosarcoma: a report of the Intergroup Rhabdomyosarcoma Studies I and II. Intergroup Rhabdomyosarcoma Committee. *J Clin Oncol* 1990; **8**: 443–52.

Douglass EC, Rowe ST, Valentine M *et al.* Variant translocations of

chromosome 13 in alveolar rhabdomyosarcoma. *Genes Chromosom Cancer* 1991; **3**: 480–2.

Ellsworth RM. Discussion of 'localised orbital rhabdomyosarcoma'. *Ophthalmology* 1987; **94**: 254.

Frayer WC, Enterline HT. Embryonal rhabdomyosarcoma of the orbit in children and young adults. *Arch Ophthalmol* 1959; **62**: 203–10.

Garrido CM, Arra A. Immunohistochemical study of embryonal rhabdomyosarcomas. *Ophthalmologica* 1986; **193**: 154–9.

Ghafoor SY, Dudgeon J. Orbital rhabdomyosarcoma: improved survival with combined pulsed chemotherapy and irradiation. *Br J Ophthalmol* 1985; **69**: 557–61.

Haik BG, Jereb B, Smith ME *et al.* Radiation and chemotherapy of parameningeal rhabdomyosarcoma involving the orbit. *Ophthalmology* 1986; **93**: 1001–9.

Harry J. Pathology of rhabdomyosarcoma. *Mod Probl Ophthalmol* 1975; **14**: 325–9.

Heyn R, Haeberlen V, Newton WA *et al.* Second malignant neoplasms in children treated for rhabdomyosarcoma. Intergroup Rhabdomyosarcoma Study Committee. *J Clin Oncol* 1993; **11**: 262–70.

Heyn RM, Holland R, Newton WA *et al.* The role of combined chemotherapy in the treatment of rhabdomyosarcoma in children. *Cancer* 1974; **34**: 2128–42.

Heyn RM, Ragab A, Raney RB Jr *et al.* Late effects of therapy in orbital rhabdomyosarcoma in children. A report from the Intergroup Rhabdomyosarcoma Study. *Cancer* 1986; **57**: 1738–43.

Himmel S, Siegel H. Congenital embryonal orbital rhabdomyosarcoma in a newborn. *Arch Ophthalmol* 1967; **77**: 662–5.

Hogan MF, Zimmerman LE. In: *Ophthalmic Pathology: An Atlas and Textbook*, 2nd edn. Philadelphia: WB Saunders, 1962: 746–51.

Jones IS, Reese AB, Krout J. Orbital rhabdomyosarcoma: an analysis of 62 cases. *Trans Am Ophthalmol Soc* 1965; **63**: 223–51.

Kahn HJ, Yeger H, Kassim O *et al.* Immunohistochemical and electron microscopic assessment of childhood rhabdomyosarcoma. *Cancer* 1983; **51**: 1897–903.

Kassel SH, Kopenhaver R, Arean VM. Orbital rhabdomyosarcoma. *Am J Ophthalmol* 1965; **60**: 811–18.

Knowles DM, Jakobiec FA, Jones IS. Rhabdomyosarcoma. In: Duane TD, ed. *Clinical Ophthalmology*. Philadelphia: Harper & Row, 1983.

Knowles DM, Jakobiec FA, Potter GD, Jones IS. Ophthalmic striated muscle neoplasms. *Surv Ophthalmol* 1976; **21**: 219–61.

Lederman M, Wybar K. Embryonal sarcoma. *Proc Roy Soc Med* 1976; **69**: 895–903.

Li FP, Fraumeni JF Jr. Rhabdomyosarcoma in children: epidemiologic study and identification of a familial cancer syndrome. *J Nat Cancer Inst* 1969; **43**: 1365–73.

Li FP, Fraumeni JF, Mulvihill JJ *et al.* A cancer family syndrome in 24 kindreds. *Cancer Res* 1988; **48**: 5358–62.

Maurer HM, Beltangady M, Gehan EA *et al.* The intergroup rhabdomyosarcoma study – I. A final report. *Cancer* 1988; **61**: 209–20.

Maurer HM, Gehan EA, Beltangady M *et al.* The intergroup rhabdomyosarcoma study – II. *Cancer* 1993; **71**: 1904–22.

Palmer NF, Sachs N, Foulkes M. Histopathology and prognosis in rhabdomyosarcoma (IRS I). *ASCO Abstracts* 1982; **C660**: 170.

Palmer NF, Sachs N, Foulkes M. Histopathology and prognosis in the second intergroup rhabdomyosarcoma study (IRS II). *ASCO Abstracts* 1983; **C897**: 229.

Porterfield JF, Zimmerman LE. Rhabdomyosarcoma of the orbit. A clinico-pathologic study of 55 cases. *Virch Arch Pathol Anat Histopathol* 1962; **335**: 324–44.

Riccardi VM. *Neurofibromatosis: Phenotype, Natural History, and Pathogenesis*, 2nd edn. Baltimore: Johns Hopkins University Press, 1992.

Rodary C, Rey A, Olive D *et al.* Prognostic factors in 281 children with nonmetastatic rhabdomyosarcoma (RMS) at diagnosis. *Med Pediatr Oncol* 1988; **16**: 71–7.

Ruymann FB, Maddux HR, Ragab A *et al*. Congenital anomalies associated with rhabdomyosarcoma. A report from the Intergroup Rhabdomyosarcoma Study Committee (representing the Children's Cancer Study Group, the Pediatric Oncology Group, the United Kingdom Children's Cancer Study Group, and the Pediatric Intergroup Statistical Center). *Med Pediatr Oncol* 1988; **16**: 33–9.

Sagerman RH. Orbital rhabdomyosarcoma: a paradigm for irradiation. *Radiology* 1993; **187**: 605–7.

Shields JA, Bakewell B, Augsburger JJ *et al*. Space occupying orbital masses in children. A review of 250 consecutive biopsies. *Ophthalmology* 1986; **93**: 379–84.

Shuangshoti S, Phonprasert C. Primary intracranial rhabdomyosarcoma producing proptosis. *J Neurol Neurosurg Psychiatry* 1976; **39**: 531–5.

Vade A, Armstrong D. Orbital rhabdomyosarcoma in childhood. *Radiol Clin N Am* 1987; **25**: 701–14.

Weichselbaum RR, Cassady JR, Albert DM, Gonder JR. Multimodality management of orbital rhabdomyosarcoma. *Int Ophthalmol Clin* 1980; **20**: 247–59.

Wharam M, Beltangady M, Hays D *et al*. Localized orbital rhabdomyosarcoma. An interim report of the Intergroup Rhabdomyosarcoma Study Committee. *Ophthalmology* 1987; **94**: 251–4.

Wybar K. Malignant disease. In: Wybar K, Taylor D, eds. *Pediatric Ophthalmology*. New York: Marcel Dekker, 1983: 417–30.

Yanoff M, Fine RS. *Ocular Pathology: a Text and Atlas*. New York: Harper & Row, 1976: 538–40.

31: Other Mesenchymal Abnormalities

Christopher Lyons and Jack Rootman

In Chapter 30, we discussed rhabdomyosarcoma since this is a relatively common and important orbital disease in childhood. It is important to note that every mesenchymal component of the orbit can give rise to sarcomatous tumours. However, these are exceedingly rare and therefore do not warrant discussion in this text. Nevertheless, they form part of the differential diagnosis of rhabdomyosarcoma.

Dysplasias

Fibrous dysplasia of the orbit

Fibrous dysplasia is a rare disorder of unknown aetiology characterized by the replacement of normal bone by a cellular fibrous stroma containing islands of immature bone and osteoid. It usually presents in childhood although its onset is extremely insidious and it may remain asymptomatic until adult life. Its growth usually ceases in the second or third decade, when 'bone maturity' is reached. It is important to distinguish it from meningioma and osteosarcoma. Rarely malignant transformation can occur, either spontaneously or following radiotherapy (Schwartz & Alpert 1964; Gross & Montgomery 1967; Huvos *et al.* 1972; Feintuch 1973).

Fibrous dysplasia may be confined to a single site (monostotic form) or, more rarely, involve multiple bony sites (polyostotic form). Polyostotic fibrous dysplasia may co-exist with cutaneous pigmentation, and endocrine abnormalities. This is known as Albright's syndrome (Albright *et al.* 1937).

Clinical features

Most patients with orbital fibrous dysplasia have the monostotic form of the disease; several contiguous bones are usually affected but the disease usually remains unilateral. The clinical features vary depending on which orbital wall is predominantly involved. The most common is the roof, resulting in proptosis and downward displacement of the globe and orbit (Gass 1965; Moore 1969; Moore *et al.* 1985; Bibby *et al.* 1994). The lacrimal fossa may be affected, mimicking a lacrimal gland tumour (McCluskey *et al.* 1993). Involvement of the maxilla (Fig. 31.1) displaces the eye upwards. If the bony nasolacrimal duct is affected there is persistent epiphora (Moore 1969; Moore *et al.* 1985). Sphenoid involvement may result in narrowing of the optic canal (Fig. 31.2) and consequent optic atrophy (Sassin & Rosenberg 1968; Moore *et al.* 1985; Jan *et al.* 1994). This was the case in 50% of the patients reported by Bibby and McFadzean (1994). The optic nerve may also be compressed by an associated sphenoid sinus mucocoele (Liakos *et al.* 1979; Weisman *et al.* 1990). Rarely, involvement of the sella turcica may result in chiasmal compression, bitemporal hemianopia or bilateral visual failure (Weyand *et al.* 1952). Other uncommon neuro-ophthalmic complications include cranial nerve palsies (Finney & Roberts 1976; Fernandez *et al.* 1980), trigeminal neuralgia (Finney & Roberts 1976) and raised intracranial pressure and papilloedema (Moore 1969; Ameli *et al.* 1981). Extensive orbitocranial involvement may also give rise to severe cosmetic deformity. Pain may occur, either localized to the orbit or as a diffuse ipsilateral headache. Visual loss was a feature in three of nine cases reported by Rootman (1988) and two of Moore's 16 cases (Moore *et al.* 1985). Malignant transformation to osteogenic sarcoma has been reported without previous radiotherapy (Rootman 1988).

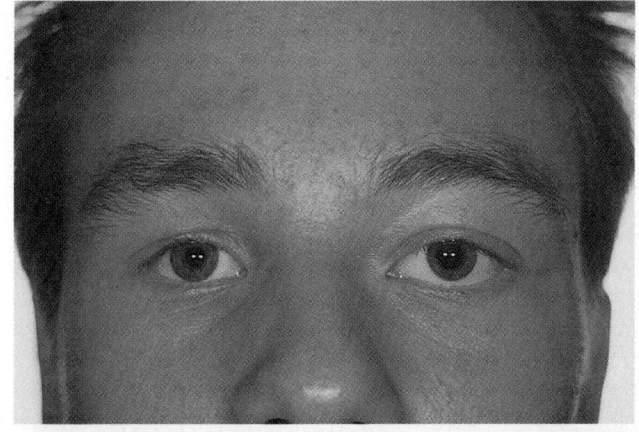

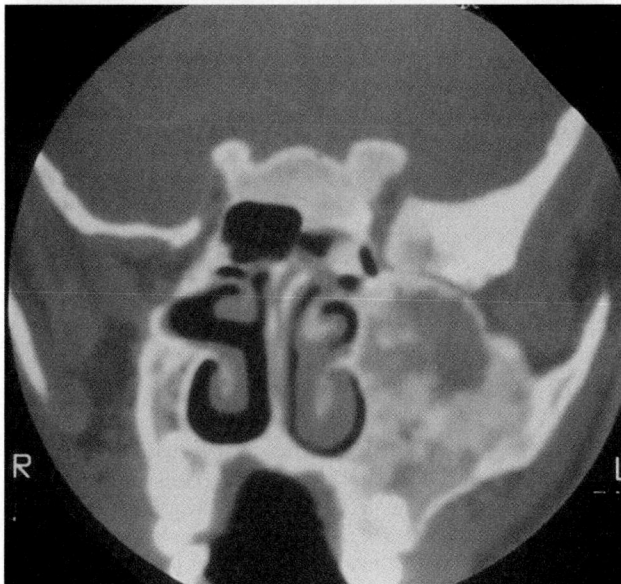

Fig. 31.1 (a) This 16-year-old presented with a history of progressive facial distortion and decreasing vision to 20/40. Compressive optic neuropathy was diagnosed secondary to fibrous dysplasia. (b) CT scan of the same case showing cystic fibrous dysplasia involving the orbital apex which was decompressed by surgically removing the maxillary component. Patient of the University of British Columbia.

The main radiographic feature of fibrous dysplasia is expansion of bone. The lesions may be sclerotic, with a dense ground-glass homogeneity, lytic, with increased lucency, or show a mixed picture with alternating areas of lucency and increased density (Fries 1957; Leeds & Seaman 1962; Jan *et al*. 1994). Fortunately most orbital cases are easily diagnosed since they are of the sclerotic type (Moore 1969). The main radiological differential diagnosis includes histiocytosis-X, hyperostotic meningioma, Paget's disease and some bone tumours. On magnetic resonance imaging (MRI), there is a correlation between T1 and T2 signal intensity and clinical and pathological activity of the lesion (Casselman *et al*. 1993). Occasionally, large cystic lesions form in the orbital wall (Moore *et al*. 1985).

These may contain blood (Fig. 31.3) and necrotic debris and can be mistaken for aneurysmal bone cysts (Rootman 1988). Computed tomography (CT) scanning is the best modality to evaluate the extent of cranial and orbital involvement. The optic canal and chiasmal region should be assessed carefully for signs of compression.

Management

Fibrous dysplasia is a benign, self-limiting condition. However, the final extent and time of arrest of the lesion is unpredictable. The aim of treatment is to prevent complications such as optic nerve compression, and minimize any cosmetic defect while waiting for spontaneous arrest to occur.

When there is little doubt about the diagnosis, as in the case of a child with a typical sclerotic lesion on X-ray, an initial period of observation and repeat radiological assessment is mandatory. If the lesion in the orbital wall is lytic or cystic, biopsy is usually necessary to confirm the diagnosis.

The recommended treatment is surgical. Outside the orbit, the risk of malignant change after radiotherapy has been reported to be high (Schwartz & Alpert 1964; Huvos *et al*. 1972). This modality is therefore not used, although malignant transformation after radiotherapy has not been reported in the orbit. Surgery is indicated for cosmetic disfigurement, intractable pain or evidence of optic nerve compression. Since dysplastic bone can be very vascular and haemorrhagic at surgery, preoperative cross-matching is advisable. Resection of dysplastic bone around the optic canal can reverse the visual loss of early compressive optic neuropathy (Rootman 1988; Weisman *et al*. 1990). Steroids may also be useful in this context (Arroyo *et al*. 1991). When decompressing the optic nerve, rongeurs rather than high speed drills should be used so trauma to the nerve can be minimized (Munro 1990). Surgery has traditionally consisted of debulking of the lesion. However, the margins of the affected bone are difficult to define clinically and recurrence after this 'limited' form of surgery is common (Bibby & McFadzean 1994). Good results have been reported with radical excision of all diseased bone and immediate facial and orbital reconstruction using bone grafts (Moore *et al*. 1985; Posnick *et al*. 1993). This is best carried out in conjunction with a craniofacial team.

Bone tumours

Reparative granuloma

Reparative granuloma and aneurysmal bone cyst are both part of a spectrum of reactive giant cell lesions, and it may be difficult to distinguish between them histologically.

Reparative granulomas tend to occur in the mandible (Cook 1965) and affect patients in the first and second

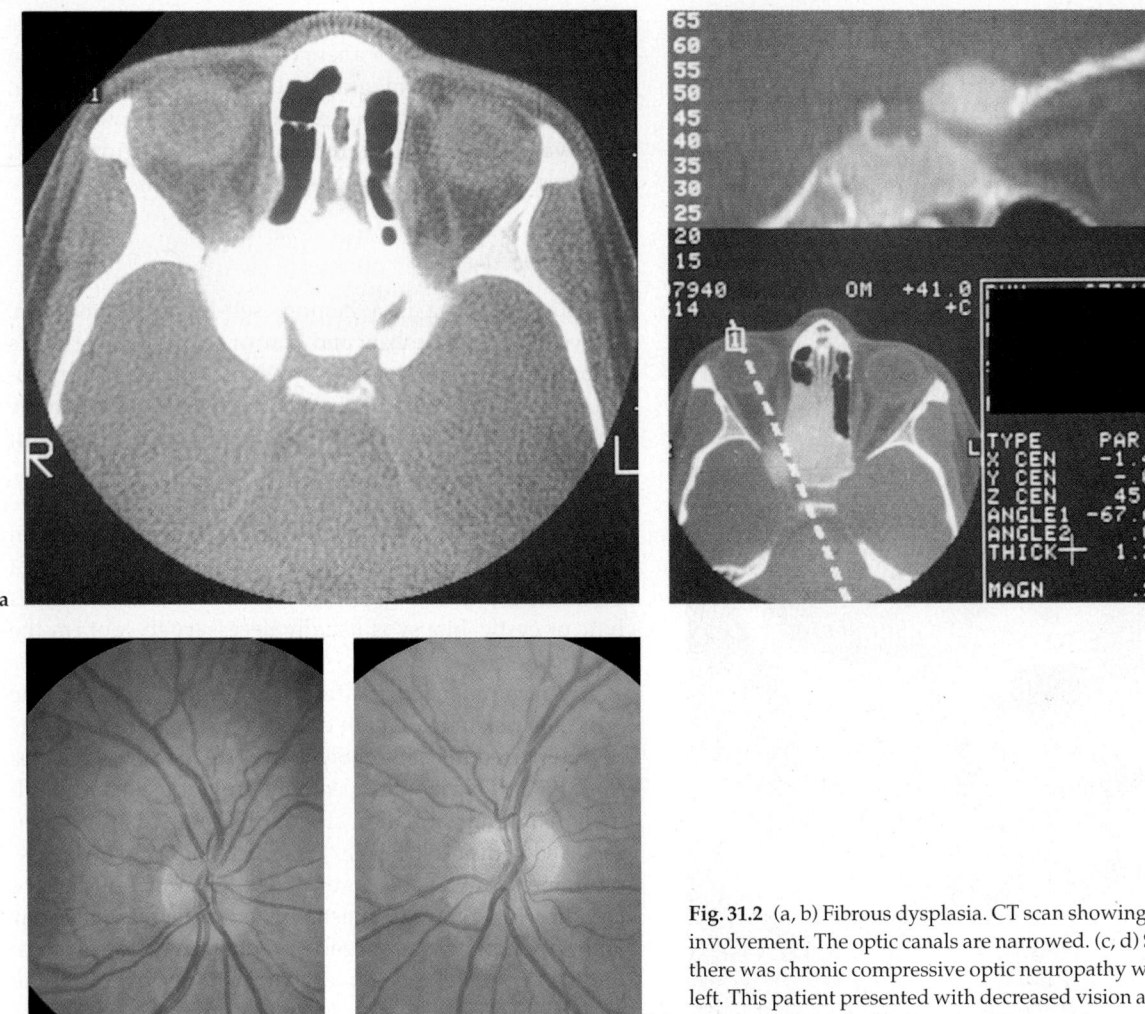

Fig. 31.2 (a, b) Fibrous dysplasia. CT scan showing sphenoid involvement. The optic canals are narrowed. (c, d) Same patient: there was chronic compressive optic neuropathy with atrophy on the left. This patient presented with decreased vision at 12 years of age and she showed no deterioration two years later with minimal residual signs or symptoms; she was not treated.

decades of life. Spread to the maxilla, ethmoid (deMello *et al.* 1980) and sphenoid bones has been recorded, with involvement of the orbit (Fig. 31.4) leading to proptosis (Sood *et al.* 1967; Hoopes *et al.* 1981). The presentation may be catastrophic if intralesional haemorrhage occurs (Rootman 1988). Histopathologically, there is a spindle cell stroma with profuse haemorrhagic and haemosiderin content. Osteoblastic giant cells are present within the stroma and new bone may be laid down at the edge of the lesion.

The course is usually benign. The treatment is by surgical curettage, after which healing occurs by new bone formation. Occasionally, the bony margins have to be resected to effect a cure.

Aneurysmal bone cyst

This uncommon lesion usually affects the metaphysis of long bones or the spine. The skull is affected in less than 1% of cases and about one-quarter of these affect the orbit

(Hunter *et al.* 1990). It is a benign lesion which can usually be differentiated from reparative granuloma by the presence of large blood-filled channels lined by multinucleate giant cells and fibroblasts. Occasionally, however, they can be solid, making this differentiation difficult. The two may also co-exist (Levy *et al.* 1975).

Aneurysmal bone cysts of the orbit (Fig. 31.5) have been reviewed by Powell and Glaser (1975) and Ronner and Jones (1983). They may occur in childhood and the great majority of cases present before the age of 20 years. The history is usually shorter than 3 months and presenting symptoms may include proptosis, diplopia, ptosis, headache, visual deterioration and nasal congestion (Hunter *et al.* 1990). Most cases involve the orbital roof and result in gradually increasing unilateral proptosis and downward displacement of the globe (Johnson *et al.* 1988). The medial and lateral orbital walls can also be involved. Like reparative granulomas, intralesional haemorrhage may occur with catastrophic onset of signs of mass effect, which may mimic orbital malignancy in early childhood

time of surgery (Powell & Glaser 1975; Ronner & Jones 1983). The prognosis is good despite a recurrence rate which can be as high as 66% (Biesecker *et al.* 1970).

Neoplasias

Juvenile ossifying fibroma of the orbit

This is an uncommon disorder which arises in the bony wall of the orbit and gives rise to slowly progressive proptosis. Although there are clinical and pathological similarities to fibrous dysplasia it is probably a distinct entity (Margo *et al.* 1985).

Most of the so-called osteomas of the orbit are juvenile ossifying as opposed to osteoid osteomas. In our own

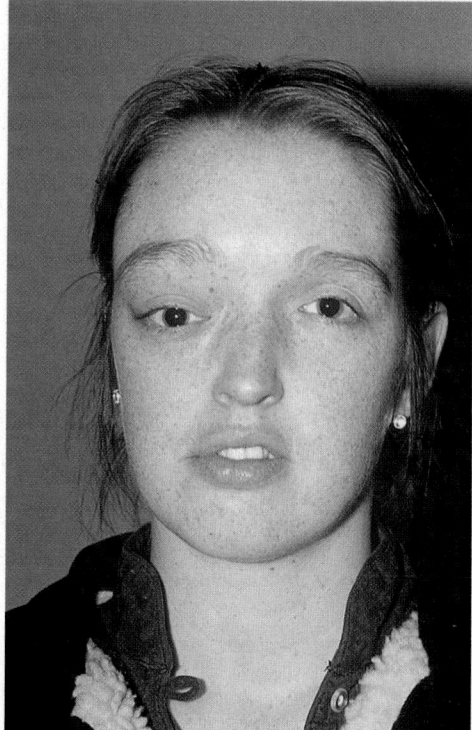

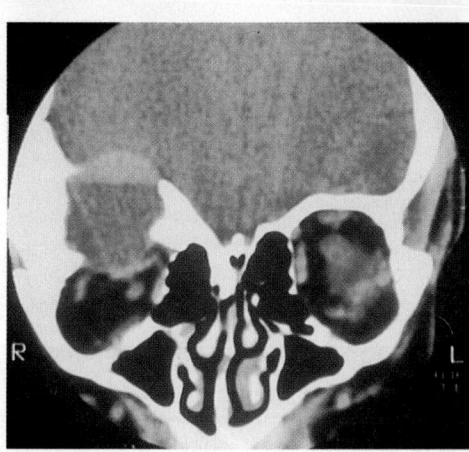

Fig. 31.3 This 22-year-old developed sudden proptosis after a history of slowly progressive facial asymmetry from early childhood. CT scan showed the fluid level of a haemorrhage within the cystic dysplastic bone. The diagnosis was fibrous dysplasia. Patient of the University of British Columbia.

(Bealer *et al.* 1993). Large cysts with intracranial extension may give rise to raised intracranial pressure and papilloedema (Constantini 1966). Optic nerve compression may also occur (Yee *et al.* 1977; Rootman 1988).

Radiologically, irregular expansion with destruction of bone is seen on CT scan, with a thin shell of bone outlining the limits of the lesion. There may be patchy enhancement of the mass or its rim. The treatment of choice is surgical excision or curettage and grafting with autogenous bone chips. Craniofacial reconstruction may be indicated at the

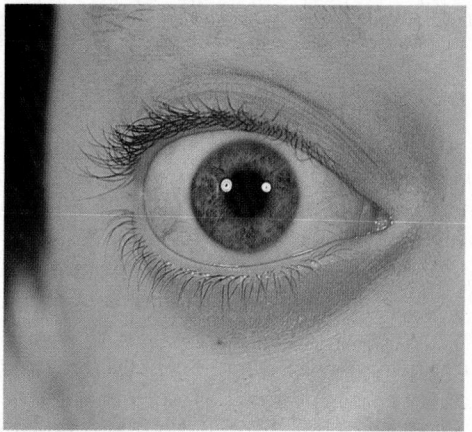

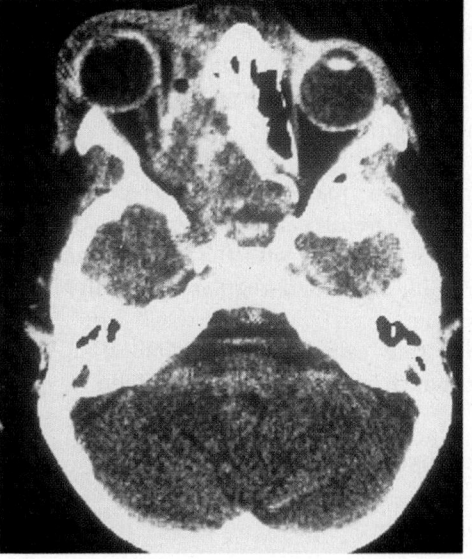

Fig. 31.4 (a, b) This 10-year-old had a 1-month history of progressive proptosis and lateral displacement of the globe. There was gradual loss of vision. Reparative granuloma was diagnosed by intranasal biopsy and the patient underwent lateral rhinotomy and excision of lesion via the ethmoid and maxillary sinuses. Patient of the University of British Columbia.

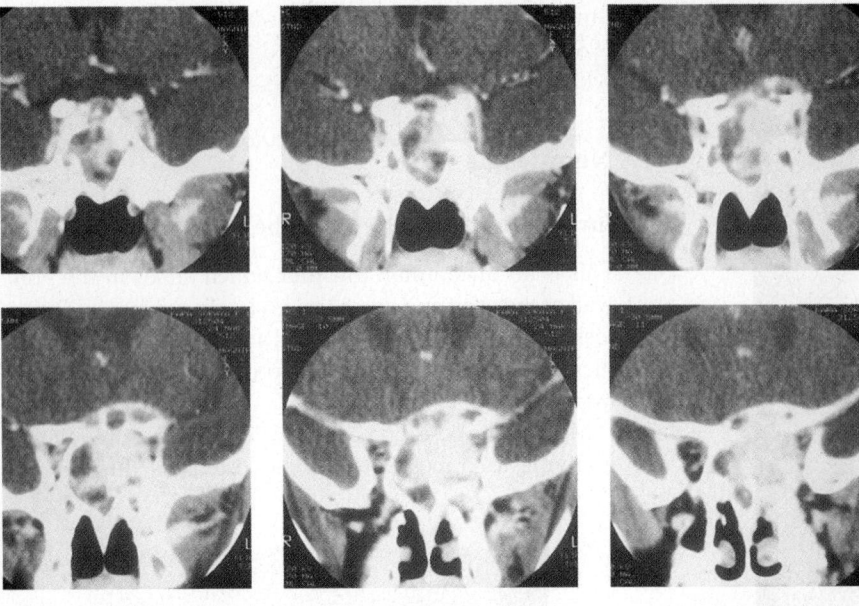

Fig. 31.5 This 12-year-old girl presented with gradual loss of vision. A sphenoid and ethmoid mass was apparent on CT. This was shown to be an aneurysmal bone cyst by intranasal biopsy and she underwent cranio-orbitotomy. Patient of the University of British Columbia.

series, the majority have presented in adolescence or early adulthood although younger cases have been reported. The usual presentation is with slowly progressive painless proptosis. The orbital roof (Fig. 31.6) or ethmoid bone are the most common sites (Blodi 1976; Margo *et al.* 1985) although rarely maxillary involvement may cause upward displacement of the globe (Shields *et al.* 1985). There may be massive enlargement with considerable morbidity and cosmetic disfigurement (Margo *et al.* 1985).

CT scan shows a homogeneous central zone with a sclerotic margin expanding surrounding bone. Histopathologically the predominant feature is a whorled, cellular, vascular stroma. The psammomatoid variant contains islands of lamellar bone surrounded by a rim of osteoid and osteoblasts which may resemble the psammoma bodies of meningioma.

Juvenile ossifying fibromas tend to be more erosive clinically and have a greater tendency to recur. The treatment of choice is careful complete excision. Unfortunately, recurrence is common with the psammomatoid variety (Margo *et al.* 1985) and regular follow-up is therefore indicated.

Extragnathic cementomas (Vivian *et al.* 1994) are tumours which behave in a similar fashion.

Other mesenchymal tumours

Osteoblastoma

This benign tumour rarely involves the orbit (Abdalla & Hosni 1966; Lowder *et al.* 1986). Clinically, it presents with mass effect. Lowder *et al.* (1986) described a 5-year-old boy who developed a firm mass in the left supero-orbital region. Radiologically, they are well circumscribed and may have a lucent centre with foci of calcification. The

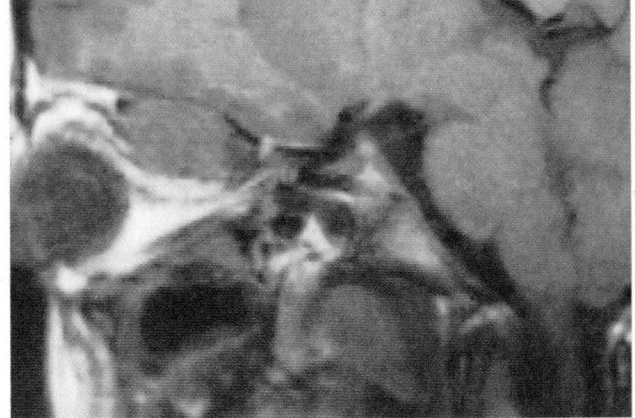

a

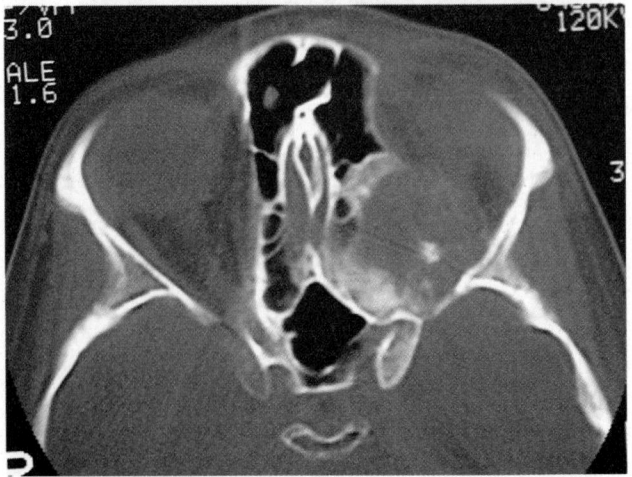

b

Fig. 31.6 (a) Ossifying fibroma. This 7-year-old child presented with progressive proptosis and downward displacement of the globe. The MRI scan shows a mass in the orbital roof displacing the levator–superior rectus complex, the globe and the optic nerve downwards. (b) Same patient. CT scan showing the sclerotic margin of the fibroma.

treatment of choice is surgical, either with curettage or more radical excision and reconstruction, although both of these may be associated with profuse bleeding due to the vascularity of the tumour. Histologically, they resemble osteoid osteomas but are larger and more vascular. The postoperative prognosis is reasonably good. These tumours are more common in the spine and the long bones where they have a 10–15% recurrence rate after curettage (Jackson 1978). Although sarcomatous transformation occasionally occurs at these sites, this has not been reported in the orbit.

Post-irradiation osteosarcoma of the orbit

Survivors of the genetic form of retinoblastoma are at greater risk of developing a second tumour (Strong & Knudson 1973; Abrahamson *et al.* 1984). Most of these tumours are osteosarcomas (Abrahamson *et al.* 1984) which may occur within the field of radiation given to treat the retinoblastoma, or at a distant site. In Abrahamson's series (1984) of 693 patients with bilateral retinoblastoma 89 developed second tumours; 58 occurred within the radiation field and 31 outside. The latent period from completion of radiotherapy to development of the second tumour ranged from 10 months to 23 years (mean 10.4 years). The prognosis of osteosarcoma of the orbit is extremely poor; most patients die within a year of diagnosis.

Infantile cortical hyperostosis (Caffey's disease)

This uncommon disorder of unknown aetiology affects infants in the first few months of life. It is characterized by sudden onset of fever, irritability and soft tissue swelling in a young infant. The soft tissue over the involved bone is swollen and tender and plain X-rays show subperiosteal new bone formation and cortical thickening. There is usually a leucocytosis and raised erythrocyte sedimentation rate. The mandible is the most common bone to be involved in which case the infants have a characteristic facial appearance with swollen cheeks. The condition is generally self-limiting and the radiological appearance reverts to normal within a few months. Involvement of the facial and skull bones may lead to periorbital oedema and even proptosis (Iliff & Ossofsky 1962; Minton & Elliot 1967). The management is generally conservative with an initial period of observation and follow-up radiological examination of the involved bones. Systemic steroids may be used for persistent disease, or to hasten remission if there is gross swelling.

Osteopetrosis

This rare disorder of bone, thought to be due to defective resorption by osteoclasts, is characterized by an increase in thickness and density of bone. This may result in narrowing of the marrow cavity and also of the bony foramina of the skull (Fig. 31.7). The bony changes result in an increased susceptibility to fracture. Three types are recognized (Shapiro 1993): (i) infantile autosomal recessive malignant osteopetrosis, which is fatal within the first few years of life if left untreated; (ii) intermediate autosomal recessive, which appears during the first decade and whose course is more benign; and (iii) autosomal dominant osteopetrosis in which life-expectancy is normal albeit with numerous orthopaedic problems. The latter is often discovered incidentally on routine X-ray and is not associated with ophthalmic complications.

The malignant form presents in infancy with failure to thrive, anaemia and thrombocytopenia; extramedullary haematopoiesis results in hepatosplenomegaly and lym-

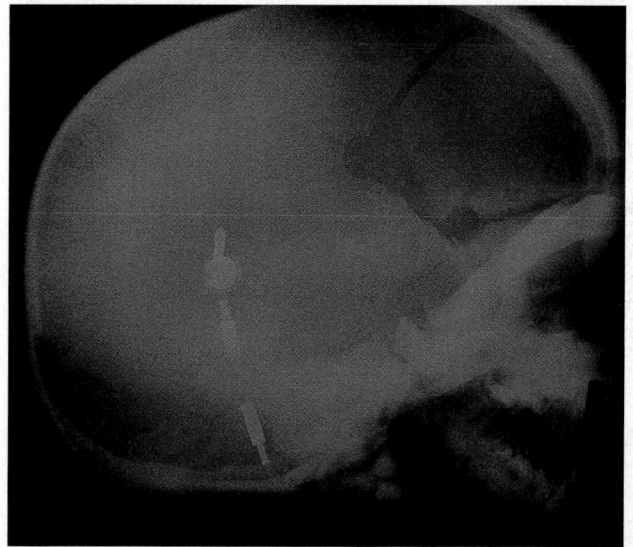

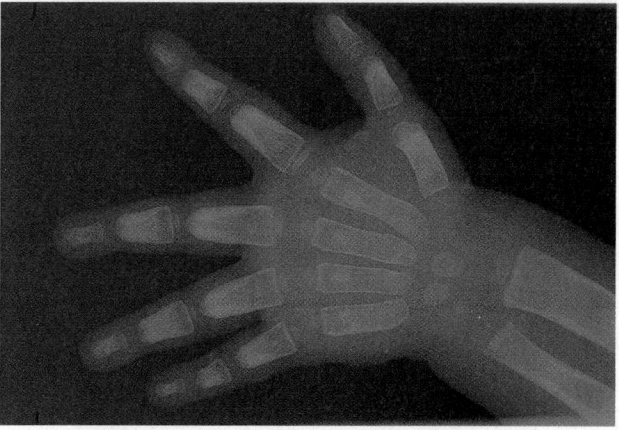

Fig. 31.7 (a) Osteopetrosis. This infant had a bilateral compressive optic neuropathy which failed to respond to optic nerve decompression. He also has a shunt *in situ*. Bone marrow transplantation has been successful in some cases. (b) X-ray of the hands showing increased density of distal ends of the phalanges (same patient).

phadenopathy. Bony involvement in the autosomal recessive forms may result in small orbits with proptosis (Bartynski *et al.* 1989), narrowing of the cranial foramina, temporal bossing and nasolacrimal duct obstruction (Ainsworth *et al.* 1993). Optic atrophy (Riser 1941; Ellis & Jackson 1962; Klintworth 1963; Hill & Charlton 1965; Aasved 1970) follows narrowing of the optic canal and optic nerve compression. Compression of other cranial nerves may result in facial palsy and deafness.

The bone density on X-ray is seen to be uniform without corticomedullary demarcation (Fig. 31.7). There is broadening of the metaphyses and pathological fractures are common.

Visual function may be preserved or improved by early decompression of the optic canal (Ellis & Jackson 1962; Al-Mefty *et al.* 1988; Haines *et al.* 1988). However, there appears to be a subgroup of patients with infantile malignant osteopetrosis in whom visual loss results from a retinal degeneration rather than optic nerve compression (Keith 1968; Hoyt & Billson 1979; Ruben *et al.* 1990). Keith (1968) reported rod and cone degeneration in one such patient. This may be clinically evident as a macular chorioretinal abnormality (Ruben *et al.* 1990) or may only be detected by electrophysiological testing (Hoyt & Billson 1979). The possibility of retinal disease should be borne in mind when evaluating a child with osteopetrosis with visual loss, particularly if optic nerve decompression is being considered!

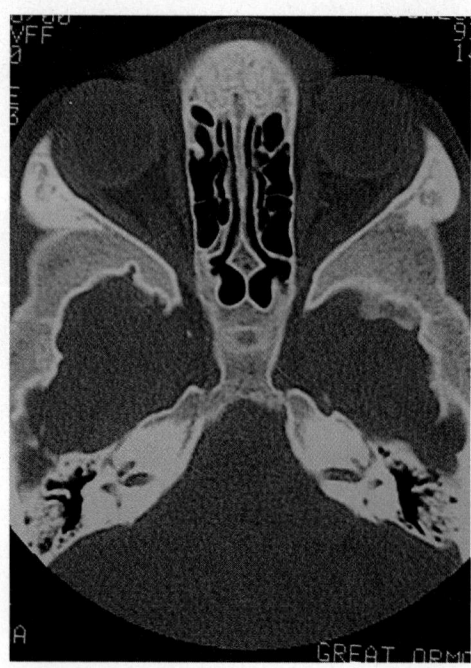

Fig. 31.8 X-linked hypophosphataemic rickets. CT scan showing increased bone density, especially of the cortical bone. There was chronic optic nerve compression which did not deteriorate over a 10-year period while it was monitored by measuring acuity, colour vision, pupil reactions, visual fields and VEPs.

Ocular involvement by a median age of 2 months was present in half of the 33 patients with autosomal recessive osteopetrosis studied by Gerritsen *et al.* (1994b). Retinal degeneration was identified in three of their patients. Other ophthalmic complications include exophthalmos (Ellis & Jackson 1962; Patel *et al.* 1992), nystagmus secondary to bilateral visual loss, and cranial nerve palsies (Klintworth 1963). Medical treatment involves high-dose calcitriol to stimulate osteoclast differentiation and bone marrow transplantation to provide monocytic osteoclast precursors (Ballet *et al.* 1977; Shapiro 1993; Gerritsen *et al.* 1994a).

Other bone dysplasias

Other bone dysplasias include craniometaphyseal dysplasia, cranioepiphyseal dysplasia, X-linked hypophosphataemic rickets (Fig. 31.8) and many others which may be characterized by bone thickening, foraminal occlusion and orbital narrowing.

References

Aasved H. Osteopetrosis from the ophthalmological point of view. A report of two cases. *Acta Ophthalmol* 1970; **48**: 771–7.

Abdalla MI, Hosni F. Osteoblastoma of the orbit. Case report. *Br J Ophthalmol* 1966; **50**: 95.

Abrahamson DH, Ellsworth RM, Kitchin D, Tung G. Second non-ocular tumours in retinoblastoma survivors. *Ophthalmology* 1984; **91**: 1351–5.

Ainsworth JR, Bryce IG, Dudgeon J. Visual loss in infantile osteopetrosis. *J Pediatr Ophthalmol Strabismus* 1993; **30**: 201–3.

Al-Mefty O, Fox JL, Al-Rodhan N, Dew JH. Optic nerve decompression in osteopetrosis. *J Neurosurg* 1988; **68**: 80–4.

Albright F, Butler AM, Hampton AO, Smith P. Syndrome characterised by osteitis fibrosa disseminata, areas of pigmentation and endocrine dysfunction, with precocious puberty in females; report of five cases. *New Engl J Med* 1937; **216**: 727–46.

Ameli NO, Rahmat H, Abbassioun K. Monostotic fibrous dysplasia of the cranial bones: report of 14 cases. *Neurosurg Rev* 1981; **4**: 71–7.

Arroyo JG, Lessel S, Montgomery WW. Steroid-induced visual recovery in fibrous dysplasia. *J Clin Neuro-ophthalmol* 1991; **11**: 259–61.

Ballet JJ, Griscelly C, Coutris C, Milhaud G, Maroteaus P. Bone marrow transplantation in osteopetrosis. *Lancet* 1977; ii: 1137.

Bartynski WS, Barnes PD, Wallman JK. Cranial CT of autosomal recessive osteopetrosis. *Am J Neuroradiol* 1989; **10**: 543–50.

Bealer LA, Cibis GW, Barker BF, Egelhoff JC, Freeman AI, Zwick DA. Aneurysmal bone cyst: report of a case mimicking orbital tumor. *J Pediatr Ophthalmol Strabismus* 1993; **30**: 199–200.

Bibby K, McFadzean R. Fibrous dysplasia of the orbit. *Br J Ophthalmol* 1994; **78**: 266–70.

Biesecker JL, Marcove RC, Huvos AG, Mike V. Aneurysmal bone cysts. A clinicopathologic study of 66 cases. *Cancer* 1970; **26**: 615–25.

Blodi F. Pathology of orbital bones: Edward Jackson memorial lecture. *Am J Ophthalmol* 1976; **81**: 1–26.

Casselman JW, De Jonge I, Neyt L, De Clercq C, D'Hont G. MRI in craniofacial fibrous dysplasia. *Neuroradiology* 1993; **35**: 234–7.

Constantini F. Aneurysmal bone cyst as an intracranial space occupying lesion: a case report. *J Neurosurg* 1966; **25**: 205–7.

Cook H. Giant cell granuloma. *Br J Oral Surg* 1965; **3**: 97.

deMello DE, Archer CR, Blair JD. Ethmoidal fibro-osseous lesion in a child: diagnostic and therapeutic problems. *Am J Surg Pathol* 1980; **4**: 595.

Ellis P, Jackson WE. Osteopetrosis: a clinical study of optic nerve involvement. *Am J Ophthalmol* 1962; **53**: 943–53.

Feintuch TA. Chondrosarcoma arising in a cartilaginous area of previously irradiated fibrous dysplasia. *Cancer* 1973; **31**: 877–81.

Fernandez E, Colavita N, Moschini M, Fileni A. 'Fibrous dysplasia' of the skull with complete unilateral cranial nerve involvement; case report. *J Neurosurg* 1980; **52**: 404–6.

Finney HL, Roberts TS. Fibrous dysplasia of the skull with progressive cranial nerve involvement. *Surg Neurol* 1976; **6**: 341–3.

Fries JW. The roentgen features of fibrous dysplasia of the skull and facial bones; a critical analysis of 39 pathologically proved cases. *Am J Roentgenol Radiol Ther Nucl Med* 1957; **77**: 71–88.

Gass JDM. Orbital and ocular involvement in fibrous dysplasia. *South Med J* 1965; **58**: 324–9.

Gerritsen EJ, Vossen JM, Fasth A *et al*. Bone marrow transplantation for autosomal recessive osteopetrosis. A report from the working party on inborn errors of the European Bone Marrow Transplant Group. *J Pediatr* 1994a; **125**: 896–902.

Gerritsen EJ, Vossen JM, Van Loo IH *et al*. Autosomal recessive osteopetrosis: variability of findings at diagnosis and during the natural course. *Pediatrics* 1994b; **93**: 247–53.

Gross CW, Montgomery WW. Fibrous dysplasia and malignant degeneration. *Arch Otolaryngol* 1967; **85**: 653–7.

Haines SJ, Erickson DL, Wirts JD. Optic nerve decompression for osteopetrosis in early childhood. *Neurosurgery* 1988; **23**: 407–50.

Hill BG, Charlton WS. Albers–Schonberg disease. *Med J Aust* 1965; **2**: 365–7.

Hoopes PC, Anderson RL, Blodi FC. Giant cell (reparative) granuloma of the orbit. *Ophthalmology* 1981; **88**: 1361.

Hoyt CS, Billson FA. Visual loss in ostopetrosis. *Am J Dis Child* 1979; **133**: 955–8.

Hunter JV, Yokoyama C, Moseley IF, Wright JE. Aneurysmal bone cyst of the sphenoid with orbital involvement. *Br J Ophthalmol* 1990; **74**: 505–8.

Huvos AG, Higginbotham NL, Miller TR. Bone sarcomas arising in fibrous dysplasia. *J Bone Joint Surg (Am)* 1972; **54**: 1047–56.

Iliff C, Ossofsky H. Infantile cortical hyperostosis: an unusual case of proptosis. *Am J Ophthalmol* 1962; **53**: 976–80

Jackson RP. Recurrent osteoblastoma: a review. *Clin Orthopedics* 1978; **131**: 229.

Jan M, Dweik A, Destrieux C, Djebbari Y. Fronto-orbital sphenoidal fibrous dysplasia. *Neurosurgery* 1994; **34**: 544–7.

Johnson TE, Bergin DJ, McCord CD. Aneurysmal bone cyst of the orbit. *Ophthalmology* 1988; **95**: 86–90.

Keith CG. Retinal atrophy in osteopetrosis. *Arch Ophthalmol* 1968; **79**: 234–41.

Klintworth GK. The neurologic manifestations of osteopetrosis (Albers–Schonberg disease). *Neurology* 1963; **13**: 512–20.

Leeds N, Seaman WB. Fibrous dysplasia of the skull and its differential diagnosis; a critical analysis of 31 pathologically proved cases. *Radiology* 1962; **78**: 570–82.

Levy WM, Miller AS, Bonakdarpor A, Aegerter E. Aneurysmal bone cyst secondary to other osseous lesions: report of 57 cases. *Am J*

Clin Pathol 1975; **64**: 1–8.

Liakos GM, Walker CB, Carruth JAS. Ocular complications in craniofacial fibrous dysplasia. *Br J Ophthalmol* 1979; **63**: 611–16.

Lowder CY, Berlin AJ, Cox W, Hahhn JF. Benign osteoblastoma of the orbit. *Ophthalmology* 1986; **93**: 1351–4.

McCluskey P, Wingate R, Benger R, McCarthy S. Monostotic fibrous dysplasia of the orbit: an unusual lacrimal fossa mass. *Br J Ophthalmol* 1993; **77**: 54–6.

Margo CE, Ragsdale BD, Perman K, Zimmerman LE, Sweet DE. Psammomatoid ossifying fibroma. *Ophthalmology* 1985; **92**: 150–9.

Minton L, Elliot J. Ocular manifestations of cortical hyperostosis. *Am J Ophthalmol* 1967; **64**: 902–7.

Moore RT. Fibrous dysplasia of the orbit. *Surv Ophthalmol* 1969; **13**: 321–34.

Moore AT, Buncic JR, Munro I. Fibrous dysplasia of the orbit in childhood. *Ophthalmology* 1985; **92**: 12–20.

Munro IR. Discussion: treatment of craniomaxillofacial fibrous dysplasia: how early and how extensive? *Plastic Reconstr Surg* 1990; **86**: 843–4.

Patel PJ, Kolawole TM, Al-Mofada S, Malabrey TM, Hulailah A. Osteopetrosis: brain ultrasound and computed tomography findings. *Eur J Pediatr* 1992; **151**: 827–8.

Posnick JC, Wells MD, Drake JM, Buncic JR, Armstrong D. Childhood fibrous dysplasia presenting as blindness: a skull base approach for resection and immediate reconstruction. *Pediatr Neurosurg* 1993; **19**: 260–6.

Powell J, Glaser J. Aneurysmal bone cysts of the orbit. *Arch Ophthalmol* 1975; **93**: 340–2.

Riser RO. Marble bones and optic atrophy. *Am J Ophthalmol* 1941; **24**: 874–8.

Ronner HJ, Jones IS. Aneurysmal bone cyst of the orbit: a review. *Ann Ophthalmol* 1983; **15**: 626–9.

Rootman J. *Diseases of the Orbit*. Philadelphia: JB Lippincott, 1988.

Ruben JB, Morris RJ, Judisch GF. Chorioretinal degeneration in infantile malignant osteopetrosis. *Am J Ophthalmol* 1990; **110**: 1–5.

Sassin JF, Rosenberg RN. Neurological complications of fibrous dysplasia of the skull. *Arch Neurol* 1968; **18**: 363–9.

Schwartz DT, Alpert M. The malignant transformation of fibrous dysplasia. *Am J Med Sci* 1964; **247**: 1–20.

Shapiro F. Osteopetrosis. Current considerations. *Clin Orthop Rel Res* 1993; **294**: 34–44.

Shields JA, Peyster RG, Handler SD, Augsburger JJ, Kapustiak J. Massive juvenile ossifying fibroma of maxillary sinus with orbital involvement. *Br J Ophthalmol* 1985; **69**: 392–5.

Sood GC, Malik SR, Gupta DK *et al*. Reparative granuloma of the orbit causing unilateral proptosis. *Am J Ophthalmol* 1967; **63**: 524.

Strong L, Knudson A. Second cancers in retinoblastoma. *Lancet* 1973; **ii**: 1086.

Vivian A, Harkness W, Kriss A, Ramani P, Paikos P, Taylor D. Extragnathic cementoma. *J Paediatr Ophthalmol Strabismus* 1994; **31**: 399–400.

Weisman JS, Hepler RS, Vinters HV. Reversible visual loss caused by fibrous dysplasia. *Am J Ophthalmol* 1990; **110**: 244–9.

Weyand RD, Craig WM, Rucker CW. Unusual lesions involving the optic chiasm. *Proc Staff Mtg Mayo Clin* 1952; **27**: 505–11.

Yee RD, Cogan DG, Thorp TR, Schut L. Optic nerve compression due to aneurysmal bone cyst. *Arch Ophthalmol* 1977; **95**: 2176–9.

32: Metastatic, Secondary and Lacrimal Gland Tumours

Christopher Lyons and Jack Rootman

Neuroblastoma and Ewing's sarcoma account for most childhood orbital metastatic disease (Albert *et al.* 1967). Other tumours occasionally metastasize to the orbit, including Wilms' tumour (Apple 1968), testicular embryonal sarcoma, ovarian sarcoma and renal embryonal sarcoma (Nicholson & Green 1981).

Jakobiec and Jones (1983) are careful to differentiate between blood-borne deposits of a malignant tumour (metastatic disease) and extension of a tumour into the orbital tissues from an adjacent structure (secondary disease). Retinoblastoma extending into the optic nerve or orbital structures is the most important source of secondary orbital disease in children, but spread of rhabdomyosarcoma from the sinuses is also relatively common and is discussed in Chapter 30.

Metastatic disease

Neuroblastoma

Neuroblastoma is the most common solid tumour of childhood, accounting for 10–15% of all paediatric cancer (De Lorimer 1969; Jakobiec & Jones 1983). It is also the most common source of orbital metastasis, accounting for 41 of 46 cases of orbital metastatic disease reported by Albert *et al.* (1967). As an orbital malignancy of childhood, it is second only to rhabdomyosarcoma in frequency of occurrence (Rootman 1988). Nevertheless, neuroblastoma

remains a rare cause of orbital disease since it accounted for only 1.5% of 214 orbital tumours reported by Porterfield (1962) and 3% of 307 orbital tumours in children quoted by Nicholson and Green (1981).

Neuroblastoma is derived from embryonic neural crest tissue anywhere within the postganglionic sympathetic nervous system. Knudson & Strong (1972) suggested that, as in the case of retinoblastoma, two genetic hits, with the loss of function of both alleles are necessary for the genesis of these tumours. Tumour karyotype analysis frequently shows deletion of the short arm of chromosome 1, but chromosome 14 has also been implicated, as has a dominantly acting oncogene, N-*myc* (Cowell 1994). This oncogene may amplify and insert itself into the genome, resulting in uncontrolled tumour growth. Amplification of this oncogene (i.e. the presence of more than three copies per haploid genome) is a better predictor of poor outcome than surgical stage (Seeger *et al.* 1988).

The adrenals are the site of primary involvement in 51% of cases, but the tumour may arise in the cervical sympathetic chain, mediastinum or pelvis (Gross *et al.* 1959; De Lorimer 1969). The tumour may present from birth to the late teens, the vast majority occurring under the age of 3 years (Davis *et al.* 1987). Localized primary orbital neuroblastoma has also been reported, but tends to occur in adults (Jakobiec *et al.* 1987; Bullock *et al.* 1989). Neuroblastoma is more common in patients with neurofibromatosis type 1 (NF1).

The systemic diagnosis is often not made until late in the disease when the patient has widespread metastases (Anonymous 1975; Musarella *et al.* 1984). Ninety per cent of patients have abnormally high levels of vanillylmandelic acid (VMA) in their urine due to catecholamine secretion by the tumour. The urinary VMA concentration can be useful both for diagnosis and to monitor treatment.

Ophthalmic features

The presence of neuroblastoma in the mediastinum or cervical sympathetic chain may first manifest with Horner's syndrome. This was the underlying diagnosis in two of 10

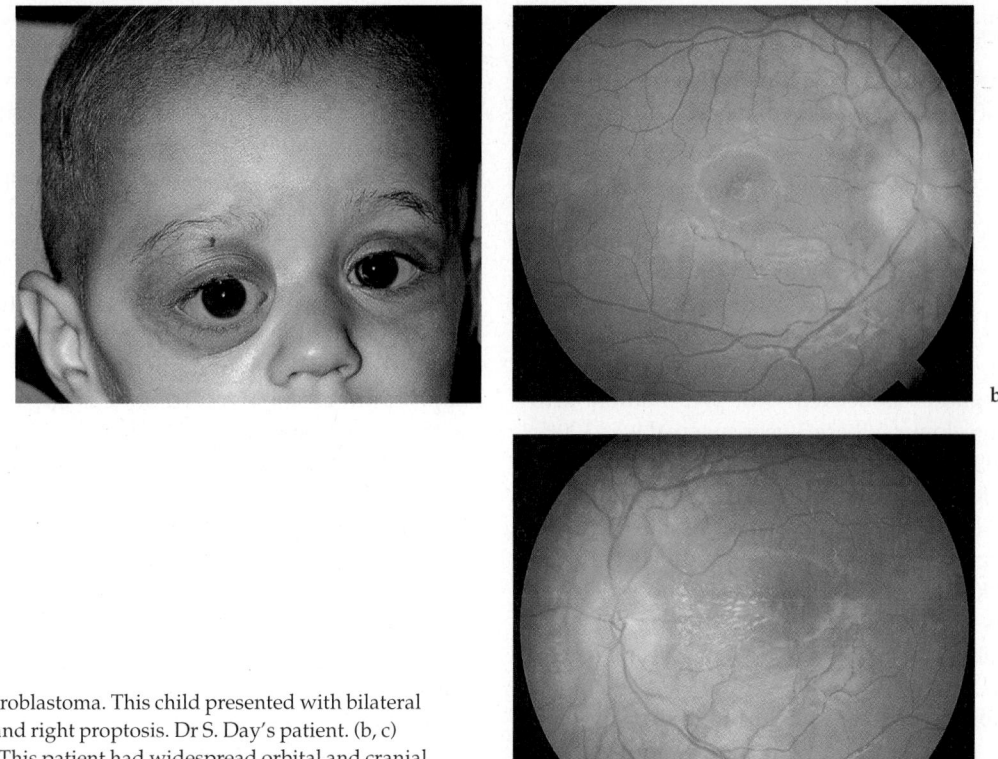

Fig. 32.1 (a) Neuroblastoma. This child presented with bilateral orbital bruising and right proptosis. Dr S. Day's patient. (b, c) Neuroblastoma. This patient had widespread orbital and cranial bone involvement with raised intracranial pressure and papilloedema.

children with Horner's syndrome reviewed by Woodruff *et al.* (1988a). Gibbs *et al.* (1992) described congenital Horner's syndrome in an infant with non-cervical neuroblastoma, suggesting that the two conditions might indicate a widespread dysgenesis of the sympathetic nervous system. Tonic pupils have also been reported as a paraneoplastic effect of adrenal neuroblastoma (West & Repka 1992; Fisher *et al.* 1994). Iris (Sekimoto *et al.* 1991) and choroidal (Cibis *et al.* 1990) metastases from abdominal neuroblastoma have also been described. The presence of opsoclonus (see Chapter 64), a striking large amplitude erratic ocular flutter also known as 'dancing eyes syndrome', with or without ataxia and myoclonus suggests occult localized neuroblastoma (Musarella *et al.* 1984). This presentation is usually associated with a good prognosis (see below), possibly because in many of these patients, only single copies of the N-*myc* oncogene are present within the tumour cells (Cohn *et al.* 1988). Nevertheless opsoclonus can also be present with multiple N-*myc* copies, signalling a poor outcome (Hiyama *et al.* 1994).

Presentation

In 93% of the 46 cases reported by Albert *et al.* (1967), the primary tumour had been diagnosed prior to presentation with orbital signs. Ninety per cent of the 60 patients with orbital metastases reviewed by Musarella *et al.* (1984) had

a primary tumour situated in the abdomen. Orbital metastases commonly present with sudden onset and rapid progression of proptosis (Fig. 32.1) which may be unilateral or bilateral. Ecchymosis (Fig. 32.2) is present in 25% of cases (Mortada 1967; Alfano 1968; Musarella *et al.* 1984). The lesion is most commonly found in the superolateral orbit and zygoma but may occur anywhere within the orbit. Bony lesions give rise to swelling of overlying tissues so periorbital swelling and ptosis may be present. This presentation may be confused with orbital cellulitis or other rapidly progressive orbital tumours such as rhabdomyosarcoma, Ewing's sarcoma, medulloblastoma,

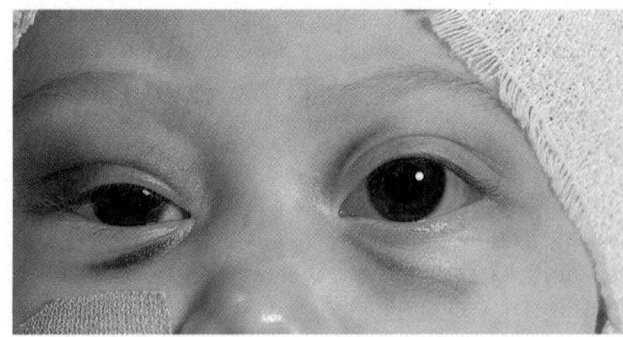

Fig. 32.2 Periorbital ecchymoses in a patient with orbital neuroblastoma.

Wilms' tumour and acute lymphoblastic leukaemia (Slamovits *et al.* 1991). A bleed into a pre-existing but clinically unsuspected lymphangioma may also present with sudden onset of proptosis with ecchymosis.

Treatment

The primary lesion is removed where possible. The prognosis is better for young patients (under 1 year is favourable), if the primary site is thoracic rather than abdominal and if there is no widespread metastatic disease at the time of diagnosis. Musarella (1984) stressed the favourable prognosis associated with presentation with opsoclonus–myoclonus, where 3-year survival was 100%. Koh *et al.* (1994) stressed that there is not always a complete resolution of the neurological symptoms in these cases and that chronic neurological and cognitive deficits are common and should be identified early. In Musarella *et al.*'s series (1984), children who presented with Horner's syndrome had a 79% 3-year survival, whilst those with orbital metastases had a 3-year survival rate of 11% only.

Orbital lesions are treated with radiotherapy and chemotherapy, in conjunction with surgery for systemic disease (Green *et al.* 1976). Disseminated disease requires aggressive high-dose chemotherapy with agents such as cisplatin, adriamycin, cyclophosphamide, vincristine, carmustine and melphalan, in some cases followed by autologous bone marrow transplantation (Green *et al.* 1976, 1981; Hartmann *et al.* 1987, 1988; Philip *et al.* 1987). Spontaneous regression of some types of neuroblastoma (stage 4S disease) is well recognized (Carvalho 1973; Schwartz *et al.* 1974). Overall, however, the prognosis for affected children remains poor.

Ewing's sarcoma

Ewing's sarcoma is a highly malignant tumour of primitive mesenchymal cells present in the bone marrow. It usually arises in the axial skeleton, but may occasionally occur in soft tissues. Primary orbital involvement or spread from contiguous structures such as the sinuses may also occur. Four per cent of primary tumours are in the head and neck, usually the maxilla or mandible, but the orbital roof may also be primarily involved (Alvarez-Berdecia *et al.* 1979). There is a marked tendency to spread to adjacent soft tissues, other bones and the lungs (Jakobiec & Jones 1983). The usual age of onset is 10–25 years, especially the first half of the second decade, and the tumour is very rare in African and Chinese people. No constitutional chromosomal abnormalities are found but a reciprocal translocation, t(11:22)(q24;q12) is present in 83% of tumours (Turc-Carel *et al.* 1988). The breakpoint on chromosome 22 results in the production of a hybrid protein which results in deregulation of other genes within

the cell and development of the malignant phenotype (Delattre *et al.* 1992).

Albert *et al.* (1967) reported five patients with Ewing's sarcoma metastatic to the orbit. Orbital presentation occurred on average 14 months after diagnosis of the primary tumour. The usual presenting signs were rapidly progressive proptosis and orbital haemorrhage. Woodruff *et al.* (1988b) reported a 6-year-old boy with primary Ewing's sarcoma of the orbit who first presented with headaches and visual loss due to optic nerve involvement.

On computed tomography (CT) scan, a 'moth-eaten' appearance of the involved bone is apparent, associated with a soft tissue mass. The histological differentiation from other round cell tumours of childhood may be difficult, but can be made on the basis of glycogen-rich cytoplasmic granules which stain with periodic acid–Schiff (PAS) and are also evident on electron microscopy. Moreover, specific genetic markers, as discussed above, may be used to aid diagnosis.

Treatment of the primary tumour is by radiotherapy with or without chemotherapy (Jaffe *et al.* 1976; Hayes *et al.* 1987). After induction chemotherapy the tumour is resected surgically. Histologically clear margins obviate the need for radiotherapy, although these tumours are very radiosensitive.

The use of new chemotherapeutic regimes with local radical radiation or surgery has improved 5-year survival from 10 to 80% or more. Since there is an appreciable risk of late recurrence or development of a second malignancy such as osteogenic sarcoma, prolonged scrupulous follow-up is indicated.

Secondary disease

Retinoblastoma

Retinoblastoma confined within the eye poses little threat to life and is a curable disease (Jakobiec & Jones 1983; Abramson 1985). The prognosis is greatly worsened by extension into the orbit or central nervous system or the presence of widespread metastatic disease. The consequences of trans-scleral involvement of the orbital tissues (orbital spread) and extension of the tumour into the optic nerve (optic nerve spread) are considered in this section.

Orbital spread

Orbital involvement with retinoblastoma was observed in 8% of patients reported by Jakobiec and Jones (1983) but in only nine out of 268 (3.5%) cases reported by Lennox *et al.* (1975).

Clinical signs (Fig. 32.3) include proptosis, a palpable orbital mass, swelling and ecchymosis. Orbital spread may be apparent as an extrascleral mass at enucleation.

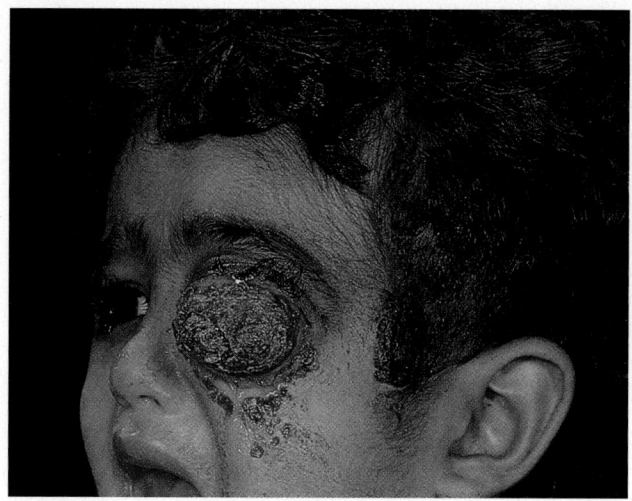

Fig. 32.3 Retinoblastoma. This sad picture of a child with extensive orbital involvement with lymphatic spread (note the pre-auricular gland involvement) is a common presentation in developing countries.

Pathological examination of an enucleated eye may reveal microscopic trans-scleral spread. Orbital disease may be signalled by a mass arising in the orbit after enucleation. Biopsy is helpful to confirm that this is indeed retinoblastoma rather than a second tumour, such as an osteosarcoma, arising in the field of previous radiotherapy (Abramson *et al.* 1984). Biopsy may be combined with removal of residual optic nerve but removal of the intracranial nerve back to the chiasm is not advised (Ellsworth 1969). The mainstay of management is a combination of radiotherapy and early adjuvant chemotherapy (Rootman *et al.* 1978).

Optic nerve spread

This is the most common route by which retinoblastoma gains access to the orbit (Henderson 1973). Following invasion of the optic nerve, the tumour may gain access to the cerebrospinal fluid and cause widespread central nervous system deposits. Optic nerve spread was identified in 12.7% of the series quoted by Jakobiec and Jones (1983) and 15% of the patients reported by Lennox *et al.* (1975). Extension into the nerve is most commonly a histological finding; removal of as much optic nerve as possible at the time of enucleation is desirable.

Treatment

Biopsy-proven orbital retinoblastoma carries 100% mortality following surgical treatment alone (Ellsworth 1974). Irradiation of the orbital lesions is effective but most patients develop widespread disease within 18 months if radiation is used alone (Abramson 1985). Present treat-

ment of biopsy-proven orbital retinoblastoma therefore involves irradiation and systemic chemotherapy with agents such as vincristine, cyclophosphamide, actinomycin D or doxorubicin (White 1983; Abramson 1985). If optic nerve involvement suggests central nervous system spread, treatment of the central nervous system with radiation or chemotherapy or both is also indicated (White 1983; Keith & Ekert 1987; Zelker *et al.* 1988).

Malignant melanoma

Intraocular melanoma very rarely occurs in infancy and childhood. Occasionally, it is seen in the neonatal period, and extensive involvement of the orbital and other facial tissues is noted at presentation (see Fig. 38.28).

Lacrimal gland tumours

The most common cause of a lacrimal gland fossa mass in childhood is dermoid cyst, since these lesions tend to occur in the upper outer quadrant of the orbit (Nicholson & Green 1981).

Primary epithelial tumours of the lacrimal gland are rare in young children (Fig. 32.4) but increase in frequency over the age of 10 years. Benign mixed tumour of the lacrimal gland is unusual and accounted for only one of the 214 childhood orbital tumours reported by Porterfield (1962). Cure is effected by complete removal of the tumour, with a tendency to recurrence if excision is incomplete. They can usually be recognized by their slow progression and the certainty of diagnosis is increased by CT scanning prior to removal (Wright 1979).

Adenoid cystic carcinoma is also uncommon in childhood, although Galliani *et al.* (1993) reported this in a 6-year-old girl and cases have been reported by Porterfield (1962), Wolter and Henderson (1969), Font and Gamel (1978), Dagher *et al.* (1980), Shields *et al.* (1986) and Rootman (1988).

These tumours have a tendency to develop rapidly and to be associated with pain and paraesthesia due to perineural invasion. The latter often extends microscopically well beyond the tumour mass and is in part responsible for the poor prognosis and recurrence after excision.

Radiologically, bone erosion and the presence of calcification in the mass are highly suggestive of malignancy. However, it is important to note that absence of erosion does not exclude malignancy; since bony remodelling occurs rapidly in childhood, localized bony expansion may be seen even with rapidly growing masses such as adenoid cystic carcinoma (Rootman 1988) whereas in adults, this sign would indicate a slow-growing mass such as pleomorphic adenoma.

These tumours may be difficult to distinguish clinically from other lacrimal lesions such as low grade infections, non-specific inflammation (Kennerdell & Dresner 1984) or

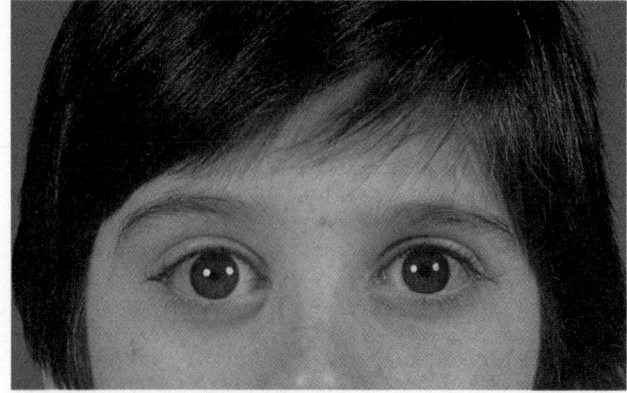

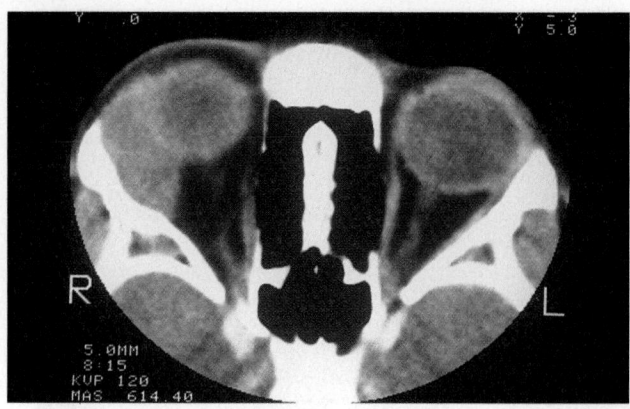

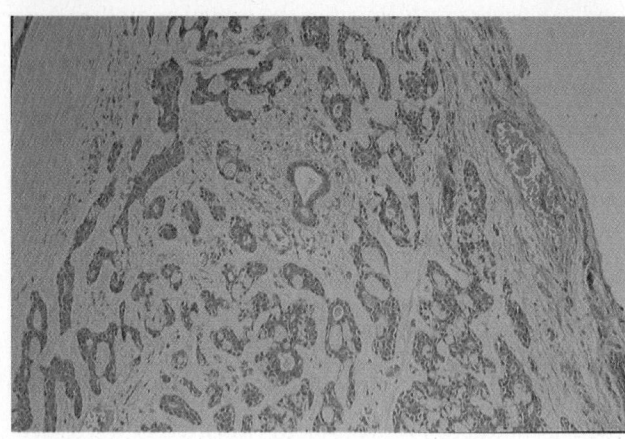

Fig. 32.4 (a) This 10-year-old boy presented with a 1-year history of gradual right orbital enlargement and upper lid swelling. There was no pain or sensory loss. CT scan showed a lacrimal gland mass excavating the frontal bone, without erosion. Even rapidly growing lesions may cause excavation in childhood. It was an adenoid cystic carcinoma of the lacrimal gland. The patient is alive and well 10 years later. Patient of the University of British Columbia.

leukaemic deposits (Kincaid & Green 1983) and biopsy may be required for confirmation.

Adenoid cystic carcinoma is highly invasive and carries a poor prognosis despite surgery, radiotherapy and chemotherapy (Krohel *et al.* 1981).

References

Abramson DH. Treatment of retinoblastoma. In: Blodi FC, ed. *Retinoblastoma*. Edinburgh: Churchill Livingstone, 1985: 86–8.

Abramson DH, Ellsworth RM, Kitchin FD, Tung G. Second nonocular tumours in retinoblastoma survivors. *Ophthalmology* 1984; **91**: 1351–5.

Albert DM, Rubenstein RA, Scheie HG. Tumour metastasis to the eye II. Clinical study in infants and children. *Am J Ophthalmol* 1967; **63**: 727–32.

Alfano JE. Ophthalmological aspects of neuroblastomatosis: a study of 53 verified cases. *Trans Am Acad Ophthalmol* 1968; **72**: 830–48.

Alvarez-Berdecia A, Schut L, Bruce DA. Localized primary intracranial Ewing's sarcoma of the orbital roof. Case report. *J Neurosurg* 1979; **50**: 811–13.

Anonymous. Neuroblastoma (editorial). *Lancet* 1975; **i**: 379–80.

Apple DJ. Wilms' tumour metastatic to the orbit. *Arch Ophthalmol* 1968; **80**: 480–3.

Bullock JD, Goldberg SH, Rakes SM *et al.* Primary orbital neuroblastoma. *Arch Ophthalmol* 1989; **107**: 1031–3.

Carvalho L. Spontaneous regression of an untreated neuroblastoma. *Br J Ophthalmol* 1973; **57**: 832–5.

Cibis GW, Freeman AI, Pang V, Roloson GJ. Bilateral choroidal neuroblastoma. *Am J Ophthalmol* 1990; **109**: 445–9.

Cohn SL, Salwen H, Heast CV *et al.* Single copies of the N-*myc* oncogene in neuroblastoma from children presenting with the syndrome of opsoclonus–myoclonus. *Cancer* 1988; **62**: 723–6.

Cowell JK. Genetics of paediatric solid tumours. *Br Med Bull* 1994; **50**: 600–23.

Dagher G, Anderson RL, Ossoinig KC *et al.* Adenoid cystic carcinoma of the lacrimal gland in a child. *Arch Ophthalmol* 1980; **98**: 1098.

Davis G, Rogers MAM, Pendergrass TW. The evidence and epidemiologic characteristics of neuroblastoma in the United States. *Am J Epidemiol* 1987; **126**: 1063–74.

De Lorimer AA. Neuroblastoma in childhood. *Am J Dis Child* 1969; **118**: 441–50.

Delattre O, Zucman J, Plougastel B *et al.* Gene fusion with an ETS DNA-binding domain caused by chromosome translocation in human tumours. *Nature* 1992; **359**: 162–5.

Ellsworth RM. Orbital retinoblastoma. *Trans Am Acad Ophthalmol* 1974; **72**: 79–86.

Ellsworth RM. The practical management of retinoblastoma. *Trans Am Ophthalmol Soc* 1969; **67**: 462–534.

Fisher PG, Wechsler DS, Singer HS. Anti-Hu antibody in a neuroblastoma-associated paraneoplastic syndrome. *Pediatr Neurol* 1994; **10**: 309–12.

Font RL, Gamel JW. Epithelial tumours of the lacrimal gland: an analysis of 256 cases. In: Jakobiec FA, ed. *Ocular and Adnexae Tumours*. Birmingham: Aesculapius, 1978.

Galliani CA, Faught PR, Ellis PD. Adenoid cystic carcinoma of the lacrimal gland in a six-year-old girl. *Pediatr Pathol* 1993; **13**: 559–65.

Gibbs J, Appleton RE, Martin J, Findlay G. Congenital Horner's syndrome associated with non-cervical neuroblastoma. *Dev Med Child Neurol* 1992; **34**: 642–4.

Green AA, Hayes FA, Husto HO. Sequential cyclophosphamide and doxorubicin for induction of complete remission in children with disseminated neuroblastoma. *Cancer* 1981; **48**: 2310–17.

Green AA, Hustu HO, Palmer R, Pinkel D. Total-body sequential segmental irradiation and combination chemotherapy for children with disseminated neuroblastoma. *Cancer* 1976; **38**: 2250–7.

Gross RE, Farber S, Martin LW. Neuroblastoma sympatheticum. A study and report of 217 cases. *Pediatrics* 1959; **23**: 1179–91.

Hartmann O, Benhamon E, Beaujean F *et al.* Repeated high-dose chemotherapy followed by purged autologous bone marrow transplantation as consolidation therapy in metastatic neuroblastoma. *J Clin Oncol* 1987; **5**: 1205–11.

Hartmann O, Pinkerton CR, Philip T *et al.* Very high-dose cisplatinum and etoposide in children with untreated advanced neuroblastoma. *J Clin Oncol* 1988; **6**: 44–50.

Hayes FA, Thompson EI, Parvely L *et al.* Metastatic Ewing's sarcoma: remission, induction and survival. *J Clin Oncol* 1987; **5**: 1199–204.

Henderson JW. *Orbital Tumours.* Philadelphia: WB Saunders, 1973: 444–94.

Hiyama E, Yokoyama T, Ichikawa T *et al.* Poor outcome in patients with advanced stage neuroblastoma and coincident opsomyoclonus syndrome. *Cancer* 1994; **74**: 1821–6.

Jaffe N, Traggis D, Sahan S, Caffady JR. Improved outlook for Ewing's sarcoma with combination chemotherapy (vincristine, actinomycin D and cyclophosphamide) and radiation therapy. *Cancer* 1976; **38**: 1925–30.

Jakobiec FA, Jones IS. Metastatic and secondary tumours. In: Duane TD, ed. *Clinical Ophthalmology*, Vol. 2. Hagerstown: Harper & Row, 1983.

Jakobiec FA, Klepach GL, Crissman JD, Spoor TC. Primary differentiated neuroblastoma of the orbit. *Ophthalmology* 1987; **94**: 255–66.

Keith CG, Ekert H. The management of retinoblastoma. *Austr NZ J Ophthalmol* 1987; **15**: 359–63.

Kennerdell JS, Dresner SC. The non-specific orbital inflammatory syndromes. *Surv Ophthalmol* 1984; **29**: 93–103.

Kincaid MC, Green WR. Ocular and orbital involvement in leukemia. *Surv Ophthalmol* 1983; **15**: 211–32.

Knudson AG, Strong LC. Mutation and cancer: neuroblastoma and pheochromocytoma. *Am J Hum Genet* 1972; **24**: 514–32.

Koh PS, Raffensperger JG, Berry S *et al.* Long-term outcome in children with opsoclonus–myoclonus and ataxia and coincident neuroblastoma. J Pediatr 1994; **125**: 712–16.

Krohel GB, Stewart WB, Chavis RM. *Orbital Disease — a Practical Approach.* New York: Grune & Stratton, 1981.

Lennox EL, Draper GJ, Sanders BM. Retinoblastoma: a study of natural history and prognosis of 268 cases. *Br Med J* 1975; **3**: 731–4.

Mortada A. Clinical characteristics of early orbital metastatic neuroblastoma. *Am J Ophthalmol* 1967; **63**: 1787–93.

Musarella MA, Chan HS, De Boer G, Gallie BL. Ocular involvement in neuroblastoma; prognostic implications. *Ophthalmology* 1984; **91**: 936–40.

Nicholson DH, Green WR. *Pediatric Ocular Tumours.* New York: Masson, 1981.

Philip T, Bernard JL, Zucker JM *et al.* High-dose chemotherapy with bone marrow transplantation as consolidation treatment in neuroblastoma: an unselected group of stage IV patients over 1 year of age. *J Clin Oncol* 1987; **5**: 266–71.

Porterfield J. Orbital tumours in children: a report of 214 cases. *Int Ophthalmol Clin* 1962; **2**: 319–35.

Rootman J. *Diseases of the Orbit: a Multidisciplinary Approach.* Philadelphia: JB Lippincott, 1988.

Rootman J, Ellsworth RM, Hofbauer J, Kitchen D. Orbital extension of retinoblastoma: a clinico-pathological study. *Canad J Ophthalmol* 1978; **13**: 72.

Schwartz AD, Dadesu-Zadel M, Lee H, Swaney JJ. Spontaneous regression of disseminated neuroblastoma. *J Pediatr* 1974; **85**: 760–3.

Seeger RC, Brodeur GM, Sather H *et al.* Association of multiple copies of the N-*myc* oncogene with rapid progression of neuroblastomas. *New Engl J Med* 1988; **311**: 1111–16.

Sekimoto M, Hayasaka S, Setogawa T, Kishi K. Presumed iris metastasis from abdominal neuroblastoma. *Ophthalmologica* 1991; **203**: 8–11.

Shields JA, Bakewell B, Augsberger JJ *et al.* Space occupying orbital diseases in children. *Ophthalmology* 1986; **93**: 379–84.

Slamovits TL, Rosen CE, Suhrland MJ. Neuroblastoma presenting as acute lymphoblastic leukaemia but correctly diagnosed after fine needle aspiration biopsy. *J Clin Neuro-ophthalmol* 1991; **11**: 158–61.

Turc-Carel C, Aurias A, Mugneret F *et al.* Chromosomes in Ewing's sarcoma. An evaluation of 85 cases and remarkable consistency of t(11;22)(q24;q12). *Cancer Genet Cytogenet* 1988; **32**: 229–38.

West CE, Repka MX. Tonic pupils associated with neuroblastoma. *J Pediatr Ophthalmol Strabismus* 1992; **29**: 382–3.

White L. The role of chemotherapy in the treatment of retinoblastoma. *Retina* 1983; **3**: 194–9.

Wolter JR, Henderson JW. Adenoid cystic carcinoma in the orbit of a child. *J Pediatr Ophthalmol Strabismus* 1969; **6**: 47.

Woodruff G, Buncic JR, Morin JD. Horner's syndrome in children. *J Pediatr Ophthalmol Strabismus* 1988a; **25**: 40–4.

Woodruff G, Thorner P, Skarf B. Primary Ewing's sarcoma of the orbit presenting with visual loss. *Br J Ophthalmol* 1988b; **72**: 786–92.

Wright JE. Symposium on orbital tumours: methods of examination. *Trans Ophthalmol Soc UK* 1979; **99**: 216–19.

Zelker M, Gonzalez G, Schwartz L *et al.* Treatment of retinoblastoma. Results obtained from a prospective study of 51 patients. *Cancer* 1988; **61**: 1530–6.

33: Histiocytic, Haematopoietic and Lymphoproliferative Disorders

Christopher Lyons and Jack Rootman

The histiocytoses are an uncommon group of disorders in which cells derived from the monocyte–phagocyte system proliferate in many different tissues of the body. They are broadly classified into two groups; in Langerhans' cell histiocytosis (LCH) (histiocytosis-X) the abnormal histiocytes are derived from Langerhans' cells and show typical inclusions on electron microscopy. The function of the Langerhans' cell is to process and present antigens to T lymphocytes (Rowden 1981). In non-Langerhans' cell histiocytosis the histiocytes have a different origin and lack the Langerhans' inclusion granules.

Three histiocyte disorders, LCH, juvenile xanthogranuloma and sinus histiocytosis, which may involve the eye and orbit, will be considered here.

Langerhans' cell histiocytosis (histiocytosis-X)

LCH is an uncommon disorder, characterized by focal proliferation of abnormal histiocytes. The destructive and space-occupying nature of these give rise to a clinical picture which varies with the tissue involved and its site. In children, the disease most commonly affects bones, especially those involved in haematopoiesis, and skin. Lesions tend also to occur in the other organs which normally contain histiocytes and macrophages such as the spleen, liver, lymph nodes and lung. The monoclonal origin of these tumours was recently demonstrated by Willman *et al.* (1994), suggesting that LCH arises from a somatic mutation in a Langerhans' cell or its precursor. The resultant clinical picture might vary according to the number of mutations within the cell, the role of immune surveillance and the site of origin of the affected cell.

Historically, the subject of histiocytosis has been complicated by confusing nomenclature. Three different histiocytic disorders were initially described. First, eosinophilic granuloma, a condition in which the histiocytic lesions were confined to bone, typically affecting children 4–7 years of age. The second, usually seen in younger patients, was a more widespread and aggressive disorder, named Hand–Schuller–Christian disease. Multifocal lesions at the skull base resulted in the triad of diabetes insipidus (from infiltration of the hypothalamus and/or posterior pituitary), exophthalmos and bony defects of the skull. The third, often affecting the youngest group of patients with LCH (frequently aged 2 years or less), was characterized by multisystem involvement including cutaneous, lymph node, visceral, ocular and orbital disease. This, the most aggressive end of the LCH spectrum, was known as Letterer–Siwe disease and was frequently fatal. The histopathological changes found in the three groups are indistinguishable (Risdall *et al.* 1983) and, since there was also considerable clinical variation and overlap between them, Lichtenstein (1953) believed these were different clinical expressions of a single disease process. He called the whole group 'histiocytosis-X', a term which emphasized the common cell of origin as well as the unknown aetiology of these disorders. The term LCH has now replaced histiocytosis-X in order to differentiate conditions in which the abnormal histiocytes are derived from the Langerhans' cell from the other histiocytic disorders. With some justification, LCH has been subdivided clinically into localized and disseminated forms, each of which may be acute or chronic.

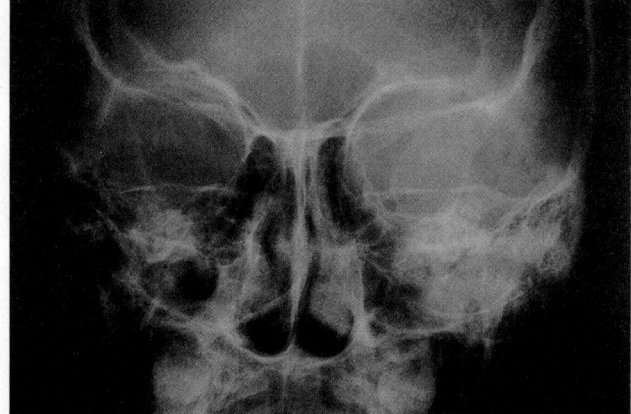

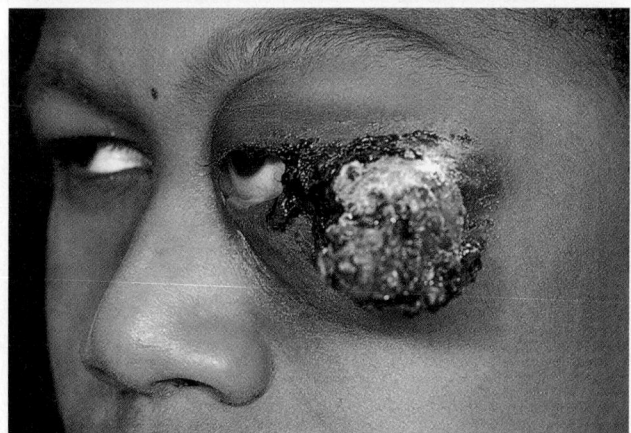

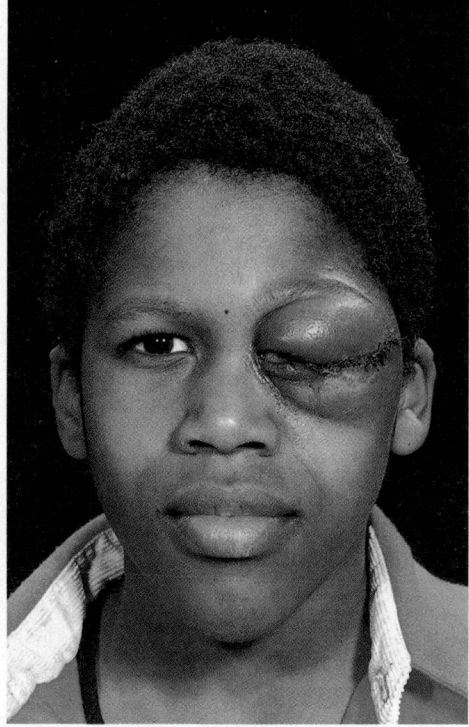

Fig. 33.1 (a) LCH with extensive bone hypertrophy around a chronic lesion. (b) Same patient with marked orbital involvement. The vision was unaffected. (c) Same patient with ulcerated skin lesion which ultimately responded to steroid injection, limited surgery and curettage.

Ophthalmic involvement

The most common cause of presentation of LCH to an ophthalmologist is orbital involvement (Fig. 33.1) (Obermann 1968; Moore *et al.* 1985), but disease of the ocular structures and brain may also precipitate ophthalmic consultation. Intraocular lesions, with infiltration of the uveal tract, are seen most frequently in infants with disseminated LCH (Lahav & Albert 1974; Epstein & Grant 1977). Intracranial involvement may give rise to visual field defects due to infiltration of the optic nerves, chiasm or tracts. Cranial neuropathy or raised intracranial pressure (Bernard & Aguilar 1969; Kepes & Kepes 1969; Goodman *et al.* 1979) are also occasional complications.

Orbital involvement

Orbital involvement occurs in about 20% of cases of LCH (Obermann 1968; Moore *et al.* 1985) and is usually seen in children with the localized form of the disease (eosinophilic granuloma). Orbital involvement is rare in patients whose disease is limited to soft tissue suggesting that, in the orbit, the lesion usually arises in the bone (Moore *et al.* 1985). There is a tendency for the parietal and frontal bones to be involved. Orbital lesions are usually situated superotemporally. The lesions have a lytic appearance, with expansion of the surrounding tissues (Figs 33.1–33.3). Occasionally, lytic bony lesions may be noted radiologically in the absence of any clinical signs.

Clinical features

The usual presentation is with unilateral or bilateral proptosis in a child with known LCH. Rarely, the proptosis may be extreme enough to precipitate luxation of the globe (Wood *et al.* 1988). Less commonly the presentation is with isolated orbital involvement in a previously healthy child, in which case the disease is usually unilateral. Initially, the course may be evanescent and relapsing. An isolated lesion of the superior orbital wall may present with unilateral ptosis. Optic nerve compression and cranial nerve palsies are rare but may be seen with extensive orbital involvement (Beller & Kornbleuth 1951; Moore *et al.* 1985). Skin tethering (Fig. 33.4) and erosion may occur (Fig. 33.4). Visual loss is unusual but may be caused by optic nerve compression (Beller & Kornbleuth 1951; Moore *et al.* 1985), optic atrophy following chronically raised intracranial pressure (Moore *et al.* 1985), chiasmal

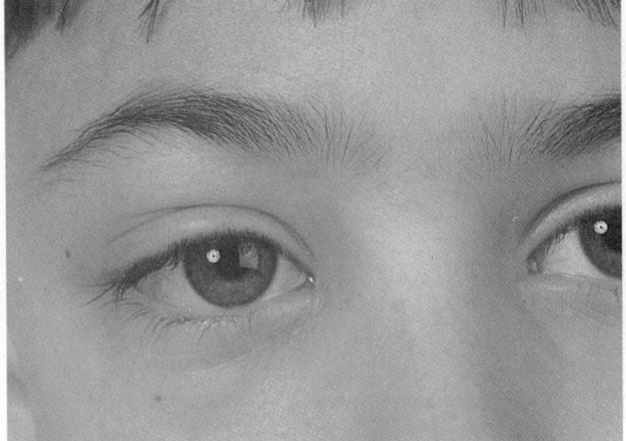

a

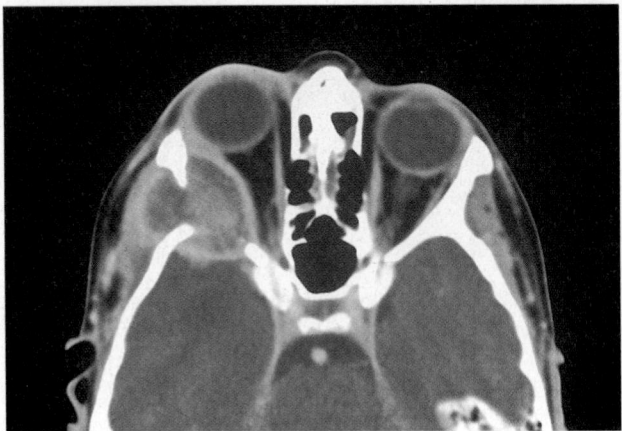

b

Fig. 33.2 (a, b) This 9-year-old boy presented with swelling and erythema of the right upper lid of 2 weeks duration. There was 4 mm proptosis. The CT scan (b) showed a mass which had eroded the posterolateral wall of the orbit, into the temporal fossa. Fine needle biopsy was consistent with LCH. The lesion was excised surgically and irrigated locally with corticosteroid. There was a good response to a tapering course of systemic prednisolone given in addition. Patient of the University of British Columbia.

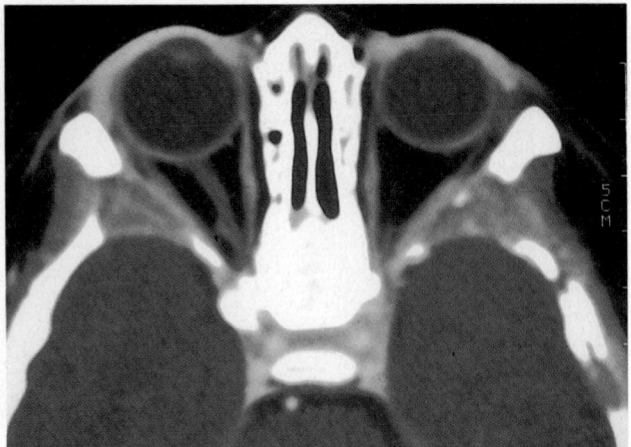

a

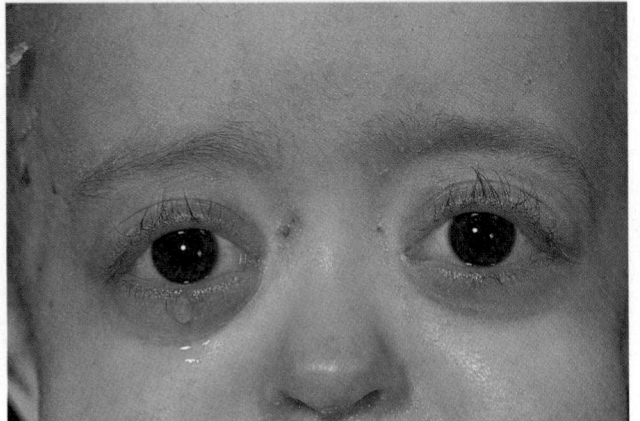

b

Fig. 33.3 (a) LCH with extensive orbital involvement with bony erosion on CT scan. (b) Patient with bilateral LCH, proptosis and obstructed nasolacrimal duct.

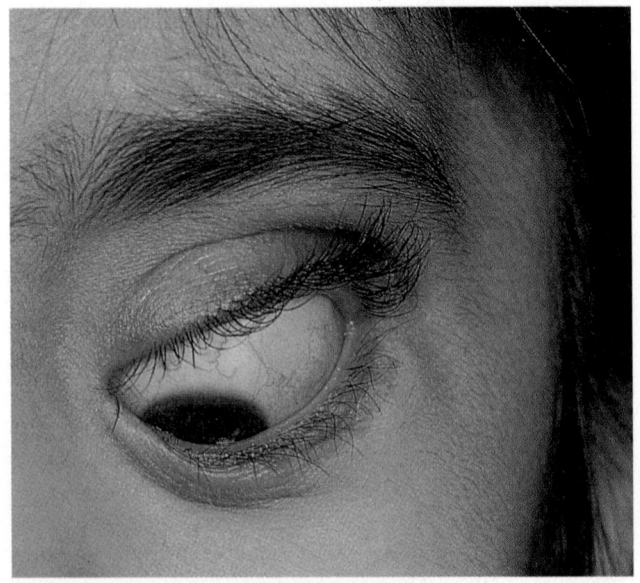

Fig. 33.4 Skin and lid tethering with orbital LCH.

disease (Bernard & Aguilar 1969; Kepes & Kepes 1969; Goodman *et al.* 1979) or intraocular infiltration (Mozziconacci *et al.* 1966; Rupp & Holloman 1970; Epstein & Grant 1977). Chronic disseminated LCH (Hand–Schuller–Christian disease) may initially present with polyuria and polydipsia, and can be associated with growth, thyroid and gonadotrophic hormone deficiencies.

Investigation

In most children with orbital involvement, plain X-rays (Fig. 33.5) will demonstrate a lytic lesion of the orbital wall and computed tomography (CT) scan or magnetic resonance imaging (MRI) will delineate the extent of intraorbital and intracranial involvement (Fig. 33.6). As the disease arises in the bone, orbital lesions usually remain

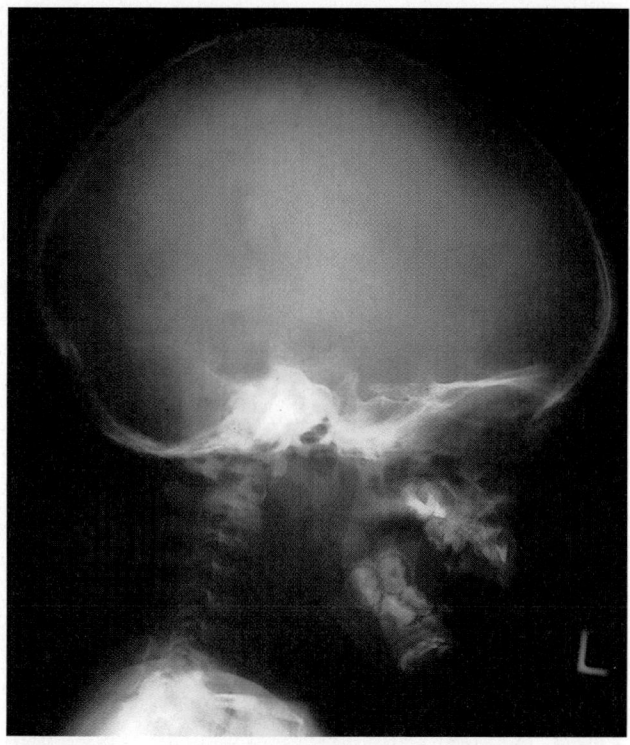

Fig. 33.5 Eosinophilic granuloma with punched-out skull lesion.

extraconal. However, they may spread into the muscle cone.

The diagnosis is confirmed by histological examination of involved tissue. In children with multisystem disease, an accessible site such as skin or a peripheral bony site should be biopsied, but in cases with solitary orbital involvement, orbital biopsy cannot be avoided. Fine needle aspiration may be useful in these circumstances. Children who present initially to the ophthalmologist should be referred to a paediatric oncologist to define the extent of any systemic involvement. Further investigations may include chest X-ray, skeletal survey, lung and liver function tests and specific gravity of early morning urine.

Examination of tissue by light microscopy reveals granulomatous infiltration consisting of histiocytes and multinucleated lipid-laden giant cells, together with eosinophils, lymphocytes, plasma cells and neutrophils. Electron microscopy of the histiocytes demonstrates the presence of typical Langerhans' granules (also known as Birbeck or racket bodies) indicating that the proliferating histiocytes are derivatives of the Langerhans' cells, part of the mononuclear–phagocyte system (Katz *et al.* 1979).

Management and prognosis

Children with LCH and ophthalmic involvement are best managed by a paediatric oncologist in collaboration with

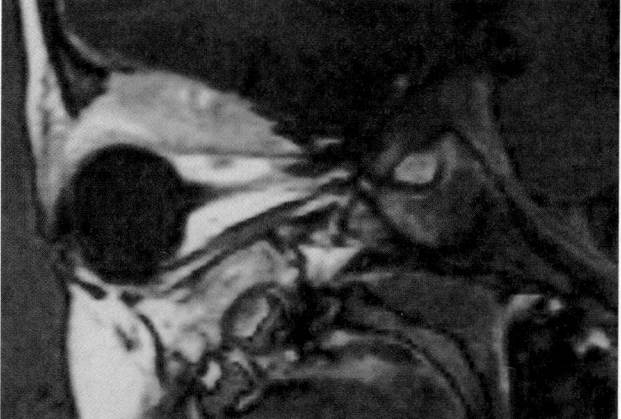

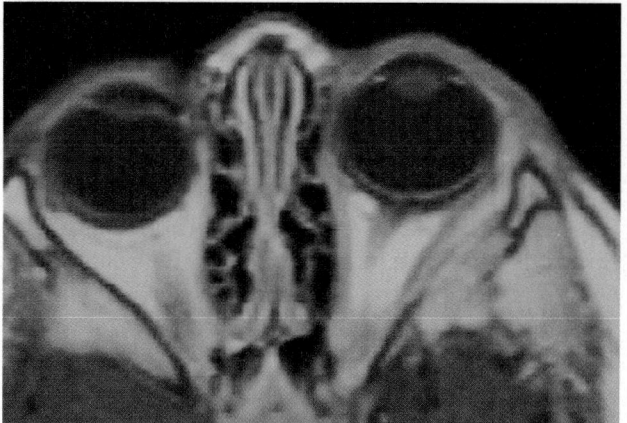

Fig. 33.6 (a, b) LCH showing extensive involvement of the left orbital bones.

the ophthalmologist. Advice from other specialities such as ENT and orthopaedic surgeons may be needed for specific problems.

The management of orbital involvement depends on whether there is single system involvement, for instance skin or bone, or multisystem disease. In cases with a single orbital lesion, biopsy and curettage is often followed by spontaneous resolution (Moore *et al.* 1985). Intralesional steroids may also be used to hasten remission (Moore *et al.* 1985; Wirtschafter *et al.* 1987; Kindy-Degnan *et al.* 1991). Cases with uncomplicated orbital involvement may be managed conservatively, but if there is marked proptosis or evidence of optic nerve compression, a short course of systemic steroids or radiotherapy may be used to induce remission. A radiation dose of 500–600 cGy is usually sufficient. The total dose should not exceed 1000 cGy because of the risk of radiation-induced malignancies occurring in later life. Cosmetically disfiguring lesions of the orbital wall may be removed surgically with curettage of the underlying bone. Orbital histiocytosis frequently results in arrested growth of the orbital walls which results in orbital shallowing. This feature is not related to the use of radiotherapy.

In patients with generalized LCH, orbital involvement will generally respond to systemic chemotherapy. Local radiotherapy may be used in addition if there is progressive proptosis or optic nerve compression. The most frequently used systemic agents are prednisolone, vincristine, vinblastine, and VP 16 which are used singly or in combination (Pritchard 1979; Moore *et al.* 1984). However, because of the tendency for spontaneous regression an initial period of observation without specific treatment is recommended in uncomplicated disease (Pritchard 1979; Moore *et al.* 1984).

Children with single system involvement, for example of the bone, have a good prognosis (Pritchard 1979; Broadbent 1986). Conversely, the prognosis is poor in multisystem or visceral disease, especially if there is involvement and failure of key organs such as the bone marrow, liver, and lungs, which may be fatal. Children under the age of 2 years have a mortality rate of 55–60% but death is rare after the age of 3 years (Lucaya 1971; Lahey 1975). Although some authors have stressed age as the most important prognostic factor (Greenberger *et al.* 1981), it is really the tendency of infants to develop multisystem disease rather than their age which dictates the poorer prognosis of children aged 2 years and under (Nezelov & Barbey 1985).

Non-Langerhans' cell histiocytosis

Juvenile xanthogranuloma

Juvenile xanthogranuloma (JXG) is a disorder of unknown aetiology in which there is abnormal proliferation of non-Langerhans' histiocytes. It is characteristically seen as a benign skin disorder in infants and young children and has a tendency to undergo spontaneous regression. This abnormality is more common among children with neurofibromatosis type 1 (NF1) (Morier *et al.* 1990) and this group could be more liable to develop leukaemias (Riccardi 1992). The skin lesions are occasionally accompanied by ocular involvement. Conversely, ocular involvement may occur without cutaneous lesions. In contrast to LCH, visceral and bony involvement are rare (Zimmerman 1965).

Histopathology

The JXG lesion consists of a mixture of lymphocytes, plasma cells, histiocytes, giant cells and occasional eosinophils. The distinctive histological feature, however, is the presence of Touton giant cells, in which a ring of nuclei in the middle of the cell enclose an area of eosinophilic cytoplasm (Fig. 33.7). An important electron microscopic feature is the absence of Langerhans' granules in the histiocytes, distinguishing these lesions from the granulomas of LCH.

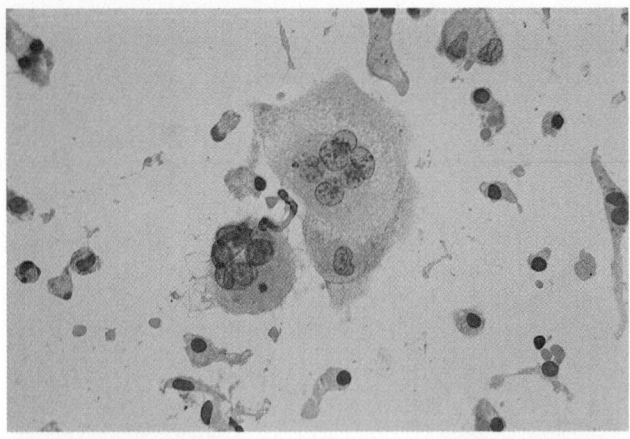

Fig. 33.7 Juvenile xanthogranuloma. Touton giant cell.

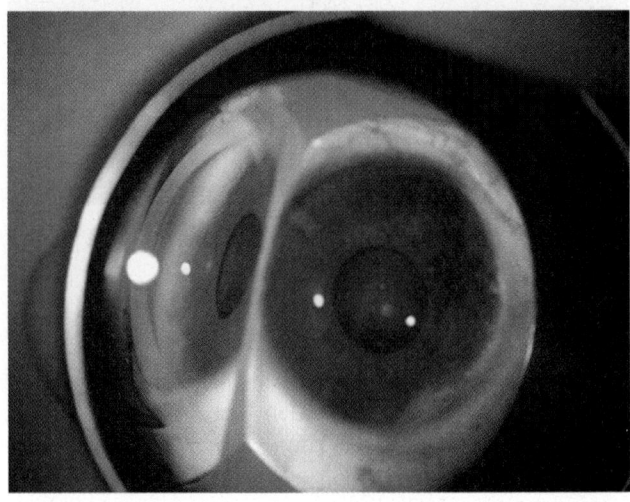

Fig. 33.8 Juvenile xanthogranuloma. Gonioscopy view showing the angle filled with yellowish xanthogranuloma material. It can also be seen in the bottom right of the picture directly.

Ocular involvement

As its name suggests, JXG predominantly occurs in infancy and early childhood; in Zimmerman's series (1965) 85% of patients with ocular involvement were less than 1 year old and 64% less than 8 months. Patients with ocular involvement may occasionally present in adult life (Brenkman *et al.* 1977; Rouhiainen *et al.* 1992). Most patients have unilateral disease although a few cases with bilateral involvement have been reported (Smith *et al.* 1969; Hadden 1975).

Uveal involvement

JXG may involve the iris (Sanders 1960; Gass 1964; Zimmermann 1965; Smith & Ingram 1968; Hadden 1975; Brenkman *et al.* 1977), ciliary body (Sanders 1960; Zimmermann 1965; Smith *et al.* 1969), or rarely the posterior choroid (Wertz *et al.* 1982). Most cases involve the iris.

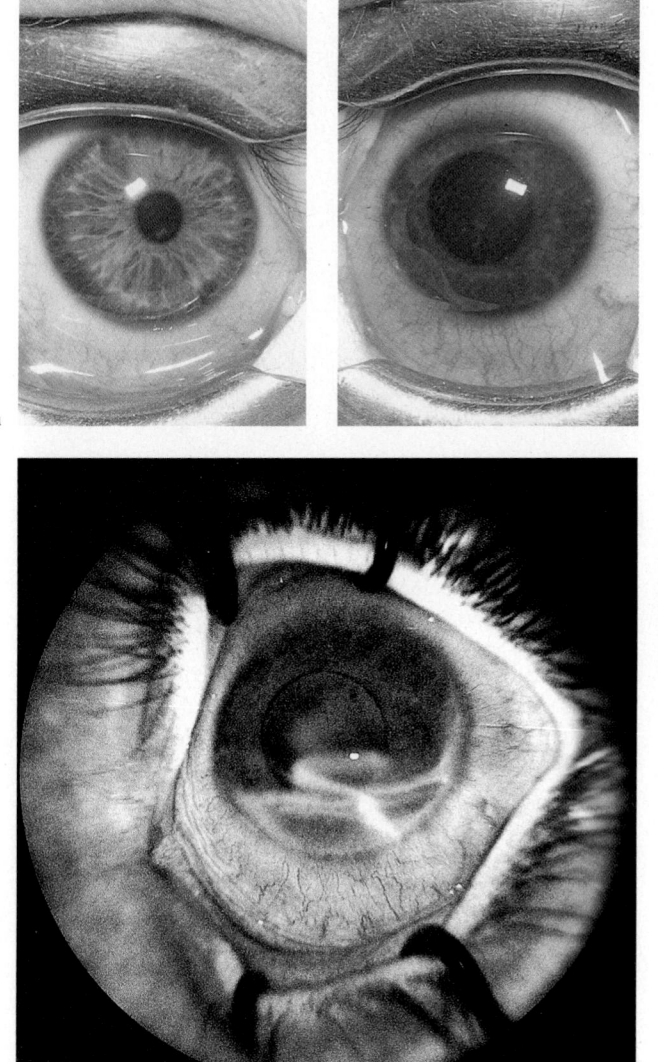

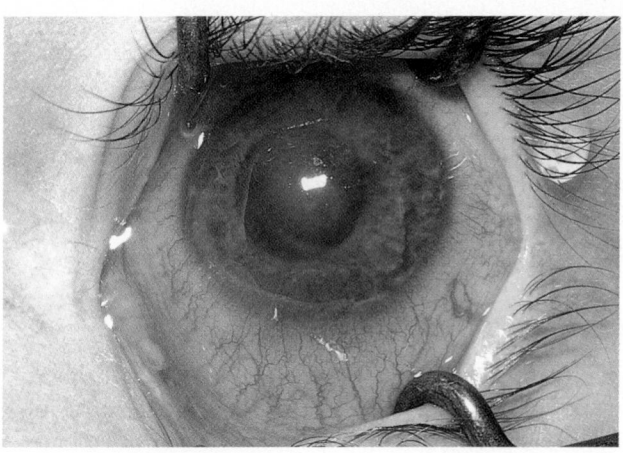

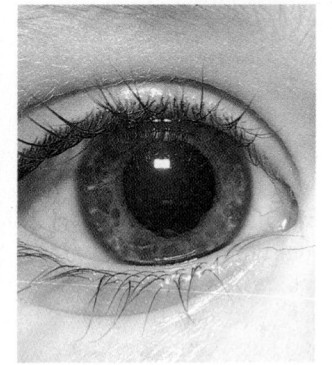

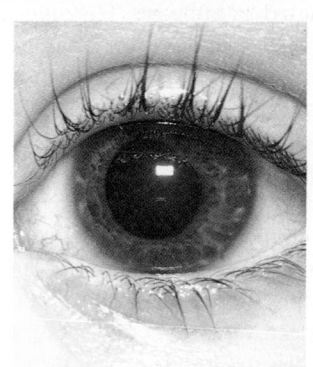

Fig. 33.9 (a–c) Presumed juvenile xanthogranuloma. The patient had presented because of recurrent left hyphaema resulting in glaucoma. There was iris vascularization with profuse fluorescein leakage but no frank mass formation. (d) One year later. After 350 cGy radiotherapy there was a very marked improvement and after a period of occlusion of the right eye the acuity was 6/6. No recurrence occurred over 9 years.

Zimmermann (1965) has reviewed the main presenting signs. Typically, a localized or diffuse yellow iris lesion (Fig. 33.8) is accompanied by spontaneous hyphaema (Fig. 33.9) in one eye of an infant. Glaucoma, with corneal oedema, ocular enlargement and circumcorneal flush is frequently present. There may be some uveitis and a xanthochromic flare. In some cases, iris heterochromia is the only presenting sign.

Although typically yellow or creamy-white, the iris lesion may occasionally be very vascular and can therefore be mistaken for a haemangioma. The main differential diagnoses of hyphaema in childhood include the following.

1 Trauma.
2 Tumour (retinoblastoma, dictyoma, LCH, leukaemia, neuroblastoma).
3 Rubeosis (secondary to retinopathy of prematurity, retinal dysplasia, persistent hyperplastic primary vitreous (PHPV)).
4 Iris arteriovenous malformation.

Management

If cutaneous lesions are present in a patient with an iris lesion, a diagnosis of JXG is best confirmed by skin biopsy. In cases without cutaneous involvement, examination of aqueous obtained through a paracentesis may show typical histiocytes. Diagnostic iris biopsy should be avoided if possible because of the risk of haemorrhage.

Several different methods of treatment have been advocated for uveal lesions, including topical and systemic steroids (Casteels *et al.* 1993), radiotherapy and surgical excision. Medical treatment is preferable because of the risk of extensive haemorrhage following excision. A reasonable approach is to try a short course of topical (Clements 1966), subconjunctival (Treacy *et al.* 1990) and/or systemic steroids (Harley *et al.* 1982) to induce remission, adding a topical beta-blocker or carbonic anhydrase inhibitor if the intraocular pressure is raised. If there is no response to steroids, radiotherapy (at a dose not exceeding 500 cGy) should be used (Harley *et al.* 1982).

Optic nerve and retinal involvement

Wertz *et al.* (1982) reported a 20-month-old infant who presented with iris heterochromia in the absence of skin lesions. Haemorrhagic infarction of the retina was accompanied by rubeosis. Histological examination of the enucleated eye revealed massive infiltration of the optic nerve, disc, retina and choroid with histiocytes. Touton giant cells, diagnostic of JXG, were also present.

Epibulbar lesions

Conjunctival (Fig. 33.10), episcleral and corneal involvement in JXG is uncommon. The presentation is either with yellowish nodules at the limbus which may grow over the cornea, or as a yellowish or pinkish subconjunctival mass which is similar in appearance to a subconjunctival lymphoma (Zimmerman 1965). Progressive lesions at this site may be treated in the same way as uveal lesions, with topical or systemic steroids or radiotherapy.

Involvement of the ocular adnexae

The typical skin lesions (Fig. 33.11) early in the course of the disease are tense pinkish papules. Later, these become

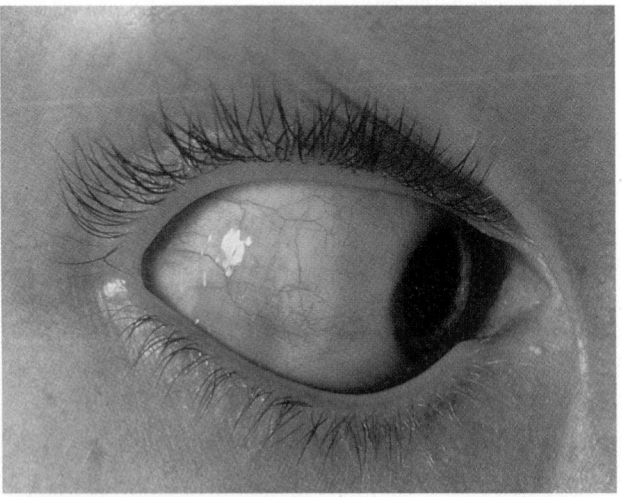

Fig. 33.10 A slowly enlarging yellowish lesion was noticed in the conjunctiva of this 15-year-old boy. Histology showed Touton giant cells, characteristic of juvenile xanthogranuloma. Patient of the University of British Columbia.

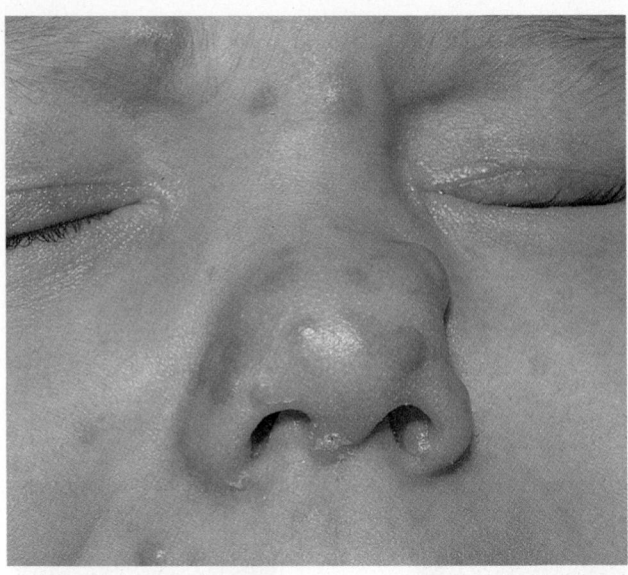

Fig. 33.11 Juvenile xanthogranuloma with skin lesions. Both eyes were glaucomatous (see Chapter 40).

softer and orange or yellow–brown in colour. Since they have a predilection for the face, neck and trunk, it is not surprising that lesions are common on the eyelids. Occasionally, a single lid lesion is the only manifestation of JXG and biopsy may be necessary to make a diagnosis. The skin lesions usually regress spontaneously within a year of their appearance but may occasionally persist for several years.

Orbital involvement in JXG is uncommon (Sanders & Miller 1965; Zimmerman 1965; Sanders 1966; Gaynes & Cohen 1967; Shields *et al.* 1990). The usual presentation is with unilateral proptosis in infancy. Most of the cases have presented within the first 6 months of life, often in the absence of cutaneous findings. The extraocular muscles may be involved, resulting in strabismus and limitation of ocular movement (Zimmerman 1965; Sanders 1966). In contrast to LCH, bony destruction is unusual but may occur (Gaynes & Cohen 1967). If there are no other systemic features it may be difficult to differentiate between JXG and histiocytosis-X clinically but light and electron microscopy are diagnostic (see p. 359).

As JXG has a tendency to undergo spontaneous remission, patients with orbital involvement should initially be observed. Patients with progressive proptosis or marked restriction of ocular motility should be given a short course of systemic steroids to induce remission (Gaynes & Cohen 1967). If there is no response to this, low-dose radiotherapy (500 cGy) should be given. The visual and systemic prognosis is usually excellent.

Sinus histiocytosis

Sinus histiocytosis is a disease of unknown aetiology predominantly affecting children and young adults. In the series reported by Foucar *et al.* (Foucar *et al.* 1979) for example, the average age was 8.6 years. There is usually massive painless cervical lymphadenopathy, often with enlargement of other lymph node groups. About 30% of patients have involvement of extranodal sites such as the orbit, upper respiratory tract, salivary gland, skin, testes and bone (Foucar *et al.* 1979). Laboratory findings include raised erythrocyte sedimentation rate, neutrophil leucocytosis and hypergammaglobulinaemia.

Patients with ophthalmic involvement usually present with unilateral or bilateral proptosis. The condition affects the soft tissues of the orbit, without bony involvement (Friendly *et al.* 1977; Foucar *et al.* 1979; Karcioglu *et al.* 1988); the tumour mass usually remains extraconal so that optic nerve compression is rare. Less commonly there is an epibulbar mass without proptosis (Karcioglu *et al.* 1988; Stopak *et al.* 1988). Progressive proptosis may lead to corneal exposure, ulceration and even endophthalmitis (Friendly *et al.* 1977; Foucar *et al.* 1979). Involvement of the lids is common and rarely there may be intraocular involvement with infiltration of the uveal tract by histiocytes (Foucar *et al.* 1979). The lack of bony and visceral involvement helps to differentiate this condition from LCH.

Histopathological examination of orbital biopsy specimens show a dense cellular infiltrate of histiocytes, lymphocytes and plasma cells surrounded by a coat of connective tissue. The histiocytes often show intracellular phagocytosed lymphocytes and plasma cells. Electron microscopy fails to demonstrate the typical cytoplasmic inclusions of Langerhans' cells, differentiating this condition from LCH.

There is no general agreement regarding the treatment of this disorder; high-dose systemic steroids, systemic chemotherapeutic agents such as vinblastine and methotrexate, and radiotherapy have all been used without consistent success. The management of orbital involvement should include frequent assessment of vision and the maintenance of adequate corneal care. Progressive proptosis causing exposure keratitis may require orbital decompression (Friendly *et al.* 1977; Foucar *et al.* 1979).

The orbital disease tends to run a chronic course with occasional recurrences, but the overall systemic prognosis is good; there was one death in Foucar *et al.*'s series (Foucar *et al.* 1979) which may have been related to complications from systemic chemotherapy.

Leukaemia

The eye, like the brain, is a relative 'pharmacological sanctuary' in the treatment of leukaemia. It is not surprising therefore that recurrent disease frequently manifests within the eye or central nervous system.

Leukaemia accounted for 11% of the 27 cases of unilat-

eral proptosis in children reported by Oakhill *et al.* (1981). It was second only to rhabdomyosarcoma in frequency of childhood malignant orbital disease in Porterfield's (1962) series. The orbit is more commonly involved in acute than chronic leukaemia and, in children, by myeloblastic than lymphoblastic tumours. Ridgway *et al.* (1976) examined 657 children with acute leukaemia and found clinical evidence of orbital involvement in 1%. Kincaid and Green (1983) found postmortem evidence of orbital involvement in 10% of 384 patients.

The clinical features of orbital leukaemic involvement include proptosis, lid oedema, chemosis and pain (Mortada 1963; Cavdar *et al.* 1971). Both orbits are involved in 2% of patients with orbital leukaemia. The proptosis may be due either to a mass of leukaemic cells or to orbital haemorrhage (Jha & Lamba 1971) which may also appear subconjunctivally and cause eyelid discoloration (Fig. 33.12) (Rosenthal 1983). Other diseases which may present with rapidly increasing proptosis, chemosis and haemorrhage must be considered in the differential diagnosis. These include rhabdomyosarcoma, neuroblastoma, Ewing's sarcoma and orbital cellulitis (Jha & Lamba 1971; Kincaid & Green 1983).

Orbital leukaemic deposits are often associated with meningeal involvement (Ridgway *et al.* 1976) and are often part of terminal disease (Porterfield 1962; Ridgway *et al.* 1976) although, in some cases, orbital signs may be the presenting feature of leukaemia and biopsy provides the systemic diagnosis. The lacrimal gland (Zimmerman & Font 1975) or, more rarely, the extraocular muscles (Kincaid & Green 1983) may be infiltrated and contiguous sinus disease is a common postmortem finding. The orbit is occasionally the site of opportunistic infection by bacteria or fungi in immunosuppressed leukaemic children (Rubinfield *et al.* 1988). Iatrogenic complications include ptosis and extraocular muscle palsy from the use of cytotoxic agents such as vincristine (Nicholson & Green 1981).

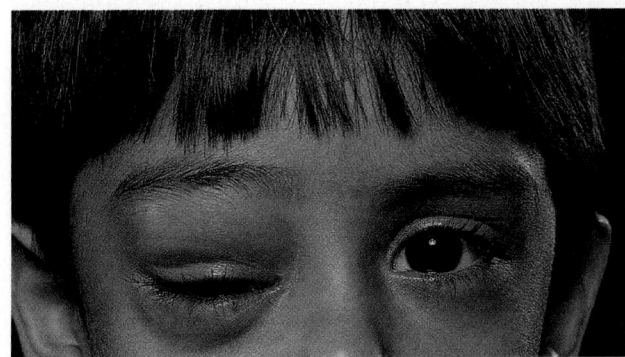

Fig. 33.12 Orbital deposit in myeloid leukaemia (chloroma). There was no abnormality in the peripheral blood film at this stage. The diagnosis was made by bone marrow aspiration at the time of orbital biopsy.

Leukaemic deposits consist of cells derived either from lymphoblasts or myeloblasts. A localized form of acute myeloblastic leukaemia has a predilection for the orbit where it presents as a rapidly expanding tumour. This was initially called 'chloroma', a reference to its greenish colour from the pigmented enzyme myeloperoxidase. The terms 'myeloblastoma' and 'granulocytic sarcoma' are now preferred. Granulocytic sarcoma may appear at any time in the course of myeloblastic leukaemia and occasionally may precede the generalized leukaemic process by weeks or months (Rajantie *et al.* 1984; Davis *et al.* 1985). Histologically, it is a poorly differentiated high grade malignancy which should be distinguished from the other round cell tumours of childhood. Its main diagnostic differential, large cell type B-cell lymphoma (also referred to as histiocytic lymphoma or reticulum cell sarcoma) is very much rarer in children. If necessary, esterase stains may be useful to identify myelocytic differentiation in granulocytic sarcoma (Jakobiec & Jones 1983).

Granulocytic sarcoma carries a poor prognosis: 19 of 32 affected patients reported by Zimmerman and Font (1975) were dead within 30 months of the onset of ophthalmic signs.

Treatment of orbital leukaemia is by systemic chemotherapy and local irradiation, although the dose and effect of the latter (reviewed by Kincaid & Green 1983) are not clearly defined. Intrathecal chemotherapy will not modify orbital disease. Orbital disease in children with acute leukaemia still carries a poor prognosis despite chemotherapy and radiotherapy (Kincaid & Green 1983).

Lymphoma

Knowles *et al.* (1983) state that they have never seen orbital lymphoma as part of systemic nodal disease in children. Bearing this in mind, the only lymphoma likely to occur in the paediatric orbit is Burkitt's lymphoma.

This is a high grade undifferentiated lymphocytic tumour which most commonly affects children in tropical Africa. It is thought that the Epstein–Barr virus acts as an oncogene in patients who have been immunologically stimulated by chronic exposure to malaria organisms (Henle & Henle 1974). The tumour affects males more commonly than females (2:1 ratio) with a median age of 7 years at presentation. In 60% of African cases, there is a maxillary tumour causing massive proptosis, but this may only appear late in the disease, since only 13% of patients present with exophthalmos. Non-African cases tend to present later (median age 11 years) with a greater propensity for abdominal involvement.

The tumour responds to chemotherapy with prolonged remission and some patients are reported to show immunological self cure (Jakobiec & Jones 1983).

References

Beller AJ, Kornbleuth W. Eosinophilic granuloma of the orbit. *Br J Ophthalmol* 1951; **35**: 220–5.

Bernard JD, Aguilar MJ. Localised hypothalamic histiocytosis X: report of a case. *Arch Neurol* 1969; **20**: 368–72.

Brenkman RF, Oosterhuis JA, Manschot WA. Recurrent haemorrhage in the anterior chamber caused by a (juvenile) xantho-granuloma of the iris in an adult. *Documenta Ophthalmol* 1977; **42**: 329–33.

Broadbent V. Favourable prognostic features in histiocytosis-X: bone involvement and absence of skin disease. *Arch Dis Child* 1986; **61**: 1219–21.

Casteels I, Olver J, Malone M, Taylor D. Early treatment of juvenile xanthogranuloma of the iris with subconjunctival steroids. *Br J Ophthalmol* 1993; **77**: 57–60.

Cavdar AO, Arcasoy A, Gozdaxoglu S *et al.* Chloroma-like manifestation in Turkish children with acute myelomonocytic leukaemia. *Lancet* 1971; **i**: 680–2.

Clements DB. Juvenile xanthogranuloma treated with local steroids. *Br J Ophthalmol* 1966; **50**: 663–5.

Davis JL, Parke DW II, Font RL. Granulocytic sarcoma of the orbit. A clinicopathologic study. *Ophthalmology* 1985; **92**: 1758–62.

Epstein DL, Grant WM. Secondary open angle glaucoma in histiocytosis X. *Am J Ophthalmol* 1977; **84**: 332–6.

Foucar E, Rusai J, Dorfman FR. The ophthalmological manifestations of sinus histiocytosis with massive lymphadenopathy. *Am J Ophthalmol* 1979; **87**: 354–67.

Friendly DS, Font RL, Rao NA. Orbital involvement in sinus histiocytosis. *Arch Ophthalmol* 1977; **95**: 2006–11.

Gass JD. Management of juvenile xanthogranuloma of the iris. *Arch Ophthalmol* 1964; **71**: 344–7.

Gaynes PM, Cohen GS. Juvenile xanthogranuloma of the orbit. *Am J Ophthalmol* 1967; **63**: 755–7.

Goodman RH, Post KD, Molitch ME *et al.* Eosinophilic granuloma mimicking a pituitary tumour. *Neurosurgery* 1979; **5**: 723–5.

Greenberger JS, Crocker AC, Wawter G *et al.* Results of treatment of 127 patients with systemic histiocytosis (Letterer–Siwe syndrome, Schuller–Christian syndrome and multifocal eosinophilic granuloma). *Medicine* 1981; **60**: 311–38.

Hadden OB. Bilateral juvenile xanthogranuloma of the orbit. *Br J Ophthalmol* 1975; **59**: 699–702.

Harley RD, Romayananda N, Chan GH. Juvenile xanthogranuloma. *J Pediatr Ophthalmol Strabismus* 1982; **19**: 33–9.

Henle W, Henle G. Epstein–Barr virus and human malignancies. *Cancer* 1974; **34**: 1368–74.

Jakobiec FA, Jones IS. Lymphomatous, plasmacytic, histiocytic and haemopoietic tumours. In: Duane TD, ed. *Clinical Ophthalmology*, Vol. 2. Hagerstown: Harper & Row, 1983.

Jha BK, Lamba PA. Proptosis as a manifestation of acute myeloid leukaemia. *Br J Ophthalmol* 1971; **55**: 844–7.

Karcioglu ZA, Allam B, Insler MS. Ocular involvement in sinus histiocytosis with massive lymphadenopathy. *Br J Ophthalmol* 1988; **72**: 793–6.

Katz SI, Tamaki K, Sachs DH. Epidermal Langerhans' cells are derived from cells originating in bone marrow. *Nature* 1979; **282**: 324–6.

Kepes JJ, Kepes M. Predominantly cerebral forms of histiocytosis X. A reappraisal of 'Gagel's hypothalamic granuloma', 'granuloma infiltrans of the hypothalamus' and 'Ayala's disease' with a report of four cases. *Acta Neuropathol (Berlin)* 1969; **14**: 77–98.

Kincaid MC, Green WR. Ocular and orbital involvement in leukaemia. *Surv Ophthalmol* 1983; **15**: 211–32.

Kindy-Degnan N, Laflamme P, Duprat G, Allaire G. Intralesional steroid in the treatment of an orbital eosinophilic granuloma. *Arch Ophthalmol* 1991; **109**: 617–18.

Knowles DM, Jakobiec FA, Jones IS. Rhabdomyosarcoma. In: Duane TD, ed. *Clinical Ophthalmology*, Vol. 2. Hagerstown: Harper & Row, 1983.

Lahav M, Albert DM. Unusual ocular involvement in acute disseminated histiocytosis X. *Arch Ophthalmol* 1974; **91**: 455–8.

Lahey ME. Histiocytosis X—an analysis of prognostic factors. *J Pediatr* 1975; **87**: 184–9.

Lichtenstein L. Histiocytosis X. Integration of eosinophilic granuloma of bone. 'Letterer–Siwe disease' and 'Schuller–Christian disease' as related manifestations of a single nosological entity. *Arch Pathol* 1953; **56**: 84–102.

Lucaya JL. Histiocytosis X. *Am J Dis Child* 1971; **121**: 289–95.

Moore AT, Pritchard J, Taylor D. Histiocytosis X: an ophthalmological review. *Br J Ophthalmol* 1985; **69**: 7–14.

Morier P, Merot Y, Paccaud D *et al.* Juvenile chronic granulocytic leukemia, juvenile xanthogranulomas, and neurofibromatosis. Case report and review of the literature. *J Am Acad Dermatol* 1990; **22**: 962–5.

Mortada A. Orbital lymphoblastomas and acute leukaemia in children. *Am J Ophthalmol* 1963; **55**: 327–31.

Mozziconacci P, Offret G, Forest A *et al.* Histiocytose X avec lesions oculaires etude anatomique. *Ann Pediatr* 1966; **13**: 348–55.

Nezelof C, Barbey S. Histiocytosis: nosology and pathobiology. *Pediatr Pathol* 1985; **3**: 1–41.

Nicholson DH, Green WR. *Pediatric Ocular Tumours*. New York: Masson, 1981: 257–60.

Oakhill A, Willshaw H, Mann JR. Unilateral proptosis. *Arch Dis Child* 1981; **56**: 549–51.

Obermann HA. Idiopathic histiocytosis: a correlative review of eosinophilic granuloma, Hand–Schuller–Christian disease and Letterer–Siwe disease. *J Pediatr Ophthalmol* 1968; **5**: 86–92.

Porterfield J. Orbital tumours in children: a report of 214 cases. *Int Ophthalmol Clin* 1962; **2**: 319–35.

Pritchard J. Histiocytosis X: natural history and management in childhood. *Clin Exp Dermatol* 1979; **4**: 421–33.

Rajantie J, Tarkkanen A, Rapola J *et al.* Orbital granulocytic sarcoma as a presenting sign in acute myelogenous leukemia. *Ophthalmologica* 1984; **189**: 158–61.

Riccardi VM. *Neurofibromatosis: Phenotype, Natural History, and Pathogenesis*, 2nd edn. Baltimore: Johns Hopkins University Press, 1992.

Ridgway EW, Jaffe N, Walton DB. Leukaemic ophthalmopathy in children. *Cancer* 1976; **38**: 1744–9.

Risdall RJ, Dehner LP, Duray P *et al.* Histiocytosis X (Langerhans' cell histiocytosis). Prognostic role of histopathology. *Arch Pathol Lab Med* 1983; **107**: 59–63.

Rosenthal AR. Ocular manifestations of leukaemia: a review. *Ophthalmology* 1983; **90**: 899–905.

Rouhiainen H, Nerdrum K, Puustjarvi T, Kosma VM. Xanthogranuloma juvenile—a rare cause of orbital swelling in adulthood. *Ophthalmologica* 1992; **204**: 162–5.

Rowden G. The Langerhans' cell. *Crit Rev Immunol* 1981; **3**: 95–180.

Rubinfield RS, Gootenberg JE, Chavis RM, Zimmerman LE. Early onset acute orbital involvement in childhood acute lymphoblastic leukaemia. *Ophthalmology* 1988; **95**: 116–20.

Rupp RH, Holloman KR. Histiocytosis X affecting the uveal tract. *Arch Ophthalmol* 1970; **84**: 468–70.

Sanders TE. Infantile xanthogranuloma of the orbit: a report of three cases. *Am J Ophthalmol* 1966; **61**: 1299–306.

Sanders TE. Intraocular juvenile xanthogranuloma (nevoxanthogranuloma): a survey of 20 cases. *Trans Am Ophthalmol Soc* 1960; **58**: 59–74.

Sanders TE, Miller JE. Infantile xanthogranuloma of the orbit. *Trans Am Acad Ophthalmol Otolaryngol* 1965; **69**: 458–64.

Shields CL, Shields JA, Buchanon HW. Solitary orbital involvement with juvenile xanthogranuloma. *Arch Ophthalmol* 1990; **108**: 1587–9.

Smith ME, Sanders TE, Bresnik GH. Juvenile xanthogranuloma of the ciliary body in an adult. *Arch Ophthalmol* 1969; **81**: 813–14.

Smith JLS, Ingram RM. Juvenile oculodermal xanthogranuloma. *Br J Ophthalmol* 1968; **52**: 696–703.

Stopak SS, Dreizen NG, Zimmerman LE, O'Neill JF. Sinus histiocytosis presenting as an epibulbar mass: a clinicopathologic case report. *Arch Ophthalmol* 1988; **106**: 1426–36.

Treacy KW, Letson RD, Summers CG. Subconjunctival steroid in the management of uveal juvenile xanthogranuloma: a case report. *J Pediatr Ophthalmol Strabismus* 1990; **27**: 126–8.

Wertz FD, Zimmerman LE, McKeown LA *et al.* Juvenile xanthogranuloma of the optic nerve, disc, retina and choroid. *Ophthalmology* 1982; **89**: 1331–5.

Willman CL, Busque L, Griffith BB *et al.* Langerhans' cell histiocytosis (histiocytosis X) a clonal proliferative disease. *N Engl J Med* 1994; **331**: 154–60.

Wirtschafter J, Nesbit M, Anderson P, McClain K. Intralesional methylprednisolone for Langerhans' cell histiocytosis of the orbit and cranium. *J Pediatr Ophthalmol Strabismus* 1987; **24**: 194–7.

Wood CM, Pearson ADJ, Craft AW, Howe JW. Globe luxation in histiocytosis. *Br J Ophthalmol* 1988; **72**: 631–4.

Zimmerman LE. Ocular lesions of juvenile xanthogranuloma: nevoxanthogranuloma. *Trans Am Acad Ophthalmol Otolaryngol* 1965; **69**: 412–42.

Zimmerman LE, Font RC. Ophthalmic manifestations of granulocytic sarcoma/myeloid sarcoma or chloroma. *Am J Ophthalmol* 1975; **80**: 975–90.

34: Craniofacial Abnormalities

Christopher Lyons

These disorders fall into three groups: (i) craniosynostoses, in which an abnormally shaped skull results from premature closure of sutures (for example Crouzon's and Apert's syndromes); (ii) the clefting syndromes, in which there is failure of apposition or fusion of tissues *in utero*; and (iii) the mandibulofacial dysostoses, a group which includes Treacher Collins and Goldenhar's syndromes.

Craniosynostosis syndromes

Normal development of the face and cranial vault requires co-ordinated growth of all the bones of the skull. Approximately one in 3000 infants are affected by a form of craniosynostosis, in which premature fusion of one or more sutures results in abnormalities of the face and cranial vault.

Genetics

Over 100 syndromes with craniosynostosis are recognized. Many of these are known to be autosomal dominantly transmitted but the cellular mechanisms leading to these malformations are still largely unknown. Recently, however, the genetic bases of Crouzon's, Pfeiffer's and Apert's syndromes have been attributed to defects in a group of genes coding for fibroblast growth factor receptors (FGFRs) (Reardon *et al.* 1994; Rutland *et al.* 1995; Wilkie *et al.* 1995). These receptors are crucial in conveying intercellular signals concerned with the proliferation, migration, differentiation and survival of cells. A genetic mutation which results in substitution of even one amino acid in these receptor structures can produce widespread and fundamental malformations. Sickle cell anaemia is a well-known example of a single amino acid substitution leading to an alteration in protein structure which has devastating results. Achondroplasia is now known to be caused by a mutation in the gene for fibroblast growth factor receptor 3 (FGFR-3) (Shiang *et al.* 1994). In Crouzon's, Pfeiffer's and Apert's syndromes, mutations have been identified in the FGFR-2 gene on chromosome 10 (10q 25.3–26). The mutations causing Crouzon's and Pfeiffer's syndromes are identical, although the latter can also be caused by a mutation of the gene coding for another fibroblast growth factor receptor, FGFR-1. Two other mutations of the FGFR-2 receptor gene cause Apert's syndrome.

It is, as yet, not clear why an abnormality in a seemingly ubiquitous receptor gives rise to these characteristic patterns of malformation. In the 14.5-day mouse embryo, FGFR-2 is found in the developing middle ears and frontal bones of the skull, a distribution consistent with the major growth disturbances of Crouzon's syndrome. It is also found in the developing limb bud, which may account for the limb abnormalities found in Apert's syndrome (Orr-Uretreger *et al.* 1993). It is not known why the same mutation gives rise to the different phenotypes of Crouzon's and Pfeiffer's syndromes. Neither is the mechanism of action of the specific FGFR defects understood; in particular, why the limbs are spared in Crouzon's and not in Pfeiffer's and Apert's syndromes.

Pathogenesis

The basic structure of the head and face is established in the first 7 weeks of embryonic life. Since most congenital craniofacial anomalies represent an arrest in the development of specific structures at one point of development, a brief reminder of the embryology of the skull and face is pertinent.

Development of the face

The mandible and maxilla are formed from the first branchial arch. As the maxilla develops around week 6, the eyes are gradually brought from the lateral surfaces of the head to face progressively more anteriorly, a process which is helped by the growth of the nose and is mostly completed by week 16. Arrest of this process results in a lateral orientation of the orbits, a defect known as exorbitism. Late in week 6, the maxillary processes cover the nasal groove and fuse with the medial nasal fold, enclosing the future nasolacrimal duct. The eyelids develop from mesodermal collections covered by surface ectoderm. Fusion of the lids occurs at week 9 and separation at week 25.

Development of the cranial vault

The vault of the skull arises from neural crest cells which condense at the site of the future crista galli, lesser wings of the sphenoid and the petrous ridges (Smith & Tondury 1978). These condensations grow to surround the enlarging brain, and the sites at which these sheets of cells meet determine the future sites of the cranial sutures. The bone of the cranium is produced from osteoblastic centres at the suture sites. Intervening dura keeps the suture open for expansion; failure to do this results in fusion or synostosis (Fig. 34.1).

Premature closure of a suture inhibits growth perpendicular to it. The skull grows in a direction parallel to the suture to accommodate the enlarging brain. Thus, premature closure of the sagittal suture results in an elongated, boat-shaped skull (scaphocephaly). If anteroposterior growth is restricted by premature fusion of the coronal suture, the head becomes short and wide (brachycephaly). If both anteroposterior and lateral growth are restricted, growth is directed vertically and the head becomes peaked (acrocephaly) or pointed (oxycephaly). When the skull is excessively high as well as short the term turricephaly (tower head) is used. Lastly, closure of any single suture may result in considerable distortion of the skull and face, with flattening of the forehead on the affected side (plagiocephaly).

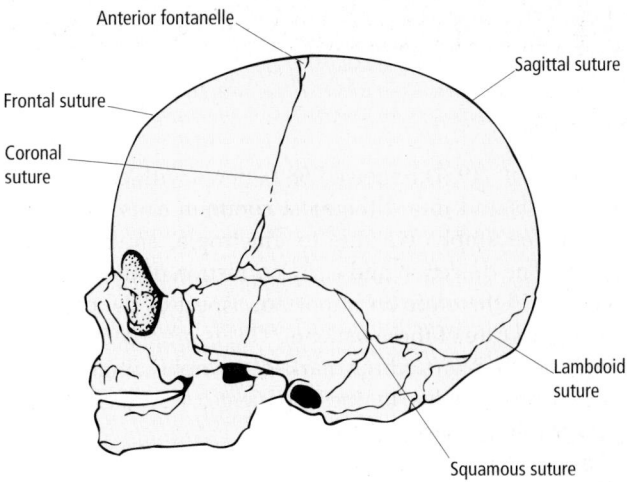

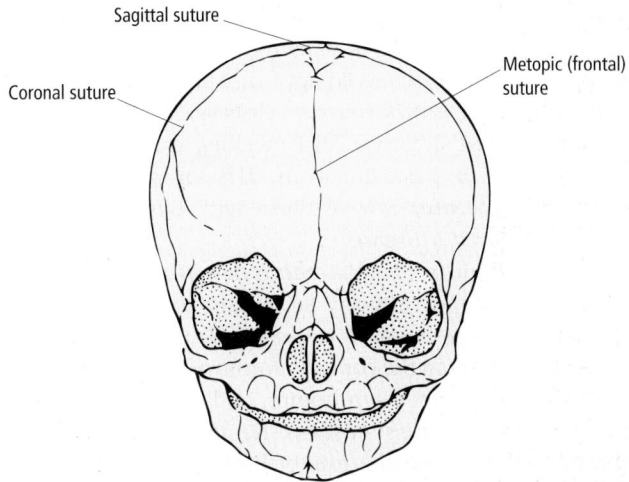

Fig. 34.1 The cranial sutures and fontanelles in an infant skull.

The bones of the skull base are formed from differentiation of cartilage surrounding the notochord. Premature closure of skull base sutures, especially sphenozygomatic and sphenoethmoidal, results in reduced midfacial growth and shallow orbits. The cartilage destined to form the bones of the base of the skull also contributes to the nasal septum which, as discussed above, plays an important role in reducing the wide interorbital distance and 'exorbitism' of the embryonic face.

Classification of craniosynostosis was reviewed by Howell (1954), Blodi (1957), Duke-Elder (1964), Cohen (1975) and Marchac and Renier (1982). Fries and Katowitz (1990) produced an excellent review of the subject.

Common ophthalmic features in craniosynostosis syndromes

The ocular manifestations of the craniosynostoses share a number of similarities. These will be discussed first, and the specific features of each of the common craniosynostoses will then be highlighted.

Amblyopia

Hertle *et al.* (1991) reviewed 58 patients with craniofacial synostosis and found the most common cause of visual loss to be amblyopia due to ametropia, strabismus or ptosis. The detection and early correction of these abnormalities is therefore an important aspect of the ophthalmological care of these patients. This is often complicated by difficulties in patching markedly exophthalmic globes, and fitting glasses in these patients, where the nasal bridge is hypoplastic (Buncic 1991).

Structural abnormalities

Visual failure due to optic atrophy is a relatively common finding. In a series of 244 patients with craniosynostosis, Dufier *et al.* (1986) observed optic disc pallor or atrophy in 50% of patients with Crouzon's disease, 34% oxycephaly and 24% Apert's disease. Disc swelling was observed at some stage in assessment in 31% of patients with Crouzon's disease, 23% of those with oxycephaly and 9.5% with Apert's disease.

The mechanism of optic nerve damage is not clearly understood. Optic atrophy secondary to chronic papilloedema is one possible cause. Hydrocephalus occurs more frequently in the complex forms of craniosynostosis — Apert's, Crouzon's syndromes, and clover-leaf skull — than in single suture synostosis (Renier *et al.* 1982). A disproportion between the rate of brain and skull growth with resultant increase in intracranial pressure has often been suggested as the cause of papilloedema (Howell 1954; Tessier 1971; Archer *et al.* 1974; Marchac & Renier 1982; Renier *et al.* 1982).

Papilloedema (Fig. 34.2) may also result from central nervous abnormalities such as Chiari malformation or stenosis of the jugular foramina. Since these could be remedied by shunting or calvarial remodelling (Archer *et al.* 1974), regular fundoscopic examination of patients with craniosynostosis is important.

Other possible mechanisms such as narrowing of the optic canals (Tessier 1971) and kinking or stretching of the optic nerves (Duke-Elder 1964) have also been suggested to explain the high incidence of optic atrophy.

Exophthalmos

Orbital shallowing, maxillary hypoplasia and retrusion of the lower forehead contribute to the exophthalmic appearance of many patients with craniofacial synostosis. Patients with Crouzon's, Pfeiffer's and clover-leaf skull syndromes are particularly severely affected (Fig. 34.3). Maxillary hypoplasia results in lower lid retraction and

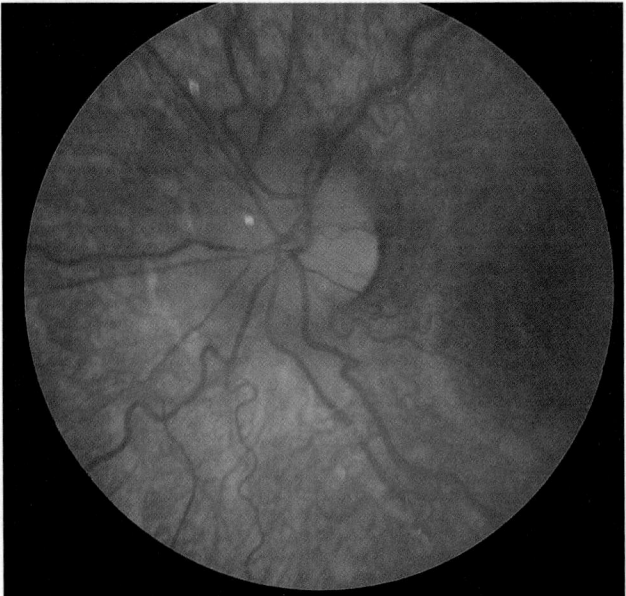

a

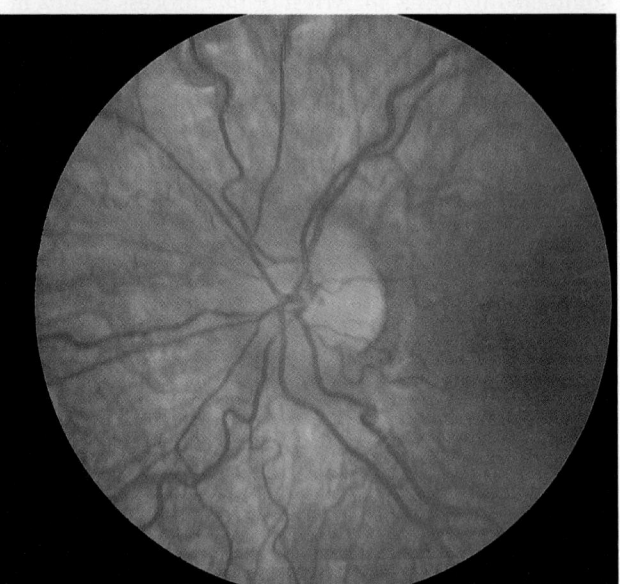

b

Fig. 34.2 (a) Crouzon's disease: left eye on 25 August 1979 showing mild papilloedema. (b) Same patient on 12 April 1983. Mild papilloedema in Crouzon's syndrome may remain stable for many years but great clinical care is needed because many develop optic atrophy.

inferior scleral show with a risk of spontaneous prolapse of the globe (Blodi 1957; Duke-Elder 1964). Lagophthalmos with exposure of the conjunctiva and cornea may be complicated by vascularization or infection, descemetocoele formation and perforation, unless preventative measures are instituted early. These may include the frequent use of topical lubricants and application of ointment at night, the temporary use of moisture chambers and, in severe cases, lateral and medial tarsorrhaphies.

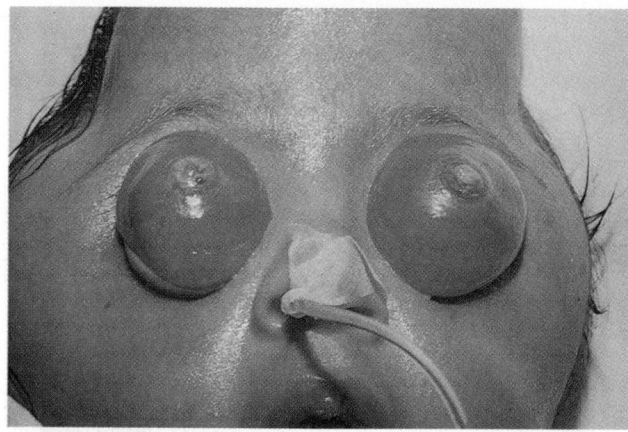

Fig. 34.3 Clover-leaf skull with trilobed flattened skull appearance, subluxated globes, exposure keratitis, and chemotic conjunctiva.

Strabismus

Dufier *et al.* (1986) identified strabismus in 73 of 200 patients (36.5%) with craniofacial anomalies, and Cheng *et al.* (1993) in 68% of 63 patients. Morax (1984) found exotropia or a vertical deviation in 89% of his series. V-pattern exotropia (Fig. 34.4) is the most commonly reported abnormality, with marked updrift of the adduct-

ing eye. When unilateral, as in plagiocephaly, the patient may present with a head tilt to the opposite side (Bagolini *et al.* 1982). A number of explanations have been suggested to account for this pattern, including divergent orbital axes or exorbitism (Dufier *et al.* 1986), shortening of the anteroposterior orbital dimensions resulting in mechanical disadvantage of the superior oblique muscle (Bagolini *et al.* 1982), and hypertelorism. All of these could contribute to the development of exodeviations. In addition, absence or abnormal insertion of one or more extraocular muscles has been described (Diamond *et al.* 1980; Dufier 1986). Cheng *et al.* (1993) observed excyclorotation of the orbits (and extraocular muscles) on the magnetic resonance imaging (MRI) and computed tomography (CT) scans of five patients with craniosynostosis. This finding was also reported in one patient by Buncic (1991). Cheng *et al.* (1993) suggested that the ocular motility findings are simply the result of Herring's law acting on muscles which are no longer truly coupled as yoke pairs due to the orbital excyclorotation. He also described one patient in whom the inferior rectus and superior oblique muscles, thought to be absent at the time of surgery, were later shown by MRI to be present, but in abnormally excyclorotated positions. Preoperative review of coronal CT scans or MRIs may be

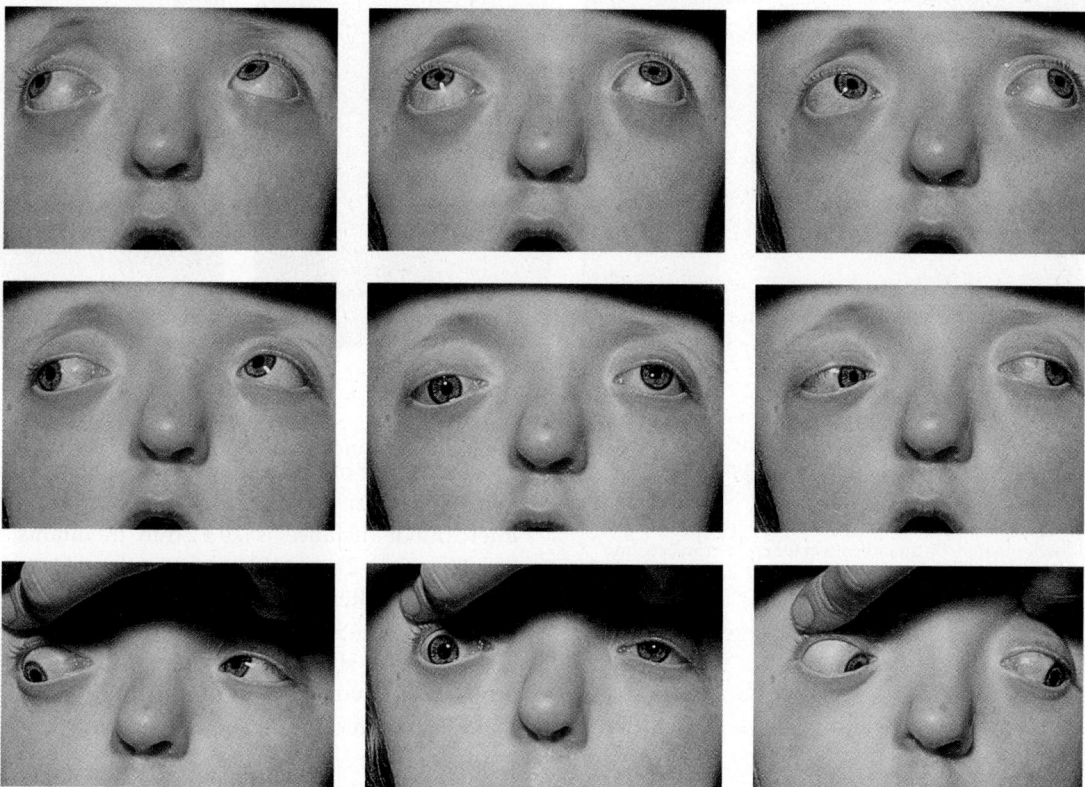

Fig. 34.4 Apert's syndrome showing a horizontal and vertical strabismus which may be associated with anomalies or absence of vertical muscles. A V-pattern exotropia is most common in Apert's syndrome. There is marked updrift of the adducting left eye.

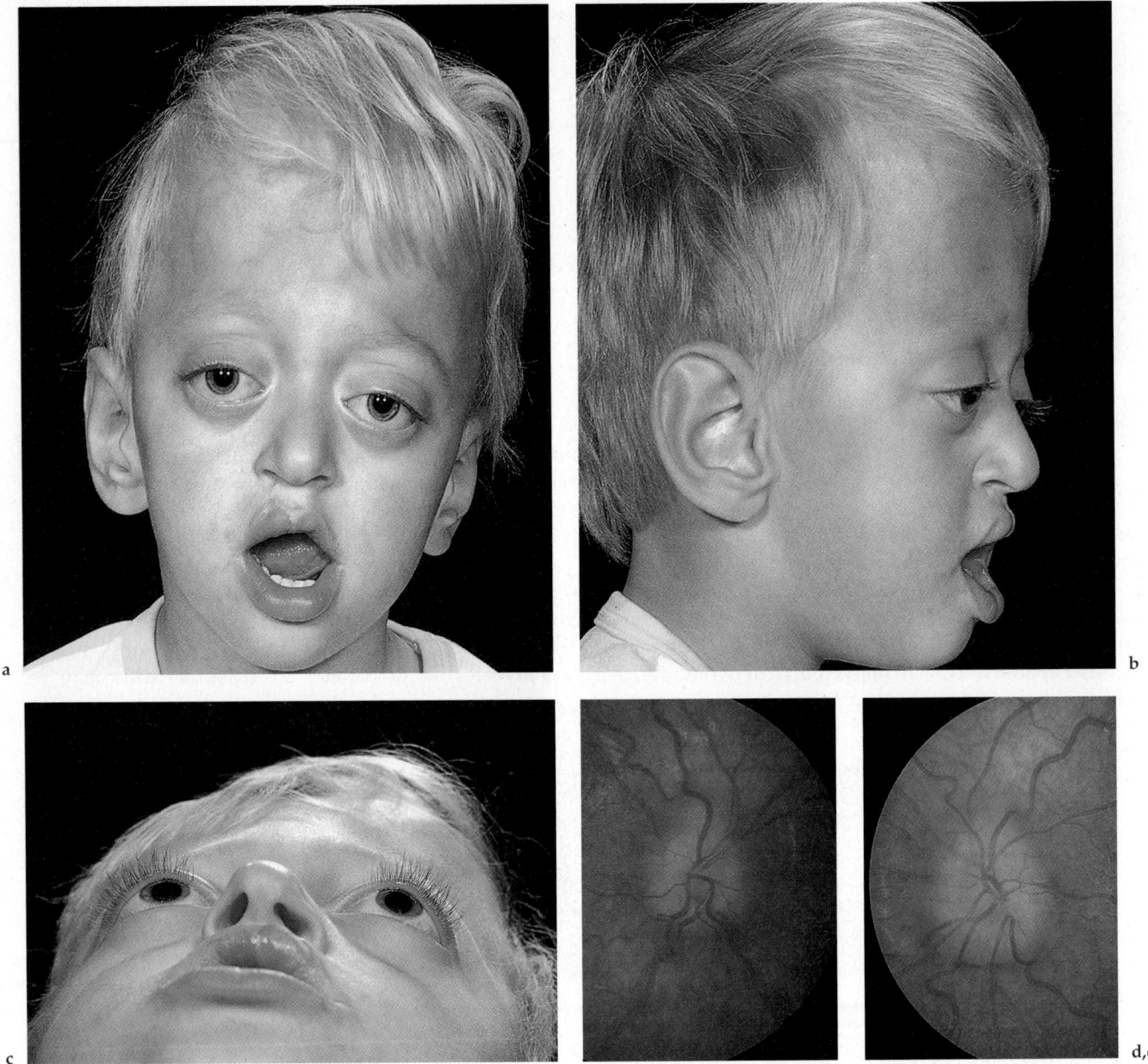

Fig. 34.5 (a–c) Oxycephaly showing the high narrow skull with increased height of the skull, shallow orbits, superior prognathism, and poorly developed superciliary ridges. (d, e). Same patient. Oxycephaly showing papilloedema secondary to craniosynostosis. Marked papilloedema may be an indication for early craniectomy.

helpful when planning strabismus surgery for these patients.

Hypertelorism

Wide separation of the orbits or hypertelorism occurred in 45% of the patients with craniosynostosis reviewed by Dufier *et al.* (1986). The diagnosis is best made on the basis of radiographic findings although telecanthus is a fairly good indicator of underlying hypertelorism in most craniofacial syndromes (Fries & Katowitz 1990). The normal intercanthal distance is 20 ± 2 mm in infants, less than 26 ± 1.5 mm in 2 year olds and less than 30 mm in adults. The normal interpupillary distance is 39 ± 3 mm at birth increasing to 48 ± 2 by the age of 2 years (Feingold & Bossert 1974). Hypotelorism (abnormal proximity of the orbits) was a common feature of trigonocephaly and it may occur in midline facial clefting (see below).

Description of conditions

Ophthalmic complications are likely in oxycephaly, and

Crouzon's and Apert's syndromes; these conditions are outlined in this section. Pfeiffer's and Carpenter's syndromes, conditions which are similar to Apert's, are also mentioned. Hypertelorism is discussed.

Oxycephaly

This condition is characterized by a high, narrow, pointed or dome-shaped skull (Mann 1957). The forehead is high (Fig. 34.5) and the superciliary ridges are poorly developed. There is hypertelorism. Proptosis is due to orbital shallowing from medial and forward displacement of the greater wing of the sphenoid and to a lesser extent the vertical orientation of the orbital plate of the frontal bone. The orbital roof is thus almost vertical, continuing the line of the forehead (Duke-Elder 1964).

There is superior prognathism (François 1975) and the palatal arch is high and narrow. The deformity results from premature synostosis of all the skull sutures, particularly the coronal suture. Intracranial hypertension is common in oxycephaly (Marchac & Renier 1982) and may give rise to visual failure, headache and vomiting. Skull X-ray may show marked digital impression reflecting chronically elevated intracranial pressure. Mental ability in these patients may fluctuate, being inversely related to intracranial pressure (Renier *et al.* 1982). Occasionally, there is a history of convulsions in infancy (Mann 1957) and the electroencephalogram (EEG) may be abnormal (Blodi 1957).

Ocular problems, including visual failure, proptosis, strabismus, restricted eye movements, and nystagmus, tend to become evident in the 2–5-year-old age group.

Crouzon's syndrome (craniofacial dysostosis)

This developmental abnormality, described by Crouzon (1912), consists of premature craniosynostosis, midfacial hypoplasia (Fig. 34.6) and exophthalmos. Although occasionally noted at birth, the synostosis usually develops during the first year of life and is complete by the age of 2 or 3 years. The shape of the calvarium is highly variable (Cohen 1975). Some affected children have no vault deformity, but the majority have anteroposterior shortening of the skull with a steep forehead and occiput, suggesting that the coronal suture is predominantly involved.

The facial appearance is more characteristic, with orbital shallowing resulting in proptosis. The orbits are also widely separated and their axes are laterally rotated (exorbitism). The bridge of the nose is flattened and its tip, as in Apert's syndrome, is often shaped like a parrot's beak (Duke-Elder 1964). The flattened appearance of the midface is emphasized by the prominence of the lower jaw. In addition, the palatal arch is often high and the mouth characteristically held half open (François 1975).

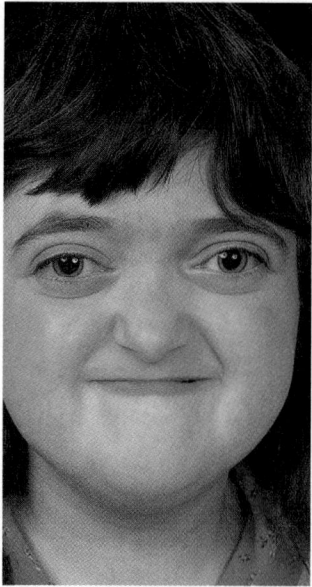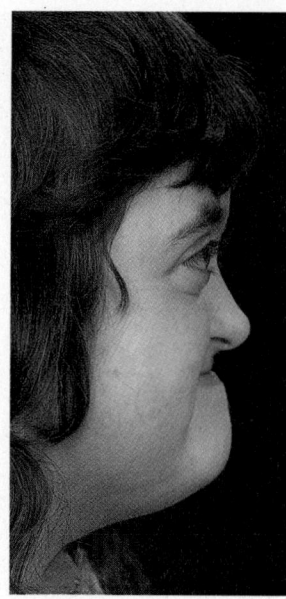

Fig. 34.6 Crouzon's disease. This girl has the features of inferior prognathism, maxillary hypoplasia, and a prominent forehead, her nose is quite straight—it often is more 'hooked' in this condition.

Orbital shallowing may be extreme, leading to severe problems with corneal exposure. Spontaneous prolapse of the globe, often provoked by a fit of coughing, is a distressing event which can be complicated by ischaemic changes as well as exposure problems. The globe should be repositioned using traction on the lids which may have to be accompanied by gentle pressure on the anaesthetized eye using a wet gauze square. It can precipitate the need to proceed with maxillary advancement surgery.

Optic nerve complications were present in 80% of Bertelson's series (1958). Intracranial hypertension may be related to herniation of the cerebellar tonsils following craniofacial surgery (Francis *et al.* 1992).

V-pattern exotropia is commonly present, as described above. Other reported associations include iris coloboma, aniridia, corectopia, microcornea, megalocornea, cataract, ectopia lentis, blue sclera, glaucoma and nystagmus. Associated abnormalities include deafness and epilepsy. Mental retardation was present in 13% of Bertelson's patients.

Inheritance is autosomal dominant with complete penetrance and variable expressivity (Cohen 1986; Kreiborg & Cohen 1990). The gene defect has been mapped to chromosome 10 (see above).

Acrocephalosyndactyly

Wheaton (1894) preceded Apert by 8 years with his description of two children with congenital cranial deformity associated with fusion of the fingers and toes. The

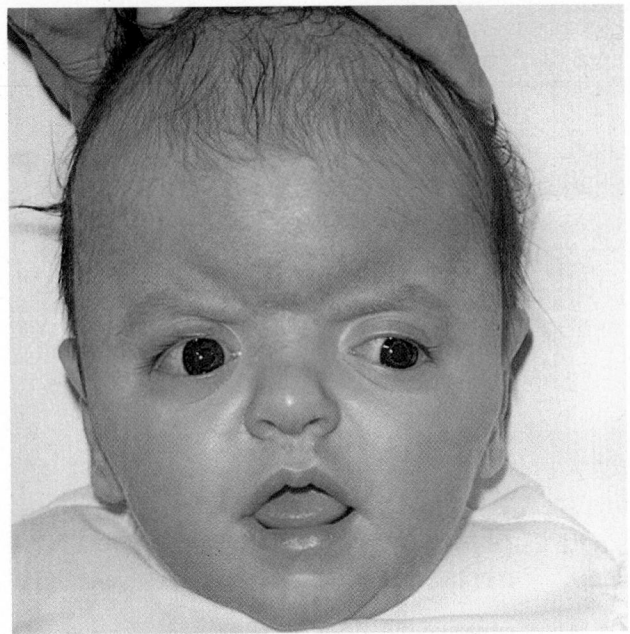

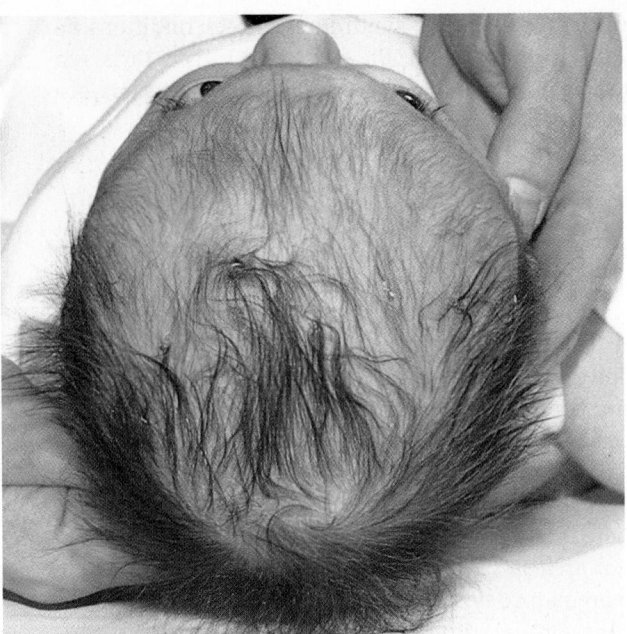

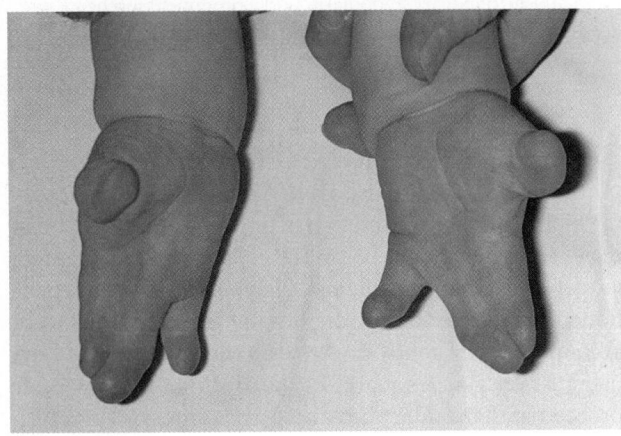

Fig. 34.7 (a–b) Apert's syndrome showing the shallow orbits, deficient supraorbital ridge, strabismus, open mouth and maxillary hypoplasia. (c) Apert's syndrome. The syndactyly usually affects the second to fifth digits of hands and feet.

association of craniofacial synostosis with syndactyly was termed 'acrocephalosyndactyly' by Apert (1906). Five types are now recognized (Temtamy & McKusick 1969). Apert's syndrome (type I), Saethre–Chotzen (type III) and Pfeiffer's syndrome (type V) are the most common. In Carpenter's syndrome (type II), craniofacial synostosis is associated with syndactyly as well as supernumerary digits Goodman's syndrome (type IV) is similar to Carpenter's.

Apert's syndrome

This condition, closely allied to Crouzon's syndrome, is characterized by craniosynostosis and symmetrical syndactyly of fingers and toes involving the second to fourth or fifth digits (Fig. 34.7).

The estimated frequency of occurrence is one in 65 000 live births (Cohen *et al.* 1992) and 4% of all cases of craniosynostosis. It is autosomal dominantly inherited, most cases arising from a new mutation made more likely by advanced paternal age. However, only nine familial cases have been documented due to the reduced fitness of affected individuals. The genetic basis of Apert's syndrome has recently been reported by Wilkie *et al.* (1995) and is discussed above.

As with Crouzon's and Pfeiffer's syndromes, patients with Apert's syndrome may first be seen in the special care nursery, with neonatal respiratory difficulties related to shortening of the nasopharyngeal space. The palate, which is usually highly arched, is also cleft in approximately one-third of cases. Other associations such as tracheo-oesophageal fistula and congenital heart disease may contribute to the neonatal problems.

The typical facial appearance includes oxycephaly (due to predominant involvement of the coronal suture), a markedly deficient supraorbital ridge which is replaced by a horizontal groove, and midfacial hypoplasia with upward tilting. The lower jaw is protuberant. Dental abnormalities are common, as are ear anomalies which may include conductive deafness.

There are few differences between the ophthalmic findings of Apert's and Crouzon's syndromes. Proptosis is often less marked in Apert's syndrome. Severe proptosis was only present in three of 33 patients with Apert's syndrome reviewed by Hanieh and David (1993). Hypertelorism is also relatively mild (Hanieh & David 1993). The palpebral fissures have an antimongoloid slant. Rare associations which have been reported include keratoconus, ectopia lentis, and congenital glaucoma. The optic discs may be normal, oedematous or atrophic.

The presence of hydrocephalus in craniosynostosis presents a challenge for the neurosurgeon, particularly the indications for surgical intervention (Humphreys 1991). Ventriculomegaly on CT scan or MRI may be secondary to hydrocephalus from aqueductal stenosis, synostosis at the skull base impeding cerebrospinal fluid flow from the fourth ventricle, or to defective cerebrospinal fluid reabsorption due to stenosis of the basal foramina impeding drainage from the venous sinuses. However, primary malformations of the central nervous system are common in Apert's syndrome (Cohen & Kreiborg 1990) and ventriculomegaly may also be due to a malformation such as agenesis of the corpus callosum rather than intracranial hypertension. Hanieh and David (1993) found true hydrocephalus to be uncommon in Apert's syndrome. When the intracranial pressure is raised, neurosurgeons may either opt for vault reshaping or shunting. Murovic *et al.* (1993) noted ventriculomegaly in 60% of 25 patients with Apert's syndrome but only opted to shunt three of these patients. They suggested that shunting is indicated only in the presence of documented progressive ventriculomegaly or ventriculomegaly in association with clinical signs of raised intracranial pressure (bulging fontanelles, papilloedema, optic atrophy, apnoea) unrelieved by cranial vault suture release, decompression and reshaping. Nevertheless, since head circumference is a poor indicator of the need for shunting in a patient with craniosynostosis and since hydrocephalus can be present without any symptoms of raised intracranial pressure, careful examination of the optic nerves is an essential part of the follow-up of patients, especially after closure of the fontanelles.

Mental retardation, often thought to be invariably associated with Apert's syndrome, is common but not always present. Normal intelligence has often been reported (Cohen *et al.* 1971; Cohen 1975) but 52% of 29 patients with Apert's syndrome reviewed by Patton *et al.* (1988) had an IQ below 70. Various theories have been postulated to account for its frequent occurrence. Premature closure of the sutures may limit brain growth and therefore intelligence. However, early craniectomy did not lead to a significant reduction in its incidence (Patton *et al.* 1988). Hydrocephalus is another possible cause and Renier *et al.* (1982) found a statistically significant relationship between intracranial pressure and IQ, although there was a great deal of variation. Lastly, low cortical neurone numbers have been reported in postmortem analysis of a macroscopically normal brain from a patient with Apert's syndrome (Crome 1961); mental retardation may be a further manifestation of the central nervous system anomalies which often accompany this syndrome (Cohen & Kreiborg 1990).

Pfeiffer's syndrome

This disorder is very much rarer than Apert's syndrome; it consists of acrocephaly, mild syndactyly, and characteristic broad thumbs (Fig. 34.8) and great toes with varus deformities. Cohen (1993) provides useful guidelines for its diagnosis. The fingers are often short with soft tissue syndactyly and X-rays may show missing phalanges or reduplicated metatarsals. There may also be vertebral abnormalities.

Although the facial and ophthalmic features are similar to Apert's syndrome, mental retardation is less common in Pfeiffer's syndrome. Transmission is autosomal dominant with complete penetrance but variable expressivity (Goodman 1977), the most extreme of which is clover-leaf skull (see below).

Identical mutations of the FGFR-2 gene can cause Pfeiffer's and Crouzon's syndrome phenotypes (Rutland *et al.* 1995). Despite this, the conditions breed true, with no cases of Crouzon's being born in families with Pfeiffer's syndrome and vice versa. Pfeiffer's syndrome can also be caused by a mutation of the gene for FGFR-1 (Muenke *et al.* 1994). It seems that the FGFR-2 mutation results in a more severe craniofacial phenotype (Rutland *et al.* 1995).

Clover-leaf skull

There is a great deal of variation in the expression of Crouzon's, Carpenter's, and Pfeiffer's syndromes. At their most marked these may present as clover-leaf skull (see Fig. 34.3) syndrome (Kleeblattschaedel) (Cohen 1975). This is much more common in Pfeiffer's than in Crouzon's syndrome and it tends to occur more commonly in sporadic than familial cases, perhaps because of the reduced fitness of the affected individual (Rutland *et al.* 1995).

The skull has a flat, trilobed appearance from synostosis of the coronal and lambdoid sutures — hence the term clover-leaf. Hydrocephalus and airway problems are common and difficult to treat (Lodge *et al.* 1993). The orbits are extremely shallow and proptosis with globe subluxation and repeated corneal damage may occur (Walters *et al.* 1973). The definitive treatment of the subluxation is by frontal bone advancement. In the first instance, however, reposition of the globes followed by moist chambers with medial and lateral tarsorrhaphies may be necessary to protect the ocular surface. Life-expectancy is limited.

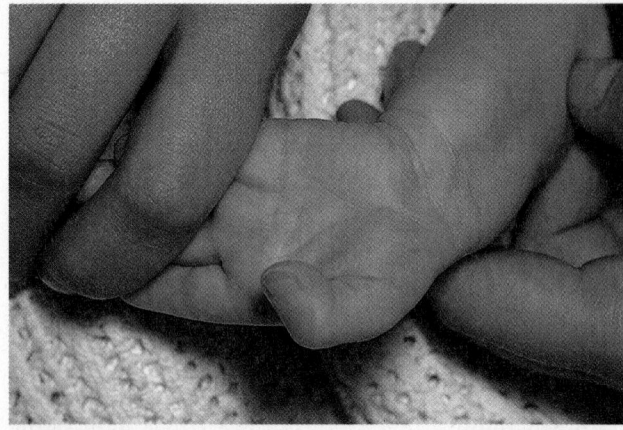

a

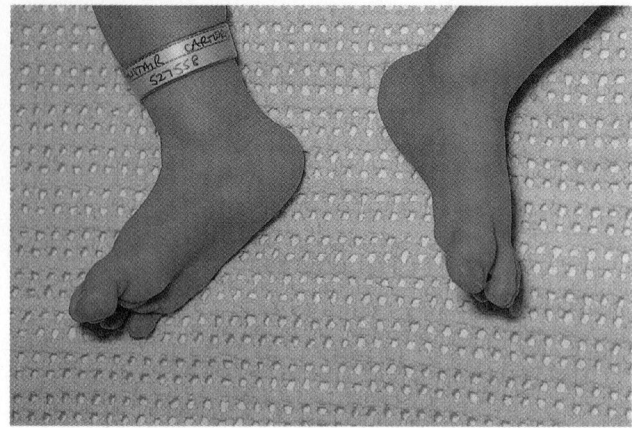

b

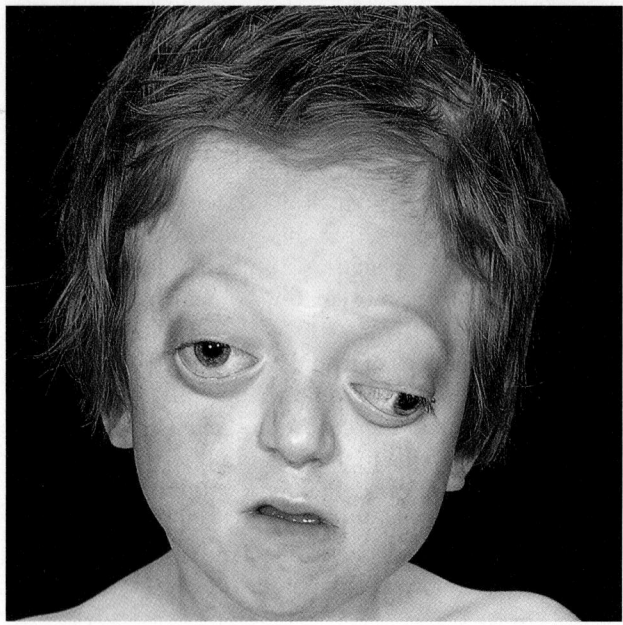

c

Fig. 34.8 (a–b) Pfeiffer's syndrome showing broad thumb and great toes. (c) Same patient. Pfeiffer's syndrome showing acrocephaly and hypertelorism.

Saethre–Chotzen syndrome

Variable skull and facial asymmetry, short fingers with cutaneous syndactyly and a low-set frontal hair-line characterize this rare syndrome. The diagnosis may be missed as the facial changes are often subtle; there is very little midfacial hypoplasia and the eyes are not proptosed. Instead, ptosis is common as are tear duct abnormalities, including bony obstruction of the nasolacrimal duct, which is present in up to 50% of cases (Fries & Katowitz 1990). The genetic defect has been mapped to the chromosome 7p2 region (Brueton *et al.* 1992).

Carpenter's syndrome

This rare syndrome consists of craniosynostosis, polysyndactyly of the feet and syndactyly of the hands, with shortening of the fingers. The craniosynostosis is severe, affecting multiple sutures and resulting in a markedly shrunken and distorted skull vault. Mental retardation is usually present. The ocular findings include hypertelorism, epicanthic folds and telecanthus (Cohen 1975).

Hypertelorism

This term describes a condition in which the two orbits are widely separated. It may be difficult to distinguish the point at which wide orbital separation ceases to be a normal variant (morphogenetic hypertelorism) and becomes a condition determined by anomalous development of the face and head, as described by Greig (embryonic hypertelorism). The latter condition involves characteristic broadening of the nasal bridge with a prominent forehead. The orbits are widely displaced and there is commonly a divergent strabismus. Visual function is usually good. François (1975) considered transmission to be either dominant (mild form) or recessive (pronounced form). Hypertelorism may also be due to other disorders including encephalocoele, or previous trauma. Hypertelorism may also be associated with facial clefting (Tessier 1971; Collin 1983).

Management of craniosynostoses

Children with craniofacial abnormalities are best managed by a team consisting of a paediatrician and ophthalmologist, together with a plastic surgeon, ENT specialist and neurosurgeon. Other specialists may need to be consulted, including oral surgeons and orthodontists, speech therapists, audiologists and psychologists. Families with an affected child should also be offered genetic counselling. The patient's progress should be monitored by periodic visits followed by multidisciplinary planning conferences.

The role of the ophthalmologist may be to co-ordinate referral to these various specialists. Generally, the main function of the ophthalmologist is to ensure that ocular structures are adequately protected, that visual development proceeds normally and that orbital anatomy is respected during reconstruction surgery. Specifically, the most important duty is to ensure that the optic discs are examined regularly and frequently.

Surgical approaches to the skull (Fig. 34.9) include decompressive osteotomy when intracranial pressure is raised early in life and, later, combined craniofacial techniques as described by Tessier (1971). The timing of this surgery remains controversial but early surgery may be indicated if vision is threatened by optic atrophy or corneal exposure.

Generally, the first step in reconstructive surgery is a forehead advancement, if this is necessary (as in Apert's syndrome). The effect of this procedure may be short-lived if it is performed in infancy, especially in Apert's syndrome. Midfacial hypoplasia can be addressed by midface advancement surgery at preschool age. This surgery results in considerable cosmetic improvement but is associated with significant morbidity if carried out earlier in life. A Le Fort III 'monobloc' maxillary osteotomy with advancement of the forehead, orbital margins, nose and maxillae results in expansion of the restricted intracranial space and improves the child's cosmesis in a single procedure. However, this procedure creates direct continuity between the nasal and intracranial spaces and therefore a risk of meningitis. Many surgeons would opt for a staged procedure in which the forehead advancement precedes the Le Fort III maxillary advancement. Finally, surgery during the teenage years is aimed at correcting any residual midfacial abnormality, including the bridge of the nose.

Facial reconstructive surgery often involves elevation of the periorbit and fracture/mobilization of the anterior two-thirds of the orbital walls. Ocular complications which may arise include intraorbital haemorrhage, direct trauma to the optic nerve or globe during surgery or pressure on these structures by a malpositioned bone graft. Although ocular alignment was found to be relatively unaffected by orbital procedures in craniofacial reconstruction (Diamond *et al.* 1980), we feel that strabismus is a relatively common finding following facial reconstruction which involves the orbits.

Clefting syndromes

The second major group of craniofacial abnormalities are known as the clefting syndromes. These result from defective apposition or failure of fusion of neighbouring structures during embryonic development. Tessier classified facial clefts in a purely descriptive manner, numbering them from 0 to 14 in clockwise rotation about the right eye. Thus, clefts involving the midline structures of the nose and forehead are numbered 0 and 1 below the level of the medial canthus and 13 and 14 above. Nasolacrimal and medial canthal clefts are numbered 2, 3, 4 below and 10, 11, 12 above and so on (Fig. 34.10).

This descriptive system gives no clue to the underlying mechanism; clefts with aetiologies as diverse as failure of embryonic closure of the nasolacrimal furrow, amniotic bands, and Goldenhar's syndrome are simply numbered according to their location relative to the eye. Nevertheless, it is a logical method of expressing a facial defect and it is widely used.

Although Tessier's system encompasses the syndromes grouped together as mandibulofacial dysostoses by François (1975), their eponymous names are so well known that, in our view, they are helpful. They include a number of congenital disorders of the face due primarily to retarded differentiation of the first branchial arch mesoderm. Treacher Collins and Goldenhar's syndrome are the most common syndromes in this category.

Treacher Collins syndrome

This syndrome was described by Treacher Collins in 1900 but is also associated with the names of Franceschetti and Zwahlen who made a detailed description in 1944. The mode of inheritance is autosomal dominant with complete penetrance but variable expressivity. The gene responsible has been mapped to the long arm of chromosome 5 (5q32–33.3) (Dixon *et al.* 1991, 1993).

The facial characteristics of Treacher Collins syndrome (Fig. 34.11) include malar hypoplasia, and hypoplastic zygomas with deficient inferolateral orbital angles. Absence of the nasofrontal angle results in a birdlike or fishlike profile. The lower jaw is hypoplastic with abnormal dentition. Choanal atresia and mandibular retrusion may cause respiratory problems. Malformations of the external ear are common and may be associated with middle or inner ear abnormalities, causing deafness. Accesso-

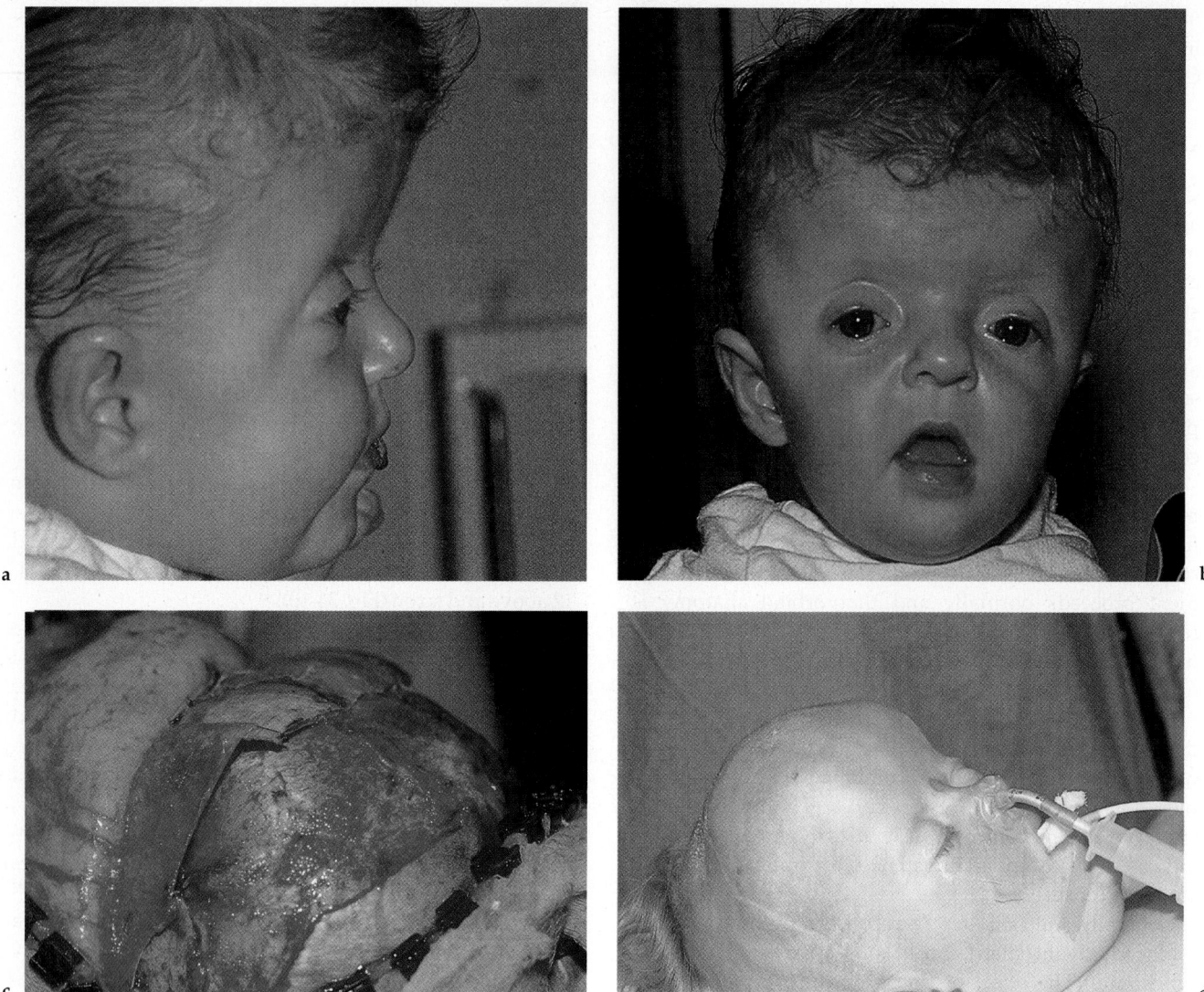

Fig. 34.9 (a–b) This 5-month-old girl with Apert's syndrome has pronounced brow and lower forehead retrusion. (c) The forehead and supraorbital margin are advanced for cosmetic purposes and to increase the intracranial volume; the vault is divided by a coronal incision and a horizontal incision divides the orbital roof and the root of the nose. (d) 15 months later turricephaly has developed due to vault expansion at the previous operative site.

ry auricular appendages as well as blind fistulae occur anywhere between the angle of the mouth and the ear.

The palpebral fissures have an antimongoloid slant and colobomas of the lateral third of the lower lid are common. These may be pseudocolobomas, where cilia, subcutaneous tissues and muscle are hypoplastic. Canthal dystopia, nasolacrimal obstruction and limbal or orbital dermoids also occur frequently (Wang *et al.* 1990; Hertle *et al.* 1993).

Treatment involves oculoplastic repair of the lid colobomas and, where appropriate, surgery to correct the under-

development of the zygoma, maxillae and mandible by bone or cartilage grafts (Tulasne & Tessier 1986). Early audiological assessment is important.

Goldenhar's syndrome

In 1952, Goldenhar described a syndrome consisting of epibulbar dermoids, pre-auricular appendages and mandibular hypoplasia (Goldenhar 1952) which was also termed hemifacial microsomia. Gorlin *et al.* (1990) expanded this to the 'oculo-auriculovertebral spectrum' to encompass the wide range of abnormalities seen with this condition. Expression is extremely variable (Gorlin *et al.* 1990) and may range from a few pre-auricular appendages only, to pronounced facial asymmetry and the 'expanded Goldenhar complex' in which vertebral, cardiac, renal and central nervous system abnormalities are present. The latter may include severe hydrocephalus, and mental retardation. Microphthalmos and cleft lip and

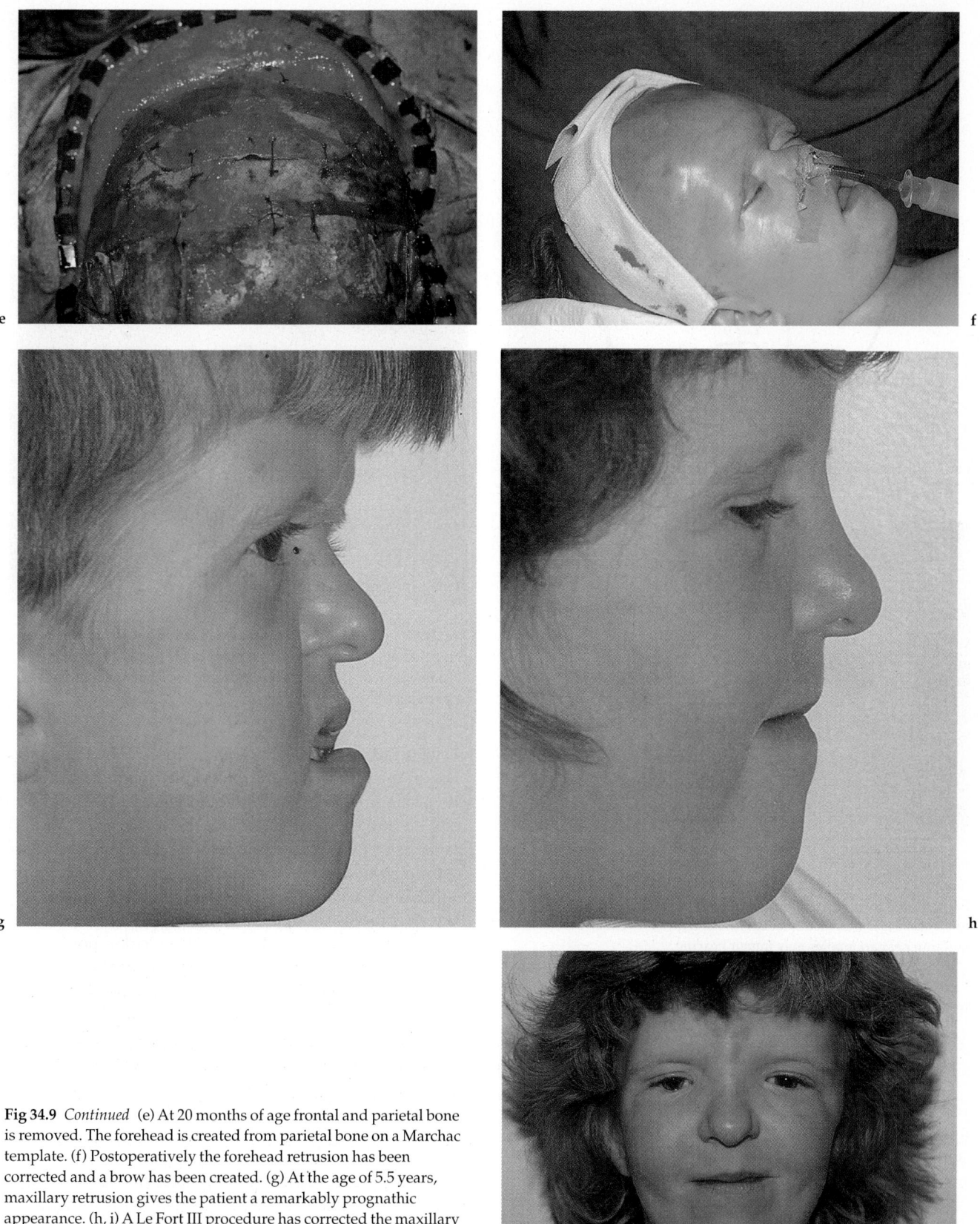

Fig 34.9 *Continued* (e) At 20 months of age frontal and parietal bone is removed. The forehead is created from parietal bone on a Marchac template. (f) Postoperatively the forehead retrusion has been corrected and a brow has been created. (g) At the age of 5.5 years, maxillary retrusion gives the patient a remarkably prognathic appearance. (h, i) A Le Fort III procedure has corrected the maxillary retrusion. Patient of Dr Don Fitzpatrick and Dr Paul Steinbok, University of British Columbia.

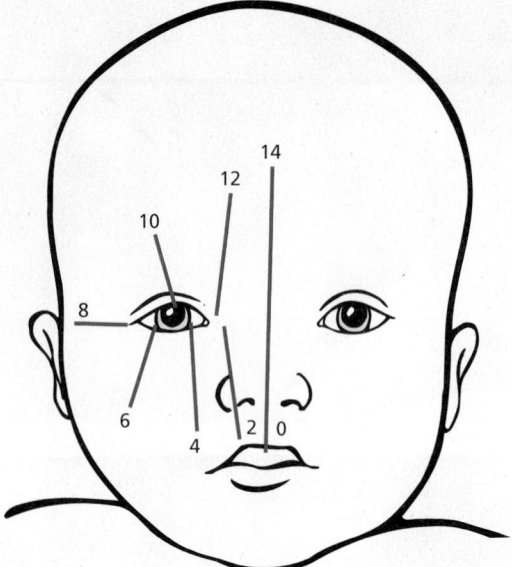

Fig. 34.10 Sites of facial clefts. Modified from Tessier (1971).

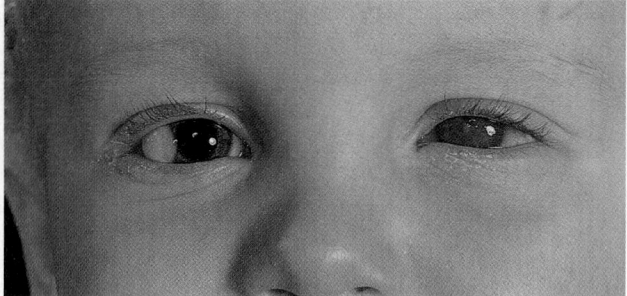 a

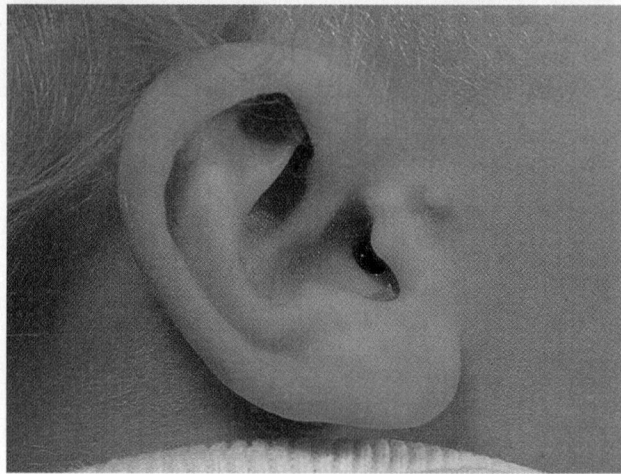 b

Fig. 34.12 (a) Goldenhar's syndrome showing limbal dermoid on the right and a keratitis due to an anaesthetic cornea on the left. (b) Same patient. Goldenhar's syndrome showing a pre-auricular appendage.

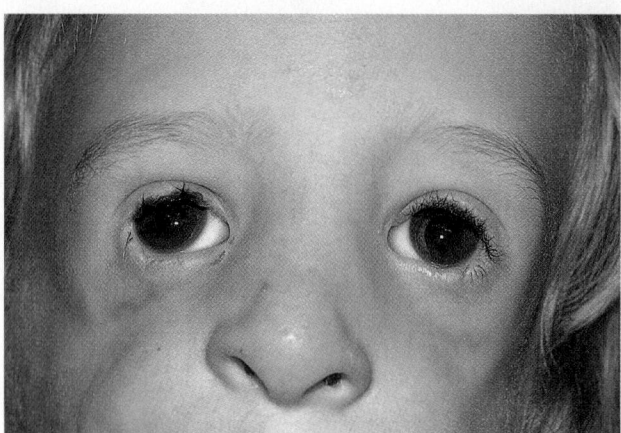

Fig. 34.11 Treacher Collins syndrome. These patients may have marked malar hypoplasia, an antimongoloid slant to the palpebral fissures, and lower lid colobomata together with mandibular hypoplasia and macrostomia. Ear malformations occur and middle and inner ear anomalies may impair hearing.

palate are common in the severe form of the complex. Most cases are sporadic but familial cases have been reported.

The facial abnormalities may be bilateral, but are usually more severe on one side. The pre-auricular appendages are usually anterior to the tragus, with or without fistulae to the ear. Vertebral, cardiac or pulmonary anomalies are common. Ocular findings include ptosis (12%), nasolacrimal duct obstruction and fistula, and coloboma of the middle third of the upper lid (20%), which is often associated with an epibulbar lesion on the ipsilateral eye. This may be a dermoid (white, solid) or dermolipoma (yellow, often conjunctival). Dermoids may

occur unilaterally (50%) or bilaterally (25%), at any location on the globe or within the orbit. The most common site is the inferotemporal limbus (Fig. 34.12). The vision may be impaired if they encroach on the visual axis or cause astigmatism and amblyopia. Dermolipomas are justly famous for the problems which result from over-enthusiastic attempts at complete excision, which may include ptosis, diplopia and dry eye (Crawford 1979; McNab *et al.* 1990; Fry & Leone 1994). Ocular motility disorders are common in Goldenhar's syndrome. Duane's syndrome, esotropia and exotropia are found in approximately one-quarter of patients (Gorlin *et al.* 1990). The syndrome shares a number of features with Treacher Collins syndrome, and combinations of the two have been reported (Goldenhar 1952; François 1975).

Midline facial clefts

These may combine midline bifid nose, cleft lip and palate and midline encephalocoele together with intracranial abnormalities (Fig. 34.13) (see Chapter 50). The signs of an underlying cleft may be rather subtle. A small notch in the upper lip or in the middle of the nose may alert the clinician to an underlying defect.

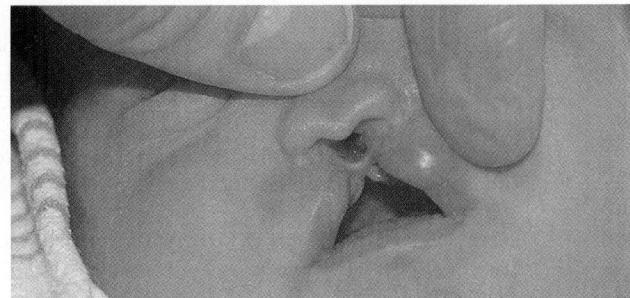

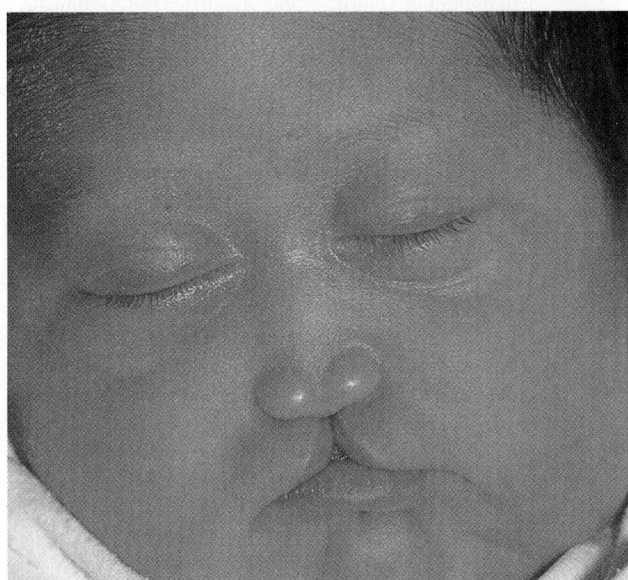

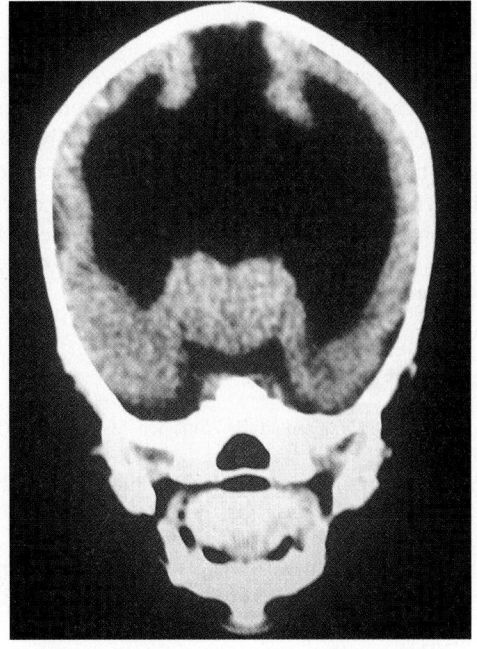

Fig. 34.13 (a) Midline facial and nose cleft. (b) Marked hypotelorism. (c) Associated severe holoprosencephaly. This would be classified as a 0/14 cleft on Tessier's (1971) classification. Patient of the University of British Columbia.

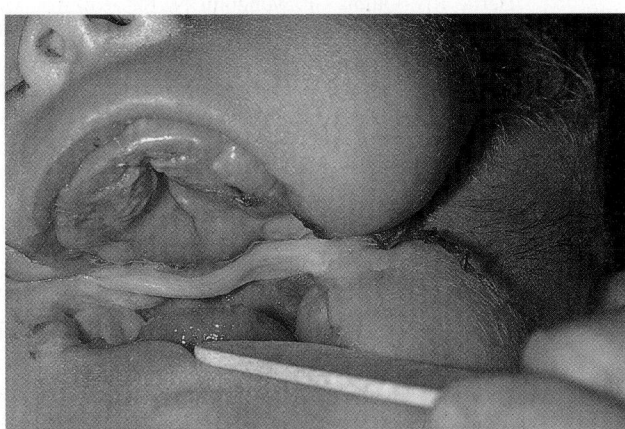

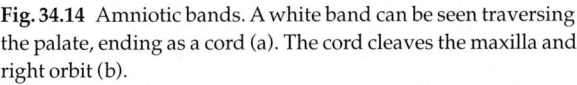

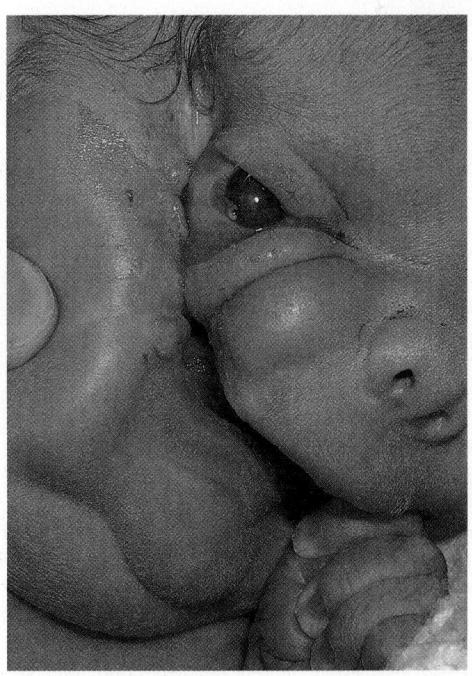

Fig. 34.14 Amniotic bands. A white band can be seen traversing the palate, ending as a cord (a). The cord cleaves the maxilla and right orbit (b).

Amniotic bands

Amniotic bands are thought to occur when bands of amnion encircle parts of the developing fetus, locally restricting growth: the clefts that result do not conform to developmental patterns. They may cause minor deformities, such as ring constriction of fingers but major craniofacial malformations may occur (Fig. 34.14). The condition is sporadic and both sexes are affected equally (Fries & Katowitz 1990).

References

Apert E. De l'acrocephalsyndactylie. *Bull Soc Med Paris* 1906; **23**: 1310–37.

Archer DB, Gordon DS, Maguire CJF, Glendhill CA. Ophthalmic aspects of craniosynostosis. *Trans Ophthalmol Soc UK* 1974; **94**: 172–96.

Bagolini B, Campos E, Chiesi C. Plagiocephaly causing superior oblique deficiency and ocular torticollis. *Arch Ophthalmol* 1982; **100**: 1093–6.

Bertelson TI. The premature synostosis of the cranial sutures. *Arch Ophthalmol (Copenh)* 1958; **5**: 47–66.

Blodi FC. Developmental abnormalities of the skull affecting the eye. *Arch Ophthalmol* 1957; **57**: 593–610.

Brueton LA, van Herwerden L, Chotai KA, Winter RM. The mapping of a gene for craniosynostosis: evidence for linkage of the Saethre–Chotzen syndrome to distal chromosome 7p. *J Med Genet* 1992; **29**: 681–5.

Buncic JR. Ocular aspects of Apert syndrome. *Clin Plastic Surg* 1991; **18**: 315–19.

Cheng H, Burdon MA, Shun-Shin GA, Czypionka S. Dissociated eye movements in craniosynostosis: a hypothesis revived. *Br J Ophthalmol* 1993; **77**: 563–8.

Cohen MM Jr. An etiologic and nosologic overview of the craniosynostosis syndromes. *Birth Defects (Series A)* 1975; **11**: 137–89.

Cohen MM Jr. Pfeiffer syndrome update, clinical subtypes, and guidelines for differential diagnosis. *Am J Med Genet* 1993; **45**: 300–7.

Cohen MM Jr. Syndromes with craniosynostosis. In: Cohen MM Jr, ed. *Craniosynostosis: Diagnosis, Evaluation and Management.* New York: Raven Press, 1986: 413–990.

Cohen MM Jr, Kreiborg S. The central nervous system in Apert syndrome. *Am J Med Genet* 1990; **35**: 36–45.

Cohen MM Jr, Kreiborg S, Lammer EJ *et al.* Birth prevalence study of the Apert syndrome. *Am J Med Genet* 1992; **42**: 655–9.

Cohen MM Jr, Pantke H, Siris E. Nosologic and genetic considerations in the aglossy adactyly syndrome. *Birth Defects (Series A)* 1971; **7**: 237–40.

Collin R. The craniofacial dysostoses. In: Wybar K, Taylor D, eds. *Pediatric Ophthalmology: Current Aspects.* New York: Marcel Dekker, 1983.

Crawford JS. Benign tumors of the eyelid and adjacent structures: should they be removed? *J Pediatr Ophthalmol Strabismus* 1979; **16**: 246–50.

Crome L. A critique of current views on acrocephaly and related conditions. *J Mental Sci* 1961; **107**: 459–74.

Crouzon MO. Dysostose cranio-faciale hereditaire. *Bull Soc Méd Hôp Paris* 1912; **33**: 545–55.

Diamond GR, Katowitz JA, Whitaker LA *et al.* Variations in extraocular muscle number and structure in craniofacial dysostosis. *Am J*
Ophthalmol* 1980; **90**: 416–18.

Dixon MJ, Dixon J, Houseal T *et al.* Narrowing the position of the Treacher Collins syndrome locus to a small interval between three new microsatellite markers at 5q32–33.1. *Am J Hum Genet* 1993; **52**: 907–14.

Dixon MJ, Haan E, Baker E *et al.* The gene for Treacher Collins syndrome maps to the long arm of chromosome 5. *Am J Hum Genet* 1991; **49**: 17–22.

Dufier JL, Vinurel MC, Renier D, Marchac D. Les complications ophthalmologiques des crâniofaciosténoses. A propos de 244 observations. *J Franç Ophtalmol* 1986; **9**: 273–80.

Duke-Elder S. Normal and abnormal development. Congenital deformities. In: Duke–Elder S, ed. *System of Ophthalmology*, Vol. III, Part 2. London: Henry Kimpton, 1964: 1037–57.

Feingold M, Bossert WH. Normal values for selected physical parameters: an aid to syndrome delineation. *Birth Defects (Series A)* 1974; **10**: 1–16.

Francis PM, Beals S, Rekate HL *et al.* Chronic tonsillar herniation and Crouzon's syndrome. *Paediatr Neurosurg* 1992; **18**: 202–6.

François J. Heredity of the craniofacial dysostoses. *Mod Probl Ophthalmol* 1975; **14**: 5–48.

Fries PD, Katowitz JA. Congenital craniofacial anomalies of ophthalmic importance. *Surv Ophthalmol* 1990; **35**: 87–119.

Fry CL, Leone CR. Safe management of dermolipomas. *Arch Ophthalmol* 1994; **112**: 1114–16.

Goldenhar M. Associations malformatives de l'oeil et del'oreille; en particulier le syndrome dermöide epibulbaire—appendices auriculaires—fistula auris congenita et ses relations avec la dysostose mandibulo-faciale. *J Genet Hum* 1952; **1**: 243.

Goodman RM. *Atlas of the Eye in Genetic Disorders.* St Louis: CV Mosby, 1977: 182.

Gorlin RJ, Cohen MM Jr, Levin LS. *Syndromes of the Head and Neck*, 3rd edn. New York: Oxford University Press, 1990.

Hanieh A, David DJ. Apert's syndrome. *Child Nervous Syst* 1993; **9**: 289–91.

Hertle RW, Quinn GE, Minguini N, Katowitz JA. Visual loss in patients with craniofacial synostosis. *J Pediatr Ophthalmol Strabismus* 1991; **28**: 344–9.

Hertle RW, Ziylan S, Katowitz JA. Ophthalmic features and visual prognosis in the Treacher Collins syndrome. *Br J Ophthalmol* 1993; **77**: 642–5.

Howell SC. The craniostenoses. *Am J Ophthalmol* 1954; **37**: 359–79.

Humphreys RP. Apert syndrome. Diagnosis and treatment of craniostenosis and intracranial anomalies. *Clin Plastic Surg* 1991; **18**: 231–5.

Kreiborg S, Cohen MM Jr. Germinal mosaicism in Crouzon syndrome. *Hum Genet* 1990; **84**: 487–8.

Lewanda AF, Cohen MM, Hood J *et al.* Cytogenetic survey of Apert syndrome. *Am J Dis Child* 1993; **147**: 1306–8.

Lodge ML, Moore MH, Hanieh A *et al.* The cloverleaf skull anomaly: managing extreme cranio-orbitofaciostenosis. *Plastic Reconstr Surg* 1993; **91**: 1–9.

McNab AA, Wright JE, Caswell AG. Clinical features and surgical management of dermolipomas. *Austral N Zeal J Ophthalmol* 1990; **18**: 159–62.

Mann I. *Developmental Abnormalities of the Eye.* London: British Medical Association, 1957.

Marchac D, Renier D. *Craniofacial Surgery for Craniosynostosis.* Boston: Little, Brown, 1982.

Morax S. Oculomotor disorders in craniofacial malformations. *J Maxillofacial Surg* 1984; **12**: 1–10.

Muenke M, Schell U, Hehr A *et al.* A common mutation in the fibroblast growth factor receptor 1 gene in Pfeiffer syndrome. *Nature*

Genet 1994; **8**: 269–74.

Murovic JA, Posnick JC, Drake JM *et al.* Hydrocephalus in Apert syndrome: a retrospective review. *Pediatr Neurosurg* 1993; **19**: 151–5.

Orr-Uretreger A, Bedford MT, Burakova T *et al.* Developmental localization of the splicing alternatives of fibroblast growth factor receptor-2 (FGFR-2). *Dev Biol* 1993; **158**: 475–86.

Patton MA, Goodship J, Hayward R, Lansdown R. Intellectual development in Apert's syndrome: a long-term follow-up of 29 patients. *J Med Genet* 1988; **25**: 164–7.

Reardon W, Winter RM, Rutland P *et al.* Mutations in the fibroblast growth factor receptor 2 gene cause Crouzon syndrome. *Nature Genet* 1994; **8**: 98–103.

Renier D, Sainte-Rose C, Marchac D, Hirsch JF. Intracranial pressure in craniostenosis. *J Neurosurg* 1982; **57**: 370–7.

Rutland P, Pulleyn LJ, Reardon W *et al.* Identical mutations in the FGFR2 gene cause both Pfeiffer and Crouzon syndrome phenotypes. *Nature Genet* 1995; **9**: 173–6.

Shiang R, Thompson LM, Zhu YZ *et al.* Mutations in the transmembrane domain of FGFR3 cause the most common genetic form of dwarfism, achondroplasia. *Cell* 1994; **78**: 335–42.

Smith DW, Tondury G. Origin of the calvaria and its sutures. *Am J Dis Child* 1978; **132**: 662–6.

Temtamy S, McKusick V. Synopsis of hand malformations with particular emphasis on genetic factors. *Birth Defects* 1969; **5**: 125–85.

Tessier P. The definitive plastic surgical treatment of the severe facial deformities of craniofacial dysostosis. *Plastic Reconstr Surg* 1971; **48**: 419–42.

Tulasne JF, Tessier PL. Results of the Tessier integral procedure for correction of Treacher Collins' syndrome. *Cleft Palate J* 1986; **23**(Suppl. 1): 40–9.

Walters EC, Hiles DA, Johnson BL. Cloverleaf skull syndrome. *Am J Ophthalmol* 1973; **76**: 716–26.

Wang FM, Millman AL, Sidoti PA, Goldberg RB. Ocular findings in Treacher Collins syndrome. *Am J Ophthalmol* 1990; **110**: 280–6.

Wheaton SW. Two specimens of congenital cranial deformity in infants associated with fusion of the fingers and toes. *Trans Pathol Soc London* 1894; **45**: 238–50.

Wilkie AOM, Slaney SF, Oldridge M *et al.* Apert syndrome results from localized mutations of FGFR2 and is allelic with Crouzon syndrome. *Nature Genet* 1995; **9**: 165–72.

35: Cystic Lesions and Ectopias

Christopher Lyons and Jack Rootman

Cystic lesions

Cystic lesions of the orbit in childhood include lacrimal ductal cyst, dermoid cysts, sinus mucocoeles, microphthalmos with cyst, encephalocoele, congenital cystic eyeball and teratoma. In some parts of the world parasitic cysts involving organisms such as *Echinococcus* and *Schistosoma* are common, but these are rare in Europe and North America (Jakobiec & Jones 1985). Haemorrhage within orbital lymphangiomas may give rise to the so-called 'chocolate' cysts. Cystic lesions of the orbital wall may be seen in fibrous dysplasia, ossifying fibroma and aneurysmal bone cyst. Cystic lesions of the orbit and bone were reviewed by Lessner *et al.* (1994).

Lacrimal ductal cyst

Lacrimal ductal cysts are rare but important since they are part of the differential diagnoses of ocular adnexal masses in childhood, particularly in the lacrimal gland region. Bullock *et al.* (1986) suggested that lacrimal cysts should be classified according to their site of origin, i.e. palpebral lobe (simple dacryops), orbital lobe, accessory glands or ectopic lacrimal gland. The first three are considered here, whilst ectopic lacrimal gland is considered below. Their differential diagnoses include dermoid, inclusion, parasitic and aneurysmal bone cysts.

Overall, lacrimal ductal cysts most commonly arise in the palpebral lobe. These tend to occur in adulthood but may be seen in the teenage years. Their onset is sometimes preceded by a history of trauma or inflammation. A smooth, transilluminating mass slowly enlarges in the lateral aspect of the upper lid (Fig. 35.1), and may be seen as a blueish cyst on lid eversion. Pain or tenderness is often a feature, spontaneously resolving as the cyst decompresses itself with a gush of tears. The association with blepharochalasis was reported by Smith and Rootman (1986). Careful surgical excision of the intact cyst is curative if the patient is symptomatic.

Cysts originating in the orbital lobe are rare but usually present in infancy or early childhood as a tense mass in the region of the lacrimal fossa. They tend to be larger than their palpebral counterparts. The cyst may enlarge, sometimes quite suddenly due to inflammation or haemorrhage, to cause marked proptosis and inferonasal displacement of the globe. Globe subluxation may occur (Duke-Elder 1964a). Deep extension into the posterior orbit may be seen on computed tomography (CT) scan. Once again, excision of the intact cyst is desirable. A lateral orbitotomy may be necessary if there is posterior extension. Histologically, ductal cysts of the palpebral lobe are lined by myoepithelium, unlike orbital lobe cysts whose lining epithelium is cuboidal.

Cysts of the accessory glands of Krause and Wolfring may also occur, resulting in swelling in the region of the fornices. These can be excised via a conjunctival approach.

Lacrimal tissue may occasionally occur ectopically within the eye and orbit, and often with an associated cystic component (see below).

Dermoid cyst

Dermoid cysts of the orbit and periorbital region are common in childhood, accounting for 3–9% of orbital masses in most series (Youseffi 1969; Crawford 1983). They are

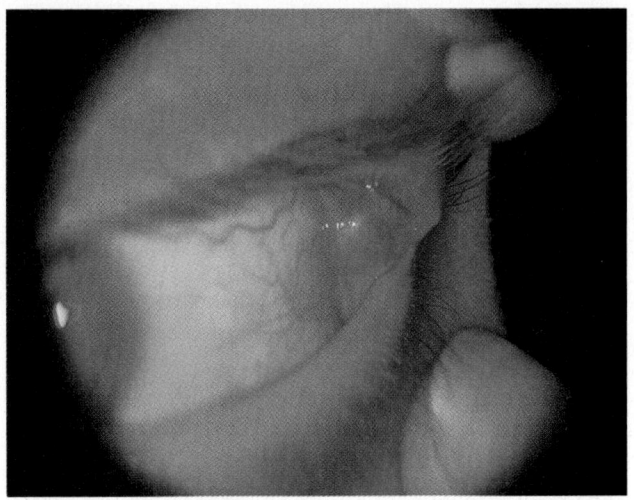

Fig. 35.1 Lacrimal ductal cyst showing as a transilluminating mass in the lateral fornix revealed by pulling the lid away from the globe. Patient of the University of British Columbia.

developmental choristomas which are thought to arise from ectodermal rests trapped at suture lines or within mesenchyme during orbital development.

Histologically, the cysts are lined by keratinized stratified squamous epithelium. Dermal appendages, including hair follicles and sebaceous glands, are found in their wall. Cyst leakage or rupture may give rise to a chronic granulomatous reaction.

Dermoids may be superficial or deep (Grove 1981). Conjunctival dermoids are unusual variants, occurring posterior to the septum. Most of the dermoids seen in childhood are superficial.

Superficial dermoids

These often present in infancy as a rounded mass, typically at the superotemporal (Fig. 35.2) margin of the orbit (Pfeiffer & Nichol 1948). They may also arise in the medial orbit (Fig. 35.3). They are painless, non-tender, firm, non-fluctuant and often immobile. Since, strictly speaking, they are outside the orbit, they cause no displacement of the globe and the orbital rim is palpable behind their pos-

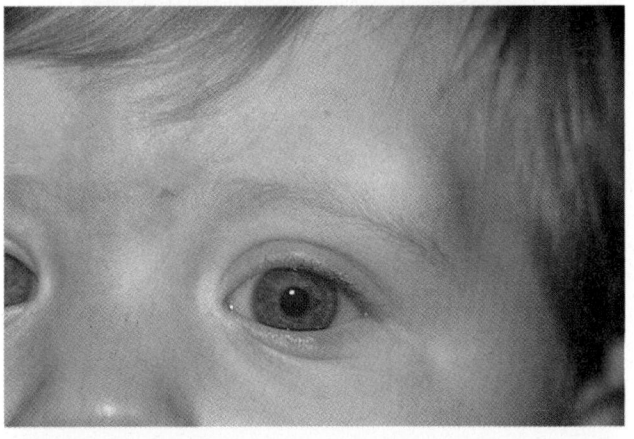

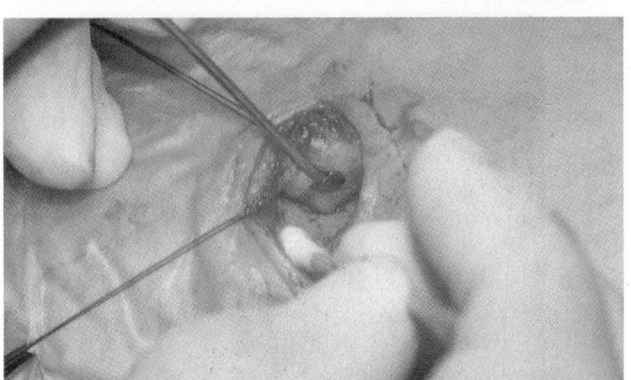

Fig. 35.2 (a) Typical superficial dermoid cyst on the brow of an 18-month-old boy. No intraorbital extension was noted preoperatively, although a small tail was seen to insert into bone at the time of surgery (b). This was divided and cauterized. The cyst was intact. Patient of the University of British Columbia.

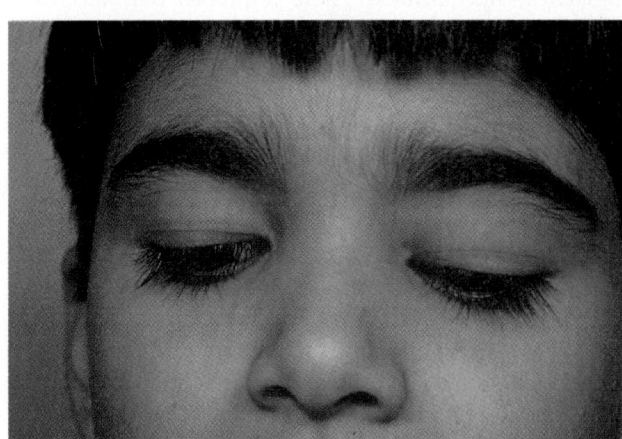

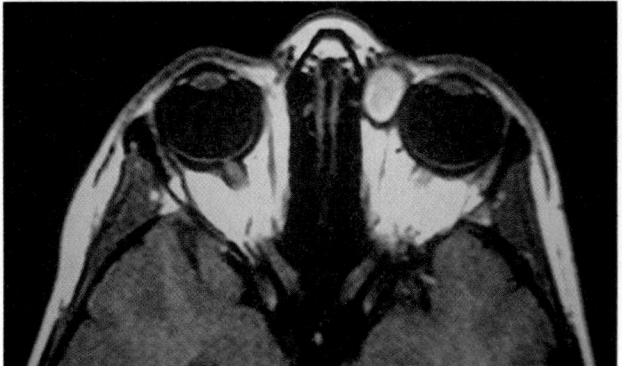

Fig. 35.3 (a, b) This 10-year-old boy had a gradually enlarging mass in his left upper lid for several years. T1-weighted MRI shows that this is situated anteriorly and its contents are isodense with orbital fat. It was a dermoid cyst and was excised completely. Patient of the University of British Columbia.

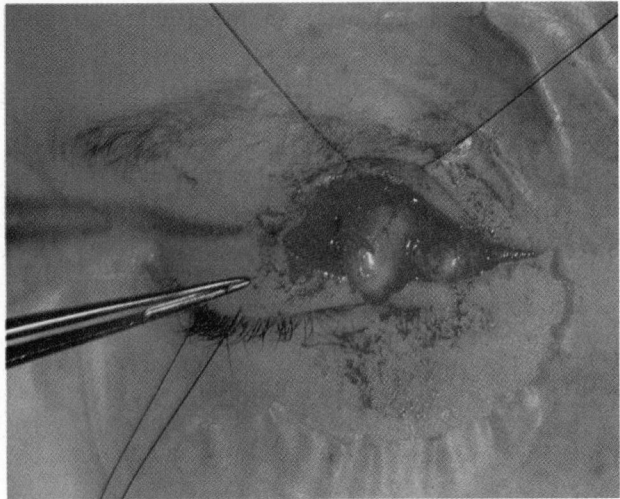

Fig. 35.4 Surgical excision of a 'dumbbell' dermoid. The intervening bone has been removed. Patient of the University of British Columbia.

terior edge. Unsuspected deep extension into the temporalis fossa, posterior orbit or even intracranial space is not an uncommon finding in the apparently superficial dermoid cysts of childhood. These 'dumbbell' dermoids may present with the typical signs of superficial dermoid but extend into the temporalis fossa through an hour-glass configuration (Fig. 35.4). This finding was present in 24 of 70 patients with outer canthus dermoids reviewed at Moorfields (Sathananthan *et al.* 1993). Very rarely, proptosis with mastication can result from pressure on a communicating cyst by temporalis contraction with chewing (Whitney *et al.* 1986).

The radiological appearance of a dermoid cyst is characteristic: on CT scan, a rounded discrete mass is seen, associated with thinning and smooth erosion of the underlying bone. The contents are often of heterogeneous density. Although fat lucency is not universally present, it was noted in 71% of the 70 patients reviewed by Sathananthan *et al.* (1993). Its presence within the cyst is often considered diagnostic (Nugent *et al.* 1987).

Direct excision of superficial dermoid cysts is relatively simple. In our opinion, it should be performed by the age of 5 years or so to avoid accidental rupture. Although excision of the intact cyst is desirable, intraoperative rupture is not disastrous if the contents and all the cyst wall are carefully removed. Failure to do so may elicit a chronic inflammatory reaction with sinus formation and persistent discharge.

Interestingly, rupture of a dermoid cyst is frequently not associated with dramatic inflammatory signs. These were present in only four of 17 patients with ruptured cysts reported by Satorre *et al.* (1991). A chronic lipogranulomatous response was more common.

Clearly, preoperative assessment of any dermoid cyst is essential to rule out the presence of deep extension from a superficial dermoid. The modality of choice for this evaluation is CT scanning with 2 mm slices through the lesion, preferably with coronal cuts.

Deep dermoids

Although these typically present in adolescence and adulthood with gradual enlargement and consequent displacement of orbital contents, they can occasionally present in infancy in a similar way (Leonardo *et al.* 1994). Typically only their smooth and rounded anterior margin can be palpated although they may extend to the orbital apex (Sherman *et al.* 1984). The lesion may not be palpable at all (Fig. 35.5), as in the intraconal dermoid cyst reported by Wilkins & Byrd (1986). Proptosis and/or globe displacement predominate in the clinical picture but ocular motility and even visual disturbances and pain may occur. Howard *et al.* (1994) recently reported two patients with dermoid cysts located within the lateral rectus muscle.

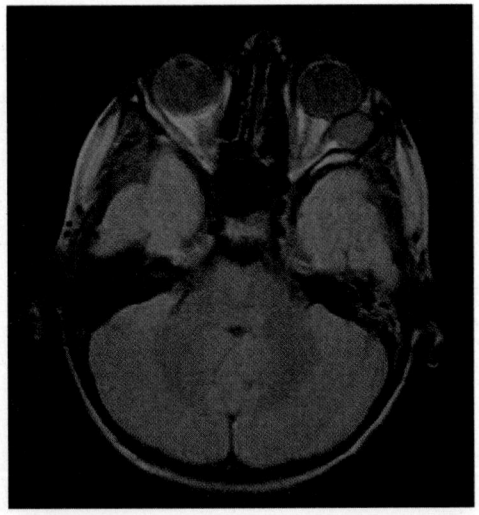

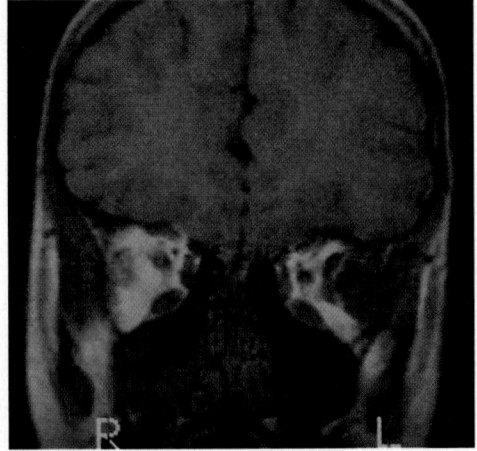

Fig. 35.5 (a, b) Orbital dermoid. MRI scan showing lateral retro-ocular lesion on the left side.

The CT findings of deep dermoids are similar to those of superficial dermoids except for the frequent presence of irregular orbital wall defects as well as sclerosis, irregular scalloping or notching of the underlying bone. The walls of large dermoid cysts may calcify.

The management of deep dermoids is complicated (Pfeiffer & Nichol 1948; Sherman *et al.* 1984; Lane *et al.* 1987) since total surgical excision is necessary to prevent complications. A careful preoperative clinical and radiological assessment is essential to plan the appropriate surgical approach, which may involve combined anterior and lateral orbitotomies (Sherman *et al.* 1984). Although it was felt that this surgery was best delayed until bone growth had ceased (Lane *et al.* 1987), the craniofacial literature suggests that delay is not necessary to safeguard facial bony growth.

Orbital encephalocoele

These rare lesions arise from an embryological defect in which neuroectoderm fails to separate from surface ectoderm. This results in a bony dehiscence with a 'cystic' herniation of dura into the orbit, either alone (meningocoele) or with brain tissue (meningoencephalocoele). They may present in association with an optic disc anomaly (Pollock *et al.* 1968); a basal encephalocoele should always be excluded in a child with an optic nerve anomaly such as coloboma or morning glory disc, especially if there is also a midline facial anomaly such as hypertelorism, cleft lip or palate (Caprioli & Lesser 1983). Children may also present with proptosis due to an orbital encephalocoele.

Orbital encephalocoeles are uncommon. They may be anterior or posterior (Duke-Elder 1964b). Anterior orbital encephalocoeles herniate through the region of the sutures dividing the frontal, ethmoid, lacrimal and maxillary bones. They usually present as a congenital cystic swelling at the medial aspect of the orbit extending onto the face. They may also present in infancy and early childhood with gradually increasing forward and lateral globe displacement. The medial canthal tendon is usually displaced in an inferolateral direction. Atypical presentations are also encountered, such as the 10 mm blueish cystic mass in the superonasal fornix of a 1-month-old patient which was found to be a meningoencephalocoele (Terry *et al.* 1993).

Classically, the size of the cyst increases on straining or crying (Mortada & E-Toraei 1960; Duke-Elder 1964a; Consul 1965; Leone & Marlowe 1970). It may be fluctuant, pulsatile, reducible with gentle pressure and it may transilluminate. Anterior encephalocoeles are important in the differential diagnoses of any medial canthal swelling, and have been mistaken for sinus mucocoeles, dermoid cysts or even nasolacrimal duct mucocoeles (Rashid *et al.* 1986). A bony defect is usually evident on X-ray and intracranial communication can be confirmed by CT scan. Three-dimensional CT reconstruction may be helpful in planning surgery (David *et al.* 1984), which is usually performed by neurosurgical and/or maxillofacial teams (Lello *et al.* 1989).

Posterior encephalocoeles herniate into the orbit via the optic foramen, orbital fissures or via a bony defect. They present with slowly progressive proptosis which may be pulsatile. Occasionally, posterior encephalocoeles may present during the teenage years or in adulthood.

Typically, the eye is displaced forwards and downwards (Duke-Elder 1964a) and the proptosis increases on straining or crying. Plain X-rays demonstrate enlarged foramina or a bony defect of the posterior orbit. CT scan delineates the size and content of the cyst. Posterior encephalocoeles are particularly associated with the sphenoid wing dysplasia of neurofibromatosis type 1 (NF1). This type of defect can also be associated with enophthalmos.

Sinus mucocoele

The paranasal sinuses are of clinical relevance to childhood orbital disease and it is important to be familiar with their development. All the sinuses are present at birth in a rudimentary form, except the frontal sinus which first appears at the age of 2 years. There are two spurts of enlargement: at the age of 6 or 7 years, coinciding with the eruption of the second dentition, and again at puberty (Last 1978). Since the frontal sinus is the source of most mucocoeles, it is not surprising that this disorder is rare in childhood. Ethmoidal sinus mucocoeles, however, may present in early life (Alberti *et al.* 1968; Robertson & Henderson 1969), particularly in association with cystic fibrosis.

A mucocoele is a cystic swelling of a paranasal sinus which results from obstruction of its ostium. The normal mucous secretions of the respiratory epithelium lining accumulate within the sinus leading it to expand gradually, with loss of its internal bony structure. With further expansion, the cystic mass transgresses the orbital wall and results in displacement of the orbital contents. It may also erode into the intracranial space (Delfini *et al.* 1993). Eventually, the cyst consists of viscous material which may be white, yellow or brown, contained within a fibrous capsule.

The usual presentation is with proptosis (Fig. 35.6) of gradual onset with lateral displacement of the globe. This may appear clinically as hypertelorism. A firm cystic noncompressible swelling may be palpable in the medial orbit; its extension above the medial canthal tendon should differentiate it from a mucocoele of the lacrimal sac. Inflammatory signs are absent. The absence of a bony skull defect, pulsatility or expansion on straining differentiate it from an encephalocoele. Sphenoid sinus mucocoeles are rare in childhood. Recently, however,

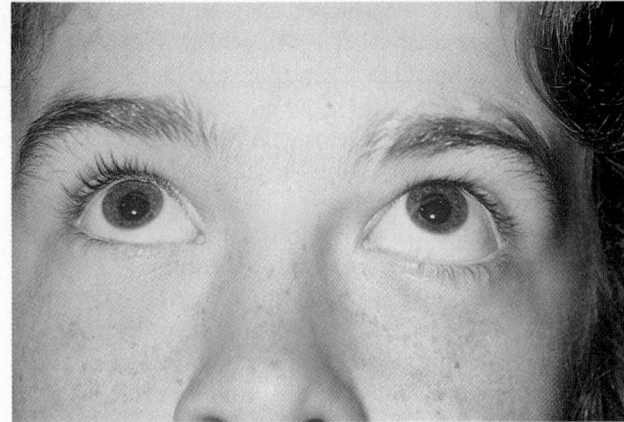

a

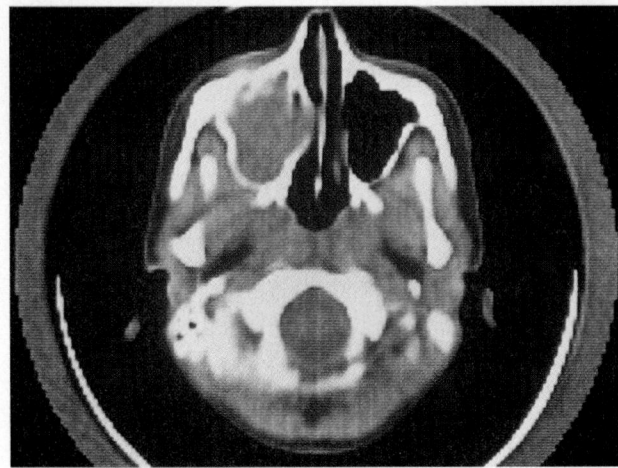

b

Fig. 35.6 (a) Post-traumatic mucocoele. At the age of 9 years, this patient sustained an orbital blow-out fracture which was repaired using a silastic sheet. He is seen here at the age of 14 years; there is proptosis and upward displacement of the globe. CT scanning showed the silastic implant had caused maxillary sinus obstruction and secondary mucocoele (b). The implant was removed and the sinus opened surgically to allow drainage into the nose. Patient of the University of British Columbia.

Casteels *et al.* (1992) reported a 10-year-old girl presenting with sudden blindness from optic nerve compression by a previously unsuspected sphenoid sinus mucocoele.

Plain X-rays will show a markedly enlarged sinus on the affected side. On CT scan, a smooth-walled cystic lesion, often containing egg-shell calcification, arises from the affected sinus. In childhood, this is most commonly the ethmoid, and expansion into the medial orbit is noted along with thinning of the orbital wall and destruction of the internal septa.

The management is surgical, aiming to completely remove the cyst walls and re-establish sinus drainage. Collaboration with an ENT surgeon is essential. Lund & Rolfe (1989) have stressed the importance of carefully repositioning the trochlea after Lynch–Howarth type fronto-ethmoidectomy for mucocoele drainage, in order to avoid postoperative superior oblique underaction. In-

complete excision of the cyst wall is frequently followed by recurrence. Other cystic lesions arising in the sinuses may also cause proptosis, including dentigerous cysts.

Microphthalmos with cyst

Incomplete closure of the fetal fissure in early development (between 7 and 14 mm stage) may result in a variety of colobomatous defects of the eye (Pagon 1981). Eyes with severe colobomas are often microphthalmic and proliferation of neuroectoderm at the lips of the persistent fetal fissure may result in the formation of an orbital cyst which communicates with the eye. The size of the cyst varies from microscopic to massive. Arrest of development before the 7 mm stage results in a congenital cystic eye or 'anophthalmos with cyst' (Dollfus 1968; Helveston *et al.* 1970). In the latter, no recognizable globe is present within the orbit.

Clinical presentation

Typically, a blueish cystic transilluminating lesion (Fig. 35.7) in the lower fornix displaces a microphthalmic or rudimentary eye under the upper lid (Waring *et al.* 1976; Weiss *et al.* 1985). Occasionally, the eye cannot be identified clinically (Waring *et al.* 1976). Rarely the cyst may be present in the upper lid and the eye is displaced downwards (Nicholson & Green 1981). Bilateral microphthalmos with cyst has been reported (Arstikaitis 1969). The cyst communicates with the eye via a narrow stalk. The microphthalmic eye usually has extremely poor vision and an associated optic nerve and retinal coloboma. The other eye may be normal or also have optic nerve or retinal coloboma (Waring *et al.* 1976; Weiss *et al.* 1985). Ocular coloboma may be associated with a variety of systemic malformations (Waring *et al.* 1976; Pagon 1981). The extent of the cystic component is best delineated by CT scan, although B-scan ultrasound can also be useful. Small asymptomatic cysts may occasionally be found incidentally on CT scan (Fig. 35.8). The glial nature of the cyst lining can be clearly demonstrated by immunohistochemistry (Lieb *et al.* 1990).

Management

In most cases no active intervention is needed (Weiss *et al.* 1985). If cyst enlargement results in an unsightly appearance it is best managed by aspiration. Recurrence is common and repeated aspiration may be necessary. When there is recurrence of the cyst after multiple aspirations, surgery may be indicated although it may be difficult to excise the cyst without sacrificing the globe.

Congenital cystic eyeball (anophthalmos with cyst)

Congenital cystic eyeball can be distinguished from

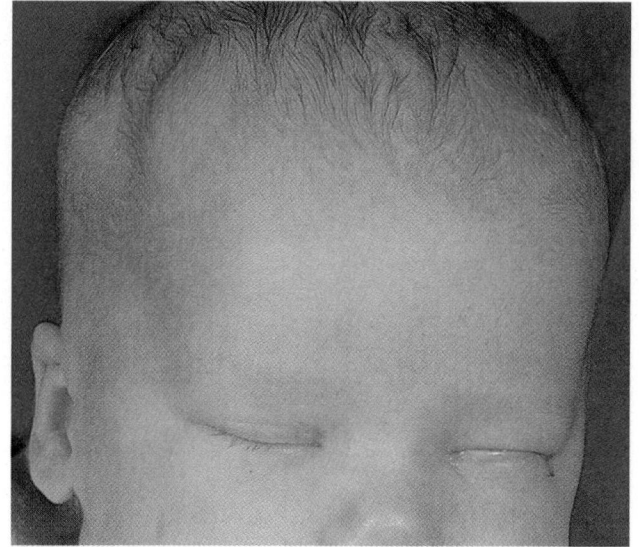

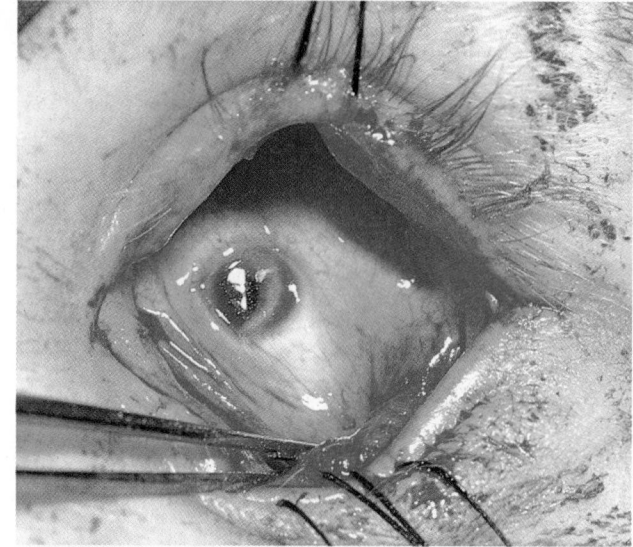

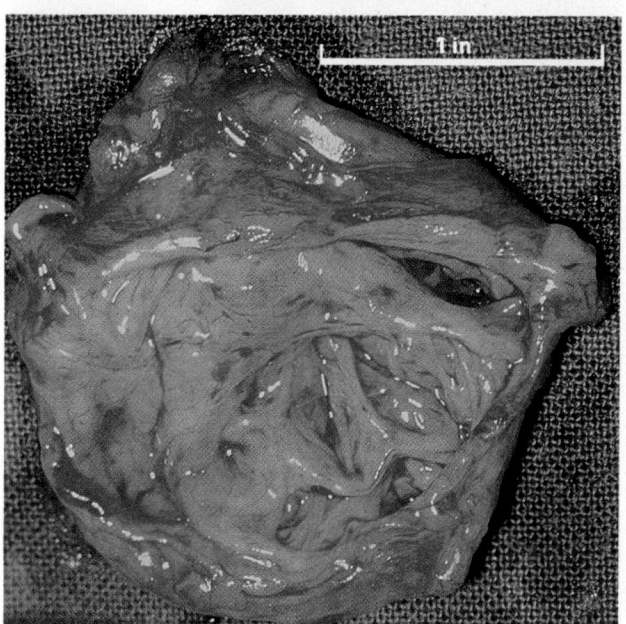

Fig. 35.7 (a) Bilateral microphthalmos, with a cyst in the lower lid of the left orbit. (b) At surgery the cyst was removed resulting in temporary collapse of the globe due to the connection between the cyst and the eye. (c) The cyst after removal showing trabeculations.

microphthalmos with cyst by the complete absence of any rudimentary globe. It presents at birth as a large cystic swelling within the affected orbit which, in contrast to microphthalmos with cyst, predominantly distends the upper lid (Dollfus *et al*. 1968; Helvenston *et al*. 1970). Histologically, multiple cavities filled with proliferating glial tissue are seen (Dollfus *et al*. 1968). These cystic orbital lesions, occurring in neonates, should be distinguished from teratomas. Their growth is generally slower, and the eye is markedly microphthalmic or absent.

The presence of an eye is thought to be important in inducing normal orbital growth. Also, if an anophthalmic socket is left 'empty' in infancy, conjunctival contraction will prevent satisfactory prosthetic fitting later. Early orbital volume replacement with an appropriate implant and/or prosthesis is therefore advocated if the globe is small or absent. Various types of socket expanders can be used to maintain the conjunctival fornices and promote normal orbital growth (Price *et al*. 1986; O'Keefe *et al*. 1987; Dootz 1992; Downes *et al*. 1992).

Orbital teratoma

Teratomas are tumours which arise from pluripotential embryonic stem cells and consist of elements derived from more than one germ cell layer. Although classically all three layers should be represented within the tumour, only mesoderm is invariably seen, and ectodermal or endodermal elements can be absent. Strictly speaking, such tumours should be called 'teratoid'. The extent of the tumour can be limited to the orbit (primary orbital teratoma) or it may involve the intracranial compartment

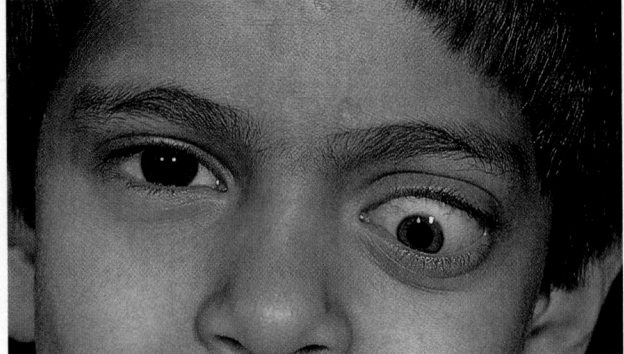

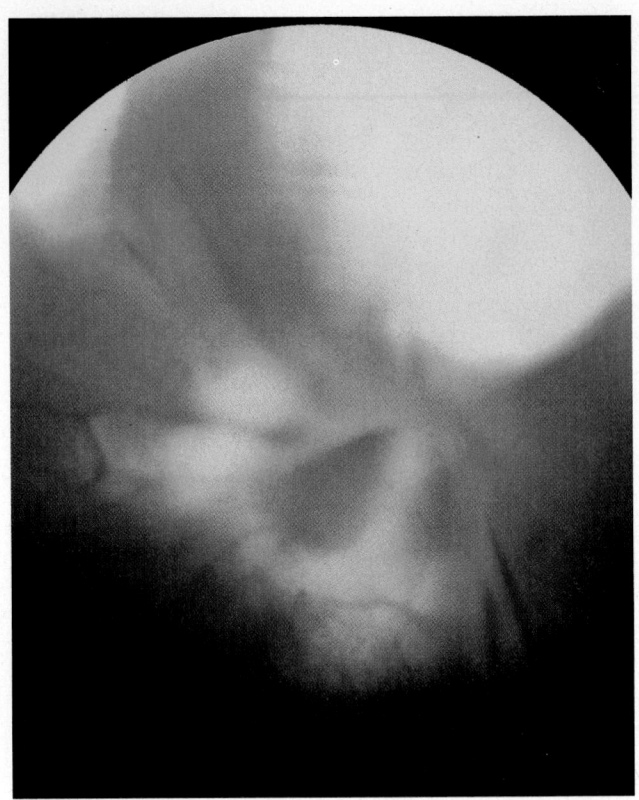

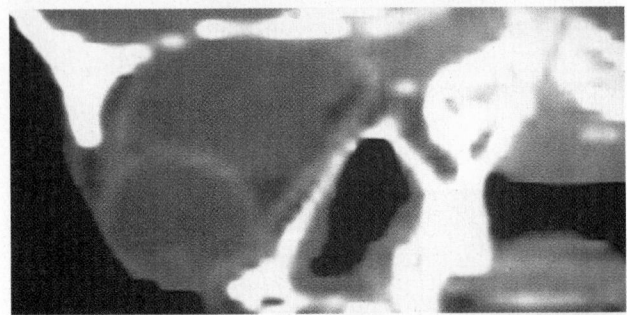

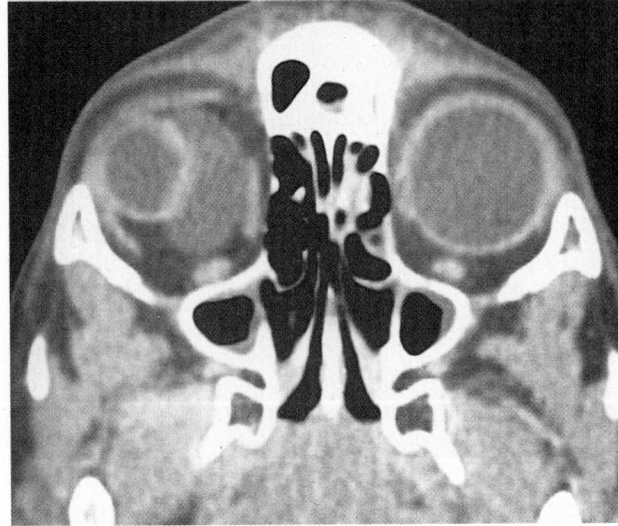

Fig. 35.8 (a) This 10-year-old boy had a small left eye and gradually increasing proptosis with downward displacement of the microphthalmic globe. (b) The left fundus showed a severe colobomatous defect. The right was normal. (c, d) CT scans showing the superior and medial orbital cyst.

and/or nasal and sinus cavities (combined orbital and extraorbital teratoma). Occasionally, a much larger primary intracranial tumour invades the orbit (secondary orbital teratoma). This usually manifests prenatally as polyhydramnios and is rarely compatible with life (Kivela & Tarkkanen 1994).

The usual presentation of a primary orbital teratoma is with unilateral, often massive proptosis in a newborn child (Hoyt & Joe 1962; Barber *et al.* 1974; Chang *et al.* 1980; Levin *et al.* 1986). Teratomas are more common in females by a ratio of 2 : 1. Surprisingly, the globe itself is usually of normal size or slightly small (Fig. 35.9) but it is surrounded by intensely chemotic conjunctiva. It is displaced by a

large cystic mass which is often fluctuant and transilluminates but may also appear solid. The mass is often intraconal, giving rise to axial displacement with indentation by the four recti. Superior or inferior teratomas can also occur. Typically there is rapid growth after birth as secretions from the epithelial elements of the tumour accumulate within its cystic spaces. Exposure keratopathy, ulceration and even perforation can complicate the resultant lagophthalmos. The tumour may stretch and adhere to the optic nerve, giving rise to secondary optic atrophy. Occasionally, teratomas grow slowly over a number of years (Levin *et al.* 1986).

On ultrasound, the tumour is of heterogeneous density

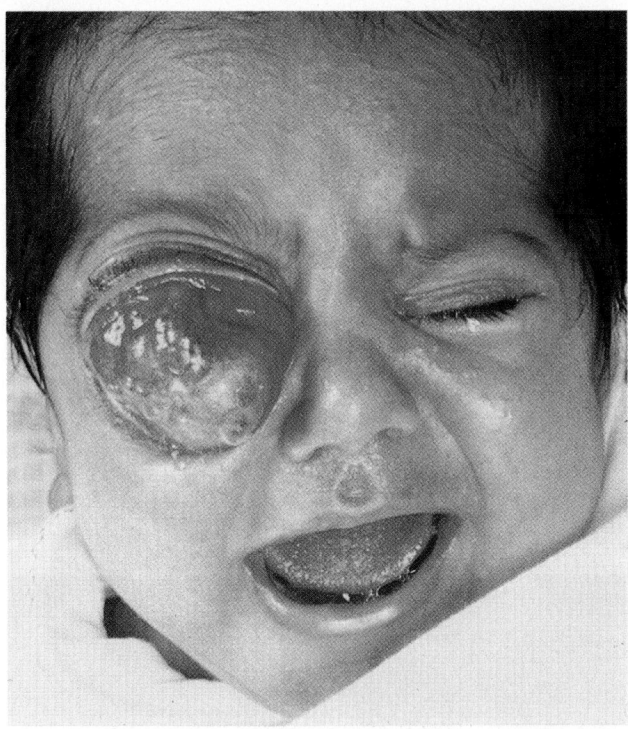

Fig. 35.9 Orbital teratoma.

and may contain foci of calcification. Plain X-rays will show an enlarged orbit on the affected side and the extent of the lesion is easily delineated on CT scan. This modality is particularly useful to exclude intracranial extension.

The treatment of choice is surgical excision within the first month, with preservation of the globe (Hoyt & Joe 1962; Barber *et al.* 1974; Levin *et al.* 1986). Many cases have been reported in whom some vision was preserved in the affected eye (Chang *et al.* 1980). Intraoperative aspiration of fluid from the cystic mass may facilitate tumour removal. Unlike teratomas arising from other sites, malignant change is very rare in the orbit (Soares *et al.* 1983). However, it is recorded in combined orbital and intracranial teratoma, where a bony defect allows the tumour to extend into the intracranial space. In these cases, a combined orbitotomy and craniotomy is necessary to remove the tumour. Total excision can be difficult, and the residual tumour can give rise to problems of late recurrence and malignancy (Garden & McManis 1986).

Parasitic cysts

Echinococcosis (hydatid cyst)

The tapeworm *Echinococcus* is an intestinal parasite of dogs and foxes. Sheep, cattle or rodents may ingest contaminated faeces and become hosts, and dogs become infected by eating their carcasses. Humans are drawn accidentally into the cycle by ingesting ova in contaminat-

ed meat, berries or faeces from poor hand hygiene. The ova hatch in the intestine, and larvae migrate throughout the body, settling in various end-organs to form slowly enlarging, fluid-filled cysts full of larvae. Due to the distribution of blood from the portal tract, there is a predilection for the right lobe of the liver. Orbital involvement is well recognized (Gomez Morales *et al.* 1988; Alparslan *et al.* 1990). Approximately 1% of infestations involve the orbit (Rootman 1988), especially the superonasal quadrant.

Most sheep- and cattle-rearing areas of the world have a high prevalence. Clinically, orbital echinococcosis presents with insidious signs of mass effect, which may be accompanied by chemosis, diplopia and restricted ocular motility. Pressure on the optic nerve can result in visual loss and optic atrophy.

The diagnosis of orbital echinococcosis is made by ultrasonography, CT (Fig. 35.10) or magnetic resonance imaging (MRI) scanning, which show a cystic mass whose wall is occasionally calcified and which contains fluid which is isodense with vitreous. Other confirmatory findings include eosinophilia on a blood film, and positive enzyme-linked immunosorbent assay (ELISA) testing for echinococcal antibodies – this has over 90% sensitivity and specificity for *Echinococcus*.

The best therapeutic approach is surgical excision of the intact cyst. Intraoperative rupture should be avoided since it may be complicated by inflammation and implantation of daughter cysts within the surgical site.

Other parasitic infestations of the orbit include cysticercosis and trichinosis, both acquired from pork.

Ectopias

Dermolipoma

These congenital lesions arise as a result of sequestration of skin within the conjunctival tissues at the time of embryonic development of the eyelids. They are frequently mistaken for true orbital dermoids. They may occur alone or as part of the Goldenhar spectrum, with lid coloboma, pre-auricular skin tags, hemifacial microsomia, palatal and hearing abnormalities. They are situated laterally on the bulbar surface and have a pink and fleshy appearance (Fig. 35.11), occasionally with hairs which can cause irritation. There may occasionally be bony tissue within the lesion (Fry & Leone 1994). They frequently extend superiorly and posteriorly and are closely associated with the lacrimal ducts as well as the levator (Eijpe *et al.* 1990). Surgery for discomfort or cosmetic problems should be performed with the microscope and should be limited to excising the hair-bearing surface tissues or the interpalpebral lesion (Rootman 1988; McNab *et al.* 1990). Care should be taken to identify the lacrimal ducts at the start of surgery, and to avoid the lateral rectus and levator

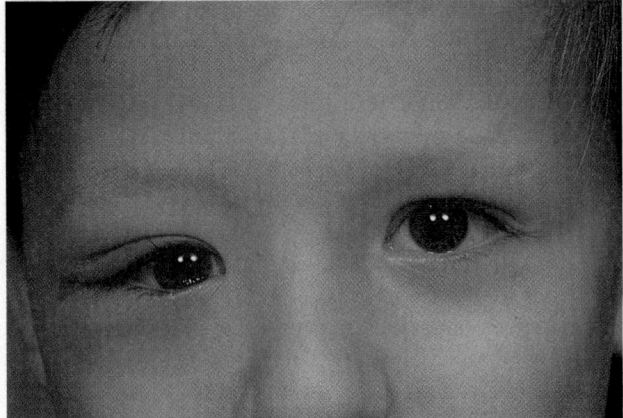

a

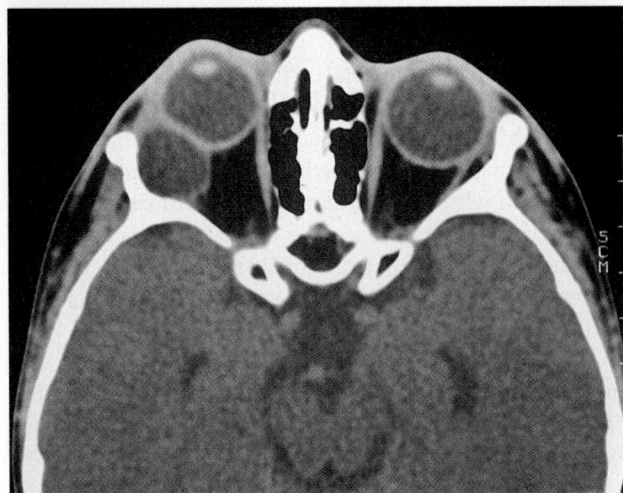

b

Fig. 35.10 (a) This 9-year-old refugee, who had no access to sanitation for 2 years, presented with a 6-month history of increasing right upper lid swelling. He has 4 mm of right proptosis, downward displacement of the globe and lateral ptosis. (b) On CT scan a cystic lesion is found situated posterolaterally to the globe; this was an echinococcal cyst which was excised intact. Patient of the University of British Columbia.

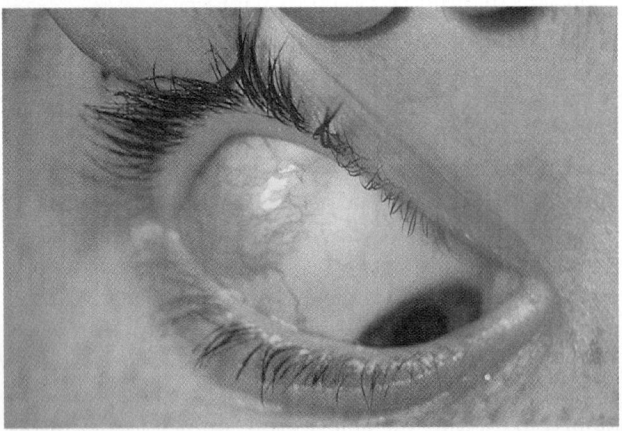

Fig. 35.11 This 16-year-old girl has a long-standing lesion in the upper fornix of the right eye which is consistent with a dermolipoma.

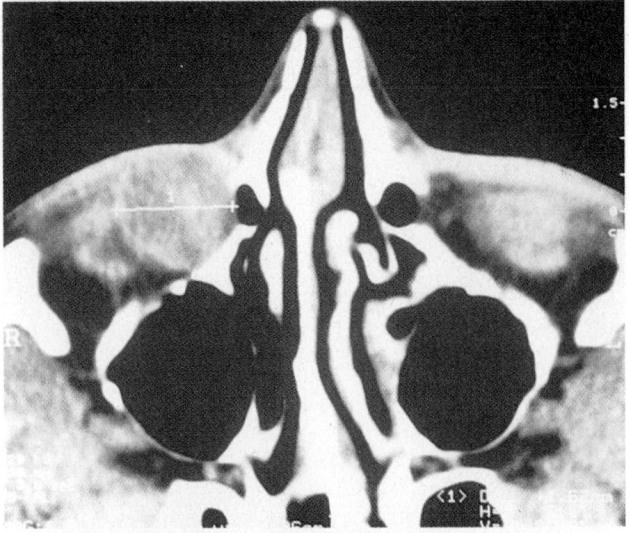

a

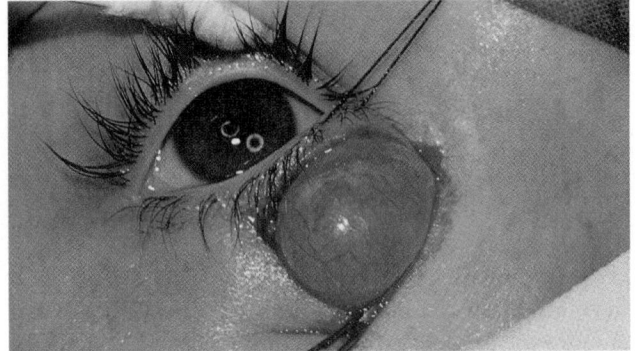

b

Fig. 35.12 (a) This child had a lower lid swelling, found to be cystic on CT scanning. A conjunctival cyst was excised via a skin incision (b). Differential diagnoses included conjunctival dermoid, ductal cyst, lymphangioma and respiratory cyst. Dr Alan McNab's patient.

muscles. There have been numerous reports of complications following attempts at complete excision of dermolipoma. These have included dry eye, restrictive symblepharon, strabismus and ptosis (Crawford 1979; Fry & Leone 1994).

Ectopic lacrimal gland

Lacrimal gland tissue may occasionally occur at ectopic sites within the orbit. Most commonly, it is found in the eyelid or conjunctiva, but it may occur on the cornea or even the iris and choroid (Hunter 1960). Green and Zimmerman (1967) reported eight such cases and since then, more have been added to the literature, often in children or teenagers. The ectopic tissue may be situated intra- or extraconally. Typically, the patients present with proptosis; double vision is a common symptom due to muscle restriction from the inflammatory response which the ectopic tissue often incites. The differential diagnosis includes true orbital neoplasms. Investigation, including

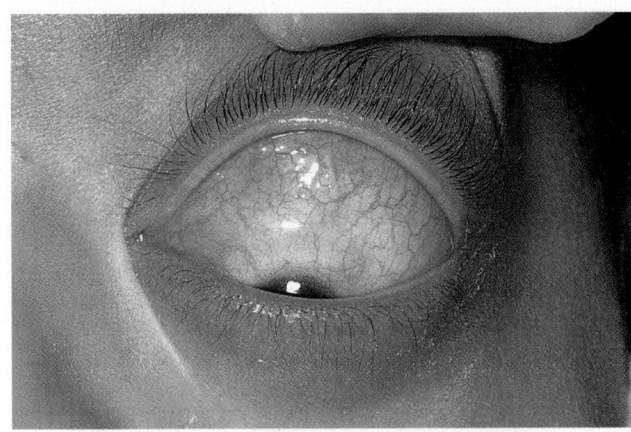

a

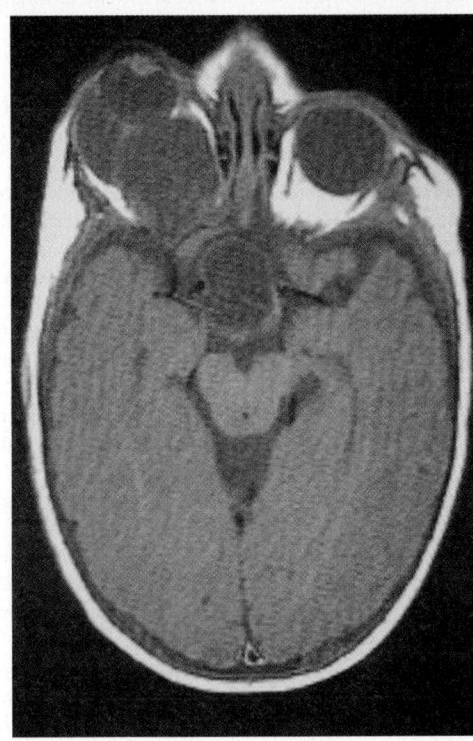

b

Fig. 35.13 (a) This 1-year-old child had a congenital proptosis with a cystic lesion seen almost surrounding the eye. (b) MRI scanning showed the cystic lesion to be contiguous with a cyst in the suprasellar cystern. Total excision revealed that this was an ectopic neural cystic hamartoma. The lesion was removed *en bloc*.

CT scan, often shows a cystic component (Rush & Leone 1981). The treatment of choice is surgical excision. If this is incomplete, proptosis may recur (Green & Zimmerman 1967). The aberrant tissue may also give rise to tumours such as pleomorphic adenoma (Boudet & Bertezene 1964) or adenocarcinoma (Green & Zimmerman 1967).

Conjunctival and inclusion cyst

Conjunctival tissue may be sequestered as a primary embryological malformation or as a result of trauma or surgery. This may occur anywhere on the conjunctiva and may be seen as a blister-like conjunctival swelling, filled with clear fluid. Occasionally, a posterior extension is present, with mass effect. Recurrence is common if the cyst is punctured and complete excision of the wall is indicated for a cure (Fig. 35.12). Histologically, this is conjunctival epithelium. Inclusion cysts may also occur on the skin of the eyelids after trauma or surgery.

Other cystic lesions

A variety of other very rare, developmental cysts of neural structures may occur (Fig. 35.13).

References

Alberti PWRM, Marshall HF, Munro-Black JI. Frontal ethmoidal mucocoele as a cause of unilateral proptosis. *Br J Ophthalmol* 1968; **52**: 833–8.

Alparslan L, Kanberoglu K, Peksayar G, Cokyuksel O. Orbital hydatid cyst: assessment of two cases. *Neuroradiology* 1990; **32**: 163–5.

Arstikaitis M. A case report of bilateral microphthalmos with cysts. *Arch Ophthalmol* 1969; **82**: 480–2.

Barber JC, Barber LF, Guerry D, Geeraets WJ. Congenital orbital teratoma. *Arch Ophthalmol* 1974; **91**: 45–8.

Boudet G, Bertezene M. Exophthalmie par adenome lacrymal en position ectopique (angiographie de l'orbite). *Bull Soc Fr Ophthalmol* 1964; **64**: 624.

Bullock JD, Fleishman JA, Rosset JS. Lacrimal ductal cysts. *Ophthalmology* 1986: **93**: 1355–60.

Caprioli J, Lesser RL. Basal encephalocele and morning glory syndrome. *Br J Ophthalmol* 1983; **67**: 349–51.

Casteels I, De Loof E, Brock P *et al.* Sudden blindness in a child: presenting symptom of a sphenoid sinus mucocele. *Br J Ophthalmol* 1992; **76**: 502–4.

Chang DF, Dallow RL, Walton DS. Congenital orbital teratoma: report of a case with visual preservation. *J Pediatr Ophthalmol Strabismus* 1980; **17**: 88–95.

Consul BN, Kulshrestha OP. Orbital meningocoele. *Br J Ophthalmol* 1965; **49**: 374–6.

Crawford JS. Benign tumors of the eyelid and adjacent structures: should they be removed? *J Pediatr Ophthalmol Strabismus* 1979; **16**: 246–50.

Crawford JS. Diseases of the orbit. In: Crawford JS, Morin JD, eds. *The Eye in Childhood*. New York: Grune & Stratton, 1983: 361–94.

David DJ, Sheffield L, Simpson D, White J. Frontoethmoidal meningoencephaloceles: morphology and treatment. *Br J Plastic Surg* 1984; **37**: 271.

Delfini R, Missori P, Iannetti G, Ciappetta P, Cantore G. Mucoceles of the paranasal sinuses with intracranial and intraorbital extension: report of 28 cases. *Neurosurgery* 1993; **32**: 901–6.

DiLoreto DA, Kennedy RA, Neigel JM, Rootman J. Infestation of extraocular muscles by cysticercus cellulosae. *Br J Ophthalmol* 1990; **70**: 751–2.

Dollfus MA, Langlois J, Clement JC, Forthomme J. Congenital cystic eyeball. *Am J Ophthalmol* 1968; **66**: 504–9.

Dootz GL. The ocularist's management of congenital microphthalmos and anophthalmos. *Adv Ophthalmic Plast Reconstr Surg* 1992; **9**: 41–56.

Downes R, Lavin M, Collin R. Hydrophilic expanders for the congenital anophthalmic socket. *Adv Ophthalmic Plast Reconstr Surg* 1992; **9**: 57–61.

Duke-Elder S. Congenital deformities of the orbit. In: Duke-Elder S, ed. *System of Ophthalmology*, Vol. 3. London: Kimpton, 1964a: 949–56.

Duke-Elder S, ed. *System of Ophthalmology*, Vol. 3, Part 2, *Normal and Abnormal Development: Congenital Deformities*. London: Henry Kimpton, 1964b: 919–21.

Eijpe AA, Koornneef L, Bras J *et al.* Dermolipoma: characteristic CT appearance. *Documenta Ophthalmol* 1990; **74**: 321–8.

Fry CL, Leone CR. Safe management of dermolipomas. *Arch Ophthalmol* 1994; **112**: 1114–16.

Garden JW, McManus J. Congenital orbital-intracranial teratoma with subsequent malignancy. *Br J Ophthalmol* 1986; **70**: 111–14.

Green WR, Zimmerman LE. Ectopic lacrimal gland tissue. Report of eight cases with orbital involvement. *Arch Ophthalmol* 1967; **78**: 318.

Grove AS Jr. Orbital disorders: diagnosis and management. In: McCord CD Jr, ed. *Oculoplastic Surgery*. New York: Raven Press, 1981: 274–7.

Helveston EM, Malone E, Lashmet MH. Congenital cystic eye. *Arch Ophthalmol* 1970; **84**: 622–4.

Howard GR, Nerad, JA, Bonavolonta G, Tranfa F. Orbital dermoid cysts located within the lateral rectus muscle. *Ophthalmology* 1994; **101**: 767–71.

Hoyt WF, Joe S. Congenital teratoid cyst. *Arch Ophthalmol* 1962; **68**: 197–201.

Hunter WS. Aberrant intraocular lacrimal gland tissue. *Br J Ophthalmol* 1960; **44**: 619.

Jakobiec FA, Jones IS. Orbital inflammations. In: Duane TD (ed.) *Clinical Ophthalmology*. Philadelphia: Harper & Row, 1985; 60–5.

Kivela T, Tarkkanen A. Orbital germ cell tumors revisited: a clinicopathological approach to classification. *Surv Ophthalmol* 1994; **38**: 541–54.

Lane CM, Erlich WW, Wright JE. Orbital dermoid cyst. *Eye* 1987; **1**: 504–11.

Last RJ. *Anatomy. Regional and Applied*. Edinburgh: Churchill Livingstone, 1978.

Lello GE, Sparrow OC, Gopal R. The surgical correction of fronto-ethmoidal meningo-encephaloceles. *J Craniomaxillofacial Surg* 1989; **17**: 293–8.

Leone CR, Marlowe JF. Orbital presentation of an ethmoidal encephalocoele. *Arch Ophthalmol* 1970; **83**: 445–7.

Leonardo D, Shields CL, Shields JA, Nelson LB. Recurrent giant orbital dermoid of infancy. *J Pediatr Ophthalmol Strabismus* 1994; **31**: 50–2.

Lessner AM, Antle CM, Rootman J, White VA, Margo CE. Cystic lesions of the orbit and radiolucent defects of bone. In: Margo CE, Hamed LM, Mames RN, eds. *Diagnostic Problems in Clinical Ophthalmology*. Philadelphia: WB Saunders, 1994: 87–98.

Levin M, Leone CR, Kincaid MC. Congenital orbital teratoma. *Am J Ophthalmol* 1986; **102**: 476–81.

Lieb W, Rochels R, Gronemeyer U. Microphthalmos with colobomatous orbital cyst: clinical, histological, immunological, and electronmicroscopic findings. *Br J Ophthalmol* 1990; **74**: 59–62.

Lund VJ, Rolfe ME. Ophthalmic considerations in front ethmoidal mucocoeles. *J Laryngol Otol* 1989; **103**: 667–9.

McNab AA, Wright JE, Caswell AG. Clinical features and surgical management of dermolipomas. *Austral N Zeal J Ophthalmol* 1990; **18**: 159–62.

Morales GA, Croxatto JO, Crovetto L, Ebner R. Hydatid cysts of the orbit. A review of 35 cases. *Ophthalmology* 1988; **95**: 1027–32.

Mortada A, E-Toraei I. Orbital meningo-encephalocoele and exophthalmos. *Br J Ophthalmol* 1960; **44**: 309–14.

Nicholson DH, Green RW. *Microphthalmos with Cyst in Pediatric Ocular Tumours*. Chicago: Year Book Medical Publishers, 1981: 219–21.

Nugent RA, Lapointe JS, Rootman J, Robertson WD, Graeb DA. Orbital dermoids: features on CT. *Radiology* 1987; **165**: 475–8.

O'Keefe M, Webb M, Pashby RC, Wagman RD. Clinical anophthalmos. *Br J Ophthalmol* 1987; **71**: 635–8.

Pagon RA. Ocular coloboma. *Surv Ophthalmol* 1981; **25**: 223–36.

Pfeiffer RL, Nichol RJ. Dermoid and epidermoid tumours of the orbit. *Arch Ophthalmol* 1948; **40**: 639–64.

Pollock JA, Newton TH, Hoyt WF. Trans-sphenoidal and transethmoidal encephalocoeles. *Radiology* 1968; **90**: 442–53.

Price E, Simon JW, Calhoun JH. Prosthetic treatment of severe microphthalmos in infancy. *J Pediatr Ophthalmol Strabismus* 1986; **23**: 22–4.

Rashid ER, Bergstrom TJ, Evans RM, Arnold AC. Anterior encephaloceles presenting as nasolacrimal obstruction. *Ann Ophthalmol* 1986; **18**: 132–6.

Robertson DM, Henderson JW. Unilateral proptosis secondary to orbital mucocoele in infancy. *Am J Ophthalmol* 1969; **68**: 845–7.

Rootman J. *Diseases of the Orbit*. Philadelphia: JB Lippincott, 1988.

Rush A, Leone CR. Ectopic lacrimal gland cyst of the orbit. *Am J Ophthalmol* 1981; **92**: 198–201.

Sathananthan N, Moseley IF, Rose GE, Wright JE. The frequency and clinical significance of bone involvement in outer canthus dermoid cysts. *Br J Ophthalmol* 1993; **77**: 789–94.

Satorre J, Antle CM, O'Sullivan R *et al.* Orbital lesions with granulomatous inflammation. *Canad J Ophthalmol* 1991; **26**: 174–95.

Sherman RP, Rootman J, La Pointe JS. Orbital dermoids: clinical presentation and management. *Br J Ophthalmol* 1984; **68**: 642–52.

Smith S, Rootman J. Lacrimal ductal cysts. Presentation and management. *Surv Ophthalmol* 1986; **30**: 245–50.

Soares E, Lopes K, Adrade J, Faleiro L, Alves J. Orbital malignant teratoma. A case report. *Orbit* 1983; **2**: 235–40.

Terry A, Patrinely JR, Anderson RL, Smithwick W 4th. Orbital meningoencephalocele manifesting as a conjunctival mass. *Am J Ophthalmol* 1993; **115**; 46–9.

Waring GO, Roth AM, Rodrigues M. Clinicopathologic correlation of microphthalmos with cyst. *Am J Ophthalmol* 1976; **82**: 714–21.

Weiss A, Martinez C, Greenwald M. Microphthalmos with cyst. Clinical presentation and computed tomographic findings. *J Pediatr Ophthalmol* 1985; **22**: 6–12.

Whitney CE, Leone CR, Kincaid MC. Proptosis with mastication: an unusual presentation of an orbital dermoid cyst. *Ophthal Surg* 1986; **17**: 295–8.

Wilkins RB, Byrd WA. Intraconal dermoid cyst. *Ophthal Reconstr Surg* 1986; **2**: 83–7.

Youseffi B. Orbital tumours in children: a clinical study of 62 cases. *J Pediatr Ophthalmol Strabismus* 1969; **61**: 177–81.

36: Inflammatory Disorders

Christopher Lyons and Jack Rootman

The orbit in childhood can be affected by a variety of inflammatory problems. As discussed in Chapter 27, these become more common in the second decade of life, when causes of orbital disease increasingly resemble those found in adulthood.

The principal causes of inflammation in our series can be divided into non-specific orbital inflammatory syndromes (NSOIS) (previously known under the umbrella term of 'inflammatory pseudotumour') and specific causes such as sarcoidosis and Wegener's granulomatosis, both of which are rare but potentially life-threatening. The incidence of thyroid orbitopathy increases with age in the teenage years, and this subject is discussed briefly.

Infective orbital cellulitis in early childhood is most commonly related to dacryocystitis or trauma. Over the age of 6 years, and particularly in the second decade, the fully formed sinuses become the most common source of orbital cellulitis (see Chapter 16).

Non-specific orbital inflammatory syndromes (inflammatory pseudotumours)

Definition

The child's orbit is occasionally the site of acute or sub-acute inflammation of unknown cause (Mottow & Jakobiec 1978; Slavin & Glaser 1982; Grossniklaus *et al.* 1985;

Rootman 1988). This entity was previously known as 'orbital inflammatory pseudotumour' (Blodi & Gass 1968), a term which, with the advent of computed tomography (CT) and magnetic resonance imaging (MRI), has been abandoned in favour of terminology describing the site of inflammation (Rootman & Nugent 1982; Jakobiec & Jones 1983). Thus, anterior, diffuse, apical, myositic and lacrimal types are recognized. Children tend to present with the anterior and diffuse types. Myositis and lacrimal inflammation are also well recognized. Apical involvement is rare. Sclerosing NSOIS is very rare in childhood.

These syndromes present acutely or subacutely with inflammatory signs. Although apparently idiopathic, they have many features of an orbital immune reaction (Kennerdell & Dresner 1984). Histologically, there is an influx of neutrophils, lymphocytes, plasma cells and macrophages. Inflammatory mediators cause oedema, vascular dilatation and pain without systemic malaise. In contrast, chronic inflammations and granulomatous diseases cause mass effect as their predominant feature without signs of acute inflammation. The common imaging feature of acute or subacute NSOIS is the presence of a poorly defined margin to the inflammatory focus, as well as contrast enhancement (Moseley & Sanders 1982; Atlas *et al.* 1987).

Anterior idiopathic orbital inflammation: acute and subacute

This is the most common type of NSOIS found in childhood. The inflammatory process is centred on the anterior orbit and adjacent globe (Fig. 36.1). Pain, proptosis, lid swelling, conjunctival injection and decreased vision are the main presenting features, with an onset over days or occasionally weeks. Of particular note in the paediatric age group is the presence of associated anterior and posterior uveitis, which can lead to erroneous treatment with topical steroid due to misdiagnosis (Rootman 1988; Bloom *et al.* 1992; Hertle *et al.* 1993). On CT scan, there is diffuse anterior orbital inflammation centred on the globe and producing scleral and choroidal thickening with or without serous retinal detachment. Characteristically, the

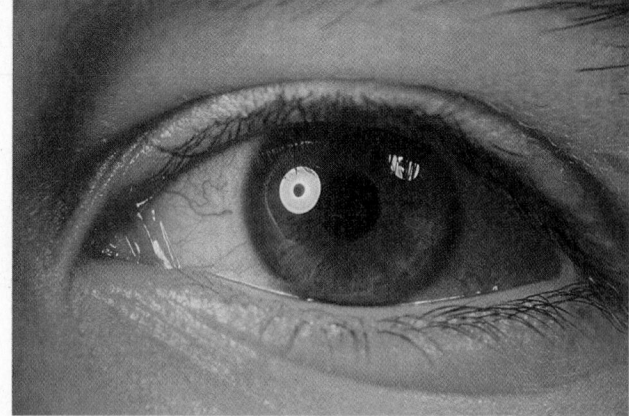

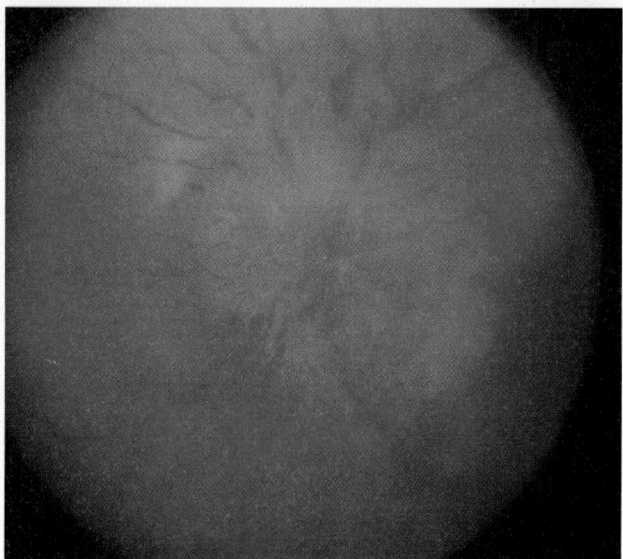

ry soft tissue changes permeate all the orbital components on CT scan, with a white-out appearance whose density is proportional to the severity of the clinical signs, and which resolves as the condition settles. Again, the T-sign is evident on ultrasonography.

Anterior and diffuse non-specific orbital inflammatory syndromes: differential diagnoses and management

The differential diagnoses include infection such as orbital cellulitis, sudden enlargement of a pre-existing lesion as in a ruptured dermoid or haemorrhage into a lymphangioma, or malignancy which, in childhood, may be rhabdomyosarcoma, neuroblastoma, Ewing's sarcoma as well as leukaemic infiltration. Anterior and diffuse NSOIS are also part of the differential diagnoses of uveitis and serous retinal detachment in childhood. Biopsy of involved orbital tissues should be considered in all but the most typical cases.

Fig. 36.1 Anterior NSOIS in a 6-year-old boy who presented with a red eye (a), pain on eye movement and decreased vision of 3 days duration. Fundoscopy (b) shows choroidal swelling and papillitis. Patient from the University of British Columbia.

junction of the globe and optic nerve is obscured on CT scan and the inflammatory changes extend along the nerve sheath. On ultrasound, there is a uniform-density infiltrate corresponding to sclerotenonitis, with accentuation of the sub-Tenon space and doubling of the optic nerve shadow which produces a T-shaped shadow (or T-sign) (Fig. 36.2). Systemically, the erythrocyte sedimentation rate is raised, and there is often cerebrospinal fluid pleocytosis (Mottow-Lippa *et al.* 1981).

Diffuse idiopathic orbital inflammation: acute and subacute

This is clinically similar to the anterior form described above, although the symptoms and clinical signs tend to be more severe (Fig. 36.3). Restriction of eye movements is more pronounced and the visual acuity is worse due to retinal detachment and/or optic neuropathy. Inflammato-

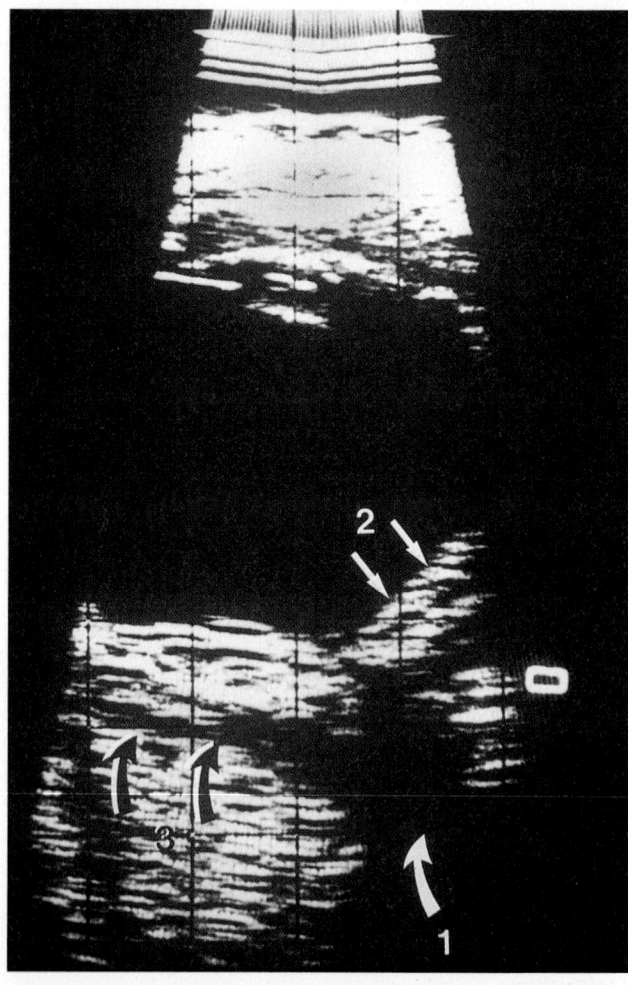

Fig. 36.2 Ultrasound scan of anterior NSOIS showing the T-sign. There is doubling of the optic nerve shadow (1), shallow retinal detachment (2) and accentuation of Tenon's space (3). Patient from the University of British Columbia.

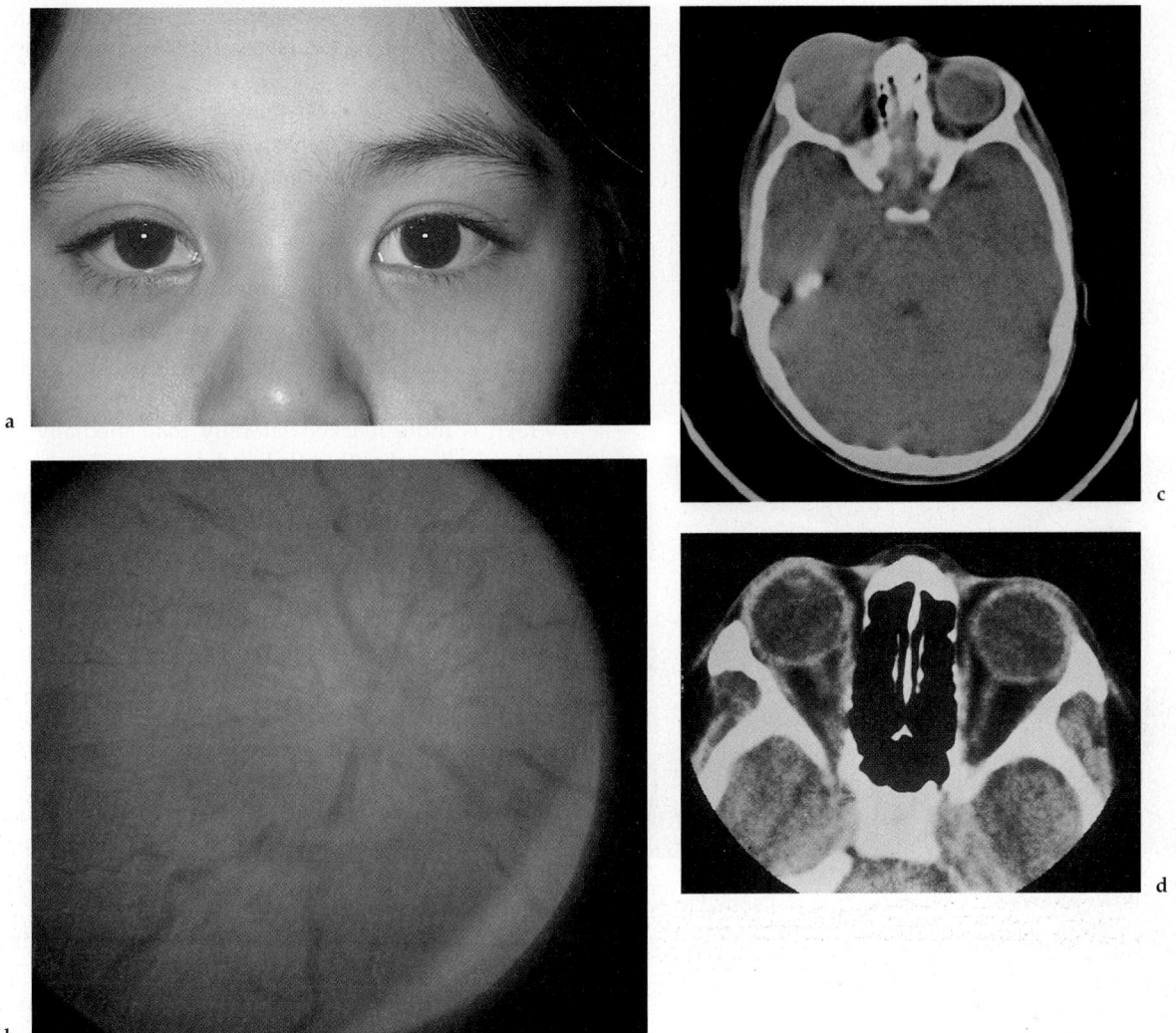

Fig. 36.3 Diffuse NSOIS in a 12-year-old girl who presented with a retrobulbar ache, associated with ptosis (a), and pain on eye movement. There was right-sided uveitis with marked disc swelling (b). On CT scanning (c), there was a 'white-out' appearance of the right orbit (similar patient) which resolved after treatment with systemic steroids (d) (same patient from the University of British Columbia).

Treatment with non-steroidal anti-inflammatory drugs such as flurbiprofen is tried first. Systemic steroids may be used in addition, or as an alternative in doses of 1–1.5 mg/kg per day. There is usually a rapid improvement in symptoms, especially pain, as well as clinical signs. Progress can be monitored by resolution of the CT and ultrasound features. This disease may run a recalcitrant course, with frequent recurrences and steroid dependence. High-dose steroid is restarted for recurrence and tapered as quickly as clinical progress will allow, usually over a few weeks. Failure to respond suggests the need for biopsy of involved tissues and the renewed search for a specific aetiology. Low-dose radiotherapy has been advo-

cated for biopsy-proven cases which do not respond to steroids.

Idiopathic orbital myositis: acute and subacute

This is characterized by pain and limitation of eye movement, diplopia, ptosis and lid oedema and conjunctival chemosis. Proptosis was present in five of six cases reported by Hankey *et al.* (1987). Ductions are limited in the direction of action of the involved muscle(s). Spasm of the affected muscle also causes restriction of the ipsilateral antagonist with a positive forced duction test. Globe retraction and narrowing of the lid fissure similar to Duane's syndrome is a frequent finding (Timms *et al.* 1989; Moorman & Elston 1995).

CT scan shows diffuse muscle enlargement with irregular margins (Fig. 36.4). The muscle enlargement frequently extends forward to involve the tendon (Trokel & Hilal 1979), in contradistinction to thyroid orbitopathy where, typically, the tendon is spared. The superior rectus–leva-

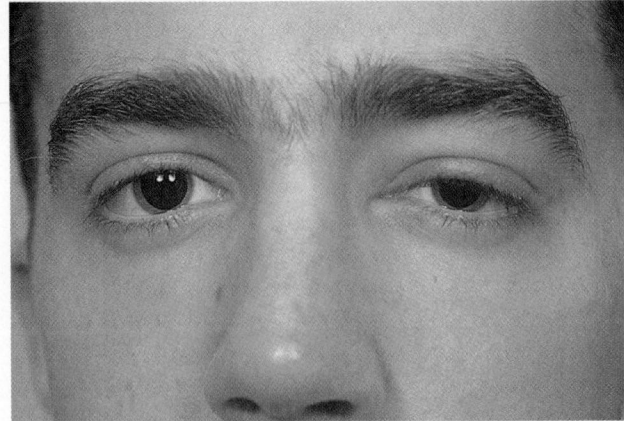

a

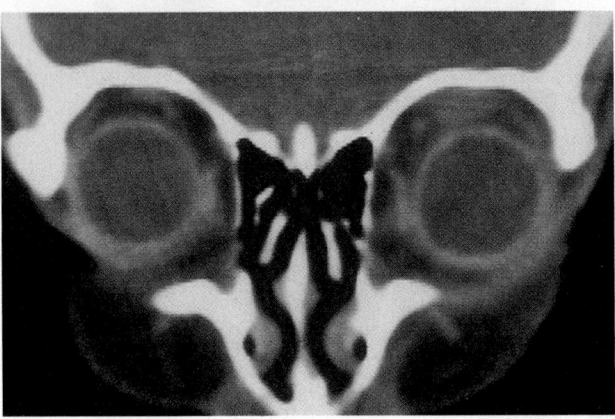

b

Fig. 36.4 Left superior rectus myositis in a 16-year-old boy. Ptosis (a), and pain limitation of upgaze with diplopia were the presenting signs; this was due to left superior rectus myositis shown as (b) a thickened muscle complex on CT scan. Patient from the University of British Columbia.

tor complex or medial rectus are the most common muscles to be involved, but any muscle can be affected, including the obliques (Wan *et al.* 1988). More than one muscle may simultaneously be involved and bilateral disease is well recognized (Slavin & Glaser 1982).

The cause of orbital myositis is unknown but a number of associations have been reported in the literature, including upper respiratory tract infection (Purcell & Taulbee 1981), Lyme disease (Seidenberg & Leib 1990), Whipple's disease (Orssaud *et al.* 1992) and other autoimmune diseases (Weinstein *et al.* 1983).

The differential diagnoses include thyroid orbitopathy, which differs from idiopathic orbital myositis in that a preceding or concurrent history of thyroid disorder is commonly present, pain is absent, the inferior recti tend to be the first muscles involved (although any muscle may be involved) and sparing of the tendon is apparent on CT scan (see above). In some cases, differentiating between these two conditions can be very difficult (Jellinek 1969) and misdiagnosis is not uncommon (Rootman 1988). Early orbital cellulitis, orbital metastasis, and trichinosis also form part of the differential diagnoses.

Non-steroidal anti-inflammatory treatment has been advocated by some (Noble *et al.* 1989), but the rapid and dramatic response to steroids is almost diagnostic. We recommend an initial dose of 0.5–1 mg/kg per day, tapering to nothing over 2–4 weeks. Delay in diagnosis and initiation of therapy is associated with recurrence and incomplete resolution of signs.

Idiopathic lacrimal inflammation: acute and subacute

Pain, tenderness and swelling over the lateral aspect of the upper lid are typical presenting features of this disorder. The lid may adopt an S-shaped configuration with ptosis which is more marked laterally than medially and the globe is often slightly displaced downward and medially. Slit-lamp examination shows superotemporal conjunctival chemosis and pouting of the lacrimal duct orifices. There is no uveitis. On CT scans, the inflammation is seen to be centred on the lacrimal gland, often extending diffusely into the lateral orbit and involving the adjacent side of the globe. The differential diagnoses include bacterial and viral dacryoadenitis, the latter often occurring in association with childhood infections such as mumps or mononucleosis. In this situation, the child is likely to be ill, and generalized lymphadenopathy or salivary gland enlargement may be noted, along with lymphocytosis. Inflammation related to leakage from a dermoid cyst and neoplasia are other rare possibilities. Lacrimal gland involvement in orbital sarcoid tends to be a chronic process, presenting with signs and symptoms of dry eyes, and is rare in childhood.

Acute or subacute lacrimal gland swellings in childhood do not need biopsy if they are related to an obvious viral illness such as mumps or if there are other findings suggestive of mononucleosis. A high index of suspicion should be retained for atypical lesions with early biopsy in patients whose signs and symptoms fail to respond to treatment.

Treatment of idiopathic lacrimal inflammation is with high-dose steroid, tapering with resolution of symptoms and signs.

Specific causes of orbital inflammation

The most common cause of orbital inflammation in childhood is infective orbital cellulitis (see Chapter 16). Other orbital inflammatory diseases encountered in childhood are comparatively rare. Nevertheless, we have seen 36 cases of thyroid orbitopathy in childhood over the last 19 years.

Wegener's granulomatosis is rare in childhood, but we have treated three affected children in the last 20 years. It is important to consider Wegener's granulomatosis in the differential diagnosis of orbital inflammation in childhood since failure to recognize this largely treatable dis-

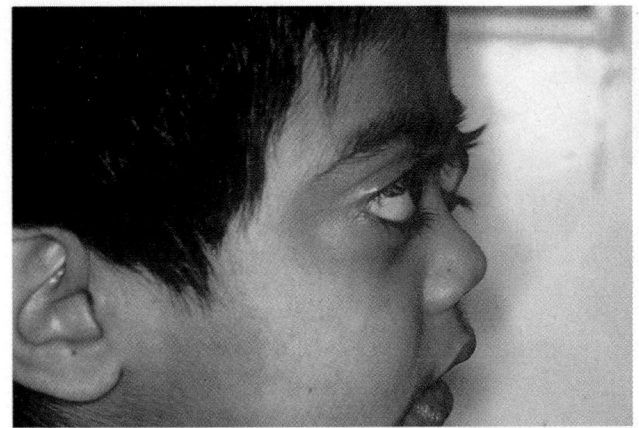

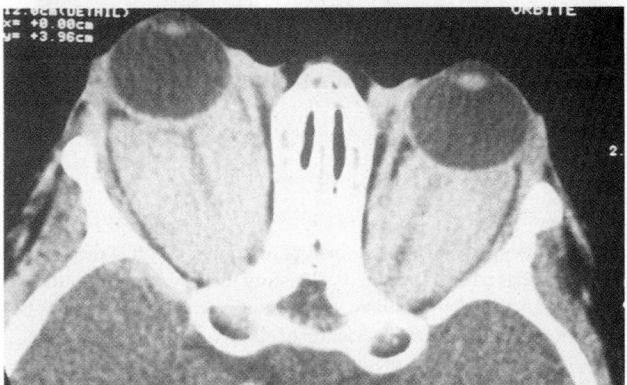

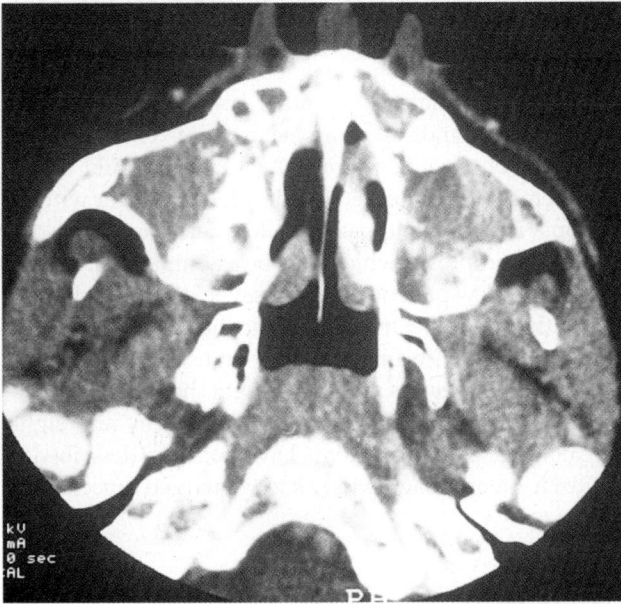

Fig. 36.5 A 7-year-old boy presented with a 3-month history of progressive bilateral proptosis (a). He has positive ANCA titres. CT (b, c) shows widespread involvement of the orbital soft tissues and maxillary sinuses. Patient from the University of British Columbia.

ease can be life-threatening. Sarcoidosis, another rare cause of orbital inflammation which may present in childhood, is also discussed.

Wegener's granulomatosis

This is a necrotizing granulomatous vasculitis which has a predilection for the airways and the kidneys. There is a limited form of the disease in which the kidneys are spared and which has a better prognosis. Before the introduction of cyclophosphamide, over 90% of affected patients died within 2 years (Hollander & Manning 1967).

Clinical features

The onset of orbital disease is often preceded by a history of subacute or chronic low grade disease, with sudden aggravation leading to presentation. The main features are proptosis, which is frequently bilateral, with ocular and facial pain which may be severe. An orbital mass is usually present (Fig. 36.5), displacing the globe. Lacrimal gland involvement with lid swelling and brawny discoloration occurred in two of our three patients with childhood or adolescent Wegener's granulomatosis. Ocular inflammation may be present with scleritis and marginal corneal infiltrates. Decreased vision is a common finding which may be related to optic neuropathy.

The orbital disease was bilateral in two patients; midline disease and lacrimal gland involvement was present in all three. All our patients had ENT symptoms in the 3 months prior to presentation, including nasal blockage, discharge or bleeds, pain over the paranasal or mastoid sinuses and hearing loss or tinnitus.

CT scans show an orbital mass with infiltrative margins obscuring the adjacent fat planes. Midline bony erosion may also be seen. Histological changes include areas of fat disruption by focal necrosis with lipid-laden macrophages, giant cells and some evidence of acute inflammatory cells. Vasculitis is often difficult to find in these specimens (Satorre *et al.* 1991). Fibrosis is a common feature. Stains for fungi and mycobacteria should be performed to exclude these causes of granulomatous inflammation.

Septra (Septrin), an antibiotic combination of trimethoprim and sulphamethoxazole, is a first-line treatment for this condition. Azathioprine is a second-line drug. Cyclophosphamide is known to be effective in Wegener's granulomatosis (Fauci *et al.* 1983) but is reserved for children who have not responded to the above, due to its oncogenic potential. Antineutrophil cytoplasmic antibodies (cANCA) are specific markers for Wegener's if there is a 'cytoplasmic' staining pattern. Their plasma level correlates with disease activity. Failure of these to return to normal after clinical improvement with treatment indicates a high risk of relapse (Power *et al.* 1995).

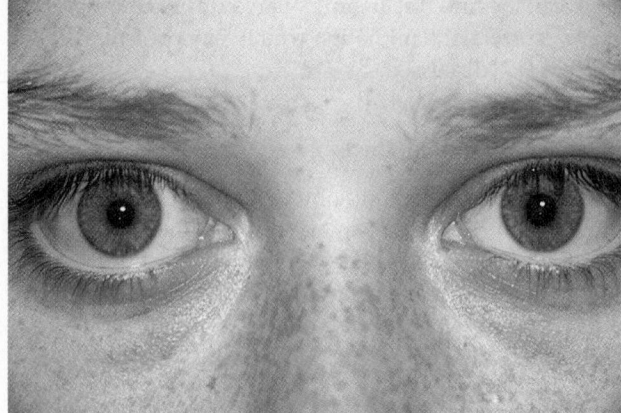

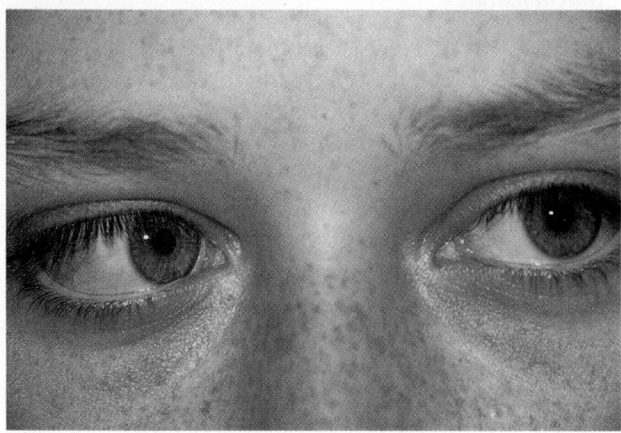

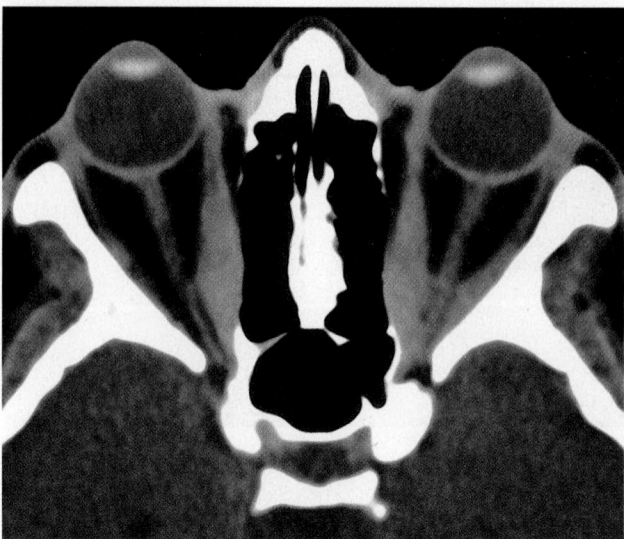

Fig. 36.6 This girl had a 6-year history of double vision at the extremes of gaze. Her past medical history included autoimmune hepatitis and hyperthyroidism, treated with radioiodine. There is lid retraction (a), lid lag, and restriction of abduction with esotropia in lateral gaze (b). Bilateral medial rectus enlargement involving the muscle belly but sparing the tendons is evident on CT scanning (c). Patient from the University of British Columbia.

Sarcoidosis

This granulomatous inflammatory disease of unknown cause is most commonly seen in the orbit as a cause of dacryoadenitis in females aged 30 years and over. Nevertheless, it occasionally affects the orbit in childhood, with optic nerve infiltration, uveitis or extraocular muscle infiltration. Cornblath *et al.* (1993) recently reported a 15-year-old white boy with pain, diplopia and ophthalmoplegia from generalized involvement of the extraocular muscles. There was diffuse enlargement of all the muscles on CT, a picture reminiscent of orbital myositis or thyroid orbitopathy. Unlike the latter (Trokel & Jakobiec 1981), the muscle insertions were enlarged on CT scan.

Thyroid orbitopathy

Approximately 2.5% of all cases of Graves' disease occur in children (Bram 1937), and about half of these develop ophthalmic signs (Young 1979; Uretsky *et al.* 1980). This was the most common cause of proptosis in children (13.6%) in one series published from the Toronto Hospital for Sick Children (1967). Neonatal thyroid orbitopathy is well recognized in the infants of hyperthyroid mothers.

There is commonly a family or past history of hyperthy-roidism; an association with other autoimmune disorders and Down's syndrome has been noted. Generally, the mean age of onset is around 12 years, with mild orbital involvement, often limited to lid oedema, with or without diplopia in extreme upgaze due to inferior rectus restriction. Mild proptosis, which may be asymmetrical, may be a feature. A few patients develop severe thyroid orbitopathy with marked restriction of ductions (see Fig. 36.6a,b) and proptosis with inflammatory signs. The severity of the orbitopathy tends to increase with the age of involvement (Uretsky *et al.* 1980). Optic neuropathy and sight-threatening corneal problems have not been described in children. Neuroimaging may show enlarged muscles (see Fig. 36.6c).

References

Atlas FW, Grossman RI, Savino PJ *et al.* Surface coil MRI of orbital pseudotumour. *Am J Roentgenol* 1987; **8**: 141–6.

Blodi FC, Gass DJM. Inflammatory pseudotumour of the orbit. *Br J Ophthalmol* 1968; **52**: 79–93.

Bloom JN, Graviss ER, Byrne BJ. Orbital pseudotumour in the differential diagnosis of pediatric uveitis. *J Pediatr Ophthalmol Strabismus* 1992; **29**: 59–63.

Bram I. Exophthalmic goiter in children: comments based upon 128 cases in patients of 12 and under. *Arch Pediatr* 1937; **54**: 419–24.

Cornblath WT, Elner V, Rolfe M. Extraocular muscle involvement in sarcoidosis. *Ophthalmology* 1993; **100**: 501–5.

Fauci AS, Haynes BF, Katz P, Wolff SM. Wegener's granulomatosis: prospective clinical and therapeutic experience with 85 patients for 21 years. *Ann Intern Med* 1983; **98**: 76–85.

Grossniklaus HE, Lass JH, Abramowsky CR, Levine MR. Childhood orbital pseudotumor. *Ann Ophthalmol* 1985; **17**: 372–7.

Hankey GJ, Silbert PL, Edis RH, Nicoll AM. Orbital myositis: a study of six cases. *Austral N Zeal J Med* 1987; **17**: 585–91.

Hertle RW, Granet DB, Goyal AK, Schaffer DB. Orbital pseudotumor in the differential diagnosis of pediatric uveitis (letter). *J Pediatr Ophthalmol Strabismus* 1993; **30**: 61.

Hollander D, Manning RT. The use of alkylating agents in the treatment of Wegener's granulomatosis. *Ann Intern Med* 1967; **67**: 393–8.

Jakobiec FA, Jones IS. Orbital inflammation. In: Duane T, ed. *Clinical Ophthalmology*, Vol. 2. Hagerstown: Harper & Row, 1983.

Jellinek EH. The orbital pseudotumour syndrome and its differentiation from endocrine exophthalmos. *Brain* 1969; **92**: 35–58.

Kennerdell JS, Dresner SC. The non-specific orbital inflammatory syndromes. *Surv Ophthalmol* 1984; **29**: 93–103.

Moorman CM, Elston JS. Acute orbital myositis. *Eye* 1995; **9**: 96–101.

Moseley IF, Sanders MD. *Computerised Tomography in Neuro-ophthalmology*. London: Chapman & Hall, 1982.

Mottow LS, Jakobiec FA. Idiopathic inflammatory orbital pseudotumour in childhood I. Clinical characteristics. *Arch Ophthalmol* 1978; **96**: 1410–17.

Mottow-Lippa L, Jakobiec FA, Smith M. Idiopathic inflammatory orbital pseudotumour in childhood II. Results of diagnostic tests and biopsies. *Ophthalmology* 1981; **88**: 565–74.

Noble AG, Tripathi RC, Levine RA. Indomethacin for the treatment of idiopathic orbital myositis. *Am J Ophthalmol* 1989; **108**: 336–8.

Orssaud C, Poisson M, Gaddeur D. Myosite orbitaire, recidive d'une maladie de Whipple. *J Franc Ophtalmol* 1992; **15**: 205–8.

Perry SR, Rootman J, White VA. The clinical and pathologic constellation of Wegener's granulomatosis of the orbit (in press).

Power WJ, Rodriguez A, Neves RA, Lane L, Foster S. Disease relapse in patients with ocular manifestations of Wegener's granulomatosis. *Ophthalmology* 1995; **102**: 154–60.

Purcell JJ Jr, Taulbee WA. Orbital myositis after upper respiratory tract infection. *Arch Ophthalmol* 1981; **99**: 437.

Rootman J. *Diseases of the Orbit: A Multidisciplinary Approach*. Philadelphia: JB Lippincott, 1988: chap. 9.

Rootman J, Nugent R. The classification and management of acute orbital pseudotumors. *Ophthalmology* 1982; **89**: 1040–8.

Satorre J, Antle M, O'Sullivan R, White VA, Nugent RA, Rootman J. Orbital lesions with granulomatous inflammation. *Canad J Ophthalmol* 1991; **26**: 174–95.

Seidenberg KB, Leib ML. Orbital myositis with Lyme disease. *Am J Ophthalmol* 1990; **109**: 471–2.

Slavin ML, Glaser JS. Idiopathic orbital myositis. A report of six cases. *Arch Ophthalmol* 1982; **100**: 1261–5.

Timms C, Russell-Eggitt IM, Taylor DSI. Simulated (pseudo-) Duane's syndrome secondary to orbital myositis. *Binocular Vis Q* 1989; **4**: 109–12.

Toronto Hospital for Sick Children, Department of Ophthalmology. *The Eye in Childhood*. Chicago: Year Book Medical Publishers, 1967: 333.

Trokel SL, Hilal SK. Recognition and differential diagnosis of enlarged extraocular muscles in computed tomography. *Am J Ophthalmol* 1979; **87**: 503–12.

Trokel SL, Jakobiec FA. Correlation of CT scanning and pathologic features of ophthalmic Graves' disease. *Ophthalmology* 1981; **88**: 553–64.

Uretsky SH, Kennerdell JS, Gutai JP. Graves' ophthalmopathy in childhood and adolescence. *Arch Ophthalmol* 1980; **98**: 1963–4.

Wan WL, Cano MR, Green RL. Orbital myositis involving the oblique muscles: an echographic study. *Ophthalmology* 1988; **95**: 1522–8.

Weinstein GS, Dresner SC, Slamovits TL, Kennerdel JS. Acute and sub-acute orbital myositis. *Am J Ophthalmol* 1983; **96**: 209–17.

Young LA. Dysthyroid ophthalmopathy in children. *J Pediatr Ophthalmol Strabismus* 1979; **16**: 105–7.

37: Vascular Disease

Christopher Lyons and Jack Rootman

Tumours

Vascular tumours of the orbit include capillary and cavernous haemangiomas, haemangiopericytomas, orbital varices, and lymphangiomas. Capillary haemangiomas are common, usually present in early childhood and characteristically undergo spontaneous regression (Margileth & Museles 1965; Haik *et al.* 1979). Cavernous haemangiomas and haemangiopericytomas are predominantly seen in adults although may rarely cause proptosis in childhood. Lymphangiomas, like capillary haemangiomas, present in early childhood, but unlike the latter do not undergo spontaneous regression and may be complicated by bouts of haemorrhage.

Capillary haemangioma (see also Chapter 21)

Capillary haemangioma is the most common orbital tumour of childhood. It occurs more frequently in females than males by a ratio of 3:2 (Haik *et al.* 1994) with no apparent familial inheritance pattern. It is distinguished from other orbital vascular lesions by its natural history, since spontaneous regression is the rule. An accurate diagnosis is therefore important in order to plan treatment which is appropriate for a self-limiting condition and occasionally to reassure the parents of a disfigured infant that no treatment is indicated.

The histopathological appearance of this vascular hamartoma varies with its clinical phase; in its early proliferative phase, the tumour consists mostly of numerous dividing endothelial cells and vascular spaces are rare. Also, it is surprisingly rich in mast cells (Glowacki & Mulliken 1982), whose function at this site has not been clearly established. Mitotic figures may be profuse at this stage, possibly leading to an erroneous diagnosis of malignancy in rapidly enlarging lesions. The characterization of poorly differentiated lesions may be helped by reticulin stains or by the identification of factor VIII, which is produced by the endothelial cells, using peroxidase or fluorescein antibody techniques (Haik *et al.* 1994). In more mature tumours, vascular spaces are larger, with fewer flattened endothelial cells. The tumour is not encapsulated and usually tends to infiltrate surrounding structures. In the involutional phase, there is often deposition of fibrous and adipose tissue around the lesion

Clinical features

Approximately one-third of capillary haemangiomas (Fig. 37.1) are present at birth, and they will all have appeared by the age of 6 months. The appearance of the tumour may be preceded by a faint telangiectatic cutaneous flush. Rapid growth lasting 3–6 months is followed by a period of stabilization. The tumour then usually regresses (Fig. 37.2). Margileth and Museles (1965) found that 30% of 336 haemangiomas had regressed by the age of 3 years, 60% by 4 years, and 76% by 7 years.

Capillary haemangiomas are most commonly situated in the upper lid or orbit (Fig. 37.3). Their appearance varies according to the depth of involvement; superficial cutaneous lesions have the red lobulated appearance which gave rise to the name 'strawberry naevus'. Subcutaneous haemangiomas are often blueish in colour. Lesions situated deep to the orbital septum may present with proptosis only with no cutaneous discoloration. Occasionally, the proptosis is severe enough to cause corneal expo-

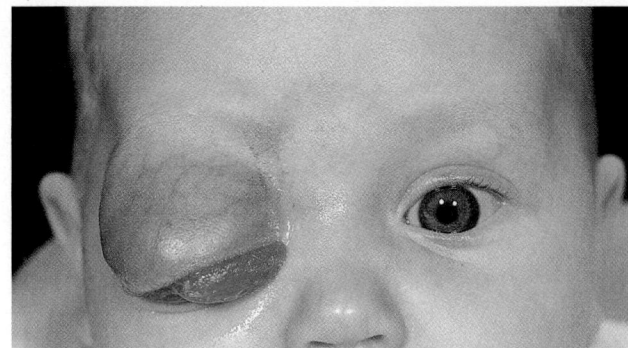

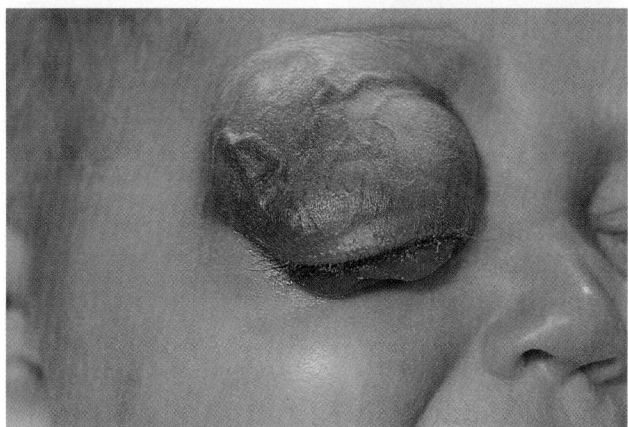

Fig. 37.1 (a) Capillary haemangioma of the anterior orbit and lid. (b) Same patient when crying showing engorgement and mild increase in size.

mus is common as a result of the interruption of binocularity.

Systemic complications of capillary haemangiomas are rare (Haik *et al.* 1994). The Kasabach–Merritt syndrome is a coagulopathy resulting from consumption of fibrinogen and platelet entrapment within a large vascular haemangioma, often in the viscera. It usually responds to treatment with platelet replacement and corticosteroids.

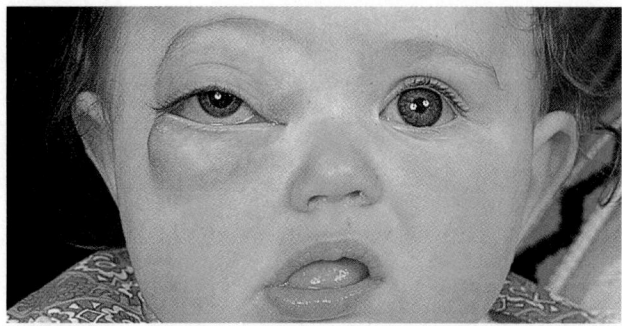

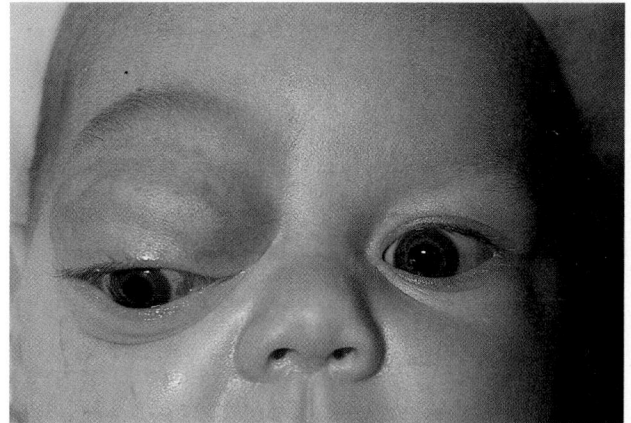

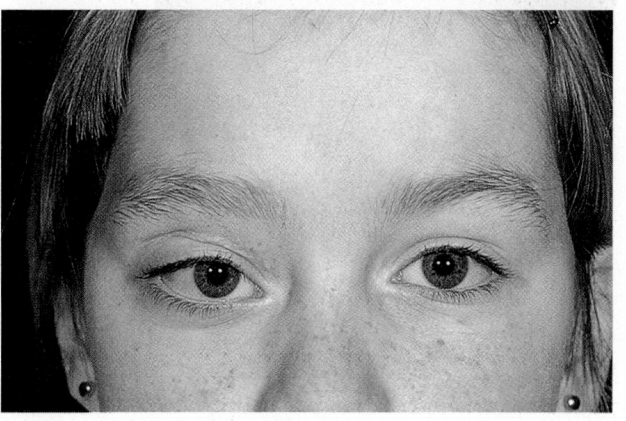

Fig. 37.2 (a) Orbital capillary haemangioma. As sometimes happens, the mother of this child on several occasions, was accused of having injured her child. (b) Orbital capillary haemangioma in a child aged 2 months. (c) Same patient as (b) aged 9 years after some spontaneous resolution and surgery. Surgery is usually not necessary and best avoided in most instances (see text).

sure. In about one-third of cases, the haemangioma involves several levels of depth (Rootman 1988). Other helpful diagnostic signs include the increase in the size of the tumour or proptosis with crying, which may be accompanied by a change in its colour to blue; the blueish discoloration of an underlying tumour, which may be seen with eyelid eversion; and, in about 30% of patients, the presence of 'strawberry' naevi at other cutaneous sites (Haik *et al.* 1979). Occasionally, enormous growth occurs obliterating facial structures (Fig. 37.4).

Amblyopia is common in patients with orbital capillary haemangiomas, with a prevalence ranging between 43 and 60% in published series of affected verbal children (Robb 1977; Stigmar *et al.* 1978; Haik *et al.* 1979). This may result from occlusion of the visual axis by a bulky tumour. More often, however, it results from distortion of the globe by tumour giving rise to corneal astigmatism. The axis of the corrective plus cylinder is directed towards the tumour. This may persist after the haemangioma has regressed (Robb 1977) but usually resolves at least partially (Morrell & Willshaw 1991). Lastly, prolonged occlusion can result in ipsilateral myopia (Hoyt *et al.* 1981) and the resultant anisometropia may be another contributory factor in the development of amblyopia. Secondary strabis-

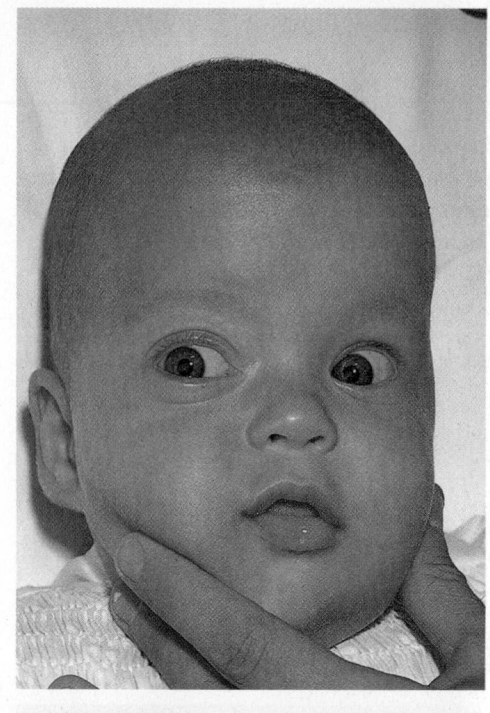

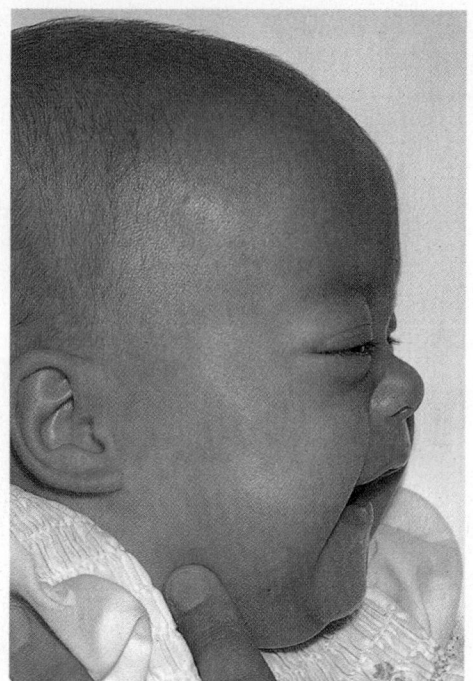

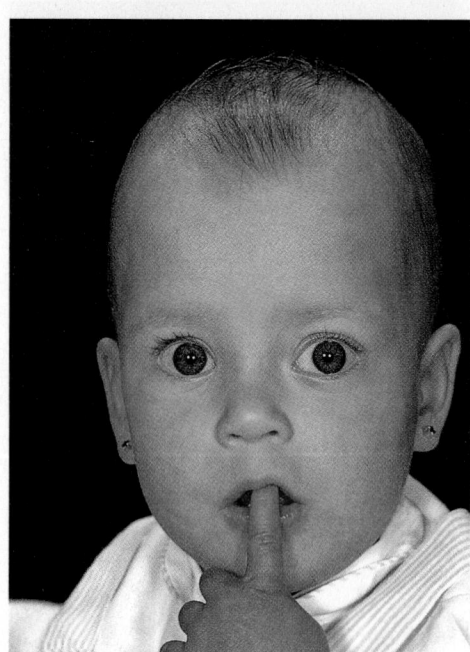

Fig. 37.3 (a, b) Right orbital capillary haemangioma in a child aged 5 months. (c) Complete resolution without treatment.

Investigation

In the majority of children presenting with proptosis, lid involvement or other cutaneous haemangiomas allow a clinical diagnosis to be made. Plain X-ray of the orbit may show enlargement of the affected side but is otherwise unhelpful. The extent of the lesion can be assessed by computed tomography (CT) scanning. A soft tissue density mass is seen to infiltrate the orbit, often crossing bound-

aries between compartments such as the muscle cone or orbital septum. Enhancement is variable, according to the vascularity of the lesion and its stage of growth or involution. T2-weighted magnetic resonance imaging (MRI) is useful to delineate the tumour since the lesion is hyperintense due its intrinsic blood flow. T1-weighted gadolinium-enhanced views with fat suppression to improve contrast give the best assessment of the anatomical relationships of the tumour. Lesions confined to the posterior

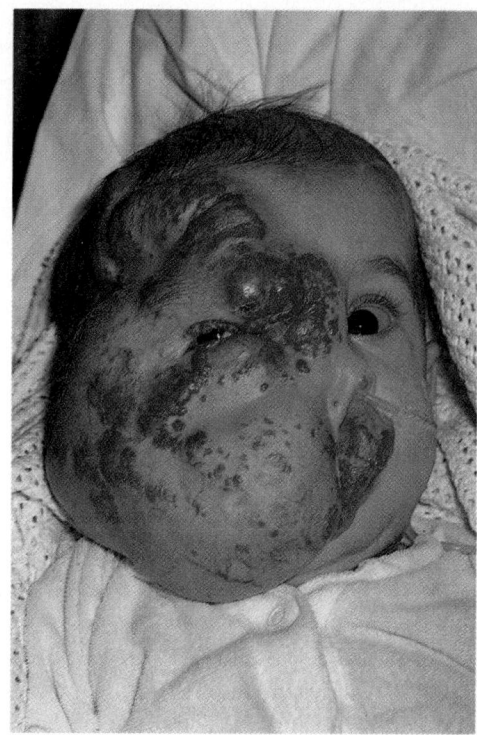

Fig. 37.4 Massive facial and orbital capillary haemangioma.

orbit, especially during a period of growth, may occasionally be mistaken for a malignant tumour such as rhabdomyosarcoma, and biopsy may then be indicated.

Management

As discussed above, most capillary haemangiomas undergo spontaneous regression and three-quarters disappear by the age of 7 years (Margileth & Museles 1965). Management should therefore be conservative if possible, with treatment of any amblyopia and significant refractive error, while awaiting spontaneous regression. The appearance of superficial pale stellate areas of scarring on a typical 'strawberry' lesion is a useful early indicator of spontaneous regression which can be reassuring to anxious parents. It should be stressed that occlusion of the contralateral eye for amblyopia therapy should always be accompanied by correction of the astigmatic error of the affected eye with appropriate glasses (Fig. 37.5).

Active treatment to reduce the size of the tumour is only indicated if there is occlusion of the visual axis or if a posterior lesion results in progressive proptosis with evidence of optic nerve compression or corneal exposure. Methods of treatment have included surgical excision, radiotherapy, injection of sclerosing agents, and local or systemic steroids (Hiles & Pilchard 1971). Kushner (1982) has reported good results with injection of local steroid into the haemangioma. We have similarly obtained good results with this technique and recommend the injection

of a combination of methylprednisolone 25–40 mg and triamcinolone 40–80 mg into the haemangioma. Tumour regression should be noted within 2–4 weeks, and further injections may be necessary. The steroid should be given by slow injection throughout the tumour while the needle is withdrawn to reduce the risk of central retinal artery embolization, a rare but devastating complication recently reported to have occurred bilaterally in one case (Ruttum *et al.* 1993). Other reported complications include local fat atrophy, eyelid necrosis and adrenal suppression with Cushingoid features (Haik *et al.* 1994). The whitish skin discoloration which is sometimes noted from superficial accumulation of depot steroid after injection is usually transient.

Systemic steroids in doses of 1.5–2.5 mg/kg per day are occasionally preferred for very large or posteriorly situated lesions, although the side-effects of growth retardation, adrenal suppression and Cushingoid changes make this form of therapy undesirable for all but the most serious cases. A rebound phenomenon has been noted after discontinuation of oral steroid, with an increase in size of the capillary haemangioma.

Sight-threatening lesions which have failed to respond to steroids may be amenable to treatment with interferon alpha 2a, although the response to this treatment may be slow (Ezekowitz *et al.* 1992). Loughnan *et al.* (1992) have reported a rapid regression of a massive steroid-unresponsive orbital capillary haemangioma after systemic injections of interferon alpha 2b.

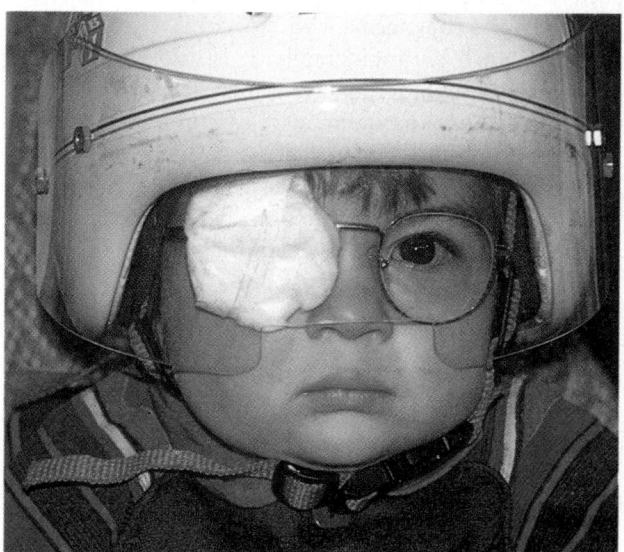

Fig. 37.5 Deep capillary haemangioma in a 6-month-old boy. A faint blueish tinge is evident in the left lower lid. There is a + 4.0 dioptre induced cylinder. Occlusion is vital in virtually every case and, in this child, his inventive parents have devised a novel method of preventing him from removing the patch. Eighteen months later the lesion had resolved, as had the cylinder. Patient from the University of British Columbia.

The carbon dioxide, argon, yttrium–aluminium–garnet (YAG) and dye lasers have all been used to treat haemangiomas. Their use is limited by the scarring they induce, although the dye laser tuned to 577 or 585 nm with a 10 ms pulse duration may allow selective thermal damage of capillary tissue with minimal scarring and accelerated regression (Garden *et al.* 1992). The use of lasers to treat these lesions is still not widely accepted. Radiotherapy and sclerosing agents should no longer be used.

Surgical excision is usually deferred until the lesion has stopped regressing, often after 6 or 7 years of age. Any residual cosmetic defect may then be corrected (Boyd & Collin 1991). Surgery is complicated by the infiltrative nature of the tumour which makes its dissection from normal orbital structures difficult. Nevertheless, good results have been reported in young patients with well-demarcated lesions both after failure to respond to other therapeutic modalities (Rootman 1988) and as a primary therapeutic approach in highly selected cases (Deans *et al.* 1992; Walker *et al.* 1994).

Haemangiopericytoma

This rare tumour, which is derived from the pericyte, is predominantly seen in adults although it has been reported to affect children as young as 20 months (Kapoor *et al.* 1978; Croxatto & Font 1982). Its pattern of behaviour is unpredictable but the usual presentation is with gradually increasing proptosis and mass effect related to a tumour which, typically, is superiorly placed. On CT scan, it is seen as a well-circumscribed lesion that shows marked homogeneous enhancement with contrast. There is a pronounced blush on angiography. It is a locally invasive tumour that can undergo distant metastasis and it is best treated by complete excision with careful preservation of the pseudocapsule. Unfortunately, as these are friable, local recurrence is common, often due to incomplete excision. Occasionally, these tumours behave very aggressively and, in these cases, exenteration may be necessary to control local tumour progression.

Lymphangioma

These vascular anomalies usually arise in childhood and are often difficult to manage. They may enlarge gradually but usually their expansion is sudden, as a result of intralesional haemorrhage. Unlike capillary haemangiomas, they do not undergo spontaneous regression. When deeply situated, they are difficult to excise surgically since their margins are poorly defined and they arborize widely throughout the orbital tissues.

Lymphangiomas accounted for 3% of the 600 orbital tumours on file at Wills Hospital in Iliff and Green's series (1979). In approximately one-third of cases, the lymphangioma is apparent at birth or within the first weeks of life (Jones 1959; Harris *et al.* 1990), and over three-quarters of patients present in the first decade of life (Iliff & Green 1979). The average age of onset in Jones' (1959) series of 29 patients was 6.2 years. A female preponderance (ratio 2–3:1) has been reported (Iliff & Green 1979; Harris *et al.* 1990).

Their frequency of occurrence within the orbit is puzzling in view of the absence of lymphatic drainage from the retroseptal tissues. It is likely that lymphangiomas arise from primitive vascular elements within the orbit (Jakobiec & Font 1986). Unlike capillary haemangiomas, they do not appear to grow by cellular proliferation. Instead, the full extent of the malformation is present at birth, insinuating itself within the normal orbital tissues (Harris *et al.* 1990). Since the vascular channels have characteristics of both lymphatic and blood vessels, the histological differentiation of lymphangiomas from orbital varices has been a source of debate. Haemodynamically, lymphangiomas and varices are part of a continuum of venous-derived lesions, which are differentiated according to the presence or lack of connection to the venous system. Whereas varices, typically, are connected and therefore expand with valsalva manoeuvre or supine posture, lymphangiomas are isolated and therefore do not. Many lesions are mixed, with various types of tumour represented within a single lesion. The extremes of the spectrum can also be differentiated histopathologically, since the lymphangiomatous element has distinctive electron microscopic features (Rootman *et al.* 1986).

Histopathologically, they consist of diaphanous, serous fluid-filled channels lined by endothelium. These have characteristics of true lymphatic channels as well as areas of dysplastic channels (Rootman 1988). Lymphoid follicles are often present in the stromal components. Haemorrhage into the tumour is common giving rise to so-called chocolate cysts.

The clinical features of lymphangiomas vary with the extent and depth of orbital involvement.

Superficial

Isolated superficial involvement is comparatively rare and may consist of multiple conjunctival cysts filled with clear or xanthochromic fluid, or a subcutaneous blueish cystic swelling of the eyelid. The latter may transilluminate and may occasionally present with an abrupt localized change in colour due to haemorrhage into a pre-existing lesion (Pang *et al.* 1984). Superficial lymphangiomas are easily accessible and, if unsightly, may be excised surgically with good results.

Deep

The hallmark of deeply situated orbital lymphangiomas is proptosis (Fig. 37.6). Deep lymphangiomas may present

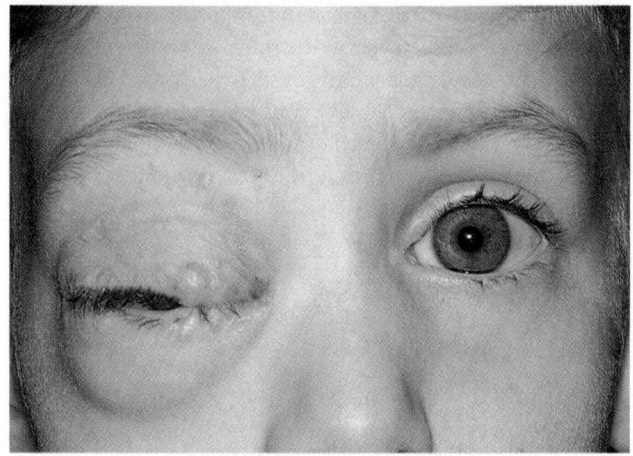

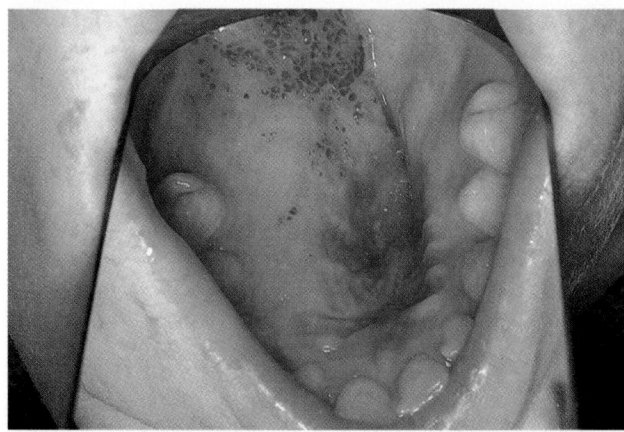

Fig. 37.6 (a) This 4-year-old boy was born after a 32-week gestation. Right proptosis developed by 4 weeks and was progressive despite orbital surgery, until the age of 3 years. It has been static since then. The diagnosis was a lymphangioma. (b) Same patient showing clear and blood-filled cystic lesions on the palate.

with gradually increasing proptosis with or without ptosis. In contrast to capillary haemangiomas the proptosis is said to be variable. An increase with upper respiratory tract infections and other generalized inflammatory states (Jones 1959) has been ascribed to lymphoid activity within the lesion. This association is poorly defined and may only be coincidental, since upper respiratory tract infections are so common in childhood. Nevertheless eight of the 15 patients questioned by Harris *et al.* (1990) reported enlargement with upper respiratory tract infection.

The most typical presentation, however, is with sudden proptosis resulting from haemorrhage into a hitherto unsuspected lesion. In these cases, the differential diagnoses include other causes of rapidly increasing proptosis such as rhabdomyosarcoma, neuroblastoma, and so on. In this situation, examination of the nasal and palatal mucosa may be helpful if it reveals the characteristic mixed clear fluid and blood-filled blebs of widespread lymphangioma (Fig. 37.6). Optic nerve compression is common with rapidly expanding blood-filled 'chocolate cyst' (Kazim *et al.* 1992) (Fig. 37.7) and can result in decreased visual acuity with disc swelling. It is an indication for urgent orbital intervention to decompress the lesion.

Combined lesions

These usually present in infancy, gradually enlarging over many years. Long-standing lesions may be associated with orbital enlargement (Fig. 37.8). The presence of telltale conjunctival and lid changes is helpful in making the diagnosis of lymphangioma. Haemorrhage into superficial lesions may result in the striking appearance of blood menisci within the conjunctival cysts. These may be accompanied by generalized recurrent subconjunctival haemorrhage and lid ecchymosis. Deep haemorrhage results in proptosis which is commonly associated with compressive optic neuropathy. Combined lesions may be large enough to simultaneously involve every orbital space and can give rise to gross proptosis and facial deformity. We have identified several patients in whom the lymphangioma passed through the superior orbital fissure and, in two cases, this configuration was associated with an intracranial bleed from separate vascular anomalies of the brain.

Investigation

CT scanning shows a soft tissue density mass with poorly defined margins and inhomogeneous enhancement after injection of contrast medium. Bony destruction is absent but large lesions can result in smooth enlargement of the orbit. The presence of a cystic component may be helpful in differentiating lymphangiomas from capillary haemangiomas. Since haemoglobin has paramagnetic qualities which change as blood denatures after haemorrhage, blood-containing 'chocolate cysts' are particularly well visualized by MRI scanning (Bond *et al.* 1992; Kazim *et al.* 1992). The age of intralesional haemorrhages can also be assessed with this modality since oxyhaemoglobin in fresh haemorrhage is hypointense on T1- and T2-weighted images, gradually becoming hyperintense as this is converted to methaemoglobin. Later still, degradation to ferritin and haemosiderin once again produces a hypointense image. Gadolinium is not particularly helpful in imaging lymphangioma.

Management

A conservative approach should be adopted if possible, since complete excision is impossible in all but the most superficial lesions and since haemorrhagic cysts tend to shrink with time. In addition, surgery itself can precipitate further haemorrhage (Henderson 1973). Wilson *et al.* (1989) have stressed that bed rest alone or with the use of

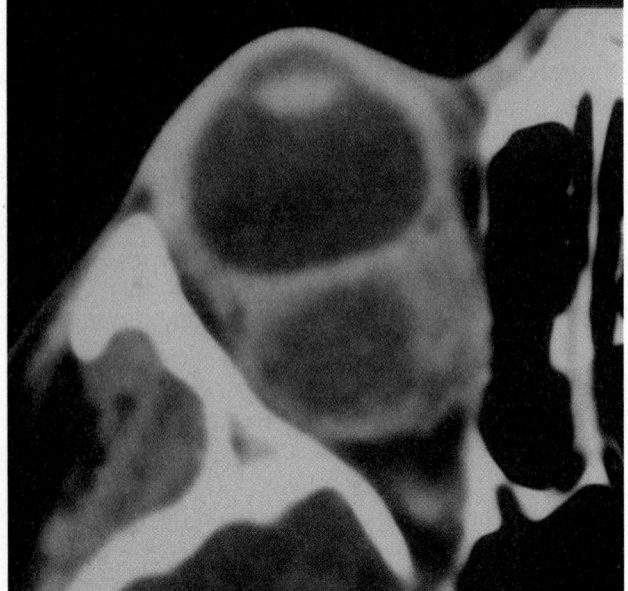

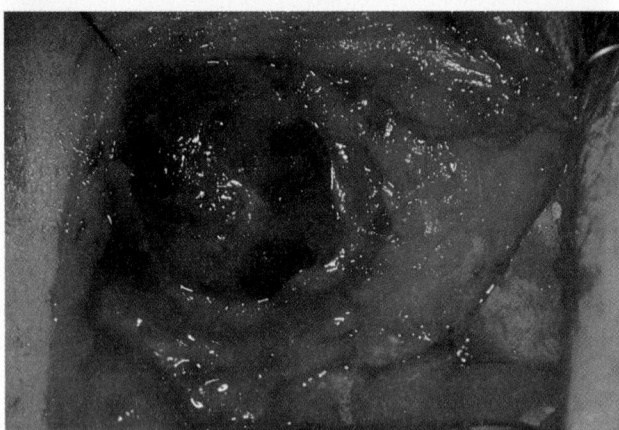

Fig. 37.7 Previously asymptomatic 8-year-old presenting with sudden onset axial proptosis overnight, decreased vision, afferent pupillary defect and optic disc swelling. (a) CT shows a cystic mass indenting the globe posteriorly. (b) At surgery, the chocolate cyst was identified and decompressed. Patient from the University of British Columbia.

cold compresses can be associated with a good outcome even in cases with acute proptosis of up to 10 mm. None of their six patients had an afferent pupillary defect, but biopsy was performed in the acute stage in three of these patients which might have contributed to the resolution of the problem.

Surgery is indicated if there is evidence of optic nerve dysfunction, corneal exposure, pain and nausea from raised orbital pressure or the risk of amblyopia from induced astigmatism or strabismus. It is possible to temporize by aspirating the cyst contents through a needle under ultrasound guidance. Poor results and frequent morbidity have been reported from attempts at subtotal excision. We feel that surgery should be aimed at excising

the offending focus of lymphangiomatous tissue as well as incision of blood cysts with release of their contents. Unlike dermoid or sebaceous cysts, excision of the whole cyst wall is not necessary to avoid recurrence. The carbon dioxide laser may be useful in reducing the haemorrhagic complications associated with conventional subtotal excision surgery (Kennerdell *et al.* 1986).

Abnormalities

Congenital orbital varices

Wright (1974) believes on the basis of venography studies that most cases of lymphangiomas described in the literature are congenital orbital varices. We feel that there is a spectrum of vascular abnormalities, ranging from the isolated lymphatic lymphangioma described above to the 'high flow varix' described below. Reports of patients with concurrent lymphangioma and orbital varices as well as patients with concurrent lymphangioma with arteriove-

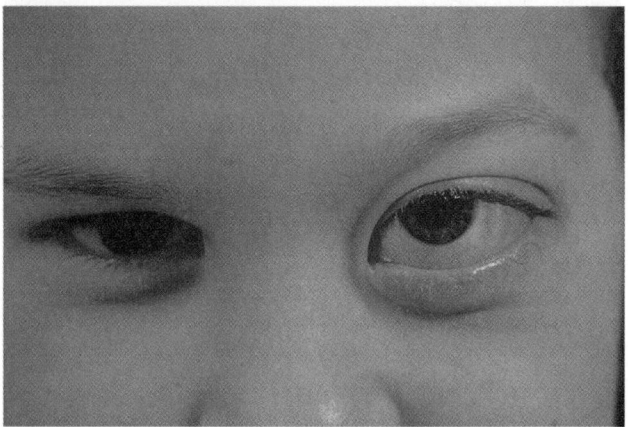

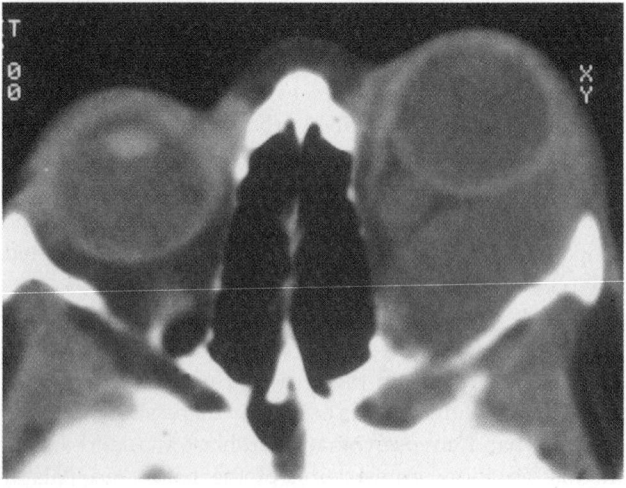

Fig. 37.8 Orbital lymphangioma. (a) Sudden onset of proptosis in the left eye of a previously asymptomatic 5-year-old child. (b) CT scan shows diffuse soft tissue density lesion arborizing through the retrobulbar tissues. Patient from the University of British Columbia.

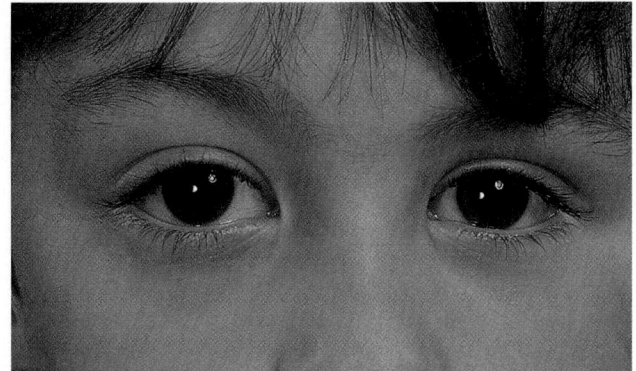

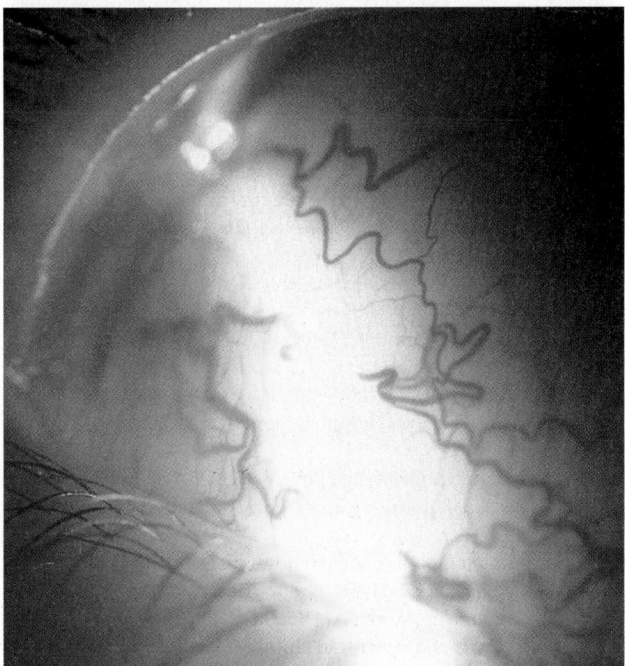

Fig. 37.9 (a) Orbital varices. A subconjunctival varix can just be seen in the right lateral fornix. (b) With the lid retracted the subconjunctival varices can be clearly seen. Patient from the University of British Columbia.

nous malformation suggest that a fundamental problem with vasculogenesis may be at the root of all these lesions. Varices may be divided into high and low flow types. Low flow varices are clinically similar to lymphangiomas, with a tendency for sudden, often recurrent haemorrhage (Kremer *et al.* 1987), whilst high flow varices expand with increased jugular vein pulse and rarely bleed.

Orbital varices grow only slowly during childhood and rarely give rise to visual problems. There is often a subconjunctival component (Fig. 37.9). Plain X-rays show enlargement of the orbit on the affected side and phleboliths are often seen. Surgical excision when indicated for cosmetic reasons may be confined to the anterior varices as attempts to excise deep orbital varicosities may result in optic nerve or other cranial nerve damage

(Wright 1974), although combined neuroradiological methods allow safe excision in experienced hands. Some orbital varices may be associated with extensive intracranial varicosities (Fig. 37.10).

Sturge–Weber syndrome (see Chapter 61)

Sturge–Weber syndrome consists of facial port-wine stain, with leptomeningeal angiomatosis. The facial lesion is classically unilateral, involving the dermatome of the ophthalmic branch of the trigeminal nerve. The maxillary and mandibular divisions may also be involved. Hypertrophy of the underlying tissues is common. This frequently causes greater disfigurement than the cutaneous discoloration. Angiomatous malformations may involve other tissues including the eye, respiratory tract and gastrointestinal tracts, ovary and pancreas. Cerebral involvement may give rise to seizures, hemiplegia and mental retardation. Not all patients, however, have the complete syndrome and there is wide variability in expression.

The ophthalmic manifestations include unilateral glaucoma, which may be congenital but is often juvenile

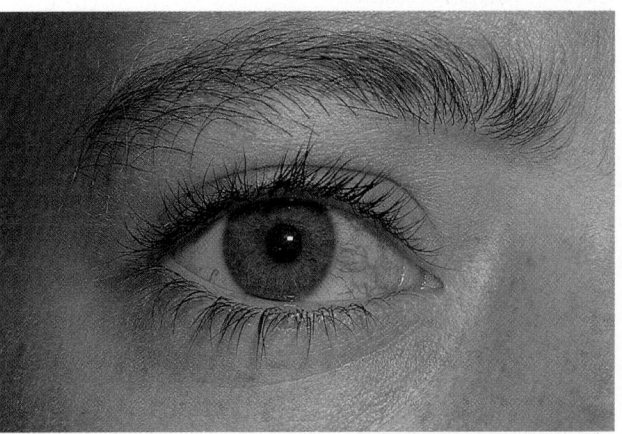

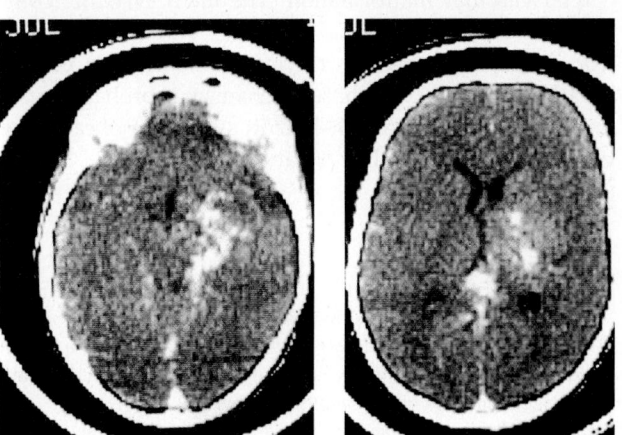

Fig. 37.10 (a) Subconjunctival varicosities in a patient with an orbital and intracranial haemangioma. (b) Contrast-enhanced CT scans showing the intracranial lesion (same patient).

(Sujansky & Conrandi 1995). Episcleral and conjunctival vascular anomalies and diffuse choroidal haemangiomas are also common. The latter may be complicated by serous retinal detachment. Orbital involvement is rare; Hofeldt *et al.* (1979) described two patients with ipsilateral naevus flammeus and a unilateral orbital vascular malformation causing proptosis. In each case there was no evidence of any intracranial lesion.

Early results of the use of pulsed dye lasers for naevus flammeus have been encouraging. In the long term, this treatment may reduce the disfiguring hypertrophy which accompanies the port-wine stain.

Rare vascular lesions of the orbit

Klippel–Trenaunay–Weber syndrome (see Chapter 61)

This rare syndrome comprises multiple cutaneous naevi associated with various angiomas of one or more limbs, which may show hypertrophy of the soft tissues. Rathbun *et al.* (1970) described a 15-year-old girl with the classical features of the syndrome who developed intermittent proptosis from an orbital varix. This was ligated and excised with good results.

Blue rubber bleb naevus syndrome

This rare syndrome usually presents in childhood. It consists of multiple blueish cutaneous cavernous haemangiomas, associated with angiomas of the gastrointestinal tract, lung, heart and central nervous system. The cutaneous lesions are soft, rubbery and compressible. Most cases are sporadic but autosomal dominant inheritance has been reported in several families. Conjunctival, iris and retinal angiomas may occur (Crompton & Taylor 1981). Rennie *et al.* (1982) have reported an adult with the syndrome who developed unilateral proptosis from an orbital vascular malformation. The main systemic complication is gastrointestinal bleeding, which may lead to iron-deficiency anaemia or even a consumption coagulopathy (Oranje 1986) whose mechanism is probably similar to that of the Kasabach–Merritt syndrome of capillary haemangiomas (Moodley & Ramdial 1993).

References

Bond JB, Haik BG, Taveras JL *et al.* Magnetic resonance imaging of orbital lymphangioma with and without gadolinium contrast enhancement. *Ophthalmology* 1992; **99**: 1318–24.

Boyd MJ, Collin JRO. Capillary haemangiomas: an approach to their management. *Br J Ophthalmol* 1991; **75**: 298–300.

Crompton JL, Taylor D. Ocular lesions in the blue rubber naevus syndrome. *Br J Ophthalmol* 1981; **65**: 133–7.

Croxatto JO, Font RL. Haemangiopericytoma of the orbit: a clinicopathologieal study of 30 cases. *Hum Pathol* 1982; **13**: 210–18.

Deans RM, Harris GJ, Kivlin JD. Surgical dissection of capillary haemangiomas. An alternative to intralesional corticosteroids. *Arch Ophthalmol* 1992; **110**: 1743–7.

Ezekowitz RAB, Mulliken JB, Folkman J. Interferon alpha–2a therapy for life-threatening hemangiomas of infancy. *N Engl J Med* 1992; **326**: 1456–63.

Garden JM, Bakus AD, Paller AS. Treatment of cutaneous hemangiomas by the flashlamp-pumped pulsed dye laser: prospective analysis. *J Pediatr* 1992; **120**: 555–60.

Glowacki J, Mulliken JB. Mast cells in hemangiomas and vascular malformations. *Paediatrics* 1982; **70**: 48–51.

Haik BG, Jakobiec FA, Ellsworth RM, Jones IL. Capillary haemangioma of the lids and orbit: an analysis of the clinical features and therapeutic results in 101 cases. *Ophthalmology* 1979; **86**: 760–89.

Haik BG, Karcioglu ZA, Gordon RA, Pechous BP. Capillary hemangioma (infantile periocular hemangioma). *Surv Ophthalmol* 1994; **38**: 399–426.

Harris GJ, Sakol PJ, Bonavolonta G, De Concillis C. An analysis of 30 cases of orbital lymphangioma. Pathophysiologic considerations and management recommendations. *Ophthalmology* 1990; **97**: 1583–92.

Henderson JW. *Orbital Tumours*. Philadelphia: WB Saunders, 1973.

Hiles D, Pilchard WA. Corticosteroid control of neonatal haemangiomas of orbit and ocular adnexae. *Am J Ophthalmol* 1971; **71**: 1003–8.

Hofeldt AJ, Zaret CR, Jakobiec FA *et al.* Orbitofacial angiomatosis. *Arch Ophthalmol* 1979; **97**: 484–8.

Hoyt CS, Stone RD, Fromer C, Billson FA. Monocular axial myopia associated with neonatal eyelid closure in human infants. *Am J Ophthalmol* 1981; **91**: 197–206.

Iliff WJ, Green WR. Orbital lymphangiomas. *Ophthalmology* 1979; **86**: 914–29.

Jakobiec FA, Font RL. Orbit. In: Spencer WH, ed. *Ophthalmic Pathology: an Atlas and Textbook*, 3rd edn, Vol. 3. Philadelphia: WB Saunders, 1986: 2533–8.

Jones IS. Lymphangiomas of ocular adnexae: an analysis of 62 cases. *Trans Am Ophthalmol Soc* 1959; **57**: 602–65.

Kapoor S, Kapoor MS, Aurora AL, Sood GC. Orbital haemangiopericytoma: a report of a 3-year-old child. *J Pediatr Ophthalmol Strabismus* 1978; **15**: 40–2.

Kazim M, Kennerdell JS, Rothfus W, Marquardt M. Orbital lymphangioma. Correlation of magnetic resonance images and intraoperative findings. *Ophthalmology* 1992; **99**: 1588–94.

Kennerdell JS, Maroon JC, Garrity JA, Abla AA. Surgical management of orbital lymphangioma with the carbon dioxide laser. *Am J Ophthalmol* 1986; **102**: 308–14.

Kremer I, Nissenkorn I, Feuerman P, Ben-Sira I. Congenital orbital vascular malformation complicated by massive retrobulbar haemorrhage. *J Pediatr Ophthalmol Strabismus* 1987; **24**: 190–3.

Kushner BJ. Intralesional corticosteroid injection for infantile adnexal hemangioma. *Am J Ophthalmol* 1982; **93**: 496–506.

Loughnan MS, Elder J, Kemp A. Treatment of a massive orbital capillary hemangioma with interferon alpha-2b: short-term results (letter). *Arch Ophthalmol* 1992; **110**: 1366–7.

Margileth AM, Museles M. Cutaneous haemangiomas in children. Diagnosis and conservative management. *J Am Med Assoc* 1965; **194**: 135–8.

Moodley M, Ramdial P. Blue rubber bleb nevus syndrome: case report and review of the literature. *Pediatrics* 1993; **92**: 160–2.

Morrell AJ, Willshaw HE. Normalisation of refractive error after steroid injection for adnexal haemangiomas. *Br J Ophthalmol* 1991; **75**: 301–5.

Oranje AP. Blue rubber bleb nevus syndrome. *Pediatr Dermatol* 1986; **3**: 304–10.

Pang P, Jakobiec FA, Iwamoto T, Hornblass A. Small lymphangiomas of the eyelids. *Ophthalmology* 1984; **91**: 1278–84.

Rathbun JE, Hoyt WF, Beard C. Surgical management of orbitofrontal varix in Klippel–Trenaunay–Weber syndrome. *Am J Ophthalmol* 1970; **70**: 109–12.

Rennie IG, Shortland JR, Mahood JM, Brown BH. Periodic exophthalmos associated with the blue rubber bleb naevus syndrome: a case report. *Br J Ophthalmol* 1982; **66**: 594–9.

Robb R. Refractive errors associated with haemangiomas of the eyelids and orbit in infancy. *Am J Ophthalmol* 1977; **83**: 52–7.

Rootman J, Hay E, Graeb D, Miller R. Orbital adnexal lymphangiomas: a spectrum of haemodynamically isolated vascular hamartomas. *Ophthalmology* 1986; **93**: 1558–70.

Rootman J. *Diseases of the Orbit: a Multidisciplinary Approach.* Philadelphia: JB Lippincott, 1988.

Ruttum MS, Abrams GW, Harris GJ, Ellis MK. Bilateral retinal embolization associated with intralesional corticosteroid injection for capillary haemangioma of infancy. *J Pediatr Ophthalmol Strabismus* 1993; **30**: 4–7.

Stigmar G, Crawford JS, Ward CM, Thomson HG. Ophthalmic sequelae of infantile haemangiomas of the eyelids and orbit. *Am J Ophthalmol* 1978; **85**: 806–13.

Sujansky E, Conradi S. Sturge–Weber syndrome: age of onset of seizures and glaucoma and the prognosis for affected children. *J Child Neurol* 1995; **10**: 49–58.

Walker RS, Custer PL, Nerad JA. Surgical excision of periorbital capillary hemangiomas. *Ophthalmology* 1994; **101**: 1333–40.

Wilson ME, Parker PL, Chavis RM. Conservative management of childhood orbital lymphangioma. *Ophthalmology* 1989; **96**: 484–9.

Wright JE. Orbital vascular anomalies. *Trans Am Acad Ophthalmol Otolaryngol* 1974; **78**: 606–16.

Youseffi B. Orbital tumours in children: a clinical study of 62 cases. *J Paediatr Ophthalmol Strabismus* 1969; **61**: 177–81.

38: The Uveal Tract

Susan Day and Andrew Narita

The uveal tract consists of iris, ciliary body and choroid, each of which has a rich vascular supply and pigment. Its colourful grape-like appearance gives rise to its name 'uvea'. The structure contains two apertures—the pupil and the region of the optic nerve.

The uveal tract's functions are diverse—its pigment acts as a filter; iris musculature forms an 'F-stop' for the eye; the ciliary body secretes aqueous, provides the skeleton for the zonular suspension of the lens as well as the power for focusing, and provides nutrition for the lens. The choroid with its rich vascular supply provides nutrition for 65% of the outer retinal layers (Alm & Bill 1972). Bruch's membrane forms a boundary between retina and choroid; abnormalities in this layer play an important role in various choroidal and retinal disorders (Feeney & Hogan 1961; Hogan 1961).

Embryology

The uveal tract includes contributions from the neural ectoderm, neural crest and mesoderm. The neural ectoderm gives rise to the iris sphincter and dilator muscles, posterior iris epithelium, pigmented and non-pigmented ciliary epithelium. Neural crest cells contribute to iris and choroidal stroma as well as ciliary smooth muscle. Mesodermal tissue forms the endothelium for the many blood vessels (Ozanics & Jakobiec 1982).

The neural ectoderm differentiation occurs within 6–10 weeks of conception whilst definition of the vasculature and pigment migration span the final two trimesters.

Iris formation commences with closure of the fetal cleft at approximately 35 days of gestation. The sphincter is first evidenced by neuroectodermal pigment at the optic cup's margin by 10 weeks of gestation (Mund *et al.* 1972) and differentiation into myofibril occurs at 11–12 weeks of gestation. The dilator forms at approximately 24 weeks gestation.

The neuroectoderm also gives rise to both pigmented and non-pigmented ciliary epithelium. Once the optic cup has invaginated, creating the inner and outer layers of neuroectoderm, pigmentation of only the outer layer occurs. At 10–12 weeks, longitudinal ridges form from the outer layer and adhere to the inner layers, and the ciliary processes form. More posteriorly, the two layers adhere to each other without folding, giving rise to the pars plana.

After the neuroectoderm invaginates, neural crest cells are derived from within the space between the neuroectoderm and surface ectoderm. Neural crest cells may be to the head and neck as mesoderm is to somites of the body, since no true somites exist in the head and neck region (O'Rahilly 1965). Tissue derived from these cells is referred to as mesectoderm and its connection to the neuroepithelium remains loose into adulthood, accounting for the porosity of the iris to particles of 50–200 mm by diffusion (Rodrigues *et al.* 1982). The ciliary smooth muscle is first evident at nearly 4 months gestation just posterior to the precursors of the iris stroma. The fibres connect anteriorly to the developing scleral spur during the fifth month, and further increase in size and structure continues after birth.

Finally, neural crest cells also give rise to pigment cell precursors of the uveal tract (in contradistinction to neuroectoderm-derived retinal pigment epithelium). Pigmented cells surrounding the optic cup are visible at 10 weeks gestation. Pigment appears in the peripapillary region after 24 weeks. Migration occurs anteriorly and is nearly complete at birth as mostly mature melanosomes (Rodrigues *et al.* 1982).

The mesoderm gives rise solely to the endothelium of blood vessels whereas the muscular and support structures of the vessels arise from neural crest cells. These two components combine to form the 'mesenchyme' or connective tissue elements of the head and neck region.

The iris vasculature primordia are present by 6 weeks gestation as loops extending over the anterior surface of the anterior chamber (tunica vasculosa lentis), in association with the development of the ciliary body vasculature. By the end of the third month, indentations are created by the radially oriented vessels. The long posterior ciliary arteries are present in the ciliary body, and their terminal branches unite with the peripheral parts of the tunica vasculosa lentis to form the major arterial circle. As the tunica vasculosa lentis regresses, a residual pupillary membrane is created. During the fifth month of gestation the major arterial circle gives rise to radial vessels and branches to the ciliary body.

The choroidal vasculature first differentiates from mesenchymal elements during the second month of gestation, with precursors of the short posterior ciliary arteries which connect posteriorly with the developing choriocapillaris at 3 months, at which time the long posterior ciliary arteries anastomose with the anterior circulation. Further differentiation with intermediate-size vessels occurs during the fourth month (Ozanics & Jakobiec 1982). The arterial and venous systems undergo further differentiation into the forerunners of the middle or Sattler's layer during the fifth month (Heimann 1970). The foveal circulation differentiates at approximately the third to fourth month (Heimann 1972).

Postnatal development

At birth, the uveal tract is well differentiated. Two features which are very well scrutinized by the parents are iris colour and pupil size. Of particular concern is the colour of the eyes. The ophthalmologist might best observe that (i) the neonate's eyes will never be lighter than they are at birth; (ii) pigmentation is usually defined by 6 months of age and always by 1 year; and (iii) it is possible for brown-eyed but heterozygous parents to have a blue-eyed child.

At birth, Caucasians often have blue eyes because there are few melanocytes present with sparse pigment. More darkly pigmented races have irides with already pigmented melanocytes. The pigmentation in all races increases over the first 6 months to 1 year of life.

Pupil size is relatively small at birth, especially in darkly pigmented eyes. As the iris dilator muscle develops postnatally, the pupil correspondingly enlarges. The pupil margin may be accentuated by a prominent ectropion uveae, creating unnecessary concern by the parents or paediatrician.

In the full-term infant, the residual pupillary membrane may rarely alter the red reflex, resulting in referral from the primary care physician for further evaluation. In the preterm infant, assessment of the degree of atrophy of the pupillary membrane and its precursor, the tunica vasculosa lentis, has been used to estimate gestational age.

The ciliary muscle is incompletely developed at birth, the increase in accommodation over 3–6 months (Howland 1982) supports further development postnatally. An autopsy study of 76 infant eyes has documented this development (Aiello *et al.* 1992) with 75% of the final adult ciliary body length being achieved by 2 years of age.

The clinically significant effects of prematurity on the development of retinal circulation are not matched by any effect on choroidal circulation. Choroidal development and pigmentation is relatively complete at birth (Rodrigues *et al.* 1982); the changing fundus pigmentation is more due to changes in the retinal pigment epithelium.

Developmental abnormalities

Albinism

Albinism is a hereditary error of metabolism within pigment cells that has widespread and variable effects on the eyes, the visual system and the skin. Albinism is a heterogeneous group of conditions which are divided clinically into oculocutaneous albinism and ocular albinism and may be inherited in a variety of ways. Histopathologically, however, all forms may be truly oculocutaneous albinism; for patients with oculocutaneous albinism, there is less melanin in each melanosome, whereas the eyes and skin of patients with ocular albinism have macromelanosomes (O'Donnell *et al.* 1976), and type IV melanosomes in the iris (McCartney *et al.* 1985).

Clinical features

The ocular involvement and clinical significance of albinism varies greatly but nystagmus and reduced vision are almost constantly present (Abadi & Pascal 1991; Cheong *et al.* 1992).

Reduced visual acuity and contrast sensitivity. The reduced acuity associated with albinism is associated with defective fundus pigmentation (Fig. 38.1) and foveal hypoplasia (Fig. 38.2); rods are present within the fovea and cones

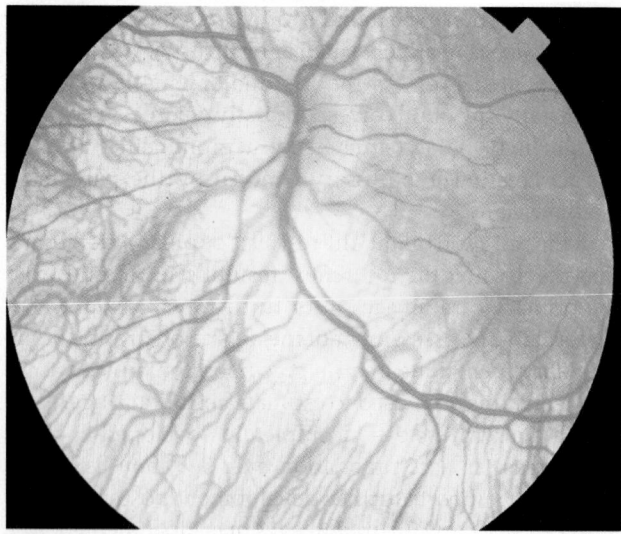

Fig. 38.1 Albinism showing marked choroidal and retinal pigmentation and foveal hypoplasia.

are distributed away from the fovea (O'Donnell 1984; Abadi & Cox 1992). Other factors that contribute to reduced acuity include nystagmus, refractive errors and amblyopia (Abadi & Pascal 1991). The pigment defect proportionally affects all parts of the uvea (Fig. 38.3).

Macular hypoplasia may be the most consistent feature of albinism. Abadi and Pascal noted four characteristic features: (i) absence of a foveal pit; (ii) reduction in the usually marked foveal pigment; (iii) lack of macular yellow pigments; and (iv) vessels crossing the macula. Subtle macular hypoplasia may be difficult to ascertain.

Very rarely, patients have normal vision, no nystagmus, and were termed as having albinoidism (Bergsma & Kaiser-Kupfer 1979); there are numerous conditions with skin, and more widespread, hypopigmentation but there is no need to call these albinoid. These patients may have symptoms of photophobia, iris transillumination and fundus hypopigmentation without being albinos!

Delayed visual maturation. Many albinos appear to have little or no vision in early infancy: they have a form of delayed visual maturation (see Chapter 3). This must be borne in mind when giving a prognosis in early infancy!

Nystagmus. Nystagmus is frequently the presenting symptom. The parents may notice the eyes wobbling, or the nystagmus may be noticed at a routine test. There is no typical waveform, and the onset of the nystagmus may not be until 3 months; the amplitude often rapidly increases, only to slowly decline over 1–3 years.

Strabismus. Both esotropia and exotropia are very common in albinos, and any binocular vision is likely to be rudimentary (Apkarian & Reits 1989).

Iris translucency. In tyrosinase-deficient oculocutaneous albinism (OCA1) the irides are pink or blue–pink (see Fig. 38.3); they can be diagnosed with the naked eye, although in many albinos slit-lamp microscopy with retroillumination is necessary. Iris translucency is rare in normal brown-eyed people, but quite common in young blue-eyed people (Jay *et al.* 1976). It is more easily detected by slit-lamp examination in a darkened room.

Photophobia. Most, but not all, albinos are photophobic to a variable degree, especially when young.

Neurophysiological changes. During embryogenesis of the neural pathways, the chiasm of an albino develops a decreased proportion of uncrossed fibres, there is abnormal layering of the lateral geniculate body (LGB), and abnormal visual pathways from the LGB to the occipital cortex (Guillery *et al.* 1975; Brodsky *et al.* 1993). It is felt that these chiasmal abnormalities may result, in part, in oculomotor abnormalities in patients with albinism. Abnormal-

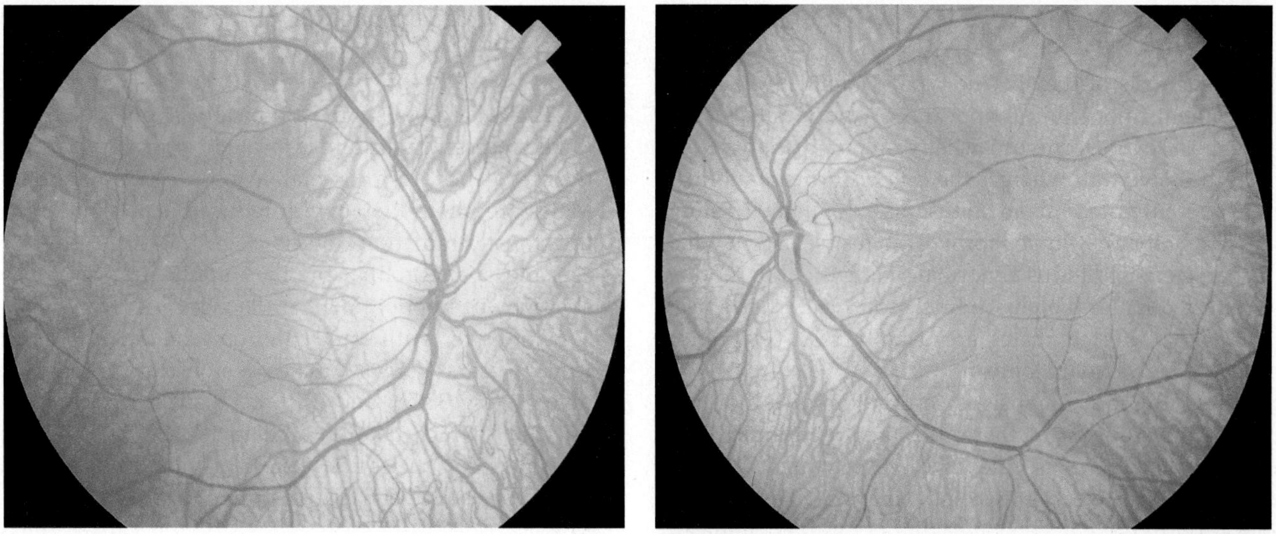

Fig. 38.2 (a, b) Albinism showing hypopigmentation and macular hypoplasia. (c) Albinism. A slit-lamp photograph where the beam is being shone through the dilated pupil: there is a marked red reflex through the sclera due to the lack of pigmentation.

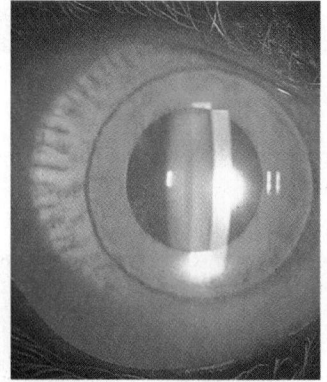
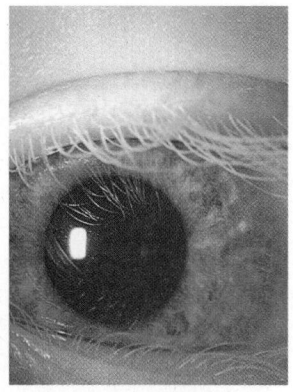
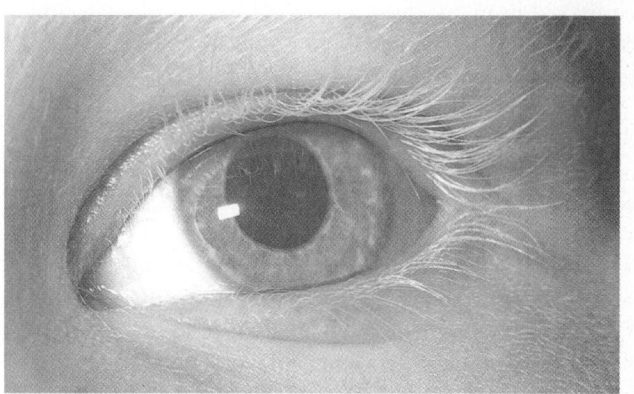

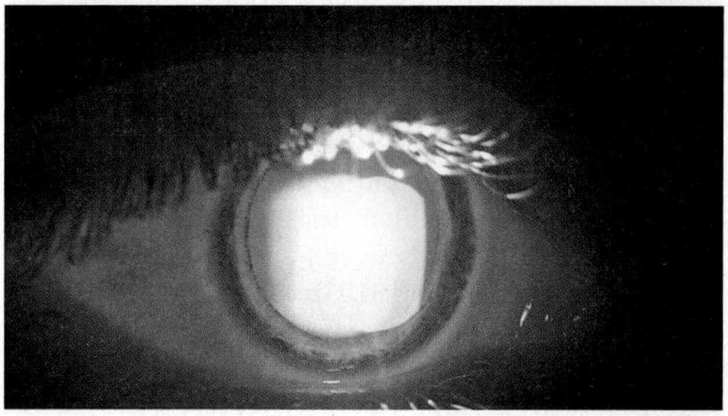

Fig. 38.3 (a) Albinism showing iris transillumination in direct light (on the right) and in retroillumination (on the left). The retroillumination picture shows details of the lens and ciliary processes seen through the transilluminant iris. (b) Albinism showing white lashes and pink–blue iris.

ities of the visually evoked potentials (VEP) reflect these anatomical variations (see Fig. 9.14) (Creel *et al.* 1974; Taylor 1978). Also the misdirection of the optic nerve fibres has been noted on positron emission tomography (PET) (Nakagawa *et al.* 1993) and, though magnetic resonance imaging (MRI) appears normal (Brodsky *et al.* 1993), functional MRI shows the cross-over anomaly (Hedera *et al.* 1994). This peculiar association between abnormal pigmentation and chiasmal 'mis-wiring' may indicate local interactions between pigmented cells and migrating retinal ganglion cells and an abnormal pleotropic gene controlling pigmentation and chiasm formation (Creel 1984).

The electroretinogram may be of larger amplitude (Russell-Eggitt *et al.* 1990).

Diagnosis

The diagnosis of the specific type of albinism is largely dependent upon clinical appearance and family history. The most severe forms are usually inherited as an autosomal recessive trait whereas the milder forms of albinism may be inherited in an autosomal dominant fashion. Additionally, an X-linked form of albinism exists in which a characteristic fundus abnormality is present in mothers of affected males (Forsius & Ericksson 1964; Charles *et al.* 1993), the affected males are usually relatively mildly affected with ocular albinism.

Generally, the diagnosis is straightforward; the iris is clearly transilluminant, there is nystagmus, a family history, and the fundus is pale. In cases in whom the signs are equivocal, electrophysiology may be most helpful, but until molecular genetic testing is routinely clinically available, some cases will defy a precise diagnosis. For instance, cases occur with iris transillumination and other defects such as ophthalmoplegia but no VEP cross-over defect; the same applies to Prader–Willi (Hered *et al.* 1988) and Angelman syndromes with hypopigmentation but not all the signs of albinos: no one sign is pathognomonic.

The hairbulb incubation test qualitatively detects tyrosinase in individuals over 5 years of age (King & Witkop 1976; O'Donnell 1984; Green 1985); those patients having little or no evidence of tyrosinase activity (usually OCA1 albinos) are termed tyrosinase-negative, those with tyrosinase activity are termed tyrosinase-positive. Although the test has been made semi-quantitative, it is equivocal in many cases and therefore of little use clinically, especially in infants, the group in which a clinical test is most needed.

The classification of albinism includes up to 10 types of oculocutaneous albinism, and four of ocular albinism (King *et al.* 1995); a simplified version is presented here.

- OA, ocular albinism.
- OA1, X-linked ocular albinism.
- AROA, autosomal recessive ocular albinism.
- OCA, oculocutaneous albinism.
- OCA1, tyrosinase-deficient oculocutaneous albinism.
- OCA1a, steely white hair, pink–blue irides, pink skin.
- OCA1b, yellow albinos.
- OCA1ts, peripheral pigmentation.
- OCA2, tyrosinase-positive oculocutaneous albinism.
- OCA3.
- ADOCA, autosomal dominant oculocutaneous albinism.
- Albinism with systemic disease.

Ocular albinism

Clinical differences exist between the different types of albinism, although variable phenotypic expression can exist within a pedigree (Castronuovo *et al.* 1991; Cheong 1992).

OA1. Ocular albinism most typically is inherited as an X-linked recessive tract and is termed Nettleship–Falls type; the prevalence is approximately one in 50 000 population. Males are photophobic with reduced acuity, nystagmus, iris transillumination defects (Fig. 38.4), foveal hypoplasia, and sparse retinal pigment epithelium (RPE); their skin may be hypopigmented. The visual acuity is usually 6/60 or better, with some children achieving 6/9 by their teenage years. Carrier females demonstrate partial iris slit defects (Fig. 38.5), and RPE disturbances peripherally (Fig. 38.6) which take on a characteristic mosaic pattern (Green 1985; Charles *et al.* 1993). Histologically, macromelanosomes have been demonstrated in the iris, ciliary and RPE as well as in skin biopsy of the carrier females (O'Donnell *et al.* 1976). Ocular albinism must be suspected

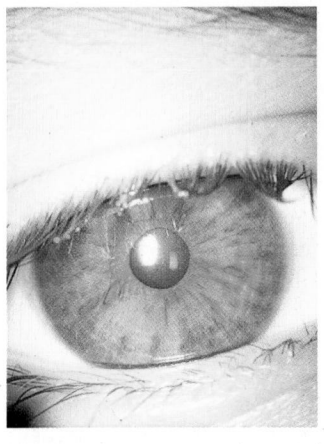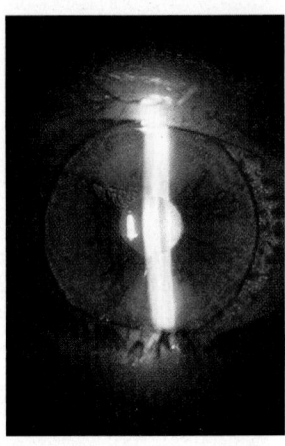

a   b

Fig. 38.4 X-linked ocular albinism in a child of Indian origin who presented with nystagmus and poor vision. (a) Showing a brown iris, but (b) marked transillumination.

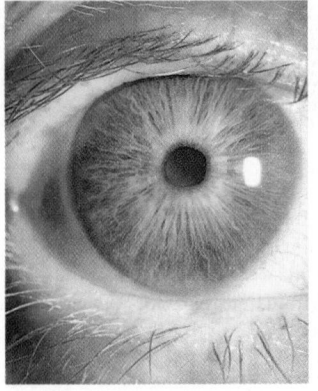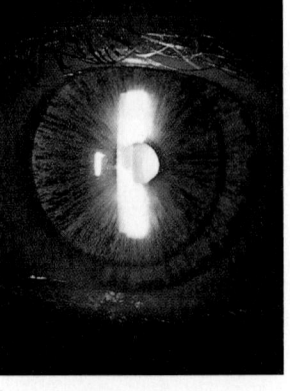

a   b

Fig. 38.5 (a) Female carrier of ocular albinism showing the iris in direct illumination. (b) The iris is transilluminant on retroillumination.

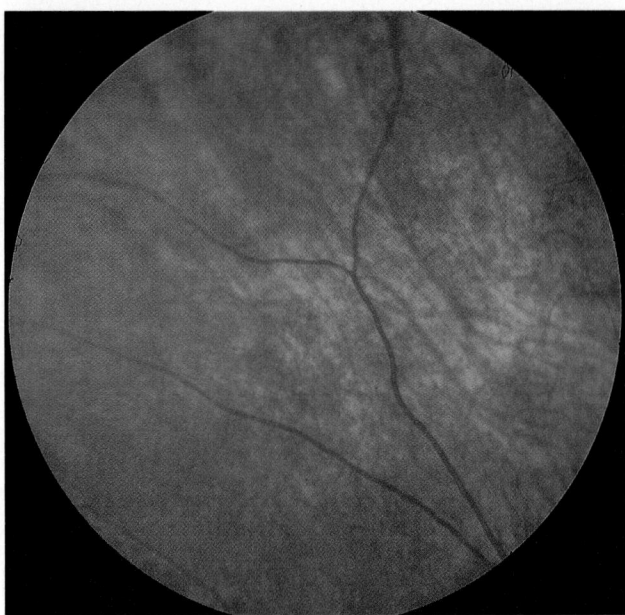

Fig. 38.6 Female carrier of X-linked ocular albinism showing the peripheral retina with mottled areas of hypopigmentation.

in any child with unexplained congenital nystagmus, even in darkly pigmented races (O'Donnell *et al.* 1978; Shiono *et al.* 1995). In one series, 20% of cases of X-linked ocular albinism had been diagnosed as having idiopathic congenital nystagmus (Charles *et al.* 1993). The OA1 gene is at Xp22.3–22.2 (Bassi *et al.* 1995).

AROA. An autosomal recessive ocular albinism has been described; some of these cases may be mild cases of oculo-cutaneous albinism (Fukai *et al.* 1995).

Aland island eye disease. This is an X-linked recessive condition, also known as Forsius–Eriksson albinism, with some features of ocular albinism, night-blindness, mild red–green colour blindness and myopia but no evidence of mis-routeing of the visual pathways and the electroretinogram is abnormal with a reduced B wave (see Chapter 44). It may be identical with incomplete congenital stationary night-blindness (Hawksworth *et al.* 1995).

Oculocutaneous albinism

Patients with oculocutaneous albinism may be 'complete' or 'incomplete', correlating to tyrosinase-negative and tyrosinase-positive hairbulb diagnostic testing.

OCA1a. Tyrosinase-negative albinos have the classical clinical picture of steely white hair, pink skin that is sensitive to sunburn, poor vision, nystagmus and pink or pink–blue eyes. Visual acuity is 2/60–6/36. It is associated with one of a variety of deletions in the large tyrosinase

gene (Giebel *et al.* 1991b) at 11q14–21. If both alleles are affected the clinical picture of OCA1a results.

OCA1b. These albinos have hair that is white at birth which becomes yellow with time, and the skin becomes pigmented. Affected patients are allelic for mutations in the tyrosinase gene (Giebel *et al.* 1991b).

OCA1ts. Siamese cats are albinos who have a thermolabile abnormal tyrosinase (Giebel *et al.* 1991a). A human equivalent has been described with yellow hair and pigmented hair on the extremities (King *et al.* 1991).

OCA2. Affected individuals have a similar phenotype to OCA1, but they have more pigment, and are tyrosinase-positive, and usually have better vision. The tyrosinase gene is normal and the deletions that give rise to the phenotype of OCA2 are in the P gene at 15q11–q13 (Durham-Pierre *et al.* 1994); uniparental deletions at this site or disomic cells are also present in patients with hypopigmentation in the Prader–Willi and Angelman syndromes.

OCA3. The first case described was of an African–American boy who was lightly pigmented and had abnormalities of tyrosinase-related protein 1 (TRP1).

ADOCA. The status of apparently dominantly inherited oculocutaneous albinism is not clear. Cases all have skin hypopigmentation, and may have iris transillumination.

Albinism with systemic disease

Chediak–Higashi syndrome. Infants with albinism and repeated infections may have the Chediak–Higashi syndrome (Bedoya *et al.* 1969). It is a rare autosomal recessively inherited multi-organ disorder which, apart from incomplete or partial oculocutaneous albinism, manifests with a proneness to recurrent bacterial infections of the skin and respiratory tract, and a mild bleeding diathesis, as well as hepatosplenomegaly and peripheral and cranial neuropathies. The pathogenesis is unknown but results in accumulation of giant lysosomes within granulocytes (Nathan 1992). Histologically, the melanocytes contain giant melanosomes that prevent the even distribution of melanin and resultant hypopigmentation.

Hermansky–Pudlak syndrome. Patients with typical (OCA2) albinism but with easy bruisability may have the rare Hermansky–Pudlak syndrome (Summers *et al.* 1988), which is inherited as an autosomal recessive trait. The underlying disorder is a platelet dysfunction with accumulation of ceroid-like pigment within leucocytes and macrophages of the bone marrow (Lee *et al.* 1992). Other associations include pulmonary fibrosis and inflammatory bowel disease due to organ infiltration with the abnormal reticuloendothelial cells (Garay *et al.* 1979). The bleeding diathesis is correctable with 1-desamino-8-D-arginine-vasopressin (Nathan 1993). Although the diagnosis is suspected on clinical grounds, consultation with appropriate subspecialists is indicated.

Cross syndrome. Albinism with mental retardation and small eyes (Cross *et al.* 1967; Lerone *et al.* 1992); it is autosomal recessive.

Albinism and short stature. Albinism, microcephaly, short stature and dysmorphism (Bitoun & Morel-Charron 1990); it is autosomal recessive.

Albinism and cerebellar ataxia. Autosomal recessive (Skre & Berg 1974; Bamezai *et al.* 1987).

Albinism with clumps of black hair (Witkop 1985).

X-linked albinism and deafness. The gene locus is at Xq26.3–q27.1 (Shiloh *et al.* 1990).

Treatment

Treatment for the ocular involvement with albinism includes symptomatic relief of photophobia with a sun hat, tinted lenses and, for those with significantly reduced vision, low vision aids (O'Donnell 1984), the detection and correction of any significant refractive errors and the treatment of any underlying amblyopia. Partial occluder contact lenses and prosthetic scleral lenses for infants with albinism and aniridia have been recommended to reduce glare (Stone 1981), but the difficulties in their use often outweigh the benefits. Genetic counselling should be offered in all cases. Although many albinos need extra help with their education, and have some psychological problems, normal attainments can be achieved irrespective of the type of albinism (Fulcher *et al.* 1995).

Coloboma

See Chapter 50.

Congenital iris and ciliary body cysts

These occur when fluid fills an epithelium-lined cyst of the iris. The two types of cyst are iris stromal cysts (Figs 38.7, 38.8) and pigment epithelial cysts (Fig. 38.9). They consist of a squamous epithelial or neuroepithelial lining, respectively (Naumann & Rummelt 1990; Paridaens *et al.* 1992; Brooks *et al.* 1993) and are probably congenital in origin (Grutzmacher *et al.* 1987).

Iris stromal cysts occur on the anterior surface of the iris, and have a transparent wall with a visible vascular lining. Pigment epithelial cysts occur at or behind the

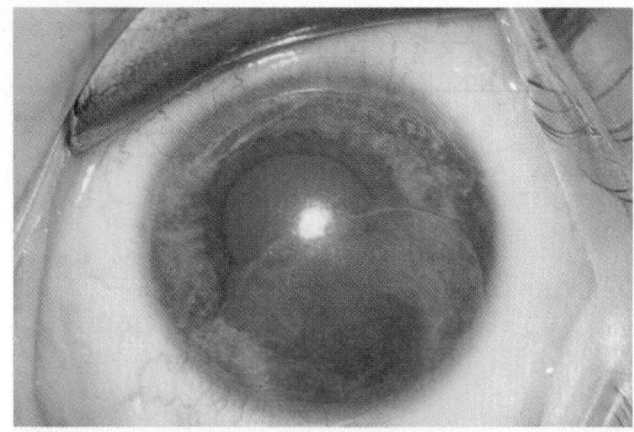

Fig. 38.7 Iris cyst. This stromal cyst recurred after local removal and eventually required a sector iridectomy.

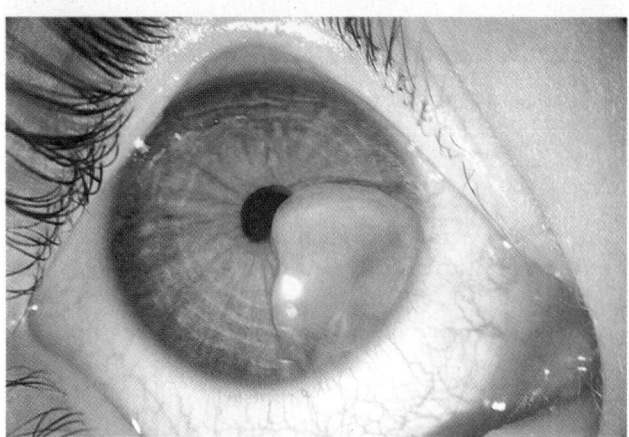

Fig. 38.8 Iris stromal cyst.

pupillary margin (Fig. 38.9) and have a non-transparent lining. If the size and location impairs the visual axis, surgical intervention may be necessary. Complications include glaucoma (Albert *et al.* 1992) and spontaneous detachment intraocularly (Watts & Rennie 1991). Iris pigment epithelial cysts are usually stationary (Shields *et al.* 1984).

Stromal cysts appear to enlarge progressively as they may recur if incompletely excised – a wide excision is recommended. Suggested treatments have included photocoagulation, injection of sclerosants (Capo *et al.* 1993) and radiation. However, surgical excision with sector iridectomy apparently gives best results (Naumann & Rummelt 1990). Pigment epithelial cysts often require no treatment, but may be treated by simple excision or puncture with a yttrium–aluminium–garnet (YAG) laser.

The differential diagnoses of iris cysts include secondary cyst formation from epithelial implantation due to surgery or penetrating trauma (Hoh *et al.* 1993), and solid iris or ciliary body tumours.

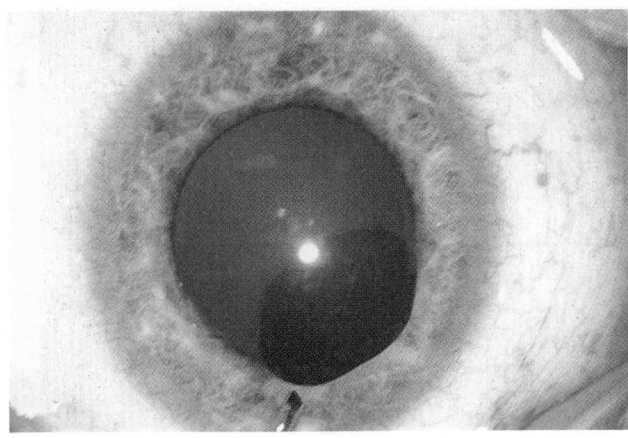

Fig. 38.9 Posterior iris cyst consisting of pigment epithelium. Cysts of this type tend not to recur after simple removal with a vitrectomy machine or puncture with a YAG laser.

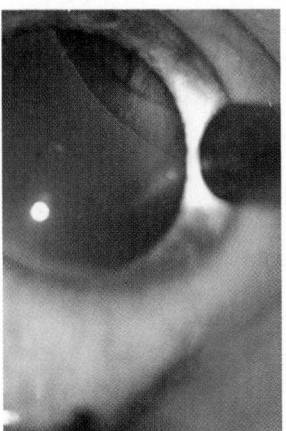
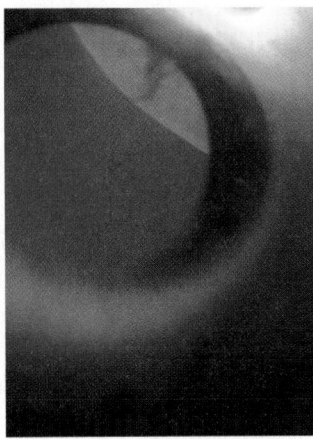

a,b

Fig. 38.10 (a) Ciliary body cyst in direct illumination. It appears brown and solid. (b) Ciliary body cyst in transillumination: it is semi-transparent and fluid filled.

Ciliary body cysts may cause astigmatism and amblyopia (see Fig. 38.10).

Brushfield's spots

These are typically found with Down's syndrome, occurring in 85% of people with trisomy 21 (Brushfield 1924). Donaldson (1961) found a 24% incidence in normal individuals; the spots were closer to the pupil margin, more numerous and distinct in Down's syndrome. He found no correlation with age or IQ. Histologically, the spots correlate with a normal to hypercellular area of iris tissue with surrounding relative stromal hypoplasia.

Persistent pupillary membranes

Persistent pupillary membranes represent an incomplete involution of the anterior tunica vasculosa lentis. The membranes are attached to the collarette (Fig. 38.11) and may be free floating, span the pupil to attach on its opposite side, or attach to the anterior surface of the lens (Figs 38.12, 38.13) with or without an associated cataract. They may bleed (Brusini & Beltrane 1983). Autosomal dominant inheritance has been reported (Merin *et al.* 1971). The membranes have been noted to occur in conjunction with other ocular anomalies including microcornea, megalocornea, microphthalmos and coloboma. (Waardenburg 1949; Cassady & Light 1957).

They may be substantial but even then may not impair vision (Mader *et al.* 1988). The vast majority of cases do not have visual consequences. However, there is a group which take on the appearances of a hyperplastic membrane (Jacobs *et al.* 1991). With these more extensive membranes (Fig. 38.14a), the red reflex may be altered, despite pharmacological dilation, and they may impair vision.

It is important to realize that the tunica vasculosa lentis does not normally involute until the beginning of the third trimester, and it may be seen in normal, but very premature babies (Fig. 38.14b,c).

The membranes may have fibrous remnants with extensive attachments to the lens (Fig. 38.15); surgical management has included attempts to improve vision with iridectomy, some of which have been unsuccessful (Levy 1957; Merin *et al.* 1971), removal of the membrane (Reynolds *et al.* 1983) and laser therapy to the persistent strands to the collarette (Kumar *et al.* 1994). On the whole, those pupillary membranes that require treatment respond to medical therapy alone, i.e. pupillary dilation and occlusion therapy (Miller & Judisch 1979).

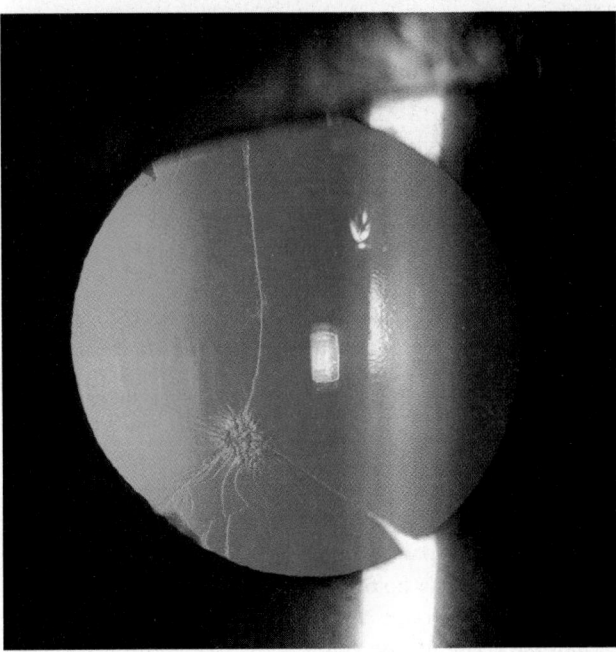

Fig. 38.11 Persistent pupillary membrane with vascularized attachments to the collarette and anterior to the lens.

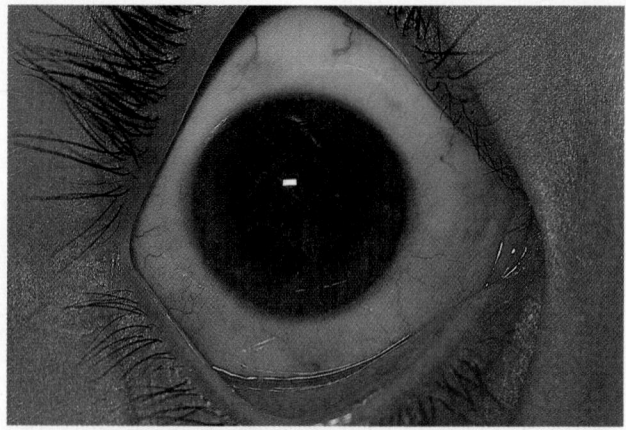

a

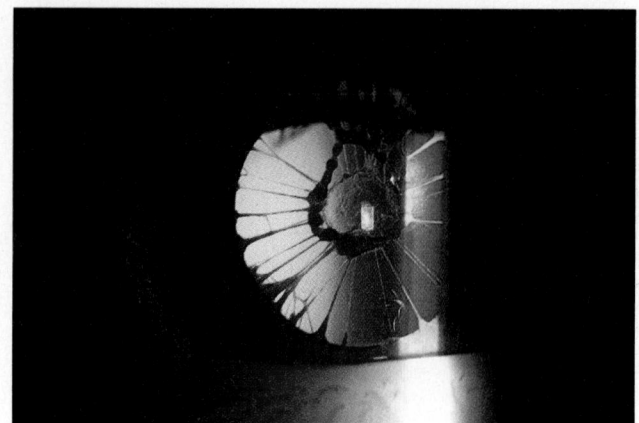

c

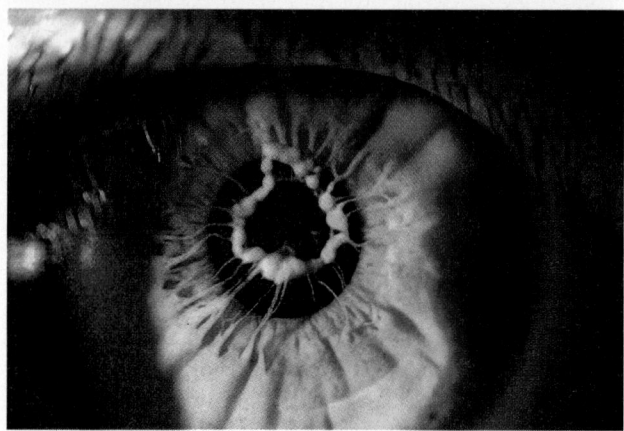

b

Fig. 38.12 (a) Hyperplastic persistent pupillary membrane. Dr John Crompton's patient. (b, c) Persistent pupillary membrane. The visual acuity was 6/12.

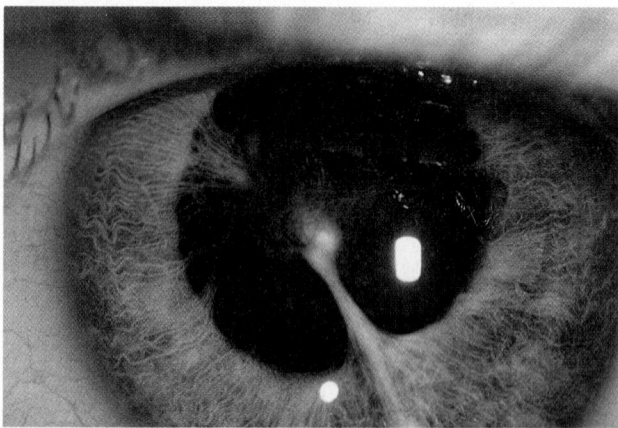

Fig. 38.13 Persistent pupillary membrane attached to the lens.

Congenital idiopathic microcoria

Microcoria is a small pupil with a diameter of less than 2 mm when the patient looks at a distant object (Duke-Elder 1964). It may be transmitted as an autosomal dominant trait (Toulemont *et al.* 1995). In this predominantly unilateral anomaly the pupil is microscopically small so that the pupil is nearly or actually obliterated (Fig. 38.16); it is often eccentric (Ackinson *et al.* 1994). It is probably

related to an abnormality of the development of the fetal pupillary membrane and its main effect is to cause amblyopia and put the eye at risk from glaucoma. An accurate refraction is essential as the condition is associated with myopia and astigmatism (Toulemont *et al.* 1995). Early surgical treatment and occlusion therapy can result in useful vision (Lambert *et al.* 1988).

Bilateral microcoria has been reported in association with microphthalmos and more posterior anomalies (Maden *et al.* 1991).

Aniridia

Aniridia represents a spectrum of disorders with iris hypoplasia. Its incidence has been estimated between 1 : 64 000 and 1 : 96 000 (Mollenbach 1947; Shaw *et al.* 1960). Both hereditary and sporadic forms exist. The usual mode of inheritance is as an autosomal dominant trait but autosomal recessive transmission is suggested in the rarer, Gillespie's syndrome, i.e. aniridia associated with mental retardation and cerebellar ataxia (Crawfurd *et al.* 1979). One-third of cases arise spontaneously and they may have the 11p13 deletion.

Aniridia may occur due to anomalous development of the neuroectoderm or neural crest cells (Spaeth *et al.* 1982).

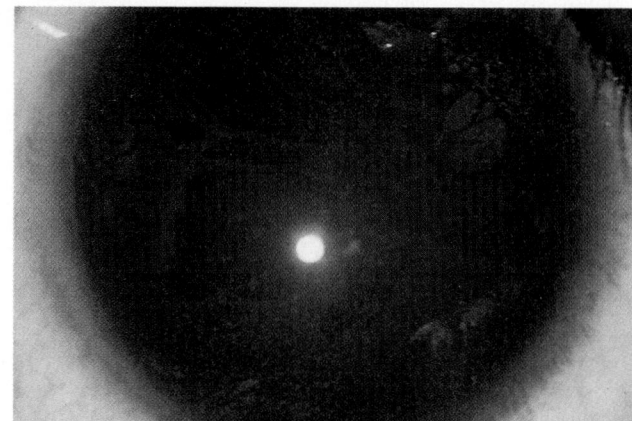

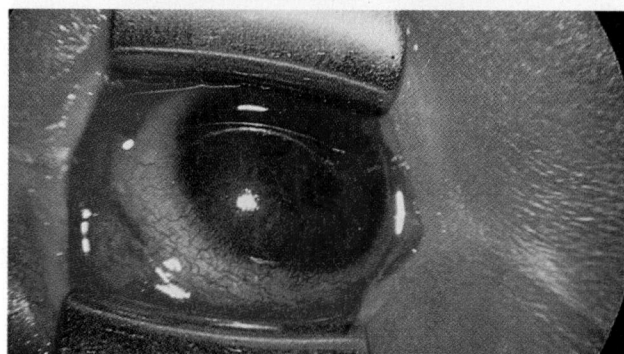

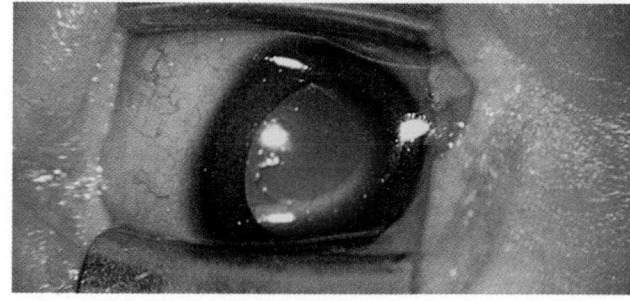

Fig. 38.14 (a) Marked persistent hyperplastic pupillary membrane. (b) Prominent tunica vasculosa lentis in a very premature baby. There is no haemorrhage. (c) Same patient as (b) 11 days later. A persistent tunica vasculosa lentis is barely visible, and disappeared to leave a perfectly normal eye. Mr Robert Morris' patient.

The neuroectoderm yields a developing optic cup rim at 12–14 weeks gestation (Mann 1964), whilst neural crest cells contribute to iris stroma formation during the second month of gestation. Aniridia has been produced experimentally in mice with maternal vitamin A deficiency (Warkany & Schraffenberger 1946; Kalter & Warkany 1959).

Histologically, the iris is reduced to a small stub (Fig. 38.17), and smooth muscle is usually absent. The angle may be poorly developed, and the retina may be present over portions of the pars plana and pars plicata of the ciliary body. Later changes include development of

peripheral anterior synechiae with corneal endothelial growth into the angle (Margo 1983). Other corneal irregularities include epithelial and Bowman's layer abnormalities (Margo 1983) and a thick fibrovascular pannus in patients with glaucoma (Mackman *et al.* 1979). The corneal pannus and conjunctivalization may represent a corneal epithelial stem cell deficiency (Nishida *et al.* 1995).

Aniridia is a bilateral condition but can show marked asymmetry between the two eyes in patients with a family

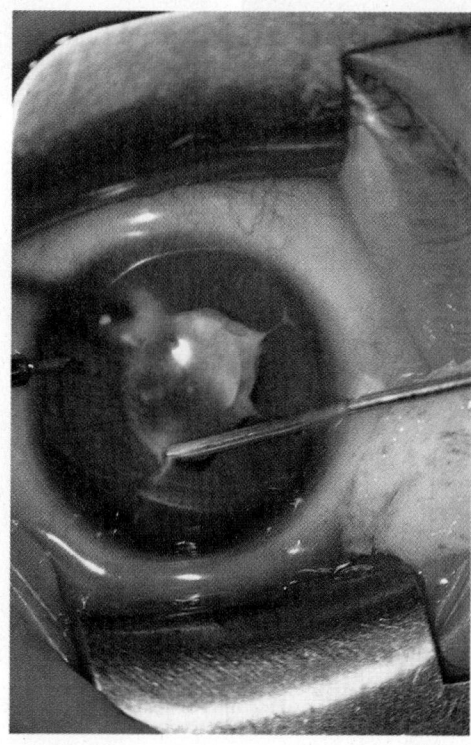

Fig. 38.15 Hyperplastic pupillary membrane stretching across the pupil attached to the collarette. It also involves the anterior capsule of the lens.

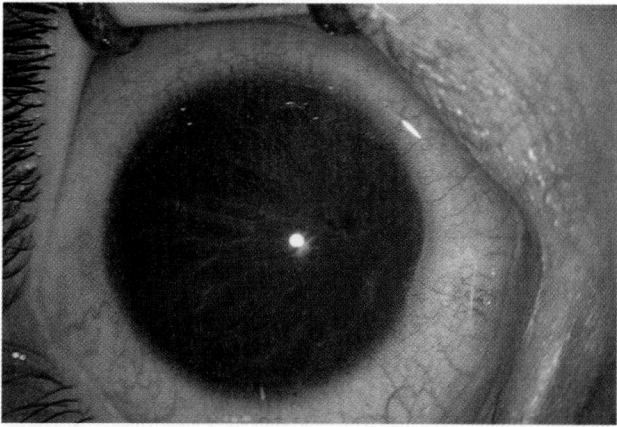

Fig. 38.16 Congenital idiopathic extreme microcoria. The pupil in this case was so small that the eye was potentially amblyopic and a pupil was created surgically.

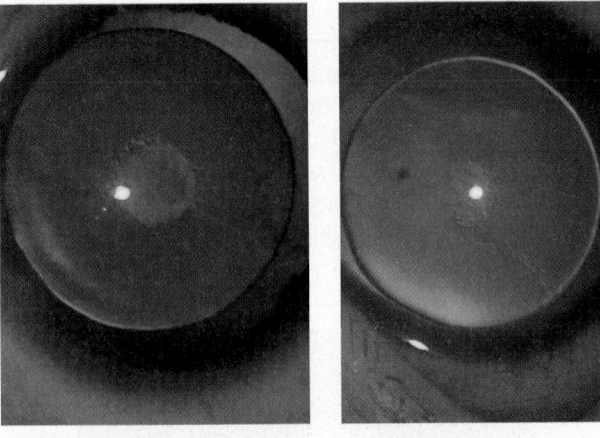

Fig. 38.17 Aniridia. No iris can be seen, revealing the zonules. There is a cataract in both eyes.

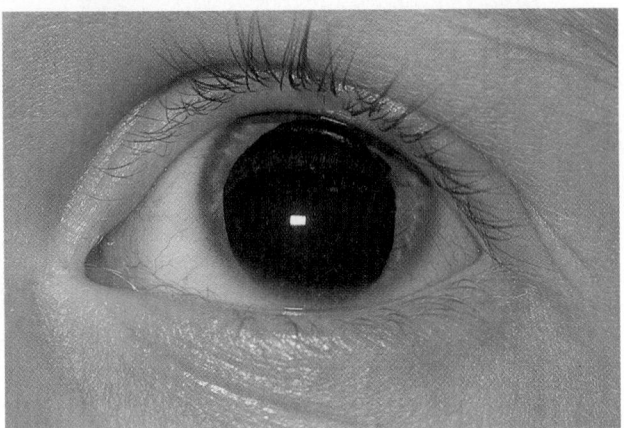

Fig. 38.18 Partial aniridia in a member of a dominant pedigree.

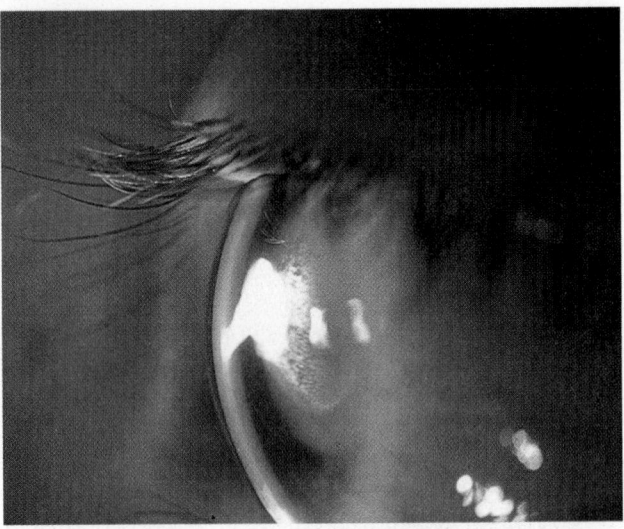

Fig. 38.19 Aniridia with a Peters' anomaly-like attachment of the cataractous lens to the posterior aspect of the cornea.

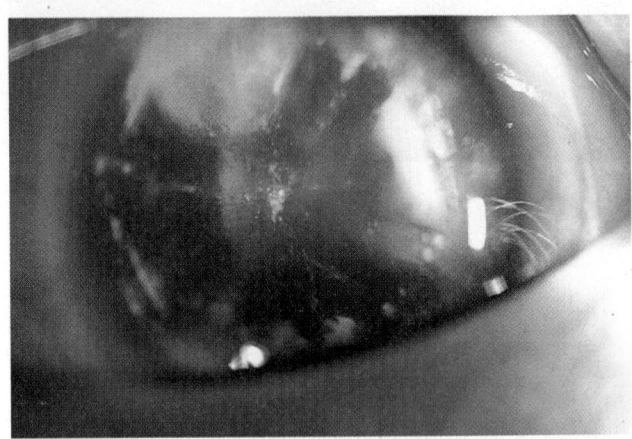

Fig. 38.20 Dominant aniridia with cataract, the onset of which was in the early teens.

history of aniridia. In the screening of other family members for evidence of aniridia, it is important to recognize the variable expressivity (Fig. 38.18) of this condition (Mintz-Hittner *et al.* 1992). Aniridia is not only associated with poor vision, glaucoma and cataract but also with systemic abnormalities. Decreased vision is usual, with multiple contributory factors including light scatter, corneal and lenticular opacities (Fig. 38.19), severe glaucoma, optic nerve hypoplasia, foveal hypoplasia and nystagmus. Pedigree studies have found approximately 60% with vision better than 6/9 (20/30) and 5% with vision worse than 6/60 (20/200) (Elsas *et al.* 1977; Hittner *et al.* 1980). Others have reported as high an incidence as 86% with vision 6/30 (20/100) or worse (Grove *et al.* 1961; Jesberg 1962). A lot of the variation in the various studies is accounted for by different inclusion criteria.

Although glaucoma is not typically present at birth, the incidence of childhood glaucoma has been reported between 6 and 75% (Grant & Walton 1974; Shaffer & Cohen 1975; Elsas *et al.* 1977; Walton 1979). The delay in the onset of glaucoma is probably due to progressive changes in the angle. The glaucoma is due either to angle anomalies leading to an open angle glaucoma or angle closure glaucoma from obstruction of the angle by the rudimentary iris stump (Nelson *et al.* 1984).

Cataract formation (Fig. 38.20) is present in 50–85% of patients by the age of 20 years (Layman *et al.* 1974; Elsas *et al.* 1977). The changes are usually progressive. Ectopia lentis (Fig. 38.21) may also occur in conjunction with aniridia (Callahan 1949; Shaw *et al.* 1960), due to an abnormality of the zonular structure (Nelson *et al.* 1984).

The corneal abnormalities are also progressive (Mackman *et al.* 1979); peripheral corneal epithelial irregularities spread to involve the entire cornea. Microcornea has also been reported in association with aniridia (David *et al.* 1978).

Optic nerve hypoplasia was found in nine of 12 patients by Layman *et al.* (1974), contributing to reduced vision.

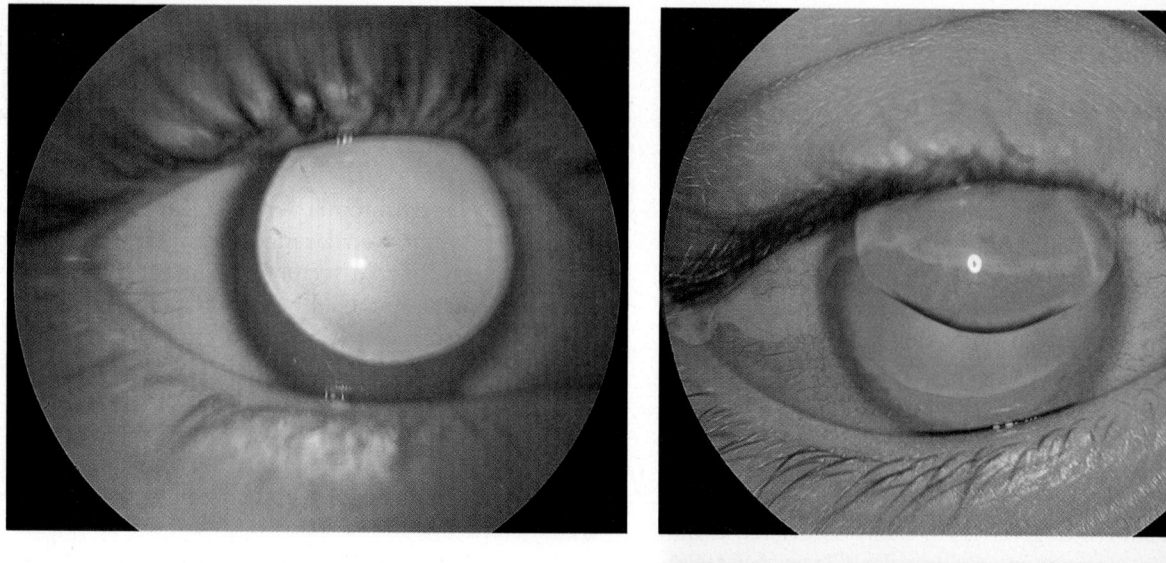

Fig. 38.21 (a) Aniridia showing the lens in transillumination on 1 November 1979. (b) Same patient. Aniridia showing the lens in retroillumination on 31 October 1985. There has been considerable subluxation. A cataract is now present and the eye is glaucomatous. (c) Same patient, 8 years later, showing peripheral corneal vascularization associated with a progressive dystrophy.

Aniridia with systemic disease

The WAGR syndrome (Wilms' tumour, aniridia, genitourinary abnormalities and mental retardation). Between one-quarter and one-third of children with sporadic aniridia will develop Wilms' tumour prior to 3 years of age (Flanagan & DiGeorge 1969; Pilling 1975; Francois *et al.* 1982). Frequently, mental retardation, genitourinary abnormalities, craniofacial abnormalities, microcephaly and growth retardation are also present. In the triad of aniridia, genitourinary abnormalities and mental retardation, in which an extensive deletion of the short arm of chromosome 11 has been demonstrated (Riccardi & Borges 1978), there is also a high incidence of bilateral Wilms' tumours (Garcia *et al.* 1976; Warburg *et al.* 1980).

There may be other systemic manifestations (Jotterand *et al.* 1990). Until the molecular genetic identification of the deletion is routinely available, patients with sporadic aniridia need to be screened for Wilms' tumour by abdominal palpation (this can also be done by the parents), or ultrasound studies every 3 months for 5 years.

Gillespie's syndrome. Aniridia with cerebellar ataxia and mental retardation (Gillespie 1965; Pendergrass 1976; Crawfurd *et al.* 1979; Wittig *et al.* 1988; Francois *et al.* 1983; Nevin & Lim 1990).

Aniridia in association with absent patellae (Mirkinson & Mirkinson 1975).

Dominant aniridia with ptosis, obesity and mental retardation (Hamming *et al.* 1986).

Aniridia, anophthalmos and microcephaly (Edwards *et al.* 1984). There may be some similarities between this condition and that of the case described by Glaser *et al.* (1994) suggesting PAX6 gene dosage effect in a child, both of whose parents had aniridia.

Gene mapping has supported the 11p13 deletion locus in patients with aniridia and Wilms' tumour. The majority of patients with the 11p13 deletion are sporadic. It now appears that chromosomes 1 and 2 do not play an important role in dominant congenital aniridia with linkage studies supporting the existence of a single map position for aniridia at the 11p13 position involving the PAX6 gene (Jordan *et al.* 1992; Glaser *et al.* 1994). PAX6 gene mutations have been shown to give rise to many associated ocular anomalies in conjunction with aniridia (Glaser *et al.* 1994).

Elevated intraocular pressure may be better tolerated in aniridic eyes (Callahan 1949; Nelson *et al.* 1984). When surgery is required, a higher percentage of patients require tube implantation (Wiggins & Tomey 1992).

Infants with aniridia and glaucoma may not have a normal Schlemm's canal, making goniotomy an unlikely choice for surgery (Callahan 1949; Barkan 1953). Walton (1979) advocated at least yearly gonioscopy to assess for the presence of increasing iris processes and angle closure with a view to prophylactic goniotomy. Laser trabeculoplasty is not helpful and trabeculectomy may be a better procedure in older patients (Nelson *et al.* 1984).

Cataract extraction in aniridia patients must also require extra preparation since the lens zonules do not support the lens in a normal fashion; the issue of intraocular lens implantation has met with some success (Johns & O'Day 1991) but, because of potential lens dislocation with time, intraocular lenses are probably not indicated in the young. Penetrating keratoplasty may help severe cases of associated corneal involvement but visual expectations must be limited. Corneal surgery in such patients has warranted caution due to the high rate of graft rejection (Kremer *et al.* 1993).

Optical correction of significant refractive errors, and a shift to an aphakic refractive error after lens subluxation may be of great help to some affected children. Even though the 'pupil' is large, cycloplegic agents must be used for refraction in young patients since active accommodation is present. The use of occluder contact lenses with a pupillary aperture has been advocated for infants (Stone 1981) but is not warranted in most cases.

Heterochromia iridis

A difference in iris colour can be congenital or acquired, the abnormal eye being either darker or lighter than the other eye, and it may be difficult to decide which is the abnormal eye. Skin pigmentation, parental eye colour, assessment of earlier photographs and the history usually resolve this question.

Congenital

Congenital heterochromia with the involved iris being darker, may point to ocular melanocytosis or oculodermal melanocytosis, or to a sector iris hamartoma syndrome. An iris pigment epithelial hamartoma creates a jet-black superficial lesion which consists of iris pigment epithelium with clumped smooth muscle cells and melanocytes (Jakobiec *et al.* 1975a; Quigley & Stanish 1978).

Horner's syndrome. Congenital Horner's syndrome results in ipsilateral hypopigmentation, miosis and ptosis (see Chapter 59).

Waardenburg's syndrome. Waardenburg's syndrome is transmitted as an autosomal dominant trait. There are two clinical types. Type 1 (Fig. 38.22) includes lateral displacement of the inner canthi, prominent root of the nose and unusual brows. Type 2 (Fig. 38.23) does not include the facial dysmorphism. Both clinical types include sensorineural deafness, a white forelock and heterochromia iridis. Fundus pigmentary heterochromia may also be present. Type 1 is caused by a mutation in the PAX3 gene located on chromosome 2q35 (Tassabehji *et al.* 1993). More recently type 2 Waardenburg's syndrome has been isolated to 3p12–p14.1, close to the homologue of the microphthalmia gene (Hughes *et al.* 1994).

Iris sector heterochromia and Hirschsprung's disease. A similar autosomal recessive syndrome is iris sector heterochromia (Fig. 38.24) and Hirschsprung's disease (Brazel *et al.* 1992), which may represent a neural crest cell lineage abnormality; such a finding must be relayed to the primary care physician (Liang *et al.* 1983).

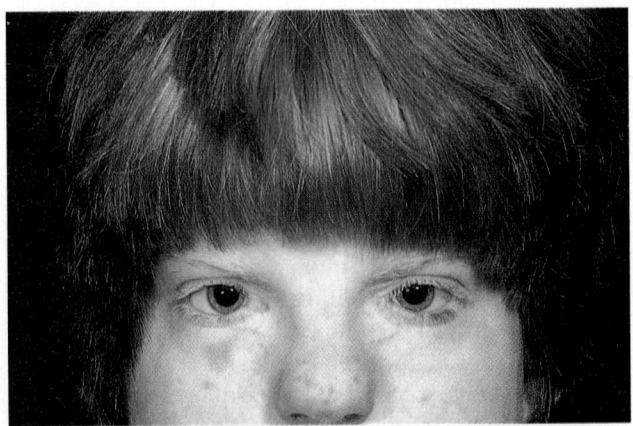

Fig. 38.22 Waardenburg's syndrome type 1 showing poliosis, lateral displacement of the inner canthi and a prominent root of the nose.

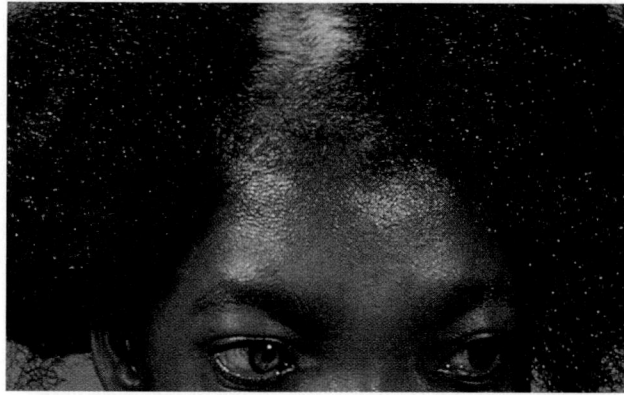

Fig. 38.23 Waardenburg's syndrome type 2 showing heterochromia and white forelock. Dr Dai Stephens' patient.

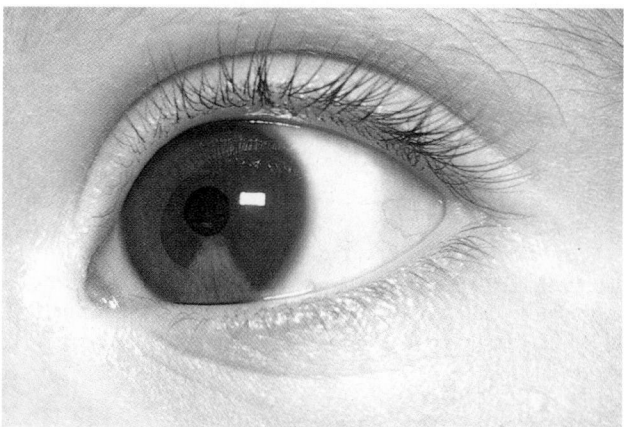

Fig. 38.24 Iris sector hypopigmentation.

Williams' syndrome

Williams' syndrome is a rare autosomal dominantly inherited disorder that has the general features of aortic valvular disease, hypercalcaemia, physical and developmental delay, elfin or pixie-like facial features with prominent lips, hyperacusis and a predisposition to developing otitis media (Morris *et al.* 1988; Klein *et al.* 1990). Ophthalmic involvement comprises a typical iris pattern (Fig. 38.26) which takes on a stellate appearance (Jensen *et al.* 1976; Holmstrom *et al.* 1990). Other ocular features include strabismus, mainly esotropia, hypermetropia and retinal vessel tortuosity (Greenberg & Lewis 1988; Morris *et al.* 1988; Kapp *et al.* 1995).

Iris ectropion and flocculi

When the posterior pigment epithelium of the iris extends onto the front of the iris it is known as ectropion uveae or,

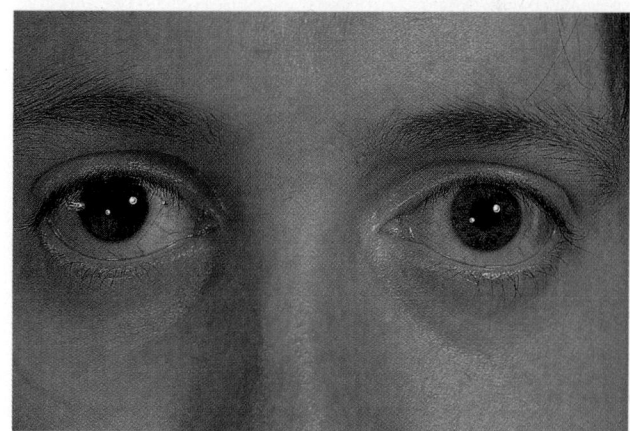

Fig. 38.25 Iris heterochromia due to an extensive naevus of the right iris.

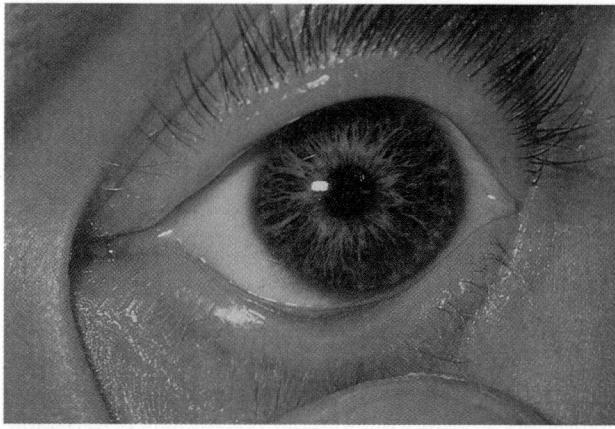

Fig. 38.26 Williams' syndrome showing the characteristic stellate iris pattern.

Acquired

Acquired heterochromia with the involved iris darker results from infiltrative processes — such as naevi (Fig. 38.25) and melanomatous tumours—and deposition of material within the iris.

Siderosis results from iron deposition within the dilator muscles of the iris (Burger & Klintworth 1974). Heterochromia may be the presenting feature of an intraocular foreign body, which may only be found on a computed tomography (CT) scan (Barr *et al.* 1984). Haemosiderosis results from deposition of iron derived from blood products, as in heterochromia from long-standing hyphaema (Sugar *et al.* 1967; Winter 1967).

With an acquired lighter coloured iris, Fuchs' heterochromic iridocyclitis must be strongly considered (see below); more rarely infiltrations such as juvenile xanthogranuloma, metastatic malignancies and leukaemia can be responsible. Acquired Horner's syndrome early in the first year of life can also lead to heterochromia.

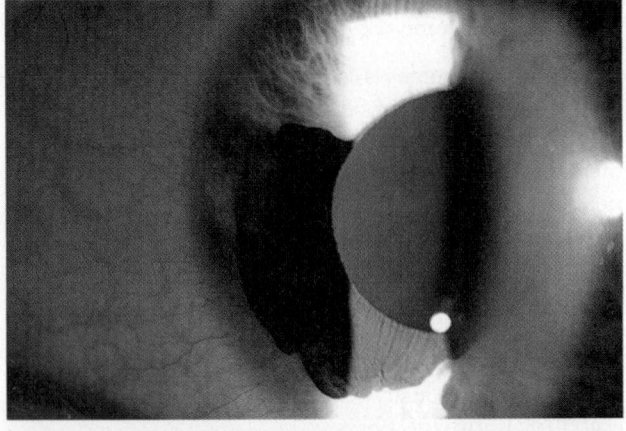

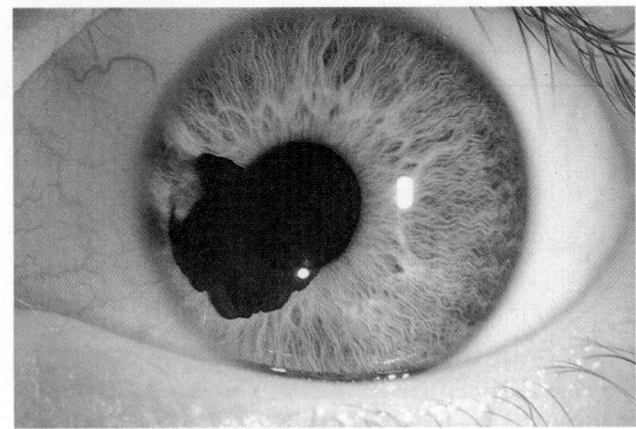

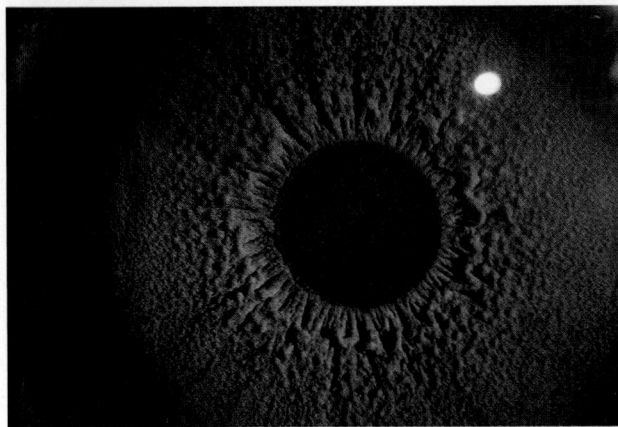

Fig. 38.27 (a) Iris ectropion. The pupil functions were normal. (b) Iris ectropion. (c) Iris mamillations. Patient of Dr A.L. Murphree and Miss N. Ragge.

more correctly, as iris ectropion (Fig. 38.27). It may be congenital (Wilson 1990). It is sometimes associated with glaucoma (see Chapter 40), neurofibromatosis type 1 (NF1) or anterior segment dysgenesis. Iris flocculi are small excrescences of pigment epithelium at the pupil margin; whilst normally isolated and of no significance, they may act as a marker for familial aortic dissection (Lewis & Merin 1995).

Uveal tumours

With the exception of iris naevi, tumours involving the uveal tract are rare in children. Presentation of tumours may be as heterochromia, glaucoma, hyphaema or decreased vision, with or without squint in the case of more posterior masses.

Iris naevi and freckles

Iris naevi consist of localized nests of melanocytes which vary in size and shape: spindle (the most common), epitheloid and polyhedral. They are common and their association with posterior choroidal melanomas is debatable (Michelson & Shields 1977). Rarely, involvement of angle structures can lead to glaucoma (Nik *et al.* 1981). Glauco-

ma has also been described in association with an aggressive form of iris naevi in children (Carlson *et al.* 1995). Iris naevi may also create an irregular pupil, be associated with a sectoral cataract, or seed into the anterior chamber. None of these has any prognostic significance, as iris naevi are benign (Shields 1983).

Iris naevi should be distinguished from iris freckles, which are on the anterior surface of the iris without altering the iris structures. Histologically, iris freckles are a cluster of normal iris melanocytes.

Iris melanosis and iris mamillations

Iris melanosis is a condition in which the iris is hyperpigmented. It is commonly associated with scleral pigmentation and choroidal hyperpigmentation; the surface of the iris is smooth. It may be familial, occurring in sibships (Joondeph & Goldberg 1989) or as an autosomal dominant trait.

Iris mamillations (Fig. 38.27c) are villiform protuberances that can cover much of the anterior surface of the iris and are sometimes associated with an iris naevus (Ragge *et al.* 1996).

The incidence of glaucoma in both conditions is uncertain, but affected people should be followed for life.

Cogan–Reese syndrome

In the Cogan–Reese syndrome, a unilateral iris naevus occurs with peripheral anterior synechiae in young people with ocular hypertension.

Iris and choroidal melanoma

These are uncommon in children (Verdager 1965). Iris melanomas are relatively non-aggressive (Ashton 1964; Arentson & Green 1975; Jakobiec & Silbert 1981), and all melanomas are rare in black people (Arentson & Green 1975). Iris melanomas present 10–20 years earlier than choroidal melanomas due to their visibility (Friedenwald *et al.* 1952). Whereas less than 10% of all malignant melanomas in the general population arise in the iris, 40–50% of such tumours arise in the iris in patients 29 years of age or younger (Apt 1963; Nicholson & Green 1981). In Shields' series, 12% of malignant uveal tumours arose from the iris in patients under 20 years of age (Shields *et al.* 1991).

Iris melanomas have a strong bias for presentation inferiorly (Cleasby 1958; Arentson & Green 1975). Due to their vascularity, their presentation may be as a hyphaema (Arentson & Green 1975).

Iris melanoma differs histologically from that of ciliary body and choroidal melanomas; approximately 60% are spindle cell, 33% are mixed cell and the remainder epitheloid. Only the spindle cell type behaves in a malignant fashion. A more detailed histological classification has been made by Jakobiec and Silbert (1981) which includes their view of appropriate treatment. The benign and malignant characteristics have been reviewed by Kersten *et al.* (1985).

The differential diagnoses of iris melanomas include juvenile xanthogranuloma (Ferry 1965), iris rhabdomyosarcoma (Naumann *et al.* 1972), iris foreign body (Ferry 1965), segmental melanosis oculi (Ferry 1965), iris abscess (Gass 1973), and Fuchs' adenoma in adults (Zaidman *et al.* 1983). Differentiation must also be made from a ciliary body mass since the prognosis differs for this location (Jakobiec & Silbert 1981; Engel *et al.* 1982; Hill *et al.* 1991).

Uveal melanomas are exceedingly rare during childhood, with two-thirds of enucleation specimens coming from people of 50 years of age or older (Paul *et al.* 1962). Childhood uveal melanomas represent between 0.6 and 1.1% of all patients with uveal melanoma (Paul *et al.* 1962; Shields *et al.* 1991). Two cases reports exist of a uveal melanoma in neonates (Fig. 38.28) (Greer 1966; Broadway *et al.* 1991) both with infants having multiple skin naevi. The slow growth of these tumours may account for their relatively late presentation due to refractive changes and lens distortion, narrowed anterior chamber, prominent episcleral vessels and slightly reduced intraocular pres-

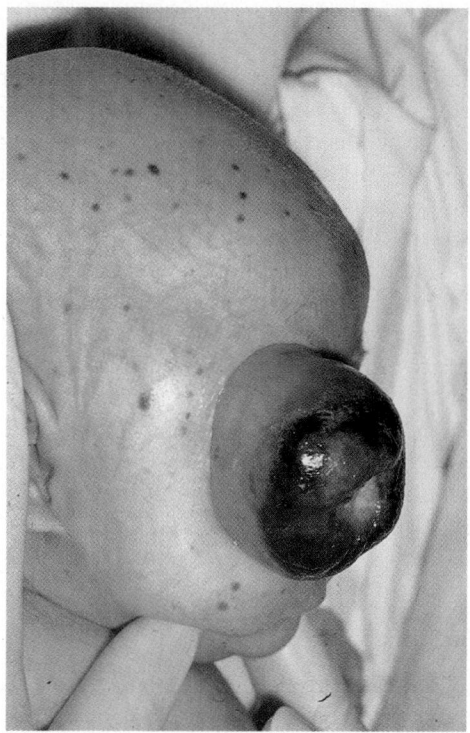

Fig. 38.28 Congenital malignant melanoma. This child was born with disseminated melanoma with the eye expanded at birth. She was still alive at follow-up 5 years later (Broadway *et al.* 1991).

sure (Foos *et al.* 1969). Later, extension into the anterior chamber, cataracts and glaucoma may be the presenting features.

Choroidal melanomas are rare in childhood but failure to consider this diagnosis may lead to a delay in treatment (Leonard *et al.* 1975; Apt 1963). There have been two reports of this tumour in two 5-year-old children (Rosenbaum *et al.* 1988). An extensive review by Shields *et al.* (1991) of 40 patients less than 20 years of age demonstrates the need to consider this rare but potentially fatal tumour. The differential diagnoses include choroidal naevi, which are characterized as having a diameter of 7 mm or less, an elevation of 2 mm or less, overlying drusen in older patients, and sparse lipofuscin; they are asymptomatic and have no or slow growth. Choroidal naevi may give rise to malignant melanoma (Nicholson & Green 1981). Photographic documentation with careful follow-up is appropriate.

Childhood uveal malignant melanomas do not seem to have a poorer prognosis than adult tumours (Barr *et al.* 1981): the 5-year mortality rate was 25% in one series of 42 patients. A more recent review has shown 5-year survival rates to be 96% (Shields *et al.* 1991). Poorer prognostic indicators include extraocular extension at the time of diagnosis, base diameter greater than 10 mm, and mixed or epitheloid cell type (Barr *et al.* 1981).

Although the enucleation of eyes with suspected malignant melanomas is controversial in adults (Apple & Blodi 1980; Zimmerman & McLean 1980), Nicholson and Green (1981) favour early enucleation in children when unequivocal growth is documented since the expected lifespan is greater, and since they have experienced failure of long-term success with irradiation of a childhood tumour.

Certain congenital disorders are felt to predispose to uveal melanomas. In addition to previously mentioned choroidal melanomas (Yanoff & Zimmerman 1967; Naumann *et al.* 1971), neurofibromatosis may be associated with a greater number of melanocytic naevi and of uveal melanomas (Yanoff & Zimmerman 1967).

Although familial occurrences of malignant melanoma are known (Walker *et al.* 1979), the inverse relationship with skin pigmentation has been much more apparent to clinicians (Scotto *et al.* 1976; Albert *et al.* 1980; Casswell *et al.* 1989).

Medulloepithelioma

Medulloepithelioma is usually a unilateral, solid or cystic tumour of the ciliary body non-pigmented epithelium; it is a congenital lesion derived from embryonic retina which occasionally includes cartilage, brain, striated muscle and other elements and are called teratomedulloepitheliomas. Ordinarily they are comprised of membranes, tubules and rosettes. The arrangement of such networks accounts for their initial designation by Fuchs (1908) as dictyomas. They may undergo malignant transformation (Zimmerman & Broughton 1978). Other structures such as the optic nerve may rarely be involved (Green *et al.* 1974).

They usually present within the first decade as a visible iris tumour, leukocoria, abnormally shaped pupil, glaucoma, hyphaema or decreased vision with or without strabismus (Apt *et al.* 1973). The average age at enucleation is 5 years (Zimmerman & Broughton 1978). Two-thirds showed malignancies and metastases occur frequently. Extraocular extension at the time of enucleation was the most important prognostic indicator with an excellent prognosis for tumour confined to the eye. Other series have implied a more benign nature (Canning *et al.* 1988).

Occurrence with other tumours has been reported including retinoblastoma and pinealoblastoma (Mamalis *et al.* 1992; Minoda *et al.* 1993).

Enucleation is the recommended treatment unless well localized anteriorly, when local excision or cryotherapy may play a role (Jakobiec *et al.* 1975b; Zimmerman & Broughton 1978). The differential diagnoses include juvenile xanthogranuloma and retinoblastoma, but the cystic nature, the origin from the ciliary body, the rather felt-like appearance and the unilaterality speak heavily for medulloepithelioma (see Chapter 42).

Choroidal and iris haemangioma

Choroidal haemangiomas may be divided into diffuse and localized lesions. The localized form is a minimally growing lesion which is usually asymptomatic. They are characteristically orange–red in colour, located usually within two disc diameters of the optic disc (Anand *et al.* 1989). They may include both capillary and cavernous components. Superficial changes, including pigmentation (Anand *et al.* 1989), have resulted in a misdiagnosis with subsequent enucleation for malignant melanoma (Jones & Cleasby 1959; Witschel & Font 1976).

The diffuse choroidal haemangiomas (tomato ketchup fundus) are associated with Sturge–Weber syndrome and carry a risk of associated glaucoma (Susac *et al.* 1974). Episcleral vascular hamartomas may be the cause of the increased intraocular pressure (Phelps 1978).

Retinal detachment may also occur and laser treatment has been advocated for this (Shields 1983). Localized haemangiomas are associated with a poor visual prognosis with subfoveal involvement. Extrafoveal tumours may be associated with a better prognosis with usage of scatter photocoagulation. For small solitary tumours, radiotherapy, using a lens-sparing technique, may be indicated. No treatment is effective for diffuse or large solitary tumours.

Iris haemangiomas are rare lesions. They have been described as occurring in conjunction with a more generalized diffuse neonatal haemangiomatosis (Naidoff *et al.* 1971; Weiss & Ernest 1976). They have also been reported in association with infants who have more typical lid haemangiomas (Ruttum *et al.* 1993).

Uveal adenoma and adenocarcinoma

Rare cases of adenomas involving the iris (Rennie *et al.* 1992) and ciliary body (Campochiaro *et al.* 1992) have been reported. Adenomas and adenocarcinomas of the iris and ciliary body may arise from the pigmented (Papale *et al.* 1984) or non-pigmented ciliary epithelium.

Adenocarcinoma of the ciliary non-pigmented epithelium in children has been documented following ocular trauma (Margo & Brooks 1991).

Choroidal osteoma

Choroidal osteomas, though typically unilateral, rarely present bilaterally (Noble 1990). The clinical presentation and course may vary (Eting & Savir 1992). They are a benign ossifying tumour of the choroid which is typically found in the peripapillary region (Fig. 38.29). There is a suggestion that the tumour tendency may be inherited as an autosomal dominant trait (Cunha 1984; Noble 1990). The exact pathogenesis is unclear. They may represent a choristoma, i.e. a primary congenital tumour of an embryonic tissue nest, or may represent a secondary calcification

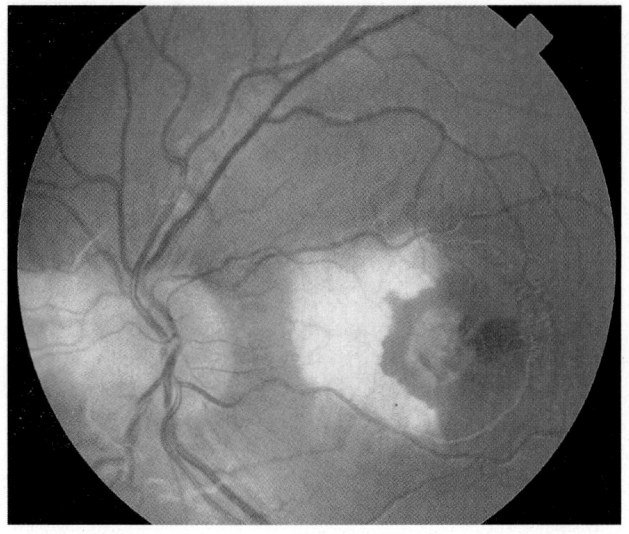

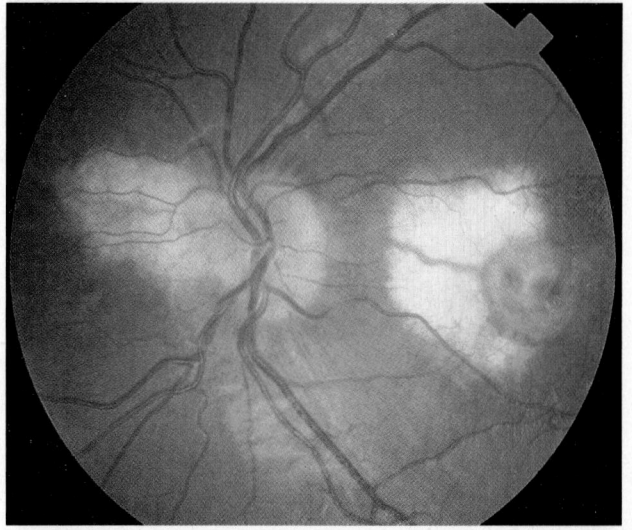

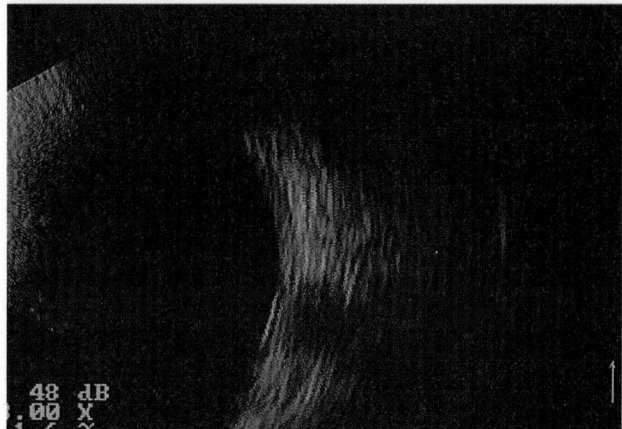

Fig. 38.29 (a) Choroidal osteoma with submacular haemorrhage. The acuity had deteriorated to 6/60. (b) Same patient 1 year later when the acuity was 6/24. (c) Same patient. Ultrasound showing increased echoes from the osteoma.

of an area affected by inflammatory disease or trauma (Fig. 38.30) (Katz & Gass 1983; Trimble & Schatz 1983). Clinically, choroidal osteomas are yellow–white in colour. B-scan ultrasonography confirms the presence of calcification. These tumours may not exhibit any growth. Complications include visual loss secondary to extension of the osteoma onto the foveal region, subretinal neovascular membrane formation and exudative retinal detachment (Avila *et al.* 1984; Grand *et al.* 1984; Eting & Savir 1992).

Iris rhabdomyosarcoma

This rare mass has been described as a light fleshy tumour of the iris (Elsas *et al.* 1991).

Juvenile xanthogranuloma

See Chapter 33.

Lisch nodules and neurofibromatosis

See Chapter 28.

Leiomyoma

Leiomyomas of the iris and ciliary body are benign slow-growing tumours of smooth muscle. They are rare tumours that are more prevalent in females.

Iris leiomyomas take on a pale or pink appearance and are well-circumscribed lesions. The presenting features may include pupillary distortion, hyphaema, with complications of secondary glaucoma and cataract formation (de Buen *et al.* 1971).

Ciliary body lesions may present as a result of enlargement onto adjacent structures. The increasing mass can result in iris distortion, secondary local cataract formation or glaucoma from angle occlusion (Meyer *et al.* 1968).

The appearances of both iris and ciliary body leiomyomas are indistinguishable from melanoma. It has been suggested that many previously diagnosed leiomyomas may in fact be melanocytic lesions (Foss *et al.* 1994). The tumours may not enlarge in size. If there is definite evidence of enlargement then surgical excision is indicated.

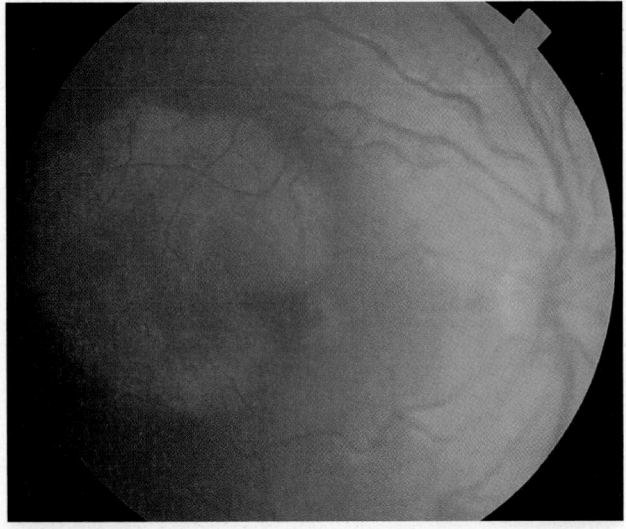

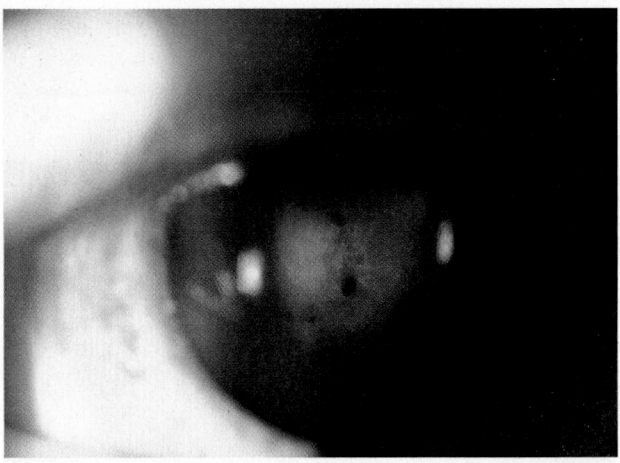

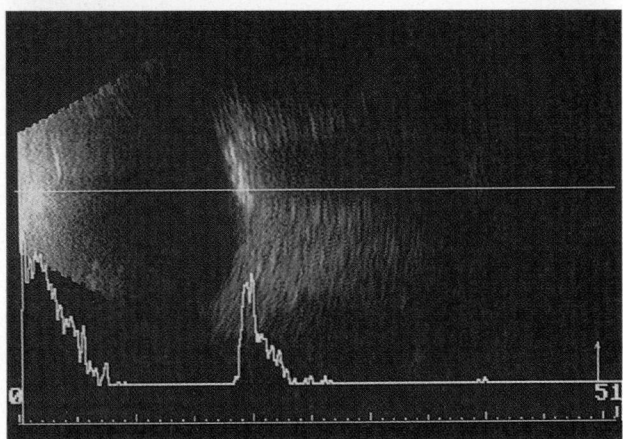

Fig. 38.30 Choroidal osteoma probably of traumatic origin. This unilateral lesion presented because of poor vision found at a routine school test. There was also a posterior subcapsular cataract (a) and the pale fundus lesion (b) had high echogenicity on ultrasound (c).

Other tumours

There have been sporadic reports of rare forms of uveal tumours both primary and secondary. These include haemangiopericytomas of the ciliary body (Brown *et al.* 1991), neuroblastoma of the choroid (Cibis *et al.* 1990) and choristoma of the iris and ciliary body (Shields *et al.* 1995).

Spontaneous hyphaema

Trauma is the leading cause of hyphaema and even when there is no history of trauma other signs of trauma, such as recessed angle or contralateral retinal haemorrhages, must be carefully sought. Non-accidental injury may also cause hyphaema.

Truly spontaneous hyphaemas can occur and indicate either underlying pathology of the uveal tract or a bleeding diathesis. Vascular tumours such as juvenile xanthogranuloma, medulloepithelioma, and retinoblastoma are important. Retinoschisis, retinopathy of prematurity, persistent hyperplastic primary vitreous, blood dyscrasias such as leukaemia, and postcontusion injury or postsurgical intervention have all been implicated (Howard 1962). In older children and adults, scurvy, purpura, severe iritis, rubeosis and migraine may also cause apparently spontaneous hyphaema (Doggart 1950).

Spontaneous hyphaemas deserve immediate concern about elevated intraocular pressure and corneal blood staining, but equal importance must be paid to determination of the underlying cause, including studies such as ultrasound and CT scanning. A careful general physical examination may reveal other clues, as might haematological screening for blood dyscrasias.

Uveal manifestations (non-inflammatory) of systemic disease

Direct leukaemic infiltration of the iris may lead to heterochromia, spontaneous hyphaema, glaucoma or hypopyon (Perry & Mallen 1979; Ninane *et al.* 1980; Kincaid & Green 1983; Schachat *et al.* 1988). However, a study of 657 children with leukaemia revealed only nine children with anterior segment abnormalities (Ridgeway *et al.* 1976).

Burkitt's lymphoma, with its close association with

Epstein–Barr virus, commonly affects children from tropical countries (Burkitt & O'Connor 1961). Although orbital involvement is most common, choroidal findings have been seen on postmortem cases (Green 1985). This tumour may gain further clinical significance since it has been reported in association with acquired immunodeficiency syndrome (Fujikawa *et al.* 1983). Although radiotherapy is most frequently used for localized tumour, favourable results may be given with the use of cyclophosphamide (Ziegler 1977).

Uveitic processes that fail to respond to routine therapy should raise the suspicion of other underlying pathological processes. Focal lesions giving rise to inflammatory diseases may include intraocular tumours, primary or secondary. Adjacent orbital inflammatory processes giving rise to a secondary uveitis, such as pseudotumours, may also need to be considered (Bloom *et al.* 1992).

Uveitis

Inflammation involving the uveal tract is called uveitis, with further differentiation based on the primary site of inflammation such as panuveitis, iritis, choroiditis, pars planitis, iridocyclitis or cyclitis.

Uveitis is felt to represent an inflammatory response to a noxious stimulant, be it biological or physical. Polymorphonuclear leucocytes and monocytes respond to the stimulant, and they release chemical factors which can either eliminate the agent, create further inflammatory response, or both (O'Connor 1983).

Uveitis may be classified on the basis of location, clinical characteristics of the inflammatory pathology, or related to the cause or severity and course. Smith and Nozik (1983) have offered a clinical approach which aids the diagnosis in 75–85% cases. Approximately 6% of all uveitis occurs in children. Juvenile rheumatoid and spondyloarthropathy associated uveitides account for the majority of paediatric uveitis (Tugal-Tutkun *et al.* 1996).

Although of no histopathological significance, the terms 'granulomatous' and 'non-granulomatous' may be used on the basis of the slit-lamp findings; in the former, symptoms are relatively mild and iris nodules as well as 'mutton fat' keratic precipitates (KPs) are present. In the latter, few KPs are present, and the symptoms are more severe, a fibrinous anterior chamber reaction may be present.

Acute anterior uveitis, non-specific features

The symptoms of pain, redness and photophobia may last days to weeks. Flare and cells are seen on slit-lamp biomicroscopy (Fig. 38.31) and cells may be deposited on the cornea as fine KP and on the lens. In severe inflammation vision is reduced (Fig. 38.32) and the eye may become hypotonic. When cells are present on slit-lamp examina-

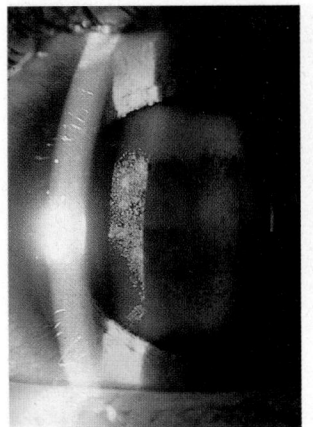
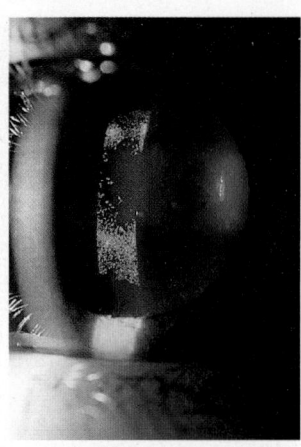
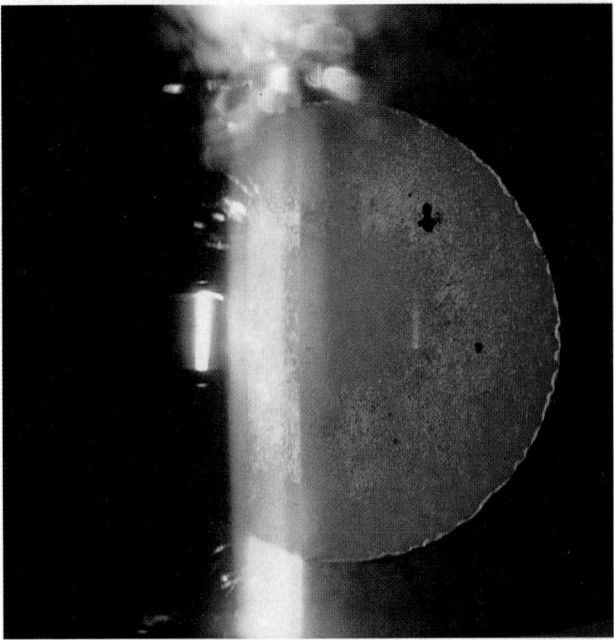

Fig. 38.31 (a) Acute anterior uveitis with fibrinous exudate on the anterior surface of the lens. (b) Acute anterior uveitis. There have been repeated attacks of acute iritis in this child and a cataract is present.

tion behind the lens, iridocyclitis is present. Slit-lamp examination should also be used to assess for corneal changes and iris transillumination defects which may be present with Fuchs' heterochromic cyclitis, and other uveitides especially varicella and traumatic uveitis.

Chronic anterior uveitis, non-specific features

This does not have severe symptoms although milder symptoms may be present for months to years. The anterior chamber cellular reaction is usually less, but flare is often prominent. Both granulomatous and non-granulomatous chronic iridocyclitis have KPs (Fig. 38.33). Synechiae, band keratopathy, secondary cataract and

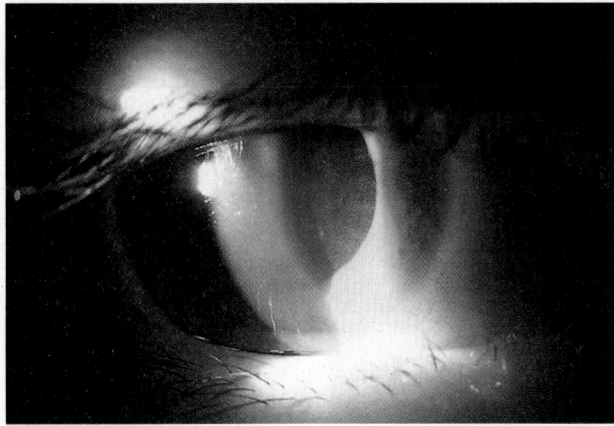

Fig. 38.32 Reiter's syndrome. There is acute uveitis and the eye is hypotonic.

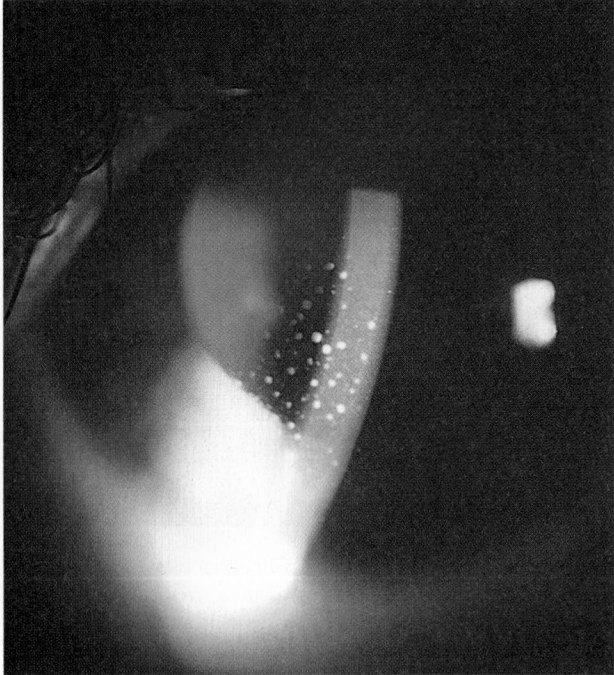

Fig. 38.33 Sarcoidosis showing 'mutton-fat' KP.

glaucoma are common and cystoid macular oedema and vitreous cells may cause decreased vision.

Specific causes of acute anterior uveitis

Traumatic acute anterior uveitis

Traumatic iridocyclitis is common in childhood. The history usually involves blunt injury to the eye. Symptoms include severe pain, photophobia and redness. It must be ascertained that pathology is limited to the anterior segment. If the iritis responds to cycloplegia with topical steroids, no further laboratory tests are necessary.

Infectious diseases

Iritis associated with childhood measles, mumps, chickenpox (Kachmer *et al.* 1990) or other viruses (Mochizuki *et al.* 1994) is typically a transient acute anterior uveitis, sometimes with keratitis. Rarer causes such as brucellosis (Gedalia *et al.* 1990), human T-cell leukaemia virus type 1 (HTLV-1) (Mochizuki *et al.* 1994) and cat-scratch disease (Golnick *et al.* 1994) have been documented in children. It has been suggested that the timing of the iritis may correspond to the viraemic phase of the illness (Edwards 1965).

Any childhood uveitis should be carefully assessed prior to the use of steroids as there may be a possible herpetic uveitis. Assessment of corneal sensitivity and the appearance of the conjunctiva are valuable clues. If herpes simplex is possible any steroid used must be covered with antiviral agents (Grayson 1983). Herpes simplex iridocyclitis may be associated with keratitis; corneal involvement is shown by fluorescein or rose Bengal staining but the iridocyclitis may recur without the corneal lesions (Hogan *et al.* 1963). Viral particles (Witmer & Iwamoto 1968) and herpes virus antigen (Patterson *et al.* 1968) have been isolated from the anterior chamber, suggesting a direct infection, but the inflammation could be due to hypersensitivity (Oh 1976).

Infectious mononucleosis has been associated with anterior uveitis as well as other forms of uveitis (Stevens *et al.* 1951; Martenet 1981).

Leprosy can present with many ocular signs. Acute iridocyclitis with keratitis occurs in the lepromatous form of the disease in the later stages, contributing significantly to blindness (Ticho & Ben-Sira 1970; Ffytche 1981).

Kawasaki's disease

Kawasaki's disease (Kawasaki *et al.* 1974; Tizard *et al.* 1991), or mucocutaneous lymph node syndrome, is a systemic vasculitis of unknown aetiology which mainly affects prepubescent children. There may be an HLA association with HLA-DR5 and HLA-A1 (Lapointe *et al.* 1982). It is characterized by an acute febrile illness with the following associations: (i) a high fever of greater than 4–5 days duration; (ii) stomatitis; (iii) palmar erythema and peripheral oedema; (iv) cervical lymphadenopathy; (v) erythema multiforme rashes; (vi) meningitis; (vii) uveitis; and (viii) myocarditis (Melish 1981). Approximately 15–20% of individuals develop secondary coronary or axillary artery aneurysms (Kato *et al.* 1975) with about a 3% mortality. Pericardial effusions are not uncommon (Tizard *et al.* 1991).

The major ocular involvement is a transient bilateral conjunctival hyperaemia without discharge in the first week of onset of the fever (Burke & Rennebohm 1981; Burns *et al.* 1985; Smith *et al.* 1989). The second most common ocular feature is an acute transient anterior uveitis seen in the acute phases of the illness (Burns *et al.* 1985). The majority of cases of uveitis are asymptomatic and self-limiting and only a few cases are severe enough to warrant topical steroidal therapy. Less common ocular findings include vitreous opacities and a mild vitritis and choroiditis (Jacob *et al.* 1982). Retinal ischaemia secondary to the vasculitis, optic nerve head oedema and a punctate keratopathy have also been documented (Font *et al.* 1983). Therapy involves a combination of high-dose aspirin and intravenous gammaglobulin which decreases the incidence of coronary complications (Newburger *et al.* 1986; Committee on Infectious Diseases 1988).

Lyme disease

Lyme disease has been associated with a host of ophthalmological manifestations, including uveitis and neuro-ophthalmic involvement (Orlin & Lauffer 1989; Kauffman & Wormser 1990; Lesser *et al.* 1990; Spalton 1990). The disease is caused by the spirochaete, *Borrelia burgdorferi*, and results in a multisystem disorder. It is spread by the tick, *Ixodes ricinus*, and is characterized by three phases: infection, dissemination and immunological reactions. The ocular features are uncommon apart from conjunctivitis and facial nerve palsy. Other ocular features include a chronic anterior uveitis, pars planitis, interstitial keratitis (Orlin & Lauffer 1989) and endophthalmitis (Kaufmann & Wormser 1990). The presence of a resistant pars planitis should prompt investigation for Lyme disease, which is readily treatable with intravenous antibiotics (Breeveld *et al.* 1993). The also has the neuro-ophthalmic manifestations of neuroretinitis, optic neuritis and ocular motor palsies (Lesser *et al.* 1990).

Systemic manifestations include a characteristic rash of erythema chronicum migrans, a radiculoneuropathy, dementia, myopathy, oligoarthropathy, meningitis and cardiac involvement.

Diagnosis is made through serological means using an enzyme-linked immunosorbent assay (ELISA) test or by direct culturing of the spirochaete.

Spondyloarthropathies

Ankylosing spondylitis

Ankylosing spondylitis is characterized by axial skeletal arthritis, but may present as a peripheral pauci-articular arthropathy (Calabro 1983). This peripheral arthropathy may precede the onset of the axial involvement by several years. There is a strong association with the histocompatibility antigen, HLA-B27, with approximately 90% of Caucasians and 50% of black patients with ankylosing spondylitis being positive. This compares with between 4 and 8% of the normal population. A similar relationship

exists with the other spondyloarthropathies. Ankylosing spondylitis is more prevalent in the male population and the mean age of onset in the paediatric age group is about 10 years.

Approximately 25% of patients with ankylosing spondylitis go on to develop an anterior uveitis. Cystoid macular oedema may limit vision in such patients (Belmont & Michelson 1982). Ocular involvement is often bilateral, and hypopyon, posterior synechiae, band keratopathy or secondary glaucoma may develop. Successful therapy includes intense topical steroids and mydriatics started early during each attack (Smith & Nozik 1983).

The course of the disease is somewhat different to juvenile rheumatoid arthritis in that patients with ankylosing spondylitis do not develop the chronic progressive form of iridocyclitis.

Reiter's syndrome

Reiter's syndrome is characterized by recurrent iridocyclitis (Fig. 38.32), mucosal mouth lesions (Fig. 38.34), polyarthritis which typically is a peripheral arthropathy, conjunctivitis, and urethritis in males older than 20 years. The iridocyclitis may be very severe with hypopyon and secondary degenerative ocular changes such as cataract and iris atrophy.

In children, the association with a urethritis is uncommon and occurs more in association with a cross-reactivity from bacterial infections of *Salmonella*, *Yersinia* and *Campylobacter* (Ostler *et al.* 1971).

Behçet's disease

Behçet's disease is an idiopathic, multisystem disorder of a vasculitic nature which is characterized by rash, usually erythema nodosum, arthritis, genital ulcerations and aphthous stomatitis. There is usually a very severe and refractory recurrent hypopyon iritis. It is rare in children, accounting for only two of 340 children with uveitis in a

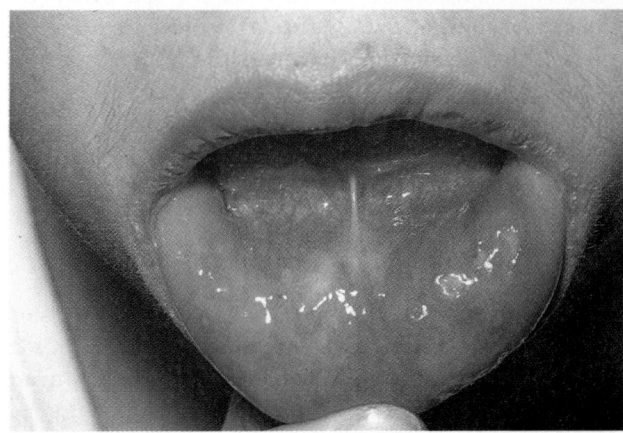

Fig. 38.34 Reiter's syndrome showing mucosal mouth lesions.

large series (Kanski & Shun-Shin 1984); it is most frequent in 20–40-year-olds (James & Spiteri 1982) with a male preponderance from Far Eastern and Mediterranean countries. Posterior segment involvement includes a retinal vasculitis with haemorrhage and vessel occlusions, exudates, exudative retinal detachments and papillitis. These patients require systemic immunosuppression with corticosteroids and/or chemotherapy.

Psoriatic arthritis

The characteristic feature of this spondyloarthropathy is that of a childhood onset arthritis associated with psoriasis. The mean age of onset of the arthropathy is 11–12 years of age. The psoriasis may predate the onset of the arthropathy, with a mean age of onset of just over 8 years of age. The arthritis is typically monoarticular and involves a large joint, especially the knees. There may be a pauci-articular onset. The arthropathy may progress to become a polyarthropathy. In one series, the incidence of iridocyclitis was found to be 8% (Shore & Ansell 1982) and is of a chronic type. Antinuclear antibody (ANA) positivity places patients at a high risk of developing an iridocyclitis (Shore & Ansell 1982).

Inflammatory bowel disease

When uveitis occurs in association with chronic inflammatory bowel disease it may be asymptomatic. In Crohn's disease approximately 6% of patients have an anterior uveitis. There is a possible relationship with colonic involvement. The onset of the uveitis does not parallel the severity of the disease process. There appear to be few significant sequelae of the ocular involvement (Hofley *et al.* 1993).

Other associations

Acute anterior uveitis has been observed to occur in association with inflammatory renal disease. In rare instances, glomerulonephritis and interstitial nephritis have been implicated (Bunchman & Bloom 1993; Nash *et al.* 1993). The associated uveitis appears to be readily responsive to topical corticosteroid therapy.

Chronic anterior uveitis

Juvenile rheumatoid arthritis (Still's disease)

Juvenile rheumatoid arthritis, juvenile chronic arthritis or Still's disease, is a common association of bilateral chronic anterior uveitis in a child aged 15 years or younger, accounting for 80% of children with uveitis in one series (Kanski & Shun-Shin 1984). By definition, the age of onset should be before 16 years of age with symptom duration

from between 6 weeks to 3 months. Pauci-articular arthritis involves four or less joints in the first 3 months with a polyarticular form involving five or more joints. The incidence of juvenile rheumatoid arthritis is variable ranging from between 1.3 and 19.6 per 100 000, depending on the type of survey and the country of origin (Ansell & Bywaters 1959; Brewer *et al.* 1977; Gare & Fasth 1992).

Children with this condition may have chronic progressive monoarticular or pauci-articular arthritis, lymphadenopathy, splenomegaly, pericarditis, pleuritis, anaemia, fever and growth retardation. Since Ohm's (1910) first report of the uveitis, its association has been further defined on the basis of clinical features, serological testing and HLA antigen typing (Arnett *et al.* 1982).

The acute febrile and polyarticular onset types tend not to be associated with iritis. With pauci-articular onset, however, eye findings are of importance. These are further subdivided into the following.

1 Pauci-articular, rheumatoid factor negative; HLA-B27 negative; positive ANA factor. Females are affected more commonly than males (Kanski 1977), and the onset is before 10 years of age. Chronic iridocyclitis with few symptoms is a significant concern. Some association with HLA-DR5 may be present (Glass *et al.* 1980).

2 Pauci-articular, ankylosing spondylitis, seronegative rheumatoid factor and ANA-positive HLA-B27; acute iridocyclitis. These patients may evolve into a polyarticular type of rheumatoid arthritis (Arnett *et al.* 1980).

3 Pauci-articular, seronegative rheumatoid, ANA, HLA-B27 negative; HLA-DW8 and HLA-DRW8 positive.

The pauci-articular forms do not tend to persist into adulthood unlike the polyarticular forms.

The incidence of iridocyclitis approaches 20% in pauci-articular disease (Bywaters & Ansell 1965; Calabro *et al.* 1970); it occurs especially in females (Kanski 1977) with a 3:1 ratio (Kanski 1989). The uveitis is typically bilateral and is usually an asymptomatic, chronic, non-granulomatous iridocyclitis. The activity of the iridocyclitis does not parallel the activity of the arthritis (Schaller *et al.* 1969). The uveitis may precede the onset of the arthritis, in which case the visual prognosis is worse than when the arthritis precedes the uveitis (Wolf *et al.* 1987).

Common complications include band keratopathy (Fig. 38.35), cataract and secondary glaucoma. Rare complications include a keratoconjunctivitis sicca and corneal melting (Kanski 1988).

Histopathology of the chronic changes includes granulomatous inflammation, plasma cells and lymphocytic inflammation (Green 1985).

The diagnosis of juvenile rheumatoid arthritis is made primarily on the basis of clinical history. Positive ANA has been found in 88% of these patients who also have chronic iridocyclitis (Schaller *et al.* 1973). HLA testing is indicated (Stastney & Fink 1979).

Because of the relatively pain-free course of iridocyclitis

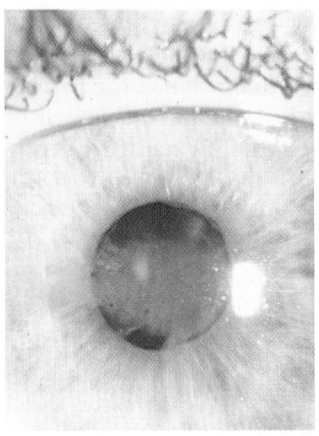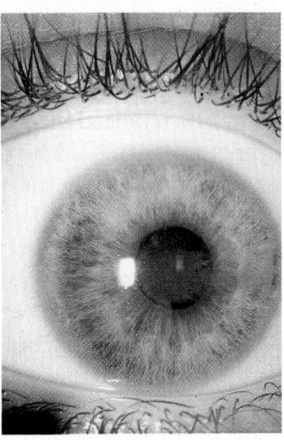

Fig. 38.35 Still's disease. This patient presented because the parents noticed a white spot on the cornea which was due to the band keratopathy associated with chronic uveitis with posterior synechiae. She had the pauci-articular form of Still's disease and later developed cataract which required surgery.

associated with juvenile rheumatoid arthritis, follow-up examinations are recommended for young patients, especially with the pauci-articular type.

A follow-up regime would involve the following time scales.
- Systemic onset, annually.
- Polyarticular, 6 monthly.
- Pauci-articular, 3 monthly.
- Positive ANA, 2 monthly.

It is recommended that screening should occur for at least 7 years after the onset of the disease (Kanski 1989).

Treatment includes mydriatics and corticosteroids topically when cells are present in the anterior chamber. Occasionally sub-Tenon's injections of steroids may be required. Systemic forms of therapy include non-steroidal anti-inflammatory agents and systemic steroids; for the most resistant forms, systemic immunosuppressive chemotherapeutic agents may need to be considered (Hemady *et al.* 1992; Foster & Barrett 1993).

Band keratopathy may require chelating agents such as ethylenediaminetetra-acetic acid (EDTA), removal by corneal scraping or laser ablation.

Cataract surgery may be complicated (Smith & Nozik 1983) and a lensectomy/vitrectomy approach is indicated (Flynn *et al.* 1988; Casteels & Taylor 1992; Kanski 1992), together with covering doses of systemic and topical steroids to prevent perioperative flare-up of the uveitis. Long-term visual outcomes associated with cataract extraction in juvenile rheumatoid arthritis may be affected by glaucoma, retinal detachment (Fig. 38.36) and macular disease (Fox *et al.* 1992).

With respect to outcomes, in one large series, 25% of patients had relatively mild uveitis with an excellent visual prognosis, 50% were well controlled on topical medica-

tion and a further 25% had a poor response to therapy and a poor visual prognosis (Kanski 1988).

Sarcoidosis

Sarcoidosis is an unusual cause of chronic anterior uveitis in children less than 15 years old (Hetherington 1982). Patients younger than 5 years present with the classic triad of uveitis (Fig. 38.37), arthropathy and skin rash as the major features (North *et al.* 1970). Other features include hepatosplenomegaly, fever, parotid swelling and hypertension. It is more common in black children (Kendig 1974) and may also involve the orbit simultaneously (Khan *et al.* 1986). Anterior uveitis occurs in 2–48% of child patients in the three largest reported series (Jasper & Denny 1968; Siltzbach & Greenberg 1968; Kendig 1974); it is often granulomatous. In a study of 26 patients of 5 years of age or less, 20 patients had anterior uveitis (Hoover *et al.* 1986). Diagnosis is made by an abnormal chest X-ray, though this may be normal in very young children (Cohen *et al.* 1981), biopsy changes of involved structures (including conjunctiva), Kveim test, the finding of a negative Mantoux test at decreasing dilutions, gallium scans and the finding of raised levels of serum angiotensin-converting enzyme (Baarsma *et al.* 1987).

The treatment of the primary uveitis as well as the sequelae is similar to that of juvenile rheumatoid arthritis

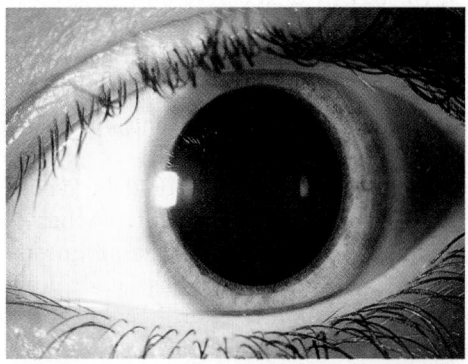

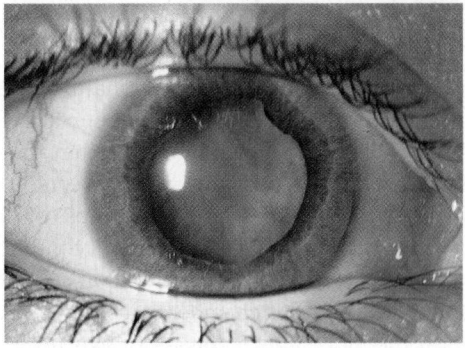

Fig. 38.36 Still's disease. Only the left eye was affected with glaucoma, cataract and uveitis. The left eye is aphakic and developed a retinal detachment.

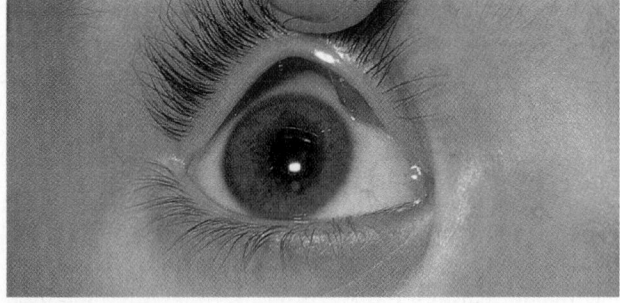

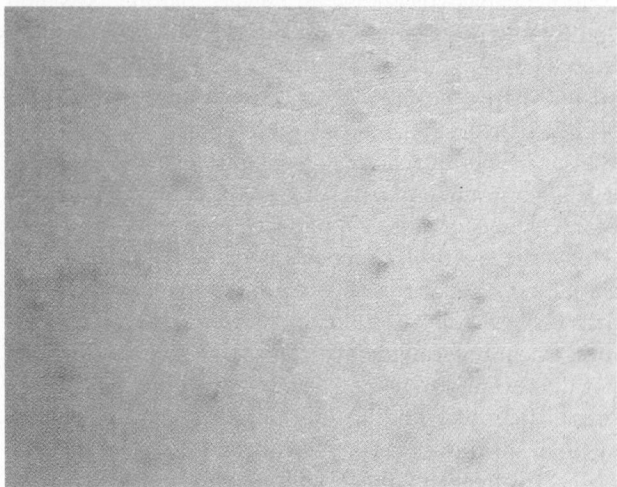

Fig. 38.37 (a) Sarcoidosis showing a very large KP just below the pupil. There are posterior synechiae and the iris is engorged. (b) Sarcoidosis. Skin nodule.

except that more consideration should be given to using systemic steroids (Kendig 1974) and chemotherapy is rarely indicated.

The early onset sarcoidosis should be distinguished from the late onset disease as they differ in their presentation, course and final outcomes. The prognosis is poor with the early onset type sarcoidosis, i.e. <4 years of age, with significant morbidity from cardiac and cerebral involvement (Hafner & Vogel 1993).

Fuchs' heterochromic iridocyclitis

Fuchs' heterochromic iridocyclitis is characterized by a chronic anterior uveitis with hypopigmentation in the involved eye (Fig. 38.38). It may occur from the second decade onwards but typically starts between 30 and 40 years of age as slow painless progressive loss of vision or of heterochromia. It is usually a unilateral condition. Slit-lamp findings include small diffuse keratic precipitates with a low grade anterior chamber reaction with minimal injection of the globe and no posterior synechiae formation, and iris transillumination defects. Other iris findings include increased visibility of the iris vasculature, patchy pigment epithelial atrophy, angle neovascularization and,

rarely, iris nodules (Rothova *et al.* 1994) on the pupillary margin or anterior iris surface. Glaucoma develops in 25–50% of patients. Cataract is a common sequela, with an up to 80% reported incidence (Jones 1991a,b). This form of events is considered by some to be the most frequently misdiagnosed form of uveitis (Smith & Nozik 1983; O'Connor 1985).

It has been considered as a degenerative disorder, and described in association with hemifacial atrophy (La Hey & Baarsma 1993) and a similar uveitis occurs in linear scleroderma (morphoea), but evidence now points to several aetiological mechanisms including an immunological disorder, perhaps related to depressed suppressor T-cell activity. It is now not thought to be associated with toxoplasmosis (La Hey *et al.* 1992). Occasionally, a positive family history is present (O'Connor 1985). An overview on pathogenetic mechanisms and associations is given by Jones (1993) and La Hey *et al.* (1994).

Patients with this condition do not usually respond favourably to steroids. Glaucoma management is often difficult with pressure control usually becoming refractory to topical therapy (La Hey *et al.* 1993).

Tuberculosis

Tuberculosis has re-emerged as a significant public health problem, with high-risk groups such as human immunodeficiency virus (HIV)-positive and other immunosuppressed individuals and immigrants from South-East Asia being at greatest risk.

Tuberculosis can cause anterior chronic granulomatous uveitis in addition to necrotizing retinochoroiditis, choroiditis and subacute endophthalmitis (Helm & Holland 1993). The incidence of tuberculosis related uveitis is low with 0.27% reported by Donahue (1967) in his survey of 10 524 affected patients. Some advocate systemic treat-

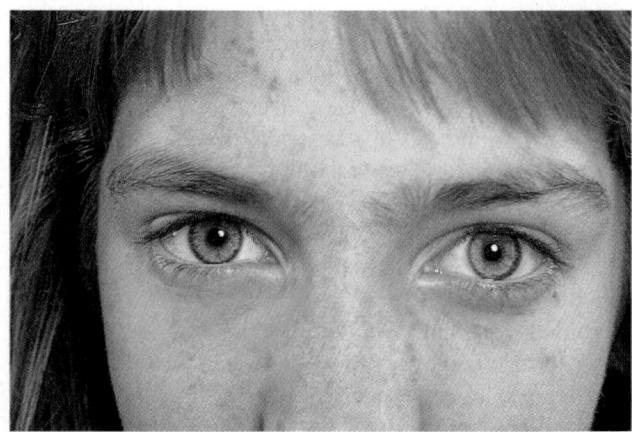

Fig. 38.38 Fuchs' heterochromic iridocyclitis. This girl presented because of mildly blurred vision in the left eye and heterochromia which her parents had noticed. She had a mild chronic anterior uveitis without synechiae and a cataract developed.

ment for tuberculosis in patients with positive skin tests and chronic granulomatous uveitis (Schlaegel & O'Connor 1981). Infants with miliary tuberculosis may have multiple focal choroidal lesions.

Syphilis

Syphilis typically results in either chorioretinitis or chronic iridocyclitis which may be immune-mediated. Iris papules or roseolae may be visible by slit-lamp examination (Schwartz & O'Connor 1980).

Anterior uveitis is rarely associated with interstitial keratitis of congenital syphilis (Spicer 1924).

Pars planitis/intermediate uveitis

Pars planitis is one of many terms (cyclitis, peripheral uveitis, peripheral cyclitis and chronic cyclitis) which describe a relatively common entity of non-infectious inflammation of the vitreous secondary to inflammation of the retina, ciliary body and vitreous. Its incidence peaks between 15 and 25 years of age. The condition is usually bilateral with unilateral disease often progressing to bilateral involvement. Patients complain of floaters and may note distorted vision if cystoid macular oedema develops. Symptoms of pain, redness and photophobia are very rare (Smith & Nozik 1983) though in the young they may present with symptoms that are very similar to an acute anterior uveitis (Giles 1989). Rarely presentation may be due to decreased vision from a vitreous haemorrhage.

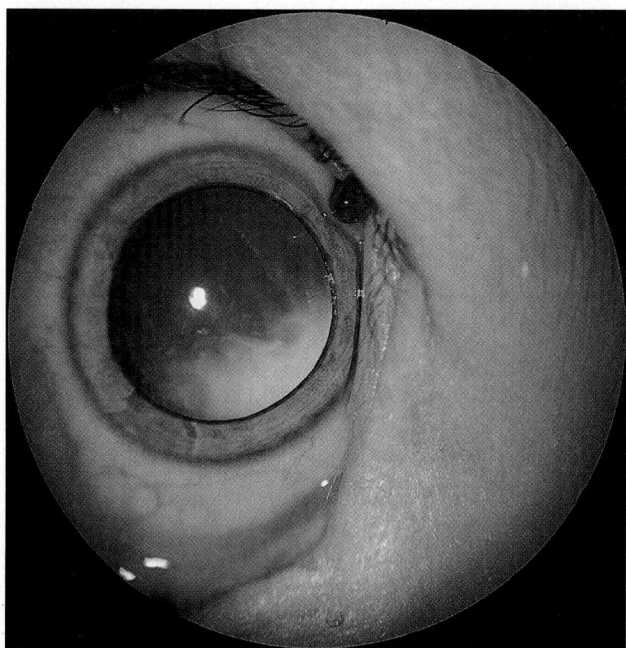

Fig. 38.39 Pars planitis in a 4-year-old girl with no systemic abnormality. The matted white exudate is present mainly in the inferior part of the pars plana.

The classic finding is 'snow-banking' (Fig. 38.39) on the inferior parts (Aaberg 1987) of the pars plana which consists of mononuclear cells (Kenyon *et al.* 1975); minimal anterior chamber reaction may be present. Posterior synechiae may be found.

Retinal findings may include vasculitis, peripapillary retinal oedema, and cystoid macular oedema. Complications include cataract, secondary glaucoma, disc neovascularization (Kalina *et al.* 1990), vitreous haemorrhage, retinal detachment, band keratopathy and cyclitic membranes. Overall, visual acuity is 6/12 (20/40) or better in almost 80% of patients with long-term follow-up.

No clear-cut cause is known, although viral and immunological causes have been suggested. Laboratory tests, including those for tuberculosis and syphilis, are usually negative. There is a suggestion that patients with pars planitis and a periphlebitis are at greater risk of developing multiple sclerosis (Malinowski *et al.* 1993).

Treatment with sub-Tenon's steroid should be considered if vision is reduced and cystoid macular oedema is present by fluorescein angiography. Topical therapy is not usually efficacious. If a patient worsens despite treatment, transconjunctival cryotherapy might be considered and immunosuppressive agents may also have a role (Verma *et al.* 1991; Josephberg *et al.* 1994).

Posterior uveitis

Posterior uveitis refers to inflammation of the choroid; differentiation of choroiditis, chorioretinitis, retinochoroiditis, retinitis and retinal vasculitis is often quite arbitrary.

Posterior uveitis may be either diffuse or focal. Active lesions often trigger an inflammatory response in the overlying vitreous. Inactive lesions may evolve into hypopigmented or hyperpigmented chorioretinal scars. The manner of presentation is dependent upon which area of the posterior pole is involved and whether the process is unilateral or bilateral. Posterior uveitides are more likely to have a causative agent as compared to anterior uveitides. Important considerations include the differential diagnosis of occult tumours including retinoblastoma, unsuspected intraocular foreign bodies, and consideration of any underlying systemic immunosuppression that may predispose the child to an infective posterior uveitis.

Infective causes

HIV retinopathy and cytomegalovirus retinitis (see Chapter 14).

Endophthalmitis (see Chapter 17).

Toxoplasmosis (see Chapter 13).

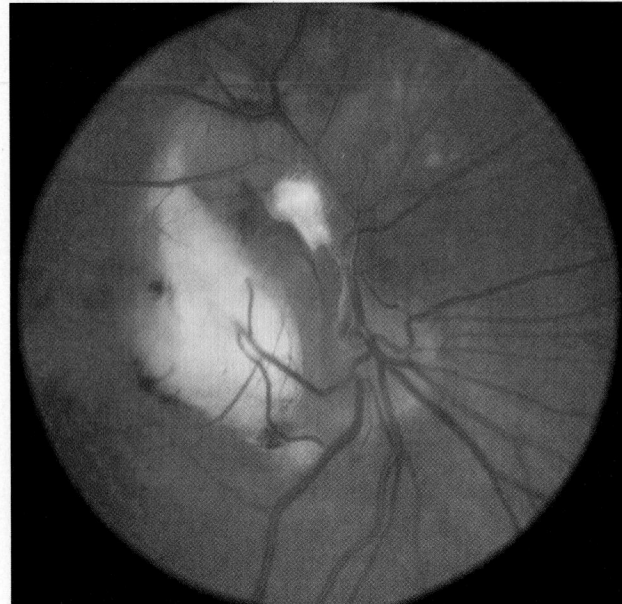

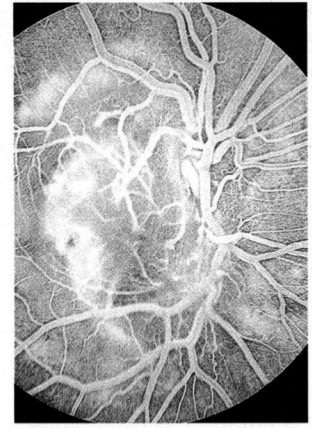
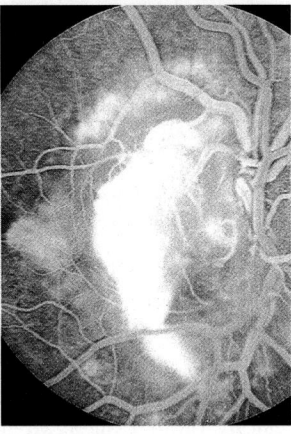

Fig. 38.40 (a) *Toxocara*. This 5-year-old child failed his school eye test and was found to have a raised peripapillary lesion between the disc and the macula in his left eye. At this stage there was minimal active inflammation. (b) Same patient. *Toxocara* lesion with minimal leakage at this late stage.

Varicella-zoster. Deegan and Duker (1994) described a young adult with focal choroiditis.

Toxocara. Toxocariasis is common in children, though ocular involvement is rare and fortunately usually unilateral, since vision may be greatly impaired in the infected eye. Its presentation shares many common features with those of unilateral retinoblastoma, making its recognition all the more important. *Toxocara* seropositivity occurs in a high proportion of asymptomatic kindergarten children (Ellis *et al.* 1986).

Three forms of ocular involvement exist: (i) endophthalmitis; (ii) macular retinochoroidal granuloma (Fig. 38.40); and (iii) peripheral retinochoroidal granuloma (Gillespie *et al.* 1993).

The condition is caused by the second stage larvae of *Toxocara canis,* and it is the disintegrating organism which evokes eosinophilia and inflammation. Dogs and cats are the natural hosts of the worm, and human infection occurs with ingestion of eggs from contaminated pets, clothes or dirt.

Patients with ocular findings do not usually give a history of systemic disease (visceral larval migrans). Onset is usually between 2 and 3 years with a mean age of onset around 7 years, and rare past 12 years of age. Males are affected more often than females. Presenting features include strabismus and leukocoria or failed screening examination at school.

Toxocara endophthalmitis presenting in individuals between 2 and 9 years of age is most often confused with retinoblastoma, as the red reflex is absent and a complete retinal detachment is present. Macular lesions, presenting slightly later, are solitary and confined to the posterior pole with few overlying vitreous cells. The lesions are usually single but multiple sites of inflammation have been recorded and may be due to the larva moving into subretinal space when it is relatively protected from the host's immunological surveillance (Lyness *et al.* 1987). Peripheral chorioretinal granulomas present later since vision is less affected. Rarely, bands of scar tissue may drag the macula and create a pseudoexotropia.

Histopathology will often fail to reveal any organisms but rather be characterized by eosinophilia and granulomatous inflammation.

Laboratory tests include the ELISA for *Toxocara;* when used appropriately, it can help diagnose the condition in over 90% of cases. Eosinophilia is not usually present. Vitreous aspiration may be helpful in differentiating from retinoblastoma (Smith & Nozik 1983) but only if retinoblastoma is *extremely* unlikely (see Chapter 42).

Treatment should only be undertaken once the possibility of retinoblastoma has been eliminated. *Toxocara* lesions are responsive occasionally to steroids, anthelminthic drugs do not seem to help. Enucleation should only be performed when the diagnosis of retinoblastoma cannot be excluded or the eye is blind and painful.

Candidiasis. Candidiasis usually presents as retinitis or vitritis in an immunodeficient child (see Chapter 14).

Tuberculosis. Tuberculosis may also present as a posterior segment inflammation and pseudoglioma in predisposed children (Saini *et al.* 1986). It is a rare cause of uveitis and if diagnosed in an otherwise healthy child, an underlying immunosuppressive disorder should be suspected and appropriate investigations ordered.

Intraocular tuberculosis is usually associated with a secondary infection rather than being a primary site of involvement (Helm & Holland 1993). Involvement of any of the posterior segment structures can occur. Ciliary body

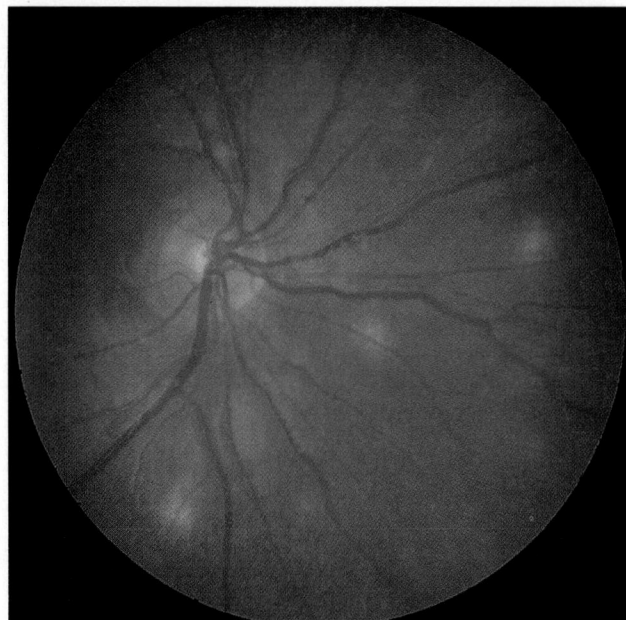

Fig. 38.41 Miliary tuberculosis with focal choroidal lesions.

tuberculosis can manifest as a low grade chronic anterior uveitis as well as vitreous opacity formation (Ni *et al.* 1982). Choroidal involvement is suggestive of haematogenous spread (Fig. 38.41) and may suggest miliary dissemination (Massaro *et al.* 1964). Choroidal tubercles are one of the most common manifestations of posterior segment tuberculosis. It may be unilateral and situated in the posterior pole, and the size may vary from one-quarter to several disc diameters. These tubercles are readily responsive to systemic therapy. The majority of choroidal tubercles do not usually incite an anterior uveitis or vitritis (Helm & Holland 1993). Retinal involvement can manifest as a periphlebitis, though it is uncommon.

The role of the paediatric ophthalmologist in patients with tuberculosis is not only in the diagnosis and monitoring of disease response to systemic therapy but more importantly in the screening for any serious and permanent vision-threatening side-effects associated with systemic therapy.

Sympathetic ophthalmia

Sympathetic ophthalmia (see Fig. 39.48) is a disorder in which the uveal tract becomes infiltrated by lymphocytes and epitheloid cells in response to injury to the fellow eye usually involving damage to the uvea. There is a high incidence associated with war injuries, with 14% of eye injuries during the US Civil War associated with sympathetic ophthalmia. It occurs very rarely following intraocular surgery — 0.007% according to one series (Liddy & Stuart 1972). It has also been associated with intraocular

tumours (Riwchun & DeCoursey 1941) and following cyclodestructive procedures (Sabates 1988).

The interval between trauma and onset of sympathetic ophthalmia has reportedly spanned 5 days (Thies 1947) to 42 years, but usually occurs between 2 weeks and 3 months after insult (Lubin *et al.* 1980).

This condition is characterized by pain, photophobia, decreased vision and worsening of the traumatized eye. Uveitis may include 'plastic' iritis (i.e. with thick viscous exudate) and choroidal infiltration as well as exudative retinal detachment. Vitiligo and poliosis may occur, showing common ground between sympathetic ophthalmia and the Vogt–Koyanagi–Harada syndrome (Schlaegel 1981).

Histopathology reveals similar changes in the 'exciting' and the 'sympathizing' eye (Easom & Zimmerman 1964). Characteristic Dalen–Fuchs' nodules represent epitheloid cells just internal to Bruch's membrane (Lubin *et al.* 1980).

The treatment for sympathetic ophthalmia prior to the advent of steroids consisted of enucleation of the injured eye (Lubin *et al.* 1980) but corticosteroids are now the primary mode of treatment (Makley & Leibold 1960).

The extensive literature on sympathetic ophthalmia includes a 30-year follow-up of a child who at 9 months perforated her cornea. After the fellow eye became red, the buphthalmic injured eye was enucleated. Recurrent inflammation with cataract and glaucoma ensued over the following 29 years in the remaining eye. The patient had ambulatory vision after a pars plana lensectomy/vitrectomy (Kinyoun *et al.* 1983).

Chronic granulomatous disease

In this rare multisystem disorder, uveitis, exudative retinal detachment and chorioretinal scarring occur (Valluri *et al.* 1995).

Sarcoidosis

Sarcoidosis tends to cause anterior uveitis in children. Posterior involvement can include chorioretinitis, periphlebitis and venous sheathing, chorioretinal nodules, vitreous cells, vitreous haemorrhage and retinal neovascularization (James *et al.* 1964) as well as optic nerve granuloma (Laties & Scheie 1972). Extraocular muscle involvement in children has been reported (Cornblath *et al.* 1993), and, rarely, a nebular interstitial keratitis (Lennarson & Barney 1995).

Diagnosis

Most cases can be diagnosed clinically or by further diagnostic studies, but if there is no diagnosis in a progressive lesion that is threatening the macula, if there is suspicion of malignancy, or where there is a possibility of treatable infection, a chorioretinal biopsy may be appropriate (Taylor *et al.* 1981; Nussenblatt 1993).

References

Aaberg T. The enigma of pars planitis. *Am J Ophthalmol* 1987; **103**: 828–30.

Abadi RV, Cox MJ. The distribution of macular pigment in human albinos. *Inv Ophthalmol Vis Sci* 1992; **33**: 494–7.

Abadi RV, Pascal E. The recognition and management of albinism. *Ophthal Physiol Opt* 1989; **9**: 3–15.

Abadi RV, Pascal E. Visual resolution limits in human albinism. *Vision Res* 1991; **31**: 1445–7.

Ackinson C, Brodsky M, Hiles D, Simon J. Idiopathic tractional corectopia. *J Pediatr Ophthalmol Strabismus* 1994; **31**: 387–90.

Aiello AL, Tran VT, Narsing AR. Postnatal development of the ciliary body and pars plana: a morphometric study in childhood. *Arch Ophthalmol* 1992; **110**: 802–5.

Albert D, Brownstein S, Kattleman B. Mucogenic glaucoma caused by an epithelial cyst of the iris stoma. *Am J Ophthalmol* 1992; **114**: 222–3.

Albert DM, Puliafito CA, Fulton AB *et al.* Increased incidence of choroidal malignant melanoma occurring in a single population of chemical workers. *Am J Ophthalmol* 1980; **89**: 323–37.

Alm A, Bill A. The oxygen supply to the retina II. Effects of high intraocular pressure and of increased arterial carbon dioxide tension on uveal and retinal blood flow in cats. *Acta Physiol Scand* 1972; **84**: 306–19.

Anand R, Augsburger JJ, Shields JA. Circumscribed choroidal haemangioma. *Arch Ophthalmol* 1989; **107**: 1338–42.

Ansell BM, Bywaters EGL. Prognosis in Still's disease. *Bull Rheum Dis* 1959; **9**: 189.

Apkarian P, Reits D. Global stereopsis in human albinos. *Vis Res* 1989; **71**: 355–67.

Apkarian P, Spekreijse H, van Swaay E, van Schooneveld M. Visual evoked potentials in Prader–Willi syndrome. *Documenta Ophthalmol* 1989; **71**: 355–67.

Apple DJ, Blodi FC. Pathologic observations and clinical approval to uveal melanoma. In: DH Nicholson, ed. *Ocular Pathology Update*. New York: Masson, 1980: 213.

Apt L. Uveal melanoma in children and adolescents. *Int Ophthalmol Clin* 1963; **2**: 403–10.

Apt LA, Heller MD, Moskovitz M, Foos RY. Dictyoma (embryonal medulloepitheliomas). Recent review and case report. *J Pediatr Ophthalmol Strabismus* 1973; **10**: 30–7.

Arentson JJ, Green WR. Melanoma of the iris. Report of 72 cases treated surgically. *Ophthalmic Surg* 1975; **6**: 23–37.

Arnett FC, Bias WB, Stevens MB. Juvenile onset chronic arthritis. Clinical and X-ray features of a unique HLA-B27 subset. *Am J Med* 1980; **69**: 369–76.

Arnett FC Jr, Widman LE, Feinstein RS. Clinical conferences at the Johns Hopkins Hospital. Juvenile rheumatoid arthritis. *Johns Hopkins Med J* 1982; **151**: 313–17.

Ashton N. Primary tumours of the iris. *Br J Ophthalmol* 1964; **48**: 650–68.

Avila MP, El-Makarbi H, Azzolini C, Jalka AE, Burns D, Weiter JJ. Bilateral choroidal osteoma and subretinal neovascularisation. *Ann Ophthalmol* 1984; **16**: 381.

Baarsma GS, La Hey E, Glasius E, de Vries J, Kijlstra A. The predictive value of serum angiotensin converting enzyme and lysozyme levels in the diagnosis of ocular sarcoidosis. *Am J Ophthalmol* 1987; **104**: 211–18.

Bamezai R, Husain SA, Misra S, Thacker AK. Cerebellar ataxia and total albinism. *Clin Genet* 1987; **31**: 178–81.

Barkan O. Goniotomy for glaucoma associated with aniridia. *Arch Ophthalmol* 1953; **49**: 1–5.

Barr CC, McLean IW, Zimmerman LE. Uveal melanoma in children and adolescents. *Arch Ophthalmol* 1981; **99**: 2133–6.

Barr CC, Vine AK, Martonyi CL. Unexplained heterochromia. Intraocular foreign body demonstrated by computed tomography. *Surv Ophthalmol* 1984; **28**: 409–11.

Bassi MT, Schiaffino MV, Renien A *et al.* Cloning the gene for ocular albinism type I from the distal short arm of the X chromosome. *Nature Genet* 1995; **10**: 13–19.

Bedoya V, Grimley PH, Dugue O. Chediak–Higashi syndrome. *Arch Pathol* 1969; **88**: 340–9.

Belmont JB, Michelson JB, Vitrectomy in uveitis associated with ankylosing spondylitis. *Am J Ophthalmol* 1982; **94**: 300–4.

Bergsma DR, Kaiser-Kupfer M. A new form of albinism. *Am J Ophthalmol* 1979; **77**: 837–44.

Bitoun P, Morel-Charron J. A hereditary syndrome association of oculocutaneous albinism, dysmorphic features and short stature. *Ophthalmol Paediatr Genet* 1990; **11**: 209–13.

Bloom JN, Graviss RE, Byrne BJ. Orbital pseudotumour in the differential diagnosis of pediatric uveitis. *J Pediatr Ophthalmol Strabismus* 1992; **29**: 59–63.

Brazel SM, Sullivan TJ, Thorner PS, Clarke MP, Hunter WS, Morin JD. Iris heterochromia as a marker for neural crest disease. *Arch Ophthalmol* 1992; **110**: 233–5.

Breeveld J, Kuiper H, Spanjaard L, Luyendijk L, Rothova A. Uveitis and Lyme borreliosis. *Br J Ophthalmol* 1993; **77**: 480–1.

Brewer EJ, Bass J, Baum J *et al.* Current proposed revision of JRA criteria. *Arthritis Rheum* 1977; **20**(Suppl.): 195.

Broadway D, Lang S, Harper J *et al.* Congenital malignant melanoma of the eye. *Cancer* 1991; **67**: 2642–52.

Brodsky MC, Glasier CM, Creel DJ. Magnetic resonance imaging of the visual pathways in human albinos. *J Pediatr Ophthalmol Strabismus* 1993; **30**: 382–5.

Brooks S, Baervaldt G, Rao N, Smith R. Primary iris stromal cysts. *J Pediatr Ophthalmol Stabismus* 1993; **30**: 194–8.

Brown HH, Brodsky MC, Hembree K, Mrak RE. Supraciliary hemangiopericytoma. *Ophthalmology* 1991; **98**: 378–82.

Brushfield T. Mongolism. *Br J Child Dis* 1924; **21**: 241–58.

Brusini D, Beltrane G. Spontaneous hyphaema from pupillary membrane. *Acta Ophthalmol* 1983; **1**: 1099–102.

Bunchman TE, Bloom JN. A syndrome of acute interstitial nephritis and anterior uveitis. *Pediatr Nephrol* 1993; **7**: 520–2.

Burger PC, Klintworth GK. Experimental retinal degeneration in the rabbit produced by intraocular iron. *Lab Invest* 1974; **30**: 9–19.

Burke MJ, Rennebohm RM. Eye involvement in Kawasaki disease. *J Pediatr Ophthalmol Strabismus* 1981; **18**: 7–11.

Burkitt D, O'Connor GT. Malignant lymphoma in African children I. A clinical syndrome. *Cancer* 1961; **14**: 258–69.

Burns JC, Joffe L, Sargent RA, Glode MP. Anterior uveitis associated with Kawasaki syndrome. *Pediatr Infect Dis* 1985; **4**: 258–61.

Bywaters EGL, Ansell BM. Monoarticular arthritis in children. *Ann Rheum Dis* 1965; **24**: 116–22.

Calabro JJ. Clinical aspects of juvenile and adult ankylosing spondylitis. *Br J Rheum* 1983; **22**(Suppl. 2): 104.

Calabro JJ, Parrino GR, Atchoo PD, Marchesano JM, Goldberg LS. Chronic iridocyclitis in juvenile rheumatoid arthritis. *Arthritis Rheum* 1970; **13**: 406–13.

Callahan A. Aniridia with ectopia lentis and secondary glaucoma, genetic, pathologic, and surgical consideration. *Am J Ophthalmol* 1949; **32**: 28–39.

Campochiaro PA, Gonzalez-Fernandez F, Newman SA, Conway BP, Feldman PS. Ciliary body adenoma in a 10-year-old girl who had a rhabdomyosarcoma. *Arch Ophthalmol* 1992; **110**: 681–3.

Canning CR, McCartney ACE, Hungerford J. Medulloepithelioma (dictyoma). *Br J Ophthalmol* 1988; **72**: 764–8.

Capo H, Palmer E, Nicholson D. Congenital cysts of the iris stroma. *Am J Ophthalmol* 1993; **116**: 228–32.

Carlson DW, Wallace LM, Folberg R. Aggressive nevus of the iris with secondary glaucoma in a child. *Am J Ophthalmol* 1995; **119**: 367–8.

Cassady JR, Light A. Familial persistent pupillary membranes. *Arch Ophthalmol* 1957; **58**: 438.

Casswell AG, McCourtney AC, Hungerford JL. Choroidal malignant melanoma in an albino. *Br J Ophthalmol* 1989; **73**: 840–6.

Casteels I, Taylor D. Cataracts in children with uveitis. *Br J Ophthalmol* 1992; **76**: 66–8.

Castronuovo S, Simon JW, Kandel GL *et al.* Variable expression of albinism within a single kindred. *Am J Ophthalmol* 1991; **111**: 419–26.

Charles SJ, Green JS, Grant JW, Yates JRW, Moore AT. Clinical features of affected males with X-linked ocular albinism. *Br J Ophthalmol* 1993; **77**: 222–7.

Cheong PYY, King RA, Bateman JB. Oculocutaneous albinism: variable expressivity of nystagmus in a sibship. *J Pediatr Ophthalmol Strabismus* 1992; **29**: 185–8.

Cibis GW, Freeman AI, Pang V *et al.* Bilateral choroidal neonatal neuroblastoma. *Am J Ophthalmol* 1990; **109**: 445–9.

Cleasby GW. Malignant melanoma of the iris. *Arch Ophthalmol* 1958; **60**: 403–17.

Cohen KL, Pfeiffer RL Jr, Powell DA. Sarcoidosis and ocular disease in a young child: a case report and review of the literature. *Arch Ophthalmol* 1981; **99**: 422–4.

Committee on Infectious Diseases, American Academy of Pediatrics. Intravenous gamma-globulin use in children with Kawasaki disease. *Pediatrics* 1988; **82**: 122.

Cornblath WT, Elner V, Rolfe M. Extraocular muscle involvement in sarcoidosis *Ophthalmology* 1993; **100**: 501–5.

Crawfurd M d'A, Harcourt RB, Shaw PA. Non-progressive cerebellar ataxia, aplasia of pupillary zone of iris, and mental subnormality (Gillespie's syndrome) affecting three members of a non-consanguineous family in two generations. *J Med Genet* 1979; **16**: 373–8.

Creel D. Problems of ocular miswiring in albinism, Duane's syndrome and Marcus Gunn phenomenon. *Int Ophthalmol Clin* 1984; **24**: 165–76.

Creel D, Witkop CJ, King RA. Asymmetric visually evoked potentials in human albinos: evidence for visual system anomalies. *Invest Ophthalmol Vis Sci* 1974; **13**: 430–40.

Cross HE, McKusick VA, Breen W. A new oculocerebral syndrome with hypopigmentation. *J Pediatr* 1967; **70**: 398–406.

Cunha SL. Osseous choristoma of the choroid. *Arch Ophthalmol* 1984; **102**: 1052–4.

David R, MacBeath L, Jenkins T. Aniridia associated with microcornea and subluxated lenses. *Br J Ophthalmol* 1978; **62**: 118–21.

de Buen S, Olivares ML, Charlin VC. Leiomyoma of the iris. Report of a case. *Br J Ophthalmol* 1971; **55**: 353–6.

Deegan W, Duker J. Unifocal choroiditis in primary varicella zoster (chickenpox). *Arch Ophthalmol* 1994; **112**: 735–6.

Doggart JH. Spontaneous hyphaema XVI. *Concil Ophthalmol Acta* 1950; **1**: 450–5.

Donaldson DD. The significance of spotting of the iris in Mongoloid Brushfield's spots. *Arch Ophthalmol* 1961; **65**: 26–31.

Donahue HC. Ophthalmologic experience in a tuberculosis sanatorium. *Am J Ophthalmol* 1967; **64**: 742–8.

Duke-Elder S. Part 2: Congenital deformities. In: Duke-Elder S, ed. *Normal and Abnormal Development*, Vol. III *System of Ophthalmology*. London: Henry Kimpton, 1964: 590–1.

Durham-Pierre D, Gardner J, Nakatsu Y *et al.* African origin of an intragenic deletion of the human gene in tyrosinase positive oculocutaneous albinism. *Nature Genet* 1994; **7**: 176–9.

Easom HA, Zimmerman LE. Sympathetic ophthalmia and bilateral phacoanaphylaxis. A clinicopathologic correlation of the sympathogenic and sympathizing eyes. *Arch Ophthalmol* 1964; **72**: 9–15.

Edwards J, Lampert R, Hammer M, Young S. Ocular defects and dysmorphic features in three generations. *J Clin Dysmorphol* 1984; **2**: 8–12.

Edwards TS. Ophthalmic complications from varicella. *J Pediatr Ophthalmol Strabismus* 1965; **2**: 37–40.

Ellis GS, Pakalnis VA, Worley G *et al. Toxocara canis* infestation: clinical and epidemiological associations with seropositivity in kindergarten children. *Ophthalmology* 1986; **93**: 1032–8.

Elsas FE, Mroczek EC, Kelly DR, Specht CS. Primary rhabdomyosarcoma of the iris. *Arch Ophthalmol* 1991; **109**: 982–4.

Elsas TJ, Maumenee IH, Kenyon KR, Yodar F. Familial aniridia with preserved ocular function. *Am J Ophthalmol* 1977; **83**: 718–24.

Engel HM, de la Cruz ZC, Jimenez-Abalahin LD, Green WR, Michels RG. Cytopreparatory techniques for eye fluid specimens obtained by vitrectomy. *Acta Cytol* 1982; **26**: 551–60.

Eting E, Savir H. An atypical fulminant course of choroidal osteoma in two siblings. *Am J Ophthalmol* 1992; **113**: 52–5.

Feeney L, Hogan M. Electron microscopy of the human choroid. *Am J Ophthalmol* 1961; **51**: 1457–83.

Ferry AP. Lesions mistaken for malignant melanoma of the iris. *Arch Ophthalmol* 1965; **74**: 9–18.

Ffytche TJ. Role of iris changes as a cause of blindness in lepromatous leprosy. *Br J Ophthalmol* 1981; **65**: 231–9.

Flanagan JC, DiGeorge AM. Sporadic aniridia and Wilms' tumour. *Am J Ophthalmol* 1969; **67**: 558–61.

Flynn HW, Davis JL, Culbertson WW. Pars plana lensectomy and vitrectomy for complicated cataracts in juvenile rheumatoid arthritis. *Ophthalmology* 1988; **95**: 1114–19.

Font RL, Mehta RS, Streusand SD *et al.* Bilateral retinal ischaemia in Kawasaki disease. *Ophthalmology* 1983; **90**: 569–77.

Foos RY, Hull SN, Straatsma BR. Early diagnosis of ciliary body melanomas. *Arch Ophthalmol* 1969; **81**: 336–44.

Forsius H, Eriksson AW. Ein neues augensyndrom mit X–chromosomaler transmission. Eine sippe mit fundus albinismus, fovea hypoplasie, nystagmus, myopie, astigmatismus und dyschromatopsie. *Klin Monatsbl Augenheilkd* 1964; **144**: 447–57.

Foss AJ, Pecorella I, Alexander RA, Hungerford JL, Garner A. Are most intraocular 'leiomyomas' really melanocytic lesions? *Ophthalmology* 1994; **101**: 919–24.

Foster CS, Barrett F. Cataract development and cataract surgery in patients with juvenile rheumatoid arthritis associated iridocyclitis. *Ophthalmology* 1993; **100**: 809–17.

Fox GM, Flynn HW, Davis JL, Culbertson W. Causes of reduced visual acuity on long-term follow-up after cataract extraction in patients with uveitis and juvenile rheumatoid arthritis. *Am J Ophthalmol* 1992; **114**: 708–14.

François J, Verschragen-Spae MR, De Sutter E. The aniridia–Wilms' tumour syndrome and other associations of aniridia. *Ophthalmol Paediatr Genet* 1982; **1**: 125–38.

Friedenwald JS, Wilder HC, Maumenee AE *et al. Ophthalmic Pathology: an Atlas and Textbook.* Philadelphia: WB Saunders, 1952.

Fuchs E. Wucherungen und geschwulste des ciliarepithels. *Albrecht Von Graefe's Arch Ophthalmol* 1908; **68**: 534–87.

Fujikawa LS, Schwartz LK, Rosenbaum EH. Acquired immunodeficiency syndrome associated with Burkitt's lymphoma presenting with ocular findings. *Ophthalmology* 1983; **90**: 50–1.

Fukai K, Holmes S, Lucchese N *et al*. Autosomal recessive ocular albinism associated with a functionally significant tyrosinase gene polymorphism. *Nature Genet* 1995; **9**: 92–5.

Fulcher T, O'Keefe M, Bowell R *et al*. Intellectual and educational attainment in albinism. *J Pediatr Ophthalmol Strabismus* 1995; **32**: 368–72.

Garay SM, Gardella JE, Farzzini EP, Goldring RM. Hermansky–Pudlak syndrome: pulmonary manifestations of a ceroid storage disorder. *Am J Med* 1979; **66**: 737.

Garcia R, Niero JA, Nistal M. Aniridia associated with gonadoblastoma in the Smith–Lemli–Opitz syndrome. *Ann Esp Pediatr* 1976; **9**: 19–24.

Gare BA, Fasth A. Epidemiology of juvenile chronic arthritis in southwestern Sweden: a 5-year prospective population study. *Pediatrics* 1992; **90**: 950–8.

Gass JDM. Iris abscess simulating malignant melanoma. *Arch Ophthalmol* 1973; **90**: 300–2.

Gedalia A, Watemberg N, Rothschild M. Childhood brucellosis in the Negev. *Harejuah* 1990; **119**: 313–15.

Giebel LB, Tripathi RK, King RA, Spritz RA. A tyrosinase gene missense mutation in temperature-sensitive type 1 oculocutaneous albinism. A human homologue to the Siamese cat and the Himalayan mouse. *J Clin Invest* 1991a; **87**: 1119–22.

Giebel LB, Tripathi RK, Strunk KM *et al*. Tyrosinase gene mutations associated with type 1B ('yellow') oculocutaneous albinism. *Am J Hum Genet* 1991b; **48**: 1159–67.

Giles CL. Pediatric intermediate uveitis. *J Pediatr Ophthalmol Strabismus* 1989; **26**: 136–9.

Gillespie FD. Aniridia, cerebellar ataxia, and oligophrenia. *Arch Ophthalmol* 1965; 73: 338–41.

Gillespie SH, Dinning WJ, Voller A, Crowcroft NS. The spectrum of ocular toxocariasis. *Eye* 1993; **7**: 415–18.

Glaser T, Jepeal L, Edwards JG, Young SR, Favor J, Mass RL. Pax 6 gene dosage effect in a family with congenital cataracts, aniridia, anophthalmia and central nervous system defects. *Nat Genet* 1994; **7**: 463–71.

Glass D, Litvin D, Wallace K, Chylack L, Garovoy M, Carpenter CB, Schur PH. Early onset pauciarticular juvenile rheumatoid arthritis associated with human leukocyte antigen DRW 5, iritis, and antinuclear antibody. *J Clin Invest* 1980; **66**: 426–9.

Golnik K, Marotto M, Fanous M *et al*. Ophthalmic manifestations of Rochalimaea species. *Am J Ophthalmol* 1994; **118**: 145–51.

Grand MG, Burgess DR, Singerman LJ, Ramsay J. Choroidal osteoma. Treatment of associated subretinal neovascular membranes. *Retina* 1984; **4**: 84.

Grant WM, Walton DS. Progressive changes in the angle in congenital aniridia, with development of glaucoma. *Am J Ophthalmol* 1974; **18**: 842–7.

Grayson M. Viral diseases. In: Grayson M, ed. *Diseases of the Cornea*. St Louis: CV Mosby, 1983: 150–98.

Green WR, Oliff WJ, Trotter RR. Malignant teratoid medulloepithelioma of the optic nerve. *Arch Ophthalmol* 1974; **91**: 451–4.

Greenberg F, Lewis RA. The Williams' syndrome: spectrum and significance of ocular features. *Ophthalmology* 1988; **95**: 1608–12.

Greer CH. Congenital melanoma of the anterior uvea. *Arch Ophthalmol* 1966; **76**: 77–8.

Grove JH, Shaw MW, Bourgue G. A family study of aniridia. *Arch Ophthalmol* 1961; **65**: 81–4.

Grutzmacher R, Lindquist T, Chittum M, Bunt-Milam A, Kalina R. Congenital iris cysts. *Br J Ophthalmol* 1987; **71**: 227–35.

Guillery RW, Okoro AN, Witkop CJ Jr. Abnormal visual pathways in the brain of a human albino. *Brain Res* 1975; **96**: 373–7.

Hafner R, Vogel P. Sarcoidosis of early onset. A challenge for the pediatric rheumatologist. *Clin Exp Rheumatol* 1993; **11**: 685–91.

Hamming NA, Miller MT, Rabb M. Unusual variant of familial aniridia. *J Pediatr Ophthalmol Strabismus* 1986; **23**: 195–200.

Hawkesworth NR, Headland S, Good P, Thomas NST, Clarke A. Aland Island eye disease: clinical and electrophysiological studies of a Welsh family. *Br J Ophthalmol* 1995; **79**: 424–30.

Hedera P, Lai S, Lerner AJ, Hopkins AL, Lewin JS, Friedland RP. Abnormal connectivity of the visual pathways in human albinos demonstrated by susceptibility-sensitised MRI. *Neurology* 1994; **44**: 1921–6.

Heimann K. The development of the choroid in man: choroidal vascular system. *Ophthalmic Res* 1972; **3**: 257–73.

Heimann K. Zur gefassentwicklump der macularen aderhautzone. *Klin Monatsbl Augenheilkd* 1970; **157**: 636–42.

Helm CJ, Holland GN. Ocular tuberculosis. *Surv Ophthalmol* 1993; **38**: 229–56.

Hemady RK, Baer JC, Foster CS. Immunosuppressive drugs in the management of progressive corticosteroid resistant uveitis associated with juvenile rheumatoid arthritis. *Int Ophthalmol Clin* 1992; **32**: 241–52.

Hered R, Rogers S, Zang Y-F, Biglan AW. Ophthalmic features of the Prader–Willi syndrome. *J Pediatr Ophthalmol Strabismus* 1988; **25**: 145–50.

Hetherington S. Sarcoidosis in young children. *Am J Dis Child* 1982; **136**: 13–15.

Hill JC, Stannard C, Bowen RM. Ciliary body malignant melanoma in a black child. *J Pediatr Ophthalmol Strabismus* 1991; **28**: 38–40.

Hittner HM, Riccardi VM, Ferrell RE, Borda RR, Justice J. Variable expressivity in autosomal dominant aniridia by clinical electrophysiologic, and angiographic criteria. *Am J Ophthalmol* 1980; **89**: 531–9.

Hofley P, Roarty J, McGinnity *et al*. Asymptomatic uveitis in children with chronic inflammatory bowel diseases. *J Pediatr Gastroenterol Nutr* 1993; **17**: 397–400.

Hogan M. Ultrastructure of the choroid. Its role in the pathogenesis of chorioretinal disease. *Trans Pacific Coast Ophthalmol Soc* 1961; **42**: 61.

Hogan MJ, Kimura SJ, Thygeson P. Pathology of herpes simplex keratoiritis. *Trans Am Ophthalmol Soc* 1963; **61**: 75–84.

Hoh H, Menage M, Dean-Hart C. Iris cyst after traumatic implantation of an eyelash into the anterior chamber. *Br J Ophthalmol* 1993; **77**: 741–2.

Holmstrom G, Almond G, Temple K, Taylor DSI, Baraitser M. The iris in Williams' syndrome. *Arch Dis Child* 1990; **65**: 987–9.

Hoover DL, Khaim JA, Giangiacomo J. Pediatric ocular sarcoidosis. *Surv Ophthalmol* 1986; **30**: 215–28.

Howard GM. Spontaneous hyphema in infancy and childhood. *Arch Ophthalmol* 1962; **68**: 615–20.

Howland AC. Infant eyes: optics and accommodation. *Curr Eye Res* 1982; **2**: 217–24.

Hughes AE, Newton VE, Liu XE, Read AP. A gene for Waardenburg syndrome type 2 maps close to the human homologue of the microphthalmia gene at chromosome 3p12–p14.1. *Nat Genet* 1994; **7**: 509–12.

Jacob J, Polomeno R, Chad Z *et al*. Ocular manifestations of Kawasaki's disease (mucocutaneous lymph node syndrome). *Canad J Ophthalmol* 1982; **17**: 199–202.

Jacobs M, Jaouni Z, Crompton J, Kriss A, Taylor D. Persistent pupillary membranes. *J Pediatr Ophthalmol Strabismus* 1991; **28**: 215–18.

Jakobiec FA, Howard GM, Devoe AG. Sector hamartoma of the iris. *Arch Ophthalmol* 1975a; **93**: 614–17.

Jakobiec FA, Howard GM, Ellsworth RM, Rosen M. Electron microscopic diagnosis of medulloepithelioma. *Am J Ophthalmol* 1975b; **79**: 321–9.

Jakobiec FA, Silbert G. Are most iris 'melanomas' really nevi? *Arch Ophthalmol* 1981; **99**: 2117–32.

James DG, Anderson R, Langley D, Ainslie D. Ocular sarcoidosis. *Br J Ophthalmol* 1964; **48**: 461–70.

James DG, Spiteri M. Systemic ophthalmology, Behçet's disease. *Ophthalmology* 1982; **89**: 1279–85.

Jasper L, Denny FW. Sarcoidosis in children with special emphasis on the natural history and treatment. *J Pediatr* 1968; **73**: 494–571.

Jay B, Carruthers J, Treplin MC, Winder AF. Human albinism. *Birth Defects* 1976; **12**: 415–26.

Jensen OA, Marberg M, Dupont A. Ocular pathology in the elfin face syndrome. *Ophthalmologica* 1976; **172**: 434–40.

Jesberg DO. Aniridia with retinal lipid deposits. *Arch Ophthalmol* 1962; **68**: 331–6.

Johns KJ, O'Day DM. Posterior chamber intraocular lenses after extracapsular cataract extraction in patients with aniridia. *Ophthalmology* 1991; **98**: 1698–702.

Jones IS, Cleasby GW. Hemangioma of the choroid, a clinicopathologic analysis. *Am J Ophthalmol* 1959; **48**: 612–20.

Jones N. Fuchs' heterochromic uveitis: a reappraisal of the clinical spectrum. *Eye* 1991a; **5**: 649–61.

Jones N. Fuchs' heterochromic uveitis: an update. *Surv Ophthalmol* 1993; **37**: 253–72.

Jones N. Glaucoma in Fuchs' heterochromic uveitis: aetiology, management and outcome. *Eye* 1991b; **5**: 662–7.

Joondeph BC, Goldberg MF. Familial iris melanosis—a misnomer? *Br J Ophthalmol* 1989; **73**: 289–94.

Jordan T, Hanson I, Zaletayev *et al.* The human pax 6 gene is mutated in two patients with aniridia. *Nature Genet* 1992; **1**: 328–32.

Josephberg RG, Kanter ED, Jaffee RM. A fluorescein angiographic study of patients with pars planitis peripheral exudation (snow banking) before and after cryopexy. *Ophthalmology* 1994; **101**: 1262–6.

Jotterand V, Boisjoly H, Hamois C *et al.* 11p13 deletion, Wilms' tumour and aniridia: unusual genetic, non-ocular and ocular features of three cases. *Br J Ophthalmol* 1990; **74**: 568–71.

Kachmer ML, Annable WL, Dimarco M. Iritis in children with varicella. *J Pediatr Ophthalmol Strabismus* 1990; **27**: 221–2.

Kalina PH, Pach JM, Bueyyner H, Robertson DM. Neovascularization of the disc in pars planitis. *Retina* 1990; **10**: 269–73.

Kalter H, Warkany J. Experimental production of congenital malformation in mammals by metabolic procedure. *Physiol Res* 1959; **39**: 69–115.

Kanski JJ. Anterior uveitis in juvenile rheumatoid arthritis. *Arch Ophthalmol* 1977; **95**: 1794–7.

Kanski JJ. Lensectomy for complicated cataract in juvenile chronic iridocyclitis. *Br J Ophthalmol* 1992; **76**: 72–5.

Kanski JJ. Screening for uveitis in juvenile chronic arthritis. *Br J Ophthalmol* 1989; **73**: 225–8.

Kanski JJ. Uveitis in juvenile chronic arthritis: incidence, clinical features and prognosis. *Eye* 1988; **2**: 641–5.

Kanski JJ, Shun-Shin GA. Systemic uveitis syndromes in childhood—an analysis of 340 cases. *Ophthalmology* 1984; **91**: 1247–51.

Kapp ME, von Norden GK, Jenkins R. Strabismus in Williams' syndrome. *Am J Ophthalmol* 1995; **119**: 355–60.

Kato H, Koike S, Yamamoto M, Ito Y, Yano E. Coronary aneurysms in infants and young children with acute febrile mucocutaneous lymph node syndrome. *J Pediatr* 1975; **86**: 892–8.

Katz RS, Gass JDM. Multiple choroidal osteoma developing in association with recurrent orbital inflammatory pseudotumour. *Arch Ophthalmol* 1983; **101**: 1724.

Kauffmann DJH, Wormser GP. Ocular Lyme disease: case report and review of the literature. *Br J Ophthalmol* 1990; **74**: 325–7.

Kawasaki T, Kosaki F, Okawa S, Shigematsu I, Yanagawa H. A new infantile acute febrile mucocutaneous lymph node syndrome (MLNS) prevailing in Japan. *Pediatrics* 1974; **54**: 271–6.

Kendig EL Jr. The clinical picture of sarcoidosis in childhood. *Pediatrics* 1974; **54**: 289–92.

Kenyon KR, Pederson JE, Green WR, Maumenee AE. Fibroglial proliferation in pars planitis. *Trans Ophthalmol Soc UK* 1975; **95**: 391–7.

Kerston RC, Tse DT, Anderson R. Iris melanoma, nevus or malignancy? *Surv Ophthalmol* 1985; **29**: 423–33.

Khan JA, Hoover DL, Giangiacoma J, Singsen BH. Orbital and childhood sarcoidosis. *J Pediatr Ophthalmol Strabismus* 1986; **23**: 190–5.

Kincaid MC, Green WR. Ocular and orbital involvement in leukemia. *Surv Ophthalmol* 1983; **27**: 211–13.

King RA, Townsend DeW, Oetting W *et al.* Temperature-sensitive tyrosinase associated with peripheral pigmentation in oculocutaneous albinism. *J Clin Invest* 1991; **87**: 1046–53.

King RA, Witkop CJ. Hairbulb tyrosinase activity in oculocutaneous albinism. *Nature* 1976; **263**: 69–71.

King RH, Hearing VJ, Cred DJ, Oetting WS. Albinism. In: Scriver CR, Beaudet AL, Sly WS, Valle D, eds. *The Metabolic and Molecular Basis of Inherited Disease*. New York: McGraw Hill 1995: 4353–90.

Kinyoun JL, Bensinger RE, Chuang EL. 30-year history of sympathetic ophthalmia. *Ophthalmology* 1983; **90**: 59–65.

Klein AJ, Armstrong BL, Greer MK, Brown FR. Hyperacusis and otitis media in individuals with Williams' syndrome. *J Speech Hear Disord* 1990; **55**: 339–44.

Kremer I, Rajpal R, Rapuano C, Cohen E, Laibson P. Results of penetrating keratoplasty in aniridia. *Am J Ophthalmol* 1993; **115**: 317–20.

Kriss A, Russell-Eggitt I, Harris CM, Lloyd IC, Taylor DSI. Aspects of albinism. *Ophthal Paediatr Genet* 1992; **13**: 89–100.

Kumar H, Sakhuja N, Sachdev MS. Hyperplastic pupillary membrane and laser therapy. *Ophthalmol Surg* 1994; **25**: 189–90.

La Hey E, Baarsma G. Fuchs' heterochromic cyclitis and retinal vascular abnormalities in progressive hemifacial atrophy. *Eye* 1993; **7**: 426–8.

La Hey E, de Jong PTVM, Kijlstra A. Fuchs' heterochromic cyclitis: review of the literature on the pathogenetic mechanisms. *Br J Ophthalmol* 1994; **78**: 307–12.

La Hey E, de Vries J, Langerhorst CT, Baarsma GS, Kijlstra A. Treatment and prognosis of secondary glaucoma in Fuchs' heterochromic cyclitis. *Am J Ophthalmol* 1993; **116**: 327–40.

La Hey E, Rothova A, Baarsma S, de Vries J, Knapen F, Kijlstra A. Fuchs' heterochromic iridocyclitis is not associated with ocular toxoplasmosis. *Arch Ophthalmol* 1992; **110**: 806–11.

Lambert SR, Amaya L, Taylor D. Congenital idiopathic microcoria. *Am J Ophthalmol* 1988; **106**: 590–4.

Lapointe N, Chad Z, Lacroix J *et al.* Kawasaki disease: association with uveitis in seven patients. *Pediatrics* 1982; **69**: 376–9.

Laties AM, Scheie HG. Evolution of multiple small tumours in sarcoid granuloma of the optic disc. *Am J Ophthalmol* 1972; **79**: 60–6.

Layman PR, Anderson DR, Flynn JT. Frequent occurrence of hypoplastic optic discs in patients with aniridia. *Am J Ophthalmol* 1974; **77**: 573–6.

Lee RG *et al.* Disorders of hemostasis. In: *Wintrobe's Clinical Hematology*, 9th edn. Pennsylvania: Lea & Febiger, 1992: 1402–3.

Lennarson P, Barney NP. Interstitial keratitis as presenting ophthalmic sign of sarcoidosis in a child. *J Pediatr Ophthalmol Strabismus* 1995; **32**: 194–6.

Leonard BC, Shields JA, McDonald PR. Malignant melanomas of the uveal tract in children and young adults. *Canad J Ophthalmol* 1975;

10: 441–9.

Lerone M, Persagno A, Taccone A *et al.* Oculocerebral syndrome with hypopigmentation (Cross syndrome). *Clin Genet* 1992; **41**: 87–9.

Lesser RL, Kornmehl EW, Pachner AR, Kattah J, Hedges III TR *et al.* Neuro-ophthalmologic manifestations of Lyme disease. *Ophthalmology* 1990; **97**: 699–706.

Levy WJ. Congenital iris lesion. *Br J Ophthalmol* 1957; **41**: 120–3.

Lewis RA, Merin LM. Iris flocculi and familial aortic dissection. *Arch Ophthalmol* 1995; **113**: 1330–1.

Liang JC, Juarez CP, Goldberg MF. Bilateral bicoloured irides with Hirschsprung's disease: a new neural crest syndrome. *Arch Ophthalmol* 1983; **101**: 69–73.

Liddy BSL, Stuart J. Sympathetic ophthalmia in Canada. *Canad J Ophthalmol* 1972; **7**: 157–9.

Lubin JR, Albert DM, Weinstein M. Sixty-five years of sympathetic ophthalmia. A clinicopathologic review of 105 cases (1913–1978). *Ophthalmology* 1980; **87**: 109–21.

Lyness R, Earley O, Logan W, Archer D. Ocular larva migrans: a case report. *Br J Ophthalmol* 1987; **71**: 396–401.

McCartney ACE, Spalton DJ, Bull TB. Type IV melanosomes of the human albino iris. *Br J Ophthalmol* 1985; **69**: 537–42.

Mackman G, Brightbell FS, Opitz JM. Corneal changes in aniridia. *Am J Ophthalmol* 1979; **87**: 497–502.

Maden A, Buyukgebiz B, Gunenc U, Cevik N. Bilateral congenital absence of pupillary aperture. *Am J Ophthalmol* 1991; **112**: 608–9.

Mader TH, Wergeland FL, Chismire KJ. Enlarged pupillary membranes. *J Pediatr Ophthalmol Strabismus* 1988; **25**: 73–5.

Makley TA, Leibold JE. Modern therapy of sympathetic ophthalmia. *Arch Ophthalmol* 1960; **64**: 809–16.

Malinowski SM, Pulido JS, Folk JC. Long-term visual outcome and complications associated with pars planitis. *Ophthalmology* 1993; **100**: 818–24.

Mamalis N, Font R, Anderson CW, Monson MC, Williams AT. Concurrent benign teratoid medulloepithelioma and pinealoblastoma. *Ophthalmic Surg* 1992; **23**: 403–8.

Mann I. *The Development of the Human Eye*. London: British Medical Association, 1964.

Margo CE. Congenital aniridia: a histopathologic study of the anterior segment in children. *J Pediatr Ophthalmol Strabismus* 1983; **20**: 192–8.

Margo CE, Brooks HL Jr. Adenocarcinoma of the ciliary epithelium in a 12-year-old black child. *J Pediatr Ophthalmol Strabismus* 1991; **28**: 232–5.

Martenet AC. Role of viruses in uveitis. *Trans Ophthalmol Soc UK* 1981; **101**: 308–11.

Martin D, Chan C-C, de Smet M *et al.* Type IV melanosomes of the human albino iris. *Br J Ophthalmol* 1985; **69**: 537–42.

Massaro D, Katz S, Sachs M. Choroidal tubercles: a clue to haematogenous tuberculosis. *Ann Intern Med* 1964; **60**: 231–41.

Melish ME. Kawasaki syndrome: a new infectious disease? *J Infect Dis* 1981; **143**: 317–24.

Merin S, Crawford JS, Cardarelli J. Hyperplastic persistent pupillary membrane. *Am J Ophthalmol* 1971; **72**: 717–19.

Michelson JB, Shields JA. The relationship of iris nevi to posterior uveal melanomas. *Am J Ophthalmol* 1977; **83**: 694–6.

Miller SD, Judisch GF. Persistent pupillary membrane: successful medical management. *Arch Ophthalmol* 1979; **97**: 1911–13.

Minoda K, Hirose T, Sugano I *et al.* Occurrence of sequential intraocular tumors: malignant medulloepithelioma subsequent to retinoblastoma. *Jpn J Ophthalmol* 1993; **37**: 293–300.

Mintz-Hittner HA, Ferrell RE, Lyons LA, Krezzer FL. Criteria to detect minimal expressivity within families with autosomal dominant aniridia. *Am J Ophthalmol* 1992; **114**: 700–7.

Mirkinson AE, Mirkinson NK. A familial syndrome of aniridia and absence of the patella. *Birth Defects* 1975; **11**: 129–31.

Mochizuki M, Tagma K, Watanabe T, Yamaguchi K. Human T lymphotropic virus type I uveitis. *Br J Ophthalmol* 1994; **78**: 149–54.

Mollenbach CJ. Congenital defects in the internal membranes of the eye. Clinical and genetic aspects. In: *Opera ex Dorno Biologiae Hereditariae Humanae Universitatis Hafniensis*, Vol. 15. Copenhagen: Ejner Munksgaard, 1947: 1–165.

Morris CA, Demsey SA, Leonard CO, Dilts C, Blackburn BL. Natural history of Williams' syndrome: physical characteristics. *J Pediatr* 1988; **113**: 318–26.

Mund ML, Rodrigues MM, Fine BS. Light and electron microscopic observations on the pigmented layers of the developing human eye. *Am J Ophthalmol* 1972; **73**: 167–82.

Naidoff MA, Kenyon KR, Green WR. Iris haemangioma and abnormal retinal vasculature in a case of diffuse congenital haemangiomatosis. *Am J Ophthalmol* 1971; **72**: 633–44.

Nakagawa Y, Kiyosawa M, Tamai M, Iro M. Positron emission tomography and 18 F-fluorodeoxyglucose for the detection of visual pathway abnormalities in albinism. *Am J Ophthalmol* 1993; **116**: 112–13.

Nash MC, Jones CL, Walker, Powell HR. Anti-neutrophil cytoplasmic antibody-associated glomerulonephritis in children. *Pediatr Nephrol* 1993; **7**: 11–14.

Nathan DG. Disorders of granulocyte function and granulopoiesis. In: *Hematology of Infancy and Childhood*, 4th edn. Philadelphia: WB Saunders, 1993: 916–19.

Naumann GOH, Font RC, Zimmerman LE. Electron microscopic verification of primary rhabdomyosarcoma of the iris. *Am J Ophthalmol* 1972; **74**: 110–17.

Naumann GOH, Hellnar K, Naumann LR. Pigmented nevi of the choroid. Clinical study of secondary changes in the overlying tissue. *Trans Am Acad Ophthalmol Otolaryngol* 1971; **75**: 110–23.

Naumann GOH, Rummelt V. Congenital nonpigmented epithelial iris cyst removed by block excision. *Graef Arch Clin Exp Ophthamol* 1990; **228**: 392–7.

Nelson LB, Spaeth GL, Nowinski TS *et al.* Aniridia, a review. *Surv Ophthalmol* 1984; **28**: 621–42.

Nevin N, Lim J. Syndrome of partial aniridia, cerebellar ataxia and mental retardation—Gillespie syndrome. *Am J Med Genet* 1990; **35**: 468–9.

Newburger JW, Takahashi M, Burns JC *et al.* The treatment of Kawasaki syndrome with intravenous gamma globulin. *N Engl J Med* 1986; **315**: 341–7.

Ni C, Paple JJ, Robinson NL, Wu BF. Uveal tuberculosis. *Int Ophthalmol Clin* 1982; **22**: 103–24.

Nicholson DH, Green WR. *Pediatric Ocular Tumours*. New York: Masson, 1981: 87–96.

Nik NA, Hidayat A, Zimmerman LE, Fine BS. Diffuse iris nevus manifested by unilateral open angle glaucoma. *Arch Ophthalmol* 1981; **99**: 125–7.

Ninane J, Taylor D, Day S. The eye as a sanctuary in acute lymphoblastic leukaemia. *Lancet* 1980; **i**: 452–3.

Nishida K, Kinoshita S, Ohashi Y, Yasuaki K, Yamamoto S. Ocular surface abnormalities in aniridia. *Am J Ophthalmol* 1995; **120**: 368–75.

Noble KG. Bilateral choroidal osteoma in three siblings. *Am J Ophthalmol* 1990; **109**: 656–60.

North AF, Font CW, Gibson WM *et al.* Sarcoid arthritis in children. *Am J Med* 1970; **48**: 449–55.

Nussenblatt R. The role of the chorioretinal biopsy in the management of posterior uveitis. *Ophthalmology* 1993; **100**: 705–14.

O'Connor GR. Doyne lecture; heterochromic iridocyclitis. *Trans Oph-*

thalmol Soc UK 1985; **109**: 219–31.

O'Connor GR. Factors related to the initiation and recurrence of uveitis. XL Edward Jackson memorial lecture. *Am J Ophthalmol* 1983; **96**: 577–99.

O'Donnell FE. Congenital ocular hypopigmentation. In: Kivlin JD, ed. *Developmental Abnormalities of the Eye*. International Ophthalmologic Clinics, 1984: 133–42.

O'Donnell FE, Green WR, Fleischman JA, Hambrick GW. X-linked ocular albinism in blacks. *Arch Ophthalmol* 1978; **96**: 1189–92.

O'Donnell FE, Hambrick GW, Green WR, Iliff WJ, Stone DL. X-linked ocular albinism: an ocularcutaneous macromelanosomal disorder. *Arch Ophthalmol* 1976; **94**: 1883–92.

Oh JO. Primary and secondary herpes simplex uveitis in rabbits. *Surv Ophthalmol* 1976; **21**: 178–84.

Ohm J. Bandformige hornhauttrubung bei einem neunjahrigen madchen und ihre Behandlung mit subkonjunktivalen Jodkaliumeinspritzungen. *Klin Monatsbl Augenheikd* 1910; **48**: 243–6.

O'Rahilly R. The optic, vestibulocochlear and terminal vomeronasal neural crest in staged human embryos. In: Rohen JW, ed. *Second International Symposium on the Structure of the Eye*. Stuttgart: Schattauer-Verlag, 1965: 557–64.

Orlin SE, Lauffer JS. Lyme disease keratitis. *Am J Ophthalmol* 1989; **107**: 678–80.

Ostler HB, Dawson CR, Schachter J, Engleman EP. Reiter's syndrome. *Am J Ophthalmol* 1971; **71**: 986–91.

Ozanics V, Jakobiec FA. Prenatal development of the eye and its adnexa. In: Jakobiec FA, ed. *Ocular Anatomy, Embryology and Teratology*. Philadelphia: Harper & Row, 1982: 11–13.

Papale JJ, Akiwama, Hirose T *et al*. Adenocarcinoma of the ciliary body pigment epithelium in a child. *Arch Ophthalmol* 1984; **102**: 100–3.

Paridaens ADA, Deuble K, McCartney ACE. Spontaneous congenital non-pigmented epithelial cysts of the iris stroma. *Br J Ophthalmol* 1992; **76**: 39–42.

Patterson A, Sommerville RG, Jones BR. Herpetic keratouveitis with herpes virus antigen in the anterior chamber. *Trans Ophthalmol Soc UK* 1968; **88**: 243–9.

Paul EV, Parnell BL, Fraker M. Prognosis of malignant melanomas of the choroid and ciliary body. *Int Ophthalmol Clin* 1962; **2**: 487–502.

Pendergrass TW. Congenital anomalies in children with Wilms' tumour. A new survey. *Cancer* 1976; **37**: 403–8.

Perry HD, Mallen FJ. Iris involvement in granulocytic sarcoma. *Am J Ophthalmol* 1979; **87**: 530–2.

Phelps CD. The pathogenesis of glaucoma in Sturge–Weber syndrome. *Ophthalmology* 1978; **85**: 276–86.

Pilling GP. Wilms' tumour in seven children with congenital aniridia. *Pediatr Surg* 1975; **10**: 87–96.

Quigley HA, Stanish FS. Unilateral congenital iris pigment epithelial hyperplasia associated with late onset glaucoma. *Am J Ophthalmol* 1978; **86**: 182–4.

Ragge NK, Acheson J, Murphree AL. Iris mamillations: their significance and associations. *Eye* 1996; **10**: 86–91.

Rennie IG, Parsons MA, Palmer CA. Congenital adenoma of the iris and ciliary body: light and electron microscopic observations. *Br J Ophthalmol* 1992; **76**: 563–6.

Reynolds JD, Hiles DA, Johnson BL, Biglan AW. Hyperplastic persistent pupillary membrane—surgical management. *J Pediatr Ophthalmol Strabismus* 1983; **20**: 149–52.

Riccardi VM, Borges W. Aniridia, cataracts, and Wilms' tumour. *Am J Ophthalmol* 1978; **86**: 577–99.

Ridgeway EW, Jaffe N, Walton DS. Leukemic ophthalmopathy in children. *Cancer* 1976; **38**: 1744–9.

Riwchun MH, De Coursey E. Sympathetic ophthalmia caused by non-perforating intraocular sarcoma. *Arch Ophthalmol* 1941; **25**: 848–58.

Rodrigues MM, Hackett J, Donohon P. Iris. In: Jakobiec FA, ed. *Ocular Anatomy, Embryology and Teratology*. Philadelphia: Harper & Row, 1982: 285–302.

Rosenbaum PS, Boniuk M, Font R. Diffuse uveal melanoma in a 5-year-old child. *Am J Ophthalmol* 1988; **106**: 601–6.

Rothova A, La Hey E, Baarsma GS, Breebaart AC. Iris nodules in Fuchs' heterochromic uveitis. *Am J Ophthalmol* 1994; **118**: 338–42.

Russell-Eggitt I, Kriss A, Taylor DSI. Albinism in childhood—a flash VEP and ERG study. *Br J Ophthalmol* 1990; **74**: 136–40.

Ruttum MS, Mittelman D, Singh P. Iris hemangiomas in infants with periorbital capillary hemangiomas. *J Pediatr Ophthalmol Strabismus* 1993; **30**: 331–3.

Sabates R. Choroiditis compatible with the histopathologic diagnosis of sympathetic ophthalmia following cyclocryotherapy of neovascular glaucoma. *Ophthalmol Surg* 1988; **19**: 176–81.

Saini JS, Mukherjee AK, Nadkarani N. Primary tuberculosis of the retina. *Br J Ophthalmol* 1986; **70**: 533–5.

Schachat AP, Jabs DA, Graham ML, Ambinder RF, Green WR, Soral R. Leukemic iris infiltration. *J Pediatr Ophthalmol Strabismus* 1988; **25**: 135–8.

Schaller J, Johnson GJ, Ansell BM, Holborrow EJ. Antinuclear antibodies (ANA) in patients with iridocyclitis and juvenile rheumatoid arthritis (JRA, Still's disease). *Arthritis Rheum* 1973; **16**: 130.

Schaller J, Kupfer C, Wedgwood RJ. Iridocyclitis in juvenile rheumatoid arthritis. *Pediatrics* 1969; **44**: 92–100.

Schlaegel TF. Uveitis of suspected viral origin. In: Duane TD, ed. *Clinical Ophthalmology*. Hagerstown: Harper & Row, 1981: 9.

Schlaegel TF, O'Connor GR. Tuberculosis and syphilis (letter). *Arch Ophthalmol* 1981; **99**: 2206–7.

Schwartz LK, O'Connor GR. Secondary syphilis with iris papules. *Am J Ophthalmol* 1980; **90**: 380–4.

Scotto J, Fraumeni JF, Lee JA. Melanoma of the eye and other non cutaneous sites. *J Natl Cancer Inst* 1976; **56**: 489–91.

Shaffer RN, Cohen JS. Visual reduction in aniridia. *J Pediatr Ophthalmol Strabismus* 1975; **12**: 220–2.

Shaw MW, Falls HF, Neel JV. Congenital aniridia. *Am J Hum Genet* 1960; **12**: 389–415.

Shields CL, Shields JA, Milite J, DePotter P, Sabbag R, Menduke H. Uveal melanoma in teenagers and children. A report of 40 cases. *Ophthalmology* 1991; **98**: 1662–6.

Shields JA. Melanocytic tumours of the iris. In: Shields JA, ed. *Diagnosis and Management of Intraocular Tumours*. St Louis: CV Mosby, 1983: 83–94.

Shields JA, Eagle R, Shields C, de Potter P, Poliak J. Natural course and histopathologic findings of lacrimal gland choristoma of the iris and ciliary body. *Am J Ophthalmol* 1995; **119**: 219–24.

Shields JA, Kline MUS, Augsburger JJ. Primary iris cysts: a review of the literature and report of 62 cases. *Br J Ophthalmol* 1984; **68**: 152–66.

Shiloh Y, Litoak G, Ziv Y *et al*. Genetic mapping of X-linked albinism–deafness syndrome to Xq26.3–q27.1. *Am J Hum Genet* 1990; **47**: 20–7.

Shiono T, Tsunoda, Chida Y, Nakazawa M, Tamai M. X-linked ocular albinism in Japanese patients. *Br J Ophthalmol* 1995; **79**: 139–43.

Shore A, Ansell B. Juvenile psoriatic arthritis. *J Pediatr* 1982; **100**: 529–35.

Siltzbach LE, Greenberg GM. Childhood sarcoidosis—a study of 18 patients. *N Engl J Med* 1968; **279**: 1239–45.

Skre H, Berg K. Cerebellar ataxia and total albinism: a kindred suggesting pleiotropism or linkage. *Clin Genet* 1974; **5**: 196–204.

Smith LB, Newburger JW, Burns JC. Kawasaki syndrome and the eye.

Pediatr Infect Dis J 1989; **8**: 116–18.

Smith RE, Nozik RA. Uveitis. In: *A Clinical Approach to Diagnosis and Management* of Uveitis. Baltimore: Williams & Wilkins, 1983.

Spaeth G, Nelson LB, Beaudoin AR. Ocular teratology. In: Jakobiec FA, ed. *Ocular Anatomy, Embryology and Teratology*. Philadelphia: Harper & Row, 1982: 1627–56.

Spalton DJ. Lyme disease. *Br J Ophthalmol* 1990; **74**: 321–3.

Spedick MJ, Beauchamp GR. Retinal and optic nerve abnormalities in albinism. *J Pediatr Ophthalmol Strabismus* 1986; **23**: 58–63.

Spicer WTH. Parenchymatous keratitis: interstitial keratitis: uveitis anterior. *Br J Ophthalmol Monograph* 1924; **1**(Suppl.): 1–63.

Stastny P, Fink CW. Different HLA-D associations in adult and juvenile rheumatoid arthritis. *J Clin Invest* 1979; **63**: 124–30.

Stevens JE, Bayrd W, Heck FJ. Infectious mononucleosis: a study of 210 sporadic cases. *Am J Med* 1951; **11**: 202–8.

Stone J. Special types of contact lenses and their use. In: Stone J, Phillips AJ, eds. *Contact Lenses* , Vol 2. London: Butterworth, 1981: 667.

Sugar HS, Kobernicke SD, Weingarten JE. Hematogenous ocular sclerosis of local cause. *Am J Ophthalmol* 1967; **64**: 749–56.

Summers CG, Knobloch WH, Witkop CJ, King RA. Hermansky–Pudlak syndrome: ophthalmic findings. *Ophthalmology* 1988; **95**: 545–55.

Susac JO, Smith JL, Scelfo R. The 'tomato catsup' fundus in Sturge–Weber syndrome. *Arch Ophthalmol* 1974; **92**: 69–70.

Tassabehji M *et al.* Mutations in the PAX 3 gene causing Waardenburg syndrome type 1 and type 2. *Nature Genet* 1993; **3**: 26–30.

Taylor D, Day S, Tiedemann K, Chessels J, Marshall WC, Constable IJ. Chorioretinal biopsy in a patient with leukaemia. *Br J Ophthalmol* 1981; **65**: 489–93.

Taylor WOG. Visual disabilities of oculocutaneous albinism and their alleviation. *Trans Ophthalmol Soc UK* 1978; **98**: 423–45.

Thies O. Gedanken uber den Ausbruch der sympathischen ophthalmie. *Klin Monatsbl Augenheilkd* 1947; **112**: 185–7.

Ticho U, Ben-Sira I. Ocular leprosy in Malawi. Clinical and therapeutic survey of 8325 leprosy patients. *Br J Ophthalmol* 1970; **521**: 107–12.

Tizard EJ, Suzuki A, Levin M, Dillon MJ. Clinical aspects of 100 patients with Kawasaki disease. *Arch Dis Childh* 1991; **66**: 185–8.

Toulemont PJ, Urvoy M, Coscus G, Lecallonec A, Cuvilliers AF. Association of congenital microcoria with myopia and glaucoma. *Ophthalmology* 1995; **102**: 193–8.

Trimble SN, Schatz H. Choroidal osteomas after intraocular inflammation. *Am J Ophthalmol* 1983; **96**: 759.

Tugal-Tutkun I, Havrlikova K, Power WJ, Foster CS. Changing patterns in uveitis of childhood. *Ophthalmology* 1996; **103**: 375–83.

Valluri S, Chu FC, Smith MC. Ocular pathologic findings of chronic granulomatous disease of childhood. *Am J Ophthalmol* 1995; **120**: 120–3.

Verdager J. Prepubertal and pubertal melanomas in ophthalmology. *Am J Ophthalmol* 1965; **60**: 1002–11.

Verma L, Kumar A, Garg S, Khosla PK, Tewari HK. Cryopexy in pars planitis. *Canad J Ophthalmol* 1991; **26**: 313–15.

Waardenburg PJ. Gross remnants of the pupillary membrane: anterior polar cataract and microcornea in a mother and her children. *Ophthalmologica* 1949; **118**: 828.

Walker JP, Weiter JJ, Albert DM *et al.* Uveal malignant melanoma in three generations of the same family. *Am J Ophthalmol* 1979; **88**: 723–6.

Walton DS. Aniridia with glaucoma. In: Chandler PA, Grant WM, eds. *Glaucoma*. Philadelphia: Lea & Febiger, 1979: 351–4.

Warburg M, Mikkelsen M, Andersen SR *et al.* Aniridia and interstitial deletion of the short arm of chromosome 11. *Metab Pediatr Ophthalmol* 1980; **4**: 97–102.

Warkany J, Schraffenberger E. Congenital malformations induced in rats by maternal vitamin A deficiency. *Arch Ophthalmol* 1946; **35**: 150–69.

Watts MT, Rennie IG. Detached iris cyst presenting as an intraocular foreign body. *J Roy Soc Med* 1991; **84**: 172–3.

Weiss MJ, Ernest JT. Diffuse congenital haemangiomata with infantile glaucoma. *Am J Ophthalmol* 1976; **81**: 216–18.

Wiggins RE, Tomey KF. The results of glaucoma surgery in aniridia. *Arch Ophthalmol* 1992; **110**: 503–5.

Wilson ME. Congenital iris ectropion and a new classification for anterior segment dysgenesis. *J Pediatr Ophthalmol Strabismus* 1990: **27**: 48–55.

Winter TC. Ocular hemosiderosis. *Trans Am Acad Ophthalmol Otolaryngol* 1967; **71**: 813–19.

Witkop CJ. Inherited disorders of pigmentations. *Clin Dermatol* 1985; **3**: 70–134.

Witmer R, Iwamoto T. Electronmicroscopic observation of herpes like particles in the iris. *Arch Ophthalmol* 1968; **79**: 331–7.

Witschel H, Font RL. Hemangioma of the choroid. A clinicopathologic study of 71 cases and a review of the literature. *Surv Ophthalmol* 1975; **20**: 415–31.

Wittig E, Moreira C, Freure-Maia N, Vianna-Morgante A. Partial aniridia, cerebellar ataxia and mental deficiency (Gillespie syndrome) in two brothers. *Am J Med Genet* 1988; **30**: 703–8.

Wolf MD, Lichter PR, Ragsdale CG. Prognostic factors in the uveitis of juvenile rheumatoid arthritis. *Ophthalmology* 1987; **94**: 1242–7.

Yanoff M, Zimmerman LE. The relationship of congenital ocular melanocytosis and neurofibromatosis to uveal melanomas. *Arch Ophthalmol* 1967; **77**: 331–6.

Zaidman GW, Johnson BL, Salamon SM, Mondino BJ. Fuchs' adenoma affecting the peripheral iris. *Arch Ophthalmol* 1983; **101**: 771–3.

Ziegler JL. Treatment results of 54 American patients with Burkitt's lymphoma are similar to the African experience. *N Engl J Med* 1977; **297**: 75–80.

Zimmerman LE, Broughton WL. A clinicopathologic and follow-up study of 56 intraocular medulloepitheliomas. In: Jakobiec FA, ed. *Ocular and Adnexal Tumours*. Alabama: Aesculapius, 1978: 181–5.

Zimmerman LE, McLean IW. A comparison of progression in the management of retinoblastomas and uveal melanomas. In: Nicholson DH, ed. *Ocular Pathology Update*. New York: Masson, 1980: 191.

39: Lens

Scott Lambert

Anatomy

The crystalline lens is a biconvex optical structure lying posterior to the iris and anterior to the vitreous humor. It is suspended by zonular fibres from the ciliary body. At birth, the lens has an equatorial diameter of 6.5 mm and an anterior–posterior depth of 3.5 mm at its poles. A collagenous capsule surrounds the lens with a monolayer of cuboidal epithelial cells on its anterior inner surface. The cuboidal cells in the equatorial region continue to develop into long spindle-shaped secondary lens fibres throughout life. The addition of secondary lens fibres in the equatorial region accentuates the elliptical shape of the lens in childhood and early adulthood. The lens achieves an equatorial diameter of 9 mm and an anterior–posterior depth of 5 mm by adulthood.

The equatorial diameter of the lens stabilizes in early adulthood, with additional growth occurring in the anterior–posterior depth of the lens thereafter. The fetal nucleus is demarcated from the embryonic nucleus by Y-shaped upright sutures anteriorly and inverted Y-shaped sutures posteriorly. Both the embryonic and fetal nuclei are present at birth. Lens fibres developing after birth become the adult nucleus and cortex. The lens nucleus consists of compacted lens fibres which are indistinguishable from one another. The lens fibres in the cortex are less densely packed and individual fibres may be identified by specular microscopy in the superficial layers (Bron & Lambert 1984).

Embryology

Lens induction occurs in response to factors present even before the presence of the optic vesicle (Grainger *et al.* 1992). The lens visibly develops initially as a thickening of the surface ectoderm overlying the optic vesicle. The thickened surface ectoderm or lens placode then invaginates to form a lens pit which subsequently becomes the lens vesicle. The posterior surface of the lens vesicle is lined by columnar epithelial cells which elongate to become the primary lens fibres. The primary lens fibres gradually fill the lumen of the lens vesicle creating a

445

nearly spherical structure. Only the anterior wall of the lens vesicle retains a monolayer of cuboidal epithelial cells which persists throughout life. Beginning at 7 gestational weeks, cuboidal epithelial cells in the equatorial region develop into secondary lens fibres. The secondary lens fibres elongate in both an anterior and posterior direction inserting over the primary lens fibres. They are thickest equatorially resulting in preferential growth of the equatorial diameter of the fetal lens. Secondary lens fibres insert anteriorly and posteriorly at Y-shaped sutures (Mann 1928).

The lens capsule forms from the deposition of basement membrane material from the lens epithelium. Zonular fibres develop from the non-pigmented epithelium of the ciliary body during the fifth gestational month.

The tunica vasculosa lentis forms from branches of the hyaloid artery posteriorly and the annular vessel laterally. It encircles the developing lens, but begins to regress during the fourth gestational month (Mann 1928) and disappears during the seventh gestational month.

Developmental anomalies

Developmental defects of the lens include a wide spectrum of anomalies ranging from primary aphakia to abnormalities in the transparency, position, shape and size of the lens.

Congenital aphakia occurs when the surface ectoderm in the developing embryo fails to form a lens placode and vesicle. Secondary aphakia occurs when the developing lens is spontaneously absorbed. Both conditions only occur in cases of maldevelopment of the remainder of the eye so that functional vision is rarely possible in these patients (Mann 1957).

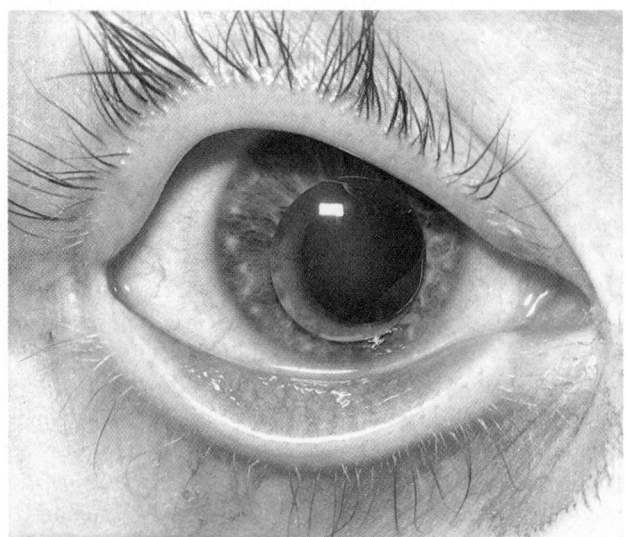

Fig. 39.1 Microspherophakia with anterior dislocation.

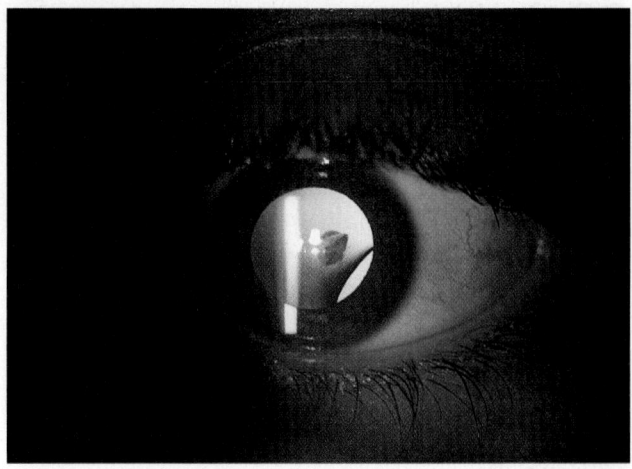

Fig. 39.2 Lens coloboma (Dr S. Day's patient).

Microspherophakia (Fig. 39.1) is a developmental abnormality in which the lens is reduced in diameter and spherical in shape. Although it may occur as an isolated hereditary abnormality, it more frequently occurs as part of the Weill–Marchesani syndrome. Microspherophakia may occur due to an arrest in the development of the secondary lens fibres or the insertion of abnormally thin secondary lens fibres.

Duplication of the lens is an extremely rare anomaly associated with metaplasia of the cornea (Evans & Hickey-Dwyer 1991) and colobomas of the iris and chorioretinal tissue (Lyford & Roy 1974; Hemady *et al.* 1993). The anomaly is believed to occur secondary to metaplastic changes in the surface ectoderm which prevent the lens placode from invaginating into a single lens vesicle.

Lens colobomas (Fig. 39.2) may be expressed as wedge-shaped defects or indentations in the lens or only a flattening of a segment of the lens in a region where the zonules have failed to develop. They may occur unilaterally as an isolated anomaly or bilaterally in association with colobomas of the uveal system. A localized lens opacity may often be found in the region of the coloboma. Most colobomas occur in the lower portion of the lens either directly inferiorly or inferotemporally.

Lenticonus (Figs 39.3–39.5) and lentiglobus are axial deformations of the anterior or posterior lens surfaces. Abnormalities of the posterior surface occur more frequently than those of the anterior surface. The refractive error through the centre of the lens may be highly myopic and astigmatic, while the peripheral lens is emmetropic. Lentiglobus is more common than lenticonus and is usually unilateral (Crouch & Parks 1978). It may be familial (Bleik *et al.* 1992; Gibbs *et al.* 1993), with an X-linked recessive inheritance (Vivian *et al.* 1995). Rarely it may occur in association with a persistent hyaloid artery remnant (Kitty & Hiles 1993).

Anterior lenticonus is frequently associated with

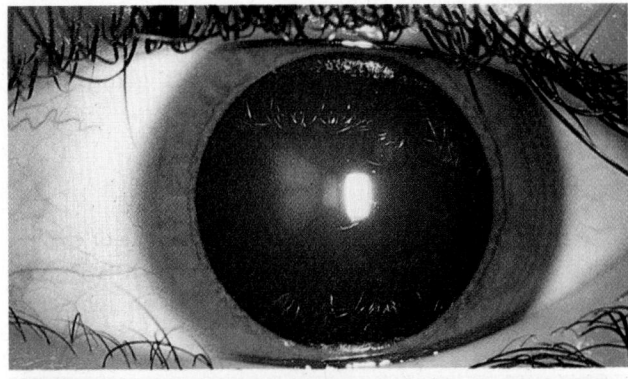

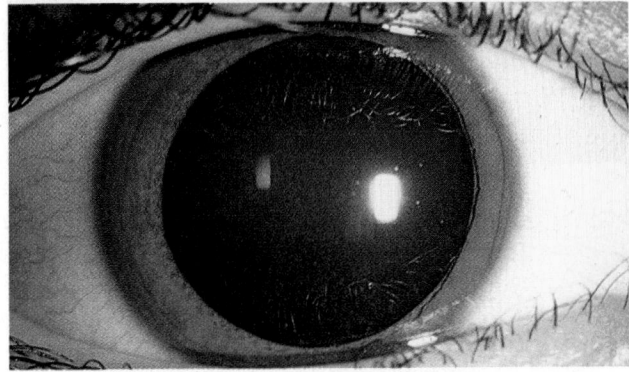

Fig. 39.3 Lenticonus with cataract. The characteristic reflex is only visible on retroillumination as in Fig. 39.4.

Alport's syndrome and may be secondary to an abnormally thin anterior capsule centrally (Streeten *et al.* 1987; Thompson *et al.* 1987; Jeffrey *et al.* 1994). It is most easily detected using retinoscopy. Alport's syndrome is inherited as an X-linked trait (Flinter *et al.* 1988) and is due to a mutation in the COL4A5 collagen gene at Xq22 (Barker *et al.* 1990). Patients with Alport's syndrome also have retinal flecks without electroretinographic changes and posterior subcapsular cataract (Jacobs *et al.* 1992).

Remnants of the tunica vasculosa lentis are residues from the vascular network which surround the lens early in fetal life. They usually consist of a vascular pigmented pupillary membrane attached to the iris at the collarette. Another vascular remnant, the epicapsular star, appears as a single spot or group of pigmented spots attached to the anterior capsule. A Mittendorf dot is a remnant of the posterior tunica vasculosa lentis and consists of a dense white spot inferonasal to the posterior pole of the lens either adherent to the posterior lens capsule or slightly posterior to it. The tunica vasculosa lentis may be seen in premature infants.

Persistent hyperplastic primary vitreous

The term persistent hyperplastic primary vitreous (PHPV) is used to describe a wide spectrum of congenital

anomalies. These abnormalities most commonly consist of a retrolental plaque (Fig. 39.6) in a microphthalmic eye with prominent blood vessels on the iris, a shallow anterior chamber, elongated ciliary processes and occasionally intralenticular haemorrhages (Reese 1955; Kazuhiko *et al.* 1986). They are unilateral in 90% of patients (Karr & Scott 1986). While the lens may be clear initially, with time they usually become cataractous. In some instances, the lens cortex and nucleus may undergo spontaneous absorption through a break in the posterior lens capsule while in others the lens becomes swollen resulting in the loss of the anterior chamber and an elevation in the intraocular pressure. The retrolental fibrovascular plaque may be vascular (Figs 39.7, 39.8) and frequently bleeds if cut surgically. In early infancy, the ciliary processes are often stretched (Fig. 39.9). Retinal involvement usually occurs secondary to contraction of the retrolental plaque resulting in traction on the vitreous base and peripheral retina.

While in many instances the posterior pole is normal, fibrous tissue arising from the remnant of the hyaloid vessels (Fig. 39.10) may occur and occasionally result in peri-

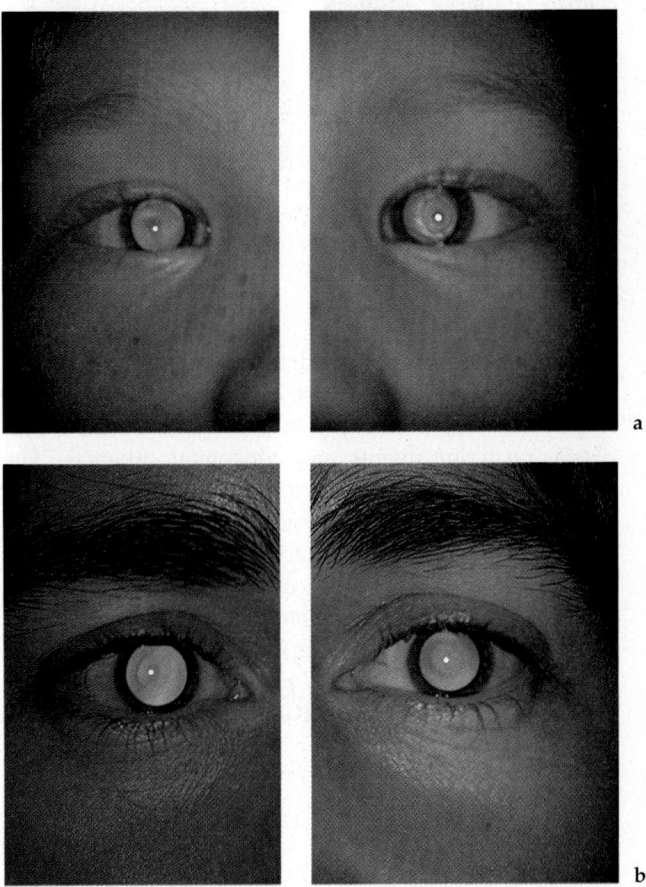

Fig. 39.4 (a) Lenticonus. Although the reflex is a dynamic phenomenon seen on retinoscopy it can be seen here as a static change in the homogeneity of the red reflex. (b) Mother of patient in Fig. 39.4a. Posterior lenticonus is more frequent in boys and may be X-linked.

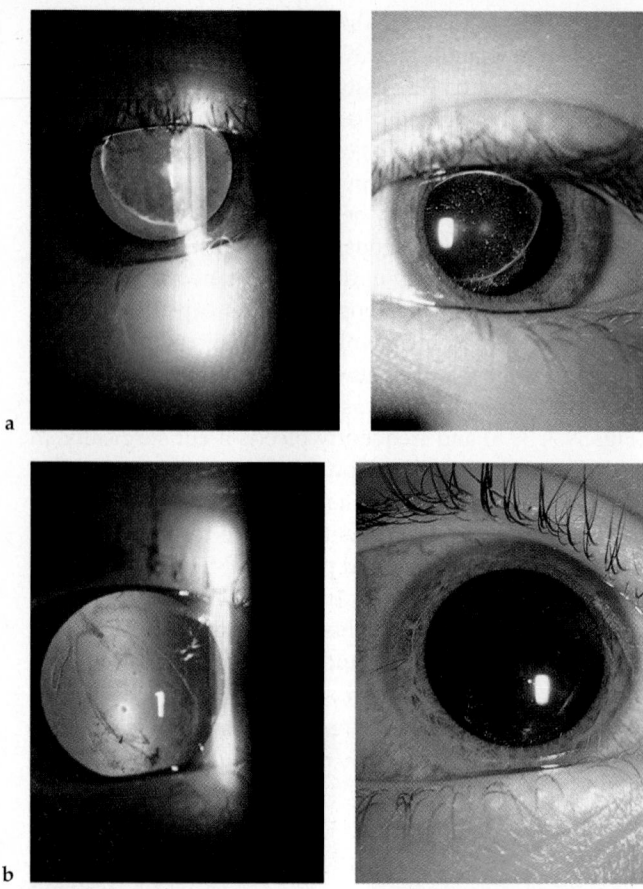

luxation or posterior dislocation of the lens. Anterior dislocation of the lens, however, often produces symptoms of pain secondary to pupil block glaucoma or corneal oedema.

Marfan's syndrome

Marfan's syndrome is the most common cause of ectopia lentis in childhood. It has an incidence of 1:10000 births without a racial or ethnic predilection. It is an autosomal

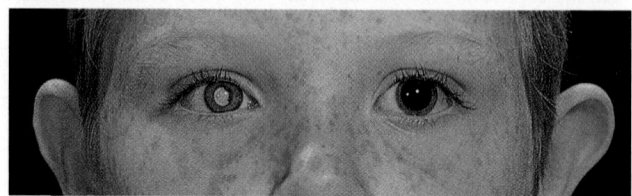

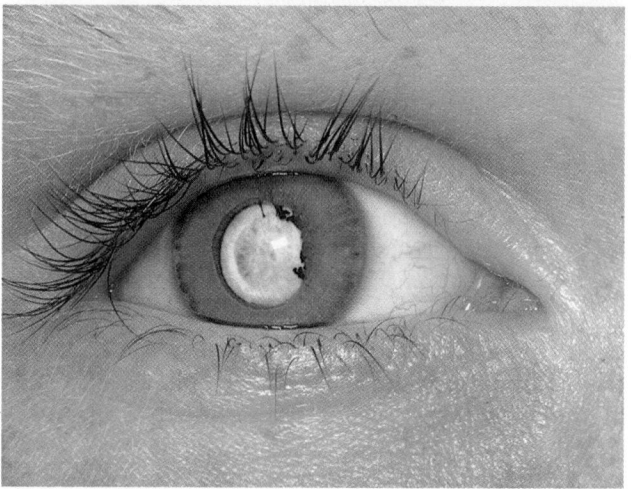

Fig. 39.5 (a) Lenticonus with posterior extension and cataract formation. (b) Postoperative photograph with retroillumination on the left showing the defect in the posterior capsule (same patient).

Fig. 39.6 (a, b) Unilateral PHPV with spontaneous reabsorption of the lens.

papillary tractional retinal detachments (Haddad *et al.* 1978). Other conditions which can mimic PHPV include: retinoblastoma, retinopathy of prematurity, retinal dysplasia, posterior uveitis and congenital cataracts. The presence of microphthalmos, a shallow anterior chamber, long ciliary processes, a cataract and a retrolental opacity with a persistent hyaloid artery are all helpful in distinguishing PHPV from these other conditions. In some instances, good visual results have been obtained in eyes with PHPV after early surgery (Karr & Scott 1986); however, most eyes with PHPV have a poor visual outcome secondary to amblyopia, glaucoma or retinal detachment.

Dislocated lenses

A subluxed lens is partially displaced from its normal position but remains within the pupillary space. In contrast, a luxated or dislocated lens is completely displaced from the pupil implying separation of all or nearly all of the zonular attachments. A reduction in visual acuity is the most common presenting symptom of sub-

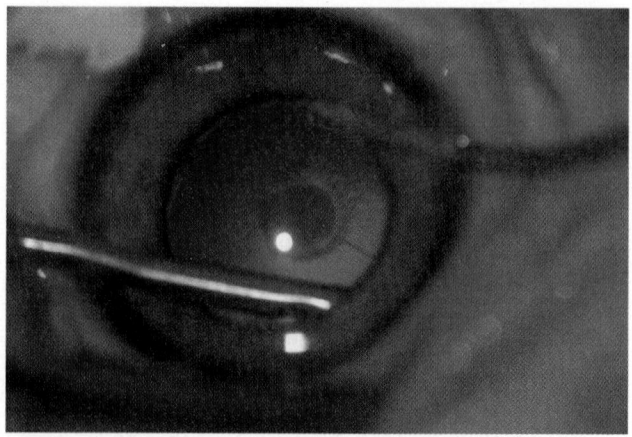

Fig. 39.7 PHPV showing a vascular lake in the membrane fed by a hyaloid artery (seen at 4 o'clock) and drained by a vein to the iris (seen at 8 o'clock).

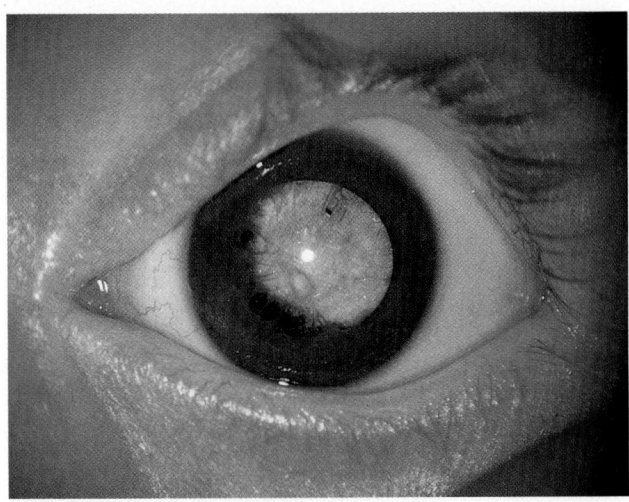

Fig. 39.8 Marked vascular PHPV with multiple vessels between the fibrous plaque, lens and the iris.

dominantly inherited disorder which has been linked to a variety of mutations of the fibrillin gene (FBN1) on chromosome 15q21.1 (Kainulainen *et al.* 1990; Dietz *et al.* 1991; Maumenee 1992; Francke & Furthmayr 1994). Fibrillin is one of the major components of extracellular microfibrils which form the matrix for elastin; it is widespread in the eye (Wheatley *et al.* 1995). Genetic heterogeneity is suggested by the finding of a second locus at 3p24.2–p25. (Collod *et al.* 1994), although the phenotype of the kindred described in this paper is questioned (Dietz *et al.* 1995).

Clinically, Marfan's syndrome is characterized by cardiac, skeletal and ocular abnormalities (Pyeritz & McKusick 1979). The cardiac abnormalities most commonly consist of dilation of the aortic root, mitral valve prolapse and aortic aneurysms. Skeletal findings include excessive height, arachnodactyly, scoliosis and chest wall deformities. The most common ocular abnormalities include ectopia lentis (Figs 39.11, 39.12), cataracts, high myopia and retinal detachment. At least two of the four criteria (family history and skeletal, cardiovascular or ocular abnormalities) should be present to make the diagnosis (Tsipouras & Devereux 1993).

Certain 'hard' manifestations such as subluxed lenses, aortic dilation and severe kyphoscoliosis are more reliable than other 'soft' signs such as myopia, mitral valve prolapse, tall stature or joint laxity (Pyeritz & McKusick 1979) (Fig. 39.13). The metacarpal index, for instance, is a poor discrimina-tor between Marfan's syndrome and constitutional tall stature (Nelle *et al.* 1994). Subluxation of the lens occurs in 60–80% of affected patients (Cross & Jensen 1973; Maumenee 1981). Lenses most commonly sublux superiorly, but may sublux in any direction (Maumenee 1981). The zonules usually remain intact but elongated, and

accommodation may be unaffected. Lens subluxation may be as subtle as a flattening or notching of one sector of the lens visible only after pupillary dilation. Maumenee observed progression of subluxation in only 7.5% of 193 patients followed longitudinally (Maumenee 1981). Although ectopia lentis is frequently not detected until later in childhood, it is probably congenital in most instances. Many patients with Marfan's syndrome also have axial myopia and are at increased risk of developing retinal detachment. Many also have strabismus (Izquierdo *et al.* 1994). There is a high intrafamilial concordance rate for the ocular findings of this syndrome (Maumenee 1981).

Homocystinuria

Homocystinuria is a disease of methionine metabolism. Classic homocystinuria (type 1) is due to a deficiency of the enzyme cystathionine-B-synthetase. Affected individuals develop elevated levels of homocystine and methionine in the blood and other tissues. A urine sodium–nitroprusside test can be used as a rapid screening test but a more definite diagnosis can be made by measuring the levels of homocystine in freshly voided urine after ingesting a bolus of methionine; this technique should be used when the clinical diagnosis is suggestive even in the absence of a positive nitroprusside test (Michalski *et al.* 1988).

Affected individuals are normal at birth. During infancy they may fail to thrive and are developmentally delayed. The diagnosis is frequently not established until years later when ectopia lentis develops (Mudd *et al.* 1985). If untreated, 90% of affected patients develop progressive ectopia lentis (Cross & Jensen 1973). Ectopia lentis has been observed in an affected child at 3 years of age, but more commonly develops in later childhood or early adulthood. In patients with a subluxed lens, the zonules are markedly abnormal with only short broken filaments remaining attached to the lens capsule (Henkind & Ashton 1965). The lens usually subluxes inferiorly or anteriorly and may dislocate into the anterior chamber (Fig. 39.14). A careful slit-lamp examination will usually reveal the irregular distribution of the lens zonules and their matted appearance on the margins of the lens (Ramsey & Dickson 1975).

Patients with homocystinuria are tall with arachnodactyly, a malar flush and fair hair (Fig. 39.15). Progressive mental retardation frequently occurs if the disorder is not treated, although affected patients may have normal intelligence (Barber & Spaeth 1969). Patients with homocystinuria are also at increased risk of having thromboembolic events including occlusion of the central retinal artery, particularly after surgical intervention (Mudd *et al.* 1985; Berg *et al.* 1990). The disorder has been estimated to occur in one in 200 000 births, but is more common among

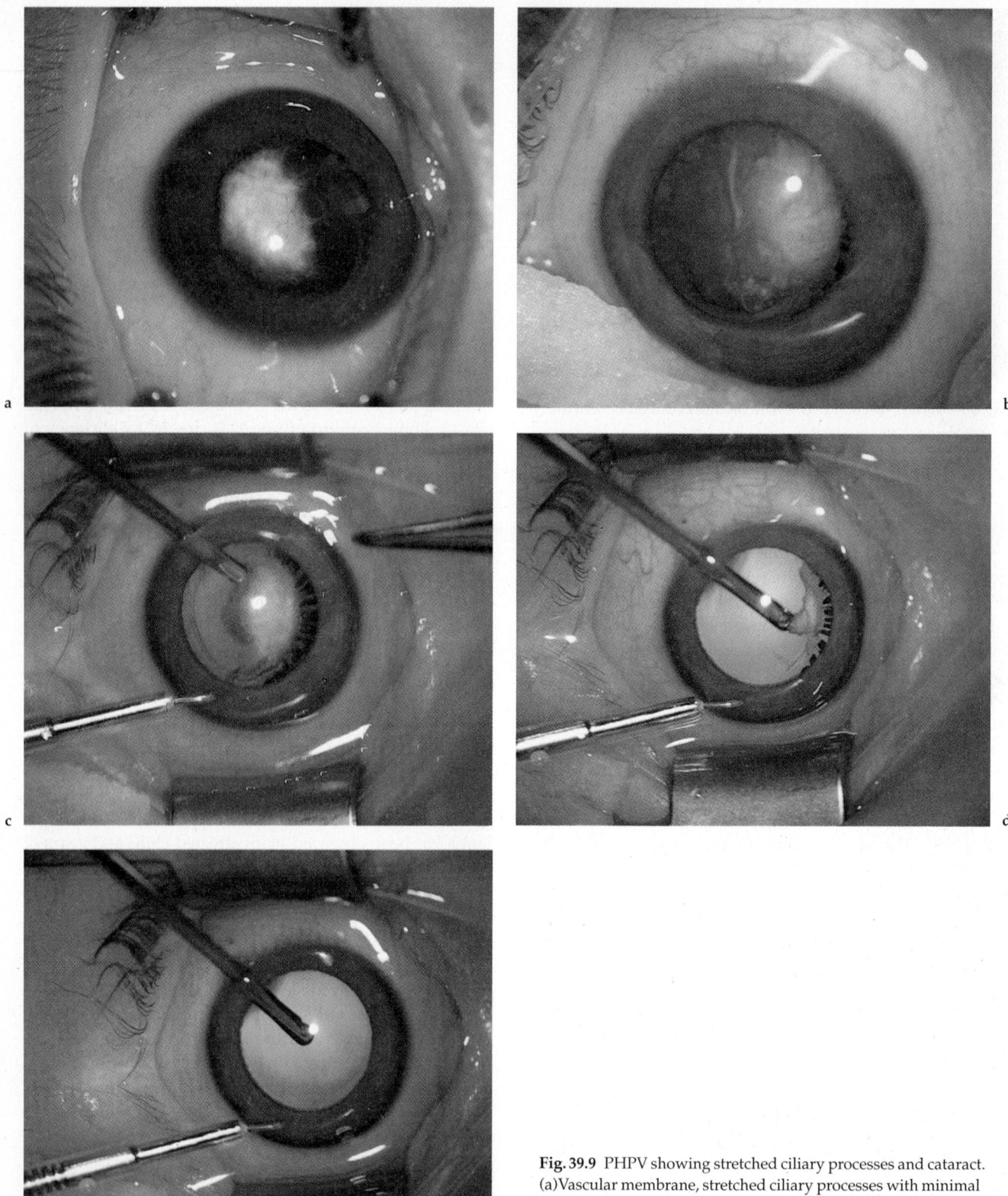

Fig. 39.9 PHPV showing stretched ciliary processes and cataract. (a)Vascular membrane, stretched ciliary processes with minimal cataract. (b) Cataract obscuring an avascular membrane. (c–e) Removal of the cataract and membrane seen in (b).

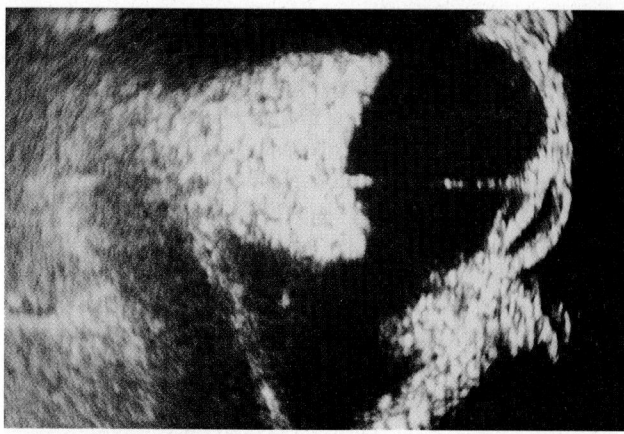

Fig. 39.10 PHPV. Ultrasound showing persistent hyaloid artery.

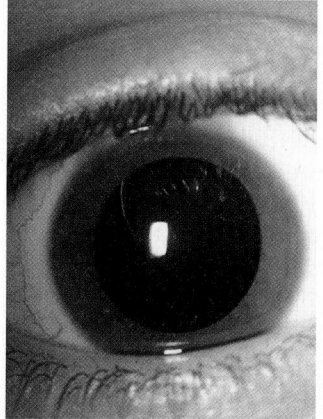 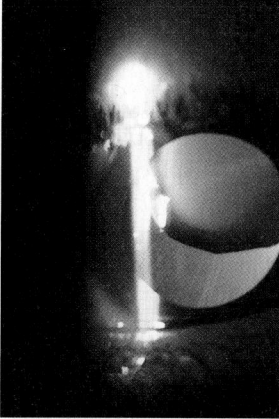

Fig. 39.11 Marfan's syndrome. Upward and nasal dislocation of the lens with intact zonules.

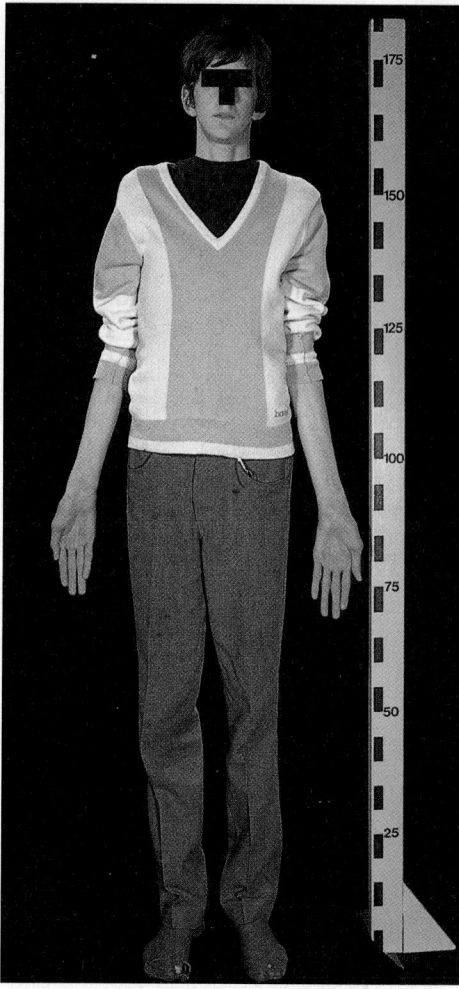

Fig. 39.13 Marfan's syndrome. At 15 years of age he is 1.75 m in height. He has very long limbs, arachnodactyly and pectus excavatum.

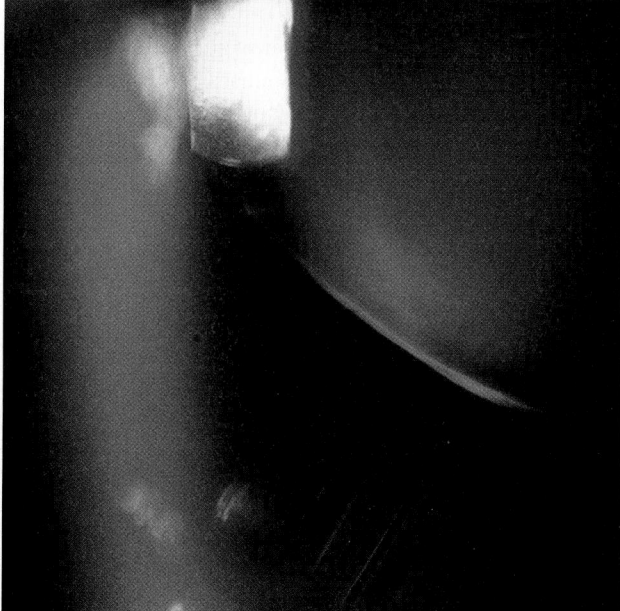

Fig. 39.12 Marfan's syndrome. Dislocated lens with intact stretched zonules.

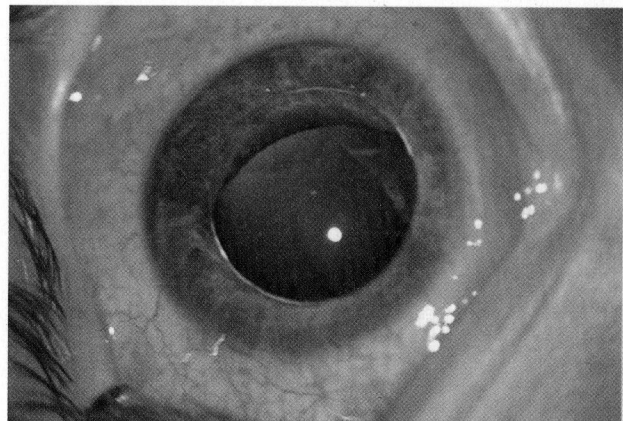

Fig. 39.14 Homocystinuria. Anterior and inferior dislocation of the lens, which is jammed in the pupil.

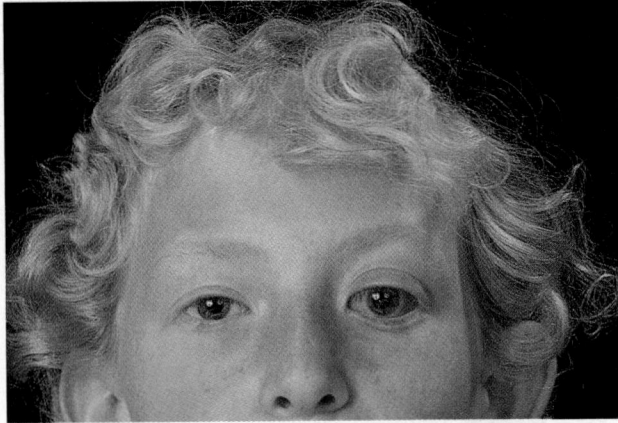

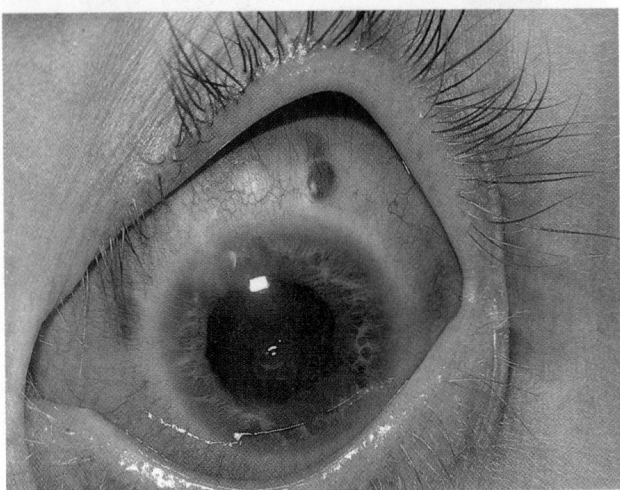

Fig. 39.15 (a, b) Homocystinuria. Fair-haired boy with chronic glaucoma following unreported anterior dislocation of the lens. Despite his age the left eye had become buphthalmic.

certain ethnic groups. In Ireland it has an incidence of one in 52 000 births.

Pyridoxine (vitamin B$_6$) acts as a co-factor with cystathione-B-synthetase and 40–50% of patients with homocystinuria show biochemical improvement after being treated with high doses of pyridoxine (200–1000 mg over 24 hours) (Shih & Efron 1970; Mudd *et al.* 1985). Patients unresponsive to pyridoxine may benefit from treatment with betaine (Smolin *et al.* 1981). A low methionine and high cysteine diet is also associated with improved metabolic control in many of these patients (Perry *et al.* 1968), which makes anaesthesia safer (Michalski *et al.* 1988). Dietary changes and pyridoxine treatment may prevent or delay lens subluxation and mental retardation if initiated early in life (Mudd *et al.* 1985; Burke *et al.* 1989a).

Weill–Marchesani syndrome

The Weill–Marchesani syndrome is a rare disorder characterized by short stature, brachycephaly, stubby fingers and toes, and spherophakia (McGavic 1959). The lens commonly dislocates into the anterior chamber resulting in pupillary block glaucoma (Willi *et al.* 1973). Patients also usually have lenticular myopia (Jensen *et al.* 1974). It is probably an autosomal recessive trait, although some pedigrees suggest an autosomal dominant inheritance with variable expressivity (Kloepfer & Rosenthal 1975).

Aniridia

Children with aniridia also commonly develop ectopia lentis. Later in life, many also develop cataracts and glaucoma. Since the removal of subluxed lens in these eyes frequently compromises the success of subsequent glaucoma filtering operations, lensectomies should be avoided in these eyes if at all possible (Callahan 1949).

Ectopia lentis et pupillae

Ectopia lentis et pupillae is a rare autosomal recessive cause of ectopia lentis characterized by the lens and pupil being displaced in opposite directions resulting in a slit- or oval-shaped pupil (Townes 1976). Affected patients may also have axial myopia, large corneas and transillumination defects of the irides (Goldberg 1988).

Trauma and glaucoma

Trauma is also a common cause of ectopia lentis (Jarrett 1967). Ectopia lentis also can occur in large eyes with uncontrolled congenital glaucoma.

Sulphite oxidase deficiency

This is an extremely rare disorder of sulphur metabolism. It is associated with dislocated lenses, progressive muscular rigidity and decerebrate posturing. Death usually occurs prior to 5 years of age (Shih *et al.* 1977).

Molybdenum co-factor deficiency

This is another rare metabolic disease with early lens dislocation, refractory seizures and urinary excretion of sulphite, xanthine, hypoxanthine and S-sulfocysteine (Lueder & Steiner 1995).

Xanthine oxidase deficiency

Xanthine oxidase deficiency, which is associated with very low levels of uric acid in the serum, has also been described as a very rare cause of dislocated lenses.

Simple ectopia lentis

Ectopia lentis may also occur as an isolated autosomal

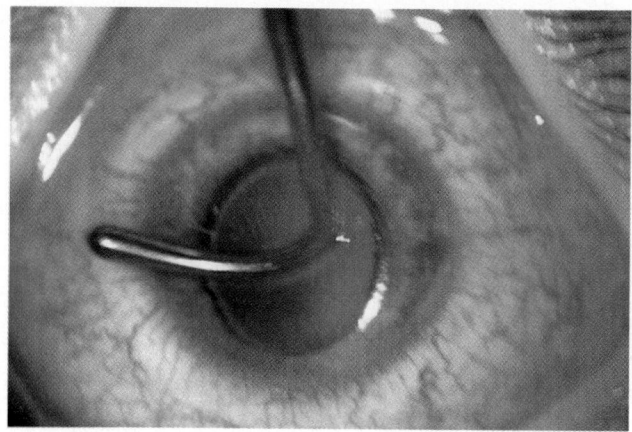

Fig. 39.16 Homocystinuria with anterior dislocation and glaucoma. This picture shows the lens being reposited under local anaesthetic with a strabismus hook.

dominant trait (Falls & Cotterman 1943; Seland 1973). Some patients have mutations of the fibrillin gene, but lack the other stigmas of Marfan's syndrome (Kainulainen *et al.* 1994). Shawaf *et al.* (1995) described ectopia lentis with spontaneous filtering blebs and dysmorphism.

Treatment of dislocated lenses

Satisfactory visual improvement can be obtained in many patients with ectopia lentis using spectacles alone (Alcorn & Maumenee 1987). If the lens is significantly subluxed and the visual acuity fails to improve with the phakic correction, aphakic correction should be instituted. Sometimes, acceptance of aphakic correction can be enhanced by pharmacologically dilating the pupils or using contact lenses.

Optical correction of a subluxed lens is most difficult when the pupil is bisected by the lens. If the child remains visually impaired with both his phakic and aphakic correction, a lensectomy (Reese & Weingeist 1987) or yttrium-aluminium-garnet (YAG) laser zonulysis should be performed (Tchah *et al.* 1989). A posteriorly dislocated lens should only be removed if it results in persistent uveitis, glaucoma or cystic retinal degeneration.

Anterior dislocation of the lens occurs most frequently with homocystinuria. It may be treated with pupillary dilatation and manual repositioning of the lens by pressure on the cornea (Fig. 39.16) and then chronic miosis (Elkington *et al.* 1973). Since patients with homocystinuria are at a higher risk of complications from general anaesthesia, lens extraction should be avoided (Berg *et al.* 1990) unless the diet is well maintained; patients should be kept well hydrated before, during and after surgery.

Serious operative and postoperative complications commonly occurred when subluxed lenses were removed before the advent of vitreous cutting instruments (Chandler 1964; Jarrett 1967; Cross & Jensen 1973); however, postoperative complications occur infrequently when using these instruments in a closed eye (Reese & Weingeist 1987; Behki *et al.* 1990; Girard *et al.* 1990; Hakin *et al.* 1992; Plager *et al.* 1992). When using a limbal approach (Fig. 39.17), the vitreous cutting instrument should be introduced in the area of greatest subluxation even if this necessitates entering the eye inferiorly (Saleh-pour *et al.* 1996). Care should be taken to prevent the lens or lens material from falling posteriorly. Subluxed and dislocated lens can also be approached by a pars plana approach (Peyman *et al.* 1979; Reese & Weingeist 1987). Occasionally, a minimally subluxed lens may be removed using an extracapsular technique, but vitreous loss is a frequent complication (Maumenee & Ryan 1969; Seetner & Crawford 1981).

Retinal detachments are the most serious postoperative complication occurring after extraction of subluxed lenses. While retinal detachments were a frequent complication with older techniques, they occur infrequently after a lensectomy with a vitreous cutting instrument (Reese & Weingeist 1987). However, longer follow-ups will be necessary to determine if this continues to be the case (Toyofuku *et al.* 1980; Jagger *et al.* 1983).

Alternatively, a subluxed lens bisecting the pupil may be moved out of the pupillary opening by lysing the lens zonules with a YAG laser (Tchah *et al.* 1989). The patient can then be given their aphakic optical correction. In a small percentage of cases, the lens may be damaged during this procedure, necessitating its later removal.

Aphakic correction

Spectacles or contact lenses are the only appropriate aphakic correction because intraocular lenses can only be suspended by what are experimental techniques, or be placed in the anterior chamber, where their presence is untried over the lifespan of a child.

Visual results

The visual results following surgery in recent years have been good, with visual improvement in nearly all cases (Hakin *et al.* 1992). A late improvement in vision occurs (Speedwell & Russell-Eggitt 1995), so disappointing early visual results may improve with time.

Cataracts

Cataracts are opacities of the crystalline lens. Because they frequently interfere with normal visual development, they represent an important problem in paediatric ophthalmology (Fig. 39.18). Up to one-third of children with bilateral congenital cataracts remain legally blind even after surgical and optical treatment (Gelbart *et al.* 1982; Parks 1982) and eyes with monocular congenital

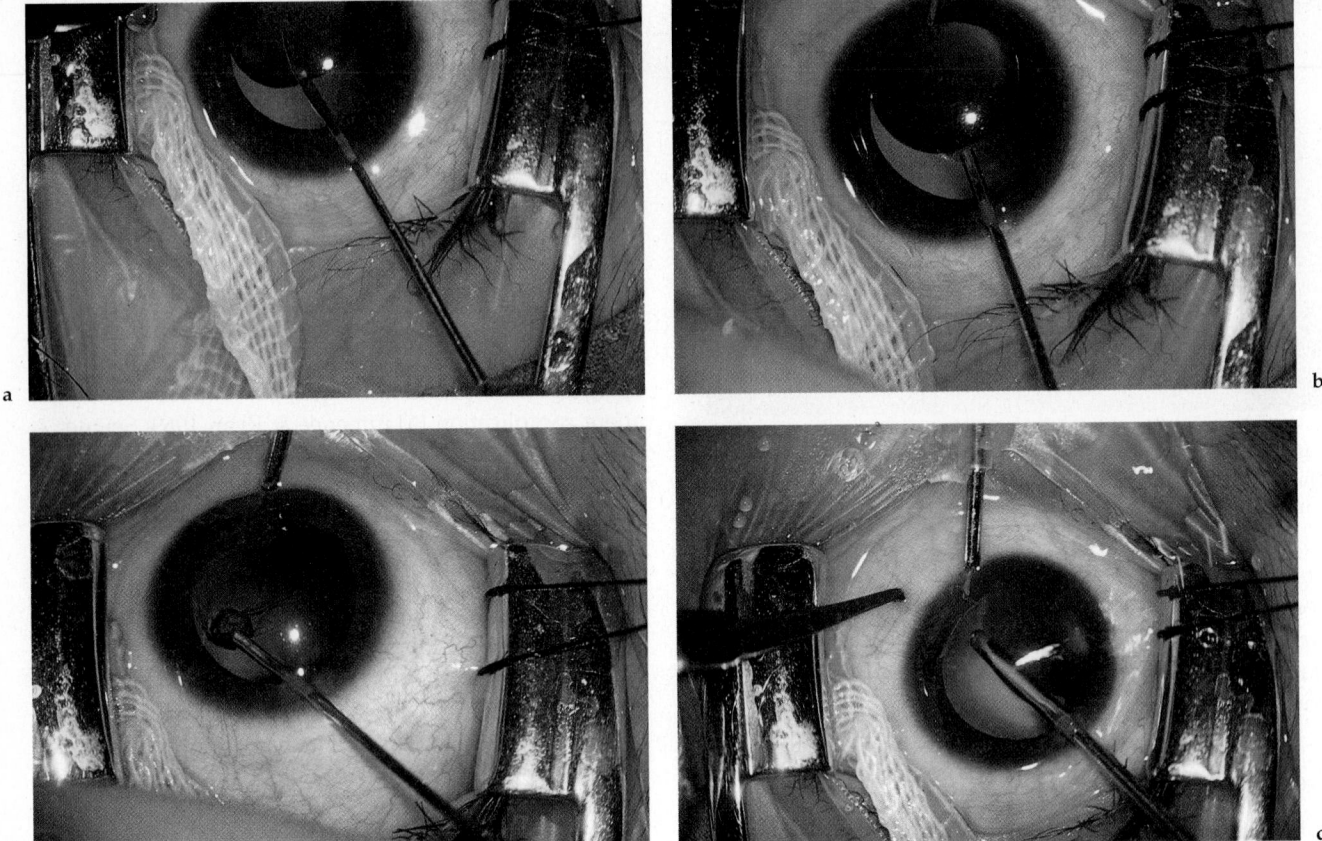

Fig. 39.17 (a) Marfan's syndrome. Lens surgery. The anterior chamber is maintained by a small cannula (not visible on this photograph) and a sharp knife is being used to penetrate the lens capsule. (b) A simple aspiration cannula is inserted into the lens. (c) All of the lens material is aspirated. (d) A vitrectomy machine is used to clear the remains of the capsule.

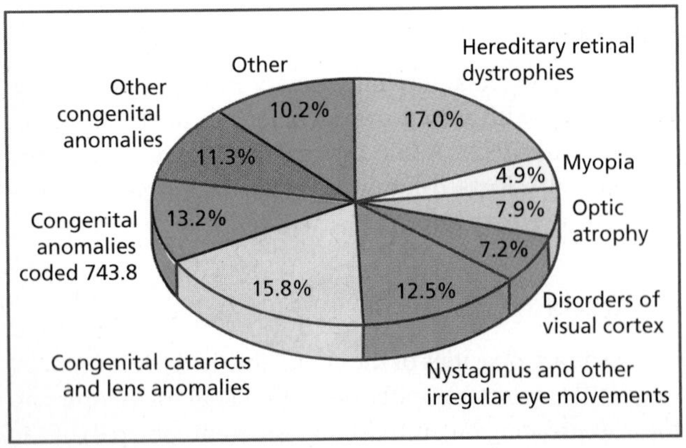

cataracts often do not develop useful vision in the affected eye (Neumann *et al.* 1993). Since early treatment is probably the most important factor in determining the visual outcome of these eyes, prompt detection and treatment of cataracts in neonates is of the utmost importance.

Aetiology

The aetiology of congenital cataracts can be established in many children by a careful preoperative assessment (Merin & Crawford 1971a; Kohn 1976). The most common aetiologies include intrauterine infections, metabolic disorders and genetically transmitted syndromes (Table 39.1). In an otherwise healthy child, an extensive preoperative evaluation is not usually necessary. A paediatrician and an ophthalmologist working together can detect most of the associated ocular and systemic diseases with only a few simple urine and blood tests.

Intrauterine infection

An intrauterine infection should be suspected in infants with dense unilateral or bilateral central cataracts. A history of a maternal illness accompanied by a rash during the pregnancy is particularly suggestive of an intrauterine

Fig. 39.18 Congenital cataract is a significant cause of visual handicap. In the developed world most cases are partially sighted as opposed to blind. This pie-chart is taken from figures for the 1980s UK Visual Handicap Registration figures.

Table 39.1 Aetiology of cataracts in childhood.

Idiopathic	*Inherited with systemic abnormalities*
Intrauterine infection Rubella (Cotlier 1978) Varicella (Lambert *et al.* 1989) Toxoplasmosis (Stagno *et al.* 1977) Herpes simplex (Nahmias *et al.* 1977)	*Chromosomal* Trisomy 21 (Catalano 1990) Turner's syndrome (Lessell & Forbes 1966) Trisomy 13 (Apple *et al.* 1970) Trisomy 18 (Mullaney 1973) Cri du chat syndrome (Farrell *et al.* 1988)
Uveitis or acquired infection Juvenile rheumatoid arthritis (Kanski 1990) Pars planitis *Toxocara canis*	*Craniofacial syndromes* COFS syndrome (Insler 1987)
Drug-induced Corticosteroids (Brocklebank *et al.* 1982) Chlorpromazine	*Renal disease* Lowe's syndrome (Tripathi *et al.* 1986) Alport's syndrome (Jacobs *et al.* 1992) Hallermann–Streiff–François (Falls & Schull 1960)
Metabolic disorders Galactosaemia (Stambolian 1988) Galactokinase deficiency Hypocalcaemia (Stambolian *et al.* 1995) Hypoglycaemia (Merin & Crawford 1972) Diabetes mellitus Mannosidosis (Letson & Desnick 1978)	*Skeletal disease* Smith–Lemli–Opitz (Cotlier & Rice 1971) Conradi's syndrome (Armaly 1957) Weill–Marchesani syndrome (Jensen *et al.* 1990) Stickler syndrome (Seery *et al.* 1990) Syndactyly, polydactyly or digital anomalies Bardet–Biedl syndrome (Green *et al.* 1989) Rubinstein–Taybi syndrome (Roy *et al.* 1968)
Trauma Accidental Laser photocoagulation (Capone & Drack 1994) Non-accidental	*Central nervous system abnormalities* Zellweger's syndrome (Folz & Trobe 1991) Meckel–Gruber syndrome (MacRae *et al.* 1972) Marinesco–Sjögren syndrome (Alter *et al.* 1962) Infantile neuronal ceroid-lipofuscinosis (Bateman & Philppart 1986)
Radiation-induced (Henk *et al.* 1993)	*Muscular disease* Myotonic dystrophy (Gold & Weingeist 1990)
Other diseases Microphthalmia (Zeiter 1963) Leber's congenital amaurosis (Lambert *et al.* 1989) Aniridia (Nelson *et al.* 1984) Retinitis pigmentosa PHPV (Haddad *et al.* 1978) Retinopathy of prematurity (McCormick 1988) Endophthalmitis (Clinch *et al.* 1989)	*Dermatological* Crystalline cataract and uncombable hair (de Jong *et al.* 1990) Cockayne's syndrome (Pearce 1992) Rothmund–Thomson (Wahl & Ellis 1965) Atopic dermatitis (Cowan & Klauder 1950) Incontinentia pigmenti (Scott 1955) Progeria (Jones 1988) Congenital ichthyosis (Jay *et al.* 1968) Ectodermal dysplasia (Jones 1989) Werner's syndrome (Petronclos 1963)
Inherited Autosomal dominant (Scott *et al.* 1994) Autosomal recessive (Forsius *et al.* 1992) X-linked (Lewis *et al.* 1992)	
Mental retardation See text	

rubella (Fig. 39.19) or varicella infection. Rubella immunoglobulin G (IgG) and IgM antibody titres should be obtained from the mother and the child. At the time of surgery, the lens aspirate can also be cultured for rubella virus. Intrauterine varicella infections may also result in congenital cataracts (Lambert *et al.* 1989b).

Metabolic disorders

Classic galactosaemia is caused by a mutation of the gene on the short arm of chromosome 9 coding for the enzyme galactose-1-phosphate uridyl-transferase (GALT). More than 60% of patients with classical galactosaemia have

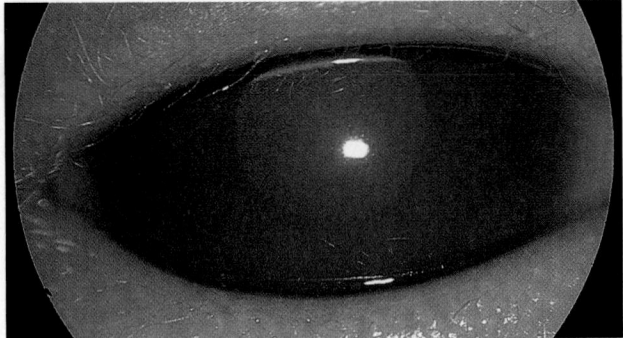

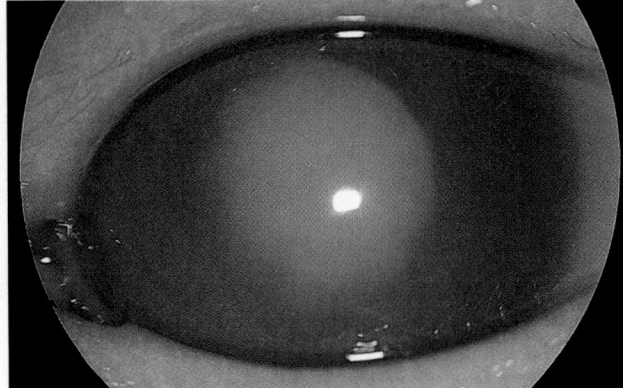

a

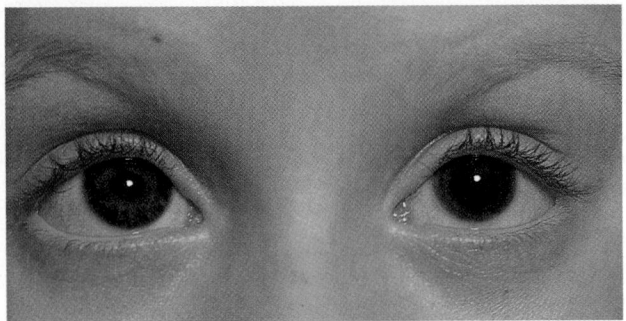

b

Fig. 39.19 (a) Congenital rubella with 'steamy' corneas and a unilateral cataract. Buphthalmos was suspected. (b) Same patient aged 6 years showing that the corneas had not enlarged. Buphthalmos does occur in congenital rubella but it is important to be sure that the intraocular pressure is raised because corneal oedema also occurs from a transient keratopathy.

a mutation on exon 6 (Q188R) of the GALT gene which causes a glutamine to be substituted for an arginine (Leslie *et al.* 1992; Elsas *et al.* 1994b). Homozygotes for this mutation have no GALT activity and present during infancy with diarrhoea, vomiting, jaundice, hepatomegaly and Gram-positive septicaemia. Classical galactosaemia occurs in one out of every 39 000 live births. Heterozygotes for classical galactosaemia are also at increased risk of developing cataracts during early adulthood. The Duarte variant is a more common mutation of the GALT gene on exon 10 (N314D). Homozygosity of the Duarte allele results in 50% GALT activity (Elsas *et al.* 1994a). Investiga-

tions are currently being conducted to determine whether this mutation can result in juvenile onset cataracts. Reducing substances are present in the urine of patients with both classical galactosaemia and galactokinase deficiency after a galactose-containing meal (milk). Enzymatic assays using erythrocytes and DNA studies can then be used to distinguish between the different types of galactosaemia.

Infants with classical galactosaemia develop 'oil droplet' cataracts (Fig. 39.20) which are not true cataracts but refractive changes in the lens nucleus which appear as a drop in the centre of the lens in retroillumination like an oil droplet floating in water. If left untreated, these oil droplet cataracts progress to lamellar (Fig. 39.21) and then total cataracts due to the accumulation of galactitol in the lens (Kinoshita *et al.* 1962). However, if galactose is eliminated from the diet of these children early in life, the cataracts may become transparent again (Beigi *et al.* 1993).

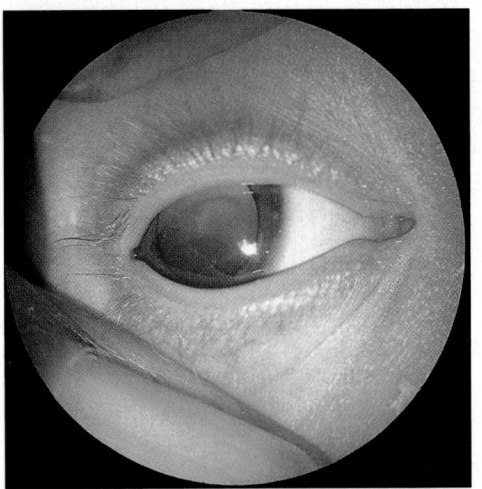

a

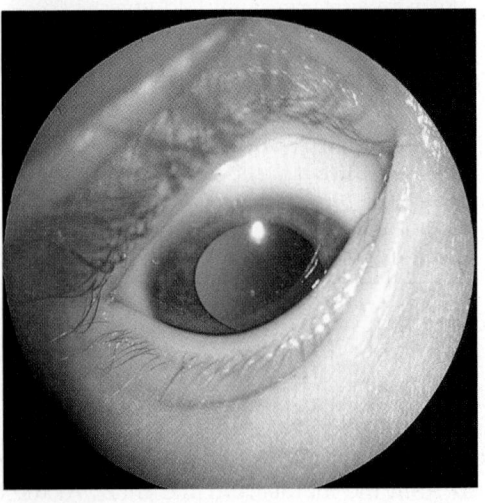

b

Fig. 39.20 (a) Galactosaemia—'oil droplet' cataract. It is a change in the refractive index in the nucleus of the lens. (b) After early dietary treatment the 'cataract' had disappeared (same patient).

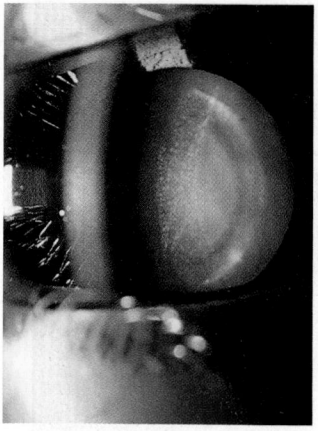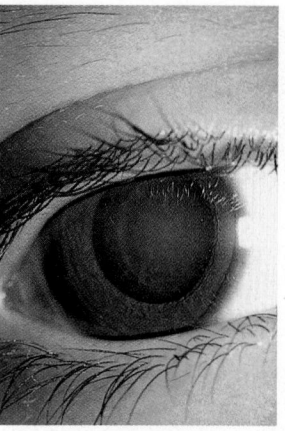

Fig. 39.21 Galactosaemia. In some cases, perhaps related to late treatment, a cataract forms which is lamellar and may cause a visual defect.

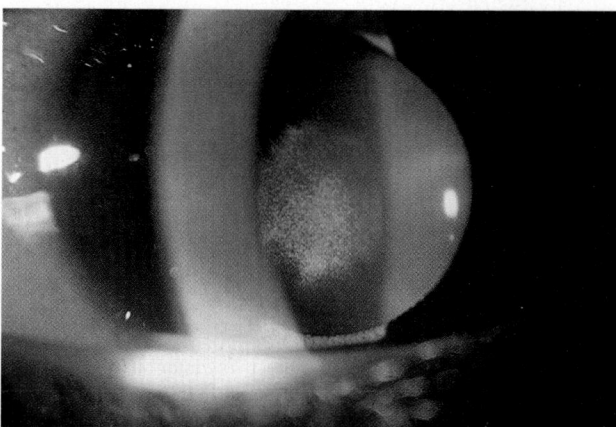

Fig. 39.22 Wilson's disease—'sunflower' cataract (Dr G. Holmstrom's patient).

Galactose-1-phosphate levels in the serum can be used to monitor dietary compliance.

An autosomal recessive syndrome with exercise-related lactic acidosis, mitochondrial cytopathy and hypertrophic cardiomyopathy without mental retardation was described in 12 children with congenital cataract from six unrelated families by Cruysberg *et al.* (1986).

In Wilson's disease there may be subcapsular 'sunflower' cataracts (Fig. 39.22).

Cerebrotendinous xanthomatosis is an autosomal recessive sterol storage disorder due to lack of mitochondrial hydroxylase; the gene is on chromosome 2. Affected children have dementia, ataxia and tendon xanthomas. Bilateral, irregular, corticonuclear, anterior polar or posterior capsular cataracts occur sometimes in the first decade (Cruysberg *et al.* 1995).

Children with hypocalcaemia usually have seizures, failure-to-thrive and irritability. Many also develop cataracts as a result of the altered permeability of the lens capsule. These cataracts generally begin as fine white punctate opacities (Fig. 39.23) scattered throughout the lens cortex which may then progress to lamellar cataracts. Serum calcium and phosphorus levels should be measured in infants with bilateral cataracts.

Cataracts occur infrequently in children with diabetes mellitus. When they do develop, they usually occur in the teenage years. They frequently begin as cortical opacities but may rapidly progress to total cataracts.

Hypoglycaemia during the perinatal period or in early infancy may result in lens opacities (Merin & Crawford 1971b). These opacities are reversible in most cases but occasionally may develop into total cataracts.

Morphologically specific cataracts occur in Fabry's disease (see Chapter 57).

Inherited cataracts

Congenital cataracts are frequently inherited as an autosomal dominant trait (Fig. 39.24) accompanied by microphthalmos. Parents and siblings should be examined using biomicroscopy for clinically insignificant cataracts since variable expressivity is a characteristic of autosomal dominantly inherited cataracts (Gibbs *et al.* 1993). In addition to intrafamilial morphological variability, there can also be marked interocular variability in the morphology of these cataracts (Scott *et al.* 1994). Anterior polar cataracts may also be inherited as an autosomal dominant trait (Traboulsi & Weinberg 1989).

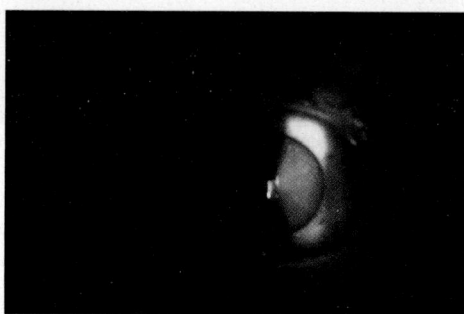

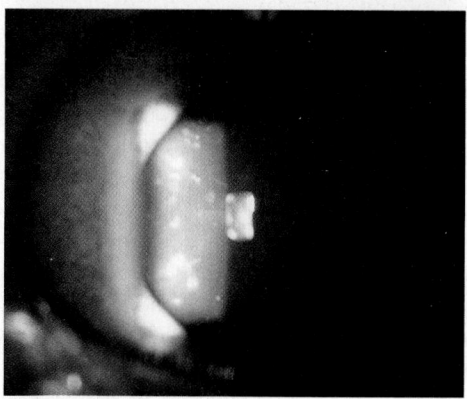

Fig. 39.23 Hypocalcaemic cataract—punctate dots.

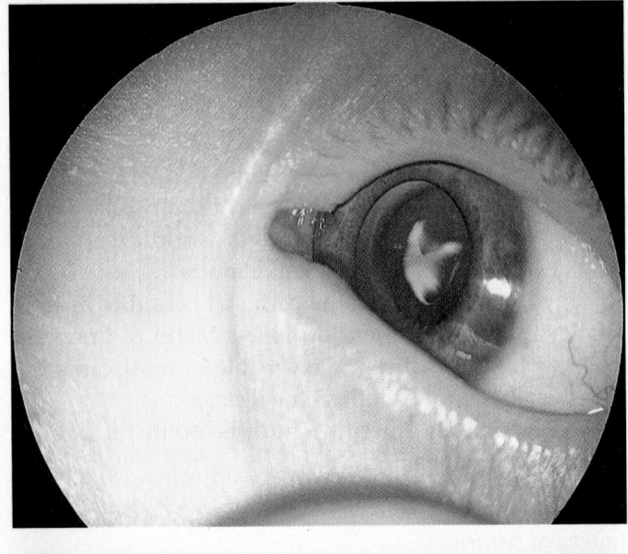

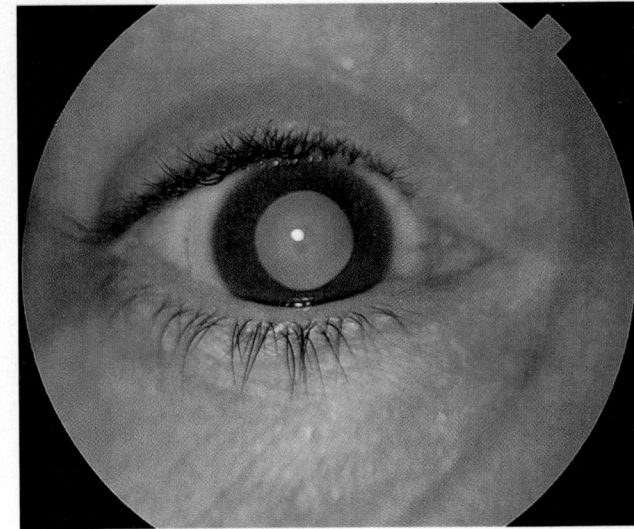

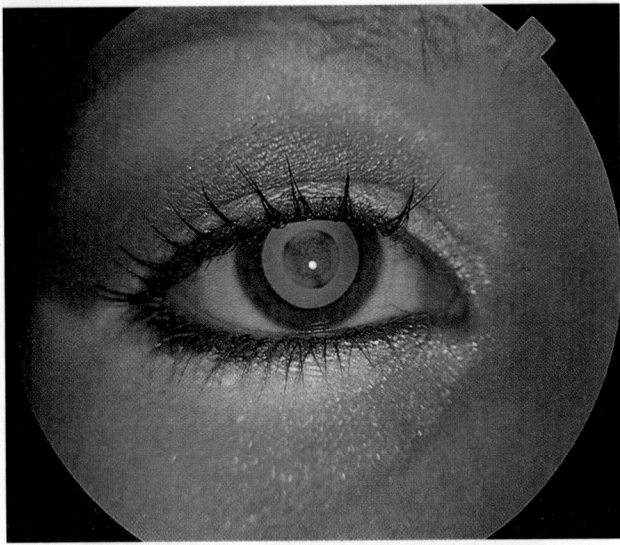

Fig. 39.24 (a) Dominant lamellar cataract. The infant had presented because his parents had seen the white spots in the pupil. (b) His asymptomatic mother, who has vision good enough to drive a car. (c) His asymptomatic grandmother who had a tiny lamellar cataract. There is considerable difference between various members of families.

Autosomal recessive inheritance is less common, but should be suspected if there is consanguinity or multiply affected offspring and unaffected parents. Galactosaemia is a notable autosomal recessive condition causing cataracts.

Lowe's syndrome (Fig. 39.25) is the most common X-linked condition causing cataracts. Children with Lowe's syndrome have hypotonia, mental retardation, aminoaciduria and an abnormal facial appearance with frontal bossing, and chubby cheeks. The lens typically has a reduced anterior–posterior diameter and posterior lentiglobus (Ginsberg *et al.* 1981; Tripathi *et al.* 1986). In addition, these eyes frequently have mesenchymal dysgenesis and glaucoma. Carriers have multiple fine peripheral cortical punctate lens opacities which can progress to visually significant cataracts (Johnson & Nevin 1976; Delleman *et al.* 1977; Cibis *et al.* 1986).

X-linked inheritance also occurs in the Nance–Horan syndrome (Fig. 39.26) in which cataract, supernumerary teeth and prominent ears with anteverted pinnae are associated with developmental delay. Obligate carriers have sutural cataracts and abnormal teeth. The gene has been mapped to Xp22.2–p22.3 (Lewis *et al.* 1992b).

The X-linked recessive Lenz syndrome may also be associated with cataracts; other features of this syndrome include microphthalmos (colobomatous in 75%), prominent simple ears and dental anomalies (Van Dorp *et al.* 1979; Baraitser *et al.* 1982; Traboulsi *et al.* 1988). Developmental delay is very frequent as are ptosis, skeletal abnormalities and urogenital anomalies and clefts.

Chromosomal and other syndromes

Cataracts are manifest in a large number of syndromes (see Table 39.1), the most common being trisomy 21. Children with trisomy 21 usually develop cataracts later in childhood, but less commonly they may develop during infancy (Cunha & Moreira 1996).

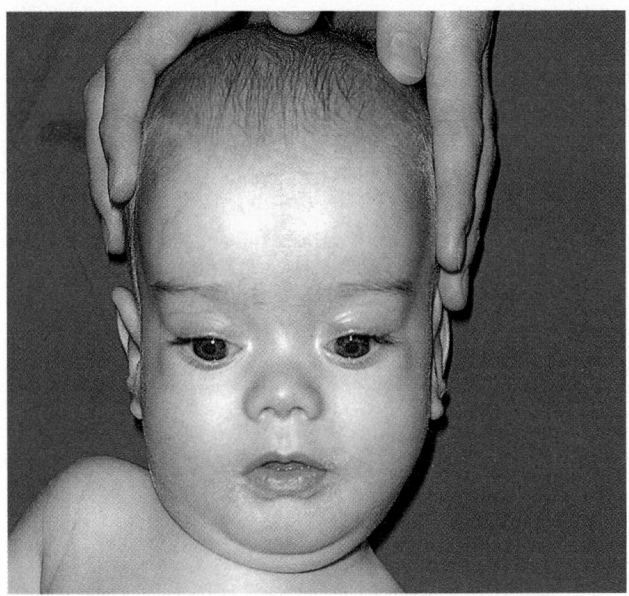

Fig. 39.25 Lowe's syndrome showing 'chubby' cheeks and rounded forehead. He has bilateral cataracts.

Cataracts have also been reported in children with reciprocal translocations of chromosomes 3 and 4 (Reese *et al.* 1987) with a familial 2;14 translocation (Moross *et al.* 1984) and the cri du chat syndrome caused by a partial deletion of the short arm of chromosome 5 (Farrell *et al.* 1988).

Cataracts may also be the presenting sign of the Hallermann–Streiff–François syndrome (Cohen 1991; Soriano & Funk 1991; Newell *et al.* 1994); it comprises the following:

1 Dyscephaly with a beak-shaped nose (Fig. 39.27) and micrognathia.
2 Short stature.
3 Hypotrichosis.
4 Dental abnormalities.
5 Blue sclerae.
6 Congenital cataract.

Cataracts with mental retardation

Cataracts occur with mental retardation in the following:

1 Martsolf's syndrome: micrognathia, brachycephaly, flat maxilla, broad sternum, talipes, clefts (Hennekan *et al.* 1988).
2 The Marinesco–Sjögren syndrome: cerebellar ataxia and myopathy (Zimmer *et al.* 1992).
3 The peroxisomal disorders, and mitochondrial cytopathies (see Chapter 44).
4 Chondrodysplasia punctata. This occurs in three main forms:
  (a) an autosomal recessive 'rhizomelic', lethal form with rhizomelia (short limbs), mongoloid eye-slant, ichthyosis, flat nasal bridge;
  (b) an X-linked dominant form: shortened leg bones;

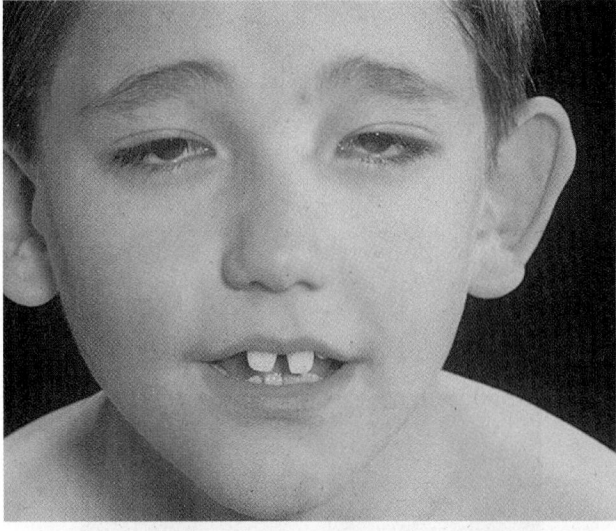

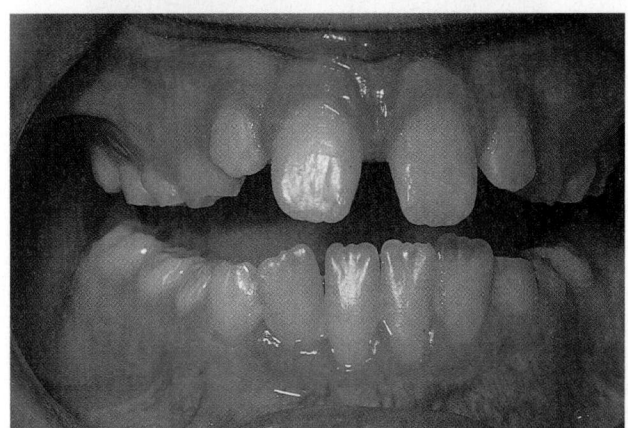

Fig. 39.26 (a) Nance–Horan syndrome showing prominent ears and teeth. (b) Nance–Horan syndrome showing supernumerary and abnormal teeth.

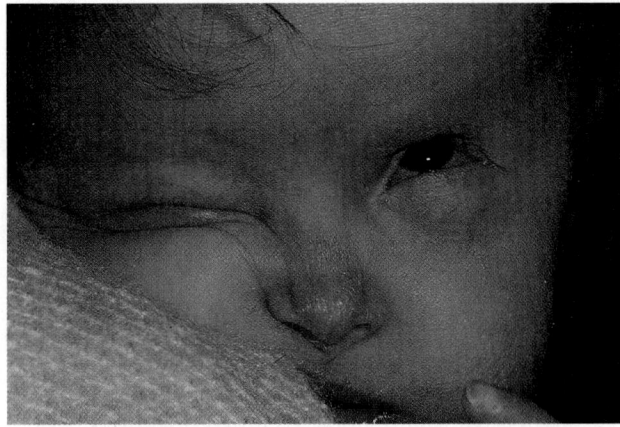

Fig. 39.27 Hallermann–Streiff–François syndrome showing a small nose with prominent veins. Baldness and progeria are common.

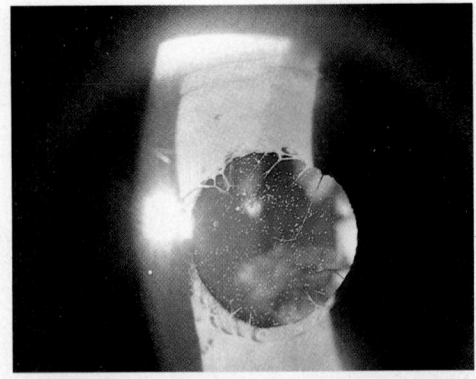

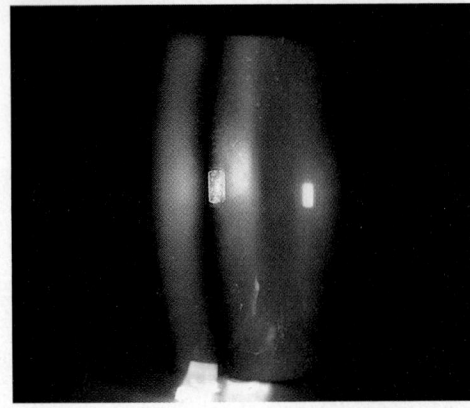

Fig. 39.28 (a) ?Dominant Conradi's syndrome in a girl with multiple dot-like cataracts. (b) Conradi's syndrome. The mother of the patient in (a) showing spoke-like peripheral cataracts.

scaly, 'orange peel' skin; alopecia. The cataracts may be sectoral, a possible lyonization effect (Happle & Kuchle 1983); and

(c) a possible autosomal dominant form similar to (b) (Fig. 39.28).

5 X-linked cataract, spasticity and mental retardation (Pfeiffer 1985).

6 Autosomal cerebro-oculofacial skeletal (Fig. 39.29) syndrome (COFS). These infants have microcephaly, joint contractures, rocker-bottom feet, micrognathia, sloping forehead and prominent nasal root (Winter *et al.* 1981; Gershoni-Baruch *et al.* 1991).

7 Czeizel–Lowry syndrome. Affected children have cataract, microcephaly, mental retardation and Perthes disease of the hip (Czeizel & Lowry 1990). It is probably autosomal recessive.

8 The Killian–Pallister mosaic syndrome. The syndrome is associated with tetrasomy of the short arm of chromosome 12, coarse facial features with a broad forehead hypertelorism, saggy cheeks and mouth, and sparse hair. The condition is diagnosed by skin chromosome studies and can be made prenatally (Bernert *et al.* 1992).

9 Progressive spinocerebellar ataxia, deafness and a peripheral neuropathy (Begeer *et al.* 1991).

10 A syndrome with proximal myopathy with facial,

ocular and bulbar weakness, hypogonadism and ataxia (Lundberg 1974).

11 IBIDS, TAY, BIDS or Pollitt's syndrome (see p. 272). In this autosomal recessive syndrome, cataract and mild to moderate mental retardation are associated with short stature and scaly skin with trichorhexis nodosa (Pollitt & Vamos 1990).

12 The Schwartz–Jampel syndrome (Schwartz & Jampel 1962; Al Gazali 1993) associated with a congenital

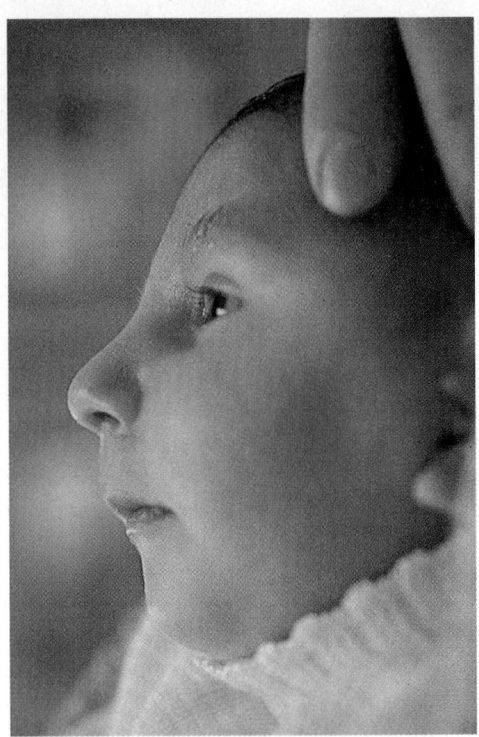

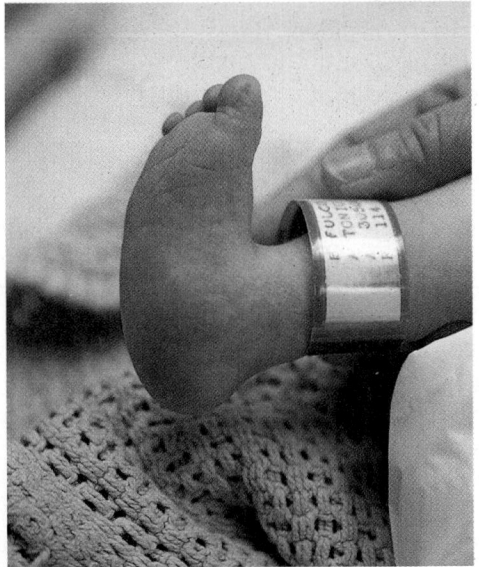

Fig. 39.29 (a) COFS syndrome showing the micrognathia, and the sloping forehead. (b) COFS syndrome. Rocker bottom feet.

myotonic myopathy, ptosis and skeletal defects with microphthalmos and cataract.

13 Cataract, mental retardation, microdontia, pectus excavation and hypertrichosis (Temtamy & Sinbawy 1991).

14 The velocardiofacial (Shprintzen) syndrome is an autosomal dominant syndrome with cardiac anomalies, a prominent nose with square tip, notched alae nasae, micrognathia and a cleft palate. These individuals have 22q11 deletions and there is an overlap with di George's syndrome (Kelly *et al.* 1993). These and some other syndromes with conotruncal cardiac defects have been given the catchy acronym CATCH 22 (Hall 1993; Wilson *et al.* 1993).

15 Cataracts and mental retardation also occur in the following conditions described elsewhere in this book: aniridia, Lowe's syndrome, Bardet–Biedl syndrome, Cockayne's syndrome, congenital varicella and rubella syndromes, vitamin A toxicity, Hallgren's syndrome, Stickler's syndrome and many other retinal and vitreous degenerations. These cataracts are usually acquired.

Steroid cataracts

Chronic corticosteroid therapy, even when given in low doses, may result in the formation of posterior subcapsular cataracts (Kaye *et al.* 1993). The progression of these cataracts may be arrested if the corticosteroids are promptly discontinued (Forman *et al.* 1977). However, since the systemic conditions that prompted the initial steroid therapy are often life-threatening (Fig. 39.32), cessation of steroid therapy may not be possible. Steroid-induced posterior subcapsular cataracts are frequently associated with little if any visual disability and may progress quite slowly (Brocklebank *et al.* 1982; Dunn *et al.* 1993). Posterior subcapsular cataracts also commonly develop in children treated with external beam radiation to the orbital region (Henk *et al.* 1993).

Uveitis

Posterior subcapsular cataracts also develop in children with uveitis secondary to juvenile rheumatoid arthritis (JRA) and pars planitis (Foster & Barrett 1993). Children with JRA-associated cataracts also characteristically develop band keratopathy and posterior synechiae (Key & Kimura 1975). Cystoid macular oedema is a common accompaniment of both conditions.

Prematurity

Transient cataracts have been noted in some premature infants (McCormick 1968). They are usually bilateral and symmetrical opacities beginning as vacuoles along the posterior lens suture. Only rarely do they persist and result in permanent lens opacities.

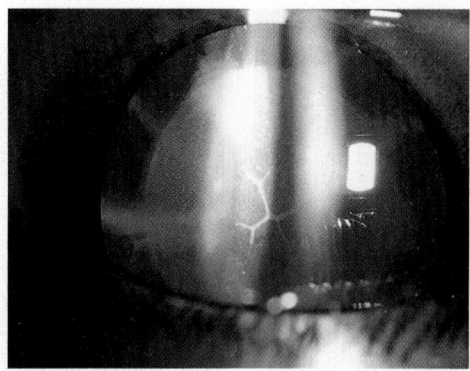

Fig. 39.30 Lamellar and sutural cataracts. The anterior suture is very prominent.

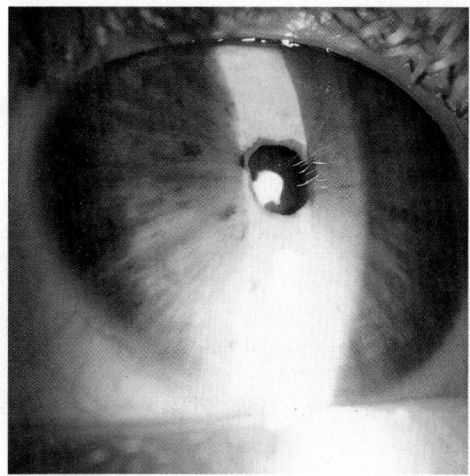

Fig. 39.31 Anterior polar cataract. The acuity is 6/6.

Morphology

Although it may be technically difficult, a slit-lamp examination is usually necessary to define the precise morphology and location of cataracts in infants and young children. Certain morphological patterns have lesser effects on vision, e.g. sutural (Fig. 39.30) (Phelps-Brown 1993), while other types are known to be less likely to progress, e.g. anterior polar cataracts (Fig. 39.31). In some instances, e.g. PHPV) the aetiology of the cataract may be deduced from its morphology alone.

The location and density of cataracts determines their amblyogenic potential (Parks *et al.* 1993). Posteriorly located cataracts (Fig. 39.32) are particularly amblyogenic and if more than 2–3 mm in diameter are rarely associated with good visual acuity if left untreated. Other relatively large anterior polar and lamellar cataracts (Figs 39.33–39.35) may be associated with surprisingly little visual disability (Jaafar & Robb 1984). The cataracts associated with posterior lenticonus are believed to be acquired in most instances and as such

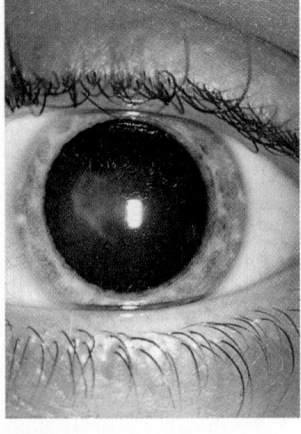
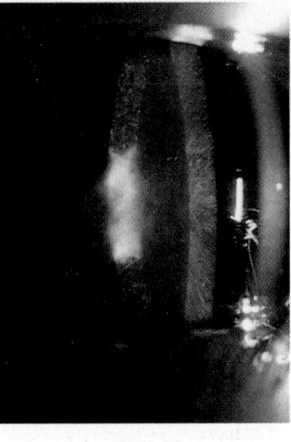

Fig. 39.32 Posterior subcapsular cataract in a child treated for leukaemia. This may be due to steroid treatment, chemotherapy or radiotherapy.

may be associated with a good visual outcome (Cheng *et al.* 1991a).

Certain types of cataracts are also frequently associated with other ocular abnormalities. For instance, nuclear cataracts are often associated with microphthalmos while autosomal dominantly inherited anterior polar cataracts are frequently associated with corneal guttata (Traboulsi & Weinberg 1989) or astigmatism (Bouzas 1991). Anterior subcapsular and anterior capsular cataracts (Fig. 39.37) are usually acquired in children with severe skin diseases (syndermatotic cataract).

Progression occurs in many cataracts and may be very rapid in some cases. Spontaneous reabsorption may occur (Smith *et al.* 1990; Soriano & Funk 1991) and is very common in PHPV.

Caerulean cataracts are progressive blue–white nuclear or cortical cataracts. The gene in one family was linked to 17q24 (Armitage *et al.* 1995). Other autosomal dominant

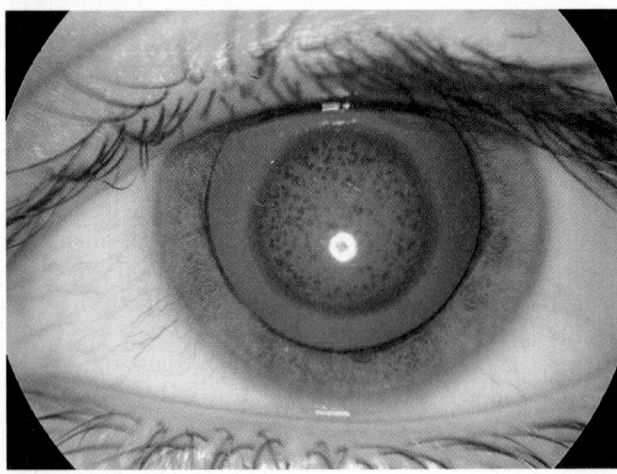

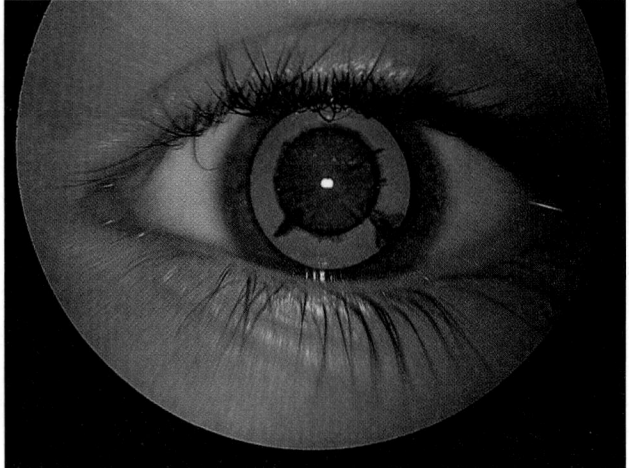

Fig. 39.34 Lamellar cataract with riders; the acuity is 6/24.

Fig. 39.33 Bilateral symmetrical lamellar cataracts in retroillumination. The acuity is 6/9 in both eyes.

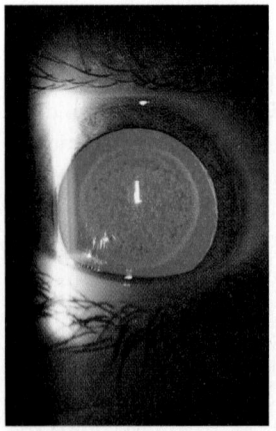
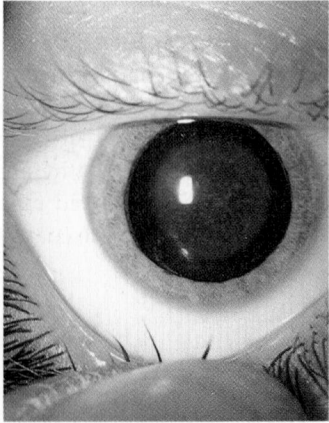

Fig. 39.35 Punctate lamellar cataracts in retroillumination and direct illumination.

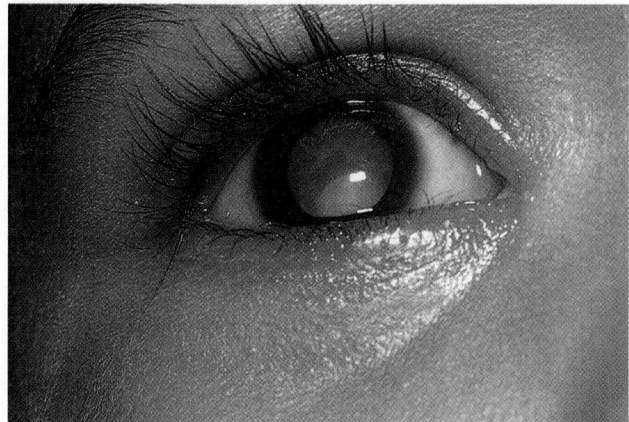
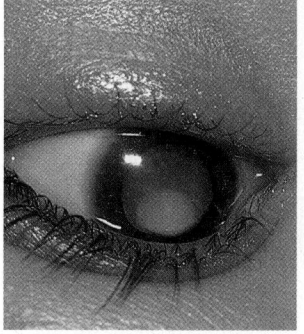
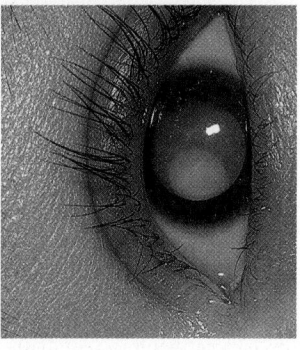

a

b,c

Fig. 39.36 Congenital cataract with liquefied cortex which allows the nucleus to move to different positions depending on posture. (a) Right way up. (b) Upside down. (c) Sideways.

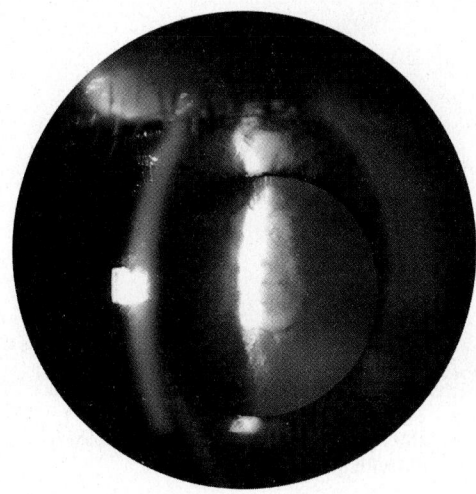

Fig. 39.37 Syndermatotic anterior capsular and subcapsular cataract in a child with eczema.

cataracts have been mapped to 1q21–q25, 2q33–36 and 16q22.1.

Wedge-shaped (Fig. 39.38) or sectional cataracts may occur with Stickler's syndrome (Seery *et al*. 1990) and Conradi's syndrome. It has been suggested that this may be a manifestation of lyonization (Happle & Kuchle 1983).

Visual effects

Because of the significant visual deprivation that occurs with both monocular and binocular cataracts in early infancy, success requires early detection and immediate referral for definitive treatment. The red light reflex should be assessed by direct ophthalmoscopy in the newborn nursery at 6 weeks and 6 months of age by a general practitioner or paediatrician. If an abnormality is detected, a prompt referral should be made to an ophthalmologist. Pupillary dilation may be necessary to detect incomplete cataracts in some children.

Children with visually significant monocular cataracts often present with strabismus which may not develop until irreparable visual loss has occurred. Rarely monocular nystagmus may be the presenting sign of a monocular congenital cataract. In most instances, visual behaviour will be unaffected by a monocular cataract, and parents are not aware of the problem. In contrast, dense binocular cataracts are usually associated with delayed development and obviously impaired visual behaviour. If manifest nystagmus does develop the visual prognosis is worse although on occasion it may be reversed by prompt treatment (Gelbart *et al*. 1982). Children with manifest nystagmus in primary gaze during the first year of life should be carefully evaluated for cataracts.

Management

Assessment

Although dense bilateral congenital cataracts should be removed as early as possible, partial cataracts should only be removed after a careful assessment of the morphology of the lens opacity and the visual behaviour of the child. Conservative management is indicated at least until the child's visual status can be accurately assessed. The visual prognosis of bilateral incomplete cataracts correlates better with the density than the size of the opacity. Hence

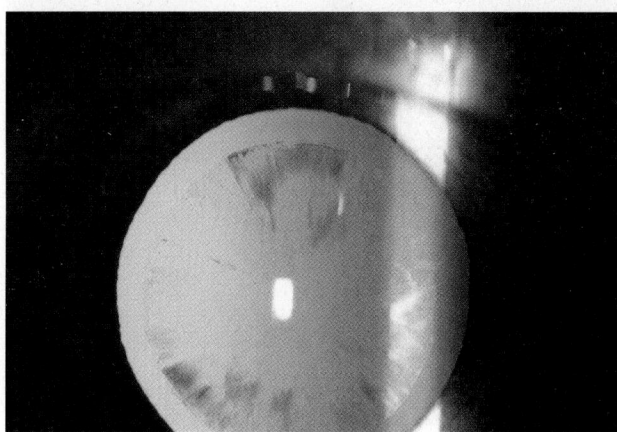

Fig. 39.38 Wedge-shaped cataracts as part of a lamellar cataract.

nuclear cataracts, although smaller in size than lamellar cataracts, may have a poorer visual prognosis. If the major blood vessels of the fundus cannot be distinguished through the central portion of the cataract, significant visual deprivation can be expected from even a moderately sized partial cataract.

The systemic investigation should usually be carried out in collaboration with a paediatrician who has an interest in dysmorphology and metabolic disease and who will carry out further tests as appropriate, such as plasma electrolytes and amino acid studies. Further investigations, such as galactose enzyme studies, can be carried out when appropriate. Clearly some cataracts, such as posterior lenticonus and unilateral PHPV, are purely ocular problems and do not require a paediatric investigation.

An attempt should be made to evaluate the integrity of the retina and optic nerve in all children with significant cataracts. If the density of the cataracts precludes an adequate view of the fundus, an ultrasound examination may be carried out prior to any surgical intervention. It is also important to assess the pupillary reflexes. An afferent pupillary defect suggests a structural defect of the optic disc or retina and is associated with a poor visual prognosis. A visual assessment should also be performed using patterns of fixation and supplemented when possible by forced choice preferential looking (Lloyd *et al.* 1994) and/or pattern visual evoked potentials. Surgery for visually significant bilateral cataracts should be carried out as soon as possible without jeopardizing the general health of the child. Only a short interval should elapse between the removal of the right and left lenses to prevent relative amblyopia (Taylor *et al.* 1979) of the fellow eye.

Surgery

The surgical treatment (Figs 39.39–39.42) of children's

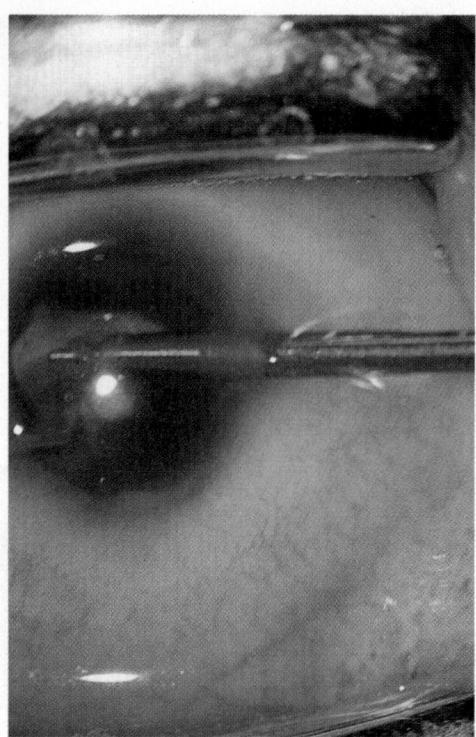

Fig. 39.40 Surgery for congenital cataract and microphthalmos. In this picture an intraocular diathermy is being used to prevent haemorrhage from vessels on the abnormal vascularized lens in this eye with a horizontal corneal diameter of 7 mm.

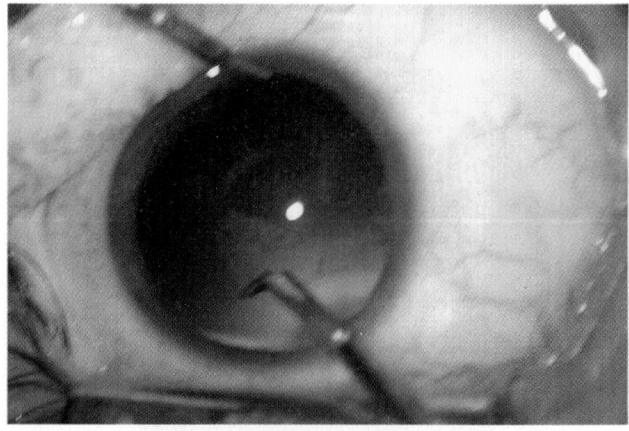

Fig. 39.41 Cataract surgery. A membrane being peeled from the posterior capsule with intraocular forceps.

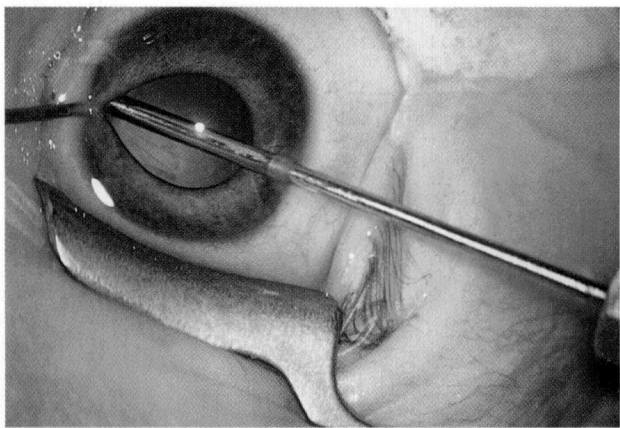

Fig. 39.39 Lensectomy showing the iris retracted by an irrigating cystitome and the vitrectomy machine removing the cortex and capsule underneath this area. Using a two-handed technique may help to get a fuller clearance of the lens and capsule.

cataracts has evolved considerably since Scheie popularized the aspiration procedure (Scheie 1960). At present, most authorities prefer to perform a lensectomy and anterior vitrectomy utilizing a closed eye system in infant eyes (Lambert *et al.* 1989). By creating a primary posterior capsulotomy or primary posterior capsulorrhexis, the number of secondary operations can be greatly reduced (Taylor 1981). Moreover, the clear visual axis thus created

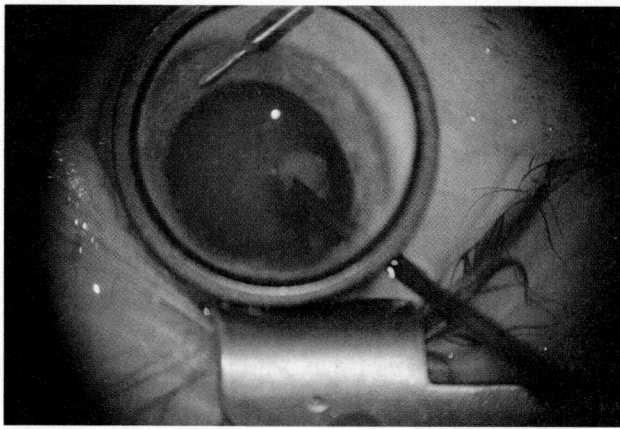

Fig. 39.42 Retrieval of soft lens material from the vitreous using a fundus viewing (Machmer) lens.

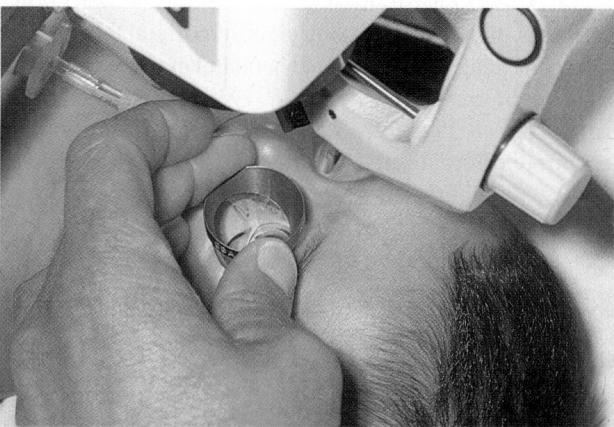

Fig. 39.43 Horizontally mounted YAG laser. Using a contact lens (in this case a gonioscopy lens) patients can be treated easily under general anaesthetic.

facilitates retinoscopy. The incidence of secondary glaucoma and retinal detachment may also be reduced by utilizing this technique (Gelbart *et al.* 1982; Parks 1982). However, since the latent period for retinal detachment is long, the incidence of retinal detachment following a lensectomy may prove to be higher with longer term follow-up (McLeod 1986).

In older children, who are less susceptible to amblyopia and in whom posterior capsular opacification is less likely to occur, a simple lens aspiration with or without the implantation of an intraocular lens is the preferred procedure. While phacoemulsification can be used to remove a paediatric cataract, aspiration alone is usually sufficient.

If the posterior capsule opacifies a YAG laser (see Fig. 39.43) can be used to create a posterior capsulotomy (Lloyd *et al.* 1992) (Fig. 39.44). It is important that the procedure not be delayed because of the danger of amblyopia developing and the increased difficulty of opening a thickened posterior capsule. Posterior capsule opacification is

due largely to proliferation and migration of residual lens epithelial cells (Apple *et al.* 1992).

Correction of aphakia

One of the major obstacles confronting ophthalmologists and the families of infants requiring cataract extraction is the optical treatment of the induced aphakia.

Contact lenses

Contact lenses remain the standard method of optically correcting unilateral aphakia during infancy (Fig. 39.45) and are commonly used to treat bilateral aphakia as well. Rigid gas-permeable contact lenses are well suited for correcting aphakia during infancy because of their wide range of available powers, low cost, ability to correct large astigmatic errors, and their greater ease of insertion and removal (Amos *et al.* 1992). Their biggest disadvantage is the greater expertise required to fit them (Saunders & Ellis 1981; Pratt-Johnson & Tillson 1985). Silicone lenses have been used in the past, but are being used less frequently because of their increased cost and greater rate of complications (Nelson *et al.* 1985). Aphakic soft lenses are relatively inexpensive and easy to fit (Epstein *et al.* 1988; Levin *et al.* 1988; Amaya *et al.* 1990), but have the disadvantage of being more difficult to insert and can only correct small astigmatic errors.

The frequent loss of lenses and the need to change regularly the lens power as the eye elongates necessitates frequent lens replacements, particularly during the first 2 years of life (Moore 1989; Amaya *et al.* 1990). Parents are strongly advised to remove the lenses if the child's eye becomes inflamed, irritated or if excessive discharge develops. Inadequate care can result in ulcerative keratitis

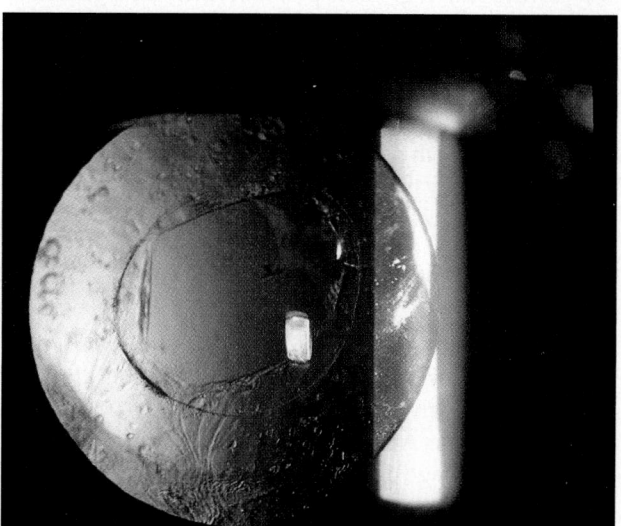

Fig. 39.44 YAG laser capsulotomy.

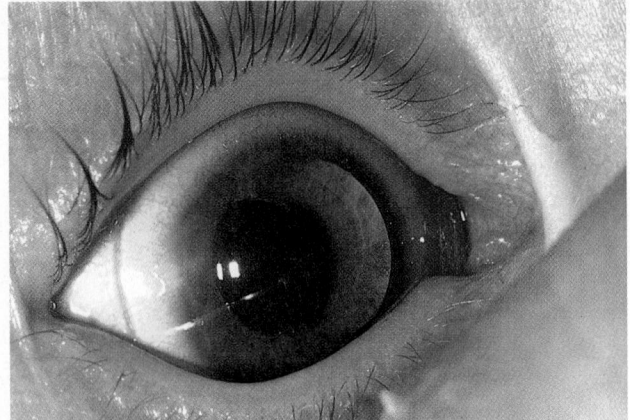

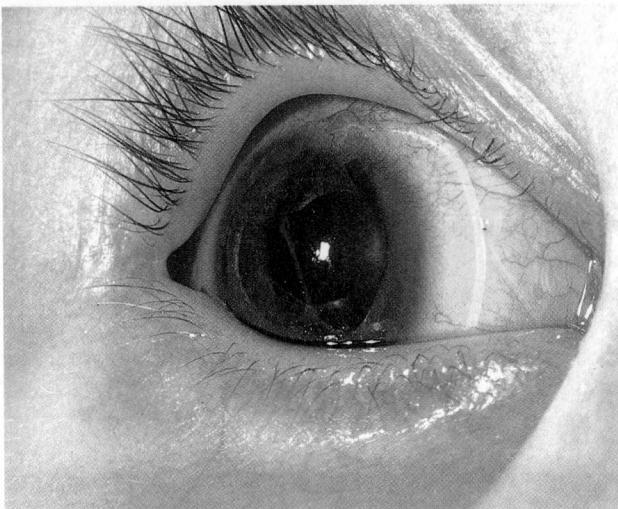

Fig. 39.45 Aphakic contact lenses are the treatment of choice in infant aphakia (see text).

Intraocular lenses

Intraocular lenses are being used increasingly to optically correct aphakia in children, with good visual results (Ben-Ezra 1990; Dahan & Salmenson 1990; Gupta *et al.* 1992; Buckley *et al.* 1993; Gimbel *et al.* 1993; Koenig *et al.* 1993; Hiles & Atkinson 1994; Crouch *et al.* 1995; Lambert *et al.* 1996). However, in most instances their use is currently contraindicated during infancy because of the difficulty of accurately predicting the most appropriate lens power to insert and the increased incidence of complications in these eyes (Burke *et al.* 1989b; Markham *et al.* 1992; Lambert *et al.* 1995). Although an intraocular lens with a standard power of 21–22 dioptres could be implanted, in most cases this would necessitate an overcorrection during the critical years of visual development (Gordon & Donzis 1985; BenEzra 1996). In addition, many infants with cataracts have microphthalmic eyes and a standard powered lens would significantly undercorrect these eyes. Also, removing the lens from a neonatal eye may retard its subsequent growth (Wilson *et al.* 1987; Tigges *et al.* 1990; Lambert *et al.* 1996). As a consequence most authorities recommend implanting an intraocular lens with a power which will slightly undercorrect a child 6 years of age or

and corneal scarring. These problems increase significantly if contact lenses are worn overnight (Schein *et al.* 1989). Poor compliance with contact lens wear is most commonly due to poor vision in the aphakic eye or poor patient cooperation rather than complications arising from use (Moore 1993). With persistence, contact lenses can be successfully worn by more than 90% of infants (Amaya *et al.* 1990; Holmstrom *et al.* 1990; Moore 1993).

Spectacles

Aphakic spectacles (Fig. 39.46) are better tolerated than contact lenses by some children with bilateral aphakia. This is particularly true of children between 18 months and 4 years of age. Aphakic spectacles sometimes have the cosmetic advantage of improving the appearance of mildly microphthalmic eyes because of the magnification they induce. In addition, a secondary strabismus may be manipulated by the prismatic effect of spectacles.

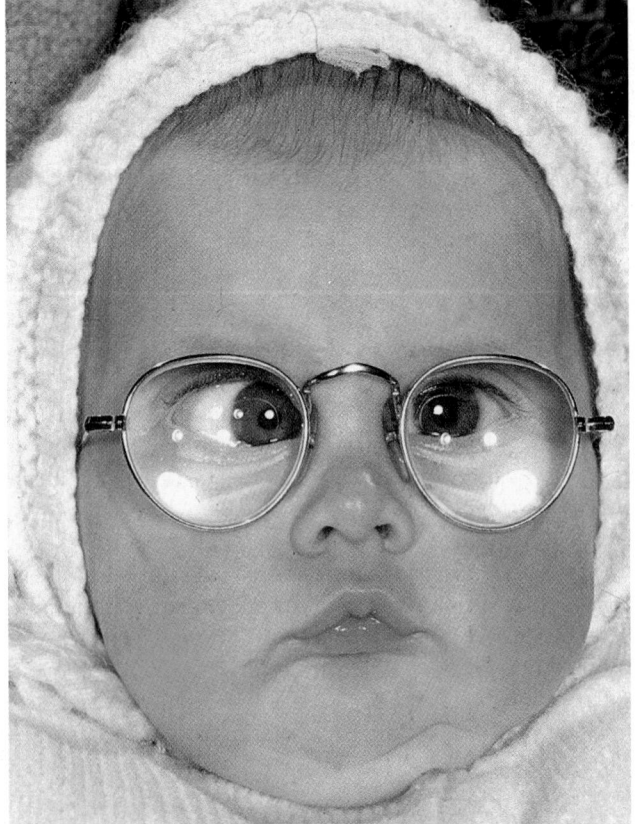

Fig. 39.46 Aphakic spectacles are safe and easily changed but have optical and cosmetic disadvantages.

these eyes many years after implantation (Bourne *et al.* 1994).

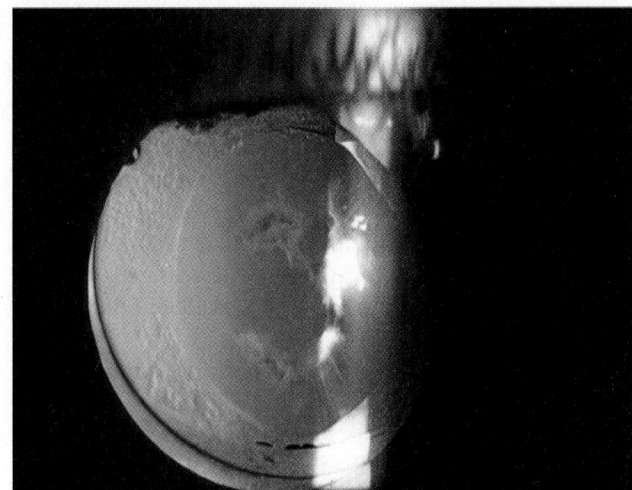

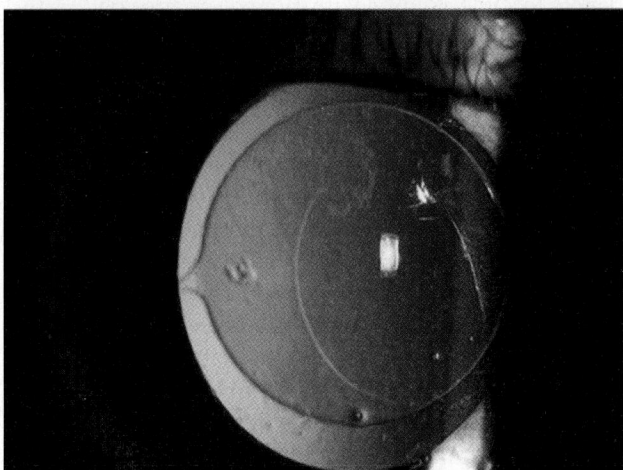

Epikeratophakia

Epikeratophakia, the use of a lamellar onlay corneal graft (Fig. 39.49), has been used to treat children who are intolerant of contact lenses or spectacles. In most children it has been performed as a monocular procedure (Arffa *et al.* 1986; Morgan *et al.* 1988; Rostron 1988; Morgan & Somers 1989). The visual results obtained with this procedure in children have generally been disappointing (Price & Binder 1987; Elsas 1990).

Management of amblyopia

No matter what form of aphakic correction is chosen, frequent re-evaluations are necessary. Each examination should include a careful analysis of fixation behaviour to screen for amblyopia. If amblyopia is suspected, occlusion

Fig. 39.47 (a) Intraocular lens. This one-piece PMMA lens is placed in the bag through a capsulorrhexis. There are a few posterior capsular opacities which will require YAG laser treatment. (b) Intraocular lens. The 5.5 mm lens has been inserted through a 4 mm capsulorrhexis.

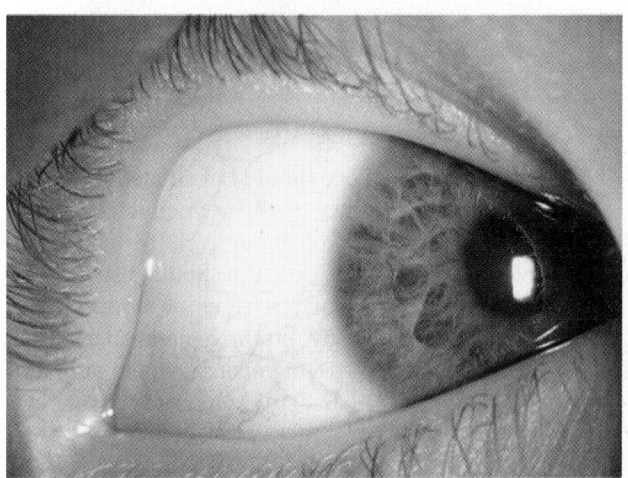

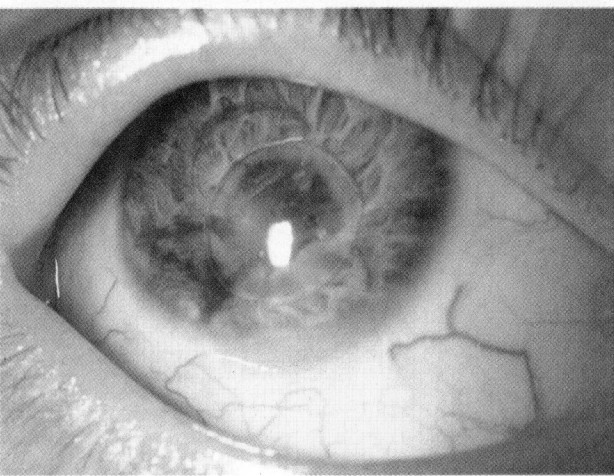

Fig. 39.48 This child had a secondary intraocular lens implant when 18 months old. By 2.5 years she had a bilateral uveitis with vision in the best eye of hand movements.

less, but fully correct a child 6 years of age or older (Hutchinson *et al.* in press). While it is generally easier to implant an intraocular lens at the same time a cataract is removed, intraocular lenses can also be implanted as a secondary procedure using the residual lens capsule for support (Dahan *et al.* 1989). Multifocal lenses (Lambert *et al.* 1994) remain experimental in children.

In older children, especially after trauma (Ellis 1992), intraocular lenses may safely be implanted. Currently an 'in-the-bag' single piece polymethylmethacrylate (PMMA) lens is the most popular method (Fig. 39.47).

Intraocular lens implantation should (as with any other optical correction) be viewed as part of the treatment of amblyopia, not as a technical feat. There are some other outstanding problems: the inflammatory response produced by an infant may be greater than in an older child (Fig. 39.48) and we still do not know what happens to

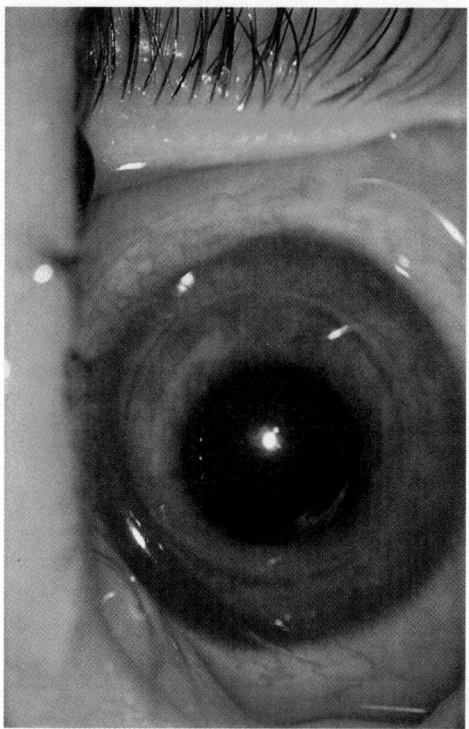

Fig. 39.49 Epikeratophakia graft.

therapy of the preferred eye should be initiated. Frequent retinoscopic measurements of the refractive error and adjustments in the power of the aphakic correction are imperative. The intraocular pressure should also be periodically assessed, particularly if signs or symptoms of glaucoma develop. This may require general anaesthesia in an infant. The importance of encouragement and support for the parents of aphakic children cannot be overem-

phasized if a successful rehabilitation programme is to be established.

Monocular cataract. The management of monocular congenital cataracts is particularly problematic. Although eyes with monocular congenital cataracts may be successfully rehabilitated on occasion (Beller *et al.* 1981; Gregg & Parks 1992), most eyes with monocular cataracts do not achieve a visual acuity compatible with reading (Kushner 1986; Robb *et al.* 1987; Birch & Stager 1988; Drummond *et al.* 1989; Neumann *et al.* 1993).

Before a decision is made to perform surgery on a monocular congenital cataract, the difficulties associated with the use of aphakic contact lenses and occlusion therapy should be described in detail to the parents. If a contact lens is not tolerated, aphakic spectacles may be of benefit to some children with monocular aphakia.

If a decision is made to perform surgery on a monocular congenital cataract, prompt surgical intervention is critical (Rogers *et al.* 1981). Most studies suggest that surgery after the first 6 weeks of life is less likely to result in good visual acuity (Vaegan & Taylor 1979; Birch & Stager 1988; Lorenz *et al.* 1994; Birch & Stager 1996). Immediate and continued optical correction of the monocular aphakia and occlusion therapy of the phakic eye is crucial in the visual rehabilitation of these eyes. The fitting of contact lenses at the time of surgery has been advocated (Vila-Coro & Mazow 1989), but this makes it difficult to tell the difference between contact lens-related inflammation and surgical complications, so many leave the optical correction for a few days postoperatively.

Occluding the fellow eye 50–70% of all waking hours throughout early childhood (Fig. 39.50) has the best visual outcomes in aphakic eyes (O'Dell *et al.* 1989; Gregg &

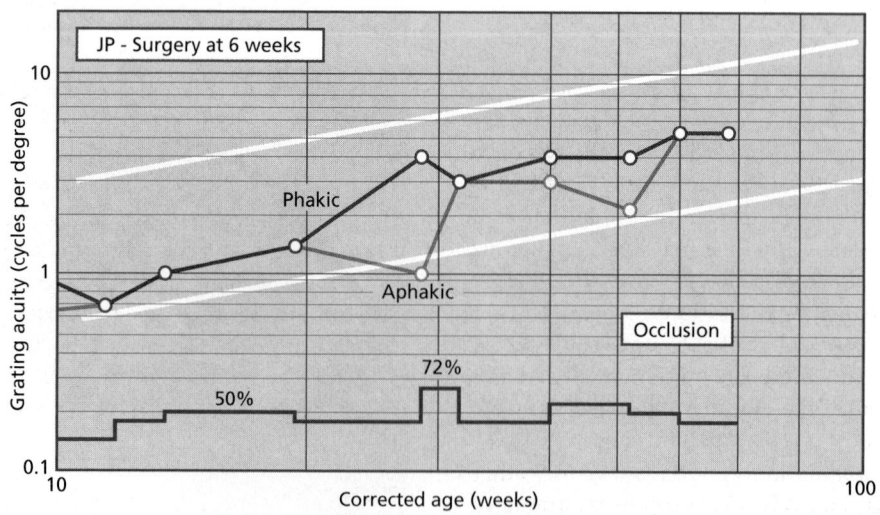

Fig. 39.50 Monocular cataract occlusion regime. The acuities of the phakic (blue) and aphakic (pink) eye have been monitored using Keeler cards (see Chapter 8). Initially the acuities in the two eyes were the same and the child was maintained on a 50% of waking hours occlusion regime. When the aphakic eye fell behind the phakic eye, the amount of occlusion (bottom line) was increased to a maximum of 72% in this case. Illustration by courtesy of Mr Chris Lloyd, Manchester, UK.

Parks 1992; Boothe *et al.* 1996). Patching with varying amounts depending on visual assessment using forced choice preferential looking may improve the results (Lloyd *et al.* 1995). Excessive patching may result in the development of subtle visual deficits in the fellow eye (Spielmann 1990; Lewis *et al.* 1992a; Lloyd *et al.* 1992; Summers & Letson 1992). Although 'binocular' vision is unusual in children treated for monocular cataracts (Lorenz *et al.* 1994), it may rarely be achieved (Greg & Parks 1992).

Bilateral and traumatic cataracts

Occlusion therapy is often not necessary in children with bilateral congenital cataracts (Lloyd *et al.* 1994) or children with unilateral traumatic cataracts who are treated promptly.

Complications of cataract surgery

A much higher incidence of complications occurs in children after cataract surgery than in adults. While some complications are preventable by meticulous attention to surgical technique and postoperative care, others arise due to the intrinsic abnormalities of these eyes or the more exuberant inflammatory response associated with surgery on an immature eye.

Amblyopia

Amblyopia is a nearly universal finding in children with congenital cataracts, and a common finding in children with developmental cataracts during the first 7 years of life. It is particularly a problem in children with monocular congenital cataracts. It arises as a consequence of the retina receiving a defocused image during the critical period of visual development. Uncorrected aphakia or induced anisometropia can exacerbate this amblyopia even after the removal of a cataract. In most cases forced visual deprivation of the fellow eye using occlusion therapy, optical defocus or atropinization is required.

Glaucoma

Glaucoma (see Chapter 40) may arise during the early postoperative period or as a late complication years later. Pupil block glaucoma has a particularly high incidence in neonates following a lensectomy. In some cases this may occur second to vitreous prolapsing forward into the anterior chamber while in other cases it may occur secondary to a pupillary membrane. Affected patients usually have ocular pain, corneal oedema and iris bombe. Performing a deep anterior vitrectomy, creating a peripheral iridectomy and dilating the pupil of an infant for several weeks after a lensectomy can prevent this complication from develop-

ing. Glaucoma is also one of the most common late complications of cataract surgery, occurring in up to one-third of all children after cataract extraction (Keech *et al.* 1989; Simon *et al.* 1991). Its prevalence is particularly high in children with microphthalmos and nuclear cataracts (Johnson & Parks 1991) and may be more frequent in eyes operated on during infancy (Mills & Robb 1994). Unlike infantile onset glaucoma, which is usually associated with readily detectable signs and symptoms such as buphthalmos, photophobia and corneal oedema, juvenile onset glaucoma is usually more protean in its manifestations. While an elevation of the intraocular pressure and optic disc cupping may be present, it is frequently difficult to obtain a reliable measurement of intraocular pressure until later in childhood. For this reason, particular attention should be paid to any cupping of the optic disc, increase in eye size, or rapid loss of hypermetropia (Egbert & Kushner 1990).

Strabismus

Strabismus is often the presenting sign of a child with a monocular cataract and is also frequently present preoperatively in children with bilateral cataracts (France & Frank 1984; Cheng *et al.* 1991b). Esotropias are more commonly observed in children with congenital cataracts while exotropias are observed more frequently in children with acquired cataracts. An even higher percentage of children develop strabismus after surgical and optical treatment of their cataracts. Strabismus is a particularly troubling problem in older children with acquired cataracts if there is a delay in the removal of the cataract or the optical correction of the induced aphakia. In some cases, these patients can develop diplopia which will persist even after the eyes are surgically aligned secondary to a disturbance of central fusion (Pratt-Johnson & Tilson 1989).

Capsular opacification

Soemmerring's rings are ubiquitous in children's eyes after cataract surgery unless the lens capsule is completely removed at the time of surgery (Kappelhof *et al.* 1987). While in most cases they remain confined to the retroiridal space, on occasion reproliferating lens material can extend into the pupillary aperture (Morgan & Karcioglu 1987; Amaya *et al.* 1990). In these instances, a re-operation is usually necessary to create a clear visual axis.

Irregular pupil

An irregular pupil is a fairly common complication of cataract surgery during infancy (Fig. 39.51). In some instances, the iris sphincter muscle is damaged intraoperatively by the vitreous cutting instrument. In other

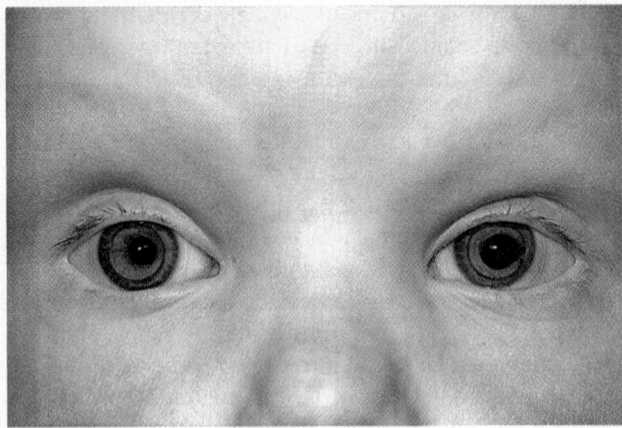

Fig. 39.51 Irregular pupil in the left eye secondary to iris damage during surgery.

instances, the iris may prolapse out of the scleral incision during surgery and become atrophic thereafter. This is particularly a problem in children with lightly coloured irides.

Strands of vitreous extending to the surgical incision may also cause peaking of the pupil. This complication may be averted by turning off the infusion line before removing the vitreous cutting instrument from the eye, maintaining a low flow of irrigating solution, and minimizing the number of times the vitreous cutting instrument is inserted and removed from the eye.

Even when the pupil remains round after cataract surgery, it frequently is less reactive to light and pharmacological dilation. Rigid pupils are particularly common in children who undergo a lensectomy during infancy.

Secondary membranes

Secondary membranes may arise from fibrin forming a pupillary membrane or opacification of the residual posterior lens capsule. If they obstruct the visual axis, they may be opened with a YAG laser or surgical discission. Because of the high incidence of these complications in infants a primary posterior capsulotomy is usually recommended coupled with atropinization of the pupil for at least 2 weeks after surgery.

Endophthalmitis

Bacterial endophthalmitis is an uncommon, but devastating complication of cataract surgery (Fig. 39.52). It occurs in 0.07–0.4% of paediatric eyes after cataract extraction (Good *et al.* 1990; Wheeler *et al.* 1992). A concurrent nasolacrimal duct obstruction, upper respiratory infection or periorbital skin disease increases the risk of this complication developing. The most common organisms causing postoperative endophthalmitis in children are *Staphylococcus aureus* and *Streptococcus pneumoniae*.

Even though most cases are diagnosed during the first 3 postoperative days, the visual prognosis still quite poor. In one series, 65% of affected eyes ended up with no light perception vision despite aggressive treatment with intravitreal and systemic antibiotics (Wheeler *et al.* 1992). While bilateral simultaneous cataract extractions may be justified in infants with increased anaesthetic risks (Guo *et al.* 1990), the risk of bilateral endophthalmitis developing in these patients is the strongest argument against this practice (Good *et al.* 1990).

Nystagmus

Nystagmus is present in 50% of children with bilateral congenital cataracts (France & Frank 1984). Nystagmus may also develop in children with monocular cataracts, although this occurs less frequently. In some cases, it may become the limiting factor in the visual rehabilitation of children after cataract extraction. Early treatment may reduce the incidence of this complication, but very early and excessive patching may make it worse.

Retinal haemorrhages and detachments

A haemorrhagic retinopathy develops in a significant percentage of infants after a lensectomy and anterior vitrectomy (Christiansen *et al.* 1993). In most cases this consists of flame-shaped haemorrhages in the posterior pole that resolve without sequelae in several weeks. Occasionally, a haemorrhage may occur in the fovea and result in a severe reduction of vision. In these cases, even after the haemorrhage has resolved, the visual acuity may remain reduced secondary to amblyopia.

Retinal detachments usually occur decades after the removal of a congenital cataract (Toyofuku *et al.* 1980). In a series by Jagger *et al.* (1983) the average interval between

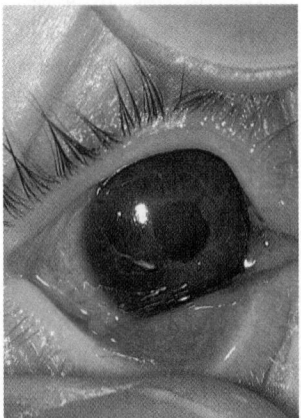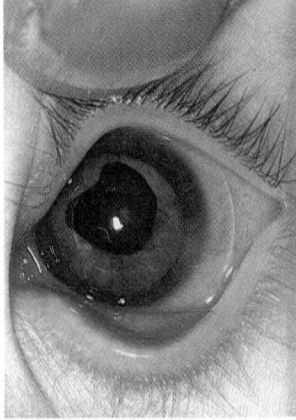

Fig. 39.52 Endophthalmitis of the right eye. This child had bilateral cataracts and microcoria. The left eye had been operated successfully and a larger pupil created. The right eye developed endophthalmitis detected during the first postoperative day.

cataract surgery and retinal detachment was 28 years (range 1–51 years). While Chrousos *et al.* (1984) only reported a 2% incidence of retinal detachment in aphakic children, the mean postoperative follow-up in their series was only 5.5 years. Retinal detachments frequently occur bilaterally and the visualization of the retinal breaks may be hampered by miotic pupils and Soemmerring's rings.

Cystoid macular oedema

Cystoid macular oedema is a common complication after cataract extraction in adults, but a rare complication in children. Poer *et al.* (1981) reported no cases of cystoid macular oedema in 25 children who underwent fluorescein angiography after cataract extraction.

Corneal oedema

Corneal oedema can occur after cataract surgery, but usually resolves within a few days. While in most cases it is probably caused by prolongation of the surgical procedure, it may occur secondary to detergent left on surgical instruments or cannulas (Nuyts *et al.* 1990). It also commonly occurs after the removal of rubella cataracts.

Visual results

The visual results after the surgical removal of paediatric cataracts have improved dramatically over the last two decades (Scheie 1960; Pratt-Johnson & Tillson 1985). Improvements in surgical results may be attributed to better surgical techniques, the availability of paediatric aphakic contact lenses, the increased implantation of intraocular lenses in children, and the improved screening of children for cataracts by paediatricians and general practitioners at an earlier age. Nevertheless, complete visual rehabilitation is rarely possible.

The visual results obtained after cataract extraction in infants and children depend on a number of factors including: (i) the age of onset of the cataracts; (ii) the age when surgery is performed; (iii) associated ocular and systemic conditions; and (iv) compliance with optical and patching therapy (Hing *et al.* 1990; Wright *et al.* 1992; Bradford *et al.* 1994). In some cases macular hypoplasia may account for relatively poor results (Howard *et al.* 1993). Children who develop cataracts after the completion of normal visual development, usually have an excellent visual prognosis.

Many children with early onset bilateral cataracts also have an excellent visual outcome if treatment is initiated immediately; however, if treatment is delayed, many of these children will remain legally blind secondary to amblyopia (Gelbart *et al.* 1982; Parks 1982; Synnove *et al.* 1986).

Early onset monocular cataracts continue to be associated with the worse visual prognosis, although even they can be associated with a good visual outcome on occasion (Cheng *et al.* 1991b; Gregg & Parks 1992; Birch *et al.* 1993; Lloyd *et al.* 1995).

Concomitant ocular abnormalities such as corneal opacities, glaucoma, retinal abnormalities and nystagmus worsen the visual prognosis of children with cataracts. Mental retardation is also associated with a poor visual prognosis. Although mental retardation *per se* is not a contraindication to cataract surgery, the postoperative care and visual rehabilitatin of these children is much more difficult. While gross stereopsis may develop on rare occasions in a child after cataract surgery, in most instances the disruption of normal binocular input to the central nervous system during the critical period of visual development precludes this outcome (Gregg & Parks 1992; Tytla *et al.* 1993).

References

Al Gazali LI. The Schwartz–Jampel syndrome. *Clin Dysmorphol* 1993; **2**: 47–54.

Alcorn DM, Maumenee IH. Optical correction and visual acuity in patients with the Marfan syndrome and dislocated lenses (abstract). *Invest Ophthalmol Vis Sci* 1987; **28**(Suppl.): 324.

Alter M, Talbert OR, Croffead G. Cerebellar ataxia, congenital cataracts and retarded somatic and mental maturation. *Neurology* 1962; **12**: 836–47.

Amaya LG, Speedwell L, Taylor D. Contact lenses for infant aphakia. *Br J Ophthalmol* 1990; **74**: 150–4.

Amos CF, Lambert SR, Ward MA. Rigid gas permeable contact lens correction of aphakia following congenital cataract removal during infancy. *J Pediatr Ophthalmol Strabismus* 1992; **29**: 243–5.

Apple DJ, Holden JD, Stallworth B. Ocular pathology of Patau's syndrome with an unbalanced DID translocation. *Am J Ophthalmol* 1970; **70**: 383–91.

Apple DJ, Solomon K, Tetz M *et al.* Posterior capsule opacification. *Surv Ophthalmol* 1992; **37**: 73–116.

Arffa RC, Marvelli TL, Morgan KS. Long-term follow-up of refractive and keratometric results of pediatric epikeratophakia. *Arch Ophthalmol* 1986; **104**: 668–70.

Armaly MF. Ocular involvement in chondrodystrophia calcificans congenita punctata. *Arch Ophthalmol* 1957; **57**: 491–502.

Armitage M, Kivlin J, Ferrell R. A progressive early onset cataract gene maps to human chromosome 17q24. *Nature Genet* 1995; **9**: 37–40.

Baraitser M, Winter RM, Taylor DSI. Lenz microphthalmia syndrome. *Clin Genet* 1982; **22**: 99–101.

Barber GW, Spaeth GL. The successful treatment of homocystinuria with pyridoxine. *J Pediatr* 1969; **75**: 463–78.

Barker DF, Hostikka S, Zhou J *et al.* Identification of 6 mutations in the COL4A5 collagen gene in Alport syndrome. *Science* 1990; **248**: 1224–6.

Bateman JB, Phillipart M. Ocular features of the Hagberg–Santavuori syndrome. *Am J Ophthalmol* 1986; **102**: 262–71.

Begeer J, Scholte F, Van Essen A. Two sisters with mental retardation, cataract, ataxia, progressive hearing loss, and polyneuropathy. *J Med Genet* 1991; **28**: 884–5.

Behki R, Noel L-P, Clarke WN. Limbal lensectomy in the management of ectopia lentis in children. *Arch Ophthalmol* 1990; **108**:

809–11.

Beigi B, O'Keefe M, Bowell R *et al*. Ophthalmic findings in classical galactosaemia—prospective study. *Br J Ophthalmol* 1993; **77**: 162–4.

Beller R, Hoyt CS, Marg E *et al*. Good visual function after neonatal surgery for congenital monocular cataracts. *Am J Ophthalmol* 1981; **91**: 559–65.

Ben-Ezra D. Intraocular lenses for unilateral paediatric aphakia. Early lenses and long term follow up. *Eur J Implant Ref Surg* 1990; **2**: 285–9.

BenEzra D. Cataract surgery and intraocular lens implantation in children. *Am J Ophthalmol* 1996; **121**: 224–5.

Berg W, Verbraak FD, Bos PJM. Homocystinuria presenting as central retinal artery occlusion and longstanding thromboembolic disease. *Br J Ophthalmol* 1990; **74**: 696–7.

Bernert J, Bartels I, Gatz G *et al*. Prenatal diagnosis of the Pallister–Killian mosaic aneuploidy syndrome. *Am J Med Genet* 1992; **42**: 747–50.

Birch EE, Stager DR. Prevalence of good visual acuity following surgery for congenital unilateral cataract. *Arch Ophthalmol* 1988; **106**: 40–3.

Birch EE, Stager DR. The critical period for surgical treatment of dense congenital unilateral cataract. *Invest Ophthalmol Vis Sci* 1996; **37**: 1532–8.

Birch EE, Swanson WH, Stager DR *et al*. Outcome after very early treatment of dense congenital unilateral cataract. *Invest Ophthalmol Vis Sci* 1993; **34**: 3687–99.

Bleik J, Traboulsi E, Maumenee I. Familial posterior lenticonus and microcornea. *Arch Ophthalmol* 1992; **110**: 1208–10.

Boothe RG, Louden T, Lambert SR. Acuity and contrast sensitivity in monkeys following neonatal intraocular lens implantation with and without part-time occlusion of the fellow eye. *Invest Ophthalmol Vis Sci* 1996; **37**: 1520–31.

Bourne WM, Nelson LR, Hodge DO. Continued endothelial cell loss 10 years after lens implantation. *Ophthalmology* 1994; **101**: 1014–23.

Bouzas A. Anterior polar congenital cataract and corneal astigmatism. *J Pediatr Ophthalmol Strabismus* 1991; **29**: 210–12.

Bradford GM, Keech RV, Scott WE. Factors affecting visual outcome after surgery for bilateral congenital cataracts. *Am J Ophthalmol* 1994; **117**: 58–64.

Brocklebank JT, Harcourt RB, Meadow SR. Corticosteroid-induced cataracts in idiopathic nephrotic syndrome. *Arch Dis Child* 1982; **53**: 30–4.

Bron AJ, Lambert S. Specular microscopy of the lens. *Ophthalmic Res* 1984; **16** (Suppl.): 209.

Buckley EG, Klombers LA, Seaber JH, Scalise-Gardy A, Mintzer R. Management of the posterior capsule during pediatric intraocular lens implantation. *Am J Ophthalmol* 1993; **115**: 722–8.

Burke JP, O'Keefe M, Bowell R *et al*. Ocular complications in homocystinuria — early and late treated. *Br J Ophthalmol* 1989a; **73**: 427–31.

Burke JP, Willshaw HE, Young JDH. Intraocular lens implants for uniocular cataracts in childhood. *Br J Ophthalmol* 1989b; **73**: 860–4.

Callahan A. Aniridia with ectopia lentis and secondary glaucoma: genetic, pathologic and surgical considerations. *Am J Ophthalmol* 1949; **32** (Part II): 28–40.

Catalano RA. Down syndrome. *Surv Ophthalmol* 1990; **34**: 385–98.

Chandler PA. Choice of treatment in dislocation of the lens: the first E.B. Dunphy Lecture. *Arch Ophthalmol* 1964; **71**: 765–86.

Cheng KP, Hiles DA, Biglan AW *et al*. Management of posterior lenticonus. *J Pediatr Ophthalmol Strabismus* 1991a; **28**: 143–9.

Cheng KP, Hiles DA, Biglan AW, Pettapiece MC. Visual results after early surgical treatment of unilateral congenital cataracts. *Ophthalmology* 1991b; **98**: 903–10.

Christiansen SP, Munoz M, Capo H. Retinal hemorrhage following lensectomy and anterior vitrectomy in children. *J Pediatr Ophthalmol Strabismus* 1993; **30**: 24–7.

Chrousos GA, Parks MM, O'Neill JF. Incidence of chronic glaucoma, retinal detachment and secondary membrane surgery in pediatric aphakic patients. *Ophthalmology* 1984; **91**: 1238–41.

Cibis GW, Waeltermann JM, Whitcraft CT *et al*. Lenticular opacities in carriers of Lowe's syndrome. *Ophthalmology* 1986; **93**: 1041–5.

Cohen MM. Hallermann–Streiff syndrome: a review. *Am J Med Genet* 1991; **41**: 488–99.

Collod G, Babron M-C, Jondeau G *et al*. A second locus for Marfan's syndrome maps to 3p24.2–25. *Nature Genet* 1994; **8**: 264–8.

Cotlier E. Congenital varicella cataract. *Am J Ophthalmol* 1978; **86**: 627–9.

Cotlier E, Rice P. Cataracts in the Smith–Lemli–Opitz syndrome. *Am J Ophthalmol* 1971; **72**: 955–9.

Cowan A, Klauder JV. Frequency of occurrence of cataract in atopic dermatitis. *Arch Ophthal* 1950; **43**: 759–68.

Cross HE, Jensen AD. Ocular manifestations in the Marfan syndrome and homocystinuria. *Am J Ophthalmol* 1973; **75**: 405–20.

Crouch ER Jr, Parks MM. Management of posterior lenticonus complicated by unilateral cataract. *Am J Ophthalmol* 1978; **85**: 503–8.

Crouch ER Jr, Pressman SH, Crouch ER. Posterior chamber intraocular lenses: long-term results in pediatric cataract patients. *J Pediatr Ophthalmol Strabismus* 1995; **32**: 210–18.

Cruysberg JRM, Sengers RCA, Pinckers A, Kubat K, van Haelst UJGM. Features of a syndrome with congenital cataract and hypertrophic cardiomyopathy. *Am J Ophthalmol* 1986; **102**: 740–9.

Cruysberg JRM, Wevers RA, van Engelen BGM, Pinckers A, van Spreaken A, Tolboom JJM. Ocular and systemic manifestations of cerebrotendinous xanthomatosis. *Am J Ophthalmol* 1995; **120**: 597–604.

Cunha R, Moreira JB. Ocular findings in Down's syndrome. *Am J Ophthalmol* 1996; **122**: 236–44.

Czeizel A, Lowry RB. Syndrome of cataract, mild microcephaly, mental retardation and Perthes-like changes in sibs. *Acta Paediatr Hung* 1990; **30**: 343–9.

Dahan E, Salmenson BD. Pseudophakia in children: precautions, technique, and feasibility. *J Cataract Refract Surg* 1990; **16**: 75–82.

Dahan E, Salmenson BD, Levin J. Ciliary sulcus reconstruction for posterior implantation in the absence of an intact posterior capsule. *Ophthalmic Surg* 1989; **20**: 776–80.

de Jong PTVM, Bleeker-Wagemakers EM, Vrensen GFJM, Broekhuyse RM, Peereboom-Wynia JDR, Delleman JW. Crystalline cataract and uncombable hair. Ultrastructural and biochemical findings. *Ophthalmology* 1990; **97**: 1181–7.

Delleman JW, Bleeker-Wagemakers EM, Van Veelen AW. Opacities of the lens indicating carrier status of the oculocerebrorenal syndrome. *J Pediatr Ophthalmol Strabismus* 1977; **14**: 205–7.

Dietz HC, Francke U, Furthmayr H *et al*. The question of heterogeneity in Marfan syndrome. *Nature Genet* 1995; **9**: 228–31.

Dietz HC, Pyeritz RE, Hall BD *et al*. The Marfan syndrome locus: confirmation of assignment to chromosome 15 and identification of tightly linked markers at 15q15–q21.3. *Genomics* 1991; **9**: 355–61.

Drummond GT, Scott WE, Keech RV. Management of monocular congenital cataracts. *Arch Ophthalmol* 1989; **107**: 1113–14.

Dunn JP, Jabs DA, Wingard J, Enger C, Vogelsang G, Santos G. Bone marrow transplantation and cataract development. *Arch Ophthalmol* 1993; **111**: 1367–73.

Egbert JE, Kushner BJ. Excessive loss of hyperopia. A presenting sign of juvenile aphakic glaucoma. *Arch Ophthalmol* 1990; **108**: 1257–9.

Elkington ARL, Freedman SS, Jay B *et al*. Anterior dislocation of the lens in homocystinuria. *Br J Ophthalmol* 1973; **57**: 325–9.

Ellis F. Intraocular lenses in children. *J Pediatr Ophthalmol Strabismus* 1992; **29**: 71–2.

Elsas FJ. Visual acuity in monocular pediatric aphakia: does epikeratophakia facilitate occlusion therapy in children intolerant of contact lens or spectacle wear? *J Pediatr Ophthalmol Strabismus* 1990; **27**: 304–9.

Elsas LJ, Dembure PP, Langley S *et al.* A common mutation associated with the Duarte galactosemia allele. *Am J Hum Genet* 1994a; **54**: 1030–6.

Elsas LJ, Langley S, Steele E. Galactosemia: a strategy to identify new biochemical phenotypes and molecular genotypes. *Am J Hum Genet* 1995; **56**: 630–9.

Epstein RJ, Fernandes A, Gammon JA. The correction of aphakia in infants with hydrogel extended-wear contact lenses. Corneal studies. *Ophthalmology* 1988; **95**: 1102–6.

Evans AK, Hickey-Dwyer MU. Cleft anterior segment with maternal hypervitaminosis. *Br J Ophthalmol* 1991; **75**: 691–2.

Falls HF, Cotterman CW. Genetic studies on ectopic lentis. *Arch Ophthalmol* 1943; **30**: 610–20.

Falls HF, Schull WJ. Hallermann–Streiff syndrome. A dyscephaly with congenital cataracts and hypotrichosis. *Arch Ophthalmol* 1960; **63**: 409–20.

Farrell JW, Morgan KS, Black S. Lensectomy in an infant with cri du chat syndrome and cataracts. *J Pediatr Ophthalmol Strabismus* 1988; **25**: 131–4.

Flinter FA, Cameron J, Chantler C, Houston I, Bobrow M. Genetics of classic Alport's syndrome. *Lancet* 1988; **ii**: 1005–7.

Folz SJ, Trobe JD. The peroxisome and the eye. *Surv Ophthalmol* 1991; **35**: 353–68.

Forman AR, Loreto JA, Tina LU. Reversibility of corticosteroid associated cataracts in children with the nephrotic syndrome. *Am J Ophthalmol* 1977; **84**: 75–8.

Forsius H, Arentz-Grastvedt B, Eriksson AW. Juvenile cataract with autosomal recessive inheritance. A study from the Aland Islands, Finland. *Acta Ophthalmol* 1992; **70**: 26–32.

Foster CS, Barrett F. Cataract development and cataract surgery in patients with juvenile rheumatoid arthritis–associated iridocyclitis. *Ophthalmology* 1993; **100**: 809–17.

France TD, Frank JW. The association of strabismus and aphakia in children. *J Pediatr Ophthalmol Strabismus* 1984; **21**: 223–6.

Francke U, Furthmayr H. Marfan's syndrome and other disorders of fibrillin. *N Engl J Med* 1994; **330**: 1384–5.

Gelbart SS, Hoyt CS, Jastrebski G *et al.* Long-term visual results in bilateral congenital cataracts. *Am J Ophthalmol* 1982; **93**: 615–21.

Gershoni-Baruch R, Ludatscher RM, Lichtig C *et al.* Cerebro-oculo-facio skeletal syndrome: further delineation. *Am J Med Genet* 1991; **41**: 74–7.

Gibbs ML, Jacobs M, Wilkie AOM, Taylor D. Posterior lenticonus: clinical patterns and genetics. *J Pediatr Ophthalmol Strabismus* 1993; **30**: 171–5.

Gimbel HV, Ferensowicz M, Raanan M, de Lucca NI. Implantation in children. *J Pediatr Ophthalmol Strabismus* 1993; **30**: 69–79.

Ginsberg J, Bove KE, Fogelson MH. Pathological features of the eye in the oculocerebrorenal (Lowe) syndrome. *J Pediatr Ophthalmol Strabismus* 1981; **8**: 16–24.

Girard LJ, Canizales R, Esnaola N, Rand WJ. Subluxated (ectopic) lenses in adults: long term results of pars plana lensectomy vitrectomy by ultrasonic fragmentation with and without a phacoprosthesis. *Ophthalmology* 1990; **97**: 462–6.

Gold DH, Weingeist TA, eds. *The Eye in Systemic Disease.* Philadelphia: JB Lippincott, 1990.

Goldberg MF. Clinical manifestations of ectopia lentis et pupillae in 16 patients. *Ophthalmology* 1988; **95**: 1080–7.

Good WV, Hing S, Irvine AR, Hoyt CS, Taylor DSI. Postoperative endophthalmitis in children following cataract surgery. *J Pediatr Ophthalmol Strabismus* 1990; **27**: 283–5.

Gordon RA, Donzis PB. Refractive development of the human eye. *Arch Ophthalmol* 1985; **103**: 785–9.

Grainger RM, Henry JJ, Saha MS, Servetnick M. Recent progress on the mechanisms of embryonic lens formation. *Eye* 1992; **6**: 117–22.

Green JS, Parfrey PS, Harnett JD *et al.* The Laurence–Moon–Biedl syndrome. *N Engl J Med* 1989; **321**: 1002–9.

Gregg FM, Parks MM. Stereopsis after congenital monocular cataract extraction. *Am J Ophthalmol* 1992; **114**: 314–17.

Guo S, Nelson LB, Calhoun J *et al.* Simultaneous surgery for bilateral congenital cataracts. *J Pediatr Ophthalmol Strabismus* 1990; **27**: 23–5.

Gupta AK, Grover AK, Gurha N. Traumatic cataract surgery with intraocular lens implantation in children. *J Pediatr Ophthalmol Strabismus* 1992; **29**: 73–8.

Haddad R, Font RL, Reeser F. Persistent hyperplastic primary vitreous. A clinicopathologic study of 62 cases and review of the literature. *Surv Ophthalmol* 1978; **23**: 123–34.

Hakin KN, Jacobs M, Rosen P, Taylor D, Cooling R. Management of the subluxed crystalline lens. *Ophthalmology* 1992; **99**: 542–5.

Hall J. CATCH 22 (editorial). *J Med Genet* 1993; **30**: 801–2.

Happle R, Kuchle HJ. Sectorial cataract: a possible example of lyonisation. *Lancet* 1983; **ii**: 919–20.

Hemady RK, Blum S, Sylvia BM. Duplication of the lens, hour-glass cornea, and cornea plana. *Arch Ophthalmol* 1993; **111**: 303.

Henk JM, Whitelocke RAF, Warrington AP *et al.* Radiation dose to the lens and cataract formation. *Int J Radiat Oncol Biol Phys* 1993; **25**: 815–20.

Henkind P, Ashton N. Ocular pathology in homocystinuria. *Trans Ophthalmol Soc UK* 1965; **85**: 21–38.

Hennekan RCM, van de Meeberg AG, van Doorne JM *et al.* Martsolf syndrome in a brother and sister: clinical features and pattern of inheritance. *Eur J Pediatr* 1988; **147**: 539–43.

Hiles DA, Atkinson CS. Intraocular lens for correction of aphakia in children. In: Cotlier E, Lambert S, Taylor D, eds. *Congenital Cataracts.* Austin, Texas: RG Landes, 1994: 165–9.

Hing S, Speedwell L, Taylor D. Lens surgery in infancy and childhood. *Br J Ophthalmol* 1990; **74**: 73–7.

Holmstrom G, Speedwell L, Taylor D. Contact lenses—still the only solution for infant aphakia. *Eur J Implant Ref Surg* 1990; **2**: 265–7.

Howard C, Smith A, Warman R. Macular hypoplasia in familial cataracts. *J Pediatr Ophthalmol Strabismus* 1993; **30**: 176–7.

Hutchinson AK, Drews-Botsch C, Lambert SR. Myopic shift following intraocular lens implantation during childhood. *Ophthalmology* (in press).

Insler MS. Cerebro–oculo–facio–skeletal syndrome. *Ann Ophthalmol* 1987; **19**: 54–5.

Izquierdo N, Traboulsi E, Enger C, Maumenee I. Strabismus in the Marfan syndrome. *Am J Ophthalmol* 1994; **117**: 632–5.

Jaafar MS, Robb RM. Congenital anterior polar cataract: a review of 63 cases. *Ophthalmology* 1984; **91**: 249–54.

Jacobs M, Jeffrey B, Kriss A, Taylor D, Sa G, Barratt M. Ophthalmologic assessment of young patients with Alport syndrome. *Ophthalmology* 1992; **99**: 1039–44.

Jagger JD, Cooling RJ, Fison LG *et al.* Management of retinal detachment following congenital cataract surgery. *Trans Ophthalmol Soc UK* 1983; **103**: 103–7.

Jarrett WH. Dislocation of the lens. A study of 166 hospitalized cases. *Arch Ophthalmol* 1967; **78**: 289–96.

Jeffrey BG, Jacobs M, Sa G, Barratt TM, Taylor D, Kriss A. An electrophysiological study in children and young adults with Alport's syndrome. *Br J Ophthalmol* 1994; **78**: 44–8.

Jensen AD, Cross HE, Paton D. Ocular complications in the Weill–Marchesani syndrome. *Am J Ophthalmol* 1974; **77**: 261–9.

Johnson DA, Parks MM. Cataracts in childhood: prognosis and complications. *Semin Ophthalmol* 1991; **6**: 201–11.

Johnson SS, Nevin NC. Ocular manifestations in patients and female relatives of families with the oculocerebrorenal syndrome of Lowe. *Birth Defects* 1976; **12**: 567–77.

Jones KL. *Smith's Recognizable Patterns of Human Malformation*, 4th edn. Philadelphia: WB Saunders, 1988.

Kainulainen K, Karttunen L, Puhakka L *et al*. Mutations in the fibrillin gene responsible for dominant ectopia lentis and neonatal Marfan syndrome. *Nature Genet* 1994; **6**: 64–9.

Kainulainen K, Pulkkinen L, Savolainen A *et al*. Location on chromosome 15 of the gene defect causing Marfan syndrome. *N Engl J Med* 1990; **323**: 935–9.

Kanski JJ. Juvenile arthritis and uveitis. *Surv Ophthalmol* 1990; **34**: 253–67.

Kappelhof JP, Vrensen GFJM, de Jong PTVM *et al*. The ring of Soemmerring in man: an ultrastructural study. *Graefe's Arch Clin Exp Ophthalmol* 1987; **225**: 77–83.

Karr DJ, Scott WE. Visual acuity results following treatment of persistent hyperplastic primary vitreous. *Arch Ophthalmol* 1986; **104**: 662–7.

Kaye LD, Kalenak JW, Price RL, Cunningham R. Ocular implications of long-term prednisone therapy in children. *J Pediatr Ophthalmol Strabismus* 1993; **30**: 142–4.

Kazuhiko U, Kumiko N, Norio O. Haemorrhage in the lens: spontaneous occurrence in congenital cataract. *Br J Ophthalmol* 1986; **70**: 593–5.

Keech RV, Tongue AC, Scott WE. Complications after surgery for congenital and infantile cataracts. *Am J Ophthalmol* 1989; **108**: 136–41.

Kelley CG, Keates RH, Lembach RG. Epikeratophakia for pediatric aphakia. *Arch Ophthalmol* 1986; **104**: 680–2.

Kelly D, Goldberg R, Wilson D *et al*. Confirmation that the velocardiofacial syndrome is associated with haplo insufficiency of genes of chromosome 22q11. *Am J Med Genet* 1993; **45**: 305–12.

Key SN III, Kimura SJ. Iridocyclitis associated with juvenile rheumatoid arthritis. *Am J Ophthalmol* 1975; **80**: 425–9.

Kinoshita JH, Merola LO, Dikmak E. The accumulation of dulcitol and water in rabbit lens incubated with galactose. *Biochem Biophys Acta* 1962; **62**: 176–8.

Kitty LA, Hiles DA. Unilateral posterior lenticonus with persistent hyaloid artery remnant (letter). *Am J Ophthalmol* 1993; **116**: 104–6.

Kloepfer HW, Rosenthal JW. Possible genetic carriers in the spherophakia–brachymorphia syndrome. *Am J Hum Genet* 1975; **7**: 398–420.

Koenig SB, Ruttum MS, Lewandowski MF, Schutz R. Pseudophakia for traumatic cataracts in children. *Ophthalmology* 1993; **100**: 1218–24.

Kohn BA. The differential diagnosis of cataracts in infants and childhood. *Am J Dis Child* 1976; **130**: 184–92.

Kushner BJ. Visual results after surgery for monocular juvenile cataracts of undetermined onset. *Am J Ophthalmol* 1986; **102**: 468–72.

Lambert SR, Drack AV. Infantile cataracts. *Surv Ophthalmol* 1996; **40**: 427–58.

Lambert SR, Amaya L, Taylor D. Treatment of infantile cataracts. *Int Ophthalmol Clin* 1989a; **29**: 51–6.

Lambert SR, Fernandes A, Drews-Botsch C *et al*. Multifocal versus monofocal correction of neonatal monocular aphakia. *J Pediatr Ophthalmol Strabismus* 1994; **31**: 195–201.

Lambert SR, Fernandes A, Drews-Botsch C, Tigges M. Pseudophakia retards axial elongation in neonatal monkey eyes. *Invest Ophthalmol Vis Sci* 1996; **37**: 451–8.

Lambert SR, Fernandes A, Grossniklaus H *et al*. Neonatal lensectomy and intraocular lens implantation: effects in Rhesus monkey. *Invest Ophthalmol Vis Sci* 1995; **36**: 300–10.

Lambert SR, Taylor D, Kriss A *et al*. Ocular manifestations of the congenital varicella syndrome. *Arch Ophthalmol* 1989b; **107**: 52–6.

Leslie ND, Immerman EB, Flach JE *et al*. The human galactose-1-phosphate uridyltransferase gene. *Genomics* 1992; **14**: 474–80.

Lessell S, Forbes AP. Eye signs in Turner's syndrome. *Arch Ophthalmol* 1966; **76**: 211–13.

Letson RD, Desnick RJ. Punctate lenticular opacities in type II mannosidosis. *Am J Ophthalmol* 1978; **85**: 218–24.

Levin AV, Edmonds SA, Nelson LB *et al*. Extended-wear contact lenses for the treatment of pediatric aphakia. *Ophthalmology* 1988; **95**: 1107–13.

Lewis RA, Nussbaum RL, Stambolian D. Mapping X-linked ophthalmic diseases: provisional assignment of the locus for X-linked congenital cataracts and microcornea (the Nance–Horan syndrome) to Xp22.2–p22.3. *Ophthalmology* 1992b; **97**: 110–20.

Lewis TL, Maurer D, Tytla ME *et al*. Vision in the 'good' eye of children treated for unilateral congenital cataract. *Ophthalmology* 1992a; **99**: 1013–17.

Lloyd IC, Dowler J, Kriss A, Russell-Eggitt IM, Taylor D. Preferential looking and the management of congenital cataract: new occlusion protocols. In: Cotlier E, Lambert S, Taylor D, eds. *Congenital Cataracts*. Austin, Texas: RG Landes, 1994: 93–102.

Lloyd IC, Dowler JGF, Kriss A *et al*. Modulation of amblyopia therapy following early surgery for unilateral congenital cataracts. *Br J Ophthalmol* 1995; **79**: 802–6.

Lloyd IC, Goss-Sampson M, Jeffrey BG *et al*. Neonatal cataract: aetiology, pathogenesis and management. *Eye* 1992; **6**: 184–96.

Lloyd IC, Kriss A, Speedwell L, Thompson DA, Russell-Eggitt I, Taylor D. Modulation of amblyopia therapy following early surgery for unilateral congenital cataracts. *Br J Ophthalmol* 1995; **79**: 802–6.

Lorenz B, Worle J, Friedl N, Boergen K-P. Monocular and binocular functional results in cases of contact lens corrected infant aphakia. In: Cotlier E, Lambert S, Taylor D, eds. *Congenital Cataracts*. Austin, Texas: RG Landes, 1994: 151–63.

Lueder GT, Steiner RD. Ophthalmic abnormalities in molybdenum cofactor deficiency and isolated sulfite oxidase deficiency. *J Pediatr Ophthalmol Strabismus* 1995; **32**: 334–7.

Lundberg PO. Hereditary myopathy, oligophrenia, cataract, skeletal abnormalities and hypergonadotrophic hypogonadism: a new syndrome. *Acta Genet Med Gemel* 1974; **23**: 245–7.

Lyford JH, Roy FH. Arhinencephaly unilateralis, uveal coloboma, and lens reduplication. *Am J Ophthalmol* 1974; **77**: 315–18.

McCormick AQ. Transient cataracts in premature infants: a new clinical entity. *Canad J Ophthalmol* 1968; **3**: 302–8.

McGavic JS. 41st Meeting of the New England Ophthalmological Society: 19 February 1958: Marchesani's syndrome. *Am J Ophthalmol* 1959; **47**: 413–14.

McLeod D. Congenital cataract surgery: a retinal surgeon's viewpoint. *Aust NZ J Ophthalmol* 1986; **14**: 79–84.

MacRae DW, Howard RO, Albert DM, Hsia YE. Ocular manifestations of the Meckel syndrome. *Arch Ophthalmol* 1972; **88**: 106–13.

Mann I. *The Development of the Human Eye*. Cambridge: Cambridge University Press, 1928.

Mann I. *Developmental Abnormalities of the Eye*. London: British Medical Association, 1957.

Markham RHC, Bloom PA, Chandra A *et al*. Results of intraocular lens implantation in paediatric aphakia. *Eye* 1992; **6**: 493–8.

Maumenee AE, Ryan SJ. Aspiration technique in the management of the dislocated lens. *Am J Ophthalmol* 1969; **68**: 808–11.

Maumenee I. The Marfan syndrome is caused by a point mutation in the fibrillin gene. *Arch Ophthalmol* 1992; **110**: 472–3.

Maumenee IH. The eye in Marfan syndrome. *Trans Am Ophthalmol Soc* 1981; **79**: 684–733.

Merin S, Crawford JS. Etiology of congenital cataracts. A survey of 386 cases. *Canad J Ophthalmol* 1971a; **6**: 178–82.

Merin S, Crawford J. Hypoglycemia and infantile cataract. *Arch Ophthalmol* 1971b; **86**: 495–8.

Michalski A, Leonard JV, Taylor DSI. The eye and inherited metabolic disease: a review. *J Roy Soc Med* 1988; **81**: 286–90.

Mills M, Robb R. Glaucoma following childhood cataract surgery. *J Pediatr Ophthalmol Strabismus* 1994; **31**: 355–61.

Moore BD. Changes in the aphakic refraction of children with unilateral congenital cataracts. *J Pediatr Ophthalmol Strabismus* 1989; **26**: 290–5.

Moore BD. Pediatric aphakic contact lens wear: rates of successful wear. *J Pediatr Ophthalmol Strabismus* 1993; **30**: 253–8.

Morgan KS, Karcioglu ZA. Secondary cataracts in infants after lensectomies. *J Pediatr Ophthalmol Strabismus* 1987; **24**: 45–8.

Morgan KS, McDonald MB, Hiles DA *et al.* The nationwide study of epikeratophakia for aphakia in older children. *Ophthalmology* 1988; **95**: 526–32.

Morgan KS, Somers M. Update on epikeratophakia in children. *Int Ophthalmol Clin* 1989; **29**: 37–47.

Moross T, Vaithilingam SS, Styles S, Garnder HA. Autosomal dominant anterior polar cataracts associated with a familial 2;14 translocation. *J Med Genet* 1984; **21**: 52–3.

Mudd SH, Skovby F, Levy HL *et al.* The natural history of homocystinuria due to cystathionine Ii synthetase deficiency. *Am J Hum Genet* 1985; **37**: 1–31.

Mullaney J. Ocular pathology in trisomy 18 (Edwards' syndrome). *Am J Ophthalmol* 1973; **76**: 246–54.

Nahmias AJ, Visintine AM, Caldwell DR, Wilson LA. Eye infections with herpes simplex viruses in neonates. *Surv Ophthalmol* 1976; **21**: 100–5.

Nelle M, Troger J, Rupprath G, Bettendorf M. Metacarpal index in Marfan's syndrome and in constitutional tall stature. *Arch Dis Child* 1994; **70**: 149–50.

Nelson LB, Cutler SI, Calhoun JH *et al.* Silsoft extended wear contact lenses in pediatric aphakia. *Ophthalmology* 1985; **92**: 1529–31.

Nelson LB, Spaeth GL, Nowinski TS, Margo CE, Jackson L. Aniridia. A review. *Surv Ophthalmol* 1984; **28**: 621–42.

Neumann D, Weissman BA, Isenberg SJ, Rosenbaum A, Bateman JB. The effectiveness of daily wear contact lenses for the correction of infantile aphakia. *Arch Ophthalmol* 1993; **111**: 927–30.

Newell SW, Hall BD, Anderson CW, Lim ES. Hallermann–Streiff syndrome with Coats disease. *J Pediatr Ophthalmol Strabismus* 1994; **31**: 123–5.

Nuyts RMMA, Edelhauser HF, Pels E *et al.* Toxic effects of detergent on the corneal endothelium. *Arch Ophthalmol* 1990; **108**: 1158–62.

O'Dell CD, Gammon JA, Fernandes A *et al.* Development of acuity in a primate model of human infantile unilateral aphakia. *Invest Ophthalmol Vis Sci* 1989; **30**: 2068–74.

Parks MM. Visual results in aphakic children. *Am J Ophthalmol* 1982; **94**: 441–9.

Parks MM, Johnson D, Reed G. Long-term visual results and complications in children with aphakia: a function of cataract type. *Ophthalmol* 1993; **100**: 826–41.

Pearce WG. Ocular and genetic features of Cockayne's syndrome. *Canad J Ophthalmol* 1972; **7**: 435–44.

Perry TL, Hansen S, Love DL *et al.* Treatment of homocystinuria with a low methionine diet, supplemental cystine and methyl donor. *Lancet* 1968; **2**: 474–8.

Petrohelos MA. Werner's syndrome. *Am J Ophthalmol* 1963; **56**: 941.

Peyman GA, Raichand M, Goldberg MF *et al.* Management of subluxated and dislocated lenses with the vitrophage. *Br J Ophthalmol* 1979; **63**: 771–8.

Pfeiffer RA. Familial congenital cataract, non-progressive neurological disorders and mental deficiency: a new X-linked syndrome. *Ophthalmol Paediatr Genet* 1985; **5**: 201–3.

Phelps-Brown N. The morphology of cataract and visual performance. *Eye* 1993; **7**: 63–7.

Plager DA, Parks MM, Helveston EM, Ellis F. Surgical treatment of subluxated lenses in children. *Ophthalmology* 1992; **99**: 1018–23.

Poer DV, Helveston EM, Ellis FD. Aphakic cystoid macular edema in children. *Arch Ophthalmol* 1981; **99**: 249–52.

Pollitt RJ, Vamos E. Trichothiodystrophy, mental retardation, short stature, ataxia and gonadal dysfunction in three Moroccan siblings. *Am J Med Genet* 1990; **35**: 566–73.

Pratt-Johnson JA, Tillson G. Hard contact lenses in the management of congenital cataracts. *J Pediatr Ophthalmol Strabismus* 1985; **22**: 94–6.

Pratt-Johnson JA, Tillson G. Intractable diplopia after vision restoration in unilateral cataract. *Am J Ophthalmol* 1989; **107**: 23–6.

Price FW, Binder PS. Scarring of a recipient cornea following epikeratoplasty. *Arch Ophthalmol* 1987; **105**: 1556–60.

Pyeritz RE, McKusick VA. The Marfan syndrome: Diagnosis and management. *N Engl J Med* 1979; **300**: 772–7.

Ramsey MS, Dickson DH. Lens fringe in homocystinuria. *Br J Ophthalmol* 1975; **59**: 338–42.

Reese AB. Persistent hyperplastic primary vitreous: the Jackson Memorial Lecture. *Am J Ophthalmol* 1955; **40**: 317–31.

Reese PD, Tuck-Muller CM, Maumenee IH. Autosomal dominant congenital cataract associated with chromosomal translocation [t(3;4)(p26.2;p15)]. *Arch Ophthalmol* 1987; **105**: 1382–4.

Reese PD, Weingeist TA. Pars plana management of ectopia lentis in children. *Arch Ophthalmol* 1987; **105**: 1202–4.

Robb RM, Mayer DL, Moore BD. Results of early treatment of unilateral congenital cataracts. *J Pediatr Ophthalmol Strabismus* 1987; **24**: 178–81.

Rogers GL, Tishler CL, Tsou BH *et al.* Visual acuities in infants with congenital cataracts operated on prior to 6 months of age. *Arch Ophthalmol* 1981; **99**: 999–1003.

Rostron CK. Epikeratophakia: clinical results and experimental development. *Eye* 1988; **2**: 56–62.

Roy FH, Summitt RL, Hiatt RL, Hughes JG. Ocular manifestations of the Rubinstein–Taybi syndrome. *Arch Ophthalmol* 1968; **79**: 272–8.

Salehpour O, Lavy T, Leonard J, Taylor D. The surgical management of nontraumatic ectopic lenses. *J Pediatr Ophthalmol Strabismus* 1996; **33**: 8–13.

Saunders RA, Ellis FD. Empirical fitting of hard contact lenses in infants and young children. *Ophthalmology* 1981; **88**: 127–30.

Scheie HG. Aspiration of congenital or soft cataracts: a new technique. *Am J Ophthalmol* 1960; **50**: 1048–56.

Schein OD, Glynn RJ, Poggio EC *et al.* The relative risk of ulcerative keratitis among users of daily-wear and extended-wear soft contact lenses. A case–control study. *N Engl J Med* 1989; **321**: 773–8.

Schwartz O, Jampel RS. Congenital blepharophimosis associated with a unique generalised myopathy. *Arch Ophthalmol* 1962; **68**: 52–7.

Scott JG, Friedmann AI, Chitters M, Peplar WJ. Ocular changes in the Bloch–Sulzberger syndrome (incontinentia pigmenti). *Br J Ophthalmol* 1955; **39**: 276–92.

Scott MH, Hejtmancik JF, Wozencraft LA *et al.* Autosomal dominant congenital cataract. Intraocular phenotypic variability. *Ophthalmology* 1994; **101**: 866–71.

Seery CM, Pruett RC, Liberfarb RM, Cohen BZ. Distinctive cataract in the Stickler syndrome. *Am J Ophthalmol* 1990; **110**: 1430–49.

Seetner AA, Crawford JS. Surgical correction of lens dislocation in children. *Am J Ophthalmol* 1981; **91**: 106–10.

Seland JH. The lenticular attachment of the zonular apparatus in congenital simple ectopia lentis. *Acta Ophthalmol* 1973; **51**: 520–8.

Shawaf S, Noureddin B, Khouni A, Traboulsi E. A family with a syndrome of ectopia lentis, spontaneous filtering blebs and craniofacial dysmorphism. *Ophthal Genet* 1995; **16**: 163–9.

Shih VE, Abroms IF, Johnson JL *et al*. Sulfite oxidase deficiency. Biochemical and clinical investigations of a hereditary metabolic disorder in sulfur metabolism. *N Engl J Med* 1977; **297**: 1022–8.

Shih VE, Efron ML. Pyridoxine-unresponsive homocystinuria. Final diagnosis of MGH Case 19 471, 1933. *N Engl J Med* 1970; **283**: 1206–8.

Simon JW, Mehta N, Simmons ST, Catalano R, Lininger L. Glaucoma after pediatric lensectomy vitrectomy. *Ophthalmology* 1991; **98**: 670–4.

Smith G, Shun-Shin AG, Bron A. Spontaneous reabsorption of a rubella cataract. *Br J Ophthalmol* 1990; **74**: 564–6.

Smolin LA, Benerenga NJ, Berlow S. The use of betaine for the treatment of homocystinuria. *J Pediatr* 1981; **99**: 467–72.

Soriano JM, Funk J. Bilateral spontaneous reabsorption of the lens—a case of Hallermann–Streiff syndrome. *Klin Mbl Augenheilkd* 1991; **199**: 195–8.

Speedwell L, Russell-Eggitt I. Improvement in visual acuity in children with ectopia lentis. *J Pediatr Ophthalmol Strabismus* 1995; **32**: 94–7.

Spielmann A. The fate of the 'sound' eye in unilateral congenital cataract. *Eur J Implant Ref Surg* 1990; **2**: 245–8.

Stagno S, Reynolds DW, Amos CS *et al*. Auditory and visual defects resulting from symptomatic and subclinical congenital cytomegaloviral and *Toxoplasma* infections. *Pediatrics* 1977; **59**: 669–78.

Stambolian D. Galactose and cataract. *Surv Ophthalmol* 1988; **32**: 33–49.

Stambolian D, Ai Y, Sikjanin D *et al*. Identification in two families with galactokinase deficiency and cataracts. *Nature Genet* 1995; **10**: 307–12.

Streeten BW, Robinson MR, Wallace R *et al*. Lens capsule abnormalities in Alport's syndrome. *Arch Ophthalmol* 1987; **105**: 1693–7.

Summers C, Letson R. Is the phakic eye normal in monocular pediatric aphakia? *J Pediatr Ophthalmol Strabismus* 1992; **29**: 324–7.

Synnove C, Hyvarinen L, Avitti R. Persistent behavioural blindness after early visual deprivation and active visual rehabilitation: a case report. *Br J Ophthalmol* 1986; **70**: 607–11.

Taylor D. Choice of surgical technique in management of congenital cataracts. *Trans Ophthalmol Soc UK* 1981; **101**: 114–17.

Taylor D, Vaegan, Morris JA *et al*. Amblyopia in bilateral infantile and juvenile cataract: relationship to timing of treatment. *Trans Ophthalmol Soc UK* 1979; **99**: 170–5.

Tchah H, Larson RS, Nichols BD *et al*. Neodymium: YAG laser zonulysis for treatment of lens subluxation. *Ophthalmology* 1989; **96**: 230–5.

Temtamy SA, Sinbawy AHH. Cataract, hypertrichosis, and mental retardation (CAHMR): a new autosomal recessive syndrome. *Am J Med Genet* 1991; **41**: 432–3.

Thompson SM, Deady JP, Willshaw HE *et al*. Ocular signs in Alport's syndrome. *Eye* 1987; **1**: 146–53.

Tigges M, Tigges J, Fernandes A *et al*. Postnatal axial eye elongation in normal and visually deprived rhesus monkeys. *Invest Ophthalmol Vis Sci* 1990; **31**: 1035–46.

Townes PL. Ectopia lentis et pupillae. *Arch Ophthalmol* 1976; **94**: 1126–8.

Toyofuku H, Hirose T, Schepens CL. Retinal detachment following congenital cataract surgery I. Preoperative findings in 114 eyes. *Arch Ophthalmol* 1980; **98**: 669–75.

Traboulsi EI, Lenz W, Gonzales-Ramos M, Siegel J, Macrae WG, Maumenee IH. The Lenz microphthalmia syndrome. *Am J Ophthalmol* 1988; **105**: 40–5.

Traboulsi EI, Weinberg RJ. Familial congenital cornea guttata with anterior polar cataracts. *Am J Ophthalmol* 1989; **108**: 123–5.

Tripathi RC, Cibis GW, Tripathi BJ. Pathogenesis of cataracts in patients with Lowe's syndrome. *Ophthalmology* 1986; **93**: 1046–51.

Tsipouras P, Devereux RB. Marfan syndrome: genetic basis and clinical manifestations. *Semin Dermatol* 1993; **12**: 219–28.

Tytla ME, Lewis TL, Maurer D *et al*. Stereopsis after congenital cataract. *Invest Ophthalmol Vis Sci* 1993; **34**: 1767–73.

Vaegen, Taylor D. Critical period for deprivation amblyopia in children. *Trans Ophthalmol Soc UK* 1979; **99**: 432–9.

Van Dorp D, Delleman JW. A family with X chromosome recessive congenital cataract, microphthalmia, a peculiar form of the ear and dental anomalies. *J Pediatr Ophthalmol Strabismus* 1979; **16**: 166–71.

Vila-Coro A, Mazou ML. Initiation of amblyopia treatment in monocular congenital cataracts (letter). *Arch Ophthalmol* 1989; **107**: 1113.

Vivian AJ, Lloyd IC, Russell-Eggitt I, Taylor D. Familial posterior lenticonus. *Eye* 1995; **9**: 119–23.

Wahl JW, Ellis PP. Rothmund–Thomson syndrome. *Am J Ophthalmol* 1965; **60**: 722–6.

Wheatley H, Traboulsi E, Flowers B *et al*. Immunohistochemical localization of fibrillin in human ocular tissues: relevance to the Marfan syndrome. *Arch Ophthalmol* 1995: **113**: 103–9.

Wheeler DT, Stager DR, Weakley Jr DR. Endophthalmitis following pediatric intraocular surgery for congenital cataracts and congenital glaucoma. *J Pediatr Ophthalmol Strabismus* 1992; **29**: 139–41.

Willi M, Kut L, Cotlier E. Pupillary-block glaucoma in the Marchesani syndrome. *Arch Ophthalmol* 1973; **90**: 504–8.

Wilson DI, Burn J, Scambler P, Goodship J. Syndrome of the month. Di George syndrome part of CATCH 22. *J Med Genet* 1993; **30**: 852–6.

Wilson JR, Fernandes A, Chandler CV *et al*. Abnormal development of the axial length of aphakic monkey eyes. *Int Ophthalmol Vis Sci* 1987; **28**: 2096–9.

Winter RM, Donnai D, Crawfurd MD'A. syndromes of microcephaly, microphthalmos, cataracts and joint contractures. *J Med Genet* 1981; **18**: 129–33.

Wright KW, Christensen LE, Noguchi BA. Results of late surgery for presumed congenital cataracts. *Am J Ophthalmol* 1992; **114**: 409–15.

Zeiter JH. Congenital microphthalmos: a pedigree of four affected siblings and an additional report of 44 sporadic cases. *Am J Ophthalmol* 1963; **55**: 910–22.

Zimmer C, Gosztonyi G, Cervos-Navarro J *et al*. Neuropathy with lysosomal charges in Marinesco–Sjogren syndrome: fine structural findings in skeletal muscle and conjunctiva. *Neuropediatrics* 1992; **23**: 329–35.

40: Childhood Glaucoma

Isabelle Russell-Eggitt

Although rare, glaucoma is very important as it is one of the pre-eminently preventable causes of childhood visual handicap. Detection and management of some forms is one of the most challenging tasks that faces a paediatric ophthalmologist, not only from the nature of the condition itself but also its occurrence in frequently unco-operative and fractious children. The rarity of glaucoma in children makes the acquisition of management skills the privilege of only a few ophthalmologists, for it is a condition in which referral to one with practical expertise is preferable.

The clinical picture independent of aetiology

Photophobia/tearing

In most cases of glaucoma presenting in the first year of life, corneal opacification and enlargement will be accompanied by photophobia (Fig. 40.1). This may be very marked with the child being miserable and burying his or her head in a pillow. The eye is sometimes red with corneal haze and tearing. If unilateral, the parents often comment that the eye 'looks a different colour' as well as being larger (Fig. 40.2). Even when the intraocular pressure is controlled, the child often remains significantly photophobic and practical measures such as sunglasses and sunhats make a great difference to their comfort.

Enlargement of the globe

If intraocular pressure is raised in a child under 2 years of age the eye may enlarge in excess of the normal increase in volume (Bluth 1983). Pathological enlargement is unusual after this age and is not even invariable in infancy. Although the term buphthalmos has often been used synonymously with trabeculodysgenesis, enlargement of the globe may occur with other glaucomas in childhood, as well as in congenital megalocornea without glaucoma. Even children with enlarged eyes may present late if the enlargement is symmetrical as the corneas are not invariably cloudy—their large eyes may be their parents' pride and joy!

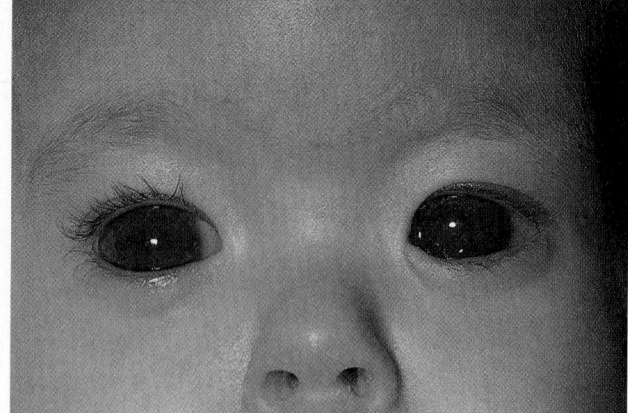

Fig. 40.1 Buphthalmos. The parents had noticed both eyes watering together with photophobia so marked that they did not take her outdoors even on a cloudy day.

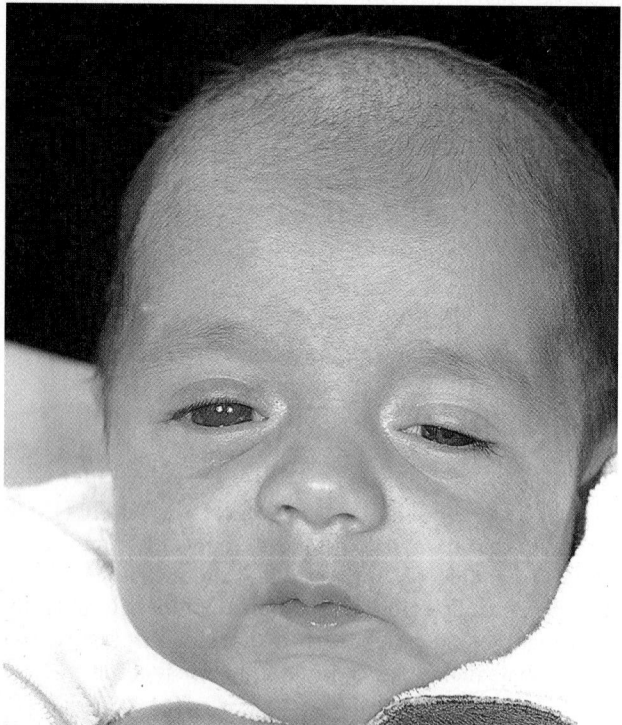

Fig. 40.2 Buphthalmos of the right eye. The parents had thought that the left eye was small.

Corneal changes

When the intraocular pressure is raised in young children the cornea usually becomes diffusely oedematous and enlarged (Fig. 40.3). When the corneal diameter increases, splits occur in Descemet's membrane and damage occurs to corneal endothelial cells (Morin & Coughlin 1980; Wenzel *et al.* 1989). Descemet's tears viewed by specular microscopy have parallel 'rail track' borders (Brooks *et al.* 1989). Endothelial cells lay down new basement mem-

brane in the region of the splits causing curvilinear areas of increased opacity, Haab's striae (Fig. 40.4), which persist even when the pressure is lowered (Waring *et al.* 1974). Corneal opacification may not always be secondary to

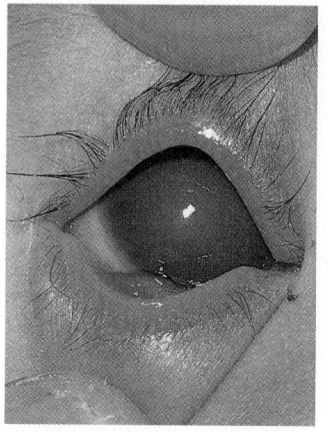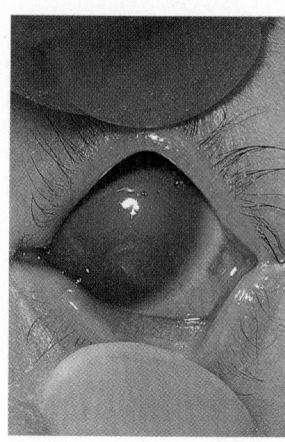

Fig. 40.3 Bilateral severe buphthalmos in a neonate with enlarged, 'steamy' corneas.

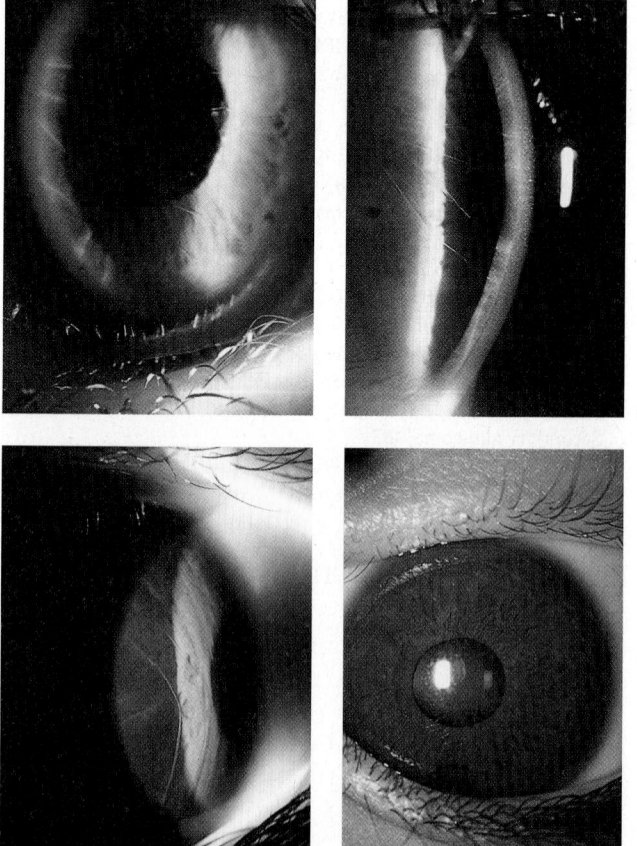

Fig. 40.4 (a) Splits in Descemet's membrane have corneal oedema at their edges for many months giving rise to linear opacities (Haab's striae) which are present even when the intraocular pressure is controlled. (b) Haab's striae.

intraocular pressure elevation in childhood. Other causes of opacification of the infant cornea include rubella embryopathy, congenital hereditary endothelial dystrophy and sclerocornea. Corneal clouding may persist for weeks after intraocular pressure control (Rice 1972). When the intraocular pressure is elevated during relapse of glaucoma the cornea is not invariably oedematous. Another useful sign may be bulging of the cornea which reverses on pressure control: this may be noticed by the parents even though it may be difficult for the ophthalmologist to see.

Optic disc cupping

Although the optic disc becomes progressively cupped (Fig. 40.5) with nerve damage, if the pressure is controlled

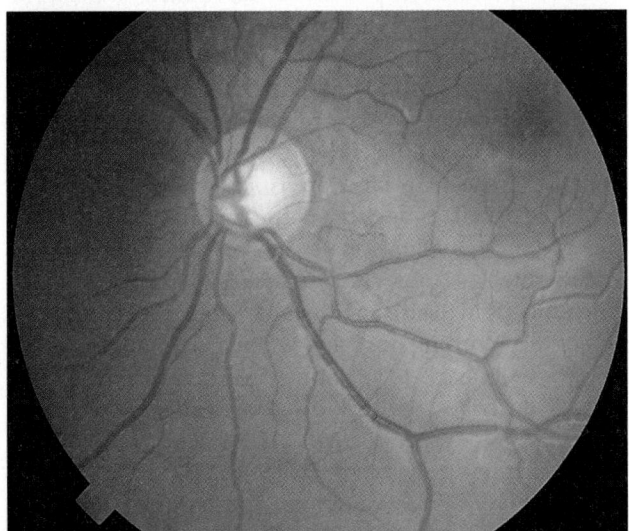

a

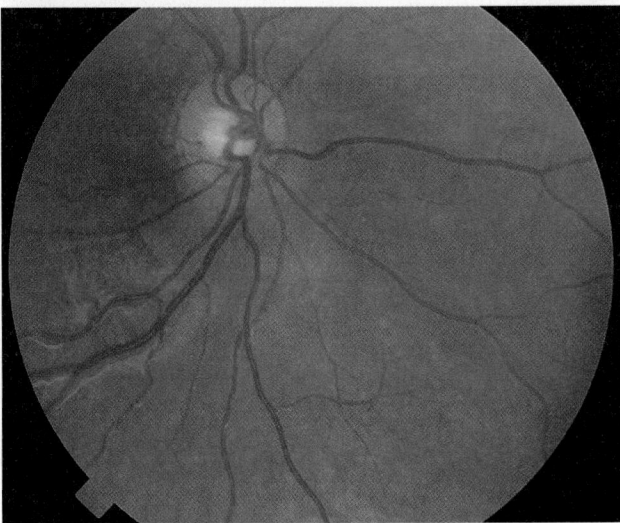

b

Fig. 40.5 (a) Cupped discs in congenital glaucoma, more marked in the left eye (a), treated successfully in infancy. Visual acuity was 6/6 in the right eye (b) but the left eye (a) had 6/12 acuity and suppression indicating that the left eye is amblyopic.

cupping may reverse in the child's eye (Iwata *et al.* 1977; Quigley 1982). The scleral canal is stretched, so there may be an increase in cupping with relative preservation of the neuroretinal rim. The normal range of optic disc cup to diameter varies with age, refractive error and racial group (Mansour 1992). Serial assessments of optic disc appearance are important in the management of glaucoma, particularly in children, when measurement of intraocular pressure may be difficult and testing of the visual field impossible.

Refractive changes and strabismus

Anisometropia and strabismus co-exist in many patients with congenital glaucoma and are important causes of ocular morbidity due to amblyopia (Rice 1972). Strabismus and amblyopia occur secondary to ametropia, anisometropia and corneal opacity. In older children, glaucoma may present with increasing myopia (Egbert & Kushner 1990). In aphakic young children, a myopic shift in refraction may be the first sign of glaucoma. Subluxation of the lens may occur with globe enlargement.

Classification

A primary glaucoma is a condition caused by an intrinsic disorder of the aqueous outflow mechanism. A secondary glaucoma is caused by disease processes in other regions of the eye and body (see Table 40.3). Both primary and secondary paediatric glaucoma disorders may be associated with important systemic conditions that need to be specifically identified.

Developmental glaucoma

Anatomical or genetic?

In the management of a childhood glaucoma, a useful classification is one based upon the mechanism of the obstruction to aqueous flow because the degree to which the angle structures are malformed affects the response to surgery. This chapter uses an anatomical classification based on that proposed by Hoskins *et al.* (1984a).

Awareness of the genetic condition is also important for the overall care of the patient and his or her family. Dissimilar expression of a gene may occur within a pedigree or even between the two eyes of one individual: for example, a variety of expression occurs with mutations in the PAX6 gene on chromosome 11 (Bateman *et al.* 1984). Mutation or deletion of a portion of this gene leads to bilateral aniridia. If the deletion is extensive the contiguous gene syndrome of Wilms' tumour susceptibility with aniridia may result. The PAX6 mutation may also cause a more complex anterior segment malformation with the cornea and lens involved: these individuals may also be at risk from renal tumours. Mutation of the PAX6 gene can also manifest as an iridotrabecular dysgenesis with the Rieger's or Peters' phenotype (see Chapter 23).

Anatomical–embryological classification

Genetics aside, the behaviour and management of the glaucoma usually depends on the clinical picture and the postulated mechanisms responsible for it (Hoskins *et al.* 1984b). Study of normal embryogenesis and of spontaneous, teratogen-induced and inherited conditions of abnormal development in humans and animals (Cook 1989) may help in the understanding and management of developmental glaucoma in infants. Much of the anterior segment of the eye, including the trabecular meshwork, is derived from neural crest tissue (Bahn *et al.* 1984; Lang & Fleischer-Peters 1989; Rodrigues & Font 1989; Tripathi & Tripathi 1989). Abnormalities associated with glaucoma may result from genetic or teratogenic interference with neural crest cell formation, migration and final differentiation (Bahn *et al.* 1984; Beauchamp & Knepper 1984). Anterior segment malformations are not always neurocristopathies, but they may be the result of just a 'knock on' effect.

Although the major developmental events leading to iridocorneal angle formation occur during the third trimester, it appears that embryonic insults during the first 3–5 weeks postfertilization can induce an abnormal sequence of events leading to anterior segment dysgenesis. For example, if the lens has not separated from the surface ectoderm completely there will be a mechanical block to neural crest tissue migration; as this would only interfere with neural crest locally there would be no associated abnormalities of other neural crest derived facial structures (see Peters' anomaly below).

Shields (1983) and Shields *et al.* (1985) propose that the Axenfeld/Rieger spectrum is due to developmental arrest with retention of primordial endothelial tissue on the iris and across the anterior chamber angle, with excessive basement membrane formation (the prominent Schwalbe's line). This endothelial tissue may contract progressively. Congenital iris ectropion may also occur by this mechanism (Wilson 1990). The maturation of the angle structures is arrested associated with this membrane, resulting in incomplete formation of the trabecular meshwork; the iris insertion remains high, with the pull of the ciliary muscle fibres tending to compress the trabecular spaces.

Histological examination by light and transmission electron microscopy of trabeculectomy specimens from eyes with congenital glaucoma have revealed a variety of abnormalities including: (i) a hypoplastic trabecular meshwork containing an abundance of abnormal collagenous tissue in the extracellular spaces; and (ii) the presence of endothelial cells overlying a continuous collagenous membrane of mesenchymal tissue in the angle (Linn 1992; Talbot *et al.* 1992; Linn *et al.* 1994). These findings provide histological support for the theory by Shields. Additional histological findings are: (i) shifting forward of ciliary muscle fibres (Linn 1992); and (ii) numerous abnormal blood vessels in the iris stroma, with a paucity of mural contractile cells (Talbot *et al.* 1992). Vascularity of the iris and 'membrane' incised at goniotomy are common clinical findings.

Trabeculodysgenesis (primary congenital glaucoma)

This is the most common form of glaucoma in children accounting for one in 10 000 births (Miller 1962), and is slightly more commonly bilateral than unilateral. The underlying disorder (Fig. 40.6) is present at birth, but the clinical signs and symptoms may be variable in their presentation (Morin *et al.* 1974).

The angle, on gonioscopic examination, may have the same appearance as in a full-term baby, even in an infant of several months: presumably the angle structures have failed to mature sufficiently to cope with aqueous flow. The iridotrabecular junction is abnormal yet the iris appears normal, as does the cornea apart from secondary changes such as splits. A pale amorphous tissue (Barkan's 'membrane') is apparent with vessels running radially extending from the iris to Schwalbe's line. Lister described this as the 'morning mist' and when incised at goniotomy this iris falls back to a normal position. Hoskins *et al.* (1984a) describes two iris insertion patterns associated with trabeculodysgenesis.

1 A flat iris insertion where the iris inserts into the trabecular meshwork either anterior or posterior to the scleral spur, the anterior stroma of the iris not appearing to extend into the angle.

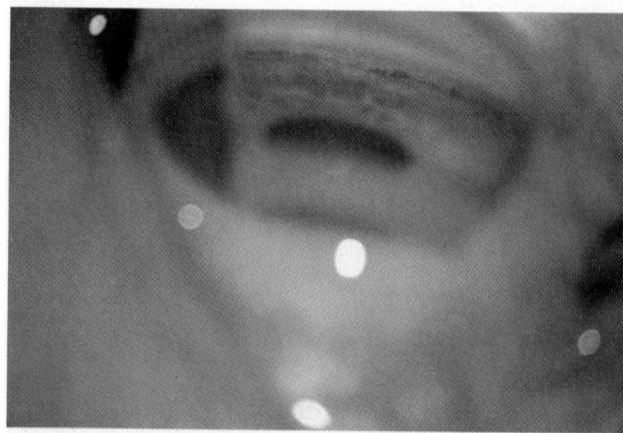

Fig. 40.6 Gonioscopy in primary congenital glaucoma. Schwalbe's line is barely visible anterior to the grey band of the iris insertion posterior to which pigment knuckles project anteriorly from the iris route through bands of fine tissue extending from the anterior surface of the iris—'Barkan's membrane'.

2 A concave iris insertion where the anterior stromal iris tissue appears to continue up over the trabecular meshwork and obscures both the ciliary body and the scleral spur.

Most cases of trabeculodysgenesis present between 3 and 6 months of age, a smaller number within a few days of birth. The latter eyes respond less well to goniotomy surgery and may have even more immature angle structures deep to the 'Barkan membrane' and even an absent or uncannulated canal of Schlemm. Glaucoma is more likely to relapse in these eyes than in those whose symptoms developed in the first few months of life or later. Catalano *et al.* (1989) showed that the eyes with the highest presenting intraocular pressures had a reduced chance of control following goniotomy. Eyes requiring multiple goniotomies in infancy are more likely to relapse than those controlled by a single procedure (Russell-Eggitt *et al.* 1992). Children presenting as late as 3 years of age usually respond well to goniotomy.

The periphery of the iris in primary congenital glaucoma frequently shows abnormalities. The stroma may be abnormally thin. In approximately 50% of cases, a forward tenting of the portion of the iris to which the uveal meshwork is attached is noted. Usually, neither the iris nor its blood vessels are attached far enough anteriorly to obscure the ciliary band or scleral spur. A number of different aberrations of angle development probably account for the development of primary congenital glaucoma. The severity and pathological mechanisms of this disorder depend in part on how early in embryogenesis the normal angle development is interrupted.

Genetics

Trabeculodysgenesis is more common in males than females in the ratio 5 : 2 (Russell-Eggitt *et al.* 1992). However, there is no evidence of X-linked inheritance. Interestingly the average normal corneal size at term is larger in females than in males, perhaps implying more advanced development. Trabeculodysgenesis may be hereditary (Moller 1977), usually autosomal recessive; the pattern of inheritance in the majority of cases is polygenic or multifactorial (Merin & Morin 1972; Jay & Rice 1978) at least in Europe and North America. In the Middle East the autosomal recessive nature is more clear and the disease appears, in consanguineous families, to be more difficult to control; it may be that the angle abnormality is more extensive. Intrauterine infection with the rubella virus may result in corneal haze which is usually transient, but more rarely there may be true developmental glaucoma with an angle indistinguishable from idiopathic trabeculodysgenesis (Weiss *et al.* 1966).

There are a few reports of typical trabeculodysgenesis being associated with an abnormal genotype. Verbraak (1992) reported congenital glaucoma in a child with partial duplication of chromosome 1 (1q41–qter) and partial deletion of chromosome 9 (9p24–pter). As this was the second report of a patient with monosomy 9p24–pter and congenital glaucoma, it was postulated that it may indicate localization of a gene involved in congenital glaucoma to this region. Nishimura *et al.* (1994) reported an individual with a 6:13 translocation and a second individual with an unbalanced translocation with a 6p deletion. Sarfarazi *et al.* (1995) assign a locus for primary congenital glaucoma to 2p21 and also give evidence of genetic heterogeneity.

Systemic associations

Most patients with trabeculodysgenesis do not have associated systemic abnormalities. Developmental glaucoma in many syndromes involves a more extensive anterior chamber abnormality with iris and/or corneal changes.

Iridotrabeculodysgenesis

This broad term includes: posterior embryotoxon, Axenfeld's anomaly, Rieger's anomaly and aniridia. These developmental abnormalities may be inherited as an autosomal dominant with considerable variation in expression in a single family. The glaucoma often does not begin until later in childhood, necessitating careful, periodic examinations, even if the intraocular pressure is initially normal.

Axenfeld–Rieger anomaly

The term posterior embryotoxon is used to describe an abnormal thickening of Schwalbe's line at the peripheral termination of Descemet's membrane. In some patients, this is an isolated abnormality without any functional implication, while in others there may be glaucoma (Waring *et al.* 1975).

Axenfeld's anomaly is a condition in which the filtration angle is largely obscured from view by attachments between the iris and a posterior embryotoxon; the trabeculum may be intermittently visible and may appear either normal or abnormal. Glaucoma is frequent.

In Rieger's anomaly (Fig. 40.7), similar abnormalities of the chamber angle are noted, but in addition hypoplasia of the anterior iris stroma occurs resulting in pupillary abnormalities (Zauberman & Sira 1970). There may be polycoria, corectopia or irregularly shaped pupils. Shields (1983) noted the overlapping of ocular and non-ocular defects in patients with Axenfeld's and Rieger's anomaly and proposed a collective term Axenfeld–Rieger (AR) syndrome.

Non-ocular features. Systemic abnormalities are most frequently associated with Rieger's anomaly (Zauberman & Sira 1970), including midface hypoplasia, telecanthus

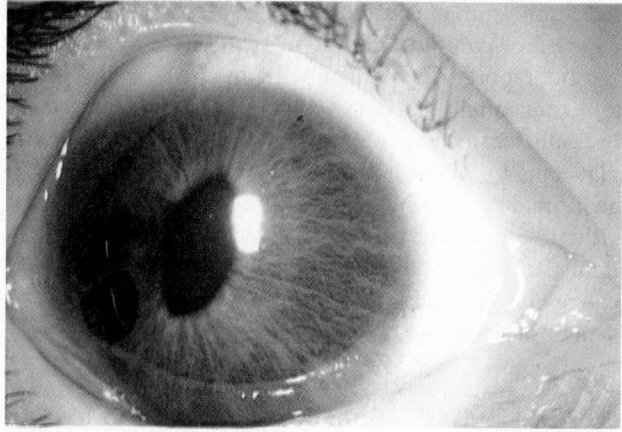

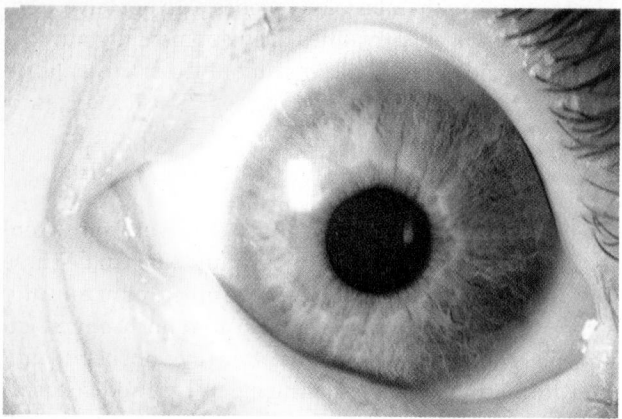

Fig. 40.7 Anterior segment dysgenesis. Bilateral glaucoma and Rieger's anomaly more marked in the left eye.

with a broad flat nasal root, dental abnormalities – absent maxillary incisor teeth, microdontia, anodontia and oligodontia (Childers & Wright 1986; Fleischer-Peters & Lang 1989) – and failure of periumbilical skin to involute or umbilical hernia (Aarskog *et al.* 1983). Less commonly, visceral defects such as congenital heart anomalies, middle ear deafness, mental retardation and cerebellar vermis hypoplasia may occur.

Ocular associations. Developmental abnormalities of the anterior segment similar to that seen in Rieger's anomaly have been reported in association with other ocular abnormalities. These reports mostly relate to single dominant pedigrees and include: (i) conjunctival xerosis and arcus lipoides (de Keizer 1991); (ii) presenile hypermature cataract (Hodes *et al.* 1993); (iii) retinal detachment (Spallone 1989); (iv) bilateral persistent hyperplastic primary vitreous (Storimans & Van-Schooneveld 1989); and (v) coloboma (Verloes & Dodinval 1990).

Genetics. In 1990 Anton reported a case of Rieger's syndrome with 46XX, t1; 4(p36; q23). Rieger's syndrome was subsequently mapped to between 4q25 and 4q27 (Vaux *et al.* 1992) and reported in a patient with an interstitial 4q26

deletion (Fryns & Van Den Berghe 1992). The gene itself has not yet been identified, but there is linkage of Rieger's syndrome to the region of the epidermal growth factor gene on chromosome 4 and evidence that autosomal dominant iris hypoplasia (Rieger's anomaly) and Rieger's syndrome are allelic (Murray *et al.* 1992; Héon *et al.* 1995). However, there may be more than one genetic defect that results in the Rieger phenotype. Families with an ocular phenotype indistinguishable to the Rieger's anomaly have been shown to have abnormalities within PAX6 on chromosome 11 (see section on aniridia below). Shohat (1991) reported a case with a deletion of chromosome 20p11.3–pter and minor facial anomalies, Rieger's anomaly, congenital heart defect, severe failure to thrive and growth hormone deficiency. Rieger's anomaly has also been reported in pericentric inversion of chromosome 6 (Heinemann *et al.* 1979) and partial deletion of the long arm of chromosome 18 (Izquierdo *et al.* 1993).

Aniridia

This can be viewed as a severe variant of iridotrabeculodysgenesis. Glaucoma occurs commonly in aniridia (Walton 1979; Nelson 1984), at any age from infancy to late in life warranting regular assessments The angle may close, which can be used as an argument for prophylactic goniotomy but which may require two procedures to be effective. There may be an associated malformation or underdevelopment of drainage angle structures. Another cause of raised intraocular pressure may be progressive angle closure by the iris vestige (Walton 1986).

Glaucoma complicating aniridia has a poor prognosis especially if present in infancy (Wiggins & Tomey 1992). There is a high incidence of surgical complications. Whilst goniotomy may be effective in controlling infantile onset glaucoma in aniridia, trabeculotomy may be safer (Hoskins *et al.* 1984b), but some authors advocate a primary drainage implant (Wiggins & Tomey 1992). Direct ablation of the ciliary processes using yttrium-aluminium-garnet (YAG) or argon laser may have a temporary pressure lowering effect (Nelson *et al.* 1984).

Genetics. The most common form of aniridia is an autosomal dominant trait although up to 20% of patients have new mutation or deletions. Most patients with the aniridia phenotype have an abnormal allele of the PAX6 gene on chromosome 11 (see Chapter 38). Abnormality with this region of chromosome 11 may result in a wide variation in anterior segment malformation (see section on Peters' anomaly). The expression of the genetic defect may vary even within one family. Aniridia is always bilateral.

Gillespie's syndrome is a rare form of aniridia associated with cerebellar ataxia, ptosis and mental retardation which is inherited as an autosomal recessive trait

Table 40.1 Syndromes that may be associated with a developmental abnormality of the drainage angle and iris, and in which screening for glaucoma is advised.

Lowe syndrome

Syndromes with cutaneous manifestations
Naevus flammeus/Sturge–Weber (if skin around the eye involved)
Cutis marmorata telangiectasia congenita (if skin around the eye involved)
Neurofibromatosis (rare association with glaucoma)
Naevus of Ota
Hypomelanosis of Ito

Other syndromes
Ackerman's syndrome (dental anomalies, lid entropion, skin syndactyly; Ackerman 1973)
Alagille's syndrome (neonatal jaundice, Axenfeld's anomaly) (Watson 1973; Romanchuk 1981; Johnson 1990; Potamis 1993)
Arthrogryposis multiplex congenita (Sakamoto *et al.* 1992)
Brook's syndrome (dental anomalies, Rieger's anomaly, choanal atresia, anal atresia, short stature with kyphoscoliosis) (Brooks 1989)
Buphthalmos in association with congenital nephrotic syndrome (Braga 1989)
Diamond–Blackfan erythroid hypoplasia (Young *et al.* 1992)
dos Santos syndrome (buphthalmos in association with multiple congenital skeletal, muscle, and cardiac abnormalities) (dos Santos 1992)
Down's (Traboulsi *et al.* 1988; Jacoby *et al.* 1990)
Empty sella Rieger's anomaly (Kleinmann 1981)
Oculodentodigital dysplasia (Dudgeon 1974; Sugar 1978; Judisch 1979)
Kneist's syndrome (skeletal dysplasia, disproportionate short stature, cleft palate and hearing loss) (Mawn 1990)
Marfan's syndrome (may be associated with Rieger anomaly) (Grin 1987)
Pierre Robin syndrome (Cosmon & Keyser 1974)
Rieger anomaly partial lipodystrophy (Aarskog 1983)
Rubinstein–Taybi syndrome (see p. 485)
SHORT syndrome (short stature, hyperextensible joints, ocular depression (deep set eyes), Rieger anomaly, teething delayed) (Brooks 1975)
Split hand/split foot syndrome (Singh 1989)
Walker–Warburg syndrome (anterior segment malformation, retinal dysplasia, lissencephaly, hydrocephalus) (Warburg 1978; Winter 1981; Attia 1986)
Wolf–Hirschhorn syndrome (Mayer & Bialasiewicz 1989; Kosma 1990)

(Gillespie 1965; Nevin & Lim 1990). The iris is hypoplastic but usually to a milder degree than in typical aniridia and there may be strands from the iris margin to a persistent pupillary membrane.

Other rare associations with aniridia are: (i) ectopia lentis and abnormal incisors (Zamzam *et al.* 1988); (ii) hypoplastic patellae (Mirkinson & Mirkinson 1975); and (iii) sensorineural deafness (Courteney-Harris & Mills 1990).

Posterior polymorphous dystrophy

Posterior polymorphous dystrophy (PPMD) of the cornea may be especially difficult to distinguish from congenital glaucoma (Cibis *et al.* 1977; Weissman *et al.* 1989), and in some instances congenital glaucoma may co-exist with PPMD. PPMD is inherited as an autosomal dominant trait with variable expression.

Syndromes associated with childhood glaucoma

A number of congenital disorders present with the malformations of the anterior segment of the eye, usually involving the cornea, angle, iris and lens. Glaucoma may occur in some of these disorders, which may conveniently be divided into those with (i) developmental anomaly of the drainage angle and peripheral anterior segment (see Table 40.1); and (ii) those with abnormal angle and central cornea (Table 40.2) (Waring *et al.* 1975).

Facial naevus flammeus

Naevus flammeus may be part of the Sturge–Weber syndrome (see Chapters 38 and 61). Mainly those patients with port-wine stain over the ophthalmic branch of the trigeminal nerve have a risk of developing glaucoma. There is a higher frequency of glaucoma in patients with

Table 40.2 Peters' anomaly may be an occasional finding in the conditions listed here.

Goldenhar syndrome (Ghose 1992)
Pfeifer's syndrome (Traboulsi 1992)
Fetal alcohol syndrome (Miller *et al.* 1981, 1984; Chan *et al.* 1991; Hinzpeter *et al.* 1992)
Brachymesomelia and Peters' anomaly (Kivlin 1986, 1993)
Multiple congenital contractures (arthrogryposis) in association with Peters' anomaly and chorioretinal colobomata (Sullivan 1992; Sullivan *et al.* 1992a)
Warburg syndrome (HARD ± E)
Without encephalocoele (reported a male infant with Warburg's syndrome without retinal dysplasia, but with Peters' anomaly and optic nerve hypoplasia)

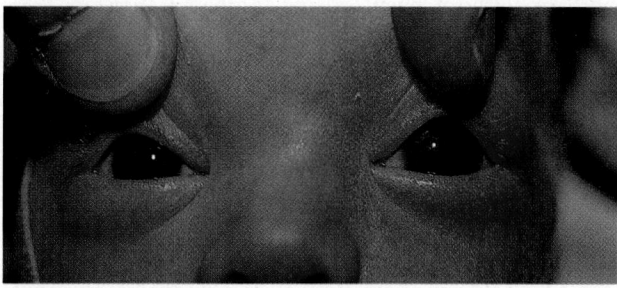

Fig. 40.8 Sturge–Weber syndrome with ipsilateral glaucoma.

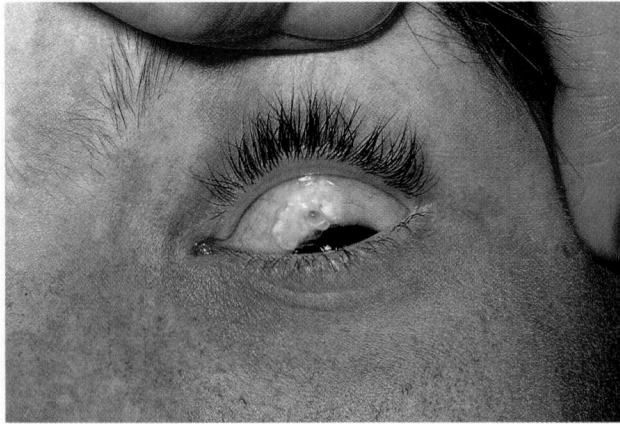

Fig. 40.9 Same patient as Fig. 40.8 aged 13 years. Filtration surgery carried out at 2 years of age. The conjunctiva, Tenon's capsule and sclera are very vascular and the surgical prognosis should be guarded.

extrafacial angioma with or without epilepsy (Bioxeda *et al.* 1993). The majority of eyes with glaucoma have conjunctival or episcleral haemangiomas (Phelps 1978; Sullivan *et al.* 1992b) and may also have choroidal lesions.

Glaucoma may present in infancy (Fig. 40.8) when the chamber angle is anomalous, but in juvenile and adult onset glaucoma the angle appears clinically normal and histology of trabeculectomy specimens gives similar findings to primary open angle glaucoma (Cibis *et al.* 1984). Cibis *et al.* (1984) postulate that premature ageing of the angle structures occurs in eyes with naevus flammeus.

Jorgensen *et al.* (1987) have demonstrated that episcleral venous pressure is raised and tonography shows a marked decrease in outflow facility presumably due to secondary damage of the trabecular meshwork.

Goniotomy may be initially effective in controlling infantile onset glaucoma in naevus flammeus, but there is a high incidence of relapse especially in early childhood (Hoskins *et al.* 1984b; Iwach *et al.* 1990). Combined trabeculotomy–trabeculectomy is advocated by some authors to tackle both postulated mechanisms of glaucoma (Board & Shields 1981; Agarwal *et al.* 1993). Trabeculectomy (Fig. 40.9) is usually advocated for juvenile and adult onset glaucoma associated with Sturge–Weber syndrome (Ali *et al.* 1990).

Intraoperative complications include choroidal effusion with or without haemorrhage (Shihab & Kristan 1983; Theodossiadis *et al.* 1985; Iwach *et al.* 1990) which may result in expulsion of intraocular tissue (Christensen & Records 1979). There is also an increased risk of postoperative choroidal detachment and/or vitreous haemorrhage.

The visual prognosis is very variable even if an early diagnosis of glaucoma is made (Sullivan *et al.* 1992b). Unfortunately, patients may still present with advanced glaucoma where screening for this high-risk group is absent.

Cutis marmorata telangiectasia congenita

Cutis marmorata telangiectasia congenita (CMTC) is a vascular disorder with livedo reticularis (a blotchy marbling of the skin); there may also be stroke-like episodes and seizures (Baxter *et al.* 1993). The skin lesion may be confused with naevus flammeus especially if near the eye as conjunctiva and sclera have a similar vascular appearance and there may be associated congenital onset glaucoma: the lesions may co-exist (Sato *et al.* 1988).

The glaucoma tends to present as buphthalmos in the first year of life, postulated as due either to a primary developmental abnormality (Sato *et al.* 1988) or to angle changes secondary to increased episcleral pressure (Miranda *et al.* 1990). CMTC may rarely present with congenital retinal detachment with a secondary neovascular glaucoma (Shields *et al.* 1990). Goniotomy may be complicated by haemorrhage. Intraocular pressure may be controlled by trabeculotomy (Mayatepek *et al.* 1991) or trabeculectomy (Miranda *et al.* 1990). There is an increased risk of intraoperative suprachoroidal haemorrhage (Kremer *et al.* 1991).

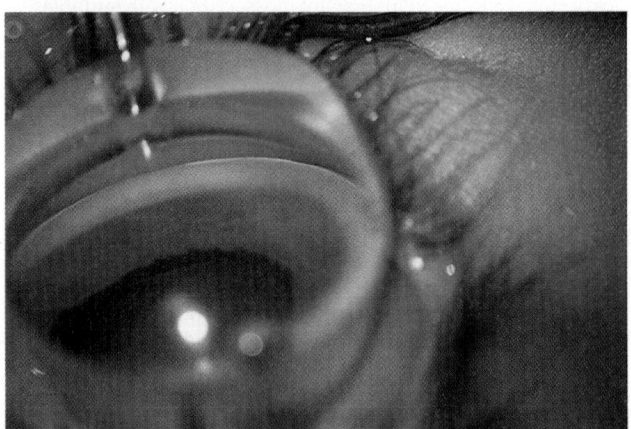

a

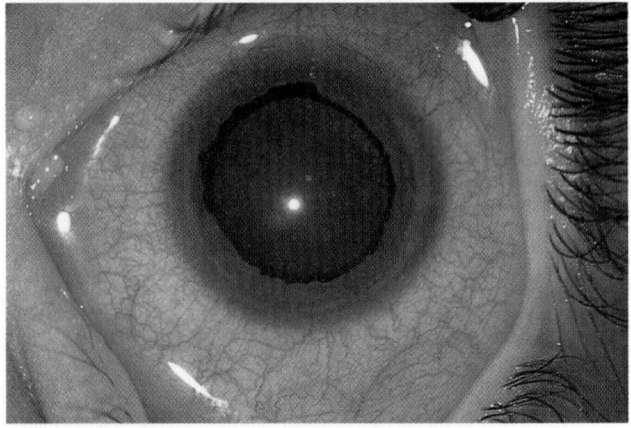

b

Fig. 40.10 Ectropion uveae and iridotrabeculodysgenesis. The hallmark of these usually unilateral cases is ectropion uveae (b). The anterior chamber angle (a) is abnormal with an anteriorly inserted iris root.

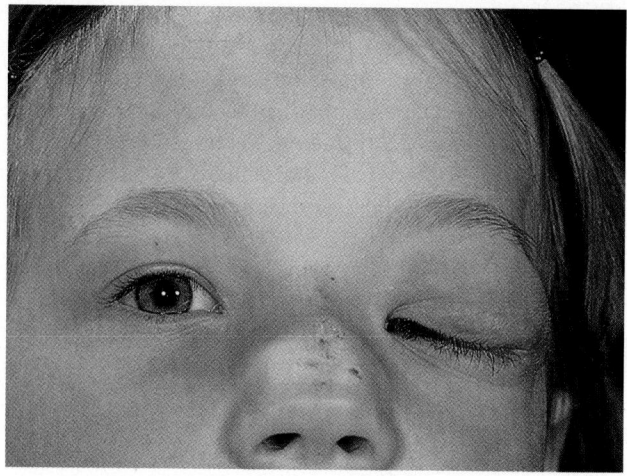

Fig. 40.11 Neurofibromatosis with a plexiform neuroma of the right upper lid associated with glaucoma.

Iris ectropion

Congenital iris ectropion (Fig. 40.10) is characterized by a non-progressive ectropion of the iris pigment epithelium, a glassy smooth cryptless iris surface, a high iris insertion, dysgenesis of the drainage angle and often glaucoma. It is probably a congenital anomaly of the neural crest-derived tissues of the anterior segment of the eye (Wilson 1990).

A rare but important condition is glaucoma associated with iridotrabecular dysgenesis and ectropion uveae – a widespread ocular defect with iris hypoplasia and anterior insertion of the iris root on gonioscopy. It is usually unilateral and not associated with systemic disorders. Response to goniotomy is not good (Dowling 1985) but some do well with trabeculectomy.

Neurofibromatosis

Congenital iris ectropion and glaucoma may occur with neurofibromatosis type 1 (von Recklinghausen); the glaucoma is often associated with ipsilateral iris ectropion (Grant & Walton 1968; Castillo *et al.* 1988) and sometimes with a choroidal neurofibroma (Reed *et al.* 1986; Burke *et al.* 1991). Commonly, there is an associated plexiform neurofibroma of the eyelid (Fig. 40.11) or orbit (Reed *et al.* 1986; Zanella & Kirchhof 1986) which is relentlessly progressive and may manifest as regional elephantiasis (Bardelli & Hadjistilianou 1989). An enlarged cornea may also be a sign of regional giantism in some cases rather than of congenital glaucoma (Hoyt & Billson 1977). The angle appearance is as in isolated iris ectropion but the presentation is typically (but not invariably) soon after birth, before Lisch nodules, skin stigmata of neurofibromatosis type 1 or any associated neurofibroma become manifest. The prognosis is very poor with many eyes being refractory to surgery and being enucleated for pain.

This may be because the glaucoma is due not only to the abnormal tissue in the angle, but also to angle closure secondary to the choroidal neurofibroma.

Naevus of Ota

Liu and Ball (1991) reported three black patients with naevus of Ota with ipsilateral open angle glaucoma and melanocytic infiltration of the outflow tracts. It is not clear whether regular glaucoma screening is warranted.

Hypomelanosis of Ito

This is a rare neurocutaneous disorder with associated ocular, facial, dental and skeletal abnormalities. Flaherty *et al.* (1991) reported a case with developmental abnormality of the anterior segment of the Axenfeld type.

Rubinstein–Taybi syndrome

Infants with the Rubinstein–Taybi syndrome have a characteristic facies: hypertelorism, antimongoloid slant and slight eyelid ptosis with long eyelashes, and broad thumbs and great toes (Fig. 40.12) (Roy *et al.* 1968; Hennekam 1990). Glaucoma is a rare association and may be infantile or juvenile in onset (Levy 1976). Fujisawa *et al.* (1990) found on histological examination of a trabeculectomy specimen from a 31-year-old with the Rubinstein–Taybi syndrome compact tissue filled with a large amount of collagen fibres with few cells in the juxtacanalicular tissue of Schlemm's canal. They concluded that this was due to underdevelopment of the angle. Other abnormalities including megalocornea, corneal opacities, cupped discs and coloboma may make the evaluation of glaucoma in Rubinstein–Taybi syndrome more difficult (Brei *et al.* 1995).

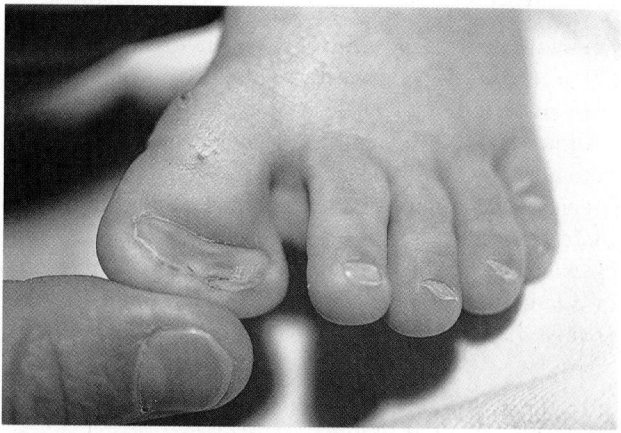

Fig. 40.12 Rubinstein–Taybi syndrome. Broad thumbs and toes are a characteristic feature (see text).

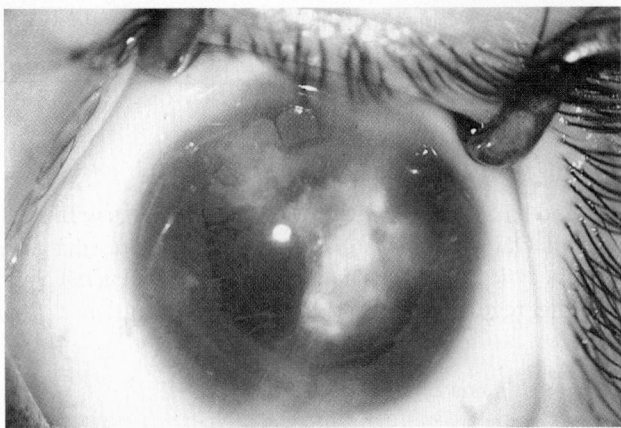

Fig. 40.13 Anterior segment dysgenesis with glaucoma (Peters' anomaly). Corneal opacities, to the posterior surface of which are attached iris strands. A cataract is hidden by the corneal opacities.

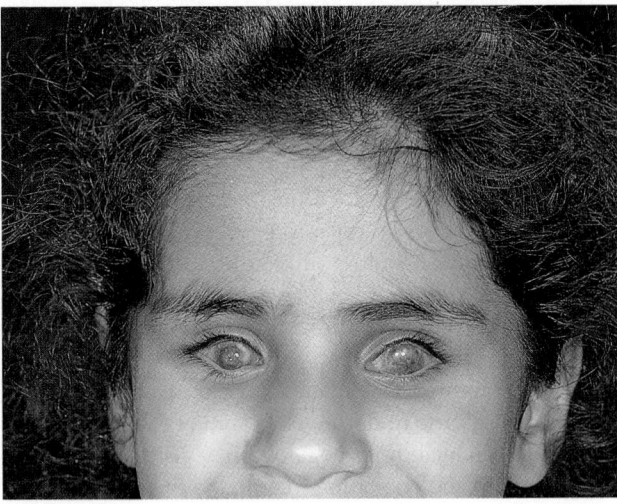

Fig. 40.14 Bilateral glaucoma with anterior segment dysgenesis.

Iridotrabeculocorneal dysgenesis: Peters' anomaly

Peters' anomaly is the term for a congenital central opacity of the cornea with relative clarity of the corneal periphery with an underlying lens defect and sometimes iris abnormalities (Fig. 40.13). This is a morphological finding rather than a distinct entity (Mayer 1992). Peters' anomaly has been associated with a variety of chromosomal anomalies (Bateman *et al.* 1984; Eiferman 1984; Cibis *et al.* 1985; Wertelecki *et al.* 1985). Inheritance may be autosomal recessive or dominant (Green & Johnson 1986; DeRespinis & Wagner 1987; Holmström *et al.* 1991) with variable expression.

Glaucoma in Peters' anomaly

Glaucoma may be present at birth (Koster & van-Balen 1985)—or develop later. The angle anomaly may be subtle:

Heath and Shields (1991) examined the trabeculectomy specimen of a 26-year-old with open angle glaucoma since childhood: the only abnormality was an abundance of broad-banded collagen fibres in the trabecular lamellae interpreted as premature ageing. Peters' anomaly may be associated with other ocular anomalies such as congenital aphakia (Harris *et al.* 1980) and cataract (Green & Johnson 1986).

Children with anterior segment dysgenesis syndromes require life-long follow-up, and the prognosis should be guarded (Fig. 40.14). Measurement of intraocular pressure is often difficult, therefore control has to be assessed using other parameters.

Surgery in Peters' syndrome

Peters' anomaly may be associated with glaucoma, particularly following penetrating keratoplasty (Eggink *et al.* 1991; Parmley *et al.* 1993; Althaus & Sundmacher 1996). Penetrating keratoplasty in infants is generally disappointing, yet the prognosis for graft clarity in Peters' anomaly is possibly better (Brown & Salamon 1983; Cameron 1993). Two out of nine cases remained clear in a report by Kampik *et al.* (1986). A clear peripheral cornea improves the prognosis in infant grafting: a clear transplant was obtained in seven of 16 eyes with Peters' anomaly with a minimum length of follow-up of 3 months (Erlich *et al.* 1991). An associated anomaly of the lens or glaucoma means the prognosis is still very poor.

A developmental anomaly of the cornea ('Peters' type') and glaucoma is often associated with systemic abnormalities some of which form well-characterized syndromes (Heon *et al.* 1992; Mayer 1992; Myles *et al.* 1992; Traboulsi & Maumenee 1992). Many of the systemic abnormalities suggest a generalized disorder of neural crest migration or differentiation such as conotruncal heart defect (Myles *et al.* 1992). Tabuchi *et al.* (1985) reported three siblings with Peters' anomaly with glaucoma and congenital heart disease (tetralogy of Fallot in one and ventricular septal defect with patent ductus arteriosus in another).

Peters' plus syndrome

van-Schooneveld *et al.* (1984) reported 11 patients with Peters' anomaly, short stature, brachymorphy, mental retardation, abnormal ears and cheilognathopalatoschisis. The condition can be relatively mild, but also even lethal in the fetal period. Frydman *et al.* (1991) suggested the eponym Krause–Kivlin syndrome for the condition, now more often known as Peters' plus syndrome, and reported three further cases: two cousins and an unrelated patient, all offspring of consanguineous parents. Cardiac and renal malformations may be present and a variable degree of mental retardation. de Almeida *et al.* (1991) reported two siblings born to a consanguineous marriage, both had

Peters' anomaly and the systemic features of the Peters' plus syndrome.

Juvenile open angle glaucoma

This rare form of glaucoma is inherited as an autosomal dominant trait. Linkage to markers on 1q has been demonstrated (Sheffield *et al.* 1993; Richards *et al.* 1994; Wiggs *et al.* 1995) and linkage to the Rieger gene on chromosome 4 has been excluded (Johnson *et al.* 1993). The drainage angle is normal on gonioscopy as is the iris. However, using light and electron microscopy on trabeculectomy specimens from eyes with juvenile glaucoma, Tawara and Inomata (1984) found a thick compact tissue consisting of cells with fine processes and extracellular substances at the anterior chamber side of Schlemm's canal and abnormal deposits of ground substances in the thick tissue. This was interpreted as immaturity of the trabecular meshwork.

Presentation is usually as a result of screening of members of families at risk; many index cases present very late because of the rarity of the condition and because acuity (the only readily measurable parameter in young children) remains normal until late. Increasing and asymmetrical myopia may be a clue, but is often missed because primary myopia is often asymmetrical and usually progressive in young people. Progressive myopia may also occur in early onset chronic angle closure glaucoma (Cherny *et al.* 1992), and a myopic shift may be a sign of glaucoma in juvenile aphakes. Open angle glaucoma presenting young is much more common in blacks than in Caucasians particularly if they are myopes (Lotufo *et al.* 1989).

Table 40.3 The main causes of secondary glaucoma in childhood.

Retrolental mass, neovascularization of the iris, pupil block and traumatic damage to the drainage angle

Retinopathy of prematurity, persistent hyperplastic primary vitreous, retinoblastoma, retinal dysplasia, congenital retinal detachment due to intrauterine infections, neurofibroma choroid, von Hippel–Lindau syndrome, uveitis (Kanski 1985), aphakia, dislocated lens (Rodman 1963), trauma

Metabolic syndromes
Marfan's syndrome (see Chapter 39)
Homocystinuria (see Chapter 39)
Weill–Marchesani syndrome (see Chapter 39)
Zellweger's syndrome (see Chapter 44)
Mucopolysaccharidoses (see Chapter 57)

Neoplasia
Retinoblastoma
Juvenile xanthogranuloma (Zimmerman 1965; Chang *et al.* 1996)
Neurofibroma choroid (see above)

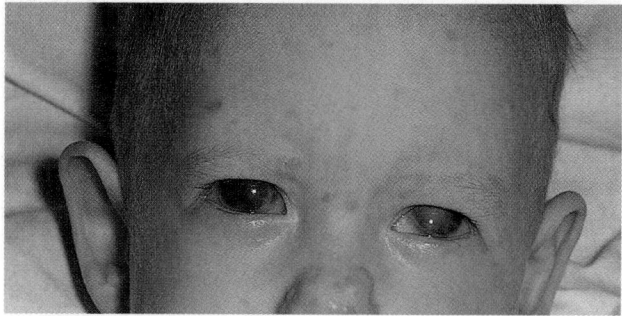

Fig. 40.15 Bilateral juvenile xanthogranuloma. Repeated haemorrhages gave rise to an intractable glaucoma in both eyes. Low-dose radiotherapy usually brings about rapid resolution.

Secondary glaucoma

Inflammatory eye disease

Glaucoma may be difficult to manage in inflammation of the eye particularly in Still's disease (see Chapter 38). Niffenegger and Walton (1994) found goniotomy helpful in glaucoma with chronic anterior uveitis (Table 40.3).

Juvenile xanthogranuloma

Xanthogranulomas are generally benign, self-limited lesions (Malone 1991), but may cause blinding glaucoma. Skin lesions (Fig. 40.15) may persist or continue to erupt for years, particularly in individuals who first develop lesions after the age of 20 years (Cohen & Hood 1989). The juvenile form is distinct from the adult form (Zelger *et al.* 1994). There is a rare association between juvenile chronic granulocytic leukaemia, juvenile xanthogranulomas, and neurofibromatosis (Morier 1990). Uveal juvenile xanthogranuloma is a rare intraocular tumour which usually occurs in very young children and may present as buphthalmos or spontaneous hyphaemia (Amoric *et al.* 1991; Murdoch *et al.* 1991). Intraocular surgery may be complicated by major haemorrhage (Casteels *et al.* 1993). Successful treatments include subconjunctival steroid (Treacy *et al.* 1990; Casteels *et al.* 1993), systemic steroids, low-dose irradiation or excision.

Ectopia lentis

Congenital ectopia lentis with secondary buphthalmos appeared to occur as an autosomal recessive trait in a Turkish family where affected members all had subluxed lenses by the age of 2 years (Bjerrum & Kessing 1991). Glaucoma is particularly frequent in homocystinuria, when the lenses are prone to dislocate anteriorly (Fig. 40.16). In buphthalmos with a grossly large eye the lens may dislocate spontaneously (Fig. 40.17).

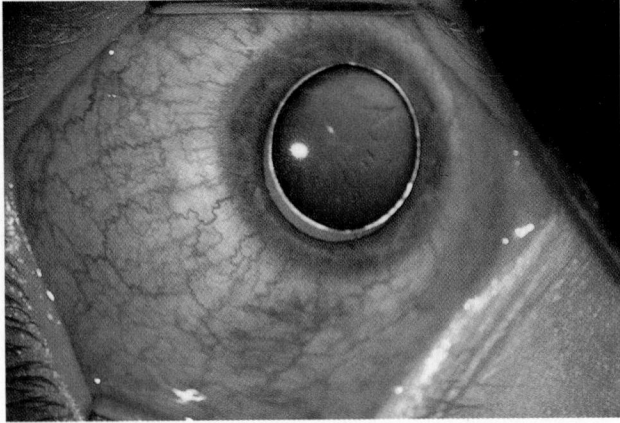

Fig. 40.16 Homocystinuria. Dislocated lens blocking the pupil and giving rise to glaucoma.

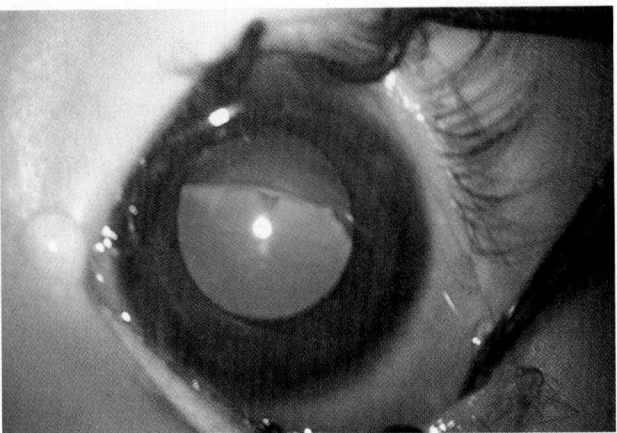

Fig. 40.17 Buphthalmos. The grossly enlarged globe is associated with a superior dislocation of the lens.

Aphakic glaucoma

Glaucoma may be an early complication of cataract surgery due to pupil block with vitreous and residual lens matter particularly in infants with pupils that do not dilate well. Congenital cataract may be associated with a primary developmental glaucoma. The cataract may even be unilateral and the glaucoma in the contralateral eye indicating that this is a genuine association rather than a complication of cataract surgery (Summers & Letson 1992). There is also the risk of open angle glaucoma which in up to 40% of eyes presents during the subsequent 5 years (Phelps & Arafat 1977; Chrousos *et al.* 1985; Robb & Petersen 1992). Parks (1993) and Asrani and Wilensky (1995) identified 'type of cataract' as a major risk factor in the development of aphakic glaucoma, with microphthalmic eyes with nuclear cataract having a worse prognosis. Blockage of the pupil by vitreous may give rise to acute glaucoma and vitreous can fill the anterior chamber

(Fig. 40.18). Screening of intraocular pressure and regular examination of optic discs is essential (but difficult) in childhood aphakia. A further presenting sign is excessive loss of hyperopia (Egbert & Kushner 1990).

Management of glaucoma in childhood

Decreased visual function occurs secondary to optic nerve damage, corneal opacification and scarring, cataracts, lens dislocation, retinal detachment (Cooling *et al.* 1980), and amblyopia. The problem of anisometropic and strabismic amblyopia is especially important in the rehabilitation of monocular congenital glaucoma. Although the prognosis for trabeculodysgenesis is good (Fig. 40.19) in most other forms of childhood glaucoma the prognosis should be guarded (Figs 40.20, 40.21).

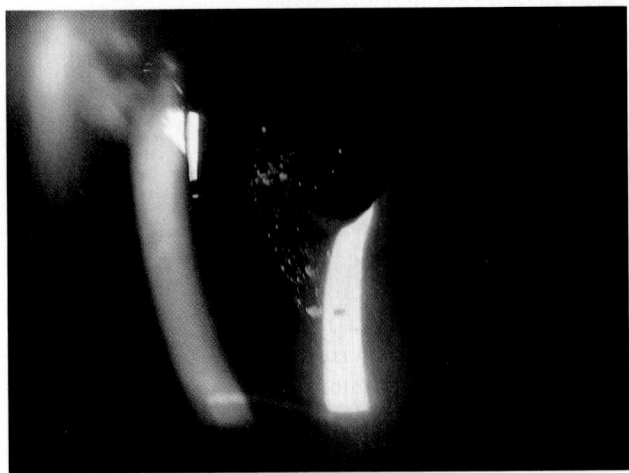

a

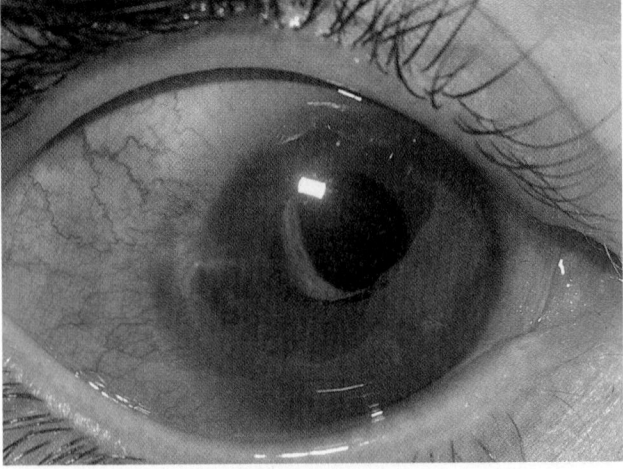

b

Fig. 40.18 (a) Aphakic glaucoma following lens aspiration in infancy. The vitreous can be seen filling the pupil and covering the anterior surface of the iris. (b) Vitrectomy brought about long-term resolution of the condition—the vitreous was adherent to the anterior iris leaf and 'bite' marks can be seen on the iris where the vitrectomy machine cut the anterior leaf.

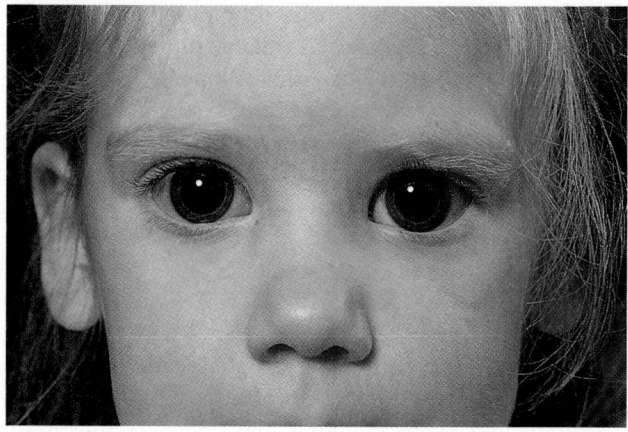

Fig. 40.19 Severe bilateral glaucoma associated with trabeculodysgenesis which responded to goniotomy alone and treatment of the amblyopia. The acuity was 6/9 in either eye with spectacles for myopia.

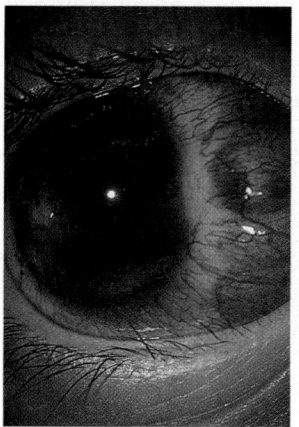
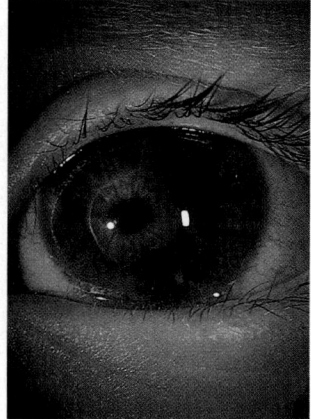

Fig. 40.20 Severe bilateral intractable glaucoma. The right eye required enucleation, the left eye became blind from optic atrophy.

Clinical assessment

The same principles of assessment of glaucoma apply independent of the aetiology. Assessment of control is multifactorial and intraocular pressure measurement particularly prone to variables, such as corneal size and clarity, depth and type of anaesthesia (Dear *et al.* 1987). Patients are regularly examined to record corneal clarity, diameter, intraocular pressure and optic disc appearance; a combination of these parameters determines whether further treatment is indicated.

Intraocular pressure in children is lower than the mean in adults (Jaafar & Kazi 1993b; Pensiero *et al.* 1992) and measurements are difficult to interpret in isolation.

It may be possible to assess intraocular pressure in the office without sedation. Small infants are kept hungry and given a bottle at the examination. Air puff tonometers, such as the Keeler Pulsair, are useful and reasonably com-

parable to Goldmann tonometry (Moseley *et al.* 1993) for intraocular pressure measurement, particularly in young aphakes. They may tend to overread in small strabismic eyes and they need regular calibration (Atkinson *et al.* 1992). The pressure measurements, however, are reproducible (Vernon 1995). In enlarged corneas with opacities large unpredictable errors in reading occur and applanation tonometry is advised, such as the Perkins or the Goldmann tonometer. Methods of sedation include oral chloral hydrate (Jaafar & Kazi 1993a) and intramuscular ketamine hydrochloride. The latter causes a rise in intraocular pressure, but advocates find that this produces a useful reading. Older children may suffer from nightmares follow-ing ketamine. Many general anaesthetic agents such as halothane lower intraocular pressure, but useful readings may be obtained early after induction prior to any intubation of the airway (Deal *et al.* 1987).

Amblyopia is a major cause of ocular morbidity, particularly in unilateral congenital glaucoma. Regular refraction should be performed with correction of any errors and occlusion therapy monitored by acuity assessment by fixation preference if strabismus is present. Congenital glaucoma can be complicated by dislocation of the lens, massive intraocular haemorrhage or rupture of the globe with minor trauma and retinal detachment (Cooling *et al.* 1980).

Medical treatment

Beta-blockers, such as timolol, have been shown to lower intraocular pressure in relapsed glaucoma due to trabecular dysgenesis, in aniridia, and in the Sturge–Weber syndrome. They are often only useful as an adjunctive therapy not usually controlling intraocular pressure when used as the sole therapy in developmental glaucomas

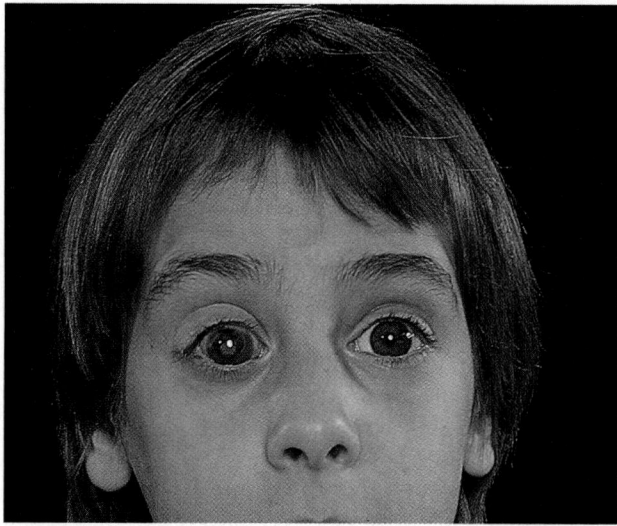

Fig. 40.21 Severe bilateral glaucoma. The right eye became blind and had to be enucleated but the left eye had normal vision.

(McMahon *et al.* 1981). Kawa *et al.* (1993) showed in bovine eyes that antiglaucoma drugs (epinephrine, timolol and levobunolol), depending on their concentrations, may profoundly influence the growth and phagocytic activity of trabecular meshwork cells. In children systemic effects of antiglaucoma medications may be serious. Punctal occlusion is recommended together with a caution not to instil more than the recommended dosage. Newer, more selective preparations such as Betoptic 0.25% may reduce risk further.

Goniotomy

If the corneal epithelium is too hazy for the angle to be viewed then topical glycerol may be applied. Very rarely, the epithelium needs to be removed in which case a cotton bud soaked in absolute alcohol should be used (aminoglycosides such as gentamicin must not be used subsequently or irreversible corneal opacity may result). This procedure, because it involves the use of a highly toxic substance, is best reserved for exceptional cases. The eye is then securely fixed using two toothed locking forceps and a reliable assistant. The globe is rotated and the microscope tilted until a clear view of the angle is achieved with the irrigating goniotomy lens on the eye. This may be difficult due to corneal splits obscuring the view of some of the angle. 'Blind' goniotomy is inadvisable. If the view is poor then trabeculotomy is preferable. A goniotomy blade is introduced into the peripheral cornea usually temporally and the tissue in the nasal angle incised for about 100° by a combination of eye rotation by the assistant and movement of the blade. In primary congenital glaucoma a correct incision will result in the iris falling back. The success of goniotomy does not seem to be closely related to the extent of incision of the trabecular tissue (Catalano *et al.* 1989). The incision usually does not require a suture.

The complications of goniotomy include intraocular infection, haemorrhage and lens touch. The latter is extremely rare in experienced hands and although a small bleed is almost invariable severe hyphaema is also rare: some surgeons use anterior chamber sodium hyaluronate (Healon) to reduce haemorrhage. Healon has been shown to reduce the incidence of hyphaemia, but not to influence glaucoma control (Catalano *et al.* 1989). Preoperative pilocarpine or intraoperative acetylcholine injected into the anterior chamber may be used to constrict the pupil reducing the risk to the lens.

Endophthalmitis is also rare, but an important consideration as many surgeons perform bilateral surgery to avoid treatment delay and extra anaesthetic. It may be advisable to keep the number of instruments and intraocular solutions to the minimum for this reason and not to use acetylcholine or viscoelastic routinely. Joos *et al.* (1993) demonstrated in the pig that an endoscope coaxially coupled to a goniotomy needle tip allows visualization of the anterior chamber angle during goniotomy despite the presence of a cloudy cornea. A suitable fine endoscope for routine human use has yet to be developed.

Goniotomy has a high success rate in congenital glaucoma due to trabeculodysgenesis: 86% of 335 eyes operated with trabeculodysgenesis and glaucoma were controlled by a single or multiple goniotomies (Russell-Eggitt *et al.* 1992).

YAG laser goniotomy

Q-switched neodymium (Nd)–YAG laser has been advocated to perform a goniotomy in eyes with infantile or juvenile onset developmental glaucoma (Yumita *et al.* 1984). Laser shots are placed anterior to the end of the iris insertion to separate the iris tissue from the trabecular band. However, although this technique may initially control intraocular pressure, long-term follow-up is less promising. The laser may induce changes in the angle. Dueker *et al.* (1990) showed that both argon laser and pulsed Nd–YAG laser to the trabecular meshwork of monkey eyes stimulated cell division in the meshwork and surrounding tissues. Argon laser is used to damage trabecular meshwork and produce glaucoma in monkey eyes in glaucoma studies (Pasquale *et al.* 1992).

Trabeculotomy

Trabeculotomy is usually performed in primary congenital glaucoma when a view of the angle is not possible and therefore goniotomy is not safe. Some surgeons advocate trabeculotomy as the primary procedure (Debnath *et al.* 1989), particularly in aniridia where goniotomy may be difficult. A limbus-based conjunctival flap is dissected in a similar fashion to the technique for trabeculectomy except that many surgeons choose to perform trabeculotomy temporally or inferiorly to preserve the superior sites for any later drainage surgery. A limbus-based rectangular or triangular lamellar scleral flap is dissected to about three-quarters depth. The plane of Schlemm's canal is where the limbus just changes to a bluish hue. A small radial incision is slowly deepened until a bead of aqueous escapes. The incision is slightly enlarged circumferentially and a Harms trabeculotome is slid through the plane and carefully rotated into the anterior chamber and then withdrawn. Ideally the second trabeculotome is inserted in the opposite direction (Harms & Dannheim 1969). Preoperative miotic will reduce the risk of lens damage.

Combined trabeculotomy–trabeculectomy

Combined trabeculotomy-trabeculectomy is advocated by some authors as this approach attempts to tackle both postulated mechanisms of glaucoma (Board & Shields 1981; Elder 1994; O'Connor 1994). This has the disadvantage in trabecular dysgenesis that the conjunctiva has been disturbed at a superior site in an eye where a primary goniotomy would have had a high chance of success, and in both surgical groups long-term relapse may occur requiring further surgery. However, this technique may be most useful in more abnormal angles where trabeculotomy can be difficult and either a combined operation is then performed as planned or a failed trabeculotomy converted into a trabeculectomy.

Trabeculectomy

There is a great tendency of blebs to fail in young people; previous surgery or laser treatment and a high preoperative pressure are poor prognostic factors (Sturmer *et al.* 1993). The prognosis is poor in early childhood, but after the age of 11 years, age and race may have little effect (Sturmer *et al.* 1993).

Peroperative measures to improve prognosis include a single dose of beta-radiation with a strontium 90 applicator (Khaw *et al.* 1991; Miller & Rice 1991), the topical cytotoxic 5-fluorouracil (5FU) and mitomycin (Fluorouracil Filtering Surgery Study Group 1993). Most 5FU regimens require repeated subconjunctival injections, which is not practical in young children (Smith *et al.* 1992). A single application of 5FU peroperatively is used in children (Mora *et al.* 1996). However, failing blebs can be rescued by fornix injection of 5FU within a few weeks of surgery.

Healing in children is different to adult eyes and these agents appear to have a less potent effect. Even mitomycin seems often not to result in a thin cystic bleb if a similar regime is followed to that advocated for high-risk glaucoma in adults (Chen *et al.* 1990). Mitomycin should be reserved for high risk eyes as major complications may occur such as endophthalmitis (Greenfield *et al.* 1996). Valtot and Denis (1990) use ultrasound (one to four ultrasound applications each of 5 seconds duration and at an intensity level of $10\,kW/cm^2$) to rescue failed blebs. Pasquale *et al.* (1992) in a study on monkey eyes showed that a single intraoperative topical application of mitomycin C produced a patent sclerostomy and hypocellular clinically effective bleb in contrast to the poor results in balanced salt solution control eyes. There is a higher risk of suprachoroidal haemorrhage in aphakic vitrectomized eyes. Intraoperative and postoperative hypotony can be reduced by using intraocular gas such as C3F8 (Furia *et al.* 1987).

Cyclocryotherapy

Frucht-Pery *et al.* (1989) treated three eyes with marked buphthalmos and congenitally opaque corneas with cyclocryotherapy. The size of the eyes became rapidly smaller during the first 2 weeks postoperatively. Pham Duy (1989), over the last 10 years, has treated over 700

glaucomatous eyes (ages not stated in abstract) using a standardized technique: six applications in the lower half of the globe, 4mm posterior to the limbus as measured from the centre of the 2.5mm diameter cryoprobe. Freezing lasted 60 seconds; the temperature of the cryoprobe in the air was –65°C and about –55°C during the application. In 85% of the treated glaucomatous eyes, it was possible to bring the intraocular pressure under control. However, in half of these eyes medical therapy was also needed.

Cyclolaser therapy

Non-contact Nd–YAG cyclophotocoagulation may be successful in lowering intraocular pressure, but there is a tendency to relapse especially in young adults (Robert *et al.* 1990; Noureddin *et al.* 1992) and children. However, applications can be repeated. Repeated laser applications may lead to generalized conjunctival reaction and this scarring could potentially influence the result of any future surgery. Sympathetic ophthalmitis has been recorded (Bechrakis *et al.* 1994). Diode laser cyclophotocoagulation may also lower intraocular pressure (Schuman *et al.* 1990; Brancato *et al.* 1995).

Drainage tube implantation

Molteno *et al.* (1984) showed that draining implants, inserted in two stages, together with the temporary administration of medication to control bleb fibrosis was a successful technique even in eyes with advanced juvenile glaucoma. Double-plate Molteno implantation more frequently affords intraocular pressure control than single-plate Molteno implantation (Molteno 1990). However, double plates are associated with greater risk of complications (Heuer *et al.* 1992). Since then one-stage implantation has been modified to reduce the risk of early hypotony. There are various methods for temporarily closing or reducing the lumen of the drainage tube in one-stage placement of Molteno tubes such as 7–0 polypropylene ligatures which are later cut by argon laser (Price & Whitson 1989) or placement within the tube of a 5–0 nylon suture to reduce the lumen temporarily (Susanna 1991). Molteno implants are more likely to fail in children than in adults (Mills *et al.* 1996). There are various techniques for placement of the implant including insertion of the tube via the pars plana rather than the usual route via a trabeculectomy-like scleral flap. A 4–0 steel guide suture may aid tube placement (Susanna 1991). Perforation of the tube plate has been suggested in an effort to increase drainage (Susanna 1991). Early complications of tube implantation include choroidal effusion, flat anterior chamber (Lotufo 1991) and endophthalmitis (Munoz *et al.* 1991). There is a greater risk of suprachoroidal haemorrhage in aphakic eyes that have undergone vitrectomy.

Postoperative hypotony should be avoided if possible particularly in tube implant surgery (Canning 1989) by injection of a slowly absorbing gas bubble such as 20% SF6. Late complications include chronic hypotony, tube–cornea touch, corneal oedema, implant extrusion, persistent hyphaemia, vitreous haemorrhage, cystoid macula oedema, opacified vitreous face, retinal detachment, traction detachment with fibrous ingrowth and phthisis (Lotufo 1991; Melamed *et al.* 1991). These complications are not necessarily directly related to Molteno surgery as these eyes usually have severe disease and multiple previous surgery. Tubes may fail to control intraocular pressure due to tube block or fibrosis of filtration bleb (Hill *et al.* 1991). Resuscitation of the bleb can be attempted using dissection of the fibrous capsule around the implant and injection of subconjunctival cytotoxic agents and intensive steroids.

Other drainage implants

Dobrogowski *et al.* (1990) described rabbit eye trials of a silastic tube implant where at a second procedure a Nd–YAG laser in the thermal mode was used to burn holes in the tube in the anterior chamber.

Trabeculodialysis

This is a procedure used in inflammatory glaucoma. A goniotomy knife is used to divide any anterior synechiae, then to incise just posterior to Schwalbe's line (Kanski & McAllister 1985).

Corneal grafting in congenital glaucoma

There are very few reports of a successful outcome following corneal grafting in congenital glaucoma (Ariyasu *et al.* 1994; Frucht-Pery *et al.* 1989). In spite of reporting a successful outcome in many paediatric penetrating keratoplasties Erlich *et al.* (1991) do not support grafting in congenital glaucoma.

References

Aarskog D, Ose L, Pande H *et al.* Autosomal dominant partial lipodystrophy associated with Rieger anomaly, short stature, and insulinopenic diabetes. *Am J Med Genet* 1983; **15**: 29–38.

Ackerman JL. Taurodont, pyramidal, and fused molar roots associated with other anomalies in a kindred. *Am J Phys Anthropol* 1973; **38**: 681–94.

Agarwal HC, Sandramouli S, Sihota R, Sood NN. Sturge–Weber syndrome: management of glaucoma with combined trabeculotomy–trabeculectomy. *Ophthalmic Surg* 1993; **24**: 399–402.

Ali MA, Fahmy IA, Spaeth GL. Trabeculectomy for glaucoma associated with Sturge–Weber syndrome. *Ophthalmic Surg* 1990; **21**: 352–5.

Althaus C, Sundmacher R. Keratoplasty in newborns with Peters' anomaly. *Ger J Ophthalmol* 1996; **5(1)**: 31–5.

Amoric JC, Stalder JF, Schmuck C, Bureau B, Litoux P. Ocular complication disclosing juvenile xanthogranuloma. Apropos of a case (English abstract). *Ann Dermatol Venereol* 1991; **118**: 629–32.

Ariyasu RG, Silverman J, Irvine JA. Penetrating keratoplasty in infants with congenital glaucoma. *Cornea* 1994; **13(6)**: 521–6.

Asrani SG, Wilensky JT. Glaucoma after congenital cataract surgery. *Ophthalmology* 1995; **102**: 863–7.

Atkinson P, Wishart P, James J, Vernon S, Reid F. Deterioration in the accuracy of the pulsair non-contact tonometer with use: need for regular calibration. *Eye* 1992; **6**: 530–4.

Attia MF, Burn J, McCarthy JH, Purohit DP, Milligan DW. Warburg (HARD ± E) syndrome without retinal dysplasia: case report and review. *Br J Ophthalmol* 1986; **70**: 742–7.

Bahn CF, Falls HF, Varley GA, Meyer RF, Edelhauser HF, Bourne WM. Classification of corneal endothelial disorders based on neural crest origin. *Ophthalmology* 1984; **91**: 558–63.

Bardelli AM, Hadjistilianou T. Buphthalmos and progressive elephantiasis in neurofibromatosis. A report of three cases. *Ophthalmic Paediatr Genet* 1989; **10**: 279–86.

Bateman JB, Maumenee IH, Sparkes RS. Peters' anomaly associated with partial deletion of the long arm of chromosome 11. *Am J Ophthalmol* 1984; **97**: 11–15.

Baxter P, Gardner Medwin D, Green SH, Moss C. Congenital livedo reticularis and recurrent stroke-like episodes. *Dev Med Child Neurol* 1993; **35**: 917–21.

Beauchamp G, Knepper P. Role of neural crest in the anterior segment development and disease. *J Pediatr Ophthalmol Strabismus* 1984; **21**: 209–14.

Bechrakis N, Muller-Stolzenburg N, Helbig H, Foerster M. Sympathetic ophthalmia following laser cyclocoagulation. *Arch Ophthalmol* 1994; **112**: 80–4.

Bioxeda P, de Misa RF, Arrazola JM, Perez B, Harto A, Ledo A. Facial angioma and the Sturge–Weber syndrome: a study of 121 cases (English abstaract). *Med Clin Barc* 1993; **101**: 1–4.

Bjerrum K, Kessing SV. Congenital ectopia lentis and secondary buphthalmos likely occurring as an autosomal recessive trait. *Acta Ophthalmol Copenh* 1991; **69**: 630–4.

Bluth K. Ultrasonic biometry in congenital glaucoma. In: Hillman JS, Le May MM, eds. *Ophthalmic Ultrasonography*. The Hague: Dr W. Junk, 1983: 267–93.

Board RJ, Shields MB. Combined trabeculotomy–trabeculectomy for the management of glaucoma associated with Sturge–Weber syndrome. *Ophthalmic Surg* 1981; **12**: 813–17.

Braga S, Monn E, Zimmermann A, Oetliker O. Congenital nephrotic syndrome with congenital buphthalmos: a new genetic entity? *Prog Clin Biol Res* 1989; **305**: 205–9.

Brancato R, Carassa RG, Bettin P, Fiori M, Trabucchi G. Contact transscleral cyclophotocoagulation with diode laser in refractory glaucoma. *Eur J Ophthalmol* 1995; **5(1)**: 32–9.

Brei TJ, Burke JM, Rubinstein JH. Glaucoma and findings simulating glaucoma in the Rubinstein–Taybi syndrome. *J Pediatr Ophthalmol Strabismus* 1995; **32**: 248–52.

Brooks JK, Coccaro PJ Jr, Zarbin MA. The Rieger anomaly concomitant with multiple dental, craniofacial, and somatic midline anomalies and short stature. *Oral Surg Oral Med Oral Pathol* 1989; **68**: 717–24.

Brown SI, Salamon SM. Wound healing of grafts in congenitally opaque infant corneas. *Am J Ophthalmol* 1983; **95**: 641–4.

Burke JP, Leitch RJ, Talbot JF, Parsons MA. Choroidal neurofibromatosis with congenital iris ectropion and buphthalmos: relationship and significance. *J Pediatr Ophthalmol Strabismus* 1991; **28**: 265–7.

Cameron JA. Good visual result following early penetrating keratoplasty for Peters' anomaly. *J Pediatr Ophthalmol Strabismus* 1993; **30**: 109–12.

Canning CR, Lavin M, McCartney AC, Hitchings RA, Gregor ZJ. Delayed suprachoroidal haemorrhage after glaucoma operations. *Eye* 1989; **3**: 327–31.

Casteels I, Olver J, Malone M, Taylor D. Early treatment of juvenile xanthogranuloma of the iris with subconjunctival steroids. *Br J Ophthalmol* 1993; **77**: 57–60.

Castillo M, Quencer RM, Glaser J, Altman N. Congenital glaucoma and buphthalmos in a child with neurofibromatosis. *J Clin Neuroophthalmol* 1988; **8**: 69–71.

Catalano RA, King RA, Calhoun JH, Sargent RA. One versus two simultaneous goniotomies as the initial surgical procedure for primary infantile glaucoma. *J Pediatr Ophthalmol Strabismus* 1989; **26**: 9–13.

Chan T, Bowell R, O'Keefe M, Lanigan B. Ocular manifestations in fetal alcohol syndrome. *Br J Ophthalmol* 1991; **75**: 524–6.

Chang MW, Frieden IJ, Good W. The risk of intraocular juvenile xanthogranuloma: survey of current practises and assessment of risk. *J Am Acad Dermatol* 1996; **34(3)**: 445–9.

Chen CW, Huang HT, Bair JS, Lee CC. Trabeculectomy with simultaneous topical application of mitomycin-C in refractory glaucoma. *J Ocul Pharmacol* 1990; **6**: 175–82.

Cherny M, Brooks AMV, Gillies WE. Progressive myopia in early onset chronic angle closure glaucoma. *Br J Ophthalmol* 1992; **76**: 758–9.

Childers NK, Wright JT. Dental and craniofacial anomalies of Axenfeld–Rieger syndrome. *J Oral Pathol* 1986; **15**: 534–9.

Christensen GR, Records RE. Glaucoma and expulsive hemorrhage mechanisms in the Sturge–Weber syndrome. *Ophthalmology* 1979; **86**: 1360–6.

Chrousos G, Parks MM, O'Neill JF. Incidence of chronic glaucoma, retinal detachment and secondary membrane surgery in paediatric aphakic patients. *Ophthalmology* 1985; **92**: 856–61.

Cibis GW, Kratchmer JH, Phelps CD, Weingeist TE. The clinical spectrum of posterior polymorphous dystrophy. *Arch Ophthalmol* 1977; **95**: 1529–33.

Cibis GW, Tripathi RC, Tripathi BJ. Glaucoma in Sturge–Weber syndrome. *Ophthalmology* 1984; **91**: 1061–71.

Cibis GW, Waeltermann J, Harris DJ. Peters' anomaly in association with ring 21 chromosomal abnormality. *Am J Ophthalmol* 1985; **100**: 733–4.

Cohen BA, Hood A. Xanthogranuloma: report on clinical and histologic findings in 64 patients. *Pediatr Dermatol* 1989; **6**: 262–6.

Cook CS. Experimental models of anterior segment dysgenesis. *Ophthalmic Paediatr Genet* 1989; **10**: 33–46.

Cooling RJ, Rice NSC, McLeod DM. Retinal detachment in congenital glaucoma. *Br J Ophthalmol* 1980; **64**: 417–21.

Cosmon B, Keyser JJ. Eye abnormalities and skeletal defects in the Pierre Robin syndrome. A balanced evaluation. *Cleft Palate J* 1974; **11**: 404–11.

Courteney-Harris RG, Mills RP. Aniridia and deafness: an inherited disorder. *J Laryngol Otol* 1990; **104**: 419–20.

de Almeida JC, Reis DF, Llerena Junior J *et al.* Short stature, brachydactyly, and Peters' anomaly (Peters' plus syndrome): confirmation of autosomal recessive inheritance. *J Med Genet* 1991; **28**: 277–9.

de Keizer RJ. Conjunctival xerosis, arcus lipoides and Rieger's disease. *Doc Ophthalmol* 1991; **78**: 265–71.

Dear G de L, Hammerton M, Hatch DJ, Taylor D. Anaesthesia and intraocular pressure in young children. *Anaesthesia* 1987; **42**: 259–65.

Debnath SC, Teichmann KD, Salamah K. Trabeculectomy versus trabeculotomy in congenital glaucoma. *Br J Ophthalmol* 1989; **73**: 608–11.

DeRespinis PA, Wagner RS. Peters' anomaly in a father and son. *Am J Ophthalmol* 1987; **104**: 545–6.

Dobrogowski MJ, Dolman PJ, Douglas GR. A new glaucoma filter implant. *Ophthalmic Surg* 1990; **21**: 481–5.

dos Santos RCS, Castro NHC, Ferraz OP, Walter-Moura J *et al.* Ophthalmological, skeletal, and cardiac abnormalities in sibs born to consanguinous parents: a new syndrome? *Am J Med Genet* 1992; **43**: 946–8.

Dowling JL Jr. Primary glaucoma associated with iridotrabecular dysgenesis and ectropion uveae. *Ophthalmology* 1985; **92**: 912–21.

Dudgeon J, Chisolm IA. Oculo–dento–digital dysplasia. *Trans Ophthalmol Soc UK* 1974; **94**: 203–10.

Dueker DK, Norberg M, Johnson DH, Tschumper RC, Feeney-Burns L. Stimulation of cell division by argon and Nd–YAG laser trabeculoplasty in cynomolgus monkeys. *Invest Ophthalmol Vis Sci* 1990; **31**: 115–24.

Egbert JE, Kushner BJ. Excessive loss of hyperopia. A presenting sign of juvenile aphakic glaucoma. *Arch Ophthalmol* 1990; **108**: 1257–9.

Eggink CA, Mooy CM, Pinckers A. Peters' anomaly: an unusual case. *Ophthalmic Paediatr Genet* 1991; **12**: 19–22.

Eiferman RA. Association of Wilms' tumor with Peter's anomaly. *Ann Ophthalmol* 1984; **16**: 933–4.

Elder MJ. Combined trabeculotomy–trabeculectomy compared with primary trabeculectomy for congenital glaucoma. *Br J Ophthalmol* 1994; **78**: 745–8.

Erlich CM, Rootman DS, Morin JD. Corneal transplantation in infants, children and young adults: experience of the Toronto Hospital for Sick Children, 1979–88. *Canad J Ophthalmol* 1991; **26**: 206–10.

Flaherty MP, Padilla CD, Sillence DO. Axenfeld anomaly in association with hypomelanosis of Ito. *Ophthalmic Paediatr Genet* 1991; **12**: 23–30.

Fleischer-Peters A, Lang GE. Missing upper incisors as cardinal symptom in Rieger's syndrome. *Dtsch Zahnarztl Z* 1989; **44**: 228–31.

Fluorouracil Filtering Surgery Study Group. Three-year follow-up of the fluorouracil filtering surgery study. *Am J Ophthalmol* 1993; **115**: 82–92.

Frucht-Pery J, Feldman ST, Brown SI. Transplantation of congenitally opaque corneas from eyes with exaggerated buphthalmos. *Am J Ophthalmol* 1989; **107**: 655–8.

Frydman M, Weinstock AL, Cohen HA, Savir H, Varsano I. Autosomal recessive Peters' anomaly, typical facial appearance, failure to thrive, hydrocephalus, and other anomalies: further delineation of the Krause–Kivlin syndrome. *Am J Med Genet* 1991; **40**: 34–40.

Fryns JP, Van Den Berghe H. Rieger syndrome and interstitial 4q26 deletion. *Genet Couns* 1992; **3**: 153–4.

Fujisawa K, Kinoshita K, Tawara A, Inomata HA. Case of Rubinstein–Taybi syndrome suspected with goniodysgenetic glaucoma (English abstract). *Nippon Ganka Gakkai Zasshi* 1990; **94**: 693–700.

Furia M, Hamard H, Denis P, Frot P, Despreaux C, Elalouf M. Value of C3F8 in the surgical treatment of serous or hematic choroidal detachment with or without retinal detachment in aphakic patients with anti-glaucoma fistula (English abstract). *Bull Soc Ophthalmol Fr* 1987; **87**: 1351–5.

Ghose S, Kishore K, Patil ND. Oculoauricular dysplasia syndrome of Goldenhar and Peters' anomaly: a new association. *J Pediatr Ophthalmol Strabismus* 1992; **29**: 384–6.

Gillespie FD. Aniridia, cerebellar ataxia, and oligophrenia in siblings. *Arch Ophthalmol* 1965; **78**: 338–41.

Grant WM, Walton DS. Distinctive gonioscopic findings in glaucoma due to neurofibromatosis. *Arch Ophthalmol* 1968; **79**: 127–34.

Green JS, Johnson GJ. Congenital cataract with microcornea and

Peters' anomaly as expressions of one autosomal dominant gene. *Ophthalmic Paediatr Genet* 1986; **7**: 187–94.

Greenfield DS, Suñer IJ, Miller MP, Kangas TA, Palmberg PF, Flynn HW Jr. Endophthalmitis after filtering surgery with Mitomycin. *Arch Ophthalmol* 1996; **114(8)**: 943–9.

Grin TR, Nelson LB. Rieger's anomaly associated with Marfan's syndrome. *Ann Ophthalmol* 1987; **19**: 380–4.

Harms H, Dannheim R. Epicritical consideration of 300 cases of trabeculotomy ab externo. *Trans Ophthalmol Soc UK* 1969; **89**: 491–9.

Harris R, Brownstein S, Little JM. Peters' anomaly with congenital aphakia. *Canad J Ophthalmol* 1980; **15**: 91–4.

Heath DH, Shields MB. Glaucoma and Peters' anomaly. A clinico-pathologic case report. *Graefes Arch Clin Exp Ophthalmol* 1991; **229**: 277–80.

Heinemann MH, Breg R, Cotlier E. Rieger's syndrome with pericentric inversion of chromosome 6. *Br J Ophthalmol* 1979; **63**: 40–4.

Hennekam RCM. Bibliography on Rubinstein–Taybi syndrome. *Am J Med Genet* 1990; (Suppl. 6): 77–83.

Héon E, Barsoum-Homsy M, Cevrette L *et al.* Peters' anomaly. The spectrum of associated ocular and systemic malformations. *Ophthalmic Paediatr Genet* 1992; **13**: 137–43.

Héon E, Shetn BP, Kalenak JW, Sunden SL, Streb LM, Taylor CM, Alward WL, Sheffield VC, Stone EM. Linkage of autosomal dominant iris hypoplasia to the region of the Rieger syndrome locus (4q25). *Hum Mol Genet* 1995; **4(8)**: 1435–9.

Heuer DK, Lloyd MA, Abrams DA *et al.* Which is better? One or two? A randomized clinical trial of single-plate versus double-plate Molteno implantation for glaucomas in aphakia and pseudophakia. *Ophthalmology* 1992; **99**: 1512–19.

Hill RA, Heuer DK, Baerveldt G, Minkler DS, Martone JF. Molteno implantation for glaucoma in young patients. *Ophthalmology* 1991; **98**: 1042–6.

Hinzpeter EN, Renz S, Loser H. Eye manifestations of fetal alcohol syndrome. *Klin Monatsbl Augenheilkd* 1992; **200**: 33–8.

Hodes BL, Noecker RJ, Prendiville KJ. Autosomal dominant inheritance of iridogoniodysgenesis and cataract. *Ophthalmology* 1993; **100**: 168–72.

Holmström GE, Reardon WP, Baraitser M, Elston JS, Taylor DS. Heterogeneity in dominant anterior segment malformations. *Br J Ophthalmol* 1991; **75**: 591–7.

Hoskins HD, Shaffer RN, Hetherington J. Anatomical classification of developmental glaucomas. *Arch Ophthalmol* 1984a; **102**: 1331–4.

Hoskins HD, Shaffer RN, Hetherington J. Goniotomy vs trabeculectomy. *J Pediatr Ophthalmol Strabismus* 1984b; **20**: 153–7.

Hoyt CS, Billson FA. Buphthalmos in neurofibromatosis: is it an expression of regional giantism? *J Pediatr Ophthalmol Strabismus* 1977; **14**: 228–32.

Iwach AG, Hoskins HD Jr, Hetherington J Jr, Shaffer RN. Analysis of surgical and medical management of glaucoma in Sturge–Weber syndrome. *Ophthalmology* 1990; **97**: 904–9.

Iwata K, Sobue K, Imai A, Sakuvai I. On the reversibility of glaucomatous disc cupping and the visual field. *Jpn J Clin Ophthalmol* 1977; **31**: 759–65.

Izquierdo NI, Maumenee IH, Traboulsi EI. Anterior segment malformations in 18q– (de Grouchy) syndrome. *Ophthal Paediatr Genet* 1993; **14**: 91–4.

Jaafar M, Kazi G. Effect of oral choral hydrate sedation on the intraocular pressure measurement. *J Paediatr Ophthalmol Strabismus* 1993a; **30**: 372–6.

Jaafar M, Kazi G. Normal intraocular pressure in children: a comparative study of the Perkins applanation tonometer and the pneumatonometer. *J Paediatr Ophthalmol Strabismus* 1993b; **30**: 284–7.

Jacoby B, Reed J, Cashwell L. Malignant glaucoma in a patient with Down's syndrome and corneal hydrops. *Am J Ophthalmol* 1990; **110**: 433–4.

Jay MR, Rice NSC. Genetic implications of congenital glaucoma. *Metab Ophthalmol* 1978; **2**: 257–8.

Johnson AT, Drack AV, Kwitek AE, Cannon RL, Stone EM, Alward WL. Clinical features and linkage analysis of a family with autosomal dominant juvenile glaucoma. *Ophthalmology* 1993; **100**: 524–9.

Johnson BL. Ocular pathologic features of arteriohepatic dysplasia (Alagille's syndrome). *Am J Ophthalmol* 1990; **110**: 504–12.

Joos KM, Alward WL, Folberg R. Experimental endoscopic goniotomy. A potential treatment for primary infantile glaucoma. *Ophthalmology* 1993; **100**: 1066–70.

Jorgensen JS, Guthoff R. Sturge–Weber syndrome: glaucoma with elevated episcleral venous pressure (English abstaract). *Klin Monatsbl Augenheilkd* 1987; **191**: 275–8.

Judisch GF, Martin-Casals A, Hanson JW, Olin WH. Oculodentodigital dysplasia: four new reports and a literature review. *Arch Ophthalmol* 1979; **97**: 878–84.

Kampik A, Lund OE, Halbig W. Penetrating keratoplasty in congenital corneal opacities. *Klin Monatsbl Augenheilkd* 1986; **188**: 188–92.

Kanski JJ, McAllister JA. Trabeculodialysis for inflammatory glaucoma in children and young adults. *Ophthalmology* 1985; **92**: 927–30.

Kawa JE, Higginbotham EJ, Chang IL, Yue BY. Effects of antiglaucoma medications on bovine trabecular meshwork cells *in vitro*. *Exp Eye Res* 1993; **57**: 557–65.

Khaw PT, Ward S, Grierson I, Rice NSC. Effect of beta radiation on proliferating human Tenon's capsule fibroblasts. *Br J Ophthalmol* 1991; **75**: 580–3.

Kivlin JD, Carey JC, Richey MA. Brachymesomelia and Peters' anomaly: a new syndrome. *Am J Med Genet* 1993; **45**: 416–19.

Kivlin JD, Fineman RM, Crandall AS, Olson RJ. Peters' anomaly as a consequence of genetic and non-genetic syndromes. *Arch Ophthalmol* 1986; **104**: 61–4.

Kleinmann RE, Kazarian EL, Raptopoulos V, Braverman LE. Primary empty sella and Rieger's anomaly of the anterior chamber of the eye. A familial syndrome. *N Engl J Med* 1981; **304**: 90–3.

Kozma C, Hunt M, Meck J, Traboulsi E, Scribanu N. Familial Wolf–Hirschhorn syndrome associated with Rieger anomaly of the eye. *Ophthalmic Paediatr Genet* 1990; **11**: 23–30.

Koster R, van-Balen AT. Congenital corneal opacity (Peters' anomaly) combined with buphthalmos and aniridia. *Ophthalmic Paediatr Genet* 1985; **6**: 241–6.

Kremer I, Metzker A, Yassur Y. Intraoperative suprachoroidal hemorrhage in congenital glaucoma associated with cutis marmorata telangiectatica congenita. *Arch Ophthalmol* 1991; **109**: 1199–200.

Lang GE, Fleischer-Peters A. Rieger syndrome as an expression of neural crest dysgenesis. *Fortschr Ophthalmol* 1989; **86**: 366–9.

Lee CF, Yue BY, Robin J, Sawaguchi S, Sugar J. Immunohistochemical studies of Peters' anomaly. *Ophthalmology* 1989; **96**: 958–64.

Levy NS. Juvenile glaucoma in the Rubinstein–Taybi syndrome. *J Pediatr Ophthalmol* 1976; **13**: 141–3.

Linn JY. Ultrastructural observations of the anterior chamber angle tissues in congenital glaucoma (English abstract). *Chung Hua Yen Ko Tsa Chih* 1992; **28**: 221–4.

Linn J, Sun W, Li E, Wang S, Bai J, Yang H. Ultrastructural observations of the anterior chamber angle tissues in congenital glaucoma (English Abstract). *Yen Ko Hsueh Pao* 1994; **10(1)**: 50–6.

Liu JC, Ball SF. Nevus of Ota with glaucoma: report of three cases. *Ann Ophthalmol* 1991; **23**: 286–9.

Lotufo D, Ritch R, Szmyd L Jr, Burris JE. Juvenile glaucoma, race, and refraction. *J Am Med Assoc* 1989; **261**: 249–52.

Lotufo DG. Postoperative complications and visual loss following Molteno implantation. *Ophthalmic Surg* 1991; **22**: 650–6.

McMahon CD, Hetherington J Jr, Hoskins HD Jr, Shaffer RN. Timolol and pediatric glaucomas. *Ophthalmology* 1981; **88**: 249–52.

Malone M. The histiocytoses of childhood. *Histopathology* 1991; **19**: 105–19.

Mansour AM. Racial variation of optic disc parameters in children. *Ophthalmic Surg* 1992; **23**: 469–71.

Mawn LA, O'Brien JE, Hedges TR. Congenital glaucoma and skeletal dysplasia. *J Pediatr Ophthalmol Strabismus* 1990; **27**: 322–4.

Mayatepek E, Krastel H, Volcker HE, Pfau B, Almasan K. Congenital glaucoma in cutis marmorata telangiectatica congenita. *Ophthalmologica* 1991; **202**: 191–3.

Mayer UM. Peters' anomaly and combination with other malformations (series of 16 patients). *Ophthalmic Paediatr Genet* 1992; **13**: 131–5.

Mayer UM, Bialasiewicz AA. Ocular findings in a 4p– deletion syndrome (Wolf–Hirschhorn). *Ophthalmic Paediatr Genet* 1989; **10**: 69–72.

Melamed S, Cahane M, Gutman I, Blumthal M. Postoperative complications after Molteno implant surgery. *Am J Ophthalmol* 1991; **111**: 319–22.

Merin S, Morin JD. Heredity of congenital glaucoma. *Br J Ophthalmol* 1972; **56**: 414–17.

Miller M, Israel J, Cuttone J. Fetal alcohol syndrome. *J Pediatr Ophthalmol Strabismus* 1981; **18**: 6–15.

Miller MH, Rice NSC. Trabeculectomy combined with beta radiation for congenital glaucoma. *Br J Ophthalmol* 1991; **75**: 584–9.

Miller MT, Epstein RJ, Sugar J *et al*. Anterior segment anomalies associated with the fetal alcohol syndrome. *J Pediatr Ophthalmol Strabismus* 1984; **21**: 8–18.

Miller SJH. Genetic aspects of glaucoma. *Trans Ophthalmol Soc UK* 1962; **81**: 425–34.

Mills RP, Reynolds A, Emond MJ, Barlow WE, Leen MM. Long-term survival of Molteno glaucoma drainage devices. *Ophthalmology* 1996; **103(2)**: 299–305.

Miranda I, Alonso MJ, Jimenez M, Tomas Barberan S, Ferro M, Ruiz R. Cutis marmorata telangiectatica congenita and glaucoma. *Ophthalmic Paediatr Genet* 1990; **11**: 129–32.

Mirkinson AE, Mirkinson NK. A familial syndrome of aniridia and absence of the patella. *Birth Defects Original Article Series* 1975; **11**: 129–31.

Moller PM. Goniotomy and congenital glaucoma. *Acta Ophthalmol* 1977; **55**: 436–42.

Molteno AC. The dual chamber single plate implant—its use in neovascular glaucoma. *Aust NZ J Ophthalmol* 1990; **18**: 431–6.

Molteno AC, Ancker E, Van Biljon G. Surgical technique for advanced juvenile glaucoma. *Arch Ophthalmol* 1984; **102**: 51–7.

Mora JS, Nguyen N, Iwach AG, Gaffney NM, Hetherington JJ, Hoskins HD, Wong PC, Tran H, Dickens CJ. Trabeculectomy with intraoperative sponge 5-fluorouracil. *Ophthalmology* 1996; **103**: 963–70.

Morier P, Merot Y, Paccaud D, Beck D, Frenk E. Juvenile chronic granulocytic leukemia, juvenile xanthogranulomas, and neurofibromatosis. Case report and review of the literature. *J Am Acad Dermatol* 1990; **22**: 962–5.

Morin JD, Coughlin WR. Corneal changes in primary congenital glaucoma. *Trans Am Ophthalmol Soc* 1980; **78**: 123–31.

Morin JD, Merin S, Sheppard RW. Primary congenital glaucoma; a survey. *Canad J Ophthalmol* 1974; **9**: 17–22.

Moseley M, Thompson J, Deutsch J *et al*. Comparison of the Keeler Pulsair 2000 non-contact tonometer with Goldmann applanation. *Eye* 1993; **7**: 127–30.

Munoz M, Tomey KF, Traverso C, Day SH, Senft SH. Clinical experience with the Molteno implant in advanced infantile glaucoma.

J Pediatr Ophthalmol Strabismus 1991; **28**: 68–72.

Murdoch IA, Dos Anjos R, Parsons JM, Calver DM. Spontaneous hyphaemia in childhood. *Eur J Pediatr* 1991; **150**: 717–18.

Murray JC, Bennett SR, Kwitek AE *et al*. Linkage of Rieger syndrome to the region of the epidermal growth factor gene on chromosome 4. *Nature Genet* 1992; **2**: 46–9.

Myles WM, Flanders ME, Chitayat D, Brownstein S. Peters' anomaly: a clinicopathologic study. *J Pediatr Ophthalmol Strabismus* 1992; **29**: 374–81.

Nelson LB, Spaeth GL, Nowinky TS, Margo CE, Jackson L. Aniridia. A review. *Surv Ophthalmol* 1984; **28**: 621–42.

Nevin NC, Lim JHK. Syndrome of partial aniridia, cerebellar ataxia, and mental retardation—Gillespie syndrome. *Am J Med Genet* 1990; **35**: 468–9.

Niffenegger AS, Walton DS. *Goniotomy for glaucoma complicating chronic anterior uveitis*. Presented as a poster at 20th American Association for Pediatric Ophthalmology and Strabismus meeting, June 1994. Vancouver: Canada.

Nishimura DY, Patil S, Alward WLM, Stone E, Sheffield VC. Mapping the breakpoints of an individual with congenital glaucoma and a 6:13 translocation. *Am J Hum Genet* 1994; **55(3)**(Suppl.): A198.

Noureddin BN, Wilson-Holt N, Lavin M, Jeffrey M, Hitchings RA. Advanced uncontrolled glaucoma. Nd:YAG cyclophotocoagulation or tube surgery. *Ophthalmology* 1992; **99**(3): 430–6; discussion 437.

O'Connor G. Combined trabeculotomy–trabeculectomy for congenital glaucoma. *Br J Ophthalmol* 1994; **78**: 735.

Parks MM, Johnson DA, Reed GW. Long-term visual results and complications in children with aphakia. A function of cataract type. *Ophthalmology* 1993; **100**: 826–40; discussion 840–1.

Parmley VC, Stonecipher KG, Rowsey JJ. Peters' anomaly: a review of 26 penetrating keratoplasties in infants. *Ophthalmic Surg* 1993; **24**: 31–5.

Pasquale LR, Thibault D, Dorman-Pease ME, Quigley HA, Jampel HD. Effect of topical mitomycin C on glaucoma filtration surgery in monkeys. *Ophthalmology* 1992; **99**: 14–18.

Pensiero S, Dapozzo S, Perissulti P, Cavallini G, Guerra R. Normal intraocular pressure in children. *J Paediatr Ophthalmol Strabismus* 1992; **29**: 79–84.

Pham Duy T. Cyclocryotherapy in chronic glaucoma. *Fortschr Ophthalmol* 1989; **86**: 214–20.

Phelps CD, Arafat NI. Open angle glaucoma following surgery for congenital cataracts. *Arch Ophthalmol* 1977; **95**: 1985–7.

Phelps CV. The pathogenesis of glaucoma in Sturge–Weber syndrome. *Ophthalmology* 1978; **85**: 276–81.

Potamis T, Fielder AR. Angle closure glaucoma in Alagille syndrome. *Ophthalmol Paediatr Genet* 1993; **14**: 101–4.

Price FW Jr, Whitson WE. Polypropylene ligatures as a means of controlling intraocular pressure with Molteno implants. *Ophthalmic Surg* 1989; **20**: 781–3.

Quigley HA. Childhood glaucoma: results with trabeculotomy and study of reversible cupping. *Ophthalmology* 1982; **89**: 219–25.

Reed D, Robertson WD, Rootman J, Douglas G. Plexiform neurofibromatosis of the orbit: CT evaluation. *Am J Neuroradiol* 1986; **7**: 259–63.

Rice NSC. Management of infantile glaucoma. *Br J Ophthalmol* 1972; **56**: 294–9.

Richards JE, Lichter PR, Boehnke M *et al*. Mapping of a gene for autosomal dominant juvenile onset open angle glaucoma to chromosome 1q. *Am J Hum Genet* 1994; **54**: 62–70.

Robert Y, Martenet AC, Milano D. Cyclophotocoagulation with the Nd–YAG laser (English abstract). *Klin Monatsbl Augenheilkd* 1990; **196**: 384–6.

Robb RM, Petersen RA. Outcome of treatment for bilateral congenital cataracts. *Ophthalmic Surg* 1992; **23**: 650–6.

Rodman HI. Chronic glaucoma with traumatic dislocation of the lens. *Arch Ophthalmol* 1963; **69**: 445–54.

Rodrigues M, Font RL. Neural crest origin of human trabecular meshwork and its implications for the pathogenesis of glaucoma. *Am J Ophthalmol* 1989; **108**: 469–70.

Rodrigues MM, Newsome DA, Krachmer JH, Sun TT. Posterior polymorphous dystrophy of the cornea: cell culture studies. *Exp Eye Res* 1981; **33**: 535–44.

Romanchuk KG, Judisch GF. Ocular findings in arteriohepatic dysplasia (Alagille's syndrome). *Canad J Ophthalmol* 1981; **16**: 94–9.

Roy SH, Sunjitt RL, Hiatt RL, Hughes J. Ocular manifestations of the Rubenstein–Taybi syndrome. *Arch Ophthalmol* 1968; **74**: 272–4.

Russell-Eggitt IM, Rice NS, Jay B, Wyse RK. Relapse following goniotomy for congenital glaucoma due to trabecular dysgenesis. *Eye* 1992; **6**: 197–200.

Sakamoto T, Tawara A, Inomata H. Goniodysgenesis of the eye with arthrogryposis multiplex congenita. *Ophthalmologica* 1992; **204**: 210–14.

Sarfarazi M, Akarsu AN, Hossain A, Turacli ME, Aktan SG, Barsoum-Homsy M, Chevrette L, Soyli BS. Assignment of a locus (GLC3A) for primary congenital glaucoma (Buphthalmos) to 2p21 and evidence for genetic heterogeneity. *Genomics* 1995; **30(2)**: 171–7.

Sato SE, Herschler J, Lynch PJ, Hodes BL, Fryczkowski AW, Schlossen HD. Congenital glaucoma associated with cutis marmorata telangiectaticacongenita two case reports. *J Pediatr Ophthalmol Strabismus* 1988; **25**: 13–18.

Schuman JS, Jacobson JJ, Puliafito CA, Noecker RJ, Reidy WT. Experimental use of semiconductor diode laser in contact transscleral cyclophotocoagulation in rabbits. *Arch Ophthalmol* 1990; **108(8)**: 1152–7.

Sheffield VC, Stone EM, Alward WLM *et al.* Genetic linkage of familial open angle glaucoma to chromosone 1q21–1q31. *Nature Genet* 1993; **4**: 47–50.

Shields CL, Shields JA, Buchanon HW. Solitary orbital involvement with juvenile xanthogranuloma. *Arch Ophthalmol* 1990; **108**: 1587–9.

Shields MB. Axenfeld–Rieger syndrome: a theory of mechanism and distinctions from the iridocorneal endothelial syndrome. *Trans Am Ophthalmol Soc* 1983; **81**: 736–84.

Shields MB, Buckley E, Klintworth GK, Thresher R. Axenfeld–Rieger syndrome. A spectrum of developmental disorders. *Surv Ophthalmol* 1985; **29**: 387–409.

Shihab ZM, Kristan RW. Recurrent intraoperative choroidal effusion in Sturge–Weber syndrome. *J Pediatr Ophthalmol Strabismus* 1983; **20**: 250–2.

Singh D, Daniel R, Verma M, Akhter Z, Beri RS. Split hand/split foot syndrome with atresia of nasolacrimal ducts and buphthalmos. *Indian Pediatr* 1989; **26**: 1053–5.

Smith MF, Sherwood MB, Doyle JW, Khaw PT. Results of intraoperative 5-fluorouracil supplementation on trabeculectomy for open angle glaucoma. *Am J Ophthalmol* 1992; **114**: 737–41.

Spallone A. Retinal detachment in Axenfeld–Rieger syndrome. *Br J Ophthalmol* 1989; **73**: 559–62.

Storimans CW, van-Schooneveld MJ. Rieger's eye anomaly and persistent hyperplasia primary vitreous. *Ophthalmic Paediatr Genet* 1989; **10**: 257–62.

Sturmer J, Broadway D, Hitchings R. Young patient trabeculectomy: assessment of risk factors for failure. *Ophthalmology* 1993; **100**: 928–39.

Sugar HS. Oculodentodigital dysplasia syndrome with angle closure glaucoma. *Am J Ophthalmol* 1978; **86**: 36–8.

Sullivan TJ, Clarke MP, Heathcote JG, Hunter WS, Rootman DS, Morin JD. Multiple congenital contractures (arthrogryposis) in association with Peters' anomaly and chorioretinal colobomata. *J Pediatr Ophthalmol Strabismus* 1992a; **29**: 370–3.

Sullivan TJ, Clarke MP, Morin JD. The ocular manifestations of the Sturge–Weber syndrome. *J Pediatr Ophthalmol Strabismus* 1992b; **29**: 349–56.

Summers CG, Letson RD. Is the phakic eye normal in monocular pediatric aphakia? *J Pediatr Ophthalmol Strabismus* 1992; **29**: 324–7.

Susanna Junior R. Modification of the Molteno implant and implant procedure. *Ophthalmic Surg* 1991; **22**: 611–13.

Tabuchi A, Matsuura M, Hirokawa M. Three siblings with Peters' anomaly. *Ophthalmic Paediatr Genet* 1985; **5**: 205–12.

Talbot EM, Pitts JF, Dudgeon J, Lee WR. A case of developmental glaucoma presenting with abdominal colic and subnormal intraocular pressure. *J Pediatr Ophthalmol Strabismus* 1992; **29**: 116–19.

Tawara A, Inomata H. Developmental immaturity of the trabecular meshwork in juvenile glaucoma. *Am J Ophthalmol* 1984; **98**: 82–97.

Theodossiadis G, Damanakis A, Koutsandrea C. Choroid effusion in an antiglaucoma operation in a child with Sturge–Weber syndrome (English abstract). *Klin Monatsbl Augenheilkd* 1985; **186**: 300–2.

Traboulsi EI, Levine E, Mets MB, Parelhoff ES, O'Neill JF, Gaasterland DE. Infantile glaucoma in Down's syndrome (trisomy 21). *Am J Ophthalmol* 1988; **105**: 389–95.

Traboulsi EI, Maumenee IH. Peters' anomaly and associated congenital malformations. *Arch Ophthalmol* 1992; **110**: 1739–42.

Treacy KW, Letson RD, Summers CG. Subconjunctival steroid in the management of uveal juvenile xanthogranuloma: a case report. *J Pediatr Ophthalmol Strabismus* 1990; **27**: 126–8.

Tripathi BJ, Tripathi RC. Neural crest origin of human trabecular meshwork and its implications for the pathogenesis of glaucoma. *Am J Ophthalmol* 1989; **107**: 583–90.

Valtot F, Denis P. The treatment of failed trabecular surgery in glaucoma with ultrasound (Sonocare). *Ophtalmologie* 1990; **4**: 142–4.

van-Schooneveld MJ, Delleman JW, Beemer FA, Bleeker-Wagemakers EM. Peters' plus: a new syndrome. *Ophthalmic Paediatr Genet* 1984; **4**: 141–5.

Vaux C, Sheffield L, Keith CG, Voullaire L. Evidence that Rieger syndrome maps to 4q25 or 4q27. *J Med Genet* 1992; **29**: 256–8.

Verbraak FD, Pogany K, Pilon JW *et al.* Congenital glaucoma in a child with partial 1q duplication and 9p deletion. *Ophthalmic Paediatr Genet* 1992; **13**: 165–70.

Verloes A, Dodinval P. Rieger anomaly and uveal coloboma with associated anomalies. Third observation of a rare oculopalato–osseous syndrome: the Abruzzo–Erikson syndrome. *Ophthalmic Paediatr Genet* 1990; **11**: 41–7.

Vernon SA. Reproducibility with the Keeler Pulsair 2000 non-contact tonometer. *Br J Ophthalmol* 1995; **79**: 554–7.

Walton DS. Aniridia with glaucoma. In: Chandler PA, Grant WM, eds. *Glaucoma*. Philadelphia: Lea & Feibiger, 1979: 351–4.

Walton DS. Aniridic glaucoma: the results of gonioscopy to prevent and treat this problem. *Trans Am Ophthalmol Soc* 1986; **84**: 59–70.

Warburg M. Hydrocephaly, congenital retinal non-attachment, and congenital falciform fold. *Am J Ophthalmol* 1978; **85**: 88–94.

Waring GO, Laibson PR, Rodriguez M. Clinical and pathologic alteration of Descemet's membrane. *Surv Ophthalmol* 1974; **18**: 325–68.

Waring GO, Rodriguez MM, Laibson PR. Anterior chamber cleavage syndrome. A stepladder classification. *Surv Ophthalmol* 1975; **20**: 3–14.

Watson GH, Miller V. Arteriohepatic dysplasia. Familial pulmonary arterial stenosis with neonatal liver disease. *Arch Dis Child* 1973; **48**:

459–66.

Wertelecki W, Dev VG, Superneau DW. Abnormal centromere–chromatid apposition (ACCA) and Peters' anomaly. *Ophthalmic Paediatr Genet* 1985; **6**: 247–55.

Weiss BI, Cooper LZ, Breen RH. Infantile glaucoma: a manifestation of congenital rubella. *J Am Med Assoc* 1966; **195**: 727–7.

Weissman BA, Ehrlich M, Levenson JE, Pettit TH. Four cases of keratoconus and posterior polymorphous corneal dystrophy. *Optom Vis Sci* 1989; **66**: 243–6.

Wenzel M, Krippendorff U, Hunold W, Reim M. Corneal endothelial damage in congenital and juvenile glaucoma. *Klin Monatsbl Augenheilkd* 1989; **195**: 344–8.

Wiggins R, Tomey K. The results of glaucoma surgery in aniridia. *Arch Ophthalmol* 1992; **110**: 503–5.

Wiggs JL, Del Bono EA, Schuman JS, Hutchinson BT, Walton DS. Clinical features of five pedigrees genetically linked to the juvenile glaucoma locus on chromosome 1q21–q31. *Ophthalmology* 1995; **102**: 1782–9.

Wilson ME. Congenital iris ectropion and a new classification for anterior segment dysgenesis. *J Pediatr Ophthalmol Strabismus* 1990; **27**: 48–55.

Winter RM, Garner A. Hydrocephalus, agyria, pseudo encephalocele, retinal dysplasia, and anterior chamber anomalies. *J Med Genet* 1981; **18**: 314–17.

Young TL, Schaffer DB, Cohen AR. Infantile glaucoma associated with the Diamond–Blackfan syndrome. *J Paediatr Ophthalmol Strabismus* 1992; **29**: 55–8.

Yumita A, Shirato S, Yamamoto T, Kitazawa Y. Goniotomy with Q-switched Nd–YAG laser in juvenile developmental glaucoma: a preliminary report. *Jpn J Ophthalmol* 1984; **28**: 349–55.

Zamzam AM, Sherherrif SMM, Phillips CI. Aniridia, ectopia lentis, abnormal incisors and mental retardation—an autosomal recessive syndrome. *Jpn J Ophthalmol* 1988; **32**: 375–8.

Zanella FE, Kirchhof B. Computer tomography findings of orbital changes within the scope of juvenile neurofibromatosis. *Klin Monatsbl Augenheilkd* 1986; **188**: 57–9.

Zauberman H, Sira IB. Glaucoma and Rieger's syndrome. *Acta Ophthalmol* 1970; **48**: 118–26.

Zelger B, Cerio R, Orchard G, Wilson-Jones E. Juvenile and adult xanthogranuloma. A histological and immunohistochemical comparison. *Am J Surg Pathol* 1994; **18**: 126–35.

Zimmerman LE. Ocular lesions of juvenile xanthogranuloma. *Trans Am Acad Ophthalmol Otolaryngol* 1965; **69**: 412–22.

41: Vitreous

Anthony Moore

The vitreous is a transparent gelatinous structure which fills the posterior four-fifths of the globe. It is firmly attached to the pars plana anteriorly and has a loose attachment to the retina and optic nerve posteriorly. In childhood there is also a firm attachment between the vitreous and posterior aspect of the lens.

The development of the vitreous body and zonule can be divided into three stages (Duke-Elder 1963). The primary vitreous is formed during the first month of development and is seen as a vascularized mesodermal tissue separating the developing lens vesicle and the neuroectoderm of the optic cup. This primary vitreous contains the branches of the hyaloid artery which continues to develop in early embryonic life but regresses during the formation of the secondary vitreous.

The secondary vitreous starts to form at 9 weeks (410 mm stage) (Spencer 1985) and continues to develop throughout embryonic life and during the rapid increase in size of the globe in early infancy. The secondary vitreous, which ultimately forms the established vitreous body, is avascular and transparent and displaces the primary vitreous which becomes condensed into a narrow band (Cloquet's canal) running from the optic disc to the posterior aspect of the lens. By the third month (70 mm stage) the secondary vitreous fills most of the developing vitreous cavity; the remnants of the primary vitreous are confined to a central area. The vitreous lying between the developing ciliary body and lens becomes clearly separated from the secondary vitreous and by the 110 mm stage well-formed fibrils run from the ciliary processes to the lens; this so-called tertiary vitreous later develops into the zonule.

Developmental anomalies of the vitreous

Persistence of the primary vitreous or part of its structure may give rise to a number of abnormalities of the vitreous which may remain in postnatal life.

Persistent hyaloid artery

Persistence of all, or more frequently part, of the hyaloid artery is one of the more common congenital abnormalities of the eye. Remnants of the hyaloid artery are seen in about 3% of normal full-term infants but are commonly seen in premature infants (Jones 1963) during examination for retinopathy of prematurity. Most of these regress and persistence of the whole artery is uncommon. Rarely

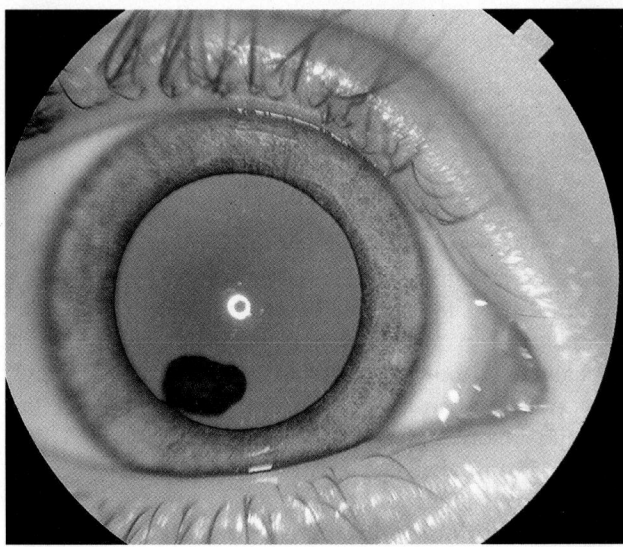

Fig. 41.1 Anterior vitreous cyst seen in retroillumination. The acuity was 6/5 and the eye otherwise healthy.

the whole artery may run from the optic disc to the posterior aspect of the lens. Posterior remnants may give rise to a single vessel running from the centre of the disc or to an elevated bud of glial tissue — the Bergmeister's papilla. Anterior remnants of the hyaloid system may be seen as a small white dot on the posterior lens capsule—the Mittendorf's dot. This does not interfere with vision and does not progress. It is often confused with a posterior cortical lens opacity.

Vitreous cysts

Cysts of the vitreous (Fig. 41.1) may be congenital or acquired; acquired cysts may be seen in association with ocular toxoplasmosis or toxocariasis, and rarely with juvenile retinoschisis (Lusky *et al.* 1988). Congenital cysts are usually found in otherwise normal eyes (François 1950; Bullock 1974; Feman & Straatsma 1974). The origin of the cysts is unknown but as blood vessels are sometimes seen within the cyst it has been suggested that they may develop from hyaloid artery remnants (François 1950). No histopathology is available.

Cysts may lie in the anterior vitreous immediately behind the lens (Hilsdorf 1965; Lisch & Rochels 1989) or in the posterior vitreous (François 1950; Bullock 1974; Feman & Straatsma 1974). They may be mobile (Bullock 1974; Elkington & Watson 1974; Feman & Straatsma 1974; Lisch & Rochels 1989) or be attached to the lens (Lisch & Rochels 1989) or optic disc (François 1950).

Persistent hyperplastic primary vitreous
(see also Chapter 39)

Persistent hyperplastic primary vitreous (PHPV), first

characterized by Reese in 1949, is a congenital abnormality of the eye caused by failure of the primary vitreous to regress. Most cases are sporadic and unilateral although there may be minor abnormalities such as a Mittendorf dot in the fellow eye. Bilateral and familial cases have been reported (Menchini *et al.* 1987; Storimans & van Schooneveld 1989; Lin *et al.* 1990) although some of these may be examples of vitreoretinal dysplasia. PHPV may occasionally be seen in association with other ocular abnormalities such as megalocornea (Burke & O'Keefe 1988), Rieger's anomaly (Storimans & van Schooneveld 1989), morning glory disc anomaly (Cennamo *et al.* 1989) and retinal vascular hypoplasia (Sneed *et al.* 1988). Bilateral persistence of the hyaloid system has been described in the oculodigitodental syndrome, a rare autosomal recessive syndrome affecting the eyes, nose, teeth and bones (Guttierez Diaz *et al.* 1982; Traboulsi *et al.* 1986).

Histopathologically, a plaque of fibrous tissue is adherent to the back of the lens and often extends from the ciliary processes in one region to another. There is a variable degree of vascularization and fat, smooth muscle and cartilaginous material may also be present in the retrolental mass (Reese 1955; Font *et al.* 1969). Liang *et al.* (1985) have reported an unusual case of a child with unilateral leucocoria who had the affected eye enucleated. Pathological examination revealed a diffuse retinoblastoma infiltrating a persistent primary vitreous; this however, is an exceptional case and should not lead one to enucleate cases of PHPV.

Pruett and Schepens (1970) have described a posterior form of PHPV. This condition usually presents with strabismus or nystagmus and the ocular abnormality is confined to the posterior segment (Rubinstein 1980). A retinal fold runs from the optic disc to the ora serrata and there is associated condensation of the vitreous and retinal detachment. It is debatable whether this condition, described by other authors as congenital retinal fold, is really a variant of PHPV or really more closely related to vitreoretinal dysplasia.

Clinical features

The typical presentation of anterior PHPV is with unilateral leucocoria, which is recognized by the paediatrician or parent soon after birth. The affected eye is microphthalmic, the anterior chamber is shallow and there may be dilated radial iris vessels. A vascularized retrolental membrane (Figs 41.2, 41.3) is present and the ciliary processes may be drawn into the fibrous tissue. Although the lens may initially be clear, a posterior cortical cataract often develops. Nystagmus may be present even in unilateral cases and strabismus is common. A persistent hyaloid artery is common (Fig. 41.4).

The condition often progresses and there may be shallowing of the anterior chamber, cataract formation and

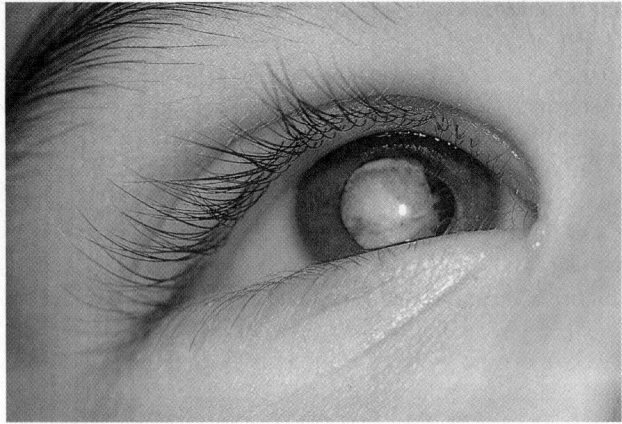

Fig. 41.2 PHPV. A yellowish, partly absorbed cataract is seen in front of a retrolental membrane with the ciliary processes stretched towards it.

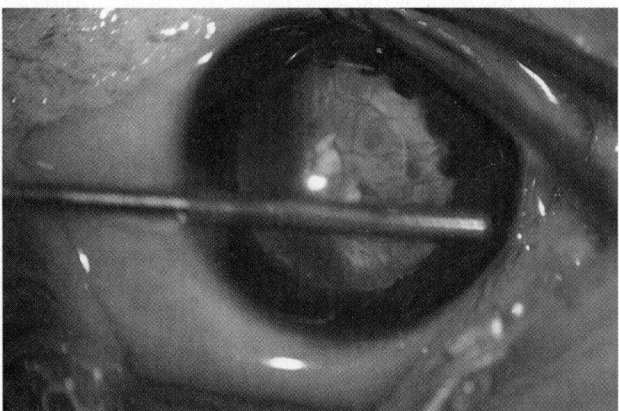

Fig. 41.3 PHPV with vascularized retrolental membrane. There was a large persistent hyaloid artery. If removed sufficiently early, and optically corrected together with occlusion of the fellow eye, useful acuity may sometimes be salvaged.

pupil block glaucoma. The lens may absorb and haemorrhage into the lens is not infrequent. Other complications include vitreous haemorrhage, retinal detachment and phthisis bulbi.

Posterior PHPV may present with leucocoria, strabismus or nystagmus. The affected eye is often microphthalmic and the lens is usually clear. Further examination usually shows a fold of condensed vitreous (Figs 41.5, 41.6) and retina running from the disc to the ora serrata and there may be an associated subtotal retinal detachment (Pruett & Schepens 1970; Pollard 1985).

The differential diagnosis of PHPV is that of leucocoria. The presence of microphthalmia and elongated ciliary processes helps to differentiate it from other causes of retrolental mass. Ultrasound and computed tomography (CT) scan are useful in differentiating PHPV from retinoblastoma where there is uncertainty about the clinical diagnosis (Goldberg & Mafee 1983).

Management

The main aim of management in PHPV is to avoid the complications of glaucoma and phthisis bulbi and allow the child to retain the eye. Enucleation should be avoided as not only is the result of a prosthesis less acceptable cosmetically but also enucleation in early infancy is associated with decreased growth of the bony orbit on the affected side and marked facial asymmetry (Kennedy 1965).

Intraocular surgery may be undertaken for visual or cosmetic reasons or to prevent glaucoma caused by anterior chamber shallowing. A limbal or pars plicata approach with vitrectomy instruments may be used to remove the lens and abnormal retrolental tissue (Stark *et al.* 1983; Pollard 1985). Intraocular scissors may be required to excise dense fibrous tissue and intraocular haemorrhage can be controlled by raising the infusion bottle or the use of intraocular diathermy. In this way it is possible to obtain a clear visual axis, deepen the anterior chamber and prevent angle closure glaucoma. A more controversial aspect of management is whether attempts should be made to

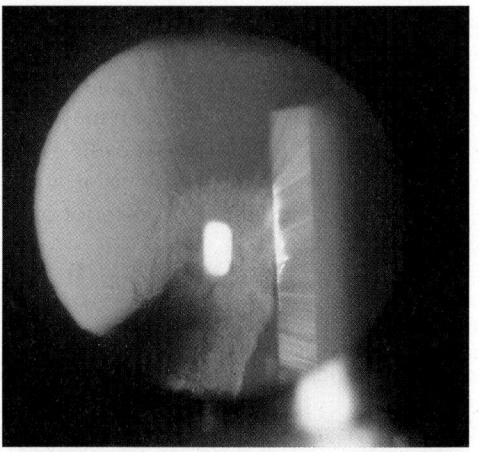

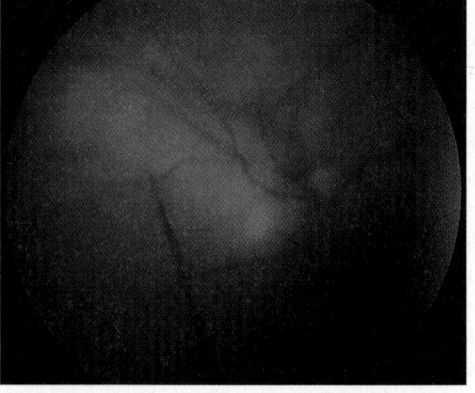

Fig. 41.4 (a) PHPV. There is a plaque on the posterior surface of the lens with strands (visible in the slit) extending to the ciliary processes. In the bottom left there is a dense condensation which goes posteriorly, extending to the optic nerve. (b) Same patient as in (a) showing the hyaloid vessel from the posterior aspect of the PHPV plaque extending towards the optic disc.

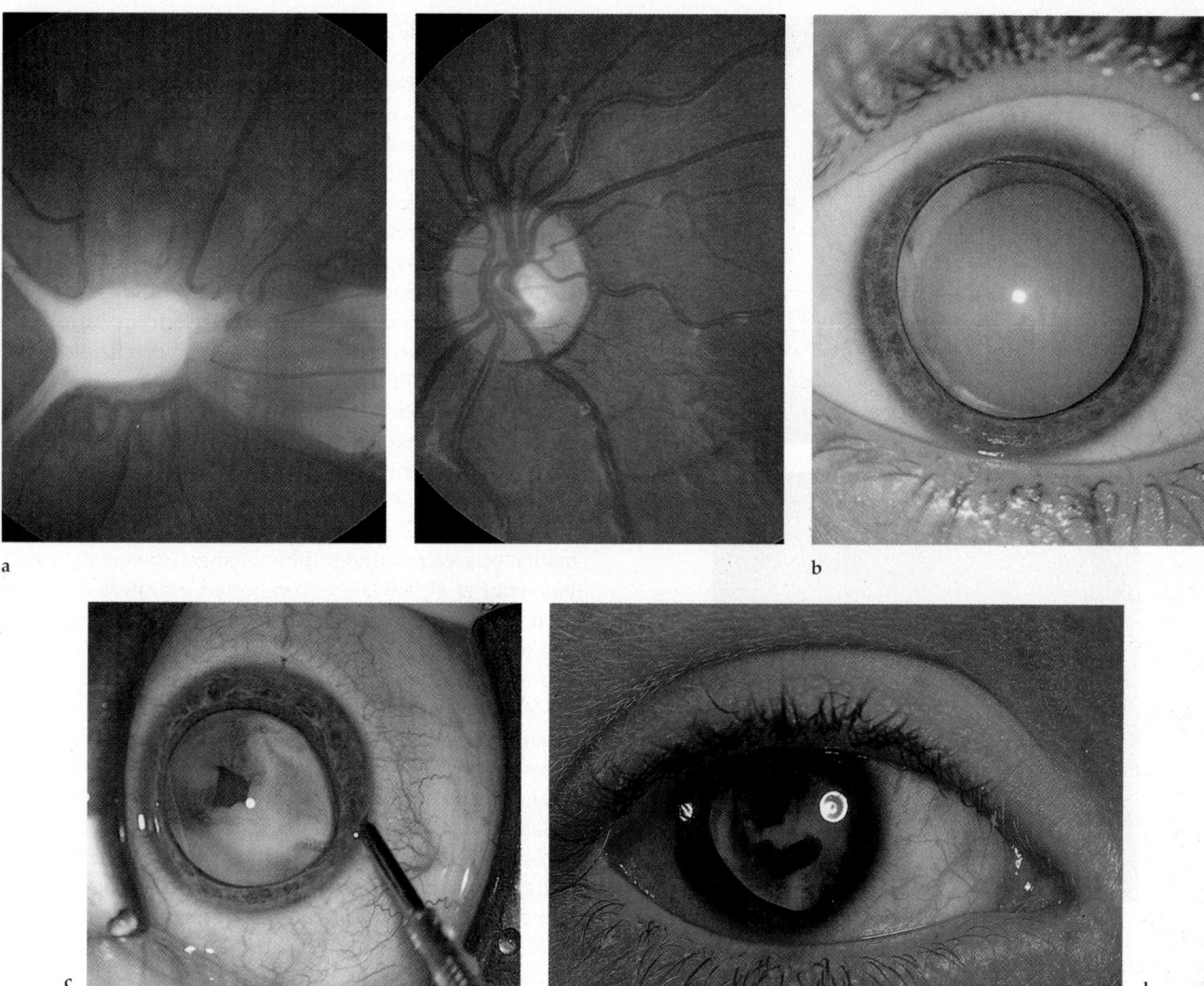

Fig. 41.5 (a) Posterior PHPV. This child presented with a right esotropia aged 1 year. There was a white fibrotic macular scar. (b) At age 2.5 years he had a dense retrolental membrane, retinal detachment, cataract and shallow anterior chamber. (c) After lensectomy, the hole in the membrane behind the cataract revealed an extensive fibrotic retinal detachment. (d) Over the next 10 years he had recurrent intraocular haemorrhage but no evidence of mass formation.

obtain a visual result by optical correction of the affected eye and a vigorous patching regime. The good results of surgery in some infants with unilateral congenital cataract (Beller *et al.* 1981; Lewis *et al.* 1986) has led to the adoption of a similar approach in the treatment in PHPV and some good visual results have been reported (Stark *et al.* 1983; Pollard 1985; Karr & Scott 1986). This aggressive approach should be reserved for those infants who present early and whose parents are sufficiently motivated to co-operate with the handling of contact lenses and intensive occlusion therapy.

Vitreoretinal dysplasia

Maldevelopment of the vitreous and retina is seen as an isolated ocular abnormality (Lahav *et al.* 1973; Ohba *et al.* 1981) or may be associated with a variety of systemic abnormalities. Several distinct syndromes such as Norrie's disease (Norrie 1927; Warburg 1961, 1963), incontinentia pigmenti (Carney & Carney 1970; Carney 1976; François 1984; Landy & Donnai 1993; Goldberg & Custis 1993) and Warburg's syndrome (Warburg 1971; Pagon *et al.* 1983) have bilateral vitreoretinal dysplasia as a common finding. It is also found in trisomy 13, trisomy 18, triploidy and in association with a variety of cerebral malformations (Fulton *et al.* 1978; Bernado *et al.* 1991). In experimental animals, certain virus infections can induce retinal dysplasia (Silverstein *et al.* 1971).

Glaucoma is a frequent complication, not rare as suggested by Preslan *et al.* (1985), but may be difficult to diag-

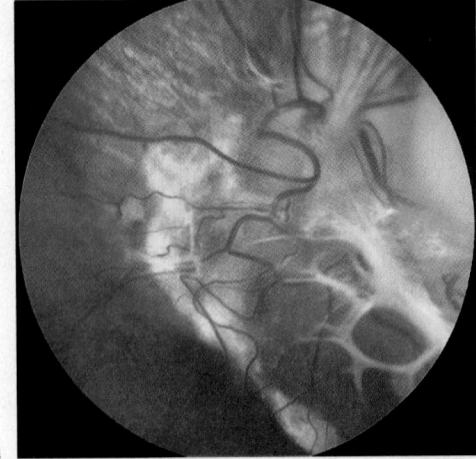

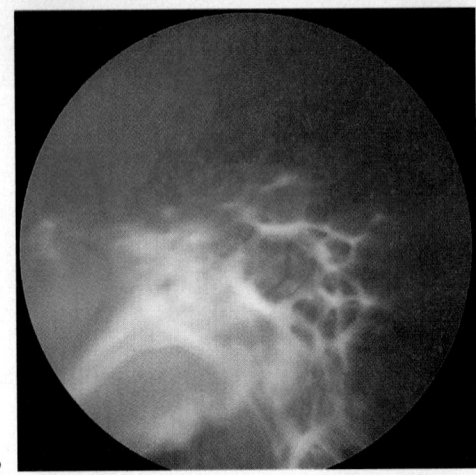

Fig. 41.6 (a, b) An extensive vitreoretinal dysplasia, possibly a form of posterior PHPV.

nose: often the rise in intraocular pressure is transient and not marked. The clues are central corneal oedema, increased corneal diameter with splits in Descemet's membrane and a shallow anterior chamber which may be obliterated first centrally then peripherally (Preslan *et al.* 1985).

The pathological findings have been reviewed by Lahav *et al.* (1973) and there appears to be no relationship between the histological findings and the various different syndromes in which retinal dysplasia is a frequent finding. The dysplastic retina contains a variety of rosettes which resemble retinoblastoma rosettes but contain Muller cells with an abnormal relationship between the retina and its pigment epithelium (Fulton *et al.* 1978).

Norrie's disease

Norrie's disease is an X-linked recessive disorder in which affected males are blind at birth or early infancy (Norrie 1927; Warburg 1961, 1963; Lieberfarb *et al.* 1985). About 25% of affected males are mentally retarded and about one-third develop cochlear hearing loss, which may develop at any time from infancy to adult life (Parving & Warburg 1977). The ocular findings include bilateral retinal folds, retinal detachment, vitreous haemorrhage and bilateral retrolental masses (vitreoretinal dysplasia). The retinal detachments are usually of early onset and have been observed *in utero* by abdominal ultrasonography (Redmond *et al.* 1993). Most cases progress to an extensive vitreoretinal mass and bilateral blindness. Angle closure glaucoma may develop in some infants and this is best managed by limbal or pars plicata lensectomy. Late signs (Fig. 41.7) include corneal opacification, band keratopathy and phthisis bulbi. Pathological examination of a vitreoretinal biopsy specimen from an infant with Norrie's disease suggests that there is an arrest of normal retinal development during the third or fourth months of gestation (Enyedi *et al.* 1991).

Carrier females do not usually show any ocular abnormality or electroretinographic change (Joos *et al.* 1994). Woodruff *et al.* (1993) have reported an affected female born to a mother who was a carrier of Norrie's disease. The female infant had a retrolental mass in the right eye and a retinal fold with a tractional retinal detachment in the left. Molecular genetic testing confirmed that she was a manifesting heterozygote (Chen *et al.* 1993c) and further investigation showed evidence of skewed X-inactivation in her peripheral blood lymphocytes suggesting that her retinal abnormalities were due to random inactivation occurring more frequently in the normal rather than the mutant X chromosome (Chen *et al.* 1993c; Black & Redmond 1994). Another female with Norrie's disease, with an X autosome translocation has been described (Ohba & Yamashita 1986).

The Norrie's disease gene was identified in 1992 (Berger *et al.* 1992; Chen *et al.* 1992) and mutations of the gene have been identified in families with Norrie's disease (Chen *et al.* 1993a,b; Wong *et al.* 1993; Zhu & Maumenee 1994). The gene has three exons (the first of which is not translated) and is expressed in both ocular and extraocular tissues (Black & Redmond 1994). The protein product is similar in structure to the mucins and also to growth factors (Meindl *et al.* 1992; Meitinger *et al.* 1993) which are known to play a role in ocular development (Matsuo *et al.* 1993). Mutations of the Norrie's disease gene may also be responsible for another rare retinal disorder, X-linked familial exudative retinopathy (see below). The identification of the Norrie's disease gene has allowed molecular genetic diagnosis of the carrier state and prenatal diagnosis (see Chapter 10).

Trisomy 13

Trisomy 13 (Patau's syndrome) was first characterized by Patau *et al.* (1960); it is the chromosomal abnormality most consistently associated with severe ocular defects. The

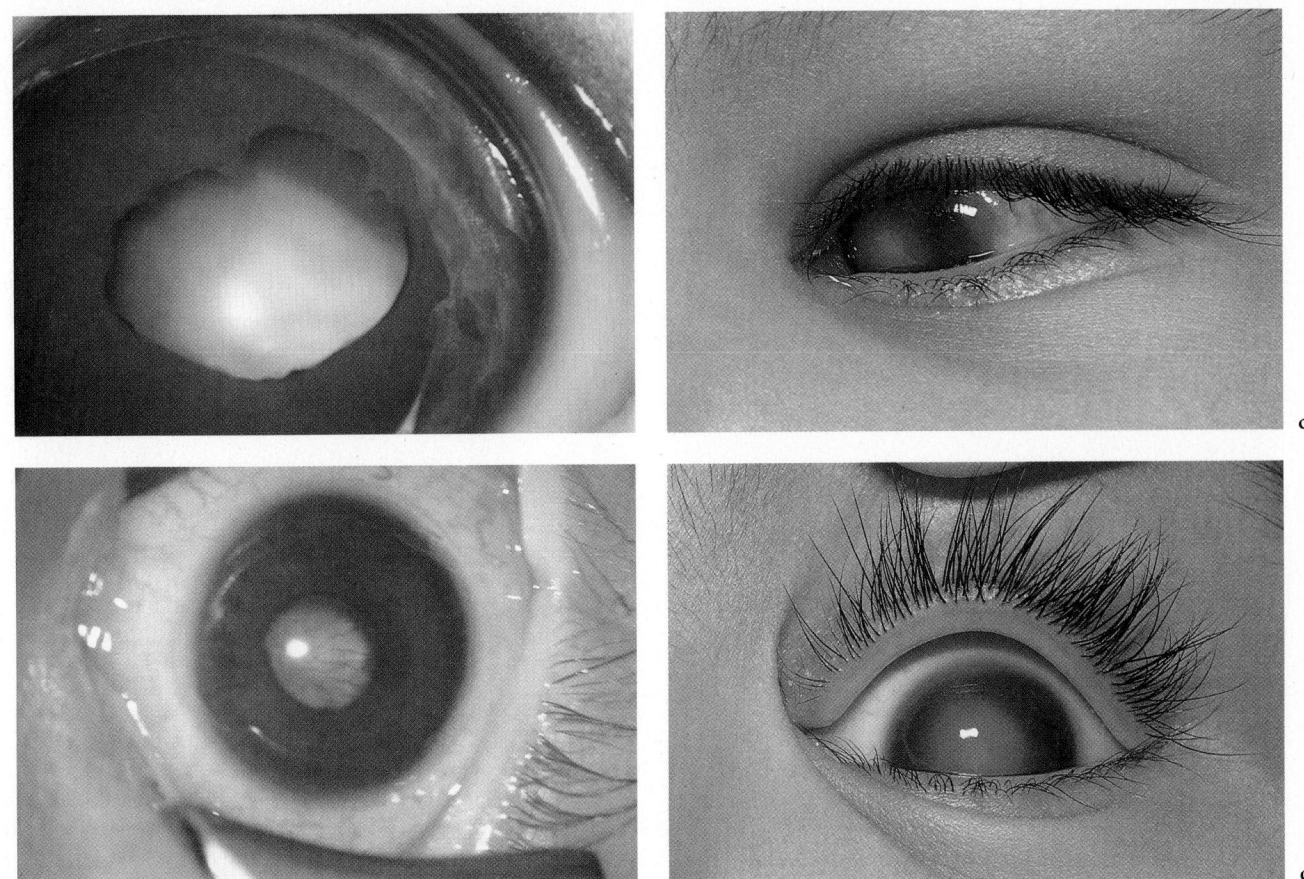

Fig. 41.7 (a) Norrie's disease showing posterior synechiae, shallow anterior chamber and retrolental white mass. (b) Norrie's disease. Brother of patient in (a) showing vascularized white retrolental mass. (c, d) Norrie's disease with flat anterior chambers and apical lens–cornea adhesions.

most common systemic abnormalities are microcephaly, cleft palate, congenital cardiac defects, polydactyly, skin haemangiomas, umbilical hernia and malformation of the central nervous system (Patau *et al.* 1960; Smith *et al.* 1963; Taylor 1968). Most affected children die within the first few months of life.

Bilateral ocular abnormalities are seen in almost all cases of trisomy 13 (Smith *et al.* 1963); the common ocular findings are detailed in Table 41.1. Affected infants often show total disorganization of vitreous and retina and histological examination of eyes obtained at postmortem has confirmed the presence of extensive retinal dyspla-sia (Sergovich *et al.* 1963; Yannoff *et al.* 1963; Cogan & Kuwabara 1964). Intraocular cartilage is frequently found (Cogan & Kuwabara 1964) and may be a characteristic abnormality.

Incontinentia pigmenti (Bloch–Sulzberger syndrome)

Incontinentia pigmenti is an uncommon familial disorder affecting the skin, bones, teeth, central nervous system and eyes. It is thought to be inherited as an X-linked dominant disorder which is usually lethal in the male, leading to a marked female predominance. The gene for the familial form of incontinentia pigmenti has been mapped by linkage studies to the Xq28 region (Sefiani *et al.* 1989; Landy & Donnai 1993). The characteristic skin lesions (Fig. 41.8) usually appear soon after birth with a linear eruption of bullae which predominantly affects the extremities. The bullae gradually resolve to leave a linear pattern of pigmentation (Carney & Carney 1970; Landy & Donnai 1993). The other systemic features have recently been reviewed by Landy and Donnai (1993).

Ocular abnormalities occur in the majority of cases and include amblyopia, strabismus, nystagmus, cataract, optic

Table 41.1 Ocular abnormalities in trisomy 13.

Microphthalmos
Coloboma of the uveal tract
Cataract
Corneal opacities
Retinal dysplasia
PHPV
Dysplastic optic nerves
Cyclopia

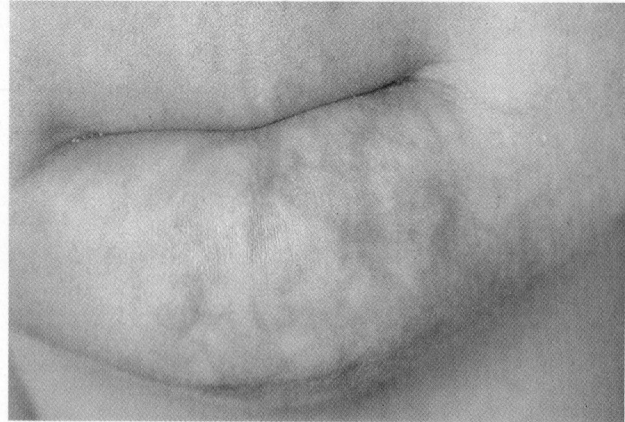

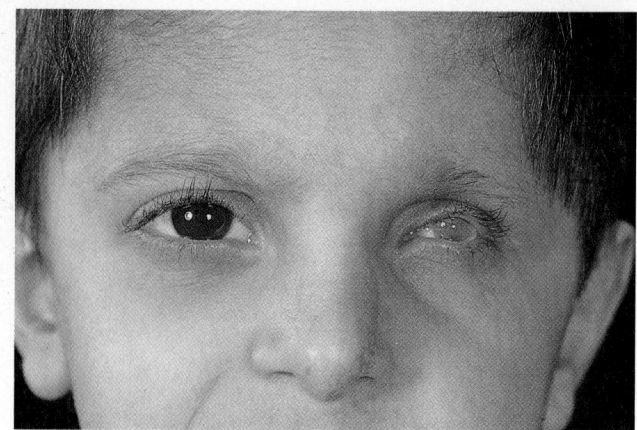

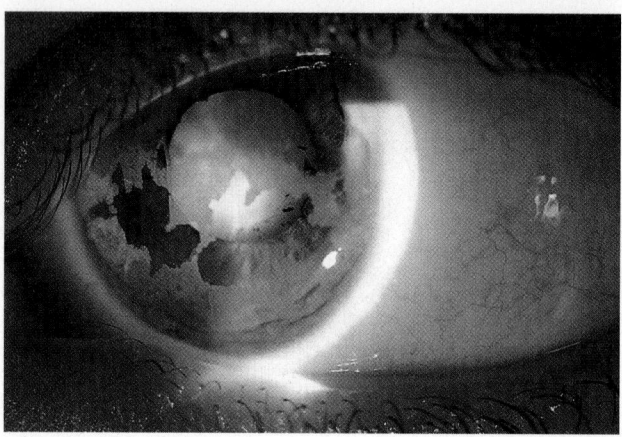

Fig. 41.8 (a) Incontinentia pigmenti showing pigmented skin lesions on chin. (b) Pigmented skin lesions on nose and phthisis bulbi of the left eye. (c) Incontinentia pigmenti. Severe vitreoretinal dysplasia with incipient phthisis bulbi, cataract and band keratopathy.

atrophy and a variety of retinal changes (Carney 1976; Weaver *et al.* 1991; Goldberg & Custis 1993; Wald *et al.* 1993). The most serious complication is retinal detachment which, if bilateral, may lead to severe visual impairment. Retinovascular abnormalities are common and include retinal vascular tortuosity, capillary closure and peripheral arteriovenous shunts (Watzke *et al.* 1976; François 1984; Spallone 1987;Weaver *et al.* 1991; Goldberg & Custis 1993; Wald *et al.* 1993). These changes are most marked in the temporal periphery and may be associated with pre-retinal fibrosis. Tractional retinal detachments are seen in a minority of patients (Catalano *et al.* 1990; Goldberg & Custis 1993; Wald *et al.* 1993). Fluorescein angiography demonstrates areas of non-perfusion in the temporal periphery (Watzke *et al.* 1976) and it is likely that these vascular anomalies may represent an early stage in the development of retinal detachment and 'pseudoglioma' (Brown 1988; Goldberg & Custis 1993; Wald *et al.* 1993). Affected females should be assessed by an ophthalmologist at regular intervals during early childhood as it is possible that early cryotherapy or photocoagulation of the retinovascular abnormalities may prevent progression of the ocular disease (Watzke *et al.* 1976; Brown 1988; Catalano *et al.* 1990; Rahi & Hungerford 1990). Established retinal detachment presents a difficult

management problem but may respond to vitreoretinal surgery (Wald *et al.* 1993).

Walker–Warburg syndrome (HARD ± E)

The acronym HARD ± E stands for hydrocephalus, agyria, retinal dysplasia, with or without encephalocoele (Fig. 41.9).

This is an autosomal recessive oculocerebral syndrome characterized by type II lissencephaly, retinal dysplasia, cerebellar malformation and congenital muscular dystrophy (Warburg 1971; Pagon *et al.* 1983; Dobyns *et al.* 1989; Rodgers *et al.* 1994). Hydrocephalus is a common feature, which is a helpful ultrasonographic sign in prenatal diagnosis. Other variable features include Dandy–Walker malformation and encephalocoele. Death often occurs in the neonatal period and survivors are severely retarded (Warburg 1971; Pagon *et al.* 1983). The ocular features in this disorder are variable and include micropthalmia, Peters' anomaly, cataract, retinal coloboma and retinal dysplasia.

Autosomal recessive vitreoretinal dysplasia

Vitreoretinal dysplasia may occur as an isolated abnor-

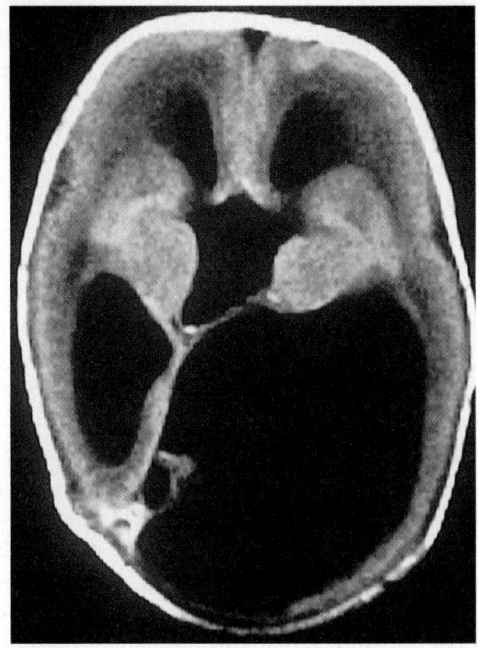

Fig. 41.9 (a) Walker–Warburg syndrome showing the eye with a shallow anterior chamber and a retrolental mass. (b) Walker–Warburg syndrome. CT scan showing hydrocephalus, lissencephaly and colpocephaly.

mality in an otherwise healthy child (Lahav *et al.* 1973; Phillips *et al.* 1973; Ohba *et al.* 1981). The usual presentation is with bilateral poor vision in early infancy and nystagmus; examination reveals a shallow anterior chamber and white retrolental mass. Progressive shallowing of the anterior chamber may lead to pupil block glaucoma which, if it fails to respond to mydriatics, may require lensectomy.

Osteoporosis–pseudoglioma–mental retardation syndrome

Neuhauser *et al.* (1976) delineated a syndrome, thought to be autosomal recessive, with osteoporosis, mental retardation and what was probably a form of vitreoretinal dysplasia. Over 20 cases have been described, and the gene

locus may be on chromosome 6 (De Paepe *et al.* 1993).

Oculopalatal–cerebral dwarfism

Frydman *et al.* (1985) described three siblings with vitreoretinal dysplasia and a number of other systemic abnormalities including microcephaly, mental retardation, cleft palate and short stature. The ocular abnormalities, which resembled those seen in PHPV, were bilateral in one child and unilateral in the other two. The parents were first cousins once removed suggesting that this rare syndrome is probably inherited as an autosomal recessive trait.

Unilateral retinal dysplasia

Lloyd *et al.* (1993) have reported an unusual family in which three affected members had unilateral retinal dysplasia without any evidence of any related systemic abnormalities. This appears to be a unique report.

Genetic counselling in the vitreoretinal dysplasias

The vitreoretinal dysplasias are a genetically heterogeneous group of disorders which result in a similar ocular abnormality; it is not possible to subdivide the disorders on the basis of the clinical or pathological ocular findings (Lahav *et al.* 1973), so that the specific diagnosis depends on the presence of associated systemic findings although the family history may suggest the likely mode of inheritance.

For the purposes of genetic counselling families fall into two groups. In the first group the diagnosis (and hence the mode of inheritance) of the affected child is clear. The second, more problematic, group are those families in which a child is born without a family history and with isolated retinal dysplasia and no associated systemic findings.

In the first group counselling is relatively straightforward. When one child has been born with a trisomy the risk of a similar affected child in a future pregnancy is about 1%, but may be higher if one of the parents has a structural chromosome abnormality or mosaicism (Steve *et al.* 1984). Such parents may be offered prenatal diagnosis. In children with the systemic features of Walker–Warburg syndrome (HARD ± E) or the osteoporosis–pseudoglioma–mental retardation syndrome the inheritance is autosomal recessive and the parents can be counselled accordingly.

In Norrie's disease there are no detectable clinical abnormalities in the carrier female to aid counselling. When there is another affected male relative the mother can be assumed to be a carrier and counselled accordingly. In isolated boys, one-third are thought to represent new mutations and in two-thirds the mothers are carriers. In the absence of any carrier tests based on DNA analysis there is an overall risk of a further son being affected of one in three. Now that the Norrie's disease gene has been identified it is possible to screen for mutations of the gene. If a mutation is identified in the child it is possible to look for the same mutation in his mother and give definite risk estimates based on molecular genetic diagnosis (see Chapter 10). Such molecular genetic techniques using mutation detection or DNA polymorphisms closely linked to the gene may be used for carrier detection or prenatal diagnosis in families with Norrie's disease (Black & Redmond 1994).

Counselling a family with an otherwise normal child born with bilateral retinal dysplasia is more difficult. Isolated retinal dysplasia is sufficiently rare that there are insufficient empirical data to aid counselling. If the affected child is female retinal dysplasia may be autosomal recessive or be non-genetic; since autosomal recessive dysplasia is rare, so long as there is no parental consanguinity the recurrence risk is likely to be low. In an affected male child the retinal dysplasia may be recessive, X-linked or non-genetic, and the risk of a subsequent affected child is higher. Molecular genetic testing if available will enable mutations of the Norrie's disease gene to be excluded.

Inherited vitreoretinal dystrophies

Goldmann–Favre disease

This rare autosomal recessive condition was first described by Favre in 1958 (Favre 1958) and since then at least 25 further cases have been reported (Lisch 1983). The usual presentation is with gradual visual loss or night-blindness and the abnormal ocular findings include liquefaction of the vitreous, macular retinoschisis and peripheral retinal pigment epithelial atrophy and pigmentation (Carr & Siegel 1970; Lisch 1983). Peripheral retinoschisis and secondary cataract may also occur. The retinal dystrophy is progressive resulting in extensive visual field loss and variable central visual loss. Fluorescein angiography may show evidence of peripheral capillary closure and vascular leakage (Fishman *et al.* 1976). The electro-oculogram (EOG) is usually subnormal and the electroretinogram (ERG) is extinguished, or markedly abnormal. Jacobsen *et al.* (1991) have studied four patients with the Goldmann–Favre syndrome using spectral ERG and have demonstrated that the short wavelength (S) cones are less affected than the mid-spectral cones. There may be some overlap between Goldmann–Favre syndrome and the enhanced S-cone syndrome where there is hypersensitivity of the short wavelength cones (Jacobsen *et al.* 1990) (see Chapter 44). Although the macular appearance may be similar, the vitreous changes, peripheral retinopathy, ERG abnormalities and mode of inheritance help differentiate this condition from X-linked juvenile retinoschisis and inherited forms of isolated foveal schisis.

Wagner's syndrome

Wagner in 1938 (Wagner 1938) described a dominantly inherited vitreoretinal dystrophy occurring in 13 affected individuals from one Swiss family. The family was subsequently re-examined by Bohringer *et al.* (1960) and Ricci (1961) and additional affected members were added to the pedigree.

Affected members are myopic (generally less than 3 dioptres) and show vitreous and retinal abnormalities. The vitreous appears optically empty apart from scattered translucent membranes: there is usually a posterior vitreous detachment with a thickened posterior hyaloid. Peripheral vascular sheathing is common and is normally associated with perivascular retinal pigment epithelial atrophy and pigment deposition. The ERG is subnormal and parallels the chorioretinal pathology. Cataract commonly develops between the ages of 20 and 30 years and is the usual cause of visual loss.

There is considerable confusion in the literature about Wagner's syndrome; in Wagner's original family there was no associated retinal detachment or systemic abnormalities and the term Wagner's syndrome should be confined to families which fit this phenotype rather than being used to describe inherited vitreoretinal degeneration, high myopia and retinal detachment in individuals without systemic abnormalities.

Wagner's disease and erosive vitreoretinopathy share some clinical features; they both have subnormal ERGs, poor night vision and field defects which are not found in COL2A1-associated Stickler's syndrome. Retinal detachment is uncommon in Wagner's, but occurs in 50% of Stickler's and erosive vitreoretinopathy. Brown *et al.* (1995) have linked Wagner's and erosive vitreoretinopathy to 5q13–14, and suggested that they are allelic disorders, distinct from COL2A1-associated Stickler's syndrome.

The relationship between the different forms of vitreoretinal degeneration will have to await further elucidation of the molecular genetic basis of these disorders.

Inherited vitreoretinal degeneration and retinal detachment

Stickler *et al.* (1965) described a large autosomal dominant pedigree in which affected members had progressive myopia, retinal detachment and a progressive arthropathy which began in childhood. Patients have a characteristic facial appearance caused by malar hypoplasia and a flattened nasal bridge and also may have sensorineural hearing loss.

Since Stickler's early report it has become clear that vitreoretinal degeneration similar to that seen in Wagner's syndrome may be associated with a variety of bone dysplasias and clefting syndromes. These disorders, which probably result from defects in collagen synthesis or metabolism, have been reviewed by Deutmann (1977) and Maumenee (1979). Maumenee (1979) has classified them into eight different types on the basis of their ocular and systemic findings. Most of these disorders carry a high risk of retinal detachment, which tends to occur at an early age, and are associated with giant retinal tears of multiple posterior retinal breaks (Billington *et al.* 1985). In some families there are the typical ocular features but systemic features are absent but in contrast to Wagner's syndrome there is a high incidence of retinal detachment. Clinical classification is on the whole unsatisfactory and the relationship between the different clinical groups will not be defined until the molecular genetic basis of these disorders is identified.

The management of the complex detachments seen in these families entails the use of closed intraocular microsurgery and silicon oil, and prophylaxis with 360° cryotherapy of the fellow eye should be considered (see Chapter 47).

Molecular genetic basis of vitreoretinal degeneration and retinal detachment

Type II collagen is a major component of secondary vitreous and articular cartilage, and mutations of the genes responsible for its structural proteins are obvious candidate genes for Stickler's syndrome and allied disorders. Francomano *et al.* (1987) first established linkage between the COL2A1 gene (which encodes for type II alpha procollagen) and Stickler's syndrome; this linkage has been confirmed in a number of other studies (Priestley *et al.* 1990; Ahmad *et al.* 1991, 1993; Brown *et al.* 1992, 1994; Korko *et al.* 1993; Snead *et al.* 1994). Several different mutations of this gene have been identified in families with Stickler's syndrome (Ahmad *et al.* 1991, 1993; Brown 1992; Brown *et al.* 1994) and a closely related disorder, Kniest's syndrome (Wilkin *et al.* 1993; Winterpacht *et al.* 1993; Bogaert *et al.* 1994). Other families, including those who have the purely ocular phenotype, do not show linkage to this gene (Knowlton *et al.* 1989; Fryer *et al.* 1990; Vintiner *et al.* 1991; Bonaventure *et al.* 1992; Snead *et al.* 1994) indicating that there is molecular genetic as well as clinical heterogeneity. Snead *et al.* (1994) have suggested that Stickler's syndrome can be divided into two types on the basis of the appearance of the vitreous on slit-lamp biomicroscopy and that families with a characteristic congenital vitreous anomaly (Stickler type 1) are associated with mutations of the COL2A1 gene, whereas those without this anomaly are not linked. Mutations of COL2A1 gene may be responsible for disease in families which have isolated ocular disease as well as those with skeletal and other systemic abnormalities suggesting that much of the variability in the phenotype is due to allelic heterogeneity (Ahmad *et al.* 1991; Brown *et al.* 1992; Ahmad *et al.* 1993, Korko *et al.*

1993). Brunner *et al.* (1994) reported linkage to chromosome 6 near the COL11A2 gene in a family with the systemic features of Stickler's syndrome but without any ophthalmological signs. The exact relationship between the different vitreoretinal disorders with high myopia and retinal detachment will have to await the identification of other genetic mutations responsible for these disorders.

Myelinated nerve fibres, vitreoretinopathy and skeletal malformations

Traboulsi *et al.* (1993) described a new syndrome characterized by a severe vitreoretinal degeneration, high myopia, myelinated nerve fibres and skeletal abnormalities occurring in a mother and her daughter. Both had severe visual impairment and roving eye movements, and electrophysiological testing in the mother showed an abnormal scotopic and photopic ERG. The ocular and systemic findings are distinct from those seen in Stickler's syndrome.

Juvenile X-linked retinoschisis

This X-linked disorder is seen almost exclusively in males. Macular abnormalities, predominantly foveal schisis, are seen in virtually all cases (Fig. 41.10) and in 50% are the only fundoscopic abnormality (Deutmann 1971, 1977; George *et al.* 1996b). The characteristic foveal retinoschisis has been described in early infancy (Pischel 1969), but most children present between the ages of 5 and 10 years either with reading difficulties or when they fail the school eye test. The visual acuity is usually in the range 6/12–6/36 at presentation and strabismus and hyperopic and astigmatic refractive errors are common. In children with subtle macular changes the condition is often misdiagnosed as strabismic or ametropic amblyopia or functional visual loss (George *et al.* 1996b). Asymptomatic individuals may be found on routine examination when a close relative has the disorder. Less commonly, sudden vitreous haemorrhage from a ruptured vessel in a vitreous veil may be the presenting sign. A small subgroup of patients present in infancy with nystagmus and strabismus and are found on fundus examination to have highly elevated bullous retinoschisis which involves the macula (Conway & Welch 1977; Kawano *et al.* 1981; George *et al.* 1995a). The bullous schisis usually regresses spontaneously leaving a flat retina with a pigment demarcation line (Fig. 41.11) which may involve the macula (Kawano *et al.* 1981; George *et al.* 1995a).

The foveal retinoschisis is easily missed unless a careful examination of the macular region is made with slit-lamp biomicroscopy. The schisis is seen as small microcysts associated with radial linear folds running out from the centre of the fovea. These changes are often better appreciated with a red-free light. In older patients the foveal schi-

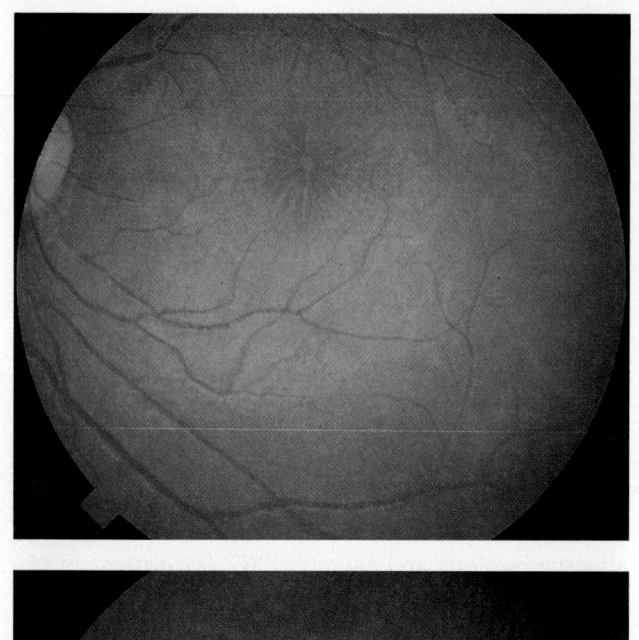

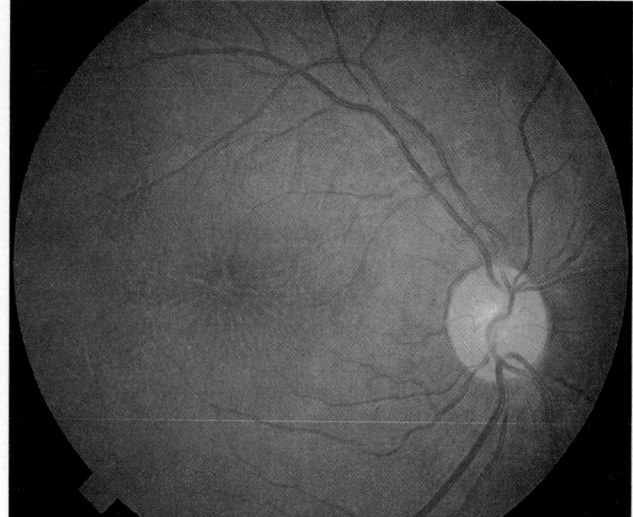

a

b

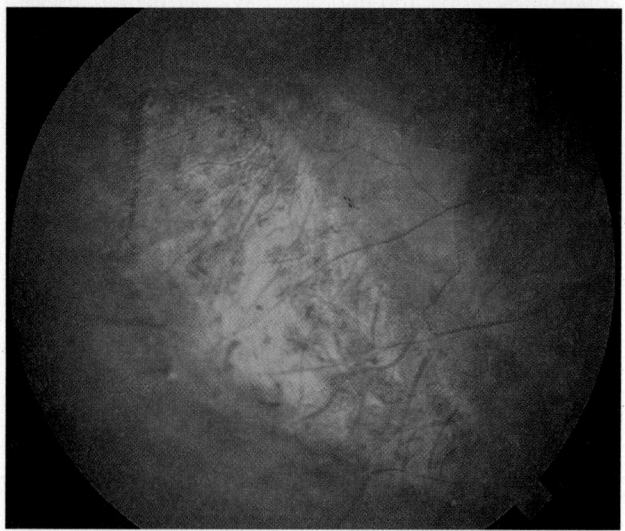

c

Fig. 41.10 (a, b) Juvenile X-linked retinoschisis. Bilateral foveal retinoschisis. (c) Same patient showing peripheral pigmentary changes in an area of schisis.

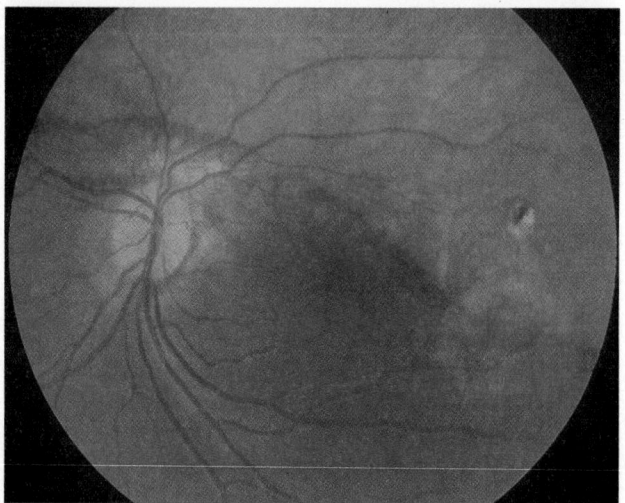

Fig. 41.11 Infantile retinoschisis showing the fundus after a bullous retinoschisis cyst has resolved leaving a flat retina with a pigment demarcation line, in this case involving the macula (Mr Anthony Moore's patient).

sis regresses leaving either a blunted foveal reflex or retinal pigment epithelial and receptor atrophy (George *et al.* 1996b). Foveal schisis may also be seen in other rare retinal dystrophies such as the Goldmann–Favre syndrome and autosomal dominant and recessive foveal schisis. These can be distinguished from X-linked retinoschisis by the mode of inheritance and different clinical and electrophysiological abnormalities (see Chapter 9).

Fifty per cent of patients with X-linked retinoschisis will also show a typical peripheral retinoschisis (Deutman 1977; George *et al.* 1996b) usually in the lower temporal quadrant (Fig. 41.12). In contrast to senile retinoschisis the split occurs in the nerve fibre layer. Inner leaf breaks are common and the thin fragmented inner layer of the schisis may give rise to membranous structures (vitreous veils) on the posterior hyaloid face (Fig. 41.13). Vessels bridging the inner leaf breaks or vitreous veils may bleed giving rise to vitreous haemorrhage. Other peripheral retinal changes (Table 41.2 on p. 508) include pigmentary

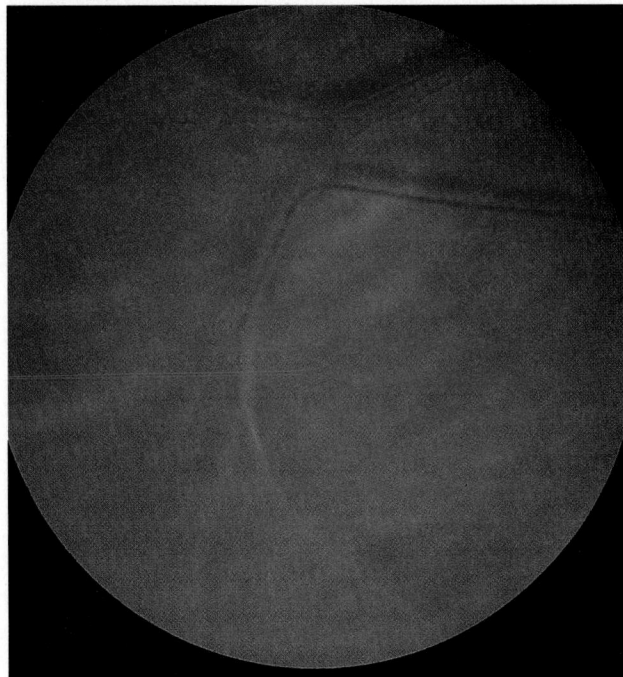

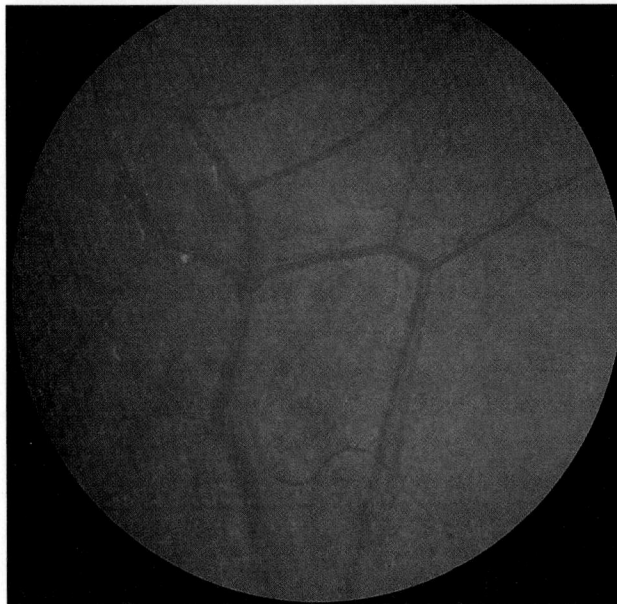

Fig. 41.12 (a, b) Juvenile X-linked retinoschisis. Peripheral schisis with vessels visible in the schitic strands. Vitreous haemorrhage is not uncommon.

retinopathy, perivascular sheathing, capillary closure, grey–white dendritiform appearance on the inner surface of the retina and even frank neovascularization (Pearson & Jagger 1989; George *et al.* 1996b). A fleck retinal appearance (Fig. 41.14) similar to fundus albipunctatus has also been described (van Schooneveld & Miyake 1994). A tapetal-like reflex is also common (Fig. 41.15) and this may show a different appearance depending on the state of

dark adaptation of the eye (Mizuo phenomenon) (de Jong *et al.* 1991; George *et al.* 1996b). Retinal detachment may complicate X-linked retinoschisis but the true incidence is not known (George *et al.* 1996b).

Fluorescein angiography is usually normal in childhood but progression of the macular changes during adult life may lead to retinal pigment epithelial atrophy and an associated hyperfluorescence. The EOG is normal but the ERG shows a reduced or absent b-wave in the presence of a normal a-wave (see Chapter 9). Other inner retinal responses such as the oscillatory potentials and scotopic threshold responses are also abnormal in X-linked retinoschisis (Peachey *et al.* 1987; Murayama *et al.* 1991). Female carriers have a normal fundus appearance and normal EOG and ERG. Arden *et al.* (1988) have demonstrated that carrier females show absence of normal

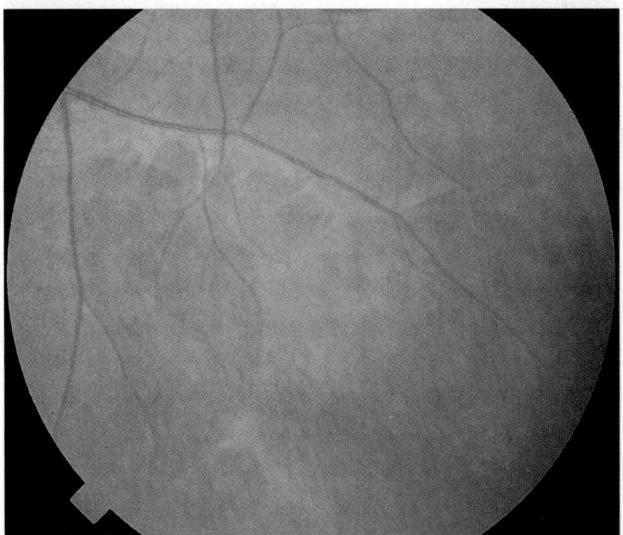

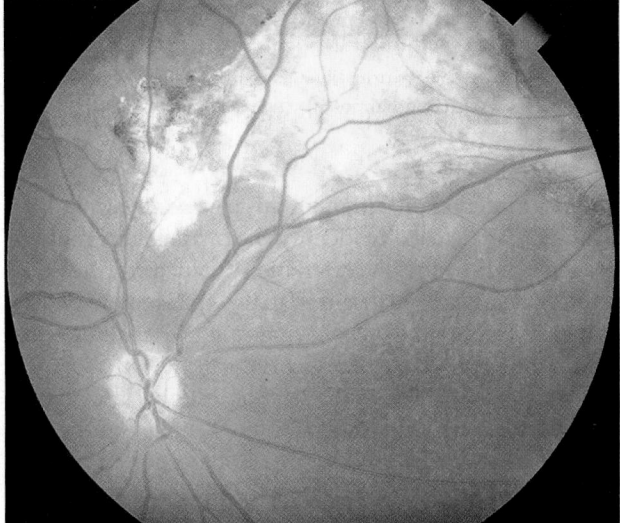

Fig. 41.13 (a) Juvenile X-linked retinoschisis. Peripheral schisis. (b) Same patient. Arcuate subretinal lesion probably due to subretinal haemorrhage.

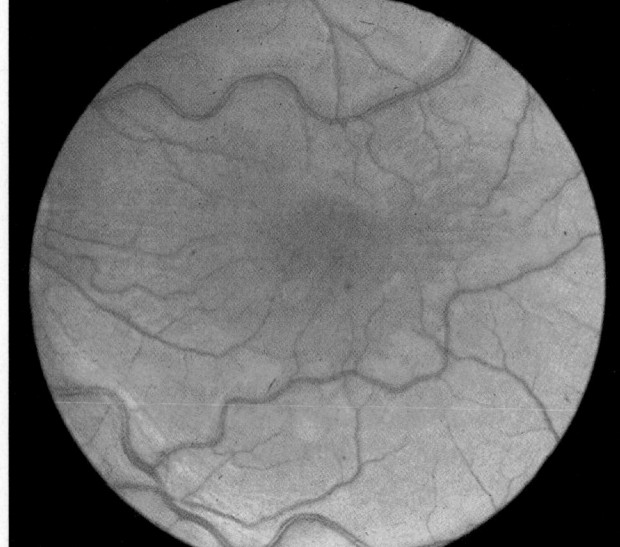

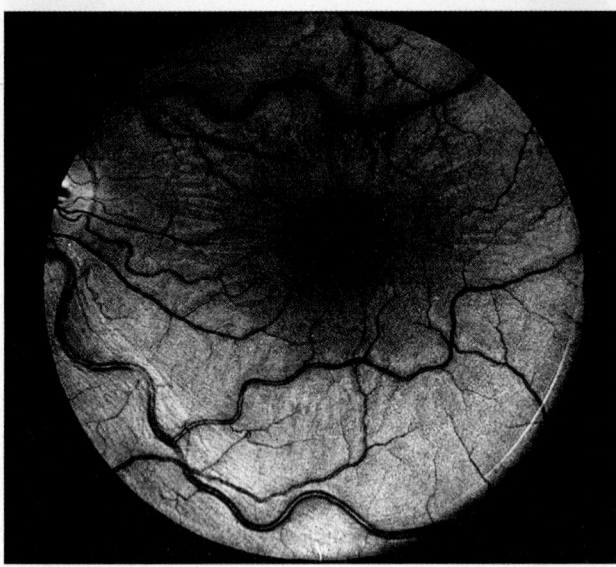

Fig. 41.14 The foveal abnormality in juvenile X-linked retinoschisis (a) is best seen with ophthalmoscopy using a red free light (b) (Mr Anthony Moore's patient).

rod–cone interaction; although this psychophysical investigation may be used to identify the carrier state, molecular genetic diagnosis is preferable. The locus for X-linked retinoschisis has been localized to the Xp22 region (Dahl & Ulf 1988; Dahl *et al.* 1988; Sieving *et al.* 1990; Alitalo *et al.* 1991b; Wieacker *et al.* 1983; George *et al.* 1996a) and there are available a large number of highly informative microsatellite markers that flank the X-linked retinoschisis locus that can be used for carrier detection. It is likely that the X-linked retinoschisis gene will be cloned within a few years.

Histopathological examination of eyes from patients with X-linked retinoschisis have shown there to be a split occurring in the nerve fibre layer (Yanoff *et al.* 1968; Man-

schot 1972). Yanoff *et al.* (1968) has suggested that the condition may be caused by a widespread defect in Muller's cells, which would be in keeping both with the histological picture and the electrophysiological evidence of abnormality of the b-wave.

The visual prognosis in this disorder is relatively good (George *et al.* 1996b). Central vision deteriorates very slowly with most patients retaining stable vision until the fifth or sixth decade when macular atrophy may develop. Peripheral fields are usually normal unless there is a peripheral retinoschisis or retinal detachment. Most patients do not require surgical treatment although vitreoretinal surgery may be indicated for persistent vitreous haemorrhage or retinal detachment. Laser photocoagulation has been successfully employed to treat the rare cases of optic disc or retinal neovascularization (Brodrick & Wyatt 1973; Pearson & Jagger 1989). The majority of children will require conservative management with correction of any high refractive errors, treatment of amblyopia and the use of low vision aids where appropriate. It is important that the parents and other family members are referred for genetic counselling.

Familial exudative vitreoretinopathy

Familial exudative retinopathy is a term used to describe a group of inherited disorders in which there is evidence of abnormal retinal vascularization which may be associated with exudation, neovascularization and tractional retinal detachment; the retinal appearances show some similarities to cicatricial retinopathy of prematurity. Two main forms of familial exudative retinopathy are recognized. The autosomal dominant form, first described by

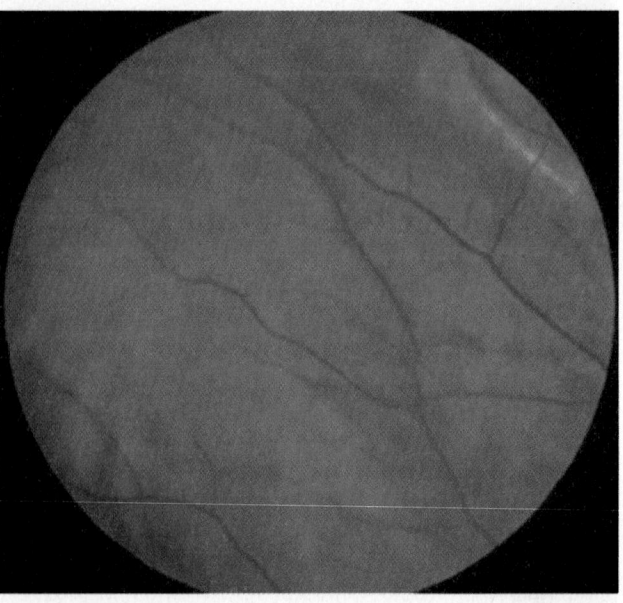

Fig. 41.15 The sheen-like reflex seen in some patients with juvenile retinoschisis (Mr Anthony Moore's patient).

Criswick and Schepens (1969), has been mapped by linkage analysis to the long arm of chromosome 11 (Li *et al.* 1992a, b). A related disorder, autosomal dominant neovascular inflammatory vitreoretinopathy, maps to the same region (Stone *et al.* 1992) although it is not clear whether the two disorders are caused by mutations of the same gene or of two different but adjacent genes. The X-linked form of familial exudative vitreoretinopathy, which has an earlier age of onset, has been shown to map to either Xp21.3 or at Xp11 (Fullwood *et al.* 1993). The latter region includes the gene for Norrie's disease, and Chen *et al.* (1993a) have recently identified a point mutation of this gene in a family with X-linked familial exudative vitreoretinopathy which appears to segregate with the disease suggesting that these two disorders are allelic (in other words different mutations of the same gene may give rise to a different but well-defined phenotype).

Autosomal dominant familial exudative vitreoretinopathy (FEVR)

Criswick and Schepens (1969) reported six children from two families with a progressive vitreoretinopathy which resembled retrolental fibroplasia. The children were otherwise normal and there was no history of prematurity or oxygen use. Gow and Oliver (1971) were able to demonstrate autosomal dominant inheritance in their family and divided the clinical course into three stages (Table 41.3). Since then many additional families have been reported

Table 41.2 Fundus abnormalities in X-linked juvenile retinoschisis (George *et al.* 1996b).

Macular changes
Foveal schisis
'Blunted' foveal reflex
Macular atrophy
Macular coloboma
Pigment line

Peripheral retinal abnormalities
Peripheral schisis
Vitreous veils
Inner leaf breaks

Vascular abnormalities
Vascular sheathing
Capillary closure
Optic disc neovascularization
Peripheral retinal neovascularization
'Dendritiform figures'
'Dragged' retinal vessels

Pigmentary retinopathy

Flecked retina

Inner retinal reflex

(Canny & Oliver 1976; Ober *et al.* 1980; Swanson *et al.* 1982; Chaudhuri *et al.* 1983; Feldman *et al.* 1983; Miyakubo *et al.* 1984; Barondes & Hamilton 1989; van Nouhuys 1991) and it is evident that there is a wide range of clinical expression. Chaudhuri *et al.* (1993) described a platelet aggregation defect which appeared to segregate with the disease in two families with autosomal dominant familial exudative vitreoretinopathy (FEVR) but this finding has not been confirmed in a subsequent study (van Nouhuys 1991) and no other systemic abnormalities have been documented.

Although eyes from patients with FEVR have been examined histopathologically (van Nouhuys 1982; Boldrey *et al.* 1985), in each case the disease was too advanced to help our understanding of the underlying pathogenesis (van Nouhuys 1982; Boldrey *et al.* 1985). Clinically there appears to be a widespread abnormality of the retinal vasculature which may be due to developmental arrest of normal vasculogenesis (van Nouhuys 1991). In the mildest form of the disease patients are usually asymptomatic but fundoscopy and fluorescein angiography reveals retinovascular abnormalities of the peripheral retina, particularly on the temporal side (Figs 41.16, 41.17). These include vascular dilatation and tortuosity, arteriovenous shunting, capillary closure and peripheral retinal neovascularization (van Nouhuys 1982; Miyakubo *et al.* 1984; van Nouhuys 1991). Optic disc neovascularization is less common (Barondes & Hamilton 1989). Vitreoretinal adhesions are frequently seen at the border between vascularized and non-vascularized retina, and other peripheral retinal changes include retinal pigmentation and intraretinal white deposits (Miyakubo *et al.* 1984). More advanced cases show evidence of vascular leakage, and cicatrization with macular ectopia, tractional retinal detachment and macular oedema (Fig. 41.18). Vitreous haemorrhage and secondary retinal rhegmatogenous retinal detachment may develop in advanced disease. Although the retinal changes may progress throughout childhood, progression is rare after the age of 20 years

Table 41.3 Classification of autosomal dominant familial exudative vitreoretinopathy (Gow & Oliver 1971).

Stage I
Mild peripheral retinal changes with abnormal vitreous traction but no evidence of retinal vascular or exudative change

Stage II
Dilated tortuous vessels between the equator and ora serrata with subretinal exudates and localized retinal detachment. Dragging of disc vessels and macular ectopia is often present

Stage III
Advanced disease with total retinal detachment and extensive vitreoretinal traction. There may be secondary cataract and rubeosis iridis

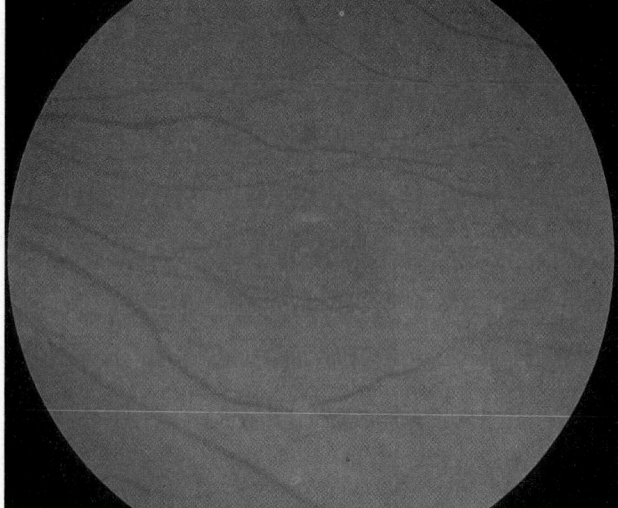

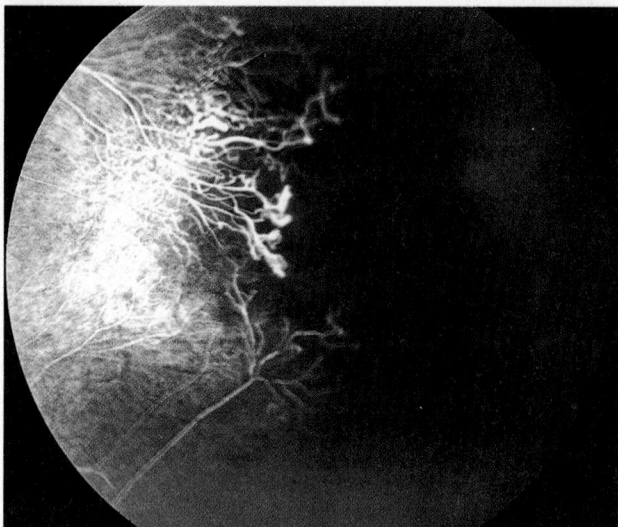

Fig. 41.16 Dominant exudative vitreoretinopathy showing minimal peripheral changes with vascular dilatation and shunting (Mr Anthony Moore's patient).

(Ober *et al.* 1980). In children who show progression from stage I disease cryotherapy of peripheral ischaemic retina may be indicated (Gow & Oliver 1971).

Although FEVR may cause severe visual impairment in childhood the majority of gene carriers are asymptomatic and have only minor retinovascular abnormalities. The gene is thought to be almost fully penetrant and in counselling families with this disorder it is important to perform a careful fundoscopic examination, preferably with fluorescein angiography, before excluding carrier status.

X-linked familial exudative retinopathy

This uncommon disorder is characterized by retinovascular abnormalities including neovascularization and cicatricial retinal detachment (Dudgeon 1979; Plager *et al.* 1992; Fullwood *et al.* 1993). The phenotype may be indis-

tinguishable from the severe form of dominant exudative vitreoretinopathy and may also resemble what has been described as congenital falciform retinal folds. Affected males have severe visual impairment of early onset and a characteristic feature is the prominent retinal folds running from the disc to the ora serrata. This disorder may be allelic with Norrie's disease (Chen *et al.* 1993a; Fullwood *et al.* 1993).

Other vitreoretinal degenerations

Autosomal dominant vitreoretinochoroidopathy

This uncommon dystrophy is characterized by abnormal chorioretinal pigmentation involving a 360° circumference between the vortex veins and the ora serrata. There are areas of hypo- and hyperpigmentation and scattered yellow dots may be seen in the peripheral retina and at the posterior pole. There is usually associated retinovascular changes with retinal arteriolar narrowing, venous occlusion and widespread vascular leakage (Kaufman *et al.* 1982; Blair *et al.* 1984; Traboulsi & Payne 1993). A sharp demarcation line is seen between the normal and abnormally vascularized retina. The vitreous is abnormal with diffuse liquefaction with areas of condensation peripherally. Presenile cataract occurs in a high proportion of cases. Fluorescein angiography shows areas of capillary dilatation and diffuse vascular leakage; peripheral neovascularization may develop in a small proportion of cases (Kaufmann *et al.* 1982). Nyctalopia is not a prominent symptom and the ERG is normal in most affected individ-

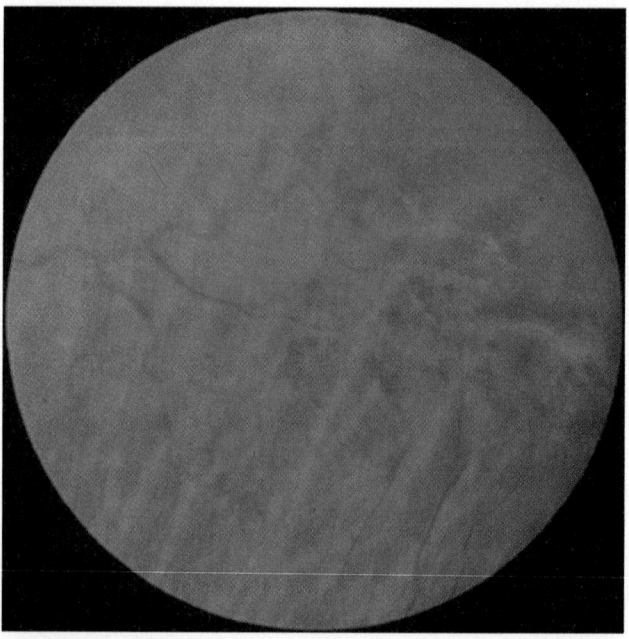

Fig. 41.17 Dominant exudative vitreoretinopathy showing peripheral vascular dilatation, tortuosity and shunting with some preretinal changes (Mr Anthony Moore's patient).

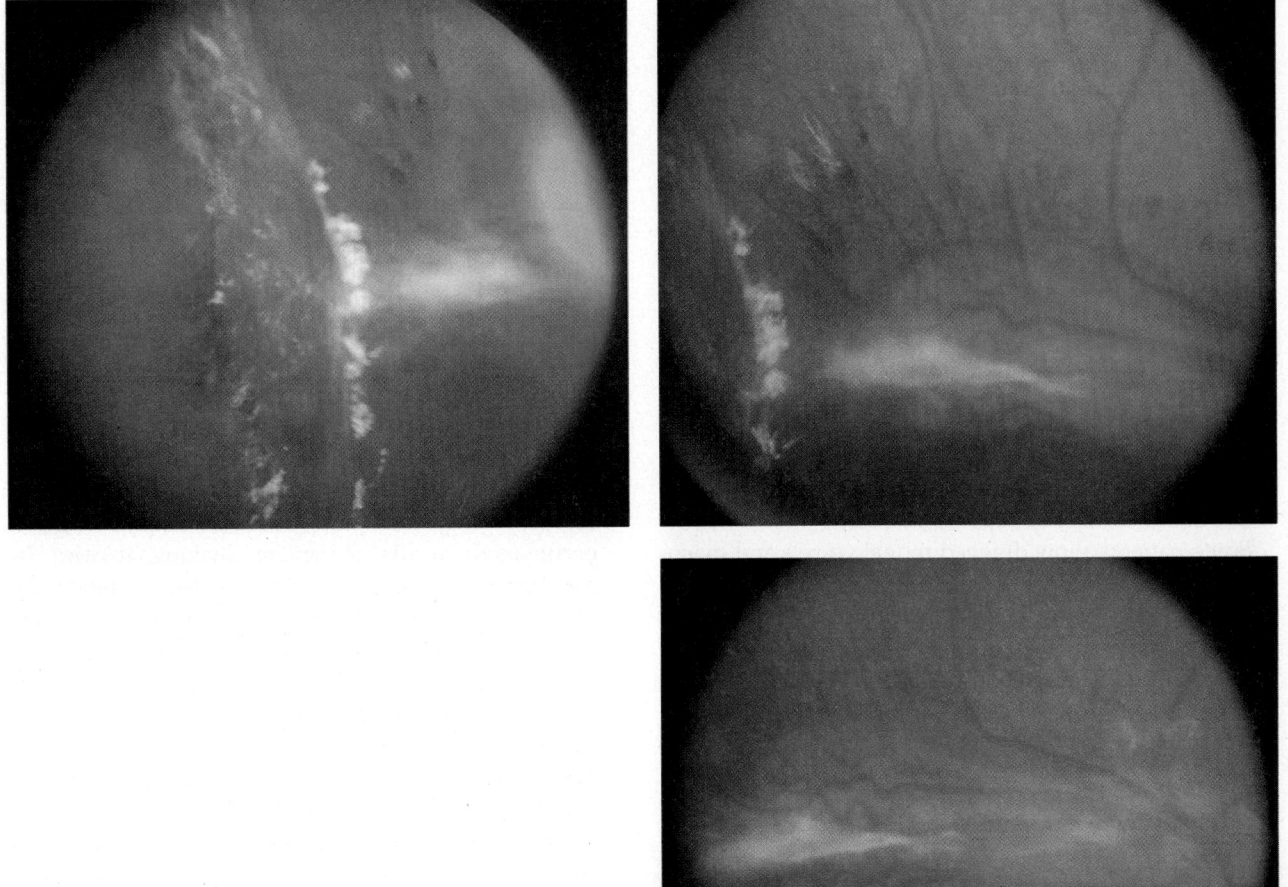

Fig. 41.18 (a–c) Dominant exudative vitreoretinopathy (Dr R. McKay's patient).

uals. The EOG is usually abnormal suggesting that there is a widespread defect in retinal pigment epithelial function (Han & Lewandowski 1992). The retinal abnormalities are present in childhood and usually progress. Visual symptoms are rare in childhood but in adult life visual loss may occur due to cataract, macular oedema and less commonly vitreous haemorrhage and retinal detachment. There are no consistent systemic abnormalities.

Autosomal dominant neovascular inflammatory vitreoretinopathy

This rare autosomal dominant disorder is characterized by anterior and posterior ocular inflammation, peripheral retinal pigment deposition, retinal vascular occlusion and neovascularization, vitreous haemorrhage and tractional retinal detachment (Bennett *et al.* 1990). Presenile cataract

is common. The ERG shows selective loss of the b-wave early in the disease which serves to differentiate this from the other forms of vitreoretinopathy with vascular closure. Night-blindness is a late feature and the ERG may become totally extinguished in advanced disease. There are no reported systemic abnormalities. The disorder has been mapped to the long arm of chromosome 11 close to the locus for autosomal dominant erosive vitreoretinopathy (Stone *et al.* 1992).

The earliest signs of the disease are vitreous cells, mild peripheral retinal ischaemia and reduced b-wave amplitudes on ERG. The condition cannot be reliably detected in childhood; Bennett *et al.* (1990) examined nine children at 50% risk of inheriting the abnormal gene and found none with definite signs of disease. The youngest affected patient was a 16-year-old boy who presented with vitreous haemorrhage due to peripheral retinal neovascularization (Bennett *et al.* 1990).

Erosive vitreoretinopathy

Erosive vitreoretinopathy is a syndrome characterized by autosomal dominant inheritance, nyctalopia, progressive field loss, vitreous abnormalities, progressive retinal pigment epithelial atrophy and combined traction and rhegmatogenous retinal detachment (Brown *et al.* 1994). ERG shows evidence of widespread rod and cone dysfunction. The earliest and most consistent abnormalities are peripheral retinal pigment epithelial atrophy, field loss and ERG abnormalities which are evident in childhood. The vitreous is syneretic with areas of condensation but without the inflammatory signs seen in autosomal dominant neovascular inflammatory vitreoretinopathy. There are no consistent systemic abnormalities.

Some patients show dragged retinal vessels and macular ectopia similar to that seen in autosomal dominant erosive vitreoretinopathy. Retinal detachment, which may be tractional or rhegmatogenous, occurs in the majority of affected adults. The visual prognosis is poor; 20% of eyes in the study of Brown *et al.* (1994) were blind from retinal detachment.

Autosomal dominant snow-flake degeneration

This disorder, first described by Hirose *et al.* (1974), is characterized by extensive 'white with pressure' change in the peripheral retina, multiple minute 'snow-flake' retinal deposits and sheathing of the peripheral retinal vessels. In older patients there may be peripheral vascular occlusion and retinal pigmentation. The vitreous is abnormal with degeneration and diffuse liquefaction. Psychophysical studies show evidence of abnormal rod and cone function and although ERG may be normal initially the b-wave amplitude is reduced in older patients (Hirose *et al.* 1980; Pollack *et al.* 1983). There is an increased risk of retinal tear formation and retinal detachment. The typical retinal changes may be seen in childhood but often do not develop until the late teens or early adult life (Robertson *et al.* 1982; Pollack *et al.* 1983). There are no associated systemic abnormalities.

Acquired disorders of the vitreous

Acquired disorders of the vitreous are uncommon in childhood and generally occur when there is vitreous opacification caused by haemorrhage or inflammation. Less commonly tumour or infection may involve the vitreous cavity.

Vitreous haemorrhage

The most common cause of vitreous haemorrhage in childhood is blunt or penetrating trauma, which occurs predominantly in older children. Other causes include haemorrhage from the retinal vessels involved in schitic areas in X-linked juvenile retinoschisis or from optic disc or peripheral retinal neovascularization that may occur in vitreoretinal dystrophies such as familial exudative vitreoretinopathy, autosomal dominant vitreoretinochoroidopathy and autosomal dominant neovascular inflammatory vitreoretinopathy. Vitreous haemorrhage may also herald the onset of retinal tear formation in Stickler's syndrome and may be an additional complication in eyes with advanced retinopathy of prematurity, PHPV or retinal dyplasia. Less commonly haemorrhage may occur in eyes with vascular abnormalities such as retinal haemangioblastomas, cavernous haemangioma (Yamaguchi *et al.* 1988), Eales' disease or Coats' disease. In young infants retinal, subhyaloid and vitreous haemorrhage may occur as a result of severe shaking injuries (nonaccidental injury), when they are usually bilateral and associated with intracranial haemorrhage. Such haemorrhages are only rarely seen in other causes of intracranial haemorrhage. Finally retinal and vitreous haemorrhage may be seen in haematological disorders such as leukaemia, thrombocytopenia, haemophilia, von Willebrand's disease and neonatal protein C deficiency (Pulido *et al.* 1987).

The management of vitreous haemorrhage is relatively straightforward in childhood and in older children who have reached the age of visual maturity. A conservative approach is preferred with surgery only indicated if the haemorrhage is persistent or if there is an associated retinal detachment which requires treatment. In infants and young children management is problematic as dense vitreous haemorrhage may lead to severe stimulus deprivation amblyopia and may also affect the process of emmetropization and lead to myopia (Miller Meeks *et al.* 1990). If after a short period of observation there is no resolution of the haemorrhage and if there is no underlying retinal abnormality that may herald a poor prognosis early vitrectomy may need to be considered despite the technical difficulties and possible complications.

Inflammatory disease of the vitreous (see Chapter 38)

Vitreous inflammatory disease is uncommon in childhood and when it does occur it is usually seen in association with juvenile pars planitis, intermediate uveitis, or less commonly retinal vasculitis. It may be seen in association with systemic sarcoidosis and in tuberculosis. Johns *et al.* (1992) have reported an unusual case of vitreous opacification caused by lymphocytic infiltration of the vitreous in X-linked immunodeficiency.

Vitritis is also commonly seen in toxoplasmic chorioretinitis and *Toxocara* infection. Bacterial infection of the vitreous is rare in childhood but may complicate penetrating trauma and less commonly intraocular surgery. Metastatic bacterial endophthalmitis and *Candida* endophthalmitis, causing vitreous opacity, may occur in sick immunosuppressed children.

Vitreous opacity due to tumour

Vitreous seeding is a well-recognized complication of retinoblastoma; clumps of tumour cells are seen floating in the vitreous chamber but rarely give rise to problems with diagnosis as there is usually a typical retinoblastoma accompanying the tumour cells in the vitreous. Occasionally when there are clumps of cells in the anterior vitreous in an inflamed eye with an opaque vitreous there may be doubt as to whether the underlying aetiology is inflammatory or neoplastic. In most cases ultrasound or CT scan of the eye will demonstrate a retinal tumour in cases of retinoblastoma although this may not be the case in the rare diffuse infiltrating forms of retinoblastoma (Morgan 1971).

Tumour cells may also be found in the vitreous in leukaemia but there is almost always associated retinal infiltration; extensive vitreous involvement is only seen in advanced disease when there is accompanying retinal and optic nerve involvement (Kincaid & Green 1983; Rosenthal 1983). Other intraocular metastatic deposits of tumour are extremely rare.

References

Ahmad NN, Ala-Korkho L, Knowlton RG *et al.* Stop codon in the procollagen II gene (COL2A1) 3 prime variable region in the family with Stickler's syndrome (arthro-ophthalmopathy). *Proc Natl Acad Sci USA* 1991; **88**: 6624–7.

Ahmad NN, McDonald-McGinn DM, Zackai EH *et al.* A second mutation in the Type II procollagen gene (COL2A1) causing the Stickler syndrome is also a premature termination codon. *Am J Hum Genet* 1993; **52**: 39–45.

Alitalo T, Kruse TA, Ahrens P, Albertsen HM, Eriksson AW, de la Chapelle A. Genetic mapping of 12 marker loci in the Xp22.3–p21.2 region. *Hum Genet* 1991a; **86**: 599–603.

Alitalo T, Kruse TA, de la Chapelle A. Refined localisation of the gene causing X-linked juvenile retinoschisis. *Genomics* 1991b; **9**: 505–10.

Arden GB, Gorin MB, Polkinghorne PJ, Jay M, Bird AC. Detection of carrier state of X-linked retinoschisis. *Am J Ophthalmol* 1988; **105**: 590–5.

Barondes MJ, Hamilton AM. Optic disc neovascularisation in dominant exudative vitreoretinopathy. *Retina* 1989; **9**: 270–5.

Beller R, Hoyt CS, Marg E, Odom JV. Good visual function after neonatal surgery for congenital monocular cataracts. *Am J Ophthalmol* 1981; **91**: 554–65.

Bennett SR, Folk JC, Kimura AE *et al.* Autosomal dominant neovascular inflammatory vitreoretinopathy. *Ophthalmology* 1990; **97**: 1125–35.

Berger W, van der Pol D, Warburg M *et al.* Mutations in the candidate gene for Norrie disease. *Hum Mol Genet* 1992; **1**: 461–5.

Bernado AI, Kirsch LS, Brownstein S. Ocular anomalies in anencephaly: a clinicopathological study of 11 globes. *Canad J Ophthalmol* 1991; **26**: 257–63.

Billington BM, Leaver PK, McLeod D. Management of retinal detachment in the Wagner–Stickler syndrome. *Trans Ophthalmol Soc UK* 1985; **104**: 875–9.

Black G, Redmond RM. The molecular biology of Norrie's disease. *Eye* 1994; **8**: 491–6.

Blair NP, Goldberg MF, Fishman GA *et al.* Autosomal dominant vitreoretino-choroidopathy (ADVIRC). *Br J Ophthalmol* 1984; **68**: 2–9.

Bogaert R, Wilkin D, Wilcox W *et al.* Expression in cartilage of a seven-aminoacid deletion in type II collagen from two unrelated individuals with Kniest dysplasia. *Am J Hum Genet* 1994; **55**: 1128–36.

Bohringer H, Dieterle P, Landrol E. Zur klinik und pathologie der degeneratio, hyaloideo-retinalis hereditaria (Wagner). *Ophthalmologica (Basel)* 1960; **139**: 330–8.

Boldrey EE, Egbert P, Gass JD, Friberg T. The histopathology of familial exudative vitreoretinopathy. A report of two cases. *Arch Ophthalmol* 1985; **103**: 238–41.

Bonaventure J, Phillipe C, Plenis *et al.* Linkage study of a large pedigree of Stickler syndrome: exclusion of COL2A1 as the mutant gene. *Hum Genet* 1992; **90**: 164–8.

Brodrick JD, Wyatt HT. Hereditary X-linked retinoschisis. *Br J Ophthalmol* 1973; **57**: 551–9.

Brown DM, Graemiger RA, Hergersberg M *et al.* Genetic linkage of Wagner disease and erosive retinopathy to chromosome 5q13–14. *Arch Ophthalmol* 1995; **113**: 671–5.

Brown DM, Kimura AE, Weingest TA *et al.* Erosive vitreoretinopathy. A new clinical entity. *Ophthalmology* 1994; **101**: 694–704.

Brown DM, Nichols BE, Weingeist TA *et al.* Procollagen II gene mutation in Stickler syndrome. *Arch Ophthalmol* 1992; **110**: 1589–93.

Brown DM, Vandenberg K, Nichols BE *et al.* Incidence of frameshift mutations in the procollagen II gene in Stickler syndrome and identification of four new mutations. *Invest Ophthalmol Vis Sci* 1994; **35**: 1717.

Brown GA. Incontinentia pigmenti: the development of pseudoglioma. *Br J Ophthalmol* 1988; **72**: 452–6.

Brunner HG, van Beersum SE, Warman SL *et al.* A Stickler syndrome gene is linked to chromosome 6 near the COL11 A2 gene. *Hum Mol Genet* 1994; **3**: 1561–4.

Bullock JD. Developmental vitreous cysts. *Arch Ophthalmol* 1974; **91**: 83–5.

Burke JP, O'Keefe M. Megalocornea and persistent hyperplastic primary vitreous masquerading as congenital glaucoma. *Acta Ophthalmol* 1988; **66**: 731–3.

Canny CLB, Oliver GL. Fluorescein angiography findings in familial exudative vitreo-retinopathy. *Arch Ophthalmol* 1976; **94**: 1114–217.

Carney RG. Incontinentia pigmenti: a world statistical analysis. *Arch Dermatol* 1976; **112**: 535–42.

Carney RG, Carney RG Jr. Incontinentia pigmenti. *Arch Dermatol* 1970; **102**: 157–62.

Carr RE, Siegel JM. The vitreo-tapeto-retinal degenerations. *Arch Ophthalmol* 1970; **84**: 436–45.

Catalano RA, Lopatynsky M, Fasman WS. Treatment of proliferative retinopathy associated with incontinentia pigmenti. *Am J Ophthalmol* 1990; **110**: 701–2.

Cennamo G, Liguori G, Pezone A, Iaccarino G. Morning glory syndrome associated with marked persistent hyperplastic primary vitreous and lens coloboma. *Br J Ophthalmol* 1989; **73**: 684–6.

Chaudhuri PR, Rosenthal AR, Goulstine DB *et al.* Familial exudative vitreoretinopathy associated with familial thrombocytopathy. *Br J Ophthalmol* 1983; **67**: 755–8.

Chen Z, Battinelli, Fielder A *et al.* A mutation in the Norrie disease gene (NDP) associated with X-linked familial vitreoretinopathy.

Nature Genet 1993a; **5**: 180–3.

Chen Z, Battinelli EM, Hendricks RW *et al.* Norrie disease gene: characterisation of deletions and possible functions. *Genomics* 1993b; **16**: 533–5.

Chen Z, Battinelli EM, Woodruff G *et al.* Characterisation of a mutation within the NDP gene in a family with a manifesting female carrier. *Hum Mol Genet* 1993c; **2**: 1727–9.

Chen Z, Hendriks RW, Jobling A *et al.* Isolation and characterisation of a candidate gene for Norrie disease. *Nature Genet* 1992; **1**: 203–8.

Cogan DG, Kuwubara T. Ocular pathology of the 13–15 trisomy syndrome. *Arch Ophthalmol* 1964; **72**: 346–53.

Conway BP, Welch RB. X-chromosomal-linked juvenile retinoschisis with haemorrhagic retinal cyst. *Am J Ophthalmol* 1977; **83**: 853–5.

Criswick VG, Schepens CL. Familial exudative vitreoretinopathy. *Am J Ophthalmol* 1969; **68**: 578–94.

Dahl N, Goonewardena P, Chotai J, Anvret M, Pettersson U. DNA linkage analysis of X-linked retinoschisis. *Hum Genet* 1988; **78**: 228–32.

Dahl N, Ulf P. Use of linked DNA probes for carrier detection and diagnosis of X-linked juvenile retinoschisis. *Arch Ophthalmol* 1988; **106**: 1414–17.

de Jong PT, Zrenner E, van Meel GJ, Keunen JEE, van Norren D. Mizuo phenomenon in X-linked retinoschisis. *Arch Ophthalmol* 1991; **109**: 1104–8.

De Paepe A, Leroy JG, Nuytinck L *et al.* Osteoporosis–pseudoglioma syndrome. *Am J Med Genet* 1993; **45**: 30–7.

Deutmann AF. Sex-linked juvenile retinoschisis. In: Deutmann AF, ed. *The Hereditary Dystrophies of the Posterior Pole of the Eye.* The Netherlands: Koninklijke Van Gorum Comp NV, 1971: 48–94.

Deutmann AF. Vitreo-retinal dystrophies. In: Krill AE, ed. *Hereditary Retinal and Choroidal Diseases*, Vol. 2. London: Harper & Row, 1977: 1043–108.

Dobyns WB, Pagon RA, Armstrong D *et al.* Diagnostic criteria for the Walker–Warburg syndrome. *Am J Med Genet* 1989; **32**: 195–210.

Dudgeon J. Familial exudative vitreoretinopathy. *Trans Ophthalmol Soc UK* 1979; **99**: 45–9.

Duke-Elder S, ed. *System of Ophthalmology*, Vol. III. London: Henry Kimpton, 1963: 141–52.

Elkington AR, Watson DM. Mobile vitreous cysts. *Br J Ophthalmol* 1974; **58**: 1103–4.

Enyedi L, de Juan E, Gaiton A. Ultrastructural study of Norrie's disease. *Am J Ophthalmol* 1991; **111**: 439–46.

Favre M. À propos de deux cas de dégénérescence hyaloideo-rétinienne. *Ophthalmologica (Basel)* 1958; **135**: 604–9.

Feldman EL, Norris J, Cleasby GW. Autosomal dominant exudative vitreoretinopathy *Arch Ophthalmol* 1983; **101**: 1532–5.

Feman SS, Straatsma BR. Cyst of the posterior vitreous. *Arch Ophthalmol* 1974; **91**: 328–9.

Fishman GA, Jampol LM, Goldberg MF. Diagnostic features of the Favre–Goldmann syndrome. *Br J Ophthalmol* 1976; **60**: 345–53.

Font RL, Yaneoff M, Zimmerman LE. Intraocular adipose tissue and persistent hyperplastic primary vitreous. *Arch Ophthalmol* 1969; **82**: 43–50.

François J. Incontinentia pigmenti (Bloch–Sulzberger syndrome) and retinal changes. *Br J Ophthalmol* 1984; **68**: 19–25.

François J. Prepapillary cysts developed from remnants of the hyaloid artery. *Br J Ophthalmol* 1950; **34**: 365–8.

Francomano C, Liberfarb RM, Hirose T *et al.* The Stickler syndrome: evidence for close linkage to the structural gene for type II collagen. *Genomics* 1987; **1**: 293–6.

Frydman M, Kauschansky A, Leshem I, Savir H. Oculo–palato-cerebral dwarfism. *Clin Genet* 1985; **27**: 414–19.

Fryer AE, Upadhyaye M, Littler M *et al.* Exclusion of COL2A1 as a candidate gene in a family with Wagner–Stickler syndrome. *J Med Genet* 1990; **27**: 91–3.

Fullwood P, Jones J, Bundey S *et al.* X-linked exudative vitreoretinopathy: clinical features and genetic linkage analysis. *Br J Ophthalmol* 1993; **77**: 168–70.

Fulton AB, Croft JL, Howard RO, Albert DM. Human retinal dysplasia. *Am J Ophthalmol* 1978; **85**: 690–8.

George ND, Yates JRW, Bradshaw K, Moore AT. Infantile presentation of juvenile X-linked retinoschisis. *Br J Ophthalmol* 1995; **79**: 653–7.

George ND, Yates JRW, Moore AT. X-linked retinoschisis. *Br J Ophthalmol* 1995b; **79**: 697–702.

George ND, Moore AT, Yates JRW. Genetic linkage analysis in British families with juvenile X-linked retinoschisis. *J Med Genet* 1996a (in press).

George NG, Yates JRW, Moore AT. Clinical features of affected males in juvenile X-linked retinoschisis. *Arch Ophthalmol* 1996b; **114**: 274–80.

Goldberg MF, Custis PH. Retinal and other manifestations of incontinentia pigmenti (Bloch–Sulzberger syndrome). *Ophthalmology* 1993; **100**: 1645–54.

Goldberg MF, Mafee M. Computerized tomography for the diagnosis of persistent hyperplastic primary vitreous. *Ophthalmology* 1983; **90**: 442–51.

Gow J, Oliver GL. Familial exudative vitreoretinopathy, an expanded view. *Arch Ophthalmol* 1971; **86**: 150–5.

Graemiger RA, Niemeyer G, Schneeberger SA, Messmer EP. Wagner vitreoretinal degeneration: follow-up of the original pedigree. *Ophthalmology* 1995; **102**: 1830–9.

Gutierrez Diaz A, Alonso MJ, Borda M. Oculodentodigital dysplasia. *Ophthalmic Paediatr Genet* 1982; **1**: 227–32.

Han D, Lewandowski M. Electro-oculography in autosomal dominant vitreoretinochoroidopathy. *Arch Ophthalmol* 1992; **110**: 1563–7.

Hilsdorf C. Uber einen fall einer einseitigen glaskorpercyste. *Ophthalmologica (Basel)* 1965; **149**: 12–20.

Hirose T, Lee KY, Schepens CL. Snowflake degeneration in hereditary vitreoretinal degeneration. *Am J Ophthalmol* 1974; **77**: 143–53.

Hirose T, Wolfe E, Schepens CL. Retinal function tests in snowflake degeneration. *Ann Ophthalmol* 1980; **12**: 1135–46.

Jacobsen SG, Marmor MF, Kemp CM *et al.* SWS (blue) cone hypersensitivity in a newly identified retinal degeneration. *Invest Ophthalmol Vis Sci* 1990; **31**: 827–38.

Jacobsen SG, Roman AJ, Roman MI *et al.* Relatively enhanced S cone function in the Goldmann–Favre syndrome. *Am J Ophthalmol* 1991; **111**: 446–53.

Johns KJ, Hummell DS, McCurley TL, Lawton A. Cellular infiltration of the vitreous in a patient with X-linked immunodeficiency with increased IgM. *Am J Ophthalmol* 1992; **113**: 183–6.

Jones HE. Hyaloid remnants in the eyes of premature babies. *Br J Ophthalmol* 1963; **47**: 39–44.

Joos K, Kimura A, Vandenburgh K, Bartley J, Stone E. Ocular findings associated with a cys39Arg mutation in the Norrie disease gene. *Arch Ophthalmol* 1994; **112**: 1574–9.

Karr DJ, Scott WE. Visual acuity results following treatment of persistent hyperplastic primary vitreous. *Arch Ophthalmol* 1986; **104**: 662–7.

Kaufman SJ, Goldberg MF, Orth DH *et al.* Autosomal dominant vitreoretino-choroidopathy. *Arch Ophthalmol* 1982; **100**: 272–8.

Kawano K, Tanaka K, Murakami F, Ohba N. Congenital hereditary retinoschisis: evolution at initial stage. *Graefe's Arch Clin Exp Ophthalmol* 1981; **217**: 315–23.

Kennedy RE. The effect of early enucleation on the orbit in animals and humans. *Am J Ophthalmol* 1965; **60**: 277–306.

Kinkaid MC, Green WR. Ocular and orbital involvement in leukemia. *Surv Ophthalmol* 1983; **27**: 211–32.

Knowlton RG, Weaver EJ, Stuyk AF *et al.* Genetic linkage analysis of hereditary arthro–ophthalmopathy (Stickler syndrome) and the type II collagen progene. *Am J Hum Genet* 1989; **45**: 681–8.

Korko J, Ritvaniemi P, Haataja *et al.* Mutations in type II procollagen gene (COL2A1) that substitutes aspartate for glycine 1–67 and that causes cataract and retinal detachment: evidence for molecular heterogeneity in the Wagner syndrome and Stickler syndrome (arthro-ophthalmopathy). *Am J Hum Genet* 1993; **53**: 55–61.

Lahav M, Albert DM, Wyand S. Clinical and histopathologic classification of retinal dysplasia. *Am J Ophthalmol* 1973; **75**: 648–67.

Landy SJ, Donnai D. Incontinentia pigmenti (Bloch–Sulzberger syndrome). *J Med Genet* 1993; **30**: 53–9.

Lewis TL, Maurer D, Brent HP. Effects on perceptual development of visual deprivation during infancy. *Br J Ophthalmol* 1986; **70**: 214–20.

Li Y, Fuhrmann C, Schwinger E *et al.* The gene for autosomal dominant familial exudative retinopathy (Criswick–Schepens) on the long arm of chromosome 11 (letter). *Am J Ophthalmol* 1992a; **113**: 712–13.

Li Y, Muller B, Fuhrmann C *et al.* The autosomal dominant familial exudative retinopathy maps on 11q and is closely linked to D11S533. *Am J Hum Genet* 1992b; **51**: 749–54.

Liang JC, Augsburger JJ, Shields JA. Diffuse infiltrating retinoblastoma associated with persistent primary vitreous. *J Pediatr Ophthalmol Strabismus* 1985; **22**: 31–3.

Lieberfarb RM, Eavey RD, De Long GR *et al.* Norrie's disease: a study of two families. *Ophthalmology* 1985; **92**: 1445–51.

Lin AE, Biglan AW, Garver KL. Persistent hyperplastic primary vitreous with vertical transmission. *Ophthalmol Pediatr Genet* 1990; **11**: 121–2.

Lisch W. Hereditary vitreoretinal degenerations. In: Straub W, ed. *Developments in Ophthalmology*, Vol. 8. Basel: Karger, 1983: 33–8.

Lisch W, Rochels R. Pathogenesis of congenital vitreous cysts. *Klin Monatsbl Augenheilk* 1989; **195**: 375–8.

Lloyd I, Colley A, Tullo A, Bonshek R. Dominantly inherited unilateral retinal dysplasia. *Br J Ophthalmol* 1993; **77**: 378–80.

Lusky M, Weinberger D, Kremer L. Vitreous cyst combined with bilateral juvenile retinoschisis. *J Paediatr Ophthalmol* 1988; **25**: 75–7.

Manschot WA. Pathology of hereditary juvenile retinoschisis. *Arch Ophthalmol* 1972; **88**: 131–8.

Matsuo T. The genes involved in the morphogenesis of the eye. *Jpn J Ophthalmol* 1993; **37**(3): 215–51.

Maumenee IH. Vitreoretinal degenerations as a sign of generalised connective tissue disease. *Am J Ophthalmol* 1979; **88**: 432–44.

Meindl A, Berger W, Meitinger T *et al.* Norrie disease is caused by mutations in an extracellular protein resembling C-terminal globular domain of mucins. *Nature Genet* 1992; **2**: 139–43.

Meitinger T, Meindl A, Bork P *et al.* Molecular modelling of the Norrie disease protein predicts cysteine knot growth factor tertiary structure. *Nature Genet* 1993; **5**: 376–80.

Menchini U, Pece A, Alberti M *et al.* Hyperplastic primary vitreous with persistent hyaloid artery in two non twin brothers. *J Franc Ophthalmol* 1987; **10**: 241–5.

Miller-Meeks MJ, Bennett SR, Keech RV, Blodi CF. Myopia induced by vitreous haemorrhage. *Am J Ophthalmol* 1990; **109**: 199–203.

Miyakubo H, Hashimoto K, Miyakubo S. Retinal vascular pattern in autosomal dominant exudative vitreoretinopathy. *Ophthalmology* 1984; **91**: 1524–30.

Morgan G. Diffuse infiltrating retinoblastoma. *Br J Ophthalmol* 1971; **55**: 600–6.

Murayama K, Kuo CY, Sieving PA. Abnormal threshold ERG response in X-linked juvenile retinoschisis: evidence for a proximal retinal origin of the human STR. *Clin Vis Sci* 1991; **6**: 317–22.

Neuhauser G, Kaveggia EG, Opitz JM. Autosomal recessive syndrome of pseudogliomatous blindness, osteoporosis and mild mental retardation. *Clin Genet* 1976; **9**: 324–32.

Norrie G. Causes of blindness in children; 25 years experience of Danish Institutes for the Blind. *Acta Ophthalmol* 1927; **5**: 357–86.

Ober RR, Bird AC, Hamilton AM, Sehmi K. Autosomal dominant exudative vitreoretinopathy. *Br J Ophthalmol* 1980; **46**: 112–20.

Ohba N, Watanabe S, Fujital S. Primary vitreoretinal dysplasia transmitted as an autosomal recessive disorder. *Br J Ophthalmol* 1981; **65**: 631–5.

Ohba N, Yamashita T. Primary vitreoretinal dysplasia resembling Norrie's disease in a female: associated with X autosome chromosomal translocation. *Br J Ophthalmol* 1986; **70**: 64–71.

Pagon R, Clarren SK, Milam FD, Hendrickson AE. Autosomal recessive eye and brain anomalies: Waarburg syndrome. *J Paediatr* 1983; **102**: 542–6.

Parving A, Warburg M. Audiological findings in Norrie's disease. *Audiology* 1977; **16**: 124–31.

Patau K, Smith DW, Therman E, Inhom SL, Wagner P. Multiple congenital anomalies caused by an extra autosome. *Lancet* 1960; **i**: 790–3.

Peachey NS, Fishman GA, Derlacki DJ, Brigell MG. Psychophysical and electroretinographic findings in X-linked juvenile retinoschisis. *Arch Ophthalmol* 1987; **105**: 513–16.

Pearson R, Jagger J. Sex-linked retinoschisis with optic disc and peripheral retinal neovascularisation. *Br J Ophthalmol* 1989; **73**: 311–13.

Phillips CL, Leighton DA, Forrester RM. Congenital hereditary nonattachment of the retina: a sibship of two. *Acta Ophthalmol* 1973; **51**: 425–33.

Pischel DK. Three brothers with juvenile retinoschisis. *Mod Probl Ophthalmol* 1969; **8**: 381–9.

Plager DA, Orgel IK, Ellis FD *et al.* X-linked recessive familial exudative vitreoretinopathy. *Am J Ophthalmol* 1992; **114**: 145–8.

Pollak A, Uchenik D, Chemmke J, Oliver M. Prophylactic laser photocoagulation in hereditary snowflake vitreoretinal degeneration: a family report. *Arch Ophthalmol* 1983; **101**: 1536–9.

Pollard Z. Treatment of persistent hyperplastic primary vitreous. *J Pediatr Ophthalmol* 1985; **22**: 180–3.

Preslan MW, Beauchamp GR, Zakcov ZN. Congenital glaucoma and retinal dysplasia. *J Pediatr Ophthalmol Strabismus* 1985; **22**: 166–70.

Priestley L, Kumar D, Sykes B. Amplification of COL2A1 3 prime variable region used for segregation analysis in a family with Stickler syndrome. *Hum Genet* 1990; **85**: 525–6.

Pruett RC, Schepens CL. Posterior hyperplastic primary vitreous. *Am J Ophthalmol* 1970; **69**: 535–43.

Pulido JS, Lingua RW, Cristol S, Byrne SF. Protein C deficiency associated with vitreous haemorrhage in a neonate. *Am J Ophthalmol* 1987; **104**: 546–7.

Rahi J, Hungerford J. Early diagnosis of the retinopathy of incontinentia pigmenti: successful treatment by cryotherapy. *Br J Ophthalmol* 1990; **74**: 377–80.

Redmond R, Vaughan J, Jay M, Jay B. *In utero* diagnosis of Norrie's disease by ultrasonography. *Ophthalmic Paediatr Genet* 1993; **141**: 1–3.

Reese AB. Persistence and hyperplasia of the primary vitreous; retrolental fibroplasia—two entities. *Arch Ophthalmol* 1949; **41**: 527–52.

Reese AB. Persistent hyperplastic primary vitreous. *Am J Ophthalmol* 1955; **40**: 317–31.

Ricci MA. Clinique et transmission héréditaire des dégénérescences vitreorétiennes. *Bull Soc Ophthalmol (Fr)* 1961; **61**: 618–32.

Robertson DM, Link TP, Riostvold JA. Snowflake degeneration of the retina. *Ophthalmology* 1982; **89**: 1513–17.

Rogers BL, Vanner LV, Pai GS, Sens MA. Walker–Warburg syndrome: report of three affected sibs. *Am J Med Genet* 1994; **49**: 198–201.

Rosenthal AR. Ocular manifestations of leukemia: a review. *Ophthalmology* 1983; **16**: 899–905.

Rubinstein K. Posterior hyperplastic primary vitreous. *Br J Ophthalmol* 1980; **64**: 105–11.

Sefiani A, Abel L, Huertz S *et al.* The gene for incontinentia pigmenti is assigned to X928. *Genomics* 1989; **4**: 427–9.

Sergovich F. The d trisomy syndrome: a case report with description of the ocular pathology. *Canad Med Assoc J* 1963; **89**: 151–7.

Sieving PA, Bingham E, Roth MS *et al.* Linkage relationships with X-linked juvenile retinoschisis with Xp22.1–p22.3 probes. *Am J Hum Genet* 1990; **47**: 616–21.

Silverstein AM, Parshall CJ, Osburn BI, Prendergast RA. An experimental virus induced retinal dysplasia in the fetal lamb. *Am J Ophthalmol* 1971; **72**: 22–34.

Smith DW, Patau K, Therman E *et al.* The D1 trisomy syndrome. *J Pediatr* 1963; **62**: 326–41.

Snead MP, Payne SJ, Barton DE *et al.* Stickler syndrome: correlation between vitreoretinal phenotypes and linkage to COL2A1. *Eye* 1994; **8**: 414–8.

Sneed PJ, Augsberger JJ, Shields JA *et al.* Bilateral vitreous hypoplasia associated with persistence of the primary vitreous: a new clinical entity? *J Pediatr Ophthalmol Strabismus* 1988; **25**: 77–85.

Spallone A. Incontinentia pigmenti (Bloch–Sulzberger syndrome) seven case reports from one family. *Br J Ophthalmol* 1987; **71**: 629–35.

Spencer WH. Vitreous. In: *Ophthalmic Pathology. An Atlas and Text-book.* London: WB Saunders, 1985: 554–6.

Stark WJ, Lindsey P, Fagadan WR, Michels RG. Persistent hyperplastic primary vitreous; surgical treatment. *Ophthalmology* 1983; **90**: 452–7.

Steve J, Steve E, Mikkelson M. Risk for chromosome abnormality at aminiocentesis following a child with a non-inherited chromosome aberration. *Prenat Diagn* 1984; **4**: 81–5.

Stickler GB, Becau PG, Farrel FS *et al.* Hereditary progressive ophthalmo-arthropathy. *Mayo Clin Proc* 1965; **40**: 433–95.

Stone EM, Kimura AE, Folk JC *et al.* Genetic linkage of autosomal dominant neovascular inflammatory vitreoretinopathy to chromosome 11q13. *Hum Mol Genet* 1992; **1**: 685–9.

Storimans CW, van Schooneveld MJ. Riegers eye anomaly and persistent hyperplastic primary vitreous. *Ophthalmol Paediatr Genet* 1989; **10**: 257–62.

Swanson D, Rush P, Bird AC. Visual loss from retinal oedema in autosomal dominant exudative vitreoretinopathy. *Br J Ophthalmol* 1982; **66**: 627–9.

Taylor AI. Autosomal trisomy syndromes: a detailed study of 27 cases of Edwards' syndrome and 27 cases of Patau syndrome. *J Med Genet* 1968; **5**: 227–52.

Traboulsi EI, Faris BM, Der Kaloustian VM. Persistent hyperplastic primary vitreous and recessive oculo–dental–osseus dysplasia. *Am J Med Genet* 1986; **24**: 95–100.

Traboulsi EI, Lim SI, Pyeritz R *et al.* A new syndrome of myelinated nerve fibres, vitreoretinopathy and skeletal malformations. *Arch Ophthalmol* 1993; **111**: 1543–5.

Traboulsi E, Payne J. Autosomal dominant vitreo-choroidopathy report of a third family. *Arch Ophthalmol* 1993; **111**: 194–6.

van Nouhuys CE. Signs, complications, and platelet aggregation in familial exudative vitreoretinopathy. *Am J Ophthalmol* 1991; **111**: 34–41.

van Schooneveld MJ, Miyake Y. Fundus albipunctatus like lesions in juvenile retinoschisis. *Br J Ophthalmol* 1994; **78**: 659–66.

Vintiner GM, Temple K, Middleton Price HR *et al.* Genetic and clinical heterogeneity of Stickler syndrome. *J Med Genet* 1991; **41**: 44–8.

Wagner H. Ein Bisher Unbekanntes Erbleiden des Auges (Degeneration Hyaloideo Retinalis Hereditaria), Beobachtet im Karifon Zurich. *Klin Monatsebl Augenheilkd* 1938; **100**: 840–56.

Wald KJ, Mehta MC, Katsumi O *et al.* Retinal detachments in incontinentia pigmenti. *Arch Ophthalmol* 1993; **111**: 614–17.

Warburg M. Norrie's disease, a new hereditary bilateral pseudotumour of the retina. *Acta Ophthalmol* 1961; **39**: 757–72.

Warburg M. Norrie's disease (atrofia bulborum hereditaria). *Acta Ophthalmol* 1963; **41**: 134–46.

Warburg M. The heterogeneity of microphthalmia in the mentally retarded. *Birth Defects* 1971; **7**: 136–54.

Watzke RC, Stevens TS, Carney RG. Retinal vascular changes of incontinentia pigmenti. *Arch Ophthalmol* 1976; **94**: 743–6.

Weaver RG, Martin T, Zanolli MD. The ocular changes of incontinentia pigmenti achromians (hypomelanosis of ITO). *J Paediatr Ophthalmol Strabismus* 1991; **28**: 160–3.

Wieacker P, Wienkert TF, Dallapicolla B, Bender K, Davies KE, Ropers HH. Linkage relationships between retinoschisis, Xg, and a cloned DNA sequence from the distal short arm of the X chromosome. *Hum Genet* 1983; **64**: 143–5.

Wilkin DJ, Weiss MA, Gruber HE *et al.* An exon skipping mutation in the type II collagen gene (COL2A1) produces Kneist dysplasia. *Am J Hum Genet* 1993; **53**: A210.

Winterpacht A, Hilbert M, Scharzeu *et al.* Kniest and Stickler dysplasia phenotype caused by collagen II gene (COL 2A1) defect. *Nature Genet* 1993; **3**: 323–6.

Wong F, Goldberg MF, Hao Y. Identification of a nonsense mutation at codon 128 of the Norrie disease gene in a male infant. *Arch Ophthalmol* 1993; **111**: 1553–7.

Woodruff G, Newbury-Ecob R, Plaha D, Young ID. Manifesting heterozygosity in Norrie's disease. *Br J Ophthalmol* 1993; **77**: 813–4.

Yamaguchi K, Yamaguchi K, Tamai M. Cavernous haemangioma of the retina in a pediatric patient. *Ophthalmologica* 1988; **197**: 127–9.

Yanoff M, Frayer WC, Scheie HG. Ocular findings in a patient with 13–15 trisomy. *Arch Ophthalmol* 1963; **70**: 372–5.

Yanoff M, Rahn EK, Zimmerman LE. Histopathology of juvenile retinoschisis. *Arch Ophthalmol* 1968; **79**: 49–53.

Zhu D, Maumenee IH. Mutation analysis of the Norrie disease gene in 11 families. *Invest Ophthalmol Vis Sci* 1994; **35**: 1265.

42: Retinoblastoma

Brenda L. Gallie and Anthony Moore

Retinoblastoma is the most common malignant ocular tumour of childhood, nonetheless it is quite rare at one in 20 000 live births (Sanders *et al.* 1988). Untreated the tumour is almost uniformly fatal but with modern methods of treatment the survival rate is over 90%. The best results are achieved when cases are referred to specialist centres where ophthalmologists, paediatric oncologists and radiotherapists collaborate in management. The tumour arises from primitive retinal cells so the majority of cases occur in children under the age of 4 years. The treatment of intraocular retinoblastoma has depended heavily on radiation for the last 30 years. Recognition of severe and life-threatening complications of radiation in these children has now led to the development of chemotherapy and focal therapy to reduce the requirement for radiation to save eyes.

Study of retinoblastoma has led to a revolutionary advance in the understanding of cancer in general. The existence of specific genes that normally act to suppress cancer was predicted from clinical studies of retinoblastoma. Studies of retinoblastoma tumours revealed that both hereditary and non-hereditary tumours develop by loss of the last normal allele of the tumour-suppressor gene. Cloning of the RB1 gene (Friend *et al.* 1986) emphasized the critical role of cell cycle regulation in cancer. Molecular identification of RB1 mutations in affected families can now potentially improve the prognosis for affected children at a greatly reduced health-care cost.

Pathogenesis of retinoblastoma

Heritable and non-heritable retinoblastoma

Close to 50% of all cases of retinoblastoma are heritable, due to a mutation in the RB1 gene, which predisposes the child to the development of retinal tumours. The majority of hereditary cases are identified by the occurrence of bilateral or multifocal tumours, but 15% of children with unilateral tumours also have a mutation of one allele of the RB1 gene in their germ cells, that will be inherited by half of their children. Less than 25% of all cases have a family history of retinoblastoma (Jay *et al.* 1988). Most children with heritable retinoblastoma do not have a family history of retinoblastoma, but the affected child has suffered a new germ-line mutation. In 10%, the mutation first arose in an ancestor, placing siblings also at risk (Bonaiti-Pellie & Briard-Guillemot 1981). Familial retinoblastoma may become more common as treatment for retinoblastoma becomes more effective. In familial cases, the predisposition to retinoblastoma is transmitted as an autosomal dominant trait (Migdal 1976).

Non-heritable retinoblastomas are caused by mutations in the same gene. In non-heritable retinoblastoma, somatic mutations in both alleles of the RB1 gene occur in a single primitive retinal cell that gives rise to a solitary, unilateral tumour; as no germ cell mutation is involved, the disease is not transmitted to offspring. However, unilateral retinoblastoma is not a guarantee of lack of heredity, since 15% have a germ-line RB1 mutation, despite having tumour in only one eye.

The spectrum of RB1 mutations

RB1 mutations that induce retinoblastoma tumours can be large rearrangements or single nucleotide changes. Deletions of chromosome 13q14 large enough to be detectable by cytogenetics are uncommon (1–3%) (Yunis & Ramsay 1978), usually associated with a variety of other congenital abnormalities including mental retardation, presumably due to loss of other genes near the RB1 locus (Wilson *et al.* 1987). The majority of mutations are submicroscopic alterations in the coding region or splice control regions of the gene: deletions, insertions or nucleotide substitutions.

The result of the mutation is usually truncation of the expected protein, which is so unstable that no mutant protein is detectable. Such mutations show high penetrance (>95% offspring affected) and expressivity (average of seven tumours per child). Two kinds of RB1 mutations cause much lower penetrance and expressivity (Lohmann *et al.* 1994): 'in frame' deletions or insertions resulting in a stable, although defective, RB protein (Gallie *et al.* 1995); and promoter mutations which result in a reduced amount of otherwise normal protein (Sakai *et al.* 1991).

The loss of both RB1 alleles induces retinoblastoma

The simple clinical observation that the children with bilateral retinoblastoma tended to be diagnosed at a younger age than those with non-hereditary retinoblastoma was analysed mathematically by Knudson (1971), leading to the prediction that two mutational events were required to produce retinoblastoma. The semi-log plot of the ages of children at diagnosis with bilateral and unilateral retinoblastoma against the proportion not yet diagnosed fitted a simple exponential suggesting that a single event (M2) was necessary for tumour development in the presence of the predisposing mutation (M1), but that unilateral cases required at least two events to form a retinoblastoma tumour.

This 'two-hit' hypothesis was expanded to suggest that the two events could be mutation of the two alleles of the predisposing gene, suggesting that such a gene could 'suppress' tumour formation in the retina when one normal allele was present (Comings 1973). The chances of two or more primitive retinal cells undergoing M2 in hereditary retinoblastomas is sufficiently large for multiple tumours to occur (Fig. 42.1). However, the chances of both M1 and M2 occurring in the same retinal cell are extremely small, so that non-hereditary cases have only a solitary tumour which presents at an older age.

The most frequent M2 event is loss of large chromosomal regions surrounding RB1, detected by loss of heterozygosity for polymorphic enzymes such as the closely linked esterase D (Godbout *et al.* 1983) or polymorphic DNA variations within or adjacent to RB1 (Cavenee *et al.* 1983). Thirty per cent of tumours arise when the second RB1 allele acquires a completely different mutation (Dunn *et al.* 1989).

The function of the retinoblastoma protein

The retinoblastoma protein (pRB) is a 110 kDa phosphoprotein that inhibits cell proliferation by altering the expression of other genes of the cell cycle through interaction with the transcription factor E2F family. DNA tumour viruses that induce cancer do so in part by binding to pRB (DeCaprio *et al.* 1988; Whyte *et al.* 1988; Dyson *et al.* 1989) through the 'pocket' region of pRB (Hu *et al.* 1990). The active form of pRB is underphosphorylated (Goodrich *et al.* 1991), and for each cell cycle to proceed, pRB is inactivated by phosphorylation by protein complexes of cyclins and cyclin-dependent kinases (Hinds *et al.* 1992). A mutant pRB that cannot be phosphorylated has increased activity in repression of transcription (Hamel *et al.* 1990) and cell proliferation (Chang *et al.* 1995).

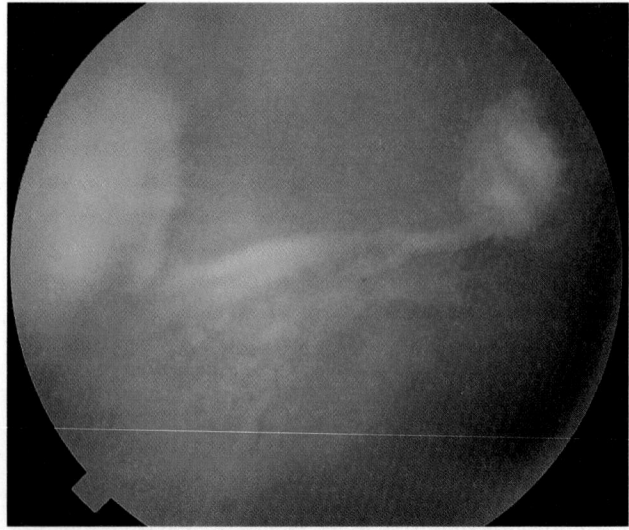

Fig. 42.1 Multifocal retinoblastoma with a tumour invading the optic disc.

Why does mutation of a cell cycle regulatory gene lead specifically to retinoblastoma? Germ-line mutation of RB1 leads to a 40 000-fold relative risk (RR) for retinoblastoma, a 500-fold RR for sarcoma (increased to 2000-fold by therapeutic radiation), and no increase in RR for leukaemia (Gallie *et al.* 1993). Although pRB is present in all cycling cells, its function in development is highly tissue-specific. Thus, mice constructed to have no RB1 gene at all, die *in utero* with failure of neuronal and haematopoietic differentiation, when many tissues have formed apparently normally. Retina may be uniquely dependent on pRB in order to terminally differentiate into adult, functioning retina. In the absence of pRB, proliferation continues, further mutations are acquired, and a retinal tumour emerges.

Histopathology

Retinoblastomas are undifferentiated malignant neuroblastic tumours, composed of cells with large hyperchromatic nuclei and scanty cytoplasm. Mitotic figures are common. In some tumours more differentiated cells form the typical Flexner–Wintersteiner rosettes in which columnar cells are uniformly arranged in a sphere around a lumen containing primitive inner segments of photoreceptors (Popoff & Ellsworth 1969).

Tumour cells often outgrow their blood supply leading to cell necrosis. True spontaneous regression of retinoblastoma is probably due to extensive tumour necrosis and may result in phthisis bulbi (Gallie *et al.* 1982b). Programmed cell death or apoptosis is also evident in the tumours, supporting the idea that the normal function of pRB is to promote differentiation over apoptosis in response to differentiation signals. Calcification is almost pathognomonic of retinoblastoma, but the origin of this calcification is not understood.

Two main patterns of retinoblastoma growth within the eye are seen. Endophytic tumours (Fig. 42.2) tend to grow forward into the vitreous and large tumours may totally fill the vitreous cavity. 'Seeds' from such tumours may float in the vitreous cavity, where they will be hypoxic and relatively resistant to therapy. When the seeds fall onto the retinal surface, they can attach and grow. Spread of tumour into the anterior chamber may lead to hypopyon, and/or secondary glaucoma, with increased risk of metastasis.

Exophytic tumours (Fig. 42.3) grow into the subretinal space leading to retinal detachment. Bruch's membrane may be breached and spread into the choroid can occur, but unless massive, this does not necessarily imply distant spread.

Diffusely infiltrating retinoblastoma (Fig. 42.4) is uncommon and, as it rarely gives rise to a solid mass or retinal detachment, it may lead to difficulty with diagnosis (Bhatnagar & Vine 1991). In an older age group, unilat-

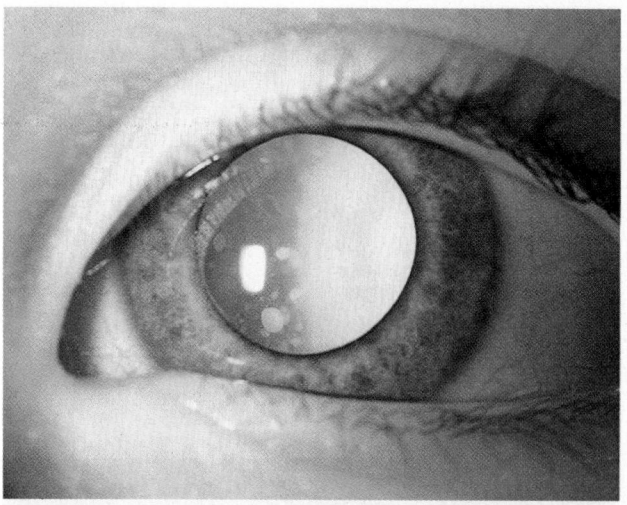

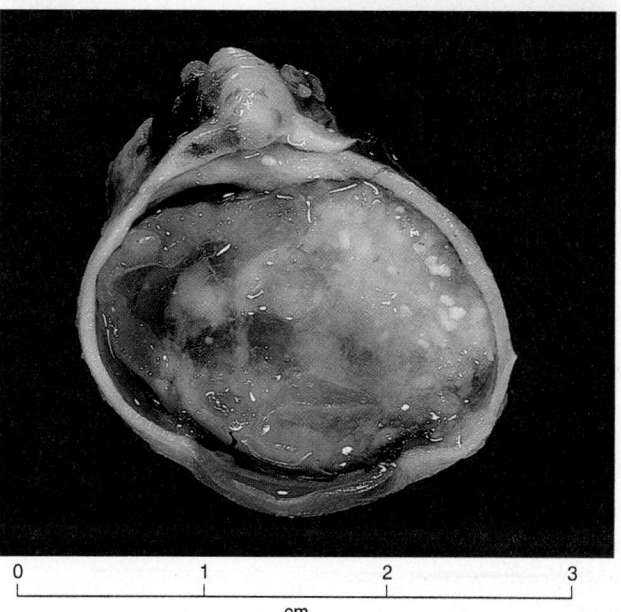

0　　　　　1　　　　　2　　　　　3
cm

Fig. 42.2 (a) Endophytic retinoblastoma. The tumour has invaded the vitreous and seeds can be seen beyond the lens. (b) Calotte of enucleated eye with tumour filling the eye (same patient).

eral hypopyon may be recognized to be retinoblastoma only on aqueous cytology. Provided tumour cells have not been spread by the aqueous tap, the prognosis after enucleation is good.

Metastasis

If metastasis occurs, it is generally evident within 18 months of the last active tumour in the eye, and is rare after 3 years (Sanders *et al.* 1988). The most common and most dangerous route of metastasis of retinoblastoma is direct extension into the optic nerve head: tumour grows to the chiasm and beyond, or into the subarach-

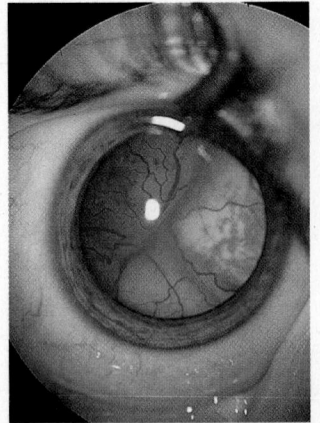
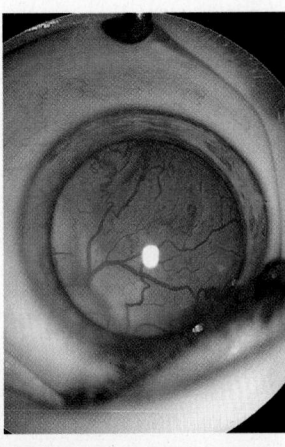

a

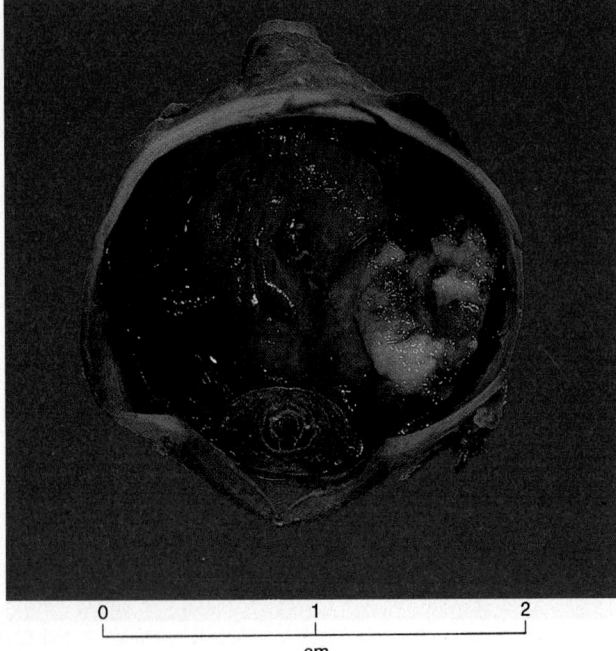

b

Fig. 42.3 (a) Exophytic retinoblastoma with retinal detachment and tumour in the subretinal space. (b) Calotte of enucleated eye with exophytic retinoblastoma.

noid space with extensive meningeal involvement (Fig. 42.5) (Messmer *et al.* 1991). Direct extension via the choroidal vessels or spread along the ciliary vessels and nerves to the orbit may occur in advanced cases and thence the tumour may spread via the meninges (Figs 42.5, 42.6).

True metastasis may occur via the choroidal circulation or aqueous drainage, particularly if glaucoma is present (Messmer *et al.* 1991; Shields *et al.* 1993a). The bone marrow is the preferred site for retinoblastoma metastasis and only terminally are bone, lymph node, and liver involved. Lung metastases are rare. If lids or anterior orbital structures are involved local spread may occur via the lymphatics (Fig. 42.7).

Other manifestations of RB1 mutations

As well as the retinal tumour, mutations of RB1 are associated with retinoma, ectopic intracranial retinoblastoma (trilateral retinoblastoma), and second non-ocular malignancies.

Retinoma

A retinoma is a non-malignant manifestation of the RB1 mutation. Three features characterize the non-progressive lesions: an elevated grey retinal mass, calcification, and surrounding pigment epithelial proliferation and pigmentation (Fig. 42.8). Fluorescein angiography may demonstrate an abnormal retinal circulation over the surface of the mass and in some cases there is associated neovascularization (Gallie *et al.* 1982b). Vitreous 'seeding' can occur with retinoma (Lueder *et al.* 1995).

Although these features are also seen after radiation treatment of retinoblastoma, retinomas are rarely documented to 'regress', appear to originate in childhood and do not progress to full malignancy. Gallie *et al.* have suggested that retinomas develop when the second 'hit' or mutation occurs in a nearly developed retinal cell that has reduced potential to acquire mutations, resulting in a benign disordered growth of the retina (Gallie *et al.* 1982a).

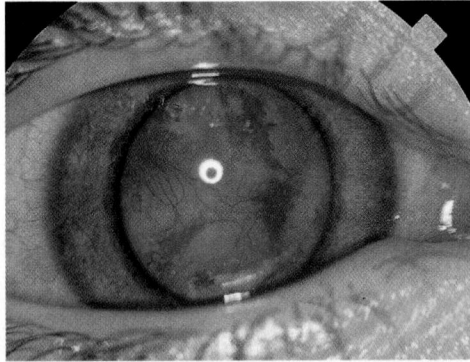

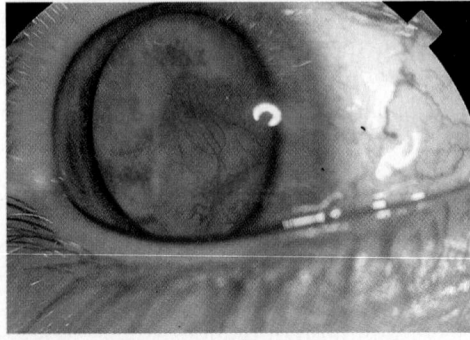

Fig. 42.4 Diffusely infiltrating retinoblastoma. The 5-year-old patient had presented with uveitis with hypopyon, retinal detachment and no calcification on the CT scan or ultrasound.

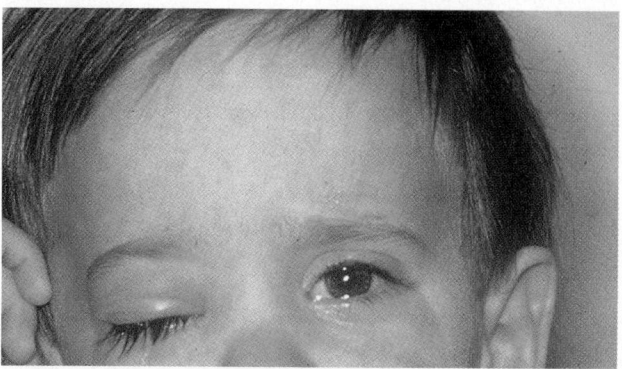

The importance of retinoma lies in its significance for genetic counselling; multiple retinomas indicate that the individual is carrying an RB1 mutation. Caution should be exercised in the follow-up of retinomas; they may show malignant characteristics after a number of years (Eagle *et al.* 1989). However, even the presence of vitreous seeding does not necessarily mean that the mass is malignant. Malignant transformation requires additional findings,

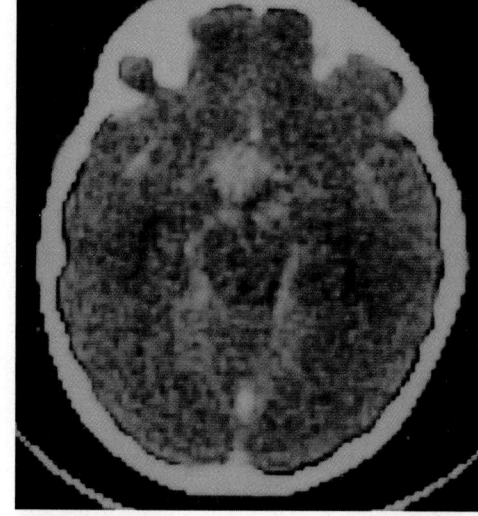

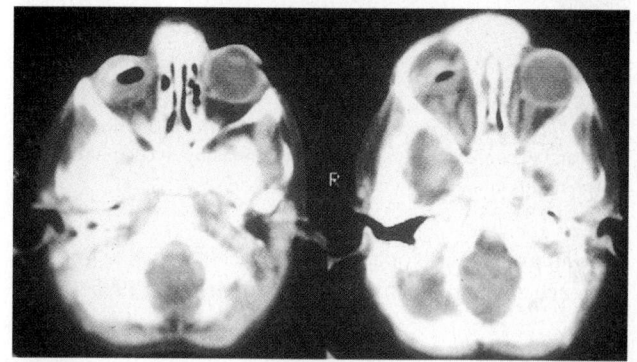

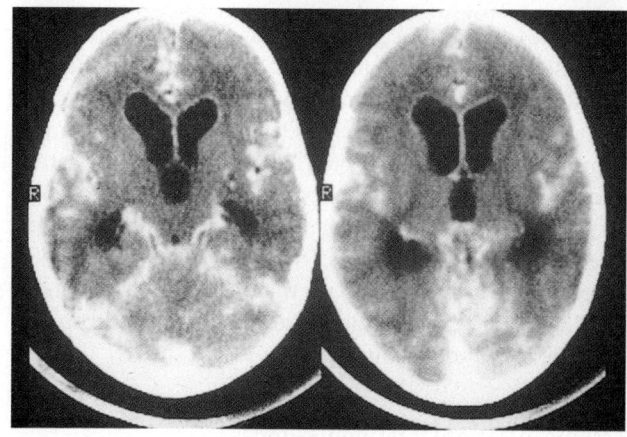

Fig. 42.5 (a) Retinoblastoma with iris invasion, glaucoma, subconjunctival and orbital extension. (b) CT scan showing optic nerve involvement. (c) CT scan showing suprasellar and cerebral extension from optic nerve invasion.

Fig. 42.6 (a) Unilateral retinoblastoma which presented as orbital cellulitis (Professor Brenda Gallie's patient). (b) Extensive intraocular necrosis and replacement of the optic nerve with tumour (Professor Brenda Gallie's patient). (c) Despite treatment, the brain was covered with meningeal retinoblastoma only 4 months later (Professor Brenda Gallie's patient).

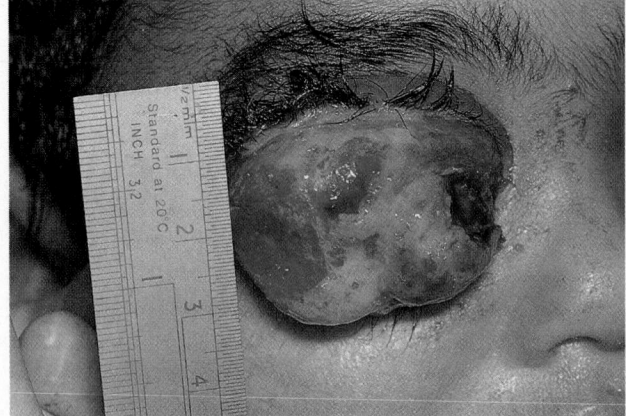

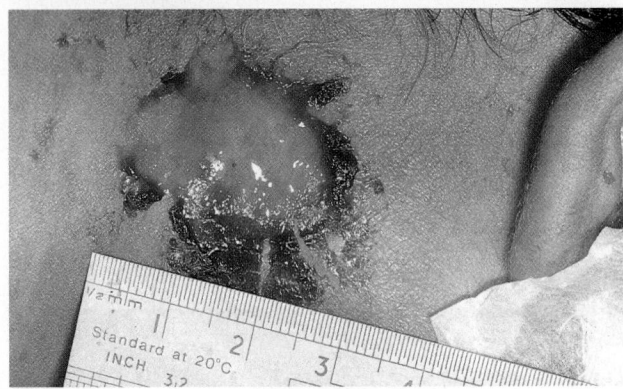

Fig. 42.7 (a) Late diagnosed retinoblastoma with destruction of the globe and orbital extension. (b) Ulcerating malignant occipital lymph nodes in same patient.

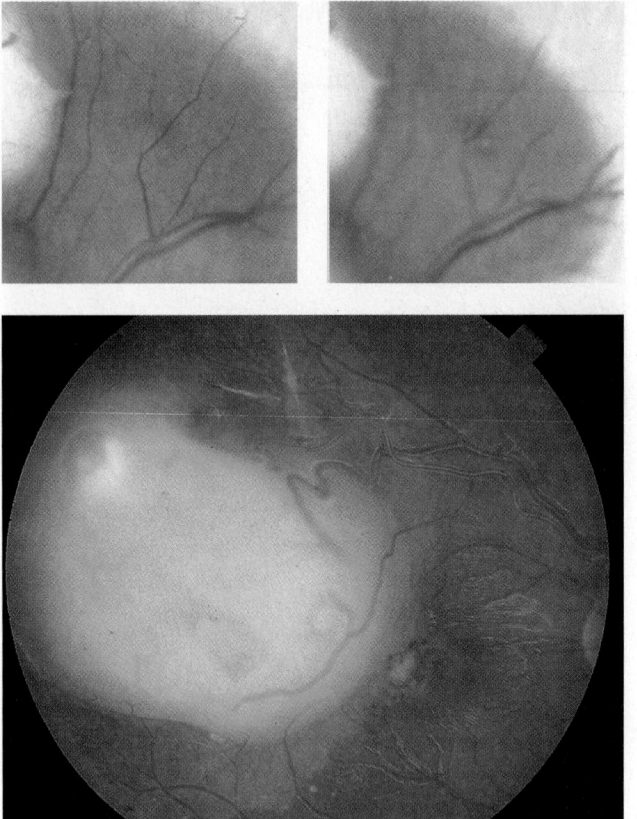

Fig. 42.8 (a) Retinoma followed for 30 years without change. Note the apparent 'seed' in the vitreous (Professor Brenda Gallie's patient). (b) Probable retinoma: this 5-year-old child failed a school vision test. The smooth mass was observed not to change over a period of 13 months; it showed minimal calcification on ultrasound studies

such as progressive opacification, increasing size and the presence of irregular fine vessels (Lueder *et al.* 1995).

Second non-ocular malignancies

Children with the hereditary form of retinoblastoma are at increased risk of developing second non-ocular malignancies (Eng *et al.* 1993), which may occur within or outside the radiation field (Fig. 42.9). Osteosarcoma is the most common tumour seen but a wide variety of other neoplasms have been reported. It is clear that radiation therapy increases the risk for a second malignancy within the radiation field (Draper *et al.* 1986; Roarty *et al.* 1988). Since these tumours are very difficult to treat, more children with RB1 mutations die of their second tumour than die of retinoblastoma.

Ectopic intracranial retinoblastoma (trilateral retinoblastoma)

The association of a midline intracranial tumour and hereditary retinoblastoma was first described by Jakobiec *et al.* (1977). The term trilateral retinoblastoma was later applied to the primary pineal tumours unassociated with

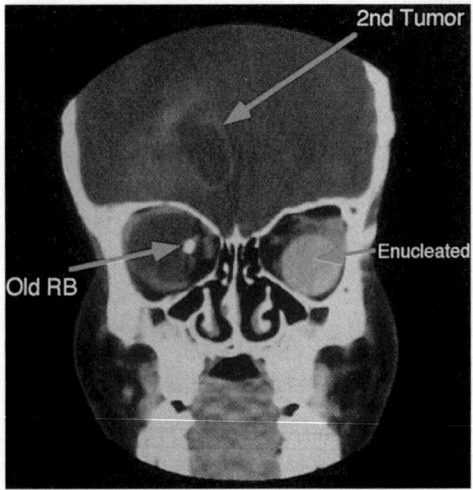

Fig. 42.9 Glioblastoma multiforme rising within the radiation field, 10 years after enucleation of the left eye and the radiation of the right eye for bilateral retinoblastoma (Professor Brenda Gallie's patient).

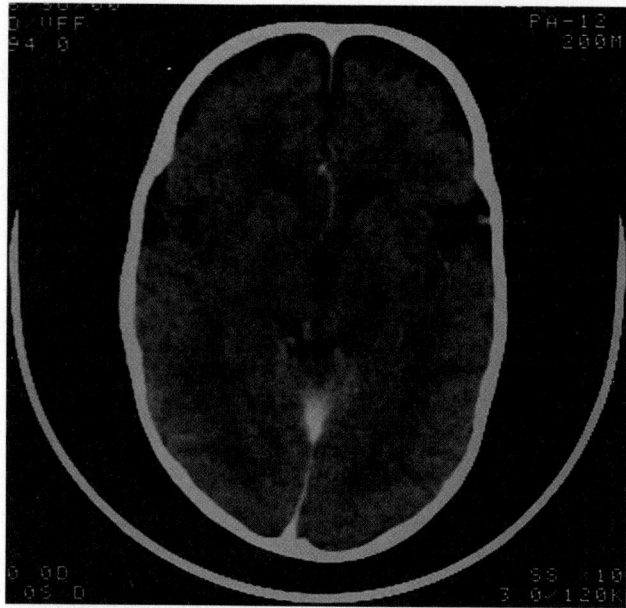

Fig. 42.10 Trilateral retinoblastoma, vascular mass in pineal region.

metastasis from retinoblastoma (Bader *et al.* 1982). The tumours are neuroblastic in origin and resemble poorly differentiated retinoblastoma. Pineal tumours may occur in 2% of cases of retinoblastoma (Kingston *et al.* 1985); since in most cases the retinoblastoma is familial or bilateral, it is assumed that the pineal gland, like the developing retina, has a risk for malignant transformation due to RB1 mutations. Affected children usually present with symptoms and signs of raised intracranial pressure and are found to have a pineal or parasellar mass on computed tomography (CT) scan (Fig. 42.10) (Nelson *et al.* 1992).

Clinical management of retinoblastoma

Presentation

Most children with retinoblastoma present with leukocoria (Tables 42.1, 42.2) (Fig. 42.11) (Ellsworth 1969). The parents will often notice an odd appearance in their child's eye or see a white pupil on a colour photograph. This appearance depends on the path of illumination being in line with the viewer's gaze, so unless the paediatrician or family physician is aware of the importance of this symptom, and specifically looks with an ophthalmoscope, the diagnosis may be missed. The parent's description is usually very accurate, and should stimulate full investigation of the eyes. Unfortunately, it is still very common for diagnosis to be significantly delayed by the primary care physician not 'hearing' the words that the parents say.

The next most common presenting sign is strabismus (esotropia or exotropia) (Ellsworth 1969; Shields 1983). The strabismus is constant and unilateral rather than alternating and the vision in the squinting eye is poor.

All young children with a constant unilateral squint should have a careful fundus examination to rule out this diagnosis.

Other presenting symptoms and signs (see Table 42.1) include painful red eye, orbital cellulitis secondary to extensive intraocular tumour necrosis (Fig. 42.12) (Shields *et al.* 1991c), unilateral mydriasis, heterochromia, hyphaema (Byrnes *et al.* 1993), hypopyon uveitis, and nystagmus due to blindness of bilateral macular involvement (Ellsworth 1969).

Retinoblastoma in close relatives of children with hereditary retinoblastoma should be found on screening examinations, long before any symptoms are present. In countries with limited medical services, many children present late, and extensive unilateral proptosis with

Table 42.1 Presenting symptoms and signs of retinoblastoma (Ellsworth 1969).

	%
White reflex	56
Strabismus	20
Glaucoma	7
Poor vision	5
Routine examination	3
Orbital cellulitis	3
Unilateral mydriasis	2
Heterochromia iris	1
Hyphaema	1
Other	2

Table 42.2 Differential diagnosis of retinoblastoma. Modified from Shields and Augsburger (1981).

Hereditary conditions	*Inflammatory conditions*
Norrie's disease	Toxocariasis
Warburg's syndrome	Toxoplasmosis
Autosomal recessive retinal dysplasia	Metastatic endophthalmitis
	Viral retinitis
Dominant exudative vitreoretinopathy	Vitritis
	Orbital cellulitis
Juvenile X-linked retinoschisis	
	Tumours
	Astrocytic hamartoma
Developmental anomalies	Medulloepithelioma
Persistent hyperplastic primary vitreous	Choroidal haemangioma
	Combined hamartoma of retina and pigment epithelium
Cataract	
Coloboma	
Congenital retinal fold	*Others*
Myelinated nerve fibres	Coats' disease
High myopia	Retinopathy of prematurity
Morning glory syndrome	Rhegmatogenous retinal detachment
	Vitreous haemorrhage
	Leukaemic infiltration of the iris

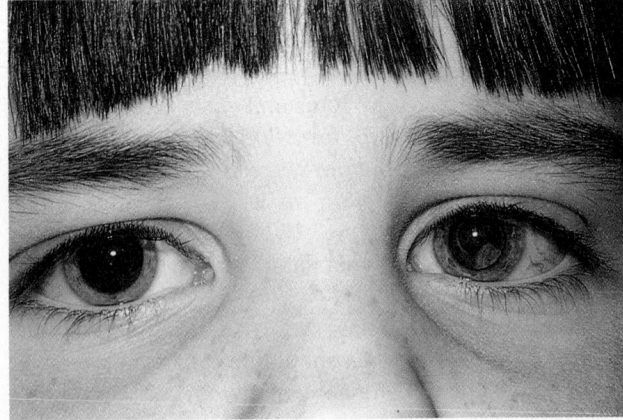

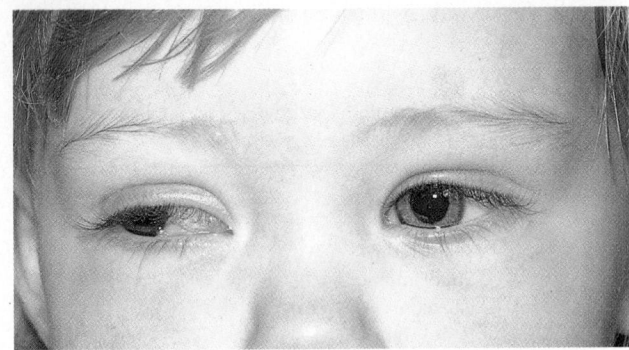

Fig. 42.11 (a) Leucocoria. For 2 years this 5-year-old's mother had noticed a strange white reflex from the pupil in certain combinations of light and positions of gaze. It was only when the tumour became visible in the vitreous through the pupil that the referral was made which led to the diagnosis of retinoblastoma. (b) Retinoblastoma presenting with strabismus. The eye is red because of anterior segment involvement and glaucoma.

orbital extension of the tumour is a common presentation (see Fig. 42.7).

Diagnosis

When a child is referred with a possible diagnosis of retinoblastoma, a careful history, and thorough ocular and systemic examination should be performed before any specialized investigations are carried out. Many other ocular conditions that simulate retinoblastoma (see Table 42.2) can thus be easily excluded.

History

Leukocoria requires that a careful history of the pregnancy, labour, delivery, birth weight and neonatal period be obtained; illnesses in early pregnancy, premature labour and oxygen use in the neonatal period may be relevant. The first observation of the leucocoria may help in establishing the differential diagnosis: an abnormality present at birth is more likely to be due to a developmental anomaly; leucocoria presents at an average age of 12 months in bilateral retinoblastoma and 24 months in unilateral retinoblastoma (Shields & Augsburger 1981). In an older infant the parents should be asked about contact with puppies and other animals. A careful family history of any eye disorder should be obtained. The fundi of both parents, the siblings and any other affected family members should also be examined.

Examination

A thorough fundus examination is performed, requiring a full general anaesthetic in infants and young children. The pupils must be widely dilated and scleral depression used in order to visualize the whole retina to the ora serrata.

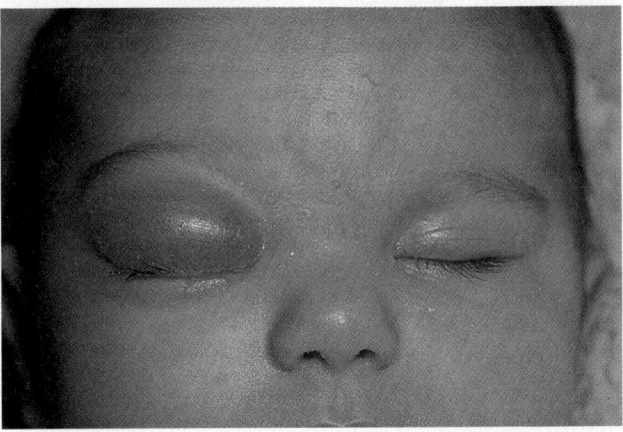

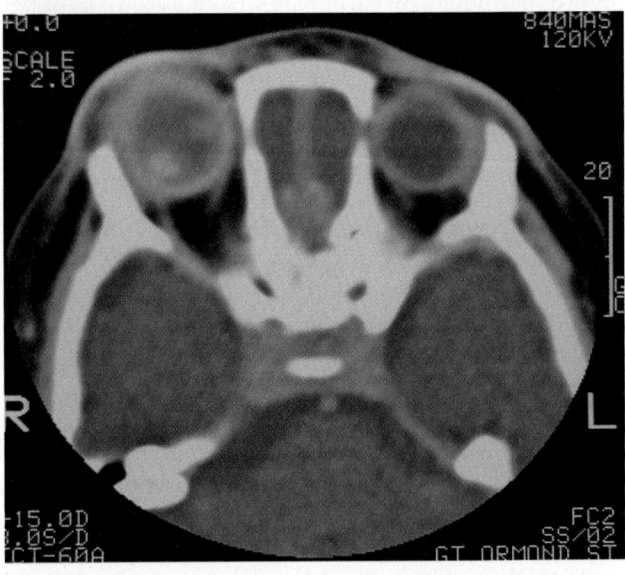

Fig. 42.12 (a) Retinoblastoma presenting as orbital cellulitis. At referral the patient was ill but apyrexial. The globe was not visible. A small non-calcified tumour was present in the left eye and a calcified retinoblastoma in the right eye. The swelling, which precluded a view of the eye, was greatly reduced by 2 days of systemic steroid treatment. (b) CT scan of same patient.

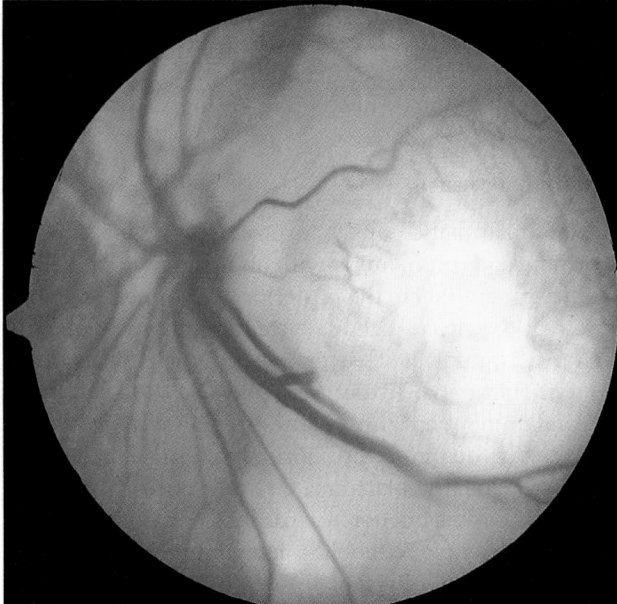

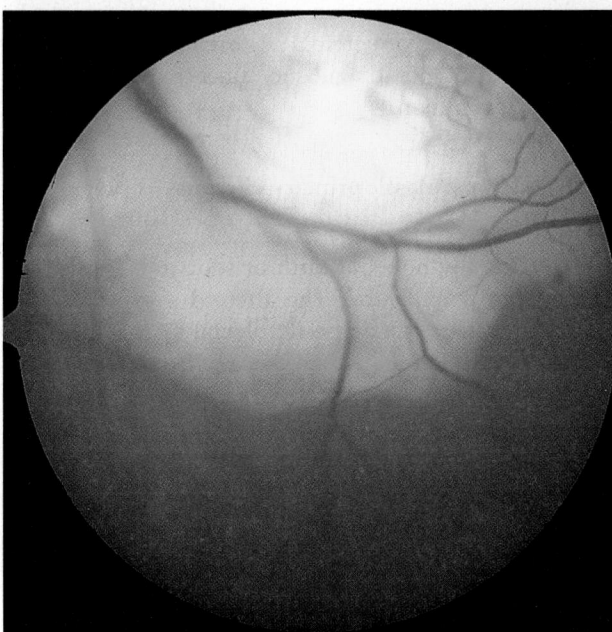

a

b

Fig. 42.13 (a, b) Retinoblastoma. Creamy raised tumour extending from the midperiphery to the optic nerve under the retina. The cut end of the optic nerve was free from tumour at enucleation.

Children presenting with suspected retinoblastoma can be divided into three broad groups. In the first group, there is a clear view of the tumour. Endophytic tumour growth gives rise to a creamy white mass (Fig. 42.13) projecting into the vitreous with large irregular blood vessels running on the surface and penetrating the tumour. Haemorrhage may be present on the surface of the tumour. Clumps of tumour cells in the vitreous (seeding) are virtually pathognomonic of retinoblastoma

(Fig. 42.14). Some tumours are surrounded by a halo of proliferating retinal pigment epithelium. Calcification within the tumour mass is common and resembles white, 'cottage cheese' (Fig. 42.15); the presence of calcification may be confirmed by ultrasound or CT scan (Fig. 42.16). Less commonly, retinoblastoma may present as an avascular white mass in the retinal periphery.

In the second group, an adequate fundus examination is not possible due to vitreous opacity or extensive retinal detachment. Other aspects of the examination may give a clue to diagnosis. Retinoblastoma occurs in normal sized

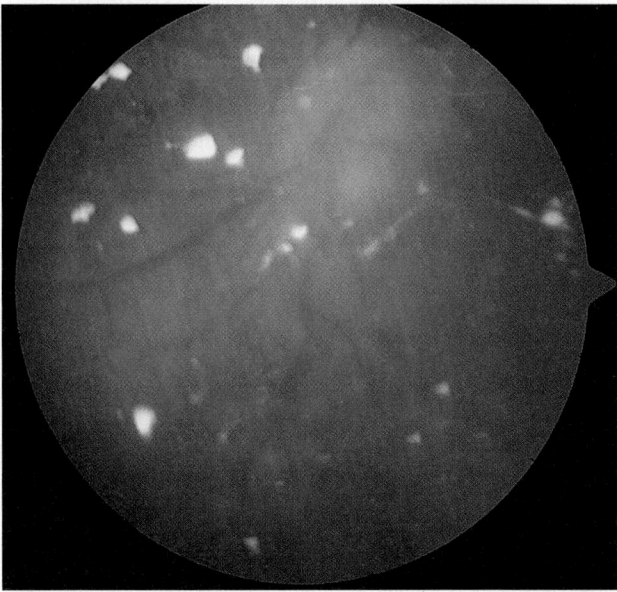

Fig. 42.14 Vitreous seeding following irradiation. The yellowish tumour particles present before treatment have become white after irradiation.

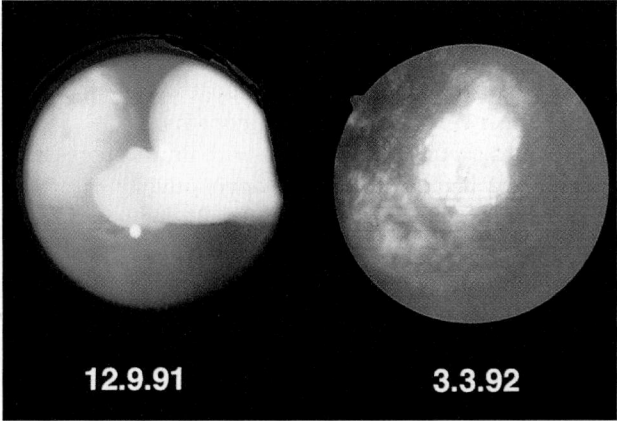

12.9.91   3.3.92

Fig. 42.15 On the left is seen the large multifocal retinoblastoma with vitreous seeds at diagnosis on 12 September 1991. On the right is seen the remnant of a quiescent scarred tumour after chemotherapy and 532 nm laser treatment on 3 March 1992 (Professor Gallie's patient).

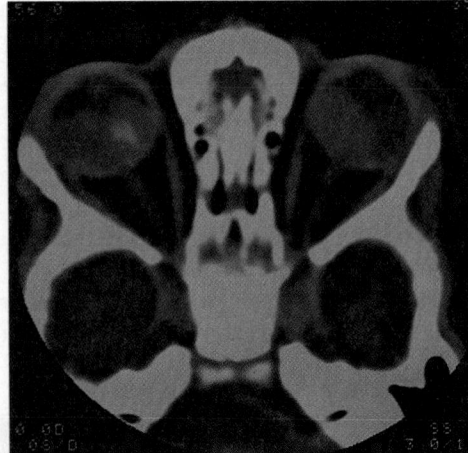

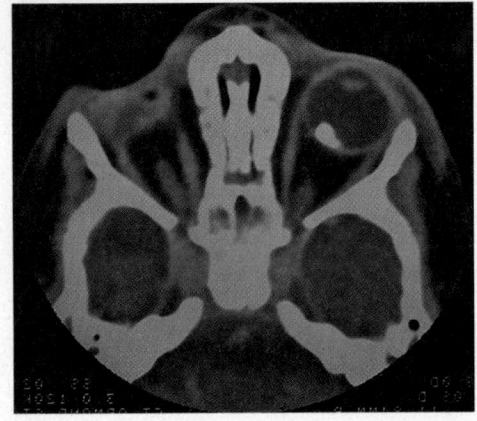

Fig. 42.16 (a) Retinoblastoma showing calcification within the tumour in both eyes. (b) After enucleation of the left eye and radiotherapy to the right eye, there is an increase in the calcification after treatment but regression in the size of the tumour.

eyes; the presence of microphthalmos makes a developmental abnormality much more likely. The other eye may give a clue to diagnosis. The presence of small tumours will confirm the diagnosis of retinoblastoma, while, for example, dragged retinal vessels and peripheral vitreoretinal changes may be seen in retinopathy of prematurity and dominant exudative vitreoretinopathy.

The third group includes cases with unusual presentation such as heterochromia, hypopyon, uveitis or orbital cellulitis. Here, diagnosis is difficult and specialized investigations may be particularly helpful, especially CT scan.

Infants with suspected retinoblastoma should be referred to a paediatrician for a careful systemic examination. Alternative diagnoses, for example the findings of typical skin lesions in tuberose sclerosis or incontinentia pigmenti, may be suggested.

Differential diagnosis

The conditions which may simulate retinoblastoma are detailed in Table 42.2. In the USA, ocular toxocariasis, persistent hyperplastic primary vitreous (PHPV) and Coats' disease are the three most common conditions confused with retinoblastoma (Shields *et al.* 1991a).

Ocular toxocariasis

Ocular inflammation due to toxocariasis presents either as a chronic endophthalmitis with an opaque vitreous, or a solitary granuloma in the posterior or peripheral retina in an otherwise healthy child; systemic symptoms or signs are rare (Duguid 1961). Several features help to differentiate retinoblastoma. Toxocariasis may show marked vitreous inflammation, with yellow–grey strands extending into the vitreous from the chorioretinal lesions; these are rarely seen in retinoblastoma. CT scan shows calcification in retinoblastoma but not in toxocariasis. Solitary granulomas may resemble retinoblastoma but often show a small translucent centre (Ellsworth 1969) (Fig. 42.17). If there is doubt about the diagnosis, a period of observation with regular fundus examination of a solitary lesion may be indicated. A positive serological test for toxocariasis is supportive, but not diagnostic, since exposure to the organism is common.

Persistent hyperplastic primary vitreous
(see Chapter 41)

PHPV is usually noted at birth or soon afterwards; it is almost always unilateral. The affected eye is microphthalmic and there is a dense retrolental mass which may be vascularized. The ciliary processes are often prominent and drawn towards the centre of the pupil. Untreated

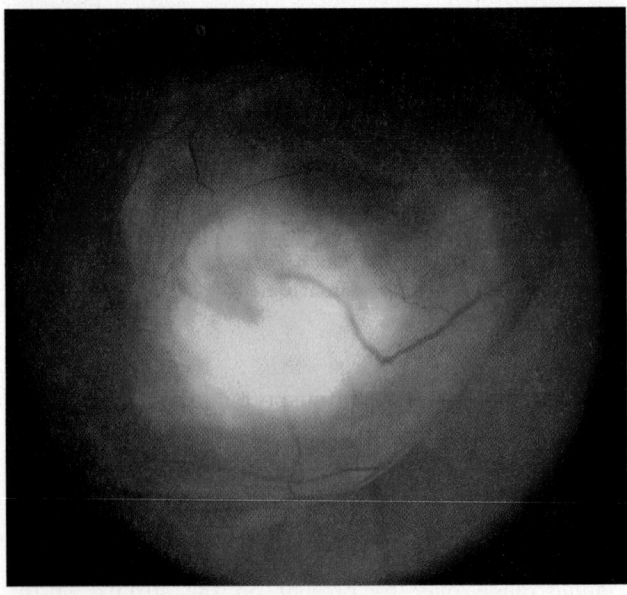

Fig. 42.17 Solitary granuloma at the macula, with a cilioretinal arteriole masquerading as a retinoblastoma.

PHPV eyes may develop pupil block glaucoma, vitreous haemorrhage, retinal detachment or phthisis bulbi; early surgery may prevent many of these complications and some reasonable visual results have been reported. As a warning, an infant with unilateral leucocoria has been reported with both PHPV and a diffuse infiltrating retinoblastoma (Liang *et al.* 1985).

Coats' disease (see Chapter 46)

Coats' disease is almost always unilateral and most commonly affects boys. Early Coats' disease may present with loss of vision or with a white pupillary reflex due to exudate accumulation at the macula. The tortuous, dilated, leaking vessels may be in the far periphery and hard to see without examination under anaesthetic. Later stages of Coats' disease develop exudative detachment with tortuous dilated telangiectatic vessels, subretinal lipid and cholesterol crystals. The colour of the 'white reflex' may be the first clue to the diagnosis: in Coats' disease it is yellow; in retinoblastoma it is white. Intraocular calcification is rare in Coats' disease. Ultrasound shows a diffuse uniform increase in the opacity of the vitreous, with no mass evident on contrast enhancement. Treatment of early Coats' disease with cryotherapy or laser coagulation may arrest the disease or result in some improvement (Ridley *et al.* 1982). In late Coats' disease, glaucoma may ultimately necessitate removal of the blind eye.

Retinal dysplasia (see Chapter 41)

Retinal dysplasia presents as a bilateral retrolental mass at birth or soon afterwards, unrelated to prematurity or oxygen use. Retinal dysplasia in trisomy 13 occurs in association with a variety of other serious systemic abnormalities. A similar ocular condition is seen in Norrie's disease, incontinentia pigmenti and Warburg's syndrome, and it may also occur as an isolated finding in an otherwise normal child. Examination under anaesthetic will reveal a shallow anterior chamber, clear lens and a relatively avascular retrolental mass without any inflammatory signs. There is no calcification on ultrasound or CT scan.

Retinopathy of prematurity (see Chapter 43)

Advanced cicatricial retinopathy of prematurity may give rise to a dense unilateral or bilateral retrolental mass. It is seen predominantly in very low birth weight infants who have been exposed to oxygen and seldom gives rise to confusion with retinoblastoma.

Metastatic endophthalmitis

Metastatic endophthalmitis results from haematogenous spread of infection from a distant infective locus such as

meningitis, endocarditis or abdominal sepsis. *Streptococcus*, *Staphylococcus* and meningococci are the organisms most commonly involved. The condition may cause marked vitreous opacification but the presence of other inflammatory signs and systemic infection usually distinguishes this condition from retinoblastoma (Shields *et al.* 1991a).

Medulloepithelioma (dictyoma) and intraocular teratoma

Medulloepithelioma arises from the ciliary epithelium and is always unilateral and may undergo glial and/or neural differentiation (Kivela & Tarrkanen 1988; Desai *et al.* 1990). It arises at a later age of onset, anteriorly from the ciliary body, and has a cystic structure (Broughton & Zimmerman 1978). These white friable tumours, sometimes with a felt-like structure (Fig. 42.18), are best treated by enucleation, since local excision is not usually successful (Canning *et al.* 1988). Life expectancy is good.

Intraocular teratoma presents at birth, may replace or destroy the globe, and is more common in females (Kivela *et al.* 1993).

Other disorders

A careful examination including a refraction will differentiate extensive myelinated nerve fibres, optic nerve coloboma, high myopia and congenital cataract, all of

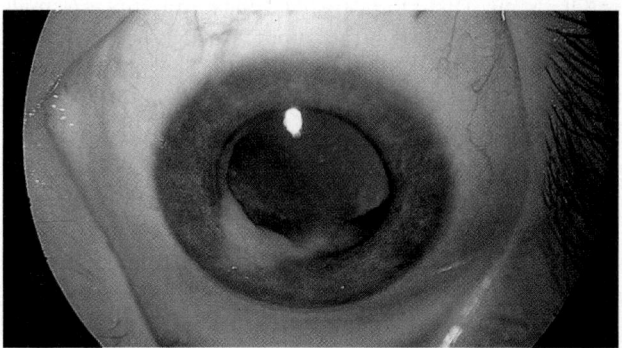

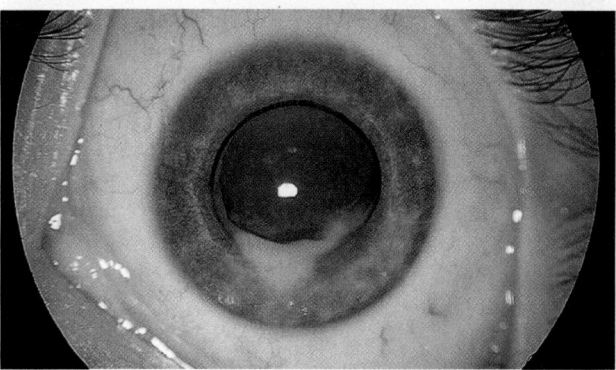

Fig. 42.18 Medulloepithelioma (dictyoma) presenting as a felt-like structure arising in the ciliary body and involving the iris.

which may show leukocoria, from retinoblastoma. Occasionally chronic granulomatous uveitis with a hypopyon may present diagnostic difficulties, especially if the posterior segment cannot be visualized. Ultrasound and CT scan are helpful in ruling out posterior segment tumour. A calcified abscess has simulated a retinoblastoma on CT scanning (Shields *et al.* 1992). If there is still doubt about the diagnosis, very careful aspiration of aqueous via a corneal paracentesis for cytology may be cautiously considered.

Management

The management of the child with retinoblastoma includes assessment to rule out metastatic spread, treatment of the ocular tumour, long-term follow-up and genetic counselling for the family, including examination of relatives at high risk of developing retinoblastoma. Management requires a team approach, with ophthalmologist, paediatric oncologist and genetic counsellor, working together, ideally with a social worker and psychologist experienced in retinoblastoma.

Investigation

Bone marrow aspiration and lumbar puncture, searching for metastatic disease, is performed during the initial examination under anaesthetic, if there is sufficient volume of tumour to require enucleation, or if the optic nerve is not visible. These tests are not done if tumours are small enough to treat the eye and avoid enucleation, and it has been suggested that they may not be useful in the usual newly diagnosed case (Mohney & Robertson 1994).

CT scan is helpful, not only in confirming the diagnosis, but also in excluding intracranial involvement or pineal tumour. Not only is the intraocular mass and pathognomonic calcification well visualized, but the optic nerves can be assessed, and the pineal region imaged. CT scanning, however, must not be taken to exclude retinoblastoma by not demonstrating calcification, especially in diffuse infiltrating retinoblastoma (Bhatnager & Vine 1991; Karr & Kalina 1991). Magnetic resonance imaging (MRI) may provide similar information, but so far is less useful in showing calcification (Mafee *et al.* 1989). It may be better at defining intracranial extension, especially in the suprasellar region and the posterior fossa. Fluorescein angiography may be helpful in distinguishing some retinoblastoma tumours from Coats' disease or dominant exudative vitreoretinopathy, but is usually unnecessary. Ultrasound may be useful in making the diagnosis of some retinoblastoma tumours (Fig. 42.19), but its major role may be in following regression of the tumour after therapy, particularly when the tumour cannot be visualized (Fig. 42.20).

Since intraocular retinoblastoma is nearly 96% curable,

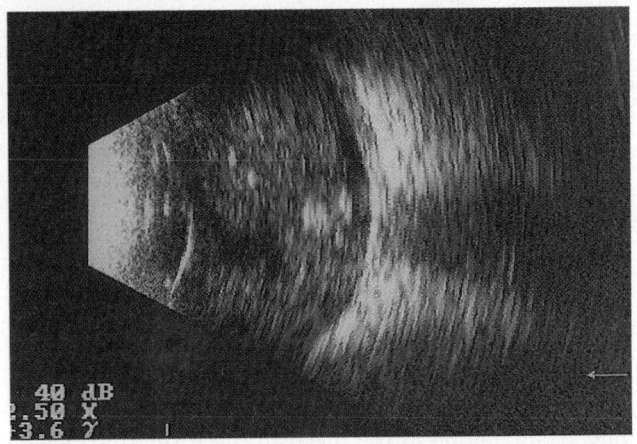

Fig. 42.19 Ultrasound of an eye filled with retinoblastoma showing flecks of calcification.

and metastatic retinoblastoma is still very difficult to cure, biopsy of retinoblastoma is contraindicated, due to the risk of spreading tumour to an extraocular location. In cases of suspected retinoblastoma with anterior segment involvement, an aqueous tap through clear cornea may be cautiously performed for cytology; vitreous biopsy should be avoided unless retinoblastoma is extremely unlikely because of the risk of extraocular spread of tumour (Stevenson *et al.* 1989).

Treatment

Enucleation

Enucleation of the eye remains a common therapy for retinoblastoma and will result in a cure if tumour is confined to the eye. Most patients with unilateral retinoblastoma present with extensive tumour in the affected eye, and once the fellow eye has been carefully examined and found to be free of tumour, enucleation is performed.

Bilateral retinoblastoma most commonly presents with one eye full of extensive tumour, and smaller tumours in the fellow eye. The worse eye, with no possibility of useful vision, is enucleated and attempts are made to save the lesser involved eye. Occasionally children are diagnosed with extensive disease in both eyes requiring bilateral enucleation. These children are already blind from the disease, although the parents may be unaware of it, and they do extremely well with only surgery. Attempts to save such severely involved eyes lead to significant short-term and long-term morbidity, and often are not in the child's own interest. Enucleation is also indicated for recurrent tumour that has already failed other treatment modalities.

Enucleation should be performed with a minimum of manipulation of the globe. A long optic nerve (8–12 mm)

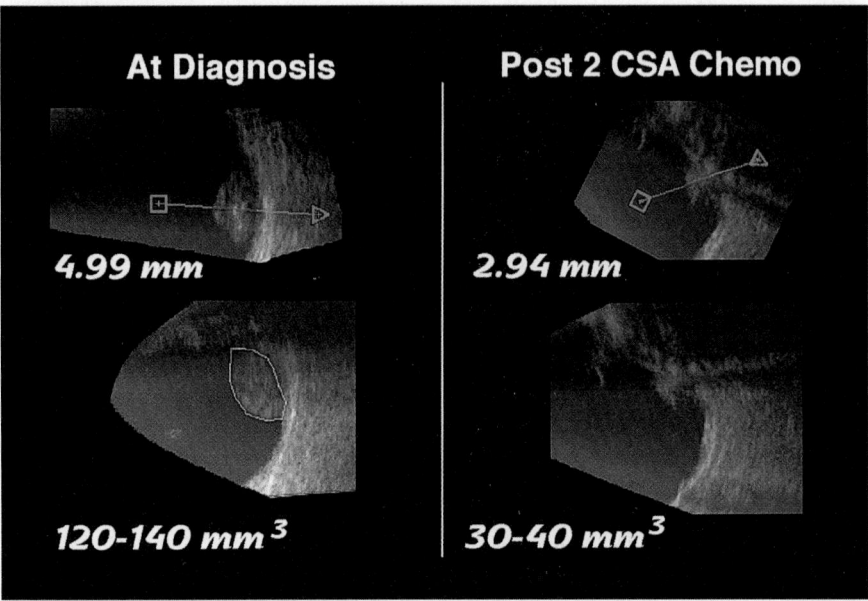

Fig. 42.20 Three-dimensional ultrasound permits accurate assessment of tumour dimensions and volume on sequential visits. Left: initial tumour. Right: regressing tumour after three doses of chemotherapy. Ultrasound processing is accomplished in three dimensions by acquiring 260 B-scan images which are realigned, reconstructed and rendered by the computer. The acquired B-scan (two-dimensional) images are over-sampled for verification of motion, location and orientation. The three-dimensional images are calibrated with three-dimensional phantoms for distance, area and volume parameters.

must be obtained in an attempt to be clear of tumour that may be invading the nerve. An orbital implant is placed, with muscles sutured to the implant to prevent its migration later out of the muscle cone. Implants designed to become vascularized, such as the hydroxyapatite implants (Shields *et al.* 1994), may give a better long-term cosmetic effect. A conformer may be placed under the eyelids for the first 10 days postoperatively, and then is replaced with the first artificial eye. The first artificial eye is nearly always imperfect, but adjustments can wait several months until healing is complete. It is important for social and family reasons to get an artificial eye in place early.

There is a trend towards conservative management (Shields *et al.* 1989; Dudgeon 1995), as more refined techniques are developed.

External beam irradiation

Radiation has been the main treatment modality for medium to large, or bilateral macular retinoblastoma tumours (Lam *et al.* 1990) for the past 30 years. Many eyes have been saved with very useful vision, but with some severe side-effects.

A total dose of 3500–4000 cGy is given in divided doses over a 3–4-week period (Harnett *et al.* 1987). A temporal portal excluding the lens is used when possible (Toma *et al.* 1995), to avoid a radiation-induced cataract, but when it is important to irradiate the ora serrata, or when vitre-

ous seeds are present, an anterior or lateral whole-eye approach may be used (Hungerford *et al.* 1995).

The first effects on the tumour are seen about 3 weeks after starting treatment, and have been classified into three patterns (Ellsworth 1969).
- Type I. The tumour regresses to a calcified mass resembling cottage cheese (Figs 42.21, 42.22).
- Type II. The tumour reduces in size, takes on a translucent fish-flesh appearance, and a ring of retinal pigment epithelial–choroidal scarring shows at the edge of the tumour. There is no calcification.
- Type III. A combination of type I and II; regression is most commonly seen.

With type II and III regression patterns it may be difficult to be sure that the tumour is inactive. These tumours must be watched closely subsequently, so that any change such as increasing opacity, globular shape change or increase in fine tumour blood vessels is noted early and treated with laser or cryotherapy. Macular tumours can regress, resulting in recovery of vision (Weiss *et al.* 1994).

The complications of external irradiation include cosmetic deformity to some extent (it is worse the younger the child is at the time of irradiation), cataract (Brooks *et al.* 1990), reduced tear effectiveness and dry-eye syndromes (Imhof *et al.* 1993), and, most importantly, second primary tumours within the radiation field in children with a germ-line RB1 mutation (Draper *et al.* 1986; Eng *et al.* 1993). Recurrence following irradiation is most

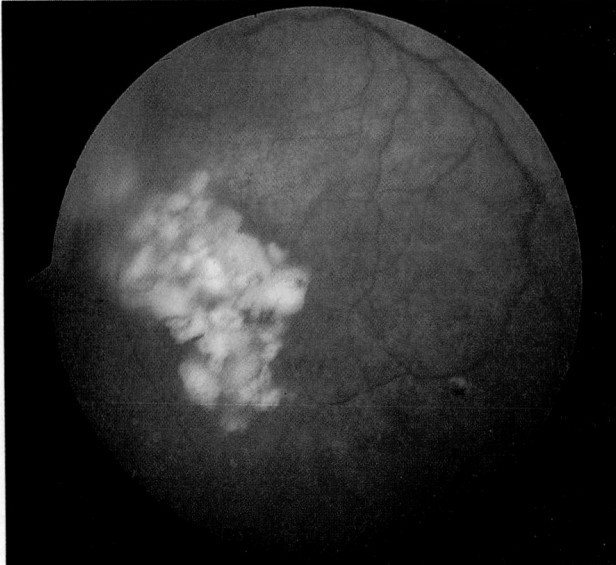

Fig. 42.21 Retinoblastoma regression following irradiation. Calcified 'cottage cheese' appearance.

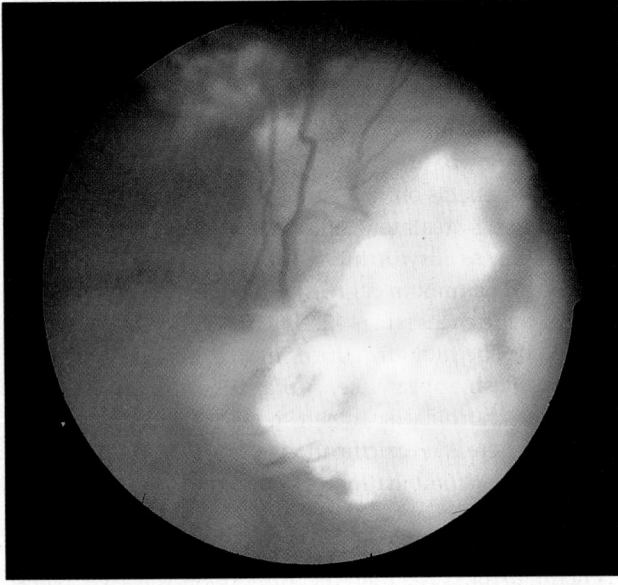

Fig. 42.22 Retinoblastoma regression following irradiation. This shows a mixed, suspicious regression but after a 4-year follow-up no recurrence was detected.

commonly seen with large tumours and vitreous seeding. Unless recurrence, post-irradiation, can be managed by chemotherapy, focal irradiation, cryotherapy or laser therapy, enucleation of the eye may be the only choice to avoid tumour spread.

The orbit is irradiated for orbital recurrence, or when histopathological examination of the enucleated globe shows involvement of the cut end of the optic nerve.

Focal irradiation

Solitary tumours less than 15 mm in diameter which are not adjacent to the disc or macula may be treated with an episcleral radioactive plaque, now most commonly iodine-125 (Stannard *et al.* 1987; Shields *et al.* 1993b). This technique may also be used to treat recurrences after chemotherapy or external beam irradiation (Shields *et al.* 1993d), where a second course of radiation to the whole eye would lead to severe radiation retinopathy or optic neuropathy. Under general anaesthesia, the tumour is localized using scleral indentation, and the plaque is sutured to the sclera and left *in situ* until the prescribed dose of radiation has been delivered to the apex of the tumour.

Chemotherapy

Systemic chemotherapy can now offer good shrinkage of intraocular tumours. Most successful protocols include carboplatin, vincristine and etoposide given every 3 weeks intravenously, followed by focal therapy with cryotherapy or laser therapy to destroy residual or recurrent tumour (Gallie *et al.* 1992). Addition of high short doses of cyclosporin A may enhance the effectiveness of the chemotherapy by blocking the multidrug resistance membrane pump, beta-glycoprotein which is commonly overexpressed in retinoblastoma tumours (Chan *et al.* 1996). Eyes with vitreous seeding require long courses of chemotherapy (greater than 6 months); the success rate in saving such eyes may be better with chemotherapy than with radiotherapy (Gallie *et al.* 1996; Chan *et al.* 1996).

Side-effects of chemotherapy include myelosuppression and hair loss, and the usual problems of chemotherapy. Unlike radiation, no cosmetic deformity results. Etoposide is reported to induce a specific leukaemia in 2% of children (Pui *et al.* 1991). Many years must pass before full effects on children with mutations of RB1 are known.

Cryotherapy

Cryotherapy is used for small anteriorly placed tumours, or more posterior tumours when visual damage will not ensue (Shields *et al.* 1993c). Since the cells are killed when they thaw, a triple freeze–thaw technique is used, with a full minute for thawing between the successive freezes (see Fig. 42.17). Cryotherapy is almost always repeated several times, months apart, until no residual active tumour remains. Cryotherapy may be used either as a primary procedure or to treat tumours that have had an inadequate response to radiation or chemotherapy. When superiorly placed, moderately sized tumours must be treated with cryotherapy, a laser barrier may be placed posterior to the tumour, to protect the retina from detachment by the serous exudate of the acute freeze.

Laser

Laser coagulation is used for small tumours, or tumours that have been initially shrunk with chemotherapy, or for recurrences following chemotherapy or radiotherapy. Most commonly a green-argon or frequency-doubled yttrium-aluminium-garnet (YAG) laser at 532 nm is used to first cut off the blood supply to a small tumour by encircling it with two confluent rows of laser burns, and later any remnant tumour within the scar is treated directly. Infrared lasers (diode or 1064 nm YAG) have also been used to advantage, to coagulate larger thicker tumours (Gallie *et al.* 1996).

Extraocular retinoblastoma

Chemotherapy has been used in patients with metastatic spread, intracranial or orbital disease. Orbital recurrences receive 4000–5000 cGy of radiation (Hungerford *et al.* 1987). Intrathecal chemotherapy has been used in meningeal spread, but with very poor results.

Prophylactic therapy

When marked choroidal invasion and involvement of the cut end of the optic nerve are noted on histopathology, extra therapy may be advised to treat the spread of tumour beyond the eye. However, lesser involvement of the optic nerve may be better managed by close follow-up and treatment only when disease is documented. Otherwise, many children may be treated unnecessarily.

Long-term follow-up

Following the initial management, assessment of the response to treatment will require frequent general anaesthetics, especially in the first year following diagnosis, when recurrence or new tumours are most likely to occur. New tumours occurred in 11% of children with retinoblastoma (Salmonsen *et al.* 1979) and were much more frequent in the peripheral retina, emphasizing the importance of a careful funduscopic examination with indentation to obtain a clear view of the periphery.

Genetic counselling for retinoblastoma

With no molecular knowledge of the RB1 mutation

Without knowledge of which RB1 allele is mutant, risk for relatives of retinoblastoma can be calculated based on population studies (Bonaiti-Pellie & Briard-Guillemot 1981; Musarella & Gallie 1987). Offspring of patients with a family history of retinoblastoma or bilateral tumours have a 50% risk of inheriting the mutant allele and 45%

Table 42.3 Risk of retinoblastoma in relatives of a bilateral or familial patient. Reproduced with permission from Musarella and Gallie (1987).

Relationship to proband	Risk of carrying the retinoblastoma mutation	Risk of developing retinoblastoma tumour
Offspring	0.5 (1×0.5)Y	0.45 $(0.9 \times 0.5)f$
Sibling	0.05 $(0.1^* \times 0.5)$	0.027 (0.54×0.05)
Offspring of unaffected sibling	0.005 $(0.1 \times 0.1 \times 0.5)$	0.0027 (0.54×0.005)
First cousin	0.0005 $(0.1 \times 0.1 \times 0.1 \times 0.5)$	0.00027 (0.54×0.0005)
Monozygotic twin	1.0	0.9 (0.9×1.0)
Dizygotic twin	0.05 (0.1×0.5)	0.027 (0.54×0.05)

Y, autosomal dominant trait; *f*, modified by factor for expressivity in proband.
* 0.1 unaffected carrier rate.

risk of developing retinoblastoma (Table 42.3). When two affected children are born to apparently normal parents, it is evident that one parent must be carrying (but not expressing) the mutant allele and hence there is also a 45% risk of any subsequent child developing retinoblastoma. The risk of other relatives inheriting the mutant allele depends on the number of intervening, apparently normal individuals; each of these has a 10% chance of carrying but not expressing the mutant allele. The risk therefore falls by a factor of 0.1 for each intervening unaffected generation.

Since 15% of patients with unilateral retinoblastoma have a germinal mutation it is evident that the offspring of individuals with unilateral retinoblastoma have a 7.5% risk of carrying the abnormal gene (Table 42.4). The probability of other relatives inheriting the abnormal gene can be calculated in a similar way (Musarella & Gallie 1987).

Infants born with such calculated risks to develop retinoblastoma are examined at regular intervals to detect early tumours to obtain the best visual result after therapy (Fig. 42.23). This includes awake examination of the full retina of infants under 3 months of age, and subsequently examination under anaesthetic every 3–6 months to the age of 3 years. Children are then followed with regular clinic examinations.

Molecular identification of the mutant RB1 allele

Polymorphic markers in and around the RB1 gene permit the mutant chromosome to be identified in familial cases (Wiggs *et al.* 1988; Cowell & Hogg 1992). However, most children do not have relatives with retinoblastoma, and frequently no informative polymorphisms can be found.

Precise RB1 mutation identification

The accurate identification of RB1 mutations will make it possible to apply the intensive screening for tumours only to the children who really have the mutation. This will be beneficial for the children and their families, and will reduce health-care expenditure. Although more than 150 RB1 mutations have been identified, service application of these techniques is only now being implemented in the clinic (Gallie *et al.* 1995).

Prognosis

With modern methods of diagnosis and treatment the prognosis of retinoblastoma is excellent; the 3-year survival for both unilateral and bilateral retinoblastoma approaches 96% (Lennox *et al.* 1975; Sanders *et al.* 1988). More patients with germ-line RB1 mutations may die of their second tumour than of retinoblastoma (Eng *et al.* 1993), but this risk may decrease as indications for radiotherapy decrease.

Poor prognostic signs for retinoblastoma include massive choroidal invasion, involvement of the optic nerve beyond the lamina cribrosa and extensive tumour (Messmer *et al.* 1991). Once there is extraocular spread, either locally or to a distant metastatic site, the prognosis is

Table 42.4 Risk of retinoblastoma in relatives of unilateral patients without a family history. Reproduced with permission from Musarella and Gallie (1987).

Relationship to proband	Risk of carrying the retinoblastoma mutation	Risk of developing retinoblastoma tumour
Offspring	0.075 $(0.15^* \times 0.5)Y$	0.057 $(0.76 \times 0.075)f$
Sibling	0.008 $(0.1 \sim \times 0.15 \times 0.5)$	0.004 (0.54×0.008)
Offspring of unaffected sibling	0.0008 $(0.1 \times 0.1 \times 0.15 \times 0.5)$	0.0004 (0.54×0.0008)
First cousin	0.00008 $(0.1 \times 0.1 \times 0.1 \times 0.15 \times 0.5)$	0.00004 (0.54×0.00008)
Monozygotic twin	0.15 (0.15×1.0)	0.081 0.54×0.15
Dizygotic twin	0.008 $(0.1 \times 0.15 \times 0.5)$	0.004 (0.54×0.008)

Y, autosomal dominant trait; *f*, modified by factor for expressivity in proband.
* 0.15 of unilateral cases carry the mutation.
~ 0.1 unaffected carrier rate.

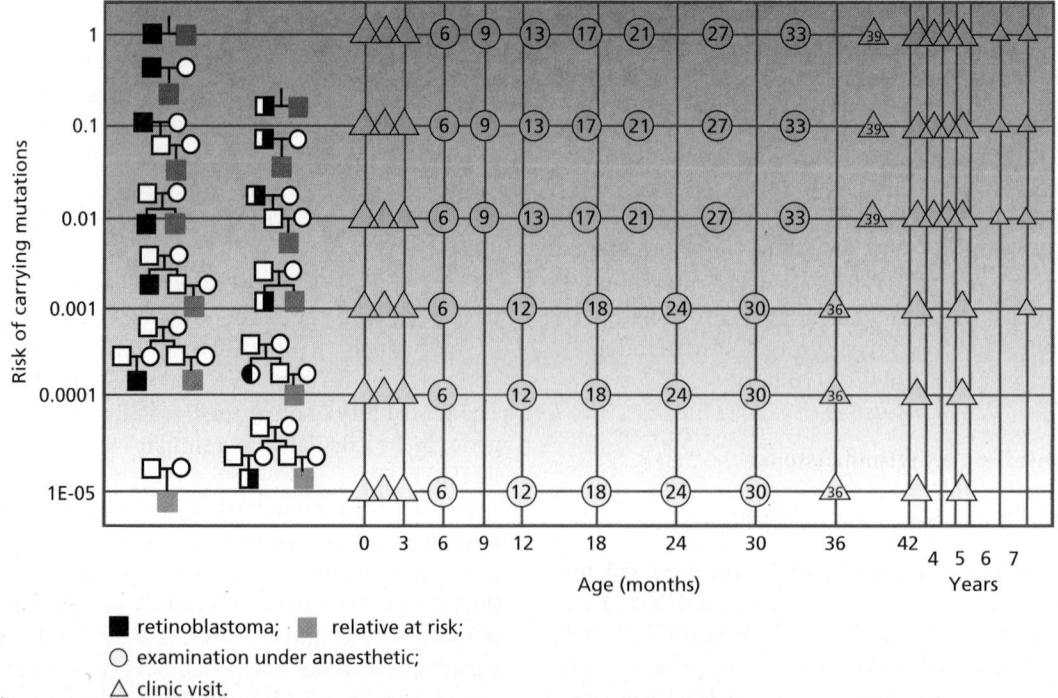

Fig. 42.23 Diagram illustrating the rationale and frequency of clinic examinations and examinations under anaesthetic from birth to 3 years of age for relatives of retinoblastoma patients who are at significant risk of also developing retinoblastoma.

extremely poor (Magramm *et al.* 1989). Most of the deaths from metastatic retinoblastoma occur in the first 3 years following treatment (Sanders *et al.* 1988); later mortality is usually due to a second primary tumour or pineal tumour.

The prognosis for vision is excellent in unilateral retinoblastoma, but depends on the size and site of the tumour in the less affected eye in bilateral cases. Small extrafoveal tumours have a good visual prognosis but when the macular region is involved, the visual result may be poor despite tumour control.

References

Bader JL, Meadows AT, Zimmerman LE *et al.* Bilateral retinoblastoma with ectopic intracranial retinoblastoma: trilateral retinoblastoma. *Cancer Genet Cytogenet* 1982; **5**: 203–13.

Bhatnagar R, Vine AK. Diffuse infiltrating retinoblastoma. *Ophthalmology* 1991; **98**: 1657–61.

Bonaiti-Pellie C, Briard-Guillemot ML. Segregation analysis in hereditary retinoblastoma. *Hum Genet* 1981; **57**: 411–19.

Brooks HL Jr, Meyer D, Shields JA, Balas AG, Nelson LB, Fontanesi J. Removal of radiation-induced cataracts in patients treated for retinoblastoma. *Arch Ophthalmol* 1990; **108**: 1701–8.

Broughton WL, Zimmerman LE. A clinicopathologic study of 56 cases of intraocular medulloepithelioma. *Am J Ophthalmol* 1978; **85**: 407–18.

Byrnes G, Shields C, Shields J, de Potter P, Eagle R. Retinoblastoma presenting with spontaneous hyphema and dislocated lens. *J Pediatr Ophthalmol Strabismus* 1993; **30**: 334–6.

Canning CR, McCartney ACE, Hungerford J. Medulloepithelioma (dictyoma). *Br J Ophthalmol* 1988; **72**: 764–7.

Cavenee WK, Dryja TP, Phillips RA *et al.* Expression of recessive alleles by chromosomal mechanisms in retinoblastoma. *Nature* 1983; **305**: 779–84.

Chan HSL, DeBoer G, Thiessen JJ, Budning A, Kingston JE, O'Brien JM, Koren G *et al.* Combining cyclosporin with chemotherapy controls intraocular retinoblastoma without radiation. *Clin Canc Res* 1996; **2**: 1499–508.

Chan HS, Thorner PS, Haddad G, Gallie BL. Multidrug-resistant phenotype in retinoblastoma correlates with P-glycoprotein expression. *Ophthalmology* 1991; **98**: 1425–31.

Chang MW, Barr E, Seltzer J *et al.* Cytostatic gene therapy for vascular proliferative disorders with a constitutively active form of the retinoblastoma gene product. *Science* 1995; **267**: 518–22.

Comings DE. A general theory of carcinogenesis. *Proc Natl Acad Sci USA* 1973; **70**: 3324–8.

Cowell JK, Hogg A. Genetics and cytogenetics of retinoblastoma. *Cancer Genet Cytogenet* 1992; **64**: 1–11.

DeCaprio JA, Ludlow JW, Figge J *et al.* SV40 large tumour antigen forms a specific complex with the product of the retinoblastoma susceptibility gene. *Cell* 1988; **54**: 275–83.

Desai VN, Lieb WE, Dorwsa LA, Eagle RC, Shields JA, Saunders R. Photoreceptor cell differentiation in intraocular medulloepithelioma. An immunohistopathologic study. *Arch Ophthalmol* 1990; **108**: 481–2.

Draper GJ, Sanders BM, Kingston JE. Second primary neoplasms in patients with retinoblastoma. *Br J Cancer* 1986; **53**: 661–71.

Dudgeon J. Retinoblastoma—trends in conservative management. *Br J Ophthalmol* 1995; **79**: 104.

Duguid IM. Features of ocular infestation by *Toxocara*. *Br J Ophthalmol* 1961; **45**: 789–96.

Dunn JM, Phillips RA, Zhu X, Becker AJ, Gallie BL. Mutations in the RB1 gene and their effects on transcription. *Mol Cell Biol* 1989; **9**: 4594–602.

Dyson N, Howley PM, Minger K, Harlow E. The human papilloma virus-16 E7 oncoprotein is able to bind to the retinoblastoma gene product. *Science* 1989; **242**: 934–7.

Eagle RC, Shields JA, Donoro L, Milner RS. Malignant transformation of spontaneously regressed retinoblastoma, retinoma, retinocytoma variant. *Ophthalmology* 1989; **96**: 1389–96.

Ellsworth RM. The practical management of retinoblastoma. *Trans Am Ophthalmol Soc* 1969; **67**: 462–534.

Eng C, Li FP, Abramson DH *et al.* Mortality from second tumours among long-term survivors of retinoblastoma. *J Natl Cancer Institute* 1993; **85**: 1121–8.

Friend SH, Bernards R, Rogelj S *et al.* A human DNA segment with properties of the gene that predisposes to retinoblastoma and osteosarcoma. *Nature* 1986; **323**: 643–6.

Gallie BL, Budning A, DeBoer G, Thiessen J, Koren G, Verjee Z, Ling V *et al.* Chemotherapy with focal therapy can cure intraocular retinoblastoma without radiation. *Arch Ophthalmol* 1996; **114**: 1321–30.

Gallie BL, Dunn JM, Hamel PA, Muncaster M, Cohen BL, Phillips RA. How do retinoblastoma tumours form? *Eye* 1992; **6**: 226–31.

Gallie BL, Ellsworth RM, Abramson DH, Phillips RA. Retinoma: spontaneous regression of retinoblastoma or benign manifestation of the mutation? *Br J Cancer* 1982a; **45**: 513–21.

Gallie BL, Hei Y-J, Dunn JM. Retinoblastoma: for the next generation. In: Cowell J, ed. *Cancer Genetics*. London: Bios, 1995; 1–29.

Gallie BL, Muncaster M, Cohen BL, Gill RM, Hamel PA, Phillips RA. Retinoblastoma mutations: initiation versus progression of cancer. In: Novak JF, ed. *Osteosarcoma Research Conference 1991*. Pittsburgh, Pennsylvania: Hogrefe & Huber, 1993: 367–73.

Gallie BL, Phillips RA, Ellsworth RM, Abramson DH. Significance of retinoma and phthisis bulbi for retinoblastoma. *Ophthalmology* 1982b; **89**: 1393–9.

Godbout R, Dryja TP, Squire J, Gallie BL, Phillips RA. Somatic inactivation of genes on chromosome 13 is a common event in retinoblastoma. *Nature* 1983; **304**: 451–3.

Goodrich DW, Wang NP, Qian Y-W, Lee EY-HP, Lee W-H. The retinoblastoma gene product regulates progression through the G1 phase of the cell cycle. *Cell* 1991; **67**: 293–302.

Hamel PA, Cohen BL, Sorce LM, Gallie BL, Phillips RA. Hyperphosphorylation of the retinoblastoma gene product is determined by domains outside the SV40 large T-binding regions. *Mol Cell Biol* 1990; **10**: 6586–95.

Harnett AN, Hungerford J, Lambert G *et al.* Modern lateral external beam (lens sparing) radiotherapy for retinoblastoma. *Ophthal Paediatr Genet* 1987; **8**: 53–61.

Hinds PW, Mittnacht S, Dulic V, Arnold A, Reed SI, Weinberg RA. Regulation of retinoblastoma protein functions by ectopic expression of human cyclins. *Cell* 1992; **70**: 993–1006.

Hu QJ, Dyson N, Harlow E. The regions of the retinoblastoma protein needed for binding to adenovirus E1A or SV40 large T antigen are common sites for mutations. *EMBO J* 1990; **9**: 1147–55.

Hungerford J, Kingston J, Plowman N. Orbital recurrence of retinoblastoma. *Ophthalmic Paediatr Genet* 1987; **8**: 63–8.

Hungerford J, Toma N, Plowman P, Kingston J. External beam radiotherapy for retinoblastoma: I. whole eye technique. *Br J Ophthalmol* 1995; **79**: 109–11.

Imhof S, Hofman P, Tan K. Quantification of lacrimal function after D-shaped field irradiation for retinoblastoma. *Br J Ophthalmol* 1993; **77**: 482–4.

Jakobiec FA, Tso MOM, Zimmerman LE, Danis P. Retinoblastoma

and intracranial malignancy. *Cancer* 1977; **39**: 2048–58.

Jay M, Cowell J, Hungerford J. Register of retinoblastoma: preliminary results. *Eye* 1988; **2**: 102–5.

Karr D, Kalina R. Computerized tomography fails to show calcification in diffuse retinoblastoma. *J Pediatr Ophthalmol Strabismus* 1991; **28**: 14–17.

Kingston JE, Plowman PN, Hungerford JL. Ectopic intracranial retinoblastoma in childhood. *Br J Ophthalmol* 1985; **69**: 742–8.

Kivela T, Merenmies L, Ilveskoski I, Tarkkanen A. Congenital intraocular teratoma. *Ophthalmology* 1993; **100**: 782–91.

Kivela T, Tarrkanen A. Recurrent medulloepithelioma of the ciliary body. Immunohistochemical characteristics. *Ophthalmology* 1988; **95**: 1565–75.

Knudson AG. Mutation and cancer: statistical study of retinoblastoma. *Proc Natl Acad Science USA* 1971; **68**: 820–3.

Lam BL, Judisch GF, Sobol WM, Blodi CF. Visual prognosis in macular retinoblastomas. *Am J Ophthalmol* 1990; **110**: 229–32.

Lennox EL, Draper GJ, Sanders BM. Retinoblastoma: a study of natural history and prognosis of 268 cases. *Br Med J* 1975; **3**: 731–4.

Liang JC, Augsburger JJ, Shields JA. Diffuse infiltrating retinoblastoma associated with persistent primary vitreous. *J Pediatr Ophthalmol Strabismus* 1985; **22**: 31–3.

Lohmann DR, Brandt B, Hüpping W, Passarge E, Horsthemke B. Distinct RB1 gene mutations with low penetrance in hereditary retinoblastoma. *Hum Genet* 1994; **94**: 349–54.

Lueder GT, Heon E, Gallie BL. Retinoma associated with vitreous seeding. *Am J Ophthalmol* 1995; **119**: 522–3.

Mafee MF, Goldberg MF, Cohen SB *et al.* Magnetic resonance imaging versus computed tomography of leukocoric eyes and use of *in vitro* proton magnetic resonance spectroscopy of retinoblastoma. *Ophthalmology* 1989; **96**: 965–75.

Magramm I, Abramson D, Ellsworth RM. Optic nerve involvement in retinoblastoma. *Ophthalmology* 1989; **96**: 217–23.

Messmer EP, Heinrich T, Hopping W, de Sutter E, Havers W, Sauerwein W. Risk factors for metastases in patients with retinoblastoma. *Ophthalmology* 1991; **98**: 136–41.

Migdal C. Retinoblastoma occurring in four successive generations. *Br J Ophthalmol* 1976; **60**: 151.

Mohney BG, Robertson DM. Ancillary testing for metastasis in patients with newly diagosed retinoblastoma. *Am J Ophthalmol* 1994; **18**: 707–11.

Musarella MA, Gallie BL. A simplified scheme for genetic counseling in retinoblastoma. *J Pediatr Ophthalmol Strabismus* 1987; **24**: 124–5.

Nelson SC, Friedman HS, Oakes WJ *et al.* Successful therapy for trilateral retinoblastoma (see comments). *Am J Ophthalmol* 1992; **114**: 23–9.

Popoff N, Ellsworth RM. The fine structure of nuclear alterations in retinoblastoma and in the developing human retina: *in vivo* and *in vitro* observations. *J Ultrastruct Res* 1969; **29**: 535–49.

Pui CH, Ribeiro RC, Hancock ML, Rivera GK, Evans WE, Raimondi SC, Head DR *et al.* Acute myeloid leukemia in children treated with epipodophyllotoxins for acute lymphoblastic leukemia. *N Engl J Med* 1991; **325**: 1682–7.

Ridley ME, Shields JA, Brown GC, Tasman W. Coats' disease: evaluation of management. *Ophthalmology* 1982; **89**: 1381–7.

Roarty JD, McLean IW, Zimmerman LE. Incidence of second neoplasms in patients with bilateral retinoblastoma. *Ophthalmology* 1988; **95**: 1583–7.

Sakai T, Ohtani N, McGee TL, Robbins PD, Dryja TP. Oncogenic germ-line mutations in Sp1 and ATF sites in the human retinoblastoma gene. *Nature* 1991; **353**: 83–6.

Salmonsen PC, Ellsworth RM, Kitchen FD. The occurrence of new retinoblastoma after treatment. *Ophthalmology* 1979; **86**: 840–3.

Sanders BM, Draper GJ, Kingston JE. Retinoblastoma in Great Britain 1969–80: incidence, treatment, and survival. *Br J Ophthalmol* 1988; **72**: 576–83.

Shields CL, Shields JA, Baez KA, Cater J, De-Potter PV. Choroidal invasion of retinoblastoma: metastatic potential and clinical risk factors (see comments). *Br J Ophthalmol* 1993a; **77**: 544–8.

Shields C, Shields J, Potter P *et al.* Plaque radiotherapy in the management of retinoblastoma: use as a primary and secondary treatment. *Ophthalmology* 1993d; **100**: 216–24.

Shields C, Shields J, de Potter P, Singh A. Problems with the hydroxyopatitic orbital implant: experience with 250 consecutive cases. *Br J Ophthalmol* 1994; **78**: 702–6.

Shields CL, Shields JA, Minelli S *et al.* Regression of retinoblastoma after plaque radiotherapy. *Am J Ophthalmol* 1993b; **115**: 181–7.

Shields JA, Augsburger JJ. Current approaches to the diagnosis and management of retinoblastoma. *Surv Ophthalmol* 1981; **25**: 347–72.

Shields J, Shields C, Eagle R, de Potter P, Douglas C. Calcified intraocular abscess simulating retinoblastoma (letter). *Am J Ophthalmol* 1992; **114**: 227–9.

Shields J, Parsons H, Shields C, Shah P. Lesions simulating retinoblastoma. *J Pediatr Ophthalmol Strabismus* 1991a; **28**: 338–40.

Shields JA, Shields CL, De-Potter P. Cryotherapy for retinoblastoma. *Int Ophthalmol Clin* 1993c; **33**: 101–5.

Shields JA, Shields CL, Parsons HM. Review: differential diagnosis of retinoblastoma. *Retina* 1991b; **11**: 232–43.

Shields JA, Shields CL, Sivalingam V. Decreasing frequency of enucleation in patients with retinoblastoma. *Am J Ophthalmol* 1989; **108**: 185–9.

Shields JA, Shields CL, Suvarnamani C, Schroeder RP, De-Potter P. Retinoblastoma manifesting as orbital cellulitis. *Am J Ophthalmol* 1991c; **112**: 442–9.

Stannard C, Sealy R, Shackleton D, Hill J, Korrubel J. The use of iodine-125 plaques in the treatment of retinoblastoma. *Ophthalmic Paediatr Genet* 1987; **8**: 89–93.

Stevenson KE, Hungerford J, Garner A. Local extraocular extension of retinoblastoma following intraocular surgery. *Br J Ophthalmol* 1989; **73**: 739–42.

Toma N, Hungerford J, Plowman P, Kingston J, Doughty D. External beam radiotherapy for retinoblastoma II. lens sparing technique. *Br J Ophthalmol* 1995; **79**: 112–17.

Weiss AH, Karr DJ, Kalina RE, Lindsley KL, Pendergrass TW. Visual outcomes of macular retinoblastoma after external beam radiation therapy. *Ophthalmology* 1994; **101**: 1244–9.

Whyte P, Buchkovich KJ, Horowitz JM *et al.* Association between an oncogene and an anti-oncogene: the adenovirus E1A proteins bind to the retinoblastoma gene product. *Nature* 1988; **334**: 124–9.

Wiggs J, Nordenskjold M, Yandell D *et al.* Prediction of the risk of hereditary retinoblastoma, using DNA polymorphisms within the retinoblastoma gene. *N Engl J Med* 1988; **318**: 151–7.

Wilson WG, Campochiaro PA, Conway BP *et al.* Deletion (13)(q14.1q14.3) in two generations: variability of ocular manifestations and definition of the phenotype. *Am J Med Genet* 1987; **28**: 675–83.

Yunis JJ, Ramsay N. Retinoblastoma and sub band deletion of chromosome 13. *Am J Dis Child* 1978; **132**: 161–3.

43: Retinopathy of Prematurity

Alistair Fielder

Retrolental fibroplasia (RLF), which is now known as retinopathy of prematurity (ROP), was first reported in 1942 by Terry (1942) who published a description of the histological findings of what would now be considered end-stage cicatricial disease. As more cases were reported, it became evident that this condition was confined to premature infants and is a disorder of the immature retinal vasculature. Retrospective studies showed it to be extremely rare before the 1940s (Terry 1945). Owens and Owens (1948) showed that the retinopathy developed postnatally in infants who had a normal fundus examination at birth. ROP subsequently became the leading cause of blindness in children in the USA and a similar epidemic of ROP was seen in certain countries in Europe during the 1940s and 1950s.

Following Campbell's (1951) suggestion that the appearance of this condition at this time might be related temporally to the introduction of oxygen therapy into the premature nursery, evidence accumulated to support the concept of a toxic effect of oxygen on the immature retinal vasculature. This clinical observation was supported experimentally (Ashton *et al.* 1953; Patz 1954; Ashton 1980) and led to the restriction of oxygen use in preterm neonates. While this resulted in a dramatic fall in incidence, ROP was not eradicated completely, and it is now clear that many factors other than oxygen may play a role in the pathogenesis of ROP (Lucey & Dangman 1984; Ben-Sira *et al.* 1988; Weakley & Spencer 1992). The history of the scientific investigation of the pathogenesis of ROP makes fascinating reading and has been comprehensively reviewed by James and Lansman (1976), Silverman (1980), Lucey and Dangman (1984) and Flynn (1987).

Retinal vascular supply

Retinal vascularization commences around 16 weeks of gestation with the centrifugal outgrowth of mesenchymal spindle cells from the optic disc. These cells migrate in sheets, with endothelial proliferation and capillary formation occurring just behind the advancing vanguard of spindle cells. These newly formed capillaries later remodel forming the mature retina vascular network (Ashton

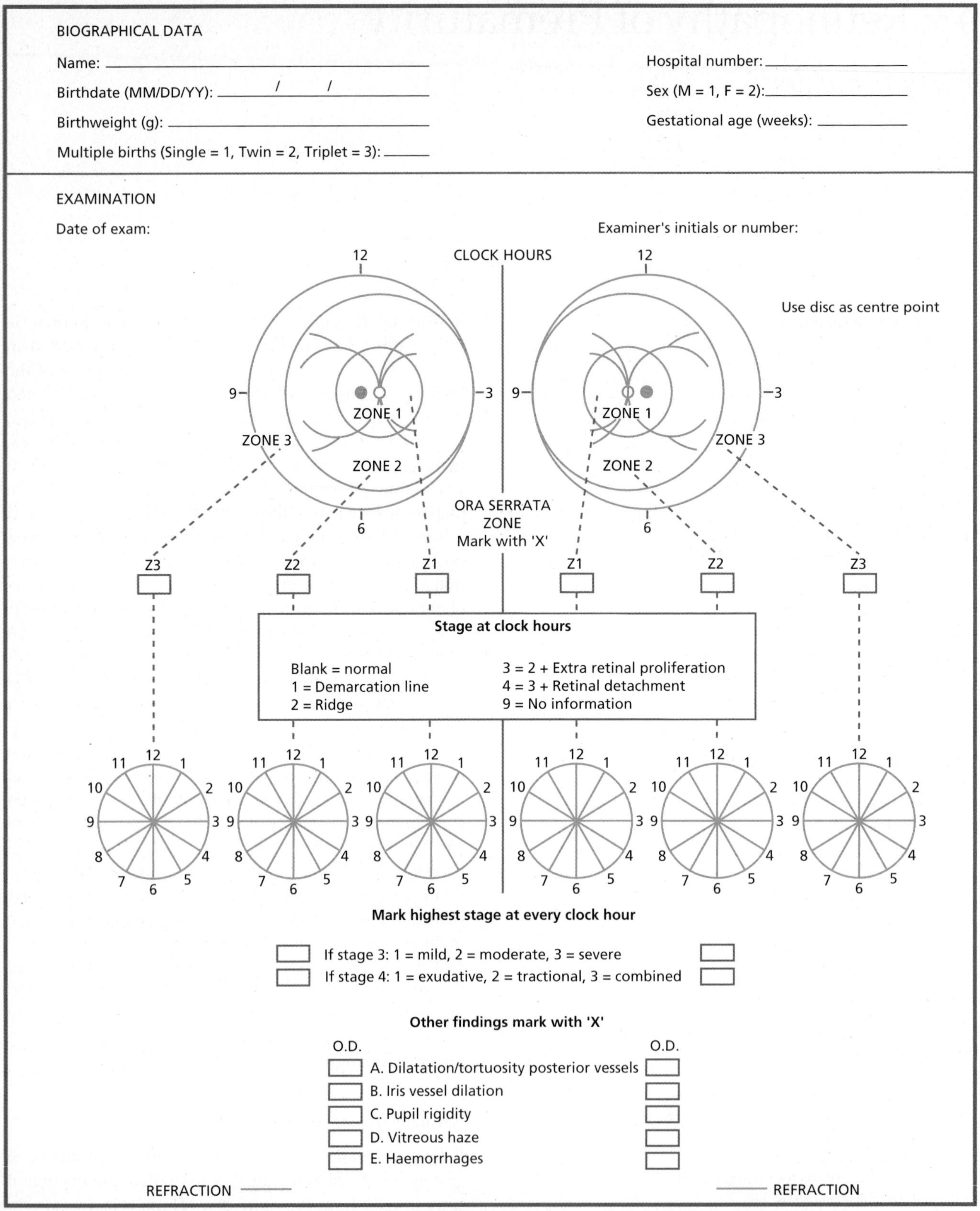

BIOGRAPHICAL DATA

Name: _____

Birthdate (MM/DD/YY): _____ / _____ / _____

Birthweight (g): _____

Multiple births (Single = 1, Twin = 2, Triplet = 3): _____

Hospital number: _____

Sex (M = 1, F = 2): _____

Gestational age (weeks): _____

EXAMINATION

Date of exam:

Examiner's initials or number:

CLOCK HOURS

Use disc as centre point

12

9 — ZONE 1 — 3   9 — ZONE 1 — 3

ZONE 3   ZONE 3

ZONE 2   ZONE 2

6   6

ORA SERRATA
ZONE
Mark with 'X'

Z3   Z2   Z1   Z1   Z2   Z3

Stage at clock hours

Blank = normal   3 = 2 + Extra retinal proliferation
1 = Demarcation line   4 = 3 + Retinal detachment
2 = Ridge   9 = No information

Mark highest stage at every clock hour

If stage 3: 1 = mild, 2 = moderate, 3 = severe
If stage 4: 1 = exudative, 2 = tractional, 3 = combined

Other findings mark with 'X'

O.D.   O.D.

A. Dilatation/tortuosity posterior vessels
B. Iris vessel dilation
C. Pupil rigidity
D. Vitreous haze
E. Haemorrhages

REFRACTION _____   _____ REFRACTION

Fig. 43.1 A chart for recording fundus details and staging ROP. Usually five stages are recorded (see text).

1970). The nasal retina is vascularized by about 32 weeks gestational age (GA) and the temporal retina by just after term (Michaelson 1948). The ophthalmoscopic appearance of the unvascularized retina is grey–white: its extent being related to the degree of immaturity. As the choroid is vascularized by 6 weeks GA (Sellhayer & Spitznas 1988) for the first 4 months or so it is the sole supply of nutrients to the retina.

The preterm retina has straight vessels (Fig. 43.2) and a fovea that is only differentiated ophthalmoscopically at around term.

Classification

The international classification of the acute stages of ROP was published in 1984 (Committee for the Classification of Retinopathy of Prematurity 1984), and in 1987 (Committee for the Classification of Retinopathy of Prematurity 1987) was expanded to include a classification of retinal detachment and the sequelae of this condition, thus replacing that of Reese *et al.* (1953). All stages of ROP are now covered by this single classification (Table 43.1) and the term RLF is no longer used. For the first time, direct comparison between centres and countries has become possible and this has stimulated an unprecedented flurry of clinical research with a major impact on clinical practice.

According to the new classification ROP is described by three features: (i) severity by stage; (ii) location by zone; and (iii) extent by clock hour of circumferential retinal involvement. A number of charts have been devised on which to record clinical findings (Fig. 43.1).

Severity of disease

ROP has been divided into five stages.

Stage 1

In stage 1 ROP there is a flat grey–white demarcation line

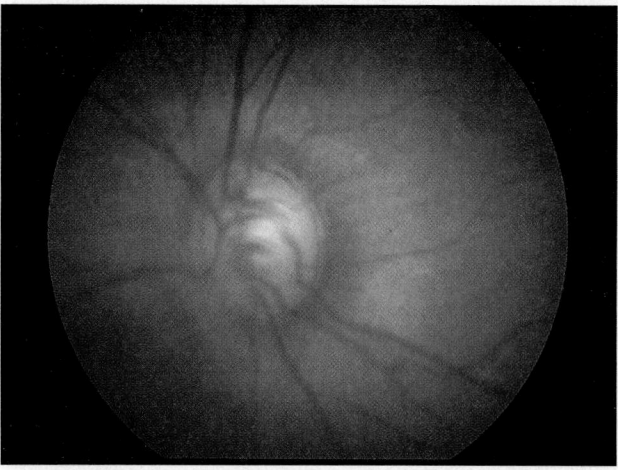

Fig. 43.2 Normal retinal vasculature and optic disc of a preterm neonate without retinopathy. Note the straightness and calibre of retinal vessels compared with Fig. 43.7. The posterior pole appears a little pale and there is a dark ring around the optic disc.

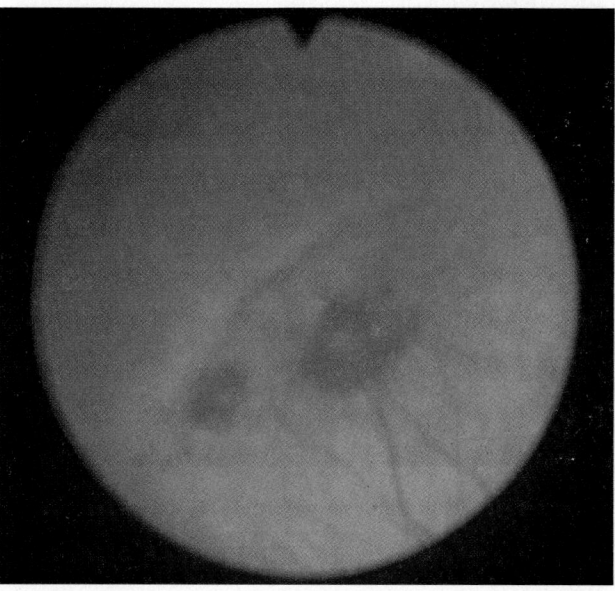

Fig. 43.3 ROP stage 1 demarcation line. The haemorrhages are perinatal and not related to the ROP (Mr E. Schulenberg's patient).

Table 43.1 Stages of ROP (from Committee for Classification of Retinopathy of Prematurity 1987).

Stage 1	Demarcation line	
Stage 2	Ridge	
Stage 3	Ridge with extraretinal fibrovascular proliferation	
Stage 4	Subtotal retinal detachment	
	extrafoveal	
	retinal detachment including fovea	
Stage 5	Total retinal detachment	
Funnel	Anterior	Posterior
	Open	Open
	Narrow	Narrow
	Open	Narrow
	Narrow	Open

separating the vascularized from non-vascularized retina. Often faint it can be difficult to identify. Retinal vessels may run up to the line but do not cross it (Fig. 43.3).

Stage 2

In stage 2 the demarcation line has increased in volume and extends out of the plane of the retina (Figs 43.4–43.6). The colour of the ridge may be white or pink and small neovascular tufts may be seen posterior to the ridge. Differentiating stage 1 and early stage 2 is not always simple.

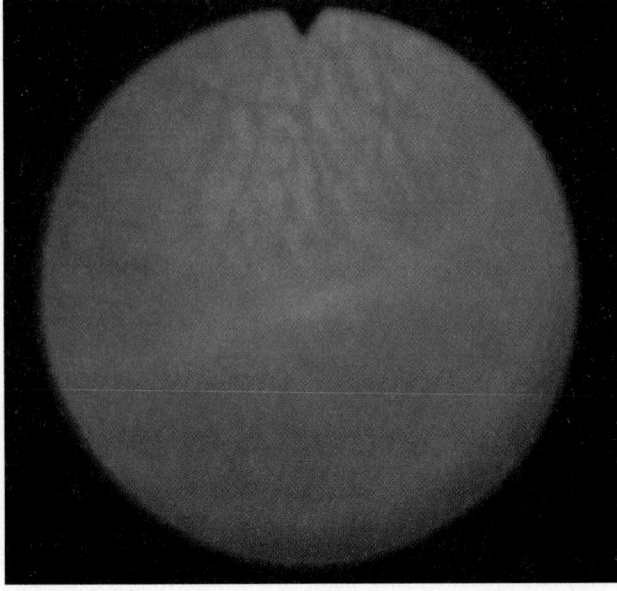

Fig. 43.4 ROP stage 2 ridge projecting (out of focus) forward into the vitreous (Mr E. Schulenberg's patient).

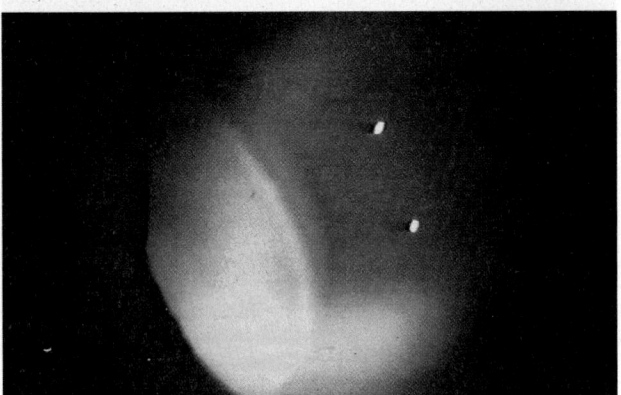

Fig. 43.5 Video ophthalmoscope picture of ROP stage 2. The thickness of the ridge can be clearly seen.

Stage 3

Stage 3 exhibits the features of stage 2, but is characterized by extraretinal neovascularization (Fig. 43.7). The new vessels may be continuous with, or disconnected from, the posterior border of the ridge, or extend into the vitreous.

Stage 4

This stage is characterized by subtotal retinal detachment, exudative or tractional, which may (stage 4b), or may not (stage 4a), involve the fovea.

Stage 5

In stage 5 there is a funnel-shaped total retinal detachment

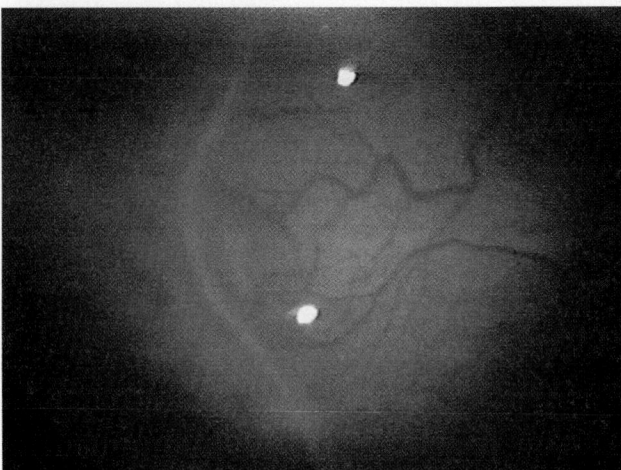

Fig. 43.6 Video ophthalmoscope view of stage 2 ROP with a well-demarcated ridge. One or two isolated frons of vessels are compatible with stage 2. Note the extensive branching of peripheral retinal vessels as they approach the ridge.

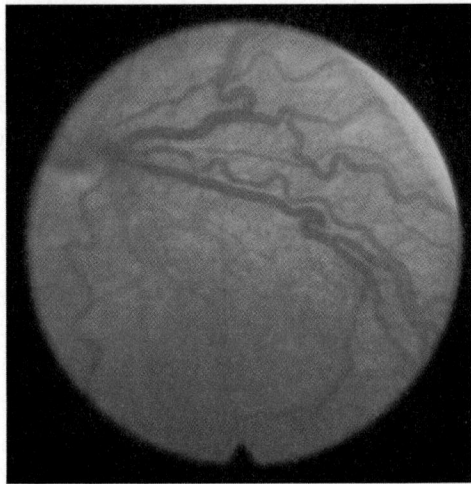

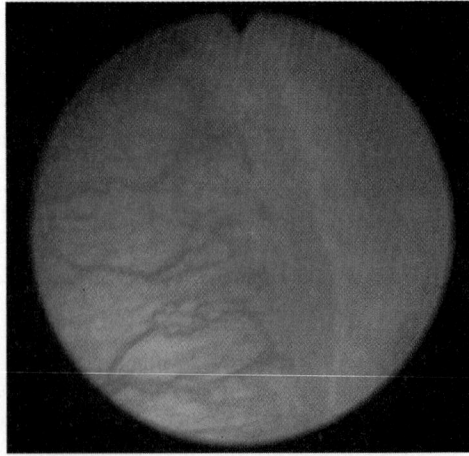

Fig. 43.7 ROP stage 3 showing marked vascular dilatation and tortuosity (top) and a ridge with new vessels (bottom) (Mr E. Schulenberg's patient).

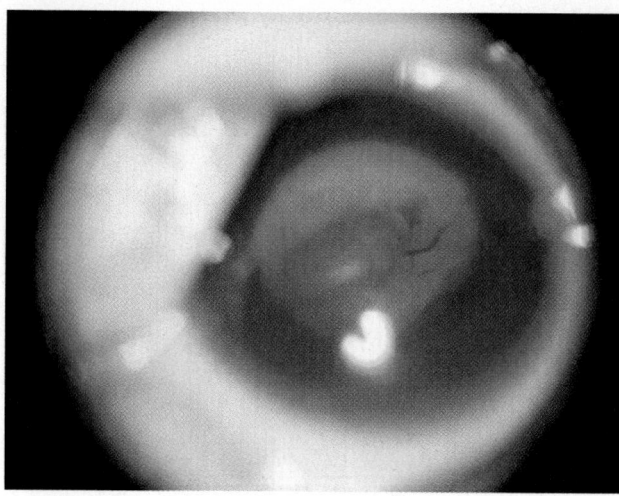

Fig. 43.8 Stage 5 funnel-shaped retinal detachment (Mr E. Schulenberg's patient).

(Fig. 43.8). This stage is further divided according to the characteristics of the funnel, whether it is open or narrowed anteriorly and posteriorly.

Plus disease

These are signs indicating ROP activity. Although plus disease can accompany any stage, if present it is likely that the condition will progress to stage 3. Plus presents with increasing severity, as tortuosity and engorgement of the posterior retinal vessels, vascular engorgement of the iris and pupil rigidity, and finally vitreous haze (Table 43.2).

Location

The retina is divided into three zones which are centred on the optic disc, in contrast to retinal neural organization which centres on the fovea. Zone 1 is a circle whose radius is twice the disc–foveal distance about 30°. Zone 2 extends from the edge of zone 1 to the ora serrata on the nasal side and encircles the anatomical equator. Zone 3 includes all retina temporally, superiorly and inferiorly which is anterior to zone 2. With no anatomical landmarks identifying zone 3, only when the nasal retina is fully vascularized can it be stated that zone 3 has been entered.

Extent

The extent of disease is described in clock hours. As the examiner looks at the eyes the 3 o'clock position is on the right, i.e. on the nasal side of the right eye and temporal side of the left eye.

Sequelae of retinopathy of prematurity

Other sequelae of severe ROP, e.g. microphthalmos,

corneal oedema, band keratopathy, posterior synechiae, angle closure glaucoma, need recording separately.

Incidence

The incidence and severity of ROP both rise with the level of immaturity. Published figures vary and the following incidence figures for any ROP for given birth weights are representative of the current situation in developed countries: < 1000 g, 53% (Keith & Kitchen 1984) and 89% (Ng *et al.* 1988); < 1250 g, 43% (Acheson & Schulenburg 1991) and 66% (Palmer *et al.* 1991); < 1300 g, 56% (Flynn *et al.* 1987a) and 75% (Ng *et al.* 1988); < 1500 g, 35% (Reisner *et al.* 1985), 48% (Schaffer *et al.* 1985) and 60% (Ng *et al.* 1988).

Stages 1 and 2 ROP resolve completely and the term severe disease is confined to stage 3 or above which may lead to visual impairment. The incidence of stage 3 ROP is as follows: < 750 g, 37–54%; 750–1000 g, 19–30%; 1000–1250 g, 3–9% (Ng *et al.* 1988; Acheson & Schulenburg 1991; Palmer *et al.* 1991; Holmstrom *et al.* 1993). For neonates < 27 weeks GA, 25–29% will develop severe ROP whereas for those at 28–31 weeks GA this is around 2–11%. The precision of these incidence and severity figures is less important than the sense that below about 1300 g birth weight infants are more likely than not to develop ROP. Severe disease is confined mainly to infants of birth weight < 1250 g and < 30 weeks GA and 6% of such neonates develop threshold ROP (see below; Schaffer *et al.* 1993).

An overview of the past 50 years shows two ROP epidemics (Patz 1980; Gibson *et al.* 1989, 1990a). The first,

Table 43.2 Cicatrical changes in retinopathy of prematurity (from Committee of Classification of Retinopathy of Prematurity 1987).

Peripheral changes	Posterior changes
Vascular	*Vascular*
Failure to vascularize peripheral retina	Vascular tortuosity
Abnormal, non-dichotomous branching of retinal vessels	Straightening of blood vessels in temporal arcade
Vascular arcades with circumferential interconnection	Decrease in angle of insertion of major temporal arcade
Telangiectatic vessels	
Retinal	*Retinal*
Pigmentary changes	Pigmentary changes
Vitreoretinal interface changes	Distortion or ectopia of macula
Thin retina	Stretching and folding of retina in macular region leading to periphery
Peripheral folds	
Vitreous membranes with or without attachment to retina	Vitreoretinal interface changes
Lattice-like degeneration	Vitreous membrane
Retinal breaks	Dragging of retina over disc
Traction/rhegmatogenous retinal detachment	Traction/rhegmatogenous retinal detachment

which commenced in the early 1940s, was brought to an end about a decade later by oxygen restriction which followed the discovery that oxygen supplementation was a factor in ROP causation. The second epidemic began in the late 1960s and is ongoing. The differences between the two epidemics merits scrutiny. During the first, the survival of neonates of <1000 g birth weight was around 5–8% and most of the babies blinded during this period were of heavier birth weight. Advances in neonatal care have largely eliminated the risk of severe ROP in these larger babies (>1000 g birth weight; Keith & Doyle 1995), but have not reduced the incidence of ROP-induced blindness in babies <1000 g birth weight. Thus these same advances which terminated the first epidemic and increased the survival of the very immature neonate (now around 50–60% <1000 g birth weight) resulted in the second epidemic which involves mainly the very immature neonate who previously was unlikely to survive. In retrospect, the first epidemic could now be considered largely preventable while currently the second is not.

How ROP affects different ethnic groups has attracted relatively little interest. One study in the UK (Ng *et al.* 1988) showed that although Asians (Indo-Pakistani) infants were not smaller than their Caucasian counterparts, and had similar incidence of acute ROP, they were significantly more likely to develop severe ROP (stage 3/4 in 14% Asians and 4% Caucasians). Afro-Caribbean infants are less likely to develop any ROP (Palmer *et al.* 1991; Schaffer *et al.* 1993).

Natural history

The past decade has seen much progress in our understanding of the natural history of ROP. This has theoretical and practical implications as it provides clues to underlying mechanisms and is vital for screening protocol design. There are four important elements in the natural history of retinopathy of prematurity: (i) age at onset; (ii) site of onset; (iii) rate of progression; and (iv) resolution.

Age at onset

ROP only affects the immature retinal vessels and does not develop after retinal vascularization is complete. Instinctively one would expect the most premature, often ill neonate, with a very immature retinal vascular system, to develop ROP sooner postnatally than his or her larger and more mature counterpart. However, this is not so (Fig. 43.9) and ROP develops over a relatively narrow postmenstrual age (PMA) range (Fielder *et al.* 1986, 1992b; Palmer *et al.* 1991; Quinn *et al.* 1992b). To quote one study (Fielder *et al.* 1992b), the onset of any ROP was between 29.7 and 45.0 weeks PMA, with 92% between 30.0 and 40.0 weeks; 81% between 30.0 and 37.8 weeks, and 75% between 30.0 and 36.0 weeks. Of the few infants (23 of 291) who devel-

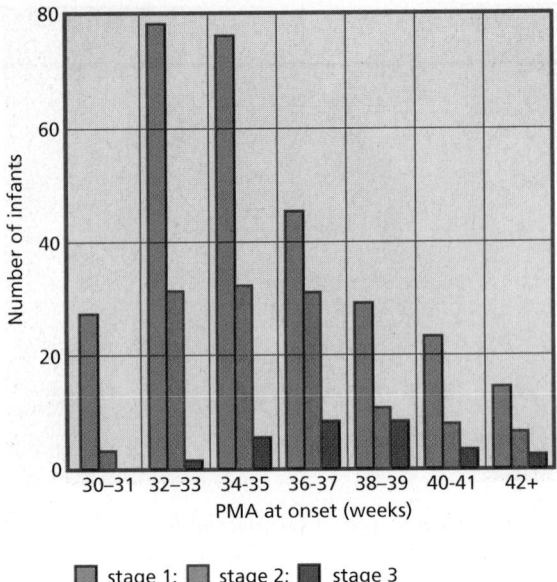

Fig. 43.9 ROP developing over narrow postmenstrual age.

oped ROP after term, none progressed to stage 3. Thus ROP onset is linked more to the stage of development of the infant than neonatal events. However, ROP is not present at birth, and this event is clearly necessary for its development. The propensity for severity is governed to a large extent by the state of retinal vascularization and this is of course influenced by neonatal events. ROP developing in a more vascularized retina has a low risk for progression to severe disease so ROP onset after 35 weeks PMA is most unlikely to reach stage 3. To counter this discussion slightly, it has been noted that onset in the most immature neonate may be hastened very slightly (Fielder *et al.* 1992b; Quinn *et al.* 1992b).

Site of onset

Traditional teaching has it that ROP commences in the temporal retina as this is the last region to vascularize. This is certainly so for the more mature neonates when the nasal retina is already vascularized. However, in the most immature neonate ROP commences preferentially in the nasal retina (Fig. 43.10) and later extends to other regions (Fielder *et al.* 1992a, b). The vertical retinal regions are less likely to be involved at onset and are only involved when ROP subsequently involves most of the circumference. The finding of ROP in these regions early in the course of the disease is a useful indicator of the possibility of future severity. The more premature the neonate, the more posterior by zone the location of the retinopathy and the greater the potential for progression. Thus zone 1 disease is very likely to progress to stage 3, but for ROP always confined entirely to zone 3 this rarely if ever happens.

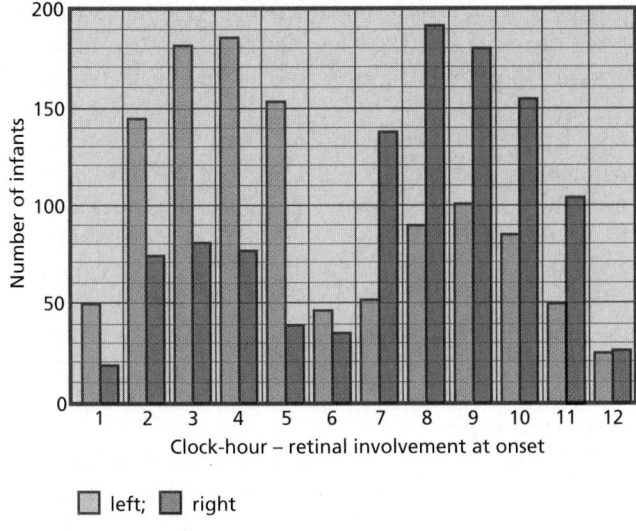

Fig. 43.10 ROP commencing in the nasal retina.

Rate of progression

As with onset, the rate of progression is also governed predominantly by the stage of development (PMA) rather than by postnatal age, or neonatal events such as oxygen therapy or illnesses (Palmer *et al.* 1991; Fielder *et al.* 1992b). Of course the latter contribute to ROP severity. The median PMA at which the various stages develop is as follows: (i) stage 1, 34 weeks; (ii) stage 2, 35 weeks; (iii) stage 3, 36 weeks, and (iv) for threshold ROP 37 weeks PMA (see Fig. 43.1).

Summary of retinopathy of prematurity natural history

ROP affects only immature retinal vessels and the greater the degree of prematurity the higher the incidence, and the greater the propensity for severe disease to develop. Intriguingly, ROP onset and progression are determined mainly by postmenstrual and not postnatal age. Furthermore, while ROP develops in the temporal retina of those infants whose vascular development has reached zone 3, for those more immature, retinopathy frequently commences in the nasal retina.

Resolution

All stages 1 and 2 ROP, provided that is the maximum stage reached, undergo complete resolution with little if any ophthalmic consequence (see below). Stage 3 may or may not resolve depending on its severity, so that when 'threshold' is reached, full resolution is unlikely and the risk of blindness is said to be close to 50% (Cryotherapy for Retinopathy of Prematurity Cooperative Group 1988).

Pathogenesis

The realization that the introduction of oxygen therapy for preterm infants played a major role in the epidemic of ROP in the 1940s and 1950s led to a period of oxygen restriction and to the anticipation of the demise of this blinding condition. Unfortunately, this proved not to be so — 'that a single manoeuvre would abolish ROP seems naive in the light of our current understanding of the condition' (Editorial 1992). Unsurprisingly, there has been an unwritten swing of clinical opinion away from the view that oxygen is the single causative factor in ROP towards almost the opposite view that oxygen plays little or no part in its development: both are incorrect. It is now evident that many factors can be involved in its pathogenesis. Currently ROP is not entirely preventable, but the evidence given below shows that meticulous medical control is vital not only for the general well-being of the baby, but also to keep ROP, especially severe ROP, to a minimum.

A review of the vast literature on this subject is outside the scope of this chapter but some of the more important factors related to the development of ROP are discussed. Several excellent articles have been published recently (Lucey & Dangman 1984; Flynn 1987; Ben-Sira *et al.* 1988; Prendiville & Schulenburg 1988; Editorial 1991, 1992; Darlow *et al.* 1992; Weakley & Spencer 1992; Gallo *et al.* 1993; Phelps 1994).

There are two current theories on the pathogenesis of this condition. The first, proposed by Ashton (1980) and Patz (1954), consists of two phases of equal importance. First, a hyperoxic phase, the phase in oxygen which causes retinal arteriolar constriction and irreversible vaso-obliteration and dissolution of the retinal capillary endothelial cells. This is followed by the second phase, on removal from the hyperoxic environment, the phase in air which is characterized by a vasoproliferative response induced by the ischaemia due to the capillary closure of the first phase.

The second theory, proposed by Kretzer and Hittner (1988), is based on the activity of the mesenchymal spindle cell precursors of the retinal capillaries. Mesenchymal spindle cells migrate centrifugally from the optic disc, and those cells canalize to form capillaries just behind the advancing vanguard. Under normal *in utero* conditions this process proceeds unimpeded, but in the relative hyperoxic extrauterine conditions, gap junctions appear between adjacent spindle cells. Gap junction formation interferes with normal migration and vascular formation and triggers the neovascular response.

Both theories invoke an oxidative insult. However, according to the 'classic' theory of Ashton and Patz, the stimulus for neovascularization is ischaemia due to capillary closure. Conversely, Kretzer and Hittner have been unable to identify retinal endothelial cell necrosis or ischaemia and have postulated therefore that angiogenic factors are synthesized by the insulted spindle cells themselves.

Risk or associated factors

Many factors have been implicated in the development of this condition, but whether each is independently significant in ROP causation or simply an associated factor indicative of a poorly neonate has on many instances yet to be determined. The enormous problem of recording, collecting and analysing data intermittently obtained from sick neonates whose state can fluctuate widely and unpredictably, from minute to minute, must not be underestimated. The definitive answer is awaited, and perhaps in the meantime the formula of Avery and Glass (1988) has some clinical sense:

Immaturity (always) + oxygen (often) + other factors (variably) = ROP.

So many 'other factors' have been reported as causally associated with ROP that they cannot be individually considered here, but they include (i) maternal factors such as complications of pregnancy or the use of beta-blockers; and (ii) fetal factors including hypercarbia, sepsis, vitamin E deficiency, intraventricular haemorrhage, recurrent apnoea, respiratory distress syndrome, surfactant, indomethacin treatment for patent ductus arteriosus, light and the type of neonatal unit. A number of these factors are considered below.

Birth weight and gestational age

The major ROP risk factor is the degree of immaturity as measured by either birth weight or GA. Although these two parameters are highly correlated, this is not invariable as in intrauterine growth retardation. Furthermore, the assessment of GA, especially for the most immature neonate is prone to inaccuracy. As stated earlier both the incidence and severity of ROP are inversely related to birth weight and GA (Kinsey *et al.* 1977; Flynn 1983; Keith & Kitchen 1984; Flynn 1987; Ng *et al.* 1988) with the first being the more powerful predictor (Darlow *et al.* 1992; Fielder *et al.* 1992b; Gallo *et al.* 1993; Schaffer *et al.* 1993).

Oxygen

Campbell (1951) was the first to suggest that supplemental oxygen was the cause for the sudden increase in the numbers of infants developing RLF in the early 1940s. Subsequently, Ashton *et al.* (1953) and Patz (1954) using animal models were able to demonstrate the toxic effect of oxygen on immature vessels. Although several controlled trials (Patz *et al.* 1952; Lanman *et al.* 1954; Kinsey *et al.* 1956) comparing high and low supplemental oxygen in prema-

ture infants later confirmed the relationship between oxygen therapy and ROP, it has not been possible over the ensuing 40 years to define safe levels of oxygen usage for clinical practice. The lower oxygen levels used in the mid–late 1950s reduced the incidence but ROP was not eliminated, and there was an increase in both neonatal mortality (Avery & Oppenheimer 1960) and neurological morbidity (McDonald 1963). Indeed Cross (1973) estimated that for each case of blindness prevented by the restriction of oxygen, about 16 infants died because of inadequate oxygenation. Although this figure has since been debated (Editorial 1992) the point is that both hypoxia and hyperoxia can have serious consequences for the preterm neonate.

With the availability of arterial blood gas monitoring, a multicentre study, using intermittent umbilical artery oxygen analysis was mounted to define the level of arterial oxygen below which ROP would not develop. Unfortunately, they failed to demonstrate any relationship between ROP and arterial blood oxygen tension (Kinsey *et al.* 1977). More recently Flynn *et al.* (1987b), in a randomized controlled trial comparing continuous transcutaneous oxygen monitoring with standard neonatal care, failed to show any reduction in ROP in the continuously monitored group, except in the older larger infants in whom ROP is less severe. However, a re-analysis of these data (Flynn *et al.* 1992) specifically studied the relationship between arterial oxygen tensions and retinopathy and found a significant association between the duration of transcutaneous $Po_2 \geq 80$ mmHg and the incidence and severity of ROP. It is worth emphasizing that this study alone used continuous rather than the intermittent monitoring employed in all other studies. Saito *et al.* (1993) concluded that extremely premature infants with widely fluctuating arterial oxygen probably have a higher risk of developing progressive ROP, confirmed by Cunningham *et al.* (1995).

After four decades of clinical research no direct relationship has been demonstrated between arterial oxygen levels and ROP. In addition, ROP may develop in preterm infants who have never received oxygen and in premature infants with cyanotic heart disease (Lucey & Dangman 1984). Furthermore, some studies have suggested a relationship between neonatal hypoxia and ROP (Lucey & Dangman 1984; Ng *et al.* 1989) and in an animal model retinal ischaemia may lead to the same retinal changes as hyperoxia (Ashton & Henkind 1965).

That hyperoxia and hypoxia may be associated with ROP is not entirely contradictory. It is postulated that while relative hyperoxia may lead to initial retinal capillary damage it is the subsequent ischaemia that acts as a stimulus for vasoproliferation. This mechanism would explain the association of recurrent apnoea and cerebral ischaemic events with ROP and provide the rationale for the administration of oxygen to treat ROP in the experimental animal (Chan-Ling *et al.* 1995), and the protocol of a current study which requires supplemental oxygen to be administered for stage 3 ROP.

Antioxidants and vitamin E

It has been suggested that the relative hyperoxic extrauterine environment causes free oxygen radical production which inhibits spindle cell migration and stimulates these cells to produce angiogenic factors responsible for ROP (Kretzer & Hittner 1988). It has been argued that vitamin E can suppress this free radical damage and this is the basis for vitamin E therapy in ROP. Certainly a suppressive effect has been shown in an animal model (Phelps & Rosenbaum 1977).

Vitamin E is a naturally occurring antioxidant important in maintaining cell integrity (Muller 1992) and the preterm neonate has low levels compared to either the adult or full-term infant (Kretzer & Hittner 1988). For this substance to be delivered to the inner retinal tissues the carrier protein interstitial retinal binding protein (IRBP) is necessary. Yet IRBP is not present in the peripheral retina until around 29 weeks gestation (Johnson *et al.* 1985a). Theoretically selenium-dependent glutathione peroxidase, which is active before 29 weeks gestation, might be the appropriate agent to offer free radical protection for the very immature neonate acting through the vitamin C antioxidant system (Kretzer & Hittner 1988). Another free-radical scavenger which may act as an antioxidant is bilirubin (Benaron & Bowen 1991) although its protective effect is not agreed (Boynton & Boynton 1989; Heyman *et al.* 1989; Gaton *et al.* 1991).

The use of vitamin E in ROP was first suggested by Owens and Owens in the late 1940s and taken up again by Johnson *et al.* (1985a, b). A flurry of clinical trials in the 1980s (Hittner *et al.* 1981; Finer *et al.* 1982; Johnson *et al.* 1985b; Phelps *et al.* 1987) demonstrated that although vitamin E does not appear to reduce the frequency of ROP it may reduce its severity. Despite these findings concern was expressed about the side-effects of vitamin E and methods of administration, including sepsis (Johnson *et al.* 1985), necrotizing enterocolitis (Johnson *et al.* 1985), retinal haemorrhage (Rosenbaum *et al.* 1985) and intraventricular haemorrhage (Phelps *et al.* 1987). Vitamin E therapy for ROP remains a controversial subject, but currently its general use as a prophylactic agent against this condition is not recommended (Muller 1992).

Exchange transfusions

Preterm infants given blood transfusions receive adult haemoglobin. As the latter binds oxygen less avidly than fetal haemoglobin the oxygen dissociation curve is shifted so that more oxygen is delivered up rendering tissues relative hyperoxic. This could increase the risk of ROP and several studies (Aranda *et al.* 1975; Bard *et al.* 1975; Clark *et al.* 1981; Shohat *et al.* 1983) have demonstrated an association between ROP and blood transfusion. However, it is still unclear whether repeated blood transfusion is an independent ROP risk factor or simply yet another indicator of a very poorly neonate. Those infants who need repeated blood transfusions are usually smaller, sicker and require a longer duration of oxygen therapy and are therefore at high risk of developing ROP anyway (Lucey & Dangman 1984).

Surfactant

The use of this agent has reduced mortality, the severity of respiratory distress syndrome and chronic lung disease in very immature neonates (Long *et al.* 1991). So far, studies (Rankin *et al.* 1992; Repka *et al.* 1993; Holmes *et al.* 1994; Axer-Siegal *et al.* 1996) have not shown any difference between treated and non-treated infants. So, although it appears unlikely that surfactant will have a direct effect on ROP, it will increase the number of very small neonates who will survive to develop ROP.

Standard of care

Infants born in large, tertiary referral neonatal units have been reported to have a lower incidence (Darlow *et al.* 1992) and severity of ROP (Schaffer *et al.* 1993). Mindful that these are the units caring for the most sick and most immature neonates, for them to have disproportionally less ROP is surprising and is attributed by Darlow *et al.* (1992) to the better quality of care they provide. Tentative support for this theory comes from the finding that in Chile ROP-induced blindness in children under 10 years of age reaches 24% (Gilbert *et al.* 1994), far higher than in most developed countries, perhaps reflecting the availability of neonatal intensive care facilities but paucity of appropriate level of resources.

Light

Early exposure to light was suggested as a causative factor in the first descriptions of this condition by Terry (1942, 1943). Studies by Hepner *et al.* (1949) and Locke and Reese (1952) did not provide supportive evidence, not surprising as at this time supplemental oxygen could well have swamped any effect of light. It was proposed that light could, by damaging retinal tissues, generate free radicals and thereby cause ROP. Interest in light re-awakened with the report by Glass *et al.* (1985) that reduction in the neonatal unit illumination reduced the incidence and severity of ROP. This finding has since been confirmed by Hommura *et al.* (1988) but not by either Ackerman *et al.* (1989) or Seiberth *et al.* (1994). Further studies are required to determine whether there is a causal relation between light exposure and ROP: it is important because although many neonatal variables are complex and defy control, here is one parameter that can easily and immediately be modified (Fielder *et al.* 1992a).

Clinical aspects

Screening

In the past, not being able to either prevent or treat ROP, the role of the ophthalmologist has been limited to one of identification alone. But now that it has been conclusively demonstrated that severe ROP can be successfully treated (Cryotherapy for Retinopathy of Prematurity Cooperative Group 1988) the ophthalmologist has a duty to screen. Recent advances in our understanding of its natural history have provided the basis for a logical and relatively simple screening protocol which is cost-effective (Javitt *et al.* 1993). There are a number of published recommendations which do not differ greatly (Palmer 1981; Biglan *et al.* 1989; Tan & Cats 1989; Schaffer 1990; Darlow & Clemett 1990; Fledelius & Rosenberg 1990; Fielder & Levene 1992; Urrea & Rosenbaum 1994; Report of a Joint Working Party 1995). Criteria for screening may well change in the future following advances in knowledge and new treatment techniques; for instance it is possible that the birth weight criterion will be reduced in the near future as severe retinopathy over 1250 g birth weight is rare (Keith & Doyle 1995).

The purpose of screening is to identify severe ROP (stage 3) which may require treatment, or in a baby due to be discharged to home or to another hospital, ROP which has the potential to become severe.

Deciding which infants should be screened

Severe ROP (stage 3 or more) is virtually confined to infants of birth weight < 1500 g and 31 weeks GA and only these babies need to be examined. There is no indication to include a sickness criterion or screen larger babies who have required prolonged oxygen therapy.

Principles of screening

Three aspects need to be taken into account: timing of the examination, severity, location by zone and extent by clock hours.

Examinations can be timed on the principle that the onset and progression of ROP are both predominantly determined by PMA rather than by neonatal events. Most important, as there is only a narrow window of opportunity for treatment — around 2 weeks — timing of examinations is critical. Onset is rare before 30 weeks PMA and ROP commencing once vascularization has entered zone 3 and/or after 36 weeks PMA is most unlikely to reach stage

3. Because of the predetermined timescale it is sometimes necessary to examine the very sick neonate who may be ventilated. The mean age for stage 3 onset is around 37 weeks PMA, but posterior (zone 1) disease may progress more rapidly ('rush' disease).

Severity is graded by the international classification for ROP. Signs of plus disease, especially in the anterior segment, are all ominous signs but it is important to remember that this is not an all-or-nothing phenomenon but a spectrum.

ROP location can indicate the likelihood of future progression. For instance, the more posterior the retinopathy the greater the propensity to become severe. Thus zone 1 retinopathy very frequently progresses to stage 3 whereas zone 3 disease does not. Also ROP frequently starts in the nasal retina in the most immature neonate and has a greater propensity to become severe than ROP with temporal onset. Similarly greater circumferential involvement is a poor prognostic sign.

Screening protocol

All infants < 1500 g birth weight and < 32 weeks GA should be examined 6–7 weeks postnatally and then every 2 weeks until 36 weeks PMA or until vascularization has progressed into zone 3 and the risk of stage 3 has passed. It is not necessary to review infants until the retina is fully vascularized. Some of the larger babies may be discharged to home before screening is due to commence. In such cases an examination before discharge is recommended as this can indicate the potential for ROP and frequently obviate the need for review so simplifying life for parents and clinician alike.

Two-weekly examinations are recommended as a routine but if ROP is severe then more frequent examinations will be required. On a practical basis a weekly visit to the neonatal unit saves the need to recall most infants discharged to home between visits. The vast majority of examinations can and should be undertaken in hospital. Visits to outpatients greatly inconvenience the family, and failure to attend at the appropriate time may have disastrous consequences. For the infant discharged to another hospital while still at risk, arrangements for the completion of the screening programme need to be made.

Methods of examination

Infants should be handled gently and it is helpful if a trained nurse is in attendance to help and to monitor the infant's well-being. The ophthalmic examination should be performed using the indirect ophthalmoscope, with a 28 dioptre lens, through dilated pupils, achieved by instilling 1 drop each of cyclopentolate 0.5% and phenylephrine 2.5% 30 minutes prior to examination and repeated once if necessary. A paediatric lid speculum and scleral indentor (for ocular rotation rather than indentation), after the instillation of sodium benoxinate 0.4% eye drops, is used by many to permit complete evaluation of the peripheral retina. While it can be argued that very peripheral disease so observed is of no clinical importance, identifying peripheral nasal retinopathy can be a clue to later progression and only by observing the state of vascularization of the nasal retina can the ophthalmologist determine whether zone 3 has been entered.

Clinical findings

The ophthalmoscopic appearance of the neonate is different in a number of respects from that of the older infant (Fielder *et al.* 1988). Before examining the retina it is important to use the 28 dioptre lens as a simple magnifier to examine the anterior segment which may contain useful information. For instance the amount of regression of the tunica vasculosa lentis is an indicator of maturity (regressing between 28 and 34 weeks GA; Hittner *et al.* 1977), and also of ROP activity as it may persist in the presence of severe disease. Transient lens vacuoles are not infrequently observed.

The retinal periphery is white–grey in its non-vascularized regions, the extent of this depending on the degree of immaturity. The optic disc frequently has a greyish and a double-ring appearance (see Fig. 43.2), almost akin to mild optic nerve hypoplasia. The macular area is relatively ill defined there being no macular or foveolar reflexes until around 36 and 42 weeks PMA, respectively (Isenberg 1986). The retinal arterioles in the early neonatal period are not tortuous, but tend to become so later, and this is in part related to ROP severity (Fielder *et al.* 1992b).

Acute phase retinopathy of prematurity

The purpose of screening is to identify severe ROP which might require treatment. First look for signs of plus disease in the posterior pole as this alerts the clinician at the outset of the examination that ROP is already present and active—even if it cannot easily be visualized. By the time the later signs of iris engorgement and pupil rigidity are apparent, ROP is well advanced and the opportunity for successful treatment may have been lost.

Only if the advancing edge of the peripheral retinal vessels can be visualized can one determine if ROP is present. Another diagnostic aid is vessels which dilate slightly rather than taper as they traverse the retina towards the periphery. Pay particular attention to the nasal and temporal peripheries. Use a scleral indentor to rotate rather than indent, but be careful that the indent does not obscure the early signs; looking to either side of the indent is helpful. In the mildest form of ROP (stage 1) a white line is seen at the junction between vascularized and non-vascularized retina and with stage 2 the line becomes thicker

and extends just out of the plane of the retina. In practice it can be difficult to distinguish stage 1 and 2. Abnormal arborization and circumferential arcading are often seen in the vessels running up to the ridge.

Acute phase ROP has a strong tendency for symmetry between the two eyes, in marked contrast to its residua which are characteristically asymmetrical (Fielder *et al.* 1992b; Quinn *et al.* 1995). The stage 3 lesion is an arteriovenous shunt which contains blood with rapid flow and marked vascular leakage on fluorescein angiography (Flynn *et al.* 1977; Kretzer & Hittner 1988) which can be seen histopathologically (Kushner *et al.* 1977). With more advanced disease new vessels grow forward into the vitreous (stage 3) and retinal detachment may be seen, which can be partial (stage 4) or total (stage 5).

Regression

All ROP stages 1 and 2 undergo complete regression (Fielder *et al.* 1992b) and in general the rate of regression is related to the severity of the acute lesion. The first sign that regression will occur is a failure of the acute changes to progress; followed by ridge thinning and break up. Later vessels grow through the ridge into the peripheral avascular retina (Flynn *et al.* 1977). When complete regression occurs the peripheral retina becomes fully vascularized. However, this does not always occur, leaving residua. Table 43.2 lists the posterior and peripheral vascular and retinal changes.

Advanced cicatricial changes involving the anterior vitreous and retina may push the lens/iris diaphragm forward and cause shallowing of the anterior chamber, glaucoma, and corneal decompensation (Fig. 43.11). In such cases lensectomy is indicated to relieve narrow angle glaucoma.

Treatment

There have been several overviews of ROP treatment to which the reader is directed for further information (e.g. Eichenbaum *et al.* 1990; Fielder 1992; Flynn & Tasman 1992; Palmer 1994; Report of a Joint Working Party 1995).

Prophylaxis

While there is no obvious prophylactic treatment on the horizon there are a number of factors which might either minimize the incidence and severity of ROP, or reduce the rate of progression to improve outcome. These have been discussed already and include the standard of neonatal care, vitamin E and light.

Acute phase retinopathy of prematurity

Cryotherapy and xenon arc photocoagulation were first

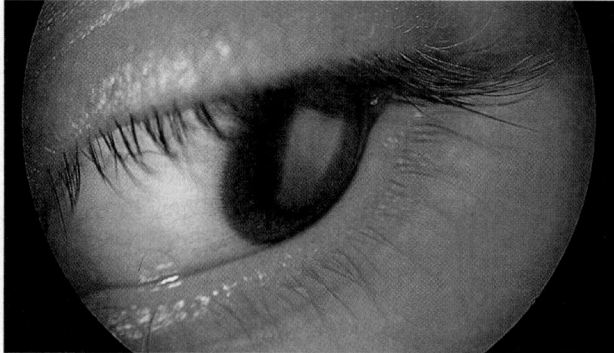

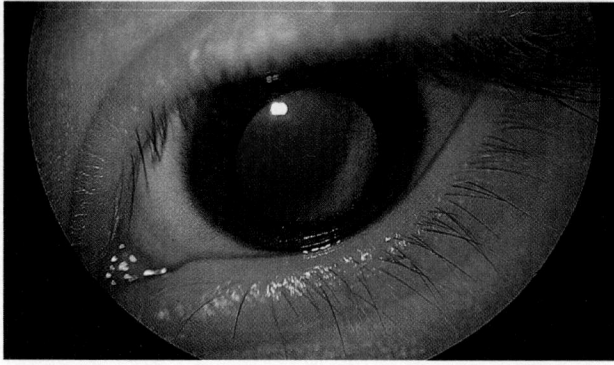

Fig. 43.11 Regressed ROP with retrolental membranes with temporal dragging of the retina; the acuity in the left eye was 6/60, the right eye saw only hand movements. Frequently, the anterior chamber becomes shallow and the eyes prone to glaucoma.

used for acute ROP in the late 1960s (reviewed in Palmer *et al.* 1985; Fielder 1992) with argon laser soon entering the picture. However, it was not until 1988 that retinal ablative therapy was proven to have a beneficial effect on severe retinopathy following the publication of the preliminary report of the US-based Multicenter Trial of Cryotherapy for Retinopathy of Prematurity (Cryotherapy for Retinopathy Cooperative Group 1988). The great impact of this study merits a detailed review here.

The Multicenter Trial of Cryotherapy for Retinopathy of Prematurity set out primarily to determine prospectively whether cryotherapy is effective in the treatment of severe acute ROP, and second to study the natural history of this condition. Study design will not be considered (Cryotherapy for Retinopathy of Prematurity Cooperative Group 1988, 1990a; Fielder & Levene 1992). All infants of ≤1250 g birth weight (*n* = 9751) were enrolled over a 23-month period commencing 1 January 1986. Ophthalmic examinations commenced at 6 weeks postnatally and were continued at fortnightly intervals until vascularization was complete. Infants who reached threshold stage (defined as five continuous or eight cumulative clock hours of stage 3 in zone 1 or 2 with plus disease) were randomly allocated to either treatment (cryotherapy) or control groups. Cryotherapy was then performed within 72 hours.

Results showed that cryotherapy produced a significant reduction in the unfavourable outcome of threshold ROP of 49.3% at 3 months (Cryotherapy for Retinopathy of Prematurity Cooperative Group 1988, 1990a), 45.8% at 12 months (Cryotherapy for Retinopathy of Prematurity Cooperative Group 1990b) and 42.5% at 3.5 years (Cryotherapy for Retinopathy of Prematurity Cooperative Group 1993), as judged by photographs and clinical examination. Not all eyes treated behaved identically: symmetrical and zone 2 disease had a significantly better outcome than zone 1 ROP. Indeed zone predicted the beneficial effect of cryotherapy better than any other parameter such as birth weight, and so on (Schaffer *et al.* 1993). At 1 year, treated infants had significantly better visual acuity (using the acuity card procedure) than controls. At 3.5 years, despite an unchanged ocular structure there was a significant reduction of favourable outcome for vision: from 37.8 to 20.1%, with 65.6% controls and 52.4% of treated infants falling into the low vision or blind category (Cryotherapy for Retinopathy of Prematurity Cooperative Group 1993). Almost certainly this does not represent a deterioration at a retinal level but simply reflects the failure for normal visual development to occur (Fielder *et al.* 1995). At $5\frac{1}{2}$ years (Cryotherapy for Retinopathy of Prematurity Cooperative Group 1996) the unfavourable outcomes as regards acuity were 47.1% in the treated group and 61.7% in controls. Unfavourable outcomes as regards structural changes were 26.9% (treated) and 45.4% (control). Of patients achieving 20/40 or better, in the untreated group 17% achieved this level whilst only 13% of the treated group reached this level.

Thus after two decades of small-scale inconclusive clinical studies, the Multicenter Trial of Cryotherapy for Retinopathy of Prematurity study has shown conclusively that cryotherapy for threshold ROP produces a significant benefit for structural status of the eye (Summers *et al.* 1992; Cryotherapy for Retinopathy of Prematurity Cooperative Group 1993) and for vision, but that normal structure is not necessarily obtained and normal acuity may well not be attained. Interestingly, in eyes which have previously had severe ROP the correlation between posterior retinal structure and visual function is good, although not invariably so (Gilbert *et al.* 1992), whereas in eyes with mild to moderate residua of ROP the prediction of function according to structure is poor, and ophthalmoscopy is no substitute for acuity measurement (Reynolds *et al.* 1993).

After the Multicenter Trial of Cryotherapy for Retinopathy of Prematurity Study

This important study has dramatically changed clinical practice worldwide and ROP screening is now mandatory. However, cryotherapy performed using the study protocol is no panacea and raises the issue of treatment criteria. Already in the immediate post-study phase, treatment cri-

teria and treatment methods are being reviewed and mod-
ifications suggested. Threshold as employed in this study
was defined as the stage where the risk of blindness if
untreated is 50%. Perhaps this threshold is set too high
and should be lowered, especially for zone 1 disease
(Fleming *et al.* 1992; Tasman 1992; Laser ROP Study Group
1994). This must be balanced against the possibility that
some eyes might be treated which would otherwise have
undergone complete spontaneous resolution.

Treatment practicalities

The issues to be considered in the rapidly changing field
of ROP treatment are dealt with very briefly here. Treatment details can be obtained from articles referenced here
(e.g. Cryotherapy for Retinopathy of Prematurity Cooperative Group 1988; Schulenburg & Acheson 1992; Report of
a Joint Working Party 1995).

Rationale and criteria for treatment

The aim of treatment is to remove, by ablating the peripheral avascular retina, the stimulus for vessel growth. The
current indication for treatment is threshold ROP as
defined (stage 3 acute ROP involving more than five contiguous or more than eight cumulative clock hours: in retinal zones 1 or 2, in the presence of plus disease). Because
of the poor outcome of treating threshold zone 1 disease,
most clinicians now treat any stage 3 in this location and
as mentioned the concept of threshold as defined here is
being questioned.

It is critical to remember that the window for treatment
occurs at the maximum of 2 weeks and treatment should
be undertaken as soon as possible — certainly within 2–3
days of threshold identification. Treatment should be performed in the neonatal unit where the baby is known; possible adverse reaction to the procedure demands full
neonatal support facilities.

Cryotherapy is painful and systemic complications can
occur (Brown *et al.* 1989), and laser treatment can take an
hour to perform. Both can be performed under either
sedation or full anaesthesia, but the important components are good analgesia and facilities for artificial ventilation. A neonatologist, or an experienced neonatal
anaesthetist, will help in this decision. Resuscitation
equipment must be available, and an intravenous line
must be in place before starting the administration of
sedation or resuscitation agents.

The pupils should be dilated but subconjunctival or
retrobulbar anaesthetic agents should not be used (Brown
et al. 1989).

Cryotherapy

Cryotherapy is applied trans-sclerally to the avascular
zone anterior to, and avoiding, the acute ROP lesion. Use a
retinal probe or one specially designed for the purpose, so
that the cryotherapy lesions are confluent. It is recommended that the entire 360° of the circumference of the
globe is treated under direct visualization. It is not usually
necessary to open the conjunctiva unless the lesion is so
posterior that the posterior section of the avascular zone
cannot be reached. Already two groups have undertaken
partial rather than the standard 360° cryoablation (Nissenkorn *et al.* 1991; Spencer *et al.* 1992).

Mydriatic (not atropine), antibiotic and sometimes
steroid eye drops are instilled for a few days postoperatively. If successful, plus disease should begin to subside
within a few days and the cryotherapy lesions appear
within a week. Re-treat as soon as it is obvious that signs
of plus are not subsiding or that regression is not occurring or is patchy, leaving active retinopathy with the
potential for traction. Temporal disease is of more concern
because of its proximity to the macula. In the absence of
active ROP it is probably not necessary to re-treat all skip
areas. Ocular complications of cryotherapy include eyelid
oedema, lacerations and haemorrhage of the conjunctiva,
pre-retinal and vitreous haemorrhage.

Laser

A resurgence of interest in laser occurred after the Multicenter Study. This has been facilitated by the introduction
of portable diode and argon lasers which can be delivered
through an indirect ophthalmoscope. This is logical and
Tasman commented (1992) that had the clinical trial of
treatment for ROP been delayed until after this development, almost certainly this modality would have been
employed. Portable indirect laser has now been used on a
number of occasions (McNamara *et al.* 1991; Landers *et al.*
1992; Capone *et al.* 1993; Goggin & O'Keefe 1993; Hunter &
Repka 1993; McNamara 1993; Clark & Hero 1994). Of particular interest is the correspondence from the Laser ROP
Study Group (1994) who undertook a meta-analysis of
four studies involving 293 eyes which compared laser
with cryotherapy and, while recognizing fundamental
flaws in such an analysis, concurred with others that laser
is at least as effective as cryotherapy. Laser can be very
accurately placed and is simpler to deliver to posterior
disease. Instead of confluence half a retinal burn space
between lesions is recommended (McNamara 1993),
although the sense of leaving more space between laser
than cryotherapy lesions eludes this author.

There are specific complications of laser. These include
corneal, iris and lens burn and the tunica vasculosa lentis
may absorb energy. Cataract formation has been reported
(Christiansen & Bradford 1995). Retinal or vitreous haemorrhage may occur, but is probably not laser-specific. Evidence so far suggests that diode red (810 nm) may be
preferable to argon green (514 nm) laser for ROP (McNa-

mara 1993). The former is more portable and requires less power. It causes less tissue destruction and as energy is less likely to be taken up by other ocular tissues, complications are less frequent.

Retinal detachment surgery

The management of stage IV and V ROP is controversial. Stage IV ROP has been successfully treated with scleral buckling in older infants (Kalina 1980; McPherson *et al.* 1982). This technique has been used in young infants (Topilow *et al.* 1990; Trese 1994) in attempts to reattach the retina and prevent progression to more severe disease. Around 67–70% of stage 4 and 40% stage 5 eyes reattached but visual outcome is unknown (Trese 1994).

For older infants both 'open sky' (Tasman *et al.* 1987) and closed vitrectomy (Machemer 1983; Chong *et al.* 1986; Trese 1986; Machemer & de Juan 1990) approaches have been used with anatomical reattachment being achieved in 40–50% of cases. Infants who developed retinal detachment in the Multicenter Study were either managed conservatively (71 eyes) or by vitrectomy (58 eyes). Reattachment was achieved in 28% of the former and none of the latter; only two eyes (both in the vitrectomy group) had any evidence of pattern vision, and that at the lowest measurable spatial frequency. In contrast Katsumi *et al.* (1991) and Hirose *et al.* (1993) reported significantly better acuities in a small number of infants following surgery for stage 5 ROP. Recently Seaber *et al.* (1995) reviewed a series of eyes which had initially responded successfully to vitrectomy. They found that retinas which were attached after surgery re-detached and the visual results were low and disappointing, although they concluded that 'there is some evidence that vitrectomized eyes function better than non-vitrectomized eyes'.

With such dismal results surgical management cannot be recommended (Knight-Nanan *et al.* 1996) and it is critical that during any discussion parents are made aware of the difference between structural and functional success.

Summary of management for retinopathy of prematurity

Infants at risk of developing severe ROP, i.e. < 1500 g birth weight and ≤ 31 weeks GA, should be screened according to recently developed protocols, and treatment for threshold disease undertaken urgently using either cryotherapy or laser. The management of infants who develop stage 4 or 5 ROP is controversial, but at present treatment has not been shown to offer a significant functional benefit. All children who have progressed to stage 3 or more require prolonged follow-up as they are at risk of developing refractive, visual and ocular motor problems. The need for review of children who as infants developed mild retinopathy (stage 2 or less) is less well defined, as their ROP is unlikely to cause clinically significant problems. However, as they are still at risk of developing a variety of problems, especially strabismus (Cryotherapy for Retinopathy of Prematurity Cooperative Group 1994), due to other associations of prematurity review of these infants is also recommended.

Outcome

Most infants with ROP undergo complete resolution without adverse effects, but this is not so for all. Generally, the incidence and severity of sequelae are related to the severity of the acute phase. Infants and children born prematurely are at risk of developing a range of ophthalmic problems, some of which are obviously the direct consequence of ROP (e.g. vitreous membrane), while the causes of others may be more complex and sometimes multifactorial (e.g. strabismus and refractive errors).

To deal first with the direct consequences of ROP: the retinal and vitreous residua (Figs 43.12–43.14) of ROP are more frequent in severe and posterior disease, but occasionally occur in mild acute ROP (Cryotherapy for Retinopathy of Prematurity Cooperative Group 1994). Retinal detachment can occur at any time of life, including after cryotherapy (Greven & Tasman 1989), although this is infrequent.

Anterior segment sequelae of severe ROP have been described (Hittner *et al.* 1979; Kelly & Fielder 1987; Summers *et al.* 1992). Microcornea/microphthalmos may be the consequence of reduced growth during the acute phase or later shrinkage due to advanced cicatrization. Other changes are largely due to changes in the anterior vitreous causing anterior displacement of the iris–lens diaphragm causing the frequent shallowing of the anterior chamber (Cryotherapy for Retinopathy of Prematurity

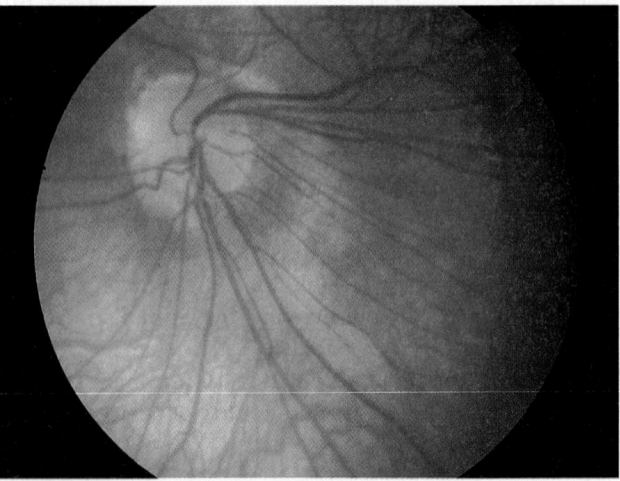

Fig. 43.12 Regressed ROP showing the retinal vessels straightened and dragged to the nasal periphery of the right eye. The fovea was intact and the acuity 6/12.

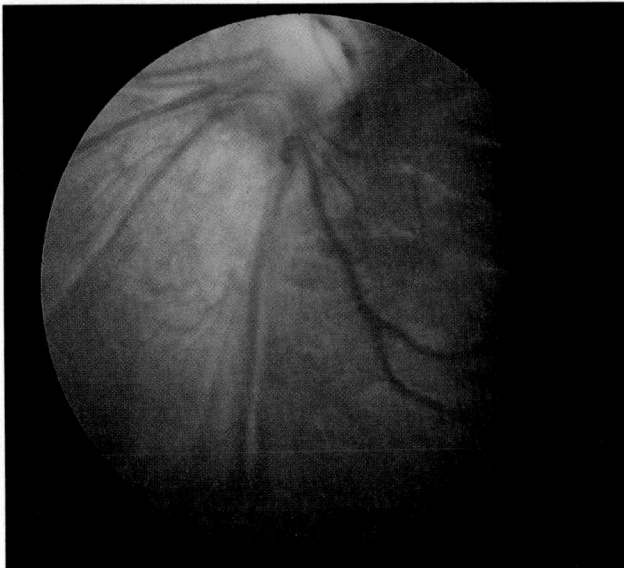

Fig. 43.13 Regressed ROP with marked nasal dragging of the vessels.

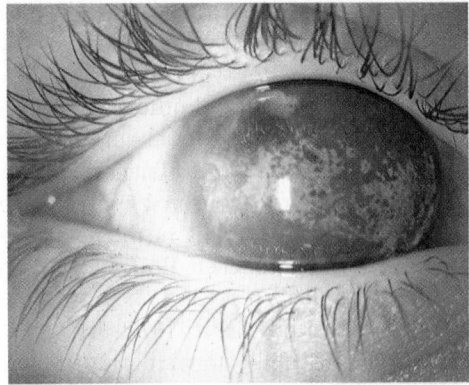

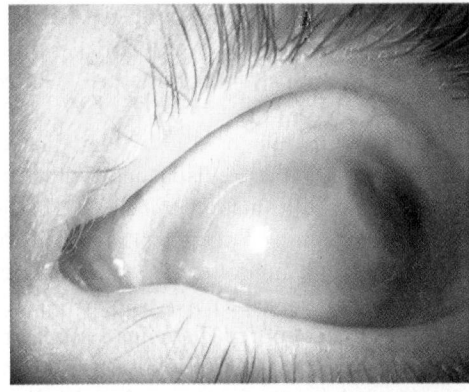

Fig. 43.15 Cicatricial ROP with bilateral obliteration of the anterior chamber and angle closure glaucoma with secondary corneal degenerative changes.

Cooperative Group 1994) and if severe, the other complications of corneal opacity and cataract (Fig. 43.15).

Other aspects of outcome are less obviously the direct result of ROP and here outcome should be seen in the context of the whole child. Two recent studies of children born at a GA of 29 weeks or less have shown that between 19% (Cooke 1994) and 23% (Johnson *et al.* 1993) sustain a severe disability, and of these 33 and 26%, respectively, had vision impairment. According to Cooke poor general outcome is independently related only to cerebral injury and without this even extremely preterm infants do well (Cooke 1994). In other words developmental outcome is related to neurological events rather than low birth weight *per se*. This statement has major limitations, especially

with regard to ROP causation, but it does make an important point: neurological events are frequent and are the major cause of disability in infants born prematurely. Against this background it is important to appreciate that the very immature neonate is more likely than not to develop ROP. Teasing out the relative contribution of neu-

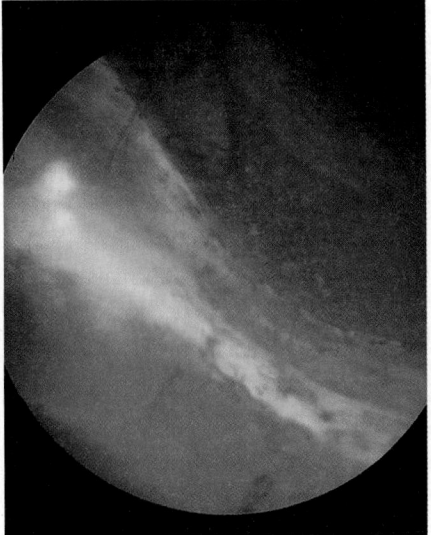

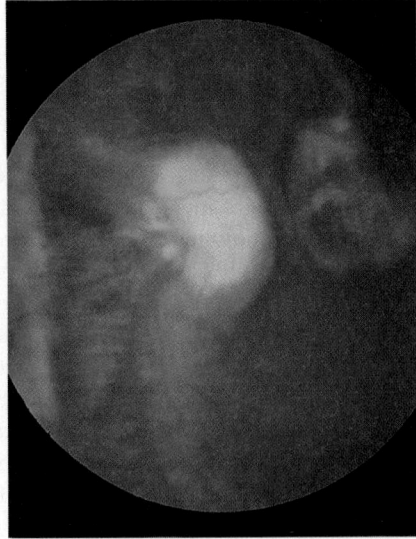

Fig. 43.14 Marked retinal dragging towards an area of chorioretinal atrophy and vitreoretinal fibrosis in the area of what was probably stage 3 zone 1 disease.

rological insult and ROP is not always possible (Laws *et al.* 1992; Page *et al.* 1993), especially as these are often interrelated.

There have been a number of studies of the visual pathway associations or complications of preterm birth (Fledelius 1976; Hittner *et al.* 1979; Tasman 1979; Hungerford *et al.* 1986; Burgess & Johnson 1991), however, relatively few include adequate data of the neonatal period (Kushner 1982; Keith & Kitchen 1983; Nissenkorn *et al.* 1983; Schaffer *et al.* 1984; Snir *et al.* 1988; Cats & Tan 1989; Gibson *et al.* 1990b; Koole *et al.* 1990; Page *et al.* 1993; Robinson & O'Keefe 1993). To date only three studies have prospectively studied infants in the neonatal period and compared the later findings with the presence and stage of acute ROP (Laws *et al.* 1992; Page *et al.* 1993; Cryotherapy for Retinopathy of Prematurity Cooperative Group 1994).

Vision impairment due to ROP is well known, but subtle deficits may also occur. Visual acuity development is normal in mild ROP (Katsumi *et al.* 1991), but significantly delayed in regressed stage 3 (Luna *et al.* 1990), a finding attributed to neurological abnormalities. Expreterm children may develop normal acuity but at a level which falls at its lower border (Fledelius 1981; Sebris *et al.* 1984), while according to McCormick *et al.* (1986) only 78% achieved normal acuity in childhood. Two studies (Laws *et al.* 1992; Mintz-Hittner *et al.* 1992) have reported, despite acuities falling within the normal range, significantly lower levels with increasing ROP severity, this trend remaining after the removal of data from eyes with cicatricial changes and those with neurological abnormalities (Laws *et al.* 1992).

The incidence of strabismus is raised between around 6% to over 30% (Kushner 1982; Keith & Kitchen 1983; McCormick *et al.* 1986; Snir *et al.* 1988; Cats & Tan 1989; Koole *et al.* 1990; Burgess & Johnson 1991; Gallo & Lennerstrand 1991; McGinnity & Bryars 1992; Page *et al.* 1993; Robinson & O'Keefe 1993) and this rises with both the incidence and severity of ROP (Laws *et al.* 1992; Cryotherapy for Retinopathy of Prematurity Cooperative Group 1994). However, strabismus is a well-known associate of neurological abnormalities especially periventricular leucomalacia (Gibson *et al.* 1990b; Pike *et al.* 1994).

The effects of mild ROP on refractive development are minimal, but with increasing severity there is a tendency towards the following: (i) myopia (see Gordon & Donzis 1986; Laws *et al.* 1992; Quinn *et al.* 1992a; Cryotherapy for Retinopathy of Prematurity Cooperative Group 1994); (ii) increasing astigmatism; (iii) axis direction away from the rule; and (iv) anisometropia. The mechanisms of myopia associated with prematurity and ROP are not fully understood, but the following mechanisms have been suggested: anomalies of corneal diameter and curvature, lens power and axial length (Cryotherapy for Retinopathy of Prematurity Cooperative Group 1994), some of these pos-

sibly related to disturbed ocular growth due to ROP. A recent publication (Algawi *et al.* 1994) reports less myopia in eyes treated by laser compared to cryotherapy. This is of interest and merits further study although the possibility that eyes are treated with laser at an earlier stage than cryotherapy must be borne in mind.

Other ophthalmic findings include nystagmus, optic atrophy and cortical visual impairment. Not all are due to ROP and they serve to highlight the fundamental problem identified earlier of not being able to differentiate different causes particularly ROP and neurological insults, to both of which the preterm neonate is especially susceptible.

Involving parents

The parents of a very preterm infant have much to cope with and they have a right to know what may befall their baby. Providing sensitive, balanced written information is essential to enable parents to be part of the decision-making process (Harrison 1993). Information is required at several stages and must be individualized to meet the requirements of the baby.

Written information and counselling

This should be available at three levels. First, for all babies who are to be screened; second, for the parents of babies with ROP which might become severe; and third for the parents of the baby with end-stage disease. For the first group, a general description of ROP is required, which correctly emphasizes that, while ROP is a frequent occurrence, over 90% acute retinopathy resolves spontaneously without adverse sequelae. Generally, in the UK, the ophthalmologist does not personally counsel the parents of all babies who are screened. Of course he or she should be prepared to speak to any parent requiring more information. For the second group, when ROP is likely to become severe, further written information should be supplied which emphasizes that treatment is available and may need to be considered. At this stage the ophthalmologist should discuss the situation with parents, mindful of the fact that severe ROP occurs just when parents are beginning to relax for the first time since their baby was born. A member of the neonatal unit staff who knows the family should be present during any discussion so that post-interview queries can be dealt with. With severe ROP always keep parents fully and frequently informed.

Unfortunately not all eyes with ROP respond satisfactorily to treatment and blindness still occurs. Ophthalmologists should not lose contact with the family, for most accept that treatment carefully performed sometimes fails, but they cannot accept what is perceived as lack of interest or care (Silverman 1980). There is still much to do and the ophthalmologist must ensure that the child gains early access to the services for the visually impaired. Registration as blind or partially sighted, if appropriate, is recommended as a positive act to ensure support, because in general terms the child not registered is less likely to receive adequate support. The need for liaison with the social and educational services cannot be overemphasized.

References

Acheson JF, Schulenburg WE. Surveillance for retinopathy of prematurity in practice: experience from one neonatal intensive care unit. *Eye* 1991; **5**: 80–5.

Ackerman B, Sherwonit E, Williams J. Reduced incidental light exposure: effect on the development of retinopathy of prematurity in low birth weight infants. *Pediatrics* 1989; **83**: 958–62.

Alan T, Hemo I, Itin A *et al.* Vascular endothelial growth factor acts as a survival factor for newly formed retinal vessels and has implications for retinopathy of prematurity. *Nature Medicine* 1995; **1**: 1024–8.

Algawi K, Goggin M, O'Keefe M. Refractive outcome following diode laser versus cryotherapy with retinopathy of prematurity. *Br J Ophthalmol* 1994; **78**: 612–14.

Aranda JV, Clark TE, Maniello R *et al.* Blood transfusions: a possible potentiating risk factor in retrolental fibroplasia. *Pediatr Res* 1975; **9**: 362.

Ashton N. Oxygen and retinal blood vessels. *Trans Ophthalmol Soc UK* 1980; **100**: 359–62.

Ashton N. Retinal angiogenesis in the human embryo. *Br Med Bull* 1970; **26**: 103–6.

Ashton N, Henkind P. Experimental occlusion of retinal arterioles. *Br J Ophthalmol* 1965; **49**: 225–34.

Ashton N, Ward B, Serpell G. Role of oxygen in the genesis of retrolental fibroplasia. A preliminary report. *Br J Ophthalmol* 1953; **37**: 513–20.

Avery GB, Glass P. Retinopathy of prematurity: progress report. *Pediatr Ann* 1988; **17**: 528–33.

Avery ME, Oppenheimer EH. Recent increase in mortality from hyaline membrane disease. *J Pediatr* 1960; **57**: 553–4.

Axer-Siegel R, Snir M, Ma'ayan A *et al.* Retinopathy of prematurity and surfactant treatment. *J Ped Ophthalmol Strabismus* 1996; **33**: 171–4.

Bard H, Cornet A, Orquin J *et al.* Retrolental fibroplasia and exchange transfusions. *Pediatr Res* 1975; **9**: 362.

Benaron DA, Bowen FW. Variation of initial serum bilirubin rise in newborn infants with type of illness. *Lancet* 1991; **338**: 78–81.

Ben-Sira I, Nissenkorn I, Kremer I. Retinopathy of prematurity. *Surv Ophthalmol* 1988; **33**: 1–16.

Biglan AW, Cheng KP, Brown DR. Update on retinopathy of prematurity. *Int Ophthalmol Clin* 1989; **29**: 1–9.

Boynton BR, Boynton CA. Retinopathy of prematurity and bilirubin. *N Engl J Med* 1989; **321**: 193.

Brown GC, Tasman WS, Naidoff M, Schaffer DB, Quinn GE, Bhutani VK. Systemic complications associated with retinal cryoablation for retinopathy of prematurity. *Ophthalmology* 1989; **97**: 855–8.

Burgess P, Johnson A. Ocular defects in infants of extremely low birth weight and low gestational age. *Br J Ophthalmol* 1991; **75**: 84–7.

Campbell K. Intensive oxygen therapy as a possible cause for retrolental fibroplasia. A clinical approach. *Med J Austr* 1951; **2**: 48–50.

Capone A, Diaz-Rohena R, Sternberg P, Mandell B, Lambert M, Lopez PF. Diode-laser photocoagulation for zone 1 threshold retinopathy of prematurity. *Am J Ophthalmol* 1993; **116**: 444–50.

Cats BP, Tan KEWP. Prematures with and without regressed retinopathy of prematurity: comparison of long-term (6–10 years) ophthalmological morbidity. *J Pediatr Ophthalmol Strabismus* 1989; **26**: 271–5.

Chan-Ling T, Gock B, Stone J. Supplemental oxygen therapy: basis for noninvasive treatment of retinopathy of prematurity. *Invest Ophthalmol Vis Sci* 1995; **36**: 1215–30.

Chong LP, Machemer R, de Juan E. Vitrectomy for advanced stages of retinopathy of prematurity. *Am J Ophthalmol* 1986; **102**: 710–16.

Christiansen SP, Bradford JD. Cataract in infants treated with argon laser photocoagulation for threshold retinopathy of prematurity. *Am J Ophthalmol* 1995; **119**: 175–80.

Clark C, Gibbs JAH, Maniello R *et al.* Blood transfusions: a possible risk factor in retrolental fibroplasia. *Acta Paediatr Scand* 1981; **70**: 535–9.

Clark DJ, Hero M. Indirect diode laser treatment for stage 3 retinopathy of prematurity. *Eye* 1994; **8**: 423–6.

Committee for the Classification of Retinopathy of Prematurity. The international classification of retinopathy of prematurity. *Br J Ophthalmol* 1984; **68**: 690–7.

Committee for the Classification of Retinopathy of Prematurity II. The classification of retinal detachment. *Arch Ophthalmol* 1987; **105**: 106–12.

Cooke RWI. Factors affecting survival and outcome at 3 years in extremely preterm infants. *Arch Dis Child* 1994; **71**: F28–31.

Cross KW. Cost of preventing retrolental fibroplasia? *Lancet* 1973; **ii**: 954–6.

Cryotherapy for Retinopathy of Prematurity Cooperative Group. Multicenter trial of cryotherapy for retinopathy of prematurity: preliminary results. *Arch Ophthalmol* 1988; **106**: 471–9.

Cryotherapy for Retinopathy of Prematurity Cooperative Group. Multicenter trial of cryotherapy for retinopathy of prematurity: 3-month outcome. *Arch Ophthalmol* 1990a; **108**: 195–204.

Cryotherapy for Retinopathy of Prematurity Cooperative Group. Multicenter trial of cryotherapy for retinopathy of prematurity: 1-year outcome. *Arch Ophthalmol* 1990b; **108**: 1408–16.

Cryotherapy for Retinopathy of Prematurity Cooperative Group. Multicenter trial of cryotherapy for retinopathy of prematurity. 3.5 year outcome—structure and function. *Arch Ophthalmol* 1993; **111**: 339–44.

Cryotherapy for Retinopathy of Prematurity Cooperative Group. The natural ocular outcome of premature birth and retinopathy. Status at 1 year. *Arch Ophthalmol* 1994; **112**: 903–12.

Cryotherapy for Retinopathy of Prematurity Cooperative Group. Multicenter trial of cryotherapy for retinopathy of prematurity: Snellen visual acuity and structural outcome at $5^1/_2$ years after randomization. *Arch Ophthalmol* 1996; **114**: 417–24.

Cunningham S, Fleck BW, Elton RA, McIntosh N. Transcutaneous oxygen levels in retinopathy of prematurity. *Lancet* 1995; **346**: 1464–5.

Darlow BA, Clemett RS. Retinopathy of prematurity: screeening and optimal use of the ophthalmologist's time. *Aust N Zeal J Ophthalmol* 1990; **18**: 41–6.

Darlow BA, Horwood LJ, Clemett RS. Retinopathy of prematurity: risk factors in a prospective population-based study. *Paediatr Perinatal Epidemiol* 1992; **6**: 62–80.

Editorial. Oxygen restriction and retinopathy of prematurity. *Lancet* 1992; **339**: 961–3.

Editorial. Retinopathy of prematurity. *Lancet* 1991; **337**: 83–4.

Eichenbaum JW, Mamelok A, Mittl RN, Orellana J. *Treatment of Retinopathy of Prematurity.* New York: Year Book Publishers, 1990.

Fielder AR. Cryotherapy of retinopathy of prematurity. In: Davidson SI, Jay B, eds. *Recent Advances in Ophthalmology*, Vol. 8. Edinburgh:

Churchill Livingstone, 1992, 129–48.

Fielder AR, Levene MI. Screening for retinopathy of prematurity. *Arch Dis Child* 1992; **67**: 860–7.

Fielder AR, Moseley MJ, Mayer DL. Response to Kushner 'Grating tests should not be used for social service purposes in preliterate children'. *Arch Ophthalmol* 1995; **115**: 970–1.

Fielder AR, Moseley MJ, Ng YK. The immature visual system and premature birth. *Br Med Bull* 1988; **44**: 1093–118.

Fielder AR, Ng YK, Levene MI. Retinopathy of prematurity: age at onset. *Arch Dis Child* 1986; **61**: 774–8.

Fielder AR, Robinson J, Shaw DE, Ng YK, Moseley MJ. Light and retinopathy of prematurity: does retinal location offer a clue? *Pediatrics* 1992a; **89**: 648–53.

Fielder AR, Shaw DE, Robinson J, Ng YK. Natural history of retinopathy of prematurity: a prospective study. *Eye* 1992b; **6**: 233–42.

Finer NN, Grant G, Schindler RF *et al*. Effect of intramuscular vitamin E on frequency and severity of retrolental fibroplasia: a controlled trial. *Lancet* 1982; **i**: 1087–91.

Fledelius HC. Ophthalmic changes from 10 to 18 years. A longitudinal study of sequels to low birthweight II. Visual acuity. *Acta Ophthalmol* 1981; **59**: 64–70.

Fledelius HC. Prematurity and the eye. Ophthalmic follow-up of children of low and normal birthweight. *Acta Ophthalmol* 1976; **128**(Suppl.): 1–245.

Fledelius HC, Rosenberg T. Retinopathy of prematurity. Where to set the screening limits? Recommendations based on two Danish surveys. *Acta Paediatr Scand* 1990; **79**: 906–10.

Fleming TN, Runge PE, Charles ST. Diode laser photocoagulation for prethreshold, posterior retinopathy of prematurity. *Am J Ophthalmol* 1992; **114**: 589–92.

Fletcher MC, Brandon S. Myopia of prematurity. *Am J Ophthalmol* 1955; **40**: 474–81.

Flynn JT. Acute proliferative retrolental fibroplasia: multivariate risk analysis. *Trans Am Ophthalmol Soc* 1983; **81**: 549–81.

Flynn JT. Retinopathy of prematurity. *Pediatr Clin North Am* 1987; **34**: 1487–516.

Flynn JT, Bancalari E, Bachynski BN *et al*. Retinopathy of prematurity. Diagnosis, severity and natural history. *Ophthalmology* 1987a; **94**: 620–9.

Flynn JT, Bancalari E, Bawol R *et al*. Retinopathy of prematurity. A randomised, prospective trial of transcutaneous oxygen monitoring. *Ophthalmology* 1987b; **94**: 630–8.

Flynn JT, Bancalari E, Snyder ES *et al*. A cohort study of transcutaneous oxygen monitoring and the incidence and severity of retinopathy of prematurity. *N Engl J Med* 1992; **326**: 1050–4.

Flynn JT, O'Grady GE, Herrera J *et al*. Retrolental fibroplasia I. Clinical observations. *Arch Ophthalmol* 1977; **95**: 217–23.

Flynn JT, Tasman W, eds. *Retinopathy of Prematurity. A Clinician's Guide*. New York: Springer-Verlag, 1992.

Gallo JE, Jacobson L, Broberger. Perinatal factors associated with retinopathy of prematurity. *Acta Paediatr* 1993; **82**: 829–34.

Gallo JE, Lennerstrand G. A population-based study of ocular abnormalities in premature children aged 5 to 10 years. *Am J Ophthalmol* 1991; **111**: 539–47.

Gaton DD, Gold J, Axer-Siegel R, Wielunsky E, Naor N, Nissenkorn I. Evaluation of bilirubin as possible protective factor in the prevention of retinopathy of prematurity. *Br J Ophthalmol* 1991; **75**: 532–4.

Gibson DL, Sheps SB, Schechter MT, Wiggins S, McCormick AQ. Retinopathy of prematurity: a new epidemic? *Pediatrics* 1989; **83**: 486–92.

Gibson DL, Sheps SB, Uh SH, Schechter MT, McCormick AQ. Retinopathy of prematurity-induced blindness: birth weight-specific survival and the new epidemic. *Pediatrics* 1990a; **86**: 405–12.

Gibson NA, Fielder AR, Trounce JQ, Levene MI. Ophthalmic findings in infants of very low birthweight. *Dev Med Child Neurol* 1990b; **32**: 7–13.

Gilbert CF, Canovas R, Kocksch de Canovas R, Foster A. Causes of blindness and severe visual impairment in children in Chile. *Dev Med Child Neurol* 1994; **36**: 326–33.

Gilbert WS *et al*. on behalf of the Cryotherapy for Retinopathy of Prematurity Cooperative Group. The correlation of visual function with posterior retinal structure in severe retinopathy of prematurity. *Arch Ophthalmol* 1992; **110**: 625–31.

Glass P, Avery GB, Kolinjavadi N *et al*. Effect of bright light in the hospital nursery on the incidence of retinopathy of prematurity. *N Engl J Med* 1985; **313**: 401–4.

Goggin M, O'Keefe M. Diode laser for retinopathy of prematurity— early outcome. *Br J Ophthalmol* 1993; **77**: 559–62.

Gordon RA, Donzis PB. Myopia associated with retinopathy of prematurity. *Ophthalmology* 1986; **93**: 1593–8.

Greven CM, Tasman W. Rhegmatogenous retinal detachment following cryotherapy in retinopathy of prematurity. *Arch Ophthalmol* 1989; **107**: 1017–18.

Harrison H. The principles for family-centered neonatal care. *Pediatrics* 1993; **92**: 643–50.

Hepner WR, Krause AC, Davis ME. Retrolental fibroplasia and light. *Pediatrics* 1949; **3**: 824–8.

Heyman E, Ohlsson A, Girschek P. Retinopathy of prematurity and bilirubin. *N Engl J Med* 1989; **320**: 256.

Hirose T, Katsumi O, Mehta MC, Schepens CL. Vision in stage 5 retinopathy of prematurity after retinal reattachment by open-sky vitrectomy. *Arch Ophthalmol* 1993; **111**: 345–9.

Hittner HM, Godio LB, Rudolph AJ *et al*. Retrolental fibroplasia: efficacy of vitamin E in a double-blind clinical study of preterm infants. *N Engl J Med* 1981; **305**: 1365–71.

Hittner HM, Hirsch NJ, Rudolph AJ. Assessment of gestational age by examination of the anterior vascular capsule of the lens. *J Pediatr* 1977; **91**: 455–8.

Hittner HM, Rhodes LM, McPherson AR. Anterior segment abnormalities in cicatricial retinopathy of prematurity. *Ophthalmology* 1979; **86**: 803–16.

Holmes JM, Cronin CM, Squires P, Myers TF. Randomised clinical trial of surfactant prophylaxis in retinopathy of prematurity. *J Pediatr Ophthalmol Strabismus* 1994; **31**: 189–91.

Holmstrom G, el Azizi M, Jacobson L, Lennerstrand G. A population-based, prospective study of the development of ROP in prematurely born children in the Stockholm area of Sweden. *Br J Ophthalmol* 1993; **77**: 417–23.

Hommura S, Usuki Y, Takei K *et al*. Ophthalmic care of very low birthweight infants. Report 4: clinical studies of the influence of light on the incidence of ROP. *Nippon Gakkai Zasshi* 1988; **92**: 456–61.

Hungerford J, Stewart A, Hope P. Ocular sequelae of preterm birth and their relation to ultrasound evidence of cerebral damage. *Br J Ophthalmol* 1986; **70**: 463–8.

Hunter DG, Repka MX. Diode laser photocoagulation for threshold retinopathy of prematurity. A randomized study. *Ophthalmology* 1993; **100**: 238–44.

Isenberg SJ. Macular development in the premature infant. *Am J Ophthalmol* 1986; **101**: 74–80.

James LS, Lansman JT, eds. History of oxygen and retrolental fibroplasia. *Pediatrics* 1976; **57**: 591–642.

Javitt J, Cas RD, Chiang Y-P. Cost-effectiveness of screening and cryotherapy for threshold retinopathy of prematurity. *Pediatrics* 1993; **91**: 859–66.

Johnson A, Townshend P, Yudkin P, Bull D, Wilkinson AR. Functional abilities at age 4 years of children born before 29 weeks of gestation. *Br Med J* 1993; **306**: 1715–18.

Johnson AT, Kretzer JL, Hittner HM *et al.* Development of the subretinal space in the preterm human eye: ultrastructural and immunocytochemical studies. *J Comp Neurol* 1985a; **232**: 497–505.

Johnson L, Bowen FW, Abbasi S *et al.* Relationship of prolonged pharmacologic serum levels of vitamin E to incidence of sepsis and necrotising enterocolitis in infants with birth weights 1500 g or less. *Pediatrics* 1985b; **75**: 619–38.

Kalina RE. Treatment of retrolental fibroplasia. *Surv Ophthalmol* 1980; **24**: 229–36.

Katsumi O, Mehta MC, Matsui Y, Tetsuka H, Hirose T. Development of vision in retinopathy of prematurity. *Arch Ophthalmol* 1991; **109**: 1394–8.

Keith CG, Doyle LW. Retinopathy of prematurity in infants weighing 1000–1499 g at birth. *J Paediatr Child Health* 1995; **31**: 134–6.

Keith CG, Kitchen WH. Ocular morbidity in infants of very low birth weight. *Br J Ophthalmol* 1983; **67**: 302–5.

Keith CG, Kitchen WH. Retinopathy of prematurity in extremely low birthweight infants. *Med J Aust* 1984; **141**: 225–7.

Kelly SP, Fielder AR. Microcornea associated with retinopathy of prematurity. *Br J Ophthalmol* 1987; **71**: 201–3.

Kinsey VE, Arnold HJ, Kalina RE *et al.* Pao2 levels and retrolental fibroplasia: a report of the co-operative study. *Pediatrics* 1977; **60**: 655–68.

Kinsey VE, Twomey JT, Hamphill FM. Retrolental fibroplasia. Co-operative study of retrolental fibroplasia and the use of oxygen. *Arch Ophthalmol* 1956; **56**: 481–529.

Knight-Nanan DM, Algawi K, Bowell R, O'Keefe M. Advanced cicatricial retinopathy of prematurity—outcome and complications. *Br J Ophthalmol* 1996; **80**: 343–5.

Koole FD, Bax PP, Samson JF, van der Lei J. Ocular examination in 9-month-old infants with very low birthweights. *Ophthalmol Paediatr Genet* 1990; **11**: 89–94.

Kretzer FL, Hittner HM. Retinopathy of prematurity: clinical implications of retinal development. *Arch Dis Child* 1988; **63**: 1151–67.

Kushner BJ. Strabismus and amblyopia associated with regressed retinopathy of prematurity. *Arch Ophthalmol* 1982; **100**: 256–61.

Kushner BJ, Essner D, Cohen IJ, Flynn JT. Retrolental fibroplasia II. Pathologic correlation. *Arch Ophthalmol* 1977; **95**: 29–38.

Landers MB, Toth CA, Semple C, Morse LS. Treatment of retinopathy of prematurity with argon laser photocoagulation. *Arch Ophthalmol* 1992; **110**: 44–7.

Lanman JT, Guy LP, Danus I. Retrolental fibroplasia and oxygen therapy. *J Am Med Assoc* 1954; **155**: 223–6.

Laser ROP Study Group. Laser therapy for retinopathy of prematurity. *Arch Ophthalmol* 1994; **112**: 154–6.

Laws D, Shaw DE, Robinson J, Jones HS, Ng YK, Fielder AR. Retinopathy of prematurity: a prospective study. Review at 6 months. *Eye* 1992; **6**: 477–83.

Locke JC, Reese AB. Retrolental fibroplasia: the negative role of light, mydriatics and the ophthalmoscopic examination in its etiology. *Arch Ophthalmol* 1952; **48**: 44–7.

Long W, Corbet A, Cotton R *et al.* A controlled trial of synthetic surfactant in infants weighing 1250 g or more with respiratory distress syndrome. *N Engl J Med* 1991; **325**: 1696–1703.

Lucey JL, Dangman B. A re-examination of the role of oxygen in retrolental fibroplasia. *Pediatrics* 1984; **73**: 82–96.

Luna B, Dobson V, Biglan AW. Development of grating acuity in infants with regressed stage 3 retinopathy of prematurity. *Invest Ophthalmol Vis Sci* 1990; **31**: 2082–7.

McCormick AQ, Tredger EM, Dunn HG, Grunau RVE. Ophthalmic disorders. In: HG Dunn, ed. *Sequelae of Low Birthweight, the Vancouver Study*, Clinics in Developmental Medicine No. 95/96. Oxford: MacKeith Press, Blackwell Scientific Publications, 1986: 127–46.

McDonald AD. Cerebral palsy in children of very low birth weight.

Arch Dis Child 1963; **38**: 579–88.

McGinnity FG, Bryars JH. Controlled study of ocular morbidity in schoolchildren born preterm. *Br J Ophthalmol* 1992; **76**: 520–4.

Machemer R. Closed vitrectomy for severe retrolental fibroplasia in infants. *Ophthalmology* 1983; **90**: 436–41.

Machemer R, deJuan E. Retinopathy of prematurity: approaches to surgical therapy. *Aust N Zeal J Ophthalmol* 1990; **18**: 47–56.

McNamara JA. Laser treatment for retinopathy of prematurity. *Curr Opinion Ophthalmol* 1993; **4**: 76–80.

McNamara JA, Tasman W, Brown GC, Federman JL. Laser photocoagulation for stage 3+ retinopathy of prematurity. *Ophthalmology* 1991; **98**: 576–80.

McPherson AR, Hittner HM, Lemos R. Retinal detachment in young premature infants with acute retrolental fibroplasia. Thirty-two new cases. *Ophthalmology* 1982; **89**: 1160–9.

Michaelson IC. The mode of development of the vascular system of the retina, with some observations on its significance for certain retinal diseases. *Trans Ophthalmol Soc UK* 1948; **68**: 137–80.

Mintz-Hittner HA, Prager TC, Kretzer FL. Visual acuity correlates with severity of retinopathy of prematurity in untreated infants weighing 750 g or less at birth. *Arch Ophthalmol* 1992; **110**: 1087–91.

Muller DPR. Vitamin E therapy in retinopathy of prematurity. *Eye* 1992; **6**: 221–5.

Ng YK, Fielder AR, Levene MI, Trounce JQ, McLellan N. Are severe retinopathy of prematurity and severe periventricular leucomalacia both ischaemic insults? *Br J Ophthalmol* 1989; **73**: 111–14.

Ng YK, Fielder AR, Shaw DE, Levene MI. Epidemiology of retinopathy of prematurity. *Lancet* 1988; **ii**: 1235–8.

Nissenkorn I, Axer-Siegel R, Kremer I, Ben-Sira I. Effect of partial cryoablation on retinopathy of prematurity. *Br J Ophthalmol* 1991; **75**: 160–2.

Nissenkorn I, Yassur Y, Mashkowski I, Sherf I, Ben-Sira I. Myopia in premature babies with and without retinopathy of prematurity. *Br J Ophthalmol* 1983; **67**: 170–3.

Owens WC, Owens EU. Retrolental fibroplasia in premature infants. *Trans Am Acad Ophthalmol Otolaryngol* 1948; **53**: 18–41.

Page JM, Schneeweiss S, Whyte HEA, Harvey P. Ocular sequelae in premature infants. *Pediatrics* 1993; **92**: 787–90.

Palmer EA. Optimal timing of examination for acute retrolental fibroplasia. *Ophthalmology* 1981; **88**: 662–8.

Palmer EA. Treatment of ROP by peripheral retinal ablation. In: SJ Isenberg, ed. *The Eye in Infancy*. Chicago: Year Book Medical Publishers, 1994: 471–7.

Palmer EA, Biglan AW, Hardy RJ. Retinal ablative therapy for active retinopathy of prematurity: history, current status and prospects. In: Silverman WA, Flynn JT, eds. *Contemporary Issues in Fetal Medicine and Neurology*, Vol. 2. *Retinopathy of Prematurity*. Oxford: Blackwell Scientific Publications, 1985: 207–28.

Palmer EA, Flynn JT, Hardy RJ. The Cryotherapy for Retinopathy of Prematurity Cooperative Group. Incidence and early course of retinopathy of prematurity. *Ophthalmology* 1991; **98**: 1628–40.

Patz A. Oxygen studies in retrolental fibroplasia IV. Clinical and experimental observations. *Am J Ophthalmol* 1954; **38**: 291–308.

Patz A. Retrolental fibroplasia (retinopathy of prematurity). *Trans Ophthalmol Soc NZ* 1980; **32**: 49–54.

Patz A, Hoeck LE, De La Cruz E. Studies on the effect of high oxygen administration in retrolental fibroplasia: a nursery observation. *Am J Ophthalmol* 1952; **35**: 1248–52.

Phelps DL. Retinopathy of prematurity. In: Isenberg SJ, ed. *The Eye in Infancy*, 2nd edn. St Louis: CV Mosby, 1994: 437–47.

Phelps DL, Rosenbaum A. The role of tocopherol in oxygen-induced retinopathy: kitten model. *Pediatrics* 1977; **59**: 998–1005.

Phelps DL, Rosenbaum A, Isenberg SJ, Leake RD, Dorey FJ. Tocopherol efficacy and safety for preventing retinopathy of prematurity: a randomised controlled double-masked trial. *Pediatrics* 1987; **79**: 489–500.

Pike MG, Holmstrom G, de Vreis LS *et al*. Patterns of visual impairment associated with lesions of the preterm infant brain. *Dev Med Child Neurol* 1994; **36**: 849–62.

Prendiville A, Schulenburg WE. Clinical factors associated with retinopathy of prematurity. *Eye* 1988; **63**: 522–7.

Quinn GE, Dobson V, Barr CC *et al*. Visual acuity in infants after vitrectomy for severe retinopathy of prematurity. *Ophthalmology* 1991; **98**: 5–13.

Quinn GE, Dobson V, Repka MX *et al*. on behalf of the Cryotherapy for Retinopathy of Prematurity Cooperative Group. Development of myopia in infants with birth weights less than 1251 g. *Ophthalmology* 1992a; **99**: 329–40.

Quinn GE, Dobson V, Repka MX *et al*. for the Cryotherapy for Retinopathy of Prematurity Cooperative Group. Correlation of retinopathy of prematurity in fellow eyes in the cryotherapy for retinopathy of prematurity study. *Arch Ophthalmol* 1995; **113**: 469–73.

Quinn GE, Johnson L, Abbasi S. Onset of retinopathy of prematurity as related to postnatal and postconceptual age. *Br J Ophthalmol* 1992b; **76**: 284–8.

Rankin SJA, Tubman TRJ, Halliday HL, Johnston SS. Retinopathy of prematurity in surfactant treated infants. *Br J Ophthalmol* 1992; **76**: 202–4.

Reese AB, King MJ, Owens WC. A classification of retrolental fibroplasia. *Am J Ophthalmol* 1953; **36**: 1333–5.

Reisner SH, Amir J, Shohat M, Krikler R, Nissenkorn I, Ben-Sira I. Retinopathy of prematurity: incidence and treatment. *Arch Dis Child* 1985; **60**: 698–701.

Repka MX, Hardy RJ, Phelps DL, Summers G. Surfactant prophylaxis and retinopathy of prematurity. *Arch Ophthalmol* 1993; **111**: 618–20.

Report of a Joint Working Party. *Retinopathy of Prematurity: Guidelines for Screening and Treatment*. London: Royal College of Ophthalmologists and British Association of Perinatal Medicine, 1995.

Reynolds J, Dobson V, Quinn GE *et al*. for the Cryotherapy for Retinopathy of Prematurity Cooperative Group. Prediction of visual function in eyes with mild to moderate posterior pole residua of retinopathy of prematurity. *Arch Ophthalmol* 1993; **111**: 1050–6.

Robinson R, O'Keefe M. Follow-up study on premature infants with and without retinopathy of prematurity. *Br J Ophthalmol* 1993; **77**: 91–4.

Rosenbaum AL, Phelps DL, Isenberg SI *et al*. Retinal haemorrhage in retinopathy of prematurity associated with tocopherol treatment. *Ophthalmology* 1985; **92**: 1012–15.

Saito Y, Omoto T, Cho Y, Hatsukawa Y, Fujimua M, Takeuchi T. The progression of retinopathy of prematurity and fluctuation in blood gas tension. *Graefe's Arch Clin Exp Ophthalmol* 1993; **231**: 151–6.

Schaffer DB. Update on retinopathy of prematurity: the examination guidelines. *Semin Ophthalmol* 1990; **5**: 100–6.

Schaffer DB, Johnson L, Quinn GE, Weston M, Bowen FW. Vitamin E and retinopathy of prematurity. *Ophthalmology* 1985; **92**: 1005–11.

Schaffer DB, Quinn GE, Johnson L. Sequelae of arrested mild retinopathy of prematurity. *Arch Ophthalmol* 1984; **102**: 373–6.

Schaffer DB, Palmer EA, Plotsky DF *et al*. on behalf of the Cryotherapy for Retinopathy of Prematurity Cooperative Group. Prognostic factors in the natural course of retinopathy of prematurity. *Ophthalmology* 1993; **100**: 230–7.

Schulenberg WE, Acheson JF. Cryosurgery for acute retinopathy of prematurity: factors associated with treatment success and failure. *Eye* 1992; **6**: 215–20.

Seaber JH, Machemer R, Eliott D, Buckley EG, deJuan E, Martin DF. Long-term visual results of children after initially successful vitrectomy for stage V retinopathy of prematurity. *Ophthalmology* 1995; **102**: 199–204.

Sebris SL, Dobson V, Hartmann EE. Assessment and prediction of visual acuity in 3–4-year old children born prior to term. *Hum Neurobiol* 1984; **3**: 87–92.

Seiberth V, Linderkamp O, Knorz MC, Liesenhoff H. A controlled trial of light and retinopathy of prematurity. *Am J Ophthalmol* 1994; **118**: 492–5.

Sellheyer K, Spitznas M. Morphology of the developing choroidal vasculature in the human fetus. *Graefe's Arch Clin Exp Ophthalmol* 1988; **226**: 461–7.

Shohat M, Reisner SH, Krikler R *et al*. Retinopathy of prematurity. Incidence and risk factors. *Pediatrics* 1983; **72**: 159–63.

Silverman WA. *Retrolental Fibroplasia: a Modern Parable*. New York: Grune & Stratton, 1980.

Snir M, Nissenkorn I, Sherf I, Cohen S, Ben-Sira I. Visual acuity, strabismus, and amblyopia in premature babies with and without retinopathy of prematurity. *Ann Ophthalmol* 1988; **20**: 256–8.

Spencer R, Hutton W, Snyder W, Fuller D, Fish G, Vaiser A, Jost B. Limiting applications of cryotherapy for severe retinopathy of prematurity. *Ophthalmic Surg* 1992; **23**: 766–9.

Stone J, Chan-Ling T, Pe'er J *et al*. Roles of vascular endothelial growth factor and astrocyte degeneration in the genesis of retinopathy of prematurity. *Invest Ophthalmol Vis Sci* 1996; **37**: 290–9.

Summers G, Dale L, Phelps MD, Tung B, Palmer E. Ocular cosmesis in retinopathy of prematurity. *Arch Ophthalmol* 1992; **110**: 1092–7.

Tan KEWP, Cats BP. Timely incidence of examination for acute retinopathy of prematurity (ROP) and its consequence for the screening strategy. *Am J Perinatol* 1989; **6**: 337–40.

Tasman W. Late complications of retrolental fibroplasia. *Ophthalmology* 1979; **86**: 1724–40.

Tasman W. Threshold retinopathy of prematurity revisited. *Arch Ophthalmol* 1992; **110**: 623–4.

Tasman W, Borrone RN, Bolling J. Open sky vitrectomy for total retinal detachment in retinopathy of prematurity. *Ophthalmology* 1987; **94**: 449–52.

Terry TL. Extreme prematurity and fibroblastic overgrowth of persistent vascular sheath behind each crystalline lens I. Preliminary report. *Am J Ophthalmol* 1942; **25**: 203–4.

Terry TL. Fibroblastic overgrowth of persistent tunica vasculosa lentis in premature infants. II: report of cases—clinical aspects. *Arch Ophthalmol* 1943; **29**: 36–53.

Terry TL. Retrolental fibroplasia in premature infants. Further studies on fibroblastic overgrowth of tunica vasculosa lentis. *Arch Ophthalmol* 1945; **33**: 203–8.

Topilow HW, Ackerman AL, Wang FM, Strome RR. Successful treatment of advanced retinopathy of prematurity. *Ophthalmic Surg* 1990; **19**: 781–5.

Trese M. Treatment of ROP by retinovitreous surgery. In: SJ Isenberg, ed. *The Eye in Infancy*. Chicago: Year Book Medical Publishers, 1994: 478–82.

Trese M. Visual results and prognostic factors for vision following surgery for stage V retinopathy of prematurity. *Ophthalmology* 1986; **93**: 574–9.

Urrea PT, Rosenbaum AT. Retinopathy of prematurity: ophthalmologist's perspective. In: SJ Isenberg, ed. *The Eye in Infancy*. Chicago: Year Book Medical Publishers, 1994: 448–70.

Weakley DR, Spencer R. Current concepts in retinopathy of prematurity. *Early Hum Dev* 1992; **30**: 121–38.

44: Inherited Retinal Dystrophies

Anthony Moore

The inherited retinal dystrophies are a genetically heterogeneous group of disorders many of which become symptomatic in childhood. They may occur as an isolated abnormality in an otherwise normal child or may be associated with other systemic abnormalities. Most are progressive but a few, notably stationary night-blindness, fundus albipunctatus, Oguchi's disease and achromatopsia, are stationary.

Classification of childhood retinal dystrophies is unsatisfactory because of heterogeneity even amongst dystrophies sharing a common mode of inheritance. Meaningful classification must await identification of the causative genetic mutations. However, these disorders can be divided according to whether they (i) are stationary or progressive; and (ii) exhibit predominantly rod involvement or predominantly cone or central receptor disease. The dystrophies presenting at birth or in the first few months of life are considered separately, as they have a different presentation and pose particularly difficult diagnostic problems.

Stationary retinal dystrophies

These include the different forms of stationary night-blindness and the stationary cone disorders.

Stationary night-blindness

Three forms of stationary night-blindness are recognized; in the various forms of congenital stationary night-blindness (CSNB) the ocular fundus is normal whereas in fundus albipunctatus and Oguchi's disease a distinctive fundus appearance is seen. There is an overlap in the phenotypes of X-linked CNSB and the Forsius–Eriksson type of X-linked ocular albinism (Åland Island eye disease) and it is probable that both disorders result from mutations at the same locus. Patients with a contiguous gene syndrome (which includes glycerol kinase deficiency, congenital adrenal hypoplasia, Duchenne muscular dystrophy (DMD) and ocular abnormalities) associated with a deletion of Xp21 have some ocular features in common with affected males with Åland Island eye disease and have similar ERG abnormalities. Furthermore, in DMD some affected males whose mutations are confined to the dystrophin gene at Xp21 have ERG abnormalities similar to those seen in CSNB. All of these disorders have a nonprogressive form of retinal dystrophy which predominantly affects the scotopic system.

Congenital stationary night-blindness

CSNB is characterized by night-blindness, variable visual loss and a normal fundus examination. It may be inherited as an autosomal dominant, autosomal recessive or X-linked disorder (Krill 1977c).

The visual acuity is normal in the dominant form (Rosenberg *et al.* 1991) whereas in the other two genetic subtypes mild central visual loss is common. Other features that may be seen in X-linked and recessive CSNB include moderate to high myopia, nystagmus, strabismus and paradoxical pupil responses (Krill 1977c; Price *et al.* 1988). Fundus examination is usually normal but some patients have pale or tilted optic discs (Heckenlively *et al.* 1983). Although most patients present with symptomatic night-blindness, occasionally in children nystagmus and visual loss are the predominant symptoms and, unless studies appropriate to night-blindness are specifically asked for when an ERG is performed, the diagnosis may be missed (Weleber & Tongue 1987; Price *et al.* 1988) (see Fig. 9.9).

As the retinal appearance is usually normal, the diagnosis depends upon demonstrating the characteristic psychophysical and electrophysiological abnormalities seen in this disorder. Most patients show a monophasic dark adaptation curve although in a few there is a recognizable rod component with a markedly elevated threshold (Krill 1977c). Cone adaptation is also abnormal, as are other measures of cone function such as flicker fusion and photopic ERG (Krill & Martin 1971).

Patients with CSNB may be divided into two groups on the basis of their ERG findings. The first group, which includes most patients with X-linked and autosomal recessive CSNB, show a near normal a-wave and a substantially reduced b-wave on testing under scotopic conditions (negative wave ERG; see Fig. 9.9). With increasing intensity of the test stimulus the amplitude of the a-wave increases but that of the b-wave is unchanged (Schubert & Bornschein 1952). The photopic b-wave, oscillatory potentials and the scotopic threshold response may also be reduced (Heckenlively *et al.* 1983; Miyake *et al.* 1986, 1994). This subgroup of CSNB can be further subdivided into two types depending on whether rod function can be demonstrated psychophysically or not (Miyake *et al.* 1986). In complete CSNB there is no psychophysical evidence of residual rod function and there is an absent scotopic b-wave and scotopic threshold response. In the incomplete form there is evidence of a rod contribution to dark adaptation and the scotopic b-wave and scotopic threshold responses are recordable (Miyake *et al.* 1986, 1994). The clinical features of the incomplete form of X-linked CSNB overlap those of the Forsius–Eriksson type of X-linked ocular albinism and the two disorders are probably caused by mutations of the same gene (see below).

Most carriers of X-linked CSNB are not night-blind and have a normal fundus examination but may show abnormal oscillatory potentials on ERG (Miyake & Kawase 1984). Manifesting heterozygotes have been described and probably represent examples of skewed X inactivation (Ruttum *et al.* 1992).

A second group of patients with CSNB (predominantly those with the autosomal dominant form) do not show a negative wave ERG, the response to the standard bright white flash of the b-wave is larger than the a-wave but the amplitude of both is reduced. Scotopic responses are very attenuated (Auerbach *et al.* 1969; Rosenberg *et al.* 1991). There is a rod contribution to the dark adaptation curve but it is slowed and the final threshold is elevated (Krill 1977c; Rosenberg *et al.* 1991).

Molecular genetics of congenital stationary night-blindness

Recently, Gal *et al.* (1994) have reported a mutation of the rod cyclic guanosine monophosphate (cGMP) phosphodiesterase beta-subunit gene in autosomal dominant stationary night-blindness. Mutations of the rhodopsin gene have also been reported in association with the dominant form of stationary night-blindness (Sieving *et al.* 1992; Dryja *et al.* 1993; Rao *et al.* 1994). In most affected families the X-linked form of CSNB (CSNB1) has been mapped to the short arm of the X chromosome to the region Xp11.3 (Musarella *et al.* 1989; Aldred *et al.* 1992). Recently, a second locus for X-linked CSNB has been mapped to the Xp21 region (Bergen *et al.* 1995) which is also the locus for a form of X-linked retinitis pigmentosa (RP3).

Åland Island eye disease

Forsius and Eriksson in 1964 first described an X-linked recessive disorder (Åland Island eye disease, AIED) characterized by reduced visual acuity, nystagmus, mild red–green dyschromatopsia and myopia. Affected males may also show iris translucency, foveal hypoplasia and decreased fundus pigmentation. Nyctalopia is common. The clinical appearance may resemble X-linked ocular albinism (XLOA) but in XLOA colour vision is usually normal and patients with AIED do not show the typical optic nerve fibre mis-routeing seen in albinism (van Dorp *et al.* 1985). The symptoms of night-blindness and the psychophysical and ERG changes seen in AIED are similar to those seen in the incomplete form of the X-linked form of CSNB (Rosenberg *et al.* 1990; Hawksworth *et al.* 1995). Both disorders map to the same region of the short arm of the X chromosome and it is likely that they are allelic (Musarella *et al.* 1989; Schwartz & Rosenberg 1991; Aldred *et al.* 1992; Glass *et al.* 1993).

Oregon eye disease

In 1989 Weleber *et al.* described a young boy with a contiguous gene deletion syndrome characterized by glycerol kinase deficiency, congenital adrenal hypoplasia, DMD and an ocular phenotype similar to that described in AIED and the incomplete form of stationary night-blindness. The scotopic responses of the ERG were absent and the responses to a bright white flash showed a negative wave form. The region of the X chromosome deleted was Xp21 which is remote from the locus for both CSNB1 and AIED ascertained from linkage studies (Musarella *et al.* 1989; Schwartz & Rosenberg 1991; Aldred *et al.* 1992; Glass *et al.* 1993). Piller *et al.* (1993) later reported four further patients with deletions of Xp21; each showed a similar abnormality on ERG. Subsequent ERG studies of patients with DMD and Becker muscular dystrophy showed that the scotopic b-wave is markedly reduced in amplitude in some patients (Pillers *et al.* 1993; Jensen *et al.* 1995). The dark-adapted cone b-wave may also be mildly reduced but light-adapted reponses are normal. Although the ERG is abnormal the ocular examination, colour vision and dark adaptation are reportedly normal (Jensen *et al.* 1995). The position and characteristics of the dystrophin gene mutation may determine if the ERG is affected (Jensen *et al.* 1995).

Pillers *et al.* (1995) have shown that dystrophin (the protein product of the DMD gene) localizes to the inner plexiform layer of the retina and may therefore be important for inner retinal function including the generation of the scotopic b-wave.

Oguchi's disease

Oguchi's disease is a rare form of stationary night-blindness in which there is a peculiar greyish or green–yellow discoloration of the fundus which reverts to normal on prolonged dark adaptation (Mizuo phenomenon). Although most cases have been reported from Japan it is seen in other races including Europeans (Krill 1977c) and American black people (Winn *et al.* 1968). It is inherited as an autosomal recessive trait.

Most patients present with poor night vision. Visual acuity is usually normal or only mildly reduced and photopic visual fields and colour vision are normal. In the light-adapted state the retina has a retractile grey–white appearance which reverts to normal after prolonged dark adaptation. In most patients exposure to light then leads to the gradual reappearance of the abnormal discoloration which may take 10–20 minutes to reach its full effect (Mizuo 1913; Carr & Gouras 1965; Krill 1977c). The abnormal appearance may be confined to the posterior pole or extend beyond the arcades.

Patients with Oguchi's disease fall into two types according to the type of abnormality seen on dark adaptation (Krill 1977c). In type 1 rod adaptation is markedly slowed; full recovery of sensitivity takes several hours and the absolute threshold is normal or only minimally elevated. In type 2 there is no recognizable rod adaptation; the abnormal retinal appearance is less marked and the Mizuo phenomenon may be absent.

Most patients with Oguchi's disease show the 'negative wave' ERG seen in CSNB. Under scotopic conditions the a-wave has a normal amplitude but the b-wave is markedly reduced or absent. In contrast to fundus albipunctatus the ERG remains abnormal even when full adaptation is complete (Carr & Gouras 1965; Krill 1977c).

Fuchs *et al.* (1995) have recently reported a homozygous deletion of nucleotide 1147 of the arrestin gene in five unrelated Japanese patients with Oguchi's disease. The mutation results in a truncated protein. Reduced activity of arrestin would be predicted to result in prolonged activation of transducin and rod phosphodiesterase on light exposure. Cyclic GMP levels would be maintained at a low level in response to even dim light exposure and the outer segment cation channels would remain closed resulting in prolonged hyperpolarization of the rod. The rods would behave as if they were light adapted and would be unresponsive to light at low levels of illumination. This would explain the pyschophysical abnormalities seen in Oguchi's disease (Fuchs *et al.* 1995).

Fundus albipunctatus

This autosomal recessive form of stationary night-blindness has a characteristic fundus appearance with multiple white dots scattered throughout the retina (see Fig. 48.2). Patients either present with night-blindness or because the abnormal retinal appearance is noted on routine fundoscopy. The visual acuity is normal and the condition non-progressive.

The deposits are discrete dull white lesions which lie at the level of the retinal pigment epithelium. They are most numerous in the midperiphery and are usually absent at the macula (Krill 1977c); the optic discs and retinal vessels are normal. Fluorescein angiography shows multiple areas of hyperfluorescence which may not conform to the deposits seen clinically (Gelber & Shah 1969; Krill 1977c). The differential diagnosis is from other causes of flecked retina (see Chapter 48).

In fundus albipunctatus both cone and rod dark adaptation is severely delayed. The rod–cone break is delayed and full rod adaptation may take several hours (Carr *et al.* 1974; Marmor 1977). The electro-oculogram (EOG) and cone–rod ERG are abnormal in the light-adapted eye but after prolonged dark adaptation may reach normal values. In contrast to Oguchi's disease and CSNB rhodopsin regeneration is slow in fundus albipunctatus (Carr *et al.* 1974).

Stationary cone disorders

The stationary cone dystrophies include the colour vision disorders where there is normal visual acuity but defective colour vision and the various forms of achromatopsia where the colour vision defect is associated with reduced vision and nystagmus.

Disorders of colour vision

Colour vision in humans is trichromatic; there are three classes of cone photoreceptors that contain visual pigments that are maximally sensitive at 560 nm (red cones), 535 nm (green cones) and 440 nm (blue cones). The genes for the protein component (opsin) of the red and green cone pigments have been identified on the long arm of the X chromosome, and the blue cone opsin gene on chromosome 7 (Nathans *et al.* 1986a, b). About 8% of men and 0.5% of women have a defect of the red–green system and these defects are associated with abnormalities of the red and green cone opsin genes. Tritanopia is an uncommon autosomal dominant disorder in which there is a specific deficiency of blue cone sensitivity associated with mutations of the blue cone opsin gene (Weitz *et al.* 1992).

This group of disorders in which there is normal central vision, a normal eye examination but abnormal colour vision will not be considered in detail here. The clinical characteristics have, however, been reviewed in detail by Krill (1977b) and the molecular pathology by Nathans (1989a,b).

Rod monochromatism (achromatopsia)

Rod monochromatism is a stationary retinal dystrophy in which there appears to be an absence of functioning cones in the retina (Sharpe *et al.* 1988). It is characterized by reduced central vision, poor colour vision, photophobia and a normal fundus examination; it occurs in typical and atypical forms (Krill 1977c).

Typical rod monochromatism

This rare disorder is inherited as an autosomal recessive trait and results in impaired vision and complete colour blindness. The incidence is approximately one in 40 000. The usual presentation is with reduced vision, nystagmus and marked photophobia in infancy. Parents often comment that vision is very much better in dim illumination, and many say that, although there may be photophobia, the most significant symptom is that the vision is poorer in bright illumination. Pupil reactions are sluggish or may show pupillary constriction in the dark—the so-called paradoxical response (Price *et al.* 1985). High hyperopic refractive errors are common and fundus examination is normal. The nystagmus although marked in infancy may improve with age and typically in late childhood there is fine rapid horizontal nystagmus. Photophobia may also improve with age.

In older children the visual acuity is usually about 6/60 and there is complete colour blindness. Peripheral visual fields are normal but a small central scotoma can often be detected. Although histopathological studies (Larsen 1921; Harrison *et al.* 1960; Falls *et al.* 1965; Glickstein & Heath 1975) have demonstrated cone-like structures in the retina, psychophysical studies show that the achromat lacks cone vision (Sharpe *et al.* 1988). The dark adaptation curve is monophasic with no evidence of a cone contribution and spectral sensitivity studies show that rods mediate threshold under both photopic and scotopic conditions (Sharpe *et al.* 1988); there is no evidence of a Purkinje shift. Electroretinography demonstrates an absence of cone responses to white light, red light (see Fig. 9.10) and flicker (Krill 1977a; Andreasson & Tornquist 1991). The scotopic ERG is normal.

The genetic mutation causing rod monochromatism is

unknown but on the basis of a chromosomal rearrangement in a single affected patient the disease locus may be on chromosome 14 (Pentao *et al.* 1992).

Incomplete typical rod monochromatism (partial achromatopsia)

The presentation and clinical findings in infancy are similar to the complete form of rod monochromatism but in later childhood and adult life the symptoms are less severe. Visual acuity is often in the range 6/24–6/36 and there may be some residual colour perception. This form is also inherited as an autosomal recessive trait (Krill 1977b). It is doubtful whether this represents a different disorder as patterns of disease resembling both the incomplete and complete subtypes are seen within the same family.

Blue cone monochromatism

Blue cone monochromatism is an X-linked recessive disorder in which affected males have normal rod and blue cone function but lack red and green cone function (Alpern *et al.* 1965; Spivey 1965; Krill 1977b). The disorder is caused by abnormalities in the red and green visual pigment genes on the long arm of the X chromosome that result in loss of function (Nathans *et al.* 1989b). Two different genetic mechanisms lead to loss of red and green cone function (Nathans *et al.* 1989b). In the first mechanism unequal homologous recombination reduces the number of pigment genes to one (similar to the dichromat) and then a second mutational event in the remaining gene results in its inactivation. The second mechanism may involve mutations which affect the function of a promoter region upstream of the red and green pigment genes.

The clinical features are similar to complete rod monochromatism but are less severe. Affected infants are photophobic and develop fine rapid nystagmus in early infancy. In contrast to rod monochromatism there is usually a myopic refractive error. The nystagmus reduces with time and is usually minimal by the late teens. The ERG findings using the standard protocol are identical to those seen in complete rod monochromatism (Spivey 1965; Andreasson & Tornquist 1991) but the two disorders may be differentiated by the mode of inheritance and findings on psychophysical testing. Specialized spectral ERG techniques may also be able to distinguish between rod monochromatism and blue cone monochromatism. Female carriers of X-linked blue cone monochromatism may have abnormal cone ERGs (Berson *et al.* 1986) and mild anomalies of colour vision (Krill 1977a). They may also show mild abnormalities on eye movement recording (Gottlob 1994).

Progressive retinal dystrophies

Rod–cone dystrophies

Leber's amaurosis (infantile rod–cone dystrophy)

Leber's amaurosis is a rod–cone dystrophy which presents at birth or the first few months of life and may be progressive in some cases. It is inherited as an autosomal recessive trait (Alstrom & Olson 1957), although it is likely that there are several different genotypes giving rise to the same clinical picture (Waardenberg & Schappert-Kimmijser 1963). Concordance in siblings is high (Lambert *et al.* 1993). It has been reported to be inherited as an autosomal dominant trait (Sorsby & Williams 1960) but this has not been confirmed. It is a common cause of blindness in children, accounting for 10–18% of children in institutions for the blind (Alstrom & Olson 1957; Schappert-Kimmijser *et al.* 1959). One gene causing this disorder has been mapped to 17p (Camuzat *et al.* 1995).

The normal presentation is with suspected blindness or poor vision with nystagmus from birth or the first few months of life. Affected infants have roving eye movements and poor pupillary responses to light. Eye-poking, the 'oculodigital' sign (Fig. 44.1), is common (Franceschetti 1947). Fundus examination and fluorescein angiography are usually normal but a variety of abnormal fundus appearances may be seen. The optic disc may be pale, the vessels thinned (Fig. 44.2) and there may be a mild peripheral pigmentary retinopathy. Less commonly there may be optic disc oedema or pseudopapilloedema (Fig. 44.3) (Flynn & Cullen 1975), a flecked retina (Fig. 44.4) (Mizuno *et al.* 1977), macular dysplasia (Fig. 44.5) (Margolis *et al.* 1977; Moore *et al.* 1985; Smith *et al.* 1990) or, less frequently, nummular pigmentation (Fig. 44.6) (Schroeder *et al.* 1987). Affected infants often have high hyperopia (Foxman *et al.* 1983; Wagner *et al.* 1985) or less commonly high myopia, suggesting that the severe visual impairment may interfere with the normal process of emmetropization.

Although the majority of patients have normal fundi in infancy, in later childhood most develop signs of a pigmentary retinopathy with optic disc pallor and retinal arteriolar narrowing (Sullivan *et al.* 1992). Rarely yellow flecks may be seen in the equatorial fundus (Chew *et al.* 1984). Other late signs which may be related to eye-poking include enophthalmos, keratoconus and cataract (Alstrom & Olson 1957; Heher *et al.* 1992). Eventual vision is in the region of 3/60 to perception of light, but only in some cases (Fig. 44.7) is deterioration demonstrable (Lambert *et al.* 1989b).

The ERG is extinguished or severely subnormal in infants with Leber's amaurosis. It is important to perform both scotopic and photopic ERGs to distinguish the disorder from CSNB and achromatopsia, which may also present in infancy with nystagmus and poor vision. The

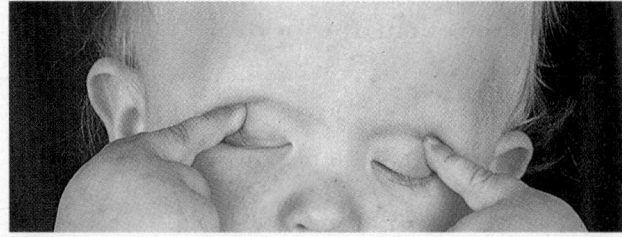

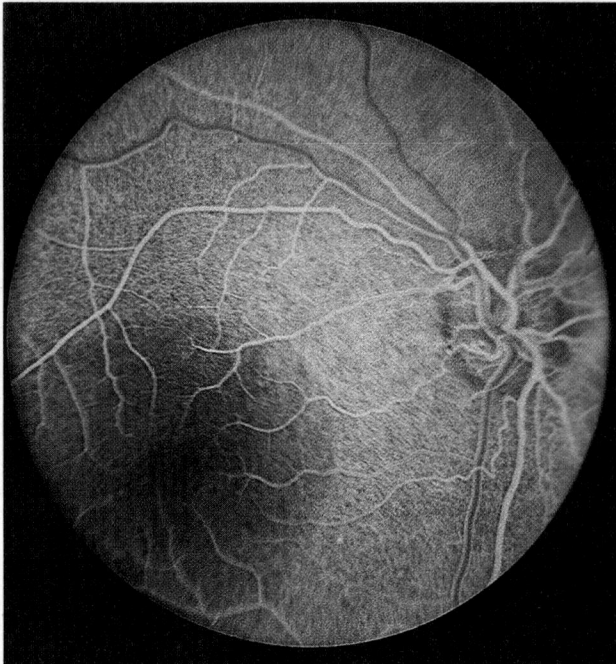

Fig. 44.1 Leber's amaurosis; (a) eye-poking, the 'oculodigital sign' is very common but of unknown cause; it results in atrophy of orbital fat and enophthalmos. (b) Normal fluorescein angiogram (same patient).

visual evoked response is usually absent but may be preserved in some infants despite an absent ERG and may indicate a better visual prognosis.

Non-ocular features

Most cases of Leber's amaurosis occur in otherwise normal infants and it may be preferable that the term Leber's amaurosis is confined to such children. However, a variety of associated systemic abnormalities including mental subnormality, neurological disorders, renal disease and hearing loss have been reported in association with a similar infantile retinal dystrophy. It is likely that the majority of these disorders are caused by different genetic mutations unrelated to that causing an isolated infantile rod–cone dystrophy.

Mental retardation and neurological disease are the most frequent of the reported associations but there is great variation in the incidence of neurological disease in

the various series (Schappert-Kimmijser 1959; Vaizey *et al.* 1977; Moore & Taylor 1984; Foxman *et al.* 1985; Lambert *et al.* 1989b). Several studies (Alstrom & Olson 1957; Nickel & Hoyt 1982) have failed to show a significantly increased incidence of such abnormalities whereas others (Schappert-Kimmijser 1959; Dekaban & Carr 1966; Dekaban 1972; Vaizey *et al.* 1977; Noble & Carr 1978) have found major neurological or developmental abnormalities in more than 25% of cases. The variation mainly reflects differences in referral patterns to the various centres but the lower incidence in more recent series (Nickel & Hoyt 1982; Lambert *et al.* 1989b) may reflect the fact that many infants with neurological disease and a retinal dystrophy are now recognized to have specific genetic conditions such as Joubert's syndrome or the peroxisomal disorders. It is also now evident that normal blind children are often hypotonic and may reach some developmental milestones later than their sighted peers; such delay is not an indication of psychomotor retardation.

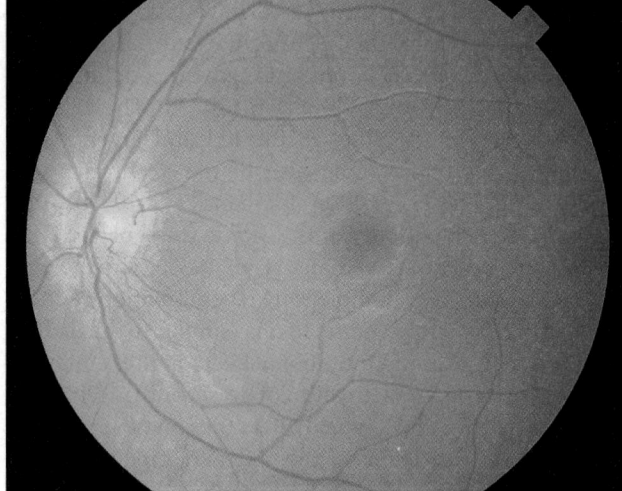

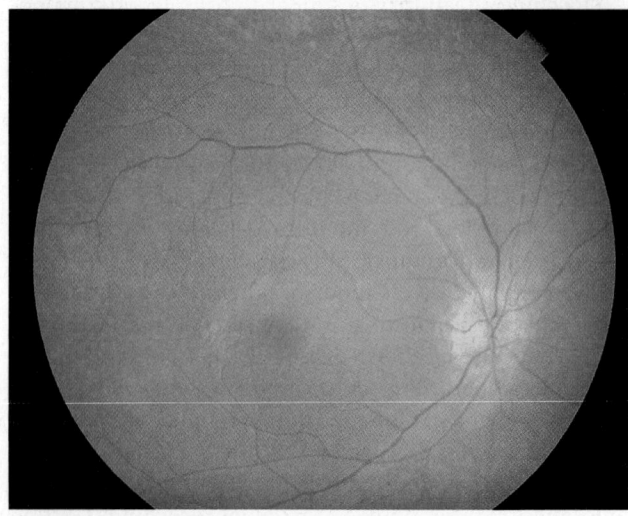

Fig. 44.2 Leber's amaurosis: blind 6-year-old, showing only mild vascular attenuation.

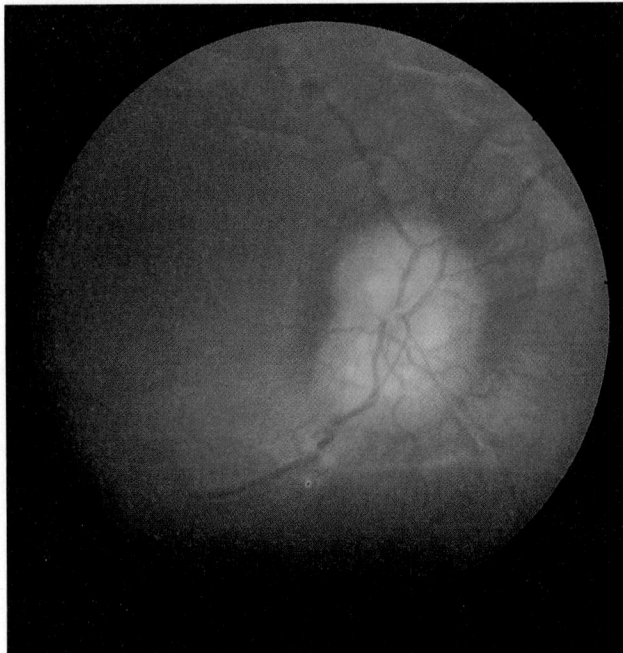

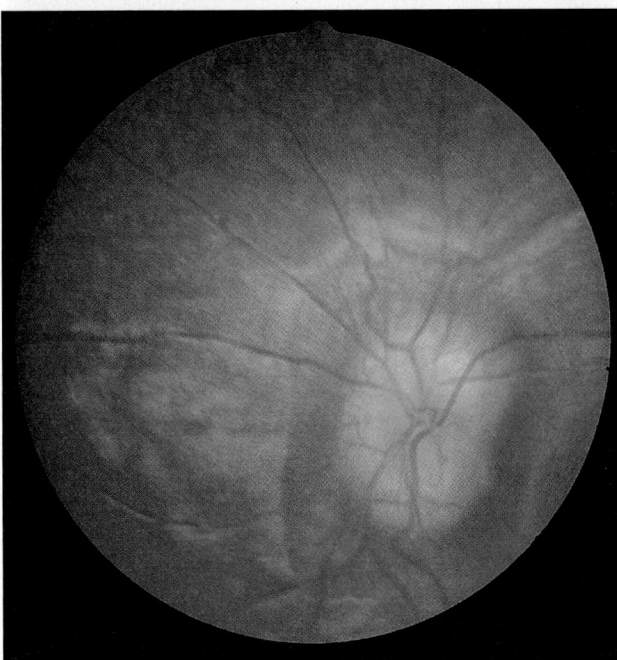

Fig. 44.3 (a, b) Leber's amaurosis—high hypermetropia and pseudopapilloedema.

Although several different abnormalities of the central nervous system (CNS) have been demonstrated on computed tomography (CT) scan the only consistent abnormality is hypoplasia of the cerebellar vermis which may be seen in 10% of infants with Leber's amaurosis (Nickel & Hoyt 1982). A retinal dystrophy and cerebellar vermis abnormalities are also seen in Joubert's syndrome, olivopontocerebellar atrophy and the carbohydrate deficient glycoprotein syndrome.

Moore and Taylor (1984) described three children with Leber's amaurosis who had a saccade palsy and head thrusts similar to that seen in ocular motor apraxia. CT scan showed cerebellar vermis hypoplasia. Although these patients did not have all the features, they are almost certainly examples of Joubert's syndrome (Joubert *et al.* 1969; King *et al.* 1984).

Sensorineural hearing loss occurs in about 5% of children with Leber's amaurosis (Lambert *et al.* 1989b); this association has not been well characterized but it is important to exclude one of the peroxisomal disorders in infants with hearing loss and a congenital retinal dystrophy.

Renal abnormalities, particularly juvenile nephronophthisis, have been reported in association with a retinal dystrophy indistinguishable from Leber's amaurosis but this association probably represents a distinct inherited disorder or group of disorders affecting both the kidney and the eye (see below).

Diagnosis

Leber's amaurosis should be suspected in any infant with poor vision, nystagmus, sluggish pupil reactions and a normal fundus examination. The diagnosis is confirmed by demonstrating an absent or severely subnormal photopic and scotopic ERG. If there are any unusual systemic features other inherited disorders such as the peroxisomal disorders or Joubert's syndrome need to be excluded.

Progressive rod–cone dystrophies (retinitis pigmentosa)

Retinitis pigmentosa (RP) is a term used for a genetically heterogeneous group of disorders characterized by night-

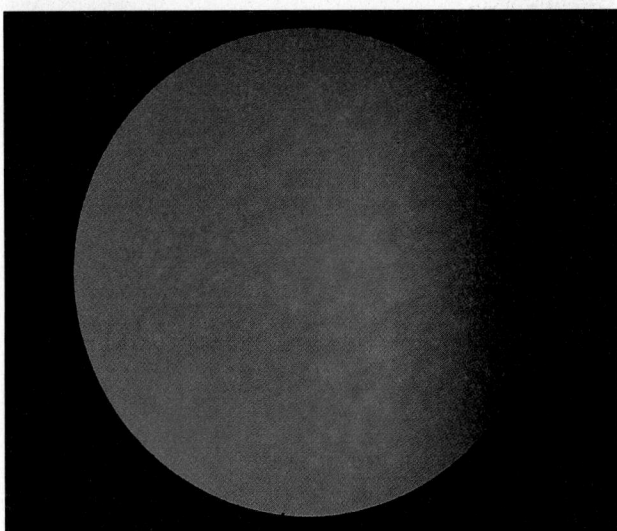

Fig. 44.4 Leber's amaurosis—flecked retina appearance.

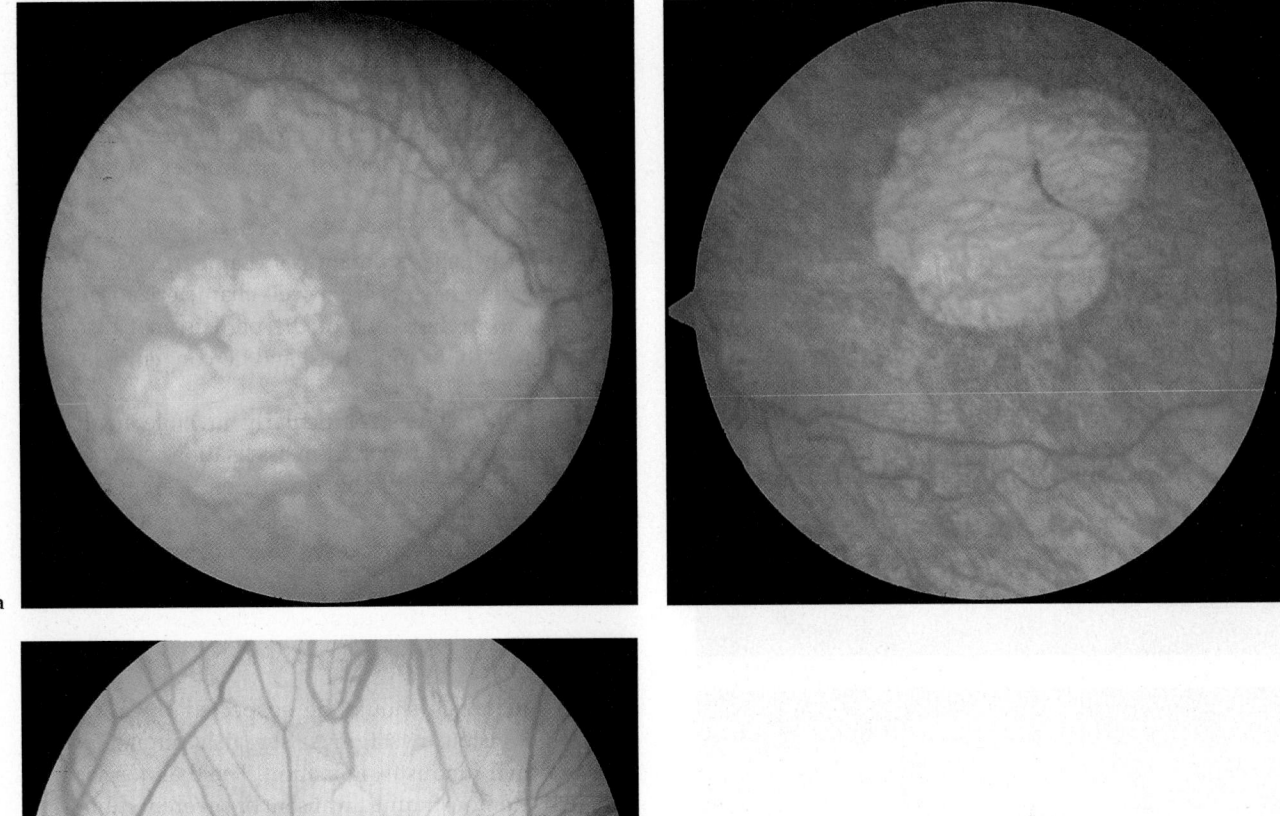

Fig. 44.5 (a, b) Leber's amaurosis—bilateral macular dysplasia. (a) Right eye and (b) left eye. (c) Congenital retinal dystrophy, probably Leber's amaurosis with macular dysplasia.

blindness, visual field loss and an abnormal or extinguished ERG. Onset is often in childhood. The disease may be confined to the eye or the retinal dystrophy may be part of a more widespread systemic disorder (Table 44.1).

Genetics

RP may be inherited as an autosomal dominant, autosomal recessive or X-linked recessive disorder. A similar retinal dystrophy may also be seen in association with mutations of mitochondrial DNA. There is genetic heterogeneity even within these classes and it is particularly marked in autosomal recessive RP (Table 44.2). The relative frequency of the different modes of inheritance differs widely in the different series (Amman *et al.* 1965; Jay 1982; Boughman & Fishman 1983; Heckenlively 1988), but

about half the patients have no family history of RP or evidence of parental consanguinity. It is unlikely that all such cases have autosomal recessive disease. Some males may have X-linked disease transmitted via asymptomatic female carriers; other cases may represent new autosomal dominant mutations or autosomal dominant disease in a family with reduced penetrance. It is also possible that some sporadic patients do not have genetic disease.

Clinical experience shows that X-linked and autosomal recessive RP tend to have an earlier onset and are more severe than dominant disease. The clinical findings may be taken into account when counselling apparently sporadic patients. A severely affected female may be considered more likely to have autosomal recessive disease whereas a severely affected male may have X-linked or autosomal recessive disease. A significant number of

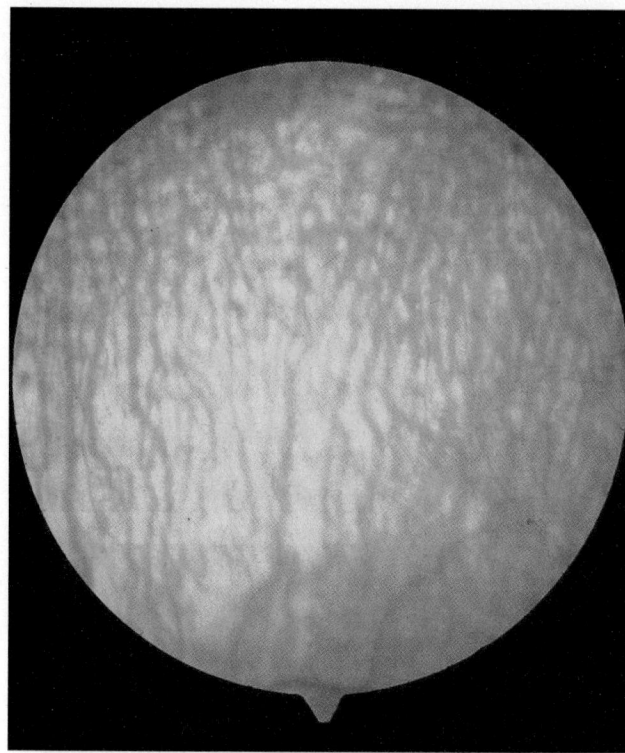

Fig. 44.6 Leber's amaurosis; nummular pigmentation.

patients with sporadic RP, however, have mild disease and a proportion of these probably have new autosomal dominant mutations. Before counselling it is clearly important to examine other family members, especially the mothers of severely affected males who may show the fundus abnormalities seen in the X-linked heterozygote.

More accurate genetic counselling hinges on identification of the causative mutations. Much progress has been made in this area in recent years and molecular genetic diagnosis is now possible in some forms of RP.

Molecular genetics

Autosomal dominant retinitis pigmentosa

There is considerable genetic heterogeneity within autosomal dominant RP. Mutations of two different genes, the rhodopsin gene on chromosome 3 (Dryja *et al.* 1990; Apfelstedt-Sylla *et al.* 1993; Bird 1995) and the peripherin/RDS gene on chromsome 6 (Farrar *et al.* 1991; Kajiwara *et al.* 1991; Fishman *et al.* 1994; Bird 1995), may give rise to autosomal dominant RP. Kajiwara *et al.* (1994) have recently reported an unusual form of RP (showing digenic inheritance) in which mutations of the peripherin/RDS gene and ROM1 (rod outer segment protein 1) gene are present within the same family. Individuals with a mutation of one gene but not the other are clinically unaffected. Affected individuals are double heterozygotes with mutations

of both the ROM1 gene and the peripherin/RDS gene. Peripherin is an outer segment protein found in rod and cone outer segment discs whilst ROM1 is only found in rods. In the rod outer segment interaction of the two proteins is important for outer segment structure and it appears that some mutations in the peripherin/RDS gene may be insufficient to cause significant photoreceptor disease unless accompanied by a defective ROM1 protein.

Four other as yet uncharacterized loci on 7p (Inglehearn *et al.* 1993), 7q (Jordan *et al.* 1993), 19q (al Maghtheh *et al.* 1994; Xu *et al.* 1995) and the pericentromeric region of chromosome 8 (Blanton *et al.* 1991), have been shown to be associated with autosomal dominant RP. Some families are not linked to any of these loci suggesting that further loci will be implicated in autosomal dominant RP.

Mutations of the rhodopsin gene account for about 25% of patients with autosomal dominant RP and more than 60 different mutations have been identified; there is considerable variation in the ocular phenotype seen with the dif-

Table 44.1 Childhood rod–cone dystrophies with systemic abnormalities.

Autosomal dominant
Olivopontocerebellar atrophy
Alagille's syndrome
Myotonic dystrophy

Autosomal recessive
Abetalipoproteinaemia
Refsum's disease
Batten's disease
Laurence–Moon syndrome
Bardet–Biedl syndrome
Usher's syndrome
Cockayne's syndrome
Mucopolysaccharidosis (I and II)
Mucolipidosis IV
Osteopetrosis
Älstrom's syndrome
Retinal dystrophy, cardiomyopathy, obesity and short stature
Peroxisomal disorders
Carbohydrate deficient glycoprotein syndrome
Hydroxyacyl-CoA dehydrogenase deficiency
Joubert's syndrome
Jeune's syndrome
Hallervorden–Spatz syndrome
Senior's syndrome
Idiopathic infantile hypercalcaemia
Chorioretinopathy and pituitary dysfunction
Cohen's syndrome

X-linked
Hunter's syndrome

Mitochondrial inheritance
Mitochondrial cytopathy

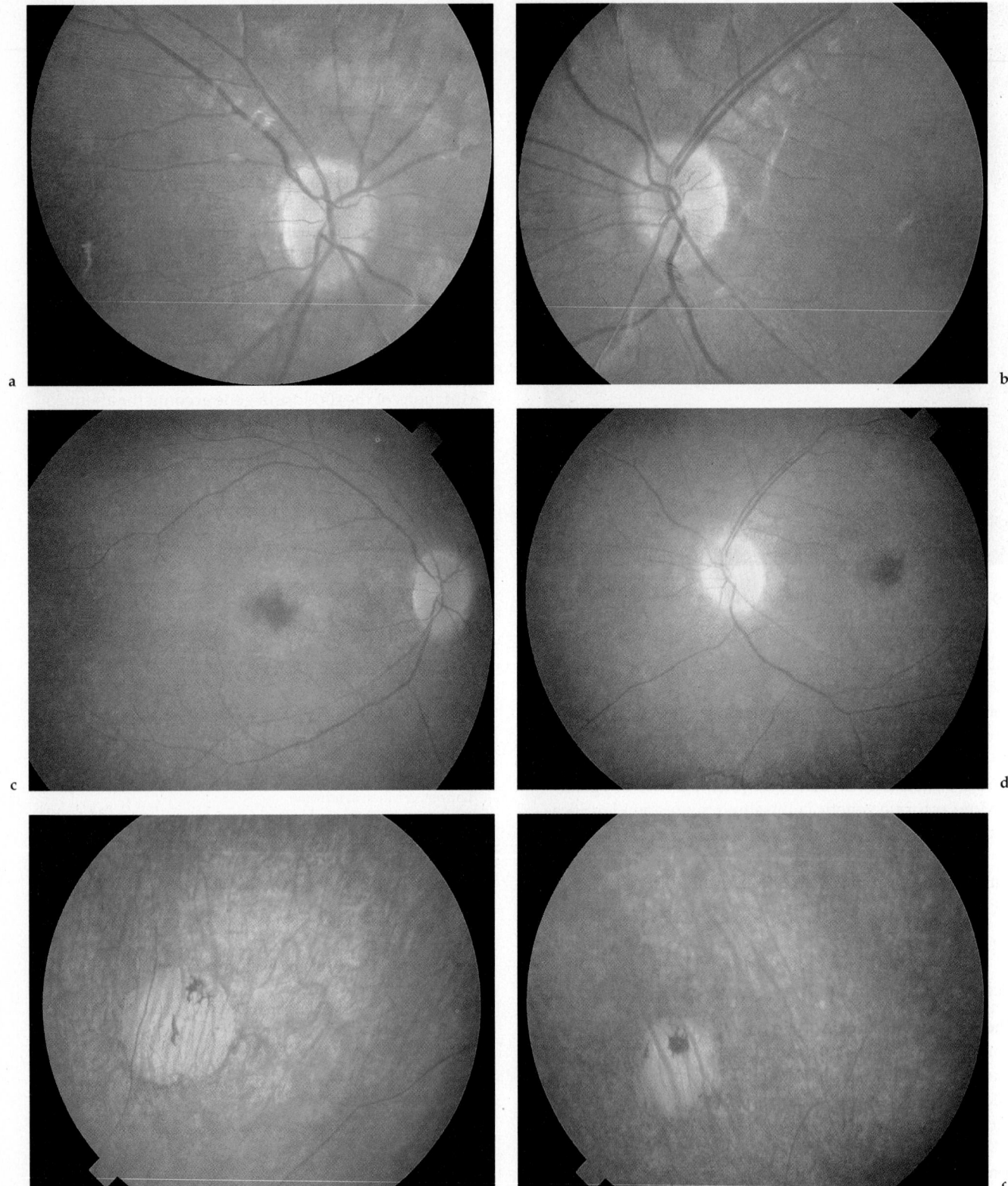

Fig. 44.7 Leber's amaurosis. (a, b) A 1-year-old showing mild pigmentary changes and slightly narrow arterioles. (c, d) Same patient 10 years later showing typical retinal pigment epithelial changes, disc pallor and arteriolar thinning with (e, f) two punched-out peripheral pigment epithelial changes.

Table 44.2 Differential diagnoses of retinitis pigmentosa.

Pigmentary retinopathy	Night-blindness
Blunt trauma	Genetic disorders
Retained intraocular FB	Congenital stationary
Congenital infection	night-blindness
Rubella	Oguchi's disease
Varicella	Fundus albipunctatus
Herpes simplex	Choroideraemia
Syphilis	Gyrate atrophy
Acquired infection	Progressive cone–rod
Measles	dystrophy
Onchocerciasis	Acquired
Metabolic	Vitamin A deficiency
Cystinosis	Desferrioxamine toxicity
Oxallosis	
Drugs	
Phenothiazines	
Chloroquine	
Desferrioxamine	
Resolved retinal detachment	
Ophthalmic artery occlusion	
Other retinal dystrophies	
Cone–rod dystrophy	
Inherited vitreoretinal dystrophies	
Unknown aetiology	
Paravenous retinochoroidal atrophy	

ferent mutations (al Maghtheh *et al.* 1993; Rosenfeld *et al.* 1994; Bird 1995; Dryja & Li 1995). Mutations of the rhodopsin gene have also been reported in dominant forms of CSNB (Sieving *et al.* 1992; Dryja *et al.* 1993; Rao *et al.* 1994) and autosomal recessive RP (Rosenfeld *et al.* 1992). The phenotypic variability is more marked with mutations of the RDS/peripherin gene where the clinical picture may resemble retinitis pigmentosa, cone–rod dystrophy, a fleck retina syndrome or macular dystrophy (see Chapters 45, 48). Mutations of the RDS/peripherin gene account for about 5% of cases of autosomal dominant RP (Rosenfeld *et al.* 1994; Bird 1995; Dryja & Li 1995). A full discussion of the relationship between the specific mutations of the rhodopsin and RDS/peripherin genes and the clinical phenotype is beyond the scope of this chapter but the reader is referred to several excellent recent reviews (al Maghtheh *et al.* 1993; Rosenfeld *et al.* 1994; Bird 1995; Dryja & Li 1995).

Autosomal recessive retinitis pigmentosa

Mutations of four different genes have been implicated in autosomal recessive RP; each was identified by using a candidate gene approach. Mutations of the rhodopsin gene (Rosenfeld *et al.* 1992), the gene coding for the beta-subunit (McLaughlin *et al.* 1993) and the alpha-subunit (Huang *et al.* 1995) of the rod cGMP phosphodiesterase and the gene for the rod cGMP-activated cation channel

(McGee *et al.* 1994; Dryja *et al.* 1995) are all associated with autosomal recessive RP. Autosomal recessive RP has also been localized to chromosome 1q in an inbred Dutch family (van Soest *et al.* 1994). The loci for the different forms of Usher's syndrome and for Biedl–Bardet syndrome have also been identified (see below) but many recessive genes causing RP remain to be discovered.

X-linked retinitis pigmentosa

Bhattacharya *et al.* (1984) were the first to localize a gene for X-linked RP to the Xp11 region of the short arm of the X chromosome using a probe L1.28. This locus has been confirmed by subsequent studies (Friedrich *et al.* 1985; Mukai *et al.* 1985; Wright *et al.* 1987) and the disorder mapping to this region has been designated RP2. Subsequently a deletion of the Xp21 region was reported in a child with RP, DMD and chronic granulomatous disease suggesting that there may be a second locus at Xp21. The second locus at Xp21.1 (RP3) has been confirmed by linkage studies (Nussbaum *et al.* 1985b; Musarella *et al.* 1988, 1990). Recently Meindl *et al.* (1996) have identified mutations in the RPGR gene in some families with RP3. The number of mutations identified so far is small and it is not yet clear whether there is heterogeneity within RP3. It is estimated that 70% of families are of the RP3 type and 30% RP2 (Teague *et al.* 1994). Kaplan *et al.* (1990, 1992) have suggested that there are differences in the phenotype between the two types of X-linked RP. Families with RP2 show early onset of night-blindness and myopia. In RP3 there is later onset of night-blindness and myopia is a variable feature. Aldred *et al.* (1994) have described three families with apparent X-linked inheritance which do not map to the RP2 or RP3 locus suggesting that there may be further genetic heterogeneity in X-linked RP.

Recognition of the X-linked carrier status. In X-linked RP the carrier state can be diagnosed with certainty only in females who have affected sons or fathers and are therefore obligate gene carriers. In other female family members carrier detection depends upon recognition of the abnormal fundus appearance seen in the heterozygote or on the results of electrophysiological, psychophysical or molecular genetic testing.

Fundus abnormalities are common in X-linked heterozygotes (Fig. 44.8). First, a prominent tapetal reflex may be seen at the posterior pole or mild pigment epithelial thinning and pigmentation may be present in the equatorial retina (Bird 1975; Berson *et al.* 1979; Fishman *et al.* 1986). Fluorescein angiography helps in confirming the peripheral pigment epithelial atrophy (Bird 1975). Bird (1975) recognized most obligate heterozygotes in his series by fundus examination whereas in Berson's series only 60% had an abnormal retinal appearance.

The ERG is often abnormal in heterozygotes with

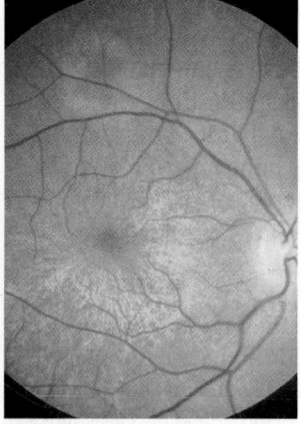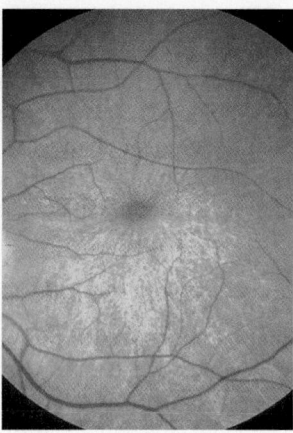

Fig. 44.8 X-linked RP carrier female showing the 'tapetal reflex' (Professor B. Jay's patient).

reduced rod and cone amplitudes and delayed cone b-wave implicit times. The proportion of obligate heterozygotes with abnormal ERG varies between series. Berson *et al.* (1979) identified 22 out of 23 obligate heterozygotes on the basis of an abnormal ERG. Fishman *et al.* (1986) similarly identified 90% of carriers by ERG testing alone and 100% when the results of the fundus examination and electrophysiological testing were combined.

Psychophysical testing has demonstrated elevated dark-adapted thresholds (Bird 1975) and reduced rod flicker sensitivity (Ernst *et al.* 1981) in X-linked heterozygotes. Rhodopsin pigment density measured by reflexion densitometry is also reduced (Bird & Hyman 1972). Vitreous fluorophotometry may also be abnormal (Gieser *et al.* 1980). Using a combination of fundoscopy, electrophysiology and in selected cases psychophysics and fluorophotometry, X-linked carriers can be identified in most cases. Molecular genetic diagnosis of female heterozygotes is possible in many families with X-linked RP.

The retinal dystrophy in the X-linked carriers appears to be progressive as older carriers may report symptoms of night-blindness and have detectable field loss and more extensive retinal pigmentation. In some reported pedigrees the carrier females may be severely affected at a relatively young age. Friedrich *et al.* (1993) reported one large family with X-linked RP in which the phenotype of the carrier females varied from a normal eye examination to a severe retinal dystrophy leading to total blindness. The severely affected females were shown to have skewed X inactivation with the X chromosome with the mutant allele active in most cells.

Clinical findings in retinitis pigmentosa

Children with RP may present with night-blindness or with symptoms associated with extensive field loss or central retinal involvement. The age of onset is extremely variable. In others there may be no symptomatic night-blindness but the child is referred because of retinal abnormalities seen on routine fundoscopy. When a parent or other close relative has RP, children may be referred early for investigation to exclude the disease.

In most cases the visual acuity is normal at presentation although later visual loss may occur as a result of posterior cortical cataract, macular oedema or macular involvement. Early visual field changes are seen as small scotomas in the midperipheral retina and are more common in the upper visual field. These field defects gradually coalesce to give the classical peripheral ring scotoma. In more advanced disease, visual fields become very constricted although there is often a small island of preserved field in the far temporal periphery. In sectorial RP, which commonly involves the lower nasal quadrant, bilateral upper temporal field loss may lead to unnecessary investigation to exclude a chiasmal lesion.

The appearance of the fundus in the early stages of RP is variable and in young children the changes may be very subtle (Fig. 44.9). The earliest change is mild pigment epithelial atrophy in the midperiphery often with small white dots at the level of the retinal pigment epithelium. Later pigment deposition is seen in the equatorial retina and there may be arteriolar narrowing and optic disc pallor. In some children abnormal pigment may be lacking (RP sine pigmento) and less commonly there may be multiple white deposits scattered throughout the retina (retinitis punctata albescens). It is unlikely that these represent different genetic subtypes as they can each be seen within the same family.

In more advanced disease the classical fundus appearance of optic disc pallor, retinal arteriolar attenuation and peripheral pigment epithelial atrophy and 'bone corpuscle' pigmentation is seen (Figs 44.10–44.13). Other changes include vitreous cells, posterior cortical cataract, optic disc drusen and macular oedema. Occasionally retinovascular changes similar to Coats' disease are seen. Persistent macular oedema may lead to the development of macular holes.

Electrophysiology and psychophysics

Electroretinography has been used for many years in the investigation of RP and the introduction of computer averaging techniques combined with the use of variable spectral stimuli and flicker has enabled rod and cone responses to be isolated (Arden *et al.* 1983). These techniques may be used in infants and young children without the need for sedation or general anaesthetic. Recently, a standard protocol has been agreed for ERG in adults and children (International Standards Committee 1989; Marmor & Zrenner 1995); however, a protocol designed specifically for small children may be more appropriate especially in preverbal or unco-operative children (see

Chapter 9). The ability to distinguish between scotopic and photopic function allows RP to be distinguished from stationary night-blindness and the cone and cone–rod disorders.

In the late stages of RP the ERG may be unrecordable although with the use of computer averaging techniques a small cone response may be found. In mild disease or early RP there is a recordable ERG which generally shows a reduction in the amplitude of the a- and b-waves and the rod-mediated b-wave implicit times are prolonged. The 30 Hz flicker responses may also be reduced in amplitude and prolonged in implicit times. Berson and Simonoff (1979) have suggested that individuals from families showing complete penetrance of the RP gene show differ-

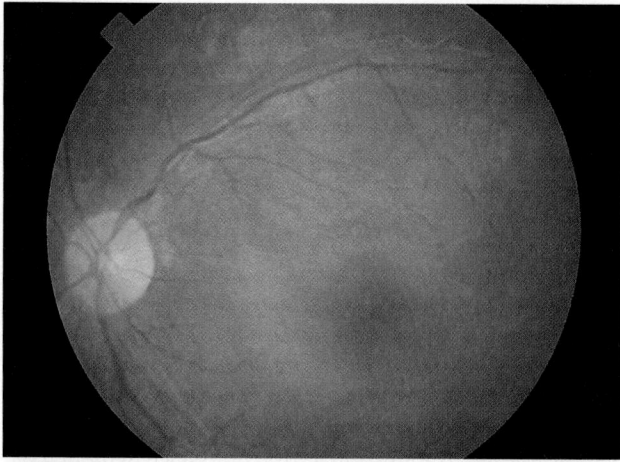

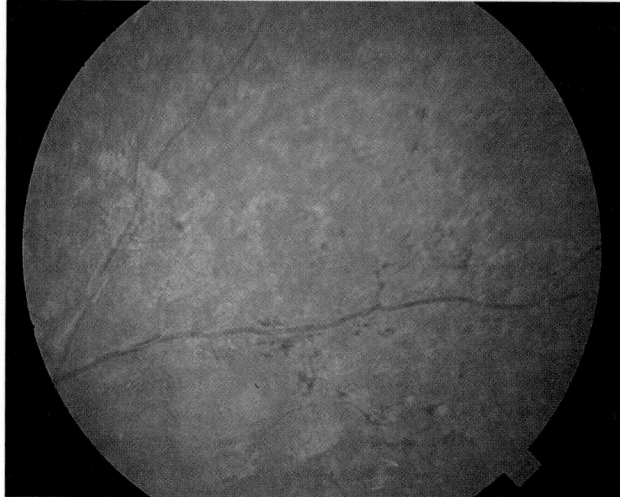

Fig. 44.9 (a, b) RP in a 6-year-old. The only symptom was night-blindness, the acuity was 6/9 in both eyes and the posterior pole is normal. Peripheral pigment clumping is present.

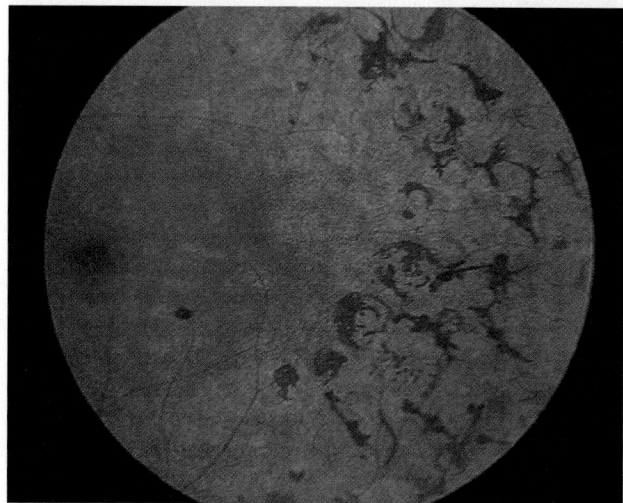

Fig. 44.11 RP. Marked pigment epithelial clumping with preservation of a relatively normal macula and good acuity.

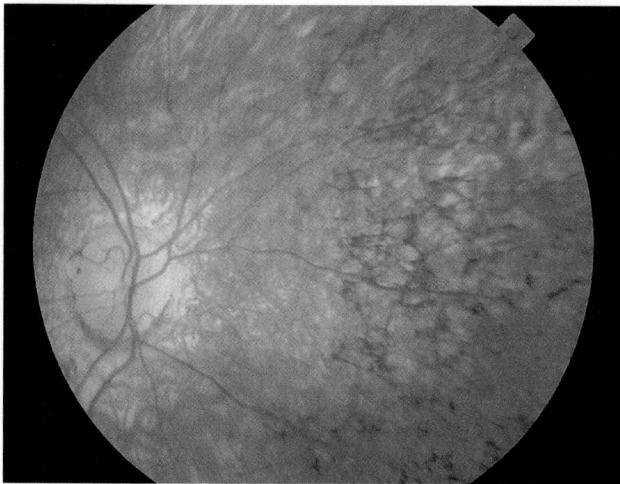

Fig. 44.10 RP. 'Bone spicule' formation in the midperiphery and arteriolar narrowing.

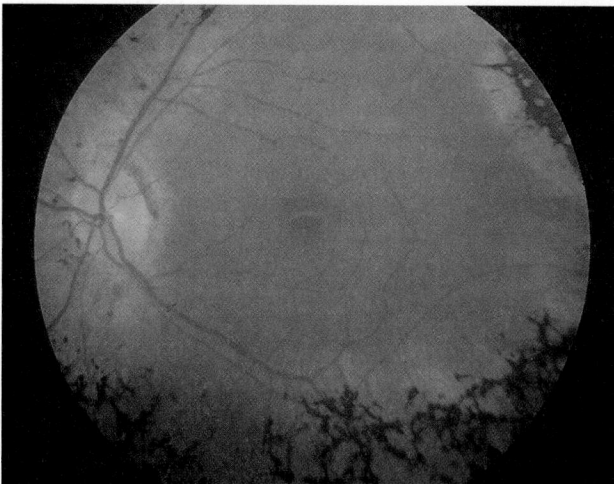

Fig. 44.12 RP showing marked 'bone spicule' formation encroaching on the posterior pole (Mr A. Moore's patient).

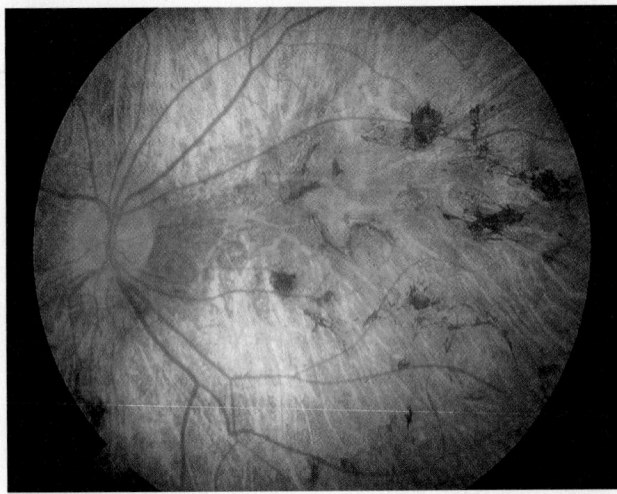

Fig. 44.13 Late stage RP showing marked pigment abnormalities and chorioretinal atrophy.

ences in cone responses from those with incomplete penetrance indicating that there may be a different underlying disease mechanism.

Although the EOG is frequently used in addition to the ERG in the assessment of patients with RP it provides little further information and has the disadvantage that it is difficult to perform in young children. In all types of RP there is a reduced or absent light rise.

Psychophysical studies in all forms of RP show elevated rod and later cone thresholds (Massof & Finkelstein 1981) and in some patients the kinetics of dark adaptation is also abnormal (Alexander & Fishman 1984a; Kemp *et al.* 1992; Moore 1992). Massof and Finkelstein (1981) subdivided patients with RP into two groups on the basis of the pattern of rod and cone dysfunction seen on dark-adapted perimetry. In type 1 disease there was early onset nightblindness and early and diffuse loss of rod function. In type 2 disease there was later onset of night-blindness and psychophysical testing showed patchy disease with some areas of retina with abnormal rod and cone function and other areas where both receptors functioned normally. Lyness *et al.* (1985) used a similar approach in studying families with autosomal dominant RP and were able to divide families into two groups termed diffuse and regional which are similar to the type 1 and 2 described by Massof and Finkelstein. The two subtypes were not seen within the same family suggesting that they may represent pure forms of disease. However, subsequent molecular genetic studies of autosomal dominant RP have not confirmed this; different mutations of the rhodopsin gene may give rise to both diffuse and regional patterns of retinal dysfunction and a similar phenotype may be seen with mutations of the RDS/peripherin gene (Bird 1995). The emphasis has now moved from attempts to subdivide RP on the basis of psychophysical and ERG testing to explor-

ing the effects of different genetic mutations on retinal function.

Sectorial retinitis pigmentosa

In sectorial RP, which is usually inherited as an autosomal dominant trait, the abnormalities are confined to one sector of the fundus, usually the lower retina. Similar sectorial involvement may occasionally be seen in the female carriers of X-linked RP and is often seen in the absence of a family history. It is important in isolated cases to examine other family members as the disorder is often asymptomatic. Dominant sector RP is often associated with mutations of the rhodopsin gene (Heckenlively *et al.* 1991; Moore *et al.* 1992). Children with sectorial RP usually have no symptoms and are referred when the abnormal fundus appearance is noted on routine fundoscopy or are found to be affected during family surveys. On Goldmann perimetry field loss is confined to one sector corresponding to the clinically involved retina. However, dark-adapted perimetry shows mild rod and cone threshold elevations in the apparently uninvolved retina indicating that there is widespread receptor disease (Massof & Finklestein 1979; Moore *et al.* 1992). Rod dark adaptation may be extremely delayed (Moore *et al.* 1992). The ERG is usually relatively well preserved with mild or moderate reductions in both rod and cone amplitudes (Berson & Howard 1971; Massof & Finklestein 1979; Moore *et al.* 1992). Disease progression is slow and confined to the clinically involved sector (Massof & Finklestein 1979; Moore *et al.* 1992). The visual prognosis is excellent.

Autosomal dominant retinitis pigmentosa with incomplete penetrance

Variability of expression is common in autosomal dominant RP but true incomplete penetrance is unusual. In some families incomplete penetrance is a notable and common occurrence and there is some evidence that in such families the disease in symptomatic individuals is of early onset and severe (Berson & Simonoff 1979; Moore *et al.* 1993; Evans *et al.* 1995b; Kim *et al.* 1995). There is evidence for genetic heterogeneity in autosomal dominant RP with incomplete penetrance; linkage has been established to 7p (Inglehearn *et al.* 1993) and 19q (al Maghtheh *et al.* 1994; Xu *et al.* 1995). Genetic counselling in families showing incomplete penetrance may be problematic because of the high incidence of asymptomatic gene carriers, and molecular genetic diagnosis can be extremely helpful (Evans *et al.* 1995b).

Unilateral retinitis pigmentosa

Unilateral RP is rare, has yet to be reported in families with RP, and is more likely to be non-hereditary and related to retinal ischaemia, inflammation or infection (Carr & Siegel 1973; Merin & Auerbach 1976). Some individuals with RP may have an asymmetric fundus appearance at presentation so that one eye appears clinically unaffected. Psychophysical testing and ERG usually demonstrate abnormal rod and cone function in the eye with a normal fundus appearance.

Differential diagnosis of retinitis pigmentosa

Other disorders may be confused with RP either because there is symptomatic night-blindness or because a similar fundus appearance (Figs 44.14–44.16) is seen (see Table 44.2). The other inherited dystrophies can usually be differentiated from RP by the clinical findings and electrophysiological testing. Although a careful history and examination may exclude many of the acquired causes of pigmentary retinopathy it is likely that some of the cases of apparently sporadic RP may be due to acquired retinal or pigment epithelial disease.

Management

In most retinal dystrophies there is no specific treatment. In Refsum's disease, abetalipoproteinaemia and gyrate atrophy the underlying biochemical defect is better understood and dietary treatment may slow progression of the retinal dystrophy. Berson *et al.* (1993) have recently reported the results of a controlled clinical trial of supplemental vitamin A in a heterogeneous group of patients with RP. There was no evidence that vitamin A treatment had any beneficial effect on visual acuity or visual field but treated patients showed less deterioration in the cone ERG amplitudes than the control group. The recorded amplitudes were extremely small and it is doubtful if this minor effect on the rate of deterioration of the ERG

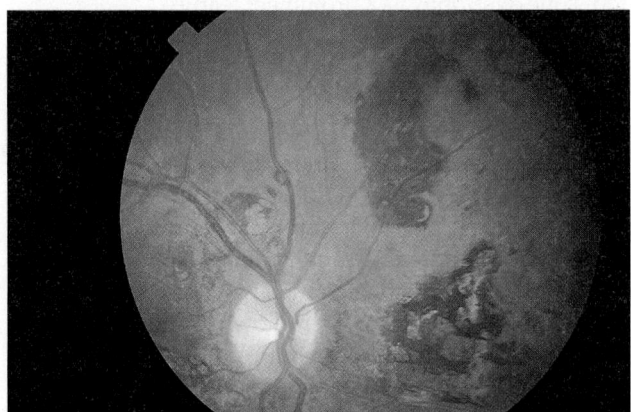

Fig. 44.14 Air-gun pellet injury with foveal retinal pigment epithelial hypertrophy. Without a definitive history the condition may be diagnosed as a previous infection or ischaemia or 'unilateral RP' (see text).

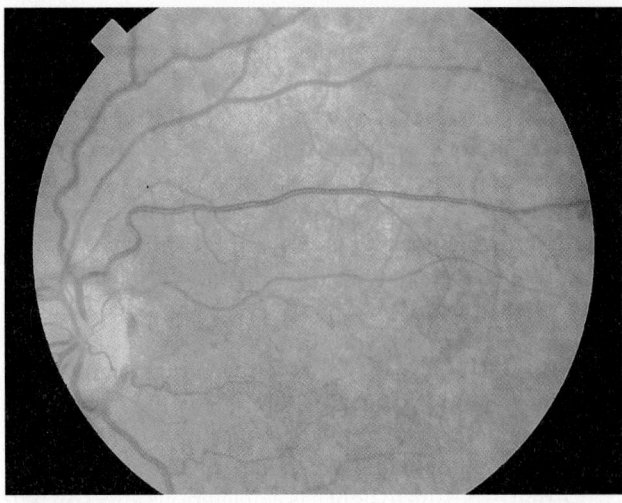

Fig. 44.15 Rubella retinopathy showing pigment mottling. Retinal function is usually good and the ERG normal whereas most retinal dystrophies with deafness have severely abnormal ERGs.

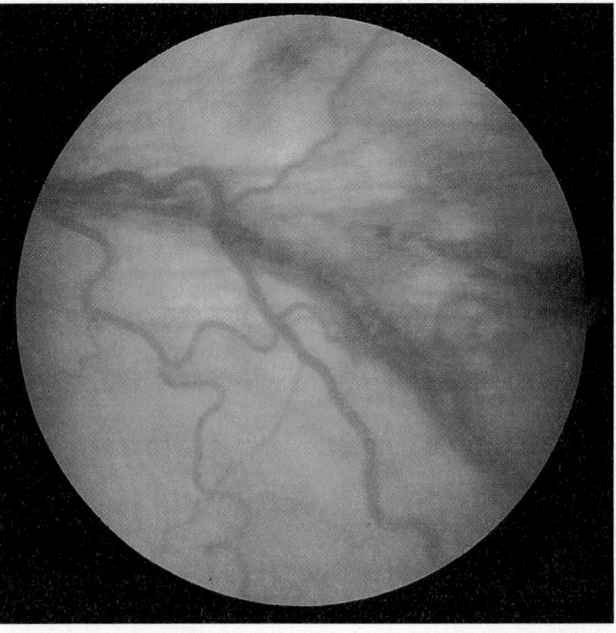

Fig. 44.16 Retinal pigment hypertrophy in a child with a resolved retinal detachment. Unless the history is known the diagnosis of sectorial RP or unilateral RP may be made.

response justifies long-term therapy (Massof & Finklestein 1993).

Although there is no specific treatment for RP, the ophthalmologist has an important role to play in the management of the child and the whole family. Once the diagnosis is established it is important that the parents and the child (if old enough) are given a full and sympathetic explanation; most parents will be especially concerned about the visual prognosis and although it is important to give an honest assessment it is better to adopt a cautiously optimistic approach. For example, they can be reassured that most children complete their education at a normal school as central vision is preserved until late in the disease.

Parents are often concerned that other children may be at risk of developing the disease; they should be offered genetic counselling and it may be appropriate to examine other family members. It is also helpful to have available the addresses of patient self-help groups such as the British, American or other RP association (see Chapter P30).

Practical help can also be given when there are visual difficulties. Many patients with RP have poor vision in bright sunlight and have problems in adapting from bright to dim illumination. Although there is no good evidence that exposure to light has a deleterious effect on retinal function in RP it would seem sensible to avoid bright sunlight and tinted lenses may be helpful in summer. Any significant refractive errors should be fully corrected. If there is macular oedema a trial of diamox (Fishman *et al.* 1989), orbital floor or systemic steroids should be given. In established oedema or macular atrophy low visual aids may be helpful. Visual loss may also develop secondary to posterior cortical cataract and although cataract surgery is often successfully performed in adults with RP it is rarely necessary in childhood.

Although at present there is no effective treatment for most patients with RP recent advances in molecular genetics, cell biology and experimental transplantation hold some hope for the future. Gene therapy, retinal and retinal pigment epithelial transplantation and intraocular growth factors have all been shown to influence photoreceptor function in dystrophic animal models, and one of these methods may prove to be of value in treating some forms of RP in the future.

Prognosis

The prognosis in RP varies according to the type of disease. In X-linked RP affected males are night-blind in early childhood, usually show extensive field loss by their teens and central visual loss in their twenties (Bird 1975). By the fourth decade most have vision reduced to less than an ability to count fingers. Autosomal recessive RP is such a heterogeneous condition that accurate prognosis is difficult. Overall disease is usually of early onset and severe. Most patients have a severely constricted visual field by their teens and may have marked central visual loss by their late twenties. Some with recessive disease do, however, follow a more benign course.

The prognosis is better in autosomal dominant RP. Although night-blindness and field loss may develop in childhood, central vision fares much better. Vision may remain normal throughout life. Many patients maintain reasonable central visual acuity until the fifth or sixth decade, although they may have extremely constricted visual fields. However, autosomal dominant RP shows wide variation, even in RP caused by mutations at the same locus (Apfelstedt-Sylla *et al.* 1995; Bird 1995). Severe, early onset forms are unusual (Lam & Judisch 1991; Richards *et al.* 1995).

True sector RP has the best prognosis of any form of the disease. Although there may be a dense scotoma in the field (usually upper) corresponding to the involved retina, involvement of the macula is uncommon.

Pigmented paravenous atrophy

This is a rare chorioretinal atrophy in which there is paravenous retinal pigment epithelial atrophy and pigment clumping (Fig. 44.17). The ERG is usually only mildly abnormal. Retinal function usually remains stable (Skalka 1979; Noble & Carr 1983; Traboulsi & Maumenee 1986) but may rarely show deterioration (Pearlman *et al.* 1975, 1978). It is more common in males and most cases are sporadic. It is usually diagnosed on routine examination in asymptomatic patients. It is uncertain whether this disorder may have a genetic basis (Traboulsi & Maumenee 1986). In one report the monozygotic twin of an affected adult was found to be normal (Small & Banks Anderson 1991) suggesting that some cases at least are non-genetic.

Rod–cone dystrophies with systemic involvement

A progressive retinal dystrophy may be seen in a wide variety of genetic disorders (see Table 44.1). They have been reviewed by Francois (1982) and Heckenlively (1988). Lambert *et al.* (1989b) have reviewed the systemic associations seen in the congenital retinal dystrophies. In this section it is proposed to give a brief account of the conditions presenting in childhood which have a progressive rod–cone dystrophy as a prominent feature.

Abetalipoproteinaemia and familial hypobetalipoproteinaemia

Abetalipoproteinaemia is a rare autosomal recessive disorder of lipoprotein metabolism. It is characterized by acanthocytosis of red cells, fat malabsorption, spinocerebellar ataxia, a retinal dystrophy and an absence of beta (low density) lipoproteins from the plasma (Francois 1982; Runge *et al.* 1986b). It has been shown that there is a complete absence of apolipoprotein B, a major component of the low density lipoproteins (Gotto *et al.* 1971); this results in defective chylomicron formation and malabsorption of the fat-soluble vitamins. The usual presentation is with failure to thrive and steatorrhoea in early infancy. The disorder is thought to be caused by an abnormality of microsomal triglyceride transfer protein (MTP) which is

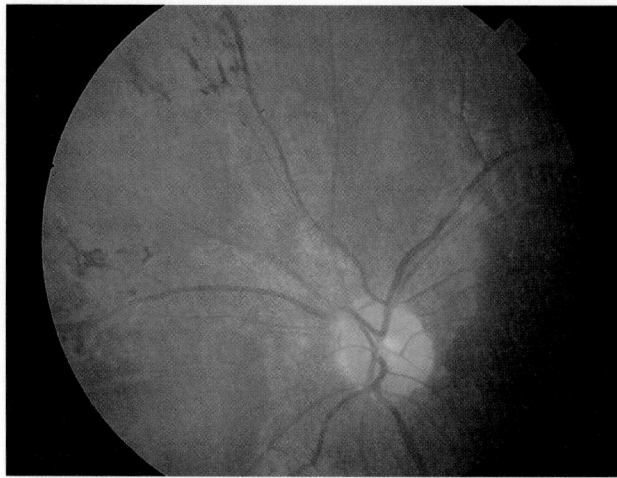

a

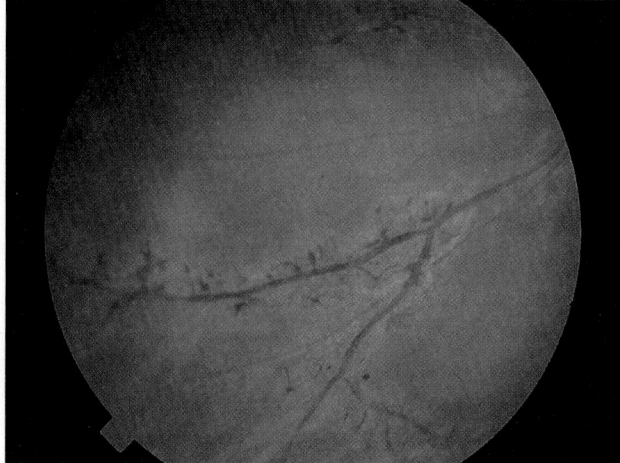

b

Fig. 44.17 (a, b) Pigmented paravenous atrophy. The veins are surrounded by a band of retinal pigment atrophy and clumping.

thought to be important for lipoprotein assembly (Wetterau *et al*. 1992; Rader & Brewer 1993).

Although the retinal dystrophy may occur at any age (Francois 1982; Judisch *et al*. 1984; Runge *et al*. 1986b) it most commonly presents in late childhood. Fundus examination may be normal in the early stages but later there may be a peripheral pigmentary retinopathy or a picture similar to retinitis punctata albescens with scattered white dots at the level of the retinal pigment epithelium (Francois 1982). The ERG may be normal initially but later becomes abnormal with scotopic responses first to be lost (Francois 1982); it is extinguished at a late stage. Treatment with large doses of vitamins A and E may prevent neurological and retinal complications (Bishihara *et al*. 1982; Runge *et al*.1986b).

Familial hypobetalipoproteinaemia (HBL) is a rare autosomal dominant disorder characterized by low plasma cholesterol levels and low levels of low density lipoproteins. The disorder is thought to be due to mutation of the apolipoprotein B gene. A variety of neurologi-

cal abnormalities and a retinal dystrophy may complicate this disorder (Brosnahan *et al*. 1994). Histopathology in an affected male suggests that there may be a defect in the renewal of photoreceptor outer segment discs (Brosnahan *et al*. 1994).

Refsum's disease

Refsum's disease is a rare autosomal recessive disorder characterized by RP, ataxia and polyneuropathy (Refsum 1946). Other abnormalities include anosmia, deafness, ichthyosis, pupillary miosis, cardiac arrhythmias and raised cerebrospinal fluid (CSF) protein. Plasma phytanic acid levels are markedly elevated. The raised phytanic acid levels are due to a phytanic acid alpha hydroxylase deficiency which can be demonstrated in skin fibroblasts.

Although symptoms may be present from late childhood the diagnosis is rarely made until early adult life. As night-blindness is a common early symptom children with sporadic or autosomal recessive RP should be screened to exclude Refsum's disease, especially if there is anosmia or ataxia (Goldman *et al*. 1985; Britton & Gibberd 1988; Claridge *et al*. 1992). Anosmia is the earliest symptom apart from RP. The diagnosis of Refsum's syndrome is often delayed and in one series the average interval between the patient presenting to the ophthalmologist and the correct diagnosis being made was 11 years (Claridge *et al*. 1992). Dietary treatment to reduce plasma phytanic acid will prevent the development of neuropathy, ataxia, cardiac arrhythmias and ichthyosis but the effect on the progression of the retinal dystrophy and deafness is less certain (Britton & Gibberd 1988; Claridge *et al*. 1992).

Usher's syndrome (see also Chapter P15)

Usher's syndrome is an autosomal recessive disorder characterized by congenital sensorineural hearing loss and RP (Usher 1935). It is the most common of the various syndromes associated with RP (Heckenlively 1988) and is estimated to have a prevalence of between three and four per 100 000 (Nuutila 1970; Boughman *et al*. 1983). Night-blindness is usually first reported in late childhood or early teens, and there is usually visual field loss and an extinguished or severely subnormal ERG at presentation. Visual acuity is good in the early stages but vision may deteriorate to 6/60 or less by the fourth decade (Heckenlively 1988).

It is evident from clinical (Merin *et al*. 1974; Fishman *et al*. 1983; Smith *et al*. 1994) and molecular genetic (Kimberling *et al*. 1990, 1992; Kaplan *et al*. 1992; Smith *et al*. 1992; Pieke *et al*. 1993; Sankila *et al*. 1995) studies that there is heterogeneity within Usher's syndrome. In type 1 Usher's syndrome there is profound deafness with no intelligible speech; vestibular responses to rotation and calorics are absent or very abnormal. The ERG is usually absent at the time of diagnosis. Ataxia, psychosis and mental retardation are variable features. In type 2 Usher's syndrome the hearing loss is more variable and in some patients it can be quite mild. The hearing loss is most apparent at high frequencies. Speech is often intelligible and vestibular responses are normal. There are rarely any other neurological problems. In type 2 Usher's syndrome the retinal dystrophy is of later onset and is less severe (Fishman *et al.* 1995); a small ERG can usually be recorded (Merin *et al.* 1974; Fishman *et al.* 1983). Smith *et al.* (1994) have described a set of minimal clinical criteria for the diagnosis of type 1 and type 2 Usher's syndrome.

A third form of Usher's syndrome (type 3) has been described which is similar to type 2 but is characterized by progressive sensorineural hearing loss (Sankila *et al.* 1995).

Ultrastructural studies of postmortem eyes in patients with Usher's syndrome type 2 have shown a substantial reduction in the number of photoreceptors which is most marked in the midperipheral retina (Berson & Adamian 1992). The remaining photoreceptors showed shortened outer segments with an abnormal configuration of the microtubules in cilia connecting the inner and outer segments. The retinal pigment epithelium was abnormal throughout the retina. Similar cilial abnormalities have been reported in nasal mucosa and spermatozoa from patients with Usher's syndrome (Arden & Fox 1979; Hunter *et al.* 1986; Barrong *et al.* 1992) and this has led to the suggestion that some forms of Usher's syndrome may be caused by a basic defect in cilial structure. This concept has been strengthened by the finding of mutations in the type VIIA myosin gene in Usher's syndrome type 1B (Weil *et al.* 1995).

Molecular genetics

Usher type 1 can be subdivided into three types on the basis of genetic linkage studies. Type 1A has been mapped to chromosome 14q (Kaplan *et al.* 1992); type 1B to 11q (Kimberling *et al.* 1992) and type 1C to 11p (Smith *et al.* 1992; Ayyagari *et al.* 1994). Type 1B accounts for the majority of cases of type 1 Usher's syndrome. Recently, Weil *et al.* (1995) used a candidate gene approach to identify mutations of the type VIIA myosin gene in five unrelated families with Usher's syndrome type 1B. This gene is homologous to the mouse deafness *shaker 1* (*sh1*) gene. Homozygotes for this gene in the mouse have evidence of vestibular dysfunction, cochlear defect, degeneration of the organ of Corti but no retinal degeneration (Gibson *et al.* 1995). Type VIIA myosin is one of a family of unconventional myosins which may be involved in cilial function (see Weil *et al.* 1995 for summary) and the genes for other members of this family may be candidate genes for other forms of Usher's syndrome.

Although most Usher type 2 families show linkage to chromosome 1q41 (USH2A) (Kimberling *et al.* 1990) some

Table 44.3 Deafness and progressive retinal dystrophy in childhood.

Usher's syndrome
Cockayne's syndrome
Alström's syndrome
Refsum's disease
Mitochondrial cytopathy
Peroxisomal disorders
MPS II and III
Leber's amaurosis
Osteopetrosis
Alport's syndrome

(USH2B) are not linked to this locus (Pieke *et al.* 1993). Usher type 3 syndrome has been mapped to chromosome 3q (USH3) (Sankila *et al.* 1995).

Differential diagnoses

In assessing children with deafness and a retinal dystrophy it is important to exclude other genetic disorders before making a diagnosis of Usher's syndrome (Table 44.3). Congenital rubella may also cause profound deafness and a pigmentary retinopathy, although the ERG is usually normal.

Peroxisomal disorders

Peroxisomes are subcellular organelles that are found in all animal cells and have an important function in the biosynthesis of certain phospholipids and in the catabolism of phytanic acid and pipecolic acid. It is now recognized that dysfunction of peroxisomes may give rise to a variety of inherited metabolic disorders (Schutgens *et al.* 1986; Michalski *et al.* 1988; Braverman *et al.* 1995). The disorders can be broadly grouped into two types (Table 44.4). In the first type a genetic mutation results in abnormal function of a single peroxisomal enzyme as occurs for example in X-linked adrenoleucodystrophy where there are mutations in the ALDP gene. In the second group of disorders there are defects in multiple peroxisome functions as occurs for example in Zellweger's syndrome (Braverman *et al.* 1995). A number of genes involved in human peroxisomal biogenesis have been identified (see Bravermann *et al.* for summary).

At least three of the peroxisomal disorders, Zellweger's syndrome, infantile Refsum's disease and neonatal adrenoleucodystrophy, may have an associated retinal dystrophy (Folz & Trobe 1991).

Zellweger's syndrome

Zellweger's (or the hepatocerebrorenal) syndrome is characterized by widespread dysmorphic features, neurologi-

Table 44.4 Peroxisomal disorders. Adapted from Braverman *et al.* (1995) and Folz and Trobe (1991).

1   Single protein disorders
      X-linked adrenoleucodystrophy (see Chapter 57)
2a Peroxisome biogenesis disorders
      Autosomal recessive
      Peroxisomes structurally abnormal and reduced in number
      (1) Zellweger's syndrome
      (2) Infantile adrenoleucodystrophy
      (3) Infantile Refsum's disease
2b Rhizomelic chondrodysplasia punctata (rhizomelic Conradi's
      disease). Peroxisomes present but may be structurally abnormal
      Cataracts (see Chapter 39)
      Shortened long bones
      Failure to thrive, very reduced lifespan
      Ichthyosis

cal abnormalities, renal cysts and hepatosplenomegaly (Schutgens *et al.* 1986; Zellweger 1987). Affected infants show marked hypotonia, psychomotor retardation, and have frequent seizures. Nystagmus is common and ocular findings include corneal clouding, cataract and a retinal dystrophy (Stanescu & Draloands 1972; Hittner *et al.* 1981; Garner *et al.* 1982; Cohen *et al.* 1983). The ERG is absent or severely subnormal (Stanescu & Draloands 1972; Hittner *et al.* 1981; Garner *et al.* 1982). Most patients die in the first year of life. Histopathological studies (Haddad *et al.* 1976; Garner *et al.* 1982; Cohen *et al.* 1983a) have demonstrated extensive photoreceptor degeneration and loss of ganglion cells with gliosis of the nerve fibre layer. Biochemical studies of postmortem eyes (Cohen *et al.* 1983a) have shown high levels of very long chain fatty acids in the ocular tissues. Inheritance is autosomal recessive and prenatal diagnosis is possible (Hajra *et al.* 1985).

Neonatal adrenoleucodystrophy

This form of adrenoleucodystrophy affects males and females equally and is thought to be inherited as an autosomal recessive trait. Affected infants are hypotonic and have severe psychomotor retardation and seizures. Clinically, adrenal insufficiency is uncommon but adrenal atrophy is frequently seen at postmortem. Affected children die between 6 months and 7 years.

Most infants show severe visual loss and nystagmus and the ocular findings include cataract, optic atrophy and a pigmentary retinopathy. Histopathology shows marked degeneration of both inner and outer segment of rods and cones and diffuse atrophy of the nerve fibre layer (Cohen *et al.* 1983b; Glasgow *et al.* 1987).

Infantile Refsum's disease

Classical Refsum's disease is an autosomal recessive dis-

order caused by defective oxidation of phytanic acid; the major features are a pigmentary retinopathy (Fig. 44.18), cerebellar ataxia and peripheral neuropathy. In 1982, Scotto *et al.* described three infants with hepatomegaly, facial dysmorphism, neurosensory deafness, a retinal dystrophy and raised plasma levels of phytanic acid. They suggested that this disorder represented infantile onset Refsum's disease.

Affected infants have poor vision and usually nystagmus from early infancy and on fundus examination have optic atrophy, narrowed vessels and a pigmentary retinopathy (Weleber *et al.* 1984). Fluorescein angiography shows widespread atrophy of the retinal pigment epithelium and choriocapillaris affecting both macula and peripheral retina (Weleber *et al.* 1984).

The ERG shows very small amplitude rod and cone responses and cone b-wave implicit times are greatly prolonged to flash and 30 Hz flicker (Weleber *et al.* 1984).

Carbohydrate deficient glycoprotein syndromes

The carbohydrate deficient glycoprotein (CDG) syndromes are a newly characterized group of autosomal recessive disorders in which there is defective glycosylation of glycoproteins (Jaeken *et al.* 1991; Jaeken & Carchon 1993). Glycoproteins have diverse functions and it is not surprising that the clinical picture is very variable; at least three subtypes are recognized. In the most common form (type 1) affected patients present either in early infancy with failure to thrive, developmental delay, hypotonia, growth retardation, facial dysmorphism and ophthalmo-

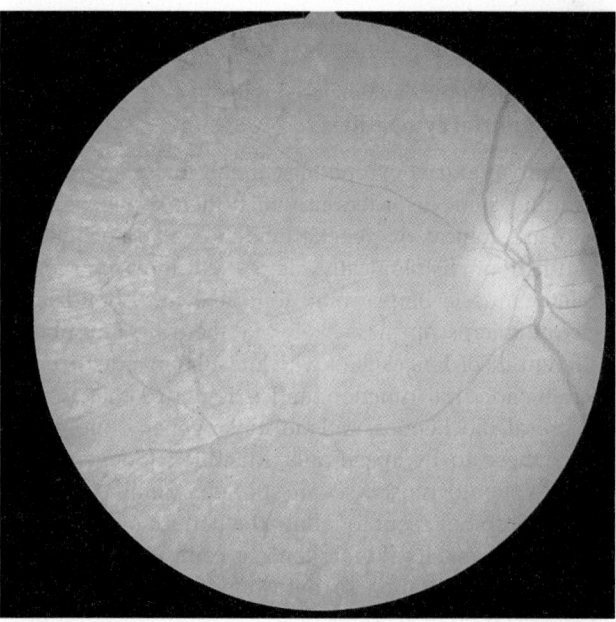

Fig. 44.18 Infantile Refsum's disease showing optic atrophy, thinned arterioles and retinal pigment abnormality.

logical abnormalities or in later childhood with predominantly neurological symptoms and signs. Mental retardation is common and there may be cerebellar ataxia, stroke-like episodes and epilepsy. Olivopontocerebellar atrophy may be a prominent feature. Other features may include cardiomyopathy (Clayton *et al.* 1992), muscle weakness and contractures, polyneuropathy and an abnormal distribution of subcutaneous fat.

Biochemical investigation reveals the defective glycosylation of a number of glycoproteins including transferrin. The detection of the abnormal serum transferrin by isoelectric focusing is a good screening test (Jaeken *et al.* 1991). In the type 2 diseases there is a deficiency in Golgi-located *N*-acetyl glucosaminyl transferase II (Jaeken *et al.* 1994).

The ophthalmological findings in this condition include a large-angle esotropia with defective abduction and a retinal dystrophy with early central visual impairment (Stromland *et al.* 1990; Andreasson *et al.* 1991). Older children may complain of night-blindness and on fundoscopy there is usually optic disc pallor and a pigmentary retinopathy similar to that seen in classical RP. The rod ERG is non-recordable at an early stage and the cone responses may show prolonged implicit times (Stromland *et al.* 1990; Andreasson *et al.* 1991; Fiumara *et al.* 1994).

Stromme *et al.* (1991) reported the postmortem findings in two patients with the CDG syndrome who died at the age of 4 months and 6 years, respectively. The CNS pathology showed evidence of extensive olivopontocerebellar atrophy and histopathology of the eyes revealed extensive photoreceptor atrophy and patchy loss of the retinal pigment epithelium. The inner retina was normal. The outer retinal changes were most marked at the posterior pole.

Retinal dystrophies associated with mitochondrial cytopathies

The mitochondrial cytopathies are an uncommon group of multisystem disorders in which there is biochemical, histopathological or genetic evidence of mitochondrial dysfunction. Histologically, ragged red fibres are seen on skeletal muscle biopsy and abnormal mitochondria on electron microscopy. It is likely that there are a number of different disorders each of which results in a disturbance of mitochondrial function, and it is hoped that in time structural, biochemical and molecular genetic studies will allow these to be specifically identified (Sengers *et al.* 1984). Although most cases are sporadic, familial cases are seen and do not seem to follow the pattern of mendelian inheritance; maternal inheritance is common and may be caused by a mutation of mitochondrial DNA (Poulton 1988; Holt *et al.* 1989; Johns 1994).

Clinical abnormalities often begin in childhood and may include lactic acidosis, anaemia, myopathy, neuro-

logical abnormalities, endocrine disturbance, renal disease, neurosensory hearing loss and a retinal dystrophy (Eggar *et al.* 1981). Cardiac conduction defects are a major cause of premature death.

A number of syndromes are recognized including the following.

1 Progressive external ophthalmoplegia (Reske-Nielsen *et al.* 1976).
2 Kearns–Sayre syndrome (Kearns & Sayre 1958).
3 Mitochondrial encephalopathy, lactic acidosis and stroke-like episodes (MELAS syndrome) (Kobayashi *et al.* 1986; Miyabayashi *et al.* 1993).

The major ophthalmological abnormalities seen in mitochondrial cytopathies are chronic external ophthalmoplegia and a retinal dystrophy (Fig. 44.19) similar to RP (Kearns & Sayre 1958; Drachman 1968). In children with a retinal dystrophy, the ERG usually shows evidence of rod and cone dysfunction with the rods being more severely affected (Ortiz *et al.* 1993). The retinal dystrophy is seen in most forms of mitochondrial syndromes and does not seem to be specific for any mitochondrial DNA mutation (Reske-Nielsen *et al.* 1976; Kobayashi *et al.* 1986; Holt *et al.* 1989; Ortiz *et al.* 1993; Rummelt *et al.* 1993; Puddu *et al.* 1993; Johns 1994). However, macular involvement seems to occur earlier in the MELAS syndrome and is associated with a poorer visual prognosis (Rummelt *et al.* 1993).

Histopathology of postmortem eyes has shown marked atrophy and degeneration of the retinal pigment epithelium and photoreceptor layer particularly at the posterior pole (Runge *et al.* 1986a; Rummelt *et al.* 1993).

Hydroxyacyl-CoA dehydrogenase deficiency (3-hydroxydicarboxylic aciduria)

This rare autosomal recessive mitochondrial enzyme disorder results in disordered fatty acid oxidation. Affected infants may present with life-threatening episodes of hypoglycaemia, muscle weakness and cardiomyopathy.

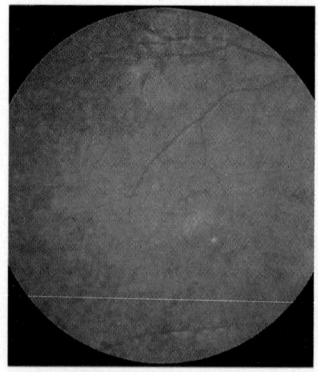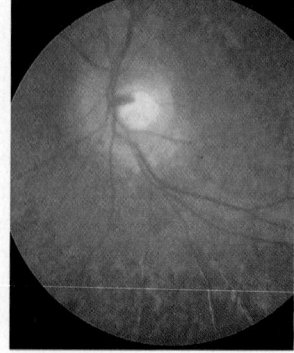

Fig. 44.19 Mitochondrial cytopathy in a 15-year-old with a very attenuated ERG and poor vision from 6 years of age. There is mild arteriolar thinning and retinal pigment epithelial defects.

Other features may include a peripheral neuropathy and rarely a generalized rod–cone dystrophy (Poll-The *et al.* 1988, 1992; Bertini *et al.* 1992).

Methylmalonic and other acidurias

Retinal degeneration has been described in a vitamin B_{12} disorder associated with methylmalonic aciduria and sulphur amino acid abnormalities (Robb *et al.* 1984).

Bardet–Biedl and Laurence–Moon syndromes
(see also Chapter P26)

The Bardet–Biedl syndrome is an autosomal recessive disorder characterized by obesity, mental retardation, postaxial polydactyly (Fig. 44.20), hypogonadism and a progressive retinal dystrophy. Renal failure, due to ureteric reflux, and hypertension are common and are the leading causes of death in this condition (Hurley *et al.* 1975).

There is a wide variability in expression of the gene so that incomplete forms are seen (Klein & Amman 1969; Schachat & Maumenee 1982). In many cases the mental retardation may be mild and if the extra digits have been excised in infancy the diagnosis may be missed unless a careful history is taken, and the hands and feet examined. Diabetes has occasionally been reported in patients with the Bardet–Biedl syndrome (Escallon *et al.* 1989; Hauser *et al.* 1990) which may lead to difficulties in differentiating the Bardet–Biedl syndrome from Alström's syndrome.

The retinal disease is seen in all cases and is a severe rod–cone dystrophy (Figs 44.21 and 44.22) with onset in childhood (Campo & Aaberg 1982) although rarely it may be present in early infancy (Runge *et al.* 1986a). Early macular involvement is common and a 'bull's eye' picture may be seen on fundoscopy and fluorescein angiography. Optic disc pallor and arteriolar narrowing are commonly observed signs but peripheral pigmentation is a variable

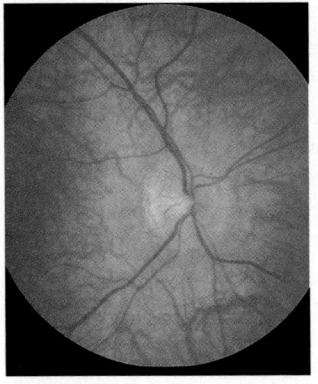
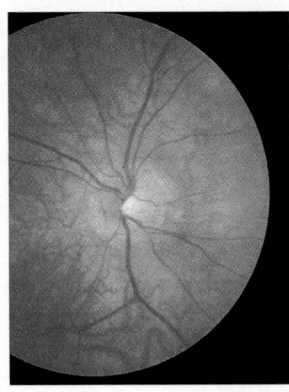

Fig. 44.21 Bardet–Biedl syndrome. The fundi show mild arteriolar narrowing despite poor vision and an attenuated ERG. The rate of visual deterioration is very variable.

feature (Campo & Aaberg 1982). The visual prognosis is poor because of the early central receptor involvement, and most patients have 6/60 vision or less by the third decade (Campo & Aaberg 1982; Jacobsen *et al.* 1990; Fulton *et al.* 1993).

Electrophysiological studies show reduced or absent ERGs with preserved VEPs in early cases (see Fig. 9.8).

In one histological study of the eyes of an infant with the Bardet–Biedl syndrome there was extensive photoreceptor degeneration at the macula with peripheral receptors having shortened outer segments (Runge *et al.* 1986a).

The Laurence–Moon syndrome is a closely related autosomal recessive disorder in which there is no obesity or polydactyly but affected patients have a short stature, hypogonadism, mental retardation, ataxia and spinal paraparesis (Laurence & Moon 1866; Campo & Aaberg 1982; Nyska *et al.* 1991). Magnetic resonance imaging (MRI) scanning of one patient showed that the paraparesis was associated with a cervical myelopathy (Nyska *et al.* 1991).

There appears to be evidence for genetic heterogeneity in the Bardet–Biedl syndrome which has been mapped to chromosome 16q (Kwitek-Black *et al.* 1993), 11q (Leppert *et al.* 1994), 3p (Sheffield *et al.* 1994) and 15q (Carmi *et al.* 1995). There is overlap in the phenotype of Bardet–Biedl syndrome and the Laurence–Moon syndrome and at present it is not known whether they are caused by mutations at the same or different genetic loci.

Albrechtsen's syndrome

Albrechtsen (1956) described siblings with hypotrichiasis, ectropolysyndactyly and a retinal degeneration.

Alström's syndrome

Alström's syndrome is an uncommon autosomal reces-

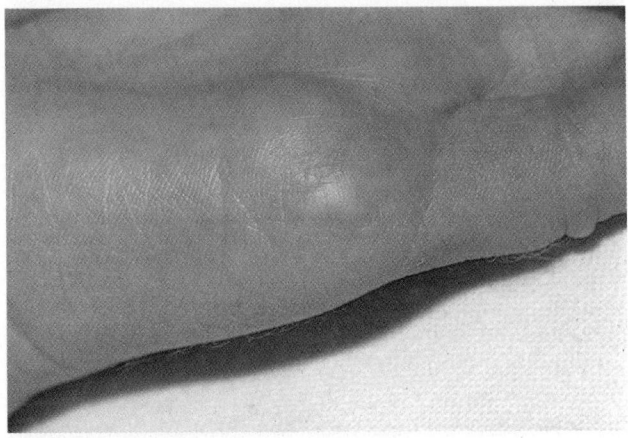

Fig. 44.20 Laurence–Moon–Biedl syndrome. Post-axial polydactyly may not be obvious if the extra digit has been removed.

sive disorder characterized by diabetes mellitus, severe nerve deafness, obesity and an early onset retinal dystrophy (Alström *et al.* 1959; Goldstein & Fialkow 1973; Sebag *et al.* 1984; Charles *et al.* 1990). Other features may include chronic renal disease, a pigmented skin lesion (acanthosis nigricans), hypothyroidism, growth hormone deficiency and, in males, hypogonadism (Goldstein & Fialkow 1973; Charles *et al.* 1990; Alter & Moshang 1993). The endocrine abnormalities appear to be caused by target hormone unresponsiveness rather than reduced levels of hormone.

Visual loss and nystagmus is usually noted in infancy but there is little published information about the ocular examination and electrophysiology at this stage. Dyer *et al.* (1994) have reported one patient with Alström's syndrome who had an ERG performed at 6 months of age. There was absent photopic responses and a markedly reduced rod response. Tremblay *et al.* (1993) reported the results of a longitudinal study of the ERG responses in four patients with Alström's syndrome; cone responses were non-recordable in early infancy but rod responses could be identified until 5 years of age. Most reported cases have been examined in later childhood when there is poor central vision, nystagmus, optic disc pallor, attenuated vessels and a pigmentary retinopathy. The ERG is usually absent at presentation (Goldstein & Fialkow 1973; Sebag *et al.* 1984). The early loss of central acuity, the presence of photophobia and the results of ERG testing in infancy suggest that Alström's syndrome is an early onset cone–rod dystrophy. Histopathology in one case revealed an absence of rods and cones (Sebag *et al.* 1984).

Alström's syndrome has some similarities with the Bardet–Biedl syndrome but can be distinguished by the absence of mental retardation and polydactyly in the former and the rarity of nerve deafness and diabetes in the latter (Goldstein & Fialkow 1973). There are also some similarities to the syndrome of Leber's amaurosis, cardiomyopathy and short stature described by Russell-Eggitt *et al.* (1989).

Infantile retinal dystrophy, cardiomyopathy, obesity and short stature

Russell-Eggitt *et al.* (1989) have described a group of children with a congenital retinal dystrophy, cardiomyopathy, obesity and short stature. Photophobia is a prominent symptom and this may represent an early onset cone–rod dystrophy. There is some overlap between this syndrome and Alström's syndrome and it is unclear at present whether they represent distinct genetic disorders.

Cockayne's syndrome

Cockayne's syndrome is a rare autosomal recessive disorder in which there is growth retardation, deafness,

presenile appearance, mental retardation, cutaneous photosensitivity, dental caries and a progressive retinal dystrophy (Coles 1969; Pearce 1972; Nance & Berry 1992). The most consistent ocular feature is a progressive retinal dystrophy with optic atrophy, arteriolar attenuation and peripheral pigmentary retinopathy (Fig. 44.23). Other reported findings include enophthalmos, corneal opacities, cataract and nystagmus (Coles 1969; Pearce 1972; Nance & Berry 1992; Traboulsi *et al.* 1992). The pupils are usually small and dilate poorly with mydriatic agents (Traboulsi *et al.* 1992). Ocular histopathology in one patient showed degeneration of all retinal layers with an intact retinal pigment epithelium (Levin *et al.* 1983).

There is wide variation in the clinical signs and severity seen in different patients suggesting that there is genetic as well as clinical heterogeneity (Nance & Berry 1992). In most cases visual and general development is normal in the first year of life following which there is slow physical and intellectual deterioration. Death occurred at a mean age of 12 years in the series reported by Nance and Berry (1992) and few patients live beyond their teens. The prognosis is worst in those patients who have prenatal growth failure, congenital structural ocular abnormalities and severe neurological dysfunction from birth.

The cause of Cockayne's syndrome is unknown but may represent a disorder of DNA repair. Fibroblasts from patients with Cockayne's syndrome show greater sensitivity to the killing effect of ultraviolet irradiation and there is deficient recovery of RNA synthesis following ultraviolet irradiation (Nance & Berry 1992).

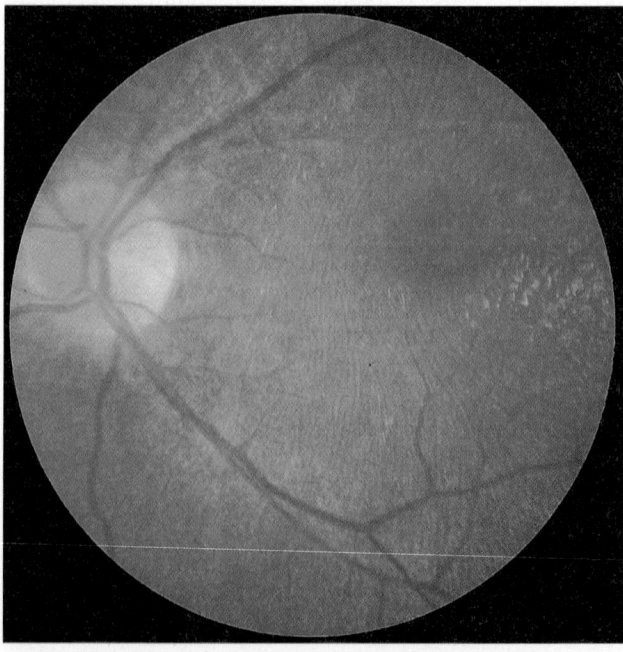

Fig. 44.22 Bardet–Biedl syndrome. Retinal dystrophy with retinal oedema.

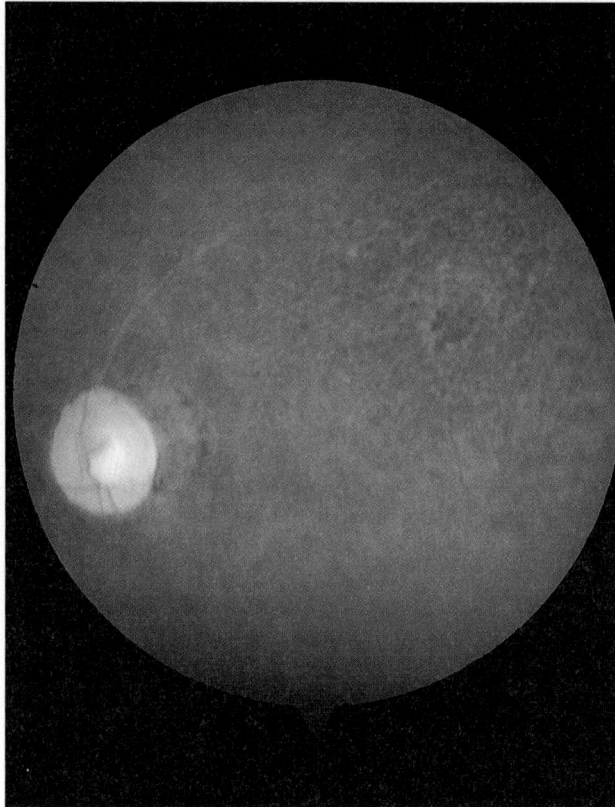

Fig. 44.23 Cockayne's syndrome. Severe retinal dystrophy and extreme arteriolar narrowing and optic atrophy.

Mucopolysaccharidoses (see Chapter 57)

A progressive retinal dystrophy may develop in all mucopolysaccharidoses (MPS) except Morquio's disease; it is especially prominent in MPS IH (Hurler's disease), MPS IS (Scheie's disease), MPS II (Hunter's syndrome) and MPS III (San Fillipo's disease). The retinal abnormality is a rod–cone dystrophy which is similar in all three types of MPS. Fundus examination may show only mild retinal abnormalities so that the ERG is the best indicator of retinal disease (Caruso *et al.* 1986). There is a wide range of severity with some patients having a normal ERG whilst in others it is severely abnormal (Caruso *et al.* 1986). The retinal and other ophthalmic features have been reviewed by François (1982) and Bateman *et al.* (1994).

Batten's disease (see Chapter 57)

Batten's disease is an autosomal recessive disorder which occurs in an infantile, late infantile and juvenile form. In the infantile and late infantile forms neurological deterioration and seizures precede the visual deterioration, which is due to a progressive retinal dystrophy. The ERG is extinguished at an early stage and there is marked optic atrophy, arteriolar attenuation and a mild pigmentary

retinopathy. A 'bull's eye' maculopathy (Table 44.5) is frequently seen (Raitta & Santavouri 1973; Francois 1982).

Juvenile Batten's disease, however, may present first to the ophthalmologist as the visual deterioration may precede the neurological signs. Visual loss usually starts between 5 and 8 years (Spalton *et al.* 1980) but this is later followed by intellectual regression, seizures and neurological deterioration. Death usually occurs by the late teens.

The earliest changes are usually seen at the macula where there may be a subtle bull's eye appearance which is more evident on fluorescein angiography. Later there is optic disc pallor, arteriolar attenuation and macular and peripheral pigmentation and atrophy (Spalton *et al.* 1980; François 1982). The ERG is substantially abnormal at an early stage (see Fig. 9.14). This diagnosis should be excluded in all children who present with visual loss between 5 and 8 years, especially if there is evidence of a mild maculopathy. In contrast to other forms of juvenile macular degeneration the scotopic and photopic ERG is absent or substantially subnormal.

The juvenile form of Batten's disease has been mapped to chromosome 16q (Gardiner *et al.* 1990).

Hallervorden–Spatz disease

Hallervorden–Spatz disease is an uncommon disorder characterized by extrapyramidal motor signs and dementia which begins in early childhood and is relentlessly progressive leading to death in early adult life (Hallervorden & Spatz 1922). A characteristic 'eye of the tiger' appearance is seen on T2-weighted images of the pallidal nuclei. It is thought to be inherited as an autosomal recessive trait. Acanthocytosis and a progressive retinal dystrophy (Fig. 44.24) are seen in a proportion of cases (Roth *et al.* 1971; Newell *et al.* 1979; Luckenbach 1983). Fundus examination may show a flecked retina and an associated bull's eye maculopathy (Newell *et al.* 1979; Luckenbach 1983); the ERG is non-recordable at an early stage (Luckenbach 1983). Postmortem studies of eyes have shown marked

Table 44.5 Bull's eye maculopathy in childhood.

Stargardt's disease
Progressive cone dystrophy
Cone–rod dystrophy
Batten's disease
Hallervorden–Spatz disease
Bardet–Biedl syndrome
Mucolipidosis IV
Fucosidosis
Drug toxicity (e.g. chloroquine)
Benign concentric macular dystrophy
Fenestrated sheen dystrophy

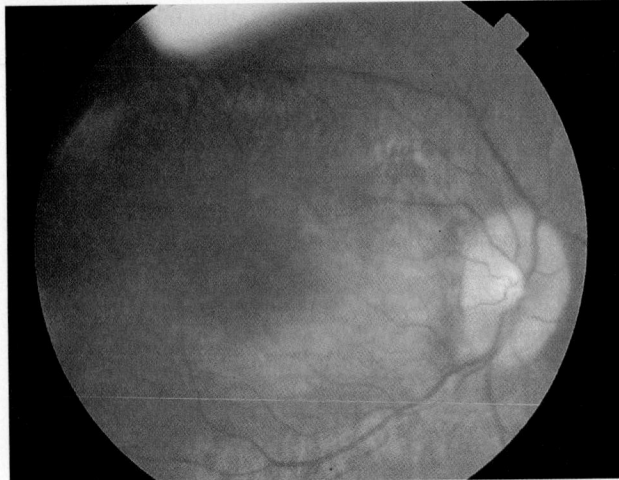

Fig. 44.24 Hallervorden–Spatz disease showing the posterior polar macular changes. The ERG showed a widespread defect.

loss of rods and cones throughout the retina (Roth *et al.* 1971; Luckenbach 1983).

Joubert's syndrome

Joubert's syndrome is an autosomal recessive disorder characterized by cerebellar vermis hypoplasia, neonatal breathing difficulties, a retinal dystrophy and ocular motor abnormalities (Joubert *et al.* 1969; Tomita *et al.* 1979; King *et al.* 1984; Lambert *et al.* 1989a). Ocular colobomas have also been described in this disorder (Lindhout *et al.* 1980; Saraiva & Baraitser 1992). The clinical features of the syndrome have been reviewed by Saraiva and Baraitser (1992) and they have suggested that patients with Joubert's syndrome can be divided into two types, those with a retinal dystrophy and those without. Rocco (1993) has pointed out the similarities between patients with Joubert's syndrome and a retinal dystrophy and the CDG syndrome and has suggested that CDG syndrome be excluded before a diagnosis of Joubert's syndrome is made in such infants.

In Joubert's syndrome the retinal dystrophy is of infantile onset and indistinguishable from Leber's amaurosis but the visual prognosis is better; vision of 6/18 or better has been recorded when the child is old enough to be formally tested (Moore & Taylor 1984; Lambert *et al.* 1988). Although fundus examination is normal in infancy, disc pallor, arteriolar attenuation and pigmentary retinopathy may develop at a later stage (Lambert *et al.* 1989a). The ERG is absent or markedly attenuated but the visual evoked response is usually preserved indicating reasonable macular function.

A wide variety of ocular motor abnormalities have been reported including nystagmus, impaired pursuit and hypometric or absent saccades. In some infants the sac-cadic palsy is severe and head thrusting similar to that seen in ocular motor apraxia may be used to aid refixation (Moore & Taylor 1984; Lambert *et al.* 1989a). Some infants show frequent hemifacial spasm (King *et al.* 1984). Joubert's syndrome should be suspected in infants with poor vision and nystagmus if there is developmental delay and a history of neonatal breathing difficulties. Electrophysiological testing will show a well-preserved visual evoked response in the presence of a substantially abnormal ERG and the finding of cerebellar vermis hypoplasia on MRI will confirm the diagnosis (Fig. 44.25).

Olivopontocerebellar atrophy and spinocerebellar degenerations

A progressive retinal dystrophy has been described in some families with olivopontocerebellar atrophy, a dominantly inherited disorder characterized by progressive cerebellar and brain stem neuronal loss (Weiner *et al.* 1967; Ryan *et al.* 1975; de Jong *et al.* 1980). The late Professor Anita Harding (Harding 1982, 1984) divided autosomal dominant cerebellar ataxias into four groups and it is the type 2 disorder (the type 3 of Konigsmark and Weiner) in her classification which is associated with a retinal dystrophy (see Fig. 44.26). The onset of cerebellar signs and visual loss is variable but has been reported in early infancy (de Jong *et al.* 1980) and childhood (Weiner *et al.* 1967; Ryan *et al.* 1975). The earlier the onset, the more severe and rapid the disease (Drack *et al.* 1992). There is optic disc pallor, arteriolar attenuation and a peripheral pigmentary retinopathy. Macular pigment epithelial atrophy and pigmentation is common (Ryan *et al.* 1975; de Jong *et al.* 1981; Traboulsi *et al.* 1988). The ERG is usually absent or severely abnormal. In the family described by To *et al.* (1993) the earliest retinal abnormality was a subnormal photopic

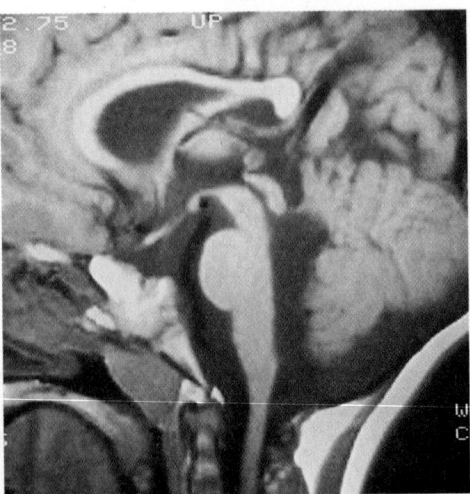

Fig. 44.25 Joubert's syndrome. MRI scan shows vermis hypoplasia with large fourth ventricle.

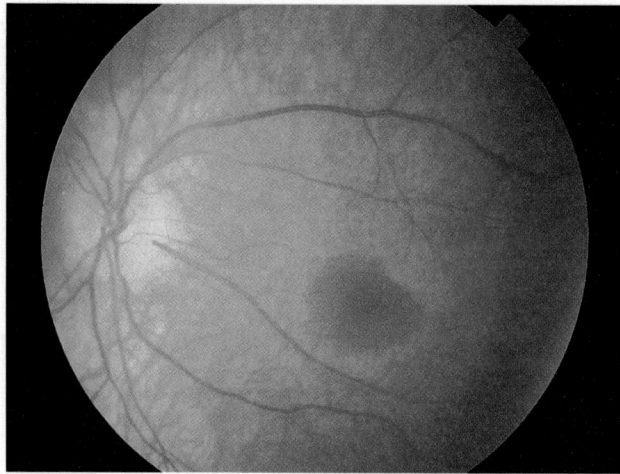

Fig. 44.26 Retinal dystrophy in a child with spinocerebellar degeneration showing widespread retinal pigment epithelial defect with preservation of the macular pigment at this early stage.

ERG; other more severely affected individuals showed subnormal scotopic and photopic responses. This suggests that the retinal abnormality seen in this disorder may be a cone–rod dystrophy. Histopathological examination of eyes obtained at postmortem have shown marked shortening of the outer segments and receptor loss which appears to start in the macular area and spread to involve the peripheral retina (Ryan *et al.* 1975; de Jong *et al.* 1980; Traboulsi *et al.* 1988; To *et al.* 1993).

Other spinocerebellar degenerations may be associated with a progressive retinal degeneration (Fig. 44.26): in one of these, the gene has been mapped to 3p (Gouw *et al.* 1995).

Alagille's syndrome (arteriohepatic dysplasia)

Alagille's syndrome is an uncommon disorder characterized by hepatic cholestasis and a variety of other systemic features including facial dysmorphism, congenital heart disease and vertebral, renal and ocular abnormalities. It is thought to be inherited as an autosomal dominant trait with variable expressivity and the disorder maps to the short arm of chromosome 20 (Snittger *et al.* 1989; Zhang *et al.* 1990). Some patients, however, have no family history. The usual presentation is with prolonged neonatal jaundice or failure to thrive. The most consistent ocular abnormality is posterior embryotoxon often with associated iris strands (Axenfeld's anomaly). Other ocular abnormalities (Fig. 44.27) include iris stromal hypoplasia, microcornea and optic nerve dysplasia (Brodsky & Cunniff 1993). Choroidal hypoplasia, a short axial length and drusen of the optic disc, which may need ultrasound studies for diagnosis, are also frequent features (Nischal *et al.* 1996). Most older patients also have a pigmentary retinopathy

and in some there is evidence of a rod–cone dystrophy on ERG (Puklin *et al.* 1981). The retinal dystrophy is not usually present in young children and may be associated with low levels of serum vitamins A and E and, although it is unclear whether the retinal abnormalities are related to hypovitaminosis, if there is evidence of reduced serum levels supplemental vitamins should be given (Alvarez *et al.* 1983).

Osteopetrosis

Osteopetrosis is a term used to describe a group of rare disorders in which there is increase in thickness and density of bone due to defective bone resorption. This results in narrowing of the bony foraminae of the skull and distortion of the marrow cavity. Several different forms are recognized but they can be broadly classified into those with childhood or adult onset. The early infantile form, which is inherited as an autosomal recessive trait, has a particularly severe phenotype. Ophthalmological complications include nystagmus, cranial nerve palsies, proptosis, papilloedema and optic atrophy. Visual loss may result from optic nerve compression due to narrowing of the optic canal, but there have been several reports of visual impairment due to a retinal dystrophy (Keith 1968; Hoyt & Billson 1979; Ruben *et al.* 1990) suggesting that in at least some infants the visual loss is retinal in origin. In those infants with a retinal dystrophy, the fundus has been reported to be normal (Hoyt & Billson 1979) or show macular atrophy and pigmentation. The ERG shows evidence of rod and cone dysfunction (Hoyt & Billson 1979; Ruben *et al.* 1990). Histopathological examination of the eyes of one patient showed evidence of retinal degeneration which was most marked posteriorly (Keith 1968).

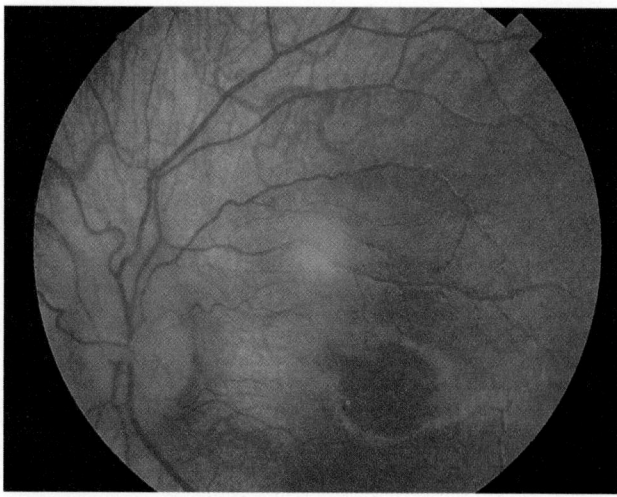

Fig. 44.27 Alagille's syndrome showing pseudopapilloedema secondary to drusen.

Jeune's syndrome (see also Chapter P26)

Jeune's syndrome is a rare autosomal recessive disorder characterized by skeletal deformities, dwarfism, nephronophthisis and in some cases a retinal dystrophy (Jeune *et al.* 1955; Oberklaid *et al.* 1977). Death may occur in childhood due to respiratory insufficiency caused by the skeletal abnormalities or chronic renal failure. The dystrophy may present in early infancy (Bard *et al.* 1978; Phillips *et al.* 1979) or only become evident in later childhood (Wilson *et al.* 1987).

Fundus examination reveals retinal arteriolar narrowing and pigment epithelial atrophy in the midperipheral retina. The ERG shows subnormal rod and cone responses (Wilson *et al.* 1987). Histopathological examination of the eyes of one patient showed extensive receptor degeneration with the rods more affected than the cones; the retinal pigment epithelium was relatively well preserved (Allen *et al.* 1979).

Myotonic dystrophy

A progressive retinal dystrophy similar to mild RP or macular pigmentary disturbances may be seen in adults with myotonic dystrophy (Mausof *et al.* 1972) but retinal involvement has not been reported in childhood.

Retinal dystrophy and juvenile nephronophthisis (Senior–Loken syndrome)

Senior *et al.* (1961) first described the association of a recessively inherited renal disease, juvenile nephronophthisis (medullary cystic disease) and a tapetoretinal degeneration. Many more cases have since been reported (Loken *et al.* 1961; Fairley *et al.* 1963; Meier & Hess 1965; Herdman *et al.* 1967; Mainzer *et al.* 1970; Abraham *et al.* 1974; Polak *et al.* 1977; Edwards & Grizzard 1981; Ellis *et al.* 1984) and it is evident that the age of onset of the retinal dystrophy is extremely variable. Some children have poor vision and

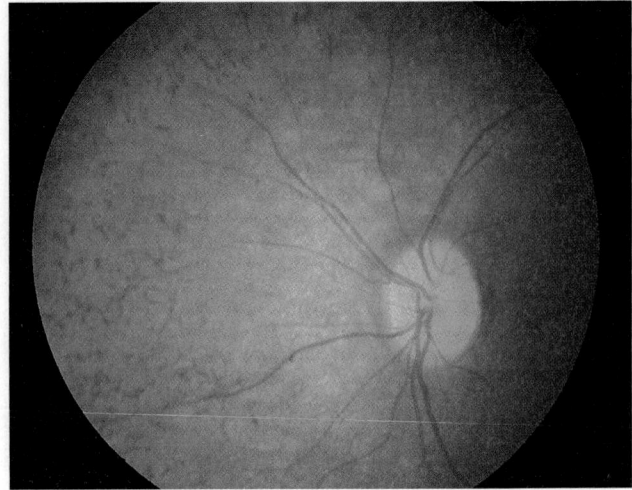

Fig. 44.29 Senior–Loken syndrome showing a pigmentary retinopathy with bone corpuscle formation.

nystagmus from birth and have a retinal dystrophy indistinguishable from Leber's amaurosis (Loken *et al.* 1961; Senior *et al.* 1961; Dekaban 1969) whilst others develop a picture similar to childhood onset RP (Fig. 44.29) with night-blindness and normal central vision (Mainzer *et al.* 1970; Abraham *et al.* 1974; Polak 1977; Edwards & Grizzard 1981). Loken *et al.* (1961) performed a histological examination of the eye of a child who was blind from infancy and who later died of chronic renal failure. They found that the photoreceptor layer was markedly abnormal with no identifiable rods; the macular region consisted of one layer of large epithelial-like cells and no normal cones could be identified.

Other associations seen in this disorder include cone-shaped epiphyses of the distal interphalangeal joints (Mainzer *et al.* 1970; Ellis *et al.* 1984), cerebellar ataxia (Mainzer *et al.* 1970), hepatic fibrosis (Stanescu *et al.* 1967) and deafness (Clarke *et al.* 1992).

In Senior–Loken syndrome asymptomatic heterozygotes may show an abnormal scotopic ERG and elevated rod thresholds when tested psychophysically (Abraham *et al.* 1974; Polak *et al.* 1977).

Idiopathic infantile hypercalciuria

Idiopathic infantile hypercalciuria is a rare autosomal recessive disorder characterized by hypercalciuria, nephrocalcinosis, nephrolithiasis and a tapetoretinal degeneration (Meier *et al.* 1979; Gil-Gilberneau *et al.* 1982). Affected children are highly myopic and fundus examination shows large oval ectatic lesions at the macula similar to macular coloboma (Meier *et al.* 1979; Gil-Gilberneau *et al.* 1982). The ERG may be mildly abnormal (Gil-Gilberneau *et al.* 1982) or show complete absence of rod responses (Meier *et al.* 1979).

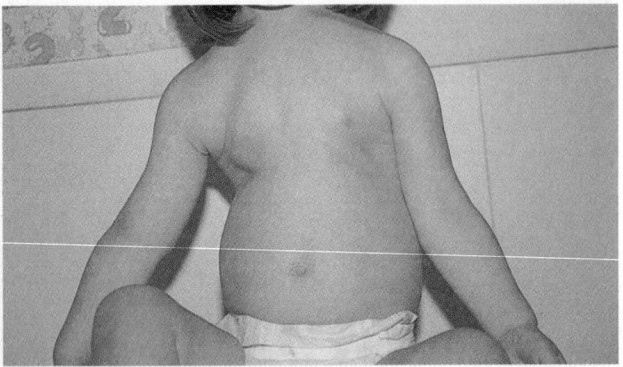

Fig. 44.28 Jeune's syndrome (asphyxiating thoracic dystrophy) showing the chest deformity.

Chorioretinopathy and pituitary dysfunction (CPD syndrome)

CPD syndrome is a rare condition characterized by severe chorioretinal degeneration beginning in infancy, hypothalamic pituitary dysfunction, trichomegaly (Fig. 44.30) with later alopecia (Patton *et al.* 1986), and variable mental retardation (Oliver & McFarlane 1965; Judisch *et al.* 1981). The inheritance is unknown. Vision is reduced often to the level of 6/60 and there is extensive atrophy of the retinal pigment epithelium and choriocapillaris (Fig. 44.31). The ERG was non-recordable in one case (Judisch *et al.* 1981).

Cohen's syndrome

Cohen's syndrome is an uncommon, autosomal recessive disorder characterized by non-progressive mental retardation, short stature, microcephaly, dysmorphic facies, hypotonia and delayed puberty (Cohen *et al.* 1973; Norio *et al.* 1984). Myopia is common and many of the reported

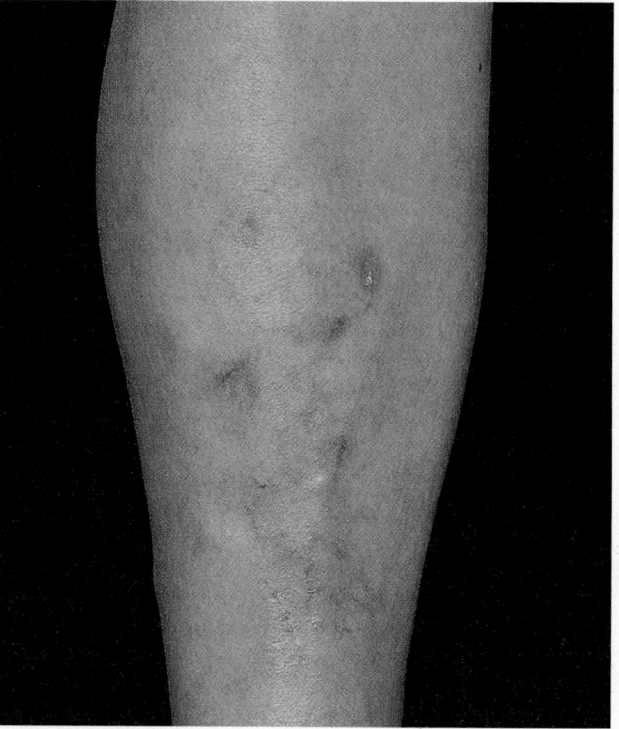

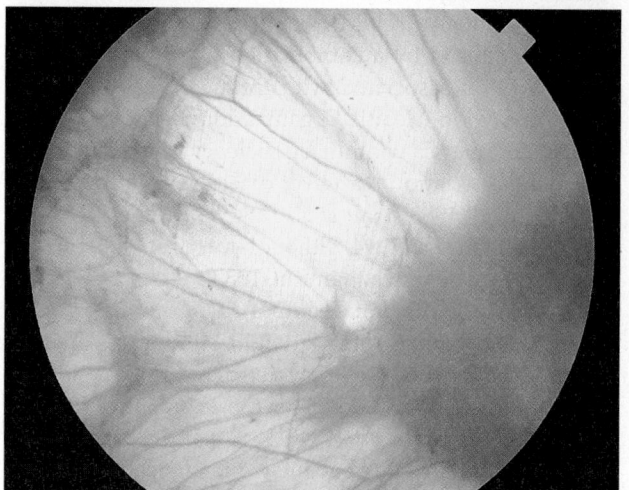

Fig. 44.31 (a) CPD syndrome in an adult male showing total alopecia. (b) CPD syndrome showing very marked retinal and choroidal atrophy.

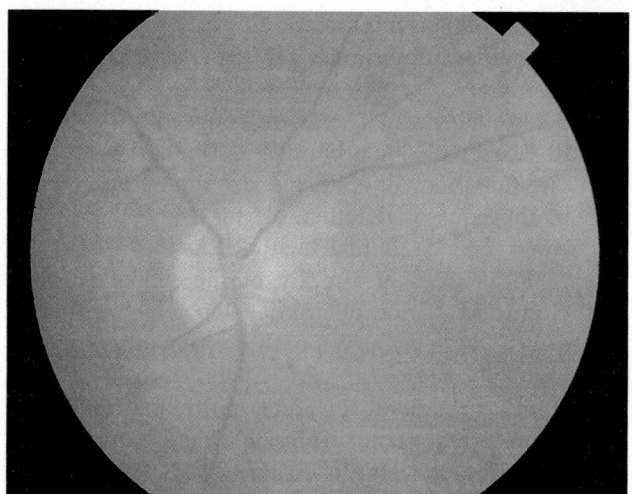

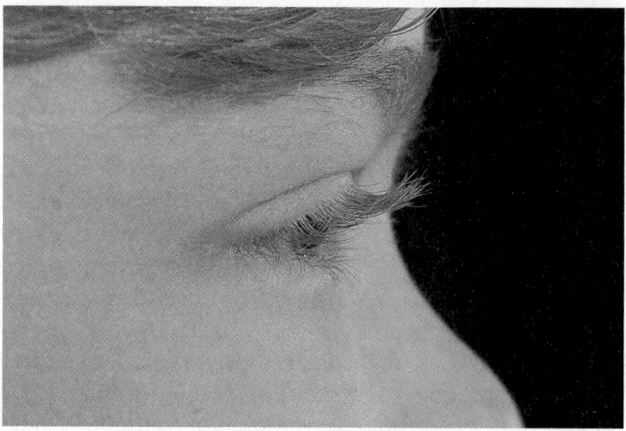

Fig. 44.30 (a) CPD syndrome showing retinal changes. The photograph is slightly out of focus but a pigmentary disturbance can be discerned. (b) CPD syndrome showing long eyelashes.

cases have had a progressive retinal dystrophy with arteriolar narrowing, retinal pigment epithelial atrophy and pigmentation. The ERG is unrecordable early in the disease (Norio *et al.* 1984). The gene has been assigned to 8q (Tahvanainen *et al.* 1994).

The association of chorioretinal degeneration, ERG abnormalities and microcephaly has been described in other families showing both autosomal recessive and autosomal dominant inheritance (Manning *et al.* 1990).

Werner's syndrome

Affected children are slender, have short stature, a beaked nose, tight atrophic skin, diabetes and poor wound healing (Kremer *et al.* 1988). A significant proportion have a progressive retinal dystrophy (Ruprecht 1989).

Microcephaly–chorioretinopathy

In the autosomal dominant form of this disease there are widespread chorioretinal lacunar defects with hyperpigmentation of the intervening retinal pigment epithelium, and retinal vascular attenuation (Parke *et al.* 1984). The microcephaly is variable, but it is usually associated with mental retardation.

In the autosomal recessive form, the visible retinal disturbance is less marked or may be non-pigmentary (Harbord *et al.* 1989).

Acquired rod–cone dystrophies

Vitamin A deficiency

Worldwide, vitamin A deficiency is the most common cause of blindness in childhood. In developing countries it is usually caused by a combination of malnutrition and malabsorption associated with frequent gastrointestinal infection (World Health Organization 1982). In Europe and North America vitamin A deficiency is rare and usually seen in association with liver disease or malabsorption (Alvarez *et al.* 1983; Walt *et al.* 1984; O'Donnell & Talbot 1987; Newman *et al.* 1994) although rarely an unusual diet may be the cause (Buchanan *et al.* 1987).

Vitamin A is an essential component of rhodopsin and it is therefore not surprising that night-blindness is an early symptom of deficiency. In early deficiency there is slowing of rod dark adaptation and later rod and cone thresholds are elevated (Walt *et al.* 1984). Peripheral fields may be constricted and in some patients white dots at the level of the pigment epithelium are seen scattered throughout the peripheral retina. The EOG and ERG responses are also abnormal (O'Donnell & Talbot 1987).

The ocular abnormalities are reversible with vitamin A supplementation if started before the disease is too advanced (Walt *et al.* 1984; O'Donnell & Talbot 1987); in some cases a lack of response to vitamin A alone (Grey 1991) may suggest a lack of other substances such as vitamin E.

Desferrioxamine toxicity

Desferrioxamine is a chelating agent used in the treatment of iron storage disorders such as transfusion siderosis (Modell 1979). Side-effects include cataract (Modell 1979), optic neuropathy (Lakhampal *et al.* 1984) and retinal degeneration (Davies *et al.* 1983; Lakhampal *et al.* 1984; Rahi *et al.* 1986). Patients with retinal toxicity develop night-blindness, peripheral field loss and a peripheral pigmentary retinopathy; dark adaptation is abnormal and the ERG shows reduced amplitude (Davies *et al.* 1983; Lakhampal *et al.* 1984). Some improvement occurs on stopping the drug.

Histological examination of the eyes of a patient with retinal toxicity showed that the retinal pigment epithelium was predominantly affected (Rahi *et al.* 1986).

Inherited chorioretinal dystrophies

Choroideraemia

Choroideraemia is an X-linked recessive disorder characterized by progressive atrophy of the retinal pigment epithelium and choriocapillaries. Affected males present in early childhood with night-blindness and develop progressive field loss but central vision is usually preserved until late in the disease. There is, however, a wide variation in clinical expression (Karna 1986). Female carriers although usually asymptomatic are easily recognized by the characteristic appearance of the peripheral retina on fundoscopy.

Affected males usually present between the ages of 5 and 10 years with night-blindness. The earliest fundus signs are fine pigment epithelial atrophy and pigmentation in the equatorial retina; at this stage the clinical appearance may be confused with RP. As the disease progresses focal areas of atrophy of the retinal pigment epithelium and choriocapillaris develop, which are particularly well demonstrated on fluorescein angiography. These areas coalesce to give a widespread atrophic appearance throughout the equatorial retina (Figs 44.32, 44.33). This later spreads to involve the peripheral and more posterior retina; the macula is spared until late in the disease. Mild myopia is common.

Visual fields initially show small midperipheral scotomas corresponding to areas of atrophy but later a typical ring scotoma develops. As the disease progresses marked constriction of the visual field occurs but there is often a small preserved island of field in the far periphery. Visual acuity remains reasonably good until the fifth to sixth decade in most patients (Karna 1986; Heckenlively 1988). The ERG is abnormal or extinguished at an early stage; in those with a preserved response rod and cone amplitudes are reduced and cone b-wave implicit times are prolonged (Heckenlively 1988).

Cases associated with deafness, hypopituitarism and mental retardation (Ayazi 1981; Rosenburg *et al.* 1987; Menon *et al.* 1989) probably represent a contiguous gene defect.

Most eyes studied histopathologically have been from patients with advanced disease but Rodrigues *et al.* (1984)

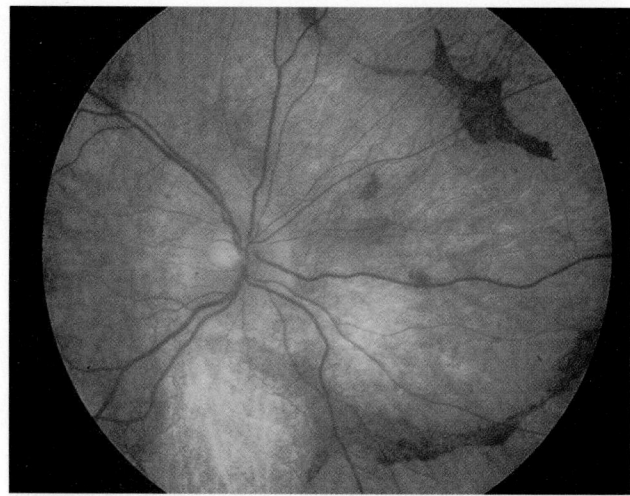

Fig. 44.32 Choroideraemia showing the marked chorioretinal changes with scalloped edges (Mr Anthony Moore's patient).

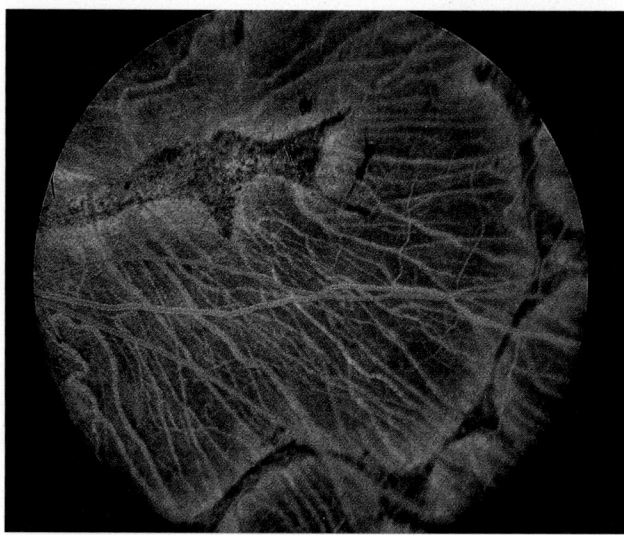

Fig. 44.33 Choroideraemia. Fluorescein angiogram showing characteristic scalloped appearance given by the surviving retinal pigment epithelium and loss of the choriocapillaries.

reported the results of the histological examination of the eyes of an 18-year-old male with early disease. This showed marked degeneration of the outer retina with loss of retinal pigment epithelium, Bruch's membrane and choriocapillaris. Biochemical studies showed reduced levels of interreceptor retinal binding protein (IRBP) and increased levels of cAMP in the retinal pigment epithelium and choroid (Rodrigues *et al.* 1984).

Female heterozygotes

Most female carriers are asymptomatic but the fundus appearance is characteristic. There is widespread fine retinal pigment epithelial atrophy and granular pigment deposition in the midperipheral retina (Fig. 44.34). The EOG and ERG are usually normal (Sieving *et al.* 1986). Elderly heterozygotes may develop nyctalopia and may show more extensive retinal pigment epithelial atrophy. The ERG may be abnormal and psychophysical testing may show elevated rod thresholds (Karna 1986).

Molecular genetics

The choroideraemia gene (CHM) was mapped to Xq21 by linkage studies (Nussbaum *et al.* 1985a) and by the detection of cytogenetic abnormalities in mentally retarded males with choroideraemia (Nussbaum *et al.* 1987; Siu *et al.* 1990). Subsequently several different mutations of a gene in this region, the CHM gene, have been identified in families with choroideraemia (Cremers *et al.* 1990; Merry *et al.* 1992; Schwartz *et al.* 1993). The CHM gene is thought to code for one of the forms of component A of Rab geronylgeronyl transferase (Seabra *et al.* 1993); the disease mechanism, however, remains to be elucidated.

Gyrate atrophy of the choroid and retina

Gyrate atrophy of the choroid and retina is a rare autosomal recessive disorder characterized by a progressive chorioretinal dystrophy, hyperornithinaemia and a deficiency of the mitochondrial enzyme ornithine aminotransferase (OAT) (Simell & Takki 1973; Takki & Simell 1974; Kennaway *et al.* 1977; Weleber & Kennaway 1988). The level of OAT activity in obligate carriers of the gene has been shown to be about 50% of normal (Valle *et al.* 1977). The human ornithine-D-aminotransferase gene was cloned in 1988 (Mitchell *et al.* 1988) and since then a large

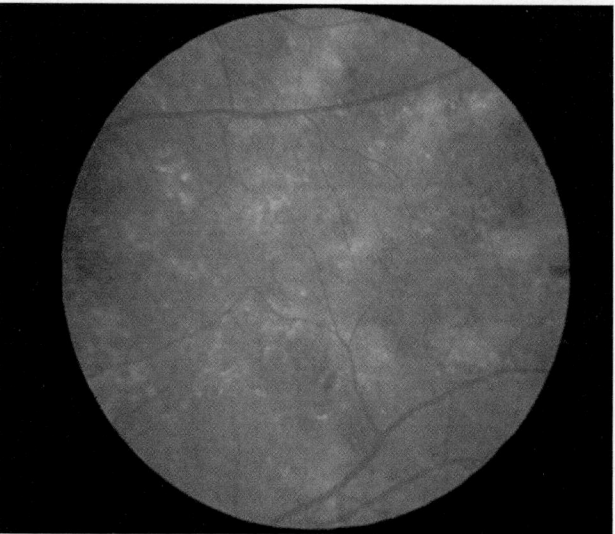

Fig. 44.34 Choroideraemia carrier: linear granular pigmented and depigmented areas in the peripheral retina (Professor B. Jay's patient).

number of different mutations of the OAT gene have been identified in patients with gyrate atrophy including some in which the OAT is pyridoxine-responsive (see McKusick 1994 for summary).

Children may present with night-blindness, progressive myopia or field loss but the diagnosis may be made in early infancy when a raised level of plasma ornithine is found in a child with a family history of gyrate atrophy (Kaiser-Kupfer *et al.* 1985). The earliest fundus changes are seen as small discrete areas of choroidal and retinal pigment epithelial atrophy in the mid- and far peripheral fundus (Takki & Simell 1976; Berson *et al.* 1978; Rinaldi *et al.* 1979; Kaiser-Kupfer *et al.* 1985; Weleber & Kennaway 1988). The adjacent fundus may show evidence of diffuse depigmentation of the retinal pigment epithelium (Fig. 44.35) and atrophic areas are particularly well

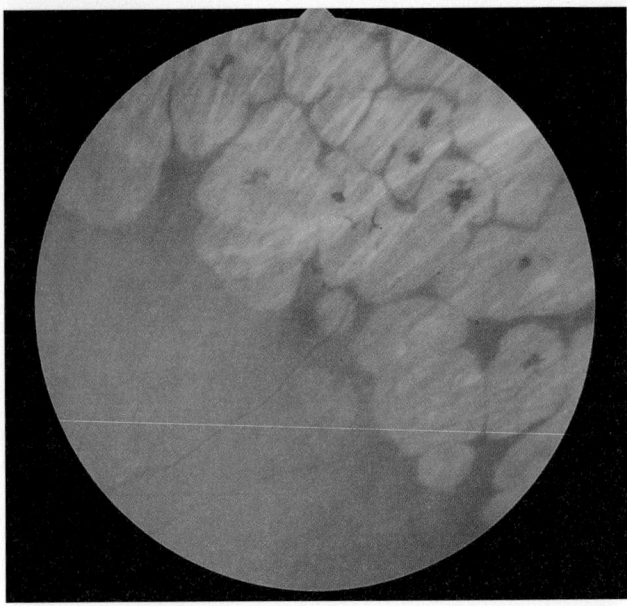

Fig. 44.36 Gyrate atrophy with hyperornithinaemia. Midperipheral coalesced atrophic areas with scalloped edge.

demonstrated on fluorescein angiography. The atrophic areas subsequently coalesce and enlarge towards the posterior pole with a characteristic scalloped appearance at the leading edge (Fig. 44.36).

Most patients have moderate to high myopia and posterior subcapsular cataracts develop in early adult life (Steel *et al.* 1992). Some develop visual loss secondary to macular oedema or atrophy (Weleber & Kennaway 1988). Most patients maintain a reasonable level of visual acuity until their forties or fifties, although with a constricted field. Visual field loss corresponds to the degree of choroidal and retinal pigment epithelial atrophy. In the early stages there are small midperipheral scotomas but progression of disease leads to marked peripheral constriction. Dark adaptation shows markedly elevated rod thresholds in areas of field corresponding to involved retina.

The EOG is subnormal in most patients with gyrate atrophy, even in young affected children (Kaiser-Kupfer *et al.* 1985). The ERG responses depend on the severity of disease; early in the disease both rod and cone amplitudes are reduced (Berson *et al.* 1978; Kaiser-Kupfer 1985) but later the ERG may be unrecordable.

Wilson *et al.* (1991) reported the results of light and electron microscopy of postmortem eyes from a patient with a pyridoxine-sensitive form of gyrate atrophy. There were focal areas of photoreceptor and retinal pigment epithelial atrophy at the posterior pole, and in the midperiphery there were areas in which there was abrupt transition from near normal to atrophic areas of retina. Electron microscopy showed abnormal mitochondria in the cornea, ciliary epithelium and ciliary muscle and in the photoreceptors. Similar mitochondrial abnormalities

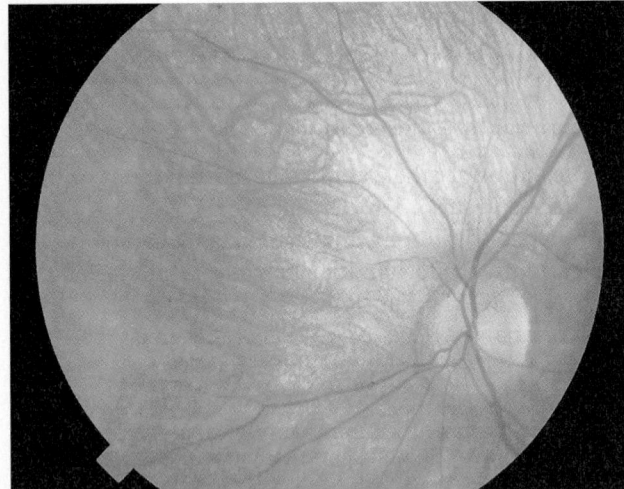

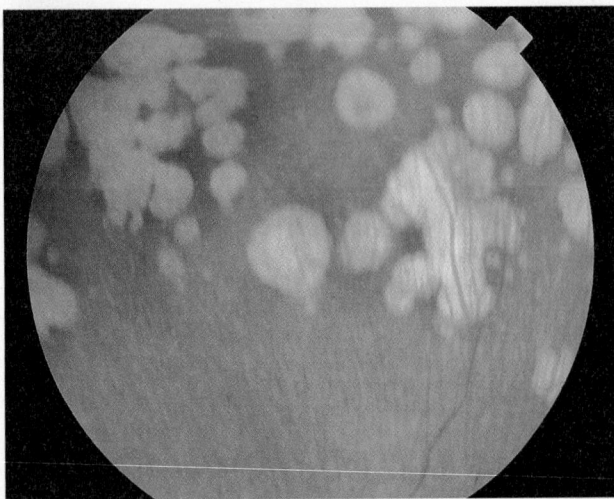

Fig. 44.35 (a, b) Gyrate atrophy with hyperornithinaemia. This 9-year-old child presented with night-blindness. The posterior pole (a) shows arteriolar narrowing and some minimal retinal pigment epithelial changes. The mid- and far periphery (b) show the typical atrophic areas.

have been reported in other tissues in patients with gyrate atrophy and are likely to be a secondary effect of the biochemical disturbance.

Non-ocular features

Although patients with gyrate atrophy show no muscle weakness, muscle biopsy shows atrophy of type 2 fibres with accumulation of tubular aggregates (Sipila *et al.* 1979). Other reported abnormalities include structural abnormalities of the hair, electroencephalographic (EEG) abnormalities and mild mental subnormality and mitochondrial abnormalities in a variety of tissues (Kaiser-Kupfer 1981; Wilson *et al.* 1991).

Biochemical findings and treatment

Patients with gyrate atrophy have a deficiency of the pyridoxal phosphate-dependent mitochondrial enzyme OAT which is responsible for the conversion of ornithine to glutamic acid. Ornithine is not present in protein and the major dietary source is arginine, which may be converted to ornithine by the arginase reaction of the urea cycle or by the glycine transamidase reaction (Valle *et al.* 1981). Ornithine is an important intermediary in the urea cycle and is necessary for the production of polyamines and in the synthesis of proline and glutamate (Weleber & Kennaway 1988).

It is not clear whether the retinal abnormalities are caused by high levels of ornithine or the reduced levels of proline and glutamate that accompany OAT deficiency. Not all patients with raised ornithine levels develop gyrate atrophy and one patient with gyrate atrophy has been reported who had normal ornithine levels and low plasma proline levels (Tada *et al.* 1983) suggesting that reduced availability of proline may be a contributory factor.

Three different approaches to treatment have been used (Weleber & Kennaway 1988). A minority of patients are responsive to pyridoxine (B$_6$) supplements and show reduced plasma ornithine levels and improvement in the ERG (Weleber & Kennaway 1988). Vitamin B$_6$ should be used initially in all patients and continued in those who show a positive response. In non-responders plasma ornithine levels may be reduced by adhering to an arginine-restricted diet (Valle *et al.* 1981) and proline supplementation has been reported to prevent retinal degeneration in some patients (Tada *et al.* 1983).

Children with gyrate atrophy are best managed in collaboration with a paediatrician with an interest in clinical biochemistry. Although the present treatment regimes are promising, more long-term studies are needed to assess whether such treatment will prevent retinal deterioration.

Cone and cone–rod dystrophies

The inherited cone dystrophies are a heterogeneous group of disorders characterized by variable photophobia, reduced central vision, abnormal colour vision and an abnormal photopic ERG (Goodman *et al.* 1963; Moore 1992). Autosomal recessive, autosomal dominant and X-linked recessive inheritance has been reported and there is heterogeneity even amongst these subtypes. The retinal dystrophy may be stationary or progressive; the stationary forms (achromatopsia) are discussed earlier in this chapter. In some forms of cone dystrophy the functional deficit is confined to the photopic system but in others, perhaps the majority, there is later evidence of rod dysfunction. The distinction between cone and cone–rod dystrophies may therefore be difficult, particularly during childhood. Most forms of cone and cone–rod dystrophy is seen in otherwise normal individuals but such dystrophies have been reported in association with other systemic abnormalities; these disorders will be discussed separately.

Progressive cone dystrophy

Clinical features

In contrast to achromatopsia, which presents in early infancy, the progressive cone dystrophies are not usually symptomatic until late childhood or early adult life (Sloan & Brown 1962; Goodman *et al.* 1963; Krill 1977a). The age of onset of visual loss and the rate of progression shows wide variability in the different families reported. Photophobia is a prominent early symptom and there is progressive loss of central vision and colour vision (Berson *et al.* 1968; Krill & Deutman 1972; Krill 1977a). Fine nystagmus is seen even in older children. A small central scotoma is frequently detected on careful visual field testing but peripheral fields remain full. The rate of visual loss is very variable but visual acuity usually deteriorates eventually to the level of 6/60 or to an ability to count fingers only.

Fundus examination (Figs 44.37, 44.38) usually shows a typical bull's eye maculopathy (Goodman *et al.* 1963; Berson *et al.* 1968; Krill & Deutman 1972; Pearlman *et al.* 1974; Krill 1977a) (see Table 44.5 for the differential diagnoses of bull's eye maculopathies). However, in some cases there may only be minor macular pigment epithelial atrophy. The optic discs show a variable degree of temporal pallor. The retinal periphery is usually normal although rarely white flecks similar to those seen in fundus flavimaculatus may be seen (Krill 1977a). Fluorescein angiography shows typical 'window' defects at the macula in the majority of cases and the so-called dark choroid sign is frequently seen (Bonnin *et al.* 1976; Uliss *et al.* 1987). A tapetal-like sheen which may change in

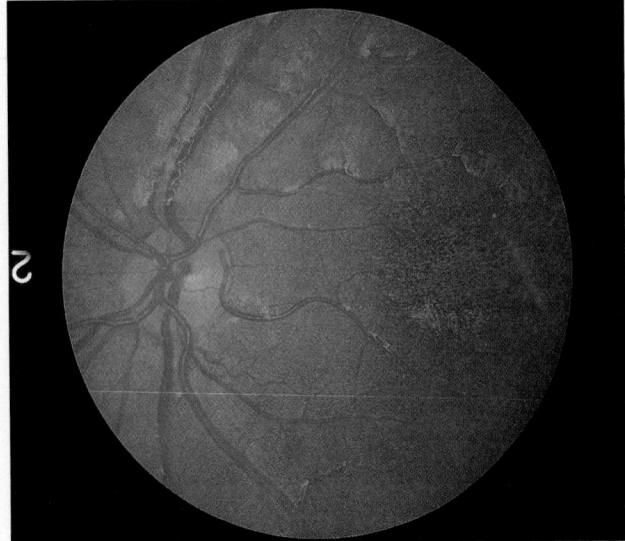

Fig. 44.37 Progressive cone dystrophy with bull's eye maculopathy.

appearance on dark adaptation (Mizuo–Nakamura phenomenom) may be seen in X-linked cone dystrophy (Heckenlively & Weleber 1986; Jacobson *et al.* 1989).

Electrophysiology and psychophysics

Dark adaptation studies show either a monophasic curve with no recognizable cone component, or a biphasic curve with elevated cone thresholds; rod-mediated thresholds are normal (Sloan & Brown 1962; Goodman *et al.* 1963; Berson *et al.* 1968; Krill 1977a). Colour vision testing and spectral sensitivity studies show variable abnormalities of the photopic responses. In some families there is generalized depression of sensitivity across all wavelengths tested (Pearlman *et al.* 1974) whilst others show more specific functional deficits in the early stages of the disease. Reichel *et al.* (1989) reported a family with X-linked cone dystrophy in which there was early loss of red cone function, and families with early loss of blue cone function have also been reported (Bresnick *et al.* 1989; Went *et al.* 1992). In advanced disease a typical rod sensitivity curve may be seen under both scotopic and photopic conditions (Goodman *et al.* 1963; Krill 1977a).

Electroretinography generally shows normal scotopic responses but absent or substantially abnormal photopic responses (Goodman *et al.* 1963; Berson *et al.* 1968; Krill 1977a). A small subgroup of patients with cone dystrophy may show supranormal scotopic responses (Gouras *et al.* 1983; Alexander & Fishman 1984b).

Obligate carriers of X-linked cone dystrophy may show evidence of cone dysfunction on electrophysiological or psychophysical testing (Heckenlively & Weleber 1986; Verdoorn & Pinckers 1988; Jacobson *et al.* 1989; Reichel *et al.* 1989; van Everdingen *et al.* 1992).

Progressive cone–rod dystrophy

In this uncommon disorder affected patients develop the typical findings of a cone dystrophy in early life but later there is evidence of rod involvement with night-blindness and peripheral field loss (Goodman *et al.* 1963; Berson *et al.* 1968; Evans *et al.* 1995a). Fundus examination shows macular atrophy in the early stages with peripheral retinal pigment epithelial atrophy, retinal pigmentation, arteriolar attenuation and optic disc pallor in the late stages of the disease. Both rod and cone thresholds are elevated on psychophysical testing and the ERG shows reduced rod and cone amplitudes (Goodman *et al.* 1963; Berson *et al.* 1968). The EOG may also be abnormal. Autosomal dominant, autosomal recessive and X-linked recessive inheritance may be seen.

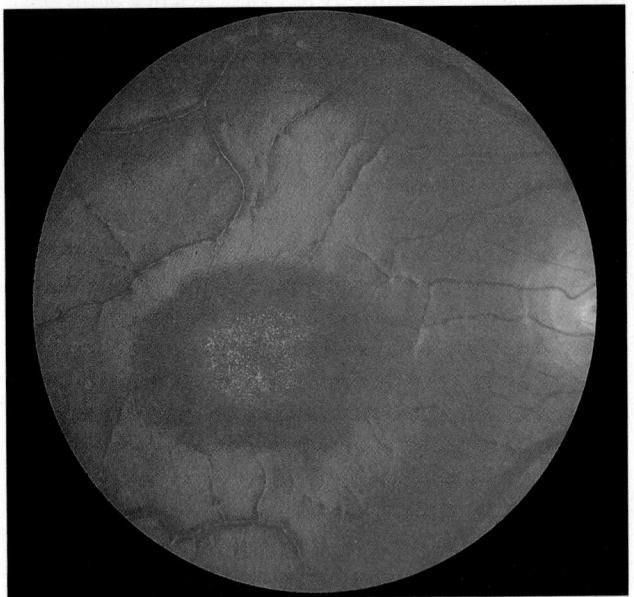

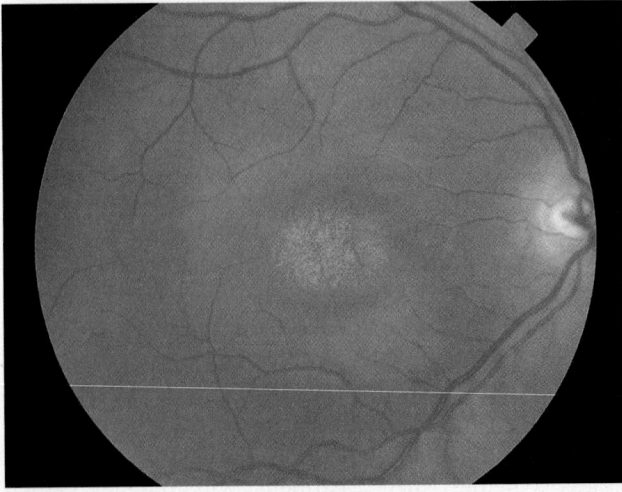

Fig. 44.38 (a) Progressive cone dystrophy in March 1982. (b) July 1985 showing minimal change (same patient)

Molecular genetics of cone and cone–rod dystrophies

Most cases of progressive cone and cone-rod dystrophy are sporadic but when familial cases are seen the most common mode of inheritance is autosomal dominant (Goodman *et al.* 1963; Berson *et al.* 1968; Krill & Deutmann 1972). Most of the sporadic cases probably represent autosomal recessive inheritance. Several well-documented families showing X-linked inheritance have been reported (Heckenlively & Weleber 1986; Verdoorn & Pinckers 1988; Jacobson *et al.* 1989; Reichel *et al.* 1989; van Everdingen *et al.* 1992).

Progressive cone dystrophy loci have been mapped to chromosomes 6q25–q26 (Tranebjaerg *et al.* 1986), Xq28 (Reichel *et al.* 1989) and Xp21–p11.1 (Meire *et al.* 1994). In the former X-linked cone dystrophy, good visual acuity is associated with predominant loss of longwave (red) cone function with normal rod function. Cone–rod dystrophy loci have been mapped to chromosomes 18q (Warburg *et al.* 1991) and 19q (Evans *et al.* 1994) and may be associated with peripherin/RDS gene mutations (Nakasawa *et al.* 1994). In addition Kylstra and Aylsworth (1993) have reported a patient with neurofibromatosis type 1 and a cone–rod dystrophy suggesting that there may be an additional locus on 17q.

Systemic associations of cone and cone–rod dystrophies

Dunya *et al.* (1993) have reported a 9-year-old boy with the cardiofaciocutaneous syndrome who had reduced vision and nystagmus; the fundus was normal but the ERG showed substantially abnormal photopic responses. The scotopic responses were normal. The cardiofaciocutaneous syndrome is a rare multisystem disorder characterized by developmental delay, growth retardation, dysmorphic facies, congenital heart defect and ectodermal dysplasia. The mode of inheritance is uncertain. Visual impairment, nystagmus and strabismus are common features (Young *et al.* 1993). In most reports the cause of the nystagmus is not detailed but the report of Dunya *et al.* (1993) suggests that the nystagmus in this syndrome may be related to an underlying cone dystrophy.

Bjork *et al.* (1956) have reported one pedigree of progressive cone–rod dystrophy in which affected members had an associated ataxia of the Pierre–Marie type. Jalili and Smith (1988) have described an autosomal recessive disorder characterized by a cone–rod dystrophy and amelogenesis imperfecta (defective tooth enamel). An early onset, autosomal recessive, cone–rod dystrophy has been described in association with trichomegaly and excessive body hair (Jalili 1989). In the syndrome of obesity, cardiomyopathy and retinal dystrophy described by Russell-Eggitt *et al.* (1989) the retinal dystrophy appears to be an early onset cone–rod dystrophy and a similar pattern of retinal disease is seen in Alstrom's syndrome.

References

Abraham FA, Yanko L, Licht A, Visroper RJ. Electrophysiologic study of the visual system in familial juvenile nephronophthisis and tapetoretinal dystrophy. *Am J Ophthalmol* 1974; **78**: 591–7.

al Maghtheh M, Gregory CY, Inglehearn CF *et al.* Rhodopsin mutations in autosomal dominant retinitis pigmentosa. *Hum Mutat* 1993; **2**: 249–55.

al Maghtheh M, Inglehearn CF, Keen TJ *et al.* Identification of a sixth locus for autosomal dominant retinitis pigmentosa on chromosome 19. *Hum Mol Genet* 1994; **3**: 351–4.

Albrechtsen B. Hypotrichiasis; syndactyly and retinal degeneration. *Acta Derm Venereol* 1956; **36**: 96–101.

Aldred MA, Kry KL, Sharp DM *et al.* Linkage analysis in X-linked congenital stationary night blindness. *Genomics* 1992; **14**: 99–104.

Aldred MA, Teague PW, Jay M. Retinitis pigmentosa families showing apparent X-linked inheritance but unlinked to the RP2 or RP3 loci. *J Med Genet* 1994; **31**: 848–52.

Alexander KR, Fishman GA. Prolonged rod adaptation in retinitis pigmentosa. *Br J Ophthalmol* 1984a; **68**: 561–9.

Alexander KR, Fishman GA. Supernormal scotopic ERG in cone dystrophy. *Br J Ophthalmol* 1984b; **68**: 69–78.

Allen AW, Moon JB, Holland KR, Minckley DS. Ocular findings in the thoracic–pelvic–phalangeal dystrophy. *Arch Ophthalmol* 1979; **97**: 489–92.

Alpern M, Lee GB, Spivey B. Π_1 cone monochromatism. *Arch Ophthalmol* 1965; **74**: 334–7.

Alström CH, Hallgren B, Nilson LB, Asander H. Retinal degeneration combined with obesity, diabetes mellitus, and neurogenic deafness. *Acta Psychiatr Scand* 1959; **34**: 1–35.

Alström CH, Olson OA. Heredo-retinopathia congenitalis. Monohybrida recessiva autosomalis. *Hereditas* 1957; **43**: 1–177.

Alter CA, Moshang T Jr. Growth hormone deficiency in two siblings with Alström syndrome. *Am J Dis Child* 1993; **147**: 97–9.

Alvarez F, Landrieu P, Laget P *et al.* Nervous and ocular disorders in children with cholestasis and vitamin A and E deficiency. *Hepatology* 1983; **3**: 410–14.

Amman F, Klein D, Franceschetti A. Genetic and epidemiological investigations on pigmentary degeneration of the retina and allied disorders in Switzerland. *J Neurol Sci* 1965; **2**: 183–96.

Andreasson S, Blennow G, Ehinger B, Stromland K. Full field electroretinograms in patients with the carbohydrate-deficient glycoprotein syndrome. *Am J Ophthalmol* 1991; **112**: 83–6.

Andreasson S, Tornquist K. Electroretinograms in patients with achromatopsia. *Acta Ophthalmologica* 1991; **69**: 711–16.

Apfelstedt-Sylla E, Kunisch M, Horn M, Rüther K, Gerding H, Gal A, Zrenner E. Ocular findings in a family with autosomal dominant retinitis pigmentosa and a frameshift mutation altering the carboxyl terminal sequence of rhodopsin. *Br J Ophthalmol* 1993; **77**: 495–501.

Apfelstedt-Sylla E, Theischen M, Rüther K, Wedermann H, Gal A, Zrenner E. Extensive intrafamilial and interfamilial phenotypic variation among patients with autosomal dominant retinal dystrophy and mutations in the human RDS/peripherin gene. *Br J Ophthalmol* 1995; **79**: 28–34.

Arden GB, Carter RM, Hogg CR *et al.* A modified ERG technique and the results obtained in X-linked retinitis pigmentosa. *Br J Ophthalmol* 1983; **67**: 419–30.

Arden GB, Fox B. Increased incidence of abnormal nasal cilia in patients with retinitis pigmentosa. *Nature* 1979; **279**: 534–6.

Auerbach E, Godel V, Rowe H. An electrophysiological and psychophysical study of two forms of congenital night-blindness.

Invest Ophthalmol 1969; **8**: 332–45.

Ayazi S. Choroideremia, obesity, and congenital deafness. *Am J Ophthalmol* 1981; **92**: 63–9.

Ayyagari R, Smith RJH, Polymeropoulos M *et al*. Linkage and haplotype analysis and physical mapping of the USH 1C gene. *Invest Ophthalmol Vis Sci* 1994; **35**: 2143.

Bard LA, Bard PA, Owens GW *et al*. Retinal involvement in thoracic–pelvic–phalangeal dystrophy. *Arch Ophthalmol* 1978; **96**: 278–81.

Barrong SD, Chaitin MH, Fliesler SJ *et al*. Ultrastructure of connecting cilia in different forms of retinitis pigmentosa *Arch Ophthalmol* 1992; **110**: 706–10.

Bateman JB, Lang GE, Maumeneee IH. Multisystem genetic disorders associated with retinal dystrophies. In: Ryan SJ, ed. *Retina*. St Louis: Mosby Year Book, 1994: 467–9.

Bergen AA, ten Brink JB, Riemslag F *et al*. Localization of a novel X-linked congenital stationary night-blindness locus: close linkage to the RP3 type retinitis pigmentosa gene region. *Hum Mol Genet* 1995; **4**: 931–5.

Berson E, Adamian M. Ultrastructural findings I. An autopsy eye from a patient with Usher's syndrome type II. *Am J Ophthalmol* 1992; **114**: 748–58.

Berson EL, Gouras P, Gunkel RD. Progressive cone degeneration dominantly inherited. *Arch Ophthalmol* 1968; **80**: 77–83.

Berson EL, Howard J. Temporal aspects of the electroretinogram in sector retinitis pigmentosa. *Arch Ophthalmol* 1971; **48**: 653–65.

Berson EL, Rosen JB, Siminoff EA. Electroretinographic testing as an aid in detection of X chromosome linked retinitis pigmentosa. *Am J Ophthalmol* 1979; **87**: 460–8.

Berson EL, Rosner B, Sandberg MA *et al*. A randomised controlled trial of vitamin A and vitamin E supplementation for retinitis pigmentosa. *Arch Ophthalmol* 1993; **111**: 761–2.

Berson EL, Sandberg MA, Maguire A. Electroretinogram in carriers of blue cone monochromatism. *Am J Ophthalmol* 1986; **102**: 254–61.

Berson EL, Schmidt SY, Shih VE. Ocular and biochemical abnormalities in gyrate atrophy of the choroid and retina. *Ophthalmology* 1978; **85**: 1018–27.

Berson EL, Simonoff EA. Dominant retinitis pigmentosa with reduced penetrance. Further studies of the electroretinogram. *Arch Ophthalmol* 1979; **97**: 1286–91.

Bertini E, Dionisis-Vici C, Garavaglia B *et al*. Peripheral sensory neuropathy, pigmentary retinopathy and fatal cardiomyopathy in long chain 3-hydroxy-acyl–CoA–dehydrogenase deficiency. *Eur J Pediatr* 1992; **151**: 121–6.

Bhattacharya SS, Wright AF, Clayton JF *et al*. Close genetic linkage between X-linked retinitis pigmentosa and a restriction fragment polymorphism identified by recombinant DNA probe. *Nature* 1984; **309**: 253–5.

Bird AC. Retinal photoreceptor dystrophies. *Am J Ophthalmol* 1995; **118**: 543–62.

Bird AC. X-linked retinitis pigmentosa. *Br J Ophthalmol* 1975; **59**: 177–99.

Bird AC, Hyman V. Detection of heterozygotes in families with X-linked pigmentary retinopathy by measurement of retinal rhodopsin concentration. *Trans Ophthalmol Soc UK* 1972; **92**: 221–8.

Bishihara S, Merin S, Cooper M *et al*. Combined vitamin A and E therapy prevents retinal electrophysiological deterioration in abetalipoproteinaemia. *Br J Ophthalmol* 1982; **66**: 767–70.

Bjork A, Lindblau U, Wadensten L. Retinal degeneration in hereditary ataxia. *J Neurol Neurosurg Psychiatr* 1956; **19**: 186–93.

Blanton SH, Heckenlively JR, Cottingham AW *et al*. Linkage mapping of autosomal dominant retinitis pigmentosa (RP1) to the pericentric region of human chromosome 8. *Genomics* 1991; **11**: 857–69.

Bonnin J, Passot M, Triolaire M. Le signe du silence choroidien dans les degenerescences tapeto-retiniennes posterieures. *Doc Ophthalmol Proc Ser* 1976; **9**: 461–3.

Boughman JA, Fishman GA. A genetic analysis of retinitis pigmentosa. *Br J Ophthalmol* 1983; **67**: 449–54.

Boughman JA, Vernon M, Shaver KA. Usher syndrome definition and prevalence from two high risk populations. *J Chronic Dis* 1983; **36**: 595–603.

Bravermann N, Dodt G, Gould SJ, Valle D. Disorders of peroxisome biogenesis. *Hum Mol Genet* 1995; **4**: 1791–8.

Bresnick GH, Smith VC, Pokorny J. Autosomal dominant inherited macular dystrophy with preferential short wavelength sensitive cone involvement. *Am J Ophthalmol* 1989; **108**: 265–76.

Britton TC, Gibberd FB. A family with heredopathia atactica polyneuritiformis (Refsum's disease). *J Roy Soc Med* 1988; **81**: 602–3.

Brodsky MC, Cunniff C. Ocular anomalies in the Alagille syndrome (arteriohepatic dysplasia). *Ophthalmology* 1993; **100**: 1767–74.

Brosnahan D, Kennedy S, Converse C, Loe W, Hammer H. Pathology of hereditary retinal degeneration associated with hypobeta-lipoproteinaemia. *Ophthalmology* 1994; **101**: 38–45.

Buchanan NM, Atta HR, Crean GJP *et al*. A case of eye disease due to dietary vitamin A deficiency in Glasgow. *Scott Med J* 1987; **32**: 52–3.

Campo RV, Aaberg TM. Ocular and systemic manifestations of the Bardet–Biedl syndrome. *Am J Ophthalmol* 1982; **94**: 750–6.

Camuzat A, Dollfus H, Rozet J-M *et al*. A gene for Leber's congenital amaurosis maps to chromosome 17p. *Hum Mol Genet* 1995; **4**: 1447–52.

Carmi R, Rokhlina T, Kwitek-Black *et al*. Use of a DNA pooling strategy to identify a human obesity syndrome locus on chromosome 15. *Hum Mol Genet* 1995; **4**: 9–13.

Carr RF, Gouras P. Oguchi's disease. *Arch Ophthalmol* 1965; **73**: 646–56.

Carr RE, Rupps H, Siegel IM. Visual pigment kinetics and adaptation in fundus albipunctatus. *Doc Ophthalmol Proc Ser* 1974; **4**: 193–204.

Carr RE, Siegel IM. Unilateral retinitis pigmentosa. *Arch Ophthalmol* 1973; **90**: 21–6.

Caruso RC, Kaiser-Kupfer MI, Muenzer J *et al*. Electroretinographic findings in the mucopolysaccharidoses. *Ophthalmology* 1986; **93**: 1612–16.

Charles SJ, Moore AT, Yates JRW, Green T, Green P. Alstrom's syndrome: further evidence for autosomal recessive inheritance and endocrinological dysfunction. *J Med Genet* 1990; **27**: 590–2.

Chew E, Deutman A, Pinckers A, DeKirk AA. Yellowish flecks in Leber's congenital amaurosis. *Br J Ophthalmol* 1984; **84**: 727–31.

Claridge KG, Gibberd FB, Sidey MC. Refsum's disease. The presentation and ophthalmologic aspects of Refsum's disease in a series of 23 patients. *Eye* 1992; **6**: 371–5.

Clarke MP, Sullivan TJ, Francis C, Baumal R, Fenton T, Pearce W. Senior–Loken syndrome. Case reports of two siblings and association with sensorineural deafness. *Br J Ophthalmol* 1992; **76**: 171–2.

Clayton PT, Winchester BG, Keir G. Hypertrophic obstructive cardiomyopathy in a neonate with the carbohydrate-deficient glycoprotein syndrome. *J Inherit Metab Dis* 1992; **15**: 857–61.

Cohen MM, Hall BD, Smith DW *et al*. A new syndrome with hypotonia, obesity, mental deficiency and facial, oral, ocular, and limb anomalies. *J Paediatr* 1973; **83**: 280–4.

Cohen SMZ, Brown FR, Martyn L *et al*. Ocular histopathologic and biochemical studies of the cerebrohepatorenal syndrome (Zellweger's syndrome) and its relationship to neonatal adrenoleukodystrophy. *Am J Ophthalmol* 1983a; **96**: 488–501.

Cohen SMZ, Green WR, De la Cruz ZC *et al*. Ocular histopathologic studies of neonatal and childhood adrenoleukodystrophy. *Am J*

Ophthalmol 1983b; **95**: 82–96.

Coles WH. Ocular manifestations of Cockayne's syndrome. *Am J Ophthalmol* 1969; **67**: 762–4.

Cremers PM, van der Pol DJR, van Kerkhof LPN *et al*. Cloning of a gene that is rearranged in patients with choroideremia. *Nature* 1990; **347**: 674–7.

Davies S, Marcus RE, Hungerford JL *et al*. Ocular toxicity of high dose intravenous desferrioxamine. *Lancet* 1983; **ii**: 181–4.

de Jong PTVM, de Jong JGY, de Jong-Ten Doeschate JMM, Delleman JW. Olivopontocerebellar atrophy with visual disturbances. An ophthalmological investigation into four generations. *Ophthalmology* 1980; **87**: 793–804.

Dekaban AS. Hereditary syndrome of congenital retinal blindness (Leber), polycystic kidneys and maldevelopment of the brain. *Am J Ophthalmol* 1969; **68**: 1029–36.

Dekaban AS. Mental retardation and neurological involvement in patients with congenital retinal blindness. *Dev Med Child Neurol* 1972; **14**: 436–44.

Dekaban AS, Carr R. Congenital amaurosis of retinal origin. Frequent association with neurological disorders. *Arch Neurol* 1966; **14**: 294–301.

Drachman DA. Ophthalmoplegia plus. The neuro-degenerative disorders associated with progressive external ophthalmoplegia. *Arch Neurol* 1968; **18**: 654–74.

Drack A, Traboulsi E, Maumenee I. Progression of retinopathy in olivopontocerebellar atrophy with retinal degeneration. *Arch Ophthalmol* 1992; **110**: 712–14.

Dryja TP, Berson EL, Rao VR, Oprian DD. Heterozygous missense mutation in the rhodopsin gene as a cause of congenital stationary night blindness. *Nature Genet* 1993; **4**: 280–3.

Dryja TP, Finn JT, Peng YW *et al*. Mutations in the gene encoding the α subunit of the rod cGMP-gated channel in autosomal recessive retinitis pigmentosa. *Proc Natl Acad Sci USA* 1995; **92**: 10177–81.

Dryja TP, Li T. Molecular genetics of retinitis pigmentosa. *Hum Mol Genet* 1995; **4**: 1739–43.

Dryja TP, McGee TL, Reichel E *et al*. A point mutation of the rhodopsin gene in one form of retinitis pigmentosa. *Nature* 1990; **343**: 364–6.

Dunya I, Hoon A, Traboulsi EI. Retinal dystrophy in the cardio-facio-cutaneous syndrome. *J Pediatr Ophthalmol Strabismus* 1993; **30**: 264–5.

Dyer DS, Wilson E, Small K, Pai GS. Alström syndrome: a case misdiagnosed as the Bardet–Biedl syndrome. *J Pediatr Ophthalmol Strabismus* 1994; **31**: 272–4.

Edwards WC, Grizzard WS. Tapeto-retinal degeneration associated with renal disease. *J Pediatr Ophthalmol Strabismus* 1981; **18**: 55–7.

Eggar J, Lake BD, Wilson J. Mitochondrial cytopathy. A multisystem disorder with ragged red fibres on muscle biopsy. *Arch Dis Child* 1981; **56**: 741–52.

Ellis DS, Heckenlively JR, Martin CL *et al*. Leber's congenital amaurosis associated with familial juvenile nephronophthisis and cone-shaped epiphyses of the hands (the Saldino–Mainzer syndrome). *Am J Ophthalmol* 1984; **97**: 233–9.

Ernst W, Clover G, Faulkner DJ. X-linked retinitis pigmentosa: reduced rod flicker sensitivity in heterozygous females. *Invest Ophthalmol Vis Sci* 1981; **20**: 812–16.

Escallon F, Traboulsi EI, Infante R. A family with the Bardet–Biedl syndrome and diabetes mellitus. *Arch Ophthalmol* 1989; **107**: 855–7.

Evans K, Duvall-Young J, Fitzke FW *et al*. Chromosome 19 cone–rod retinal dystrophy. Ocular phenotype. *Arch Ophthalmol* 1995a; **113**: 195–201.

Evans K, Fryer A, Inglehearn C *et al*. Genetic linkage of cone–rod retinal dystrophy to chromosome 19q and evidence for segregation distortion. *Nature Genet* 1994; **6**: 210–13.

Evans K, Moore AT, Jubb C *et al*. Bimodal expressivity in autosomal dominant retinitis pigmentosa genetically linked to chromosome 19q. *Br J Ophthalmol* 1995b; **99**: 841–6.

Fairley KF, Leighton PW, Kincaid-Smith P. Familial visual defects associated with polycystic kidney and medullary sponge kidney. *Br Med J* 1963; **1**: 1060–3.

Falls HF, Wolter JR, Alpern M. Typical total monochromacy. *Arch Ophthalmol* 1965; **74**: 610–16.

Farrar GJ, Kenna P, Jordan SA *et al*. A three-base-pair deletion in the peripherin–RDS gene in one form of retinitis pigmentosa. *Nature* 1991; **354**: 478–80.

Fishman GA, Anderson RJ, Lam BL, Derlacki DJ. Prevalence of foveal lesions in type 1 and type 2 Usher syndrome. *Arch Ophthalmol* 1995; **113**: 770–3.

Fishman GA, Gilbert LD, Fiscella RG *et al*. Acetazolamide for treatment of chronic macular oedema in retinitis pigmentosa. *Arch Ophthalmol* 1989; **107**: 1445–52.

Fishman GA, Kumar A, Joseph ME *et al*. Usher's syndrome: ophthalmic and neuro-otologic findings suggesting genetic heterogeneity. *Arch Ophthalmol* 1983; **101**: 1367–74.

Fishman GA, Stone E, Gilbert L, Vanenburgh K, Sheffield V, Heckenlively J. Clinical features of a previously undescribed codon 216 mutation in the peripherin/retinal degeneration slow gene in autosomal dominant retinitis pigmentosa. *Ophthalmology* 1994; **101**: 1409–21.

Fishman GA, Weinburg AB, McMahon TT. X-linked recessive retinitis pigmentosa: clinical characteristics of carriers. *Arch Ophthalmol* 1986; **104**: 1329–35.

Fiumara A, Barone R, Buttitta P *et al*. Carbohydrate deficient glycoprotein syndrome type 1: ophthalmic aspects in four Sicilian patients. *Br J Ophthalmol* 1994; **78**: 845–6.

Flynn JT, Cullen RF. Disc oedema in congenital amaurosis of Leber. *Br J Ophthalmol* 1975; **59**: 497–502.

Folz S, Trobe J. The peroxisome and the eye. *Surv Ophthalmol* 1991; **35**: 353–69.

Forsius H, Eriksson AW. Ein neues augensyndrom mit X-chromosomaler transmission. *Klin Monatsbl Augenheilkd* 1964; **144**: 447–57.

Foxman SG, Heckenlively JR, Bateman JB, Wirtschafter JD. Classification of congenital and early onset retinitis pigmentosa. *Arch Ophthalmol* 1985; **103**: 1502–6.

Foxman SG, Wirtschafter JD, Letson RD. Leber's congenital amaurosis and high hypermetropia: a discrete entity. In: Henkind P, ed. *ACTA XXIV International Congress Ophthalmology*, Vol. 1. Philadelphia: JB Lippincott, 1983: 55–8.

Franceschetti A. Rubeole pendant la grossesse et cataracte congenitale chez l'enfant: accompagne du phenomene digitooculaire. *Ophthalmologica* 1947; **114**: 332–9.

François J. Metabolic tapetoretinal degenerations. *Surv Ophthalmol* 1982; **26**: 293–333.

Friedrich U, Warburg M, Jorgensen AL. X-inactivation pattern in carriers of X-linked retinitis pigmentosa: a valuable means of prognostic evaluation. *Hum Genet* 1993; **92**: 359–63.

Friedrich U, Warburg M, Wiezacker P *et al*. X-linked retinitis pigmentosa: linkage with the centromere and a cloned DNA sequence from the proximal short arm of the X chromosome. *Hum Genet* 1985; **71**: 93–9.

Fuchs S, Nakazawa M, Maw M *et al*. A homozygous 1 base pair deletion in the arrestin gene is a frequent cause of Ogouchi's disease in Japanese. *Nature Genet* 1995; **10**: 360–2.

Fulton AB, Hansen RM, Glynn RJ. Natural course of visual functions in the Bardet–Biedl syndrome. *Arch Ophthalmol* 1993; **111**: 1500–6.

Gal A, Orth U, Baehr W *et al*. Heterozygous missense mutation in the rod cGMP phosphodiesterase beta subunit gene in autosomal dominant stationary night blindness. *Nature Genet* 1994; **7**: 64–8.

Gardiner M, Sandford A, Deadman M *et al.* Batten disease (Spielmeyer–Vogt disease, juvenile onset neuronal ceroid–lipofuscinosis) gene (CLN3) maps to human chromosome 16. *Genomics* 1990; **8**: 387–90.

Garner A, Fielder AR, Primavesi R, Steven A. Tapetoretinal degeneration in the cerebro–hepato–renal (Zellweger) syndrome. *Br J Ophthalmol* 1982; **66**: 422–31.

Gelber PJ, Shah A. Fluorescein study of albipunctate dystrophy. *Arch Ophthalmol* 1969; **81**: 164–9.

Gibson F, Walsh J, Mburu P. A type VII myosin encoded by the mouse deafness gene *shaker –1. Nature* 1995; **374**: 62–4.

Gieser DK, Fishman GA, Cunha-Vaz J. X-linked retinitis pigmentosa and vitreous fluorophotometry: a study of female heterozygotes. *Arch Ophthalmol* 1980; **98**: 307–10.

Gil-Gilberneau J, Galain A, Callis L, Rodrigo C. Infantile idiopathic hypercalciuria, high congenital myopia and atypical macular coloboma: a new oculorenal syndrome. *J Pediatr Ophthalmol Strabismus* 1982; **19**: 7–11.

Glasgow BJ, Brown HH, Hannah JB, Foos RY. Ocular pathologic findings in neonatal adrenoleucodystrophy. *Ophthalmology* 1987; **94**: 1054–60.

Glass IA, Good P, Coleman MP *et al.* Genetic mapping of cone and rod dysfunction (Åland eye disease) to the proximal short arm of the human X chromosome. *J Med Genet* 1993; **30**: 1044–50.

Glickstein M, Heath GG. Receptors in the monochromat eye. *Vision Res* 1975; **15**: 633–6.

Goldman JM, Clemens ME, Gibberd JB, Billimoria JD. Screening of patients with retinitis pigmentosa for heredopathia atactica polyneuritiformis (Refsum's disease). *Br Med J* 1985; **290**: 1109–10.

Goldstein JL, Fialkow PJ. The Alström syndrome. Report of three cases with further delineation of the clinical, pathophysiological and genetic aspects of the disorder. *Medicine* 1973; **52**: 53–71.

Goodman G, Ripps H, Siegel IM. Cone dysfunction syndromes. *Arch Ophthalmol* 1963; **70**: 214–31.

Gottlob I. Eye movement abnormalities in carriers of blue cone monochromatism. *Invest Ophthalmol Vis Sci* 1994; **35**: 3556–60.

Gotto AM, Levy RI, John K, Fredrickson DS. On the protein defect in Abetalipoproteinemia. *N Engl J Med* 1971; **284**: 813–15.

Gouras P, Eggers HM, Mackay C. Cone dystrophy, nyctalopia and supernormal rod responses. A new retinal degeneration. *Arch Ophthalmol* 1983; **101**: 718–24.

Gouw LG, Kaplan CD, Haines JH *et al.* Retinal degeneration characterizes a spinocerebellar ataxia mapping to chromosome 3p. *Nature Genet* 1995; **10**: 89–93.

Grey RHB. Visual field changes following hepatic transplantation in a patient with primary biliary cirrhosis. *Br J Ophthalmol* 1991; **75**: 377–81.

Haddad R, Font RL, Friendly DS. Cerebro–hepato–renal syndrome of Zellweger. Ocular histopathologic findings. *Arch Ophthalmol* 1976; **94**: 1927–30.

Hajra AK, Datta NS, Jackson LG *et al.* Prenatal diagnosis of Zellweger cerebro–hepato–renal syndrome. *N Engl J Med* 1985; **312**: 445–6.

Hallervorden J, Spatz H. Eigenartige erkrankung im extrapyramidalen system mit besonderer betelligung des globus pallidus unter der substantia Nigra. *Z Neurol Psychiatr* 1922; **79**: 254–62.

Harbord MG, Lambert SR, Kriss A, Brett AM, Baraitser M, Supramanian G. Autosomal recessive microcephaly, mental retardation with non-pigmentary retinopathy with a distinctive electroretinogram. *Neuropediatrics* 1989; **20**: 139–41.

Harding AE. The clinical features and classification of the late onset autosomal dominant cerebellar ataxias. A study of 11 families including descendants of the Drew family of Walworth. *Brain* 1982; **105**: 1–28.

Harding AE. *The Hereditary Ataxias and Related Disorders.* Edinburgh: Churchill Livingstone, 1984: 150.

Harrison R, Hoefnagel D, Hayward JN. Congenital total colour blindness, a clinicopathological report. *Arch Ophthalmol* 1960; **64**: 685–92.

Hauser C, Rojas C, Roth A *et al.* A patient with features of both Bardet–Biedl and Alström syndromes. *Pediatrics* 1990; **149**: 783–5.

Hawksworth NR, Headland S, Good P, Thomas NST, Clarke A. Åland eye disease: clinical and electrophysiological studies of a Welsh family. *Br J Ophthalmol* 1995; **79**: 424–30.

Heckenlively JR. *Retinitis Pigmentosa.* Philadelphia: JB Lippincott, 1988.

Heckenlively JR, Martin DA, Rosenbaum AL. Loss of electroretinographic oscillatory potentials, optic atrophy, and dysplasia in congenital stationary night-blindness. *Am J Ophthalmol* 1983; **96**: 526–34.

Heckenlively JR, Rodrigues JA, Daiger SP. Autosomal dominant sectoral retinitis pigmentosa, two families with transversion mutation in codon 23 of rhodopsin. *Arch Ophthalmol* 1991; **104**: 89–91.

Heckenlively JR, Weleber RG. X-linked recessive cone dystrophy with tapetal-like sheen. *Arch Ophthalmol* 1986; **104**: 1322–8.

Heher KL, Traboulsi EI, Maumenee IH. The natural history of Leber's congenital amaurosis. Age-related findings in 35 patients. *Ophthalmology* 1992; **99**: 241–5.

Herdman RC, Good R, Vernier RL, Anderson LA. Medullary cystic disease in two siblings. *Am J Med* 1967; **43**: 335–44.

Hittner HM, Kretzer FL, Mehta RS. Zellweger's syndrome: lenticular opacities indicating carrier status and lens abnormalities characteristic of homozygotes. *Arch Ophthalmol* 1981; **99**: 1977–82.

Holt IJ, Harding AE, Cooper JM *et al.* Mitochondrial myopathies, clinical and biochemical features of 30 patients with major deletions of muscle mitochondrial DNA. *Ann Neurol* 1989; **26**: 699–708.

Hoyt CS, Billson FA. Visual loss in osteopetrosis. *Am J Dis Child* 1979; **133**: 955–8.

Huang SH, Pittler SJ, Huang X *et al.* Autosomal recessive retinitis pigmentosa caused by mutations in the α subunit of rod cGMP phosphodiesterase. *Nature Genet* 1995; **11**: 468–71.

Hunter DG, Fishman GA, Mehta RS, Kretzer FL. Abnormal sperm and photoreceptor axonemes in Usher's syndrome. *Arch Ophthalmol* 1986; **104**: 385–9.

Hurley R, Dery P, Nogrady M, Drummond K. The renal lesion of Laurence–Moon–Biedl syndrome. *J Pediatr* 1975; **87**: 206–9.

Inglehearn CF, Carter SA, Keen TJ *et al.* A new locus for autosomal dominant retinitis pigmentosa on chromosome 7p. *Nature Genet* 1993; **4**: 51–3.

International Standardisation Committee. Standard for clinical electroretinography. *Arch Ophthalmol* 1989; **107**: 816–19.

Jacobson DM, Thompson S, Bartley JA. X-linked progressive cone dystrophy. Clinical characteristics of affected males and female carriers. *Ophthalmology* 1989; **96**: 885–95.

Jacobson SG, Borruat F, Apathy P. Patterns of rod and cone dysfunction in Bardet–Biedl syndrome. *Am J Ophthalmol* 1990; **109**: 676–89.

Jaeken J, Carchon H. The carbohydrate deficient glycoprotein syndrome: an overview. *J Inherit Metab Dis* 1993; **16**: 813–20.

Jaeken J, Scaater H, Carchon H, De Cock P, Codderville B, Spik G. Carbohydrate deficient glycoprotein syndrome type II: a deficiency in Golgi localised N-acetyl-glucosaminyl-transferase II. *Arch Dis Child* 1994; **71**: 123–7.

Jaeken J, Stibler H, Hagberg H, eds. The carbohydrate deficient glycoprotein syndrome. A new inherited multisystem disorder with severe nervous system involvement. *Acta Paediatr Scand* 1991; **375**(Suppl.): 5–71.

Jalili IK. Cone–rod congenital amaurosis associated with congenital hypertrichosis: an autosomal recessive condition. *J Med Genet* 1989; **26**: 504–10.

Jalili IK, Smith NJD. A progressive cone–rod dystrophy and amelogenesis imperfecta: a new syndrome. *J Med Genet* 1988; **25**: 738–40.

Jay M. On the heredity of retinitis pigmentosa. *Br J Ophthalmol* 1982; **66**: 405–16.

Jensen H, Warburg M, Sjo O *et al.* Duchenne muscular dystrophy: negative electroretinograms and normal dark adaptation. Reappraisal of assignment of X-linked congenital stationary night blindness. *J Med Genet* 1995; **32**: 348–51.

Jeune M, Beraud C, Canon R. Dystrophie thoracique asphyxiante de caractere familial. *Arch Fr Pediatr* 1955; **12**: 886–91.

Johns DR. mtDNA mutations and ophthalmological disease. In: Wiggs JL, ed. *Molecular Genetics of Ocular Disease*. New York: Wiley–Liss, 1994: 201–8.

Jordan SA, Farrar GJ, Kenna P *et al.* Localization of an autosomal dominant retinitis pigmentosa gene to chromosome 7q. *Nature Genet* 1993; **4**: 54–8.

Joubert M, Eisenring J, Robb JP, Andermann F. Familial agenesis of the cerebellar vermis. *Neurology* 1969; **19**: 813–25.

Judisch GF, Lowry B, Hanson JW. Chorioretinopathy and pituitary dysfunction. The CPD syndrome. *Arch Ophthalmol* 1981; **99**: 253–61.

Judisch GF, Rhead WJ, Miler DK. Abetalipoproteinemia. *Ophthalmologica* 1984; **189**: 73–9.

Kaiser-Kupfer M, Kuwabara T, Askanas V *et al.* Systemic manifestations of gyrate atrophy of the choroid and retina. *Ophthalmology* 1981; **88**: 302–6.

Kaiser-Kupfer M, Ludwig IH, de Monasterio FM *et al.* Gyrate atrophy of the choroid and retina. Early findings. *Ophthalmology* 1985; **92**: 394–401.

Kajiwara K, Berson EL, Dryja TP. Digenic retinitis pigmentosa due to mutations at the unlinked peripherin/RDS and ROM 1 loci. *Science* 1994; **264**: 1604–8.

Kajiwara K, Hahn LB, Mukai S *et al.* Mutations in the human retinal degeneration slow gene in autosomal dominant retinitis pigmentosa. *Nature* 1991; **354**: 480–2.

Kaplan J, Bonneau D, Frezal J *et al.* Clinical and genetic heterogeneity in retinitis pigmentosa. *Hum Genet* 1990; **85**: 635–42.

Kaplan J, Gerber S, Bonneau D *et al.* A gene for Usher syndrome type 1 (USH1A) maps to chromosome 14q. *Genomics* 1992; **14**: 979–87.

Karna J. Choroideremia: a clinical and genetic study of 84 Finnish patients and 126 female carriers. *Acta Ophthalmol* 1986; **176**(Suppl.): 1–68.

Kearns TP, Sayre GP. Retinitis pigmentosa, external ophthalmoplegia and complete heart block. Unusual syndrome with histologic study in one of two cases. *Arch Ophthalmol* 1958; **60**: 280–9.

Keith CG. Retinal atrophy in osteopetrosis. *Arch Ophthalmol* 1968; **79**: 234–41.

Kemp CM, Jacobson SG, Faulkner DJ. Two types of visual dysfunction in autosomal dominant retinitis pigmentosa. *Invest Ophthalmol Vis Sci* 1988; **29**: 1235–41.

Kemp CM, Jacobsen SG, Roman AJ *et al.* Abnormal rod adaptation in autosomal dominant retinitis pigmentosa with Pro-23-His rhodopsin mutation. *Am J Ophthalmol* 1992; **113**: 165–74.

Kennaway NG, Weleber RG, Buist NRM. Gyrate atrophy of the choroid and retina: deficient activity of ornithine ketoacid aminotransferase in cultured skin fibroblasts. *N Engl J Med* 1977; **297**: 1180.

Kim RY, Fitzke FW, Moore AT *et al.* Autosomal dominant retinitis pigmentosa mapping to chromosome 7p exhibits variable expression.

Br J Ophthalmol 1995; **79**: 23–7.

Kimberling WJ, Moller CG, Davenport S *et al.* Linkage of Usher syndrome type 1B (USH1B) to the long arm of chromosome 11. *Genomics* 1992; **14**: 988–94.

Kimberling WJ, Weston MD, Moller C *et al* Localisation of Usher syndrome type II to chromosome 1q. *Genomics* 1990; **7**: 245–9.

King MD, Dudgeon J, Stephenson JBP. Joubert's syndrome with retinal dysplasia; neonatal tachypnoea as the clue to a genetic brain–eye malformation. *Arch Dis Child* 1984; **59**: 709–18.

Klein D, Amman F. The syndrome of Lawrence–Moon–Biedl–Bardet and allied diseases in Switzerland. Clinical genetic and epidemiological studies. *J Neurol Sci* 1969; **9**: 479–89.

Klystra JA, Aylsworth AS. Cone–rod retinal dystrophy in a patient with neurofibromatosis type 1. *Canad J Ophthalmol* 1993; **28**: 79–80.

Kobayashi M, Morishita H, Sugiyama N *et al.* Mitochondrial encephalopathy, lactic acidosis and stroke like episodes syndrome and NADH CoQ reductase deficiency. *J Inherit Metab Dis* 1986; **9**: 301–4.

Kremer I, Ingber A, Ben-Sira I. Corneal metastatic calcification in Werner's syndrome. *Am J Ophthalmol* 1988; **106**: 221–7.

Krill AE. Cone degenerations. In: Krill AE, ed. *Hereditary Retinal and Choroidal Disease*, Vol II. London: Harper & Row, 1977a: 335–90.

Krill AE. Congenital colour vision defects. In: Krill AE, ed. *Hereditary Retinal and Choroidal Disease*, Vol II. London: Harper & Row, 1977b: 355–90.

Krill AE. Congenital stationary night-blindness. In: Krill AE, ed. *Hereditary Retinal and Choroidal Disease*, Vol. II. London: Harper & Row, 1977c: 391–417.

Krill AE, Deutman AF. Dominant macular degeneration. The cone dystrophies. *Am J Ophthalmol* 1972; **73**: 352–9.

Krill AE, Martin D. Photopic abnormalities in congenital stationary night-blindness. *Invest Ophthalmol Vis Sci* 1971; **107**: 625–36.

Kwitek-Black AE, Carmi R, Duyk DM *et al.* Linkage of Bardet–Biedl syndrome to chromosome 16q and evidence for non-allelic heterogeneity. *Nature Genet* 1993; **5**: 392–6.

Kylstra JA, Aylsworth AS. Cone–rod retinal dystrophy in a patient with neurofibromatosis type 1. *Canad J Ophthalmol* 1993; **28**: 79–80.

Lakhampal V, Schockett SS, Jiji R. Desferrioxamine (Desferol) induced toxic retinal pigmentary degeneration and presumed optic neuropathy. *Ophthalmology* 1984; **91**: 443–51.

Lam B, Judisch GF. Early onset autosomal dominant retinitis pigmentosa with severe hyperopia. *Am J Ophthalmol* 1991; **111**: 454–7.

Lam B, Vandenburgh K, Sheffield V, Stone E. Retinitis pigmentosa associated with a dominant mutation in codon 46 of the peripherin/RDS gene (arginine-46-stop). *Am J Ophthalmol* 1995; **119**: 65–71.

Lambert SR, Kriss A, Gresty M, Benton S, Taylor D. Joubert syndrome. *Arch Ophthalmol* 1989a; **107**: 109–13.

Lambert SR, Kriss A, Taylor D, Coffey R, Pembrey M. Leber's congenital amaurosis: a follow-up diagnostic reappraisal of 75 patients. *Am J Ophthalmol* 1989b; **107**: 624–31.

Lambert S, Sherman S, Taylor D, Kriss A, Coffey R, Pembrey M. Concordance and recessive inheritance of Leber's congenital amaurosis. *Am J Med Genet* 1993; **46**: 275–7.

Larsen H. Demonstration microskopischer praparate von einem monochromatischen auge. *Ophthalmologica* 1921; **46**: 228–9.

Laurence JZ, Moon RC. Four cases of retinitis pigmentosa occurring in the same family and accompanied by general imperfections of development. *Ophthalmic Rev* 1866; **2**: 32–41.

Leppert M, Baird L, Anderson KL *et al.* Bardet–Biedl syndrome is linked to DNA markers on chromosome 11q and is genetically heterogeneous. *Nature Genet* 1994; **7**: 108–12.

Levin PS, Green WR, Victor DI, Maclean AL. Histopathology of the eye in Cockayne's syndrome. *Arch Ophthalmol* 1983; **101**: 1093–97.

Lindhout D, Barth PG, Valk J, Boen-Tan TN. The Joubert syndrome associated with bilateral chorioretinal colobomas. *Eur J Paediatr* 1980; **134**: 173–6.

Loken AC, Hanssen O, Halvorsen S, Jolster NJ. Hereditary renal dysplasia and blindness. *Acta Paediatr Scand* 1961; **50**: 177–84.

Luckenbach MW, Green R, Miller M *et al*. Ocular clinicopathologic correlation of Hallervorden–Spatz syndrome with acanthocytosis and pigmentary retinopathy. *Am J Ophthalmol* 1983; **95**: 369–82.

Lyness AL, Ernst W, Quinlan MP *et al*. A clinical, psychophysical and electroretinographic survey of patients with autosomal dominant retinitis pigmentosa. *Br J Ophthalmol* 1985; **69**: 326–39.

McGee TL, Lin D, Berson EL *et al*. Defects in the rod cGMP-gated channel gene in patients with retinitis pigmentosa. *Invest Ophthalmol Vis Sci* 1994; **35**: 1716.

McKusick VA. Mendelian inheritance in man. Ornithine aminotransferase deficiency. In: *A Catalog of Human Genes and Genetic Disorders*, 11th edn. Baltimore: Johns Hopkins University Press, 1994: 2087–90.

McLaughlin ME, Sandberg MA, Berson EL, Dryja TP. Recessive mutations in the gene encoding the beta-subunit of rod phosphodiesterase in patients with retinitis pigmentosa. *Nature Genet* 1993; **4**: 130–4.

Mainzer F, Saldino RM, Ozononoff MB, Minagi H. Familial nephropathy associated with retinitis pigmentosa, cerebellar ataxia and skeletal abnormalities. *Am J Med* 1970; **49**: 556–62.

Manning FJ, Bruce AM, Berson EL. Electroretinograms in microcephaly with chorioretinal degeneration. *Am J Ophthalmol* 1990; **109**: 457–63.

Margolis S, Scher BM, Carr RE. Macular colobomas in Leber's congenital amaurosis. *Am J Ophthalmol* 1977; **83**: 27–31.

Marmor MF. Defining fundus albipunctatus. *Doc Ophthalmol Proc Ser* 1977; **13**: 227–34.

Marmor MF, Zrenner E. For the International Society for Clinical Electrophysiology of Vision. Standard for clinical electroretinography (1994 update). *Doc Ophthalmol* 1995; **89**: 199–216.

Massoff RW, Finklestein D. Supplemental vitamin A retards loss of ERG amplitude in retinitis pigmentosa (editorial; comment). *Arch Ophthalmol* 1993; **111**: 751–4.

Massof RW, Finkelstein D. Two forms of autosomal dominant primary retinitis pigmentosa. *Doc Ophthalmol* 1981; **51**: 289–346.

Massoff RW, Finkelstein D. Vision threshold profiles in sector retinitis pigmentosa. *Arch Ophthalmol* 1979; **97**: 1899–904.

Mausof FE, Burns CA, Burian HM. Morphological and functional retinal changes in myotonic dystrophy unrelated to quinine therapy. *Am J Ophthalmol* 1972; **74**: 1141–3.

Meier DA, Hess JW. Familial nephropathy with retinitis pigmentosa: a new oculorenal syndrome in adults. *Am J Med* 1965; **39**: 58–69.

Meier W, Blumberg A, Imahom W *et al*. Idiopathic hypercalciuria with bilateral macular colobomata: a new variant of ocular renal syndrome. *Helv Paediatr Acta* 1979; **34**: 257–69.

Meindl A, Dry K, Herrman K *et al*. A gene (RPGR) with homology to the RCC1 guanine nucleotide exchange factor is mutated in X-linked retinitis pigmentosa (RP3). *Nature Genetics* 1996; **13**: 35–42.

Meire FM, Bergen AAB, De Rouck A, Leys M, Dellman JW. X-linked cone dystrophy: localisation of the gene locus to Xp21–p11.1 by linkage analysis. *Br J Ophthalmol* 1994; **78**: 103–8.

Menon RK, Ball WS, Sperling MA. Choroideremia and hypopituitarism: an association. *Am J Med Genet* 1989; **34**: 511–13.

Merin S, Abraham FA, Auerbach E. Usher's and Hallgren's syndromes. *Acta Genet Med* 1974; **23**: 49–55.

Merin S, Auerbach E. Retinitis pigmentosa. *Surv Ophthalmol* 1976; **20**: 303–45.

Merry DE, Janne PA, Landers JE *et al*. Isolation of a candidate gene for choroideremia. *Proc Natl Acad Sci USA* 1992; **89**: 2135–9.

Michalski A, Leonard JV, Taylor DSI. The eye and inherited metabolic disease. *J Roy Soc Med* 1988; **81**: 286–90.

Mitchell GA, Looney JE, Brody LC *et al*. Human ornithine-delta-aminotransferase:cDNA cloning and analysis of the structural gene. *J Biol Chem* 1988; **263**: 14288–95.

Miyabayashi S, Hanamizu M, Nakamura R, Hayashi R-I, Tada K. Clinical and biochemical phenotype of the MELAS mutation. *J Inherit Metab Dis* 1993; **16**: 886–92.

Miyake Y, Horiguchi M, Terasaki H, Kondo M. Scotopic threshold response in complete and incomplete types of congenital stationary night blindness. *Invest Ophthalmol Vis Sci* 1994; **35**: 3770–5.

Miyake Y, Kawase Y. Reduced amplitude of oscillatory potentials in female carriers of X-linked recessive congenital stationary night-blindness. *Am J Ophthalmol* 1984; **98**: 208–15.

Miyake Y, Yagasaki K, Horiguchi M *et al*. Congenital stationary night-blindness with negative electroretinogram. *Arch Ophthalmol* 1986; **104**: 1013–20.

Mizuno K, Takei Y, Sears ML *et al*. Leber's congenital amaurosis. *Am J Ophthalmol* 1977; **83**: 34–42.

Mizuo G. On a new discovery in dark adaptation in Ogouchi's disease. *Acta Soc Ophthalmol Jap* 1913; **17**: 148–50.

Modell B. Advances in the use of iron-chelating agents for the treatment of iron overload. *Prog Hematol* 1979; **11**: 267–312.

Moore AT. Cone and cone–rod dystrophies. *J Med Genet* 1992; **29**: 289–90.

Moore AT, Fitzke F, Jay M *et al*. Autosomal dominant retinitis pigmentosa with apparent incomplete penetrance: a clinical, psychophysical, electroretinographic, and molecular genetic study. *Br J Ophthalmol* 1993; **77**: 473–9.

Moore AT, Fitzke FW, Kemp CM *et al*. Abnormal dark adaptation kinetics in autosomal dominant sector retinitis pigmentosa due to a rod opsin mutation. *Br J Ophthalmol* 1992; **76**: 465–9.

Moore AT, Taylor DSI. A syndrome of congenital retinal dystrophy and saccade palsy—a subset of Leber's amaurosis. *Br J Ophthalmol* 1984; **68**: 421–31.

Moore AT, Taylor DS, Harden A. Bilateral macular dysplasia ('colobomata') and congenital retinal dystrophy. *Br J Ophthalmol* 1985; **69**: 691–9.

Mukai S, Dryja TP, Bruns GAP *et al*. Linkage between the X-linked retinitis pigmentosa locus and the L.128 locus. *Am J Ophthalmol* 1985; **100**: 225–9.

Musarella MA, Anson-Cartwright L, Seal SM *et al*. Multipoint linkage analysis and heterogeneity testing in twenty X-linked retinitis pigmentosa families. *Genomics* 1990; **8**: 286–96.

Musarella MA, Burghes A, Anson-Cartwright L *et al*. Localization of the gene for X-linked recessive type of retinitis pigmentosa (XLRP) to Xp21 by linkage analysis. *Am J Hum Genet* 1988; **43**: 484–94.

Musarella MA, Weleber RG, Murphey WH *et al*. Assignment of the gene for complete X-linked congenital stationary night blindness (CNSB1) to chromosome Xp11.3 *Genomics* 1989; **5**: 727–37.

Nakasawa M, Kikawa E, Chida Y, Tamai M. Asn 244 His mutation in the peripherin RDS gene causing autosomal dominant cone–rod degeneration. *Hum Mol Genet* 1994; **3**: 1195–6.

Nance MA, Berry SA. Cockayne syndrome: review of 140 cases. *Am J Med Genet* 1992; **42**: 68–84.

Nathans J. The genes for colour vision. *Sci Am* 1989a; **260**: 42–9.

Nathans J, Davenport CM, Maumenee IH *et al*. Molecular genetics of blue cone monochromacy. *Science* 1989b; **245**: 831–8.

Nathans J, Piantadida TP, Eddy RI *et al*. Molecular genetics of inherited variation in human colour vision. *Science* 1986a; **232**: 203–10.

Nathans J, Thomas D, Hogness DS. Molecular genetics of human vision: the genes encoding blue, green, and red pigments. *Science* 1986b; **232**: 193–203.

Newell FW, Johnson RO, Huttenlocher PR. Pigmentary degeneration of the retina in the Hallervorden–Spatz syndrome. *Am J Ophthalmol* 1979; **88**: 467–71.

Newman N, Capone A, Leeper H *et al*. Clinical and subclinical ophthalmic findings with retinol deficiency. *Ophthalmology* 1994; **101**: 1077–83.

Nickel B, Hoyt CS. Leber's congenital amaurosis. Is mental retardation a frequently associated defect? *Arch Ophthalmol* 1982; **100**: 1089–92.

Nischal K, Aclimandos W, Hingorani *et al*. A new sign in Alagille's syndrome. *Europ J Ophthalmol* 1995; **5**(Suppl.): 50.

Noble KG, Carr RE. Leber's congenital amaurosis. A retrospective study of 33 cases and a histopathological study of one case. *Arch Ophthalmol* 1978; **96**: 818–21.

Noble KG, Carr RE. Pigmented paravenous chorioretinal atrophy. *Am J Ophthalmol* 1983; **96**: 338–44.

Norio R, Raitta C, Lindahl E. Further delineation of the Cohen syndrome; report on chorioretinal dystrophy, leukopenia and consanguinity. *Clin Genet* 1984; **25**: 1–14.

Nussbaum RL, Lesko JG, Lewis RA *et al*. Isolation of anonymous DNA sequences from within a submicroscopic X-chromosomal deletion in a patient with choroideremia, deafness, and mental retardation. *Proc Nat Acad Sci* 1987; **84**: 6521–5.

Nussbaum RL, Lewis RA, Lesko JG, Ferrel R. Choroideremia is linked to the restriction fragment length polymorphism DXYS1 at Xq13–21. *Am J Hum Genet* 1985a; **37**: 473–81.

Nussbaum RL, Lewis RA, Lesko JG, Ferrel R. Mapping of X-linked ophthalmic disease II. Linkage relationship of X-linked retinitis pigmentosa to X chromosomal short arm markers. *Hum Genet* 1985b; **70**: 45–50.

Nuutila A. Dystropia retinae pigmentosa–dysacusis syndrome (DRD): a study of the Usher or Hallgren syndrome. *J Hum Genet* 1970; **118**: 57–88.

Nyska M, Mozes G, Howard J *et al*. Quadriparesis in the Laurence–Moon–Bardet–Biedl syndrome. *Paraplegia* 1991; **29**: 350–4.

Oberklaid F, Danks DM, Mayne V, Campbell P. Asphyxiating thoracic dysplasia. Clinical, radiological, and pathological information on 10 patients. *Arch Dis Child* 1977; **52**: 758–65.

O'Donnell MO, Talbot JF. Vitamin A deficiency in treated cystic fibrosis: case report. *Br J Ophthalmol* 1987; **71**: 787–90.

Oliver GL, McFarlane DC. Congenital trichomegaly with associated pigmentary degeneration of the retina, dwarfism and mental retardation. *Arch Ophthalmol* 1965; **74**: 169–71.

Ortiz MG, Newman NJ, Shoffner JM *et al*. Variable retinal and neurologic manifestations in patients harbouring the mitochondrial DNA 8993 mutation. *Arch Ophthalmol* 1993; **111**: 1525–30.

Parke JT, Riccardi JM, Leeves RA *et al*. A syndrome of microcephaly and retinal pigment abnormalities without mental retardation in a family with coincidental autosomal dominant hyperreflexia. *Am J Med Genet* 1984; **17**: 585–94.

Patton MA, Harding AE, Baraitser M. Congenital trichomegaly, pigmentary retinal degeneration and short stature. *Am J Ophthalmol* 1986; **101**: 490–1.

Pearce WG. Ocular and genetic features of Cockayne's syndrome. *Canad J Ophthalmol* 1972; **7**: 435–44.

Pearlman JT, Heckenlively JR, Bastek JV. Progressive nature of pigmented paravenous retinochoroidal atrophy. *Am J Ophthalmol* 1978; **85**: 215–17.

Pearlman JT, Kamin DF, Kopelois SM, Saxton J. Pigmented paravenous retinochoroidal atrophy. *Am J Ophthalmol* 1975; **80**: 630–5.

Pearlman JT, Owen G, Brounley DW. Cone dystrophies with dominant inheritance. *Am J Ophthalmol* 1974; **77**: 293–303.

Pentao L, Lewis RA, Ledbetter DH *et al*. Maternal uniparental isodisomy of chromosome 14: association with autosomal recessive rod monochromacy. *Am J Hum Genet* 1992; **50**: 690–9.

Phillips CI, Stokoe NL, Bartholomew RS. Asphyxiating thoracic dystrophy (Jeune's disease) with retinal aplasia. A sibship of two. *J Pediatr Ophthalmol Strabismus* 1979; **16**: 279–83.

Pieke Dahl S, Kimberling WJ, Gorin MB *et al*. Genetic heterogeneity of Usher syndrome type II. *J Med Genet* 1993; **30**: 843–8.

Pillers DA, Bulman DE, Weleber RG *et al*. Dystrophin expression in the human retina is required for normal function as defined by electroretinography. *Nature Genet* 1995; **4**: 82–6.

Pillers DA, Seltzer WK, Powell BR *et al*. Negative-configuration electroretinogram in Oregon eye disease. Consistent phenotype in Xp21 deletion syndrome. *Arch Ophthalmol* 1993; **111**: 1558–63.

Polak BCP, Hogewind BL, Van Lith FHM. Tapetoretinal degeneration associated with recessively inherited medullary cystic disease. *Am J Ophthalmol* 1977; **84**: 645–51.

Poll-The BT, Billette de Villemeur T, Abitbol M *et al*. Metabolic pigmentary retinopathies: diagnosis and therapeutic attempts. *Eur J Pediatr* 1992; **151**: 2–11.

Poll-The BT, Bonnefont JP, Ogier H *et al*. Familial hypoketotic hypoglycemia associated with peripheral neuropathy, pigmentary neuropathy and C6–C14 hydroxy dicarboxylic aciduria: a new defect of fatty acid oxidation? *J Inherit Metab Dis* 1988; **11**(Suppl. 2): 183–5.

Poulton J. Mitochondrial DNA and genetic disease. *Arch Dis Child* 1988; **63**: 883–5.

Price MJ, Judisch GF, Thompson HS. X-linked congenital stationary night blindness with myopia and nystagmus without clinical complaints of nyctalopia. *J Pediatr Ophthalmol Strabismus* 1988; **25**: 33–6.

Price MJ, Thompson HS, Judisch FG *et al*. Pupillary constriction to darkness. *Br J Ophthalmol* 1985; **69**: 205–11.

Puddu P, Barboni P, Mantovani V *et al*. Retinitis pigmentosa, ataxia and mental retardation associated with mitochondrial DNA mutation in an Italian family. *Br J Ophthalmol* 1993; **77**: 84–8.

Puklin JE, Rielly CA, Simon RM, Cotlier E. Anterior segment and retinal pigmentary abnormalities in arteriohepatic dysplasia. *Ophthalmology* 1981; **88**: 337–47.

Rader DJ, Brewer HB. Abetalipoproteinaemia. New insights into lipoprotein assembly and vitamin E metabolism from a rare genetic disease. *J Am Med Assoc* 1993; **270**: 865–9.

Rahi AHS, Hungerford JL, Ahmed AI. Ocular toxicity of desferrioxamine: light microscopic, histochemical, and ultrastructural findings. *Br J Ophthalmol* 1986; **70**: 373–81.

Raitta C, Santavouri P. Ophthalmological findings in infantile type of so-called neuronal ceroid lipofuscinosis. *Acta Ophthalmol* 1973; **51**: 755–63.

Rao VK, Cohen GB, Oprian DD. Rhodopsin mutation G90D and a molecular mechanism for congenital night blindness. *Nature* 1994; **367**: 639–42.

Refsum S. Heredopathia atactica polyneuritis formis: a familial syndrome not hitherto described. A contribution to the clinical study of hereditary disorders of the nervous system. *Acta Psychiatr Scand* 1946; **38**(Suppl.): 1–303.

Reichel E, Bruce AM, Sandberg MA, Berson EL. An electroretinographic and molecular genetic study of X-linked cone degeneration. *Am J Ophthalmol* 1989; **108**: 540–7.

Reske-Nielsen E, Lou HC, Lowes M. Progressive external ophthalmoplegia. Evidence for a generalised mitochondrial disease with a defect in pyruvate metabolism. *Acta Ophthalmol* 1976; **54**: 553–73.

Richards JE, Scott KM, Sieving PA. Disruption of conserved rhodopsin disulfide bond Ley Cys 187 Tyr mutation causes early and severe autosomal dominant retinitis pigmentosa. *Ophthalmology* 1995; **102**: 669–77.

Rinaldi E, Stoppoloni GP, Savastano S *et al*. Gyrate atrophy of choroid associated with hyperornithinemia: report of the first case in Italy. *J Pediatr Ophthalmol Strabismus* 1979; **16**: 133–5.

Robb RM, Dauton B, Fulton AB, Levy ML. Retinal degeneration in vitamin B$_{12}$. *Am J Ophthalmol* 1984; **97**: 691–6.

Rocco MD. On Saraiva and Baraitser and Joubert syndrome. *Am J Med Genet* 1993; **46**: 732.

Rodrigues MM, Ballintine EJ, Wiggert B *et al*. Choroideremia: a clinical electron microscopic and biochemical report. *Ophthalmology* 1984; **91**: 873–83.

Rosenberg T, Haim M, Piczenik Y *et al*. Autosomal dominant stationary night blindness. A large family rediscovered. *Acta Ophthalmol* 1991; **69**: 694–703.

Rosenberg T, Niebatir E, Yang MM. Choroideremia, congenital deafness and mental retardation in a family with an X-chromosomal deletion. *Ophthalmol Paediatr Genet* 1987; **8**: 139–43.

Rosenberg T, Schwartz M, Simonsen SE. Aland eye disease (Forsius Eriksson Miyake syndrome) with probability established in a Danish family. *Acta Ophthalmol* 1990; **68**: 281–91.

Rosenfeld PJ, Cowley GS, McGee TL, Sandberg MA, Berson EL, Dryja TP. A null mutation in the rhodopsin gene causes rod photoreceptor dysfunction and autosomal recessive retinitis pigmentosa. *Nature Genet* 1992; **1**: 209–13.

Rosenfeld PJ, McKusick VA, Amberger JS, Dryja TP. Recent advances in the gene map of inherited eye disorders: primary hereditary diseases of the retina, choroid and vitreous. *J Med Genet* 1994; **31**: 903–15.

Roth AM, Hepler RS, Mukoyama M *et al*. Pigmentary retinal dystrophy in Hallervorden–Spatz disease. Clinico-pathologic report of a case. *Surv Ophthalmol* 1971; **16**: 24–35.

Ruben JB, Morris RJ, Judisch GF. Chorioretinal degeneration in infantile malignant osteoporosis. *Am J Ophthalmol* 1990; **110**: 1–5.

Rummelt V, Folberg R, Ionasecu V *et al*. Ocular pathology of MELAS syndrome with mitochondrial DNA nucleotide 3243 point mutation. *Ophthalmology* 1993; **100**: 1757–66.

Runge P, Calver D, Marshall J, Taylor D. The histopathology of mitochondrial cytopathy and the Laurence–Moon–Biedl syndrome. *Br J Ophthalmol* 1986a; **70**: 782–96.

Runge P, Muller DPR, McAllister J *et al*. Oral vitamin E can prevent the retinopathy of abetalipoproteinaemia. *Br J Ophthalmol* 1986b; **70**: 166–73.

Ruprecht KW. Ophthalmological aspects in patients with Werner's syndrome. *Arch Geront Geriatr* 1989; **9**: 263–70.

Russell-Eggitt I, Taylor DSI, Clayton PT *et al*. Leber's congenital amaurosis — a new syndrome with cardiomyopathy. *Br J Ophthalmol* 1989; **73**: 250–4.

Ruttum MS, Lewandowski MF, Bateman JB. Affected females in X-linked congenital stationary night blindness. *Ophthalmology* 1992; **99**: 747–52.

Ryan SJ, Knox DL, Green WR, Konigsmark BW. Olivopontocerebellar degeneration. Clinicopathologic correlation of the associated retinopathy. *Arch Ophthalmol* 1975; **93**: 169–75.

Sankila EM, Pakarinen L, Sistonen P *et al*. Assignment of an Usher type III (USH3) gene to chromosome 3q. *Hum Mol Genet* 1995; **4**: 93–8.

Saraiva JM, Baraitser M. Joubert syndrome: a review. *Am J Med Genet* 1992; **43**: 726–31.

Schachat AP, Maumenee IH. Bardet–Biedl syndrome and related disorders. *Arch Ophthalmol* 1982; **100**: 285–8.

Schappert-Kimmijser J, Henkes HE, van den Bosch J. Amaurosis congenita (Leber). *Arch Ophthalmol* 1959; **61**: 211–18.

Schroeder R, Mets M, Maumenee I. Leber's congenital amaurosis. Retrospective review of 43 cases and a new fundus finding in two cases. *Arch Ophthalmol* 1987; **105**: 356–9.

Schubert G, Bornschein H. Beitrag zur analyse des menschlichen elektroretinograms. *Ophthalmologica* 1952; **123**: 396–412.

Schutgens RBH, Heymans HSA, Wanders RJA *et al*. Peroxisomal disorders; a newly recognized group of genetic diseases. *Eur J Pediatr* 1986; **144**: 430–40.

Schwartz M, Rosenberg T. Aland eye disease: linkage data. *Genomics* 1991; **10**: 327–32.

Schwartz M, Rosenberg T, van der Hurk JAJM *et al*. Identification of mutations in Danish choroideremia families. *Hum Mutat* 1993; **2**: 43–7.

Scotto JM, Hadehouel M, Odieve M *et al*. Infantile phytanic acid storage disease. A possible variant of Refsum's disease: three cases including ultrastructural studies of the liver. *J Inherit Metab Dis* 1982; **5**: 83–90.

Seabra MC, Brown MS, Goldstein JL. Retinal degeneration in choroideremia: deficiency of Rab geranylgeranyl transferase. *Science* 1993; **259**: 377–81.

Sebag J, Albert DM, Craft JL. The Alstrom syndrome, ophthalmic histopathology and retinal ultrastructure. *Br J Ophthalmol* 1984; **68**: 494–501.

Sengers RCS, Stadhouders AM, Trijbels JMF. Mitochondrial myopathies. Clinical, morphological and biochemical aspects. *Eur J Pediatr* 1984; **141**: 192–207.

Senior B, Friedmann AI, Braudo JL. Juvenile familial nephropathy with tapetoretinal degeneration. *Am J Ophthalmol* 1961; **52**: 625–33.

Sharpe LT, van Norrend D, Nordby K. Pigment regeneration, visual adaptation and spectral sensitivity in the achromat. *Clin Vis Sci* 1988; **3**: 9–17.

Sheffield VC, Carmi R, Kwitek–Black *et al*. Identification of a Bardet–Biedl syndrome locus on chromosome 3 and evaluation of an efficient approach to homozygosity mapping. *Hum Mol Genet* 1994; **3**: 1331–5.

Sieving PA, Niffenneger JH, Berson EL. Electroretinographic findings in selected pedigrees with choroideremia. *Am J Ophthalmol* 1986; **101**: 361–7.

Sieving PA, Richards JE, Bingham EL *et al*. Dominant congenital complete nyctalopia and Gly90Asp rhodopsin mutation. *Invest Ophthalmol Vis Sci* 1992; **33**: 1397.

Simell O, Takki K. Raised plasma ornithine and gyrate atrophy of the choroid and retina. *Lancet* 1973; **1**: 1031–3.

Sipila I, Simell O, Rapola J *et al*. Gyrate atrophy of the choroid and retina with hyperornithinemia, tubular aggregates and type 2 fibre atrophy in muscle. *Neurology* 1979; **29**: 996–1005.

Siu VM, Gonder JR, Jung JH *et al*. Choroideremia associated with an X-autosomal translocation. *Hum Genet* 1990; **84**: 459–64.

Skalka HW. Hereditary pigmented paravenous retinochoroidal atrophy. *Am J Ophthalmol* 1979; **87**: 286–91.

Sloan LL, Brown DJ. Progressive retinal degeneration with selective involvement of the cone mechanism. *Am J Ophthalmol* 1962; **54**: 629–41.

Small K, Banks Anderson W. Pigmented paravenous retinochoroidal atrophy: discordant expression in monozygotic twins. *Arch Ophthalmol* 1991; **109**: 1408–10.

Smith D, Vestreicher J, Musarella M. Clinical spectrum of Leber's congenital amaurosis in the second to fourth decades of life. *Ophthalmology* 1990; **97**: 1156–62.

Smith RJH, Berlin CI, Hejtmancik JF *et al*. Clinical diagnosis of Usher's syndromes. *Am J Med Genet* 1994; **50**: 32–8.

Smith RJ, Lee EC, Kimberling WJ *et al*. Localisation of two genes for Usher's syndrome type 1 to chromosome 11. *Genomics* 1992; **7**:

250–6.

Snittger S, Hofers C, Heidemann P *et al.* Molecular and cytogenetic analysis of an interstitial 20p deletion associated with syndromic intrahepatic ductular hypolplasia (Alagille syndrome). *Hum Genet* 1989; **83**: 239–44.

Sorsby A, Williams CF. Retinal aplasia as a clinical entity. *Br Med J* 1960; **1**: 293–7.

Spalton DJ, Taylor DSI, Sanders MD. Juvenile Batten's disease: an ophthalmological assessment of 26 patients. *Br J Ophthalmol* 1980; **64**: 726–32.

Spivey BE. The X-linked inheritance of atypical monochromatism. *Arch Ophthalmol* 1965; **74**: 327–33.

Stanescu B, Draloands L. Cerebro–hepato–renal (Zellweger's) syndrome: ocular involvement. *Arch Ophthalmol* 1972; **87**: 590–2.

Stanescu B, Michaels J, Proesmans W, Van Damme B. Retinal involvement in a case of nephronophthisis associated with liver fibrosis (Senior–Boichis syndrome). *Birth Defects* 1967; **12**: 463–9.

Steel D, Wood C, Richardson J, McCarthy J. Anterior subcapsular plaque cataract in hyperornithinaemia gyrate atrophy — a case report. *Br J Ophthalmol* 1992; **76**: 762–3.

Strömland K, Hagberg B, Kristiansson B. Ocular pathology in the disialotransferrin developmental deficiency syndrome. *Ophthalmol Paediatr Genet* 1990; **11**: 309–13.

Stromme P, Maehlen J, Strom EH, Torvic A. Post mortem findings in two patients with the carbohydrate deficient glycoprotein syndrome. *Acta Paediatr Scand* 1991; **375**(Suppl.): 55–62.

Sullivan T, Lambert S, Buncic JR, Musarella M. The optic disc in Leber's congenital amaurosis. *J Pediatr Ophthalmol Strabismus* 1992; **29**: 246–9.

Tada K, Saito T, Hayasaha S, Mizuno K. Hyperornithinemia with gyrate atrophy: pathophysiology and treatment. *J Inherit Metab Dis* 1983; **6**: 105–6.

Tahvanainen G, Noris R, Karila E *et al.* Cohen syndrome gene assigned to the long arm of chromosome 8 by linkage analysis. *Nature Genet* 1994; **7**: 201–4.

Takki K, Simell O. Genetic aspects of gyrate atrophy of the choroid and retina with hyperornithinemia. *Br J Ophthalmol* 1974; **58**: 907–16.

Takki K, Simell O. Gyrate atrophy of the choroid and retina with hyperornithinemia. *Birth Defects* 1976; **12**: 373–84.

Teague PW, Aldred MA, Jay M *et al.* Heterogeneity analysis in 40 X-linked retinitis pigmentosa families. *Am J Med Genet* 1994; **55**: 105–11.

To KW, Adamian M, Jakobiec FA, Berson EL. Olivopontocerebellar atrophy with retinal degeneration. *Ophthalmology* 1993; **100**: 15–23.

Tomita H, Ohno K, Tamai A. Joubert syndrome associated with Leber's congenital amaurosis. *Brain Dev* 1979; **11**: 459–65.

Traboulsi EI, de Becker I, Maumenee IH. Ocular findings in Cockayne's syndrome. *Am J Ophthalmol* 1992; **114**: 579–83.

Traboulsi EI, Maumenee IH. Hereditary pigmented paravenous chorioretinal atrophy. *Arch Ophthalmol* 1986; **104**: 1636–40.

Traboulsi EI, Maumenee IH, Green WR *et al.* Olivopontocerebellar atrophy with retinal degeneration. A clinical and ocular histopathologic study. *Arch Ophthalmol* 1988: **106**: 801–6.

Tranebjaerg L, Sjo O, Warburg M. Retinal cone dysfunction and mental retardation associated with a *de novo* balanced translocation 1;6(q44;q27). *Ophthalmol Paediatr Genet* 1986; **7**: 167–73.

Tremblay F, La Roche RG, Shea SE, Ludman MD. Longitudinal study of the early electroretinographic changes in Alstrom's syndrome. *Am J Ophthalmol* 1993; **115**: 657–65.

Uliss A, Moore AT, Bird AC. The dark choroid in posterior retinal dystrophies. *Ophthalmology* 1987; **94**: 1423–8.

Usher CH. On a few hereditary eye affections. *Trans Ophthalmol Soc UK* 1935; **55**: 164–245.

Vaizey MJ, Sanders MD, Wybar KC, Wilson J. Neurological abnormalities in congenital amaurosis of Leber. Review of 30 cases. *Arch Dis Child* 1977; **52**: 399–402.

Valle D, Kaiser-Kupfer MI, Del Valle LA. Gyrate atrophy of the choroid and retina: deficiency of ornithine aminotransferase in transformed lymphocytes. *Proc Natl Acad Sci USA* 1977; **74**: 5159.

Valle D, Walser M, Brusilow S *et al.* Gyrate atrophy of the choroid and retina: Biochemical considerations and experience with an arginine restricted diet. *Ophthalmology* 1981; **88**: 325–30.

van Dorp DB, Eriksson AW, Delleman JW *et al.* Aland eye disease—no albino misrouting. *Clin Genet* 1985; **28**: 526–31.

van Everdingen , Went LN, Keunen JE, Oosterhuis JA. X-linked progressive cone dystrophy with specific attention to carrier detection. *J Med Genet* 1992; **29**: 291–4.

van Soest, van den Born LI, Gal A *et al.* Assignment of a gene for autosomal recessive retinitis pigmentosa (RP12) to chromosome 1q31–q32.1 in an inbred and genetically heterogeneous disease population. *Genomics* 1994; **22**: 499–504.

Verdoorn C, Pinckers A. X-linked cone dystrophy. *Doc Ophthalmol* 1988; **70**: 195–8.

Waardenburg PJ, Schappert-Kimmijser J. On various recessive biotypes of Leber's congenital amaurosis. *Acta Ophthalmol* 1963; **41**: 317–20.

Wagner RS, Caputo AR, Nelson L, Zanoni D. High hyperopia in Leber's congenital amaurosis. *Arch Ophthalmol* 1985; **103**: 1507–9.

Walt RP, Kemp CM, Lyness L *et al.* Vitamin A treatment for nightblindness in primary biliary cirrhosis. *Br Med J* 1984; **288**: 1030–1.

Warburg M, Sjo O, Fledelius HC. Deletion mapping of a retinal cone–rod dystrophy: assignment to 18q211. *Am J Med Genet* 1991; **39**: 288–93.

Weil D, Blanchard S, Kaplan J *et al.* Defective myosin VIIA gene responsible for Usher syndrome type 1B. *Nature* 1995; **374**: 60–1.

Weiner LP, Koenigsmark BW, Stoll J, Magladery JW. Hereditary olivopontocerebellar atrophy with retinal degeneration. Report of a family through six generations. *Arch Neurol* 1967; **16**: 364–76.

Weitz CJ, Miyake Y, Shinzato K. Human tritanopia associated with two amino acid substitutions in the blue sensitive opsin. *Am J Hum Genet* 1992; **50**: 498–507.

Weleber RG, Kennaway NG. Clinical trial of vitamin B6 for gyrate atrophy of the choroid and retina. *Ophthalmology* 1981; **88**: 316–24.

Weleber RG, Kennaway NG. Gyrate atrophy of the choroid and retina. In: Heckenlively JR, ed. *Retinitis Pigmentosa*. Philadelphia: JB Lippincott, 1988: 198–220.

Weleber RG, Pillers DM, Powell BR, Hanna CE, Magenis RE, Buist NRM. Aland eye disease (Forsius–Eriksson syndrome) associated with contiguous deletion syndrome at Xp21. *Arch Ophthalmol* 1989; **107**: 1171–9.

Weleber RG, Tongue AC. Congenital stationary night blindness presenting as Leber's congenital amaurosis. *Arch Ophthalmol* 1987; **105**: 360–4.

Weleber RG, Tongue AC, Kennaway NG *et al.* Ophthalmic manifestations of infantile phytanic acid storage disease. *Arch Ophthalmol* 1984; **102**: 1317–21.

Went LN, van Schooneveld MJ, Oosterhuis JA. Late onset dominant cone dystrophy with early blue cone involvement. *J Med Genet* 1992; **29**: 295–8.

Wetterau JR, Aggerbeck LP, Bouma M-E *et al.* Absence of microsomal triglyceride transfer protein in individuals with abetalipoproteinemia. *Science* 1992; **258**: 99–101.

Wilson DJ, Weleber RLG, Beals RK. Retinal dystrophy of Jeune's syndrome. *Arch Ophthalmol* 1987; **105**: 651–7.

Wilson DJ, Weleber RG, Green WR. Ocular clinico-pathological study of gyrate atrophy. *Am J Ophthalmol* 1991; **111**: 24–33.

Winn S, Tasman JW, Spaeth G *et al*. Ogouchi's disease in negroes. *Arch Ophthalmol* 1968; **81**: 501–7.

World Health Organization (WHO). *Control of Vitamin A Deficiency and Xerophthalmia. Technical Report Series No. 676 (2)*. Geneva: WHO, 1982.

Wright AF, Bhattacharya SS, Clayton JF *et al*. Linkage relationships between X-linked retinitis pigmentosa and nine short arm markers: exclusion of disease locus from Xp21and localisation between DX57 and DX514. *Am J Hum Genet* 1987; **41**: 635–44.

Wroblewski J, Wells J, Eckstein A *et al*. Ocular findings associated with a three base pair deletion in the peripherin–RDS gene in autosomal dominant retinitis pigmentosa. *Br J Ophthalmol* 1994; **78**: 831–6.

Xu S, Nakazawa M, Tamai M, Gal A. Autosomal dominant retinitis pigmentosa locus on 19q in a Japanese family. *Br J Ophthalmol* 1995; **32**: 915–16.

Young TI, Ziylan S, Schaffer DB. The ophthalmologic manifestations of the cardio-facio-cutaneous syndrome. *J Pediatr Ophthalmol Strabismus* 1993; **30**: 48–52.

Zellweger H. The cerebro-hepato-renal syndrome and other peroxisomal disorders. *Dev Med Child Neurol* 1987; **29**: 821–9.

Zhang F, Deleuze JF, Aurias *et al*. Interstitial deletion of the short arm of chromosome 20 in arteriohepatic dysplasia (Alagille syndrome). *J Pediatr* 1990; **116**: 73–7.

45: Inherited Macular Dystrophies

Anthony Moore and Kevin Evans

Macular abnormalities are seen in a large number of different inherited disorders which can be broadly divided into four groups (Noble 1986). First, there is a heterogeneous group of disorders that primarily affect the macula, and are not associated with any other anomaly. Second, macular abnormalities may be seen in more generalized retinal dystrophies, particularly in the cone and cone–rod dystrophies. Third, ocular disorders, for example albinism and aniridia, have associated hypoplasia of the fovea, which may also be seen as an isolated abnormality. Fourth, macular abnormalities are seen in a variety of inherited systemic disorders. The age of onset of macular dystrophies varies widely and in this chapter only those macular disorders which are seen in childhood will be considered.

Primary hereditary macular dystrophies

This group of disorders is characterized by early onset of bilateral visual loss, usually in the first or second decade of life, and bilateral, generally symmetrical, macular abnormalities. Many different disorders have been described (Deutman 1971; Gass 1987). Most are rare and have been incompletely characterized so that classification is unsatisfactory; they may, however, be subdivided on the basis of the mode of inheritance (Table 45.1) or the anatomical site of the primary disease (Noble 1986). A more satisfactory classification will have to await the discovery of the causative mutations. Although many of the macular dystrophies have been mapped to chromosomal loci (Table 45.2), in most cases the causative mutations have yet to be identified. Three dominant macular dystrophy families have been found to have peripherin/RDS gene mutations (Wroblewski *et al.* 1994).

Table 45.1 Primary hereditary macular dystrophies.

X-linked
X-linked juvenile retinoschisis

Autosomal recessive
Stargardt's disease
Familial foveal retinoschisis

Autosomal dominant
Vitelliform dystrophy
North Carolina macular dystrophy
Progressive bifocal chorioretinal dystrophy
Dominant macular dystrophy with flecked retina
Pattern dystrophies
Benign concentric annular dystrophy
Fenestrated sheen macular dystrophy
Dominant foveal hypoplasia
Dominant cystoid macular oedema

Mitochondrial
Stargardt-like retinopathy

Generalized choroidoretinal dystrophy with macular involvement

Central areolar choroidal dystrophy

This condition presents in late childhood, initially with minimal foveal granularity progressing to well-circumscribed, posterior polar, chorioretinal atrophy. Visual acuity is initially good but can decrease to 6/60 or worse. Fluorescein angiography reveals macular pigment epithelial transmission defects and abnormal patchy hyperfluorescence in the periphery. Minor electro-oculogram (EOG), electroretinogram (ERG) and colour vision deficits have been documented and autosomal dominant and recessive pedigrees have been described (Chopdar 1993).

Pigment epithelial disorders

Stargardt's disease (fundus flavimaculatus)

Stargardt's disease is an autosomal recessive disorder

Table 45.2 Molecular genetics of macular dystrophies.

Macular dystrophy	Inheritance	Mutation/locus	MIM	Reference
Macular dystrophy	AD	*RDS*	179605	Wells *et al.* (1993)
Cone dystrophy	AD	6p25–26	180020	Tranebjaerg *et al.* (1986)
	AD	17q	—	Balciuniene *et al.* (1995)
	XL	Xp21.1–11.3	304020	Meire *et al.* (1994)
Stargardt's disease (fundus flavimaculatus)	AR	1p21p–13	248200	Kaplan *et al.* (1993)
	AD	*RDS*	179605	Weleber *et al.* (1993)
	AD	6cen–14q	600110	Stone *et al.* (1994)
	AD	13q34	153900	Zhang *et al.* (1994)
Best's disease	AD	11q13	153700	Nicholas *et al.* (1994)
Atypical vitelliform macular dystrophy	AD	8q24	153840	Ferrel *et al.* (1983)
Adult vitelliform macular dystrophy	AD	*RDS*	179605	Wells *et al.* (1993)
North Carolina macular dystrophy	AD	6q14–16.2	136550	Small *et al.* (1993)
Progressive bifocal chorioretinal atrophy	AD	6q	—	Kelsall *et al.* (1995)
Dominant cystoid macular dystrophy	AD	7p15–21	153880	Kremer *et al.* (1994)
Pattern dystrophy	AD	*RDS*	179605	Kim *et al.* (1994)
Butterfly dystrophy	AD	*RDS*	179605	Nichols *et al.* (1993b)
Cone-rod dystrophy	AD	17q11	162200	Warburg *et al.* (1991)
		18q21	600674	Kylstra *et al.* (1993)
		19q13.4	120970	Evans *et al.* (1994)
Central areolar choroidal dystrophy	AD	*RDS*	179605	Hoyng *et al.* (1995)
Juvenile retinoschisis	XL	Xp22	312700	Gellert *et al.* (1988)
				George *et al.* (1995)

AD, autosomal dominant; AR, autosomal recessive; XL, X-linked; *RDS*, peripherin/*RDS* mutation (chromosome 6p12); MIM, McKusick's Mendelian inheritance in man reference number.

characterized by visual loss and macular atrophy, usually presenting in late childhood (Stargardt 1909). Many patients develop white flecks at the level of the retinal pigment epithelium and there is overlap with the clinical appearances described in fundus flavimaculatus. It is now evident that Stargardt's disease and fundus flavimaculatus represent different expressions of the same autosomal recessive disorder (Fishman 1976; Noble & Carr 1979; Isashiki & Ohba 1985; Weleber 1994). Families with a similar phenotype, but showing autosomal dominant inheritance (Cibis *et al.* 1980; Mansour 1992; Stone *et al.* 1994; Zhang *et al.* 1994) or mutations of mitochondrial DNA (Heher & Johns 1993) are clearly different disorders from the macular dystrophy first described by Stargardt (1909) and will be considered separately.

Clinical features

The usual presentation is with insidious, bilateral loss of visual acuity with only mild colour vision deficits, in the first two decades of life. In the earliest stages there may only be minimal ophthalmoscopic abnormalities and in such cases fluorescein angiography is particularly helpful in confirming the diagnosis. The earliest fundoscopic abnormality is a mild pigmentary disturbance or pigment epithelial atrophy at the macula (Fig. 45.1) but later there is more widespread atrophy often with a so-called 'beaten bronze' appearance. With progression there is extensive atrophy of the retina, retinal pigment epithelium, and choriocapillaris (Fishman 1976). In most cases yellow–white 'fish-tail' flecks may be seen at the posterior pole or peripheral retina; less commonly the peripheral flecks may precede the development of macular involvement (Fishman 1976; Noble & Carr 1979; Isashiki & Ohba

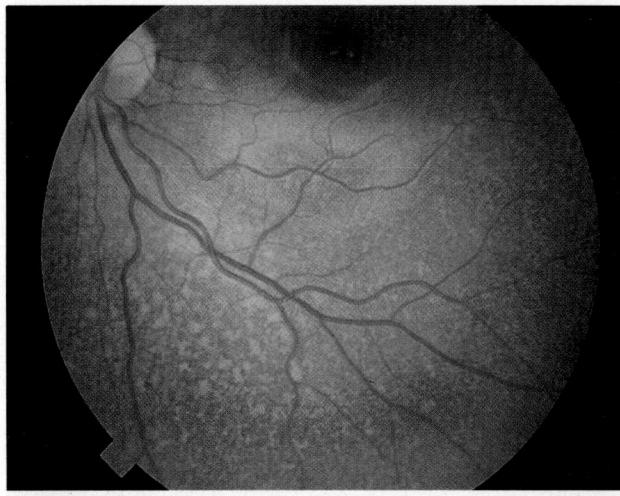

Fig. 45.2 Fundus flavimaculatus. Peripheral 'fish-tail' lesions.

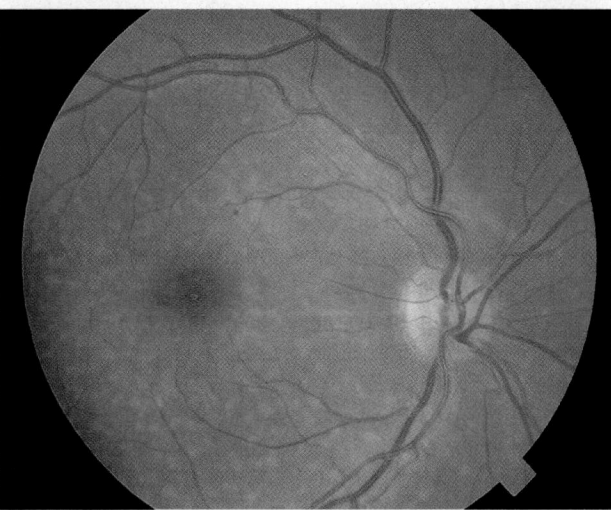

Fig. 45.3 Fundus flavimaculatus—fish-tail lesions and a mild maculopathy.

1985) (Figs 45.2, 45.3). Although visual acuity may be only mildly reduced at the outset, there is gradual deterioration usually to the level of 6/60 or finger counting (Hadden & Gass 1976). In the early stages there is a relative central scotoma which becomes absolute in time; peripheral fields remain full unless there is extensive peripheral involvement. Psychophysical testing may show prolongation of rod dark adaption but individuals with Stargardt's disease rarely report night-blindness (Fishman *et al.* 1991). Colour vision is usually normal early in the disease but becomes abnormal as central atrophy progresses (Noble & Carr 1979).

Fluorescein angiography

Fluorescein angiography is particularly useful in patients

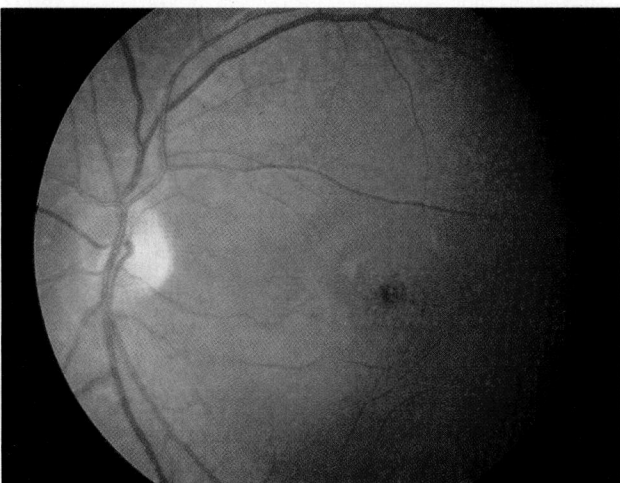

Fig. 45.1 Stargardt's disease. Early macular changes consist of pigment epithelial atrophy and clumping. Note the peripheral fish-tail lesions.

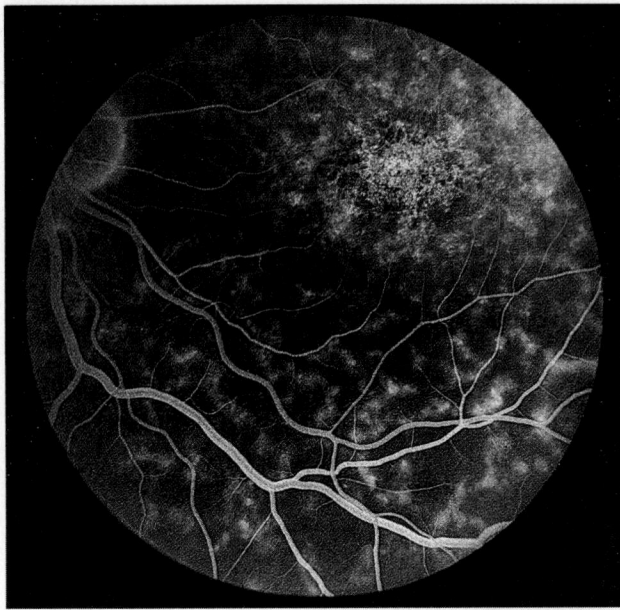

Fig. 45.4 Stargardt's disease. Fluorescein angiogram showing 'dark choroid' and transmission defects (Mr A. Moore's patient).

with early disease. The peripheral flecks usually mask underlying choroidal fluorescence early in the disease but later there is widespread patchy hyperfluorescence due to pigment epithelial atrophy (Fig. 45.4). A so-called 'dark choroid', in which there is absence of the normal choroidal fluorescence due to an abnormal absorbing layer at the level of the retinal pigment epithelium, is a common finding in Stargardt's disease (Bonnin *et al.* 1976; Fish *et al.* 1981; Uliss *et al.* 1987). This can also be an occasional feature of cone dystrophy but is not seen in families with dominant macular dystrophy similar to Stargardt's disease nor in acquired macular disease (Uliss *et al.* 1987). The fundus in patients with this sign often has a dark red or magenta appearance. A 'dark choroid' on fluorescein angiography may precede fundoscopic evidence of macular atrophy.

Electrophysiology

The flash ERG is normal in most patients but the pattern ERG is usually abnormal at an early stage. The EOG is initially normal but may become subnormal late in the disease (Noble & Carr 1979).

Genetics

Molecular genetic linkage analyses in a large number of families have localized the genetic defect to chromosome 1p21–p13 suggesting that the recessive form of the disease is genetically homogeneous (Kaplan *et al.* 1993).

Differential diagnosis

In patients with predominant macular involvement the differential diagnosis includes other forms of juvenile onset macular dystrophies, particularly progressive forms of cone dystrophy. Where there are peripheral flecks without significant macular involvement, the condition must be distinguished from other forms of the flecked retina syndrome (see Chapter 48). In most cases where there is macular atrophy and white flecks the diagnosis is straightforward. Some cases of progressive cone dystrophy may also show white flecks in the posterior or peripheral retina, but the early loss of colour vision and the electrophysiological evidence of widespread cone dysfunction serve to differentiate cone dystrophy from Stargardt's disease. Some dominant retinal dystrophies may show a similar phenotype but can be clearly distinguished from Stargardt's disease by the mode of inheritance.

Dominantly inherited macular dystrophy with flecked retina

Cibis *et al.* (1980) described a large family with dominantly inherited retinal dystrophy characterized by macular atrophy and multiple yellow pisciform subretinal deposits. The fundoscopic appearance was very similar to Stargardt's disease. The macular abnormalities were present in childhood but the peripheral retinal deposits developed in adult life. The dark choroid characteristic of autosomal recessive Stargardt's disease is not seen. The normal ERG and EOG seen in the most affected individuals serve to differentiate this disorder from dominantly inherited cone dystrophy. Other similar pedigrees have been reported (Bither & Berns 1988; Mansour 1992; Stone *et al.* 1994; Zhang *et al.* 1994) and recently two different dominantly inherited pedigrees with a similar phenotype have been assigned to chromosome 6q (Stone *et al.* 1994) and 13q34 (Zhang *et al.* 1994). In addition, a peripherin/RDS mutation at codon 153/154 has been identified in a family expressing a range of phenotypes, including fundus flavimaculatus (Weleber *et al.* 1993).

Mitochondrial DNA mutation and Stargardt-like retinopathy

Heher and Johns (1993) have reported three individuals with a retinal dystrophy similar to Stargardt's disease who have evidence of a mitochondrial DNA mutation at nucleotide position 15257. This is a primary mutation associated with Leber's hereditary optic neuropathy (LHON). The sibling of one individual developed the more classical optic neuropathy seen in LHON. Macular dystrophies have not been reported with other primary LHON mutations, but several other disorders caused by mitochondrial DNA mutations — such as Kearns–Sayre syndrome and mitochondrial myopathy — have an associated generalized retinal dystrophy (see Chapter 44).

Vitelliform dystrophy (Best's disease)

Vitelliform dystrophy is an autosomal dominant disorder which shows a wide range of clinical expression. Many obligate gene carriers have normal vision and a normal fundus examination and in symptomatic cases the disease is often asymmetrical with an extremely variable age of onset (Braley & Spivey 1964; Mohler & Fines 1981; Godel *et al.* 1986). The macula may be abnormal in the first few weeks of life (Barkmann 1961) or patients may present with a typical lesion in the fifth decade (Deutmann 1971).

Clinical features

The clinical appearances are extremely variable (Figs 45.5–45.9) and have been classified into stages 0–IVc (Deutmann 1971; Mohler & Fines 1981) which are summarized in Table 45.3. Although most patients develop bilat-

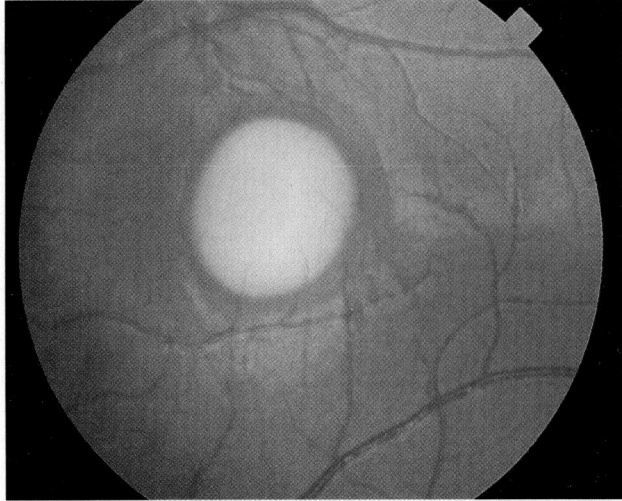

Fig. 45.6 Best's disease. Classical vitelliform lesion (stage 2) resembling an egg yolk 'sunny side up'.

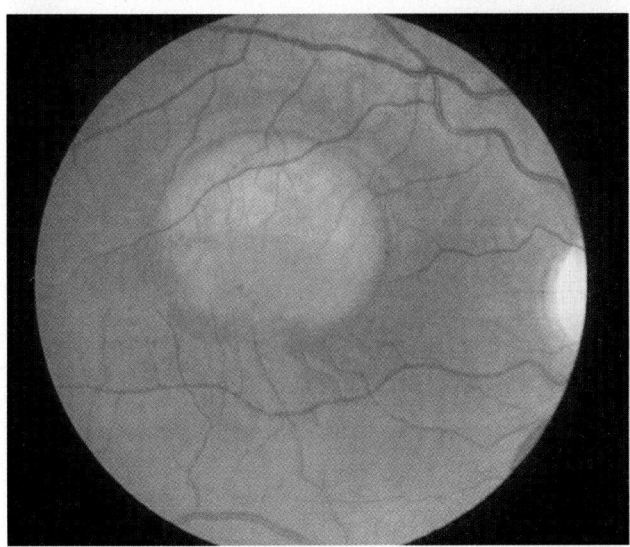

Fig. 45.5 Best's disease. Vitelliform lesion (Mr A. Moore's patient).

Table 45.3 Classification of vitelliform dystrophy. Modified from Mohler and Fine (1981).

Stage	Macular appearance
0	Normal fundus (abnormal EOG)
I	Minor retinal pigment epithelium changes
II	Typical vitelliform lesion
IIa	'Scrambled egg' appearance
III	Pseudohypopyon stage
IVa	Atrophic retinal pigment epithelium
IVb	Fibrous scar tissue
IVc	Choroidal neovascularization

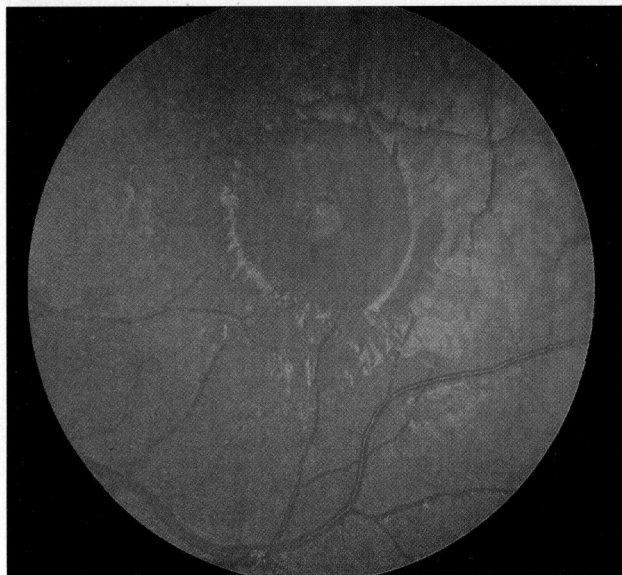

Fig. 45.7 Best's disease. 'Ruptured' vitelliform lesion.

eral disease the onset of visual loss and stage of disease may vary in the two eyes. In the mildest form, stage 0, the fundus appearance is normal but the EOG is subnormal. Visual acuity is usually normal and the long-term visual prognosis of patients with stage 0 is excellent (Mohler & Fines 1981). In stage I there are mild macular pigment epithelial abnormalities which show as window defects on fluorescein angiography (Godel *et al.* 1986). The classical vitelliform lesion (stage II) is seen as a round or oval opaque yellow subretinal deposit that resembles an egg yolk ('sunny side up'). Less commonly multiple peripheral vitelliform lesions may be seen throughout the fundus (Godel *et al.* 1986). Colour vision is usually normal in the

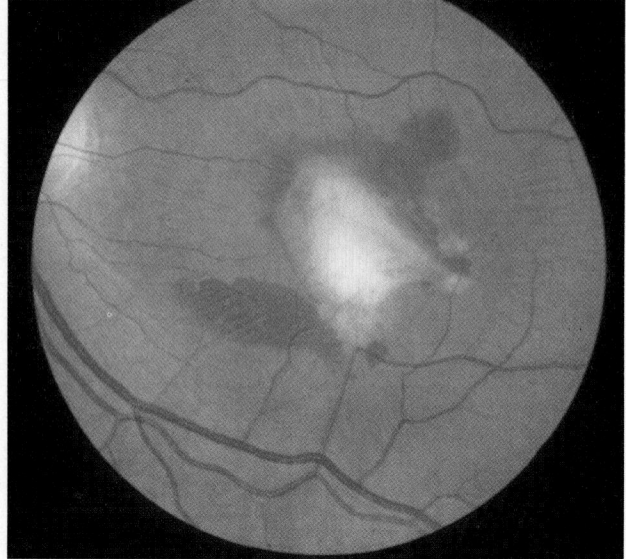

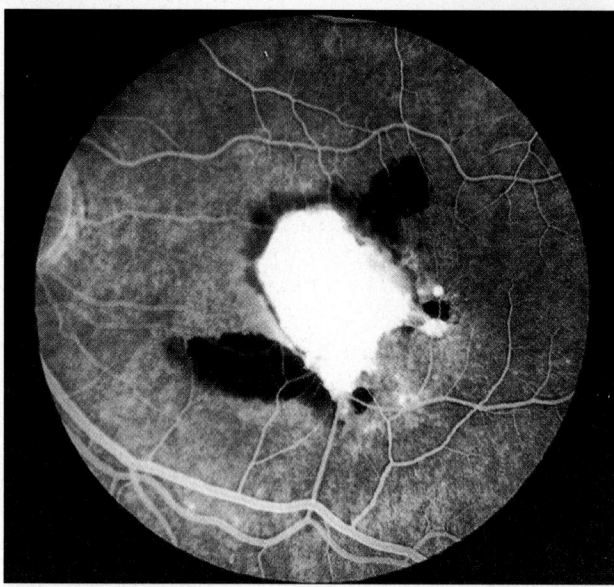

Fig. 45.8 (a) Best's disease. Vitelliform lesion with choroidal neovascularization and subretinal haemorrhage. (b) Fluorescein angiogram (same patient as Fig. 45.5) (Mr A. Moore's patient).

early stages but may become abnormal when macular atrophy occurs (Deutman 1971). Dark adaptation is normal in contrast to Stargardt's disease (Baca *et al.* 1994).

The typical vitelliform lesion is seen only transiently; resorption or rupture of the vitelliform cyst leads to the so-called scrambled egg appearance (stage IV) and later there is pigment epithelial atrophy with or without subretinal fibrosis. Choroidal neovascularization, although an important cause of visual loss, is uncommon (Mohler & Fines 1981; Godel *et al.* 1986). Rarely macular holes and retinal detachment may complicate Best's disease (Schachat *et al.* 1985; Glacet-Bernard & Coscas 1993; Soliman 1994).

The nature of the yellow material is not known with certainty. Clinically and histologically the abnormal material appears to be lipofuscin or lipofuscin-like, within the pigment epithelium and under the sensory retina (Franghieh *et al.* 1982; Weingeist *et al.* 1982). This material may partially resorb to form a pseudohypopyon (stage III) and the level of this may change on tilting the head (Kraushar *et al.* 1982).

Fluorescein angiography

Fluorescein angiographic abnormalities are first seen in stage I disease where there are multiple small areas of hyperfluorescence at the macula corresponding to areas of pigment epithelial atrophy. The abnormal yellow material in the typical lesion blocks the underlying choroidal fluorescence so that macular or peripheral lesions are seen as

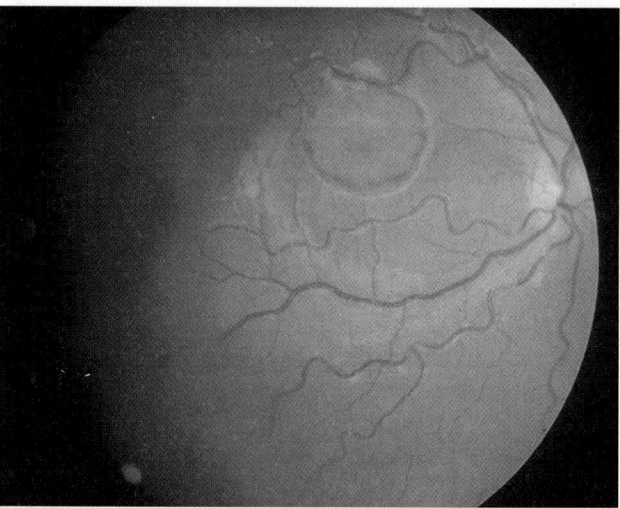

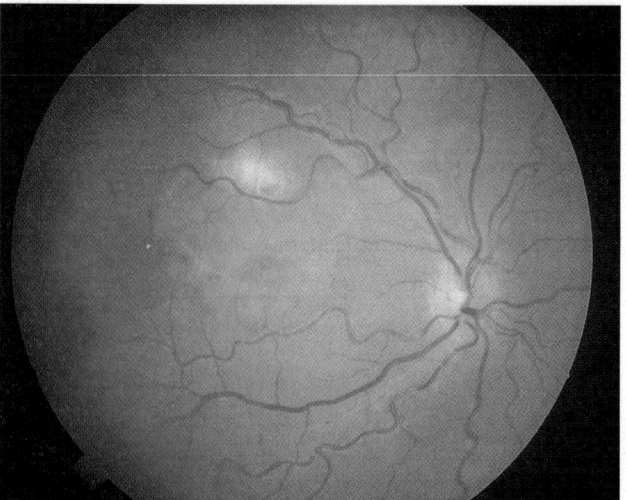

Fig. 45.9 (a, b) Changes in a vitelliform lesion over 4.5 years. The vitelliform lesion in (a) has partly dispersed and there is a subretinal scar.

round areas of hypofluorescence (Curry & Moorman 1968; Godel *et al.* 1986). In the pseudohypopyon stage the upper half of the lesion often shows hyperfluorescence due to pigment epithelial atrophy whilst the lower half may hypofluoresce. In the later stages of the disease areas of pigment epithelial atrophy and neovascularization are clearly demonstrated on angiography.

Electrophysiology

Classically, the EOG is subnormal in all individuals carrying the abnormal gene and has been used as a predictive test in genetic counselling (Deutman 1969). However, Weber *et al.* (1994) on the basis of molecular genetic haplotype analysis have identified one individual who carries the disease haplotype but is symptomless with a normal fundus appearance and normal EOG. Confirmation of the reliability of EOG in this condition will therefore need to await future mutation analysis of the Best's disease gene. Although the finding of an abnormal EOG in most cases suggests that there is a widespread disorder of the pigment epithelium, peripheral visual fields, dark adaptometry and ERG are normal.

Molecular genetics

Best's disease has been mapped to chromosome 11q13 in a number of pedigrees (Nichols *et al.* 1994; Weber *et al.* 1994). A condition termed atypical vitelliform macular dystrophy has been mapped to chromosome 8q24 (Ferrel *et al.* 1983). Affected patients have lesions similar to those seen in typical Best's disease but these tend to be smaller and more widespread. Patients with the atypical form have normal EOG responses. Macular vitelliform lesions have also been described in families with peripherin/RDS gene mutations (Wells *et al.* 1993).

Visual prognosis

The overall visual prognosis in this disorder is good (Mohler & Fines 1981; Godel *et al.* 1986; Clement 1991; Fishman *et al.* 1993). Although patients with stage 0 and I disease may progress to a typical vitelliform lesion most do not (Mohler & Fines 1981) so the visual prognosis in these groups is excellent. Patients with stage II disease do progress but most maintain good acuity in at least one eye for many years (Mohler & Fines 1981; Fishman *et al.* 1993). Patients with atrophic maculae (stage IV) have the worst prognosis but even then deterioration is slow and since the disease is often asymmetrical the visual prognosis overall is good. Fishman *et al.* (1993) studied 47 patients with vitelliform dystrophy who had stage II–IV disease and found that the majority of patients under the age of 40 had a visual acuity of 20/40 or better. However, only 20% of patients older than 40, and no patient older than 50,

had a visual acuity of 20/40 or better—a level of acuity sufficient to pass the driving standard in the UK and most American states. Most patients do, however, retain reasonable reading vision in at least one eye throughout their working life.

North Carolina macular dystrophy

Disorders previously described as dominant progressive foveal dystrophy (occasionally seen with aminoaciduria) (Lefler *et al.* 1971; Frank *et al.* 1974), central pigment epithelial and choroidal degeneration (Leveille *et al.* 1982) and central areolar pigment epithelial dystrophy (Fetkenhaur *et al.* 1976; Hermsen & Judisch 1984) have now been reclassified as this single, dominant, completely penetrant, stationary condition with high variation in expressivity (Small *et al.* 1992). The dystrophy is of early onset and may represent a failure in the development of the macular region (Small *et al.* 1992). Affected children may be asymptomatic with normal visual acuity or have severe acuity loss down to 3/60 with large central scotomas. Macular drusen are seen in the most mildly affected individuals (grade 1 disease) which may also appear confluent (grade 2). In grade 3 disease, lesions resembling macular staphylomas or colobomas are seen and are associated with severe acuity loss. Visual prognosis in grades 1 and 2 is good unless complicated by subretinal neovascularization. Previous reports of progressive pathology have now been discounted (Small *et al.* 1991). EOG, ERG and colour vision assessments are normal. Molecular genetic linkage analysis has localized the causative gene to chromosome 6q14–q16.2 (Small *et al.* 1993). Holz *et al.* (1995) have described a family in which different individuals expressed a range of phenotypes including North Carolina macular dystrophy. Molecular genetic analysis excluded linkage to the chromosome 6q locus suggesting that this phenotype is genetically heterogeneous.

Progressive bifocal macular dystrophy

Waheed and Wyse (1968) have described an autosomal dominant retinal dystrophy seen in a large Scottish family. The fundus abnormalities are evident in the first few weeks of life when a large oval area of atrophy is seen extending from the optic disc to temporal to the macula (Fig. 45.10). Only a few large choroidal vessels are seen in the base of the lesion. Later a similar area of atrophy involving retina, pigment epithelium and choroid develops on the nasal side of the disc. There is slow progression of the atrophic areas and a peripheral pigmentary retinopathy is often present. Most patients are myopic with a manifest nystagmus. Although central vision is poor some peripheral vision is maintained throughout life. We have examined one child from this family who

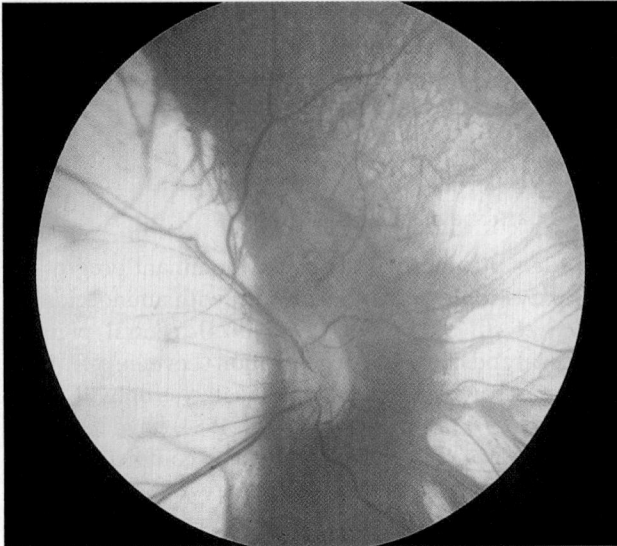

Fig. 45.10 Bifocal chorioretinal atrophy. Large oval areas of atrophy extending nasal and temporal to the optic disc (Professor A.C. Bird's patient).

developed a giant retinal tear and total retinal detachment. Recent molecular genetic data suggest that this condition may be allelic with North Carolina macular dystrophy (Kelsall *et al.* 1995).

Benign concentric macular dystrophy

Deutman (1974) has described one family with a dominantly inherited macular dystrophy in which affected members have a ring of pigment epithelial atrophy surrounding the macula. Fluorescein angiography showed a 'bull's eye' maculopathy. The macular abnormality may be seen in childhood and the visual acuity at presentation is good. Later there may be nyctalopia, reduced colour vision and a peripheral pigmentary retinopathy; the ERG shows evidence of a more widespread cone and rod dystrophy (Van der Biesen *et al.* 1985). The visual prognosis is relatively good, distinguishing this condition from other cone–rod dystrophies.

Fenestrated sheen macular dystrophy

Fenestrated sheen macular dystrophy is an autosomal dominant disorder characterized by slow visual deterioration and a characteristic macular appearance. Although the macular abnormalities are apparent in childhood, visual symptoms do not start until the fifth or sixth decade. The earliest macular abnormality is seen as a refractile green–yellow sheen at the macula with multiple red spots which represent 'windows' in the sheen which allow the normal choroidal appearance to show through.

Later there may be a 'bull's eye' area of retinal pigment epithelial atrophy at the fovea. The ERG and EOG are normal until late in the disease (Sneed & Sieving 1991).

Dominant cystoid macular oedema

Several pedigrees of dominantly inherited cystoid macular oedema have been described (Deutman *et al.* 1976; Notting & Pinckers 1977; Fishman *et al.* 1979). Variable visual loss and specifically blue–green colour vision deficit may be seen in childhood. Other findings include hyperopia, wrinkling of the internal limiting membrane and a mild peripheral pigmentary disturbance. The ERG is normal but the EOG is abnormal in older patients suggestive of a pigment epithelial disorder (Pinckers *et al.* 1983). Histopathological studies indicate that Müller cells are the primary cells involved in this condition (Loeffler *et al.* 1992). Kremer *et al.* (1994) have mapped a dominant cystoid macular oedema locus to chromosome 7p15–p21.

Pattern dystrophies of the retinal pigment epithelium

The pattern dystrophies are a group of disorders characterized by mildly reduced visual acuity associated with subretinal deposition of yellow, grey or pigmented material in various configurations (Fig. 45.11) (Gass 1987; Pinckers 1988). The ERG is usually normal although the EOG may show a reduced light rise. Although these dystrophies often first present in adult life many have been seen in childhood. The disorders are usually classified by the pattern of the pigment epithelial abnormality but different patterns may be seen within the same family so it is not clear how many distinct nosological entities there are (Pinckers 1988).

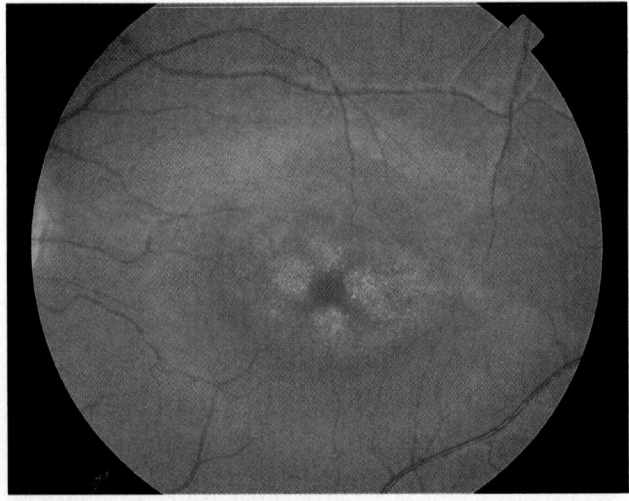

Fig. 45.11 Pattern dystrophy.

Butterfly-shaped dystrophy

This autosomal dominant macular dystrophy is first evident in late childhood. It usually presents with mild visual disturbance and fundus examination shows bilateral butterfly-shaped pigmentation at the level of the pigment epithelium. The abnormal pigment blocks the underlying choroidal fluorescence on angiography (Deutman *et al.* 1970). Visual acuity is normal or mildly reduced and colour vision, peripheral visual fields and dark adaptation are normal. The visual prognosis is good.

Reticular dystrophy

This rare form of pattern dystrophy was first reported by Sjögren in 1950, and several subsequent pedigrees have been reported (Deutman & Rumke 1969; Chopdar 1976; Kingham *et al.* 1978). It may be inherited as an autosomal dominant or autosomal recessive trait (Gass 1987).

Reticular dystrophy may first appear in early childhood (Deutman & Rumke 1969; Kingham *et al.* 1978). In these early stages there is an accumulation of pigment granules at the fovea and later a typical reticular pattern which extends out to the periphery. The appearance resembles a 'fishnet with knots'. Visual acuity is usually normal (Deutman & Rumke 1969; Kingham *et al.* 1978). The ERG is normal but the EOG may show a reduced light rise (Kingham *et al.* 1978). Dark adaptation may show elevated rod thresholds (Kingham *et al.* 1978).

Macroreticular (spider) dystrophy, an autosomal dominant condition, is similar to the reticular dystrophy described by Sjögren but with a much more striking, coarser pattern of pigmentation, of later onset and usually associated with significant loss of visual acuity (Mesker *et al.* 1970).

Fundus pulverulentus

This rare disorder is characterized by normal visual acuity, a symmetrical granular mottled pigmentation at the posterior pole and non-progression (Fig. 45.12). It has been reported in two generations of a family and may be inherited as an autosomal dominant trait (Slezalk & Hommer 1969).

Pattern dystrophies with peripherin/RDS mutations

A number of mutations (encoding premature termination codons) of the *peripherin/RDS* gene within different families have been associated with pattern dystrophy phenotypes (Nichols *et al.* 1993a, b; Weleber *et al.* 1993; Kim *et al.* 1995). In these families there is progressive visual loss and both the EOG and flash ERG are abnormal. Dark adaptation is also abnormal. These phenotypes are therefore more severe than those usually seen in pattern dystrophy

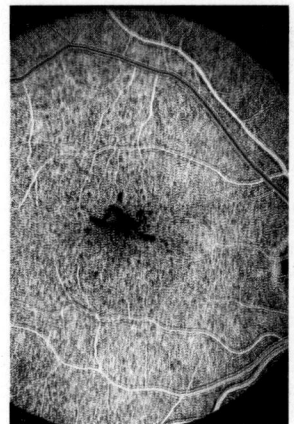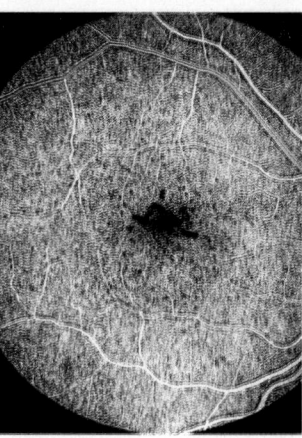

Fig. 45.12 Fundus pulverulentus. Fluorescein angiogram showing mottled and clumped pigment epithelium at the posterior pole (Professor A.C. Bird's patient).

and this should be taken into account in the genetic counselling of such families.

Other dominantly inherited macular dystrophies

Several different dominantly inherited macular dystrophies may be seen which do not fit any of the classically described phenotypes. In general, they are only very slowly progressive and the visual prognosis is good. The presence of well-preserved colour vision and normal ERG serves to differentiate these disorders from the inherited cone and cone–rod dystrophies.

Macular abnormalities in the generalized receptor dystrophies

Cone dystrophy

Cone dystrophies may be subdivided into stationary and progressive forms. Progressive cone dystrophy usually presents in the first two decades of life with reduced central vision, poor colour vision and variable nystagmus and photophobia. Fundus examination usually shows a bilateral 'bull's eye' maculopathy often with a degree of temporal pallor of the optic disc. On fluorescein angiography there is usually a central area of hyperfluorescence related to the pigment epithelial atrophy (Fig. 45.13) and there may be absence of the normal choroidal fluorescence ('dark choroid'). The ERG shows absent or diminished cone responses but a well-preserved scotopic response. Cone dystrophy may be distinguished from other causes of 'bull's eye' maculopathy by the early loss of colour vision and specific abnormality of the cone ERG (see Chapter 9). Progressive cone dystrophy loci have been mapped to chromosomes 6q25–q26 (Tranebjaerg *et al.* 1986), 17p12–13 (Balciuniene *et al.* 1995), Xq28 (Reichel *et*

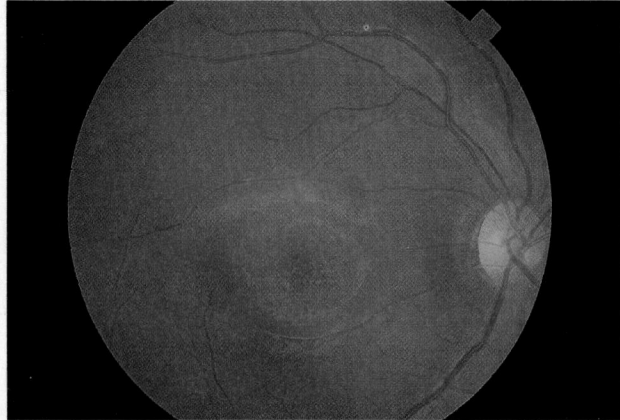

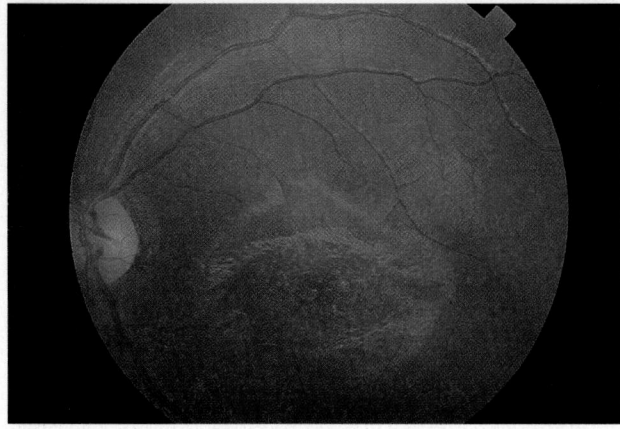

Fig. 45.13 (a, b) Progressive cone dystrophy. This 10-year-old child presented with progressive loss of visual acuity and colour vision and had defective cone function on ERG.

al. 1989) and Xp21–p11.1 (Meire *et al.* 1994). In the former X-linked cone dystrophy, good visual acuity is associated with predominant loss of longwave (red) cone function with normal rod function. In the latter case, progressive rod dysfunction in elder male affected members would suggest that this locus more correctly identifies an X-linked cone–rod dystrophy.

Cone–rod dystrophy

The cone–rod dystrophies present in a similar way to the cone dystrophies; differentiation is important, however, since visual prognosis in cone–rod dystrophy is worse. This differentiation may be based on electrophysiological responses. In cone–rod dystrophy, the abnormal photopic responses are accompanied by reduced scotopic responses. Initially there is loss of acuity and colour vision in childhood with later night-blindness and peripheral field loss. In the early stages, there is pigment epithelial atrophy confined to the macula but later there is peripheral pigment epithelial atrophy, retinal arteriolar narrowing and optic atrophy. Initially there is minimal peripheral

intraretinal pigmentation but classical bone spicule pigmentation may develop later (Evans *et al.* 1995). Cone–rod dystrophies may be subdivided into those with separate posterior polar and peripheral retinal foci of disease (Rabb *et al.* 1986) and those expressing an 'inverse retinitis pigmentosa' pattern of disease which spreads centrifugally from the macula into the periphery. Dominant and recessive inheritance patterns are seen and cone–rod dystrophy loci have been mapped to chromosomes 18q21.1 (Warburg *et al.* 1991), 18q (Kylstra & Aylsworth 1993) and 19q (Evans *et al.* 1994) and may be associated with peripherin/RDS gene mutations (Jacobson *et al.* 1994; Nakazawa *et al.* 1994). An Arg 46 stop peripherin/RDS mutation has been associated with the inverse retinitis pigmentosa-type picture of disease (Apfelstedt-Sylla *et al.* 1995).

Rod–cone dystrophy

In most rod–cone dystrophies macular atrophy is seen at a late stage although macular oedema may be seen at any time (see Chapter 44). Chronic macular oedema may be complicated by the development of a macular hole. However, in some patients, for example those with the Bardet–Biedl syndrome, macular involvement may be seen early in the disease. Early night-blindness, peripheral field loss and a reduced rod ERG preceding loss of central acuity, however, means that these disorders are rarely confused with the primary macular dystrophies.

Macular dysplasia ('coloboma')

Bilateral macular dysplasia (coloboma) has been described in association with a variety of inherited retinal dystrophies including Leber's amaurosis (Leighton & Harris 1973; Margolis *et al.* 1977; Moore *et al.* 1985), retinitis pigmentosa (Friedman & Gombos 1971), cone–rod dystrophy (Heckenlively *et al.* 1988), Joubert's syndrome (Lewis *et al.* 1994) and idiopathic infantile hypercalciuria, an autosomal recessive disorder with renal abnormalities, high myopia and a rod–cone dystrophy (Meier *et al.* 1979; Gil-Gilberneau *et al.* 1982). It has also been described in association with skeletal abnormalities (Sorsby 1935; Phillips & Griffiths 1969; Thompson & Baraitser 1988). Satorre *et al.* (1980) described a family with dominantly inherited macular colobomas. In contrast to North Carolina macular dystrophy, there was no variability of expression, each affected member had poor visual acuity and fundoscopy showed evidence of an oval area of atrophy at the macula with absence of the retinal pigment epithelium and choriocapillaris. No ERG was performed so it is unclear whether there was an associated generalized rod–cone dystrophy

In patients with macular dysplasia the retinal lesions are seen as sharply demarcated areas of retinal pigment epithelial and choroidal atrophy at the posterior pole;

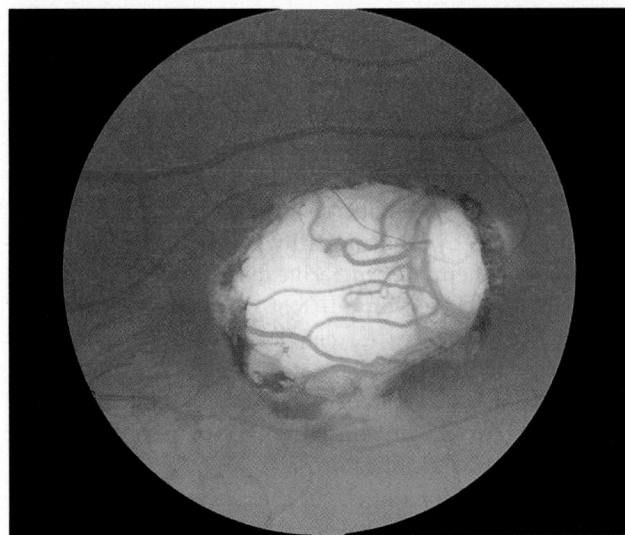

Fig. 45.14 Small macular coloboma with large choroidal vessels in its base.

there may be pigmentation at the edge of the lesion and a few large choroidal vessels may cross bare sclera at the base of the coloboma (Figs 45.14, 45.15). Scleral ectasia is often present. The macular appearance does not appear to change with time. The ophthalmoscopic appearance may resemble North Carolina macular dystrophy or congenital toxoplasmosis-related chorioretinal scarring.

Inner retinal disorders

X-linked juvenile retinoschisis (see Chapter 41)

X-linked juvenile retinoschisis (XLRS) is the most common macular dystrophy affecting male children. Affected males usually present at school age when reduced vision is detected at school screening examinations or when difficulties with reading or distance vision are noted. Other children may present with strabismus or less commonly with sudden onset of vitreous haemorrhage. Macular abnormalities are seen in all affected patients but may be very subtle in children and the condition is commonly misdiagnosed (Deutman 1971; George *et al.* 1995). The characteristic macular change in XLRS is foveal schisis which is seen as small superficial cysts radiating out from the fovea in a wheel-like fashion. It is best seen using red-free light. Foveal schisis is most common in younger patients; in older patients the typical radiating striae regress leaving an indistinct foveal reflex and later macular retinal pigment epithelial atrophy with or without pigmentary disturbance (Deutmann 1971; George *et al.* 1996a, b). Fluorescein angiography is usually normal in the early stages but 'window defects' may be seen in older patients with retinal pigment epithelial atrophy.

Peripheral retinoschisis is present in around 50% of patients (Deutman 1971; Kellner *et al.* 1990; George *et al.* 1996a, b). The splitting occurs in the superficial layers of the retina and retinal vessels may lie in the outer or inner leaf or traverse the schisis cavity. Inner leaf breaks are common and membranous remnants on the posterior hyaloid face, so-called vitreous veils, are commonly seen (Forsius *et al.* 1962; George *et al.* 1996b). Other peripheral retinal changes include perivascular sheathing, microvascular abnormalities, retinal neovascularization (Pearson & Jagger 1989; de Jong *et al.* 1991) and a silvery grey inner retinal reflex (de Jong *et al.* 1991). High, mainly hyperopic refractive errors are common and strabismus is present in about 20% of affected individuals (George *et al.* 1996a, b).

The visual prognosis in XLRS is relatively good unless complications such as vitreous haemorrhage or retinal detachment ensue. The vision and macular appearance change very little during childhood but vision may deteriorate in the fourth or fifth decade when retinal pigment epithelium atrophy occurs.

Electrophysiology

The flash ERG is abnormal in all individuals with XLRS even in those individuals where the ophthalmoscopic abnormalities are confined to the fovea. Characteristically there is a reduced scotopic and photopic b-wave. Other signals derived from the inner retina such as the oscillatory potentials and the scotopic threshold response are also abnormal (Peachey *et al.* 1987; Murayama *et al.* 1991). The a-wave is normal in the early stages of the disease indicating that the photoreceptors are not primarily involved but older affected individuals may show reduced amplitudes of the a-wave (Miyake *et al.* 1993) and a reduced light rise of the EOG (Tanino *et al.* 1985) reflecting secondary

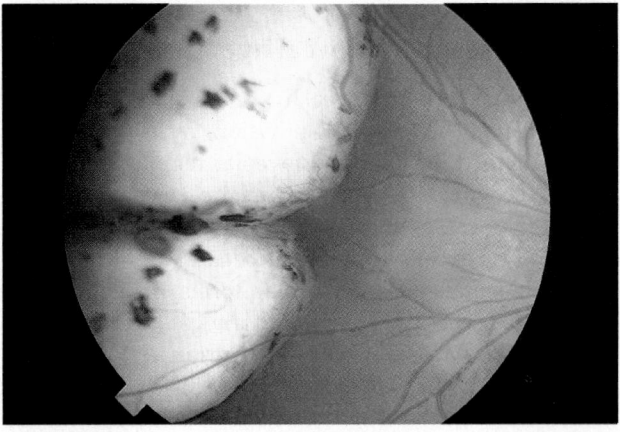

Fig. 45.15 Macular coloboma. Large ectatic bilobed macular lesion with pigment clumps in its base and one large central and a few other small choroidal vessels crossing it. Surprisingly, the acuity in this eye was 6/36.

involvement of photoreceptors and retinal pigment epithelium.

Molecular genetics

The locus for XLRS has been localized to the Xp22 region of the distal short arm of the X chromosome; there is no evidence of genetic heterogeneity (Alitalo *et al.* 1988; Dahl *et al.* 1988; Sieving *et al.* 1990; George *et al.* 1996a). A large number of highly polymorphic microsatellite markers are available in this region which can be used for carrier detection in at-risk females in families with XLRS.

Differential diagnosis

Foveal schisis may also be seen in Goldmann–Favre syndrome (see Chapter 41) and also rarely as an autosomal recessive or dominantly inherited disorder. The autosomal recessive inheritance, severe nyctalopia, pigmentary retinopathy and reduced a- and b-waves on the ERG help to differentiate XLRS from Goldmann–Favre syndrome. The characteristic ERG changes and the family history will usually help to distinguish XLRS from isolated foveal schisis.

Familial foveal retinoschisis

Yassur *et al.* (1982) have described a dominantly inherited form of retinoschisis. All affected family members had peripheral retinoschisis and peripheral retinal pigment epithelial atrophy. In three cases there was a typical macular retinoschisis. Most patients had a normal ERG. Lewis *et al.* (1977) described three (female) siblings with mild visual loss and bilateral macular retinoschisis indistinguishable from that seen in the X-linked disorder. The ERG was normal in two of the cases and mildly abnormal in the third.

Ocular disease and foveal hypoplasia

In the various forms of foveal hypoplasia there is reduced vision, usually normal colour vision, nystagmus and a poorly defined macular and foveolar region; there is no readily recognized foveolar or luteal pigment and blood vessels may cross the presumed macular region (Oliver *et al.* 1987). Foveal hypoplasia is seen in aniridia and in both oculocutaneous and ocular forms of albinism; it may also be seen in the different forms of achromatopsia and as an isolated abnormality (Curran & Robb 1976; Yoshizumi *et al.* 1979; O'Donnell & Pappas 1982; Oliver *et al.* 1987). Most cases of isolated foveal hypoplasia are sporadic but a dom-inant pedigree has been reported (O'Donnell & Pappas 1982).

Macular abnormalities and inherited systemic disorders

Macular abnormalities may be seen in a variety of other inherited disorders. A cherry red spot due to the accumulation of abnormal material in the ganglion cells is seen in several neurometabolic disorders (see Chapter 57). In addition bull's eye maculopathy is a frequent finding in certain of the neurodegenerative disorders especially Batten's disease, Hallervorden–Spatz disease and olivopontocerebellar atrophy. A macular dystrophy has been described with cerebellar ataxia and saccade palsy (Enevoldson *et al.* 1994). These neurometabolic disorders are covered in detail in other chapters.

Macular abnormalities are also seen in several other inherited conditions such as the Sjögren–Larsson syndrome, cystinosis and oxalosis which are discussed in the differential diagnosis of the flecked retina syndromes (see Chapter 48).

References

Alitalo T, Forsius H, Karna J *et al.* Linkage relationships and gene order around the locus for X-linked retinoschisis. *Am J Hum Genet* 1988; **43**: 476–83.

Apfelstedt-Sylla E, Theischen M, Rüther K *et al.* Extensive intrafamilial and interfamilial phenotypic variation among patients with autosomal dominant retinal dystrophy and mutations in the human RDS/peripherin gene. *Br J Ophthalmol* 1995; **79**: 28–34.

Baca W, Fishman GA, Alexander KR, Glenn AM. Dark adaptation in patients with Best vitelliform macular dystrophy. *Br J Ophthalmol* 1994; **78**: 430–2.

Balciuniene J, Johansson K, Sanderen O *et al.* A gene for autosomal dominant progressive cone dystrophy (CORDS) maps to chromosome 17p12–13. *Genomics* 1995; **30**: 221–6.

Barkman Y. Clinical study of central tapetoretinal degeneration. *Acta Ophthalmol* 1961; **39**: 663–71.

Bither PP, Berns EA. Dominant inheritance of Stargardt's disease. *J Am Optom Assoc* 1988; **59**: 112–17.

Bonnin P, Passet M, Tricolaire-Cotten M. Le signe du silence choroidien dans les degenerescences tapeto-retienes posterieures. *Doc Ophthalmol Proc Ser* 1976; **9**: 461–3.

Braley AE, Spivey BE. Hereditary vitelline macular degeneration. *Arch Ophthalmol* 1964; **72**: 743–62.

Chopdar A. Reticular dystrophy of the retina. *Br J Ophthalmol* 1976; **60**: 342–4.

Chopdar A. A variant of central areolar choroidal dystrophy. *Ophthal Paediatr Genet* 1993; **14**: 151–64.

Cibis GN, Meorey M, Harris DJ. Dominantly inherited macular dystrophy with flecks (Stargardt). *Arch Ophthalmol* 1980; **98**: 1785–9.

Curran RE, Robb RM. Isolated foveal hypoplasia. *Arch Ophthalmol* 1976; **94**: 48–50.

Curry AF, Moorman LT. Fluorescein photography of vitelliform macular degeneration. *Arch Ophthalmol* 1968; **79**: 705–9.

Deutman AF. Benign concentric angular dystrophy. *Am J Ophthalmol* 1974; **78**: 384–96.

Deutman AF. Electro-oculography in families with vitelliform dystrophy of the fovea. Detection of the carrier state. *Arch Ophthalmol* 1969; **81**: 305–16.

Deutman AF. *The Hereditary Dystrophies of the Posterior Pole of the Eye.* Netherlands: Van Georcum, 1971.

Deutman AF, Pinckers AJLG, De Kerk AL. Dominantly inherited cystoid macular edema. *Am J Ophthalmol* 1976; **82**: 540–8.

Deutman AF, Rumke AML. Reticular dystrophy of the retinal pigment epithelium. *Arch Ophthalmol* 1969; **82**: 4–9.

Deutman AF, Van Blommenstein, Henkes HE *et al.* Butterfly-shaped dystrophy of the fovea. *Arch Ophthalmol* 1970; **83**: 558–69.

de Jong PT, Zrenner E, van Meel GJ, Keunen JEE, van Norren D. Mizuo phenomenon in X-linked retinoschisis. *Arch Ophthalmol* 1991; **109**: 1104–8.

Enevoldson TP, Sanders MD, Harding AE. Autosomal dominant cerebellar ataxia with pigmentary macular dystrophy: a clinical and genetic study of eight families. *Brain* 1994; **117**: 445–60.

Evans K, Duvall-Young J, Fitzke FW *et al.* Chromosome 19q cone–rod retinal dystrophy, ocular phenotype. *Arch Ophthalmol* 1995; **113**: 195–201.

Evans K, Fryer A, Inglehearn C *et al.* Genetic linkage of cone–rod retinal dystrophy to chromosome 19q and evidence for segregation distortion. *Nature Genet* 1994; **6**: 210–13.

Ferrell RE, Hittner HM, Antoszyk JH. Linkage of atypical vitelliform macular dystrophy (VMD-1) to the soluble glutamate pyruvate transaminase (GPT1) locus. *Am J Hum Genet* 1983; **35**: 78–84.

Fetkenhaur CL, Gurney N, Dobbie JG, Chromokos E. Central areolar pigment epithelial dystrophy. *Am J Ophthalmol* 1976; **81**: 745–53.

Fish G, Grey R, Sehmi KS, Bird AG. The dark choroid in posterior retinal dystrophies. *Br J Ophthalmol* 1981; **65**: 359–63.

Fishman GA. Fundus flavimaculatus. *Arch Ophthalmol* 1976; **94**: 2061–7.

Fishman GA, Farbman JS, Alexander KR. Delayed rod dark adaption in patients with Stargardt's disease. *Ophthalmology* 1991; **98**: 957–62.

Fishman GA, Goldberg MF, Trautmann JC. Dominantly inherited cystoid macular oedema. *Am J Ophthalmol* 1979; **11**: 21–7.

Forsius H, Vainio-Mattila B, Eriksson A. X-linked retinoschisis. *Br J Ophthalmol* 1962; **46**: 678–81.

Frangieh GT, Green R, Fine SL. A histopathologic study of Best's macular dystrophy. *Arch Ophthalmol* 1982; **100**: 1115–21.

Frank RH, Landers MD, Williams RJ, Sidbury JB. A new dominant progressive foveal dystrophy. *Am J Ophthalmol* 1974; **78**: 913–16.

Friedman J, Gombos GM. Bilateral macular coloboma keratoconus and retinitis pigmentosa. *Am J Ophthalmol* 1971; **3**: 664–6.

Gass JDM. Heredodystrophic disorders affecting the pigment epithelium and retina. In: Gass JDM, ed. *Stereoscopic Atlas of Macular Disease*, 3rd edn. St Louis: CV Mosby, 1987: 255–331.

Gellert G, Petersen J, Kraczak M, Zoll B. Linkage relationship between retinoschisis and four marker loci. *Hum Genet* 1988; **79**: 382–4.

George NDL, Yates JRW, Moore AT. Juvenile X-linked retinoschisis. *Br J Ophthalmol* 1995; **79**: 697–702.

George NDL, Payne SJ, Bill R, Barton D, Moore AT, Yates JRW. Improved genetic mapping of X-linked retinoschisis. *J Med Genet* 1996; **33**: 919–22.

George NDL, Yates JRW, Moore AT. Clinical features of affected males in juvenile X-linked retinoschisis. *Arch Ophthalmol* 1996b; **114**: 274–80.

Gil-Gilberneau J, Galan A, Callis L, Rodrigo C. Infantile idiopathic hypercalciuria, high congenital myopia and atypical macular coloboma: a new oculo-renal syndrome. *J Pediatr Ophthalmol* 1982, **19**: 7–11.

Glacet-Bernard A, Coscas G. Full thickness macular hole and retinal detachment complicating Best's disease. *Eur J Ophthalmol* 1993; **3**: 53–4.

Godel V, Chaine G, Regenbogen L, Coscas G. Best's vitelliform macular dystrophy. *Acta Ophthalmol* 1986; **175**: 5–31.

Hadden BO, Gass JDM. Fundus flavimaculatus and Stargardt's disease. *Am J Ophthalmol* 1976; **82**: 527–39.

Heckenlively JR, Foxman SG, Parelhoff EG. Retinal dystrophy and macular coloboma. *Doc Ophthalmol* 1988; **68**: 257–71.

Heher KL, Johns DR. A maculopathy associated with the 15257 mitochondrial DNA mutation. *Arch Ophthalmol* 1993; **111**: 1495–9.

Hermsen VM, Judisch GM. Central areolar pigment epithelial dystrophy. *Ophthalmologica (Basel)* 1984; **189**: 69–72.

Holz FG, Evans K, Gregory CY, Bhattacharya SS, Bird AC. Autosomal dominant macular dystrophy simulating North Carolina macular dystrophy. *Arch Ophthalmol* 1995; **113**: 178–84.

Hoyng CB, Heutink P, Deutman AF, Oostra BA. A mutation in codon 142 in central areolar choroidal dystrophy. *Invest Ophthalmol Vis Sci* 1995; **36**(Suppl.): 3817.

Isashiki Y, Ohba N. Fundus flavimaculatus. *Br J Ophthalmol* 1985; **69**: 522–4.

Jacobson SG, Kemp CM, Cideciyan AV *et al.* Spectrum of functional phenotypes in RDS gene mutations. *Invest Ophthalmol Vis Sci* 1994; **35**(Suppl.): 1044.

Kellner U, Brummer S, Foerster MH, Wessing A. X-linked congenital retinoschisis. *Graefe's Arch Clin Exp Ophthalmol* 1990; **228**: 432–7.

Kelsall R, Godley B, Evans K *et al.* Localisation of the gene for progressive bifocal chorioretinal atrophy (PBCRA) to chromosome 6q. *Am J Hum Genet* 1995; **4**: 1653–6.

Kaplan J, Gerber S, Larget-Piet D *et al.* A gene for Stargardt's disease (fundus flavimaculatus) maps to the short arm of chromosome 1. *Nature Genet* 1993; **5**: 308–11.

Kim RY, Dollfus H, Keen TJ *et al.* Autosomal dominant pattern dystrophy of the retina associated with a four base pair insertion at codon 140 in the peripherin/RDS gene. *Arch Ophthalmol* 1995; **113**: 451–5.

Kingham JD, Fenzyl RE, Willerson D, Aberg TM. Reticular dystrophy of the pigment epithelium: a clinical and electrophysiological study of three generations. *Arch Ophthalmol* 1978; **96**: 1177–84.

Klystra JA, Aylsworth AS. Cone–rod retinal dystrophy in a patient with neurofibromatosis type 1. *Canad J Ophthalmol* 1993; **28**: 79–80.

Kraushar MF, Margolis S, Morse P, Nugent ME. Pseudohypopyon in Best's vitelliform macular dystrophy. *Am J Ophthalmol* 1982; **94**: 30–7.

Kremer H, Pinckers A, van den Helm B *et al.* Localisation of the gene for dominant cystoid macular dystrophy on chromosome 7p. *Hum Mol Genet* 1994; **3**: 299–302.

Lefler WH, Wadsworth JAC, Sidbury JB Jr. Hereditary macular degeneration and aminoaciduria. *Am J Ophthalmol* 1971; **71**: 224–30.

Leighton D, Harris R. Retinal aplasia in association with macular coloboma, keratoconus and cataract. *Clin Genet* 1973; **4**: 270–4.

Leveille AS, Morse PH, Kiernan JP. Autosomal dominant central pigment epithelial and choroidal degeneration. *Ophthalmology* 1982; **89**: 1407–13.

Lewis RA, Lee GB, Martinyi CL *et al.* Familial foveal retinoschisis. *Arch Ophthalmol* 1977; **95**: 1190–6.

Lewis SME, Roberts EA, Marion MA *et al.* Joubert syndrome with congenital hepatic fibrosis — an entity in the spectrum of oculo-encephalo-hepato-renal disorders. *Am J Hum Genet* 1994; **52**: 419–26.

Loeffler KU, Li Z-L, Fishman GA, Tso MOM. Dominant inherited cystoid macular edema, a histopathological study. *Ophthalmology* 1992; **99**: 1385–92.

Mansour AM. Long-term follow-up of dominant macular dystrophy with flecks (Stargardt). *Ophthalmologica* 1992; **205**: 138–43.

Margolis S, Sher BM, Garr RE. Macular coloboma in Leber's congenital amaurosis. *Am J Ophthalmol* 1977; **83**: 27–31.

Meier W, Blumberg A, Imahorn W *et al*. Idiopathic hypercalciuria with bilateral macular colobomata: a new variant of oculorenal syndrome. *Helv Paediat Acta* 1979; **34**: 257–69.

Meire FM, Bergen AAB, De Rouck A, Leys M, Dellman JW. X-linked cone dystrophy: localisation of the gene locus to Xp21–p11.1 by linkage analysis. *Br J Ophthalmol* 1994; **78**: 103–8.

Mesker RP, Osterhas JA, Dellerman JW. A retinal lesion resembling Sjögren's dystrophia reticularis laminae pigmentosae retinae. In: *Perspective in Ophthalmology*. Amsterdam: Excerpta Medica, 1970; **II**: 40–5.

Miyake Y, Shiroyama N, Ota I, Horiguchi M. Focal macular electroretinogram in X-linked congenital retinoschisis. *Invest Ophthalmol Vis Sci* 1993; **34**: 512–15.

Mohler CW, Fines SL. Long-term evaluation of patients with Best's vitelliform dystrophy. *Ophthalmology* 1981; **88**: 688–91.

Moore AT, Harden A, Taylor DSI. Bilateral macular dysplasia (colobomata) and congenital retinal dystrophy. *Br J Ophthalmol* 1985; **69**: 691–9.

Murayama K, Kuo CY, Sieving PA. Abnormal threshold ERG response in X-linked juvenile retinoschisis: evidence for a proximal retinal origin of the human STR. *Clin Vis Sci* 1991; **6**: 317–22.

Nakazawa M, Kikawa E, Chida Y, Tamai. Asn 244 His mutation of the peripherin/RDS gene causing autosomal dominant cone–rod retinal degeneration. *Hum Mol Genet* 1994; **3**: 1195–6.

Nichols BE, Bascom R, Litt M, McInnes R, Sheffield AC, Stone EM. Refining the locus for Best vitelliform macular dystrophy and mutation analysis of the gene ROM1. *Am J Hum Genet* 1994; **54**: 95–103.

Nichols BE, Drack AV, Vandenburgh K *et al*. A two base pair deletion in the RDS gene associated with butterfly-shaped pigment dystrophy of the fovea. *Hum Mol Genet* 1993a; **2**: 601–3.

Nichols BE, Sheffield VC, Vandenburgh K *et al*. Butterfly-shaped pigment dystrophy of the fovea caused by a point mutation in codon 167 of the RDS gene. *Nature Genet* 1993b; **3**: 202–7.

Noble KG. Hereditary macular dystrophies. In: Renie WA, ed. *Goldberg's Genetic and Metabolic Eye Disease*. Boston/Toronto: Little, Brown, 1986: 439–64.

Noble KG, Carr RE. Stargardt's disease and fundus flavimaculatus. *Arch Ophthalmol* 1979; **97**: 1281–5.

Notting JGA, Pinckers AJLG. Dominant cystoid macular oedema. *Am J Ophthalmol* 1977; **83**: 234–41.

O'Donnell FE Jr, Pappas HR. Autosomal dominant foveal hypoplasia and pre-senile cataracts: a new syndrome. *Arch Ophthalmol* 1982; **100**: 279–81.

Oliver MD, Dotan SA, Chemke I, Ahraham FA. Isolated foveal hypoplasia. *Br J Ophthalmol* 1987; **71**: 926–30.

Peachey NS, Fishman GA, Derlacki DJ, Brigell MG. Psychophysical and electroretinographic findings in X-linked juvenile retinoschisis. *Arch Ophthalmol* 1987; **105**: 513–16.

Pearson R, Jagger J. Sex-linked retinoschisis with optic disc and peripheral retinal neovascularisation. *Br J Ophthalmol* 1989; **73**: 311–13.

Phillips CI, Griffiths DL. Macular abnormality and skeletal abnormality. *Br J Ophthalmol* 1969; **53**: 346–9.

Pinckers A. Patterned dystrophies of the retinal pigment epithelium. A review. *Ophthalmol Paediatr Genet* 1988; **9**: 77–114.

Pinckers A, Deutman AF, Lion F, Aan de Kerk AL. Dominant cystoid macular dystrophy. *Ophthalmol Paediatr Genet* 1983; **3**: 157–67.

Rabb MF, Tso MO, Fishman GA. Cone–rod dystrophy. A clinical and histopathologic report. *Ophthalmology* 1986; **93**: 1443–51.

Reichel E, Bruce AM, Sandberg MA, Berson EL. An electroretino-

graphic and molecular genetic study of X-linked cone degeneration. *Am J Ophthalmol* 1989; **108**: 540–7.

Satorre J, Lopez JM, Ats-Due JM, Pinera P. Dominant macular coloboma. *J Pediatr Ophthalmol Strabismus* 1980; **27**: 148–52.

Schachat AP, Green WR, Patz A. Macular hole and retinal detachment in Best's disease. *Retina* 1985; **5**: 22–5.

Sieving PA, Bingham EL, Roth MS *et al*. Linkage relationship of X-linked juvenile retinoschisis with Xp22.1–p22.3 probes. *Am J Hum Genet* 1990; **47**: 616–21.

Sjogren H. Dystrophica reticularis laminae pigmentosa retinale. An earlier described hereditary eye disease. *Acta Ophthalmol (KBH)* 1950; **28**: 279–95.

Slezalk H, Hommer K. Fundus pulverulentus. *Von Graefe Arch Klin Exp Ophthalmol* 1969; **178**: 177–82.

Small KW, Hermsen V, Gurney N, Fetenhour CL, Folk JC. North Carolina macular dystrophy and central areolar pigment epithelial dystrophy. One family, one disease. *Arch Ophthalmol* 1992; **110**: 515–18.

Small KW, Killian J, McLean WL. North Carolina dominant progressive foveal dystrophy, how progressive is it? *Br J Ophthalmol* 1991; **75**: 401–6.

Small KW, Weber J, Roses A, Pericak-Vance P. North Carolina macular dystrophy (MCDR1). A review and refined mapping to 6q14–q16.2. *Ophthalmol Paediatr Genet* 1993; **14**: 143–50.

Sneed SR, Sieving PA. Fenestrated sheen macular dystrophy. *Am J Ophthalmol* 1991; **112**: 1–7.

Soliman MM. Vitelliform macular dystrophy: a cause of holes with retinal detachment. *Eye* 1994; **8**: 484–7.

Sorsby A. Congenital coloboma of the macula: together with an account of the familial occurrence of bilateral macular coloboma in association with apical dystrophy of hands and feet. *Br J Ophthalmol* 1935; **19**: 65–90.

Stargardt K. Über familiäre, progressive Degeneration in der Makulagegend des Auges. *Graefes Arch Clin Exp Ophthalmol* 1909; **71**: 534–50.

Stone EM, Nichols BE, Kimura AE *et al*. Clinical features of a Stargardt-like dominant progressive macular dystrophy with genetic linkage to chromosome 6q. *Arch Ophthalmol* 1994; **112**: 765–72.

Tanino T, Katsumi O, Hirose T. Electrophysiological similarities between two eyes with X-linked recessive retinoschisis. *Doc Ophthalmol* 1985; **60**: 149–61.

Thompson EM, Baraitser M. Sorsby syndrome: a report on further generations of the original family. *J Med Genet* 1988; **25**: 313–21.

Tranebjaerg L, Sjo O, Warburg M. Retinal cone dysfunction and mental retardation associated with a *de novo* balanced translocation 1;6(q44;q27). *Ophthalmol Paediatr Genet* 1986; **7**: 167–73.

Uliss A, Moore AT, Bird AC. The dark choroid in posterior retinal dystrophies. *Ophthalmology* 1987; **94**: 1423–8.

Van der Biesen PR, Deutman AF, Pinckers AJL. Evolution of benign concentric annular dystrophy. *Am J Ophthalmol* 1985; **100**: 73–8.

Waheed A, Wyse CT. Progressive bifocal chorioretinal atrophy. *Br J Ophthalmol* 1968; **52**: 742–50.

Warburg M, Sjo O, Fledelius HC. Deletion mapping of a retinal cone–rod dystrophy: assignment to 18q211. *Am J Med Genet* 1991; **39**: 288–93.

Weber BHF, Walker D, Müller B. Molecular evidence for non-penetrance in Best's disease. *J Med Genet* 1994; **31**: 388–92.

Weingeist TA, Kobrin JL, Watzke RC. Histopathology of Best's macular dystrophy. *Arch Ophthalmol* 1982; **100**: 1108–14.

Weleber RG. Stargardt's macular dystrophy. *Arch Ophthalmol* 1994; **112**: 752–4.

Weleber RG, Carr RE, Murphey WH *et al*. Phenotypic variation including retinitis pigmentosa, pattern dystrophy and fundus flavimaculatus in a single family with a deletion of codon 153 or 154 of the peripherin/RDS gene. *Arch Ophthalmol* 1993; **111**: 1531–42.

Wells J, Wroblewski J, Keen J *et al*. Mutations in the human retinal degeneration slow (RDS) gene can cause either retinitis pigmentosa or macular dystrophy. *Nature Genet* 1993; **3**: 213–18.

Wroblewski JJ, Wells JA, Eckstein A *et al*. Macular dystrophy associated with mutations at codon 172 in the human retinal degeneration slow gene. *Ophthalmology* 1994; **101**: 12–22.

Yassur Y, Nissenkeorn I, Ben Sira I *et al*. Autosomal dominant inheritance of retinoschisis. *Am J Ophthalmol* 1982; **94**: 338–43.

Yoshizumi MO, Thomas JV, Hirose T. Foveal hypoplasia and bilateral 360 degrees retinal rosettes. *Am J Ophthalmol* 1979; **87**: 186–92.

Zhang K, Bither PP, Park R *et al*. A dominant Stargardt's macular dystrophy locus maps to chromosome 13q34. *Arch Ophthalmol* 1994; **112**: 759–64.

46: Congenital and Vascular Abnormalities of the Retina

Anthony Moore

Congenital hamartomatous lesions of the retina and retinal pigment epithelium

Congenital hypertrophy of the retinal pigment epithelium

Congenital hypertrophy of the retinal pigment epithelium (CHRPE) is usually seen as a solitary, well-circumscribed, brown or black (Gass 1989), slightly raised lesion about 1–2 disc diameters in size (Fig. 46.1). There is often a depigmented halo surrounding the lesion and areas of depigmentation (lacunae) may be present within it (Buettner 1975; Purcell & Shields 1975; Gass 1987; Chamot *et al.* 1993). They are most commonly seen as an incidental finding during routine fundus examination and can be found in any area of the retina. Careful perimetry will reveal a relative scotoma in the area of visual field corresponding to the lesion (Buettner 1975). They may show a gradual increase in size on long-term follow-up (Chamot *et al.* 1993).

On fluorescein angiography there is masking of the underlying choroidal fluorescein by the hypertrophied retinal pigment epithelium but there may be areas of hyperfluorescence within the lesion related to the depigmented lacunae. Retinovascular abnormalities overlying the lesion are common and are probably secondary to retinal pigment epithelium and receptor atrophy (Cleary *et al.* 1976; Cohen *et al.* 1993).

Histopathologically the lesion is composed of a single layer of hypertrophied retinal pigment epithelial cells containing large pigment granules. In addition there is atrophy of the retinal photoreceptors overlying the lesion (Buettner 1975; Traboulsi *et al.* 1990).

Although most individuals have no systemic abnormality (Shields *et al.* 1992), multiple bilateral CHRPEs have been reported in association with adenomatous polyposis coli (Blair & Trempe 1980; Traboulsi *et al.* 1988; Romania *et al.* 1989; Polkinhorne *et al.* 1990; Burn *et al.* 1991; Moore *et al.* 1992) and with microcephaly (Parke *et al.* 1984).

Familial adenomatous polyposis coli, Gardener's and Turcot's syndromes

Familial adenomatous polyposis coli (FAP) is an autosomal dominant disorder characterized by the development of multiple adenomatous polyps throughout the colon. Malignant transformation of the polyps occurs so family members are screened regularly by colonoscopy and total colectomy is performed when polyps have developed. Some individuals develop other systemic abnormalities including osteomas, desmoid tumours and epidermoid cysts, when they are said to have Gardener's syndrome (Gardener & Richards 1953; Gardener 1962). In Turcot's syndrome there is evidence of polyposis coli in association with neuroepithelial tumours of the central nervous system (Turcot *et al.* 1959; Munden *et al.* 1991). There is now general agreement that FAP, Gardener's syndrome

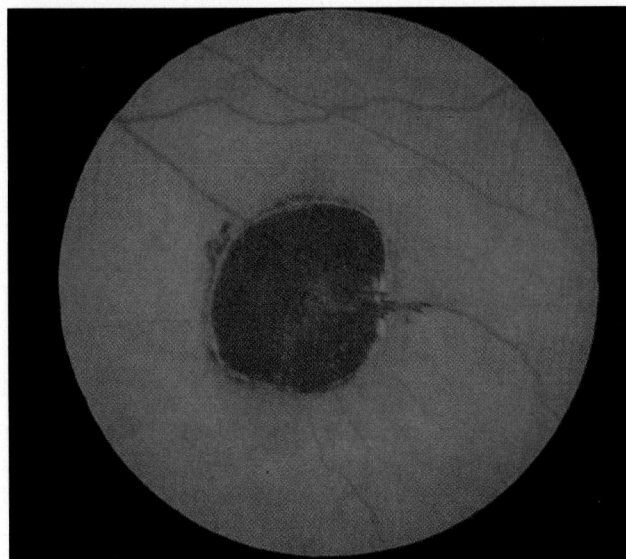

Fig. 46.1 Congenital hypertrophy of the retinal pigment epithelium. Slightly raised jet black lesion in the midperiphery with an associated small visual field defect (Professor A.C. Bird's patient).

and Turcot's syndrome represent variation in phenotypic expression of a single dominantly inherited genetic disorder.

CHRPEs are seen in individuals with FAP including those with and without extracolonic manifestations. Since the retinal lesions are congenital in onset rather than acquired (Aiello & Traboulsi 1993) they may be used as markers for the genetic mutation in at-risk family members (Traboulsi *et al.* 1988; Romania *et al.* 1989; Polkinhorne *et al.* 1990; Burn *et al.* 1991; Moore *et al.* 1992; Hicky-Dwyer & Willoughby 1993). The CHRPEs seen in FAP are multiple, bilateral and often atypical in appearance; they may be pigmented, non-pigmented or mixed and do not always have the characteristic round or oval shape seen in CHRPEs in normal individuals. Histopathological examination of the eyes of one individual with FAP and multiple CHRPEs demonstrated a widespread disturbance of melanogenesis of the retinal pigment epithelium (Traboulsi *et al.* 1990). Some of the lesions showed a similar histological appearance to solitary CHRPEs seen in normal individuals whilst other lesions in the same eye showed hamartomatous malformations of the retinal pigment epithelium.

Since CHRPEs may be seen in the normal population, in individuals with FAP or their relatives, a total number of CHRPEs over three in both eyes is taken to be abnormal and indicative that the individual has inherited the faulty gene. The interpretation of the finding of a normal fundus examination in an at-risk relative is not straightforward. Not all individuals with FAP have such retinal lesions; the incidence of CHRPEs in FAP varies from 60 to 88% in different series (Traboulsi *et al.* 1988; Romania *et al.* 1989;

Polkinhorne *et al.* 1990; Burn *et al.* 1991; Moore *et al.* 1992; Hodgson *et al.* 1994). There are significant interfamilial differences in the ocular findings (Moore *et al.* 1992) and it is important to know the ocular status of affected family members before using the presence or absence of CHRPEs to predict the genetic status. In families where multiple CHRPEs occur it is rare for an individual with FAP to have a normal fundus examination. There are, however, other families where CHRPEs do not occur and in these families a normal fundus examination in an at-risk individual cannot be used to predict genetic status. The identification of the FAP gene (Groden *et al.* 1991; Kinzler *et al.* 1991) has allowed more reliable molecular genetic presymptomatic diagnosis. Recently, Wallis *et al.* (1994) have demonstrated that the presence or absence of CHRPEs in FAP is dependent on the site of the gene deletions and the length of the truncated protein product. FAP kindreds with mutations at or before codon 283 do not have CHRPEs and the fundoscopic findings in a particular family may be used to aid mutation detection.

Grouped pigmentation of the retinal pigment epithelium

Congenital grouped pigmentation of the retinal pigment epithelium (bear track pigmentation) is an uncommon disorder in which there are multiple pigmented lesions in the fundus which resemble animal footprints (Fig. 46.2). They are usually sporadic, unilateral and grouped into one sector of the fundus (Gass 1987); familial cases have only rarely been reported (De Jong & Delleman 1988; Renardel de Lavalette *et al.* 1991). Fluorescein angiography shows masking of the underlying choroidal fluorescence. Histopathologically they are similar to CHRPE (Shields & Tso 1975; Regillo *et al.* 1993) with increased concentration of pigment granules in otherwise normal retinal pigment epithelial cells. Gass (1987) has described a condition of grouped albinotic pigment epithelial spots, closely related to bear track pigmentation in which there are scattered non-pigmented lesions in the fundus. Affected patients are asymptomatic and dark adaptation studies, electro-oculography (EOG) and electroretinography (ERG) are all normal.

Congenital hyperplasia of the retinal pigment epithelium

Localized hyperplasia of the retinal pigment epithelium is usually seen on routine fundus examination as a darkly pigmented small well-circumscribed lesion in the peripheral retina. It is usually solitary and extends from the retinal pigment epithelium through into the retina. Fluorescein angiography shows early non-fluorescence but may show some hyperfluorescence late in the angiogram (Gass 1987).

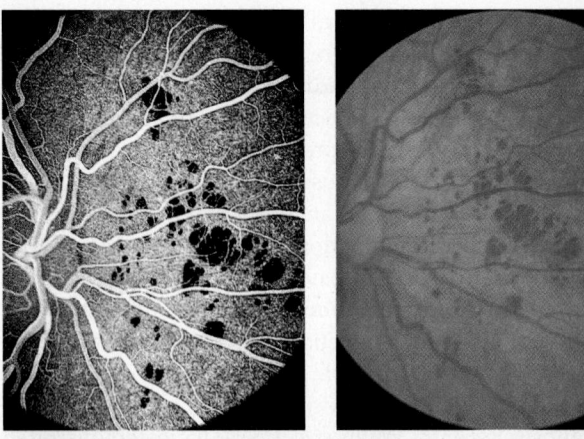

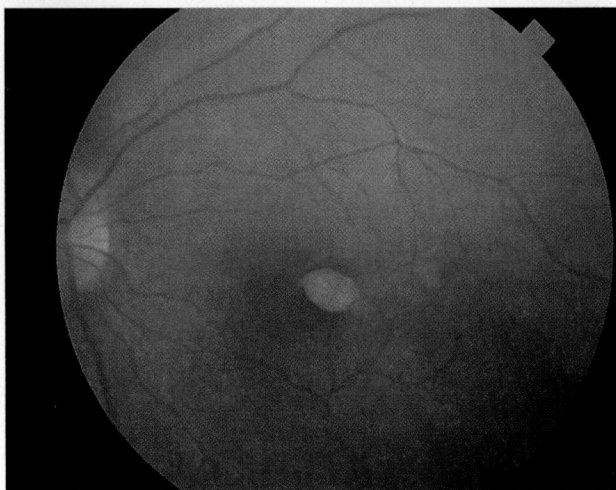

Fig. 46.2 (a) Congenital grouped pigmentation ('bear track'). Unilateral, multiple brown patches in the retinal pigment epithelium of no functional significance. Fluorescein angiography shows masking of the underlying choroidal fluorescence (Professor A.C. Bird's patient). (b) Hypopigmented naevus.

The lesions of this form of congenital hyperplasia are not thought to progress and are not associated with any systemic abnormalities.

Hypopigmented naevi

Hypopigmented spots (see Fig. 46.2b) are usually seen as an isolated lesion. Other similar lesions may represent amelanotic naevi (Roseman & Gass 1992).

Combined hamartoma of the retina and retinal pigment epithelium

Gass in 1973 described a series of patients with benign fundus lesions affecting the juxtapapillary, macular or peripheral retina which he believed were hamartomatous disorders of the retina and retinal pigment epithelium. There have been many further reports of similar abnor-

malities (Laqua & Wessing 1979; Flood *et al.* 1983; Schachat *et al.* 1984; Cosgrove *et al.* 1986). Although they have not been seen in the newborn they have been reported in early infancy (Schachat *et al.* 1984) and it is likely that they are truly congenital in origin. Most cases are sporadic and non-genetic (Gass 1987) but similar hamartomatous retinal abnormalities have been described in neurofibromatosis type 2 (Cotlier 1977; Landau *et al.* 1990; Good *et al.* 1991; Sivalingam *et al.* 1991; Bouzas *et al.* 1992) when they may be bilateral and are occasionally seen in several family members (Bouzas *et al.* 1992). Histological examination of enucleated eyes of sporadic cases has shown thickened disorganized retina with proliferation of the retinal pigment epithelium and glial tissue (Cardell & Starbuck 1961; Vogel *et al.* 1969).

Although they are rare it is important to recognize these lesions as their appearance may be confused with intraocular tumours such as retinoblastoma or choroidal melanoma and inappropriate treatment given (Gass 1973). They are more frequent in neurofibromatosis type 2 (Good *et al.* 1991).

Clinical features

The usual presentation is with unilateral visual loss, or, in young children especially, strabismus (Schachat *et al.* 1984; Gass 1987). Less commonly the retinal abnormality is found on routine fundus examination. Visual acuity is extremely variable and depends on the degree of macular involvement. In one large series (Schachat *et al.* 1984) 45% of patients had vision of 6/12 or better but 40% had 6/60 or worse. The hamartomas may involve the disc or macula and peripheral retina (Gass 1987). Peripapillary hamartomas (Fig. 46.3) are seen as slightly elevated diffuse partly pigmented tumours involving the nerve head and adjacent retina. Wrinkling of the internal limiting membrane and epiretinal membranes are commonly seen. Fluorescein angiography shows marked vascular tortuosity (Fig. 46.4) and an abnormal capillary circulation which may leak in the late phase.

Macular and peripheral retinal hamartomas have a similar appearance; the retina is thickened and hyperpigmented with very tortuous retinal vessels. There is usually associated epiretinal membrane formation and surface traction and less commonly choroidal neovascularization may develop at the edge of the lesion (Gass 1987).

The vision remains stable in most patients but visual loss may develop from exudative detachment, from increasing macular distortion due to surface traction or less commonly from associated vitreous haemorrhage (Kahn *et al.* 1984; Wang & Bruckner 1984). The hamartomas may occasionally show signs of growth (Cardell & Starbuck 1961; Rosenberg & Walsh 1984; Schachat *et al.* 1984).

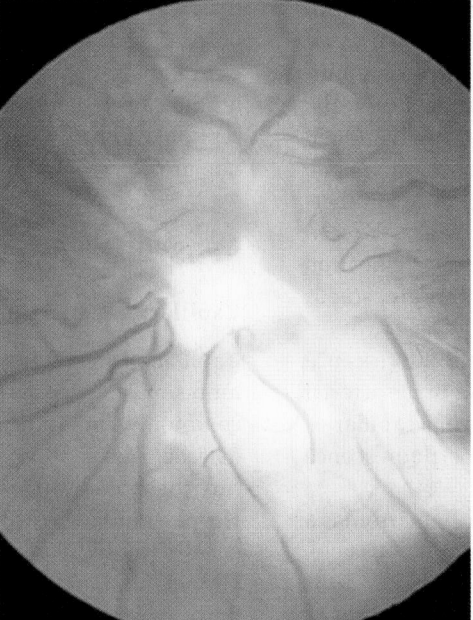
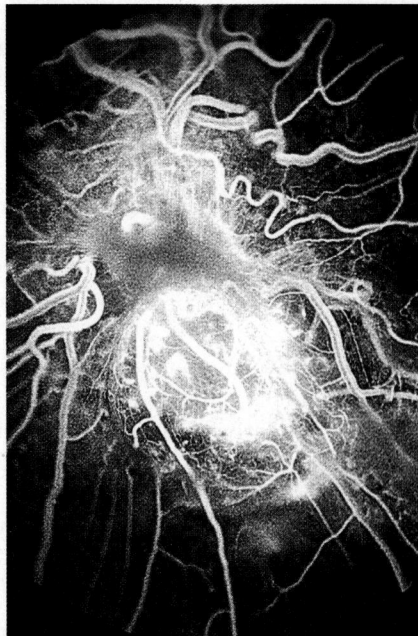

Fig. 46.3 Combined hamartoma of the retina and retinal pigment epithelium. Elevated peripapillary lesion with retinal traction and exudative detachment. The fluorescein angiogram of the same patient shows marked vascular tortuosity and distortion (Professor A.C. Bird's patient).

Management

In young children with strabismus a course of intensive occlusion therapy should be tried, as despite the appearance of the retina, the vision will sometimes improve (Schachat *et al.* 1984). In most cases no surgical treatment is indicated although macula distortion due to epiretinal membrane may be relieved by intraocular microsurgery, sometimes with good visual results (Schachat *et al.* 1984).

Astrocytic hamartoma

Retinal phakomas or astrocytic hamartoma are a common finding in tuberous sclerosis, occurring in about 40% of cases (Williams & Taylor 1985). Less commonly they are seen in neurofibromatosis (Martyn & Knox 1972), retinitis pigmentosa (Robertson 1972) or as an isolated abnormality (Foos *et al.* 1965; Ramsay *et al.* 1979; Gass 1987). In tuberous sclerosis they are often multiple, may be bilateral and are found at the optic nerve head or peripheral retina (Williams & Taylor 1985). Astrocytic hamartomas are thought to arise from the retinal ganglion cell layer and histopathologically consist of elongated astrocytes with small oval nuclei; the mass is usually vascular and may contain calcium (Ulbright *et al.* 1984; Green 1985). The tumour tissue stains positively for glial fibrillary acidic protein indicating that these lesions are of glial cell origin (Ulbright *et al.* 1984). Although these tumours may grow slowly they do not spread outside the eye. They may rarely be complicated by rubeotic glaucoma (Copeto *et al.* 1982), vitreous haemorrhage (Atkinson *et al.* 1973; Kroll *et al.* 1981; Copeto *et al.* 1982) and retinal detachment (Reeser *et al.* 1978); such cases may lead to considerable difficulties in diagnosis.

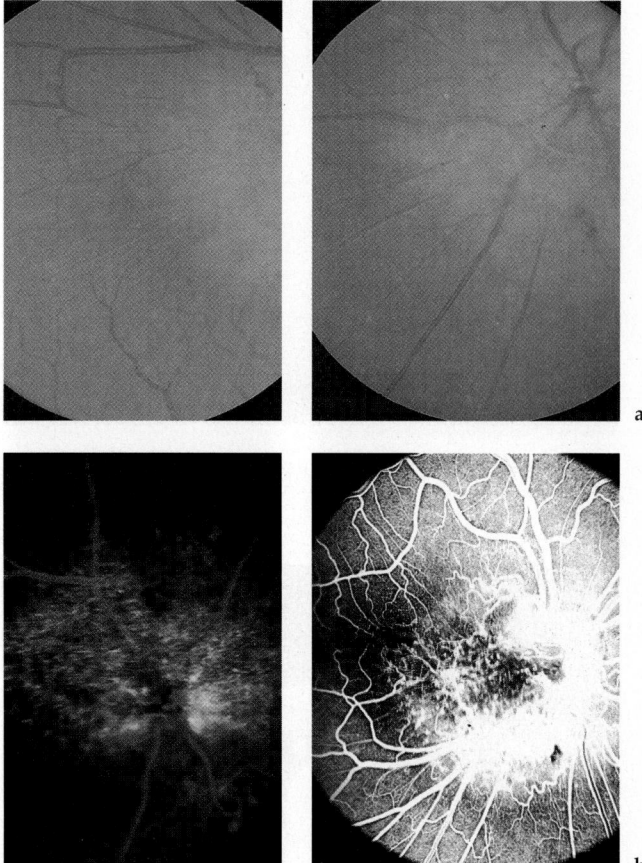

a

b

Fig. 46.4 (a) Combined hamartoma of the retina and retinal pigment epithelium. This patient has a marked elevation of the optic disc with radial retinal traction, wrinkled internal limiting membrane and retinal pigment epithelium changes around the disc. (b) Fluorescein angiogram showing the capillary beading and late leakage (Professor A.C. Bird's patient).

In infants and young children the retinal lesions are seen as translucent grey–white, minimally elevated tumours which may easily be missed unless careful indirect ophthalmoscopy is performed. In older children the more typical raised white 'mulberry' tumours (Fig. 46.5) are more common. The early translucent lesions are thought to evolve with time into the more typical 'mulberry' phakomas and intermediate stages may be seen (Nyboer *et al.* 1976; Williams & Taylor 1985). Calcification of the lesions may become evident during the later stages (Fig. 46.6).

Fluorescein angiography often shows autofluorescence of the phakomas in the control pictures, and in the arterial phase there is early filling of the often abnormal capillaries within the lesion. Most show late hyperfluorescence (Williams & Taylor 1985; Gass 1987).

In the majority of patients with astrocytic hamartomas a careful search will reveal other stigmata of tuberous scle-

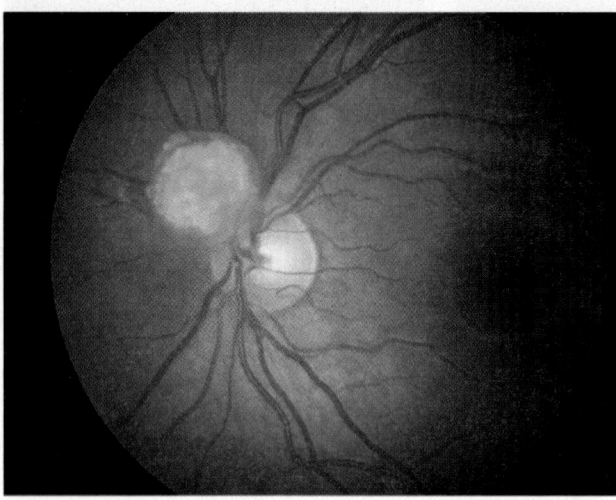

Fig. 46.5 Astrocytic hamartoma in a patient who did not have tuberous sclerosis.

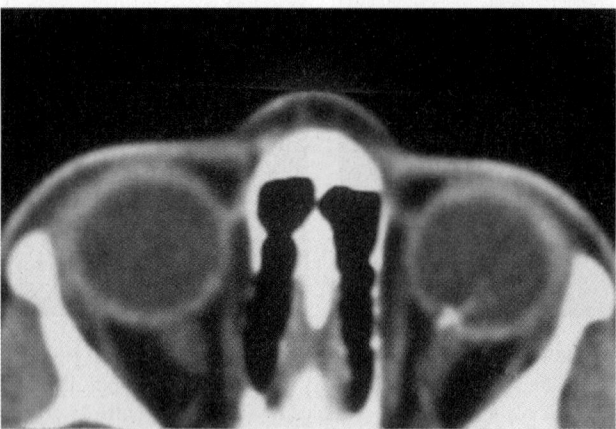

Fig. 46.6 Same patient as Fig. 46.5 showing the calcification in the hamartoma shown on CT scan.

rosis (see Chapter 61). The early lucent retinal lesions may be confused with a small retinoblastoma and if there is doubt about the diagnosis it is reasonable to observe the lesion closely for a period; the more rapid growth of retinoblastoma will help differentiate it from an astrocytic hamartoma.

Congenital vascular abnormalities

Capillary haemangioma

Capillary haemangiomas of the optic disc or peripheral retina may be seen as an isolated finding but are seen more commonly in individuals with von Hippel–Lindau disease. The clinical appearance and angiographic features of sporadic angiomas and those associated with von Hippel–Lindau disease are indistinguishable. The presence of multiple retinal angiomas is diagnostic of von Hippel–Lindau disease. In patients with a single angioma, the presence of another manifestation of von Hippel–Lindau disease or a positive family history is sufficient to confirm the diagnosis of von Hippel–Lindau disease. Histopathologically they are defined as haemangioblastomas!

von Hippel–Lindau disease (see also Chapter 61)

von Hippel–Lindau disease is a dominantly inherited cancer syndrome which exhibits a wide range of clinical expression. The most frequent complications are retinal, cerebellar and spinal haemangioblastomas and renal cell carcinoma (Melmon & Rosen 1964; Horton *et al.* 1976; Hardwig & Robertson 1984; Maher *et al.* 1990; Maher & Moore 1992). Other visceral complications include phaeochromocytoma and renal, pancreatic and epididymal cysts. Retinal haemangioma is the most common and earliest manifestation of von Hippel–Lindau disease and over 80% of patients with von Hippel–Lindau disease will develop one or more retinal haemangiomas during their lifetime (Maher *et al.* 1990).

The gene causing von Hippel–Lindau disease has recently been identified and appears to function as a tumour-suppressor gene of the retinoblastoma type (Latif *et al.* 1993). Somatic von Hippel–Lindau gene mutations have been implicated in the pathogenesis of non-familial clear cell renal cell carcinoma analogous to the role of retinoblastoma type 1 mutations in sporadic retinoblastoma (Foster *et al.* 1994; Gnarra *et al.* 1994; Shuin *et al.* 1994). It is as yet uncertain whether a similar mechanism may explain the development of the solitary sporadic retinal angioma seen in some otherwise normal individuals.

Clinical features of retinal haemangiomas

The usual presentation is with blurred vision but in some

the retinal lesions are found during examination of asymptomatic family members (Moore *et al.* 1991). The retinal haemangioblastomas are most commonly seen in the midperiphery, although papillary or peripapillary lesions are found (Welch 1970; Hardwig & Robertson 1984; Moore *et al.* 1991). The tumours are of two main types. Exophytic tumours arise from the outer retinal layers and grow inwards. They are uncommon, are more often seen in the peripapillary area and may present with optic disc swelling or exudative detachment of the macula (Gass & Braunstein 1980; Yimoyines *et al.* 1982; Kremer *et al.* 1988). They may be misdiagnosed as peripapillary choroiditis, papilloedema, or a peripapillary disciform.

The true nature of the lesion is usually demonstrated on stereofluorescein angiography; the deep angioma fills early in the arterial phase and may show a dual circulation from both the ciliary and inner retinal circulations (Gass & Braunstein 1980; Yimoyines *et al.* 1982).

Endophytic tumours which arise from the inner retinal layers are more common and give rise to the typical well-circumscribed elevated vascular lesion growing forwards into the vitreous cavity. They may be seen at the disc or more commonly in the peripheral retina, where they are often bilateral. Peripheral angiomas often show enlarged feeding and draining vessels and there may be rapid arteriovenous shunting through the lesion. Small tumours are seen as tiny capillary dilatations which may be easily missed on ophthalmoscopy but are readily apparent on fluorescein angiography (Salazara & Lamiell 1980; Moore *et al.* 1991). Visual loss may occur as a result of exudative or tractional retinal detachment, vitreous haemorrhage, macular oedema or epiretinal membrane formation causing macular distortion.

Screening of at-risk family members may reveal asymptomatic small angiomas in the peripheral retina or on the optic disc (Salazara & Lamiell 1980; Moore *et al.* 1991). Fluorescein angiography is helpful in confirming the vascular nature of these lesions.

Histopathology

Histopathological examination of eyes with untreated haemangiomas (Goldberg & Duke 1968; Jakobiec *et al.* 1976; Nicholson *et al.* 1976; Wing *et al.* 1981; Ismail *et al.* 1985; Grossnicklaus *et al.* 1992) shows that the lesions are composed of a fine network of capillaries and small blood vessels which penetrate most of the thickness of the retina. The blood vessels are fenestrated and lack the normal tight junctions so that extensive leakage of fluid occurs, resulting in chronic oedema and atrophy of the surrounding retina. The endothelial-lined channels within the tumour are separated by numerous interstitial 'foam' cells. Despite numerous histological and immunohistochemical studies the cellular origin of the foam cells remains controversial. The histological appearance of the

retinal and central nervous system vascular tumours in von Hippel–Lindau disease is identical and they are best classified as haemangioblastomas.

Management

The treatment of retinal angiomas depends on the type of lesion, its size and location. Small peripheral endophytic lesions can be successfully treated with argon laser and xenon photocoagulation (Sellors & Archer 1969; Apple *et al.* 1974; Goldberg & Koenig 1974; Lane *et al.* 1989). Intravenous fluorescein may be given in association with argon laser treatment in order to increase laser uptake (Lane *et al.* 1989). Larger tumours, which often have associated detachment, are best treated with cryotherapy using a triple freeze–thaw technique but several treatments may

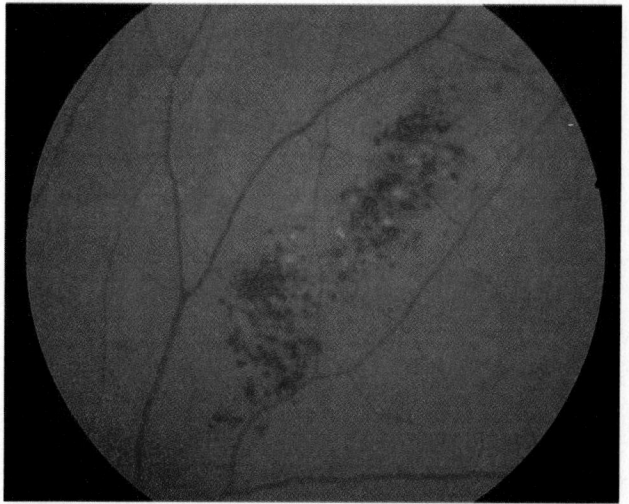

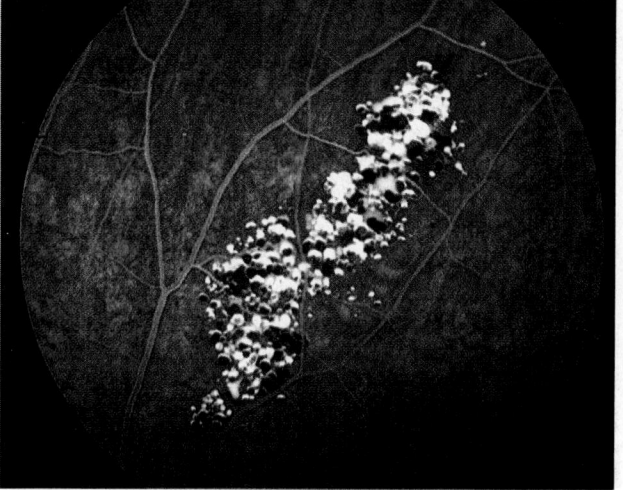

Fig. 46.7 (a) Cavernous haemangioma of the retina. There is a grape-like cluster of aneurysmal dilatations in the superior retina. (b) Fluorescein angiogram of the same patient showing slow flow and pooling. (Mr Anthony Moore's patient.)

be needed (Sellors & Archer 1969; Welch 1970; Watzke 1973; Annersley *et al.* 1977). Large peripheral tumours not responding to photocoagulation or cryotherapy may be treated with local plaque or external beam radiotherapy (Balazs *et al.* 1990) or local excision (Peyman *et al.* 1983).

Treatment of optic disc and peripapillary haemangiomas is not indicated unless there is already visual loss and signs of progression. Such tumours are particularly difficult to treat; although laser photocoagulation offers the best hope of causing tumour regression without damaging the nerve fibre layer (Yimoyines *et al.* 1982; Kremer *et al.* 1988) the results of treatment are disappointing. An alternative approach is to use external beam radiotherapy using the newer lens-sparing techniques (Plowman & Harnett 1988) but experience of this therapy is limited.

The prognosis, following treatment, is best for small peripheral tumours and it is important that all patients with von Hippel–Lindau disease undergo regular screening so that angiomas are detected at a stage when treatment is likely to be successful (Maher *et al.* 1990; Moore *et al.* 1991). The prognosis is less good for symptomatic peripapillary tumours and large peripheral tumours with associated retinal detachment at presentation. Although most angiomas will respond to treatment some eyes show relentless progression and visual loss despite all forms of treatment (Hardwig & Robertson 1984).

Cavernous haemangioma

Cavernous haemangioma is a rare vascular hamartoma which may involve the optic nerve head or peripheral retina (Gass 1971; Lewis *et al.* 1975; Goldberg *et al.* 1979; Messmer *et al.* 1983). Although it has been reported in childhood most cases are seen in young adults; it is more common in females and is usually unilateral (Lewis *et al.* 1975). In some cases there may be additional cutaneous and intracranial haemangiomas (Gass 1971; Lewis *et al.* 1975; Goldberg *et al.* 1979; Brown & Shields 1985; Pancurak *et al.* 1985). Goldberg *et al.* (1979) and Pancurak *et al.* (1983) have reported families in which several family members have retinal or central nervous system haemangiomas.

The cavernous haemangioma is seen as a grape-like cluster of aneurysmal dilatations arising near a retinal vein (see Figs 46.7 and 46.8); there is often associated fibrous tissue and small haemorrhages are sometimes seen on the surface of the lesion. There are no prominent feeder vessels as seen in von Hippel's disease although the draining vein may be dilated (Messmer *et al.* 1983). Visual acuity usually remains good unless the haemangioma is close to the macula (Gass 1971; Lewis *et al.* 1975; Messmer *et al.* 1983). Rarely bleeding from the abnormal vessels may give rise to recurrent vitreous haemorrhage.

Cavernous haemangiomas fill slowly and often incompletely on fluorescein angiography (Fig. 46.8) and there is no evidence of any arteriovenous shunting or extravascular leakage (Brown & Shields 1985). This is in keeping with the histological appearance which demonstrates similar anatomy to normal retinal vessels (Messmer *et al.* 1984). Growth of the tumour is rare and treatment is only indicated if there is recurrent vitreous haemorrhage when cryotherapy or photocoagulation may be used to cause tumour regression (Brown & Shields 1985; Gass 1987).

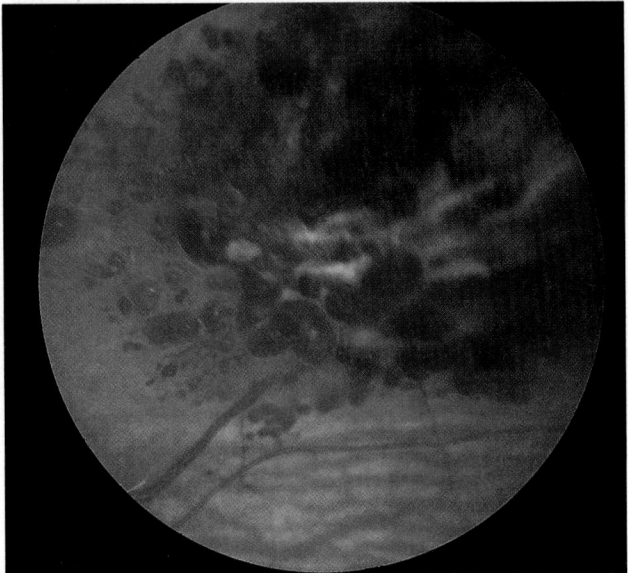

a

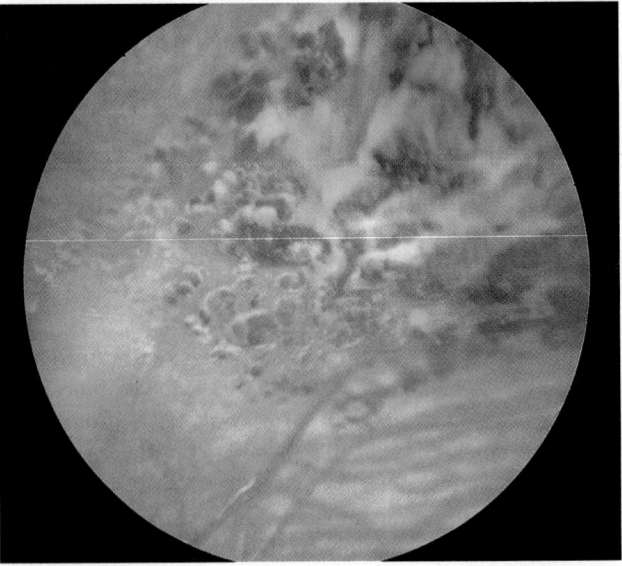

b

Fig. 46.8 (a) Cavernous haemangioma of the retina. This 11-month-old child presented with a squint, but with patching the eye acuity remained at 6/18. The grape-like cluster of abnormal vessels was adjacent to the macula and regressed over 3 years. (b) Photograph taken a few minutes after fluorescein injection. The pooling of fluorescein occurs due to the very slow blood flow. No leakage occurred.

Congenital retinal macrovessels (racemose haemangioma; retinal arteriovenous malformations)

In this uncommon disorder a large retinal vessel, usually a vein, runs from the disc to the macular region and supplies the retina above and below the horizontal raphe (Archer *et al.* 1973; Brown *et al.* 1982). Fluorescein angiography often shows arteriovenous communications and areas of capillary non-perfusion. Archer *et al.* (1973) have divided this disorder into three groups depending on the extent of the arteriovenous anastomosis. In the first group there is a small arteriovenous anastomosis which occurs across a capillary complex; although venous pressure is raised it is well compensated and vision remains good. In the second group there is direct arteriolar venous communication and high flow between the arterial and venous side of the circulation. This leads to secondary changes such as arteriolar and venous dilatation and capillary non-perfusion in neighbouring vessels. The third group consists of patients with complex large vessel anastomoses. Many vessels in the fundus may be widely dilated and vision is often poor.

The vascular abnormalities are thought to be congenital in origin and are usually non-progressive. They may rarely give rise to ocular complications including retinal, subhyaloid and vitreous haemorrhage, venous occlusion, retinal neovascularization and neovascular glaucoma (Mansour *et al.* 1989; Schatz *et al.* 1993). Treatment is not usually necessary but retinal neovascularization or rubeotic glaucoma may respond to panretinal photocoagulation (Schatz *et al.* 1993).

The retinal arteriovenous malformations may be associated with similar facial and intracranial vascular malformations. In Wyburn–Mason syndrome (Bonnet *et al.* 1937; Wyburn-Mason 1943) there are large vessel arteriovenous anastomoses of the retinal circulation (Fig. 46.9) with similar vascular malformations of the midbrain and cerebrum.

Familial retinal arteriolar tortuosity

This uncommon autosomal dominant disorder is characterized by variable tortuosity of the retinal arterioles and, frequently, associated macular or posterior pole retinal haemorrhages (Beyer 1958; Goldberg *et al.* 1972; Boyton & Purnell 1977; Bartlett & Price 1983; Wells & Kalina 1985). The arteriolar tortuosity is apparent in childhood (Wells & Kalina 1985) and may become more marked with age. The macular haemorrhages, which lie superficially in the nerve fibre layer, or in the subhyaloid space, may occur spontaneously or follow minor trauma or physical exercise (Goldberg 1985). Although the haemorrhages may be recurrent there is complete resolution with recovery of normal vision. Fluorescein angiography shows no abnormality apart from the arteriolar tortuosity and there

are no associated systemic abnormalities (Wells & Kalina 1985).

Inherited retinal venous beading

Meredith (1987) was the first to describe a dominantly inherited disorder in which affected family members had prominent segmental venous beading. Conjunctival venous anomalies were present in some family members and two also had evidence of renal disease and hearing loss. Two further families with similar retinal abnormalites have since been reported (Stewart & Gittner 1988; Piquet *et al.* 1994); neither had any systemic disorder. Although all affected family members show the typical segmental venous abnormality there is a wide range of clinical expression. Microvascular abnormalities including arteriolar narrowing, capillary closure, vascular leakage, microaneurysm formation and retinal neovascularization are evident in some affected individuals. Visual loss may occur as a result of macular oedema or exudates, venous occlusion or vitreous haemorrhage. The underlying cause of the vascular abnormality is unknown.

Coats' disease

Coats' disease is characterized by congenital retinal telangiectasis and exudative retinal detachment (Coats 1908). It usually presents in late childhood, occurs predominantly in males and is unilateral and sporadic in over 90% of cases (Morales 1965; Manschot & De Bruijn 1967; Egerer *et al.* 1974). The average age of presentation is about 8 years (Morales 1965; Ridley *et al.* 1982) when the usual presenting features are unilateral visual loss or strabismus. Infants or younger children may present with leucocoria or a painful blind eye (Judisch & Apple 1980; Ridley *et al.* 1982; McGettrick & Loeffler 1987). Retinal telangiectasis similar to Coats' disease has also been described in patients with retinitis pigmentosa (Khan *et al.* 1988).

Fundus examination shows aneurysmal dilation (Fig. 46.10) and telangiectasis of the retinal vessels with associated subretinal exudation. There may be extensive retinal detachment with relatively solid yellow exudate and refractile cholesterol crystals in the subretinal space (Fig. 46.11); the subretinal fluid often has a greenish hue. Fluorescein angiography shows aneurysmal dilation of the arterioles, capillaries and veins in the affected area often with associated capillary non-perfusion (Gass 1987). Leakage from the dilated vessels is common.

Histopathological examination of enucleated eyes shows aneurysmal dilation of the retinal vessels with thickening and hyalinization of their walls. The subretinal space contains exudate, cholesterol and foamy, melanin-containing cells which may be derived from the retinal pigment epithelium (Tripathi & Ashton 1971).

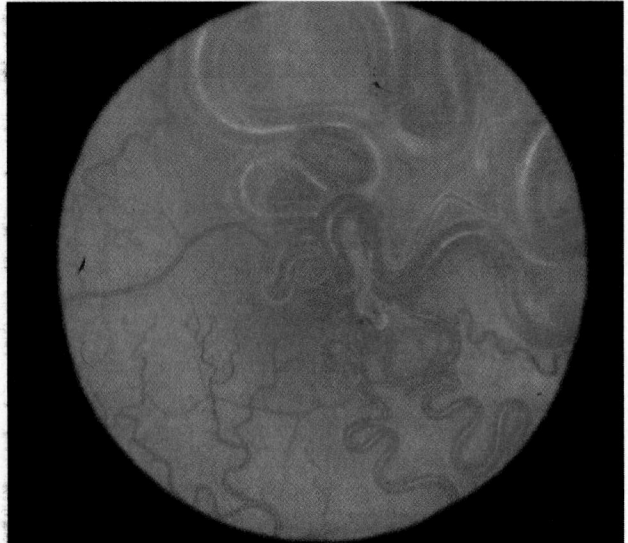

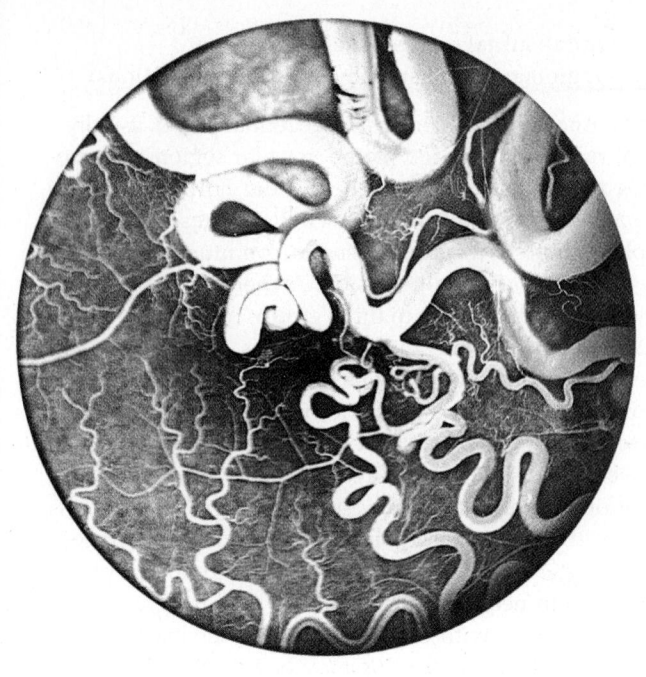

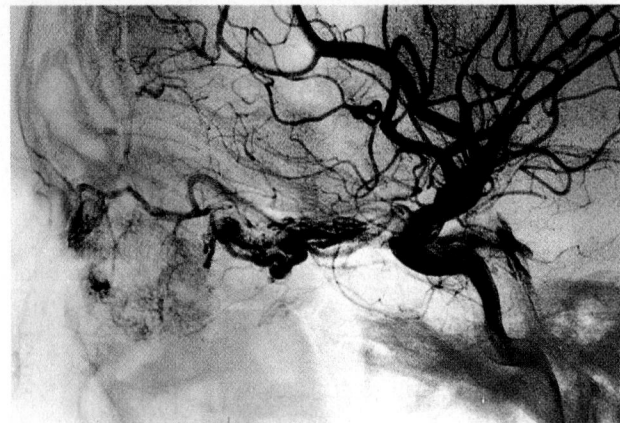

Fig. 46.9 (a) Congenital retinal macrovessels. The acuity was 6/18. (b) The fluorescein angiogram showed no leakage. (c) Carotid angiogram showing cerebral vascular malformation.

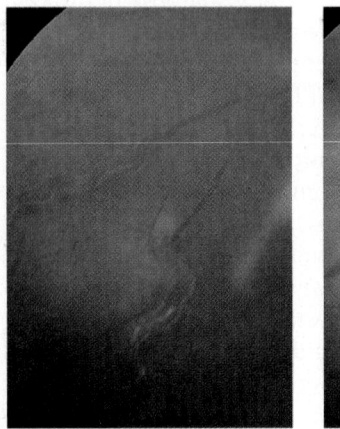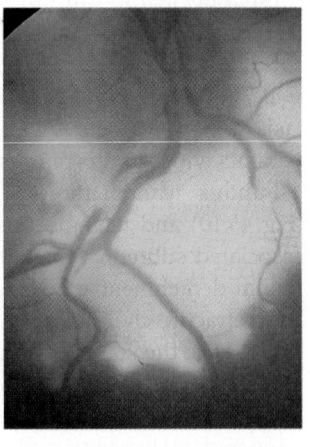

Fig. 46.10 (a) Coats' disease. Aneurysmal dilatation of the retinal arterioles. (b) Coats' disease. Exudative retinal detachment with subretinal solid exudate.

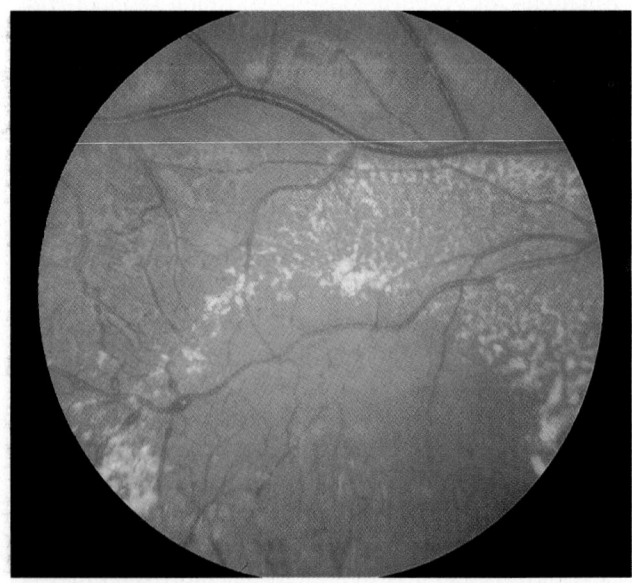

Fig. 46.11 In the inferior and temporal fundus of this child with Coats' disease a number of dilated retinal vessels can be seen. There is a serous retinal detachment and subretinal exudates.

Untreated, most cases show progression (Morales 1965) leading to total retinal detachment, neovascular glaucoma and phthisis bulbi. Judisch and Apple (1980) reported an unusual case in which an infant with Coats' disease developed an orbital cellulitis secondary to extensive ocular inflammation.

Treatment of the abnormal vessels with photocoagulation or cryotherapy may halt progression of the disease and in early cases result in reabsorption of the exudate and improvement in vision (Ridley *et al.* 1982; McGettrick & Loeffler 1987). The differential diagnosis of Coats' disease includes other causes of leucocoria and exudative retinal detachment in childhood (see Chapter 42). The presence of retinal vascular abnormalities, subretinal exudate and cholesterol crystals usually serves to differentiate this disorder from other conditions.

Retinopathies similar to Coats' disease associated with systemic disease

Coats' disease is usually unilateral and sporadic and seen in otherwise normal children. A similar retinopathy has, however, been described in association with other systemic abnormalities. Tolmie *et al.* (1988) described two female siblings with bilateral Coats' disease, intracranial calcification, sparse hair and dysplastic nails and suggested that this may represent a distinct genetic disorder. Nail and hair abnormalities and a bilateral retinopathy similar to Coats' disease have also been described in association with aplastic anaemia and central nervous system abnormalities (Revesz *et al.* 1992; Kajtar & Mehes 1994). Bilateral Coats' disease has also been described in association with congenital plasminogen deficiency type 1 (Patrassi *et al.* 1993), Cornelia de Lang syndrome (Folk *et al.* 1981) and the Hallerman–Streiff syndrome (Newell *et al.* 1994). Retinal vascular abnormalities and exudative retinal detachment similar to Coats' disease has been described in facioscapulohumeral muscular dystrophy (Small 1968; Taylor *et al.* 1982; Gurwin *et al.* 1985; Desai & Sabates 1990). Fitzsimons *et al.* (1987) performed fluorescein angiography in 75 individuals with this rare autosomal dominant disorder and found retinal capillary abnormalities (including telangiectasia, capillary closure, vascular leakage and microaneurysm formation) in 56. However, visual loss was rare. The vascular abnormalities may be seen in childhood and may occur before there are any clinical signs of muscle disease (Fitzsimons *et al.* 1987). A Coats-like retinopathy has also been reported in scapuloperoneal muscular dystrophy (Dickey & Dailey 1991), and in hemifacial atrophy (Gass *et al.* 1991).

Other congenital abnormalities

Other congenital abnormalities of the retina including myelinated nerve fibres, coloboma, and Aicardi's syndrome are discussed in Chapter 50. Albinism is covered in Chapter 38 and foveal hypoplasia and macular dysplasia (coloboma) are discussed in Chapter 50.

References

Aiello L, Traboulsi E. Pigmented fundus lesions in a pre-term infant with familial adenomatous polyposis. *Arch Ophthalmol* 1993; **111**: 302–3.

Annersley WH, Leonard BC, Shields JA, Tasman WS. Fifteen year review of treated cases of retinal angiomatosis. *Trans Am Acad Ophthalmol Otolaryngol* 1977; **83**: 446–53.

Apple DJ, Goldberg MF, Wyhinny GJ. Argon laser treatment of von Hippel–Lindau retinal angiomas II. Histopathology of treated lesions. *Arch Ophthalmol* 1974; **92**: 126–30.

Archer DM, Deutman A, Ernst JT, Krill AE. Arteriovenous communication of the retina. *Am J Ophthalmol* 1973; **75**: 224–41.

Atkinson A, Sanders MD, Wong V. Vitreous haemorrhage in tuberous sclerosis. *Br J Ophthalmol* 1973; **57**: 773–9.

Balazs E, Berta A, Rosza L *et al.* Hemodynamic changes after ruthenium irradiation of Hippel's angiomatosis. *Ophthalmologica* 1990; **200**: 128–32.

Bartlett WJ, Price J. Familial retinal arteriolar tortuosity with retinal haemorrhage. *Am J Ophthalmol* 1983; **95**: 556–8.

Beyer EM. Familiare Tortuositas der kleinen Wetzhautarterien mit Makulablutung. *Klin Monatsbl Augenheilkd* 1958; **132**: 532–9.

Blair NP, Trempe CL. Hypertrophy of the retinal pigment epithelium associated with Gardener's syndrome. *Am J Ophthalmol* 1980; **90**: 661–7.

Bonnet P, Dechaume J, Blanc E. L'aneurisme cirsoide de la retine (aneurysme racemeux). Ses relations avec l'aneurysme cirsoide de la faceet avec l'aneurysme cirsoide du cerveau. *J Med Lyon* 1937; **18**: 165–78.

Bouzas EA, Parry DM, Eldridge R, Kaiser-Kupfer MI. Familial occurrence of combined pigment epithelial and retinal hamartoma in neurofibromatosis type 2. *Retina* 1992; **12**: 103–7.

Boyton JR, Purnell EW. Congenital tortuosity of the retinal arteries. *Arch Ophthalmol* 1977; **95**: 893.

Brown GC, Donoso LA, Magargal LE *et al.* Congenital retinal macrovessels. *Arch Ophthalmol* 1982; **100**: 1430–6.

Brown GC, Shields JA. Tumours of the optic nerve head. *Surv Ophthalmol* 1985; **29**: 239–64.

Buettner H. Congenital hypertrophy of the retinal pigment epithelium. *Am J Ophthalmol* 1975; **79**: 177–89.

Burn J, Chapman P, Delhanty J *et al.* The UK northern region genetic register for familial adenomatous polyposis coli: age at onset, congenital hypertrophy of the retinal pigment epithelium, and DNA markers in risk calculation. *J Med Genet* 1991; **28**: 289–96.

Cardell BS, Starbuck MJ. Juxtapapillary hamartoma of the retina. *Br J Ophthalmol* 1961; **45**: 672–7.

Chamot L, Zografos L, Klainguti G. Fundus changes associated with congenital hypertrophy of the retinal pigment epithelium. *Am J Ophthalmol* 1993; **115**: 154–61.

Cleary PE, Gregor Z, Bird AC. Retinal vascular changes in congenital hypertrophy of the retinal pigment epithelium. *Br J Ophthalmol* 1976; **60**: 499–503.

Coats G. Forms of retinal disease with massive exudation. *Roy London Ophthalmol Rep* 1908; **17**: 440–525.

Cohen S, Quentel G, Guiberteau B, Coscas G. Retinal vascular changes in congenital hypertrophy of the retinal pigment epithelium. *Ophthalmology* 1993; **100**: 471–4.

Copeto JR, Lubin JR, Albert DM. Astrocytic hamartoma in tuberous sclerosis mimicking necrotizing retinochoroiditis. *J Pediatr Ophthalmol Strabismus* 1982; **19**: 306–13.

Cosgrove JM, Sharpe DM, Bird AC. Combined hamartoma of the retina and retinal pigment epithelium: the clinical spectrum. *Trans Ophthalmol Soc UK* 1986; **105**: 106–13.

Cotlier E. Café-au-lait spots of the fundus in neurofibromatosis. *Arch Ophthalmol* 1977; **95**: 1990–3.

De Jong PT, Delleman JW. Familial grouped pigmentation of the retinal pigment epithelium. *Br J Ophthalmol* 1988; **72**: 439–41.

Desai U, Sabates F. Long-term follow-up of facioscapulohumeral muscular dystrophy and Coats' disease. *Am J Ophthalmol* 1990; **110**: 568–9.

Dickey JB, Daily MJ. Retinal telangiectasia in scapuloperoneal muscular dystrophy. *Am J Ophthalmol* 1991; **112**: 348–9.

Egerer I, Tasman W, Tomer TL. Coats' disease. *Arch Ophthalmol* 1974; **92**: 109–12.

Fitzsimons RB, Gurwin EB, Bird AC. Retinal vascular abnormalities in facioscapulohumeral muscular dystrophy. A general association with genetic and therapeutic implications. *Brain* 1987; **110**: 631–48.

Flood TP, Orth DH, Aaberg TM, Marcus DF. Macular hamartomas of the retinal pigment epithelium and retina. *Retina* 1983; **3**: 164–70.

Folk JC, Genovese FN, Biglan AW. Coats' disease in a patient with the Cornelia de Lange syndrome. *Am J Ophthalmol* 1981; **91**: 607–10.

Foos RY, Straatsma BR, Allen RA. Astrocytoma of the optic nerve head. *Arch Ophthalmol* 1965; **74**: 319–26.

Foster K, Prowse A, van der Berg A *et al.* Somatic mutations of the von Hippel–Lindau disease tumour suppressor gene in non-familial clear cell renal carcinoma. *Hum Mol Genet* 1994; **3**: 2169–73.

Gardener EJ. Follow-up study of a family group exhibiting autosomal dominant inheritance for a syndrome including intestinal polyps, osteomas, fibromas and epidermal cysts. *Am J Hum Genet* 1962; **14**: 376–90.

Gardener EJ, Richards RC. Multiple cutaneous and subcutaneous lesions occurring simultaneously with hereditary polyposis and osteomatosis. *Am J Hum Genet* 1953; **5**: 139–47.

Gass JDM. Cavernous haemangioma of the retina: a neuro-cutaneous syndrome. *Am J Ophthalmol* 1971; **71**: 799–814.

Gass JDM. Focal congenital anomalies of the retinal pigment epithelium. *Eye* 1989; **3**: 1–19.

Gass JDM. Retinal and pigment epithelial hamartomas. In: Gass JDM, ed. *Stereoscopic Atlas of Macular Diseases*. St Louis: CV Mosby, 1987: 605–52.

Gass JDM. An unusual hamartoma of the pigment epithelium and retina simulating choroidal melanoma and retinoblastoma. *Trans Am Ophthalmol Soc* 1973; **71**: 175–85.

Gass JDM, Braunstein R. Sessile and exophytic capillary haemangiomas of the juxtapapillary retinal and optic nerve head. *Arch Ophthalmol* 1980; **98**: 1790–7.

Gass JDM, Harbin TS, Del Piero E. Exudative stellate neuroretinopathy and Coats' syndrome in patients with progressive hemifacial atrophy. *Eur J Ophthalmol* 1991; **1**: 2–11.

Gnarra JR, Tory K, Weng Y *et al.* Mutations in the VHL tumour suppressor gene in renal carcinoma. *Nature Genet* 1994; **7**: 85–90.

Goldberg MF. Retinal arteriolar tortuosity. Discussion of paper by Wells and Kalina. *Ophthalmology* 1985; **92**: 1021–4.

Goldberg MF, Duke JR. von Hippel–Lindau disease. Histopathologic findings in a treated and an untreated eye. *Am J Ophthalmol* 1968; **66**: 693–705.

Goldberg MF, Koenig S. Argon laser treatment of von Hippel–Lindau retinal angiomas. *Arch Ophthalmol* 1974; **92**: 121–5.

Goldberg RE, Pheasant TR, Shields JA. Cavernous haemangioma of the retina. *Arch Ophthalmol* 1979; **97**: 2321–4.

Goldberg MF, Pollack IP, Green WR. Familial retinal arteriolar tortu-

osity with retinal haemorrhage. *Am J Ophthalmol* 1972; **73**: 183–91.

Good W, Brodsky M, Edwards M, Hoyt W. Bilateral retinal hamartomas in neurofibromatosis type 2. *Br J Ophthalmol* 1991; **75**: 190.

Green WR. Congenital variations and abnormalities of the retina. In: Spencer WH, ed. *Ophthalmic Pathology: An Atlas and Textbook*. Philadelphia: WB Saunders, 1985: 607–47.

Groden J, Thliveris A, Samowitz W *et al.* Identification and characterisation of the familial adenomatous polyposis coli gene. *Cell* 1991; **66**: 589–600.

Grossnicklaus HE, Thomas JW, Vigneswaran N, Jarrett WH. Retinal hemangioblastoma. A histologic, immunohistochemical, and ultrastructural evaluation. *Ophthalmology* 1992; **99**: 140–5.

Gurwin EB, Fitzsimons RB, Sehmi KS, Bird AC. Retinal telangiectasis in facioscapulohumeral muscular dystrophy with deafness. *Arch Neurol* 1985; **103**: 1695–700.

Hardwig P, Robertson DM. Von Hippel–Lindau disease: a familial often fatal phakomatosis. *Ophthalmology* 1984; **91**: 263–70.

Hicky-Dwyer M, Willoughby C. Assessment of the value of congenital hypertrophy of the retinal pigment epithelium as an ocular marker for familial adenomatous polyposis coli. *Eye* 1993; **7**: 562–4.

Hodgson SV, Bishop DT, Jay B. Genetic heterogeneity of congenital hypertrophy of the retinal pigment epithelium (CHRPE) in families with familial adenomatous polyposis. *J Med Genet* 1994; **31**: 55–8.

Horton WA, Wong V, Eldridge R. Von Hippel–Lindau disease: clinical and pathological manifestations in nine families with 50 affected members. *Arch Int Med* 1976; **136**: 769–77.

Ismail SMI, Jasani B, Cole G. Histogenesis of haemangioblastomas: an immunocytochemical and ultrastructural study in a case of von Hippel–Lindau disease. *J Clin Pathol* 1985; **38**: 417–21.

Jakobiec FA, Font RL, Johnson FB. Angiomatosis retinae. An ultrastructural study and lipid analysis. *Cancer* 1976; **38**: 2042–56.

Judisch GF, Appel DJ. Orbital cellulitis in an infant secondary to Coats' disease. *Arch Ophthalmol* 1980; **98**: 2004–6.

Kajtar P, Mehes K. Bilateral Coats' retinopathy associated with aplastic anemia and mild dyskeratotic signs. *Am J Med Genet* 1994; **49**: 374–7.

Khan D, Goldberg MF, Jednock N. Combined retina–retinal pigment epithelial hamartoma presenting as a vitreous haemorrhage. *Retina* 1984; **4**: 40–3.

Khan JA, Ide CA, Strickland MP. Coats' type retinitis pigmentosa. *Surv Ophthalmol* 1988; **32**: 317–32.

Kinzler K, Nilbert MC, Su LK *et al.* Identification of FAP locus genes from chromosome 5q21. *Science* 1991; **253**: 661–4.

Kremer J, Gilad E, Ben-Sira I. Juxta-capillary exophytic capillary haemangioma treated with krypton yellow (568 nm) laser photocoagulation. *Ophthalmic Surg* 1988; **19**: 743–7.

Kroll AS, Reiken PD, Robb RM, Albert DM. Vitreous haemorrhage complicating retinal astrocytic hamartoma. *Surv Ophthalmol* 1981; **26**: 31–8.

Landau K, Dossetor FM, Hoyt WF, Muci-Mendoza R. Retinal hamartomas in neurofibromatosis type 2. *Arch Ophthalmol* 1990; **108**: 328–9.

Lane CM, Turner G, Gregor ZJ, Bird AC. Laser treatment of retinal angiomatosis. *Eye* 1989; **3**: 33–8.

Laqua H, Wessing A. Congenital retinal pigment epithelial malformation previously described as hamartoma. *Am J Ophthalmol* 1979; **87**: 34–42.

Latif F, Tory K, Gnarra J *et al.* Identification of the von Hippel–Lindau disease tumour suppressor gene. *Science* 1993; **206**: 1317–20.

Lewis RA, Cohen MH, Wise GN. Cavernous haemangioma of retina and optic disc. *Br J Ophthalmol* 1975; **59**: 422–4.

McGettrick PM, Loeffler KN. Bilateral Coats' disease in an infant (a clinical, light and electron microscopic study). *Eye* 1987; **1**: 136–45.

Maher ER, Moore AT. von Hippel–Lindau disease. *Br J Ophthalmol* 1992; **76**: 743–5.

Maher ER, Yates JR, Benjamin C, Harries R, Moore AT, Ferguson-Smith MA. Clinical features and natural history of von Hippel-Lindau disease. *Quart J Med* 1990; **77**: 1151–63.

Manschot WA, De Bruijn WC. Coats' disease: definitions and pathogenesis. *Br J Ophthalmol* 1967; **51**: 145–57.

Mansour AM, Wells CG, Jampol L, Kalima RE. Ocular complications of arteriovenous communications of the retina. *Arch Ophthalmol* 1989; **107**: 232–6.

Martyn LJ, Knox DL. Glial hamartoma of the retina in generalized neurofibromatism (Von Recklinghausen's disease). *Br J Ophthalmol* 1972; **56**: 487–91.

Melmon KL, Rosen SW. Lindau's disease: review of the literature and study of a large kindred. *Am J Med* 1964; **36**: 595–617.

Meredith T. Inherited retinal venous beading. *Arch Ophthalmol* 1987; **105**: 949–53.

Messner E, Font RL, Laqua H *et al.* Cavernous haemangioma of the retina. Immunohistochemical and ultrastructural observations. *Arch Ophthalmol* 1984; **102**: 413–18.

Messmer E, Laqua H, Wessing A *et al.* Nine cases of cavernous haemangioma of the retina. *Am J Ophthalmol* 1983; **45**: 383–90.

Moore AT, Maher ER, Koch DJ, Charles SJ. Incidence and significance of congenital hypertrophy of the retinal pigment epithelium in familial polyposis coli. *Ophthalmol Paediatr Genet* 1992; **13**: 67–71.

Moore AT, Maher ER, Rosen P *et al.* Ophthalmological screening for von Hippel–Lindau disease. *Eye* 1991; **5**: 723–8.

Morales AG. Coats' disease: natural history and results of treatment. *Am J Ophthalmol* 1965; **60**: 855–65.

Mottow-Lippa L, Tso MO, Peyman GA, Chejfec G. von Hippel angiomatosis. A light, electron microscopic, and immunoperoxidase characterisation. *Ophthalmology* 1983; **90**: 848–55.

Munden PM, Sobol WM, Weingeist TA. Ocular findings in Turcot's syndrome (glioma polyposis). *Ophthalmology* 1991; **98**: 111–14.

Newell SW, Hall BD, Anderson CW, Lim S. Hallerman–Streiff syndrome with Coats' disease. *J Pediatr Ophthalmol Strabismus* 1994; **31**: 123–5.

Nicholson DH, Green WR, Kenyon KR. Light and electron microscopic study of early lesions in angiomatosis retinae. *Am J Ophthalmol* 1976; **82**: 193–204.

Nyboer JH, Robertson DM, Gomez MR. Retinal lesions in tuberous sclerosis. *Arch Ophthalmol* 1976; **94**: 1277–80.

Pancurak J, Goldberg MF, Fenkel M, Crowell RM. Cavernous haemangioma of the retina: genetic and central nervous system involvement. *Retina* 1985; **5**: 215–20.

Parke JT, Riccardi VM, Lewis AR, Ferrel RE. A syndrome of microcephaly and retinal pigmentary abnormalities without mental retardation in a family with coincidental autosomal dominant hyperreflexia. *Am J Med Genet* 1984; **17**: 585–94.

Patrassi GM, Sartori MT, Piermarocchi S *et al.* Unusual thrombotic type retinopathy (Coats' disease) associated with congenital plasminogen deficiency type 1. *J Int Med* 1993; **234**: 619–23.

Peyman GA, Rednam KR, Mottow-Lipa L, Flood T. Treatment of large von Hippel tumours by eye wall resection. *Ophthalmology* 1983; **90**: 840–7.

Piquet B, Gross-Jendroska M, Holz FG, Bird AC. Inherited venous beading. *Eye* 1994; **8**: 84–8.

Plowman PN, Harnett AN. Radiotherapy in benign orbital disease I. Complicated retinal angiomas. *Br J Ophthalmol* 1988; **72**: 286–8.

Polkinhorne PJ, Ritchie S, Neale K *et al.* Pigmented lesions of the retinal pigment epithelium and familial adenomatous polyposis. *Eye* 1990; **4**: 216–22.

Purcell JJ, Shields JA. Hypertrophy with hyperpigmentation of the retinal pigment epithelium. *Arch Ophthalmol* 1975; **93**: 122–6.

Ramsay RL, Kin Youn JL, Hill CW *et al.* Retinal astrocytoma. *Am J Ophthalmol* 1979; **88**: 32–6.

Reeser FH, Aaberg TM, van Horn DL. Astrocytic hamartoma of the retina not asssociated with tuberous sclerosis. *Am J Ophthalmol* 1978; **86**: 688–98.

Regillo CD, Eagle RC, Shields JA *et al.* Histological findings in congenital grouped pigmentation of the retina. *Ophthalmology* 1993; **100**: 400–5.

Renardel de Lavalette VW, Cruysberg JRM, Deutman AF. Familial grouped pigmentation of the retina. *Am J Ophthalmol* 1991; **112**: 406–9.

Revesz T, Fletcher S, Algazali LI *et al.* Bilateral retinopathy, aplastic anemia, and central nervous system abnormalities — a new syndrome. *J Med Genet* 1992; **29**: 673–5.

Ridley ME, Shields JA, Brown GC, Tasman W. Coats' disease evaluation of management. *Ophthalmology* 1982; **89**:1381–7.

Robertson DM. Hamartomas of the optic disc with retinitis pigmentosa. *Am J Ophthalmol* 1972; **74**: 526–31.

Romania A, Zakov N, McGannon E *et al.* Congenital hypertrophy of the retinal pigment epithelium in familial adenomatous polyposis. *Ophthalmology* 1989; **96**: 879–84.

Roseman R, Gass JDM. Solitary hypopigmented nevus of the retinal pigment epithelium in the macula. *Arch Ophthalmol* 1992; **110**: 1358–9.

Rosenberg PR, Walsh JB. Retinal pigment epithelial hamartoma — unusual manifestation. *Br J Ophthalmol* 1984; **68**: 439–42.

Salazar FG, Lamiell JM. Early identification of retinal angiomas in a large kindred with von Hippel disease. *Am J Ophthalmol* 1980; **89**: 540–5.

Schachat AP, Shields JA, Fine SL *et al.* Combined hamartomas of the retina and retinal pigment epithelium. *Ophthalmology* 1984; **91**: 1609–15.

Schatz H, Chang LF, Ober RR *et al.* Central retinal vein occlusion associated with retinal arteriovenous malformation. *Ophthalmology* 1993; **100**: 24–30.

Sellors PJH, Archer D. The management of retinal angiomatosis. *Trans Ophthalmol Soc UK* 1969; **89**: 529–43.

Shields J, Shields C, Pankajkumar S *et al.* Lack of association among typical congenital hypertrophy of the retinal pigment epithelium, adenomatous polyposis and Gardener's syndrome. *Ophthalmology* 1992; **99**: 1709–13.

Shields JA, Tso MOM. Congenital grouped pigmentation of the retina: histopathologic description and report of a case. *Arch Ophthalmol* 1975; **93**: 1153–5.

Shuin T, Kondo K, Torigoe S *et al.* Frequent somatic mutations and loss of heterozygosity of the von Hippel–Lindau tumour suppressor gene in human renal cell carcinoma. *Cancer Res* 1994; **54**: 2852–5.

Sivalingam A, Augsberger J, Perlango G *et al.* Combined hamartoma of the retina and retinal pigment epithelium in a patient with neurofibromatosis type 2. *J Pediatr Ophthalmol Strabismus* 1991; **28**: 320–2.

Small RG. Coats' disease and muscular dystrophy. *Trans Am Acad Ophthalmol Otolaryngol* 1968; **72**: 225–31.

Stewart MW, Gittner KA. Inherited venous beading. *Am J Ophthalmol* 1988; **106**: 675–81.

Taylor DA, Carrol JE, Smith ME *et al.* Facioscapulohumeral dystrophy associated with hearing loss and Coats' syndrome. *Ann Neurol* 1982; **12**: 395–8.

Tolmie JL, Browne BH, McGettrick PM, Stephenson JBP. A familial syndrome with Coats' reaction retinal angiomas, hair and nail defects and intracranial calcification. *Eye* 1988; **2**: 297–303.

Traboulsi EI, Maumenee IH, Krush AJ *et al.* Pigmented ocular fundus lesions in the inherited gastrointestinal polyposis syndromes and in hereditary non polyposis colorectal cancer. *Ophthalmology* 1988; **95**: 964–69.

Traboulsi EI, Murphy SF, de la Cruz ZC *et al.* A clinicopathological study of the eyes in familial aenomatous polyposis with extracolonic manifestations (Gardener's syndrome). *Am J Ophthalmol* 1990; **110**: 550–61.

Tripathi R, Ashton N. Electron microscopical study of Coats' disease. *Br J Ophthalmol* 1971; **55**: 289–301.

Turcot J, Despres JP, St Pierre F. Malignant tumours of the central nervous system associated with familial polyposis of the colon: report of two cases. *Dis Colon Rectum* 1959; **2**: 465–8.

Ulbright TM, Fulling KH, Helveston EM. Astrocytic tumours of the retina. Differentiation of sporadic tumours from phacomatosis associated tumours. *Arch Pathol Lab Med* 1984; **108**: 160–3.

Vogel MH, Zimmerman LE, Gass JDM. Proliferation of the juxtapapillary retinal pigment epithelium simulating malignant melanoma. *Doc Ophthalmol* 1969; **26**: 461–81.

Wallis YL, McDonald F, Hulten M *et al.* Genotype–phenotype correlation between position of constitutional APC gene mutations and CHRPE expression in familial adenomatous polyposis. *Hum Genet* 1994; **94**: 543–8.

Wang CL, Bruckner AJ. Vitreous haemorrhage secondary to juxtapapillary hamartoma of the retina. *Retina* 1984; **4**: 44–7.

Watzke RC. Cryotherapy for retinal angiomatosis: a clinico pathologic report. *Doc Ophthalmol* 1973; **34**: 405–11.

Welch RB. von Hippel–Lindau disease: the recognition and treatment of early angiomatosis retinae and the use of cryosurgery as an adjunct to surgery. *Trans Am Ophthalmol Soc* 1970; **68**: 367–424.

Wells CG, Kalina RE. Progressive inherited retinal arteriolar tortuosity with spontaneous retinal haemorrhages. *Ophthalmology* 1985; **92**: 1015–21.

Williams R, Taylor D. Tuberous sclerosis. *Surv Ophthalmol* 1985; **30**: 143–54.

Wing GL, Weiter JJ, Kelly PJ *et al.* Von Hippel–Lindau disease. Angiomatosis of the retina and central nervous system. *Ophthalmology* 1981; **88**: 1311–14.

Wyburn-Mason R. Arterial–venous aneurysm of midbrain and retina, facial naevi and mental changes. *Brain* 1943; **66**: 165–203.

Yimoyines DJ, Topilow HW, Abedin S, McMeel JW. Bilateral peripapillary exophytic retinal haemangioblastomas. *Ophthalmology* 1982; **89**: 1388–92.

47: Retinal Detachment in Childhood

Martin Snead and Anthony Moore

Retinal detachment is rare in childhood and often leads to difficulty with diagnosis and management. The presentation is usually late and the disease advanced at the time of diagnosis. Furthermore, detachments often occur in developmentally abnormal eyes which makes surgical management particularly difficult. Although rare, a surprisingly large number of disorders may give rise to detachment in childhood (Table 47.1). Detachments may be rhegmatogenous, exudative, tractional or a combination of these. In addition retinoblastoma or other tumours may give rise to a 'solid' detachment. Congenital retinal detachment, or so-called congenital non-attachment of the retina (Foos *et al.* 1968), is now recognized as part of the spectrum of vitreoretinal dysplasia which may have a variety of causes (see Chapter 41).

Rhegmatogenous retinal detachment

Most cases of rhegmatogenous retinal detachment in children are related to trauma or developmental abnormalities of the eyes (Tasman 1967; Daniel *et al.* 1974b), including high myopia.

Traumatic retinal detachment

Traumatic retinal detachment is seen most commonly in older children and is usually caused by blunt trauma (Verdaguer 1982; Johnson 1991) where retinal tears may be found in approximately 2–5% (Eagling 1974; Kearns 1991); a cause in infancy is non-accidental injury (Mushin & Morgan 1979). Penetrating injuries and retained intraocular foreign bodies are less frequent causes (Percival 1972).

Blunt ocular trauma

Retinal detachment due to blunt trauma is most commonly caused by a disinsertion at, or anterior to, the ora serrata (Daniel *et al.* 1974b; Johnson 1991) and characterized by an accompanying festoon of avulsed pars plana epithelium (Hagler 1980). There is a greater preponderance for superior quadrant involvement in contrast to non-traumatic dialysis (Hagler 1980; Ross 1991). Although the dialysis may be very extensive and superficially resemble a giant retinal tear, the vitreous gel characteristically remains attached to the posterior flap so that independent mobility is not a feature, and such cases usually respond well to conventional scleral buckling techniques. A further distinguishing feature is the absence of radial extensions, which frequently occur at the apices of giant retinal tears. Subretinal fluid recruitment is slow so that unless the ora serrata is routinely inspected after blunt trauma, diagnosis may be delayed by several weeks until macular involvement ensues (Johnson 1991).

Ragged impact necrosis breaks account for about one-fifth of retinal breaks seen in blunt trauma (Johnson 1991). Retinal vessel and retinal pigment epithelial disruption may be confirmed on fundus fluorescein angiography: the retinal detachment usually presents within 6 weeks (Johnson 1991). These breaks are often large, postequatorial and irregular making closure by conventional scleral buckling problematic so that internal tamponade

Table 47.1 Retinal detachment in children.

Rhegmatogenous
Inherited disorders
X-linked retinoschisis
Stickler's syndrome
Familial exudative vitreoretinopathy
Other vitreoretinal dystrophies (see Chapter 41)
Incontinentia pigmenti
Clefting syndromes
EEC syndrome
Ehlers–Danlos syndrome
Marfan's syndrome
Spondyloepiphyseal dysplasia congenita
Smith–Magenis syndrome

Developmental anomalies
Myopia
Congenital cataract
Congenital glaucoma
Ocular coloboma
Optic nerve anomalies
Retinopathy of prematurity
Persistent hyperplastic primary vitreous
Non-traumatic retinal dialysis

Trauma
Blunt trauma
Penetrating eye injuries
Intraocular foreign body
Non-accidental injury

Infection
Cytomegalovirus retinitis

Tractional retinal detachment
Retinopathy of prematurity
Incontinentia pigmenti
Familial exudative vitreoretinopathy
Other vitreoretinal dystrophies (see Chapter 41)
Trauma
Toxocariasis

Exudative retinal detachment
Retinopathy of prematurity
Coats' disease
Retinitis pigmentosa
Facioscapulohumeral dystrophy
Capillary haemangioma
Posterior scleritis
Haradas disease
Choroidal haemangioma

Solid retinal detachment
Retinoblastoma
Astrocytic hamartoma
Dictyoma

is often preferred (Han *et al.* 1990). Giant retinal tears account for a minority of retinal breaks due to blunt trauma (Johnson 1991). They respond well to vitrectomy and internal tamponade although the visual prognosis is often limited by associated ocular damage (Aylward *et al.* 1993).

Penetrating ocular trauma

Penetrating injury is an uncommon cause of detachment in childhood and may rarely follow inadvertent perforation of the globe at strabismus surgery (Basmadjian *et al.* 1975). Intraocular foreign bodies are rarely seen although penetrating injuries from air-gun pellets are typically seen in older children and adolescents and have a poor prognosis (Moore *et al.* 1987).

Retinal perforation or incarceration from penetrating trauma rarely causes acute rhegmatogenous retinal detachment. The associated corneoscleral wound provides access for extrinsic fibroblasts so that the more common sequel is late retinal detachment complicated by combined tractional and rhegmatogenous components (Aylward *et al.* 1993). Vitrectomy and internal tamponade with or without relieving retinectomy may be required (Bonnet & Fleury 1991). A dialysis may also develop following penetrating trauma with vitreous loss when it tends to occur on the opposite side of the eye to the penetrating wound (Scott 1977).

Non-traumatic retinal dialysis

Non-traumatic retinal dialysis accounts for approximately 10% of all juvenile retinal detachment (Hagler 1980; Verdaguer 1982) and in 97% of cases affects the inferotemporal quadrant (Verdaguer 1982). There is a 2/3 male propensity (Verdaguer 1982) and the vast majority of patients are hypermetropic or emmetropic (Scott 1977; Hagler 1980; Ross 1991). Although retinal detachment due to dialysis is rarely bilateral (Hagler 1980; Ross 1991) a careful examination of the ora reveals oral abnormalities, in the form of a 'frill' or flat dialysis, in the fellow eye in up to 30% of cases (Heatley 1972; Scott 1977; Verdaguer 1982) suggesting that there is a predisposing weakness in the ora serrata. Detachments associated with dialysis progress slowly and usually present when the macula becomes detached (Chignell 1973). Although the anatomical success rate of surgery is high, visual function may remain poor due to the long-standing nature of the detachment.

Aphakic detachment

See Chapter 39.

Familial retinal detachment

Retinal detachment may be seen in a variety of inherited systemic disorders in which there is ocular involvement (Table 47.2). In most cases there is associated high myopia

Table 47.2 Inherited disorders associated with an increased risk of retinal detachment.

Disorder	McKusick no.	Locus/gene	Systemic features
Coloboma	120200	Unknown; likely to be several different loci	Many different systemic disorders may be associated with ocular coloboma
Congenital falciform folds	221900	Unknown	Nil
Dominant exudative vitreoretinopathy	133780	11q13	Nil
Incontinentia pigmenti	308300	(1)Xp11.21 (2)Xq28	Fatal in males; skin vesicles and pigment; alopecia; hypodontia; mental retardation
Juvenile X-linked retinoschisis	312700	Xp22.2 Fibrillin gene (FBN1)	Nil
Marfan's syndrome	154700	15q15–q21.3	Tall thin habitus; dolichocephaly; high arch palate; crowded teeth; emphysema/pneumothorax; aortic dissection/dilation; cardiac valvular prolapse; kyphoscoliosis; arachnodactyly and joint laxity
Spondyloepiphyseal dysplasia congenita	183900	COL2A1 12q13	Short-trunk dwarfism; cleft palate; platyspondyly; short neck; cervical subluxation; scoliosis; kyphosis; barrel chest; pectus carinatum
Smith–Magenis syndrome	182290	17p11.2	Mental retardation; hyperactive
Stickler's syndrome (type 1)	108300	COL2A1 12q13	Flat midface; high arch/cleft palate; sensorineural and conductive deafness; joint laxity; arthritis
Stickler's syndrome (type 2)	184840	1p21	Flat midface; high arch/cleft palate; sensorineural and conductive deafness; joint laxity; arthritis

although in some conditions, for example incontinentia pigmenti and familial exudative vitreoretinopathy (FEVR), there is an underlying retinovascular abnormality. Infrequently a true detachment may complicate juvenile X-linked retinoschisis (Verdaguer 1982; Schulman *et al.* 1985; George *et al.* 1995b).

High myopia and retinal detachment is seen in Marfan's syndrome, Ehlers–Danlos syndrome (Pemberton *et al.* 1966), Smith–Magenis syndrome (Finucane *et al.* 1993), Stickler's syndrome (Billington *et al.* 1985), spondyloepiphyseal dysplasia (Ikegawa *et al.* 1993) and in association with midfacial clefting syndromes (Delaney *et al.* 1963; Daniel *et al.* 1974a) and the EEC syndrome (Marshall 1958; Feiler-Ofry *et al.* 1980; Wald *et al.* 1993a). The detachments are often complex, frequently with associated giant tears (Scott 1980; Billington *et al.* 1985).

Marfan's syndrome

Marfan's syndrome is a dominantly inherited disorder of fibrillin production with a prevalence of approximately one in 20 000 (Pyeritz & McKusick 1979). The fibrillins are high molecular weight extracellular glycoproteins, and mutations in the fibrillin gene on chromosome 15 (FBN1) cause Marfan's syndrome and dominant ectopia lentis (Kainulainen *et al.* 1990; Dietz *et al.* 1991; Maslen *et al.* 1991). Mutations in a second fibrillin gene on chromosome 5 are responsible for congenital contractural arachnodactyly (Tsipouras *et al.* 1992). Recent work has confirmed fibrillin to be widespread in lens capsule, iris, ciliary body and sclera (Wheatley *et al.* 1995).

The association of rhegmatogenous retinal detachment with Marfan's syndrome is well recognized and has been reported in 8–50% of cases (Jarrett 1967; Maumenee 1981); approximately 75% of these occur below 20 years of age (Maumenee 1981). Although there is a significant association with myopia, this is characteristically developmental, and no case of myopia was found under 3 years of age in one large series (Maumenee 1981). This is in contrast to the congenital non-progressive myopia found in type 1 Stickler's syndrome (Scott 1980, 1989; Snead 1996). In Marfan's syndrome the pupils characteristically dilate poorly because of a structural iris abnormality (Wheatley *et al.* 1995) and when combined with lens subluxation and weak scleral architecture the repair of retinal detachment in Marfan's syndrome patients can provide a formidable surgical challenge. Pars plana lensectomy and internal tamponade are often required (Greco & Ambrosino 1993) and appropriate equipment for such procedures should always be available when managing these patients.

Stickler's syndrome

In Stickler's syndrome, myopia is common (76–85%;

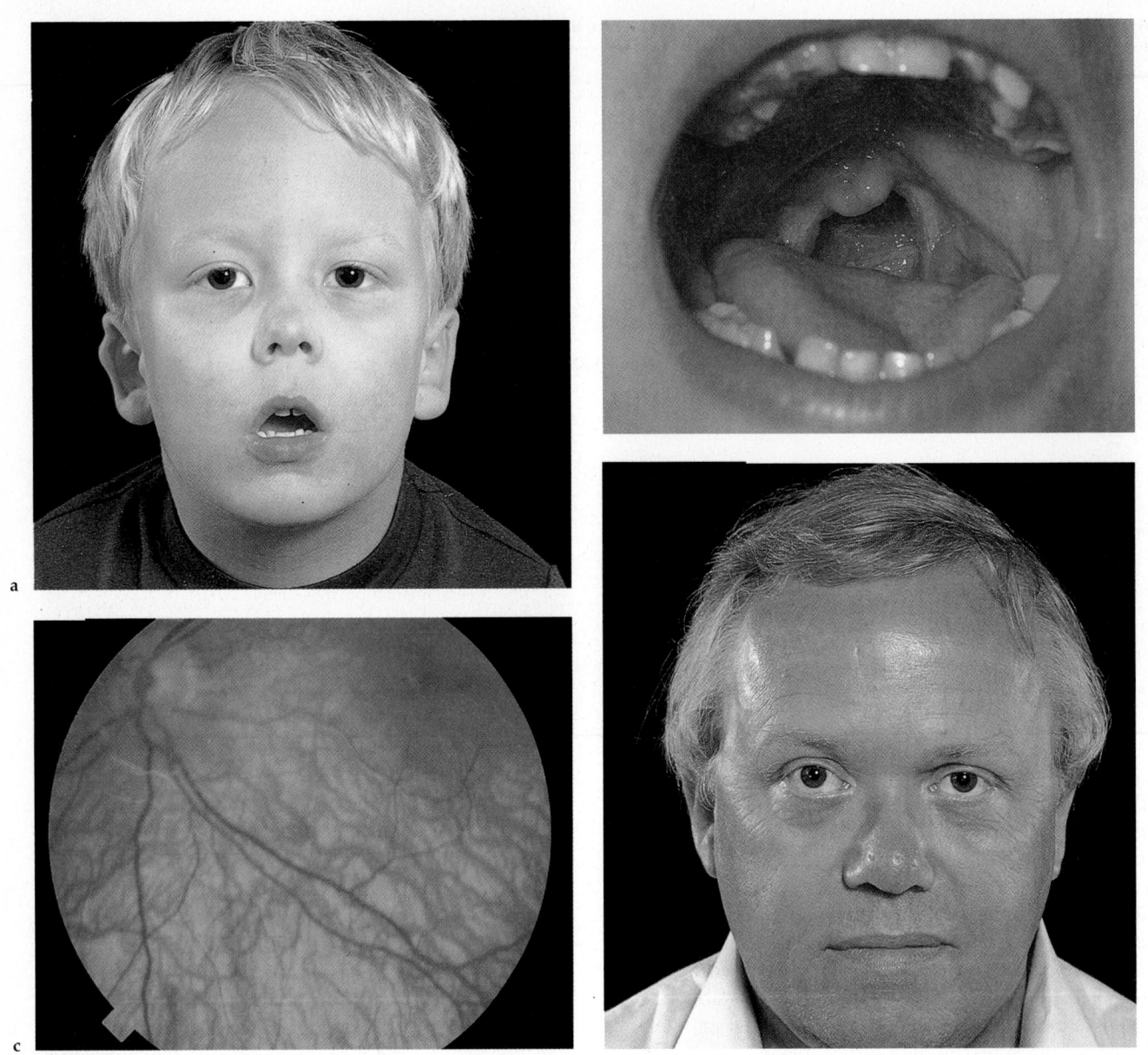

Fig. 47.1 (a) Stickler's syndrome. This boy has a flattened nasal bridge, malar hypoplasia, myopia and spondyloepiphyseal dysplasia. (b) Cleft soft palate (same patient). (c) High myopia. He also had vitreoretinal changes. (d) Father of the boy in (a) showing characteristic facies.

Liberfarb *et al.* 1981; Billington *et al.* 1985), of varying degrees, and often severe (Knobloch & Leyer 1979). Scott (1980) drew attention to several distinguishing features of the congenital myopia in Stickler's syndrome. The myopia is of high degree, non-progressive and presentation or diagnosis is usually below the age of 4 years. In addition there are no disc changes of pathological or developmental myopia. Although progressive myopia

had been noted in Stickler's original pedigree (Stickler *et al.* 1965, 1967) and by others (Spallone 1987b), the congenital non-progressive nature of the myopia as a feature of Stickler's syndrome patients was further emphasized by Wang *et al.* (1990). Congenital axial myopia of high degree was described in three Stickler's syndrome patients all examined within the first 2 months of life (Wang *et al.* 1990). It is inherited as an autosomal dominant trait (Fig. 47.1).

Cataract is another common feature of Stickler's syndrome: the quoted incidence varies from 30 to 80% according to the age range of the patients studied. In one series only 12% of patients over 50 years of age had clear lenses but most series for all ages seem to be in fairly close agree-

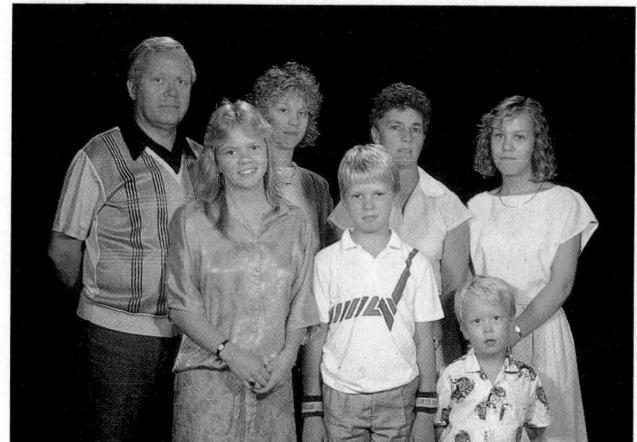

e

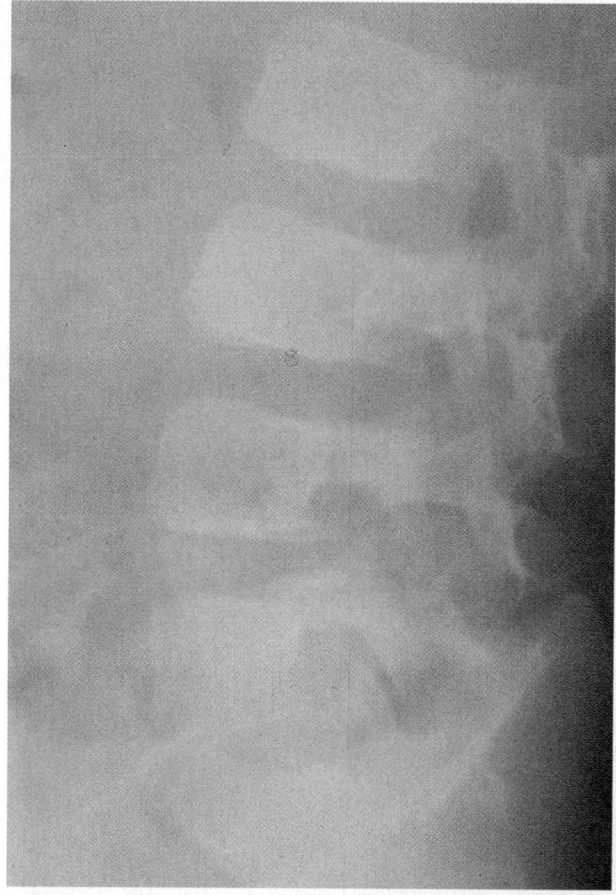

f

Fig. 47.1 *cont'd.* (e) Family of the boy in (a) showing high incidence of the characteristic facies. (f) Spondyloepiphyseal dysplasia in Stickler's syndrome: the vertebral bodies are rounded and flattened, the disc space narrowed.

ment with an incidence of approximately 45–50% (Gellis *et al.* 1976; O'Donnell *et al.* 1976; Liberfarb & Hirose 1981, 1982; Weingeist *et al.* 1982; Billington *et al.* 1985; Spallone 1987b; Seery *et al.* 1990).

Although Marshall (1958) described ectopia lentis (Fig. 47.2) in two patients with hereditary vitreoretinal disease, this has not been a feature of any subsequent accounts other than that of Spallone (1987b), who reported this finding in 12.8% of subjects.

The most comprehensive study on cataract in Stickler's syndrome (Seery *et al.* 1990) draws attention to the highly characteristic 'wedge' or 'fleck' cataracts of these patients, accounting for 43% of all cataract types. This is not significantly related to retinal detachment, in contrast to other cataract types which show significant association (Scott 1979, 1982). The strong association between the 'bird', 'wedge' or 'semilunar' cataract and Stickler's syndrome has been noted by others (Weingeist *et al.* 1982; Scott 1989).

Vitreoretinal changes and retinal detachment are the most serious ocular associations of this disorder (Liberfarb & Hirose 1982) and abnormalities of vitreous structure have long been regarded as the ophthalmic hallmark of Stickler's syndrome. Optical emptiness, liquefaction, vitreous bands and syneresis are common descriptions but contribute little to the understanding of the pathogen-

esis and even imply a degenerative and progressive disorder. Scott (1980, 1989) first reported the congenital vitreous anomalies pathognomonic of subgroups of these patients, and Stickler's syndrome has been subclassified into those with type 1 congenital vitreous anomaly linked to mutations in the gene encoding type 2 procollagen, and type 2 Stickler's syndrome in which this gene has been excluded (Snead *et al.* 1994; Richards *et al.* 1996). The exact biochemical and pathological nature of this congenital vitreous anomaly remains, at present, unknown but a glial cell origin has been suggested on the basis of cilia, microvilli and cytoplasmic filaments (Miyashita *et al.* 1994).

Rhegmatogenous retinal detachment is the most serious ocular complication of Stickler's syndrome. There is a propensity for giant retinal tear formation in childhood (Scott 1980; Billington *et al.* 1985) but a wide variety of retinal breaks have been noted. Younger patients tend to have very little retinal abnormality and lattice degeneration and pigmentation, when present, is minimal (Knobloch & Leyer 1979; Scott 1989). The incidence of retinal detachment varies between series, reflecting specialty referral patterns, and ranges from 10 to 48% (Marshall 1958; O'Donnell *et al.* 1976; Maumenee 1979; Billington *et al.* 1985; Seery *et al.* 1990). The reason why patients with

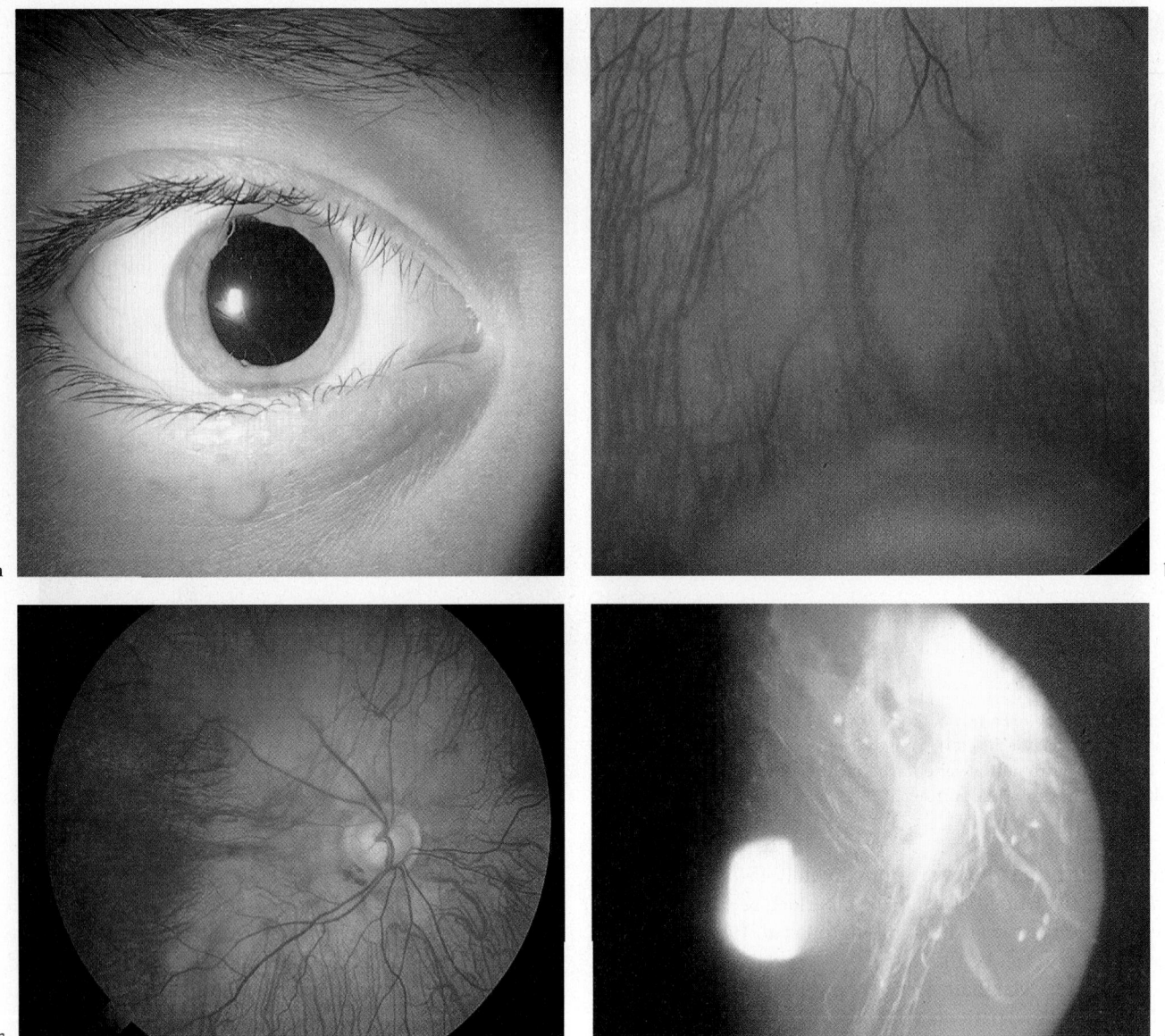

Fig. 47.2 Stickler's syndrome. (a) External eye showing iris defect following spontaneous lens subluxation (−25 dioptre myopia). (b) Fundus showing dislocated lens inferiorly. (c) Fundus showing myopic changes and defocused areas due to vitreous opacities. (d) Vitreous opacities and strands. The vitreoretinal problems in these children makes them very susceptible to retinal detachment.

Stickler's syndrome are so susceptible to retinal detachment is unknown. There is no association between retinal detachment and the presence of wedge or fleck cataract (Seery *et al.* 1990). Weingeist *et al.* (1982) alluded to a possible structural anomaly both within the vitreous and between neurosensory retina and retinal pigment epithelium predisposing these patients to retinal detachment even in the absence of clinically identifiable 'retinal degeneration'.

Abnormalities in the electroretinogram (ERG) have been related to the severity of myopia (Weingeist *et al.* 1982). Those with severe myopia can show a marked decrease in amplitude of the scotopic b-wave (Weingeist *et al.* 1982). Whether this relates to any underlying structural retinal abnormality in these patients other than that for myopia is unknown (Mantyjarvi & Tupp 1995).

Spallone (1987b) reports vascular abnormalities in the temporal retinal periphery causing leakage and exudate and in conjunction with the ectopia lentis unique to his series amongst the many reported, it is possible that these patients represent a separate subgroup.

Patients with Stickler's syndrome have variable micrognathia, cleft uvula, cleft palate, glossoptosis, a depressed nasal bridge and midface hypoplasia (Figs 47.1, 47.3). Most affected patients have spondyloepiphyseal dysplasia which may be symptomatic (Fig. 47.4).

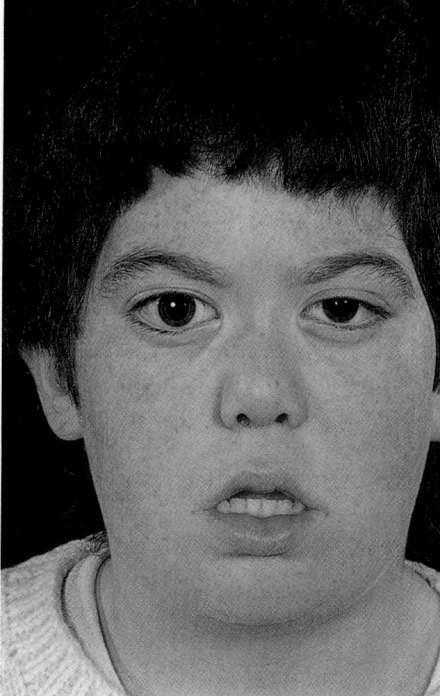
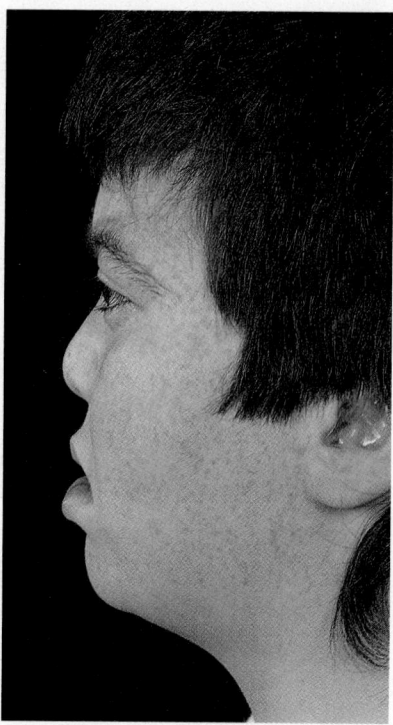

Fig. 47.3 Stickler's syndrome. These children have a flat nasal bridge, midfacial hypoplasia and deafness (note hearing aid). Micrognathia, cleft soft palate, and dental abnormalities may also be present.

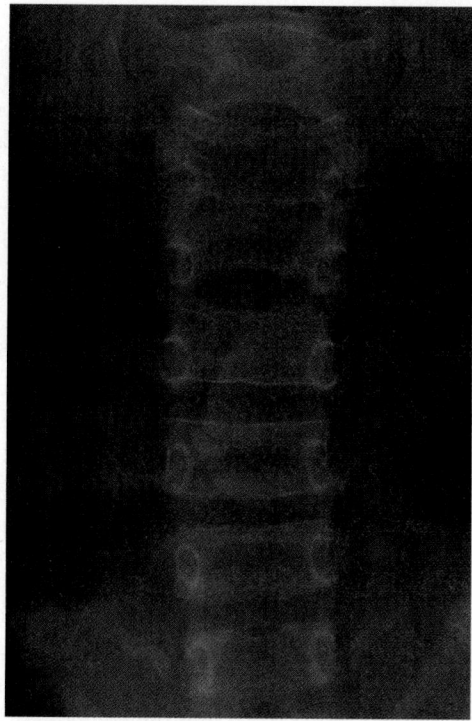

Fig. 47.4 Stickler's syndrome. Flat vertebrae as a radiological sign of spondyloepiphyseal dysplasia. These children may be born with an arthropathy and muscular hypotonia.

Kniest's syndrome

Kniest's syndrome has many similarities to Stickler's syndrome; it is autosomal dominantly inherited, and there is severe, early onset symptomatic spondylometaphyseal dysplasia, cleft palate, a flat nasal bridge, and hearing defects. Maumenee and Traboulsi (1985) described seven affected children with congenital severe myopia, vitreoretinal degeneration; four developed rhegmatogenous retinal detachments, one had dislocated lenses and two had cataracts.

Other spondyloepiphyseal dysplasias

The spondyloepiphyseal dysplasias (SED) are a heterogeneous subgroup of the skeletal dysplasias whose cardinal features are abnormal epiphyses, flattened vertebral bodies and variable ocular involvement (Rimoin & Lachman 1983). There are two principal variants: (i) SED tarda with X-linked inheritance presenting at puberty; and (ii) SED congenita with autosomal dominant inheritance presenting at birth.

Anderson *et al.* (1990) reported linkage to the gene encoding type 2 procollagen in a pedigree with SED congenita associated with cleft palate and this association was confirmed by Ramesar and Beighton (1992). Tiller *et al.* (1990) characterized the COL 2A1 mutation in an isolated individual with SED which resulted in the addition of 15 amino acids to the triple helical domain of the A1 chains of type 2 collagen.

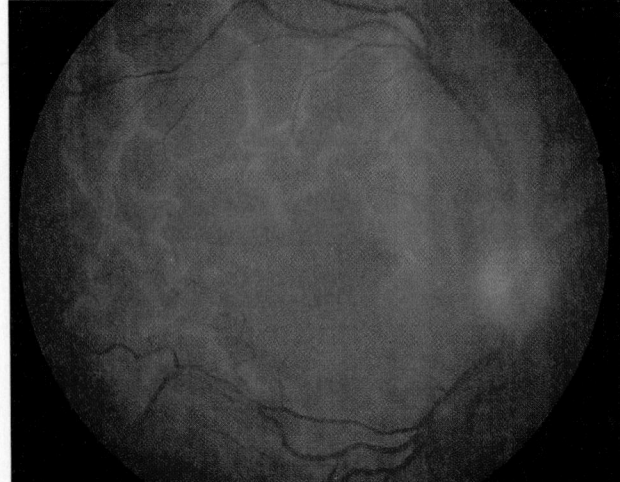

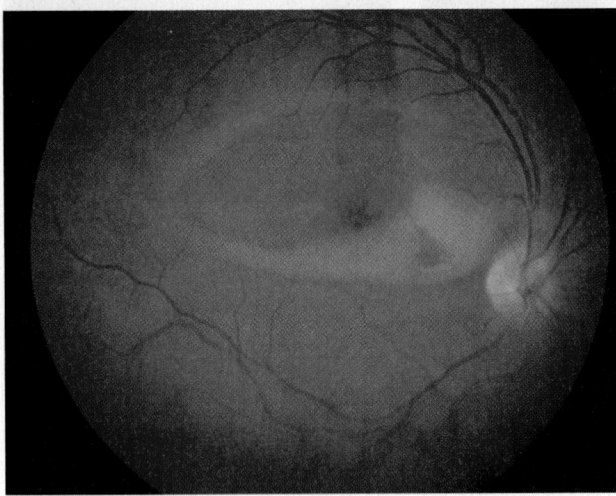

Fig. 47.5 (a) Total retinal detachment in a patient with X-linked retinoschisis and communicating inner and outer leaf breaks (Mr J.D. Scott's patient). (b) Postoperative fundus photograph of patient shown in (a), following vitrectomy and internal tamponade with 5000 cs liquid silicone. Foveal schisis can be seen underlying the silicone reflex. Visual acuity 6/24 and N5 (Mr J.D. Scott's patient).

In parallel with the type 1 Stickler's syndrome patients the known association between type 2 collagen defects and SED congenita may partly explain the high incidence of ocular complications. Myopia has been reported in 50% and rhegmatogenous retinal detachment in 20% of patients (Ikegawa *et al.* 1993).

X-linked retinoschisis

X-linked retinoschisis is an uncommon cause of retinal detachment in childhood accounting for 2.5–5% of all paediatric retinal detachments (Daniel *et al.* 1974b; Verdaguer 1982). The incidence of retinal detachment varies in the different series but it may occur in up to 16% of affected males (George *et al.* 1996). Vitreous haemorrhage is another cause of visual loss. Peripheral retinoschisis is found in approximately 50% of cases (Swartz *et al.* 1984) and can be complicated by retinal detachment by various mechanisms. A full thickness retinal break occurring *de novo* or a communication between outer and inner leaf defects in the schisis wall (Regillo *et al.* 1993) may lead to rhegmatogenous retinal detachment. Full thickness breaks may be managed effectively by scleral buckling procedures provided complete break closure can be satisfactorily achieved. Where communication exists between inner and outer leaf breaks (Fig. 47.5) an internal approach may be required to effect and maintain closure (Regillo *et al.* 1993).

Occasionally X-linked retinoschisis can be complicated by cyst formation which may develop haemorrhage into the cavity (Regillo *et al.* 1993) or even be so bullous as to obscure the visual axis (Schulman *et al.* 1985). There is some evidence that spontaneous resolution can occur (Kawano *et al.* 1981; George *et al.* 1995) but prolonged delay may compromise the visual prognosis so that some authors have advocated surgical drainage and deroofing of the cyst by internal means (Schulman *et al.* 1985).

Other vitreoretinal dystrophies

There are a number of uncommon vitreoretinal dystrophies such as autosomal dominant vitreoretinochoroidopathy, autosomal dominant neovascular inflammatory vitreoretinopathy, erosive retinopathy and snowflake degeneration in which there is an increased risk of rhegmatogenous retinal detachment. These disorders are discussed in Chapter 41.

Detachment in developmental anomalies of the eye

Ocular colobomas

Eyes with ocular colobomas are at a significantly increased risk of detachment and account for approximately 0.5% of paediatric retinal detachments (Daniel *et al.* 1974b; McDonald *et al.* 1991); giant retinal tears are seen in association with lens colobomas (Hovland *et al.* 1968) and rhegmatogenous detachment may develop in eyes with choroidal coloboma, when small retinal breaks may be found in thinned retina overlying the coloboma (Jesberg & Schepens 1961; Hanneken *et al.* 1991). Histopathological studies show the intercalary membrane to consist of hypoplastic inner retina with reversal and duplication of outer neuroblastic layers at the coloboma margin (Schubert 1995). This marginal duplication has been proposed as a 'locus minoris resistentiae' providing adhesion. The retinal pigment epithelium is absent within the coloboma,

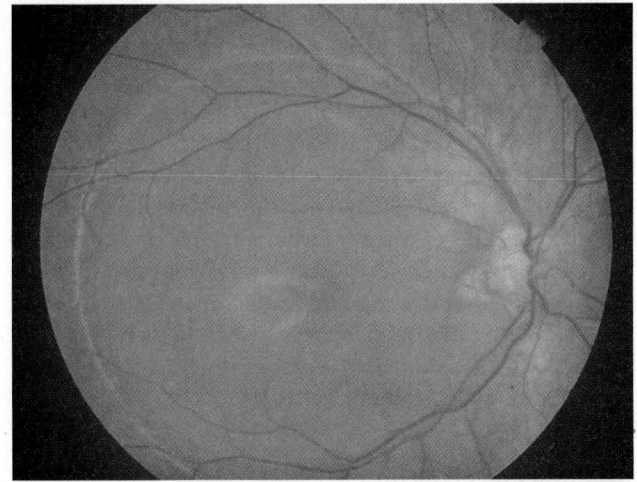

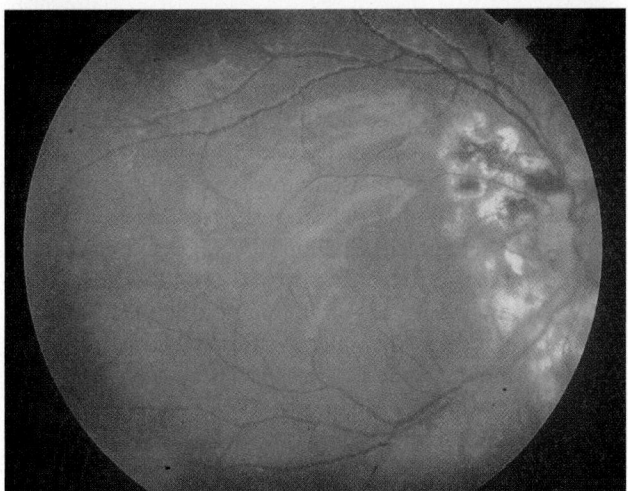

Fig. 47.6 (a) Long-standing serous macular detachment linked to optic disc pit. Visual acuity was 1/60 (Mr P.M. Jacobs' patient). (b) Postoperative fundus photograph of patient shown in (a), following vitrectomy, argon laser and gas tamponade. Visual acuity was 6/60 (Mr P.M. Jacobs' patient).

which has important implications for the production of a permanent chorioretinal adhesion.

Where retinal breaks occur away from the colobomatous area then they may be managed by conventional buckling techniques provided the sclera is of sufficient quality to take a suture and the break can be adequately closed (Corcostegui *et al.* 1992). More usually, the retinal break overlies the colobomatous area so that identification and closure with adequate retinopexy may be impossible without internal tamponade (McDonald *et al.* 1991). Retinal breaks over a coloboma are often small and may be multiple and their localization can be aided peroperatively by the identification of 'schlieren' during internal drainage. Argon laser photocoagulation may be applied around the border of the colobomatous area (McDonald *et*

al. 1991) and where this includes the papillomacular bundle this may be applied prior to retinal reattachment to minimize nerve fibre damage (Snead *et al.* 1991).

Nevertheless, the effectiveness of any retinal adhesion is dependent on maintaining retinal tamponade and stability during its formation and this can be compromised by the abnormal configuration of the colobomatous globe. Redetachment may occur in up to 30% of cases (Gopal *et al.* 1991), so that permanent internal tamponade may be required.

Spontaneous reattachment of the retina has been occasionally reported in retinal detachment associated with the morning glory anomaly (see Chapter 50) and optic nerve coloboma (Bochow *et al.* 1991).

Optic disc pits

The association of serous macular detachment and optic disc pits has long been recognized (Sugar 1967; Gass 1969). Similar findings with the morning glory disc abnormality indicate that these two conditions are variations of the same basic abnormality (Irvine *et al.* 1986). The vitreous is characteristically attached (Bonnet 1991; Snead *et al.* 1991; Akiba *et al.* 1993) and there is only a single report of an associated retinal break (von Fricken & Dhungel 1984). It has been suggested that up to 45% of optic disc pits may be complicated by serous retinal detachment (Cox *et al.* 1988; Sobol *et al.* 1990) and although spontaneous resolution has been reported in some cases (Sugar 1967; Hamada & Ellsworth 1971), the visual prognosis is poor if the detachment persists beyond 6 months (Sobol *et al.* 1990). In the light of this there has been an increasing trend towards early surgical treatment and various modalities have been tried.

Photocoagulation alone has met with mixed success. In some series no patients were successfully reattached with laser alone (Kapel *et al.* 1983; Bonnet 1991) and in others (Annersley *et al.* 1978; Abujamra *et al.* 1984; Cox *et al.* 1988; Schatz & McDonald 1988) the limited success has to be balanced against the only long-term natural history study which showed eventual spontaneous reattachment in 25% of cases (Sobol *et al.* 1990). The combination of argon laser photocoagulation with internal tamponade either with or without vitrectomy (Fig. 47.6) appears to offer greater chance of successful retinal reattachment albeit at greater risk of operative morbidity (Annersley *et al.* 1978; von Fricken & Dhungel 1984; Cox *et al.* 1988; Schatz & McDonald 1988; Bonnet 1991; Snead *et al.* 1991; Lincoff *et al.* 1993).

Retinal detachment may also occur in eyes with anterior or posterior persistent hyperplastic primary vitreous (see Chapter 41). Other ocular abnormalities associated with an increased risk of retinal detachment include congenital cataract (Kanski *et al.* 1974), congenital glaucoma (Cooling *et al.* 1980) and retinopathy of prematurity.

Tractional retinal detachment

Traction on the retina leading to detachment is rare in childhood; it may complicate primary retinovascular disease such as retinopathy of prematurity, FEVR, the inherited vitreoretinal degenerations (see Chapter 41) or incontinentia pigmenti or may develop following penetrating trauma, or intraocular inflammation associated with, for example, ocular toxocariasis. Such traction may lead to retinal detachment directly or cause retinal breaks and subsequent rhegmatogenous detachment. Proliferative vitreoretinopathy (PVR) may also complicate unsuccessful rhegmatogenous detachment repair and extensive vitreoretinal fibrosis is a common result of failed detachment surgery.

Retinopathy of prematurity

Retinopathy of prematurity accounts for approximately 2% of all paediatric retinal detachments (Daniel *et al.* 1974b). These may be broadly classified into those with early (within 1 year) and late (after 1 year) presentation.

The incidence of early retinal detachment following advanced retinopathy of prematurity has been substantially reduced by better screening and prophylactic cryotherapy (see Chapter 43). However, the visual results following vitreoretinal surgery for those which do progress to retinal detachment have been very disappointing (Quinn *et al.* 1991; Hirose *et al.* 1993; Seaber *et al.* 1995). Of the 129 eyes from the cryotherapy for retinopathy of prematurity (CRYO-ROP) studies which progressed to retinal detachment less than 2% retained any patterned vision at lowest measurable threshold either with or without treatment (Quinn *et al.* 1991). Seaber *et al.* (1995) have recently published their results of vitreoretinal surgery in 51 eyes of 33 patients with stage 5 retinopathy of prematurity; at a median follow-up of 61 months 15 eyes were blind, 27 had varying degrees of light perception and nine eyes had some crude form vision. Five children in the latter group used their sight to help navigate. The major and often multiple surgical challenges posed (the redetachment rate is high) need to be carefully weighed against a partial and spontaneous retinal reattachment in perhaps 10% of cases (Kalina 1991; Martin & de Juan 1992). There is a strong argument that vitreoretinal surgery in stage 5 retinopathy of prematurity should only be performed within the confines of a randomly controlled trial of surgery in this disorder.

The prognosis for retinal reattachment and the visual outcome are more favourable in eyes which have not progressed to stage 5 (Greven & Tasman 1990; Zilis *et al.* 1990; Sternberg *et al.* 1992). Lens-sparing techniques have been advocated for pathology confined posterior to the equator (Maguire & Trese 1993). Preservation of the crystalline lens with surgical access to the vitreous base in the neonatal eye requires adequate visualization of the pars plicata and this can be substantially enhanced by use of the operating indirect ophthalmoscope.

Late retinal detachment following treated or untreated retinopathy of prematurity is a well-recognized phenomenon. Detachments are most commonly rhegmatogenous (Greven & Tasman 1989) but may be tractional in approximately one-third of cases (Machemer 1993) or a combination of the two. The average age at presentation is 6 years (Tasman 1979) and although reattachment is frequently possible with vitreoretinal surgery (Machemer 1993), the prognosis relates more to the pre-existing visual potential prior to retinal detachment.

Incontinentia pigmenti

Incontinentia pigmenti is an X-linked dominantly inherited disorder causing death in males and dermatological, dental, central nervous system and ocular abnormalities in females. Ocular abnormalities occur in approximately one-third of patients, usually within the first year of life (Catalano 1990) and consist mainly of vascular abnormalities with abnormal peripheral perfusion and retinal pigment epithelial defects (Spallone 1987a) together with an isolated report of foveal hypoplasia (Goldberg & Custis 1992). The affected eye is often microphthalmic (Catalano 1990) and complications can arise from late tractional retinal detachment. Limited success has been achieved using complex vitreoretinal techniques (Wald *et al.* 1993b) and attention has been focused on prophylaxis. Although prophylactic cryotherapy to the peripheral avascular retina has been reported to arrest vascular proliferation and thereby prevent late tractional detachment (Rahi & Hungerford 1990) this has not been universally successful and direct vessel ablation has been suggested (Catalano *et al.* 1990).

Congenital falciform folds

An association between congenital falciform retinal folds and retinal detachment has been described (Warburg 1979; Swartz *et al.* 1984). These eyes are often microphthalmic and histology shows malformative retinal rosettes, persistent hyperplastic primary vitreous and occasionally vascular proliferation. It has been postulated that a retinal fold devoid of the influence of retinal pigment epithelium fails to acquire the potential for secreting secondary vitreous (Warburg 1979). These cases are rare. If retrolental adhesion is minor then it may be possible to establish a surgical plane so that retinal reattachment can be achieved, but the visual prognosis remains poor.

Exudative retinal detachment

Exudative detachment although uncommon has a wide

variety of causes in childhood, including Coats' disease, retinoblastoma, retinopathy of prematurity, ocular toxocariasis, choroidal haemangioma, capillary haemangioma, posterior scleritis and Harada's disease. If there is doubt about the diagnosis computed tomographic (CT) scan or ultrasound and a careful examination under anaesthetic (EUA) should be performed to rule out retinoblastoma. Treatment is usually directed at the underlying cause, for example laser photocoagulation of Coats' disease or retinal haemangiomas.

Management

In infants and young children with suspected retinal detachment it is important to carry out a thorough examination under general anaesthetic so that the cause of the detachment can be determined and treatment planned. In cases where no retinal breaks are found, scleral transillumination, ultrasound and CT scan are helpful in excluding intraocular tumour or posterior scleral thickening. Fluorescein angiography is helpful in highlighting retinovascular abnormalities in selected cases, for example in Coats' disease, FEVR and choroidal haemangioma. In non-traumatic rhegmatogenous detachment with high myopia a careful ocular and physical examination and, on occasion, paediatric referral will help exclude systemic disorders such as Marfan's and Stickler's syndromes.

Retinal detachment is rare in childhood and often associated with complex intraocular pathology. Such cases are therefore best referred to specialist centres with experience of dealing with vitreoretinal disorders in children. Even when treated in those centres, the prognosis is often poor (de Juan 1993; Ferrone *et al.* 1994).

References

Abujamra S, De Souza EC, Da Cunha SL. Pitting of the optic disc. *Rev Bras Oftalmol* 1985; **43**: 169–73.

Akiba J, Kakahashi A, Hikichi T, Trempe CL. Vitreous findings in cases of optic nerve pits and serous macular detachment. *Am J Ophthalmol* 1993; **116**: 38–41.

Anderson IJ, Goldberg RB, Marion RW, Upholt WB, Tsipouras P. Spondyloepiphyseal dysplasia congenita: genetic linkage to type 2 collagen (COL 2A1). *Am J Hum Genet* 1990; **46**: 896–901.

Annersley W, Brown G, Bolling J, Goldberg R, Fischer D. Treatment of retinal detachment with congenital optic disc pit by krypton laser photocoagulation. *Graefe's Arch Clin Exp Ophthalmol* 1978; **225**: 311–14.

Aylward GW, Cooling RJ, Leaver PK. Trauma-induced retinal detachment associated with giant retinal tears. *Retina* 1993; **13**: 136–41.

Basmadjian G, Labelle P, Dumas J. Retinal detachment after strabismus surgery. *Am J Ophthalmol* 1975; **79**: 305–9.

Billington BM, Leaver PK, McLeod D. Management of retinal detachment in the Wagner–Stickler syndrome. *Trans Ophthalmol Soc UK* 1985; **104**: 875–9.

Bochow TW, Olk RJ, Knupp JA, Smith ME. Spontaneous reattachment of the retina in an infant with microphthalmos and an optic

nerve coloboma. *Am J Ophthalmol* 1991; **112**: 347–8.

Bonnet M. Serous macular detachment associated with optic nerve pits. *Graefe's Arch Clin Exp Ophthalmol* 1991; **229**: 526–32.

Bonnet M, Fleury J. Management of retinal detachment after penetrating eye injury. *Graefe's Arch Clin Exp Ophthalmol* 1991; **229**: 539–42.

Catalano RA. Incontinentia pigmenti. *Am J Ophthalmol* 1990; **110**: 696–700.

Catalano RA, Lopatynsky M, Tasman WS. Treatment of proliferative retinopathy associated with incontinentia pigmenti. *Am J Ophthalmol* 1990; **110**: 701–2.

Chignell AH. Retinal dialysis. *Br J Ophthalmol* 1973; **57**: 572–7.

Cooling RJ, Rice NSC, McLeod D. Retinal detachment in congenital glaucoma. *Br J Ophthalmol* 1980; **64**: 407–21.

Corcostegui B, Guell JL, Garcia-Arumi J. Surgical treatment of retinal detachment in the choroidal colobomas. *Retina* 1992; **12**: 237–41.

Cox MS, Witherspoon CD, Morris RE, Flynn HW. Evolving techniques in the treatment of macular detachment caused by optic nerve pits. *Ophthalmology* 1988; **95**: 889–96.

Daniel R, Kanski J, Glasspool MG. Hyalo-retinopathy in the clefting syndrome. *Br J Ophthalmol* 1974a; **58**: 96–102.

Daniel R, Kanski JJ, Glasspool MG. Retinal detachment in children. *Trans Ophthalmol Soc UK* 1974b; **94**: 5–34.

de Juan E. The treatment of pediatric retinal detachment. *Arch Ophthalmol* 1993; **111**: 599–600.

Delaney WV, Podedworny W, Havener WH. Inherited retinal detachment. *Arch Ophthalmol* 1963; **69**: 44–50.

Dietz HC, Cutting GR, Pyeritz RE *et al.* Marfan syndrome caused by a recurrent *de novo* missense mutation in the fibrillin gene. *Nature* 1991; **352**: 337–9.

Eagling EM. Ocular damage after blunt trauma to the eye: its relationship to the nature of the injury. *Br J Ophthalmol* 1974; **58**: 126–40.

Feiler-Ofry V, Geidel V, Nemet P, Lazar M. Retinal detachment in median cleft-face syndrome. *Br J Ophthalmol* 1980; **64**: 121–3.

Ferrone P, McCuen B, deJuan E, Machemer R. The efficacy of silicone oil for complicated retinal detachments in the pediatric population. *Arch Ophthalmol* 1994; **112**: 773–7.

Finucane BM, Jaeger ER, Kurtz MB, Weinstein M, Scott CI. Eye abnormalities in the Smith–Magenis contiguous gene deletion syndrome. *Am J Med Genet* 1993; **45**: 443–6.

Foos RY, Kiechler RJ, Allen RA. Congenital non-attachment of the retina. *Am J Ophthalmol* 1968; **65**: 202–10.

Gass JDM. Serous detachment of the macula secondary to congenital pit of the optic nerve head. *Am J Ophthalmol* 1969; **67**: 821–41.

Gellis SS, Feingold M, Hermann J, Myers F. The Stickler syndrome (hereditary arthro-ophthalmopathy). *Am J Dis Child* 1976; **130**: 65–6.

George NDL, Bradshaw K, Yates JRW, Moore AT. Infantile presentation of X-linked retinoschisis. *Br J Ophthalmol* 1995; **79(7)**: 653–7.

George NDL, Yates JRW, Moore AT. Clinical features in affected males with X-linked retinoschisis. *Arch Ophthalmol* 1996; **114(3)**: 274–80.

Goldberg MF, Custis PH. Retinal and other manifestations in nine cases of incontinentia pigmenti (Bloch–Sulzberger syndrome). *Inv Ophthalmol Vis Sci* 1992; **33**: 1084.

Gopal L, Kini MM, Badrinath SS, Sharma T. Management of retinal detachment with choroidal coloboma. *Ophthalmology* 1991; **98**: 1622–7.

Greco GM, Ambrosino L. Treatment of retinal detachment in Marfan syndrome. *Ann Ophthalmol* 1993; **25**: 72–6.

Greven C, Tasman W. Rhegmatogenous retinal detachment following cryotherapy in retinopathy of prematurity. *Arch Ophthalmol* 1989; **107**: 1017–18.

Greven C, Tasman W. Scleral buckling in stages 4B and 5 retinopathy of prematurity. *Ophthalmology* 1990; **97**: 817–20.

Hagler WS. Retinal dialysis: a statistical and genetic study to determine pathogenic factors. *Trans Am Ophthalmol Soc* 1980; **68**: 686–733.

Hamada S, Ellsworth RM. Congenital retinal detachment and the optic disc anomaly. *Am J Ophthalmol* 1971; **71**: 460–3

Han DP, Mieler WF, Schwartz DM, Abrams GW. Management of traumatic retinal detachment with pars plana vitrectomy. *Arch Ophthalmol* 1990; **108**: 1281–6.

Hanneken A, deJuan E, McCuen BW. The management of retinal detachments associated with choroidal colobomas by vitreous surgery. *Am J Ophthalmol* 1991; **111**: 271–6.

Heatley J. El desprenimiento temporal inferior del adulto joven. In: Girard L, ed. *Proceedings of the IXth Pan American Conference on Ophthalmology* 1972: 137.

Hirose T, Katsumi O, Mehta M, Schepens CL. Vision in stage 5 retinopathy of prematurity after retinal reattachment by open sky vitrectomy. *Arch Ophthalmol* 1993; **111**: 345–9.

Hovland KR, Schepens GL, Freeman HM. Developmental giant retinal tears associated with lens coloboma. *Arch Ophthalmol* 1968; **80**: 325–31.

Ikegawa S, Iwaya T, Taniguchi K, Kimizuka M. Retinal detachment in spondyloepiphyseal dysplasia congenita. *J Pediatr Orthopaediatr* 1993: **13**: 791–2.

Irvine AR, Brookes Crawford J, Sullivan J. The pathogenesis of retinal detachment with the morning glory disc and optic pit. *Retina* 1986; **6**: 146–50.

Jarrett WH Jr. Dislocation of the lens: a study of 166 hospitalised cases. *Arch Ophthalmol* 1967; **78**: 289–96.

Jesberg DO, Schepens CL. Retinal detachment associated with coloboma of the choroid. *Arch Ophthalmol* 1961; **65**: 163–73.

Johnson PB. Traumatic retinal detachment. *Br J Ophthalmol* 1991; **75**: 18–21.

Kainulainen K, Pulkkinen L, Savolainen A, Kaitila I, Peltonen L. Location on chromosome 15 of the gene defect causing Marfan syndrome. *N Engl J Med* 1990; **323**: 935–9.

Kalina RE. Treatment of retinal detachment due to retinopathy of prematurity (editorial). *Ophthalmology* 1991; **98**: 3–4.

Kanski JJ, Elkington AR, Daniel R. Retinal detachment after congenital cataract surgery. *Br J Ophthalmol* 1974; **58**: 92–104.

Kapel J, Otradovel J, Dotrelova D. Maculopathies associated with congenital pits of the optic disc. *Czesk Oftalmol* 1983; **39**: 9–17.

Kawano K, Tanaka K, Murakami F, Ohba N. Congenital hereditary retinoschisis: evolution at the initial stage. *Albrecht von Graefe Archiv fur Klin Exp Ophthalmol* 1981; **217(4)**: 315–23.

Kearns P. Traumatic hyphaema: a retrospective study of 314 cases. *Br J Ophthalmol* 1991; **75**: 137–41.

Knobloch WH, Layer JM. Clefting syndromes associated with retinal detachment. *Am J Ophthalmol* 1979; **73**: 517–30.

Liberfarb RM, Hirose T. The Wagner–Stickler syndrome. *Birth Defects Original Article Series* 1982; **18**: 525–38.

Liberfarb RM, Hirose T, Holmes LB. The Wagner–Stickler syndrome: a study of 22 families. *J Pediatr* 1981; **99**: 394–9.

Lincoff H, Yannuzzi L, Singerman L, Kreissig I, Fisher Y. Improvement in visual function after displacement of the retinal elevations emanating from optic pits. *Arch Ophthalmol* 1993; **111**: 1071–9.

Machemer R. Late traction detachment in retinopathy of prematurity or ROP-like cases. *Graefe's Arch Clin Exp Ophthalmol* 1993; **231**: 389–94.

McDonald AR, Lewis H, Brown G, Sipperley JO. Vitreous surgery for retinal detachment associated with choroidal coloboma. *Arch Ophthalmol* 1991; **109**: 1399–402.

Maguire AM, Trese MT. Visual results of lens-sparing vitreoretinal surgery in infants. *J Pediatr Ophthalmol Strabismus* 1993; **30**: 28–32.

Mantyjarvi M, Tuppurainen K. Colour vision and dark adaptation in high myopia without central retinal degeneration. *Br J Ophthalmol* 1995; **79**: 105–8.

Marshall D. Ectodermal dysplasia. *Am J Ophthalmol* 1958; **45**: 143–56.

Martin DF, De Juan E. Spontaneous retinal reattachment in stage 5 retinopathy of prematurity. *Arch Ophthalmol* 1992; **110**: 453–4.

Maslen CL, Corson GM, Maddox BK, Glanville RW, Sakai LY. Partial sequence of a candidate gene for Marfan syndrome. *Nature* 1991; **352**: 334–7.

Maumenee IH. The eye in Marfan syndrome. *Trans Am Ophthalmol Soc* 1981; **69**: 684–733.

Maumenee IH. Vitreoretinal degeneration as a sign of generalised connective tissue diseases. *Am J Ophthalmol* 1979; **88**: 432–49.

Maumenee IH, Traboulsi EI. The ocular findings in Kniest dysplasia. *Am J Ophthalmol* 1985; **100**: 155–60.

Miyashita K, Tokunaga M, Akiyama K et al. Electron microscopic study on the vitreous membrane of the Stickler syndrome. *Nippon Ganka Gakkai Zashi* 1994; **98**: 86–91.

Moore AT, McArtney A, Cooling RJ. Eye injuries associated with the use of air weapons. *Eye* 1987; **1**: 422–9.

Mushin A, Morgan G. Ocular injury in the battered baby syndrome. Report of two cases. *Br J Ophthalmol* 1979; **55**: 343–7.

O'Donnell JJ, Sirkin S, Hall BD. Generalised osseous abnormalities in the Marshall syndrome. *Birth Defects* 1976; **12**: 299–314.

Pemberton JW, Freeman HM, Schepelos CL. Familial retinal detachment and the Ehlers–Danlos syndrome. *Arch Ophthalmol* 1966; **76**: 87–94.

Percival SPB. Late complications from posterior segment intraocular foreign bodies, with particular reference to retinal detachment. *Br J Ophthalmol* 1972; **56**: 462–8.

Pyeritz RE, McKusick VA. The Marfan syndrome: diagnosis and management. *N Engl J Med* 1979; **300**: 772–7.

Quinn GE, Dobson V, Barr CC et al. Visual acuity in infants after vitrectomy for severe retinopathy of prematurity. *Ophthalmology* 1991: **98**: 5–13.

Rahi J, Hungerford JR. Early diagnosis of the retinopathy of incontinentia pigmenti. Successful treatment by cryotherapy. *Br J Ophthalmol* 1990; **74**: 377–9.

Ramesar R, Beighton P. Spondyloepiphyseal dysplasia in a Cape Town family: linkage with the gene for type 2 collagen (COL 2A1). *Am J Med Genet* 1992; **43**: 833–8.

Regillo CD, Tasman WS, Brown GC. Surgical management of complications associated with X–linked retinoschisis. *Arch Ophthalmol* 1993: **111**: 1080–6.

Richards AJ, Pope FM, Yates JRW, Scott JD, Snead MP. A family with Stickler syndrome type 2 has a mutation in the COL11A1 gene resulting in the substitution of glycine 97 by valine in $\alpha 1$(XI) collagen. *Hum Mol Genet* 1996; **5**: 1339–43.

Rimoin DL, Lachman RS. In: Emery AEH, Rimoin DL, eds. *Principles and Practice of Medical Genetics*. New York: Churchill Livingstone, 1983: 703–35.

Ross WH. Retinal dialysis: lack of evidence for a genetic cause. *Canad J Ophthalmol* 1991; **26**: 309–12.

Schatz H, McDonald R. Treatment of retinal detachment associated with optic nerve pit or coloboma. *Ophthalmology* 1988; **95**: 178–86.

Schubert HD. Schisis-like retinal detachment associated with choroidal colobomas. *Graefe's Arch Clin Exp Ophthalmol* 1995; **233**: 74–9.

Schulman J, Peyman GA, Jedncock N, Larson B. Indications for vitrectomy in congenital retinoschisis. *Br J Ophthalmol* 1985; **69**: 482–6.

Scott JD. Congenital myopia and retinal detachment. *Trans Ophthal*

Soc UK 1980; **100**: 69–71.

Scott JD. Lens changes in retinal detachment. *Trans Ophthal Soc UK* 1979; **99**: 241–3.

Scott JD. Lens epithelial proliferation in retinal detachment. *Trans Ophthal Soc UK* 1982; **102**: 385–9.

Scott JD. Prevention and perspective in retinal detachment. Duke–Elder lecture. *Eye* 1989; **3**: 491–515.

Scott JD. Retinal dialysis. *Trans Ophthalmol Soc UK* 1977; **97**: 533–5.

Seaber JH, Machemer R, Eliot D *et al.* Long-term visual results after initially successful vitrectomy for stage 5 retinopathy of prematurity. *Ophthalmology* 1995; **102**: 199–204.

Seery CM, Pruett RC, Liberfarb RM, Cohen BZ. Distinctive cataract in the Stickler syndrome. *Am J Ophthalmol* 1990; **110**: 143–8.

Snead MP. Hereditary vitreopathy. *Eye* 1996; **10**: 653–63.

Snead MP, James N, Jacobs PM. Vitrectomy, argon laser, and gas tamponade for serous retinal detachment associated with an optic disc pit. *Br J Ophthalmol* 1991; **75**: 381–2.

Snead MP, Payne SJ, Barton DE *et al.* Stickler syndrome: correlation between vitreo-retinal phenotypes and linkage to COL 2A1. *Eye* 1994; **8**: 609–14.

Sobol WM, Blodi CF, Folk JC, Weingeist TA. Long-term visual outcome in patients with optic nerve pit and serous retinal detachment of the macula. *Ophthalmology* 1990; **97**: 1539–42.

Spallone A. Incontinentia pigmenti (Bloch–Sulzberger syndrome): seven case reports from one family. *Br J Ophthalmol* 1987a; **7**: 629–34.

Spallone A. Stickler's syndrome: a study of 12 families. *Br J Ophthalmol* 1987b; **71**: 504–9.

Sternberg P, Lopez PF, Lambert HM, Aabberg TM, Capone A. Controversies in the management of retinopathy of prematurity. *Am J Ophthalmol* 1992; **113**: 198–202.

Stickler GB, Belau PG, Farrell FJ *et al.* Hereditary progressive arthro-ophthalmopathy. *Mayo Clin Proc* 1965; **40**: 433–55.

Stickler GB, Pugh DG. Hereditary progressive arthro-ophthalmopathy II. Additional observations on vertebral abnormalities, a hearing defect, and a report of a similar case. *Mayo Clin Proc* 1967; **42**: 495–500.

Sugar HS. Congenital pits in the optic disc and their equivalents (congenital colobomas and coloboma-like excavations) associated with submacular fluid. *Am J Ophthalmol* 1967; **63**: 298–307.

Swartz M, Sanborn GE, Johnston RL, Miller KN, Gilmore G. Congenital retinal malformations. *Int Ophthalmol Clin* 1984; **24**: 123–31.

Tasman W. Late complications of retrolental fibroplasia. *Trans Am Acad Ophthalmol Otolaryngol* 1979; **86**: 1724–40.

Tasman W. Retinal detachment in children. *Trans Am Acad Ophthalmol Otolaryngol* 1967; **71**: 455–60.

Tiller GE, Rimoin DL, Murray LW, Cohn DH. Tandem duplication within a type 2 collagen gene (COL 2A1) exon in an individual with spondyloepiphyseal dysplasia. *Proc Natl Acad Sci USA* 1990; **87**: 3889–93.

Tsipouras P, Del Mastro R, Sarfarazi M *et al.* The international Marfan syndrome collaborative study genetic linkage of the Marfan syndrome, ectopia lentis, and congenital contractural arachnodactyly to the fibrillin genes on chromosomes 15 and 5. *N Engl J Med* 1992; **326**: 905–9.

Verdaguer J. Juvenile retinal detachment. *Arch Ophthalmol* 1982; **93**: 145–56.

von Fricken M, Dhungel R. Retinal detachment in the morning glory syndrome: pathogenesis and management. *Retina* 1984; **4**: 97–9.

Wald K, Hirose T, Topilow H. Ectodermal dysplasia, ectrodactyly and clefting syndrome and bilateral retinal detachment. *Arch Ophthalmol* 1993a; **111**: 734.

Wald KJ, Mehta MC, Katsumi O, Sabates NR, Hirose T. Retinal detachments in incontinentia pigmenti. *Arch Ophthalmol* 1993b; **111**: 614–17.

Wang FM, Scott IA, Goldberg RB. Congenital myopia in Stickler's hereditary arthro-ophthalmopathy. *Am J Ophthalmol* 1990; **110**: 435–6.

Warburg M. Retinal malformations. Doyne Memorial lecture. *Trans Ophthal Soc UK* 1979; **99**: 272–83.

Weingeist TA, Hermsen V, Hanson JW, Bumsted RM, Weinstein SL, Olin WH. Ocular and systemic manifestations of Stickler's syndrome: a preliminary report. *Birth Defects Original Article Series* 1982; **18**: 539–60.

Wheatley HM, Traboulsi EI, Flowers BE *et al.* Immunohistochemical localisation of fibrillin in human ocular tissues. *Arch Ophthalmol* 1995; **113**: 103–9.

Zilis JD, De Juan E, Machemer R. Advanced retinopathy of prematurity. *Ophthalmology* 1990; **97**: 821–6.

48: Flecked Retina Syndromes

Anthony Moore

Many disorders may give rise to multiple white or yellow deposits scattered throughout the retina leading to the appearance of a flecked retina (Table 48.1). Most are inherited but some acquired disorders such as vitamin A deficiency and certain medications may cause a similar appearance. This chapter reviews the differential diagnosis of the flecked retina. Some of the disorders, for example Bietti's crystalline dystrophy, dominant drusen and those associated with systemic medication, are only rarely seen in childhood but are included for completeness.

Stargardt's disease (fundus flavimaculatus)

This disorder, which is inherited as an autosomal recessive trait, is characterized by the presence of multiple yellow–white 'fish-tail' flecks scattered throughout the posterior pole and peripheral retina. There is normally associated macular atrophy. The flecks (Fig. 48.1) lie at the level of the retinal pigment epithelium. Fluorescein angiography may show patchy hypofluorescence early in the disease due to masking of the underlying choroidal fluorescence by the white flecks. Later in the disease there

is usually widespread hyperfluorescence due to widespread retinal pigment epithelial atrophy. A dark choroid is a common angiographic finding (Bonnin *et al.* 1976; Uliss *et al.* 1980). The electroretinogram (ERG) and electro-oculogram (EOG) are usually normal until late in the disease but the pattern ERG is commonly reduced in amplitude at an early stage in those patients with macular atrophy. Although some affected individuals may show delayed dark adaptation on psychophysical testing (Fishman *et al.* 1991), patients rarely complain of night-blindness. This disorder is discussed in detail in Chapter 45.

Autosomal dominant flecked retina disorders

A number of families with a fundus appearance similar to Stargardt's disease but showing autosomal dominant inheritance have been reported (Bither & Berns 1988; Cibis *et al.* 1980; Mansour 1992; Stone *et al.* 1994; Zhang *et al.* 1994). Two families show linkage to two different chromosomal loci, 6q (Stone *et al.* 1994) and 13q (Zhang *et al.* 1994). Weleber *et al.* (1993) have reported a mutation of the peripherin/RDS gene in a family with a dominantly inherited retinal dystrophy with a very variable phenotype which includes a fundus appearance similar to fundus flavimaculatus. These disorders are discussed in Chapter 44.

Fundus albipunctatus

Fundus albipunctatus is an autosomal recessive form of stationary night-blindness in which there are multiple yellow–white dots deposited at the level of the pigment epithelium (Fig. 48.2). There is no associated retinal pigmentation or retinal pigment epithelial atrophy. Fluorescein angiography shows patchy hyperfluorescence which does not appear to correlate with the distribution of the deposits (Krill 1977; Margolis *et al.* 1987). Visual acuity and visual fields are normal. The ERG and EOG may be abnormal when tested routinely, but revert to normal on prolonged dark adaptation. Dark adaptation is markedly delayed but normal rod thresholds are reached eventually

Table 48.1 Flecked retina syndromes.

Inherited	Acquired
Stargardt's disease	Type II mesangiocapillary glomerulonephritis
Fundus albipunctatus	Drug deposition (rare in childhood)
Kandori's flecked retina syndrome	Tamoxifen
Retinitis punctata albescens	Methoxyfluorane
Benign familial flecked retina syndrome	Anaesthesia
Dominant drusen	Canxanthine
Bietti's crystalline dystrophy	Talc
Abetalipoproteinaemia	Vitamin A deficiency
Alport's syndrome	
Oxalosis	
Cystinosis	
Sjögren–Larsson syndrome	

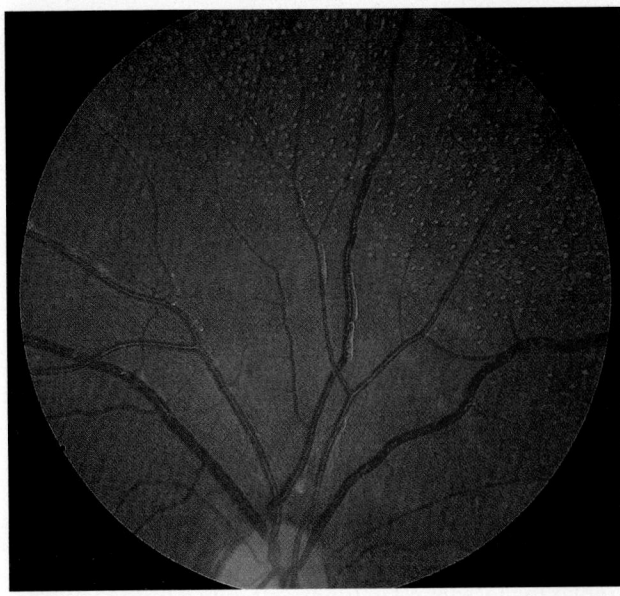

Fig. 48.2 Fundus albipunctatus. The child complained of night-blindness, but had normal acuity, colour vision and visual fields.

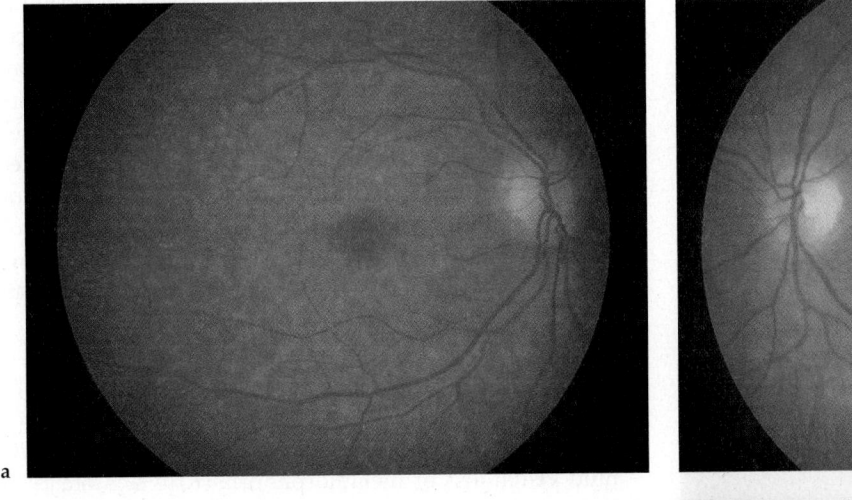

a

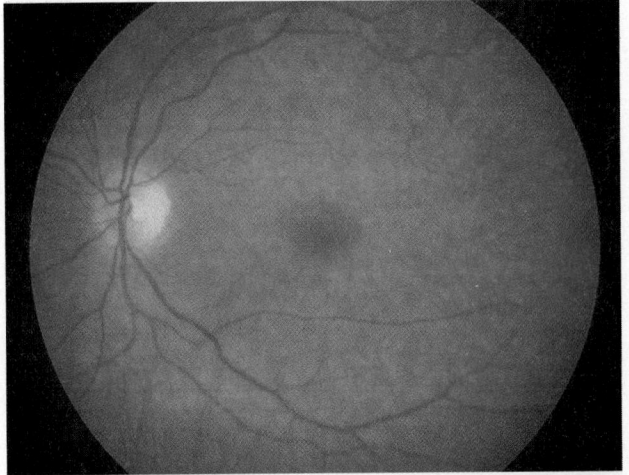

b

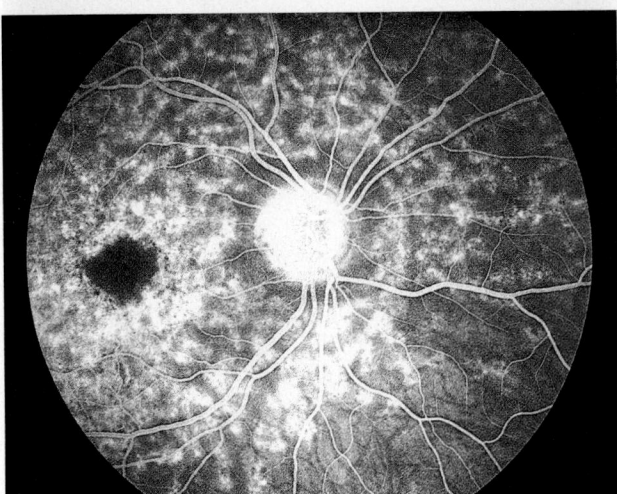

c

Fig. 48.1 (a, b) Fundus flavimaculatus showing multiple yellow–white 'fish-tail' flecks at the posterior pole. (c) Fluorescein angiogram of right eye showing patchy hyperfluorescence due to widespread pigment epithelial atrophy (Mr Anthony Moore's patient).

(Carr *et al.* 1974; Margolis *et al.* 1987). Fundus reflectometry shows that regeneration of rhodopsin is markedly slowed (Margolis *et al.* 1987).

The presence of night-blindness with normal visual acuity, visual fields and prolonged dark adaptation help to differentiate this disorder from other flecked retina syndromes.

Kandori's flecked retina syndrome

Kandori *et al.* (1972) have described a rare stationary dystrophy characterized by onset in childhood, mild slowing of dark adaptation, normal vision and visual fields and midperipheral deposition of yellow flecks. These flecks lie at the level of the retinal pigment epithelium and hyperfluoresce on fluorescein angiography. The macula is not involved. ERG and EOG are normal and the condition is non-progressive. The psychophysical findings are very similar to those found in fundus albipunctatus.

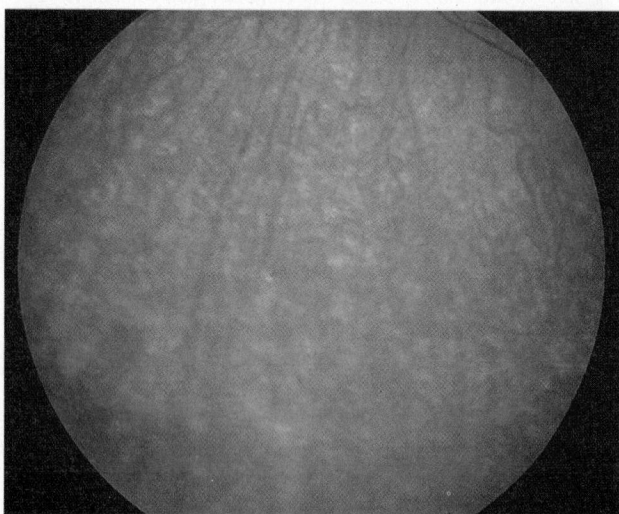
a

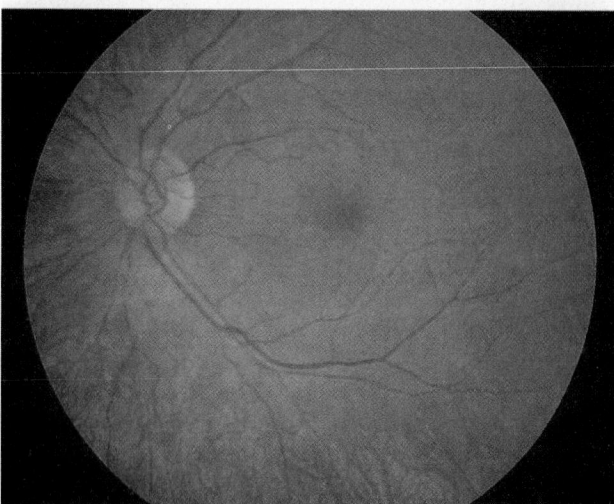
b

Fig. 48.3 (a, b) Flecked retinal appearance (retinitis punctata albescens) in a patient with retinitis pigmentosa.

Retinitis punctata albescens

Some patients with retinitis pigmentosa have multiple white dots scattered throughout the retina rather than the usual pigment deposition (Fig. 48.3). It is doubtful whether this represents a unique subtype of retinitis pigmentosa as it may be seen in patients from families where other family members have the classical fundus picture. Also the retinal appearance in patients with these white deposits may evolve to give rise to the more classical pigmentary retinopathy later in the disease. It may be distinguished from fundus albipunctatus by its progressive nature, visual field loss and ERG and EOG abnormalities.

Flecked retina associated with other retinal dystrophies

Some forms of cone dystrophy may show white deposits at the level of the retinal pigment epithelium in addition to retinal pigment epithelial atrophy at the macula. The early loss of colour vision and abnormal cone ERG help to distinguish this disorder from Stargardt's disease. Miyake *et al.* (1992) have described five unrelated patients who had a fundus appearance similar to fundus albipunctatus but in addition there was poor colour vision, a 'bull's eye' macular dystrophy and electrophysiological evidence of a cone dystrophy. A fundus appearance similar to fundus albipunctatus has also been described in juvenile X-linked retinoschisis (van Schooneveld & Miyake 1994). A flecked retina syndrome has also been described in association with a mutation of mitochondrial DNA at nucleotide position 15257 (Heher & Johns 1993). This is a primary mutation associated with Leber's hereditary optic neuropathy.

Dominant drusen

This dominant disorder usually presents in adult life with mild visual loss or metamorphopsia (Krill & Klein 1965; Deutman & Jansen 1970; Piguet *et al.* 1995). Multiple drusen are seen scattered throughout the fundus (Fig. 48.4) but are most numerous at the posterior pole (Deutman & Jansen 1970; Krill 1977). Fluorescein angiography shows widespread patchy hyperfluorescence which either corresponds to drusen or associated retinal pigment epithelial atrophy. The abnormal gene shows a marked variability of expression so that some affected family members have only a few drusen whilst others have multiple drusen and associated retinal pigment epithelial atrophy. The ERG is usually normal but the EOG may be abnormal late in the disease. Fundus abnormalities have been detected in early childhood (Deutman & Jansen 1970; Krill 1977) but since this disorder is asymptomatic in childhood it is rarely diagnosed in children and seldom gives rise to difficulties in diagnosis.

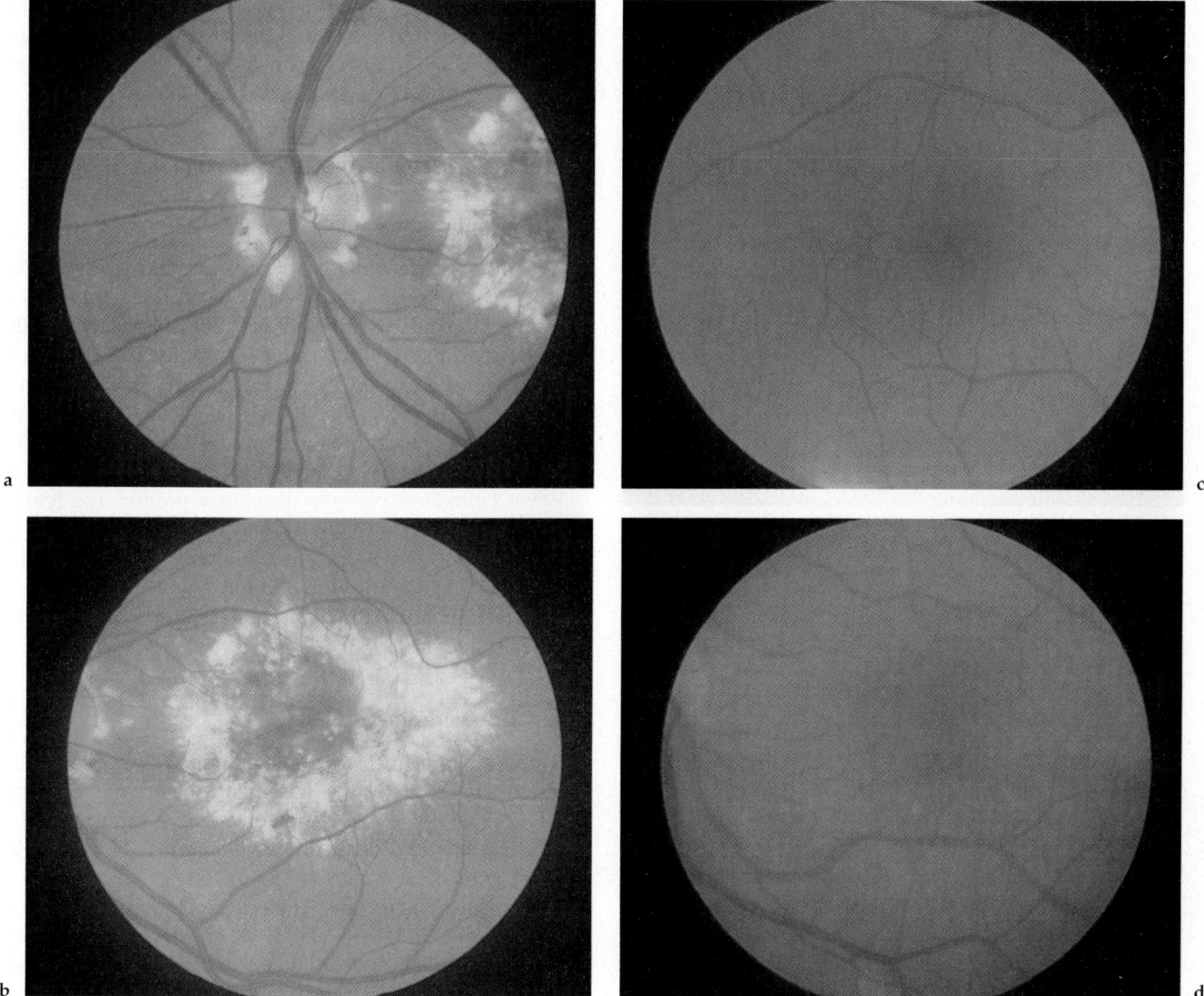

Fig. 48.4 (a, b) Dominant drusen. Dense multiple drusen at the posterior pole of the left eye. (c, d) The mother of the patient whose fundus is shown in a,b has much fewer drusen visible. Drusen increase with time but there is a marked variation in expression between family members (Mr Anthony Moore's patients).

Benign familial flecked retina syndrome

Aish and Dajani (1980) have described a flecked retina syndrome occurring in seven out of 10 siblings born to parents who were first cousins. The visual acuity, peripheral visual fields and dark adaptation were all normal. The flecks, first seen in infancy, were discrete white–yellow lesions at the level of the pigment epithelium and were scattered throughout the fundus. Fluorescein angiography showed multiple areas of hyperfluorescence which did not appear to correlate with the flecks. Although there are many similarities to fundus flavimaculatus the lack of

macular involvement in all of the seven affected siblings and the good visual prognosis suggest that this disorder may be different.

Bietti's crystalline retinal dystrophy

This rare autosomal recessive disorder is characterized by the deposition of small crystals in the peripheral cornea and the retina (Bietti 1937; Fujiwara *et al.* 1982; Wilson *et al.* 1989; Bernauer & Daicker 1992). A similar crystalline retinopathy has been reported in the absence of peripheral corneal changes (Grizzard *et al.* 1978). Patients usually become symptomatic in the third decade of life and this disorder has only recently been reported in childhood (Fujiwara *et al.* 1982).

The retinal crystals are more numerous at the posterior pole (Fig. 48.5) and there is generally widespread and progressive atrophy of the choriocapillaris and retinal pig-

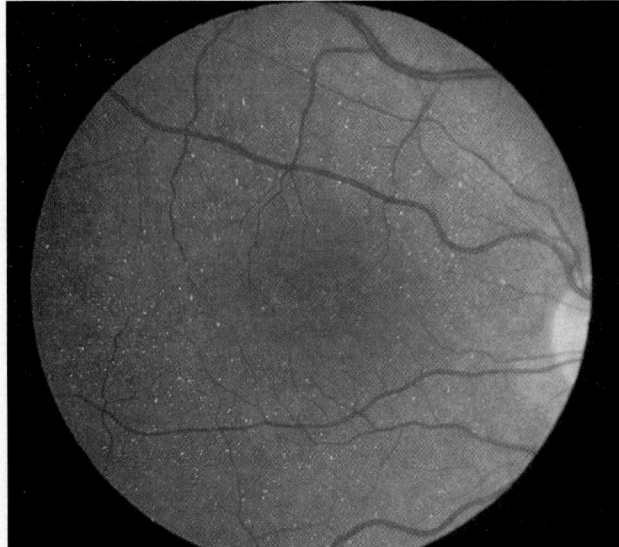

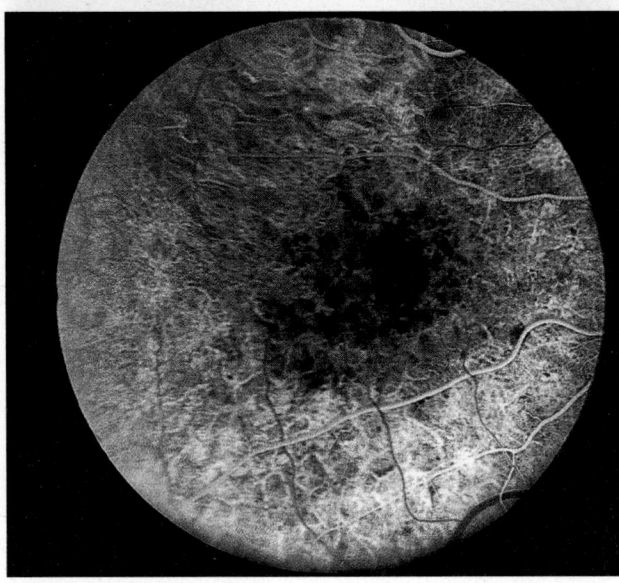

Fig. 48.5 (a, b) Bietti's crystalline retinal dystrophy. There are numerous crystals at the posterior pole and the fluorescein angiogram (b) shows choroidal and retinal pigment atrophy (Mr Anthony Moore's patient).

ment epithelium (Bernauer & Daicker 1992). There is usually progressive field loss and electrodiagnostic testing shows reduction of the EOG Arden ratio and decreased scotopic and photopic responses of the ERG (Wilson *et al.* 1989).

Histological examination of tissue from corneal and conjunctival biopsies from affected patients has shown lipid non-cholesterol inclusions, and similar inclusions are present in circulating lymphocytes, suggesting that there may be an underlying disorder of lipid metabolism (Wilson *et al.* 1989; Kaiser-Kupfer *et al.* 1995). Richards *et al.* (1991) have reported an autosomal dominant crystalline

retinal dystrophy which is very similar to Bietti's crystalline dystrophy; none of the children in this family who were examined showed any evidence of retinal abnormalities.

Flecked retina and systemic disease

Abetalipoproteinaemia

Abetalipoproteinaemia is a rare autosomal recessive disorder characterized by fat malabsorption, absence of serum beta lipoprotein, abnormally shaped red cells, ataxic neuropathy, and a retinal dystrophy. The disorder is thought to be caused by an abnormality of microsomal triglyceride transfer protein (MTP), which is thought to be important for lipoprotein assembly (Wetterau *et al.* 1992; Rader & Brewer 1993; Sharp *et al.* 1993; Shoulders *et al.* 1993). Untreated patients develop a progressive retinal dystrophy, often with white dots deposited at the level of the pigment epithelium. The ERG and EOG are usually abnormal. Treatment with vitamin A and E may prevent the development of the retinal abnormalities (Bishara *et al.* 1982; Runge *et al.* 1986).

Alport's syndrome

Alport's syndrome is an uncommon X-linked disorder caused by a defective basement membrane collagen (Flinter *et al.* 1988). It is characterized by chronic renal failure and bilateral sensorineural deafness (Gubler *et al.* 1981), and ocular abnormalities include cataract, lenticornus, corneal arcus and a fleck retinopathy (Polak & Hogewind 1977; Perrin *et al.* 1980; Zylberman *et al.* 1980; Govan 1983; Gelisken *et al.* 1988). Retinal changes are seen in the majority of patients (Govan *et al.* 1983; Gelisken *et al.* 1988) but may vary in their extent. The retinal flecks are pale yellow and multiple and lie at the level of the retinal pigment epithelium. They generally hyperfluoresce on fluorescein angiography (Govan *et al.* 1983; Gelisken *et al.* 1988). The visual fields are usually normal and although the ERG and EOG have been reported to be abnormal in some patients (Polak & Hogewind 1977; Zylberman *et al.* 1980) the majority show normal responses (Jeffrey *et al.* 1994).

Type 2 mesangiocapillary glomerulonephritis

Mesangiocapillary glomerulonephritis (MCGN) is a form of glomerulonephritis in which there is a characteristic electron dense deposit in the glomerular capillary basement membrane. A similar deposit may be demonstrated in Bruch's membrane in affected patients (Duvall-Young *et al.* 1989a,b). Patients with type 2 MCGN may show drusen-like deposits at the posterior pole which hyperfluoresce on fluorescein angiography (Duvall-

Young *et al.* 1989a). There are usually no symptoms and visual acuity remains good. The EOG may show a reduced light rise, but the ERG reponses are normal (O'Brien *et al.* 1993). It is likely that a similar pathological process affects both the glomerular capillaries and the choriocapillaris and Bruch's membrane. The fundus abnormalities have not yet been reported in children.

Primary hereditary oxalosis

Primary hereditary oxalosis is a rare autosomal recessive disorder of glyoxylate metabolism resulting in increased serum and urinary levels of oxalate. As serum levels rise calcium precipitates with oxalate to form insoluble crystals which are deposited in many different tissues. Renal involvement leads to chronic renal failure which is the major cause of death.

Two different types of the disorder have been described each with a specific enzyme deficiency. In type 1 hyperoxaluria there is a deficiency of the enzyme alpha-ketoglutarate:glyoxylate carboligase, and its absence leads to increased production of oxalic acid. In type 2 disease a deficiency of D-glyceric dehydrogenase results in increased synthesis of oxalic acid. The ocular abnormalities are confined to type 1 disease (Fielder *et al.* 1980; Zak & Buncic 1983; Meredith *et al.* 1984).

Hereditary oxalosis usually presents in early childhood and affected children may show multiple yellow crystals deposited at the level of the retinal pigment epithelium. The deposits are more numerous at the posterior pole (Fig. 48.6) and with time hyperplasia of the retinal pigment epithelium may develop giving rise to a ring of hyperpigmentation around the macula (Zak & Buncic 1983; Meredith *et al.* 1984). Fluorescein angiography in one case showed hypofluorescence related to the pigmentation and peripheral areas of ring-shaped hyperfluorescence surrounding a central area of hypofluorescence — presumably related to the crystal deposition (Meredith *et al.* 1984). Histopathological examination of involved eyes have shown deposition of oxalate in the retinal pigment epithelium (Fielder *et al.* 1980; Meredith *et al.* 1984).

Oxalate crystal deposition may also occur in secondary hyperoxaluria resulting from methoxyfluorane anaesthesia (Bullock & Albert 1975), when a similar flecked retinopathy is seen.

Sjögren–Larsson syndrome

The Sjögren–Larsson syndrome (SLS) is a rare autosomal recessive disorder characterized by mental retardation, spastic diplegia and congenital ichthyosis (Sjögren & Larsson 1957). Affected patients have impaired fatty acid oxidation caused by reduced activity of fatty aldehyde dehydrogenase (Rizzo 1993). The gene for SLS has recent-

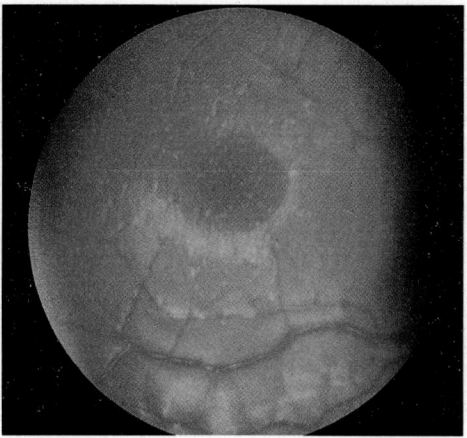

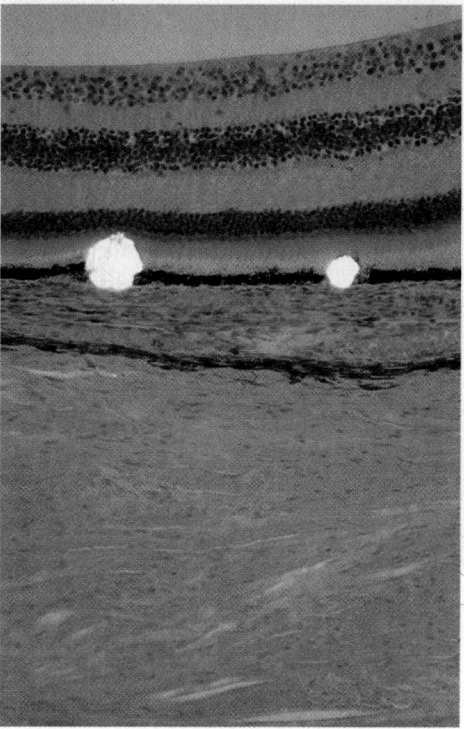

Fig. 48.6 Oxalosis type 1. Crystal deposition at the level of the retinal pigment epithelium (Professor A. Fielder's patient).

ly been mapped to chromosome 17 (Pigg *et al.* 1994). Fundus examination shows glistening yellow dots (Fig. 48.7) in the macular and paramacular area (Gilbert *et al.* 1968; Jagell *et al.* 1980). Fluorescein angiography shows patchy hyperfluorescence at the macula due to pigment epithelial atrophy (Gilbert *et al.* 1968). ERG and EOG are normal (Gilbert *et al.* 1968; Jagell 1980).

Histopathological examination of the eyes from one case showed increased lipofuscin levels in the pigment epithelium in the macular area but no evidence of any other retinal or subretinal deposits (Nillson & Jagell 1987).

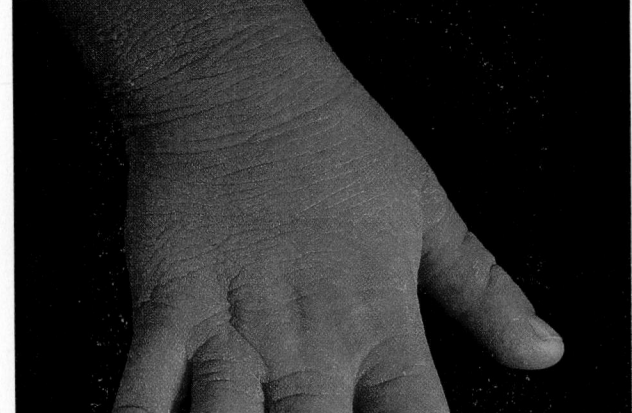

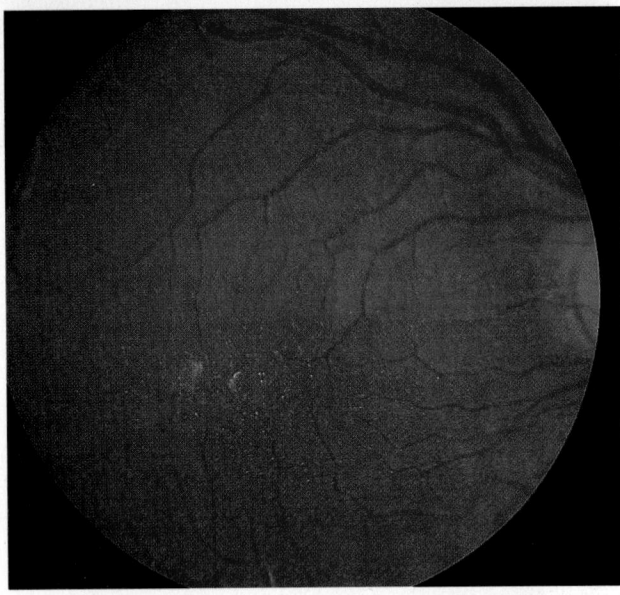

Fig. 48.7 (a, b) Sjögren–Larsson syndrome. Ichthyosis and macular crystal deposition.

Flecked retina syndrome and ring chromosome 17

There have been three reports (Oho *et al.* 1974; Charles *et al.* 1991; Gass 1994) of a fleck retinopathy (Fig. 48.8) occurring in mentally retarded children with a ring chromosome 17. Other associated features include seizures, short stature and café-au-lait spots. The yellow deposits resemble drusen but do not hyperfluoresce on angiography (Charles *et al.* 1991).

Breadcrumb-flecked retina syndrome

Protzko *et al.* (1992) have described a unique case of a young girl with developmental delay, mental subnormality and seizures who was found, on routine examination, to have a bilateral flecked retinopathy. The flecks were bilateral, multiple and were seen to be located in the deep retina anterior to the retinal pigment epithelium. They

were yellow–white in colour and the authors describe them as having the appearance of breadcrumbs. ERG and fluorescein angiography were normal.

Crystalline retinopathies

Deposits of crystals or other substances in the retina which give rise to a similar fundus appearance may occur in a number of different disorders (see Table 48.1). Oxalate crystal deposition may occur in primary oxalosis (Fielder *et al.* 1980; Zak & Buncic 1983; Meredith *et al.* 1984) or occur in association with methoxyfluorane anaesthesia (Bullock & Albert 1975), when a similar flecked retinopathy is seen. Crystalline deposition has also been reported in cystinosis (Read *et al.* 1973), SLS (Gilbert *et al.* 1968), autosomal

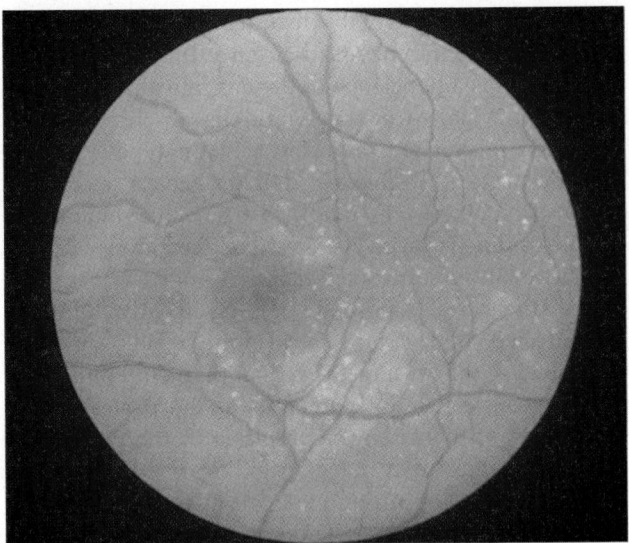

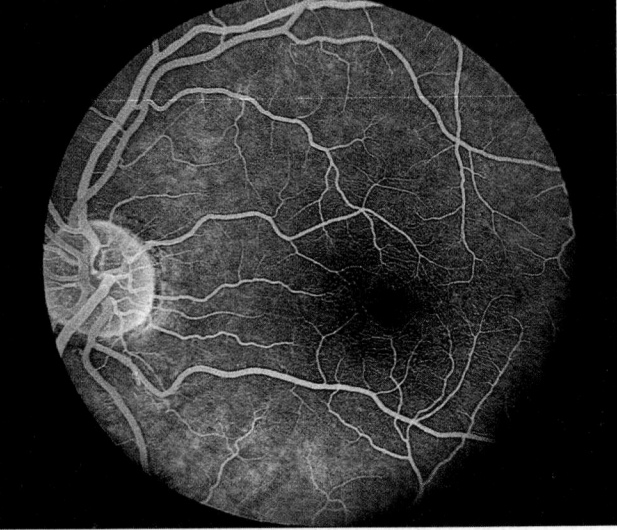

Fig. 48.8 (a, b) Flecked retina and ring chromosome 17. Posterior polar drusen-like flecks with minimal changes on fluorescein angiography (see Charles *et al.* 1991).

dominant crystalline retinopathy (Richards *et al.* 1991) and in Bietti's crystalline dystrophy (Grizzard *et al.* 1978). Retinal accumulation of certain systemic medications such as tamoxifen (Kaiser-Kupfer & Lippman 1978; Kaiser-Kupfer *et al.* 1981; McKeown *et al.* 1981) and canxanthine (Daicker *et al.* 1985) may give rise to a similar retinopathy but are unlikely to be seen in childhood. Crystalline retinal deposits may also occur in talc retinopathy, an uncommon condition affecting intravenous drug abusers (O'Brien & Schroedl 1991).

Vitamin A deficiency

Night-blindness is an early symptom of vitamin A deficiency. Chronic deficiency may lead to changes in the retinal appearance, often with grey–white flecks at the level of the retinal pigment epithelium. At this stage there is usually peripheral field loss and a reduced photopic and scotopic ERG. Dark adaptation is abnormal with an elevated final threshold and often a delayed recovery of sensitivity after exposure to light (Walt *et al.* 1984). The fleck retinopathy may disappear and visual function improve after treatment with vitamin A (Bor & Fells 1971; Walt *et al.* 1984). Nutritional deficiency is the most common cause of vitamin A deficiency worldwide, but is rarely the cause in Europe and North America. It may, however, be seen in patients with liver disease, for example in cystic fibrosis or primary biliary cirrhosis, or in malabsorption syndromes (Bor & Fells 1971; Walt *et al.* 1984).

References

Aish SFS, Dajani B. Benign familial fleck retina. *Br J Ophthalmol* 1980; **64**: 652–9.

Bernauer W, Daicker B. Bietti's corneal-retinal dystrophy. A 16-year progression. *Retina* 1992; **12**: 18–20.

Bietti G. Ueber familiares Vorkommen von Retinitis pigmentosa albescens (verbinden mit Dystrophia marginalis crystillinea corneae) Glizern des Glaskverpers und anderen degenerativen Augenveranderungen. *Klin Monatsbl Augenkeilde* 1937; **99**: 737–56.

Bishara S, Merin S, Cooper M *et al.* Combined vitamin A and E therapy prevents retina electrophysiological deterioration in abetalipoproteinemia. *Br J Ophthalmol* 1982; **66**: 767–70.

Bither PP, Berns EA. Dominant inheritance of Stargardt's disease. *J Am Optom Assoc* 1988; **59** :112–17.

Bonnin P, Passet M, Tricolaire-Cotten M. Le signe du silence choroidien dans les degenerescences tapeto-retienes posterieures. *Doc Ophthalmol Proc Ser* 1976; **9**: 461–3.

Bor F, Fells P. Reversal of the complications of self induced vitamin A deficiency. *Br J Ophthalmol* 1971; **55**: 210–14.

Bullock JD, Albert DM. Flecked retina appearance secondary to oxalate crystals frcom methoxyfluorane anesthesia. *Arch Ophthalmol* 1975; **93**: 26–31.

Carr RE, Ripps H, Siegel DM. Visual pigment kinetics and adaptation in fundus albipunctatus. *Doc Ophthalmol* 1974; **4**: 193–204.

Charles SJ, Moore AT, Dyson HM, Willat L. Flecked retina associated with ring chromosome. *Br J Ophthalmol* 1991; **75**: 125–7.

Cibis GN, Meorey M, Harris DJ. Dominantly inherited macular dystrophy with flecks (Stargardt). *Arch Ophthalmol* 1980; **98**: 1785–9.

Daicker B, Schiedt K, Adnet JJ, Bermond P. Canthaxanthine retinopathy. An investigation by light and electron microscopy and physiochemical analysis. *Graefe's Arch Klin Exp Ophthalmol* 1985; **225**: 189–201.

Deutman AF, Jansen LM. Dominantly inherited drusen of Bruch's membrane. *Br J Ophthalmol* 1970; **54**: 373–82.

Duvall-Young J, Short CD, Raines MF *et al.* Fundus changes in mesangiocapillary glomerulonephritis type II. Clinical and fluorescein angiographic findings. *Br J Ophthalmol* 1989a; **73**: 900–6.

Duvall-Young J, MacDonald MK, McKecknie NM. Fundus changes in (type 2) mesangiocapillary glomerulonephritis simulating drusen: a histopathological report. *Br J Ophthalmol* 1989b; **73**: 297–302.

Fielder AR, Garner A, Chambers TL. Ophthalmic manifestations of primary oxalosis. *Br J Ophthalmol* 1980; **64**: 782–8.

Fishman GA, Farbman JS, Alexander KR. Delayed rod dark adaption in patients with Stargardt's disease. *Ophthalmology* 1991; **98**: 957–62.

Flinter FA, Cameron JS, Chantler C *et al.* Genetics of classic Alport's syndrome. *Lancet* 1988; **ii**: 1005–7.

Fujiwara H, Nishikion T, Kano M. Two cases of crystalline retinopathy. *Jpn J Ophthalmol* 1982; **36**: 301–6.

Gass JDM. Flecked retina associated with café-au-lait spots, microcephaly, epilepsy, short stature and ring 17 chromosome. *Arch Ophthalmol* 1994; **112**: 738–9.

Gelisken O, Hendrikse F, Schroeder CH, Burden JMH. Retinal abnormalities in Alport's syndrome. *Acta Ophthalmol* 1988; **66**: 713–17.

Gilbert WR, Jr, Smith JL, Nyhan WL. The Sjögren–Larsson syndrome. *Arch Ophthalmol* 1968; **80**: 308–16.

Govan JA. Ocular manifestations of Alport's syndrome. *Br J Ophthalmol* 1983; **67**: 493–503.

Grizzard WS, Deutman AF, Nijhuis F *et al.* Crystalline retinopathy. *Am J Ophthalmol* 1978; **86**: 81–8.

Gubler M, Levy M, Brcoyer M *et al.* Alport's syndrome: a report of 58 cases and a review of the literature. *Am J Med* 1981; **70**: 493–505.

Heher KL, Johns DR. A maculopathy associated with the 15257 mitochondrial DNA mutation. *Arch Ophthalmol* 1993; **111**: 1495–9.

Jagell S, Polland W, Sandgren O. Specific changes in the fundus typical for the Sjogren–Larsson syndrome. *Acta Ophthalmol (Kbh)* 1980; **58**: 321–30.

Jeffrey BG, Jacobs MSG, Barratt TM, Taylor D, Kriss A. An electrophysiological study on children and young adults with Alport's syndrome. *Br J Ophthalmol* 1994; **78**: 44–8.

Kaiser-Kupfer MI, Chan C, Markello T *et al.* Clinical biochemical and pathologic correlations in Bietti's crystalline dystrophy. *Am J Ophthalmol* 1994; **118**: 569–82.

Kaiser-Kupfer MI, Kuppfer C, Rodrigues MM. Tamoxifen retinopathy. A clinico-pathological report. *Ophthalmology* 1981; **88**: 89–93.

Kaiser-Kupfer MI, Lippman ME. Tamoxifen retinopathy. *Cancer Treatment Rep* 1978; **62**: 315–20.

Kandori F, Tamai A, Kurimoto S, Fukunaga K. Fleck retina. *Am J Ophthalmol* 1972; **73**: 673–85.

Krill AE. Flecked retina diseases. In: Krill AE, ed. *Hereditary Retinal and Choroidal Diseases*, Vol. 2. Hagerstown: Harper & Row, 1977: 739–823.

Krill AE, Klein BA. Flecked retina syndrome. *Arch Ophthalmol* 1965; **74**: 496–508.

McKeown CA, Schwartz M, Blau J *et al.* Tamoxifen retinopathy. *Br J Ophthalmol* 1981; **65**: 177–9.

Mansour AM. Long-term follow-up of dominant macular dystrophy with flecks (Stargardt). *Ophthalmologica* 1992; **205**: 138–43.

Margolis S, Siegel IM, Ripps H. Variable expressivity in fundus albipunctatus. *Ophthalmology* 1987; **94**: 1416–22.

Meredith TA, Wright JD, Gammon JA *et al.* Ocular involvement in primary hyperoxaluria. *Arch Ophthalmol* 1984; **102**: 584–7.

Miyake Y, Shiroyama N, Sugita S *et al.* Fundus albipunctatus associated with cone dystrophy. *Br J Ophthalmol* 1992; **76**: 375–9.

Nillson SE, Jagell S. Lipofuscin and melanin content of the retinal pigment epithelium in a case of Sjögren–Larsson syndrome. *Br J Ophthalmol* 1987; **71**: 224–7.

O'Brien CO, Duvall-Young J, Brown M *et al.* Electrophysiology of type II mesangiocapillary glomerulonephritis with associated fundus abnormalities. *Br J Ophthalmol* 1993; **77**: 778–80.

O'Brien RJ, Schroedl BL. Talc retinopathy. *Optometry Vis Sci* 1991; **68**: 54–7.

Oho K, Suzuki Y, Fuji I *et al.* A case of ring chromosome E17 46XX.r(17) (p13–q25). *Jpn J Hum Genet* 1974; **19**: 235–42.

Perrin D, Jungers P, Grunfeld JP *et al.* Perimacular changes in Alport's syndrome. *Clin Nephrol* 1980; **23**: 163–7.

Peterson RA, Peterson VS, Rubb RA. Vitamin A deficiency with xerophthalmia and night blindness in cystic fibrosis. *Am J Dis Child* 1968; **116**: 662–5.

Pigg M, Jagell S, Weissenback J *et al.* The Sjögren–Larsson gene is close to D175805 as determined by linkage analysis and allelic association. *Nature Genet* 1994; **8**: 361–4.

Piguet B, Haimovici R, Bird AC. Dominantly inherited drusen represent more than one disorder: a historical review. *Eye* 1995; **9**: 34–41.

Polak BCP, Hogewind BL. Macular lesions in Alport's syndrome. *Am J Ophthalmol* 1977; **84**: 532–5.

Protzko EE, Schatz H, Raymond W *et al.* Breadcrumb-flecked retinopathy. *Retina* 1992; **12**: 21–3.

Rader DJ, Brewer HB. Abetalipoproteinaemia. New insights into lipoprotein assembly and vitamin E metabolism from a rare genetic disease. *J Am Med Assoc* 1993; **270**: 865–9.

Read J, Goldberg MF, Fishman G *et al.* Nephropathic cystinosis. *Am J Ophthalmol* 1973; **76**: 791–6.

Richards B, Brodstein DE, Nussbaum JJ *et al.* Autosomal dominant crystalline dystrophy. *Ophthalmology* 1991; **98**: 658–65.

Rizzo WB. Sjögren–Larsson syndrome. *Semin Dermatol* 1993; **12**: 210–18.

Runge P, Muller DPR, McAllister J *et al.* Oral vitamin E supplements can prevent the retinopathy of abetalipoproteinemia. *Br J Ophthalmol* 1986; **70**: 166–73.

Sharp D, Blinderman L, Combs K *et al.* Cloning and gene defects in microsomal triglyceride transfer protein associated with abetalipoproteinemia. *Nature* 1993; **365**: 65–9.

Shoulders CC, Brett DJ, Bayliss JD *et al.* Abetalipoproteinemia is caused by defects of the gene encoding the 97 kDa subunit of a microsomal triglyceride transfer protein. *Hum Mol Genet* 1993; **2**: 2109–16.

Sjögren T, Larsson T. Oligophrenia in combination with congenital ichthyosis and spastic disorders. *Acta Psychiatr Scand* 1957; **32**: 1–113.

Stone EM, Nichols BE, Kimura AE *et al.* Clinical features of a Stargardt-like dominant progressive macular dystrophy with genetic linkage to chromosome 6q. *Arch Ophthalmol* 1994; **112**: 765–72.

Uliss A, Moore AT, Bird AC. The dark choroid in posterior retinal dystrophies. *Ophthalmology* 1987; **94**: 1423–8.

van Schooneveld M, Miyake Y. Fundus albipunctatus-like lesions in juvenile retinoschisis. *Br J Ophthalmol* 1994; **78**: 659–61.

Walt RP, Kemp CM, Lyness L *et al.* Vitamin A treatment for nightblindness in primary biliary cirrhosis. *Br Med J* 1984; **288**: 1031–2.

Weleber RG, Carr RE, Murphey WH *et al.* Phenotypic variation including retinitis pigmentosa, pattern dystrophy and fundus flavimaculatus in a single family with a deletion of codon 153 or 154 of the peripherin/RDS gene. *Arch Ophthalmol* 1993; **111**: 1531–42.

Wetterau JR, Aggerbeck LP, Bouma M-E *et al.* Absence of microsomal triglyceride transfer protein in individuals with abetalipoproteinemia. *Science* 1992; **258**: 999–1001.

Wilson DJ, Weleber RG, Klein ML *et al.* Bietti's crystalline dystrophy. A clinico-pathological correlative study. *Arch Ophthalmol* 1989; **107**: 213–221.

Zak TA, Buncic R. Primary hereditary oxalosis retinopathy. *Arch Ophthalmol* 1983; **101**: 78–80.

Zhang K, Bither PP, Park R *et al.* A dominant Stargardt's macular dystrophy locus maps to chromosome 13q34. *Arch Ophthalmol* 1994; **112**: 759–64.

Zylberman R, Silverstone BZ, Brandes E *et al.* Retinal lesions in Alport's syndrome. *J Pediatr Ophthalmol* 1980; **17**: 255–60.

49: Miscellaneous Retinal Disorders

Andrew Webster

Acquired retinal vascular disorders

Diabetic retinopathy

Diabetic retinopathy is uncommon in children with insulin-dependent diabetes mellitus (IDDM) but can occur during and after puberty, with the percentage glycosylated haemoglobin being an important risk factor. In a cohort of 194 diabetic Finnish children below the age of 17 years, background retinopathy was observed in 10.8% of cases. No cases showed pre-proliferative or proliferative disease and no retinopathy was observed in the subset of 90 pre-pubescent children (Falck *et al.* 1993). This is in agreement with previous studies (Burger *et al.* 1986; Weber *et al.* 1986). However, one study did detect background diabetic retinopathy in four pre-pubescent children (Murphy *et al.* 1990). From a practical point of view regular screening for treatable disease may be safely confined to the post-pubertal age group and fortunately retinopathy severe enough to require treatment is rare in childhood.

Although the risk of developing diabetic retinopathy increases with increasing duration of disease, years of diabetes before puberty are much less influential than those after the onset of puberty. One large epidemiological study showed there was no significant difference in the prevalence of both retinopathy and nephropathy for a given duration of post-pubertal diabetes in children of pre-pubertal compared to post-pubertal onset of disease. This suggested that pre-pubertal diabetes experience has minimal influence on the development of these complications (Kostraba *et al.* 1989). However, a further large study, in which the determination of the age of onset of retinopathy was more accurate, did show a small yet significant increase in the prevalence of retinopathy in children with pre-pubertal onset diabetes compared with those with post-pubertal onset for a given duration of post-pubertal diabetes (McNally *et al.* 1993).

The diabetes control and complications trial (DCCT) has demonstrated that intensive treatment of IDDM delays the onset and slows the progression of retinopathy, nephropathy and neuropathy in a cohort of young adults (DCCT Research Group 1993). This is also true when the subset of adolescent diabetics is analysed separately (DCCT Research Group 1994). However, extrapolation of this observation to the diabetic pre-pubescent child should be made with caution. Significant hypoglycaemia, when tighter control is attempted, would be more likely to occur in such younger children whose exercise and eating habits are erratic. Such risks may not be justified particularly as the effect of pre-pubescent diabetes on long-term prognosis is relatively small (Geffner 1994).

Sickle cell disease

Sickle cell disease is a group of conditions in which the pathogenesis is attributed to abnormal sickle-shaped red blood cells apparent on examination of a blood film as first described by Hendrick (1910). Such cells are thought to cause an increase in blood viscosity and fragility resulting in haemolytic anaemia and vessel occlusion in susceptible tissues. The discovery of the molecular basis for the disease was the first demonstration of a specific molecular defect causing a clinical entity and is a milestone in molecular biology (Pauling 1949; Ingram 1956). It is known that a number of mutant beta-globin genes underlie the disease including beta^s (Glu 6 Val), beta^c (Glu 6 Lys) and beta^{Thal} (numerous mutations; Thein 1993) (Sergeant 1985). Ocular abnormalities may be seen in patients who are homozygotes or mixed heterozygotes of such genes: sickle cell disease, sickle cell haemoglobin C disease, sickle cell beta-thalassaemia and rarely also in sickle cell trait (Welch & Goldberg 1966).

A number of ocular abnormalities can occur in children and young adults with sickle cell disease and include conjunctival microvascular abnormalities (Paton 1961, 1962), iris atrophy, vitreous haemorrhage, transient red dots on the optic disc (Goldbaum 1978b), macular branch arteriolar occlusions and subsequent retinal depressions (Knapp 1972; Goldbaum 1978a), angioid streaks (Nagpal *et al.* 1976; Hamilton *et al.* 1981) and macular holes (Raichand 1978). Intraretinal haemorrhages ('salmon patch' haemorrhages) can occur at the junction of perfused and non-perfused retina and may resolve forming schitic retinal cavities and refractile bodies (Asdourian *et al.* 1975). Dark chorioretinal scars (curiously known as 'sun-burst patches') occur in sickle cell disease, sickle cell haemoglobin C disease and rarely sickle cell trait (Welch & Goldberg 1966) and may be the sequel to such haemorrhages (Asdourian *et al.* 1975). Retinal venous tortuosity is reported to be more common in sickle cell disease and sickle cell haemoglobin C disease compared to normals (Welch & Goldberg 1966) but is a difficult sign to define accurately.

Traumatic hyphaema may present particular clinical difficulties in children who either have sickle cell disease or sickle cell trait (Goldberg 1979). Goldberg reported four patients (including two children) with persistently raised intraocular pressure after hyphaema (three sickle cell trait, one sickle cell haemoglobin C disease). He showed that there was a greater proportion of sickled cells in the anterior chamber compared with venous blood and proposed that such cells might be more likely to obstruct trabecular aqueous outflow. Michelson *et al.* (1972) reported two young sickle cell trait individuals who suffered central retinal artery occlusion after a short period of raised intraocular pressure, and Acacio and Goldberg (1973) reported central retinal artery occlusion in a child with sickle cell disease. Therefore in sickle cell disease and sickle cell trait, traumatic hyphaema is more likely to be complicated by glaucoma and there is an increased risk of retinal vascular occlusions. The glaucoma may respond poorly to conventional treatment and early paracentesis may be required to prevent complications.

Proliferative sickle cell retinopathy (PSR) can cause visual morbidity in sickle cell patients and occurs following vascular occlusion and arteriovenous shunt formation as described and classified by Goldberg (1971). Enigmatically, although sickle cell disease is much more severe in its systemic manifestations than sickle cell haemoglobin C disease, the reverse is the case for PSR in that the prevalence and severity of PSR is much higher in sickle cell haemoglobin C disease (Welch & Goldberg 1966; Condon & Sergeant 1972; Fox *et al.* 1991). The neovascular lesions in PSR often resemble 'sea fans' and occur at the junction of vascular and avascular retina. Such lesions can cause vitreous haemorrhage, retinal traction and retinal detachment and the consequent visual morbidity is difficult to treat successfully. In a longitudinal natural history study many PSR lesions spontaneously regressed and new lesions were rare after 40 years of age (Fox *et al.* 1991). The first stage of sickle cell retinopathy, peripheral vascular closure (Goldberg 1971), begins at an early age and in one study (Talbot *et al.* 1988) was present in 50% of children with sickle cell disease and sickle cell haemoglobin C disease at the age of 6 years, and in 90% by age 12 years. Although vessel closure may be extensive in older children, PSR lesions are rare in childhood (Talbot *et al.* 1988). A recent study suggests that both sickle cell disease and the development of PSR lesions may be associated with an irregular pattern of retinal capillaries at the anterior edge of vascular retina (Penman *et al.* 1994) and this may indicate which patients are most in need of careful follow-up. Although PSR lesions rarely develop before adolescence, follow-up of children into adolescence is important particularly in view of the marginal benefit of both feeder vessel (Jacobson *et al.* 1991) and local scatter laser photocoagulation (Farber *et al.* 1991) in two recent controlled trials. Although of benefit, such treatment does not prevent new PSR lesions occurring. It remains to be seen whether 360° scatter photocoagulation would be useful in this regard.

Radiation retinopathy and bone marrow transplant retinopathy

Radiation retinopathy is most commonly seen in adults who have received radiotherapy for ocular, adnexal, nasopharyngeal or paranasal sinus tumours but may occur in children treated for retinoblastoma or orbital tumours (MacFaul & Bedford 1970; Brown *et al.* 1982; Amoaku & Archer 1990a; Parsons *et al.* 1994). It may complicate both focal plaque and external beam therapy. The first reports of retinopathy occurring following ocular irradiation were in children treated with implantation of radon seeds for 'glioma retinae' (retinoblastoma) by Moore and Stallard in the 1930s (Stallard 1933, 1936; Moore 1935).

Damage occurs predominantly to the retinal vasculature. Early fundal changes include capillary closure, telangiectasia and microaneurysms particularly within the macular area. Later changes include retinal haemorrhages, cotton-wool spots, exudates and retinal oedema. Visual impairment is variable but can be severe and complete. Neovascularization of the retina or iris and subsequent vitreous haemorrhage or rubeotic glaucoma can also occur rarely (Brown *et al.* 1982; Amoaku & Archer 1990a). The earliest retinal changes are well delineated by fluorescein angiography (Hayreh 1970; Amoaku & Archer 1990b). The histology has been studied in monkeys (Irvine & Wood 1987), rats (Archer *et al.* 1991) and human eyes (Archer *et al.* 1991). The earliest changes appear to be endothelial loss, with relative sparing of pericytes (the opposite to the microscopic changes of diabetic retinopathy), capillary wall thickening, microaneurysm formation and vessel occlusion. Retinopathy does not usually appear until after at least 1 year following irradiation and often many years can elapse before it is evident. The reason for this latent period is not clear. It may be due to the slow turnover of endothelial cells in response to neighbouring endothelial cell death. Such dividing cells, having incurred DNA damage during previous irradiation, would then die in mitosis (Archer 1993). Latent periods vary between different studies, with means of 18.7 months (Brown *et al.* 1982), 2.5 years (Parsons *et al.* 1994) and 4.7 years (Amoaku & Archer 1990a) for external radiation.

The probability of developing retinopathy increases with higher total radiation dose to the retina, hypofractionation of doses in external beam therapy, diabetes (Viebahn *et al.* 1991; Parsons *et al.* 1994) and concomitant chemotherapy. The threshold dose is unknown, although retinopathy is thought to be unlikely after an external dose to the retina of less than 2500 cGy in fractions of less than 200 cGy (Archer 1993). In the treatment of children for retinoblastoma, one study documented a maculopathy occurring in seven of 18 eyes with posteriorly located tumours treated by plaque therapy (Ehlers & Kaae 1987) and an ischaemic retinopathy in 10 of 44 eyes with retinoblastoma treated by external beam irradiation (Coucke *et al.* 1993). This latter study suggested that the development of retinopathy was related to high total dose and hypofractionation. More recently, lower total doses and increased fractionation mean that ischaemic retinopathy may now be an uncommon complication of treatment of retinoblastoma with external irradiation (Hungerford *et al.* 1995; Toma *et al.* 1995). Choroidal new vessels have been reported in two cases many years after local radon seed implantation for retinoblastoma (Archer *et al.* 1993).

A similar retinopathy can occur in patients following bone marrow transplantation and is of importance in children treated in this way for acute leukaemias. Cotton-wool spots occurring in bone marrow transplant recipients were first described in 1983 (Gratwohl *et al.* 1983; Gloor *et al.* 1985). The retinopathy associated with bone marrow transplantation is morphologically similar to radiation retinopathy, showing capillary drop-out, cotton-wool spots and retinal haemorrhages (Fig. 49.1) although telangiectasis may be less of a feature. There are a number of proposed factors which may contribute to retinal ischaemia in these patients; these factors include hyperviscosity secondary to leukaemia itself (Rosenthal 1983), chemotherapy (Lopez *et al.* 1991), total body irradiation (Bernauer *et al.* 1991; Lopez *et al.* 1991), graft-versus-host disease (Coskucan *et al.* 1994) and graft-versus-host disease prophylaxis treatment (Bernauer *et al.* 1991; Webster *et al.* 1995). A large prospective study (Bernauer *et al.* 1991) reported the development of such an

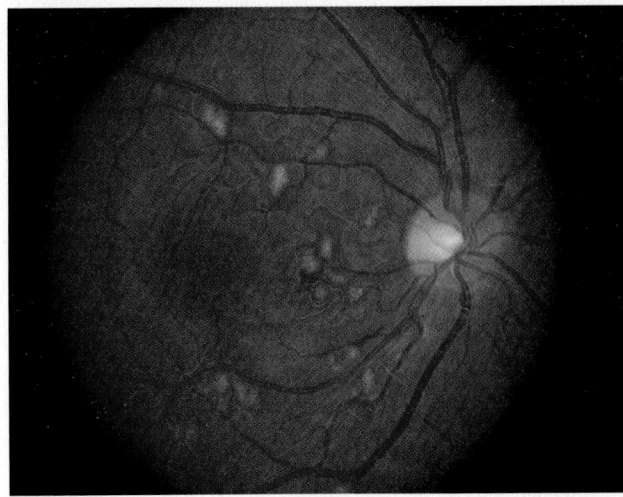

Fig. 49.1 Bone marrow transplant retinopathy showing multiple cotton-wool spots and a small perifoveal haemorrhage.

ischaemic retinopathy in 13 of 127 patients within 6 months of bone marrow transplant. Significantly, the retinopathy was only seen in patients receiving both total body irradiation (for malignancies) and cyclosporin A (following allografts) suggesting that these two factors were important.

Although bone marrow transplant retinopathy differs from radiation retinopathy in its early onset and low radiation dose (if any) the early histological changes may be similar (Webster *et al.* 1995). Other posterior segment complications of bone marrow transplantation include retinal and vitreous haemorrhage secondary to thrombocytopenia and opportunistic infections such as *Candida* uveitis and *Toxoplasma*, cytomegalovirus and herpetic retinitis (Coskucan *et al.* 1994).

Retinal vasculitis

Retinal vasculitis is characterized by inflammatory changes in retinal vessels with leakage, sheathing, irregularity of vessel diameter, haemorrhages and exudates. Retinal cotton-wool spots (Fig. 49.2) are often seen and cotton-wool spots and neovascularization represent the effects of ischaemia. There are almost invariably signs of posterior uveitis and vitritis. Retinal vasculitis occurs in the following.

1 Idiopathic retinal vasculitis is rare in childhood.
2 Retinal vasculitis with haemorrhages (Eale's disease), usually occurs in young men, but may occasionally be encountered in older children. The peripheral small vessels are closed and there is neovascularization. It has an unclear association with tuberculosis.
3 Systemic lupus erythematosus, polymyositis and other collagenoses.
4 Sarcoidosis.

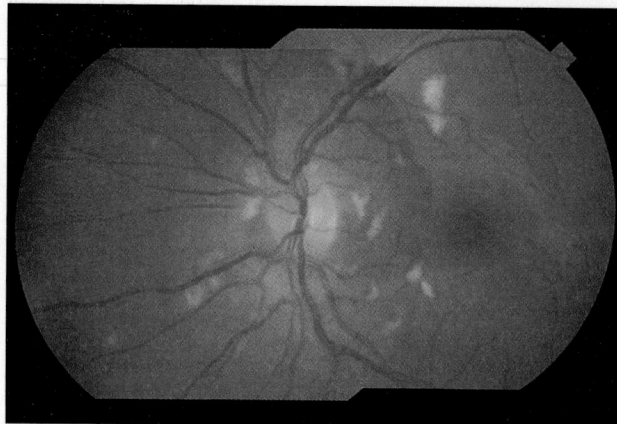

Fig. 49.2 Retinal vasculitis in systemic lupus erythematosus showing multiple cotton-wool spots.

5 Behçet's disease.
6 Human immunodeficiency virus (HIV) and acquired immunodeficiency syndrome (AIDS) (see Chapter 14).

Frosted branch periphlebitis

Frosted branch periphlebitis or angiitis is a rare retinal disorder of unknown aetiology which can affect children and young adults. It presents in previously healthy patients with sudden visual loss, which is often bilateral, and redness of the eye(s). Signs include conjunctival injection, anterior uveitis, vitreous cells, sheathing of the retinal vasculature, particularly the retinal veins, retinal exudates and haemorrhage, macular oedema and exudative macular detachment (see Fig. 49.3). Presenting visual acuity is often counting fingers but can be more subtly reduced (Browning 1992). Prognosis is good and vision usually returns to near normal after 1–2 months. Fluorescein angiography demonstrates late leakage and staining of the retinal veins. The electroretinogram (ERG) can be markedly reduced and this can persist after visual recovery (Wantanabe *et al.* 1987).

The first report of this condition was in a boy of 6 years in Japan (Ito *et al.* 1976). Subsequently there have been five further cases reported from Japan (cited in Wantanabe *et al.* 1987). Of a total of 16 cases reported in the literature the mean age is 18.0 years (range 3–33 years) and includes 10 females and three unilateral cases (Wantanabe *et al.* 1987; Kleiner *et al.* 1988; Sugin *et al.* 1991; Vander & Masciulli 1991; Browning 1992; Hamed *et al.* 1992; Nakai & Saika 1992; Atmaca & Gunduz 1993). Complications include macular scarring, vein occlusion (Sugin *et al.* 1991) and retinal fibrosis (Atmaca & Gunduz 1993). The cause is unknown and investigation of cases has been negative for sarcoid, tuberculosis, syphilis, HIV and multiple sclerosis. Most patients have been treated with high-dose systemic steroids and such treatment has been recommended

(Sugin *et al.* 1991). However, two cases have subsequently been reported in which full recovery over a similar time course has occurred with the use of only topical steroid (Vander & Masciulli 1991; Hamed *et al.* 1992). This may suggest that the natural course of the disease is good irrespective of whether or not corticosteroids are used.

Recently, a number of adults with AIDS have shown a similar fundal appearance to frosted branch periphlebitis in eyes affected by cytomegalovirus retinitis (Geier *et al.* 1992; Rabb *et al.* 1992; Secchi *et al.* 1992; Spaide *et al.* 1992). The signs of frosted branch periphlebitis improve on treatment with anticytomegalovirus drugs and steroids combined or with anticytomegalovirus drugs alone (Rabb *et al.* 1992). Interestingly a case of cytomegalovirus retinitis and frosted branch periphlebitis has been reported in a patient who was immunosuppressed following a heart transplant and who was not HIV positive (Cortina *et al.* 1994). This suggests that cytomegalovirus retinitis (not AIDS) is the common factor in these patients and that cytomegalovirus may cause the periphlebitis directly or incite an autoimmune mechanism. It remains to be seen whether infection by another, as yet uncharacterized, virus is similarly responsible for frosted branch periphlebitis in the cases that show no evidence of cytomegalovirus disease.

Angioid streaks

Angioid streaks are seen as irregular linear streaks of variable pigmentation which radiate out from the peripapillary retina into the more peripheral fundus (Fig. 49.4). The streaks can vary in colour and thickness and have a tendency to involve the macular area (Shields *et al.* 1975). On fluorescein angiography they can be hypofluorescent dur-

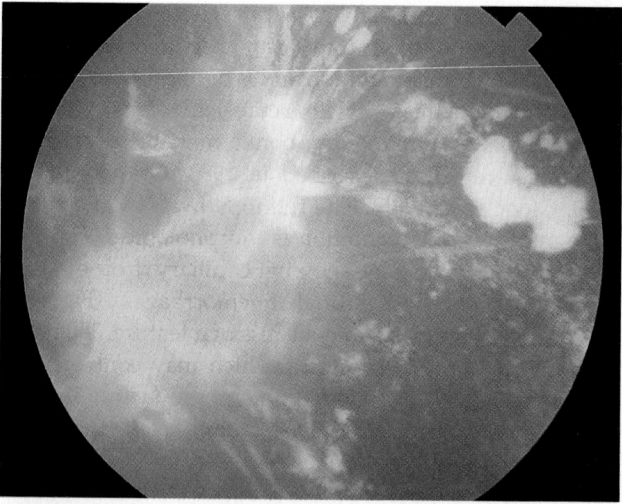

Fig. 49.3 Frosted branch periphlebitis showing sheathing of the retinal vessels, both arteries and veins. Multiple subretinal exudates. This girl was affected in the left eye only. She had no systemic disease.

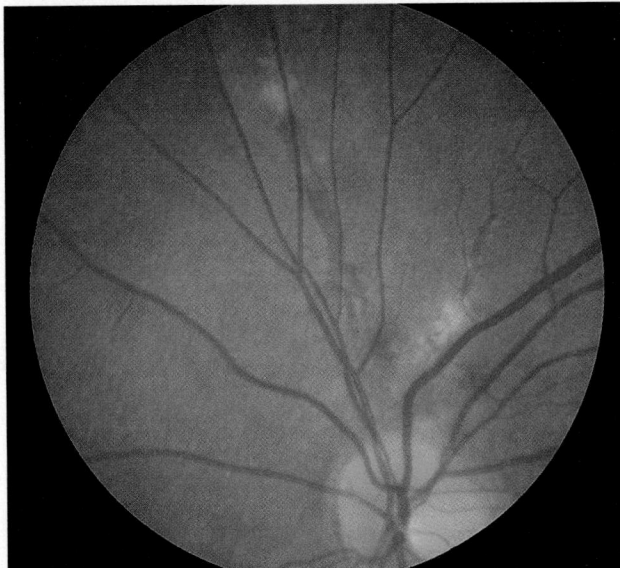

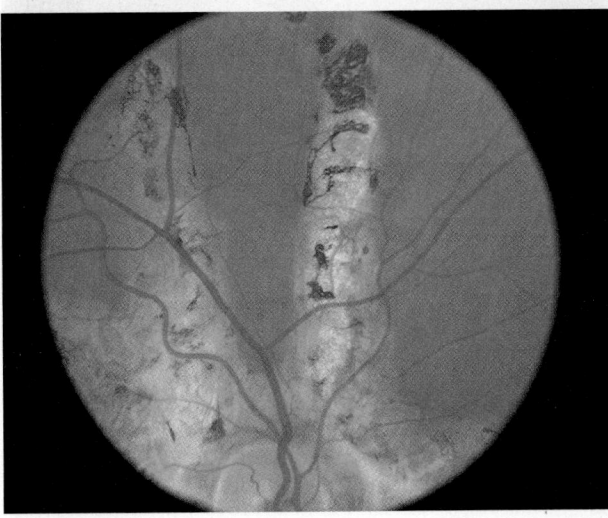

Fig. 49.4 (a) Angioid streaks in a 10-year-old girl with abetalipoproteinaemia. The streaks, which represent breaks in Bruch's membrane, radiate and taper from the optic disc, in this instance above the disc at 11.30 and 1 o'clock. (b) Angioid streaks in an adult with pseudoxanthoma elasticum. Choroidal neovascularization and haemorrhages occur at the margins of the streaks.

ing the early stages of an angiogram but then usually develop hyperfluorescence (Federman *et al.* 1975). Indocyanine green may be better at elucidating angioid streaks and associated lesions than fluorescein (Quaranta *et al.* 1995). Histology of these lesions is rare but they are thought to represent breaks in Bruch's membrane (Lawton Smith *et al.* 1964).

The systemic associations of angioid streaks are varied and curious (Table 49.1). They include pseudoxanthoma elasticum (PXE) (Pope 1974a, b) and Paget's disease (Gass & Clarkson 1973) although the latter has been contested

by a large study (Dabbs & Skjodt 1990) and a critical detailed review of previous reports (Clarkson 1991; Smith 1990). Angioid streaks are also, unarguably, associated with a number of haematological disorders including sickle cell anaemia (Nagpal *et al.* 1976; Hamilton *et al.* 1981), beta-thalassaemia minor (Kinsella & Mooney 1988), spherocytosis (McLane *et al.* 1984), beta-thalassaemia major and intermedia (Aessopos *et al.* 1992), sickle cell beta-thalassaemia (Aessopos *et al.* 1994) and abetalipoproteinaemia (Runge *et al.* 1986). Furthermore, evidence of systemic PXE has been demonstrated in individuals with sickle cell and sickle cell C disease, beta-thalassaemia (Aessopos *et al.* 1992) and sickle cell beta-thalassaemia (Aessopos *et al.* 1994). Linkage disequilibrium between the beta-globin gene cluster and a putative gene for PXE (as yet uncharacterized), which may be located on chromosome 16 next to the cluster, has been proposed to explain this curious association of angioid streaks, PXE and sickle cell disease (Hamilton *et al.* 1981). However, linkage disequilibrium is unlikely as it is known from haplotype analysis that the sickle cell mutation has arisen independently many times (Sergeant 1985) and is not likely to have done so contiguously with uncommon putative PXE mutations. Moreover, beta-thalassaemia is genetically heterogeneous involving many different types of mutation around the beta-globin locus (Thein 1993) and so linkage disequilibrium would not explain the association in this disease.

Iron deposition in Bruch's membrane secondary to haemolytic anaemia and increased iron turn-over has been proposed as an explanation (Singerman 1984) although the true pathogenetic explanation of this association remains to be elucidated.

Angioid streaks are uncommon before the age of 30 years generally (Clarkson & Altman 1982) and in sickle cell disease (Hamilton *et al.* 1981) but are occasionally seen in children (Krill *et al.* 1973). In PXE patients, a subtle speckling of the parafoveal macular area, particularly

Table 49.1 Angioid streaks: associated systemic disorders.

Pseudoxanthoma elasticum
Paget's disease of bone
Haematological disorders
    sickle cell anaemia
    beta-thalassaemia minor
    spherocytosis
    beta-thalassaemia major and intermedia
    sickle cell beta-thalassaemia
    abetalipoproteinaemia
Ehlers–Danlos syndrome
Acromegaly
Hyperparathyroidism
Hyperphosphataemia
Lead poisoning

temporally, is a common finding and has been called *peau d'orange* (Lawton Smith *et al.* 1964). It precedes the formation of angioid streaks (Krill *et al.* 1973; Schneiderman & Kalina 1994) and is seen in children. Presumed also to be an abnormality of Bruch's membrane, the lesions appear to be hypofluorescent (Federman *et al.* 1975). In contrast to other Bruch's membrane disorders such as Sorsby's dystrophy, individuals do not have abnormal dark adaptation (Holz *et al.* 1994). Angioid streaks can cause visual morbidity with the occurrence of subretinal neovascular membranes and their sequelae but this is rare in children. However, a case has been reported of a 15-year-old suffering a subretinal haemorrhage which preceded the appearance of angioid streaks which were apparent 5 years later (Schneiderman & Kalina 1994).

Idiopathic epiretinal membrane

Epiretinal membranes (macular pucker, cellophane maculopathy, macular fibrosis, premacular gliosis) can occur secondary to other ocular disease (Appiah & Hirose 1989) or as a primary finding in an otherwise healthy eye (Fig. 49.5). Such idiopathic epiretinal membranes usually occur in adults or elderly individuals (Wise 1975a; Sidd *et al.* 1982; Appiah *et al.* 1988), the mean age being 64.6 years in one large review (324 patients: Appiah *et al.* 1988). Metamorphopsia and reduction of visual acuity can occur, which is often mild but may progress. There is usually a separated posterior hyaloid membrane in the involved eye (Wise 1975a, c; Appiah *et al.* 1988). Visual acuity often improves following vitrectomy and membrane peel (Michels 1984). Histology shows a proliferation of glial cells on the inner retinal surface (Belhorn *et al.* 1975).

Idiopathic epiretinal membranes are rare in children and young adults but have been reported (Barr & Michels 1982; Kimmel *et al.* 1989; Smiddy *et al.* 1992; Webster & Jordan 1994). Wise (1975b) proposed that such membranes were a result of persistent embryonic material rather than an acquired process as in adults. Reports of membranes occurring in eyes with evidence of persistent primary vitreous on the lens and optic disc (Webster & Jordan 1994) supports this view. Spontaneous peeling of such membranes in children has been reported (Smiddy *et al.* 1992) and documented photographically (Mulligan & Daily 1992).

Idiopathic epiretinal membrane is a feature of neurofibromatosis type 2 (NF2) and has been found in seven out of nine (Kaye *et al.* 1992) and four out of six (Landau & Yasargil 1993) young affected individuals. The apparent high sensitivity of this sign for NF2, its low prevalence in normal young people and the known high new mutation rate in NF2 (Evans *et al.* 1992a) suggests that the ophthalmologist should consider this disorder when finding an apparent idiopathic retinal membrane in a child or young adult. Screening for other manifestations of this disorder,

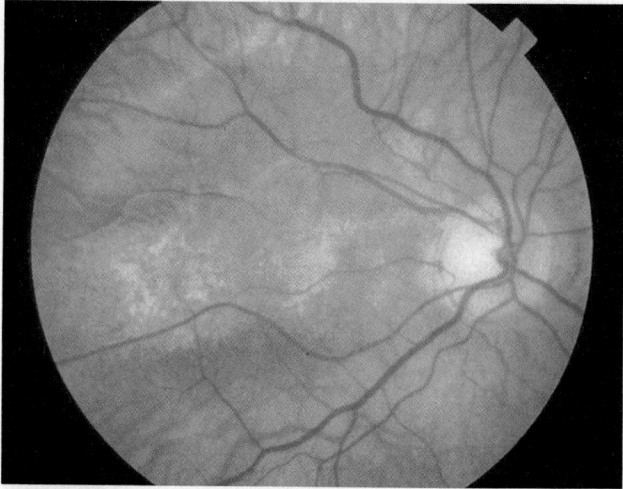

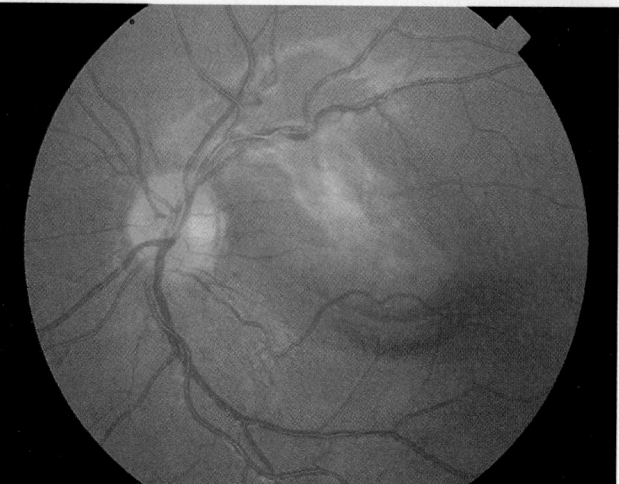

Fig. 49.5 (a) Pre-retinal fibrosis in a child with neurofibromatosis type 2. A faint white area in the superior temporal arcade can be seen slightly distorting the retinal vessels. (b) Pre-retinal fibrosis. There is a marked pre-retinal fibrous membrane causing traction on the superior and inferior temporal vessels with a subretinal disturbance.

such as acoustic neuromas and meningiomas, even in an asymptomatic patient without a family history, is therefore important, as such tumours may be more effectively treated if detected at an early presymptomatic stage (Evans *et al.* 1992b; Briggs *et al.* 1994).

Lipaemia retinalis

Lipaemia retinalis is a rare ocular finding in which the blood column within retinal arteries and veins appears pale and creamy-white in colour (see Fig. 49.6). In mild cases, this colour change is more obvious in small peripheral retinal vessels (Vinger & Sachs 1970). It occurs in subjects who have a markedly raised serum level of the two larger lipoproteins: chylomicrons and very low density lipoproteins (VLDL). The creamy-white colour of *in vivo*

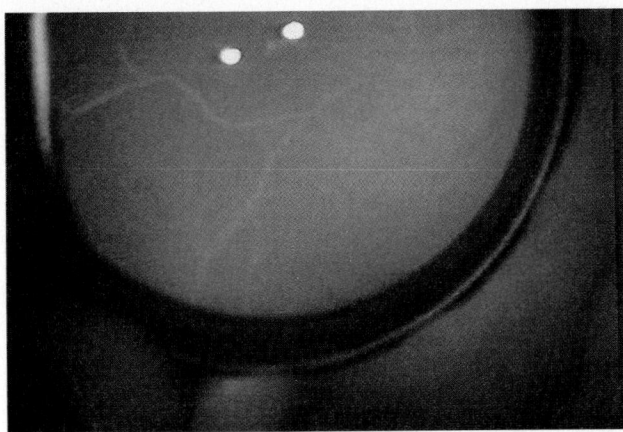

Fig. 49.6 Lipaemia retinalis in an infant with chylomicronaemia.

and *in vitro* blood and serum is due to reflection of light from these relatively large lipoprotein particles. Raised serum levels of the smaller low density lipoproteins (LDLs) or high density lipoproteins (HDLs) do not cause this sign. Because chylomicrons and VLDLs transport mainly triglycerides, lipaemia retinalis occurs in association with serum hypertriglyceridaemia, which is thought to be over the level of 2500 mg/dl (Vinger & Sachs 1970) or 1000 mg/dl (Shaeffer & Levy 1985) (normal < 200 mg/dl) when the ocular sign is evident.

Chylomicrons are produced in intestinal cells and mediate transport of the non-polar triglycerides within the aqueous serum. They enter the lymphatics of the intestine and thereafter the blood stream via the thoracic duct. VLDLs are synthesized in the liver and also predominantly contain and transport triglycerides. The main route of disposal of these two lipoproteins relies on the enzyme lipoprotein lipase situated on endothelial cells in certain tissues. This enzyme requires the protein apolipoprotein C-II, which is present within the lipoproteins, as an essential co-factor. Consequently, lipaemia retinalis, particularly when presenting in a child, may be associated with familial deficiency of lipoprotein lipase (Havel & Gordon 1960; Ram *et al.* 1993) or apolipoprotein C-II (Breckenridge *et al.* 1978). Hypertriglyceridaemia and subsequent lipaemia retinalis can occur in the diabetic child (Martinez *et al.* 1992), and can also be secondary to renal disease, obesity, hypothyroidism and alcoholism in adults. It may be a feature of those familial hyperlipidaemias that have hypertriglyceridaemia as a component (I, III, IV and V— Fredrickson's classification (Fredrickson *et al.* 1967)).

Lipaemia retinalis does not impair vision. However, complications and associated findings include 'eruptive' xanthomas (papular yellow lesions with a red base occurring on extensor surfaces or the eyelids), hepatosplenomegaly, bouts of abdominal pain, pancreatitis and if accompanied by hypercholesterolaemia (i.e. mixed hyperlipidaemia), increased risk of atheroma. To

prevent complications, it is important to exclude and treat a primary cause, particularly diabetes in children. Treatment aimed at lowering serum triglycerides is often successful and can be achieved by dietary fat restriction either alone or combined with lipid lowering drugs (Shaeffer & Levy 1985).

Cystoid macular oedema

Cystoid macular oedema (CME) caused by leakage from the perifoveolar capillaries is uncommon in childhood. It may be seen in retinovascular diseases such as radiation retinopathy, Coats' disease or diabetes, in the inherited rod–cone dystrophies and in inflammatory disorders such as juvenile pars planitis or anterior and posterior uveitis. Rarely it may be part of a dominantly inherited disorder (Deutman *et al.* 1976; Kremer *et al.* 1994).

CME may also complicate intraocular surgery in children (Hoyt & Nickel 1982). Although postoperative aphakic CME was seen in over 30% of infants who had lensectomy and anterior vitrectomy in the study of Hoyt and Nickel (1982), this high incidence has not been confirmed in other studies (Poer *et al.* 1981; Gilbard *et al.* 1983; Pinchoff *et al.* 1988; Green *et al.* 1990). There appears to be no greater risk of developing CME following one type of surgical procedure than another and the incidence of postoperative CME in cataract surgery in infancy is clearly less than seen in adults (Pinchoff *et al.* 1988).

Lamellar macular holes

Lamellar macular holes may be idiopathic or occur after trauma or other causes of macular oedema. They are associated with a variable visual loss and are seen as a sharp edged circular perifoveal lesion (Fig. 49.7). Unlike full thickness holes, they do not require treatment.

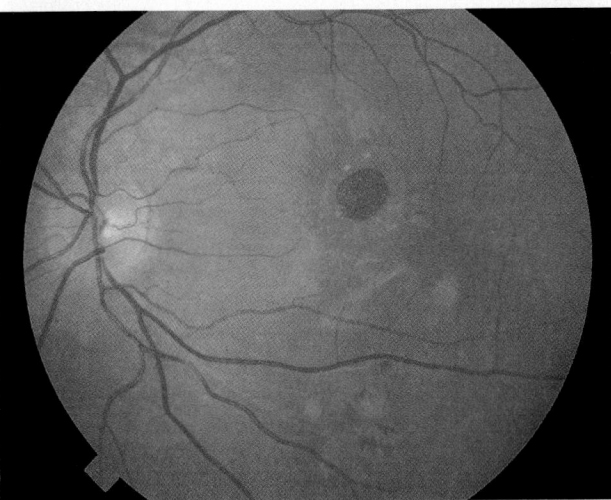

Fig. 49.7 Lamellar macular hole in a patient who had suffered blunt trauma to the eye.

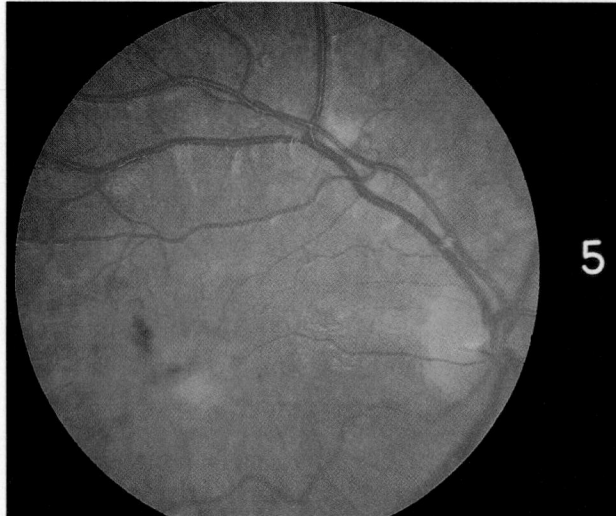

Fig. 49.8 Disciform degeneration in rubella retinopathy. This 7-year-old boy had a cataract in the left eye, was deaf and noticed a reduction of vision in his right eye. The background pigment mottling usually associated with rubella can be seen surrounding the macula, which shows a serous detachment, haemorrhage and a disciform lesion. The acuity fell to 6/60 but recovered to 6/12 over 4 months.

Table 49.2 Aetiology of choroidal neovascularization in childhood. Modified from Wilson and Mazur (1988).

Trauma
Choroidal rupture

Inflammatory lesions
Congenital rubella
Toxoplasmosis
Toxocariasis
Presumed ocular histoplasmosis syndrome
Chronic uveitis

Inherited retinal dystrophies
Vitelliform dystrophy
Choroideraemia
Fundus flavimaculatus

Others
Angioid streaks
Optic nerve drusen
Optic nerve pits
Choroidal osteoma
Choroidal haemangioma
Combined retinal pigment epithelium–retinal hamartomas

Disciform macular degeneration

Choroidal neovascularization is uncommon in childhood but can be seen following traumatic choroidal rupture (Smith *et al.* 1974), with intraocular infections such as congenital rubella (Fig. 49.8) (Deutman & Grizzard 1978;

Orth *et al.* 1980), congenital toxoplasmosis (Fine *et al.* 1981; Cotlier & Friedman 1982), and toxocariasis or in association with one of the inherited retinal dystrophies, most commonly Best's disease (see Chapter 45). Choroidal neovascularization has been reported in a boy with Sturge–Weber syndrome and choroidal haemangioma (Ruby *et al.* 1992) although this may be due to laser therapy. The aetiology, clinical features, and management of choroidal neovascularization in childhood has been reviewed by Wilson and Mazur (1988) (see Table 49.2).

References

Acacio I, Goldberg MF. Peripapillary and macular vessel occlusions in sickle cell anaemia. *Am J Ophthalmol* 1973; **75**: 861–6.

Aessopos A, Savvides P, Samatelos G *et al.* Pseudo elasticum-like skin lesions and angioid streaks in beta-thalassaemia. *Am J Hematol* 1992; **41**: 159–64.

Aessopos A, Voskaridou E, Kavoulkis E *et al.* Angioid streaks in sickle thalassaemia. *Am J Ophthalmol* 1994; **117**: 589–92.

Amoaku WMK, Archer DB. Cephalic radiation and retinal vasculopathy. *Eye* 1990a; **4**: 195–203.

Amoaku WMK, Archer DB. Fluorescein angiographic features, natural causes and treatment of radiation retinopathy. *Eye* 1990b; **4**: 657–67.

Appiah AP, Hirose T. Secondary causes of premacular fibrosis. *Ophthalmology* 1989; **96**: 389–92.

Appiah AP, Hirose T, Kado M. A review of 324 cases of idiopathic premacular gliosis. *Am J Ophthalmol* 1988; **106**: 533–5.

Archer DB. Doyne Lecture. Responses of retinal and choroidal vessels to ionising radiation. *Eye* 1993; **7**: 1–13.

Archer DB, Amoaku WMK, Gardiner TA. Radiation retinopathy: clinical, histopathological, ultrastructural and experimental correlations. *Eye* 1991; **5**: 239–51.

Archer DB, Amoaku WM, Kelly G. Choroidoretinal neovascularisation following radon seed treatment of retinoblastoma. *Br J Ophthalmol* 1993; **77**: 95–9.

Asdourian G, Nagpal KC, Goldbaum MH, Patrianasos D, Goldberg MF, Rabb M. Evolution of the retinal black sunburst in sickling hemoglobinopathies. *Br J Ophthalmol* 1975; **59**: 710–16.

Atmaca LS, Gunduz K. Acute frosted retinal periphlebitis. *Acta Ophthalmol* 1993; **71**: 856–9.

Barr CC, Michels RG. Idiopathic non-vascularized epiretinal membranes in young patients: report of six cases. *Ann Ophthalmol* 1982; **14**: 335–41.

Belhorn MB, Friedman AH, Wise GN, Henkind P. Ultrastructure and clinicopathologic correlation of idiopathic preretinal macular fibrosis. *Am J Ophthalmol* 1975; **79**: 366–73.

Bernauer W, Gratwohl A, Keller A, Daicker B. Microvasculopathy in the ocular fundus after bone marrow transplantation. *Ann Int Med* 1991; **115**: 925–30.

Breckenridge WC, Little JA, Steiner G, Choro A, Poapst M. Hypertriglyceridemia associated with deficiency of apolipoprotein C-II. *N Engl J Med* 1978; **298**: 1265–73.

Briggs RJ, Brackmann DE, Baser ME, Hitselberger WE. Comprehensive management of bilateral acoustic neuromas. Current perspectives. *Arch Otolaryngol Head Neck Surg* 1994; **120**: 1307–14.

Brown GC, Shield JA, Sanborn G, Augsburger JJ, Savino PJ, Schatz NJ. Radiation retinopathy. *Ophthalmology* 1982; **89**: 1494–501.

Browning DJ. Mild frosted branch periphlebitis. *Am J Ophthalmol* 1992; **114**: 505–6.

Burger W, Hovener G, Ousterhus D *et al.* Prevalence and development of retinopathy in children and adolescents with type I (insulin dependent) diabetes mellitus. A longitudinal study. *Diabetologica* 1986; **29**: 17–22.

Clarkson JG. Paget's disease and angioid streaks: one complication less? (letter, comment). *Br J Ophthalmol* 1991; **75**: 511.

Clarkson JG, Altman RD. Angioid streaks. *Surv Ophthalmol* 1982; **26**: 235–46.

Condon PI, Sergeant GR. Ocular findings in homozygous sickle cell disease in Jamaica. *Am J Ophthalmol* 1972; **73**: 533–43.

Cortina P, Diaz M, Espana E, Almenar L, Lopez-Aldeguer J. Acute frosted retinal periphlebitis associated with cytomegalovirus retinitis in a heart transplant patient (letter). *Retina* 1994; **14**: 463–4.

Coskucan NM, Jabs DA, Dunn JP *et al.* The eye in bone marrow transplantation IV. Retinal complications. *Arch Ophthalmol* 1994; **112**: 372–9.

Cotlier AM, Friedman AH. Subretinal neovascularization in ocular toxoplasmosis. *Br J Ophthalmol* 1982; **66**: 524–8.

Couke PA, Schmid C, Balmer A, Mirimanoff RO, Thames ID. Hypofractionation in retinoblastoma: an increased risk of retinopathy. *Radiother Oncol* 1993; **28**: 157–61.

Dabbs TR, Skjodt K. Prevalence of angioid streaks and other ocular complications of Paget's disease of bone. *Br J Ophthalmol* 1990; **74**: 579–82.

DCCT Research Group. Effect of intensive diabetes treatment on the development and progression of long-term complications in adolescents with insulin-dependent diabetes mellitus. *J Pediatr* 1994; **125**: 177–88.

DCCT Research Group. Effect of intensive treatment of diabetes on the development and progression of long-term complications in insulin-dependent diabetes mellitus. *N Engl J Med* 1993; **329**: 977.

Deutman AF, Grizzard WS. Rubella retinopathy and subretinal neovascularization. *Am J Ophthalmol* 1978; **85**: 82–7.

Deutman AF, Pinckers AJLG, De Kerk AL. Dominantly inherited cystoid macular oedema. *Am J Ophthalmol* 1976; **82**: 540–8.

Ehlers N, Kaae S. Effects of ionizing radiation on retinoblastoma and on the normal ocular fundus in infants: a photographic and fluorescein angiographic study. *Acta Ophthalmol (Copenh)* 1987; **65**(Suppl. 181): 1–84.

Evans DGR, Huson SM, Donnai D *et al.* A genetic study of type 2 neurofibromatosis in the UK I. Prevalence, mutation rate, fitness, and confirmation of maternal transmission effect on severity. *J Med Genet* 1992a; **29**: 841–6.

Evans DGR, Huson SM, Donnai D *et al.* A genetic study of type 2 neurofibromatosis in the UK II. Guidelines for genetic counselling. *J Med Genet* 1992b; **29**: 847–52.

Falck AA, Kaar ML, Laatikainen LT. Prevalence and risk factors of retinopathy in children with diabetes. A population-based study on Finnish children. *Acta Ophthalmol* 1993; **71**: 801–9.

Farber MD, Jampol LM, Fox P *et al.* A randomized clinical trial of scatter photocoagulation of proliferative sickle retinopathy. *Arch Ophthalmol* 1991; **109**: 363–7.

Federman JL, Shields JA, Tomer TL. Angioid streaks II. Fluorescein angiographic features. *Arch Ophthalmol* 1975; **93**: 951–62.

Fine SL, Owens SL, Haller JA *et al.* Choroidal neovascularization as a late complication of ocular toxoplasmosis. *Am J Ophthalmol* 1981; **91**: 318–22.

Fox PD, Vessey SJ, Farshaw ML, Sergeant GR. Influence of genotype on the natural history of untreated proliferative sickle retinopathy—an angiographic study. *Br J Ophthalmol* 1991; **75**: 229–31.

Fredrickson DS, Levy RI, Lees RS. Fat transport in lipoproteins. An integrated approach to mechanisms and disorders. *N Engl J Med* 1967; **276**: 148–56.

Gass JDM, Clarkson JG. Angioid streaks and disciform macular detachment in Paget's disease (osteitis deformans). *Am J Ophthalmol* 1973; **75**: 576–88.

Geffner ME. Reviewing the Diabetes Control and Complications Trial: one member of the 'control panel' speaks. *J Pediatr* 1994; **125**: 228–9.

Geier SA, Nasemann J, Klauss V, Kronawitter U, Goebel FD. Frosted branch angiitis in a patient with the acquired immunodeficiency syndrome (letter). *Am J Ophthalmol* 1992; **113**: 203–5.

Gilbard SM, Peyman G, Goldberg M. Evaluation of cystoid maculopathy after pars plicata lensectomy vitrectomy for congenital cataracts. *Ophthalmol* 1983; **90**: 1201–6.

Gloor B, Gratwohl A, Hahn H *et al.* Multiple cotton-wool spots following bone marrow transplantation for treatment of acute lymphatic leukaemia. *Br J Ophthalmol* 1985; **69**: 320–5.

Goldbaum MH. Retinal depression sign indicating a small retinal infarct. *Am J Ophthalmol* 1978a; **86**: 45–55.

Goldbaum MH, Jampol LM, Goldberg MF. The disc sign in sickling hemoglobinopathies. *Arch Ophthalmol* 1978b; **96**: 1597.

Goldberg MF. Classification and pathogenesis of proliferative sickle cell retinopathy. *Am J Ophthalmol* 1971; **71**: 649–65.

Goldberg MF. The diagnosis and treatment of secondary glaucoma after hyphema in sickle cell patients. *Am J Ophthalmol* 1979; **87**: 43–9.

Gratwohl A, Gloor B, Hahn H, Speck B. Retinal cotton-wool patches in bone marrow transplant recipients (letter). *N Engl J Med* 1983; **308**: 1101.

Green BF, Morin JD, Brent HP. Pars plicata lensectomy/vitrectomy for developmental cataract extraction: surgical results. *J Pediatr Ophthalmol Strabismus* 1990; **27**: 229–32.

Hamed LM, Fang EN, Fanous MM, Mames R, Friedman S. Frosted branch angiitis: the role of systemic corticosteroids. *J Pediatr Ophthalmol Strabismus* 1992; **29**: 312–13.

Hamilton AM, Pope FM, Condon PI *et al.* Angioid streaks in Jamaican patients with homozygous sickle cell disease. *Br J Ophthalmol* 1981; **65**: 341–7.

Havel RJ, Gordon RS. Idiopathic hyperlipidemia: metabolic studies in an affected family. *J Clin Invest* 1960; **39**: 1777–90.

Hayreh SS. Post-radiation retinopathy: a fluorescein fundus angiographic study. *Br J Ophthalmol* 1970; **54**: 705–14.

Hendrick JB. Peculiar elongated and sickle-shaped red corpuscles in a case of severe anaemia. *Arch Intern Med* 1910; **6**: 517.

Holz FG, Jubb C, Fitzke FW, Bird AC, Pope FM. Dark adaptation and scotopic perimetry over 'peau d'orange' in pseudoxanthoma elasticum (letter). *Br J Ophthalmol* 1994; **78**: 79–80.

Hoyt CS, Nickel D. Aphakic cystoid macular oedema. Occurrence in infants and children after transpupillary lensectomy and anterior vitrectomy. *Arch Ophthalmol* 1982; **100**: 746–8.

Hungerford JL, Toma NM, Plowman PN, Kingston JE. External beam radiotherapy for retinoblastoma I. Whole eye technique. *Br J Ophthalmol* 1995; **79**: 109–111.

Ingram VM. A specific chemical difference between the globins of normal human and sickle-cell haemoglobin. *Nature* 1956; **178**: 792–4.

Irvine AR, Wood S. Radiation retinopathy as an experimental model for ischaemic proliferative retinopathy and rubeosis iridis. *Am J Ophthalmol* 1987; **103**: 790–7.

Ito Y, Nakamo M, Kyo N, Takeuchi M. Frosted branch angiitis in a child. *Jpn J Clin Ophthalmol* 1976; **30**: 797.

Jackobson MS, Gagliano DA, Cohen SB *et al.* A randomised clinical trial of feeder vessel photocoagulation of sickle cell retinopathy. *Ophthalmology* 1991; **98**: 581–5.

Kaye LD, Rothner AD, Beauchamp GR, Meyers SM, Estes ML. Ocular findings associated with neurofibromatosis type II. *Ophthalmology* 1992; **99**: 1424–9.

Kimmel AS, Weingeist TA, Blodi CF, Wells MD. Idiopathic premacular gliosis in children and adolescents. *Am J Ophthalmol* 1989; **108**: 578–81.

Kinsella FP, Mooney DJ. Angioid streaks in beta thalassaemia minor. *Br J Ophthalmol* 1988; **72**: 303–5.

Kleiner RC, Kaplan HJ, Shakin JL, Yannuzzi LA, Croswell HH Jr, McLean WC Jr. Acute frosted retinal periphlebitis. *Am J Ophthalmol* 1988; **106**: 27–34.

Knapp JW. Isolated macular infarction in sickle cell disease. *Am J Ophthalmol* 1972; **73**: 857–8.

Kostraba JN, Dorman JS, Orchard TJ *et al.* Contributions of diabetes duration before puberty to development of microvascular complications. *Diabetes Care* 1989; **12**: 686–93.

Kremer H, Pinkers A, van den Helm B *et al.* Localisation of the gene for dominant cystoid macular dystrophy on chromosome 7p. *Hum Mol Genet* 1994; **3**: 299–302.

Krill AE, Klien BA, Archer DB. Precursors of angioid streaks. *Am J Ophthalmol* 1973; **76**: 875–9.

Landau K, Yasargil GM. Ocular findings in neurofibromatosis type 2. *Br J Ophthalmol* 1993; **77**: 646–9.

Lawton Smith J, Gass JDM, Justice J. Fluorescein fundus photography of angioid streaks. *Br J Ophthalmol* 1964; **48**: 517.

Lopez PF, Sternberg P, Dabbs CK, Vogler WR, Crocker I, Kalin NS. Bone marrow transplant retinopathy. *Am J Ophthalmol* 1991; **112**: 635–46.

MacFaul PA, Bedford MA. Ocular complications after therapeutic irradiation. *Br J Ophthalmol* 1970; **54**: 237–47.

McLane KG, Grizzard WS, Kousseff GB, Hartmann RC, Sever RJ. Angioid streaks associated with hereditary spherocytosis. *Am J Ophthalmol* 1984; **97**: 444–9.

McNally PG, Raymond NT, Swift PG, Hearnshaw JR, Burden AC. Does the prepubertal duration of diabetes influence the onset of microvascular complications? *Diabetic Med* 1993; **10**: 906–8.

Martinez KR, Cibis GW, Tauber JT. Lipemia retinalis—photoessay. *Arch Ophthalmol* 1992; **110**: 1171.

Michels RG. Vitrectomy for macular pucker. *Ophthalmology* 1984; **91**: 1384–8.

Michelson PE, Pfaffenbach D. Retinal artery occlusion following trauma in youths with sickle-trait haemoglobinopathy. *Am J Ophthalmol* 1972; **74**: 494–7.

Moore FR. Presidential address. *Trans Ophthalmol Soc UK* 1935; **55**: 3–26.

Mulligan TG, Daily MJ. Spontaneous peeling of an idiopathic epiretinal membrane in a young patient. *Arch Ophthalmol* 1992; **110**: 1367–8.

Murphy RP, Nanda M, Plotwick L, Enger C, Vitale S, Patz A. The relationship of puberty to diabetic retinopathy. *Arch Ophthalmol* 1990; **108**: 215.

Nagpal KC, Asdourian G, Goldbaum M *et al.* Angioid streaks and sickle cell haemoglobinopathies. *Br J Ophthalmol* 1976; **63**: 31–4.

Nakai A, Saika S. A case of frosted branch retinal angiitis in a child. *Ann Ophthalmol* 1992; **24**: 415–17.

Orth DH, Fishman GA, Segall M *et al.* Rubella maculopathy. *Br J Ophthalmol* 1980; **64**: 201–5.

Parsons JT, Bova FJ, Fitzgerald CR, Mendenhall WM, Million RR. Radiation retinopathy after external-beam irradiation: analysis of time–dose factors. *Int J Radiat Oncol Biol Phys* 1994; **30**: 765–73.

Paton D. The conjunctival sign of sickle cell disease. *Arch Ophthalmol* 1961; **66**: 90–4.

Paton D. The conjunctival sign of sickle cell disease—further observations. *Arch Ophthalmol* 1962; **68**: 627–32.

Pauling L, Itala HA, Singer SJ, Wells IC. Sickle cell anaemia: a molecular disease. *Science* 1949; **110**: 543–8.

Penman AD, Talbot JF, Chuang EL, Thomas P, Sergeant GR, Bird AC. New classification of peripheral retinal vascular changes in sickle cell disease. *Br J Ophthalmol* 1994; **78**: 681–9.

Pinchoff BS, Ellis FD, Helveston EM, Sato SE. Cystoid macular oedema in paediatric aphakia. *J Pediatr Ophthalmol Strabismus* 1988; **25**: 240–7.

Poer DV, Helveston EM, Ellis FD. Aphakic cystoid macular oedema in children. *Arch Ophthalmol* 1981; **99**: 249–52.

Pope FM. Autosomal dominant pseudoxanthoma elasticum. *J Med Genet* 1974a; **11**: 152–7.

Pope FM. Two types of autosomal recessive pseudoxanthoma elasticum. *Arch Dermatol* 1974b; **110**: 209–12.

Quaranta M, Cohen SY, Krott R, Sterkers M, Soubrane G, Coscas GJ. Indocyanine green videoangiography of angioid streaks. *Am J Ophthalmol* 1995; **119**: 136–42.

Rabb MF, Jampol LM, Fish RH, Campo RV, Sobol WM, Becker NM. Retinal periphlebitis in patients with acquired immunodeficiency syndrome with cytomegalovirus retinitis mimics acute frosted retinal periphlebitis. *Arch Ophthalmol* 1992; **110**: 1257–60.

Raichand M, Dizon RV, Nagpal KC, Goldberg MF, Rabb NF, Goldbaum MH. Macular holes associated with proliferative sickle retinopathy. *Arch Ophthalmol* 1978; **96**: 1592–6.

Ram J, Pandav SS, Jain S, Arora S, Gupta A, Sharma A. Reversal of lipaemia retinalis with dietary control. *Eye* 1993; **7**: 763–5.

Rosenthal AR. Ocular manifestations of leukemia—a review. *Ophthalmology* 1983; **90**: 899–905.

Ruby AJ, Jampol LM, Goldberg MF, Schroeder R, Anderson-Nelson S. Choroidal neovascularisation associated with choroidal hemangiomas. *Arch Ophthalmol* 1992; **110**: 658–61.

Runge P, Muller DRP, McAllister J, Calver D, Mayo JK, Taylor D. Oral vitamin E supplements can prevent the retinopathy of abetalipoproteinaemia. *Br J Ophthalmol* 1986; **70**: 166–73.

Schneiderman TE, Kalina RE. Subretinal hemorrhage precedes development of angioid streaks. *Arch Ophthalmol* 1994; **112**: 1622–3.

Secchi AG, Tognon MS, Turrini B, Carniel G. Acute frosted retinal periphlebitis associated with cytomegalovirus retinitis. *Retina* 1992; **12**: 245–7.

Sergeant GR. *Sickle Cell Disease.* Oxford: Oxford University Press, 1985.

Shaefer EJ, Levy RI. Pathogenesis and management of lipoprotein disorders. *N Engl J Med* 1985; **312**: 1300–10.

Shields JA, Federman JL, Tomer TL, Annesley WH. Angioid streaks I. Ophthalmoscopic variations and diagnostic problems. *Br J Ophthalmol* 1975; **59**: 257.

Sidd RJ, Fine SL, Owens SL, Patz A. Idiopathic preretinal gliosis. *Am J Ophthalmol* 1982; **94**: 44–8.

Singerman LJ. Angioid streaks associated with hereditary spherocytosis. *Am J Ophthalmol* 1984; **98**: 647–8.

Smiddy WE, Michels RG, Gilbert HD, Green WR. Clinicopathological study of idiopathic macular pucker in children and young adults. *Retina* 1992; **12**: 232–6.

Smith R. Paget's disease and angioid streaks: one complication less? (editorial). *Br J Ophthalmol* 1990; **74**: 577–8.

Smith RE, Kelley JS, Harbin TS. Late macular complications of choroidal rupture. *Am J Ophthalmol* 1974; **77**: 650–8.

Spaide RF, Vitale AT, Toth IR, Oliver JM. Frosted branch angiitis associated with cytomegalovirus retinitis. *Am J Ophthalmol* 1992: **113**: 522–8.

Stallard HB. Glioma retinae treated with radon seeds. *Br Med J* 1936; 962–4.

Stallard HB. Radiant energy as (a) a pathogenic and (b) a therapeutic agent in ophthalmic disorders. *Br J Ophthalmol Monogr* 1933; **6**(Suppl.): 1–126.

Sugin SL, Henderly DE, Friedman SM, Jampol LM, Doyle JW. Unilateral frosted branch angiitis. *Am J Ophthalmol* 1991; **111**: 682–5.

Talbot JF, Bird AC, Maude GH. Sickle cell retinopathy in Jamaican children: further observations from a cohort study. *Br J Ophthalmol* 1988; **72**: 727–32.

Thein SL. Beta-thalassaemia. *Baillière's Clinical Haematology*, Vol. 6(1). Baillière Tindall, 1993: 151–75.

Toma NM, Hungerford JL, Plowman PN, Kingston JE, Doughty D. External beam radiotherapy for retinoblastoma II. Lens sparing technique. *Br J Ophthalmol* 1995; **79**: 112–17.

Vander JF, Masciulli L. Unilateral frosted branch angiitis (letter). *Am J Ophthalmol* 1991; **112**: 477–8.

Viebahn M, Barricks ME, Osterloh MD. Synergism between diabetic and radiation retinopathy: a case report and review. *Br J Ophthalmol* 1991; **75**: 629–32.

Vinger PF, Sachs BA. Ocular manifestations of hyperlipoproteinemia. *Am J Ophthalmol* 1970; **70**: 563–73.

Wantanabe Y, Takeda N, Adachi Usami E. A case of frosted branch angiitis. *Br J Ophthalmol* 1987; **71**: 553–8.

Weber B, Burger W, Hartmann R *et al.* Risk factors for the development of retinopathy in children and adolescents with type I (insulin dependent) diabetes mellitus. *Diabetologica* 1986; **29**: 23–9.

Webster AR, Anderson JR, Richards EM, Moore AT. Ischaemic retinopathy occurring in patients receiving bone marrow allografts and campath-1G: a clinicopathological study. *Br J Ophthalmol* 1995; **79**: 687–91.

Webster AR, Jordan K. Epiretinal membranes occurring in two young adults with evidence of persistent primary vitreous. *Eye* 1994; **8**: 706–8.

Welch RB, Goldberg MF. Sickle cell haemoglobin and its relation to fundus abnormality. *Arch Ophthalmol* 1966; **75**: 353–62.

Wilson ME, Mazur DO. Choroidal neovascularization in children. Report of five cases and a literature review. *J Pediatr Ophthalmol Strabismus* 1988; **25**: 23–9.

Wise GN. Clinical features of idiopathic preretinal macular fibrosis. Schoenberg lecture. *Am J Ophthalmol* 1975a; **79**: 349–57.

Wise GN. Congenital preretinal macular fibrosis. *Am J Ophthalmol* 1975b; **79**: 363–5.

Wise GN. Relationship of idiopathic preretinal macular fibrosis to posterior vitreous detachment. *Am J Ophthalmol* 1975c; **79**: 358–62.

50: Optic Nerve: Congenital Abnormalities

David Taylor and Ann Stout

Congenital anomalies of the optic disc are important causes of visual handicap in the West and may give useful clues to underlying neurological disease. Brodsky (1994a) has given a useful review.

Normal optic disc in infancy

There are no absolute criteria for normality of the optic disc in infancy but there are important differences between an adult's and an infant's optic disc. It is best to examine the optic disc with the pupil dilated and using both the indirect and the direct ophthalmoscope taking as much time as possible.

The infant disc appears to be about the same size on ophthalmoscopy as that of an adult; in fact it is 50% of adult size by 20 weeks of gestation, 75% by birth and 95% by 1 year of age (Rimmer *et al.* 1993). The main differences are its colour, the vascular pattern and the size of the physiological cup. The disc, especially in early infancy, is comparatively pale; the fluorescein angiographic appearance is the same as in older children, making vascular changes unlikely as the cause of the relative pallor. The disc is myelinated at birth, but there may be some difference in the size or optical qualities of the axonal myelin and supporting tissue. The relative whiteness of the infant optic disc makes it easy to misdiagnose optic atrophy and extra information can be gained from examination of the nerve fibre layer of the retina about a half a disc diameter away from the edge of the disc. Normally, the retinal vessels stand out just above the level of the internal limiting membrane, which is seen as the surface sheen on the retina. In optic atrophy, the retinal nerve fibres decrease in number leaving the vessels standing up above the internal limiting membrane. This is best seen by the use of parallax in which the ophthalmoscope is moved from side to side to observe the change in the light reflex over the retinal vessels.

In infancy, the physiological cup in the optic disc is smaller than in older children; it is also difficult to see due to lack of sharp definition of its edge. From twin studies the cup to disc ratio is largely genetically determined (Teikari & Airaksinen 1992). The retinal vessels may be more tortuous especially in neonates. In the newborn, retinal haemorrhages may occur near or on the disc although they are not necessarily of serious pathological significance (von Barsewisch 1979).

Grey disc ('myelogenous dysgenesis')

Beauvieux (1926) described a grey appearance of the optic disc in neonates, usually in those born prematurely. He suggested that this may be due to 'myelogenous dysgenesis'. Initially, vision appeared defective but improved within a few weeks or months. Several subsequent case reports confirmed the occurrence of this phenomenon and it is now enshrined in the ophthalmological literature, although it does not seem often to be recognized in recent years. It may be that the cases described are analogous to infants with delayed visual maturation (see Chapter 3).

In practice it is reasonable to take a confident line with the parents, especially if there are no other central nervous system signs and if the electrophysiological tests are shown to improve. The literature on the grey disc and experience with delayed visual development both suggest a good outcome.

Pigmentation in and around the optic disc

Disc pigmentation

Congenital pigmentation of the optic disc is rare, although variations of the pigment border of the optic disc are seen quite frequently. Mann (1957) described three types.
1 Dense plaques of pigment overlying a sector of the disc and sometimes extending over the retina: these may be of ectodermal origin, but are more likely to be mesodermal in origin if they surround the optic disc.
2 Linear pigment markings concentric with the disc margin (Fig. 50.1a).

3 Lace-like veils of pigment associated with the central retinal vessels and probably of mesodermal origin, like the choroidal pigment.
4 Pigmentation following inflammation (Taylor & Ffytche 1976 (Fig. 50.1b)).

Shields (1980) has drawn attention to the occurrence of a slate-grey crescent, usually temporal or inferotemporal, in the optic disc which occurs particularly in pigmented races which may be confused with a cupped disc. This is either a congenital anomaly or acquired during the early growth of the eye.

Melanocytomas occasionally occur in children, giving jet black pigmentation to the disc and surrounding tissue together with disc oedema (Haas *et al.* 1986).

In Aicardi's syndrome (Aicardi *et al.* 1965; Hoyt *et al.* 1978) infantile spasms occur with severe retardation, ectopic cerebral grey matter (Fig. 50.2), absence of the corpus callosum, and characteristic lacunar defects in the reti-

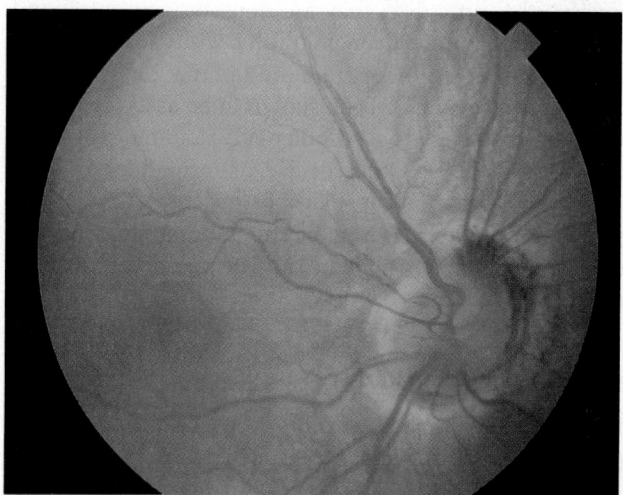

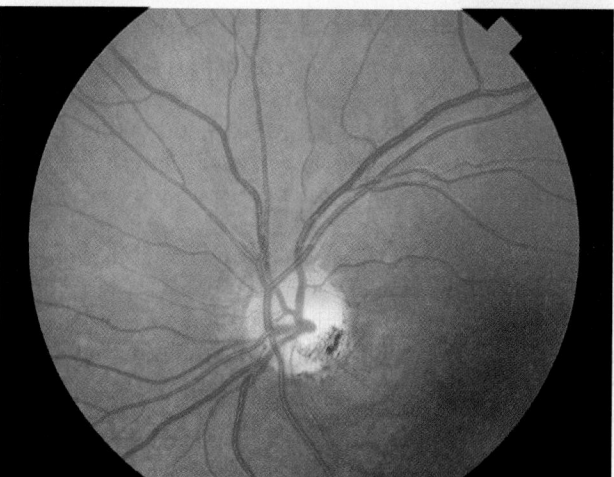

Fig. 50.1 (a) Optic disc pigmentation. Linear pigmentation concentric with the optic disc margin. (b) Optic disc pigmentation following optic neuritis.

na. These 'punched-out' defects may have anomalous reti-na and retinal pigment epithelium at their margins (Font *et al*. 1991). It occurs in girls but at least one male (47XXY) has been reported (Hopkins *et al*. 1979). *De novo* X muta-tion seems a likely explanation for the occurrence of the condition in girls and the rarity of affected family mem-bers. Molina *et al*. (1989), however, described the condition in two siblings. The optic disc may be anomalous with grey pigmentation adjacent to and involving the optic disc, usually associated with a somewhat elevated glial anomaly of the disc. The disc may be hypoplastic and associated with scleral ectasia (Carney *et al*. 1993).

A somewhat dysplastic optic disc, heavily pigmented, was described in a child with an orbital dermolipoma, cleft palate and polydactyly (Wolter *et al*. 1971).

Retinal pigment epithelial changes involving the optic disc

Retinal pigment epithelial hamartomas (Fig. 50.3) may involve the optic disc; they are densely pigmented and vascular on fluorescein angiography, with radiating folds into and dragging the surrounding retina. These hamar-tomatous lesions have been shown to be associated with neurofibromatosis type 2 (Cotlier 1977; Landau *et al*. 1990; Good *et al*. 1991). Other ocular abnormalities in NF2 include posterior subcapsular lens opacities, optic nerve sheath meningiomas, epiretinal membranes, Lisch nod-ules, optic disc glioma, medullated nerve fibres and uveal pigmented tumours (Ragge 1993).

Pigmented anomalous discs

Pigmentation, sometimes quite dense, occurs in some colobomatous and other dysplastic optic discs (Fig. 50.4).

'Congenital optic atrophy'

'Congenital optic atrophy' is not a diagnosis, but a clinical sign. Optic atrophy is distinct from optic disc hypoplasia in that the optic disc is of normal size and outline in the former, and small and misshapen in the latter. The dam-age in optic atrophy occurs after the optic disc has become fully formed.

The appearance of atrophy is due to a combination of a partial loss of the capillaries in the optic disc and loss of the refracting properties of the nerve fibres and other optic nerve tissue. The reflex from the internal limiting mem-brane of the retina highlights the vessels, which stand out indicating loss of the nerve fibre layer; the change may be diffuse or localized.

Most children who have had perinatal anoxia sufficient-ly severe to cause optic atrophy have more widespread cerebral damage (Fig. 50.5), but there are some instances where the visual pathway, especially the optic nerves, appears to be relatively selectively affected. In very pre-mature infants who have suffered early hypoxic insults there may be a combination of hypoplasia and atrophy.

Regional differences in the atrophy of an optic nerve head may indicate the presence of an associated field defect. For instance, if there is a horizontal band of optic atrophy there may well be a temporal hemianopia in that eye (see Chapter 52). Focal optic atrophy may be associat-ed with localized field defects.

Congenital vascular anomalies of or around the optic disc

Cilioretinal arteries

These are usually single, occasionally multiple, retinal vessels that arise from the ciliary circulation and appear to bend around the very margin of the optic disc (Fig. 50.6). Usually small, they are occasionally large, supplying a large proportion of the retina. Occasionally they arise in an optic disc pit. They are usually of no significance but may become selectively occluded causing infarction of the area of retina they supply or they may supply an area of retina that is spared in a central retinal artery occlusion. They may be detected by fluorescein angiography in up to 50% of the population (Justice & Lehman 1976). They occur frequently in patients with optic disc drusen (Erkki-la 1976). In patients with dysplastic discs the cilioretinal vessels may be multiple (Barosso *et al*. 1991).

Opticociliary veins and other venous abnormalities

These are veins which connect the intraocular retinal venous system via the choroidal veins to the vortex veins.

They are occasionally found in high myopia or in other-wise anomalous optic disc and are usually of no signifi-cance. They occur after chronic obstruction of the central retinal vein due to shunting of blood from the retinal to the choroidal veins via the peripapillary capillary plexus (Fig. 50.6b). The capillaries enlarge and become venous channels. Disc edge veins of Kraupa are rare anomalies where blood flows from the retina via a single large vein at the disc margin (Barroso *et al*. 1992).

Situs inversus

These are tilted optic discs occurring usually in high myopes with posterior staphylomas (Fig. 50.7) in which the vessels are distorted by being dragged towards the staphyloma.

Haemangiomas of the optic disc

Capillary haemangiomas are rare tumours, occurring

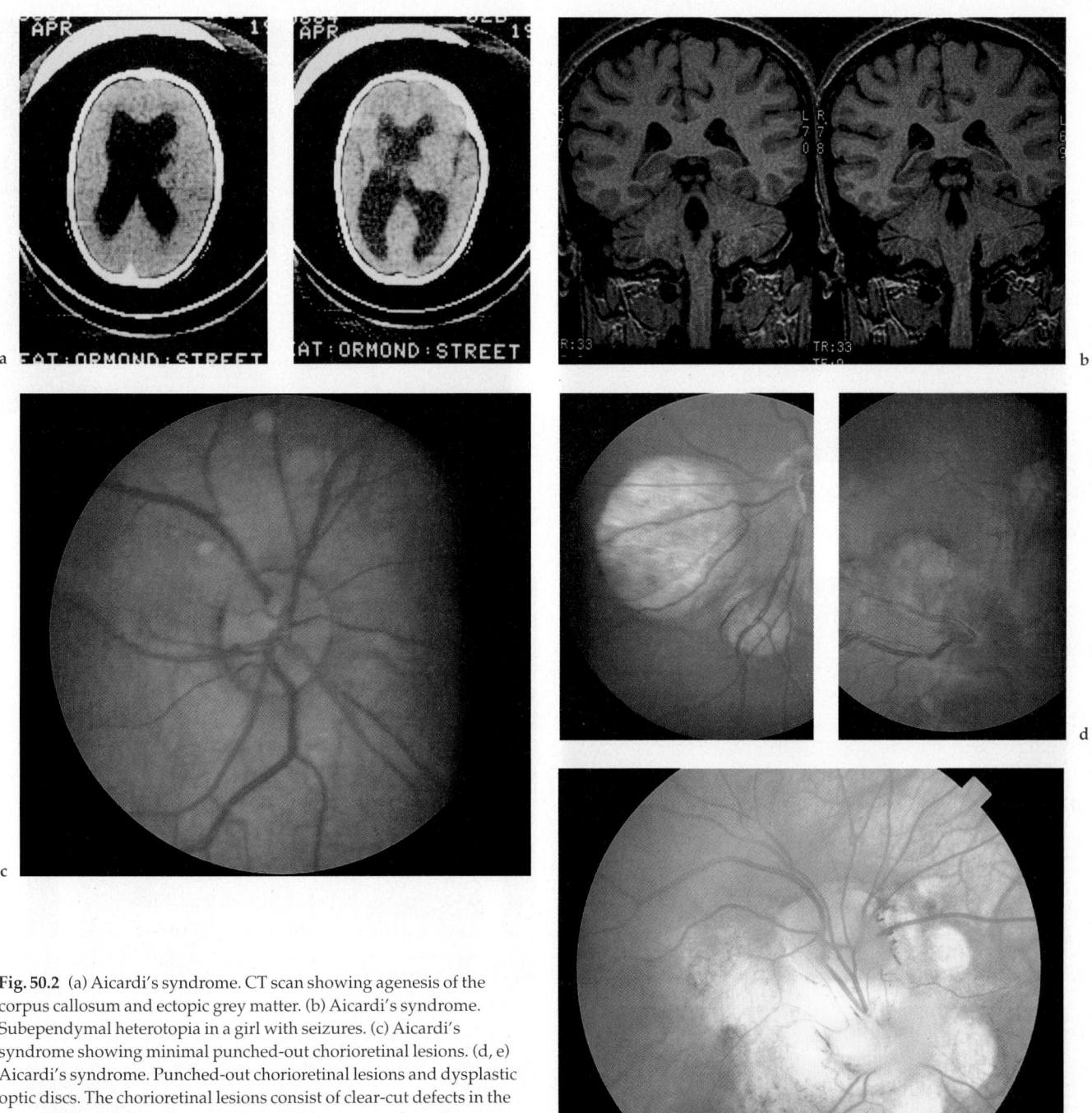

Fig. 50.2 (a) Aicardi's syndrome. CT scan showing agenesis of the corpus callosum and ectopic grey matter. (b) Aicardi's syndrome. Subependymal heterotopia in a girl with seizures. (c) Aicardi's syndrome showing minimal punched-out chorioretinal lesions. (d, e) Aicardi's syndrome. Punched-out chorioretinal lesions and dysplastic optic discs. The chorioretinal lesions consist of clear-cut defects in the retinal pigment epithelium with the neural retina overlying it intact and the underlying choroid being abnormal allowing sclera to show through more clearly.

either alone (Fig. 50.8) or in association with the von Hippel–Lindau syndrome.

They may be sharply defined, reddish, spherical knobs of tumour or diffuse orange-coloured tumours that may involve the juxta-papillary retina (Gass & Braunstein 1980). Visual loss with symptoms of blurring and distortion can occur from the formation of exudates and intraretinal or subretinal fluid.

From the literature, untreated tumours seem to show

growth and to be associated with a high incidence of visual complications; treatment, however, is fraught with problems. Schindler *et al.* (1975) believed (in the days before computed tomography (CT) scan) that an isolated disc haemangioma, diagnosed by fluorescein angiography was not an indication for further neuroradiological studies since without associated retinal lesions they are not usually part of a systemic syndrome. The advent of non-invasive scanning means that it is safer to investigate

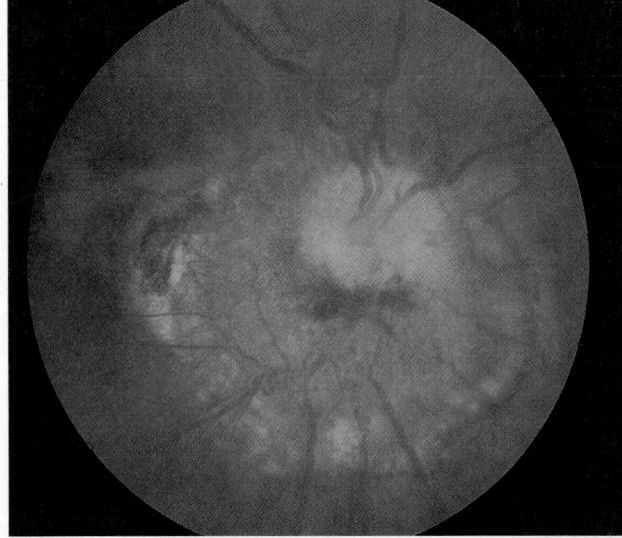

Fig. 50.3 Retinal pigment epithelial hamartoma involving the optic disc with pigmentation.

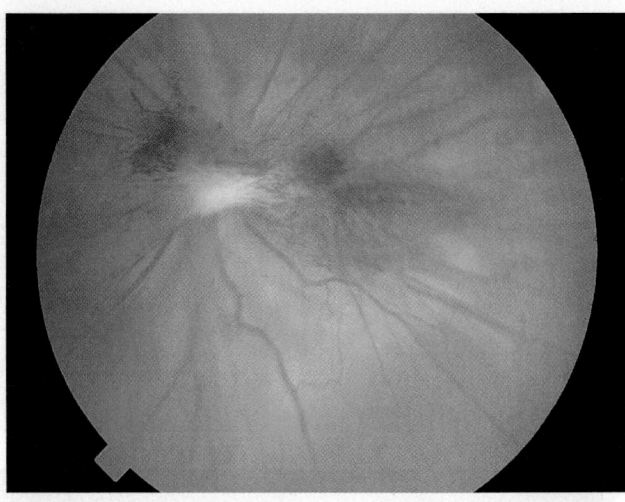

Fig. 50.4 An anomalous dysplastic disc with a surrounding pigment epithelial defect.

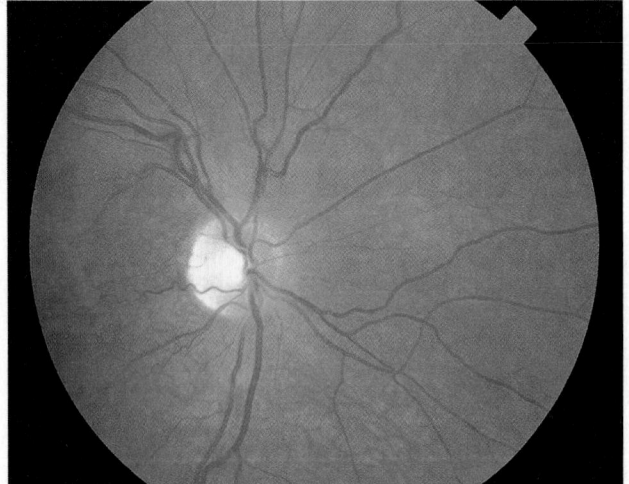

a

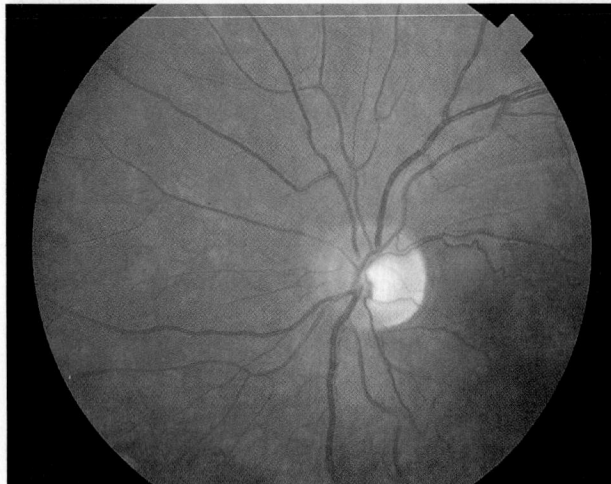

b

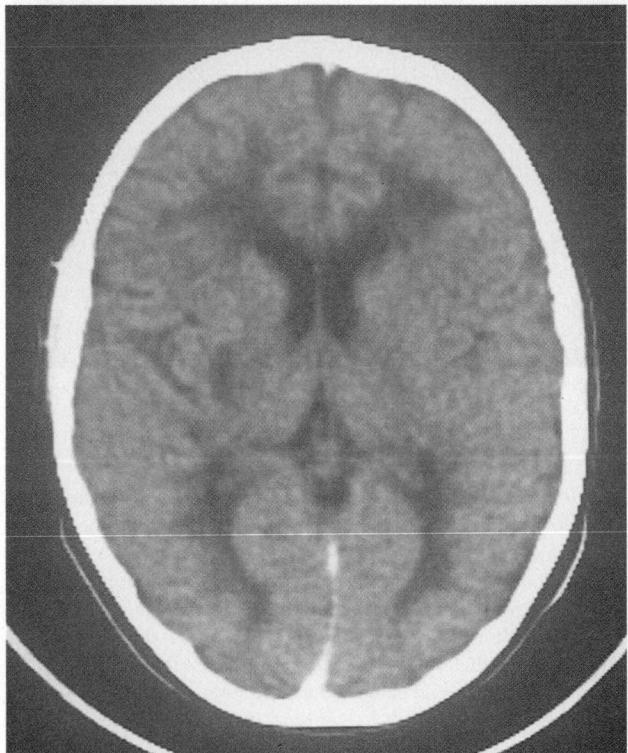

c

Fig. 50.5 (a, b) Bilateral optic atrophy in a child who had had profound perinatal anoxia. (c) Widespread periventricular lucency (same patient). When optic atrophy occurs after perinatal anoxia, there is usually damage to other areas or the central nervous system.

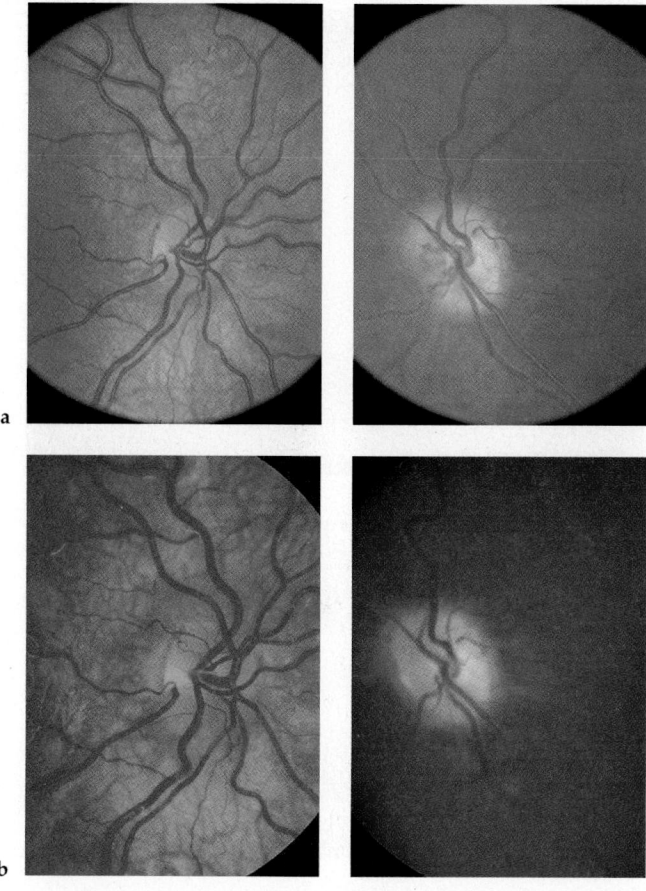

Vitreous haemorrhage may occur, associated with trauma (Yap & Buettner 1992).

Bergmeister's papilla most frequently appears as a small blue–white or grey conical elevation in front of the optic disc. It has no functional or pathological significance. Sometimes the glial element can be quite large, but the retinal vessels are not involved. They may be part of a more widespread hyaloid vascular abnormality (Fig. 50.11).

Rarely, vascular loops (Fig. 50.12), sometimes corkscrew in shape, project forwards from the optic disc, occasionally quite far into the vitreous cavity where they sometimes

Fig. 50.6 (a) Cilioretinal arteries and opticociliary veins. In the right eye there is a cilioretinal artery in the inferotemporal quadrant. This patient had a chiasmal and left optic nerve glioma and the left eye shows opticociliary shunt vessels. (b) The right eye now shows papilloedema in the upper and lower pole of the optic disc which conforms with the temporal defect in this eye (known as twin peaks papilloedema). The left eye has a totally atrophic optic nerve and the shunt vessels have disappeared (same patient 2 years later).

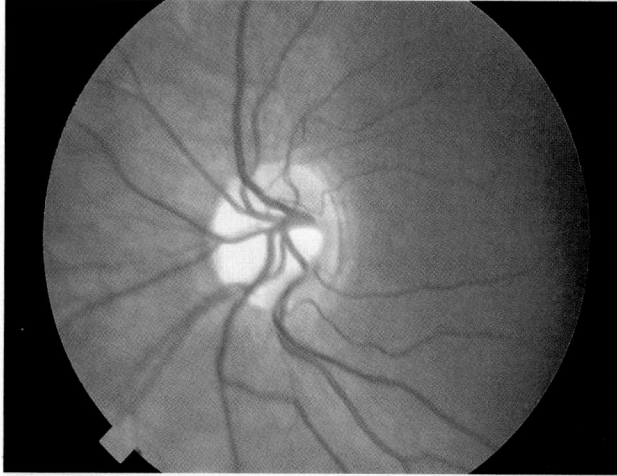

Fig. 50.7 Situs inversus (see text).

these patients and this should be carried out as part of screening for von Hippel–Lindau disease (see Chapter 61).

Cavernous haemangiomas are lobulated, dark-red hamartomas usually involving both disc and peripapillary retina. They may be familial (autosomal dominant) (Goldbert *et al.* 1979) and associated with intracranial abnormalities. They may bleed spontaneously (Haller & Knox 1993).

Bergmeister's papilla and pre-papillary vascular loops

These not uncommon abnormalities are remnants of the hyaloid vessels and their glial supporting structures (Figs 50.9, 50.10), which regress between the seventh and ninth month of gestation (Apple *et al.* 1982). They may therefore be seen in premature babies as a normal feature.

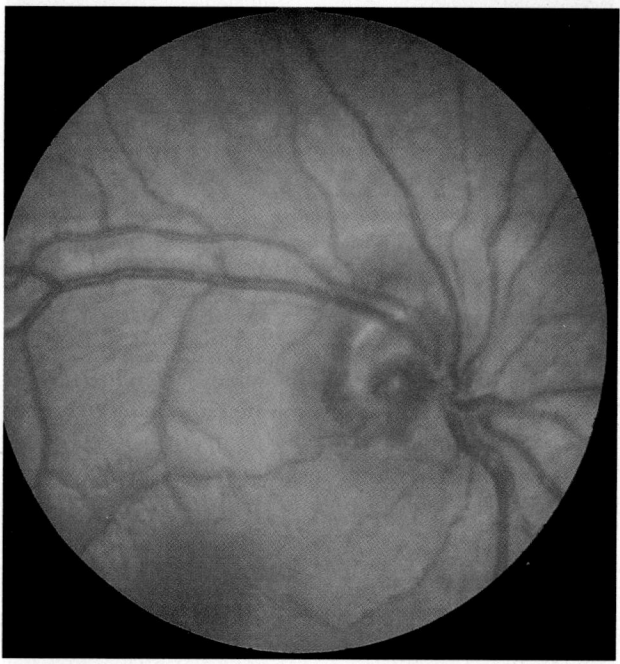

Fig. 50.8 Optic disc haemangioma in a normal child, who presented with a squint.

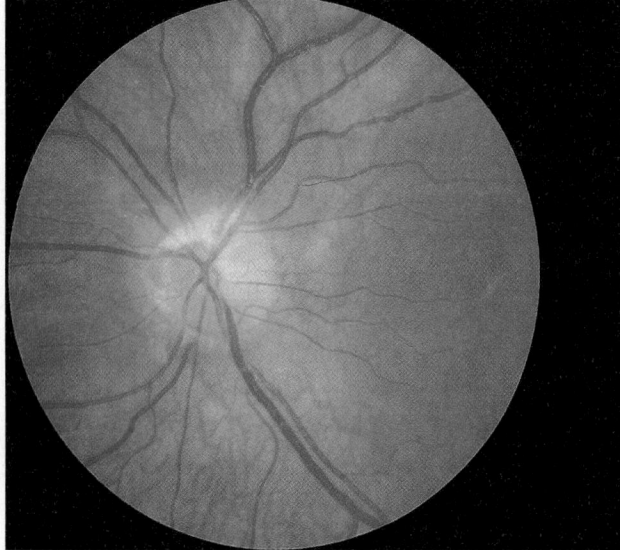

Fig. 50.9 Bergmeister's papilla in a patient suspected of having raised intracranial pressure with headaches. There was no other abnormality found.

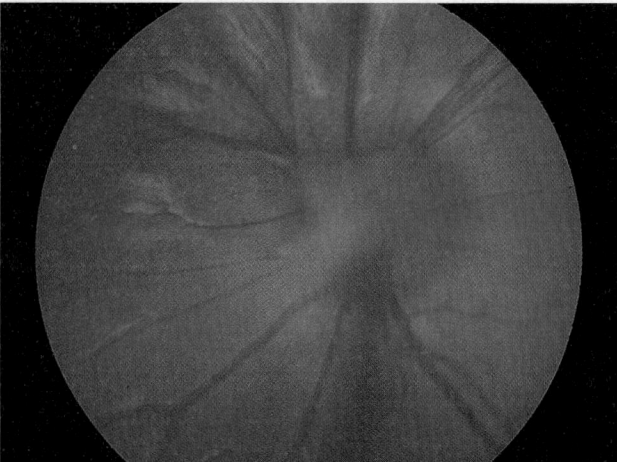

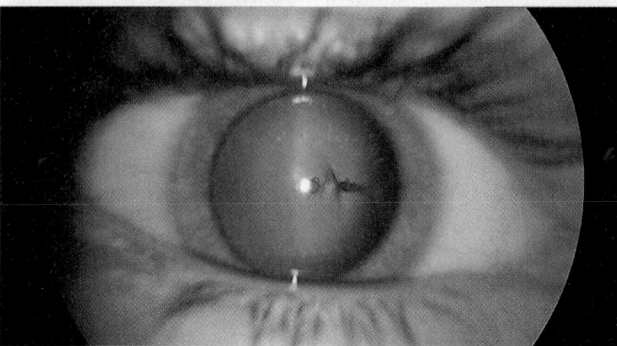

Fig. 50.11 (a) A glial vascular anomaly associated with a persistent hyaloid artery and retinal abnormalities. (b) The hyaloid artery can be seen extending to the posterior surface of the lens (same patient).

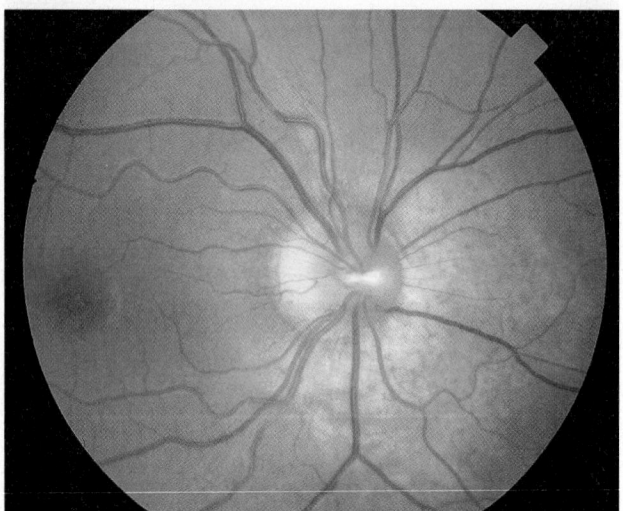

Fig. 50.10 Bergmeister's papilla showing a more or less solid glial elevation above the optic disc.

pulsate with each heartbeat (Degenhart *et al.* 1981). Generally of no local pathological or systemic significance, they have been documented to obstruct in adults with disastrous consequences for the (usually inferior) retinal arteriole which they may supply (Brown *et al.* 1979). Purely venous loops also occur (Degenhart *et al.* 1981).

Other vascular anomalies

Patients with Down's syndrome have an unusual number of vessels crossing the optic disc, sometimes in a spoke-like arrangement (Williams *et al.* 1973). Children with

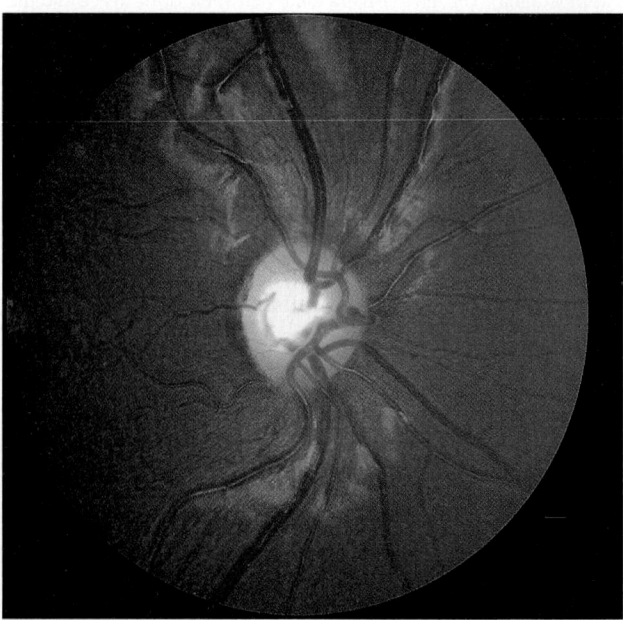

Fig. 50.12 Cork-screw prepapillary vascular loop.

Down's syndrome may have transient disc swelling of unknown cause (Catalano & Simon 1990). The disc vessels are also abnormal in the Wyburn–Mason syndrome (see Chapter 61) and in the Klippel–Trenaunay–Weber syndrome (asymmetrical limb hypertrophy with mixed haemangiomas of skin and deep tissue, sometimes with arteriovenous fistulae) where affected patients may have telangiectatic vessels around the disc (O'Connor & Smith 1978). A variety of other unusual arteriovenous malformations and tortuous vessels have also been described (Kottow 1978).

Myelinated nerve fibres

Myelination of the optic nerve begins during fetal life at the lateral geniculate body and reaches the optic disc around the time of birth. Normally the myelin does not extend anterior to the cribriform plate, but in about 1% of the population (Straatsma *et al.* 1981) the myelination may reach the retina. The most common appearance, slightly more frequent in males, is of a unilateral, feathery white opacity usually adjacent to (Fig. 50.13) but occasionally away from the optic disc. There may be a field defect related to the size and site of the myelinated fibres, but generally central vision is normal. Although most often they occur in normal eyes, they have been found with a variety of ocular malformations. There is an association between widespread myelinated fibres (Fig. 50.14), high myopia and amblyopia (Levy & Ernest 1974; Straatsma *et al.* 1981). Although the prognosis for the amblyopia is usually very poor even in compliant children, occasional good results have been reported (Summers *et al.* 1991). Myelinated fibres may atrophy after an optic neuropathy, with resolu-

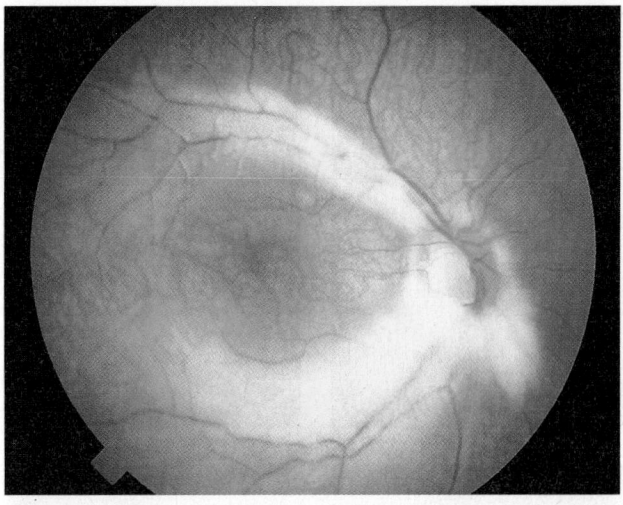

Fig. 50.14 Extensive myelinated nerve fibres associated with amblyopia and high myopia (see text).

tion of at least part of the myelinated area (Schachat & Miller 1981), and have been recorded to develop in postnatal life (Baarsma 1980; Ali *et al.* 1994). Patients with myelinated fibres are usually otherwise normal, though an association has been reported with craniofacial dysostoses (Franceschetti 1938) and in the Gorlin autosomal dominant multiple basal cell carcinoma syndrome (DeJong *et al.* 1985). Traboulsi *et al.* (1993) described a mother and daughter with a severe vitreoretinal degeneration, high myopia and extensive myelination. Their electroretinograms (ERG) were abnormal. The daughter also had limb reduction deformities. The cause and origin of myelinated nerve fibres is uncertain (Bellhom *et al.* 1979; Straatsma *et al.* 1981).

Drusen

Drusen (hyaline bodies) of the optic discs is probably the result of a congenital anomaly of the optic discs, either a vascular anomaly (Sachs *et al.* 1977) or due to the smallness of the optic nerve head (Rosenberg *et al.* 1979; Mullie & Sanders 1985) giving rise to a disturbance of axoplasmic transport with axonal degeneration (Spencer 1978). Rare in childhood, they may become quite common in the elderly and were found in between 3.4 (Lorentzen 1966) and 20 (Friedman *et al.* 1975) per 1000. Drusen may be composed of axoplasmic products (Avendano *et al.* 1980; Woodford & Tso 1980) giving rise to the appearance of a swollen optic disc, often mistaken for papilloedema. Drusen are bilateral in 75% of cases (Lorentzen 1966).

Children with drusen usually present with non-specific complaints not directly related to the optic disc itself (Erkkila 1974). Occasionally the presentation is related to haemorrhagic or other complications.

Drusen may be inherited as an autosomal dominant

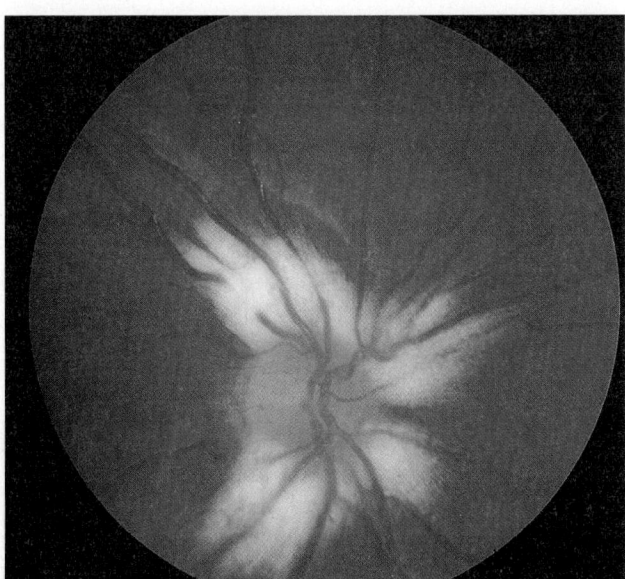

Fig. 50.13 Myelinated nerve fibres adjacent to the optic disc.

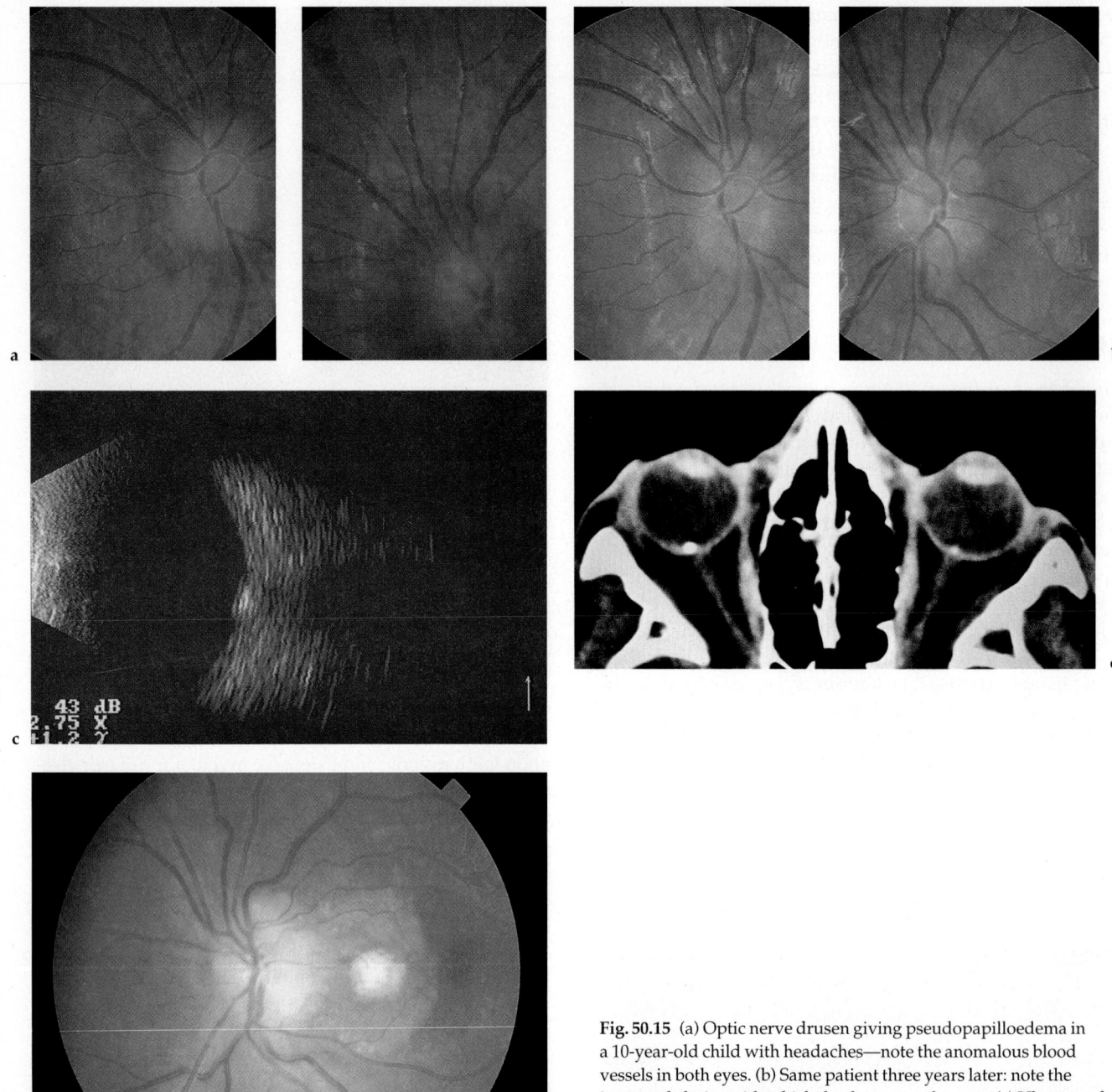

Fig. 50.15 (a) Optic nerve drusen giving pseudopapilloedema in a 10-year-old child with headaches—note the anomalous blood vessels in both eyes. (b) Same patient three years later: note the increased clarity with which the drusen can be seen. (c) Ultrasound showing echogenicity of calcified drusen. (d) CT scan showing high signal from calcified drusen. (e) Peripapillary disciform lesion following a haemorrhage related to drusen.

trait (Lorentzen 1966) and both parents should be examined when the anomaly is suspected.

In childhood the drusen are not usually visible at first, but the disc has a 'lumpy' appearance (Fig. 50.15). There is frequently an anomalous vascular pattern (Erkkila 1974), including the presence of trifurcations of vessels (Rosenberg *et al.* 1979). The optic disc capillaries are not dilated and do not leak fluorescein as they do in true papilloedema. The drusen may exhibit autofluorescence and glow

when illuminated with a blue light before the injection of fluorescein. The peripapillary nerve fibres are normal in drusen, but enlarged in true papilloedema. Haemorrhages are not uncommon and are most often crescentic, appearing at the edge of the disc, in the subretinal layer, but most types of disc haemorrhage can occur (Harris *et al.* 1981), including small linear superficial disc haemorrhages (Sanders *et al.* 1971). Disciform lesions also occur (Fig. 50.15e).

Visual field defects may be detected in older children and these may be progressive (Savino *et al.* 1979), but loss of acuity should only with caution be attributed to the drusen. The field defects include enlarged blind spots (Hoover *et al.* 1988) and, when the drusen are visible, nerve fibre bundle defects (Savino *et al.* 1979) and inferior nasal defects. The buried drusen of childhood become exposed in the late teens (Hoover *et al.* 1988).

In many cases there seems to be a slowly progressive optic neuropathy with a relatively good prognosis in the absence of serious haemorrhagic complications. Drusen occur in patients with retinitis pigmentosa (Robertson 1972) and other degenerative eye diseases but are not associated with tuberous sclerosis (in which the 'giant drusen' are a form of hamartoma) or with other phakomatoses. They have been described in hypotelorism (Awan 1977), mandibulofacial dysostoses (Collier 1958) and many ocular diseases (François & Veriest 1958).

The calcium in drusen can be detected by ultrasound (Kheterpal *et al.* 1995), or CT scanning (Frisen *et al.* 1978) (Fig. 50.15c,d) and is characteristically punctate, well defined and confined to the disc (Bec *et al.* 1984). Ultrasound is the less expensive and less invasive option.

The differential diagnosis between drusen and true papilloedema is very difficult in many cases: not many experienced neuro-ophthalmologists would claim infallibility, here more than in other areas!

Pseudopapilloedema (conditions mimicking papilloedema)

Only rarely are patients with myelinated nerve fibres (MNF) (Fig. 50.16) referred to an ophthalmologist in the mistaken belief that they have papilloedema, because the condition is now so widely recognized, but it can be very difficult in patients who have both MNF and raised intracranial pressure. Drusen, however, is often testing, even for experienced ophthalmologists most of whom have personal reasons for humility in this area! Substantially hypermetropic eyes may have small crowded optic discs and in myopes with a tilted optic disc or situs inversus the nasal edge may be indistinct due to an overlaying of the retina across the disc margin. Glial anomalies and Bergmeister's papilla (see Fig. 50.10) may also give rise to the false appearance of swelling. All of these conditions have a normal peripapillary plexus and normal nerve fibre layer, and they may have venous pulsation at the disc which, even if it is unilateral, means that raised intracranial pressure is unlikely.

Papilloedema in children

Papilloedema is optic disc swelling associated with raised

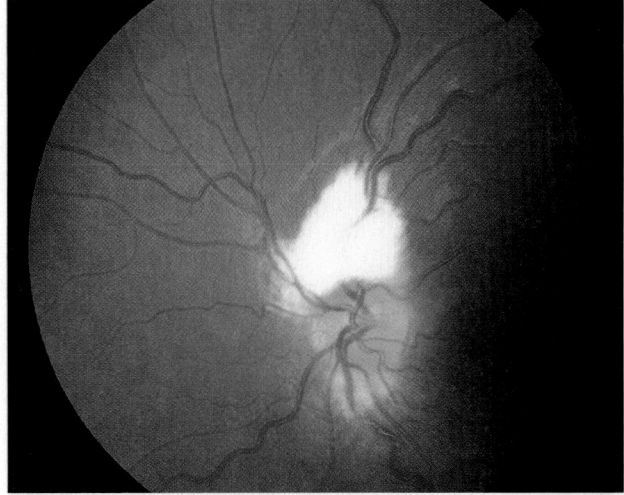
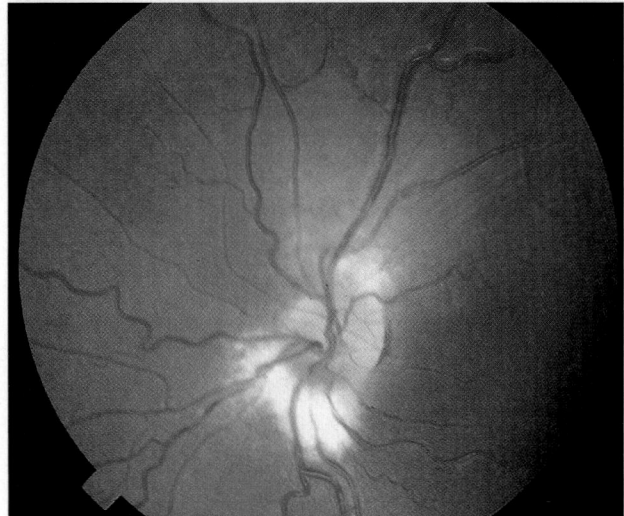

Fig. 50.16 Bilateral peripapillary myelinated nerve fibres in a patient with hydrocephalus which was mistaken for papilloedema.

intracranial pressure. The vision is usually normal, even when the discs are markedly swollen although in later or very severe cases there may be a progressive loss of visual function (Fig. 50.17). The swelling comprises congested neurones and dilated blood vessels and these spread into the surrounding tissues causing retinal disturbance and choroidal folds. A hypermetropic refractive error is induced by the raised retina, and enlargement of the blind spot is noted on visual field testing (Corbett *et al.* 1988). An enlarged blind spot also occurs in optic nerve infiltration, developmental anomalies, trauma, as part of a centrocaecal scotoma or as an event of presumed retinal origin in an otherwise normal optic disc (Fletcher *et al.* 1988). If visual loss is progressive nerve fibre bundle field defects and peripheral constriction occur.

The earliest signs of papilloedema (Fig. 50.18) include a blurring of the disc margins, an elevated disc, a dilated

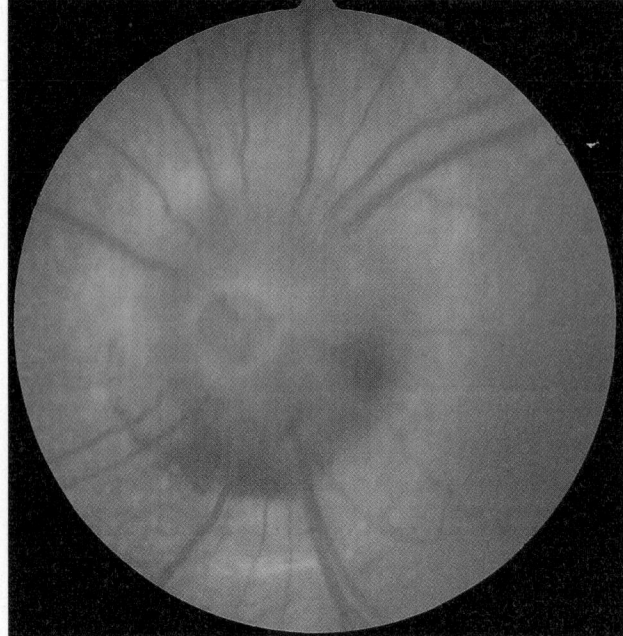

Fig. 50.17 Anomalous optic disc (unilateral) in a patient presenting with headaches suspected of having unilateral papilloedema by the referring doctor.

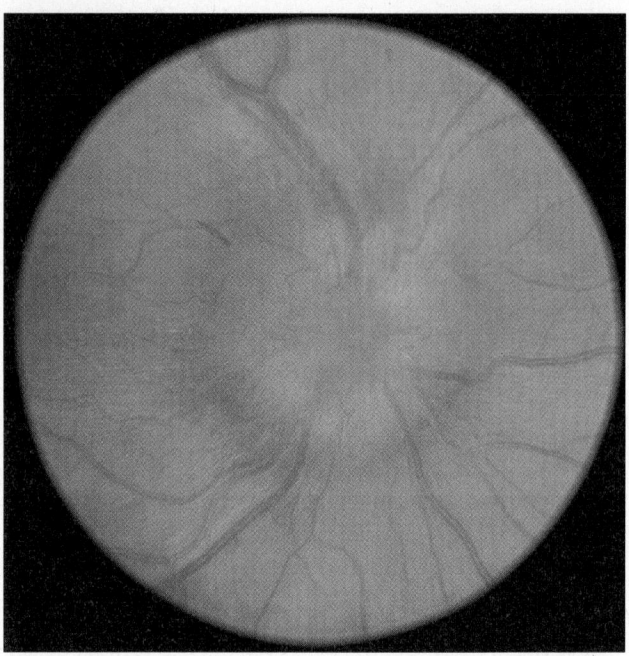

Fig. 50.19 Papilloedema secondary to raised intracranial pressure—note the elevated disc, swollen nerve fibre layer, dilated veins and small haemorrhages radiating around the disc.

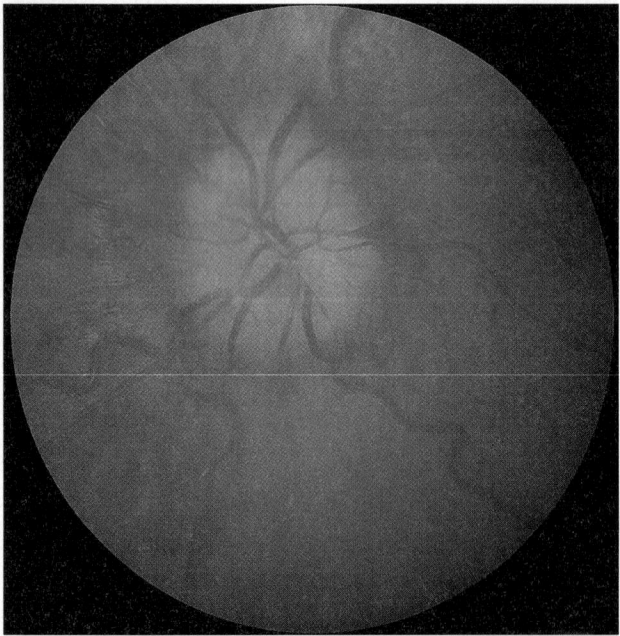

Fig. 50.18 Papilloedema in a patient with craniosynostosis—note the elevated optic disc and tortuous dilated veins.

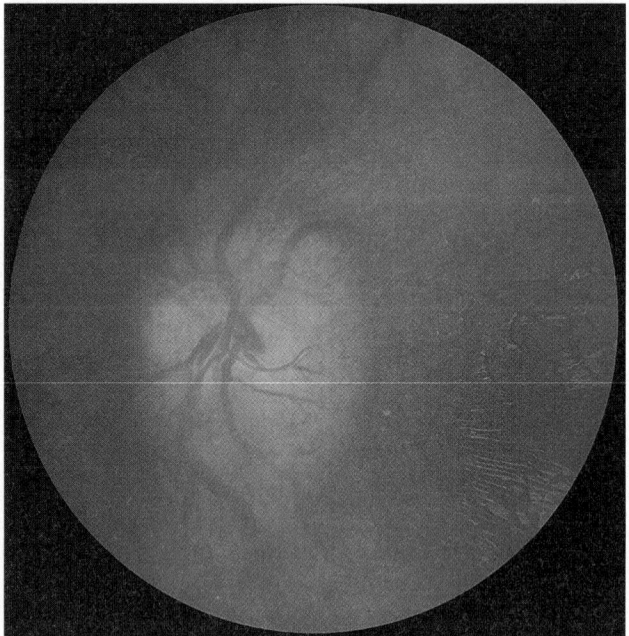

Fig. 50.20 Papilloedema in a patient with neurofibromatosis and a chiasmal glioma. The swelling of the optic disc with dilated veins, haemorrhages, a few exudates and dilated capillaries, is most marked in the upper and lower poles. This eye has a temporal hemianopia and the fibres that are swollen are those subserving the intact nasal field. The horizontal band of relative lack of swelling is in the area of the disc that is atrophic from loss of nerve fibres. The superior poles, although also atrophic, are covered by the fibres from the intact nasal field.

peripapillary capillary plexus, dilated retinal veins with absent pulsation at the optic disc, and swollen nerve fibre bundles.

Splinter haemorrhages (Fig. 50.19), a more markedly

elevated disc (Fig. 50.20), nerve fibre infarcts ('cotton-wool spots'), exudates and macular star formation (Fig. 50.21) follow. The retinal and disc capillaries become more engorged and tortuous and haemorrhages more widespread (Fig. 50.22).

Children with a chronic but mildly raised intracranial pressure (as in craniosynostosis) may have papilloedema for many years without loss of vision, the predominant clinical dilemma being the decision of whether the papilloedema is or will be associated with neuronal loss. If the

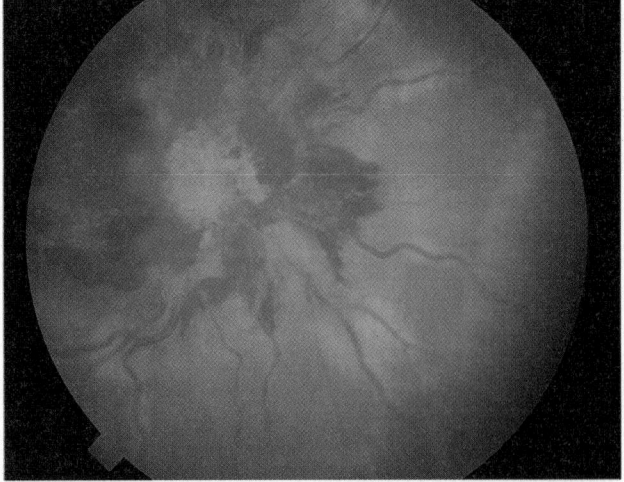

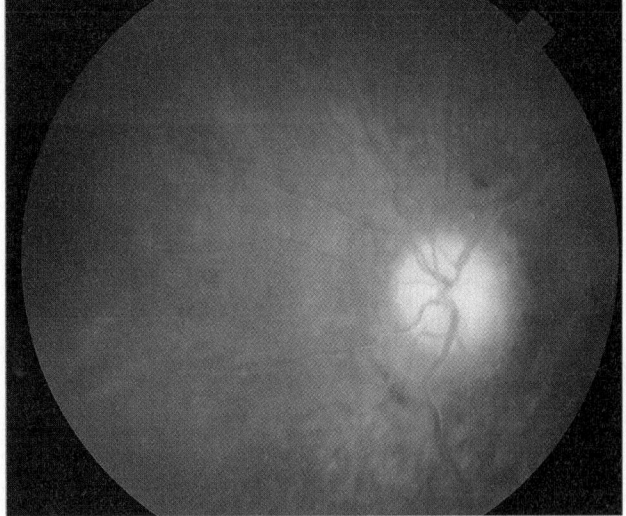

Fig. 50.22 (a) Severe papilloedema with widespread haemorrhages. (b) The optic nerve has decompensated and there is marked consecutive optic atrophy. The eye is blind. The 7-year-old child had severe papilloedema due to a posterior fossa tumour (same eye).

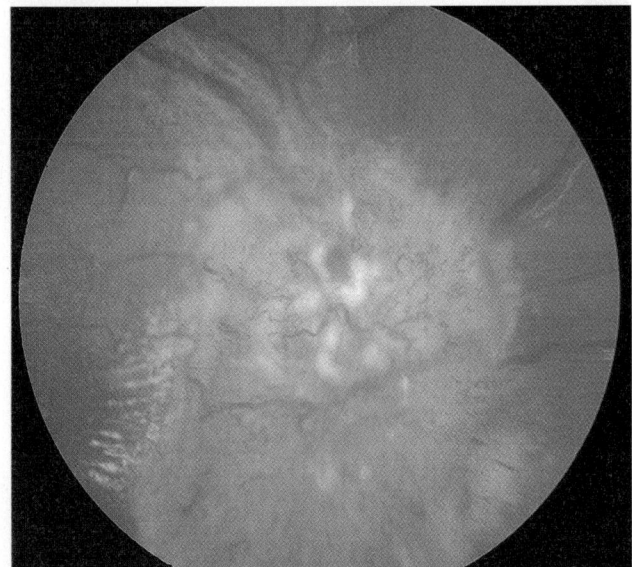

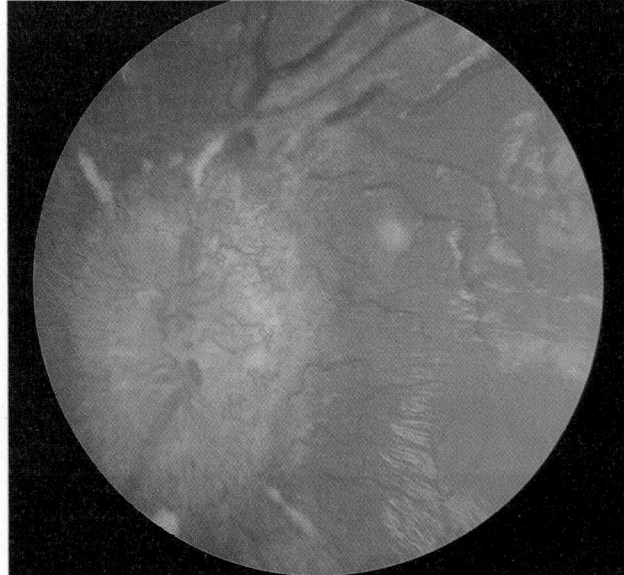

Fig. 50.21 (a) Severe papilloedema with gross elevation, haemorrhages, exudates, macular star, dilated veins and cotton-wool spots on the optic disc. (b) Same patient. The left eye is less affected. Asymmetry is frequent in papilloedema and may be due to anomalous optic nerve sheaths.

intracranial pressure is very high there is a progressive loss of neurones, accompanied by increasingly frequent visual symptoms. Optic atrophy (see Fig. 50.22) ensues as the neurones die, the disc becoming flat again after a period of being swollen and pale.

The symptoms are those of headache and episodic visual loss in the form of posture-related obscurations which consist of seconds long black-outs or grey-outs. In many children, for instance with long-standing shunted hydrocephalus in which the shunt is malfunctioning, there are very few symptoms of progressive visual loss. When there is likely to be visual loss reliance needs to be placed on acuity, colour vision and visual field examinations supplemented by serial pattern visual evoked potential (VEP) studies, CT scanning and intracranial pressure monitoring but so often the child is unco-operative and difficult to test that it is inevitable that some patients will be less than optimally managed. For management of papilloedema see Chapters 53 and P17.

Swollen optic disc in childhood

Bilateral

1 Papilloedema:
  • raised intracranial pressure;
  • hydrocephalus;
  • benign intracranial hypertension (pseudotumour cerebri).
2 Hypertension.
3 Papillitis (optic neuritis).
4 Bilateral cases of unilateral causes of unilateral disc oedema or pseudopapilloedema.

Unilateral

1 Pseudopapilloedema:
  • drusen;
  • myelinated nerve fibres;
  • hypermetropia;
  • myopia;
  • glial anomalies.
2 Tumours:
  • haemangioma;
  • mulberry tumour of tuberous sclerosis (Fig. 50.23);
  • retinal hamartoma (see Fig. 50.3);

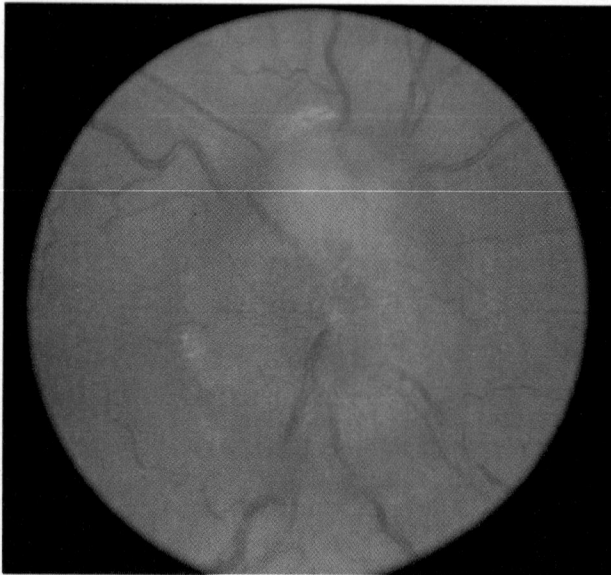

Fig. 50.23 Papilloedema in a child with tuberous sclerosis and hydrocephalus. Note that at the superior pole there is a phakoma which gave rise to a form of pseudopapilloedema in addition to the papilloedematous swelling of the optic disc.

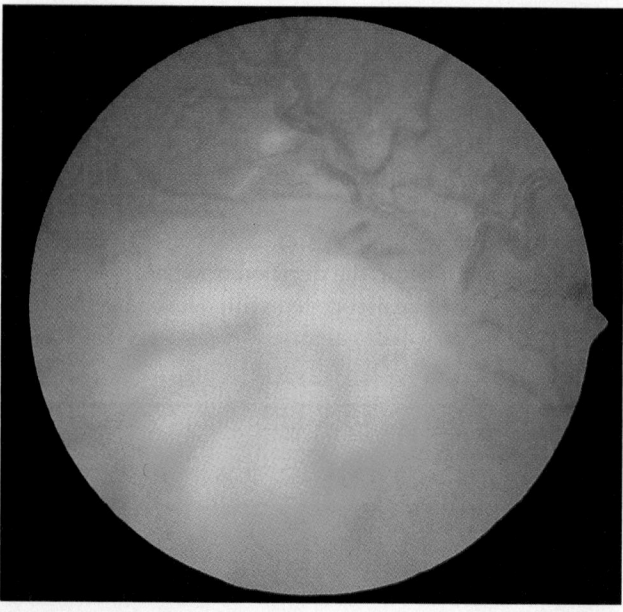

Fig. 50.24 Optic nerve involvement with glioma.

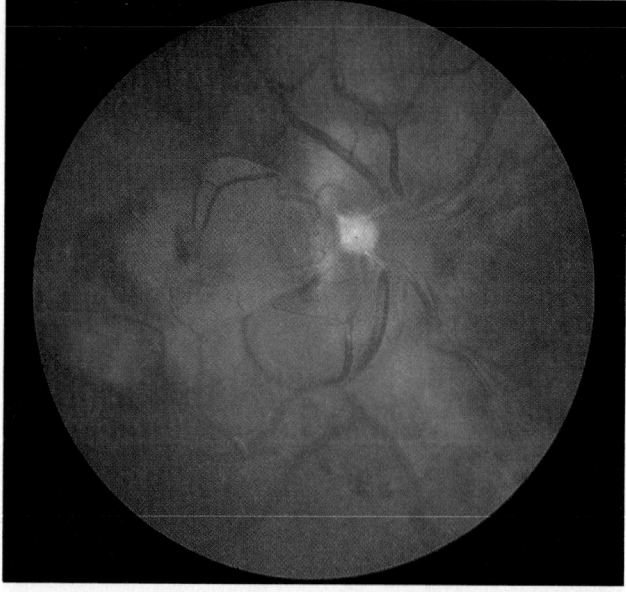

Fig. 50.25 *Toxocara* involving the optic disc. At presentation there was a marked uveitis and swelling of the optic disc obscuring all details.

  • retinoblastoma;
  • optic nerve glioma with or without disc invasion (Fig. 50.24);
  • leukaemia;
3 Uveitis:
  • *Toxocara* involving the disc (Fig. 50.25);
  • swollen disc secondary to intraocular inflammation and hypotony (Fig. 50.26);
4 Ischaemic optic neuropathy.

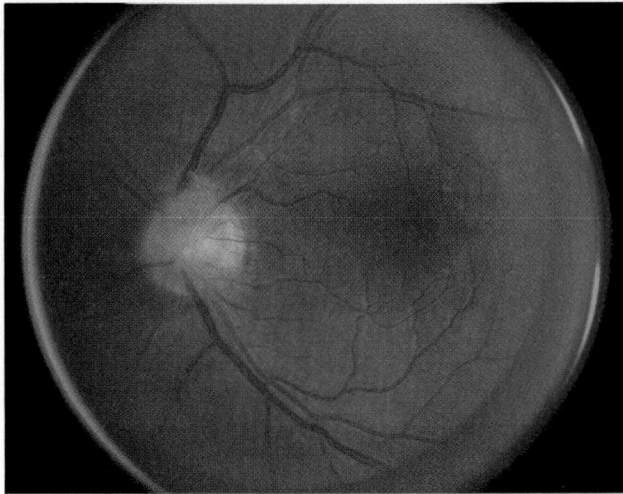

Fig. 50.26 Uveitis with optic disc swelling.

5 Papillitis.
6 Papilloedema.

Papilloedema may be highly asymmetrical due to unilateral acquired or congenital lesions preventing papilloedema in one optic disc.

Optic nerve aplasia

Optic nerve aplasia is a very rare condition in which the optic nerve and, most importantly, its vessels are absent (Yanoff *et al.* 1978). Many of the reported cases have been found on pathological examination for associated ocular anomalies (Hotchkiss & Greene 1970; Weiter *et al.* 1977) including microphthalmos (Margo *et al.* 1992), retinal dysplasia, coloboma, sclerocornea and cataract. Clinical descriptions of true optic nerve aplasia are few (Duke-Elder 1964; Renelt 1972) and clinicopathological correlation (Yanoff *et al.* 1978) even rarer, but they show that the condition is usually unilateral, and is often associated with other central nervous system defects (Blanco *et al.* 1992). The eyes are blind and have no direct pupil reaction to light. The fundus, apart from the absence of disc, vessels and retina, may appear normal or there may be other defects including lacunar retinal defects (Fig. 50.27) (Renelt 1972; Little *et al.* 1976).

Optic nerve hypoplasia

The paucity of early reports (Cords 1923; Ridley 1938; Boyce 1941; Scheie & Adler 1941; Jerome & Forster 1948; Somerville 1962; Edwards & Laydon 1970) suggested that optic nerve hypoplasia was a very rare congenital anomaly, but paediatric ophthalmologists in hospital practice see several new cases each year and it is a significant cause of blindness in childhood, possibly with an increasing incidence (Jan *et al.* 1977; Hoyt & Good 1992).

Presentation

Bilateral severe optic nerve hypoplasia presents as blindness in early infancy with roving eye movements and sluggish pupil reactions. Lesser degrees of bilateral hypoplasia may cause minor visual defects or squint at any time in childhood and may even be found without symptoms at a routine test. Unilateral optic nerve hypoplasia (Figs 50.28, 50.29) usually presents as a squint with a relative afferent pupil defect and unsteady fixation in the affected eye. The eye movement defect may resemble 'see-saw' nystagmus (Davis & Schoch 1975). Amblyopia may contribute to the poor visual acuity and especially if the discs are not markedly hypoplastic the vision may improve with patching (Kushner 1984). Astigmatism may be a frequent association.

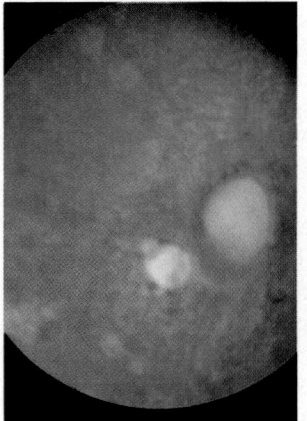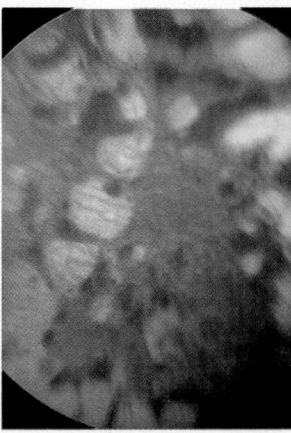

Fig. 50.27 Optic nerve aplasia with chorioretinal defects. In the right eye (left picture) there was an optic nerve aperture visible, but none was found in the left eye (right picture).

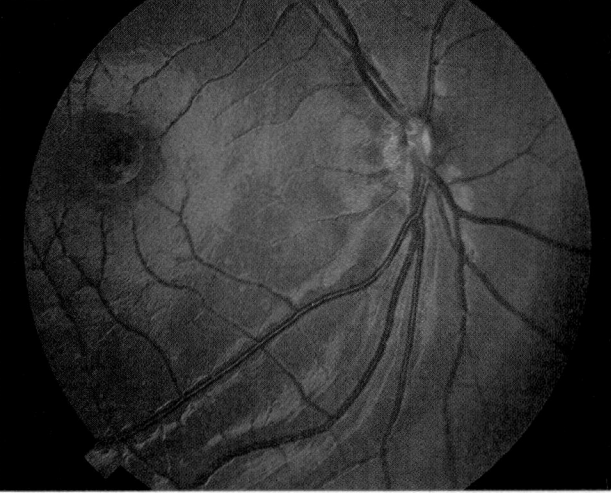

Fig. 50.28 Severe optic nerve hypoplasia with profound retinal nerve fibre layer atrophy.

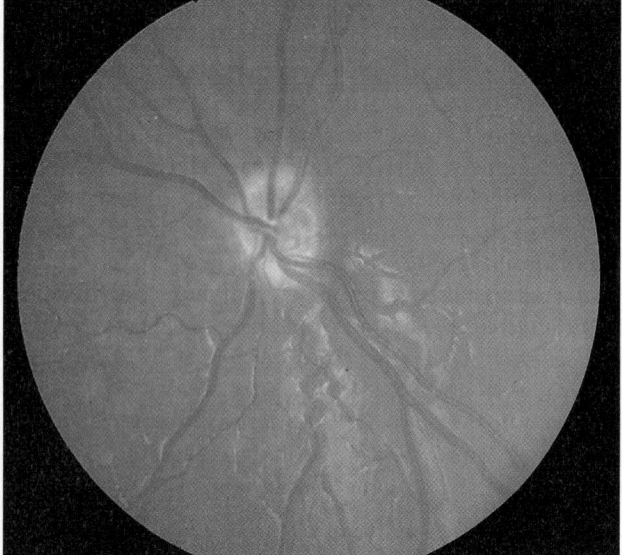

Fig. 50.29 Severe optic nerve hypoplasia with a wide surround of white sclera given by a larger defect in the retinal pigment epithelium than the hypoplastic optic nerve itself. This child had previously been diagnosed as having optic atrophy, but direct ophthalmoscopy revealed the true nature of the disorder.

Affected patients may present because of failure to thrive in infancy or as a result of a variety of endocrine disorders (Skarf & Hoyt 1984; Stanhope *et al.* 1984), such as hypothyroidism, growth hormone deficiency, or neonatal hypoglycaemia.

Hypoplastic discs occur more frequently in males than females, and probably without racial predilection (Zion 1976). The parents of children with optic disc hypoplasia tend to be young primiparae (Elster & McArnarney 1979; Purdy & Friend 1979). Less frequently, children present because of the abnormalities from the associated brain defects.

Small optic discs, not necessarily hypoplastic, may be a significant predisposing factor for ischaemic optic neuropathy, even in young children (see Chapter 51).

Ophthalmoscopic appearance

The recognition of optic disc hypoplasia should alert the doctor to the associated problems which may arise during development. The diagnosis in the extreme case is not usually difficult; the true disc substance is minute and often only identifiable as a slightly pink–yellow area from which the retinal vessels emerge. This area is surrounded by an area of exposed sclera which is roughly circular and appears to represent the area of the gap in the retinal pigment epithelium that is present when the disc is of normal size. Sometimes there is proliferation of the retinal pigment epithelium on this normally white ring, but more usually there is a small rim of pigment around part of the

margin of the white area. The temporal retinal vessels are often rather straighter than is usual in childhood, although Walton and Robb (1970) noticed that some of their cases had tortuous vessels. The retinal nerve fibre layer is variably thinned (Figs 50.28–50.31) (Whinery & Blodi 1963; Manor & Korkzyn 1976), and if the hypoplasia is segmental this thinning is also segmental. It is the white ring of sclera that is so often confused for a normal sized, but atrophic disc and this mistake is more easily made by those who use only indirect ophthalmoscopy.

The chief difficulty in diagnosis arises when optic disc hypoplasia is anything less than extreme. Frisen & Holmegaard (1978) pointed out that there was a very wide variation in the appearance of hypoplastic optic discs and that their effect on vision is also widely variable; hypoplasia is a non-specific manifestation of damage to the visual

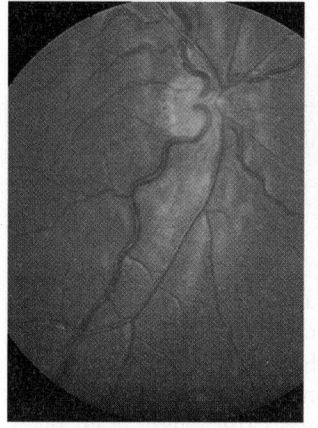 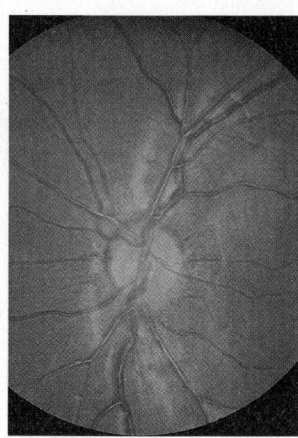

Fig. 50.30 Unilateral optic nerve hypoplasia. Although unilateral, even if there is no CT scan abnormality, these children must be followed throughout their childhood for growth defects (see text).

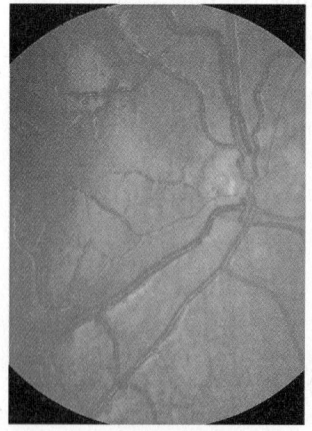 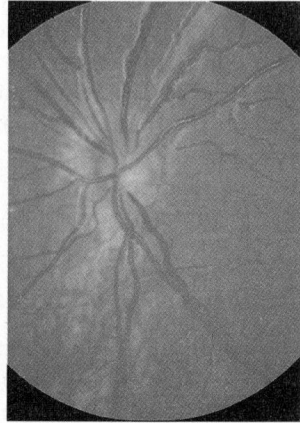

Fig. 50.31 Bilateral asymmetrical optic nerve hypoplasia, which presented at birth as strabismus and nystagmus. The right eye is blind, but the left eye, despite significant optic nerve hypoplasia, has 6/9 acuity and a useful visual field: in 1995 the patient passed her driving test.

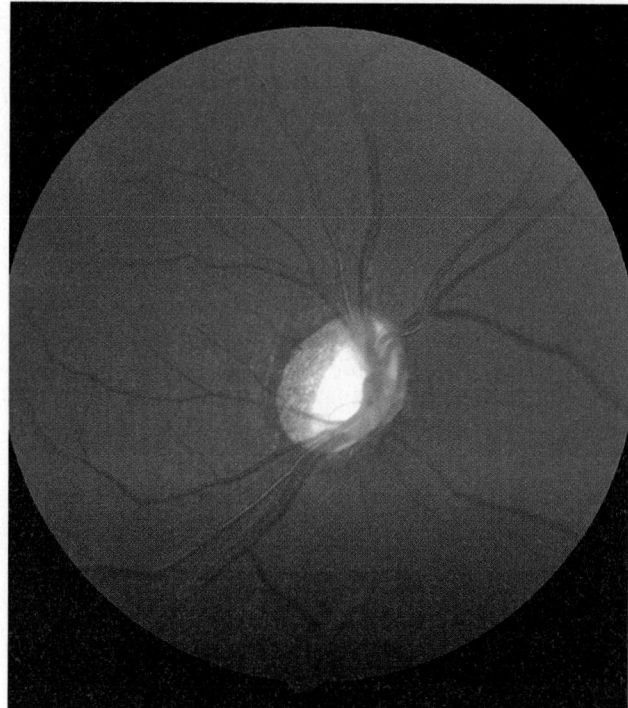

Fig. 50.32 A small irregular optic nerve that is hypoplastic.

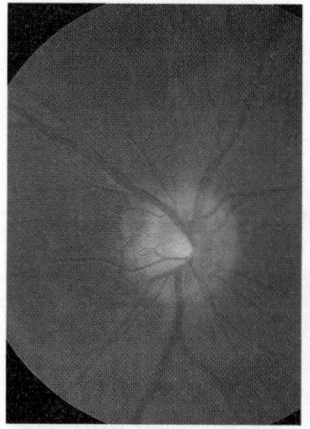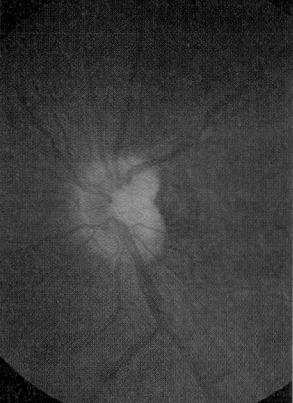

Fig. 50.33 Bilateral segmental optic nerve hypoplasia associated with a bitemporal hemianopia.

system that was sustained at any time before its full development. Notches occur in the disc (Figs 50.32, 50.33) and nerve fibre layer defects are associated with a relative smallness and irregularity in the outline of the disc in the fellow eye. A peripapillary white ring, the so-called 'double ring sign', may also be an indication of prenatal damage but should be used in the context of changes in the disc as a whole; by itself it is not pathognomonic of optic nerve hypoplasia. Changes may often be very subtle in the less affected optic disc, but may be useful additional clues. The ophthalmoscopic diagnosis is subjective, but some

objectivity can be introduced by comparing ratios of vessel size and optic disc size or the disc–macula to disc diameter ratio (Alvarez *et al.* 1988; Zeki *et al.* 1991). The technique of photogrammetry (Romano 1989) may be helpful.

Tilted disc (segmental hypoplasia)

Dorrell (1978) pointed out that the familiar tilted disc, in which the optic disc is D-shaped, is accompanied by a defect in the retinal nerve fibre layer adjacent to the flat arm of the 'D', usually inferiorly. He found that nearly half of the patients he tested had non-refractive visual abnormalities associated with the defect, and he pointed out the prenatal origin of the condition suggesting that it represents a form of segmental hypoplasia. These true visual field defects (Rucker 1946; Graham & Wakefield 1973; Young *et al.* 1976; Dorrell 1978) are frequently superotemporal (Brazitikos *et al.* 1990) and this must be remembered in the evaluation of the visual fields when there is no neurological cause found for the defect. The occurrence of suprasellar tumours in patients with tilted optic discs has been considered fortuitous (Rucker 1946; Riise 1975; Young *et al.* 1976; Keane 1977), but the association may be more than fortuitous (Fig. 50.34) as indicated by the developmental nature of the tumours and the frequency of the association (Taylor 1982). The concurrence of X-linked night-blindness (Fig. 50.35), myopia and tilted optic discs (Pinckers *et al.* 1978) has been reported.

Situs inversus

Situs inversus is a more widespread defect in which the vessels emerging from the optic disc are so distorted that, together with the appearance resulting from the tilt *per se*, the disc appears to be rotated through approximately 180°. Fuchs (1882) considered this anomaly to be related to coloboma. In patients with these bilateral dysplastic optic discs, upper bitemporal relative visual field defects may occur, which cross the midline. There may be an associated posterior staphyloma below the disc. In most cases the apparent field defect disappears with appropriate optical correction of the myopia caused by the staphyloma.

Optic nerve hypoplasia in central nervous system defects

Hoyt and Rios-Montenegros (1972) described a case in which trans-synaptic degeneration from a cerebral lesion gave rise to a characteristic pattern of optic disc hypoplasia which reflected the field defect that the lesion caused; they called this appearance homonymous hemioptic hypoplasia. The occurrence of specific patterns of hypoplasia results from local defects throughout the central nervous system. Novakovic *et al.* (1988) suggest the

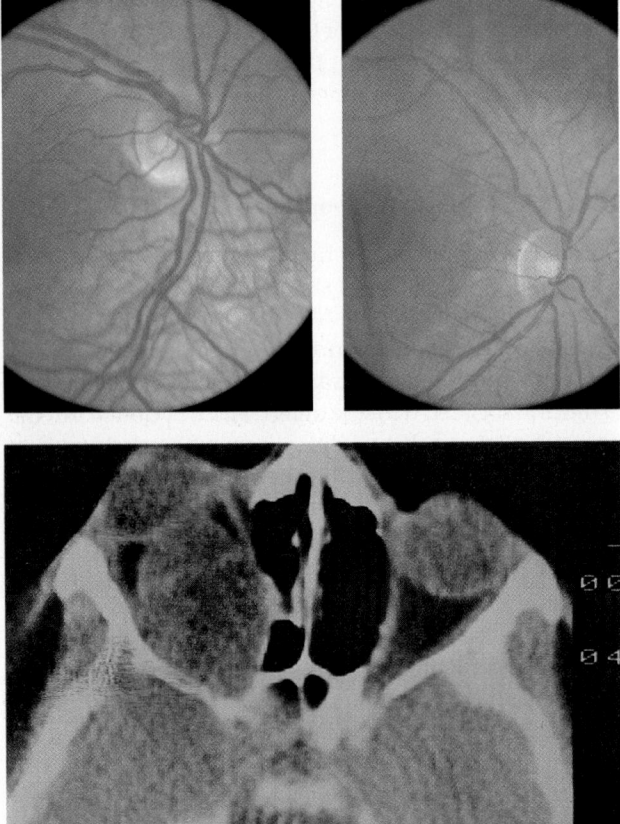

Fig. 50.34 Left optic nerve glioma with segmental hypoplasia of the optic nerve.

site of the 'insult' in optic nerve hypoplasia is reflected in the pattern of disc hypoplasia. For instance the appearance of segmental optic disc hypoplasia related to a macular coloboma means the site of the injury is in the eye, whilst optic disc hypoplasia of a 'figure of eight' shape in patients with suprasellar tumour suggests a chiasmal site. The optic disc hypoplasia therefore results from an early injury at any site in the developing nervous system.

Vision and associated features

Severe hypoplasia causes blindness, but in lesser degrees a variety of abnormalities have been described, with some patients having clinically normal vision (Gardner & Irvine 1972; Peterson & Walton 1977; Björk *et al.* 1978) although field defects in those cases with good acuity are common (Peterson & Walton 1977). The final vision may to a certain extent be predicted from VEPs and estimation of optic disc size (Borchert *et al.* 1995).

Frisen *et al.* (1978) pointed out that the diagnostic hallmarks of visual field defects due to hypoplasia are that they are static and that there are ophthalmoscopic correlates of the field defects. Patients with a diffuse deficit of

nerve fibres have more or less concentric visual field contraction and often a lowered acuity, but when the lack of nerve fibres is focal, the field defects are also focal.

Temporal visual field defects (Seeley & Smith 1971; Davis & Schoch 1975; Buchanan & Hoyt 1981) have been described, and this may indicate a chiasmal location of the primary anomaly (Frisen 1978).

Retrochiasmal lesions associated with hypoplastic discs may also have appropriate homonymous field defects. If unilateral these are clear-cut, but if the defect is bilateral the homonymous character is usually lost. Central visual field defects (Ewald 1967; Seeley & Smith 1971) and binasal defects (Missiroli 1947) also occur.

The flash ERG is usually normal in optic disc hypoplasia but may be enlarged. Colour vision is usually decreased roughly in proportion to the acuity defect.

Other features

Roving eye movements and unsteady fixation associated with poor vision, and see-saw nystagmus have been described (Davis & Schoch 1975), again suggesting a chiasmal abnormality. There may be abnormal optokinetic nystagmus (Hoyt & Rios-Montenegros 1972). A variety of different types of strabismus have been described, usually in patients with poor vision. The optic canal is not necessarily small (Walton & Robb 1970) but small optic nerves are found on CT scanning (Sanders 1980) or magnetic resonance imaging (MRI) (Brodsky *et al.* 1990).

Pathology

A few pathological studies have been carried out (Man-

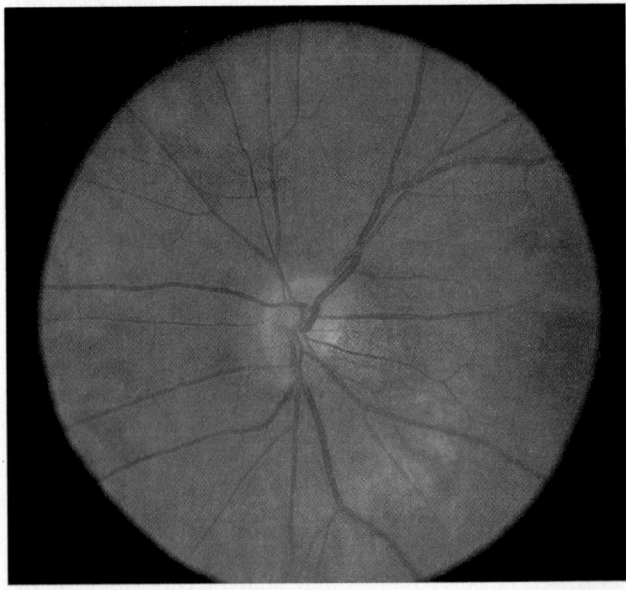

Fig. 50.35 A tilted optic disc in a patient with myopia and congenital stationary night-blindness.

schot 1971, 1972; Anderson *et al.* 1972; Boniuk & Ho 1979). Whinery and Blodi (1963) showed an absence or reduction of ganglion cells and their axons, small optic discs and nerves with abnormal glial tissue. Other parts of the neuroretina were normal and apart from incidental anomalies the eyes were otherwise normal.

Pathogenesis

The wide variety of associated central neurodevelopmental anomalies might lead one to conclude that the loss of ganglion cells was secondary to a retrograde degeneration along the visual pathway and the cases of homonymous hemioptic hypoplasia are a dramatic example of this. However, the occurrence of unilateral optic disc hypoplasia and of partial or segmental optic disc hypoplasia must mean that the site in those cases is anterior in the visual system (Novakovic *et al.* 1988). Optic disc hypoplasia is therefore probably a non-specific abnormality resulting from a prenatal insult to any part of the visual system (Fig. 50.36).

The timing of this 'insult' has been of some interest, most authors agreeing that the abnormality has occurred by the tenth week of gestation (Boniuk *et al.* 1979). The retina does not clearly appear until 30 days and therefore the 'insult' must occur after this time. It is, however, difficult to extrapolate from these various pieces of evidence and it is only possible to conclude that the defect occurs early in prenatal development.

A relationship between optic disc hypoplasia and colobomas has been suggested (Brown 1982).

Family history and genetics

Familial cases have been described (Missiroli 1947; Kytila & Miettinen 1961; Hackenbruch *et al.* 1975; Benner *et al.* 1990) but they are rare and not all necessarily genetic and in the absence of a recurrent environmental cause (such as drugs or alcohol) a very low recurrence risk can be given. Optic disc hypoplasia, and its systemic associations should therefore be regarded as sporadic in their occurrence. An exception to this rule is in aniridia, which has a familial occurrence and is associated with optic disc hypoplasia (Layman *et al.* 1974), although usually the optic disc is small rather than truly hypoplastic. Optic nerve hypoplasia may occur in the fetal alcohol syndrome (Stromland 1987; Chan *et al.* 1991), which may affect several children of alcoholic mothers.

Associated anomalies and aetiological factors

Although optic disc hypoplasia may appear to be the result of an isolated event, it occurs in association with certain other developmental anomalies (Fig. 50.37). Associations with hydranencephaly (Manschot 1971, 1972;

Herman *et al.* 1988), anencephaly (Anderson *et al.* 1972; Manschot 1972; Boniuk 1979), aniridia (Hoyt *et al.* 1972; Layman *et al.* 1974), congenital hemiplegia with hemianopia (Hoyt *et al.* 1972), porencephaly (Greenfield *et al.* 1980), cerebral atrophy (Rogers *et al.* 1981) and colpocephaly (Garg 1982) have been described. Quinine taken by the mother as an abortifacient early in pregnancy has been associated with optic nerve hypoplasia in the infant (McKinna 1966), as has maternal anticonvulsant (Hoyt & Billson 1978), LSD (Chan *et al.* 1978) and crack cocaine (Good *et al.* 1992). Viral infection has been implicated in cattle (Bistner *et al.* 1973). Diabetic mothers have babies with a higher incidence of neurological anomalies, including optic disc hypoplasia (Patel *et al.* 1975; Peterson & Walton 1977; Donat 1981; Kim *et al.* 1989). In children of diabetic mothers the superior half of the disc may be most affected (see Fig. 50.37), the so-called superior segmental optic hypoplasia (Kim *et al.* 1989). Optic nerve hypoplasia occurs in children with the fetal alcohol syndrome (Strömland 1987; Chan *et al.* 1991) and in mice (Cook *et al.* 1987).

Septo-optic dysplasia

In 1941 Reeves described a patient with what was probably optic nerve hypoplasia and absence of the septum pellucidum, but the first clear description of the syndrome of absence of the septum pellucidum and optic disc hypoplasia was by De Morsier (1956). Hoyt *et al.* (1970) were the first to clearly demonstrate hypopituitarism in patients with septo-optic dysplasia and since then a variety of hormonal defects have been described ranging from isolated growth hormone, adrenocorticotrophic or antidiuretic hormone deficiency to panhypopituitarism (Kaplan *et al.* 1970; Ellenburger & Runyan 1970; Billson & Hopkins 1972; Brook *et al.* 1972; Harris & Haas 1972; Benoit-Gonin *et al.* 1978; Krause-Brucker 1980). Hypothyroidism is probably the most common abnormality (Skarf & Hoyt 1984; Stanhope *et al.* 1984).

Abnormalities of the septum pellucidum alone may affect spatial task performances (Griffiths & Hunt 1984) but most affected children with only a septum pellucidum defect are healthy and grow well (Brodsky 1991).

Pathology in a case (Patel *et al.* 1975) showed an absent posterior lobe of the pituitary gland, with an abnormal hypothalamus. The pituitary defects may occur in optic disc hypoplasia even without evidence of absence of the septum pellucidum (Krause-Brucker 1980).

Whilst many patients have optic nerve hypoplasia with only an abnormal septum pellucidum or pituitary stalk (Kaufman *et al.* 1989) and hypopituitarism, the associated spectrum of deformities (Fig. 50.38) may vary widely in severity (Zeki *et al.* 1992) up to holoprosencephaly. In holoprosencephaly a variable midline facial defect is associated with a single cerebral ventricle, and absence of the corpus callosum and septum pellucidum; there is also a

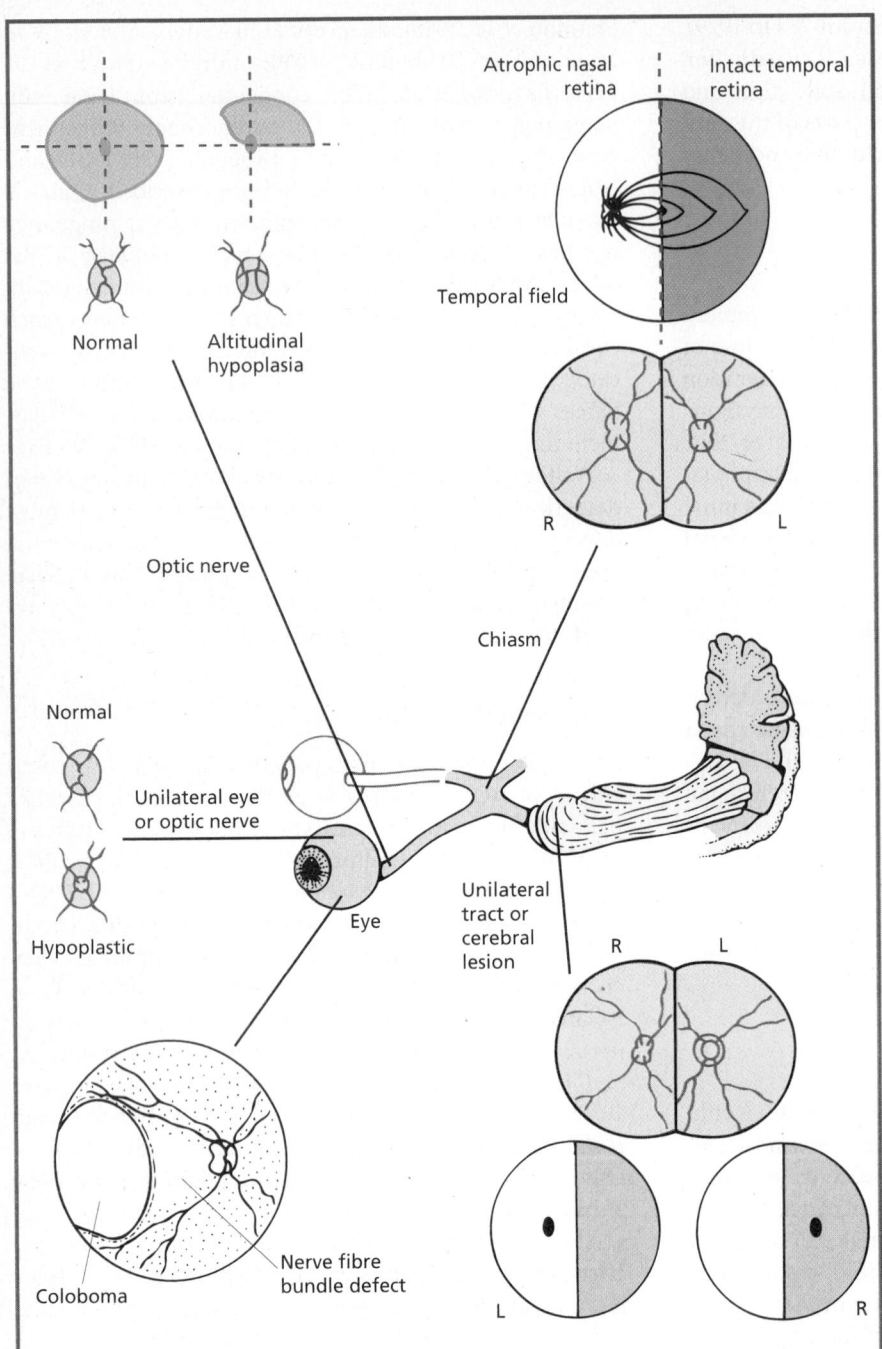

Fig. 50.36 Lesions at any site in the developing nervous system will cause optic nerve hypoplasia if their onset is early enough. Retinal defects may cause a macular coloboma with a segmental optic nerve hypoplasia. Unilateral eye or optic nerve defects cause purely unilateral hypoplasia. Unilateral retinal or anterior optic nerve defects may cause an altitudinal hypoplasia. Chiasmal defects may cause a 'figure of eight' optic disc that is hypoplastic, and tract or cerebral lesions will cause homonymous hemioptic hypoplasia (Novakovic *et al.* 1988).

wide variety of similar brain defects (Ellenberger & Runyan 1970; Jelliger & Gross 1973; Hale & Rice 1974; Donat 1981).

Pathological studies in holoprosencephaly have shown absence of the olfactory apparatus, which forms a link with Kallmann's syndrome (Kallmann *et al.* 1943) in which hypopituitarism and anosmia are associated with forebrain abnormalities (Lightman 1988).

Practical management

1 Since optic disc hypoplasia may be bilateral and highly asymmetrical, apparently unilateral optic disc hypoplasia should be considered to be bilateral in terms of the investigation of the patient.

2 Patients found to have optic disc hypoplasia in the first 4 years of life should be considered for neuroradiological

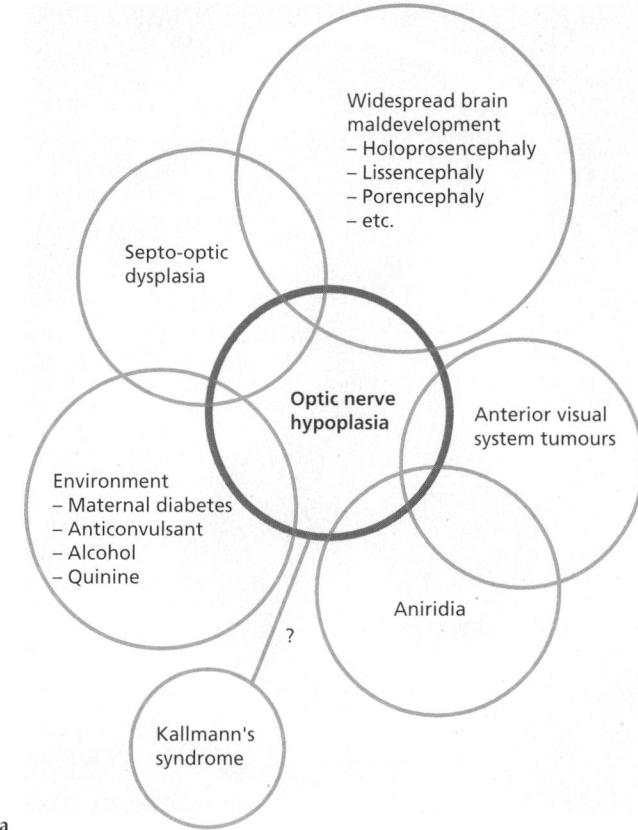

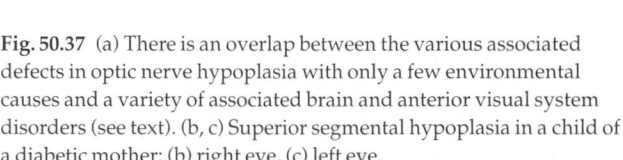

a

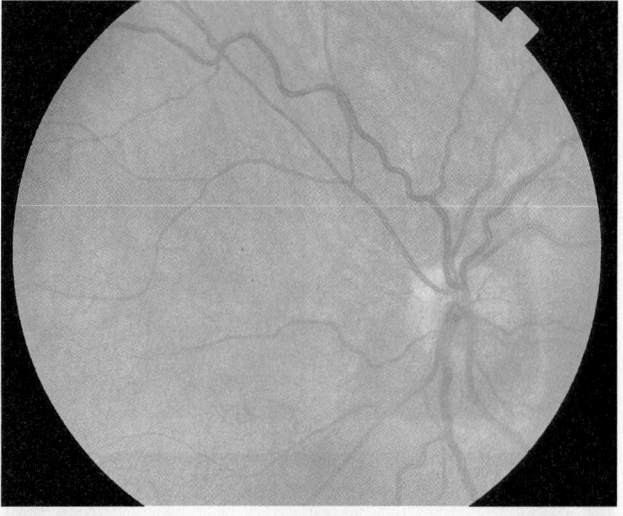

b

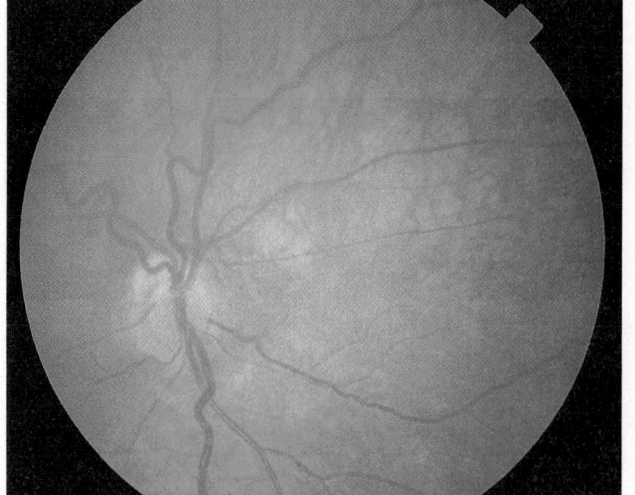

c

Fig. 50.37 (a) There is an overlap between the various associated defects in optic nerve hypoplasia with only a few environmental causes and a variety of associated brain and anterior visual system disorders (see text). (b, c) Superior segmental hypoplasia in a child of a diabetic mother: (b) right eye, (c) left eye.

studies to confirm or exclude associated cerebral malformations and other defects; those in whom they are present need to be under the care of a paediatrician, or endocrinologist. MRI spectroscopy may reveal anomalies in the hypothalamus which may predict hormonal problems, and the finding on MRI of callosal dysgenesis may be a good predictor of neurological problems (Brodsky & Glasier 1993). Whether or not cerebral abnormalities are found, weight and height must be monitored carefully (Skarf & Hoyt 1984)—this is probably the responsibility of the child's paediatrician or primary physician. After 4 years of age if the child's general development is proceeding normally it is not necessary to perform advanced neuroradiology but it is still necessary to measure height and weight regularly (Lambert *et al.* 1987a).

3 Developmental delay may occur in patients with optic disc hypoplasia without structural brain defects (Skarf & Hoyt 1984).

4 In looking for optic disc hypoplasia, a direct ophthalmoscopic examination is preferable, and an examination under anaesthetic should rarely be necessary.

5 A child with optic disc hypoplasia may also be amblyopic in that eye; the vision may be improved by timely and vigorous occlusion (Kushner 1984).

6 The condition is not inherited but familial clusters may occur, probably due to environmental reasons.

Optic disc anomalies associated with midline brain and facial defects

Optic disc hypoplasia has been described in association with midline brain defects, facial clefts and other related defects, but other optic disc anomalies do occur in these disorders. Such cases are uncommon (Van Noyhuys & Bruyn 1964; Walsh & Hoyt 1969; Goldhammer & Smith 1975; Corbett *et al.* 1990; Bullard *et al.* 1981; Caprioli & Lesser 1983) but have substantial diagnostic implications.

The patients may present with squint in childhood (Fig. 50.39) or with poor vision, or the visual aspects may be overshadowed by the effects of an associated pituitary

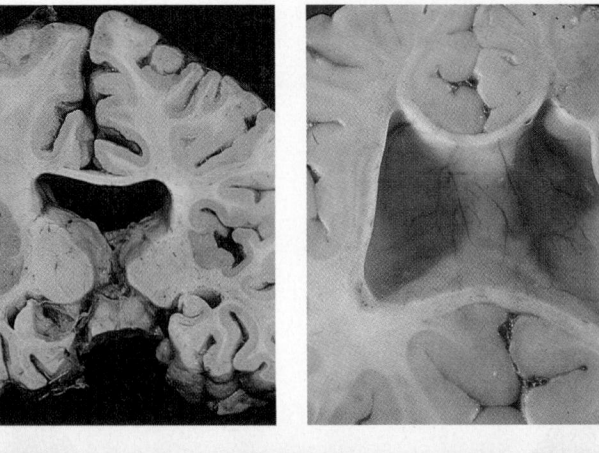

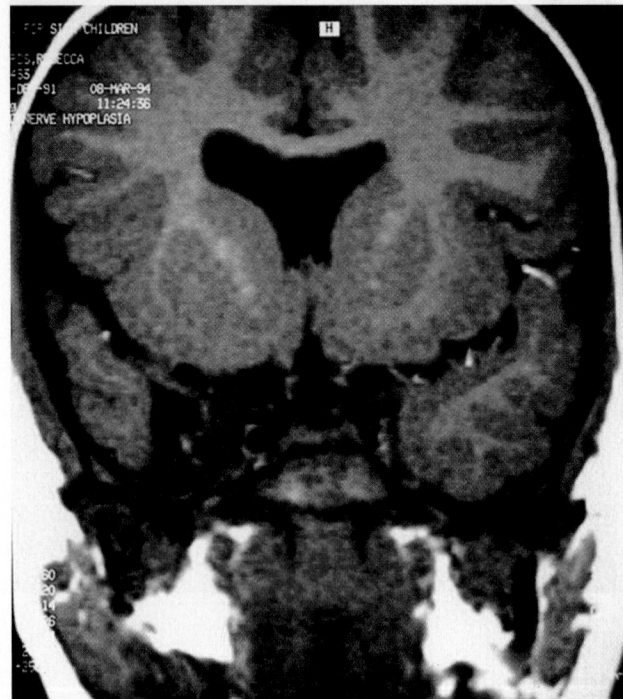

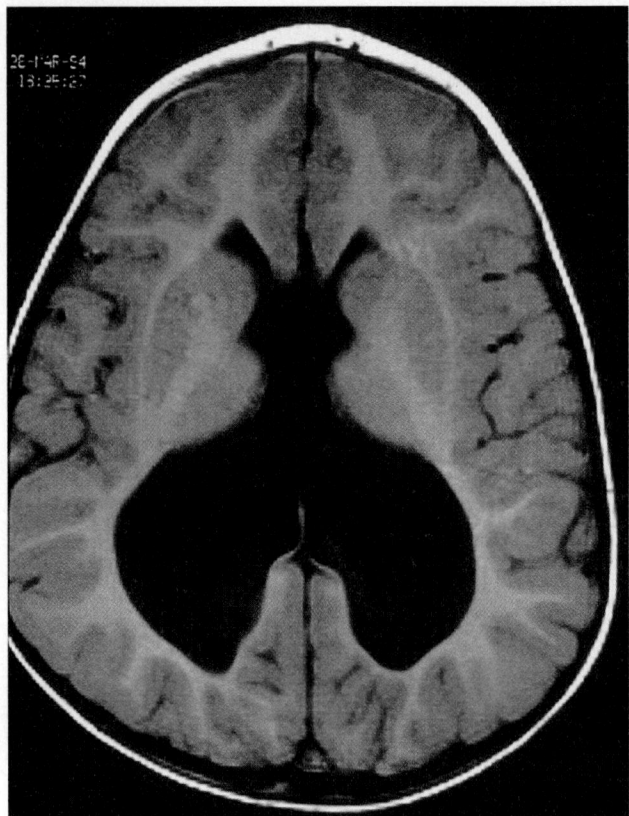

Fig. 50.38 (a) Midline brain defects ranging from holoprosencephaly, abnormal or absent septum pellucidum, to agenesis of the corpus callosum occur in association with optic nerve hypoplasia. (b) Lobar holoprosencephaly. (c) Septo-optic dysplasia with schizencephaly.

or hypothalamic defect causing failure to grow. Often there are facial clefts or a midline harelip, a bifid nose, or hypertelorism, though these manifestations may be subtle. Recurrent cerebrospinal fluid rhinorrhoea was the presentation in one case (Bullard *et al.* 1981) and a pulsatile nasal tumour that elicited unwarranted (and hazardous!) surgery in another (Goldhammer & Smith 1975). All of the optic disc anomalies were of a dysplastic type, either frankly colobomatous or having other anomalies including optic disc pits, a Morning Glory anomaly, megalopapilla or hypoplasia. 'Cryptophthalmos' (Goldhammer & Smith 1975) and microphthalmos (Walsh & Hoyt 1969) have also been described. All these conditions may result from failure in proper development and closure of the fetal fissure (see below) and may be related to colobomas even though rarely typical (Brodsky *et al.* 1995).

Optic disc anomalies with isolated maldevelopment of the anterior visual pathways

Optic disc anomalies with bitemporal hemianopia may be found in a syndrome of apparently isolated maldevelopment of the anterior visual pathways (Taylor 1982) with no abnormalities found on neuroradiological investigation.

Coloboma and related anomalies

A coloboma (Greek for curtailed or mutilated) results from an abnormality of the closure of the fetal fissure of the embryonic optic cup which occurs around 6–8 weeks postconception (15 mm) (Apple *et al.* 1982). Closure starts at the equator and extends anteriorly and posteriorly;

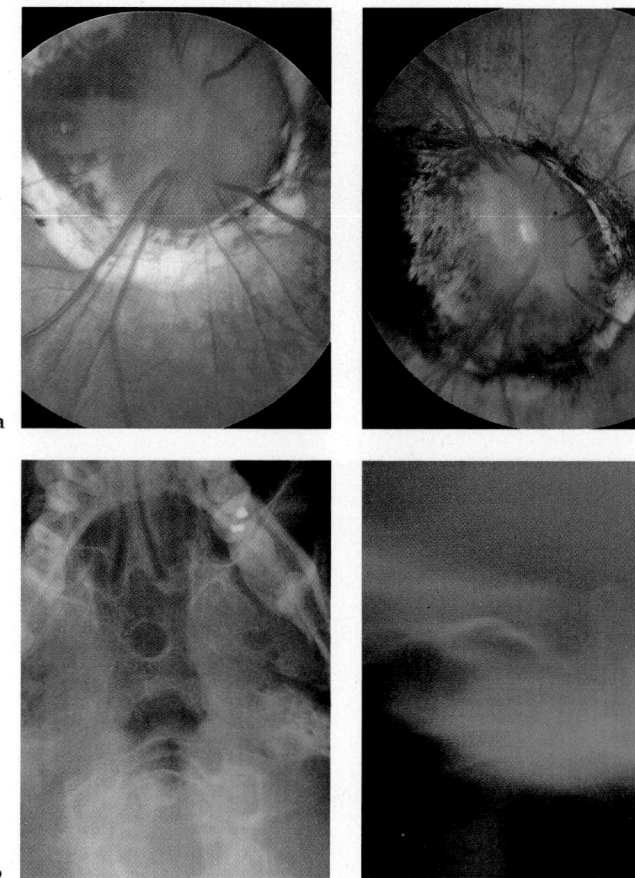

Fig. 50.39 (a) The optic discs of this child, who presented with a squint and growth defect, are dysplastic. (b) The radiological studies show that there is a defect in the floor of the pituitary fossa associated with a midline meningocoele.

Table 50.1 A phenotypic classification of colobomatous defects devised by Warburg (1993).

Typical
Coloboma of the iris
Complete (keyhole)
Partial
    peripheral
    notch in the pupil
    pigment epithelium defect
    heterochromia of the iris

Coloboma of the ciliary body

Coloboma of the choroid
Type 1
    partial
    complete
Type 2
    with macular involvement
    without macular involvement
Type 3
    cystic
    non-cystic

Coloboma of the optic nerve
Typical
    cystic
    non-cystic
'Special'
    pits
    Pedler's coloboma
    Morning Glory
    optic nerve hypoplasia

Atypical
Coloboma outside the fetal fissure

Macular coloboma

inadequate closure may create a defect of any size from the margin of the pupil to the optic disc. Iris colobomas (Fig. 50.40a, b), retinochoroidal colobomas and optic disc colobomas probably represent a spectrum of clinical manifestations of a common disease process. Microphthalmos and anophthalmos may be extreme manifestations of the same disorder, not least because they occur in syndromes with colobomas in other members of the family (Savell & Cook 1976) and may occur unilaterally with a coloboma in the other eye. Although the term coloboma is also classically applied to a whole variety of notches, holes or other defects in the iris or choroid it should perhaps be reserved for those anomalies associated with fetal fissure closure defects — 'typical' colobomas. Colobomas that do not originate in a defect of fetal fissure closure lie outside the inferonasal quadrant and are designated atypical. Some atypical disc colobomas may have a similar origin to the typical form and other optic disc anomalies. Colobomas are generally rare, occurring in about 0.25% of 12000 patients examined ophthalmoscopically (Vossius 1885).

Visual effects

Colobomas involving the choroid usually create scotomas in proportion to their size. Optic nerve colobomas may cause visual defects which cannot be ascertained merely by the appearance of the disc. Due to associated myopic astigmatism, amblyopia is often a major factor. Pattern VEPs can be used to assess vision but will not differentiate visual loss due to a nerve defect from superimposed amblyopia. Refraction is often hampered by an irregular red reflex and nystagmus, but adequate optical correction is critical to maximize vision.

A classification

For the clinician, a phenotypic classification may be most helpful, such as Warburg's (1993) classification (Table 50.1).

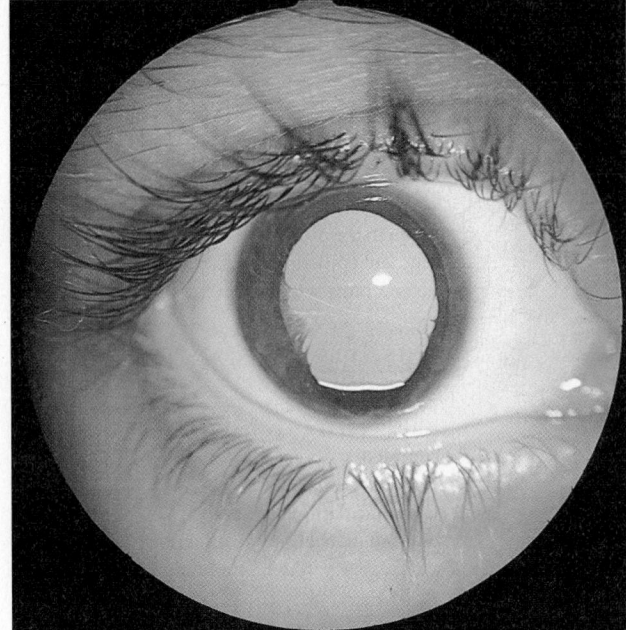

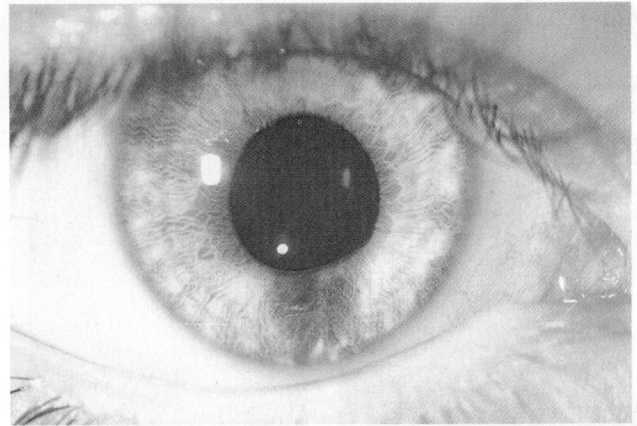

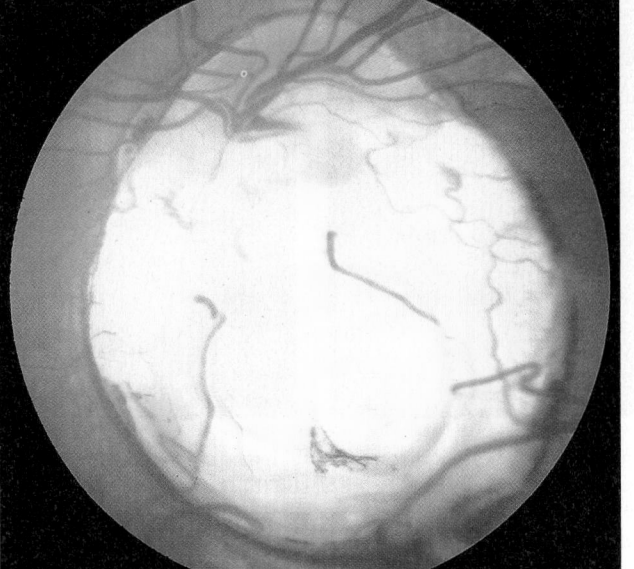

Fig. 50.40 (a) Complete iris coloboma. The edge of the lens is visible in the cleft. (b) Partial thickness iris coloboma. (c) Typical widespread optic nerve coloboma with associated retinal coloboma which gave rise to poor central vision.

Genetics

Most cases of coloboma without systemic associations are sporadic or dominantly inherited with variable expressivity (Duke-Elder 1964). Unless the subtle manifestations (Savell & Cook 1976) are taken into account several generations may appear to be missed. Autosomal recessive (McMillan 1921; François 1968; Warburg 1993; Zlotogora *et al.* 1994) and X-linked (Goldberg & McKusick 1971) inheritance may occur, but much less frequently. Microphthalmos, which may be found in families with colobomas, possibly occurs less frequently in first born than in subsequent children (Nakajima *et al.* 1979). All first-degree relatives of patients with colobomas should be screened for coloboma.

Presentation

Children with colobomas present either as a result of the appearance of the iris or the presence of a small eye, or

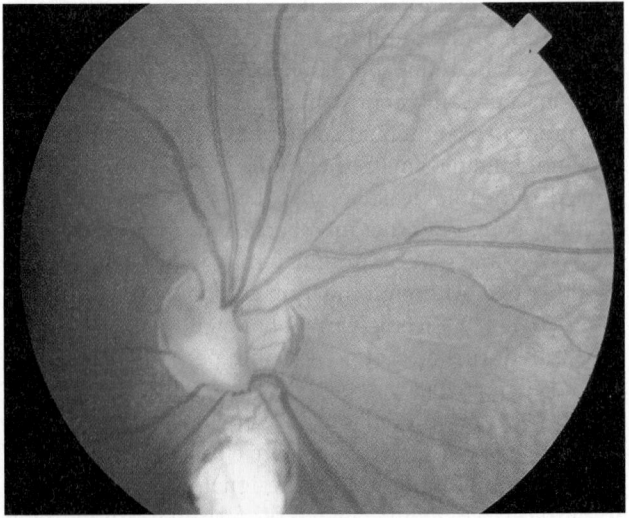

Fig. 50.41 An anomalous optic disc associated with a chorioretinal coloboma in a child with the CHARGE association with preserved central visual functions.

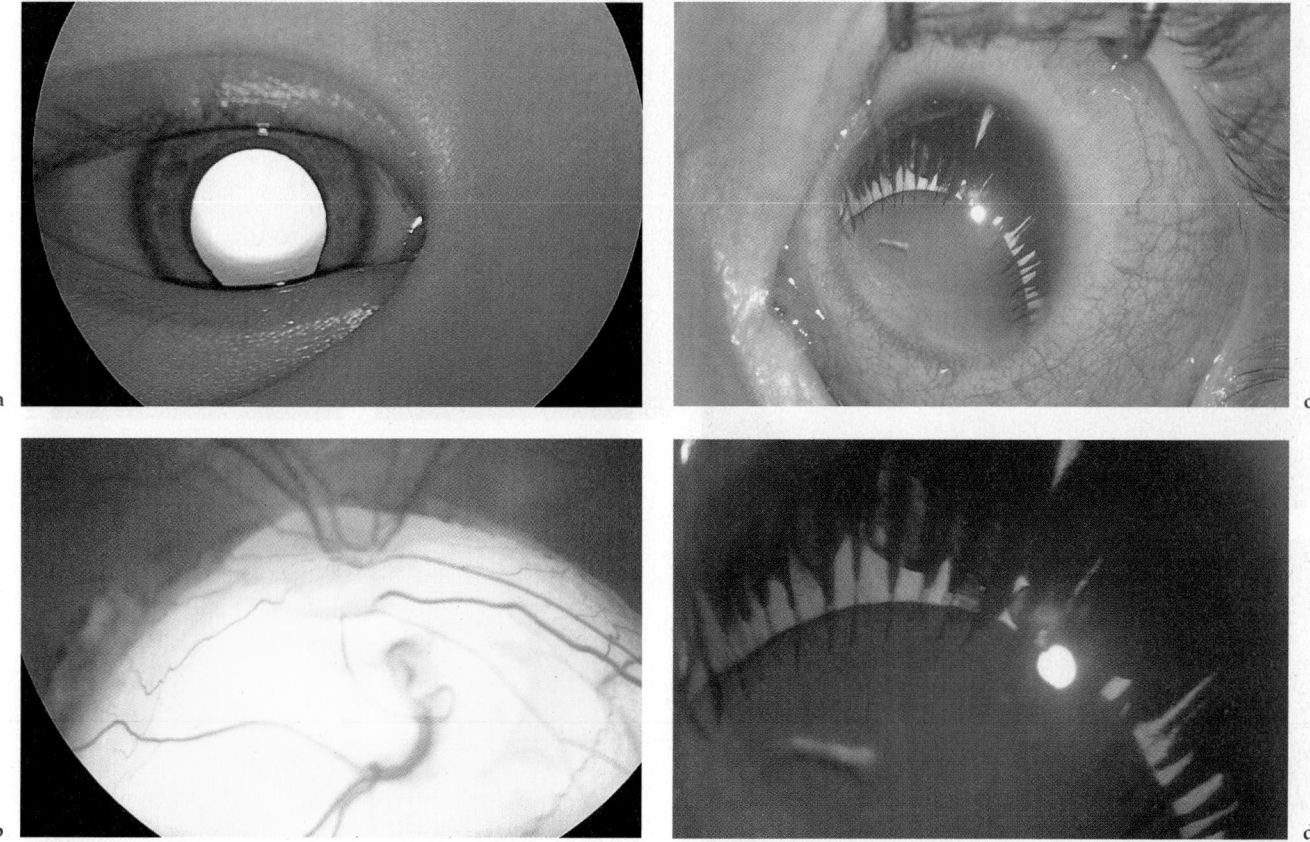

Fig. 50.42 (a,b) This child with a gross right optic nerve and chorioretinal coloboma presented because of the microphthalmos and the white reflex that the mother could see when she was feeding the child. (c) Colobomatous microphthalmos in this child, as often happens in severely affected eyes, shows a downward dislocation of the lens with stretching of the ciliary processes. (d) Same patient; it is notable that the ciliary processes stretch, not the zonule fibres. Compare with Fig. 39.12.

because of apparently poor vision, or especially if unilateral, with a squint. Sometimes the systemic associations of colobomas are the presenting features or the coloboma may only be discovered on routine examination.

Ophthalmoscopic appearance

The typical optic disc coloboma (Figs 50.40–50.42), associated with an inferonasal chorioretinal defect, is familiar to all ophthalmologists. They range from a hugely excavated disc with a cavity so large that it may appear as a retrobulbar swelling on a CT scan (Fig. 50.43 a, b) to a subtle change in the retinal pigment epithelium (Figs 50.43c, 50.44).

Colobomas of the disc are not invariably associated with choroidal or iris defects but it is important to look for subtle manifestations of these, such as an inferonasal area of transillumination of the iris, a notch in the pupil margin, heterochromia of the iris (Drews 1973) or segmental melanosis oculi (Matzkin *et al.* 1970). A notch in the lens, inferonasal lens opacities, or pigment specks on the lens surface may be additional clues (Mann 1957).

Retinal vessels pass over the colobomatous area and large choroidal vessels may be visible in the base of the coloboma. The defect may have a smooth surface but usually bulges posteriorly and may be thinned by crater-like areas.

Some developmentally abnormal optic discs, known as axial colobomas, have a disc surrounded by a rim of choroidal atrophy or thinning, with a central area of glial tissue. Vessels radiate from the edge of this disc. The occurrence of this in one eye with colobomatous microphthalmos in the other is a strong indication that the basic abnormality is a fetal fissure defect.

Brown (1982) has described a case with an optic disc coloboma in one eye and a small optic disc in the other eye; he suggested that optic disc hypoplasia and coloboma may represent a spectrum of defects with similar cause.

It is important to look for subtle phenotypic expressions since their diagnostic and genetic implications are the

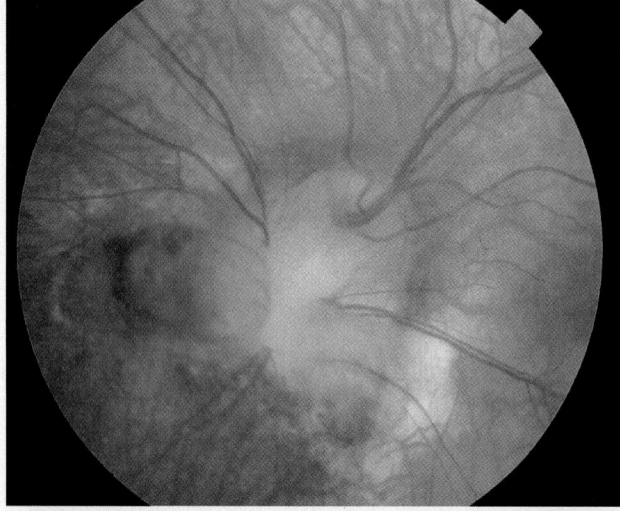

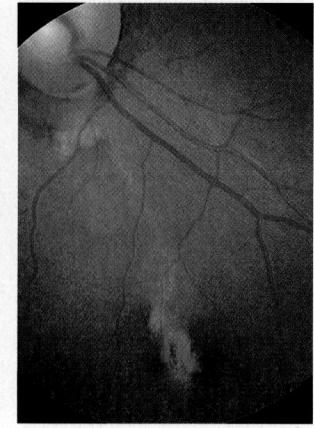

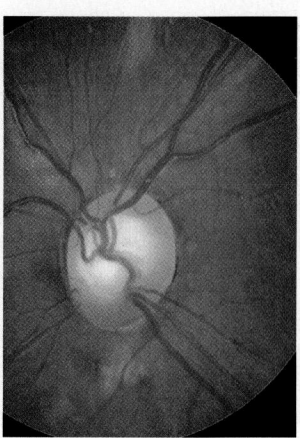

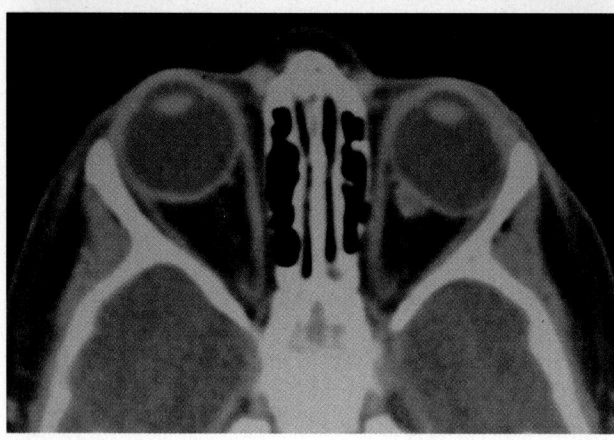

Fig. 50.43 (a) Large coloboma with retrobulbar extension. (b) Same patient showing the cystic retrobulbar extension on the CT scan. (c) This slightly anomalous optic nerve in a child with the CHARGE association is associated with a mild chorioretinal defect indicating the basic colobomatous nature of the defect.

same as the most gross manifestations and the liability of a patient to have systemic disease is not dependent on the severity of the expression.

Optic disc pits

Optic disc pits (Weiter *et al.* 1977) may be of a similar aetiology to colobomas and may occur in one eye with optic disc coloboma either in the same eye or in the other eye (Sugar 1967; Brown *et al.* 1980; Corbett *et al.* 1990). They are holes of variable sizes (Fig. 50.45) that usually occur temporally near the margin of the disc, although 20% may occur centrally (Apple *et al.* 1982). The pit is a herniation of neuroectodermal tissue into a defect in the optic nerve substance, surrounded by a connective tissue capsule contiguous with the meninges (Apple *et al.* 1982). They may be associated with visual field defects. Up to 60% of patients will develop central serous retinopathy (Apple *et al.* 1982) with associated visual symptoms (Kranenberg 1960; Theodossiadis 1977; Rubinstein & Ali 1978). The origin of subretinal fluid in humans with central serous retinopathy associated with a pit is still

uncertain (Brown & Tasman 1983). Possible fluid sources include the choriocapillaris, cerebrospinal fluid and liquid vitreous (Chang 1976; Chia Lee Lin *et al.* 1984). Although often following a benign course, subretinal neovascularization and other complications may occur (Borodick *et al.* 1984; Theodoniadis *et al.* 1993), and some authors advocate aggressive treatment in selected cases (Schatz & McDonald 1988) such as gas internal tamponade and laser treatment for patients with outer layer or inner layer serous detachments (Lincoff *et al.* 1993).

Intraocular abnormalities with colobomas

Various intraocular abnormalities may occur in association with colobomas. A preserved hyaloid vascular system has been described (Bell 1971) as well as an anomalous Cloquet's canal (Akiba *et al.* 1993) and lens notches are not infrequent. Vitreous striae and cataract occurred in one patient (Dascoffe *et al.* 1975). Glial tissue with abnormal dysplastic retina near the optic disc (Fig. 50.46) was described histopathologically (Takahashi *et al.* 1979). Mul-

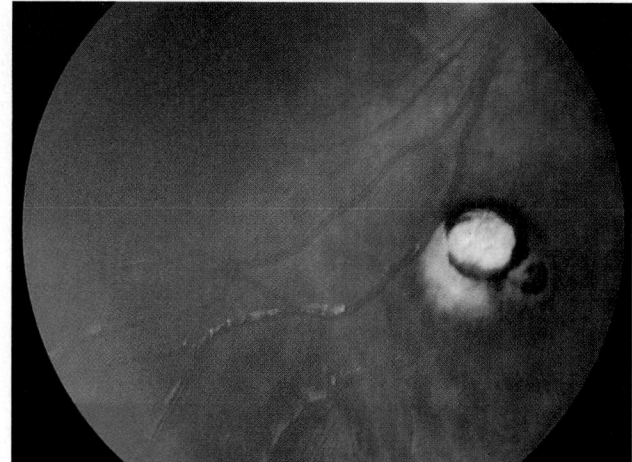

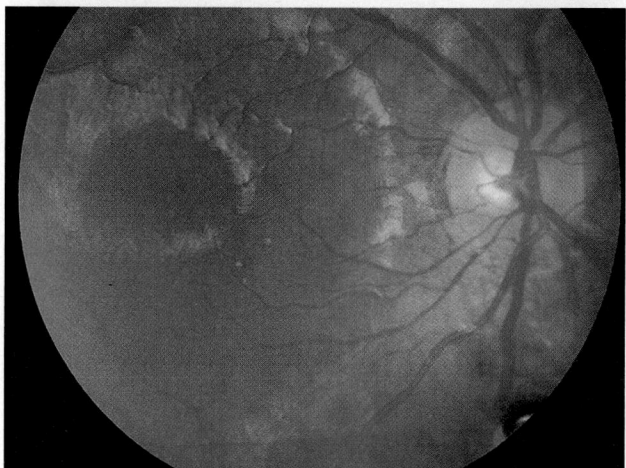

Fig. 50.44 A chorioretinal coloboma in a patient with the CHARGE association.

laney (1978) classified intraocular colobomatous malformations, unassociated with systemic disease, into five groups on histopathological grounds. She drew widely from the literature and her paper serves as a useful review.

Group 1

This group includes lesions with heterotopic intraocular tissue including the following.

1 Lacrimal tissue.

2 Cartilage with ossification.

3 Adipose and smooth muscle tissue (Pedler 1961; Willis *et al.* 1972). These cases had a variety of intraocular tissue, usually adipose or glial; in one subgroup (Willis *et al.* 1972) seven eyes were removed for suspected tumour.

Smooth muscle may be present which may be the basis for the accounts of periodic contraction of colobomas in man and animals (Wise *et al.* 1966; Sugar & Beckman 1969; Kral & Svarc 1971; Tanaka 1977; Foster 1991).

Episodic visual loss has been described (Longfellow *et*

al. 1962; Graether 1963; Seybold & Rosen 1977). The mechanism may be a sphincter-like constriction of the optic nerve entrance by the smooth muscle (Mullaney & Fitzpatrick 1973). One case (Tanaka 1977) showed a three-times-a-minute transient elevation of the optic disc which was thought to be due to rhythmic contraction of smooth muscle around a circular colobomatous cyst.

Group 2

This group includes colobomas associated with cysts. Intraocular cysts associated with colobomatous malformations are rare (Mullaney & Fitzpatrick 1973).

Patients with orbital cysts with colobomas and colobomatous microphthalmos (Von Arlt 1858; Waring *et al.* 1976) usually present first because of the ocular abnormality and the cyst presents because of its later enlargement.

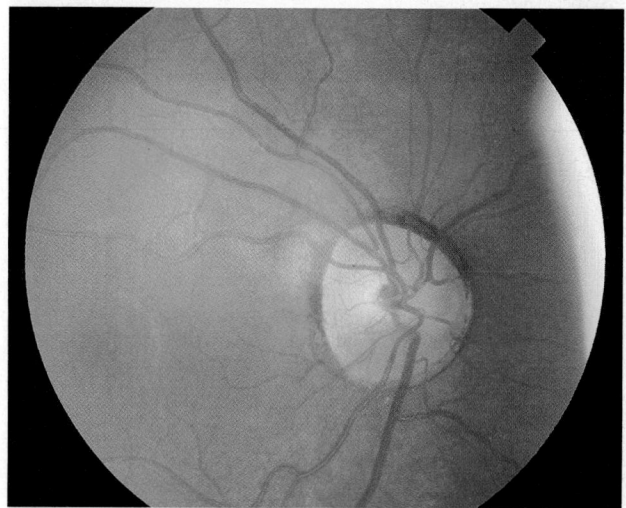

a

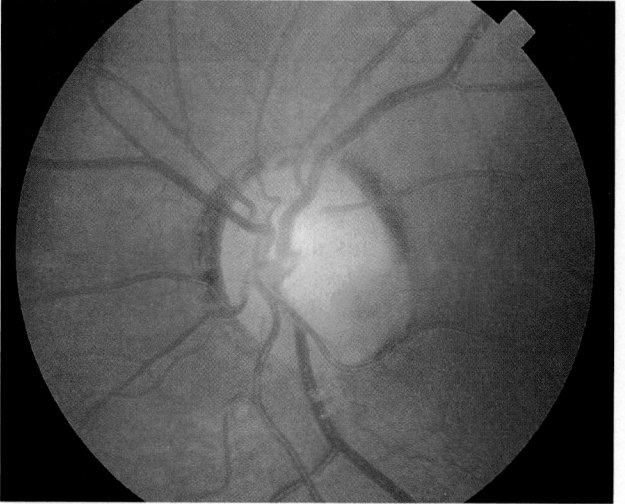

b

Fig. 50.45 (a) Optic disc pit. Right eye showing nasal pit. There were no visual symptoms. (b) Left eye showing temporal optic disc pit associated with cystoid macular oedema.

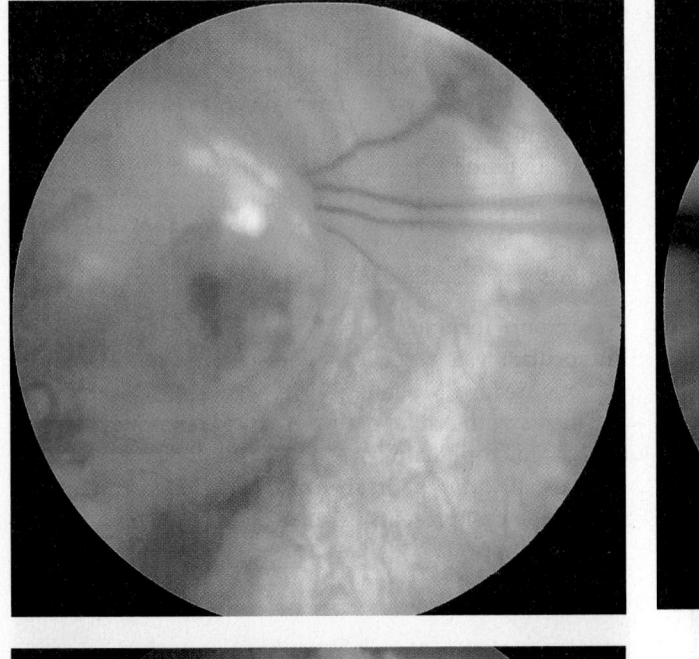

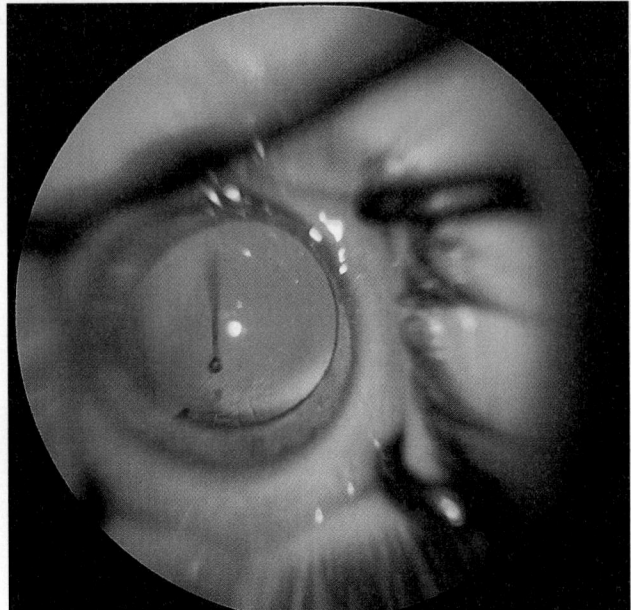

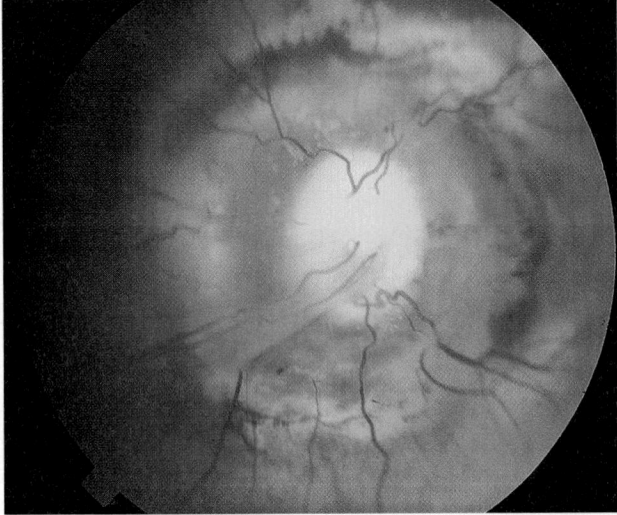

Fig. 50.46 (a) CHARGE association. Gross colobomatous defect of the disc. (b) Same patient showing preserved hyaloid system. (c) Gross colobomatous disc with peripapillary abnormalities and a retinal fold.

The cysts appear as a swelling in the lower lid which enlarges on crying (see Figs 35.7–35.9), or as a thin-walled cyst adjacent to the globe; occasionally it may cause a gradual proptosis. The cyst may communicate with the microphthalmic eye. This must be remembered during surgical removal of the cyst since decompression of the cyst may cause an alarming decompression of the eye and, if functionless, the microphthalmic eye may need to be removed. The cysts contain cerebrospinal fluid (Wiggins *et al.* 1991). Porges *et al.* (1992) described five members of a highly inbred kinship with microphthalmos with cysts; ultrasound was effective in prenatal diagnosis.

Group 3

This group includes neoplasms occurring along the line of closure of the fetal fissure including glioneuroma and medulloepithelioma.

Group 4

Group 4 includes colobomatous malformations associated with prenatal infections, particularly cytomegalovirus (Hittner *et al.* 1976). It is difficult to associate clearly these relatively common disorders.

Group 5

This group includes intraocular malformations not directly associated with the coloboma (Foos *et al.* 1968; Bell 1971; Lyford & Roy 1974; Dascoffe *et al.* 1975; Grey & Rice 1976; Weiter *et al.* 1977; Takahashi *et al.* 1979). These include

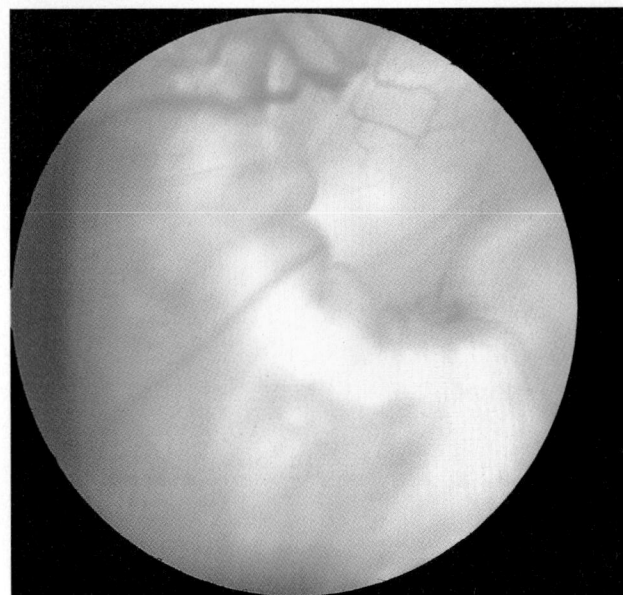

Fig. 50.47 Coloboma of the optic disc with overlay of the peripapillary retina (Pedler's coloboma; see text).

buphthalmos, accessory pupils, lens anomalies and reduplication, optic nerve aplasia, hyaloid vascular anomalies, dysplastic retina and vitreous striae.

Ocular complications and associations of colobomas

The presence of an optic disc coloboma should not blind the ophthalmologist to the presence of other eye malformations, in particular to glaucoma resulting from an anterior chamber anomaly which also causes excavation of the optic disc. Retinal detachment (Savell & Cook 1976), subretinal neovascularization (Brodsky *et al.* 1991), and disciform degeneration may all occur as complications of colobomas of the choroid.

Double optic discs

The earlier literature suggested that a true duplication of the optic disc occurs (Duke-Elder 1964). The second optic disc lies below the main disc and has its own set of retinal vessels, but it may be joined to the main disc by an arteriolar or a venular connection.

The optic nerve itself may be duplicated (Collier 1958), or split by an abnormal artery (Slade & Weekley 1957). Most double discs appear to be a part of the colobomatous malformation (Duke-Elder 1964; Brink & Larsen 1977; Junge 1978) but the accessory disc is not always below as would be expected in this case (Elbrechtz 1975). Doubling of the optic canal may occur (Lamba 1969). Two brothers with thoracic dystrophy and a renal dystrophy were described by Gallet *et al.* (1973), one of whom had a double

optic disc. Brink and Larsen (1977) suggested that the presence of doubling can only be characterized as true doubling (implying two separate nerves each with its own set of nerve fibres, perhaps subserving nasal and temporal vision separately) if it fulfils the following criteria: the absence of a field defect, a largely separate vascular supply to each disc, and double nerves demonstrable by CT scanning.

Pedler's coloboma

Pedler's coloboma (coloboma of the optic disc with overlay of the peripapillary retina; Fig. 50.47) is the description coined by Cogan (1978) who described the appearance of a uniocular peripapillary lobulated mass in a child of 9 months of age. Histopathological studies showed a scleral canal that was about twice the normal size. The central portion of the nerve head was occupied by loosely arranged vascular connective tissue and the peripapillary retina was bunched up to three times the normal thickness, and folded on itself. There was hyperplastic pigment epithelium and glial tissue between the optic nerve and sclera. This case seems to be similar to those described by other authors including Pedler (Seefelder 1909; Pedler 1961; Hogan & Zimmerman 1962; Rack & Wright 1966; Hamada & Ellsworth 1971; Willis *et al.* 1972; Tanaka 1977). Congenitally detached retinas may be found but these may not require surgery since they tend to reattach spontaneously (Hamada & Ellsworth 1971). The presence of muscle in the anomaly is suggested by periodic contractions occasionally observed (Tanaka 1977; Cennamo *et al.* 1983). The elevated appearance of the disc differentiates it from the Morning Glory disc but may lead to enucleation for suspected tumour.

Peripapillary staphyloma

In this condition the area of the sclera around the optic disc is ectatic and relatively myopic due to localized increased length of the eyeball. There is often a certain amount of glial tissue in the disc, and the vessels radiate out from the edge of the disc. Hayreh and Cullen (1972) described a case with a long history of undiagnosed visual loss due to a serous detachment of the retina around an atypical coloboma. The colobomatous nature of the problem is in many cases attested to by the thinning of the choroid being usually inferior to the disc, the usually inferior site of the staphyloma, and by the occurrence of this anomaly in syndromes usually associated with typical coloboma. Not all cases are below the disc, however, suggesting multiple aetiologies (Fig. 50.48a, b).

Morning Glory anomaly

This is an unusual coloboma consisting of a posteriorly

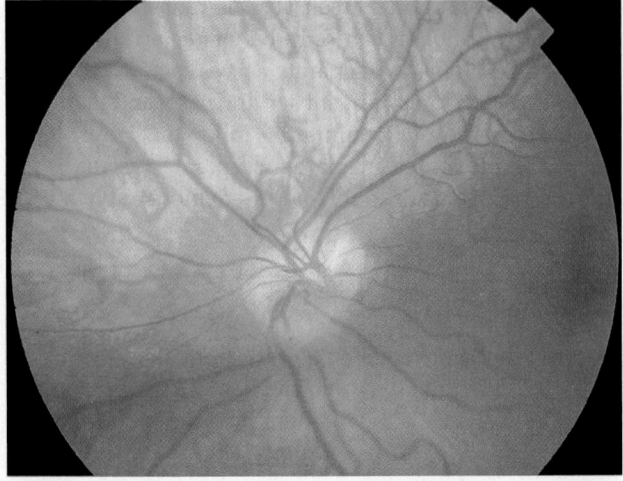

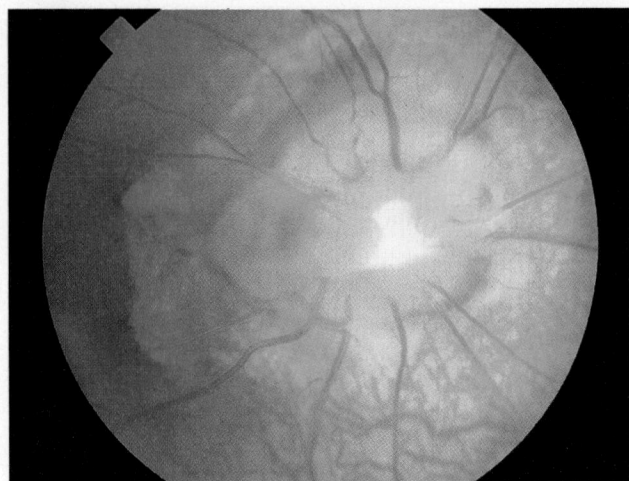

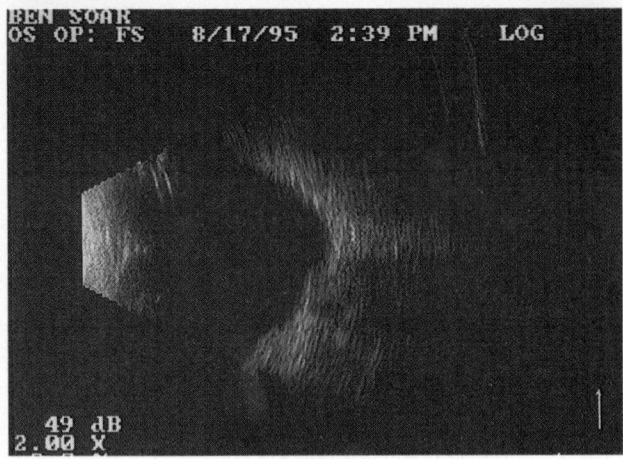

Fig. 50.48 (a, b) Peripapillary staphyloma of the fundus above the optic disc shown by the pale area above the disc (a) and on ultrasound (b). Morning Glory anomaly (c). There is a glial anomaly with a persistent hyaloid system and the retinal vessels radiate from around the optic disc. At birth the peripapillary retina was detached. It settled spontaneously.

displaced disc inside a funnel-shaped staphylomatous defect with an associated glial tuft (Fig. 50.48c). The peripapillary area is elevated with an associated annulus of pigmentary clumping. The disc may be large with a persistent hyaloid system and associated persistent hyperplastic primary vitreous (Traboulsi & Maumenee 1992). Vessels radiate out from the edge of the disc. The vision in the affected eye is usually very poor (Krause 1972; Jensen & Kalina 1976), often due to associated amblyopia from myopic astigmatism (Apple *et al.* 1982). It was probably first described by Handemann (1929) and the term Morning Glory syndrome (after the flower) was coined by Kindler (1970) 40 years later. Systemic associations are rare, but should be considered; basal encephalocoeles (Goldhammer & Smith 1975), microtia (Yamaguchi 1975; Grune & Fechner 1978), Duane's retraction syndrome (Kawano & Fujita 1981), endocrine and central nervous system anomalies (Eustis *et al.* 1994), and a variety of ocular defects (Kindler 1970; Odagiri & Ito 1975; Jensen & Kalina 1976; Steinkuller 1980; Brown & Tasman 1983) have been described. Retinal arteriovenous communications may be not uncommon (Brodsky & Sloan Wilson 1995). Sometimes there is a widespread retinal detachment earli-

er in life which may settle spontaneously (Hamada & Ellsworth 1971) or with treatment where this is deemed necessary (Chang *et al.* 1984; Haik *et al.* 1984). The detachment is non-rhegmatogenous and thought to be due to traction from the abnormal glial tissue on the disc. The ERG amplitude is low in proportion to the defect (Guiseppe 1986). The diagnosis should be made carefully (its euphonic name is attached incorrectly to many disc anomalies). Morning Glory disc is usually unilateral and non-genetic (Brodsky 1994): its nosology and relationship to typical coloboma are uncertain.

Systemic associations of colobomatous defects

In the earlier literature the association of colobomatous defects with the general health and development of the patient was barely mentioned, perhaps because ophthalmologists were not aware that they are required to look beyond the palpebral fissures! Several surveys have, however, emphasized the systemic aspects (François 1968; James *et al.* 1974; Pagon 1981; Warburg 1993).

Whilst colobomas are probably most frequently seen by

Table 50.2 Systemic associations of coloboma.

Chromosomal syndromes frequently associated with coloboma
Trisomy 13: Patau's syndrome (Taylor 1968; Warburg 1970; Hoepner & Yanoff 1972; Saraux 1972)
Cat-eye syndrome: tri- or tetrasomy 22pter (Sehachenman *et al.* 1965; Cory 1974; Bofinger 1977; Weleber 1977; Schinzel *et al.* 1981)
4p- syndrome: Wolf–Hirschhorn (Smith 1976; Jay 1977)
Triploidy (Fulton 1977)

Chromosomal syndromes uncommonly associated with coloboma
Trisomy 18: Edward's syndrome (Taylor 1968; Mullaney & Fitzpatrick 1973)
Trisomy 22 (Smith 1976; Jay 1977; Pagon 1981; Antle *et al.* 1990)
Monosomy 9 (Sakuma & Sakuma 1976)
13q- (Allderdice *et al.* 1969)
11q-: Jacobsen's syndrome (Schinzel *et al.* 1977)
18q-: deGrouchy syndrome (Yanoff *et al.* 1970)
18r (Jay 1977)
13r (Jay 1977)
Trisomy 4p (Lurie & Samochvalov 1994)

Systemic anomalies due to a single gene defect
CHARGE association (Evans & McLachlan 1971; James *et al.* 1974; Ho *et al.* 1975; Hall 1979; Hittner 1979; Lillquist 1980; Pagon 1981; Russell-Eggitt *et al.* 1990)
Lenz microphthalmia syndrome (Lenz 1955; Hermann & Opitz 1969; Goldberg & McKusick 1971)
Focal dermal hypoplasia: Goltz's syndrome (Willetts 1974; Thomas *et al.* 1977; Temple *et al.* 1990)
Meckel–Gruber syndrome (Meckel 1822; Opitz & Howe 1969; Salonen 1984; various authors 1994)
Joubert's syndrome (Benner & Gooskens 1985; Laverda *et al.* 1985; Lindhout & Barth 1985; Van Dorp *et al.* 1991)
Branchio-oculofacial syndrome (Legius 1990; Lin *et al.* 1991; Hing *et al.* 1992)
Basal cell naevus syndrome: Gorlin's syndrome (Gorlin & Sedano 1971)
Warburg syndrome: HARD ± E syndrome (Pagon *et al.* 1978; Warburg 1978)
Aicardi's syndrome (Hoyt *et al.* 1978; Chiu *et al.* 1992)

Systemic anomalies of unknown aetiology
Epidermal naevus syndrome: sebaceous naevus of Jadassohn, Soloman's syndrome, Fuerstein–Mimms syndrome (Jadassohn

1895; Marden 1966; Bianchine 1970; Soloman 1975; Barth 1977; Burch *et al.* 1980; Wilkes *et al.* 1981; Insler & Daulin 1987; Katz *et al.* 1987; Campbell & Patterson 1992)
Rubinstein–Taybi syndrome: broad thumbs syndrome (Roy *et al.*; Rubinstein 1969)
Goldenhar syndrome: oculoauricular vertebral dysplasia (Limaye 1972)
Amniotic band syndrome: limb–body wall complex (Hashemi *et al.* 1991; Jensen *et al.* 1993)
MOMO syndrome (Moretti-Ferreira 1993)
Treacher Collins–Franceschetti syndrome (Saraux 1966; Cordier *et al.* 1968)
The oralfacial-digital syndrome (Stevens & Marsh 1994)
Midline facial defects (Temple *et al.* 1990)

Brain defects (Warburg 1971; James *et al.* 1974; Jacobs & Taylor 1991)
Dandy–Walker cyst (Chemke *et al.* 1975; Orcutt & Bunt 1982)
Basal encephalocoele (Goldhammer & Smith 1975)
Arrhinencephaly (Lyford & Roy 1974)

Teratogens
Thalidomide (Smithells 1973; Stromland & Miller 1993)
Retinoic acid (Warburg 1992)
Alcohol (Hinzpeter *et al.* 1992)
Cocaine (Good *et al.* 1992)

Other reported but likely coincidental associations
Laurence–Moon–Biedl (Blumel *et al.* 1959; Klein & Amman 1969)
Stickler's syndrome (Say *et al.* 1977)
Incontinentia pigmenti (Maumenee 1974)
Ellis–van Creveld (McGregor 1954)
Hallerman–Streiff (François 1958)
Pierre–Robin anomaly (Smith & Stowe 1961)
Crouzon's syndrome (Ballantyne 1937; Howell 1974)
Kartagener's syndrome (Segal *et al.* 1963)
Klinefelter's syndrome (François *et al.* 1970; Hashmi & Karsenas 1976; Epstein *et al.* 1984)
Tuberous sclerosis (Lagos & Gomez 1967; Nevin & Pearce 1968)
Noonan's syndrome (Ascaso 1993)
Kallman's syndrome (Levy & Knudtzon 1993)
Peters' anomaly (Traboulsi & Maumenee 1992)
Mobius syndrome (Huerva *et al.* 1992)
Congenital cytomegalovirus (Hittner *et al.* 1976)

the ophthalmologist as an isolated defect they may occur either as part of a chromosomal syndrome or as part of a more widespread disorder (Jacobs & Taylor 1991). Warburg estimated that 100 different genetic traits may be associated with microphthalmos and/or coloboma, and suggested that any patient with these, mental retardation, and two other malformations would have a high chance of chromosomal abnormalities. The fact that some congenital disc anomalies have a low recurrence rate is equally important. In general there is no difference between the ocular aspects of the colobomatous manifestations seen in the various systemic syndromes.

Table 50.2 lists various associations with coloboma. Several of these are discussed in detail below.

Chromosomal syndromes frequently associated with coloboma

Trisomy 13 (Patau's syndrome)

This is recognized by the combination of a severe colobomatous defect and retinal dysplasia, with a cleft lip and palate, severe cardiac anomalies which cause nearly 80% of affected children to die within a year, and a variety of other defects. The chromosomal defect is a trisomy (an extra chromosome) 13.

The colobomas usually involve iris, choroid and disc and they may be very large. The child may be clinically anophthalmic, microphthalmic or have normally sized eyes. Anterior segment cleavage syndromes also occur and the lens may have posterior lenticonus and cataract. There may be dysplastic retina with cartilage, persistent hyperplastic primary vitreous, congenital retinal folds and detachment (Warburg 1970; Hoepner & Yanoff 1972; Saraux 1972).

Cat-eye syndrome (tri- or tetrasomy 22pter)

As the name implies, iris colobomas are very frequent in this syndrome (Schachenmann *et al.* 1965). The affected children are mildly mentally deficient; they may have anal atresia, microphthalmos, telecanthus, down-slanting palpebral fissures, epicanthal folds and squint. This is an abnormal small extra chromosome which may be a deleted part of chromosome 22 which appears as a dicentric marker chromosome (Cory & Jamison 1974; Bofinger & Soukup 1977; Weleber *et al.* 1977). Other features include pre-auricular pits or tags or microtia. Clinical suspicion must be high for this syndrome because the phenotype varies widely within families (Schinzel *et al.* 1981).

4p- syndrome (Wolf–Hirschhorn syndrome)

These profoundly mentally defective children have a characteristic face with a 'fish-like' mouth, coloboma, epicanthic folds, hypertelorism and strabismus (Smith 1976; Jay 1977).

Triploidy

Although one of the most common chromosomal aberrations at conception, most affected fetuses abort spontaneously. A few cases have been described in premature babies and even fewer in full-term gestation babies who do not survive. Mosaics may survive to teenage years but less often have coloboma. Findings include a triangular face with an abnormal nose, cleft lip and palate, microphthalmos and ptosis (Fulton 1977).

Chromosomal syndromes uncommonly associated with coloboma

Trisomy 18 (Edward's syndrome)

Although the incidence of trisomy 18 (Edward's syndrome) is higher than trisomy D, coloboma is much less frequent (Taylor 1968). Affected infants are very feeble with characteristic facies, severe mental retardation, and cardiac defects. Coloboma, short palpebral fissure, epican-

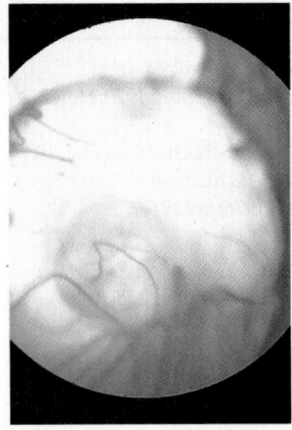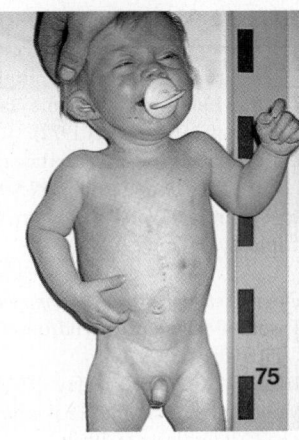

Fig. 50.49 Optic nerve coloboma in a child with tracheo-oesophageal fistula.

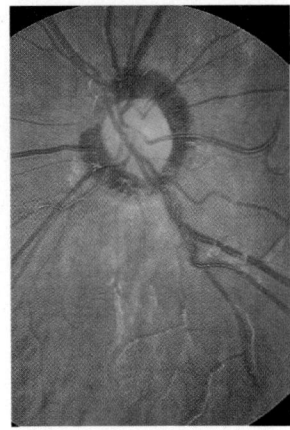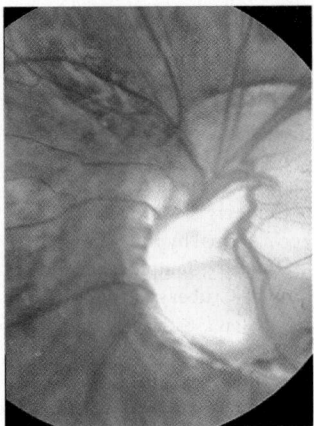

Fig. 50.50 CHARGE association. It is frequent that the optic discs in this syndrome are colobomatous, but often atypical. In this case the right optic disc is hypoplastic with a pigmented surround.

thus, ptosis, cataract and microphthalmos occur (Mullaney 1973).

Coloboma also occurs in monosomy 9 (Sakuma & Sakuma 1976), 11q- (Schinzel *et al.* 1977), 13q- (Allderdice *et al.* 1969) which is also associated with retinoblastoma, 18 deletion syndrome (Yanoff *et al.* 1970), trisomy 4p (Lurie & Samochvalor 1994), and trisomy 22 (Smith 1976; Jay 1977; Pagon 1981). The occurrence of colobomas with a systemic defect may warrant chromosome studies.

Coloboma as a part of a multisystem disorder due to single gene defects

CHARGE association (Pagon's syndrome)

Although the association between coloboma, choanal atresia and other systemic defects occurred in ophthalmological (James *et al.* 1974), otolaryngological (Evans &

MacLachlan 1971), and genetic (Ho *et al.* 1975) literature it was overlooked for many years.

CHARGE (Pagon *et al.* 1980) is a mnemonic for coloboma, heart defect, atresia choanae, retarded growth and development, genital anomalies, and ear anomalies and deafness. A patient only needs four of these major findings to fit the diagnosis (Figs 50.49, 50.50). The other anomalies that occur with the CHARGE association include facial palsy, micrognathia, cleft palate and pharyngeal incompetence (Hall 1979). Tracheo-oesophageal fistula (Hall 1979; Lillquist *et al.* 1980; Pagon 1981) and renal anomalies (Pagon 1981) can be found.

Pagon (1981) found coloboma in 16 of 19 patients ranging from iris colobomas to anophthalmos. The severity of the eye defect does not correlate with the degree of mental deficit, nor does the external ear anomaly correlate with the degree of deafness. Typical colobomas occur in about 82% of cases of the CHARGE association but they may be quite subtle (Russell-Eggitt *et al.* 1990).

The inheritance seems largely sporadic, and chromoso-

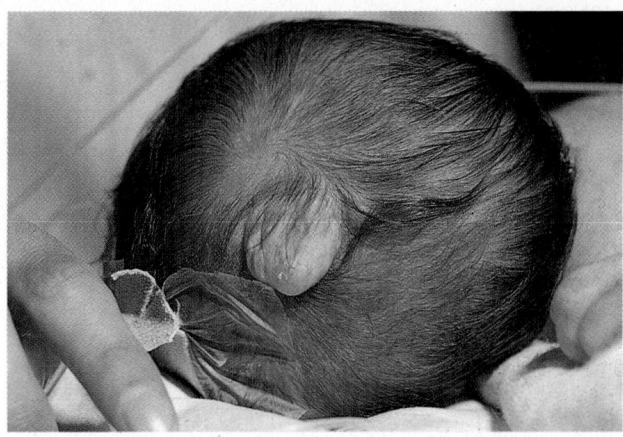

Fig. 50.52 Meckel–Gruber syndrome with occipital encephalocoele.

mal studies have been normal. There is no history of consanguinity to suggest autosomal recessive inheritance. Familial cases have been reported (Hittner *et al.* 1979), and occasional autosomal dominant inheritance has occurred. Pagon (1981) reported a patient with a normal father except for microphthalmos with coloboma, and another family with an affected mother and daughter. CHARGE association does bear phenotypic resemblance to cat-eye syndrome and DiGeorge's syndrome, both involving rearrangement of chromosome 22 (Russell-Eggitt *et al.* 1990), and one of Pagon's patients had DiGeorge's syndrome. There is also some overlap with the VACTERL syndrome (vertebral anomalies, anal atresia, cardiac defects, tracheo-oesophageal fistula, renal and ray anomalies), which lacks coloboma. The recurrence risk for most families is low, but chromosomal studies are warranted (Russell-Eggitt *et al.* 1990).

Lenz microphthalmia syndrome

Lenz (1955) first described an X-linked pedigree with microphthalmos, microcephaly, vertebral, dental, renal and urogenital anomalies, congenital heart disease and digital defects. He noted that while the proband did not have a coloboma the maternal uncle did, illustrating variable expression. Goldberg and McKusick (1971) reported four affected males in a non-consanguinous pedigree with colobomatous microphthalmos, short stature, and protruding simple ears. Hermann and Opitz (1969) described a possible maternal carrier state with short stature, microcephaly, and coarse iris features. There is often a history of multiple abortions in carriers, and affected males have never reproduced, reducing familial recurrences.

Focal dermal hypoplasia (Goltz's syndrome)

This syndrome (Fig. 50.51) of mesodermal dysgenesis

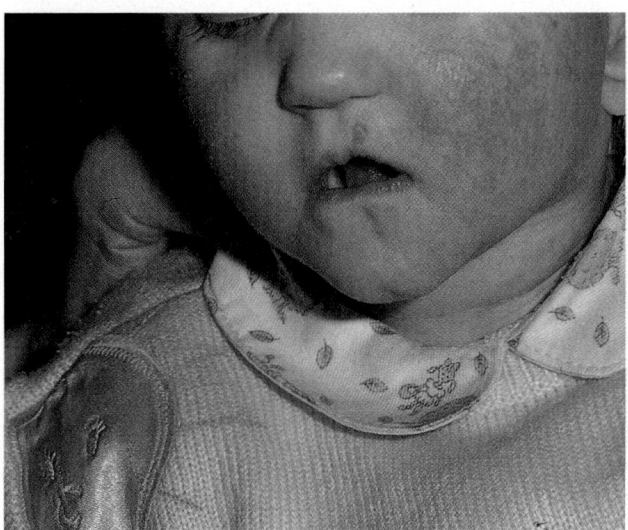

a

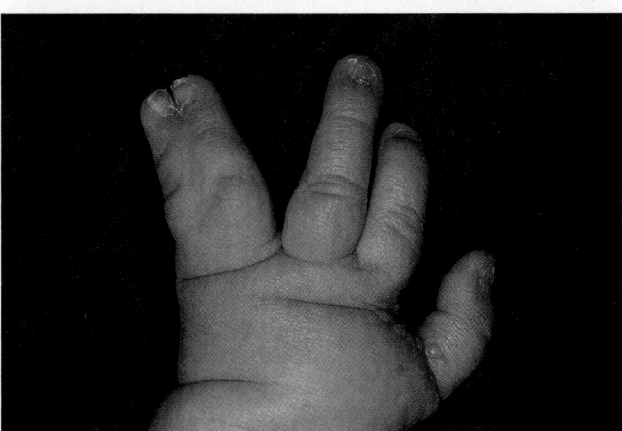

b

Fig. 50.51 (a) Goltz's syndrome showing the atrophic skin lesions. This child had bilateral optic nerve colobomas and marked left microphthalmos. (b) Goltz's syndrome showing polysyndactyly.

results in dermal hypoplasia (100%), bony defects (82%), dental anomalies (51%), ocular findings (40%) and mental retardation (12%) (Thomas *et al.* 1977). Coloboma occurs more often than microphthalmos. The skin findings are striking with pink atrophic macular areas, pinkish brown nodules of fat herniation through the dermis, and raspberry papillomas (Temple *et al.* 1990b). Of more than 200 reported cases, 88% are female, and it is thought to be X-linked dominant lethal, with a high miscarriage rate in females. Most cases are sporadic (Temple *et al.* 1990b).

Meckel–Gruber syndrome

This is a severe disorder of presumed autosomal recessive inheritance; affected infants usually have a very short lifespan. Findings include, in order of decreasing frequency, abnormal kidneys, encephalocoele (usually occipital; Fig. 50.52), polydactyly, cleft palate and micrognathia, abnormal urinary tracts, microphthalmia or coloboma, and congenital heart disease (Meckel 1822; Opitz & Howe 1969; Salonan 1984; Various Authors 1994).

Joubert's syndrome

In 1980 Lindhout *et al.* described a male with findings of Joubert's syndrome (hyperpnoea, rhythmic tongue protrusions, developmental delay, delayed visual evoked response (VER) and aplasia of the cerebellar vermis). He also had bilateral choroidal colobomas; the eyes of his parents were normal. The author noted that vermis hypoplasia also represents a fusion defect. The association of colobomas and Joubert's syndrome was also discussed by several authors who found eight reported cases, all male (Benner & Gooskins 1985; Laverda *et al.* 1985; Lindhout & Barth 1985). Van Dorp *et al.* (1991) reported another patient whose aborted sister had retinal colobomas; he felt the association was non-random.

Branchio-oculofacial syndrome

The branchio-oculofacial syndrome is an autosomal dominant syndrome with variable expression. Patients have aplastic or hemangiomatous cervical skin lesions with or without branchial sinuses, malformed ears, cleft lip and palate and coloboma/microphthalmos (Legius 1990; Lin 1991).

Basal cell naevus syndrome (Gorlin's syndrome)

Colobomas may be one of the earlier findings in this syndrome, with the characteristic basal cell carcinomas developing later. Inheritance is autosomal dominant with high penetrance and variable expression. Other features can include a characteristic face with frontal bossing, prominent supraorbital ridges, hypertelorism, mandibular

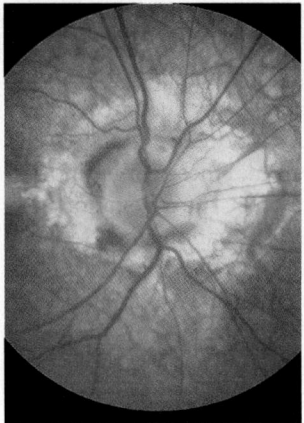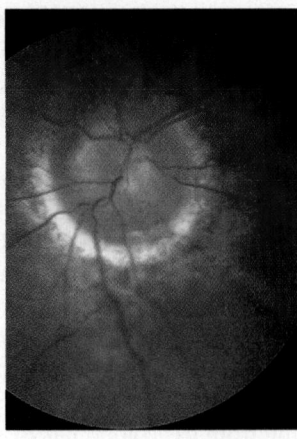

Fig. 50.53 Epidermal naevus syndrome showing the anomalous optic disc.

cysts, male hypogonadism and ovarian fibromas (Gorlin & Sedano 1971).

Coloboma associated with systemic anomalies of unknown aetiology

Epidermal naevus syndrome

This is also known as the sebaceous naevus of Jadassohn, Soloman's syndrome, or Fuerstein–Mimms syndrome. Patients have a non-dermatomal linear pigmented naevus, a variety of other skin defects, skeletal anomalies and usually severe retardation secondary to various brain defects (Jadassohn 1895; Marden 1966; Bianchine 1970; Soloman 1975; Burch 1980). Eye abnormalities (Barth 1977) include ptosis, conjunctival dermoids (Wilkes *et al.* 1981), lid colobomas (Insler & Daulin 1987) and other anterior segment anomalies. Fundus abnormalities have been described including colobomas, anomalous discs (Fig. 50.53), peripapillary staphyloma, Coats' disease (Burch *et al.* 1980), pseudopapilloedema (Campbell & Patterson 1992), osseous choristoma of the choroid (Lambert *et al.* 1987) and optic nerve hypoplasia (Katz *et al.* 1987).

Coloboma with brain defects

A variety of brain defects have been described together with coloboma: Dandy–Walker cyst (Orcutt & Bunt 1982), basal encephalocoele (Goldhammer & Smith 1975), arrhinencephaly (Lyford & Roy 1974), and others (Warburg 1971; James *et al.* 1974; Chemke *et al.* 1975).

Coloboma associated with teratogens

Thalidomide is the archetypical teratogen with damage known to occur between 20 and 36 days of gestation (Stromland & Miller 1993). This time-frame is slightly before optic fissure closure, so it is not surprising that colobomas are one of the manifestations. Smithells (1973) reviewed 154 patients with thalidomide embryopathy and found five with coloboma. Cocaine is another potential teratogen; one of 13 infants exposed *in utero* had coloboma, three others had optic nerve hypoplasia (Good *et al.* 1992). Fetal alcohol syndrome has also been associated with optic nerve hypoplasia, and more rarely, coloboma.

Other reported associations with coloboma

Pagon (1981) has carried out a useful survey of other disorders which have occurred with, but are probably not causally related to, colobomas. See Table 50.2 for a complete list of these and references. Other reported associations include MOMO syndrome with macrosomia, obesity and macrocephaly (Moretti-Ferreira *et al.* 1993), Noonan's syndrome (Ascaso *et al.* 1993), Kallman's syndrome (Levy & Knudtzon 1993) and midline facial defects (Temple *et al.* 1990). A family with a mutation of the PAX 2 gene had a combination of coloboma, renal anomalies and vesicoureteral reflux (Sanayusin *et al.* 1995); the colobomas were not completely typical.

Genetic implications of optic disc anomalies

With a low recurrence risk to subsequent children of the same parents

- Optic disc hypoplasia/aplasia.
- Aicardi's syndrome.
- Morning Glory syndrome (Fig. 50.54).
- Myelinated nerve fibres.
- Vascular anomalies (except von Hippel–Lindau).
- Glial anomalies.

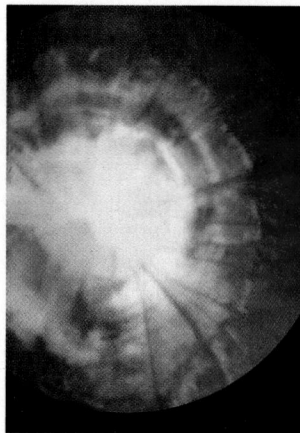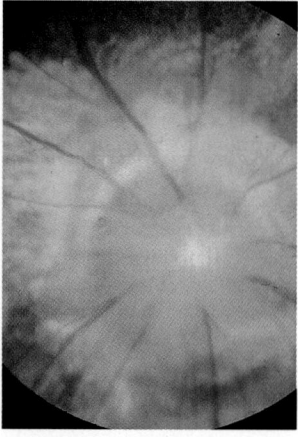

Fig. 50.54 Morning Glory syndrome (see p. 685). These two typical cases are unilateral and show vessels that radiate from the discs with an elevated peripapillary area and persistent hyaloid system.

With genetic implications

- Drusen (sometimes dominant).
- von Hippel–Lindau disease (dominant).
- Phakoma in tuberous sclerosis (dominant).
- Coloboma (i) dominant; (ii) recessive; (ii) X-linked recessive—Lenz microphthalmic syndrome; and (iv) X-dominant—Goltz's syndrome.

As a sign of chromosomal disease

See Warburg and Friedrich (1987)
- Down's syndrome—excess vessels.
- Coloboma: (i) trisomy 13, 18, 22; (ii) 22 deletion (cat-eye syndrome); (iii) triploidy; (iv) 4p-; (v) monosomy 9; (vi) 11p-; and (vii) 13q-.

References

Aicardi J, Lefebvre J, Lerique-Loechlin AA. A new syndrome: spasm in flexion, callosalagenesis ocular abnormalities. *Electroencephalogr Clin Neurophysiol* 1965; **19**: 609–10.

Akiba J, Yoshida A, Ohta I, Igarashi H, Kakehashi A. Anomalous Cloquet's canal in a case of optic nerve head coloboma associated with extensive retinal detachment. *Br J Ophthalmol* 1993; **77**: 381–2.

Ali B, Logani S, Kozlov K, Arnold A, Bateman B. Progression of retinal nerve fibre myelination in childhood. *Am J Ophthalmol* 1994; **118**: 515–17.

Allderdice PW, Davis JG, Miller OJ *et al.* The 13q– deletion syndrome. *Am J Hum Genet* 1969; **21**: 499–512.

Alvarez E, Wakakura M, Khan Z, Dulton GN. The disc–macula distance to disc–diameter ratio: a new test for confirming optic nerve hypoplasia in young children. *J Pediatr Ophthalmol Strabismus* 1988; **25**: 151–6.

Anderson SR, Bro-Rasmussen F, Tygstrup I. Anencephaly related to ocular development and malformation. *Am J Ophthalmol* 1972; **74**: 967–75.

Antle CM, Pantzar JT, White VA. The ocular pathology of trisomy 22: report of two cases and review. *J Pediatr Ophthalmol* 1990; **27**: 310–14.

Apple DJ, Rabb MF, Walsh PM. Congenital anomalies of the optic disc. *Surv Ophthalmol* 1982; **27**: 3–41.

Ascaso FJ, DelBuey MA, Huerva V, Latre B, Palomer A. Noonan's syndrome with keratoconus and optic disc coloboma. *Eur J Ophthalmol* 1993; **3**: 101–3.

Avendano J, Rodrigues MM, Hackett JJ, Gaskins R. Corpora amylacea of the optic nerve and retina; a form of neuronal degeneration. *Invest Ophthalmol Vis Sci* 1980; **19**: 550–4.

Awan KJ. Hypoteleorism and optic disc anomalies: an ignored ocular syndrome. *Ann Ophthalmol* 1977; **9**: 771–7.

Baarsma GS. Acquired medullated nerve fibres. *Br J Ophthalmol* 1980; **64**: 651–2.

Ballantyne AJ. Dysostosis cranio-facialis. *Proc Roy Soc Med* 1937; **30**: 280–5.

Baraitser M, Winter RM, Taylor DSI. The Lenz microphthalmos syndrome. *Clin Genet* 1982; **22**: 99–101.

Barroso L, Hoyt W, Narahara M. Disc edge veins of Kraupa: rare exit anomalies of the retinal vein. *Br J Ophthalmol* 1992; **76**: 442–3.

Barroso LH, Ragge NK, Hoyt WF. Multiple cilioretinal arteries and dysplasia of the optic disc. *J Clin Neuro-ophthalmol* 1991; **11**: 278–9.

Barth PG. Organoid nevus syndrome (linear nevus sebaceous of Jadassohn): clinical and radiological study of a case. *Neuropediatrics* 1977; **8**: 418–28.

Beauvieux J. La pseudo-atrophie optique des nouveau nés dysgenesie myelinique des voies optique. *Ann Oculist (Paris)* 1926; **163**: 82–92.

Bec P, Adam P, Mathis A, Alberge Y, Roulleau J, Arne JHL. Optic nerve head drusen: high resolution CT approach. *Arch Ophthalmol* 1984; **102**: 680–2.

Beener FA, Gooskens R. Chorioretinal coloboma and Joubert syndrome (reply). *J Pediatr* 1985; **107**: 158–9.

Bell RW. Case of total preservation of hyaloid artery with pupillary membrane, cataract, retinal and uveal coloboma and microphthalmos. *Ann Ophthalmol* 1971; **3**: 589–91.

Bellhom RW, Hirano A, Henkind P, Johnson PT. Schwann cell proliferations mimicking medullated retinal nerve fibres. *Am J Ophthalmol* 1979; **87**: 469–73.

Benner JD, Preslan MW, Gratz E, Joslyn J, Schwartz M, Kelman S. Septo-optic dysplasia in two siblings. *Am J Ophthalmol* 1990; **109**: 632–8.

Benoit-Gonin JJ, David M, Feit JP *et al.* La dysplasie septo-optique avec déficit en hormone antidiurétique et insuffisance surrénale centrale. *Nouv Presse Med* 1978; **37**: 3327–31.

Bianchine JW. The naevus sebaceous of Jadassohn. *Am J Dis Child* 1970; **120**: 223–8.

Billson F, Hopkins IJ. Optic nerve hypoplasia and hypopituitarism. *Lancet* 1972; **i**: 905.

Bistner S, Rubin L, Aguine G. Development of the bovine eye. *Am J Vet Res* 1973; **34**: 7–12.

Björk A, Laurell C-G, Laurell U. Bilateral optic nerve hypoplasia with normal visual acuity. *Am J Ophthalmol* 1978; **86**: 524–9.

Blanco R, Salvador F, Galan A, Gibernav J. Aplasia of the optic nerve: report of three cases. *J Pediatr Ophthalmol Strabismus* 1992; **29**: 228–31.

Blumel J, Kniker WT. Laurence–Moon–Bardet–Biedl syndrome. Review of the literature and a report of five cases including a family group with three affected males. *Texas Rep Biol Med* 1959; **17**: 391–410.

Bofinger MK, Soukup SW. Cat eye syndrome. *Am J Dis Child* 1977; **131**: 893–7.

Boniuk V, Ho PK. Ocular findings in anencephaly. *Am J Ophthalmol* 1979; **88**: 613–17.

Borchert M, McCulloch D, Rother C, Stout AV. Clinical assessment, optic disk measurements, and visual evoked potential in optic nerve hypoplasia. *Am J Ophthalmol* 1995; **120**: 605–12.

Borodick GE, Gragoudas ES, Edward WO, Brockhurst RJ. Peripapillary subretinal neovascularisation and serous macular detachment: association with congenital optic nerve pits. *Arch Ophthalmol* 1984; **102**: 229–32.

Boyce DC. Hypoplasia of the optic nerve. *Am J Ophthalmol* 1941; **34**: 888–9.

Brazitikos P, Safran A, Simona F, Zulauf M. Threshold perimetry in tilted disc syndrome. *Arch Ophthalmol* 1990; **108**: 1698–701.

Brink JK, Larsen FE. Pseudodoubling of the optic disc. *Acta Ophthalmol* 1977; **55**: 862–70.

Brodsky M. Congenital optic disc anomalies. *Surv Ophthalmol* 1994a; **39**: 89–112.

Brodsky M. Morning Glory disc anomaly or optic disc coloboma? *Arch Ophthalmol* 1994b; **112**: 153.

Brodsky M. Septo-optic dysplasia: a reappraisal. *Semin Ophthalmol* 1991; **6**: 227–32.

Brodsky MC, Ford RE, Bradford JD. Subretinal neovascular membrane in an infant with a retino-choroidal coloboma. *Arch Ophthalmol* 1991; **109**: 1650–1.

Brodsky M, Glasier C. Optic nerve hypoplasia: clinical significance of associated central nervous system abnormalities on magnetic resonance imaging. *Arch Ophthalmol* 1993; **111**: 66–74.

Brodsky MC, Glasier C, Pollock S, Angtuago E. Optic nerve hypoplasia: identification by magnetic resonance imaging. *Arch Ophthalmol* 1990; **108**: 1562–8.

Brodsky MC, Hoyt WF, Hoyt CS, Miller NS, Lam BL. Atypical retinochoroidal coloboma in patients with dysplastic optic discs and trans-sphenoidal encephalocele: report of five cases. *Arch Ophthalmol* 1995; **113**: 624–8.

Brodsky MC, Sloan Wilson R. Retinal arteriovenous communications in the Morning Glory disc anomaly. *Arch Ophthalmol* 1995; **113**: 410–11.

Brook GD, Sanders MD, Hoare RD. Septo-optic dysplasia. *Br Med J* 1972; **3**: 811–13.

Brown GC. Optic nerve hypoplasia and colobomatous defects. *J Pediatr Ophthalmol Strabismus* 1982; **19**: 90–3.

Brown GC, Magargal LE, Augsburger JJ. Pre-retinal arterial loops and retinal arterial occlusion. *Am J Ophthalmol* 1979; **87**: 646–51.

Brown GC, Shields JA, Goldberg RE. Congenital pits of the optic nerve head II. Clinical studies in humans. *Am Acad Ophthalmol* 1980; **87**: 51–65.

Brown GC, Tasman WS. *Congenital Anomalies of the Optic Disc*. New York: Grune & Stratton, 1983.

Buchanan TAS, Hoyt WF. Temporal visual field defects associated with nasal hypoplasia of the optic disc. *Br J Ophthalmol* 1981; **65**: 636–40.

Bullard DE, Crockard HA, McDonald WI. Spontaneous cerebrospinal fluid rhinorrhoea associated with dysplastic optic discs and a basal encephalocoele. *J Neurosurg* 1981; **54**: 807–10.

Burch JV, Leveille AS, Morse PH. Ichthyosis hystrix (epidermal nevus syndrome) and Coats' disease. *Am J Ophthalmol* 1980; **89**: 25–30.

Burde R. Optic disc risk factors for non-arteritic anterior ischaemic optic neuropathy. *Am J Ophthalmol* 1993; **116**: 759–64.

Campbell S, Patterson A. Pseudopapilloedema in the linear naevus syndrome. *Br J Ophthalmol* 1992; **76**: 372–4.

Caprioli J, Lesser RL. Basal encephalocoele and Morning Glory syndrome. *Br J Ophthalmol* 1983; **67**: 349–51.

Carney S, Brodsky M, Good W, Glasier C, Greibel, M, Cunniff C. Aicardi syndrome: more than meets the eye. *Surv Ophthalmol* 1993; **37**: 419–24.

Catalano R, Simon JW. Optic disc elevation in Down's syndrome. *Am J Ophthalmol* 1990; **110**: 28–32.

Cennamo G, Liguori G, Pezone A, Iaccarino G. Morning Glory syndrome associated with marked persistent hyperplastic primary vitreous and lens colobomas. *Br J Ophthalmol* 1989; **73**: 684–7.

Cennamo G, Sammartino A, Fioretti F. Morning Glory syndrome with contractile peripapillary staphyloma. *Br J Ophthalmol* 1983; **67**: 346–7.

Chan CC, Fishman M, Egbert PR. Multiple ocular anomalies associated with maternal LSD ingestion. *Arch Ophthalmol* 1978; **96**: 282–4.

Chan T, Bowell R, O'Keefe M, Lanigan B. Ocular manifestations in fetal alcohol syndrome. *Br J Ophthalmol* 1991; **75**: 524–6.

Chang M. Pits and crater-like holes of the optic disc. *Ophthalmol Semin* 1976; **1**: 21–76.

Chang S, Barrett GH, Ellsworth RM, St Louis L, Berrocal JA. Treatment of total retinal detachment in Morning Glory syndrome. *Am J Ophthalmol* 1984; **97**: 596–606.

Chemke J, Czernobilsky B, Mundel G, Barishak YR. A familial syndrome of central nervous system and ocular malformations. *Clin Genet* 1975; **7**: 1–7.

Chia Lee Linn C, Tso MOM, Vygantes CM. Coloboma of optic nerve associated with serous maculopathy. *Arch Ophthalmol* 1984; **102**: 1651–5.

Chiu NC, Shen EY, Fang SR. Aicardi's syndrome in a female infant with a family history of miscarried male siblings. *J Formosan Med Assoc* 1992; **91**: 624–6.

Cogan DG. Coloboma of optic nerve with overlay of peripapillary retina. *Br J Ophthalmol* 1978; **62**: 347–50.

Collier M. Les doubles papilles optiques. *Bull Soc Ophthalmol* 1958; **90**: 328–52.

Cook CS, Nowotny AZ, Sulik KK. Fetal alcohol syndrome. *Arch Ophthalmol* 1987; **105**: 1576–82.

Corbett JJ, Jacobson DM, Maver RC, Thompson HS. Enlargement of the blind spot caused by papilloedema. *Am J Ophthalmol* 1988; **105**: 261–6.

Corbett JJ, Savino PJ, Schatz NJ. Cavitary developmental defects of the optic disc: visual loss associated with pits and colobomas. *Arch Neurol* 1990; **37**: 210–13.

Cordier J, Triclon P, Thiriet M, Babut M, Raspiller A. Weyer's oculo-vertebral syndrome. *Rev Oto-neuro Ophthalmol* 1968; **40**: 204–11.

Cords R. Einseitige kleinheit der papille. *Klin Mbl Augenheilkd* 1923; **71**: 414–18.

Cory C, Jamison DL. The cat eye syndrome. *Arch Ophthalmol* 1974; **92**: 259–62.

Cotlier E. Café-au-lait spots of the fundus in neurofibromatosis. *Arch Ophthalmol* 1977; **95**: 1990–2.

Dascoffe JC, Woillez M, Dhoine G. Association of hereditary vitreous striae, iris, coloboma and cataract. *Bull Soc Ophthalmol Fr* 1975; **75**: 335–7.

Davis GU, Schoch JP. Septo-optic dysplasia associated with see-saw nystagmus. *Arch Ophthalmol* 1975; **93**: 137–9.

Degenhart W, Brown GC, Augsburger JJ. Prepapillary vascular loops. *Ophthalmology* 1981; **88**: 1126–31.

DeJong P, Bistervels B, Cosgrove J, DeGrip G, Leys A, Goffin M. Medullated nerve fibres. A sign of multiple basal cell nevi (Gorlin's) syndrome. *Arch Ophthalmol* 1985; **103**: 1833–7.

De Morsier G. Études sur les dysraphies crànio-encephaliques III. Agénésie du septum lucidum avec malformation du tractus optique. La dysplasie septo-optique. *Schweitz Arch Neurol Psychiatr* 1956; **77**: 267–92.

Donat JFG. Septo-optic dysplasia in an infant of a diabetic mother. *Arch Neurol* 1981; **38**: 580–91.

Dorrell D. The tilted disc. *Br J Ophthalmol* 1978; **62**: 16–20.

Drews RC. Heterochromia iridum with coloboma of the optic disc. *Arch Ophthalmol* 1973; **900**: 437–43.

Duke-Elder S. *System of Ophthalmology: Normal and Abnormal Development. Congenital Deformities*, Vol. III, Part 2. London: H. Kimpton, 1964.

Edwards WC, Layden WE. Optic nerve hypoplasia. *Am J Ophthalmol* 1970; **70**: 950–9.

Elbrechtz HC. Über eine doppelle papille im auge. *Klin Mbl Augenheilkd* 1975; **166**: 389–91.

Ellenberger C, Runyan TE. Holoprosencephaly with hypoplasia of the optic nerves, dwarfism and agenesis of the septum pellucidum. *Am J Ophthalmol* 1970; **70**: 960–7.

Elster AB, McAnarney ER. Maternal age re: septo-optic dysplasia. *J Pediatr* 1979; **94**: 162.

Epstein RJ, Mets MB, Wond PWK, Mizen TR. Uveal colobomas and Klinefelter's syndrome. *Am J Ophthalmol* 1984; **98**: 241–3.

Erkkila H. Optic disc — congenital anomaly. *Graefe's Arch Klin Exp Ophthalmol* 1976; **199**: 1–10.

Erkkila H. Optic disc drusen in children. *Graefe's Arch Klin Exp Ophthalmol* 1974; **189**: 1–7.

Eustis H, Sanders M, Zimmerman T. Morning Glory syndrome in children: association with endocrine and central nervous system anomalies. *Arch Ophthalmol* 1994; **112**: 204–7.

Evans JNG, MacLachlan RF. Choanal atresia. *J Laryngol Otol* 1971; **85**(Suppl.): 903–29.

Ewald RA. Unilateral hypoplasia of the optic nerve: radiologic and electroretinographic findings. *Am J Ophthalmol* 1967; **63**: 763–7.

Fletcher WA, Imes RK, Goodman D, Hoyt WF. Acute idiopathic blind spot enlargement. A big blind spot syndrome without optic disc edema. *Arch Ophthalmol* 1988; **106**: 44–9.

Font R, Marines H, Cartwright J, Bauserman S. Aicardi syndrome: a clinicopathologic case report including electron microscopic observations. *Ophthalmology* 1991; **98**: 1727–31.

Foos FY, Kiechler RJ, Allen RA. Congenital non-attachment of the retina. *Am J Ophthalmol* 1968; **65**: 202–11.

Foster J. Contractile optic disc coloboma. *Arch Ophthalmol* 1991; **109**: 472–7.

Franceschetti A. Fibres à myeline de la rétine et dyscranie. *Bull Soc Ophthalmol Fr* 1938; **51**: 573–7.

François J. Colobomatous malformations of the ocular globe. *Int Ophthalmol Clin* 1968; **8**: 797–816.

François J. *Heredity in Ophthalmology*. St Louis: CV Mosby, 1961.

François J. A new syndrome, dyscephalia with birdface and dental anomalies, nanism, hypotrichosis, cutaneous atrophy, microphthalmia and congenital cataract. *Arch Ophthalmol* 1958; **60**: 842–62.

François J, Hruby K. Uber seltene beobachtungen von hypoplasie der netzhaut. *Klin Mbl Augenheilkd* 1970; **157**: 605–10.

François J, Matton-Van Leuven M Th, Gombault Ph. Uveal coloboma and true Klinefelter syndrome. *J Med Genet* 1970; **7**: 213–23.

François J, Verriest G. Les druses de la papille. *Acta Neurol Belg* 1958; **51**: 327–55.

Friedman AH, Gartner S, Modi SS. Drusen of the optic disc: a retrospective study of cadaver eyes. *Br J Ophthalmol* 1975; **59**: 413–21.

Frisen L. Visual field defects due to hypoplasia of the optic nerve. *Doc Ophthalmol* 1979; **19**: 81–6.

Frisen L, Holmegaard L. Spectrum of optic nerve hypoplasia. *Br J Ophthalmol* 1978; **62**: 7–15.

Frisen L, Scholdstrom G, Svendsen P. Drusen in the optic nerve head: verification in the optic nerve head. *Arch Ophthalmol* 1978; **9**: 1611–14.

Fuchs E. Beitrag zu den angenborenen Anomalien des schnerven. *Graefe's Arch Ophthalmol* 1882; **28**: 139–69.

Fulton AB, Howard RO, Albert DM, Hsia YE, Packman S. Ocular findings in triploidy. *Am J Ophthalmol* 1977; **84**: 859–67.

Gallet J-P, Olivier C, Sanut S. Dystrophie thoracique, malformation oculaire et nèphropathie tubulo-interstitielle chez deux freres. *Ann Pediatr* 1973; **20**: 813–22.

Gardner HB, Irvine AE. Optic nerve hypoplasia with good visual acuity. *Arch Ophthalmol* 1972; **88**: 255–8.

Garg BP. Colpocephaly. *Arch Neurol* 1982; **39**: 243–6.

Gass JDM, Braunstein B. Sessile and exophytic capillary angiomas of the juxtapapillary retina and optic nerve head. *Arch Ophthalmol* 1980; **98**: 1790–7.

Goldberg MF, McKusick VA. X-linked colobomatous microphthalmos and other congenital anomalies. *Am J Ophthalmol* 1971; **71**: 1128–33.

Goldberg RE, Pleasant TR, Shields JA. Cavernous haemangioma of the retina. A four generation pedigree with neurocutaneous manifestations and an example of bilateral retinal involvement. *Arch Ophthalmol* 1979; **97**: 2321–4.

Goldhammer Y, Smith JL. Optic nerve anomalies in basal encephalocoeles. *Arch Ophthalmol* 1975; **93**: 115–18.

Good W, Brodsky M, Edwards M, Hoyt WF. Bilateral retinal hamartoma in neurofibroma type 2. *Br J Ophthalmol* 1991; **75**: 190.

Good WV, Ferriero DM, Golabi M, Kobori JA. Abnormalities of the visual system in infants exposed to cocaine. *Ophthalmology* 1992; **99**: 341–6.

Gorlin RJ, Sedano HO. The multiple nevoid basal cell carcinoma syndrome revisited. *Birth Defects* 1971; **7**: 140–7.

Graether JM. Transient amaurosis in one eye with simultaneous dilatation of retinal veins: in association with a congenital anomaly of the optic nerve head. *Arch Ophthalmol* 1963; **70**: 342–5.

Graham MV, Wakefield GJ. Bitemporal visual field defects associated with anomalies of the optic discs. *Br J Ophthalmol* 1973; **57**: 307–14.

Greenfield PS, Wilcox LM, Weiter JJ *et al.* Hypoplasia of the optic nerve in association with porencephaly. *J Pediatr Ophthalmol Strabismus* 1980; **17**: 75–8.

Grey RHB, Rice NSC. Congenital duplication of the lens. *Br J Ophthalmol* 1976; **60**: 673–6.

Griffiths P, Hunt S. Specific spatial defect in a child with septo-optic dysplasia. *Dev Med Child Neurol* 1984; **26**: 391–400.

Grune HJ, Fechner PU. Über das Morning Glory syndrom. *Klin Monatsbl Augenheilkd* 1978; **172**: 114–15.

Guiffre G. Morning Glory syndrome: clinical and electrofunctional study of three cases. *Br J Ophthalmol* 1986; **70**: 229–36.

Guiseppe G. Morning Glory syndrome: clinical and electrofunctional study of three cases. *Br J Ophthalmol* 1986; **70**: 229–36.

Haas BD, Jakobiec FA, Iwamoto T, Cox M, Bernacki EG, Pokorny JL. Diffuse choroidal melanocytoma in a child. *Ophthalmology* 1986; **93**: 1632–8.

Hackenbruch Y, Meerhoff E, Besio R, Cardoso H. Familial bilateral optic nerve hypoplasia. *Am J Ophthalmol* 1975; **79**: 314–20.

Haik BG, Greenstein SH, Smith ME, Abramson DH, Elsworth, RM. Retinal detachment in the Morning Glory syndrome. *Ophthalmology* 1984; **91**: 1638–47.

Hale BR, Rice P. Septo-optic dysplasia: clinical and embryological aspects. *Dev Med Child Neurol* 1974; **16**: 812–20.

Hall BD. Choanal atresia and association multiple anomalies. *J Pediatr* 1979; **95**: 395–8.

Haller JA, Knox DL. Vitrectomy for persistent vitreous hemorrhage from a cavernous hemangioma of the optic disk (letter). *Am J Ophthalmol* 1993; **116**: 106–7.

Hamada S, Ellsworth RM. Congenital retinal detachment and the optic disc anomaly. *Am J Ophthalmol* 1971; **71**: 460–4.

Handemann M. Erbliche, vermutlich angenborene zentrale gliose Entartung des Sehnerven mit besonderer. Beteilung der Zentralgefasse. *Klin Mbl Augenheilkd* 1929; **83**: 145–54.

Harris MJ, Fine SL, Owens SL. Hemorrhagic complications of optic nerve drusen. *Am J Ophthalmol* 1981; **92**: 70–6.

Harris RJ, Haas L. Septo-optic dysplasia with growth hormone deficiency (de Morsier syndrome). *Arch Dis Child* 1972; **47**: 973–6.

Hashemi K, Traboulsi EI, Chavis R, Scribanu N, Chrousos GA. Chorioretinal lacuna in the amniotic band syndrome. *J Pediatr Ophthalmol* 1991; **28**: 238–9.

Hashmi MS, Karseras AG. Uveal colobomata and Klinefelter syndrome. *Br J Ophthalmol* 1976; **60**: 661–4.

Hayreh SS, Cullen JF. Atypical minimal peri-papillary choroidal colobomata. *Br J Ophthalmol* 1972; **56**: 86–96.

Herman DC, Bartley GB, Bullock JD. Ophthalmic findings of hydranencephaly. *J Pediatr Ophthalmol Strabismus* 1988; **25**: 106–12.

Herrmann J, Opitz JM. The Lenz microphthalmia syndrome. *Birth Defects* 1969; **5**: 138–43.

Hing AV, Torack R, Dowton SB. A lethal syndrome resembling branchio-oculo-facial syndrome. *Clin Genet* 1992; **41**: 74–8.

Hinzpeter EN, Renz S, Loser H. Eye manifestations of fetal alcohol syndrome (German). *Klin Monatsbl Augenheilk* 1992; **200**: 33–8.

Hittner HM, Desmond MM, Montgomery JR. Optic nerve manifesta-tions of human congenital cytomegalovirus infection. *Am J Ophthalmol* 1976; **81**: 661–5.

Hittner HM, Hirsch NJ, Kreh GM, Rudolph AJ. Colobomatous microphthalmia, heart disease, hearing loss and mental retardation: a syndrome. *J Pediatr Ophthalmol Strabismus* 1979; **16**: 122–8.

Ho CK, Kaufman RL, Podos SM. Ocular colobomata, cardiac defect, and other anomalies: a study of seven cases including two sibs. *J Med Genet* 1975; **12**: 289–93.

Hoefnagel D, Keenan ME, Cullen FH. Heredofamilial bilateral anophthalmia. *Arch Ophthalmol* 1963; **69**: 760–6.

Hoepner J, Yanoff M. Ocular anomalies in trisomy 13–15. *Am J Ophthalmol* 1972; **74**: 729–37.

Hogan MJ, Zimmerman LE. *Ophthalmic Pathology*, 2nd edn. Philadelphia: WB Saunders, 1962.

Hoover D, Robb R, Petersen R. Optic disc drusen in children. *J Pediatr Ophthalmol Strabismus* 1988; **25**: 191–6.

Hopkins IJ, Humphrey I, Keigh CG. The Aicardi syndrome in a 47XXY male. *Aust Paediatr J* 1979; **15**: 278–80.

Hotchkiss ML, Green WR. Optic nerve aplasia and hypoplasia. *J Pediatr Ophthalmol* 1970; **16**: 225–40.

Howell SC. The craniostenoses. *Am J Ophthalmol* 1974; **37**: 359–79.

Hoyosaki S, Yamaguchi K, Mizuno K, Miyabayashi S, Narisawa K, Taka K. Ocular findings in childhood lactic acidosis. *Arch Ophthalmol* 1986; **104**: 1656–8.

Hoyt CS, Billson FA. Maternal anticonvulsants and optic nerve hypoplasia. *Br J Ophthalmol* 1978; **62**: 3–6.

Hoyt CS, Billson F, Ouvrier R. Ocular features of Aicardi's syndrome. *Arch Ophthalmol* 1978; **96**: 291–5.

Hoyt C, Good W. Do we really understand the difference between optic nerve hypoplasia and atrophy? *Eye* 1992; **6**: 201–4.

Hoyt WF, Kaplan SL, Grumbach MM, Glaser J. Septo-optic dysplasia and pituitary dwarfism. *Lancet* 1970; **i**: 93.

Hoyt WF, Rios-Montenegros EN, Berens MM, Eckelhoff RJ. Homonymous hemioptic hypoplasia. Fundoscopic features in standard and red-free illumination in three patients with congenital hemiplegia. *Br J Ophthalmol* 1972; **56**: 537–45.

Huerva J, Ascaso FJ, Palomar MT *et al.* Mobius syndrome and bilateral chorioretinal coloboma (French). *Ann Pediatr* 1992; **39**: 313–16.

Insler M, Daulin L. Ocular findings in linear sebaceous naevus syndrome. *Br J Ophthalmol* 1987; **71**: 268–72.

Jacobs M, Taylor D. The systemic and genetic significance of congenital optic disc anomalies. *Eye* 1991; **5**: 470–5.

Jadassohn J. Bemerkungen zur Histologie der systematisiten naevi under über 'Talgdrusen' Naevi. *Arch Dermatol Syph* 1895; **33**: 355–7.

James PML, Karseras AG, Wybar KC. Systemic associations of uveal coloboma. *Br J Ophthalmol* 1974; **58**: 917–21.

Jan JE, Robinson GC, Kinnis C, MacLeod PJM. Blindness due to optic atrophy and hypoplasia in children: an epidemiological study (1944–74). *Dev Med Child Neurol* 1977; **19**: 353–63.

Jay M. *The Eye in Chromosome Duplications and Deficiencies.* New York: Marcel Dekker, 1977.

Jelliger K, Gross H. Congenital telencephalic defects. *Neuropaediatrics* 1973; **4**: 446–52.

Jensen OA, Hagerstrand I, Brun A, Lofgren O. Limb–body wall complex with anophthalmos and choroidal coloboma. *Pediatr Pathol* 1993; **13**: 505–7.

Jensen PE, Kalina RE. Congenital anomalies of the optic disc. *Am J Ophthalmol* 1976; **82**: 27–31.

Jerome B, Forster JW. Congenital hypoplasia (partial aplasia) of the optic nerve. *Arch Ophthalmol* 1948; **89**: 669–72.

Jones M, de Sa L, Good W. Atypical iris colobomata and Pfeiffer's syndrome. *J Pediatr Ophthalmol Strabismus* 1993; **30**: 266–7.

Junge J. Über eine doppelte papille im Augenkolobom. *Klin Mon*

Augenheilkd 1978; **172**: 748–50.

Justice J, Lehman RP. Cilioretinal arteries. *Arch Ophthalmol* 1976; **94**: 1355–8.

Kallmann FJ, Schoenfeld WA, Barrera SE. Genetic aspects of primary eunuchoidism. *Am J Ment Defic* 1943; **48**: 203–28.

Kaplan SL, Grumbach MM, Hoyt WF. A syndrome of hypopituitary dwarfism, hypoplasia of the optic nerves and malformation of the prosencephalon. *Pediatr Res* 1970; **4**: 480–6.

Katz B, Wiley CA, Lee VW. Optic nerve hypoplasia and the syndrome of nevus sebaceous of Jadassohn. *Ophthalmology* 1987; **94**: 1570–6.

Kaufman LM, Miller MT, Mafee MF. Magnetic resonance imaging of pituitary stalk hypoplasia. *Arch Ophthalmol* 1989; **107**: 1485–90.

Kawano K, Fujita S. Duanes retraction syndrome associated with Morning Glory syndrome. *J Pediatr Ophthalmol Strabismus* 1981; **18**: 51–4.

Keane JR. Suprasellar tumours and incidental optic disc anomalies. *Arch Ophthalmol* 1977; **95**: 2180–3.

Kheterpal S, Good P, Beale D, Kritzinger E. Imaging of optic disc drusen: a comparative study. *Eye* 1995; **9**: 67–9.

Kim RY, Hoyt WF, Lessell S, Narahara MH. Superior segmental optic hypoplasia: a sign of maternal diabetes. *Arch Ophthalmol* 1989; **107**: 1312–15.

Kindler P. Morning Glory syndrome: unusual congenital optic disc anomaly. *Am J Ophthalmol* 1970; **69**: 376–84.

Klein D, Ammann F. The syndrome of Laurence–Moon–Bardet–Biedl and allied diseases of Switzerland. *J Neurol Sci* 1969; **9**: 479–513.

Kottow MH. Congenital malformations of the retinal vessels with primary optic nerve involvement. *Ophthalmologica (Basel)* 1978; **176**: 86–90.

Kral K, Svarc D. Contractile peripapillary staphyloma. *Am J Ophthalmol* 1971; **71**: 1090–2.

Kranenberg EW. Crater-like holes in the optic disc and central serous retinopathy. *Arch Ophthalmol* 1960; **64**: 912–24.

Krause U. Three cases of the Morning Glory syndrome. *Acta Ophthalmol* 1972; **50**: 188–98.

Krause-Brucker W, Gardner DW. Optic nerve hypoplasia associated with absent septum pellucidum and hypopituitarism. *Am J Ophthalmol* 1980; **89**: 113–20.

Kushner BJ. Functional amblyopia associated with abnormalities of the optic nerve. *Arch Ophthalmol* 1984; **102**: 683–5.

Kytila J, Miettinen P. On bilateral aplasia of the optic nerve. *Acta Ophthalmol* 1961; **39**: 416–19.

Lagos JC, Gomez MR. Tuberous sclerosis: reappraisal of a clinical entity. *Mayo Clin Proc* 1967; **42**: 26–49.

Lamba PA. Doubling of the papilla. *Acta Ophthalmol (Kbh)* 1969; **47**: 4–9.

Lambert HM, Sipperley JO, Shore JW, Dieckert JP, Evans R, Lowd DR. Linear nevus sebaceous syndrome. *Ophthalmology* 1987b; **94**: 278–83.

Lambert SR, Hoyt CS, Narahara MH. Optic nerve hypoplasia. *Surv Ophthalmology* 1987a; **32**: 1–9.

Landau K, Dosseter F, Hoyt WF, Muci-Mendoza R. Retinal hamartoma neurofibromatosis 2 (case report). *Arch Ophthalmol* 1990; **108**: 328–9.

Laverda M, Clementi M, Tenconi R. Chorioretinal coloboma and Joubert syndrome (reply). *J Pediatr* 1985; **107**: 158.

Layman PR, Anderson DR, Flynn JT. Frequent occurrence of hypoplastic optic discs in patients with aniridia. *Am J Ophthalmol* 1974; **77**: 513–16.

Legius E, Fryns JP, Van Den Berghe H. Dominant branchial cleft syndrome with characteristics of both branchio-oto-renal and branchio-oto-facial syndrome. *Clin Genet* 1990; **37**: 347–50.

Lenz W. Recessive sex-linked microphthalmos with multiple defor-

mities (German). *Z Kinderheik* 1955; **77**: 384–90.

Levy CM, Knudtzon J. Kallman syndrome in two sisters with other developmental anomalies also affecting their father. *Clin Genet* 1993; **43**: 51–3.

Levy NS, Ernest JT. Retinal medullated nerve fibres. *Arch Ophthalmol* 1974; **91**: 330–1.

Lightman S. Kallmann's syndrome. *J Roy Soc Med* 1988; **81**: 315–17.

Lillquist K, Warburg M, Anderson SR, Hagerstrand I. Colobomata of the iris, ciliary body and choroid in an infant with oesophagotracheal fistula and congenital heart defects. An unknown malformation complex. *Acta Paediatr Scand* 1980; **69**: 427–30.

Limaye SR. Coloboma of the iris and choroid and retinal detachment in oculoauricular dysplasia (Goldenhar syndrome). *Ear Eye Nose Throat Monogr* 1972; **51**: 28–31.

Lin AE, Losken HW, Jaffe R, Biglan AW. The branchio-oculo-facial syndrome. *Cleft Palate Craniofacial J* 1991; **28**: 96–102.

Lincoff H, Yannuzzi L, Singerman L, Kreissig I, Fisher Y. Improvement in visual function after displacement of the retinal elevations emanating from optic pits. *Arch Ophthalmol* 1993; **111**: 1071–9.

Lindhout D, Barth PG. Chorioretinal coloboma and Joubert syndrome (correspondence). *J Pediatr* 1985; **107**: 158–9.

Lindhout D, Barth PG, Valk J, Boen-Tan TN. The Joubert syndrome associated with bilateral chorioretinal coloboma. *Eur J Pediatr* 1980; **134**: 173–6.

Little LE, Whitmore PV, Wells TW. Aplasia of the optic nerve. *J Pediatr Ophthalmol* 1976; **13**: 84–8.

Longfellow DW, Davis FS, Walsh FB. Unilateral intermittent blindness with dilatation of retinal veins. *Arch Ophthalmol* 1962; **67**: 554–5.

Lorentzen SE. Drusen of the optic disc. *Acta Ophthalmol* 1966; **90**(Suppl.): 1–66.

Lurie IW, Samochvalov VA. Trisomy 4p and ocular defects. *Br J Ophthalmol* 1994; **78**: 415–17.

Lyford JH, Roy FH. Arrhinencephaly unilateralis, uveal coloboma and lens reduplication. *Am J Ophthalmol* 1974; **7**: 315–18.

McGregor M. Chondroectodermal dysplasia (Ellis–van Creveld syndrome): colobomata of the iris. *Proc Roy Soc Med* 1954; **47**: 540.

McKinna AJ. Quilune induced hypoplasia of the optic nerve. *Canad J Ophthalmol* 1966; **1**: 261–5.

McKusick V. *Mendelian Inheritance in Man*. Baltimore: Johns Hopkins University Press, 1978: 14.

McMillan L. Anophthalmos and maldevelopment of the eyes; four cases in the same family. *Br J Ophthalmol* 1921; **5**: 121–2.

Mann I. *Developmental Abnormalities of the Eye*. London: British Medical Association Press, 1957.

Manor RS, Korczyn AD. Retinal red-free light photographs in two congenital conditions. *Ophthalmologica* 1976; **173**: 119–27.

Manschot WA. Eye findings in hydranencephaly. *Ophthalmologica* 1971; **162**: 151–9.

Manschot WA. The optic nerve in hydranencephaly and anencephaly. In: Stanley Cant J, ed. *The Optic Nerve*. London: H. Kimpton, 1972.

Marden PM, Venters HD. A new neurocutaneous syndrome. *Am J Dis Child* 1966; **112**: 79–81.

Margo C, Hamed L, Fang E, Dawson W. Optic nerve aplasia. *Arch Ophthalmol* 1992; **110**: 1610–13.

Matzkin GM. Coloboma at the optic nerve entrance and melanosis oculi. *J Pediatr Ophthalmol* 1970; **4**: 222–4.

Maumenee IH. Genetic counseling. In: Goldberg MF, ed. *Genetic and Metabolic Eye Disease*. Boston: Little Brown, 1974: 604.

Meckel JR. Beschreibung zweier durch sehr ahnliche bildungsabweichung entsteller Gerchwister. *Dtsch Arch Physiol* 1822; **7**: 99–172.

Mellor D, Fielder A. Dissociated visual development: electrodiagnostic studies in infants who are 'slow to see'. *Dev Med Child Neurol* 1980; **22**: 327–35.

Missiroli G. Una nuova sindrome congenita a carattere falungliare, ipoplasia del nervo ottico e emianopsia binasale. *Boll Occul* 1947; **26**: 683–91.

Molina JA, Mateos F, Merino M *et al.* Aicardi's syndrome in two sisters. *J Paediatr* 1989; **115**: 282–3.

Moretti-Ferreira D, Koiffmann CP, Listik M, Sehan N, Wajntal A. Macrosomia, obesity, macrocephaly and ocular abnormalities (MOMO syndrome) in two unrelated patients: delineation of a newly recognized overgrowth syndrome. *Am J Med Genet* 1993; **46**: 555–8.

Mullaney J. Complex sporadic colobomata. *Br J Ophthalmol* 1978; **62**: 384–8.

Mullaney J. Ocular malformation in trisomy 18 (Edwards' syndrome). *Am J Ophthalmol* 1973; **76**: 246–54.

Mullaney J, Fitzpatrick C. Idiopathic cyst of the iris stroma. *Am J Ophthalmol* 1973; **76**: 64–8.

Mullie MA, Sanders MD. Scleral canal size and optic nerve head drusen. *Am J Ophthalmol* 1985; **99**: 356–60.

Nakajima A, Fujiki K, Tanabe U. Birth order and parental age in microphthalmos and other ocular conditions. *Am J Ophthalmol* 1979; **88**: 461–8.

Nevin NC, Pearce WG. Diagnostic and genetical aspects of tuberous sclerosis. *J Med Genet* 1968; **5**: 273–80.

Novakovic P, Taylor DSI, Hoyt WF. Localising patterns of optic nerve hypoplasia — retina to occipital lobe. *Br J Ophthalmol* 1988; **72**: 176–83.

O'Connor PS, Smith JL. Optic nerve variant in the Klippel–Trenaunay–Weber syndrome. *Ann Ophthalmol* 1978; **10**: 131–4.

Odagiri Y, Ito T. The Morning Glory syndrome. *J Clin Ophthalmol* 1975; **69**: 483–6.

Opitz JM, Howe JJ. The Meckel syndrome. *Birth Defects* 1969; **5**: 167–79.

Orcutt JC, Bunt AH. Anomalous optic discs in the patient with a Dandy–Walker cyst. *J Clin Neuro Ophthalmol* 1982; **2**: 42–3.

Pagon R. Ocular coloboma. *Surv Ophthalmol* 1981; **25**: 223–36.

Pagon RA, Chandler JDV, Collier WR. Hydrocephalus, agyria, retinal dysplasia, encephalocele (HARD ± E) syndrome: an autosomal recessive condition. *Birth Defects* 1978; **15**: 233–41.

Pagon RA, Graham JM, Sybert VP. The CHARGE association. *Clin Res* 1980; **28**: 118A.

Pagon RA, Graham JM, Zonana J, Yong S-L. Coloboma, congenital heart disease and choanal atresia with multiple anomalies: an association. *J Pediatr* 1981; **99**: 223–7.

Patel H, Tze WJ, Crichton JU, McCormick AQ, Robinson GC, Dolman CL. Optic nerve hypoplasia with hypopituitarism. *Am J Dis Child* 1975; **129**: 175–80.

Pedler C. Unusual coloboma of the optic nerve entrance. *Br J Ophthalmol* 1961; **45**: 803–8.

Peterson RA, Walton DS. Optic nerve hypoplasia with good acuity and visual field defects: a study of infants of diabetic mothers. *Arch Ophthalmol* 1977; **95**: 254–8.

Pinckers A, Lion F, Notting JGA. X-chromosomal recessive nightblindness and tilted disc anomaly. *Ophthalmologica* 1978; **176**: 160–3.

Porges Y, Gershoni-Baruch R, Leibu R *et al.* Hereditary microphthalmos with colobomatous cyst. *Am J Ophthalmol* 1992; **114**: 30–4.

Purdy F, Friend JCM. Maternal factors in SOD (letter). *J Pediatr* 1979; **95**: 661.

Rack JH, Wright GF. Coloboma of the optic nerve entrance. *Br J Ophthalmol* 1966; **50**: 705–9.

Ragge N. Clinical and genetic patterns of neurofibromatosis 1 and 2.

Br J Ophthalmol 1993; **77**: 662–72.

Reese AB. Congenital melanomas. *Am J Ophthalmol* 1974; **77**: 798–808.

Reeves DL. Congenital absence of the septum pellucidum. *Johns Hopkins Hosp Bull* 1941; **69**: 61–7.

Renelt P. Beitrag zur echten Papillenaplasie. *Graefe's Arch Klin Exp Ophthalmol* 1972; **184**: 94–8.

Ridley H. Aplasia of the optic nerves. *Br J Ophthalmol* 1938; **22**: 669–71.

Riise D. The nasal fundus ectasia. *Acta Ophthalmol (Kbh)* 1975; **26**(Suppl.): 1–108.

Rimmer S, Keating C, Chou T *et al.* Growth of the human optic disc and nerve during gestation, childhood and early adulthood. *Am J Ophthalmol* 1993; **116**: 748–53.

Robertson DM. Hamartomas of the optic disc with retinitis pigmentosa. *Am J Ophthalmol* 1972; **74**: 526–31.

Rogers GL, Brown D, Gray I, Bremer D. Bilateral optic nerve hypoplasia associated with cerebral atrophy. *J Pediatr Ophthalmol Strabismus* 1981; **18**: 18–22.

Romano PE. Simple photogrammetric diagnosis of optic nerve hypoplasia. *Arch Ophthalmol* 1989; **107**: 824–7.

Rosenberg MA, Savino PJ, Glaser JS. A clinical analysis of pseudopapilloedema: population, laterality, acuity, refractive error, ophthalmoscopic characteristics. *Arch Ophthalmol* 1979; **97**: 65–70.

Roy FH, Summitt RL, Hiatt RL *et al.* Ocular manifestations of the Rubinstein–Taybi syndrome. *Arch Ophthalmol* 1968; **79**: 272–8.

Rubinstein JH. The broad thumbs syndrome — progress report 1968. *Birth Defects* 1969; **5**: 25–40.

Rubinstein K, Ali M. Complications of optic disc pits. *Trans Ophthalmol Soc UK* 1978; **98**: 195–200.

Rucker CW. Bitemporal defects in the visual fields resulting from developmental anomalies of the optic discs. *Arch Ophthalmol* 1946; **35**: 546–54.

Russell-Eggitt IM, Blake KP, Taylor DSI, Wyse RKH. The eye in CHARGE association. *Br J Ophthalmol* 1990; **74**: 421–6.

Sachs JG, O'Grady RB, Choromokos E, Leestma J. The pathogenesis of optic nerve drusen: a hypothesis. *Arch Ophthalmol* 1977; **95**: 425–8.

Sakuma Y, Sakuma F. A case of monosomy 9 mosaicism with multiple congenital anomalies. *Folia Ophthalmol Jap* 1976; **27**: 987–91.

Salonen R. The Meckel syndrome: clinicopathological findings in 67 patients. *Am J Med Genet* 1984; **18**: 671–89.

Sanayusin P, Schimmenti LA, McNoe LA *et al.* Mutation of the PAX2 gene in a family with optic nerve colobomas, renal anomalies and vesicoureteral reflux. *Nature Genet* 1995; **9**: 358–64.

Sanders MD. CT scanning in diagnosis of orbital disease. *J Roy Soc Med* 1980; **73**: 284–7.

Sanders TE, Gay AJ, Newman M. Hemorrhagic complications of drusen of the optic disc. *Am J Ophthalmol* 1971; **71**: 204–17.

Saraux H. Types et contratypes en pathologie chromosomique. *Bull Mem Soc Fr Ophthalmol* 1972; **85**: 8–16.

Saraux H, Lefebvre M. Weyers et Thiers oculovertebral syndrome. *Bull Soc Fr Ophthalmol* 1966; **66**: 485–7.

Savell J, Cook JR. Optic nerve colobomas of autosomal dominant heredity. *Arch Ophthalmol* 1976; **94**: 395–400.

Savino PJ, Glaser JS, Rosenberg MA. A clinical analysis of pseudopapilloedema: visual field defects. *Arch Ophthalmol* 1979; **97**: 71–5.

Say B, Berry J, Barber N. The Stickler syndrome (hereditary arthroophthalmopathy). *Clin Genet* 1977; **12**: 179–82.

Schachat AP, Miller NR. Atrophy of myelinated retinal nerve fibres after acute optic neuropathy. *Am J Ophthalmol* 1981; **92**: 854–6.

Schachenmann G, Schmid W, Fraccaro M *et al.* Chromosomes in coloboma and anal atresia. *Lancet* 1965; **ii**: 290.

Schatz H, McDonald HR. Treatment of sensory retinal detachment associated with optic nerve pit or coloboma. *Ophthalmology* 1988;

95: 178–87.

Scheie HG, Adler FH. Aplasia of the optic nerve. *Arch Ophthalmol* 1941; **26**: 61–70.

Schindler RF, Sarin LK, MacDonald PR. Hemangiomas of the optic disc. *Canad J Ophthalmol* 1975; **10**: 305–18.

Schinzel A, Auf der Maur P, Moser H. Partial deletion of long arm of chromosome 11 [del (11) (q23)]: Jacobsen syndrome. *J Med Genet* 1977; **14**: 438–44.

Schinzel A, Schmid W, Fraccaro M et al. The 'cat-eye syndrome': dicentric small marker chromosome probably derived from 22 (tetrasomy 22pter–q11) associated with a characteristic phenotype. *Hum Genet* 1981; **57**: 148–58.

Seefelder R. Über anomalien im Bereiche der sehnerven und der Netzhaut normaler fotaler augen, ein Beitrag zur Gliomfrage. *Graefe's Arch Ophthalmol* 1909; **69**: 463–78.

Seeley RL, Smith JL. Visual field defects in optic nerve hypoplasia. *Am J Ophthalmol* 1971; **73**: 882–9.

Segal P, Kikiela M, Mrzyglod S et al. Kartagener's syndrome with familial eye changes. *Am J Ophthalmol* 1963; **55**: 1043–9.

Seybold ME, Rosen PN. Peripapillary staphyloma and amaurosis fugax. *Ann Ophthalmol* 1977; **9**: 1137–41.

Shields MB. Gray crescent in the optic nerve head. *Am J Ophthalmol* 1980; **89**: 238–44.

Skarf B, Hoyt CS. Optic nerve hypoplasia in children. *Arch Ophthalmol* 1984; **102**: 62–8.

Slade HW, Weekley RD. Diastasis of the optic nerve. *J Neurosurg* 1957; **14**: 571–4.

Smith DW. *Recognizable Patterns of Human Malformation.* Philadelphia: WB Saunders, 1976.

Smith JL, Stowe FR. The Pierre Robin syndrome (glossoptosis, micrognathia, cleft palate): a review of 39 cases with emphasis on associated ocular lesions. *Pediatrics* 1961; **27**: 128–33.

Smithells RW. Defects and disabilities of thalidomide children. *Br J Med* 1973; **1**: 269–72.

Soloman LM. Epidermal nevus syndrome. *Mod Prob Pediatr* 1975; **17**: 27–30.

Somerville F. Uniocular aplasia of the optic nerve. *Br J Ophthalmol* 1962; **46**: 51–5.

Spencer WH. Drusen of the optic disc and aberrant axoplasmic transport. *Ophthalmology* 1978; **85**: 21–39.

Stanhope R, Preece MA, Brook CGD. Hypoplastic optic nerves and pituitary dysfunction. *Arch Dis Child* 1984; **59**: 111–14.

Steinkuller PG. The Morning Glory disc anomaly: case report and a review of the literature. *J Pediatr Ophthalmol* 1980; **17**: 81–7.

Stevens J, Marsh J. Ocular anomalies in the oral-facial-digital syndrome. *J Pediatr Ophthalmol Strabismus* 1994; **31**: 397–8.

Straatsma BR, Foos RY, Heckenlively JR, Taylor GN. Myelinated retinal nerve fibres. *Am J Ophthalmol* 1981; **91**: 25–38.

Stromland K. Ocular involvement in the fetal alcohol syndrome. *Surv Ophthalmol* 1987; **31**: 277–84.

Stromland K, Miller MT. Thalidomide embryopathy: revisited 27 years later. *Acta Ophthalmol* 1993; **71**: 238–45.

Sugar HS. Congenital pits of the optic disc. *Am J Ophthalmol* 1967; **63**: 298–307.

Sugar HS, Beckman H. Peripapillary staphyloma with respiratory pulsation. *Am J Ophthalmol* 1969; **68**: 895–7.

Summers CG, Romig L, Lavoie JD. Unexpected good results after therapy for anisometropic amblyopia associated with unilateral peripapillary myelinated nerve fibers. *J Pediatr Ophthalmol Strabismus* 1991; **28**: 134–7.

Takahashi T, Murase T, Hiramatsu K, Asakura S, Okada S. The clinicopathological findings on two cases of coloboma of the optic disc. *Folia Ophthalmol Jap* 1979; **30**: 957–6.

Tanaka Y. Contractile coloboma of the optic nerve entrance. *Jpn J Clin Ophthalmol* 1977; **31**: 625–30.

Taylor AI. Autosomal trisomy syndromes: a detailed study of 27 cases of Edward's syndrome and 27 cases of Patau's syndrome. *J Med Genet* 1968; **5**: 227–52.

Taylor D. Congenital tumours of the anterior visual system with dysplasia of the optic discs. *Br J Ophthalmol* 1982; **66**: 455–63.

Taylor D, Ffytche T. Pigmented optic disc and field defect in chicken pox. *J Pediatr Ophthalmol Strabismus* 1976; **13**: 80–3.

Teikari J, Airaksinen J. Twin study on cup/disc ratio of the optic nerve head. *Br J Ophthalmol* 1992; **76**: 218–20.

Temple IK, Brunner H, Jones B, Burn J, Baraitser M. Midline facial defects with ocular colobomata. *Am J Med Genet* 1990a; **37**: 23–7.

Temple IK, MacDowall P, Baraitser M, Atherton DJ. Focal dermal hypoplasia (Goltz syndrome). *J Med Genet* 1990b; **27**: 180–7.

Theodossiadis G. Evolution of congenital pit of the optic disc with macular detachment in photocoagulated and non-photocoagulated eyes. *Am J Ophthalmol* 1977; **84**: 620–31.

Theodossiadis G, Koutsandrea C, Theodossiadis P. Optic nerve pit with serous macular detachment resulting in rhegmatogenous retinal detachment. *Br J Ophthalmol* 1993; **77**: 385–6.

Thomas JV, Yoshizumi MO, Beyer CK, Craft JL, Albert DM. Ocular manifestations of focal dermal hypoplasia syndrome. *Arch Ophthalmol* 1977; **95**: 1997–2001.

Traboulsi E, Lim J, Pyeritz R, Goldberg H, Haller J. A new syndrome of myelinated nerve fibers, vitreoretinopathy and skeletal malformations. *Arch Ophthalmol* 1993; **111**: 1543–5.

Traboulsi EI, Maunenee IH. Peters' anomaly and associated congenital malformations. *Arch Ophthalmol* 1992; **110**: 1739–42.

Traboulsi EI, O'Neill JF. The spectrum in the morphology of the so-called Morning Glory disc anomaly. *J Pediatr Ophthalmol Strabismus* 1988; **25**: 93–9.

Van Dorp DB, Palan A, Kwee ML, Barth PG, Van der Harten JJ. Joubert syndrome: a clinical and pathological description of an affected male and a female fetus from the same sibship. *Am J Med Genet* 1991; **40**: 100–4.

Van Noyhuys JM, Bruyn GW. Nasopharyngeal trans-sphenoidal encephalocoele, crater-like hole in the optic disc and agenesis of the corpus callosum. *Psychiatr Neurol Neurochir* 1964; **67**: 243–58.

Various authors. The Meckel Symposium. *Am J Med Genet* 1994; **18**: 649–711.

Von Arlt CF. Aux der k.k. Ges Aertze zu Wien 1858: 445.

Von Barsewisch B. *Perinatal Retinal Haemorrhages.* Berlin: Springer-Verlag, 1979.

Vossius A. Beitrag zur Lehre von den angenborenen Conis. *Klin Monatsbl Augenheilkd* 1885; **23**: 137–57.

Walsh FB, Hoyt WF. In: *Clinical Neuro-Ophthalmology,* 3rd edn. Baltimore: Williams & Wilkins, 1969: 716.

Walton DS, Robb RM. Optic nerve hypoplasia—a report of 20 cases. *Arch Ophthalmol* 1970; **84**: 572–8.

Warburg M. Classification of microphthalmos and coloboma. *J Med Genet* 1993; **30**: 664–9.

Warburg M. Focal dermal hypoplasia: ocular and general manifestations with a survey of the literature. *Acta Ophthalmol (Kbh)* 1970; **48**: 525–36.

Warburg M. The heterogeneity of microphthalmia in the mentally retarded. *Birth Defects* 1971; **7**: 130–54.

Warburg M. Hydrocephaly, congenital retinal non-attachment and congenital falciform fold. *Am J Ophthalmol* 1978; **85**: 88–94.

Warburg M. Update of sporadic microphthalmos and coloboma: non-inherited anomalies. *Ophthal Pediatr Genet* 1992; **13**: 111–22.

Warburg M, Friedrich U. Coloboma and microphthalmos in chromosomal aberrations. *Ophthal Paediatr Genet* 1987; **8**: 105–18.

Warburg M, Mikkelsen M. A case of 13–15 trisomy or Bartholin–Patau's syndrome. *Acta Ophthalmol (Kbh)* 1963; **41**: 321–3.

Waring GO, Roth AM, Rodrigues M. Microphthalmos with cyst. *Am J Ophthalmol* 1976; **82**: 714–22.

Weiter JJ, McLean IW, Zimmerman LE. Aplasia of the optic nerve and disc. *Am J Ophthalmol* 1977; **83**: 56–76.

Weleber RG, Walknowska J, Peakman D. Cytogenetic investigation of the cat-eye syndrome. *Am J Ophthalmol* 1977; **84**: 477–86.

Whinery RD, Blodi FC. Hypoplasia of the optic nerve: a clinical and histopathologic correlation. *Trans Am Acad Ophthalmol Otol* 1963; **67**: 733–8.

Wiethe T. Ein Fall von angeborener Difformität der Sehnerven papille. *Arch Augenheilkunde* 1882; **11**: 14–20.

Wiggins RE, von Noorden G, Boniuk M. Optic nerve coloboma with cyst: a case report and review. *J Pediatr Ophthalmol Strabismus* 1991; **28**: 274–7.

Wilkes SB, Campbell BJ, Waller RR. Ocular malformation in association with ipsilateral facial nevus of Jadassohn. *Am J Ophthalmol* 1981; **92**: 344–52.

Willetts GS. Focal dermal hypoplasia. *Br J Ophthalmol* 1974; **58**: 620–4.

Williams EJ, McCormick AQ, Tischler B. Retinal vessels in Down's syndrome. *Arch Ophthalmol* 1973; **89**: 269–71.

Willis R, Zimmerman LE, O'Grady R, Smith RS, Crawford B. Heterotopic adipose tissue and smooth muscle in the optic disc. *Arch Ophthalmol* 1972; **88**: 139–46.

Wise JB, MacLean AL, Gass JDM. Contractile peripapillary staphyloma. *Arch Ophthalmol* 1966; **75**: 626–30.

Wisek GN, Henkind P, Alterman M. Optic disc drusen and subretinal hemorrhage. *Trans Am Acad Ophthalmol Otolaryngol* 1974; **8**: 211–19.

Wolter JR. Johnson FD, Lewis RA. Papilla nigra associated with dermolipoma of the orbit, cleft palate, and an extra thumb. *J Pediatr Ophthalmol* 1971; **8**: 119–22.

Woodford B, Tso MOM. An ultrastructural study of the corpora amylacea of the optic nerve head and retina. *Am J Ophthalmol* 1980; **90**: 492–502.

Yamaguchi Y. Congenital anomalies of the optic nerve head—report of two cases. *Folia Ophthalmol Jpn* 1975; **26**: 1070–4.

Yanoff M, Rorke LB, Allman MI. Bilateral optic system aplasia with relatively normal eyes. *Arch Opthalmol* 1978; **96**: 97–101.

Yanoff M, Rorke LB, Niederer BS. Ocular and cerebral abnormalities in chromosome 18 deletion defect. *Am J Ophthalmol* 1970; **70**: 391–402.

Yap E-Y, Buettner H. Traumatic rupture of a persistent hyaloid artery (letter). *Am J Ophthalmol* 1992; **114**: 225.

Young SE, Walsh FB, Knox DL. The tilted disc syndrome. *Am J Ophthalmol* 1976; **82**: 16–23.

Zeki SM. Optic nerve hypoplasia and astigmatism: a new association. *Br J Ophthalmol* 1990; **74**: 297–300.

Zeki S, Dudgeon J, Dutton G. Reappraisal of the ratio of disc to macula/disc diameter in optic nerve hypoplasia. *Br J Ophthalmol* 1991; **75**: 538–41.

Zeki S, Hollman A, Dutton G. Neuroradiological features of patients with optic nerve hypoplasia. *J Pediatr Ophthalmol Strabismus* 1992; **29**: 107–12.

Zion V. Optic nerve hypoplasia. *Ophthal Semin* 1976; **1**: 171–96.

Zlotogora J, Legum C, Raz J, Ben-Ezra D. Autosomal recessive colobomatous microphthalmos. *Am J Med Genet* 1994; **49**: 261–2.

51: Optic Neuropathies

David Taylor

Childhood optic neuritis

Optic neuritis is rare in childhood but of significance because of its quite stunning presentation and the importance of the differential diagnosis. It probably occurs throughout childhood but is rarely recognized in toddlers because any visual defect has to be very profound, and in both eyes, before the child is obviously abnormal to the parents. The most frequent age at presentation is 7 years, it occurs more frequently in girls than boys and is usually bilateral (Taylor & Cuendet 1986).

The onset may appear to be sudden but it may, in retrospect, have been developing over a few days with increasing visual difficulty. Smaller children often do not present until they are profoundly affected, with some children complaining that they want lights put on in bright daylight, or that they have been woken by their parents while it is still night time. Other children are referred with the diagnosis of ataxia which is in fact due to blindness. The loss of acuity is usually profound, there is a central scotoma (Fig. 51.1) or diffuse visual field loss and the colour vision is profoundly affected. There is an afferent pupil defect which may be apparent to the parents, if the optic neuritis is bilateral and severe, as dilated pupils even in bright light. The optic discs are swollen in 87% of cases (Fig. 51.2), markedly so in 53% (Taylor & Cuendet 1986). Haemorrhages around the disc are rare (Figs 51.3, 51.4) and exudates unusual. Fluorescein angiography of the discs in the acute phase shows dilated capillaries and late leakage. When the optic disc is not swollen the condition is known as retrobulbar neuritis; if it is, it may be called papillitis.

The visual prognosis is generally excellent (Heirons & Lyle 1959; Kennedy & Carroll 1960; Meadows 1969; Taylor & Cuendet 1986) although many patients have residual retinal nerve fibre atrophy. Treatment with high doses of systemic steroids sometimes brings about a dramatic and rapid improvement in the vision (Farris & Pickard 1990), but there is not yet conclusive evidence that the long-term visual prognosis is improved by this treatment. Patients usually improve within several days without any treatment, and the main effect of the steroids seems to be to speed the improvement, which is particularly beneficial when the child is profoundly affected.

In contrast to optic neuritis in adults, the systemic prognosis is also good. Eighty per cent of children in one series (Taylor & Cuendet 1986) had no subsequent neurological signs and no recurrence of their optic neuritis. Other series

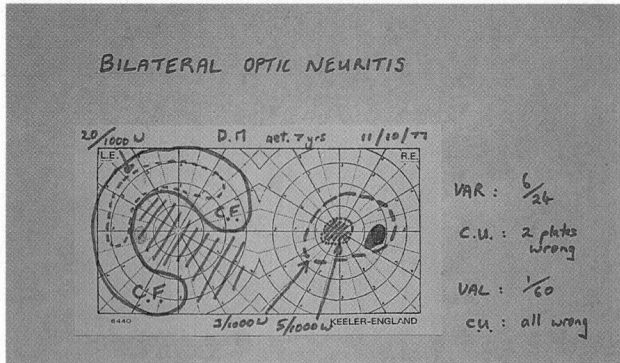

Fig. 51.1 Optic neuritis in a 7-year-old boy. Sudden onset of visual loss to 6/24 acuity right eye, 1/60 left eye, central scotomas and colour vision loss.

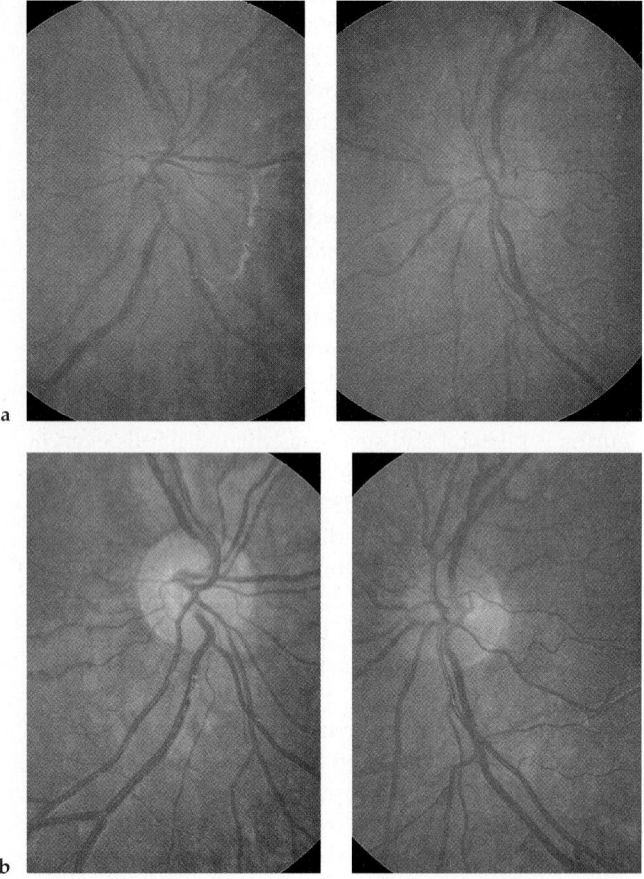

Fig. 51.2 (a) Bilaterally swollen optic discs. (b) Normal optic discs 2 months later. Complete visual recovery. Same patient as Fig. 51.1.

have reported a somewhat higher incidence of neurological problems, including multiple sclerosis (Kennedy & Carter 1961; Parkin *et al.* 1984). The incidence of neurological problems varies with the method of selection of patients and has been as high as 50% (Haller & Patzold 1979).

Patients with suspected optic neuritis should preferably be managed jointly with a neurologist, and further investigations should include computed tomography (CT) or magnetic resonance imaging (MRI) scan, cerebrospinal fluid studies, sinus X-ray and routine haematology. MRI studies reflect not only the expected inflammatory changes in the optic nerves but have also shown more widespread but asymptomatic brain white matter disease. The MRI changes may be more frequent in patients with bilateral optic neuritis (even if asynchronous), at least in adults (Beck *et al.* 1993). Visual evoked responses are useful in the acute stage because they are always abnormal (Taylor & Cuendet 1986) but a surprising difference from adults is that even pattern responses are often normal on follow-up.

The aetiology of childhood optic neuritis may be different from adult cases, possibly due to an infectious or parainfectious syndrome.

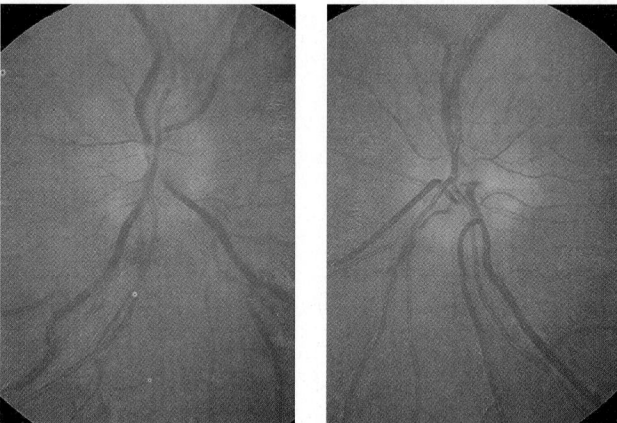

Fig. 51.3 Bilateral optic neuritis with swollen optic discs and a few peripapillary nerve fibre haemorrhages.

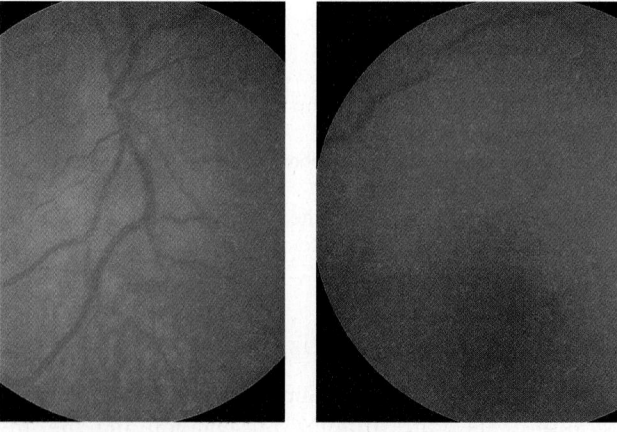

Fig. 51.4 Unilateral optic neuritis with paramacular pre-retinal haemorrhage.

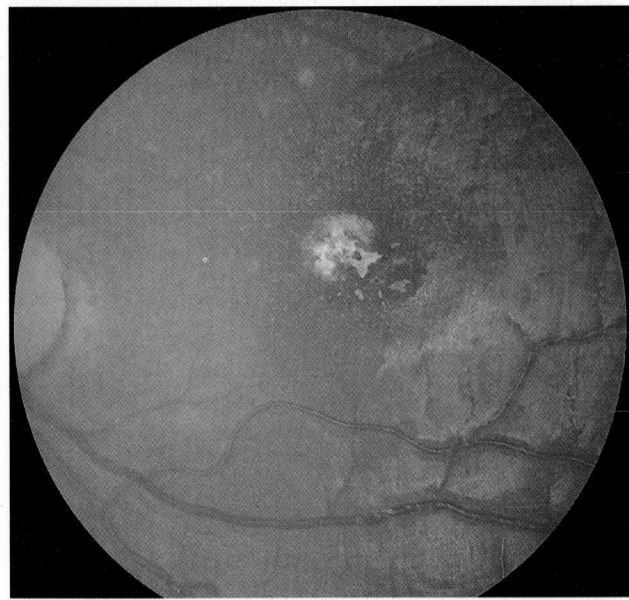

Fig. 51.5 Optic neuritis with remains of macular 'star'—the acuity is 6/9. There are similarities between childhood optic neuritis and neuroretinitis.

Neuroretinitis

The symptoms of this condition are virtually the same as in patients with optic neuritis; the difference is in the finding of a macular star (Fig. 51.5) which is a collection of intraretinal lipids in a spoke-like arrangement around the fovea, determined by the macular anatomy. It seems likely that the star is merely the sign that there is a very brisk serous exudate from the optic disc and it may well be that it is a similar condition to childhood optic neuritis but that a different part of the neurone is affected (Taylor & Cuendet 1986). The prognosis is good (Dreyer *et al.* 1984; Maitland & Miller 1984). Neuroretinitis has been described in association with toxoplasmosis (Fish *et al.* 1993), cat-scratch disease (Ulrich *et al.* 1992) and it may be recurrent and responsive to steroids (Purvin & Chiron 1994), a further similarity to optic neuritis.

Optic neuritis in infectious diseases

Exanthemas

Optic neuritis in childhood is often preceded by a non-specific illness but occasionally it is clearly related to one of the common childhood infectious illnesses, chickenpox being the most commonly reported (Purvin *et al.* 1988). Visual symptoms usually follow the rash by a few days, and although the visual loss may be profound, visual recovery is usually very good, despite the presence of residual optic atrophy (Sellost *et al.* 1983). Varicella may also cause visual loss by central retinal artery occlusion (Friedburg & Miale 1994).

Optic neuritis may be associated with rubella, measles, mumps or other vaccination (Kazarian & Gager 1979; Kline *et al.* 1982). Optic neuritis and encephalitis with a good prognosis have been described in an 8-year-old with Epstein–Barr virus infection (Straussberg *et al.* 1993). Optic neuritis has been reported with Lyme borelliosis (Arnold & Schriever 1993). Papillitis associated with toxoplasmosis may not be associated with marked visual loss, and may not have other foci to suggest toxoplasmosis (Folk & Lobes 1984).

Paranasal sinus disease

Symptoms of optic neuritis or a chiasmal syndrome (see Chapter 52) may occur in patients with acute or chronic ethmoiditis. The optic canal is extremely close to, or even runs in a bony strut through the ethmoid air cells and the optic nerve may be affected by compression, ischaemia or 'toxic' local effects. Sinus X-rays are indicated in all cases of optic neuritis in childhood even in the absence of clinical sinusitis. Treatment is with high doses of antibiotics together with systemic steroids. Casteels *et al.* (1992) described a signal case of a 10-year-old child with an asymptomatic sphenoid mucocoele who developed headaches, became blind in the right eye the next day and gradually lost vision in the left over 5 days. Subsequently, there was a partial recovery.

Optic neuropathy of malnutrition

It has long been known that patients on near-starvation diets are liable to an optic neuropathy, and it is common for hunger-strikers to go through an initially reversible, blinding optic neuropathy before death.

Hoyt and Billson (1979a) described two children who had a thiamine-reversible optic neuropathy whilst on a ketogenic diet. Chronic malnutrition is a possible cause of optic neuropathy in any child on an unusual diet, with many gut diseases, from a developing country or from the less privileged sectors of developed countries.

Optic neuropathy in leukaemia and systemic neoplasms

Optic nerve involvement in leukaemia has long been recognized as a serious complication, especially in acute lymphatic leukaemia, associated with bone marrow involvement in preterminal patients (Rosenthal *et al.* 1975). Chemotherapy and radiotherapy may have made this prognosis less than totally hopeless (Rosenthal 1983).

Optic nerve compression, not infrequently bilateral, also occurs in histiocytosis-X, neuroblastoma (Manschot 1969) and the leukaemias and non-Hodgkin's lymphomas. Rarely patients presenting with clinical optic neuritis may have tumour compression as the cause but

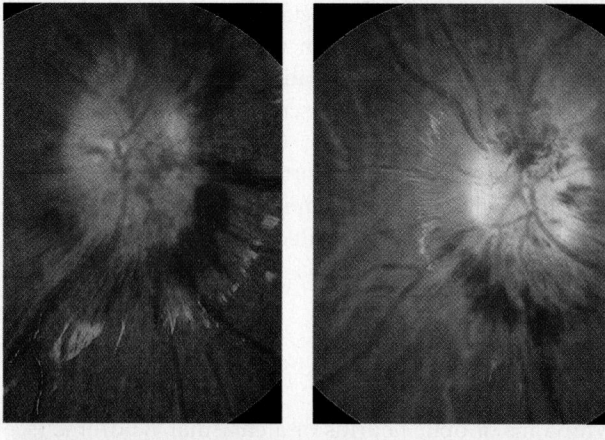

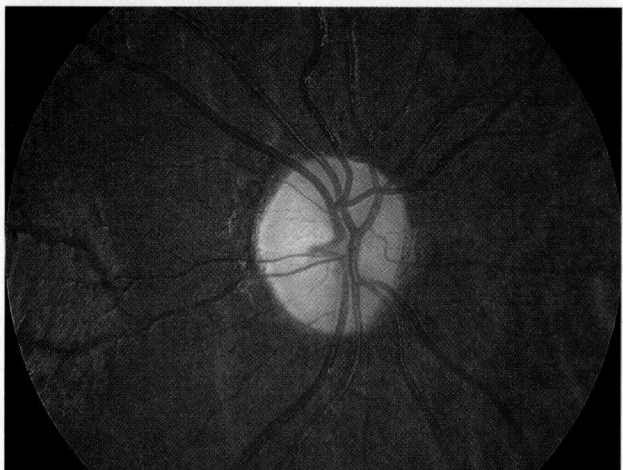

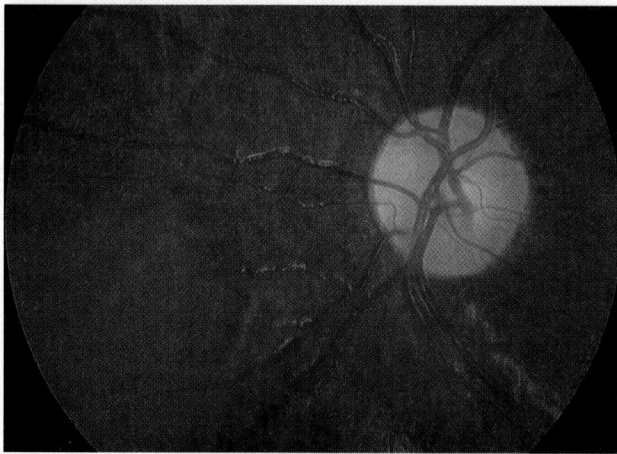

Fig. 51.6 (a) Acute optic neuropathy in a child with treated neuroblastoma on no therapy for 6 months. There was a bilateral central scotoma, acuities of 1/60 right eye, 4/60 left eye and colour vision loss. The cerebrospinal fluid and neuroradiological studies were normal. (b) Same patient 3 months later. The optic neuropathy settled on corticosteroid treatment only and the acuity (despite the obvious optic atrophy) has remained normal for 10 years.

the tumour may be corticosteroid responsive producing a temporarily satisfying response to treatment (Hirst *et al.* 1980). Children with neuroblastoma may present with acute visual loss from meningeal infiltration and rapid action must be taken (chemotherapy, irradiation and systemic steroids) to prevent the blindness which so frequently follows, whether it be from compression or ischaemia (Manschot 1969).

Optic neuritis may rarely occur as a remote effect of tumours (Fig. 51.6) or with direct involvement (Fig. 51.7).

Radiation optic neuropathy and encephalopathy occur often some weeks or months after the treatment (Shukovsky & Fletcher 1972; Oliff *et al.* 1978; Brown *et al.* 1982).

Compressive optic neuropathy

Optic atrophy from compression occurs from trauma, neoplasm, bone disease (Fig. 51.8), orbital tumours and infections. In osteopetrosis there may be early onset optic nerve compression by narrowing of the optic canal; poor vision may be the presenting sign in these children (Ainsworth *et al.* 1993). Surgical decompression of the optic canal may be successful in preventing visual loss (Haines *et al.* 1988) and may be indicated before or during bone marrow transplantation, the effects of which may take considerable time. Neurophysiological studies are a helpful adjunct because some cases have a retinal dystrophy (Keith 1968; Hoyt & Billson 1979b) and visual evoked potentials (VEPs) can be used to monitor progress (see Chapter 9). Optic disc compression/decompression by eye-poking may result in chronic disc oedema which resolves when the trauma ceases (Fig. 51.9). Catalano and Simon (1990) described transient optic disc swelling in patients with Down's syndrome.

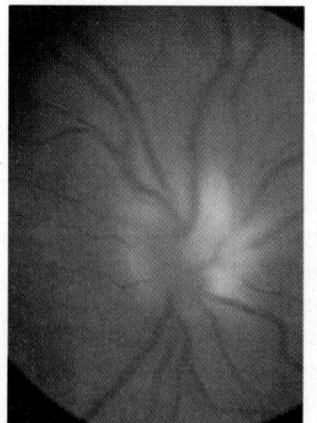
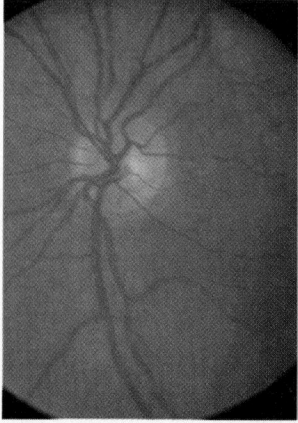

Fig. 51.7 Optic neuropathy from optic nerve glioma with optic disc involvement.

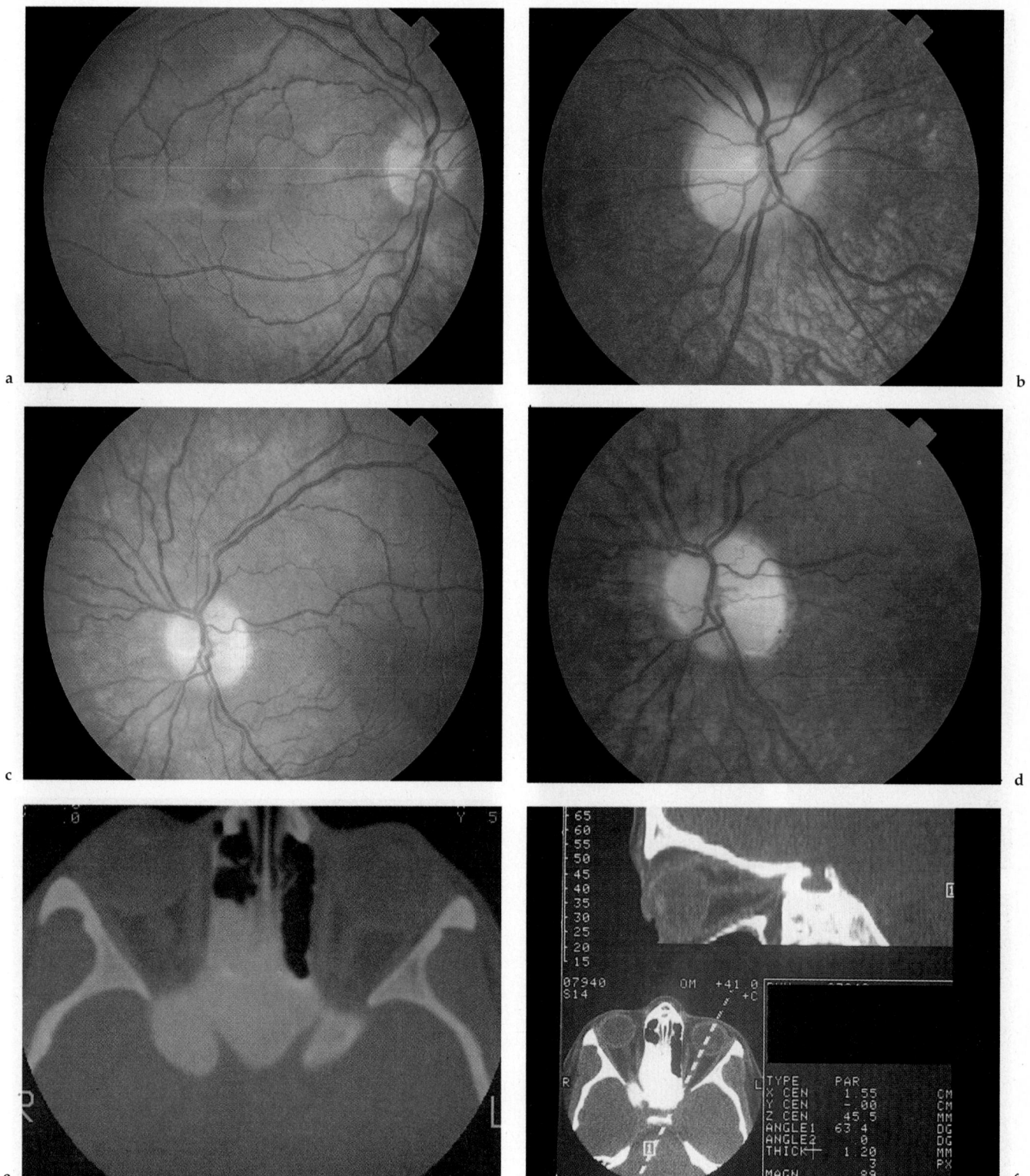

Fig. 51.8 Bilateral compressive optic neuropathy in a child with fibrous bone dysplasia. In the left eye (c) the acuity loss was arrested at 6/60 after optic canal decompression. In the right eye (a) the acuity was 6/9. The same patient 5 years later (b,d). The vision was unchanged. (e) Fibrous dysplasia giving a chronic compressive optic neuropathy. Although the optic canal was very narrow (f) there was no further visual loss after the age of 14 years.

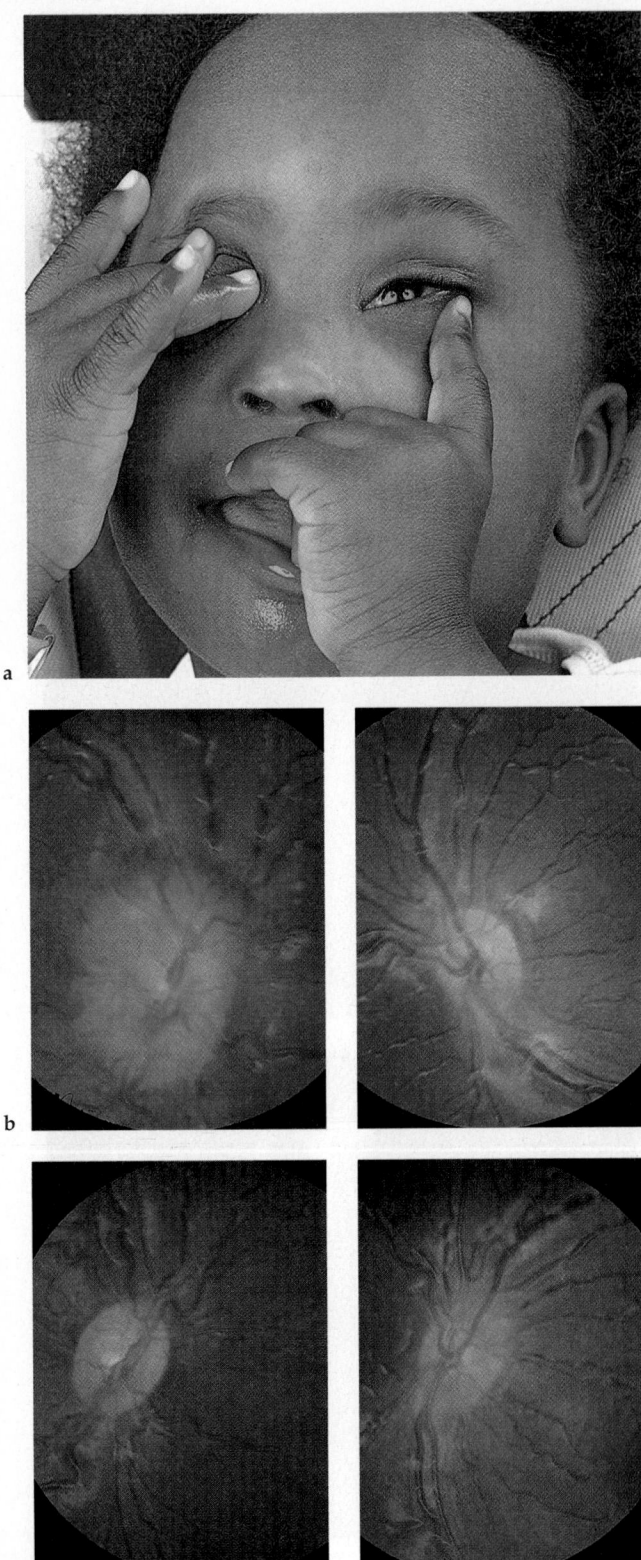

Fig. 51.9 (a) Child with severe Down's syndrome who relentlessly poked the right eye. (b) Right optic disc oedema. (c) After 2 weeks of using elbow restraints to stop the eye-poking the optic disc oedema had resolved.

Traumatic optic neuropathy

Soft tissue trauma

Blunt orbital trauma (Fig. 51.10) may cause a functional optic nerve transection if the optic nerve is compressed at the orbital apex or if there is a marked orbital haematoma. Optic disc pallor takes several weeks to appear. Eye trauma may cause secondary optic atrophy.

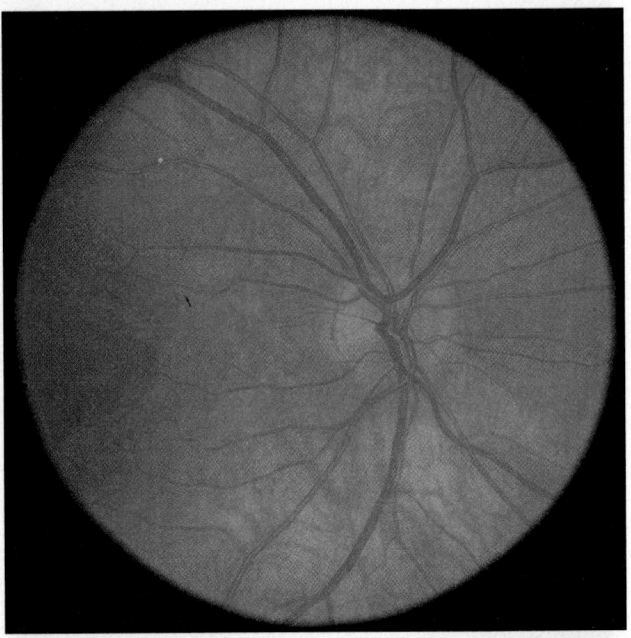

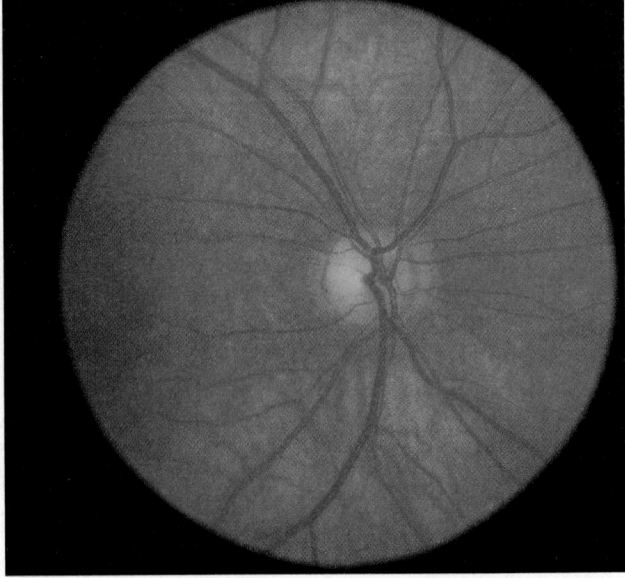

Fig. 51.10 (a) Right optic disc 4 hours after the eye was blinded by a billiards cue being accidentally thrust into the orbit of a 10-year-old boy. (b) Same patient 6 weeks later at the first appearance of optic atrophy.

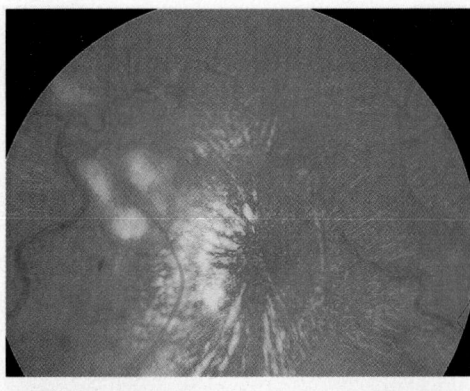

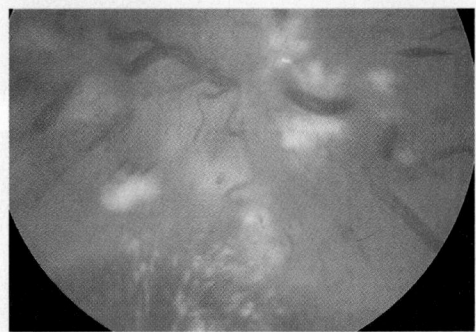

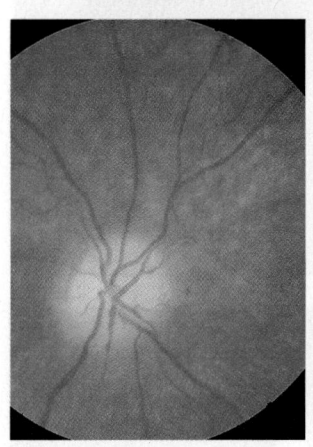
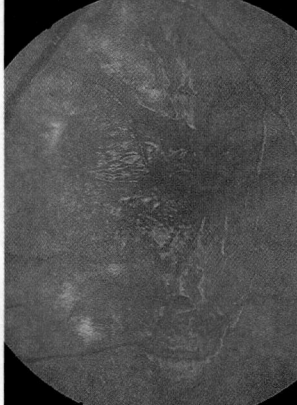

Fig. 51.11 (a) Optic neuropathy in malignant hypertension in an 11-year-old boy with reflux nephropathy. The vision had suddenly dropped associated with a gut haemorrhage. This was the presenting symptom. (b) Same patient showing the profound optic atrophy that subsequently occurred.

Skull fracture

Fractures of the sphenoid bone resulting from frontal trauma may cause a sudden blindness in one or rarely both eyes. The optic nerve defect is often discovered too late for treatment either because it is unilateral and, because the child is restless, the relative afferent pupil defect is difficult to detect, or in bilateral cases because the other effects of trauma, including lid swelling, are the overwhelming signs. If detected early high-dose systemic steroids (Seiff 1990) and optic canal decompression may help (Anderson

et al. 1982; Joseph *et al.* 1990). Although surgical treatment is not universally accepted as being effective, with modern scanning techniques the site of the injury is more readily identified and the most suitable approach, transcranial or extracranial, may be selected (Seiff 1991). Recovery may be prolonged. Feist *et al.* (1987) described a 16-year-old who had a shot-gun injury who had no perception of light for 2 weeks, but who eventually recovered to 20/100 by 4 months.

Ischaemic optic neuropathy

Ischaemic optic neuropathy occurs as a result of hypertension (Fig. 51.11) (Taylor *et al.* 1981), vasculitis as in patients with autoimmune diseases such as polyarteritis nodosa, systemic lupus or primary Sjögren's syndrome (Berman *et al.* 1990), or in anomalous optic discs in profoundly anaemic patients (Burde 1993) (Fig. 51.12).

Toxic optic neuropathy

In any child presenting with an unexplained optic neuropathy, that is with acuity and colour vision loss and a central scotoma, a careful history of drug and heavy metal ingestion must be taken.

Antituberculous drugs

Ethambutol, streptomycin, and isoniazid have been recorded as having a direct effect on optic nerve neurones. Their use in tuberculosis meningitis (Fig. 51.13) affecting

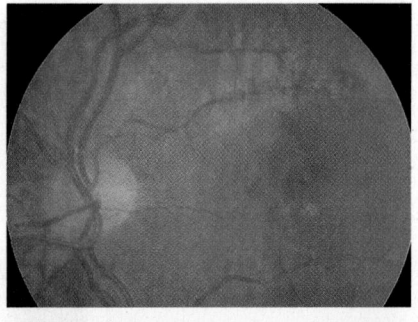

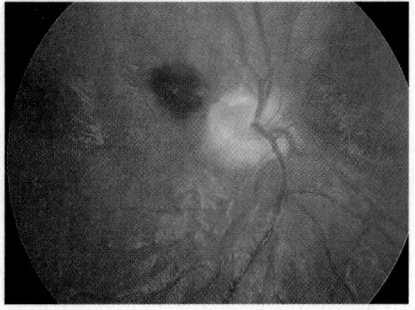

Fig. 51.12 Ischaemic optic neuropathy in the anomalous optic disc of the right eye of a patient with profound anaemia.

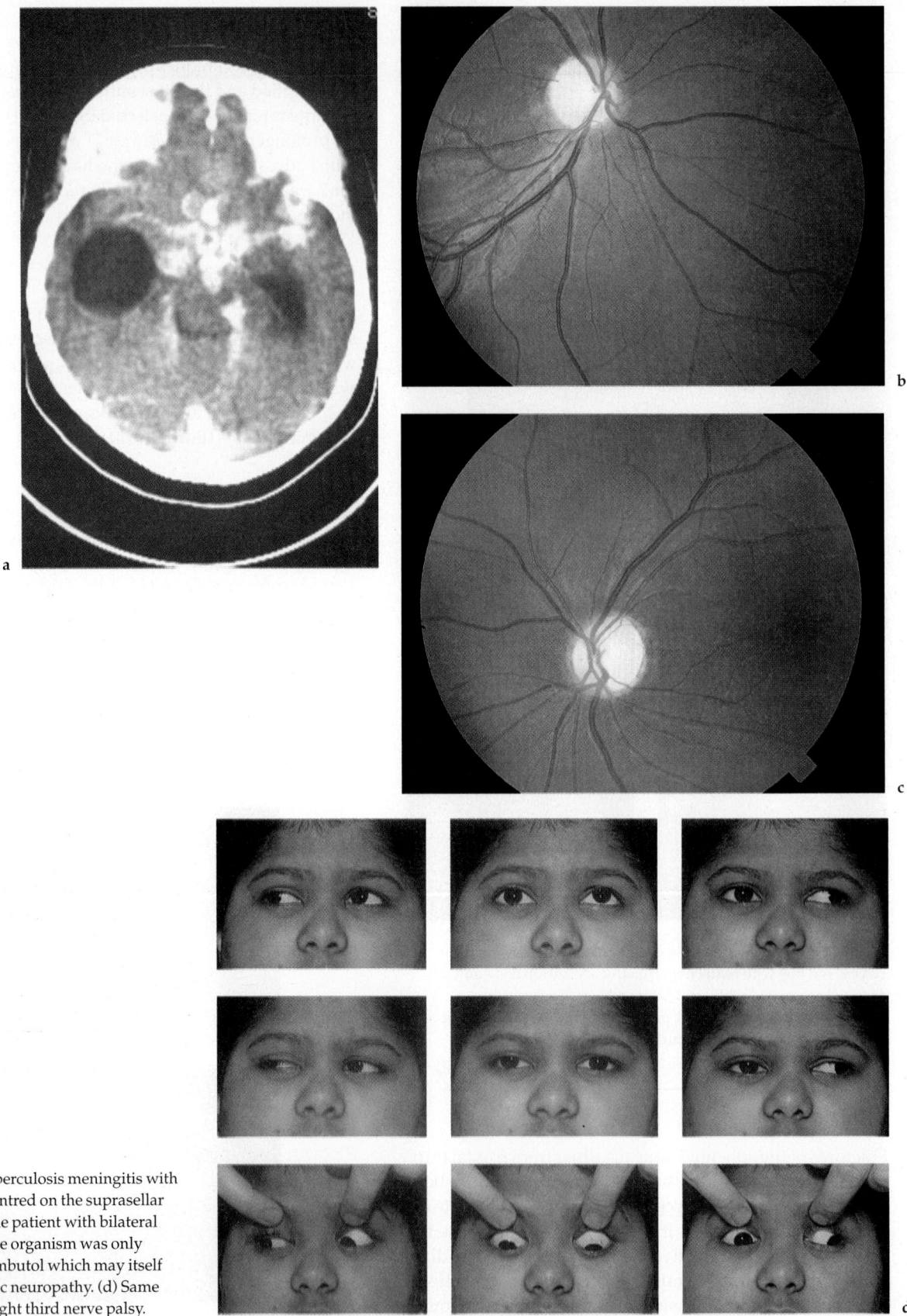

Fig. 51.13 (a) Tuberculosis meningitis with cystic changes centred on the suprasellar region. (b, c) Same patient with bilateral optic atrophy. The organism was only sensitive to ethambutol which may itself cause a toxic optic neuropathy. (d) Same patient: partial right third nerve palsy.

the chiasm and optic nerves calls for fine judgement as to the cause of further visual loss.

Desferrioxamine

High-dose desferrioxamine given for certain refractory anaemias may cause an optic neuropathy (Lakhanpal *et al.* 1984) or retinal pigmentation (Davies *et al.* 1983).

Cardiac drugs

Amiodarone causes largely asymptomatic cornea verticillas (Orlando *et al.* 1984) and retinal changes which are unusual but usually symptomatic (Ingram *et al.* 1982). A papillopathy with preserved acuity has been described (Gittinger & Asdourian 1987). Propranolol may give an optic neuropathy (Parrish & Todorov 1981) and digitalis is also suspected.

Hydroxyquinolines

Iodochlorhydroxyquin (dioquinol) when used as an antidiarrhoeal and diiodohydroxyquin (iodoquinol) may both give optic atrophy; the former in the form of subacute myelo-optic neuropathy (SMON) (Oakley 1973) and the latter as chronic optic atrophy (Behrens 1974).

Antibiotics

Chloramphenicol and sulphonamides (and their hypoglycaemic derivatives, tolbutamide and chlorpropamide) may give rise to an optic neuropathy which is reversible if treated early.

Antineoplastic agents

Carmustine (BCNU) and vincristine both give an optic neuropathy (Fraunfelder & Meyer 1983).

Others

Heavy metals, lead in particular, methanol, hexachlorophene (Slamovits *et al.* 1980) and solvents (such as carbon tetrachloride, carbon disulphide, trichlorethylene or toluene) should also be suspected in undiagnosed optic neuropathy.

Hereditary optic neuropathies

Dominant optic atrophy

This is the most common hereditary optic atrophy (Fig. 51.14). It is inherited as an autosomal dominant trait (Kjer 1959; Brodrick 1974; Kivlin *et al.* 1983), but penetrance may be low. The onset is very insidious with chil-dren often presenting in their first decade as a result of school eye tests. The acuity is symmetrically and often not severely affected (Smith 1972), 6/9–6/24 being most common and 6/36 or worse acuity being unusual. Careful examination of relatives is necessary because they may be very little disabled by their condition (see Fig. 51.14), and sometimes unaware of it. Flash electroretinography (ERG) is usually normal but may show a reduction in the scotopic response (Johnston *et al.* 1975). Pattern ERGs show a reduced amplitude of the negative component (Berninger *et al.* 1991). Blue cone ERGs differentiate dominant optic atrophy from congenital tritanopia – in the latter the blue cone ERG is absent (Miyake *et al.* 1985). Pattern VEPs may show reduced amplitude (Berninger *et al.* 1991). The acuity may deteriorate in time, but if it does it is very gradual and not to a marked degree (Eliott *et al.* 1993).

Careful visual field testing may show a subtle centrocaecal scotoma when the acuity is poor, the peripheral fields are full. When the acuity is good there is often a blue–yellow colour vision defect; when the acuity is poor there is a more profound and widespread colour defect. Nystagmus does not occur with typical dominant optic atrophy even on the rare occasions when it is detected in infancy.

The histopathological finding of ganglion cell loss with loss of myelin and nerve fibres within the optic nerve may suggest the disease is primarily a ganglion cell degeneration (Johnston *et al.* 1975). The loss of ganglion cells is most marked in the macular region and nerve fibre loss is most marked in the papillomacular bundle (Johnston *et al.* 1975) which accords with the frequent clinical finding of temporal segment disc pallor with a well-defined margin to the nerve fibre layer loss.

The affected patients are usually entirely normal apart from their eyes, but mental retardation has very occasionally been described (Kjer 1959; Johnston *et al.* 1975). However, the suspicion of systemic disease should signal caution to the wary clinician.

A similar but separate condition in which bilateral optic atrophy occurred in association with abnormal b-waves on the ERG studies in presumed dominant pedigrees was described by Weleber and Miyake (1992).

Dominant optic atrophy has been mapped to 3q (Eiberg *et al.* 1994).

Leber's optic neuropathy

Leber's optic neuropathy is unusual in childhood. It is characterized by the onset, between the late teens and the thirties, of a bilateral asynchronous (separated by a few months) loss of central vision occurring over a few days or weeks (Fig. 51.15). This is very profound and is accompanied by a large central scotoma and colour blindness. The visual defect is usually but not necessarily permanent and despite residual optic atrophy and visual defects the

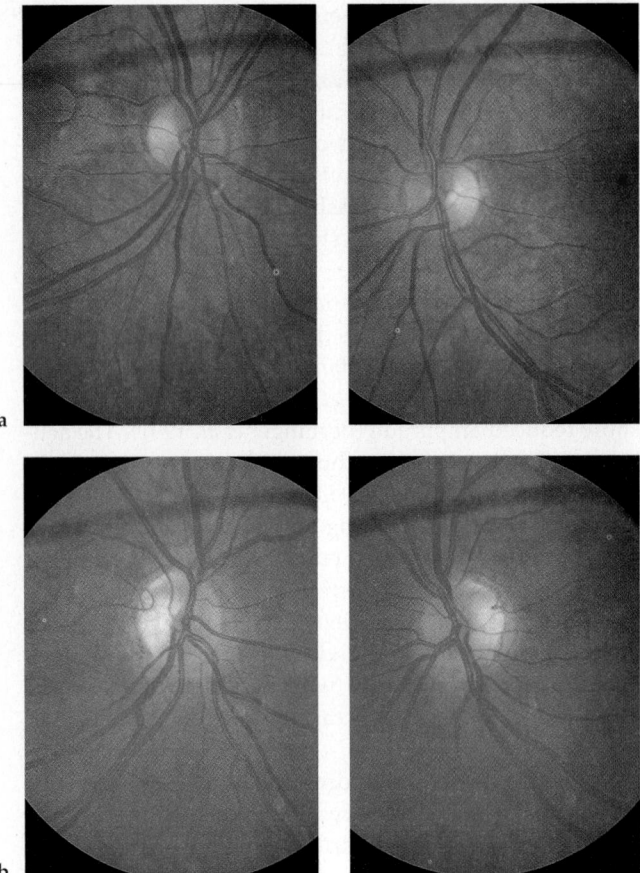

Fig. 51.14 (a) Dominant optic atrophy in a 6-year-old. He had failed the school test because his acuity was 6/12. He had normal red–green discrimination but defective blue–yellow. (b) The optic discs of the asymptomatic mother of the boy in (a). She had 6/9 acuity.

improvement in acuity over 2 years may be very useful (Lessell *et al.* 1983). In the presymptomatic phase there may be seen a telangiectatic microangiopathy (dilated telangiectatic vessels) of the peripapillary capillaries, which do not leak fluorescein (Nikoskelainen *et al.* 1984). If the acute phase occurs, the optic disc becomes swollen and the peripapillary nerve fibre bundles are easily seen (Smith *et al.* 1973); haemorrhages are unusual and not marked. Inheritance is similar to but different from X-linked recessive disease and is via a mitochondrial inheritance mechanism (see Chapter 10), through a mitochondrial DNA mutation (Wallace *et al.* 1988; Holt *et al.* 1989). Males are mainly but not exclusively affected (Franks & Sanders 1990) but they do not transmit the disease (as opposed to X-linked recessive disease where they transmit it through their daughters). Females can transmit the disease to their sons or their daughters, both having the telangiectatic microangiopathy (Nikoskelainen *et al.* 1987).

It is now known that there are a number of point mutations of mitochondrial DNA which may all give rise to varying clinical pictures of optic nerve and other system dysfunction. Another source of variation is the occurrence of heteroplasmy in at least the 11778 (Holt *et al.* 1989; Lott *et al.* 1990; Smith *et al.* 1993) and the 3460 (Black *et al.* 1996) mutations. A heteroplasmic tissue is one which contains two or more mitochondrial genotypes, normal and abnormal.

The 11778 mutation is the most frequently found (Johns 1990; Nikoskelainen *et al.* 1991) with a male predominance of 80% (Newman *et al.* 1991) and an age of onset of 8–60 years, usually without non-ocular abnormalities. Visual recovery occurs in 5% of patients with the 11778 mutation compared with 27% in the 14484, 22% in the 3460, and 29% in the 15257 mutation (Johns *et al.* 1993a,c; Mackey 1994). Patients with the 15257 mutation may have a maculopathy with or without optic neuropathy, and its role in Leber's optic neuropathy is not yet clear – it may not even be pathological. The role of secondary mutations is probably not important (Nikoskelainen *et al.* 1996).

Evidence has indicated an association with a disorder in cyanide metabolism (Hulme-Adams 1966; Wilson *et al.* 1971; Cagianut *et al.* 1981; Freeman 1988; Berninger *et al.* 1989). Associated cardiac (Nikoskelainen *et al.* 1987) and myopathic (Uemura *et al.* 1987) lesions have been described. That other factors than just the DNA mutation are important is suggested by marked discordance of the clinical picture between two identical twins (Johns *et al.* 1993b).

Optic atrophy in juvenile diabetes

Optic atrophy rarely occurs in diabetic children from the effects of the retinopathy but it may occur as part of a specific syndrome, the Wolfram–Tyrer syndrome (Wolfram 1938; Tyrer 1943) or DIDMOAD (diabetes insipidus, diabetes mellitus, optic atrophy and deafness) syndrome. It is characterized by four main symptoms (François 1975).

1 Optic atrophy of onset between 2 and 24 years, usually before 15 years (Figs 51.16, 51.17). The vision becomes very bad but blindness is rare. The visual fields are constricted and the patient is colour blind. Diabetic retinopathy is rare, perhaps reflecting the loss of nerve fibres. There is no acute stage, the atrophy is relentlessly progressive and the discs do not swell.

2 Juvenile diabetes mellitus, which is usually diagnosed before the optic atrophy.

3 Diabetes insipidus, which is usually undiagnosed until the children have persistent polyuria despite adequate control of the diabetes mellitus (Pilley & Thompson 1976). It usually responds to treatment with vasopressin (Bretz *et al.* 1970).

4 There is a bilateral symmetrical, initially partial and affecting high tones, progressive deafness that may need audiometry for presymptomatic detection.

Pigmentary changes at the posterior pole have been described occasionally (Rose *et al.* 1966; Rorsman & Soder-

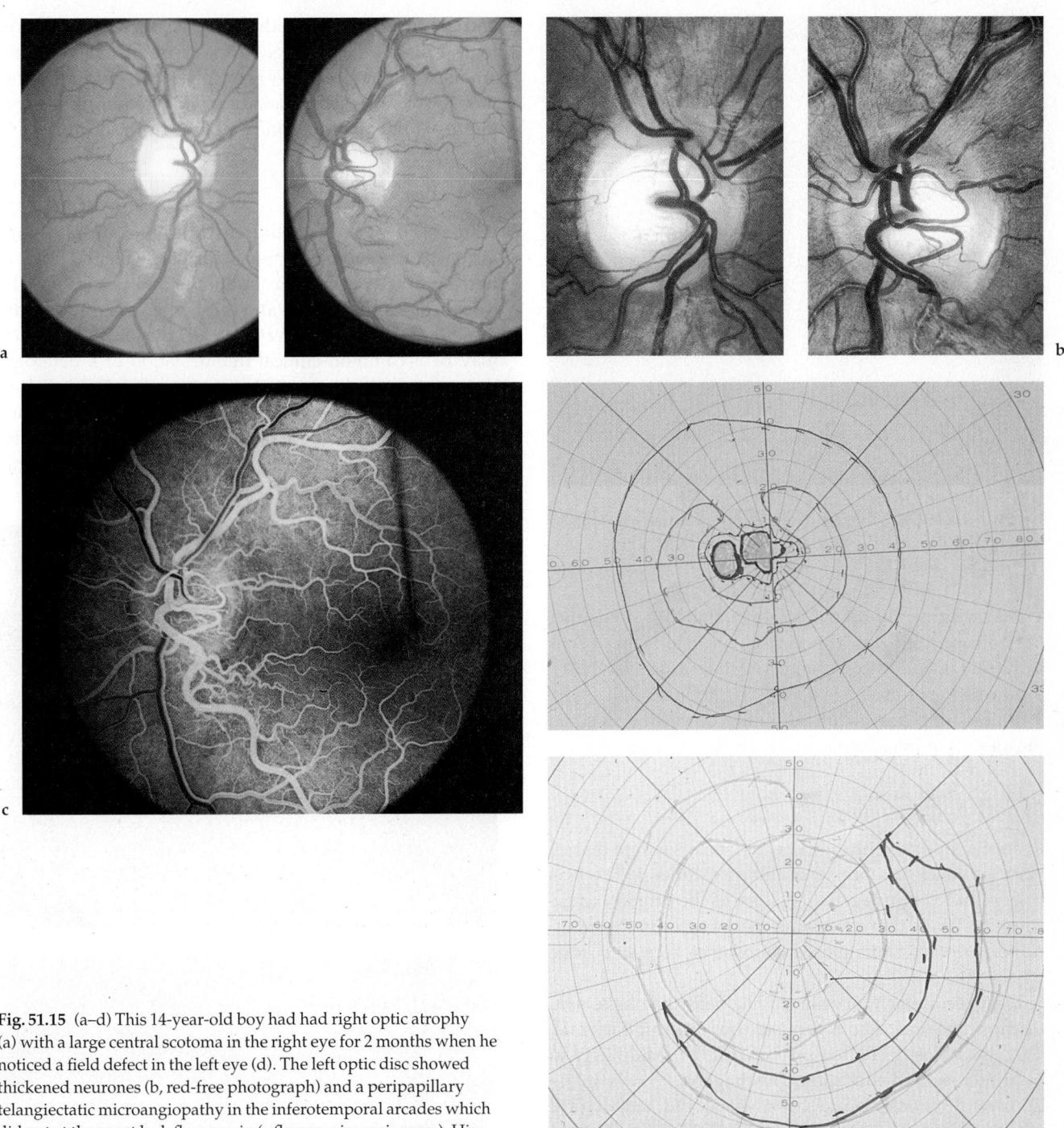

Fig. 51.15 (a–d) This 14-year-old boy had had right optic atrophy (a) with a large central scotoma in the right eye for 2 months when he noticed a field defect in the left eye (d). The left optic disc showed thickened neurones (b, red-free photograph) and a peripapillary telangiectatic microangiopathy in the inferotemporal arcades which did not at the onset leak fluorescein (c fluorescein angiogram). His brother and uncle were also affected by Leber's optic neuropathy.

strom 1967) and ERG may indicate a more widespread abnormality of the retina than just that due to ganglion cell degeneration (Niemeyer & Marquardt 1972).

Anosmia, tonic pupils and optic disc cupping are less frequent findings (Lessell & Rosman 1977). It is inherited as an autosomal recessive trait and the gene has been linked to 4p (Polymeropoulos *et al.* 1994).

There are other associations between optic atrophy and diabetes mellitus (Rose *et al.* 1966): (i) Friedreich's ataxia;

(ii) Refsum's disease; and (iii) Laurence–Moon–Biedl syndrome.

Swollen optic discs in diabetic children

Papilloedema occurs in diabetes as a result of any of the usual causes not directly related to diabetes, but diabetics more frequently have papilloedema for three specific reasons.

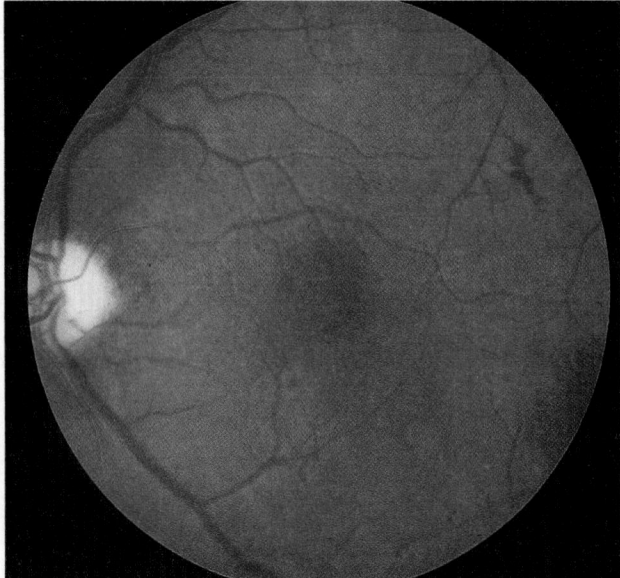

Fig. 51.16 DIDMOAD. There is optic atrophy and a diabetic retinal haemorrhage.

1 Transient papilloedema with visual loss, and ensuing optic atrophy but with a good visual prognosis may occur as a result of optic disc ischaemia (Lubow & Makley 1971).
2 Severe hypertension in diabetic nephropathy.
3 Raised intracranial pressure may occur due to sinus thrombosis or infections.

Recessive optic atrophy

Recessive optic atrophy is extremely rare—so rare that its very existence has been questioned (Moller 1992). It is important to exclude retinal disease as the primary cause since it is likely that a large number of cases in the literature represent undiagnosed autosomal recessive cone dystrophy.

The onset is early, or at birth. The baby may have nystagmus. The optic disc is very pale but otherwise normal. The visual defect is often severe with the child likely to need non-sighted education. The diagnosis is only made by careful clinical, neurophysiological and radiological exclusion of other causes. Often a family history is lacking but consanguinity in the parents and subsequent affected siblings suggest the diagnosis and heredity (Fig. 51.18).

Optic atrophy in heredodegenerative neurological disease

That optic atrophy occurred in some neurological diseases was known in the last century; Habershon (1887) referred to optic atrophy in patients with diseases of the spinal cord, locomotor ataxia and epilepsy, as well as insanity and sexual abuse or excesses. Although not frequently encountered by most ophthalmologists, hereditary neurological diseases are a significant cause of optic atrophy amongst young people (Harding 1984), adding enormously to an existing handicap and requiring a great depth of understanding and empathy by the doctor.

Behr's disease

Behr (1909) described children with optic atrophy, poor vision, squint and nystagmus with ataxia, mental retardation, spasticity, urinary incontinence and pes cavus. The disease affects both sexes and is inherited as an autosomal recessive trait (Landrigan *et al.* 1973; François 1976a), but it may be a common clinical manifestation of a heterogeneous group of disorders (Horoupian *et al.* 1979). Pathologically there is loss of central optic nerve axons (Fig. 51.19) and widespread neural loss especially in thalamic nuclei (Horoupian *et al.* 1979). The visual and systemic

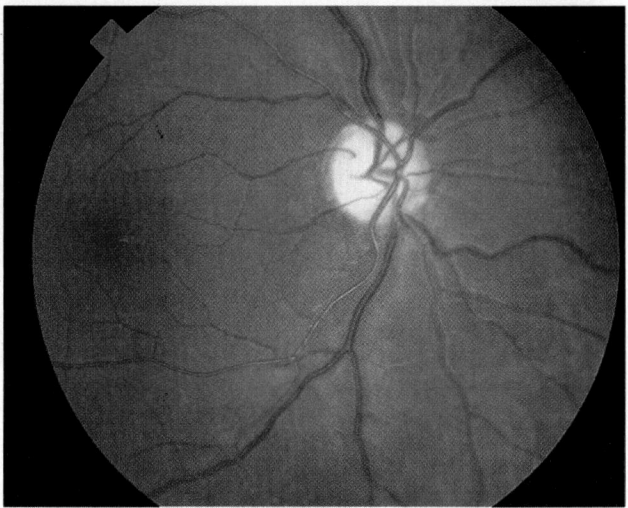

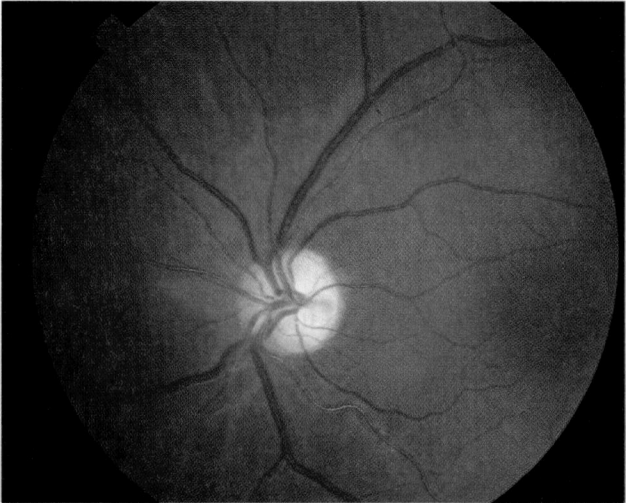

Fig. 51.17 DIDMOAD. Bilateral optic atrophy with profound visual loss.

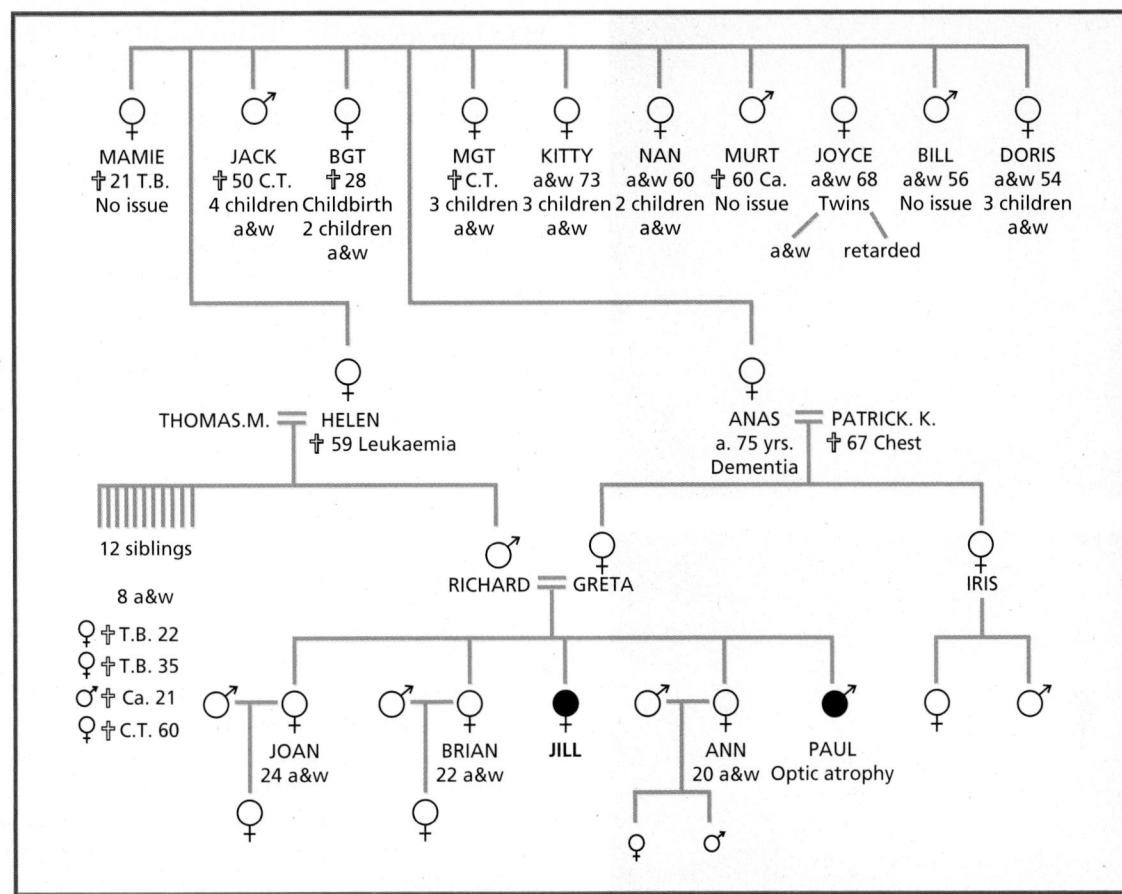

Fig. 51.18 Recessive optic atrophy. Profound optic atrophy occurred in two siblings of a consanguineous marriage. The ERG was normal to flash stimuli.

prognosis should be cautious. Sheffer *et al.* (1992) described three patients who were found to have 3-methylglutaconic aciduria and it is not infrequent that the diagnosis has to be revised.

Friedreich's ataxia

Friedreich's ataxia, and the closely related ataxia of Charlevoix–Saguenay, are characterized (Barbeau 1978) by the following.

1 Genetics: autosomal recessive.

2 Clinical: onset is before the end of puberty. Ataxia, first of lower limbs, then all four limbs, is relentlessly progressive, usually with muscle wasting.
- Dysarthria.
- Abnormal vibration and position sense in lower limbs.
- Absent deep tendon reflexes in lower limbs.
- Progressive kyphoscoliosis and pes cavus within 2 years of onset.

3 Preclinical: hypertrophic progressive cardiomyopathy.

- Abnormal sensory nerve conduction in lower more than upper limbs.
- Essentially normal motor nerve conduction and electromyography.

4 Neuro-ophthalmic abnormalities: optic atrophy occurs frequently in Friedreich's ataxia (Livingstone *et al.* 1981), and a presymptomatic phase may be observed clinically or revealed by visual evoked cortical responses (Carroll *et al.* 1980). Symptomatic, progressive optic neuropathy (Fig. 51.20) that may be disabling occurs in a significant proportion of patients.

Eye movement defects, related to the cerebellar defect, are common and occur in patients without a significant visual defect (Kirkham *et al.* 1979). They include downbeat nystagmus, gaze paretic and rebound nystagmus, asymmetrical saccades, reduced vestibulo-ocular reflex (VOR) suppression or unsteady fixation (Zee *et al.* 1976). The finding of decreased VOR responses may be helpful in the differential diagnosis from patients with parenchymal cerebellar disease who usually have increased VORs (Furman *et al.* 1983).

Olivopontocerebellar atrophy

Both autosomal recessive and autosomal dominant hered-

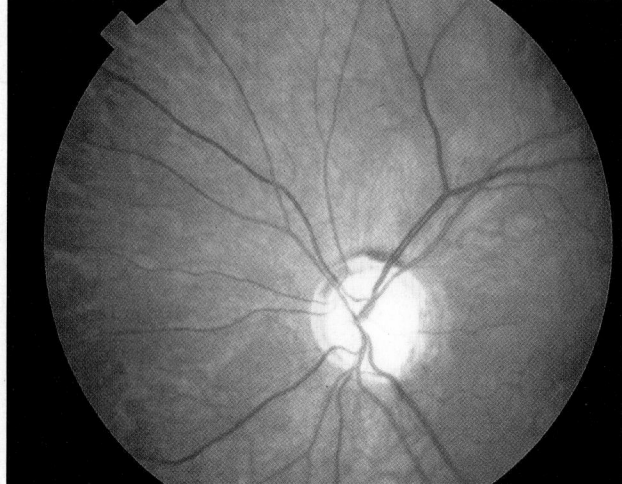

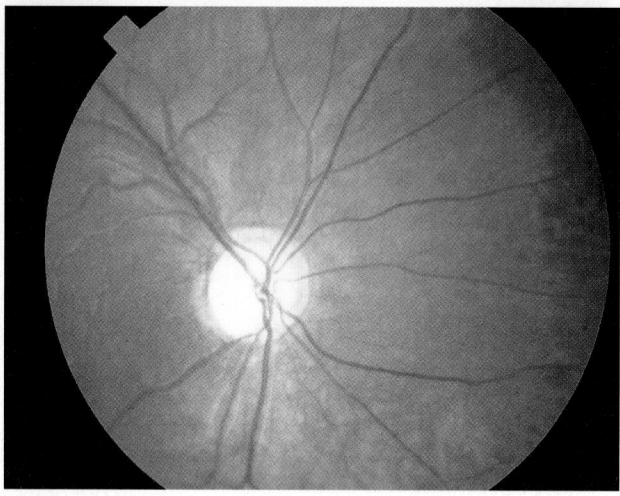

Fig. 51.19 Bilateral optic atrophy in a patient with Behr's disease.

ity has been proposed in various studies of this syndrome in which there is a variably early onset of progressive ataxia, tremor, dysarthria and visual difficulties which are largely due to a retinal degeneration (Weiner *et al.* 1967) but which may in some cases be due to an optic neuropathy as evidenced by presymptomatic changes in the VEP (Hammond & Wilder 1983).

Charcot–Marie–Tooth disease (peroneal muscular atrophy)

This is a motor neuropathy predominantly affecting the legs; it is usually inherited as an autosomal dominant trait with an onset in late childhood. Affected children have distal wasting of the legs, pes cavus and foot drop. The hands are only mildly affected and progression is very slow. Optic atrophy, starting in the teens, with loss of acuity and central scotomas is an unusual but recognized complication (Hoyt 1960). Similar cases together with deafness have been described (Rosenberg & Chutorian 1967).

PEHO syndrome

PEHO is an acronym for progressive encephalopathy with oedema, hypsarrhythmia and optic atrophy (Salonen *et al.* 1991).

These children have a severe encephalopathy with early onset. They are hypotonic, have convulsions associated with hypsarrhythmia, hyperreflexia, profound mental retardation and optic atrophy. They have puffy oedema, especially of the extremities, and they are dysmorphic with a narrow forehead, puffy cheeks and receding chin. They have epicanthic folds and strabismus. They die in the first decade and the condition is probably autosomal recessive.

Leucodystrophies

Metachromatic leucodystrophy

This occurs in late infantile, intermediate and juvenile forms which present with gait disorders, a peripheral neuropathy, behavioural problems and intellectual deterioration. The diagnosis is suspected after finding metachromatic material in the urine and confirmed by the finding of decreased levels of aryl sulphatase A in white blood cells. Optic atrophy is frequent (Libert *et al.* 1979; Taylor 1983) and may result in severely impaired vision (François 1979).

Adrenoleucodystrophy

This X-linked recessive disease occurs in 5–9-year-old

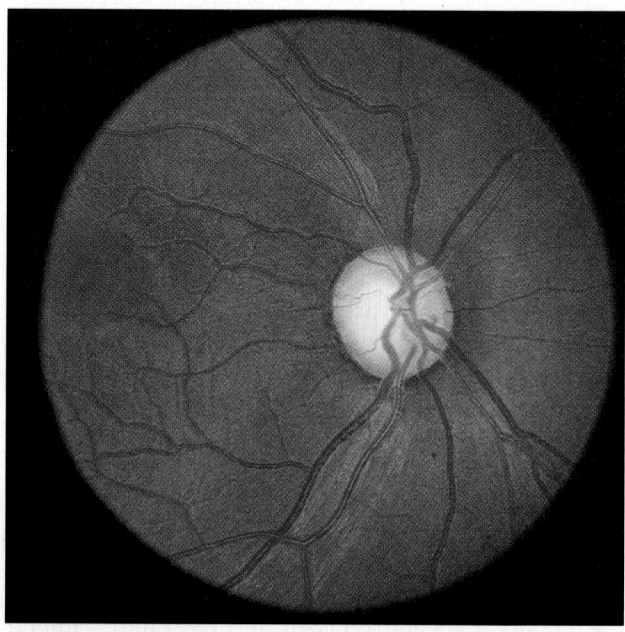

Fig. 51.20 Optic atrophy in a 10-year-old with Friedreich's ataxia. Marked grooves can be seen in the arcuate bundles.

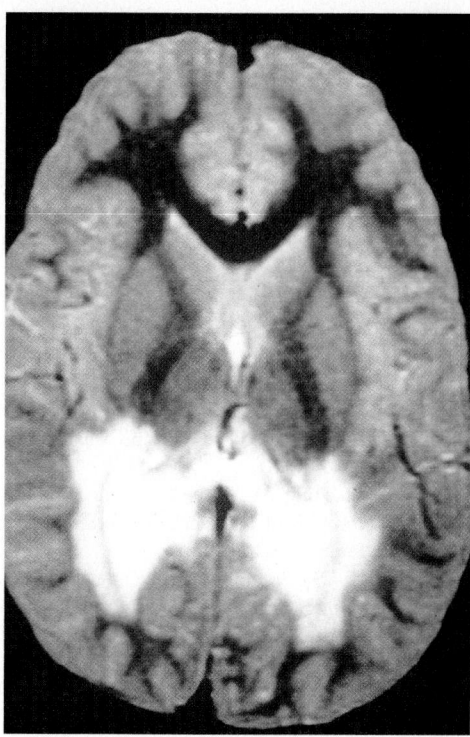

Fig. 51.21 X-linked adrenoleucodystrophy, Addison–Schilder disease. MRI scan showing posterior periventricular white matter disease. These boys usually present in the first decade with poor vision and developmental regression. Later they develop optic atrophy (see Chapter 57).

boys who have subtle behavioural changes, intellectual deterioration, symptoms of adrenal insufficiency, and a usually severe visual problem which is due to a relatively selective visual cortical defect (Fig. 51.21) but optic atrophy also occurs (Wray *et al.* 1976a).

Krabbe's leucodystrophy (globoid cell leucodystrophy)

The onset is usually in early infancy with rapidly progressive apathy, irritability and neurological regression with clinical evidence of a peripheral neuropathy. Optic atrophy occurs early but is usually overshadowed by the neurological deterioration (François 1975).

Menke's disease

Boys with this X-linked syndrome have psychomotor retardation, progressive spasticity and seizures, and abnormal ('kinky' or 'steely') hair. Plasma copper and caeruloplasmin levels are low. Retinal abnormalities are frequent, with a macular dystrophy, mottled retinal pigment epithelium and tortuous vessels (Taylor 1983) and optic atrophy which probably occurs as an additional feature to, rather than the result of, a retinal degeneration (Seelenfreund *et al.* 1968; Wray *et al.* 1976b).

Neuronal storage diseases and the mucopolysaccharidoses

Batten's disease, clinical Tay–Sachs disease and other gangliosidoses, Neimann–Pick disease type A, infantile Gaucher's disease, and some of the mucopolysaccharidoses; and sialidosis mucolipidoses (cherry red spot–myoclonus syndrome) may all have diffuse affection of their ganglion cells resulting in a cherry red spot. Ganglion cell death eventually results in optic atrophy. In the mucopolysaccharidoses optic atrophy occurs from glaucoma, retinal degeneration, optic nerve involvement directly, compression by thickened bone at the optic canal or hydrocephalus.

Optic atrophy in familial dysautonomia

As these children are now living longer, it has become evident that optic atrophy may account for a proportion of their visual loss, as further evidence of central nervous system involvement (Rizzo *et al.* 1986). Nineteen eyes of 12 patients had abnormal pattern VERs; the latency increased with age (Diamond *et al.* 1987).

References

Ainsworth J, Bryce I, Dudgeon J. Visual loss in infantile osteopetrosis. *J Pediatr Ophthalmol Strabismus* 1993; **30**: 201–3.

Anderson RL, Danje WR, Gross CE. Optic nerve blindness following blunt forehead trauma. *J Am Acad Ophthalmol* 1982; **89**: 445–55.

Arnold R, Schriever G. Lyme amaurosis in a child. *J Pediatr Ophthalmol Strabismus* 1993; **30**: 268–70.

Barbeau A. Quebec Cooperative Study of Friedreich's ataxia. Cooperative Study, phase 2: statement of the problems. *Canad J Neurol Sci* 1978; **5**: 57–9.

Beck R, Kupersmith M, Cleary P, Katz B, The Optic Neuritis Study Group. Fellow eye abnormalities in acute unilateral optic neuritis: experience of optic neuritis treatment trial. *Ophthalmology* 1993; **100**: 691–8.

Behr C. Die komplizierte, hereditar-familiare Optikusatrophie des Kindesathers. *Klin Monatsbl Augenheilkd* 1909; **47**: 138–60.

Behrens MM. Optic atrophy in children after di-iodohydroxyquin therapy. *J Am Med Assoc* 1974; **228**: 693–4.

Berman JL, Kashii S, Trachtman M, Burde R. Optic neuropathy and central nervous system disease secondary to Sjögren's syndrome in a child. *Ophthalmology* 1990; **97**: 1606–10.

Berninger TA, Jaeger W, Krastel H. Electrophysiology and colour perimetry in dominant infantile optic atrophy. *Br J Ophthalmol* 1991; **75**: 49–53.

Berninger TA, Meyer L, Seiss E, Schon O, Goebel F-D. Leber's hereditary optic atrophy: further evidence for a defect in cyanide metabolism. *Br J Ophthalmol* 1989; **73**: 314–16.

Black GCM, Morten K, Laborde A, Poulton J. Leber's hereditory optic neuropathy: heteroplasmy is likely to be significant in the expression of IHON in families with the 3460 NDI mutation. *Br J Ophthalmol* 1992; **76**: 502–4.

Bretz GW, Baghadassarian SA, Graber JD, Zacherle B, Norum RA, Blizzard RM. Coexistence of diabetes mellitus and insipidus and optic atrophy in two male siblings. *Am J Med* 1970; **48**: 398–403.

Brodrick JD. Hereditary optic atrophy with onset in early childhood. *Br J Ophthalmol* 1974; **58**: 817–24.

Brown GC, Shields JA, Sanborn G, Augsburger JJ, Savino PJ, Schatz N. Radiation optic neuropathy. *J Am Acad Ophthalmol* 1982; **89**: 1489–93.

Burde R. Optic disc risk factors for non-arteritic anterior ischaemic optic neuropathy. *Am J Ophthalmol* 1993; **116**: 759–64.

Cagianut B, Rhyner K, Furrer W, Schnebli HP. Thiosulphate–sulphur transferase (rhodanese) deficiency in Leber's hereditary optic atrophy. *Lancet* 1981; **ii**: 981–2.

Carrol WM, Kriss A, Baraitser M, Barrett G, Halliday AM. The incidence and nature of visual pathway involvement in Friedreich's ataxia, a clinical and visual evoked potential study of 22 patients. *Brain* 1980; **103**: 413–34.

Casteels I, De Loof E, Brock P, Jorissen M, Dralands L, Misotten L, Wilms G. Sudden blindness in a child: presenting symptom of a sphenoid sinus mucocele. *Br J Ophthalmol* 1992; **76**: 502–4.

Catalano R, Simon JW. Optic disc elevation in Down's syndrome. *Am J Ophthalmol* 1990; **110**: 28–32.

Davies D, Marcys RE, Hungerford JL, Miller MH, Arden GB, Huchns ER. Ocular toxicity of high-dose intravenous desferrioxamine. *Lancet* 1983; **ii**: 181–4.

Diamond GA, D'Amico RA, Axelrod FB. Optic nerve dysfunction in familial dysautonomia. *Am J Ophthalmol* 1987; **104**: 645–9.

Dreyer RF, Hopen G, Gass JDM, Smith JL. Leber's idiopathic stellate neuroretinitis. *Arch Ophthalmol* 1984; **102**: 1140–5.

Eiberg H, Kjer B, Kjer P *et al*. Dominant optic atrophy (OPA1) mapped to chromosome 3q region 1. *Hum Mol Genet* 1994; **2**: 977–80.

Eliott D, Traboulsi E, Maumenee I. Visual prognosis in autosomal dominant optic atrophy (Kjer type). *Am J Ophthalmol* 1993; **115**: 360–7.

Farris BK, Pickard DJ. Bilateral post-infectious optic neuritis and intravenous steroid therapy in children. *Ophthalmology* 1990; **97**: 339–45.

Feist RM, Kline LB, Morris RE, Witherspoon CD, Michelson MA. Recovery of vision after presumed direct optic nerve injury. *J Am Acad Ophthalmol* 1987; **94**: 1567–70.

Fish R, Hoskins J, Kline L. Toxoplasmosis neuroretinitis. *Ophthalmology* 1993; **100**: 1177–82.

Folk JC, Lobes LA. Presumed toxoplasmosis papillitis. *Ophthalmology* 1984; **91**: 64–8.

François J. Les atrophies optiques hereditaires. *J Genet Hum* 1976a; **24**: 183–200.

François J. Ocular manifestations in demyelinating diseases. *Adv Ophthalmol* 1979; **39**: 1–36.

François J. Ocular manifestations in inborn error of carbohydrate and lipid metabolism. In: *Krabbe's Disease*, Part II, Section G. Basel: Karger, 1975: 98–100.

François J. Optico-oto-diabetic syndrome. *Ophthalmologica (Basel)* 1976b; **173**: 345–51.

Franks WA, Sanders MD. Leber's hereditary optic neuropathy in women. *Eye* 1990; **4**: 482–6.

Fraunfelder FT, Meyer SM. Ocular toxicity of antineoplastic agents. *Ophthalmology* 1983; **90**: 1–3.

Freeman AG. Optic neuropathy and chronic cyanide intoxication: a review. *J Roy Soc Med* 1988; **81**: 103–6.

Friedburg MA, Miale AJ. Monocular blindness from central retinal artery occlusion associated with chickenpox (letter). *Am J Ophthalmol* 1994; **117**: 117–18.

Furman JM, Perlman S, Baloh RW. Eye movements in Friedreich's ataxia. *Arch Neurol* 1983; **40**: 343–46.

Gittinger JW, Asdourian GK. Papillopathy caused by amiodarone. *Arch Ophthalmol* 1987; **105**: 349–51.

Habershon SH. Hereditary optic atrophy. *Trans Ophthalmol Soc UK* 1887; **8**: 1–47.

Haines SJ, Erickson DL, Wirtschafter JD. Optic nerve decompression for osteopetrosis in early childhood. *Neurosurgery* 1988; **23**: 470–5.

Haller P, Patzold U. Die Optikusneuritis im Kindersalter. *Fortschr Neurol Psychiatr* 1979; **47**: 209–16.

Hammond EJ, Wilder BJ. Evoked potentials in olivoponto-cerebellar atrophy. *Arch Neurol* 1983; **40**: 366–9.

Harding AE. *The Hereditary Ataxias and Related Disorders*. London: Churchill Livingstone, 1984.

Heher K, Johns D. A maculopathy associated with the 15257 mitochondrial DNA mutation. *Arch Ophthalmol* 1993; **111**: 1495–9.

Heirons R, Lyle TK. Bilateral retrobulbar neuritis. *Brain* 1959; **82**: 56–67.

Hirst LW, Miller NR, Kumar AJ, Udvarhelyi GB. Medulloblastoma causing a corticosteroid-responsive optic neuropathy. *Am J Ophthalmol* 1980; **89**: 437–42.

Holt IJ, Miller DH, Harding AE. Genetic heterogeneity and mitochondrial DNA heteroplasmy in Leber's hereditary optic neuropathy. *J Med Genet* 1989; **26**: 739–43.

Horoupian DS, Zuker DK, Solomon M, Peterson HDC. Behr syndrome; a clinicopathological report. *Neurology* 1979; **29**: 323–7.

Hoyt CS, Billson FA. Optic neuropathy in ketogenic diet. *Br J Ophthalmol* 1979a; **63**: 191–4.

Hoyt CS, Billson FA. Visual loss in osteopetrosis. *Am J Dis Child* 1979b; **133**: 955–8.

Hoyt WF. Charcot–Marie–Tooth disease with optic atrophy. *Arch Ophthalmol* 1960; **64**: 145–8.

Hulme-Adams J, Blackwood W, Wilson J. Further clinical and pathological observations on Leber's optic atrophy. *Brain* 1966; **89**: 15–22.

Ingram DV, Jaggarao NSV, Chamberlain DA. Ocular changes resulting from therapy with amiodarone. *Br J Ophthalmol* 1982; **66**: 676–80.

Johns DR. The molecular genetics of Leber's hereditary optic neuropathy. *Arch Ophthalmol* 1990; **108**: 1405–8.

Johns D, Heher K, Miller N, Smith K. Leber's hereditary optic neuropathy: clinical manifestations of the 14484 mutation. *Arch Ophthalmol* 1993a; **111**: 495–8.

Johns D, Smith K, Miller N, Sulewski M, Bias W. Identical twins who are discordant for Leber's hereditary optic neuropathy. *Arch Ophthalmol* 1993b; **111**: 1491–4.

Johns D, Smith K, Savino P, Miller N. Leber's hereditary optic neuropathy: clinical manifestations of the 15257 mutation. *Ophthalmology* 1993c; **100**: 981–6.

Johnston PB, Gaster RN, Smith VC, Tripathi RC. A clinicopathologic study of autosomal dominant optic atrophy. *Am J Ophthalmol* 1975; **88**: 868–75.

Joseph MP, Lessell S, Rizzo J, Momose KJ. Extracranial optic nerve decompression for traumatic optic neuropathy. *Arch Ophthalmol* 1990; **108**: 1091–3.

Kazarian EL, Gager WE. Optic neuritis complicating measles, mumps and rubella vaccination. *Am J Ophthalmol* 1979; **86**: 544–7.

Keith CG. Retinal atrophy in osteopetrosis. *Arch Ophthalmol* 1968; **79**: 234–41.

Kennedy C, Carroll FD. Optic neuritis in children. *Arch Ophthalmol* 1960; **63**: 747–55.

Kennedy C, Carter W. Relation of optic neuritis to multiple sclerosis in children. *Pediatrics* 1961; **28**: 377–87.

Kirkham TH, Guitton D, Katsarkis A, Kline LB, Andermann E. Oculomotor abnormalities in Friedreich's ataxia. *Canad J Neurol Sci* 1979; **6**: 167–72.

Kivlin JD, Lovrien EW, Bishop DT, Maumenee IH. Linkage analysis in dominant optic atrophy. *Am J Hum Genet* 1983; **35**: 1190–5.

Kjer P. Infantile optic atrophy with dominant mode of inheritance. *Acta Ophthalmol (Kbh)* 1959; (Suppl.) 54.

Kline LB, Margulies SL, Oh SJ. Optic neuritis and myelitis following rubella vaccination. *Arch Neurol* 1982; **39**: 443–5.

Lakhanpal V, Schocket SS, Rouben J. Desferoxiamine-induced toxic retinal pigmentary degeneration and presumed optic neuropathy. *Ophthalmology* 1984; **91**: 443–51.

Landrigan PJ, Berenberg W, Bresnan M. Behr's syndrome. *Dev Med Child Neurol* 1973; **15**: 41–7.

Lessell S, Gise RL, Krohel GB. Bilateral optic neuropathy with remission in young men. *Arch Neurol* 1983; **40**: 2–6.

Lessell S, Rosman NP. Juvenile diabetes mellitus and optic atrophy. *Arch Neurol* 1977; **34**: 759–65.

Libert J, Van Hoof F, Toussant D, Roozitalab H, Kenyon K, Green R. Ocular findings in metachromatic leucodystrophy. *Arch Ophthalmol* 1979; **97**: 1495–504.

Livingstone IR, Mastaglia FL, Edis R, Howe JW. Visual involvement in Friedreich's ataxia and hereditary spastic ataxia. A clinical and visual evoked response study. *Arch Neurol* 1981; **38**: 75–9.

Lott MT, Voljavec AS, Wallace DC. Variable genotype of Leber's hereditary optic neuropathy patients. *Am J Ophthalmol* 1990; **109**: 625–32.

Lubow M, Makley TA. Pseudopapilloedema of juvenile diabetes mellitus. *Arch Ophthalmol* 1971; **85**: 417–22.

Mackey D. Three subgroups of patients from the UK with Leber hereditary optic neuropathy. *Eye* 1994; **8**: 431–6.

Maitland CG, Miller NR. Neuroretinitis. *Arch Ophthalmol* 1984; **102**: 1146–50.

Manschot WA. Transverse ischaemic optic nerve necrosis in neuroblastoma. *Arch Ophthalmol* 1969; **89**: 707–9.

Meadows SP. Retrobulbar and optic neuritis in childhood and adolescence. *Trans Ophthalmol Soc UK* 1969; **89**: 603–38.

Miyake Y, Yagasaki K, Ichikawa H. Differential diagnosis of congenital tritanopia and dominantly inherited optic atrophy. *Arch Ophthalmol* 1985; **103**: 1496–501.

Molina JA, Mateos F, Merino M *et al.* Aicardi's syndrome in two sisters. *J Pediatr* 1989; **115**: 282–3.

Moller H. Recessively inherited, simple optic atrophy: does it exist? *Ophthal Paediatr Genet* 1992; **13**: 31–2.

Newman N, Lott M, Wallace D. The clinical characteristics of pedigrees of Leber's hereditary optic neuropathy with the 11778 mutation. *Am J Ophthalmol* 1991; **111**: 750–63.

Niemeyer C, Marquardt JL. Wolfram–Tyrer syndrome. *Invest Ophthalmol* 1972; **2**: 617–24.

Nikoskelainen E, Hoyt WF, Nummelin K, Schatz H. Fundus findings in Leber's hereditary optic neuroretinopathy. *Arch Ophthalmol* 1984; **102**: 981–9.

Nikoskelainen EK, Huoponen K, Juvonen V, Lamminen T, Nummelin K, Savontaus M-L. Ophthalmologic findings in Leber hereditary optic neuropathy with special reference to mtDNA mutations. *Ophthalmology* 1996; **103**: 504–14.

Nikoskelainen E, Savontaus M-L, Wanni O, Katila MJ, Nummelin KU. Leber's hereditary optic neuroretinopathy, a maternally inherited disease. *Arch Ophthalmol* 1987; **105**: 665–72.

Nikoskelainen E, Vilkki J, Huoponen K, Savontaus M-L. Recent advances in Leber's hereditary optic neuroretinopathy. *Eye* 1991; **5**: 291–4.

Oakley GP. The neurotoxicity of the halogenated hydroxyquinolines. *J Am Med Assoc* 1973; **225**: 395–8.

Oliff A, Bleyer WA, Poplack DG. Acute encephalopathy after initiation of cranial irradiation for meningeal leukaemia. *Lancet* 1978; **ii**: 13.

Orlando RG, Dangel ME, School SF. Clinical experience and grading of amiodarone keratopathy. *Ophthalmology* 1984; **91**: 1184–8.

Parkin PJ, Heirons R, McDonald WI. Bilateral optic neuritis. A long-term follow-up. *Brain* 1984; **107**: 951–64.

Parrish DO, Todorov AB. Transient bilateral visual reduction and mydriasis after propranolol treatment. *Ann Neurol* 1981; **10**: 583.

Pilley SJF, Thompson HS. Familial syndrome of diabetes insipidus, diabetes mellitus, optic atrophy and deafness (DIDMOAD) in childhood. *Br J Ophthalmol* 1976; **60**: 294.

Polymeropoulos M, Swift RG, Swift M. Linkage of the gene for Wolfram syndrome with markers on the short arm of chromosome 4. *Nature Genet* 1994; **8**: 95–7.

Purvin V, Chioron G. Recurrent neuroretinitis. *Arch Ophthalmol* 1994; **112**: 365–71.

Purvin V, Hrisomalos N, Dunn N. Varicella optic neuritis. *Neurology* 1988; **38**: 501.

Rizzo JF, Lessell S, Liebman S. Optic atrophy in familial dysautonomia. *Am J Ophthalmol* 1986; **102**: 463–7.

Rorsman AR, Soderstrom N. Optic atrophy and juvenile diabetes mellitus with familial occurrence. *Acta Med Scand* 1967; **182**: 419–25.

Rose FC, Fraser GR, Friedman AI. The association of juvenile diabetes mellitus and optic atrophy: clinical and genetic aspects. *Q J Med* 1966; **35**: 385–405.

Rosenberg RN, Chutorian A. Familial opticoacoustic nerve degeneration and polyneuropathy. *Neurology* 1967; **117**: 827–32.

Rosenthal AR. Ocular manifestations of leukemia: a review. *Ophthalmology* 1983; **90**: 899–905.

Rosenthal AR, Egbert PR, Wilbur JR, Probert JC. Leukemic involvement of the optic nerve. *J Pediatr Ophthalmol Strabismus* 1975; **12**: 84–93.

Salonen R, Somer M, Haltia M, Lorentz M, Norio R. Progressive encephalopathy with edema, hypsarrhythmia and optic atrophy (PEHO syndrome). *Clin Genet* 1991; **39**: 287–93.

Seelenfreund MH, Gartner S, Vinger F. The ocular pathology of Menke's disease. *Arch Ophthalmol* 1968; **80**: 718–23.

Seiff SR. High dose corticosteroids for treatment of vision loss due to indirect injury to the optic nerve. *Ophthalmic Surg* 1990; **21**: 389–95.

Seiff S. Therapy for traumatic optic neuropathy (letter). *Arch Ophthalmol* 1991; **109**: 610.

Sellost RG, Selhorst JB, Harbison EC. Parainfectious optic neuritis. *Arch Neurol* 1983; **40**: 347–50.

Sheffer R, Zlotogora J, Elpeleg O, Raz J, Ben-Ezra D. Behr's syndrome and 3-methylglutaconic aciduria. *Am J Ophthalmol* 1992; **114**: 494–7.

Shukovsky LJ, Fletcher GH. Retinal and optic nerve complications in a high dose irradiation technique of ethmoid sinus and nasal cavity. *Radiology* 1972; **104**: 629–34.

Slamovits TL, Burde RM, Klingele TG. Bilateral optic atrophy caused by chronic oral ingestion and topical application of hexachlorophene. *Am J Ophthalmol* 1980; **89**: 676–9.

Smith DP. Diagnostic criteria in dominantly inherited optic juvenile optic atrophy. *Am J Ophthalmol* 1972; **49**: 183–94.

Smith JL, Hoyt WF, Susac JO. Ocular fundus in acute Leber's optic neuropathy. *Arch Ophthalmol* 1973; **90**: 349.

Smith K, Johns D, Heher K, Miller N. Heteroplasmy in Leber's hereditary optic neuropathy. *Arch Ophthalmol* 1993; **111**: 1486–90.

Straussberg R, Amir J, Cohen H, Savir H, Vasrsano I. Epstein–Barr virus infection associated with encephalitis and optic neuritis. *J Pediatr Ophthalmol Strabismus* 1993; **30**: 262–3.

Taylor D. Ophthalmological features of some human hereditary disorders with demyelination. *Bull Soc Belge Ophthalmol* 1983; **208**: 405–13.

Taylor D, Cuendet F. Optic neuritis in childhood. In: Hess RF, Plant GT, eds. *Optic Neuritis*. Cambridge: Cambridge University Press,

1986: 73–85.

Taylor D, Ramsay J, Day S, Dillon M. Infarction of the optic nerve head in children with accelerated hypertension. *Br J Ophthalmol* 1981; **65**: 152–60.

Tyrer J. A case of infantilism with goitre, diabetes mellitus, mental defect, and primary optic atrophy. *Med J Aust* 1943; **2**: 398–401.

Uemura A, Osame M, Nakagawa M, Nakahara K, Sameshima M, Obba N. Leber's hereditary optic neuropathy: mitochondrial and biochemical studies on muscle biopsies. *Br J Ophthalmol* 1987; **71**: 531–6.

Ulrich GG, Waecker NJ, Meister SJ, Peterson TJ, Hooper DG. Cat-scratch disease associated with neuroretinitis in a 6-year-old girl. *Ophthalmology* 1992; **99**: 246–9.

Wallace DC, Singh OG, Lott MT *et al*. Mitochondrial DNA mutation associated with Leber's hereditary optic atrophy (abstract). *Am J Hum Genet* 1988; **43**: Abstract 0392.

Weiner LP, Konigsmark BW, Stoll J, Magladery JW. Hereditary olivo-pontocerebellar atrophy with retinal degeneration. *Arch Neurol* 1967; **16**: 364–76.

Weleber R, Miyake Y. Familial optic atrophy with negative electroretinograms. *Arch Ophthalmol* 1992; **110**: 640–5.

Wilson J, Linnell JC, Matthews DM. Plasma cobalamins in neuro-ophthalmological diseases. *Lancet* 1971; **i**: 259–61.

Wolfram DJ. Diabetes mellitus and simple optic atrophy among siblings. Report of four cases. *Mayo Clin Proc* 1938; **13**: 715–18.

Wray SH, Cogan DG, Kuwabara T, Schaumberg HH, Powers JM. Adrenoleukodystrophy with disease of the eye and optic nerve atrophy. *Am J Ophthalmol* 1976a; **82**: 480–5.

Wray SH, Kuwabara T, Sanderson P. Menke's kinky hair disease: a light and electron microscopic study of the eye. *Invest Ophthalmol Vis Sci* 1976b; **15**: 128–38.

Zee DS, Yee RD, Cogan DG, Robinson DA, Engel WK. Oculomotor abnormalities in hereditary cerebellar ataxia. *Brain* 1976; **99**: 207–34.

52: Chiasmal Defects

David Taylor

Anatomy

The optic nerves and chiasm and the optic tracts extend posteriorly and upwards from the optic canals at an angle of about 45%. The anatomical relationships are not significantly different from those in the adult (Hoyt 1970). The chiasm lies in the suprasellar cistern, above the diaphragma sellae from which it is separated by several millimetres, especially posteriorly, by its oblique course. The anterior cerebral arteries and the anterior communicating arteries lie anteriorly and above the chiasm and optic nerves. The carotid arteries lie laterally with the posterior communicating artery passing underneath the optic tracts. The chiasm lies in the floor of the anterior end of the third ventricle which is above it (expansion of the third ventricle in hydrocephalus is a potent cause of visual damage from chiasmal compression). Posteriorly lies the hypothalamus and the pituitary stalk, the tuber cinerum and the mamillary bodies. The optic nerves emerge from the optic canals where they are fixed; the length of the intracranial portion of the optic nerve varies so that the position of the chiasm in relation to the tuberculum sellae and other structures is different; when the optic nerves are short the chiasm is said to be prefixed, when long it is said to be postfixed.

Development

In humans, the chiasm appears within the first month of life (Barber *et al.* 1954). The precursor of the chiasm appears as a thickening of the floor of the forebrain lying between the optic stalks at the junction of the telencephalon and the diencephalon. Retinal ganglion cells grow down the optic stalks and enter the floor of the third ventricle where they decussate to form the optic chiasm. The highly specific pattern of axon crossing is fundamental to visual processing; its formation occurs in two phases (Sretavan & Reichardt 1993). As the first retinal axons meet in the midline at the ventral diencephalon they form an X-shaped chiasm; subsequent axons grow into either the ipsilateral or contralateral optic tract. Each axon is tipped by a morphological specialization called a growth cone which allows the axon to sense and respond to signals in the embryonic brain environment (Sretavan *et al.* 1995).

At first there is a substantial overproduction of neurones which later die back, a process known as apoptosis (Provis *et al.* 1985). The lumen of the optic stalk is initially open and in communication with the forebrain cavity. It closes by the end of the second month of gestation, when it elongates and the fetal fissure is formed. Closure of the fetal fissure in the optic stalk begins distally and proceeds towards the brain. After closure, the nerve fibres fill the whole nerve. The chiasm reaches its definitive form by the fourth month of gestation.

Signs and symptoms

In all children, but especially in small infants, chiasmal disease often presents late because, particularly if the process is chronic, the child compensates well and is not suspected of having poor vision until there is a substantial and bilateral visual defect. It is often only when the last remaining vision of the second eye to be affected finally snuffs out that the small child will be noticed to have poor vision by the parents.

The hallmark of chiasmal disease is the bitemporal hemianopia. In young children, formal visual field testing is not possible but it is still vital to carry out visual field testing even by such apparently crude techniques as the ability to count fingers on either side, or the observation of a child and his response to fingers wiggling, or toys being shown to him in both sides of the visual field of one eye, since these may detect the characteristic bitemporal hemianopia (see Chapter 8). Lesions from below, usually from the pituitary gland, the surrounding bone or sometimes from the pituitary stalk, for instance craniopharyngiomas, have to grow large before signs of chiasmal compression appear. Inferior lesions compress the lower nasal fibres first and give an upper bitemporal field defect. Similarly lesions from above tend to cause initially an inferior defect. By the time a compressive lesion has caused defects there is usually gross thinning of the chiasm and the pattern of appearance of the field defects is not usually clear-cut.

In a child in whom acuity can be measured, there is often an acuity defect. Chiasm splitting lesions, such as trauma, do not affect acuity greatly because the nasal field and the nasal half of the fovea is not affected, but most frequently there is also involvement of the optic nerve or widespread involvement of both crossing and non-crossing fibres in the chiasm, and it is this that gives rise to the acuity defect. Most frequently one eye has a very severe acuity defect and the other is relatively spared, except for a field defect. In very chronic lesions, there is often a most impressive preservation of a high level of acuity in the face of fundoscopic evidence of a profound loss of neurones.

With widespread abnormalities or optic nerve involvement there is a significant colour vision defect. This is best tested for by pseudo-isochromatic plates though in the small child it is often difficult and only gross colour vision defects are detectable.

Stereopsis tends to remain intact in children with pure defects of the decussating fibres (Fisher 1986).

Children with chiasmal disease may present with nystagmus, especially if the onset is early in their life. The classic form of nystagmus is known as see-saw nystagmus. Most patients, however, have a less clear-cut abnormality with a compound nystagmus with vertical, horizontal and rotary components (see Chapter 63). The presence of this sort of nystagmus in a child demands appropriate investigations.

Optic atrophy frequently occurs when there is substantial loss of neurones in the chiasm. Although often there is a generalized loss of neurones, sometimes there may be a characteristic pattern due to the loss of the fibres subserving the defunct temporal fields and the relative preservation of those fibres which subserve the intact nasal field

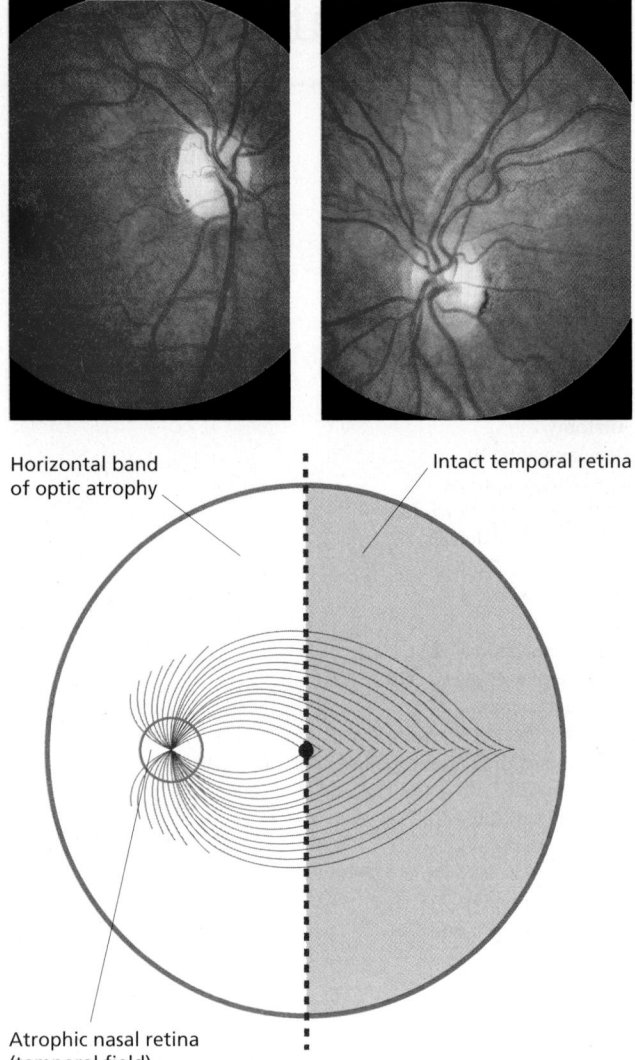

(b)

Fig. 52.1 (a) Craniopharyngioma. The right eye has bare perception of hand movements but the left has an absolute temporal hemianopia, normal colour vision and 6/5 acuity. The left optic disc shows band atrophy—there is all-round loss of the nerve fibres that subserve the defunct temporal visual field but preservation of those that subserve the intact nasal field which are inserted into the upper and lower segments of the disc. (b) The origin of the band of atrophy is due to the fact that the horizontal band or bow-tie area is the visible area of atrophy where temporal field fibres alone are inserted into the disc.

(Fig. 52.1). These, because of the temporal retinal location of their ganglion cells, have to arch over the macula and are inserted into the upper and lower quadrants of the optic disc. In cases of developmental chiasmal defects and tumours there are often optic disc defects (Figs 52.2, 52.3), for instance hypoplasia or coloboma, and the presence of one of these defects should alert the practitioner to the

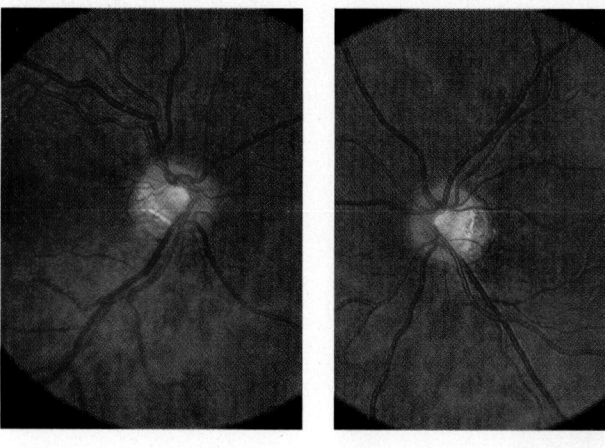

Fig. 52.2 Craniopharyngioma. Bilateral segmental hypoplasia or 'tilted' optic disc. Bitemporal hemianopia with 6/5 acuity right eye (–4.0) and 6/4 left eye (–4.50).

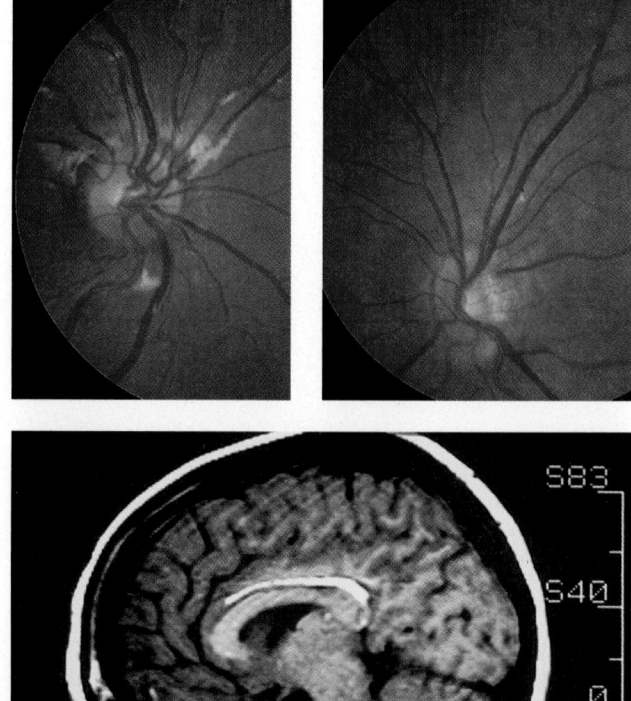

Fig. 52.3 (a) Dysplastic tilted left optic disc in a patient with a midline facial defect. (b) MRI of corpus callosum lipoma in a patient with a midline facial defect.

possibility of a chiasmal defect (Taylor 1982; Zeki *et al.* 1992).

Because of the proximity of the hypothalamus and pituitary gland, endocrine and growth defects may occur.

Some children with hypothalamus-involving tumours have a combination of emaciation with loss of subcutaneous fat (Fig. 52.4), accelerated growth in length relative to weight and personality changes with euphoria and hyperactivity: this is the diencephalic or Russell–Silver syndrome. It is important therefore that the paediatric ophthalmologist should have available facilities for measuring (Fig. 52.5) and weighing a child and entering his weight and height on an appropriate chart. Other symptoms include abnormal temperature regulations and diabetes insipidus.

In older children there may be odd complaints of visual sensory defects that often sound rather non-organic. These may be due to the bitemporal hemianopia especially if it is absolute with intact acuity. The child may complain of things disappearing because there is a segment of blindness caused by the overlapping temporal fields further away than the point of regard in which objects are not seen. Similarly, the intact nasal fields abut one another and because there are no corresponding retinal points there is little to keep the two together so they may complain of things sliding in their vision (Nachtigaller & Hoyt 1970).

Further investigations

Clinical suspicion of an underlying chiasmal pathology, and the subsequent clinical evaluation are the vital starting points in the investigation; the further investigations consist of endocrine studies, neurophysiological evaluation (see Chapter 9) and neuroimaging. Neurophysiological studies are totally risk-free and inexpensive; their main role is in detection of a crossover defect in a child (particularly a preverbal child) with a non-specific defect and in the quantitative and qualitative assessment of the visual defect, including serial studies to detect progression.

Neuroimaging, particularly magnetic resonance imaging (MRI) (Hupp & Kline 1991; Tang *et al.* 1994), gives anatomical evaluation but cannot assess function. MRI is the method of choice but, particularly for evaluation of bone changes and calcification, computed tomography (CT) may also be useful.

Developmental defects

Unilateral anophthalmos or optic nerve aplasia produces an asymmetrical chiasm (Margo *et al.* 1992) and bilateral anophthalmos is usually associated with absence of optic nerves, chiasm and lateral geniculate bodies (Recordon & Griffiths 1936; Haberland & Perou 1969; Penner & Schlelch 1976). Sometimes there are remnants of the optic nerve and chiasm (Calgianut & Theiler 1976). Bilateral optic nerve aplasia is also associated with an absent chiasm.

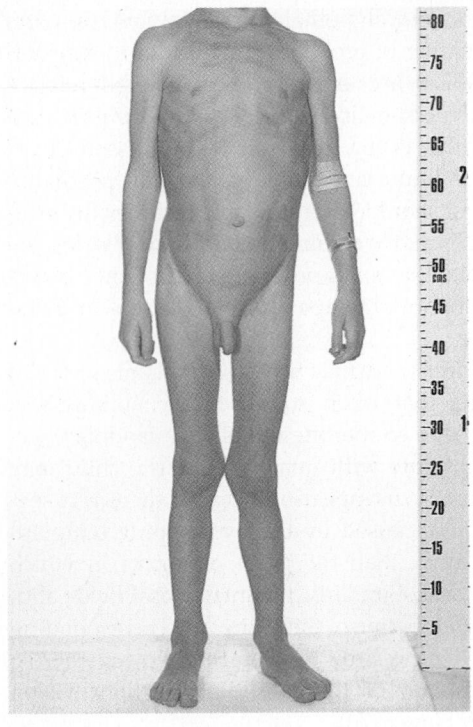
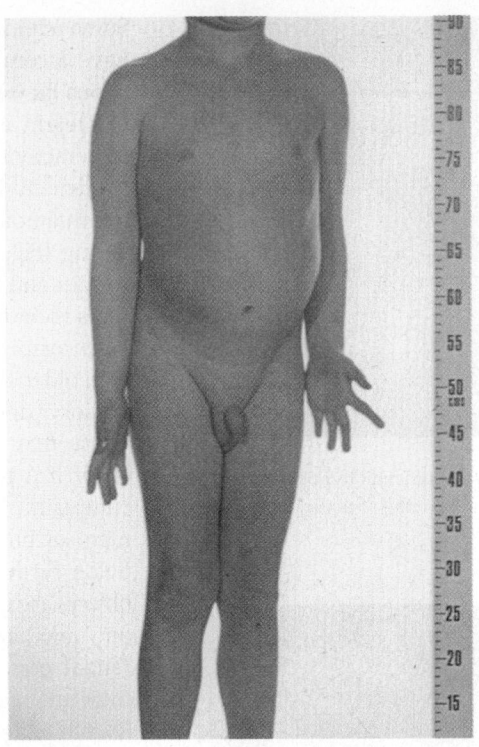

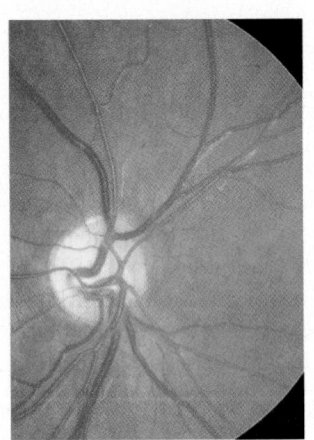
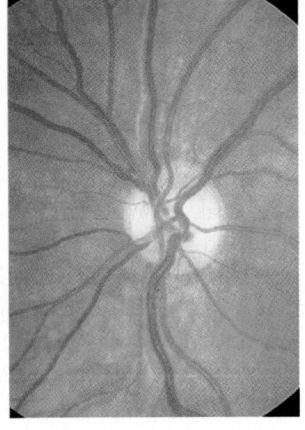

Fig. 52.4 (a) Chiasmal glioma. This boy presented with poor vision and recent weight loss. Photograph on 12 February 1973. (b) Photograph on 31 January 1974 showing rapid growth in weight and height. Weight and growth rate fluctuation are common in chiasmal glioma. (c) Bilateral band atrophy. (Same patient a–c).

Achiasmia

Associated with widespread brain developmental defects, a congenital absence of the chiasm occasionally occurs. The chiasmal lesion is demonstrated by visual evoked potentials (VEPs) (Apkarian *et al.* 1994) or by MRI (Fig. 52.6) (El Gammal *et al.* 1990).

A chiasmal spur is an anomaly found incidentally at postmortem (Ellis *et al.* 1900). The significance of this anomaly, which consists of a spur projecting anteriorly between the two optic nerves, is not known but the above authors speculated that it may represent the fibres that would have made up the anterior knee of von Willebrand.

Chiasmal anomalies as evidenced by clinical findings or by abnormalities on neuroimaging have been described in patients with midline defects, for instance septo-optic dysplasia, or midfacial defects, or basal encephalocoeles. The chiasm may be abnormal in the various midline facial (Fig. 52.7) and skull clefting syndromes that are associated with hypertelorism which may also have midline brain anomalies.

A condition of isolated maldevelopment of the anterior visual pathways occurs as the association of an anomalous optic disc with evidence of a chiasmal defect, for instance a bitemporal hemianopia, in otherwise normal people (Taylor 1983).

Trauma

Occasionally, following closed head trauma, the child develops a bitemporal hemianopia often absolute, i.e. with an intact nasal field and a sharply defined border

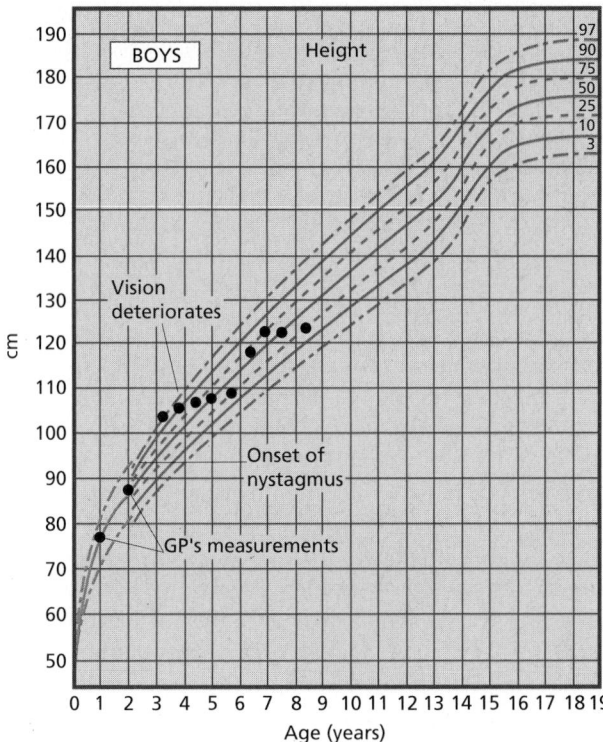

Fig. 52.5 Height growth record of a child with chiasmal glioma showing height growth rate fluctuation. Paediatric ophthalmology clinics need to have these charts available.

(Heinz *et al.* 1994). It is associated with other vision defects such as poor acuity and colour vision if there is also damage to the non-crossing fibres or optic nerve. Other defects result from damage to surrounding structures which may lead to diabetes insipidus, anosmia, cerebrospinal fluid rhinorrhoea, growth defects and mood changes.

Tumours

Chiasmal glioma

Chiasmal glioma, optic nerve glioma and hypothalamic glioma are closely related tumours, often one indistinguishable from the other and showing common histopathological features and clinical behaviour. All occur with increased frequency in neurofibromatosis and up to one-half of patients with chiasmal or optic glioma have this disease (Imes & Hoyt 1986). It may occur in association with the Beckwith–Wiedemann syndrome of macrosomia, macroglossia, encephalocoele, hemihypertrophy, hepatomegaly and advanced bone age (Weinstein *et al.* 1986).

Children with chiasmal glioma present in a variety of ways. Small children often present with a compound nystagmus and typically this is see-saw in nature (see Chapter 63). But any child with a compound nystagmus with

rotary, vertical and horizontal elements should be suspected of having a chiasmal lesion (Schulman *et al.* 1979). Visual loss is often profound before its presence is noticed by parents of young children but in older children the visual defect may be noticed by the child himself or detected by preschool or school visual testing. Some optic gliomas may be large but without gross visual defect (Goodman *et al.* 1975). Chiasmal glioma may reveal itself by its effects on growth and development. An unusual presentation is that of head bobble — the bobble-headed doll syndrome (see Chapter 63)—this is usually an indication that the child also has hydrocephalus.

The diagnosis can be made easier by visual field testing or by visual field analysis on visual evoked cortical potential testing. Plain X-rays are seldom used now but the classical finding is an expanded and pear-shaped sella turcica, with chronic bone changes and without calcification. Often one or both optic foramina are enlarged, especially if there is an optic nerve component to the tumour. CT scanning (Fletcher *et al.* 1986) shows three diagnostic patterns (Fig. 52.8).

1 A tube-like thickening of optic nerve and chiasm.

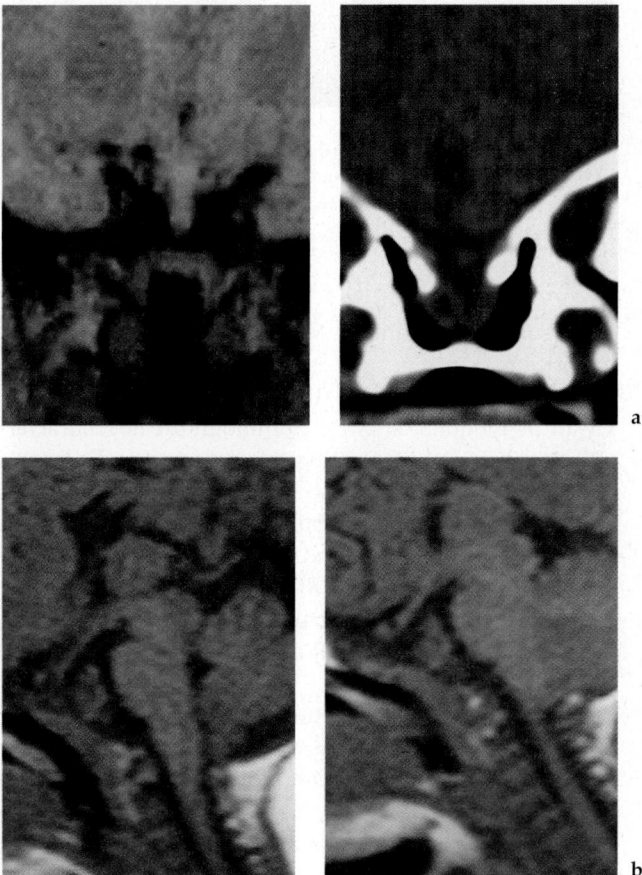

Fig. 52.6 Achiasmia showing an encephalocoele through the cribriform plate (a) and separate optic nerves (b). The cuts are taken either side of the midline and two separate optic nerves can be seen.

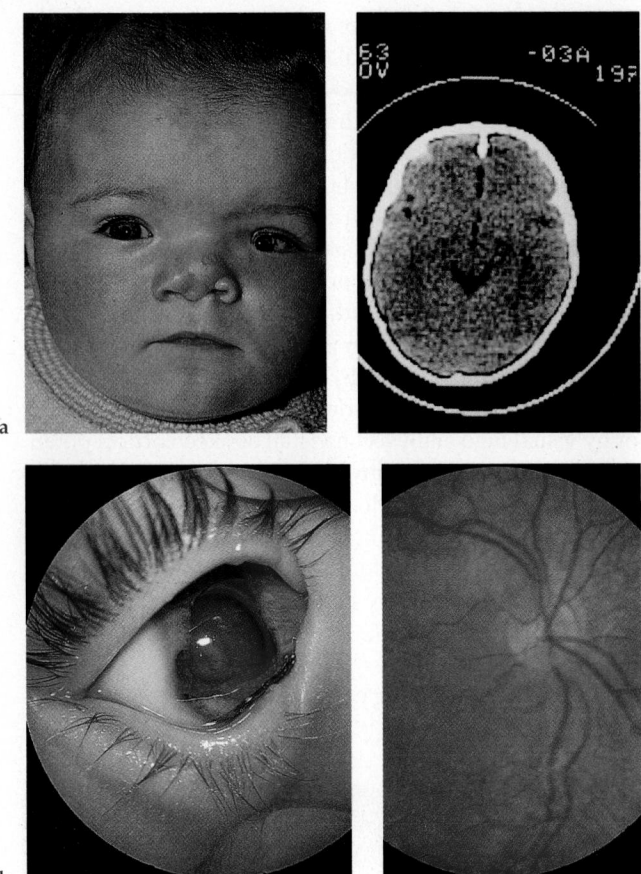

a

b

Fig. 52.7 (a) Minor midline facial defect with small intracranial lipoma. (b) Left eye has a marginally small optic disc. The right eye has iris coloboma, cataract and optic nerve hypoplasia. (Same patient).

2 A suprasellar tumour with contiguous optic nerve expansion.

3 A suprasellar tumour with optic tract involvement.

Cystic or 'globular' suprasellar tumours are not characteristic and may require histological confirmation. Fletcher's group demonstrated growth by CT scanning in three out of 22 cases and all were globular types. MRI scanning better delineates the extent and nature of the tumour (Holman *et al.* 1985). CT and MRI scanning will both show whether there is hydrocephalus. Tumours may evolve in areas thought to be normal on initial CT and even MRI scans (Listernick *et al.* 1992).

The histopathological nature of optic gliomas has long been the subject of a discussion that is important because of its relevance to treatment. Optic gliomas are benign tumours that are generally thought of as being hamartomas (Hoyt & Baghdassarian 1969).

They undergo enlargement by an accumulation of mucosubstance, by local invasion, by induction of hyperplasia in adjacent glial cells, or by growth of cell 'rests' already present in adjacent optic nerve or chiasm (Ander-

son & Spencer 1970). Malignant gliomas do occur but are very rare and mainly in adults. Meningeal spread in children, however, is not unknown (Civitello *et al.* 1988; Bruggers *et al.* 1991) and spread through a ventriculoperitoneal shunt has been recorded (Trigg *et al.* 1983).

Hoyt and Baghdassarian (1969) reviewed the clinical course of 36 optic gliomas, 29 of which were chiasmal. Some of these patients were reviewed in 1971 (Glaser *et al.* 1971) and in 1986 (Imes & Hoyt 1986). The 1971 follow-up showed a very stable course but the later follow-up by Imes and Hoyt showed that 57% of the 29 patients with chiasmal gliomas were dead, although only 18% from the direct effects of the glioma. The patients were more at risk from other tumours, thus reflecting the high proportion of patients who had neurofibromatosis. Imes and Hoyt's 12 survivors had not had radiation therapy whereas 11 of 16 patients who died had.

The biological behaviour of optic gliomas determines the way in which they should be managed. Spontaneous visual improvement may take place even in the absence of MRI changes (Liu & Lessell 1992). Many authors have reported at least reasonable long-term prognosis that does not seem to be improved by treatment (Borit & Richardson 1982; Rush *et al.* 1982; Imes & Hoyt 1986) and although radiotherapy may decrease the size of the tumour (Fletcher *et al.* 1986) and some say improve the vision of treated patients (Roberson & Till 1974; Brand & Hoover 1979; MacCarty *et al.* 1970; Flickenger *et al.* 1988; Kovalic *et al.* 1990) its use should be advocated only with caution because of the serious side-effects at therapeutic doses (Weiss *et al.* 1987; Pierce *et al.* 1990; Jenkin *et al.* 1993). The author's personal policy is to recommend radiotherapy only when there has been a rapid and recent increase in size of the tumour with recent visual loss. Chemotherapy (Civitello *et al.* 1988; Packer *et al.* 1988; Petronio *et al.* 1991) is as yet of uncertain benefit but with newer agents the outlook is promising and may allow deferment of damaging radiotherapy in the particularly susceptible younger child (Petronio *et al.* 1991).

Surgery is not indicated except to treat hydrocephalus in exophytic tumours (Housepian & Chi 1993) or if there is a cystic tumour with serious doubts about the possibility of alternative pathology when biopsy and cyst aspiration may be indicated.

Follow-up after diagnosis usually involves periodic review of the visual fields, acuity, colour vision and optic discs, neurophysiological studies where available and CT or MRI scanning, the frequency needed being judged on the apparent clinical course of the disease.

Craniopharyngioma

These cystic tumours grow slowly and do not usually present until the child is 3 or 4 years old or later but they may present even in old age. Because of its origin from the pitu-

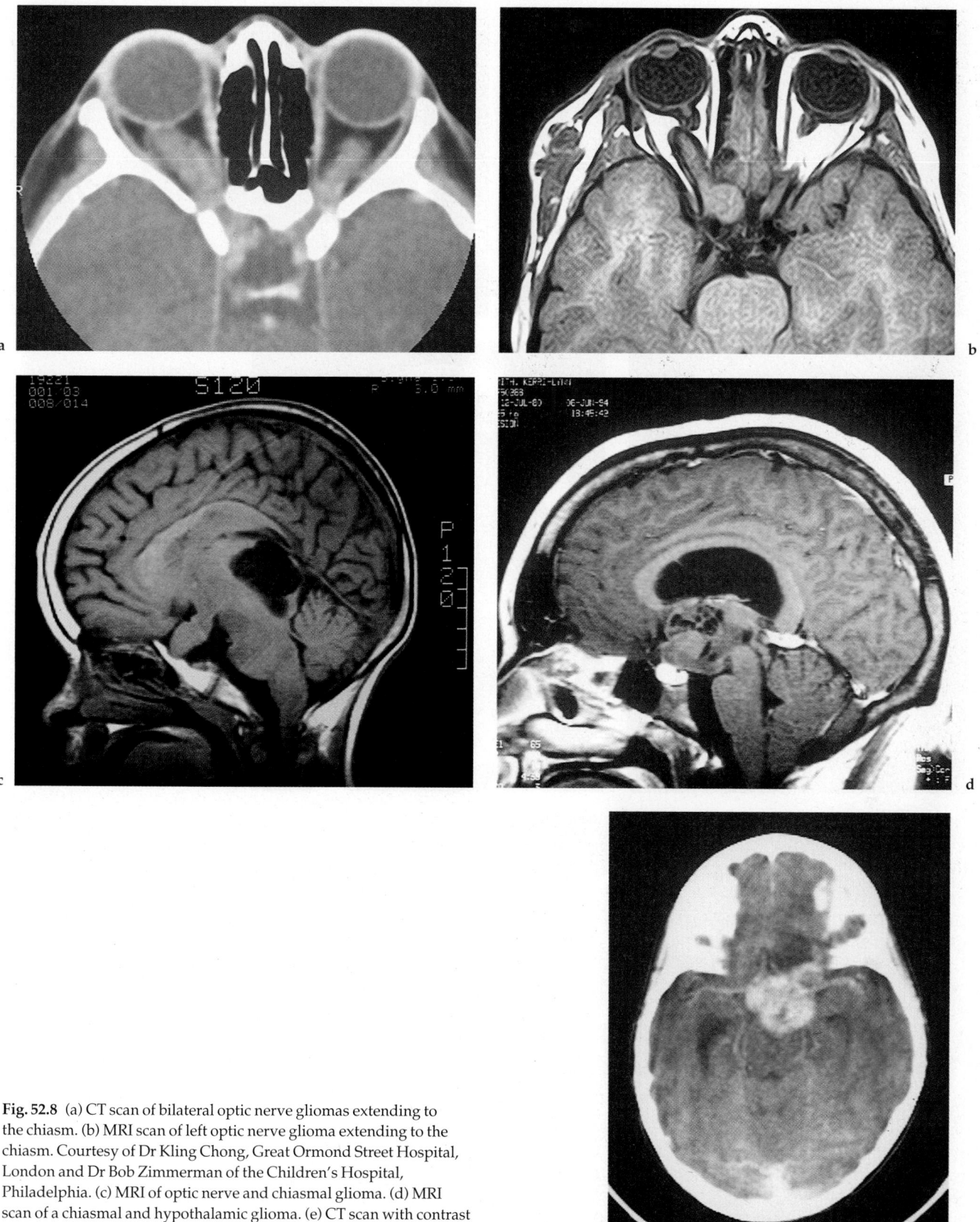

Fig. 52.8 (a) CT scan of bilateral optic nerve gliomas extending to the chiasm. (b) MRI scan of left optic nerve glioma extending to the chiasm. Courtesy of Dr Kling Chong, Great Ormond Street Hospital, London and Dr Bob Zimmerman of the Children's Hospital, Philadelphia. (c) MRI of optic nerve and chiasmal glioma. (d) MRI scan of a chiasmal and hypothalamic glioma. (e) CT scan with contrast of a cystic chiasmal glioma.

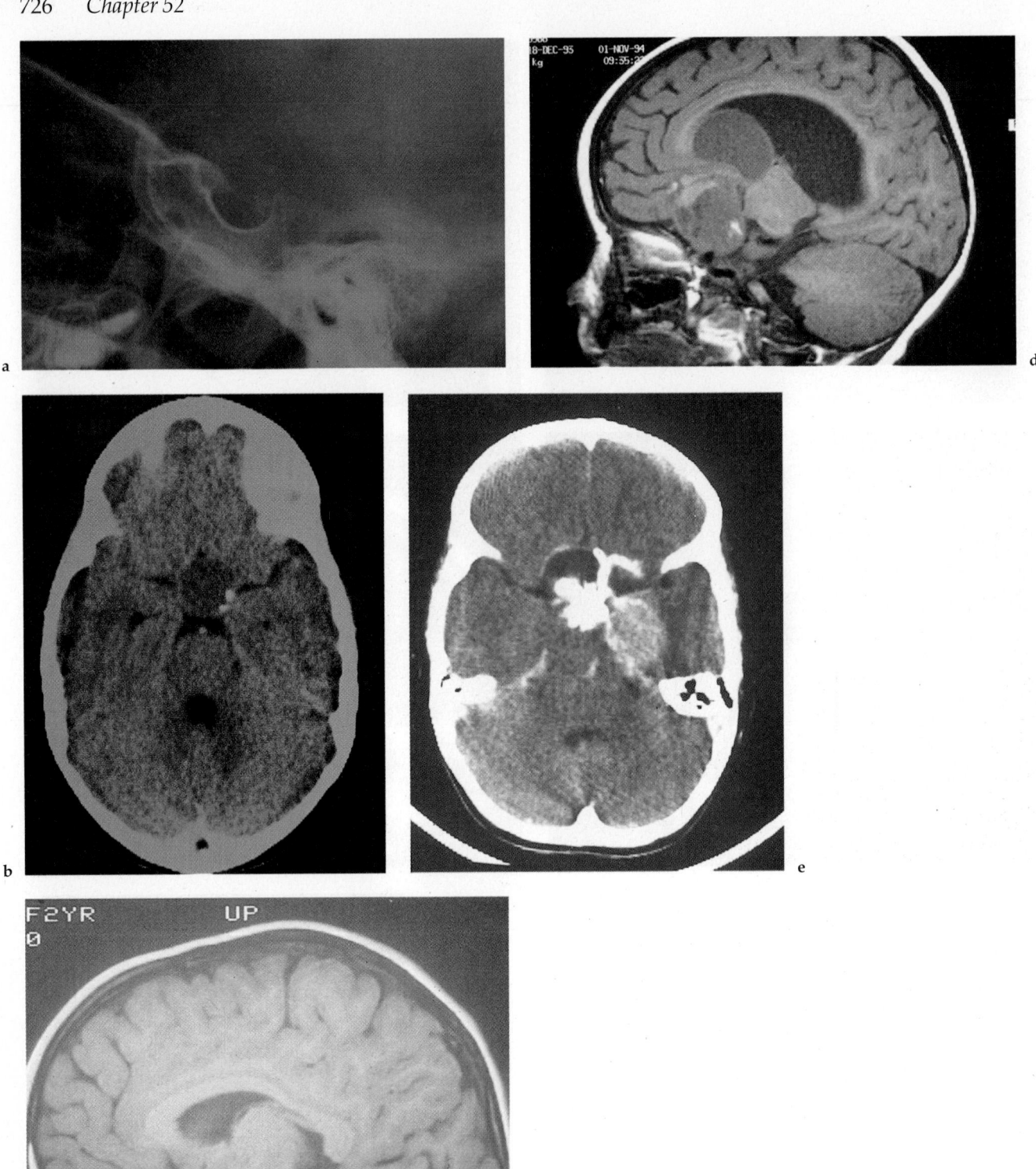

Fig. 52.9 (a) Expanded pituitary fossa shown on plain X-ray with some calcification due to a craniopharyngioma. (b) CT scan of a small cystic craniopharyngioma with calcification in its wall. (c) MRI of small craniopharyngioma. (d) MRI scan of a large cystic craniopharyngioma with calcification in its wall. There is hydrocephalus. (e) CT scan of a heavily calcified craniopharyngioma which extends out into the middle cranial fossa.

itary stalk the tumour tends to compress the chiasm in any direction but classically from behind and above. Hypothalamic disturbances are frequent and the loss of vision may be profound. Young children tend to develop symptoms of hypothalamic disturbance or hydrocephalus, whilst older children (first decade) are more likely to present with visual disturbance, squint or nystagmus (Figs 52.9 and 52.11). The diagnosis is made by CT or MRI scanning (Fig. 52.9). Calcification occurs in virtually every case in childhood and the tumours are often cystic. Pre- and postoperative endocrine assessment and management is essential. The tumours are usually treated by surgery with or without radiotherapy; total removal is sometimes possible.

Dysgerminoma

The clinical clue to the presence of a dysgerminoma is

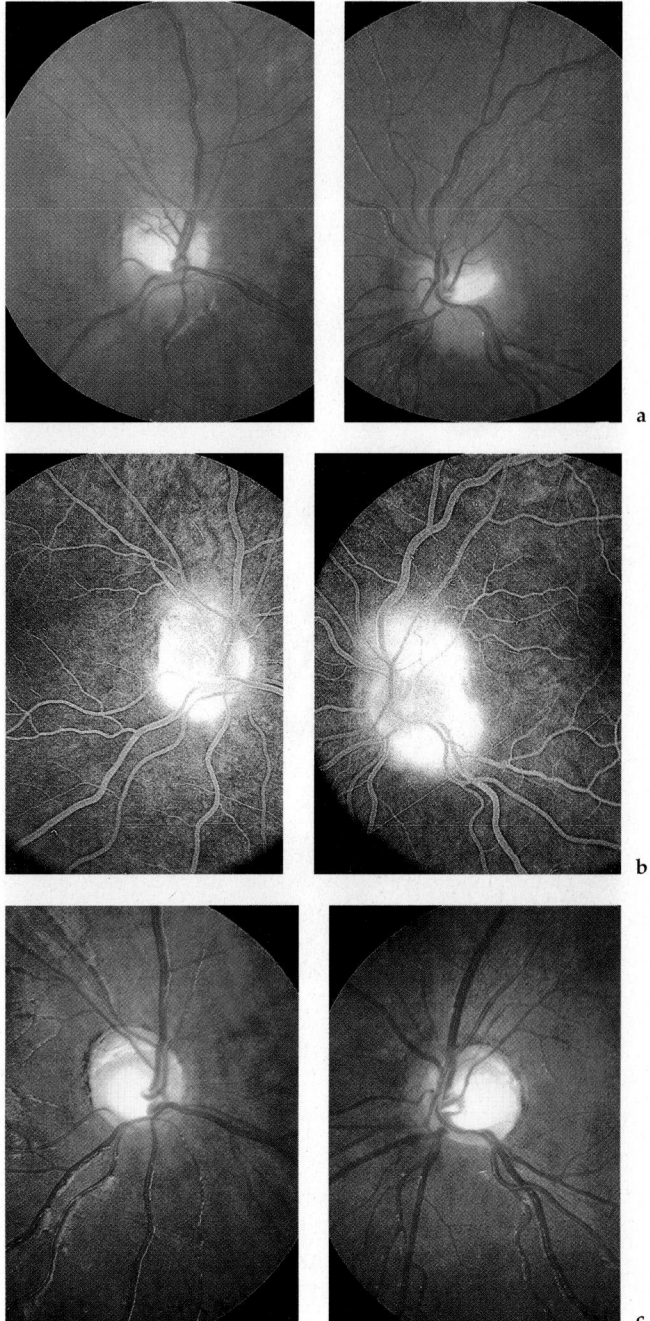

Fig. 52.11 (a, b) Craniopharyngioma showing bilobed papilloedema during a period of raised intracranial pressure. (c) Same patient 1 year later showing atrophic dysplastic discs.

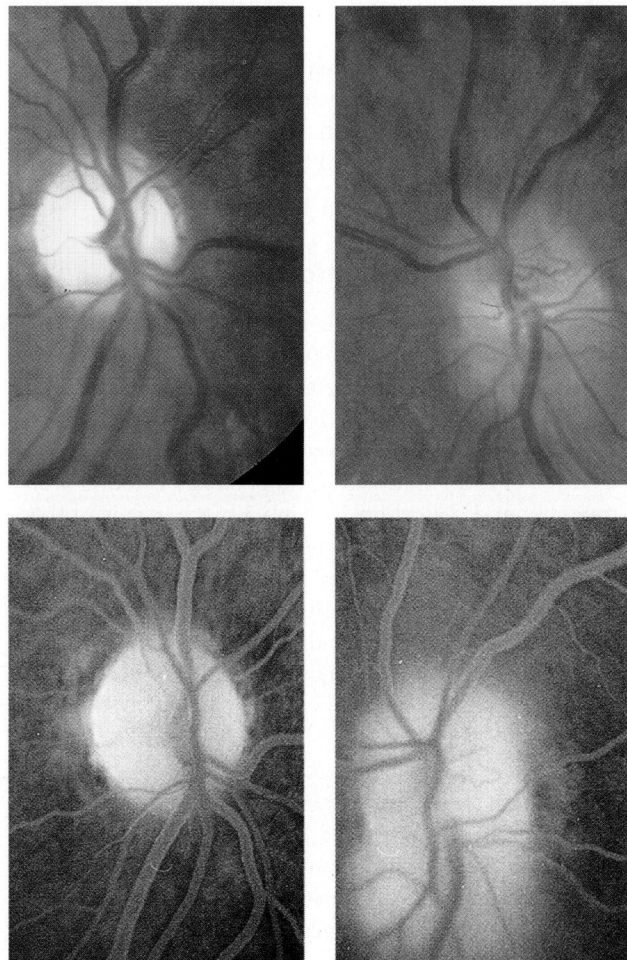

Fig. 52.10 Chiasmal glioma causing hydrocephalus and hypothalamic disturbances. Blind right eye showing minimal papilloedema. The left eye shows papilloedema at the upper and lower poles where intact nerve fibres exist (see Fig. 52.1b). This is known as bilobed or 'twin peaks' papilloedema.

when diabetes insipidus is a symptom at presentation together with chiasmal defects, including acuity and visual field loss and hypothalamic or pituitary disturbances (Jennings *et al.* 1985; Bowman & Farris 1990). The tumours are often not large (Fig. 52.12) (Takeuchi *et al.* 1978) and occur in older children or young adults (Carmins & Mount 1977).

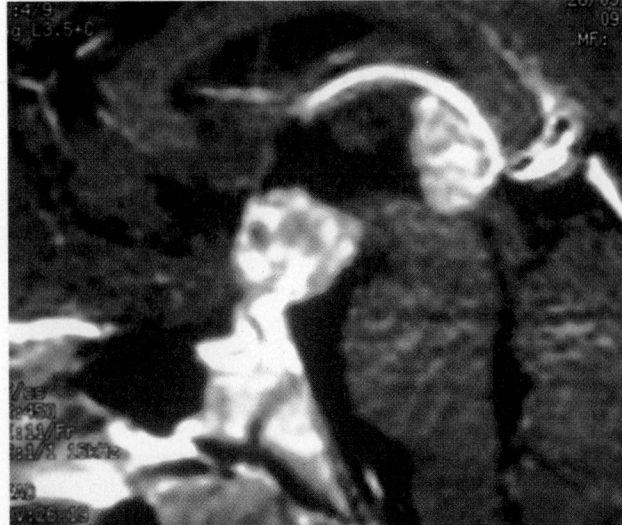

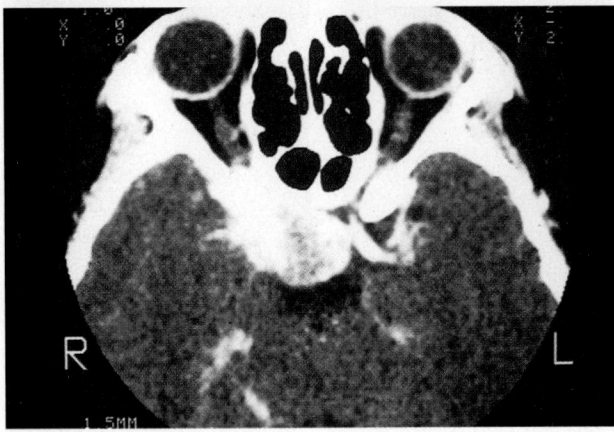

Fig. 52.12 Dysgerminoma. These tumours are often small and associated with diabetes insipidus in children.

Other chiasmal tumours

These include metastatic neuroblastoma, arachnoid cysts, choristomas (Kazim *et al.* 1992) such as ependymomas, epidermoid tumours, leukaemic deposits, ectopic pinealomas, teratomas and pituitary gland tumours. These are all rare and do not usually have specific presenting features (Till 1975), but their radiological and associated clinical features together may be suggestive of the underlying pathology.

Granulomas and chronic inflammatory disorders

The chiasm and surrounding structures may be involved in abnormalities of the skull base as in histiocytosis-X (see Chapter 33), in particular the Hand–Schuller–Christian variant of this condition, which tends to present with diabetes insipidus and visual defects. Sarcoidosis, juvenile xanthogranulomas and pseudotumours similar to those found in adults with the Tolosa–Hunt syndrome may also affect the chiasmal area.

Infections

Tuberculous meningitis, hydatid disease and cysticercosis together with fungal disorders (especially in debilitated, immunodeficient children, or those affected by AIDS) may all affect the suprasellar cistern with damage to the chiasm and surrounding structures.

Sphenoid sinus disease

In children whose sinuses have developed, a chiasmal syndrome or even rapid blindness may result from the formation and expansion of a mucocoele (Goodwin & Glaser 1978), even in the absence of symptomatic sinus disease (Casteels *et al.* 1992).

Chiasmal neuritis

Chiasmal neuritis is rare, may or may not be associated with demyelinating disease and presents with a chiasmal syndrome (Fig. 52.13a) with visual loss and bitemporal hemianopia. It is diagnosed by MRI scanning (Newman *et al.* 1991).

Third ventricle distention

In hydrocephalic patients, distention of the third ventricle may cause chiasmal damage and bitemporal or more widespread visual field defects (Sinclair & Doff 1931), with sometimes profound vision loss due to stretching or compression of the optic nerves and chiasm, to which may be added cortical blindness from posterior cerebral artery stretching and distortion. The exact mechanisms of these defects are not certain but their occurrence due to a distended ventricle is not significantly in doubt. A unilateral visual defect has been described due to compression of one optic nerve against the internal carotid artery (Calogero & Alexander 1971).

Vascular anomalies

Aneurysm is an extremely rare cause of chiasmal defects in children (Roche *et al.* 1988; Meyer *et al.* 1989) and does not produce specific symptoms or signs. In children symptomatic intracranial aneurysms are sometimes large and may be associated with polycystic kidneys, coarctation of the aorta, and Marfan's and Ehlers–Danlos syndromes.

Multiple aneurysms (usually small) may also occur in 'mycotic' aneurysms with subacute bacterial endocarditis and Moya-moya disease (Schoenberg *et al.* 1985; Waga & Tochio 1985; Noda *et al.* 1987): these mostly affect cerebral hemispheres.

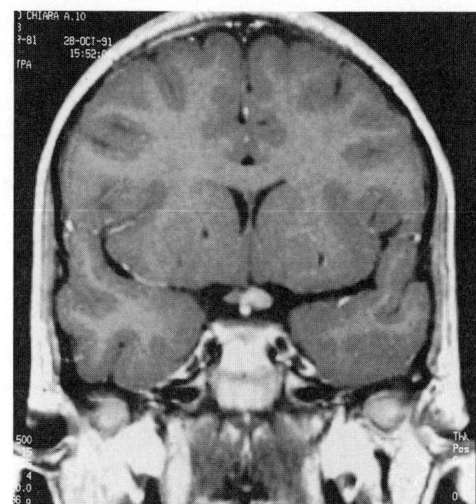

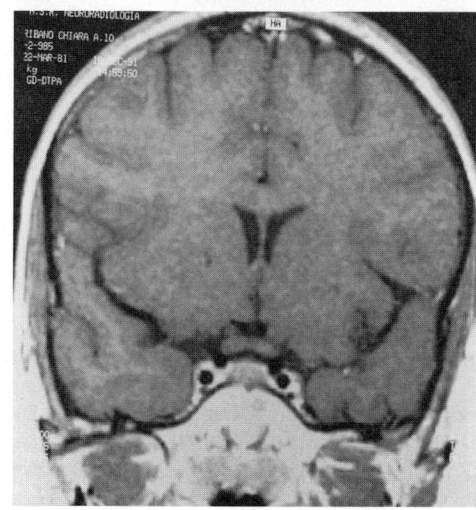

Fig. 52.13 (a) Chiasmal neuritis. MRI scan showing an expanded chiasm with high signal. (b) Same patient 2 months later showing resolution (Dr Paolo Nucci's patient).

Arteriovenous malformation may sometimes be symptomatic (Gibo *et al.* 1989; Steinberg *et al.* 1990).

Angiomas of the optic chiasm are also rare and produce symptoms by recurrent haemorrhages (Fermaglich *et al.* 1978; Hasler *et al.* 1989). Spontaneous haematomas of the optic chiasm have also been described (Riishede & Seedorff 1974). Perhaps the so-called spontaneous haematoma is related to a pre-existing angiomatous defect.

Empty sella syndrome

When the diaphragma sellae is defective and cerebrospinal fluid is found in the pituitary fossa on a CT scan, this is known as the empty sella syndrome. This may occur for no apparent reason or be associated with surgery, radiotherapy or the presence of an arachnoid cyst. Chiasmal visual field defects occasionally occur and rarely the visual defect may be substantial. Many cases follow hydrocephalus or benign intracranial hypertension (Jaffer *et al.* 1979).

References

Anderson DR, Spencer W. Ultrastructural and histochemical observations of optic nerve gliomas. *Arch Ophthalmol* 1970; **83** 324–38.

Apkarian P, Bour L, Barth PG. A unique achiasmatic anomaly detected in non-albinos with misrouted retinal-fugal projections. *Eur J Neurosci* 1994; **6**: 501–7.

Barber AN, Ronstrom GN, Muelling RH. Development of the visual pathway; optic chiasm. *AMA Arch Ophthalmol* 1954; **52**: 447–56.

Borit A, Richardson EP. The biological and clinical behaviour of pilocytic astrocytomas of the optic pathways. *Brain* 1982; **105**: 161–88.

Bowman CB, Farris BK. Primary chiasmal germinoma: a case report and review of the literature. *J Clin Neuroophthalmol* 1990; **10**: 9–17.

Brand WN, Hoover SV. Optic glioma in children review of 16 cases given megavoltage radiation therapy. *Child Brain* 1979; **5**: 459–66.

Bruggers C, Friedman H, Phillips P *et al.* Leptomeningeal dissemination of optic pathway gliomas in three children. *Am J Ophthalmol* 1991; **111**: 719–24.

Calgianut B, Theiler K. Zur aplaise der sehnerven. *Graefe's Arch Klin Exp Ophthalmol* 1976; **200**: 93–8.

Calogero JA, Alexander E. Unilateral amaurosis in a hydrocephalic child with an obstructed shunt. *J Neurosurg* 1971; **34**: 236–8.

Carmins AB, Mount LA. Primary suprasellar atypical teratoma. *Brain* 1974; **97**: 447–62.

Casteels I, de Loof E, Brock P *et al.* Sudden blindness in a child: presenting symptoms of a sphenoid sinus mucocoele. *Br J Ophthalmol* 1992; **76**: 502–4.

Civitello LA, Packer RJ, Rorke LB, Siegel PA, Sutton LN, Schut L. Leptomeningeal dissemination of low grade gliomas in childhood. *Neurology* 1988; **38**: 562–70.

El Gammal T, Brooks B, Harbour R, Kline L, Jacobi P. MR of uncommon congenital and vascular lesions of the intracranial visual pathways. *Neuroradiology* 1990; **32**: 488–91.

Ellis HA, Parish DJ, Hughes B. The chiasmal spur: an anomaly of the human optic chiasm. *J Pathol Bact* 1900; **81**: 529–32.

Fermaglich J, Kattah J, Manz H. Venous angioma of the optic chiasm. *Ann Neurol* 1978; **4**: 470–1.

Fisher N. The optic chiasm and the corpus callosum: their relationship to binocular vision. *J Pediatr Ophthalmol Strabismus* 1986; **23**: 126–31.

Fletcher WA, Imes RK, Hoyt WF. Chiasmal gliomas: appearance and long-term changes demonstrated by computerized tomography. *J Neurosurg* 1986; **65**: 154–9.

Flickenger JC, Torres C, Deutsch M. Management of low grade gliomas of the optic nerve and chiasm. *Cancer* 1988; **61**: 635–42.

Gibo H, Watanabe N, Kobayashi S, Sugita K. Removal of an arteriovenous malformation in the optic chiasm. *Surg Neurol* 1989; **31**: 142–8.

Glaser JS, Hoyt WF, Corbett J. Visual morbidity with chiasmal glioma. *Arch Ophthalmol* 1971; **85**: 3–12.

Goodman SJ, Rosenbaum AL, Hasso A, Itabashi H. Large optic nerve glioma with normal vision. *Arch Ophthalmol* 1975; **93**: 991–5.

Goodwin J, Glaser JS. Chiasmal syndrome in sphenoid sinus mucocoele. *Ann Neurol* 1978; **4**: 440–4.

Haberland O, Perou M. Primary bilateral anophthalmia. *J Neuropathol Exp Neurol* 1969; **28**: 337–51.

Hasler W, Zentner J, Wilhelm H. Cavernous angiomas of the anterior visual pathway. *J Clin Neuroophthalmol* 1989; **9**: 160–4.

Heinz G, Nunery W, Grossman C. Traumatic chiasmal syndrome associated with midline basilar skull fractures. *Am J Ophthalmol* 1994; **117**: 90–6.

Holman RE, Grimson BS, Drayer BP, Buckley EG, Brennan MW. Magnetic resonance imaging of optic gliomas. *Am J Ophthalmol* 1985; **100**: 596–601.

Housepian EM, Chi TL. Neurofibromatosis and optic pathways gliomas. *J Neuro-oncol* 1993; **15**: 51–5.

Hoyt WF. Correlative functional anatomy of the optic chiasm. *Clin Neurosurg* 1970; **17**: 189–202.

Hoyt WF, Baghdassarian SB. Optic glioma of childhood. *Br J Ophthalmol* 1969; **53**: 793–8.

Hupp S, Kline L. Magnetic resonance imaging of the optic chiasm. *Surv Ophthalmol* 1991; **36**: 207–16.

Imes RK, Hoyt WF. Childhood chiasmal gliomas: update on the fate of patients in the 1969 San Francisco study. *Br J Ophthalmol* 1986; **70**: 179–82.

Jaffer KA, Obbens EAMT, El Gammal TA. Empty sella: review of 79 cases. *J South Med* 1979; **72**: 294–6.

Jenkin D, Angyalfi S, Becker L *et al.* Optic glioma in children: surveillance, resection or irradiation. *Int J Radiation Oncol Biol Phys* 1993; **25**: 215–25.

Jennings MT, Gelman R, Hochberg F. Intracranial germ-cell tumours: natural history and pathogenesis. *J Neurosurg* 1985; **63**: 155–67.

Kazim M, Kennerdell J, Maroun J, Rothfus W, Marquardt M. Choristoma of the optic nerve and chiasm. *Arch Ophthalmol* 1992; **110**: 236–9.

Kovalic JJ, Grisby PW, Shepard MJ, Fineberg BB, Thomas PR. Radiation therapy for gliomas of the optic nerve and chiasm. *Int J Radiation Oncol Biol Phys* 1990; **18**: 927–32.

Listernick R, Charrow J, Greenwald M. Emergence of optic pathways gliomas in children with neurofibromatosis type 1 after normal neuroimaging. *J Pediatr* 1992; **121**: 584–9.

Liu G, Lessell S. Spontaneous visual improvement in chiasmal gliomas. *Am J Ophthalmol* 1992; **114**: 193–201.

MacCarty CS, Boyd AS Jr., Childs DS Jr. Tumours of the optic nerve and optic chiasm. *J Neurosurg* 1970; **33**: 439–44.

McFadzean RM. The empty sella syndrome—a review of 14 cases. *Trans Ophthalmol Soc UK* 1983; **103**: 537–42.

Margo C, Hamed L, Fang L, Dawson W. Optic nerve aplasia. *Arch Ophthalmol* 1992; **110**: 1610–13.

Meyer FB, Sundt TM, Fode NC, Morgan MK, Forbes GS, Mellinger JF. Cerebral aneurysms in childhood and adolescence. *J Neurosurg* 1989; **70**: 420–5.

Nachtigaller H, Hoyt WF. Storungen des Seheindruckes bei bitemporaller Hemianopsie und verscheibung der Schachsen. *Klin Monatbsbl Augenheilkd* 1970; **156**: 821–32.

Newman NJ, Lessell S, Winterkorn JMS. Optic chiasmal neuritis. *Neurology* 1991; **41**: 1203–10.

Noda S, Hayasaka S, Setogawa T, Matsumoto S. Ocular symptoms of moya-moya disease. *Am J Ophthalmol* 1987; **103**: 812–17.

Onus K, Lala V, Zimmer J, Juan CZ, Auruskin TW. Primary empty sella syndrome in a child. *J Paediatr* 1977; **90**: 425–7.

Packer RJ, Sutton LN, Bilaniuk LT *et al.* Treatment of chiasmatic–hypothalamic gliomas of childhood with chemotherapy. An update. *Ann Neurol* 1988; **23**: 79–91.

Penner H, Schlelch HG. Anophthalmie und begleitende fehibildungen. *Klin Padiatr* 1976; **188**: 320–30.

Petronio J, Edwards MSB, Prados M *et al.* Management of chiasmal and hypothalamic gliomas of infancy and childhood with chemotherapy. *J Neurosurg* 1991; **74**: 701–8.

Pierce S, Barnes PD, Loeffler JS, McGinn C, Tarbell NJ. Definitive radiation therapy in the management of symptomatic patients with optic glioma. *Cancer* 1990; **65**: 45–52.

Provis JM, Vandriel P, Billson F, Russell P. Human fetal optic nerve: overproduction and elimination of retinal axons during development. *J Comp Neurol* 1985; **238**: 92–100.

Recordon E, Griffiths GM. A case of primary bilateral anophthalmia. *Br J Ophthalmol* 1936; **22**: 353–61.

Riishede J, Seedorff HH. Spontaneous haematoma of the optic chiasma. *Acta Ophthalmol* 1974; **52**: 317–22.

Roberson C, Till K. Hypothalamic gliomas in children. *J Neurol Neurosurg Psychiatr* 1974; **30**: 1047–52.

Roche JL, Choux M, Czorny A *et al.* L'aneurysme artériel intracranien chez l'enfant: etude cooperative. A propos de 43 observations. *Neurochirurgie* 1988; **34**: 243–51.

Rush JA, Young BR, Campbell RJ, MacCarty CS. Optic glioma: long-term follow-up of 85 histopathologically verified cases. *Ophthalmology* 1982; **89**: 1213–19.

Schoenberg BS, Mellinger JF, Schoenberg DG. Moya-moya disease in children. *J South Med* 1978; **71**: 237–41.

Schulman JA, Shults WT, McAndrew Jones J. Monocular vertical nystagmus as an initial sign of chiasmal glioma. *Am J Ophthalmol* 1979; **87**: 87–9.

Sinclair AHH, Doff NM. Hydrocephalus-simulating tumour in the production of chiasmal and other parahypophyseal lesions. *Trans Ophthalmol Soc UK* 1931; **51**: 232–41.

Sretavan DW, Pure E, Siegel MW, Reichardt LF. Disruption of retinal axon ingrowth by ablation of embryonic mouse optic chiasm neurons. *Science* 1995; **269**: 98–101.

Sretavan DW, Reichardt LF. Time-lapse video analysis of retinal ganglion cell axon path-finding at the mammalian optic chiasm: growth cone guidance using intrinsic chiasm cues. *Neuron* 1993; **10**: 761–77.

Steinberg GK, Marks MP, Shuer LM, Sogg RL, Enzmann DR, Silverberg CD. Occult vascular malformations of the optic chiasm: magnetic resonance imaging diagnosis and surgical laser resection. *Neurosurgery* 1990; **27**: 466–70.

Takeuchi J, Handa H, Nagatal I. Suprasellar germinoma. *J Neurosurg* 1978; **49**: 41–8.

Tang RA, Kramer LA, Schiffman J, Woon C, Hayman LA, Pardo G. Chiasmal trauma: clinical and imaging considerations. *Surv Ophthalmol* 1994; **38**: 381–3.

Taylor D. Chiasmal disease in young children. In: Wybar KC, Taylor D, eds. *Paediatric Ophthalmology: Current Aspects*. New York: Dekker, 1983: 255–65.

Taylor D. Congenital tumours of the anterior visual system with dysplasia of the optic discs. *Br J Ophthalmol* 1982; **66**: 455–63.

Till K. *Paediatric Neurosurgery for Paediatricians and Neurosurgeons.* Oxford: Blackwell Scientific Publications, 1975.

Trigg ME, Swanson JD, Letellier MA. Metastasis of an optic glioma through a ventriculoperitoneal shunt. *Cancer* 1983; **52**: 599–602.

Waga S, Tochio H. Intracranial aneurysm association with moya moya disease. *Surg Neurol* 1985; **23**: 237–43.

Weinstein JM, Backonja M, Houston LW *et al.* Optic glioma associated with the Beckwith–Wiedemann syndrome. *Paediatr Neurol* 1986; **2**: 308–10.

Weiss L, Sagerman RH, King GA, Chung CT, Dubowy RL. Controversy in the management of optic nerve glioma. *Cancer* 1987; **59**: 1000–10.

Zeki S, Hollman A, Dutton G. Neuroradiological features of patients with optic nerve hypoplasia. *J Pediatr Ophthalmol Strabismus* 1992; **29**: 107–12.

53: Hydrocephalus

Anthony Moore

Hydrocephalus is a condition in which there is enlargement of the cerebral ventricles secondary to an imbalance between production and reabsorption of cerebrospinal fluid. Cerebrospinal fluid is produced mainly by the choroid plexus of the cerebral ventricles and then passes through the ventricular system to reach the subarachnoid space. Reabsorption into the vascular circulation occurs via the arachnoid villi.

Hypersecretion is rare and most cases of communicating hydrocephalus are due to impaired reabsorption. In non-communicating hydrocephalus the obstruction to the cerebrospinal fluid circulation occurs within the ventricular system and the ventricles proximal to the level of the block are dilated.

In communicating hydrocephalus reabsorption of cerebrospinal fluid from the subarachnoid space is impaired. Arrested hydrocephalus is a term used to describe a condition in which the hydrocephalic process has stopped spontaneously and although there may be some residual clinical signs, such as enlarged head size, the condition is non-progressive.

Normal pressure hydrocephalus, in which there are signs of progressive hydrocephalus with normal cerebrospinal fluid pressure, is usually unilateral in childhood, but may be a challenging problem (Stein *et al.* 1971) requiring intracranial pressure monitoring.

Aetiology

Hydrocephalus may be congenital or acquired (Table 53.1). It is one of the most frequent congenital abnormalities of the central nervous system and is usually associated with a structural central nervous system abnormality. Congenital hydrocephalus is a common complication of spina bifida. Acquired hydrocephalus may follow meningitis, intracranial haemorrhage (Fig. 53.1) or tumour and intrauterine infections such as toxoplasmosis (Fig. 53.2) and cytomegalovirus.

Post-haemorrhagic hydrocephalus is particularly common in premature infants (Phillips *et al.* 1989; Fernell *et al.* 1990, 1993). The immature central nervous system of premature infants is particularly susceptible to cerebrovascular damage (Allan 1990; Leviton & Paneth 1990) and intracranial haemorrhage is common, particularly in smaller infants and may be associated with focal infarction of the white matter. The haemorrhages arise from the subependymal germinal matrix, a fine vascular gelatinous structure lying beneath the ependyma along the length of the ventricular region and containing cells which will form mature glial cells that will later populate the cortex. The germinal matrix is present from 10 weeks gestational age and has disappeared by term. The capillaries of the germinal matrix are fragile and the preterm cerebrovascular system has a limited capacity to autoregulate; it is very vulnerable to changes in systemic blood pressure.

The metabolic and other stresses lead to changes in blood flow to the germinal matrix resulting in intraventricular or parenchymal haemorrhage or infarction.

Intraventricular haemorrhage may be complicated by secondary hydrocephalus which develops as a result of obstruction of the cerebrospinal fluid pathways and arachnoid villi by multiple blood clots or secondary basal cistern arachnoiditis. Although the incidence of post-haemorrhagic hydrocephalus in preterm infants may be declining as neonatal care improves (Phillips *et al.* 1989) this group of children represent a significant proportion of

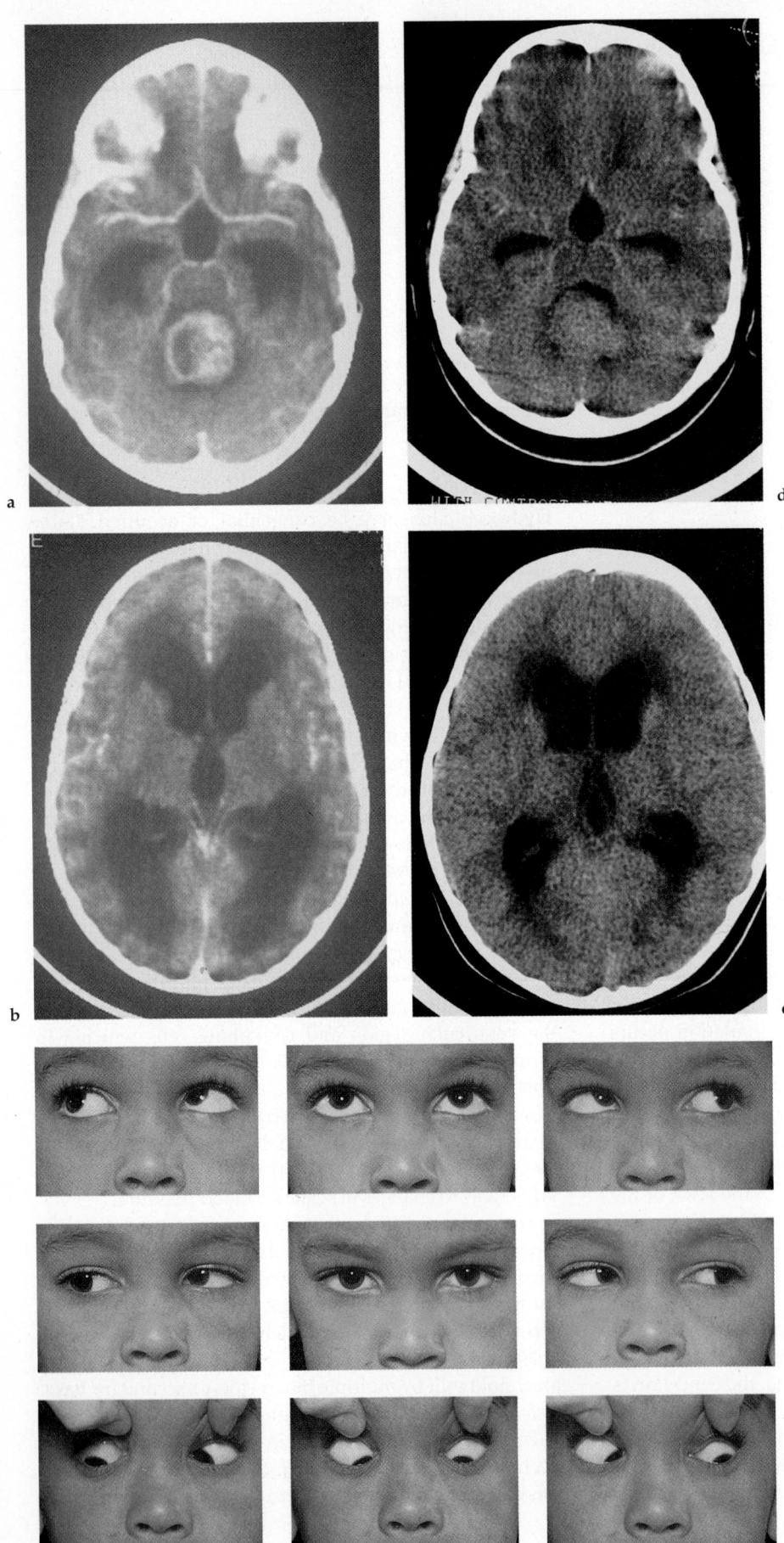

Fig. 53.1 (a) Fourth ventricular ependymoma contrast CT scan showing the fourth ventricle mass and hydrocephalus. There is extensive periventricular oedema (b). The child presented with diplopia due to a bilateral fourth nerve palsy (c). (d) Medulloblastoma. Contrast-enhanced CT scan showing the posterior fossa mass and dilated ventricles (e). This child presented as a recent onset concomitant strabismus without adequate explanation.

Table 53.1 Aetiology of hydrocephalus.

Congenital
Aqueduct stenosis
Arnold–Chiari malformation
Dandy–Walker syndrome
Porencephalic cysts
Arachnoid cysts

Acquired
Meningitis
Intracranial haemorrhage
Tumours
Intrauterine infection

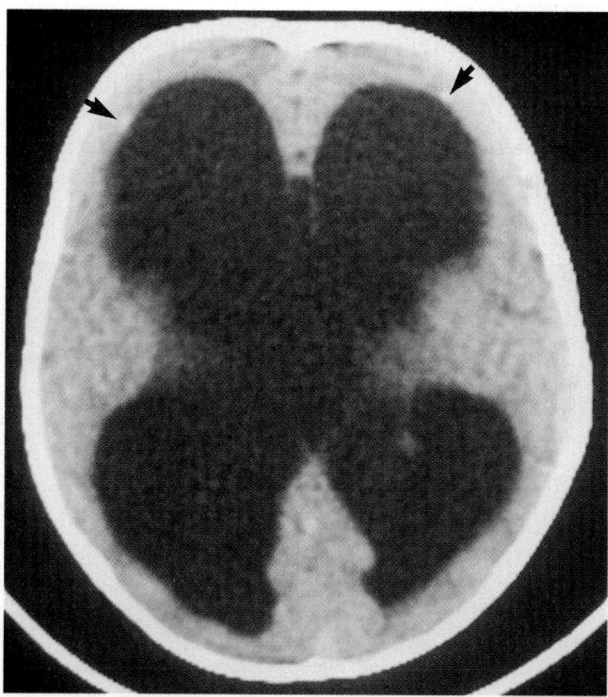

Fig. 53.2 A 10-month-old child with toxoplasmosis chorioretinitis and hydrocephalus. His toxoplasmosis dye test was positive at a 1 : 512 dilution. Note the calcification in the frontal lobes bilaterally (arrows).

infants presenting with ophthalmological abnormalities associated with hydrocephalus.

Clinical features

The clinical presentation of hydrocephalus depends on the age of the child and whether the raised intracranial pressure has an acute or more gradual onset (Brown 1991). In infants in whom the cranial sutures have not closed, there is a progressive increase in skull growth with separation of the sutures. The fontanelle is tense and scalp veins are dilated due to compression of the cortical veins and

sinuses. If the ventricles are greatly enlarged and the cerebral mantle sufficiently thin, the skull may transilluminate (Fig. 53.3). In addition the infant will be irritable and may show signs of failure to thrive or developmental delay. Papilloedema is said to be uncommon in infantile hydrocephalus, but the 'setting sun sign', where the lids are retracted and both eyes deviate downwards in the presence of an upgaze paresis, is only seen in infants (Fig. 53.4).

In later childhood the usual presentation is with symptoms and signs of raised intracranial pressure, either with an acute or chronic onset. Bilateral papilloedema is usual-

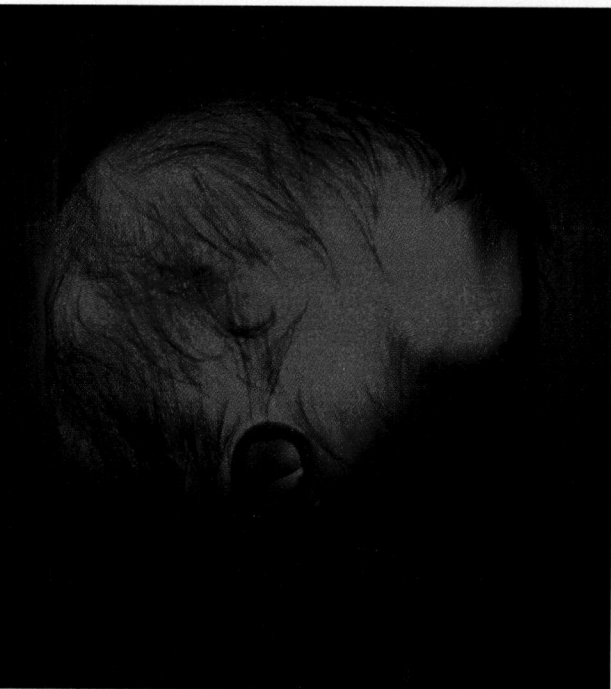

Fig. 53.3 Transillumination of the skull in severe hydrocephalus.

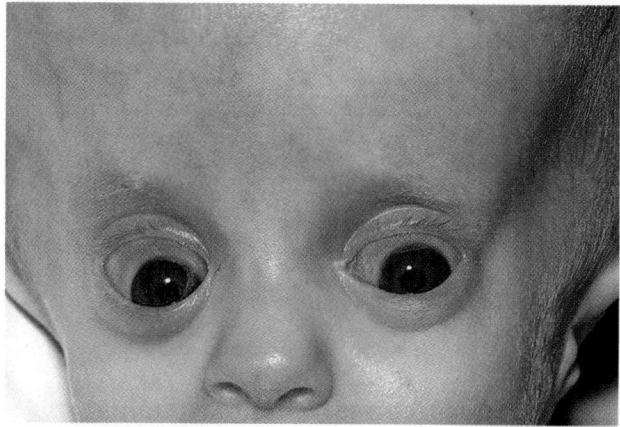

Fig. 53.4 Setting sun sign. This consists of downward deviation of the eyes, an upgaze palsy, and lid retraction.

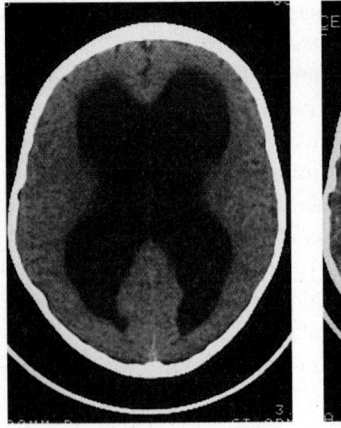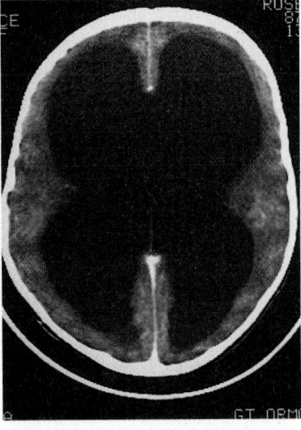

Fig. 53.5 Hydrocephalus. On the right the ventricles are huge with a thin cortical mantle. On the left is the same child after shunting.

ly present and there may be unilateral or bilateral sixth nerve paresis or impairment of vertical gaze.

Management

There have been several major advances in the management of childhood hydrocephalus in recent years (Di Rocco 1991). The advent of computed tomography (CT) (Fig. 53.5) and magnetic resonance imaging (MRI) scanning has greatly simplified the investigation of these children and allowed the site and cause of the obstruction to be easily identified.

Furthermore, repeat scans after surgery allow the size of the cerebral ventricles to be monitored radiologically without the need for more invasive techniques. Real-time ultrasound scanning is an alternative means of imaging the ventricular system which is particularly useful in preterm infants who have sustained intraventricular haemorrhage (Levene 1981). Techniques for intracranial pressure monitoring have also improved and are helpful in the management of older children with acquired, complicated forms of hydrocephalus (Leggate & Minns 1991).

Another major advance has been the introduction of valves (Fig. 53.6) such as the Spitz–Holter and Pudenz which are designed to give unidirectional flow of cerebrospinal fluid from the ventricles into the vascular system, usually the right atrium (Fig. 53.7), or peritoneal cavity. Such cerebrospinal fluid shunt procedures have greatly improved the prognosis in hydrocephalus but are still subject to complications such as infection or shunt malfunction, necessitating further surgical revision (Di Rocco 1991).

Ocular complications of hydrocephalus

Raised intracranial pressure in hydrocephalus may result in damage to the visual pathway and visual loss may fol-

low optic atrophy or cortical damage (Smith *et al.* 1966; Lorber 1967; Arroyo 1985; Gaston 1991). Disturbances of ocular motility such as gaze palsies, nystagmus and strabismus are common (Rabinowitz 1974; Rabinowitz & Walker 1975; Gaston 1991). In children with hydrocephalus ophthalmological abnormalities may be related directly to the the raised intracranial pressure or ventricular enlargement but may also be caused by other associated intracranial abnormalities such as congenital structural anomalies, tumour, infection or hypoxic ischaemic events. This account will concern itself with the ophthalmological abnormalities which are common to all forms of hydrocephalus, regardless of aetiology.

Optic nerve

Papilloedema

Papilloedema is said to be uncommon in infantile hydrocephalus as the skull is still able to expand but there have

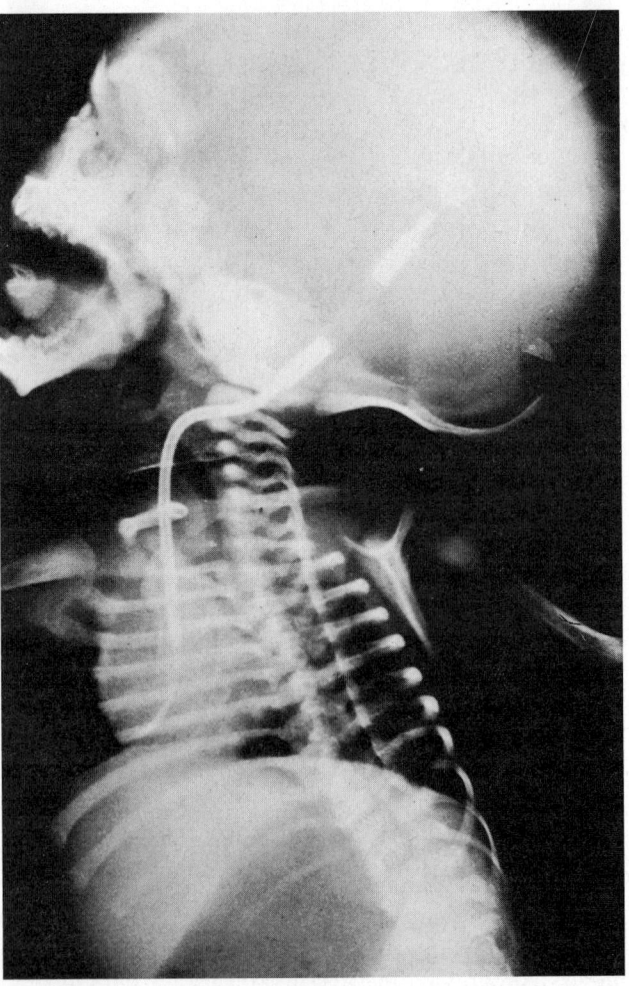

Fig. 53.6 X-ray of a ventriculo-atrial shunt system *in situ*. Ventriculoperitoneal shunts are more frequently used today.

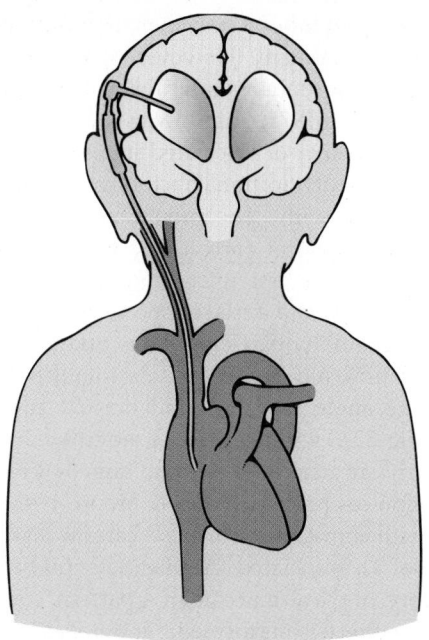

Fig. 53.7 Diagram of shunt system. The valve which can be pumped lies against the skull.

been few studies of optic nerve change in this young age group. Ghose (1983) reviewed the optic nerve changes in 200 consecutive cases of congenital hydrocephalus examined before shunt surgery. The optic disc was normal in 56%, optic atrophy was present in 29% and 5.5% had papilloedema. A further 7% had incipient or suspected papilloedema. This study suggests that optic disc oedema is more common than previously thought in infantile hydrocephalus.

In older children with acquired hydrocephalus or shunt malfunction marked papilloedema is common and may be associated with peripapillary haemorrhage or exudate.

Optic atrophy

Optic atrophy is common in all forms of hydrocephalus and is a major cause of visual morbidity (Rabinowitz 1974; Ghose 1983; Gaston 1991). Ghose (1983) found that 17% of infants with hydrocephalus had optic atrophy and a further 7% had temporal pallor of the optic disc before shunt surgery. A similar figure was reported by Gaston (1991). Rabinowitz (1974) reported that 30% of children in his study had optic atrophy. Such children are especially vulnerable to further episodes of raised intracranial pressure which may result in visual loss from damage to an already compromised optic disc. They present further problems in assessment as raised intracranial pressure may not result in optic disc swelling in the presence of atrophy and the diagnosis of shunt malfunction may be more difficult. Children with hydrocephalus who have significant optic

atrophy have a higher incidence of visual impairment and of associated severe neurological defect than those with normal optic discs (Gaston 1991). They also have a poorer prognosis for life (Gaston 1991).

Optic atrophy complicating hydrocephalus may result from several mechanisms (Table 53.2). Raised intracranial pressure may result in arterial compression (Lindenberg 1955) and ischaemia of the optic nerve. Shift of the brain stem following shunt surgery may cause traction on the optic nerves and chiasm (Emery & Levick 1966) and optic atrophy may also follow optic nerve (Calgero & Alexander 1977) or chiasmal compression by an enlarged third ventricle (Tamler 1964; Osher *et al.* 1978; Humphrey *et al.* 1982). Optic atrophy may also develop secondary to long-standing papilloedema. It is also possible in young infants that optic atrophy may follow retrograde trans-synaptic neuronal degeneration in the visual pathway secondary to damage to the visual cortex.

Chiasmal disorders

The close anatomical relationship between the third ventricle and the optic chiasm means that the optic chiasm may be distorted by a pathologically enlarged third ventricle. Most cases with evidence of chiasmal dysfunction in hydrocephalus have aqueduct stenosis. Chiasmal compression may result in optic atrophy (Osher *et al.* 1978; Humphrey *et al.* 1982) and field defects including bilateral central scotoma or bitemporal hemianopia (Humphrey *et al.* 1982). There may be some improvement in visual acuity and fields after a shunt procedure.

Visual cortical abnormalities

Bilateral visual loss or homonymous hemianopic field defects may result from ischaemic damage to the visual cortex in hydrocephalus (Smith *et al.* 1966; Lorber 1967; Rabinowitz 1974; Arroyo *et al.* 1985; Gaston 1991). Field loss extensive enough to be detected by confrontation testing has been reported in 5–10% of children (Rabinowitz 1974; Gaston 1991) but the true extent of field defects is likely to be much higher as formal perimetry was not possible in the majority of the children studied. The mechanism of visual pathway damage is uncertain but may be related to compression of the posterior cerebral arteries at the edge of the tentorium cerebelli (Lindenberg 1955;

Table 53.2 Causes of optic atrophy in hydrocephalus.

Optic nerve ischaemia
Optic nerve or chiasmal traction
Chiasmal compression
Consecutive optic atrophy
Trans-synaptic neuronal degeneration

Arroyo *et al.* 1985). Visual loss may be associated with shunt malfunction or shunt infections and cortical blindness is usually seen in children who have had multiple shunt revisions. The visual loss may be reversible in some cases if prompt treatment is given (Lorber 1967). Such children may have associated optic atrophy, but the presence of normal pupil reactions and visual loss out of proportion to the degree of optic atrophy allows a diagnosis of cortical blindness to be made. Visual evoked potential measurements and CT scan are helpful in confirming the diagnosis. Premature infants with post-haemorrhagic hydrocephalus have a high incidence of neurological abnormalities including visual pathway damage which is due to a combination of raised intracranial pressure and associated periventricular leukomalacia (Leviton & Paneth 1990; Allan 1990; Fernell *et al.* 1993; Ventriculomegaly Trial Group 1994).

Ocular motor abnormalities

The common disorders of ocular motility seen in hydrocephalus are strabismus, supranuclear gaze palsies and nystagmus.

Strabismus

Strabismus is the most common ocular complication of hydrocephalus occurring in 40–75% of patients (Rothstein *et al.* 1974; Clements & Kaushal 1970; Rabinowitz & Walker 1975; Gaston 1991). Most have horizontal deviations with esotropia being four times more common than exotropia (Rabinowitz 1974).

Esotropia

The esotropia may be incomitant or concomitant. Incomitant deviations may follow unilateral or bilateral sixth nerve palsy. The VIth nerve is especially vulnerable to episodes of raised intracranial pressure. Usually a full recovery of function occurs after shunt surgery and corrective squint surgery is rarely necessary.

Most patients with hydrocephalus have concomitant esotropia (Clements & Kaushal 1970; Rabinowitz 1974; France 1975; Gaston 1991). In ex-premature infants the esotropia often develops within the first 6 months of life and may be indistinguishable from typical infantile esotropia (Charles & Moore 1992). In older children there is a high incidence of A pattern deviations (France 1975; Rabinowitz & Walker 1975; Gaston 1991) which in half the cases is associated with bilateral superior oblique overaction (Fig. 53.8). The strabismus is usually alternating and amblyopia is uncommon. The mechanism of the development of comitant squint in hydrocephalus is uncertain. Wybar (1976) has suggested that the high incidence of strabismus is related to unilateral or bilateral sixth nerve

palsies in early childhood and that with time the squint becomes more comitant. However, only a minority of infants with hydrocephalus have recognizable lateral rectus palsies (France 1975; Rabinowitz & Walker 1975) and the relative frequency of associated superior oblique overaction suggests that additional factors may be important.

Most children with concomitant esotropia will ultimately require surgical correction. However, hyperopic refractive errors are not uncommon in hydrocephalus (Gaston *et al.* 1991) and a trial of spectacle wear and treatment of any amblyopia should be undertaken before surgery is considered. Hydrocephalic infants who present with a large angle esotropia and normal lateral rectus function (Fig. 53.9) within the first 6 months of life respond well to early surgical intervention; bimedial recession is the operation of choice (Charles & Moore 1992). In older children with comitant esotropia a careful search should be made for an associated 'A' phenomenon before planning surgery. In the absence of an A pattern, conventional horizontal surgery is performed but if present the type of surgery depends on whether or not there is associated superior oblique overaction. When this is present horizontal surgery is combined with bilateral superior oblique posterior tenotomies. In the absence of superior oblique overaction the horizontal surgery is combined with vertical displacement of the horizontal recti, the medial rectus being moved upwards one insertion width and the lateral rectus moved down by a similar amount.

Exotropia

Exotropia in hydrocephalus is usually associated with severe bilateral visual loss and optic atrophy or follows surgical overcorrection of an esotropia (Rabinowitz & Walker 1975; Gaston *et al.* 1991). Rarely it may be associated with a third nerve palsy (France 1975; Rabinowitz & Walker 1975).

Vertical deviations

Vertical deviations are less commonly seen in hydrocephalus and when present are associated with a third nerve palsy, skew deviation or asymmetrical oblique muscle dysfunction (Rabinowitz & Walker 1975; Gaston 1991).

Gaze palsies

In uncontrolled hydrocephalus two distinct types of vertical gaze palsies rnay be seen (Swash 1976). In young infants the so-called 'setting sun' sign with bilateral upper lid retraction and downward deviation of the eyes and a vertical gaze palsy affecting both saccadic and pursuit systems is seen. It is a poor prognostic sign and is often accompanied by visual loss and severe optic atrophy (Rabinowitz 1974). It usually completely resolves follow-

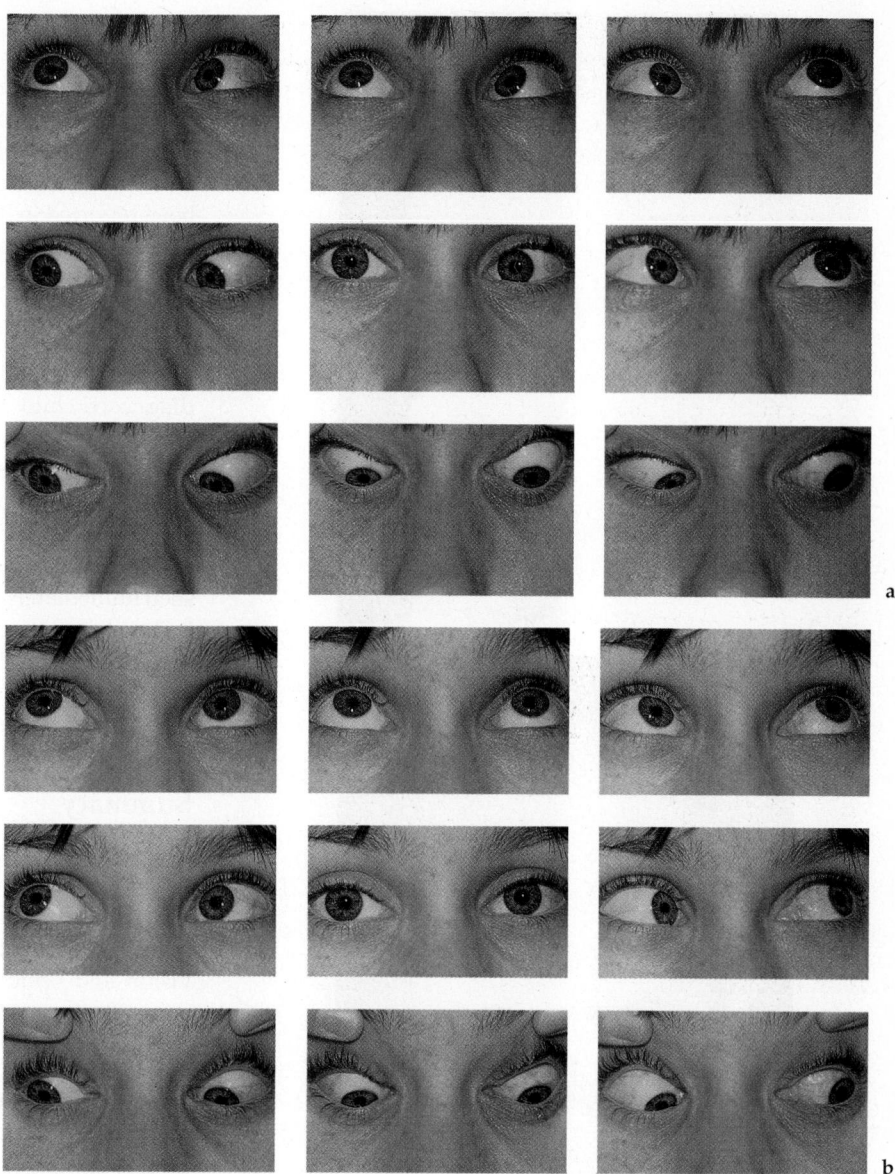

Fig. 53.8 (a) 'A' pattern esotropia in a child with hydrocephalus. Note the overaction of the superior obliques. (b) Following horizontal surgery and disinsertion of the posterior fibres of the superior oblique muscle. (Mr Anthony Moore's patient.)

ing shunt surgery but may recur during episodes of shunt malfunction (Gaston 1991).

In older children with later onset of hydrocephalus or shunt malfunction, a different clinical picture is seen. Episodes of raised intracranial pressure may result in the Sylvian aqueduct (Parinaud's) syndrome with impaired upgaze, light-near dissociation of the pupils, and convergence retraction nystagmus (Shallat *et al.* 1973; Swash 1976; Osher *et al.* 1978; Gaston 1991). The ocular motor abnormalities usually resolve after shunt surgery but may reappear during shunt malfunction (Shallat *et al.* 1973).

Disorders of vertical gaze in hydrocephalus occur more frequently in aqueduct stenosis than in other forms of non-communicating hydrocephalus (Swash 1976) and are rarely seen in communicating hydrocephalus. There is a close anatomical relationship between the vertical gaze

centres of the midbrain and the Sylvian aqueduct and third ventricle. Acquired Sylvian aqueduct syndrome is thought to result from distortion of the periaqueductal structures by an enlarged rostral aqueduct and dilated suprapineal recess of the third ventricle (Swash 1976). Conversely, the 'setting sun' sign is thought to be caused by pressure on the decussating fibres in the posterior commissure by an enlarged third ventricle. In each case decompression of the third ventricle will usually result in recovery of normal vertical gaze. Horizontal gaze palsies are rarely seen in hydrocephalus, but patients with the Arnold–Chiari malformation may develop internuclear ophthalmoplegia (Woody & Reynolds 1985).

Another rare abnormality seen in hydrocephalus is the bobble-headed doll syndrome (Kirkham 1977). In this condition there are flexion–extension movements of the

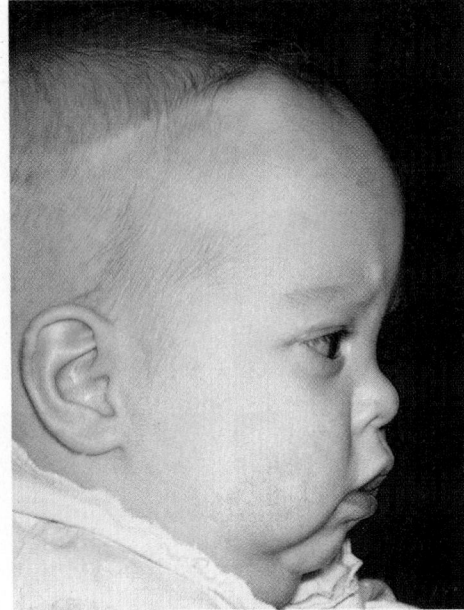

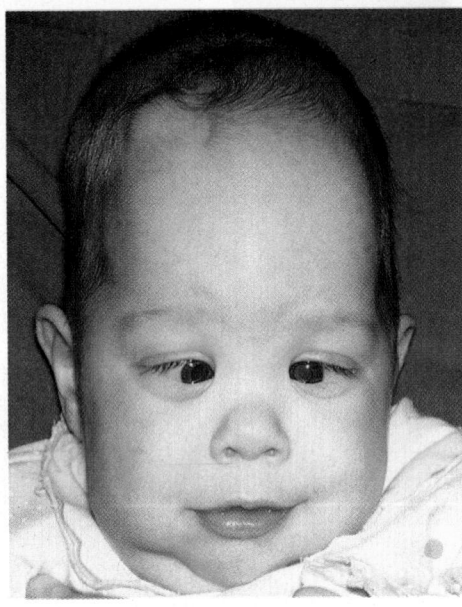

Fig. 53.9 (a, b) Large angle esotropia with full lateral rectus function in a child with hydrocephalus. In (a) the shunt tubing is just visible as a ridge on the skin of the head (Mr Anthony Moore's patient).

head and neck on the trunk at a rate of about two to three per second. The condition is almost always associated with a hugely enlarged third ventricle caused by tumour and usually resolves after shunt surgery (Table 53.3).

Nystagmus

Nystagmus occurs in about 3–5% of children with hydrocephalus (Rabinowitz 1974; Gaston 1991) and may have a variety of causes. Pendular nystagmus may follow bilater-

al visual loss from optic atrophy and gaze-evoked nystagmus may be associated with a recovering sixth nerve palsy. Children with hydrocephalus and associated posterior fossa abnormalities may develop nystagmus secondary to cerebellar dysfunction. Down-beat nystagmus is seen in the Arnold–Chiari malformation but has also been reported in hydrocephalus complicating intracranial haemorrhage (Phadke *et al.* 1981).

Advice for parents

The ophthalmologist should warn the parents of a newly diagnosed child with hydrocephalus that, although most children with the disease have only a few problems, all are at risk of losing vision and developing squints. Any squint that appears gradually — say over a period of weeks — should be seen promptly by an ophthalmologist and any squint appearing over a period of days or less should be seen immediately by an ophthalmologist or neurosurgeon because it may herald a blocked shunt, especially if accompanied by headache, nausea, vomiting and, in the smaller child, misery. Visual symptoms should prompt immediate referral to an ophthalmologist.

Summary

Children with hydrocephalus who have had shunt surgery should, where possible, be followed up by both neurosurgeon and ophthalmologist. In the older child a regular assessment of visual acuity, visual fields, colour vision and optic discs should be performed so that an episode of raised intracranial pressure associated with shunt malfunction is detected early. This is especially important in children with optic atrophy who may not develop papilloedema and in whom the discs are vulnerable to further episodes of raised intracranial pressure. Infants with blocked shunts may also fail to develop papilloedema but may show signs of reduced vision, poor pupillary reactions or vertical gaze palsy.

Children with hydrocephalus may lose vision from optic atrophy, chiasmal compression or damage to the visual cortex. Although blindness is not common in this condition, the relative frequency of childhood hydrocephalus means that it is a significant cause of visual handicap.

Table 53.3 Complications of an enlarged third ventricle.

Optic nerve compression (Calgero 1971)
Chiasmal syndrome (Tamler 1964; Humphreys *et al.* 1982)
Parinaud's syndrome (Shallat *et al.* 1973; Swash 1976; Osher *et al.* 1978)
Setting sun sign (Swash 1976)
Bobble-headed doll syndrome (Kirkham 1977)

References

Allan WC. The IVH complex of lesions: cerebrovascular injury in the pre-term infant. *Neurol Clin* 1990; **8**: 529–51.

Arroyo H, Jan J, McCormick A, Farrel K. Permanent visual loss after shunt malfunction. *Neurology* 1985; **35**: 25–9.

Brown JK. Pathological effects of raised intracranial pressure in problems of intracranial pressure in childhood. In: Minns, RA ed. *Problems of Intracranial Pressure in Childhood*. McKeith Press. *Clin Develop Med* 1991; **113/4**: 38–76.

Calgero JA, Alexander E. Unilateral amaurosis in a hydrocephalic child with an obstructed shunt. *J Neurosurg* 1971; **34**: 236–40.

Charles SJ, Moore AT. Infantile esotropia in normal infants and those with neurodevelopmental disorders. *Eye* 1992 ; **6**: 603–6.

Clements DB, Kaushal K. A study of the ocular complications of hydrocephalus and myelomeningocele. *Trans Ophthalmol Soc UK* 1970; **90**: 383–90.

Di Rocco C. A survey of the treatment of infantile hydrocephalus in problems of intracranial pressure in childhood. In: Minns, RA ed. *Problems of Intracranial Pressure in Childhood*. McKeith Press. *Clin Dev Med* 1991; **113/4**: 349–77.

Emery JL, Levick RK. The movement of the brain stem and vessels around the brain stem in children with hydrocephalus and the Arnold–Chiari deformity. *Ann Radiol (Paris)* 1966; **314**: 141–7.

Fernell E, Hagberg G, Hagberg B. Infantile hydrocephalus: the impact of enhanced pre-term survival. *Acta Paediatr Scand* 1990; **79**: 1080–6.

Fernell E, Hagberg G, Hagberg B. Infantile hydrocephalus in pre-term infants — a nationwide Swedish cohort study, 1979–88. *Acta Paediatr Scand* 1993; **82**: 45–8.

France TJ. The association of 'A' pattern strabismus with hydrocephalus. In: Moore S, Mein J, Stockbridge L, eds. *Transactions of the Third International Orthoptic Congress*. Miami: Symposia Specialists, 1975: 287–92.

Gaston H. Ophthalmic complications of hydrocephalus and spina bifida. *Eye* 1991; **5**: 279–90.

Ghose S. Optic nerve changes in hydrocephalus. *Trans Ophthalmol Soc UK* 1983; **103**: 217–20.

Humphrey PRD, Moseley IF, Ross Russell RW. Visual field defects in obstructive hydrocephalus. *J Neurol Neurosurg Psychiatr* 1982; **45**: 251–5.

Kirkham TA. Optic atrophy in the bobble-headed doll syndrome. *J Pediatr Ophthalmol* 1977; **14**: 199–301.

Leggate JRS, Minns RA. Intracranial pressure monitoring — current methods in problems of intracranial pressure in childhood. In: Minns, RA ed. *Problems of Intracranial Pressure in Childhood*. McKeith Press. *Clin Dev Med* 1991; **113/4**: 123–40.

Levene M. Measurement of the growth of the lateral ventricles in preterm infants with real time ultrasound. *Arch Dis Child* 1981; **56**: 900–4.

Leviton A, Paneth N. White matter damage in preterm newborns — an epidemiological perspective. *Early Hum Dev* 1990; **24**: 1–22.

Lindenberg R. Compression of brain arteries as a pathogenetic factor for tissue necrosis and their areas of predilection. *J Neuropathol Exp Neurol* 1955; **14**: 223–43.

Lorber J. Recovery of vision following prolonged blindness in children with hydrocephalus or following pyogenic meningitis. *Clin Pediatr* 1967; **6**: 699–703.

Osher RH, Corbett JJ, Schatz NJ. Neuro-ophthalmological complications of enlargement of the third ventricle. *Br J Ophthalmol* 1978; **62**: 536–42.

Phadke JG, Hern JEC, Blaiklock CT. Downbeat nystagmus as a false localising sign due to communicating hydrocephalus (letter). *J Neurol Neurosurg Psychiatr* 1981; **44**: 459.

Phillips AGS, Allan WC, Tito AM, Wheeler LR. Intraventricular haemorrhage in preterm infants: declining incidence in the 1980s. *Pediatrics* 1989; **84**: 797–801.

Rabinowitz IM. Visual function in children with hydrocephalus. *Trans Ophthalmol Soc UK* 1974; **94**: 353–65.

Rabinowitz IM, Walker JW. Disorders of ocular motility in children with hydrocephalus. In: Moore S, Mein J, Stockbridge L, eds. *Transactions of the Third International Orthoptics Congress*. Miami: Symposia Specialists, 1975: 279–86.

Rothstein TB, Romano PE, Shoch D. Myelomeningocele. *Am J Ophthalmol* 1974; **77**: 690–3.

Shallat RF, Paul RP, Jerva MJ. Significance of upward gaze palsy (Parinaud's syndrome) in hydrocephalus due to shunt malfunction. *J Neurosurg* 1973; **38**: 717–21.

Smith JL, Walsh HTJ, Shipley T. Cortical blindness in congenital hydrocephalus. *Am J Ophthalmol* 1966; **62**: 251–5.

Stein BM, Fraser RA, Tenner MS. Normal pressure hydrocephalus — complication of posterior fossa surgery in children. *Pediatrics* 1971; **49**: 50–7.

Swash M. Disorders of ocular movement in hydrocephalus. *Proc Roy Soc Med* 1976; **69**: 480–4.

Tamler E. Primary optic atrophy from acquired dilatation of the third ventricle. *Am J Ophthalmol* 1964; **57**: 827–8.

Ventriculomegaly Trial Group. Randomised trial of early tapping in neonatal post-haemorrhagic ventricular dilatation: results at 30 months. *Arch Dis Child* 1994; **70**: F129–36.

Woody RC, Reynolds JD. Association of bilateral internuclear ophthalmoplegia and myelomeningocoele with Arnold–Chiari malformation type II. *J Clin Neuro-ophthalmol* 1985; **5**: 124–6.

Wybar K. Disorders of ocular motility in hydrocephalus in early childhood. In: Fells P, ed. *Second Congress of International Strabismological Association*. Marseilles: Diffusion Générale de Libraire, 1976: 366–70.

54: Brain Problems

Scott Lambert

Disorders affecting the posterior visual pathway

Brain problems are a major cause of visual defect in the Western world and are all the more important because of the multiplicity of the defects ('additional defects multiply, not add onto existing defects'). Moreover, although children with cerebral disorders show a wide range of cognitive visual disorders these remain unclassified and ill understood (Dutton 1994).

Developmental and structural defects

The congenital abnormalities which affect the posterior visual pathway are best understood in the context of the developmental stages in which they occur. During the first month of embryogenesis, a neural plate is formed which invaginates into the neural groove and then fuses into a neural tube. A disturbance of the rostral closure of the neural groove often results in occipital encephalocoeles. Seventy-five to eighty per cent of encephalocoeles occur in the occipital region. They are usually filled with portions of the occipital lobe.

During the second month of gestation, the forebrain or prosencephalon is cleaved transversely into the telencephalon and diencephalon and sagittally into the cerebral hemispheres and lateral ventricles. Derangements in this process may result in holoprosencephaly, which is characterized by a single cerebral structure with a common ventricle. The most severe form of holoprosencephaly is the alobar form (Fig. 54.1) when there is a complete failure to form separate hemispheres; this is often associated with facial defects, facial dysmorphism, cyclopia and often with microcephaly. In the semi-lobar

form only the anterior ventricles fail to form separately, and in the lobar holoprosencephaly (see Fig. 54.1) there are well-formed ventricles that remain connected anteriorly and inferiorly usually at the frontal. There may be a variety of associated defects, such as agenesis of the corpus callosum, vascular anomalies and schizencephaly (Fig. 54.2) in which there is a cleft across the brain substance. In type 1 schizencephaly (so-called fused lip) there is a grey matter track between the ventricles; in the type 2 (open lip) the cleft allows direct communication between pia and ependyma. Since the face and optic vesicles are formed during the same developmental period, holoprosencephaly is often associated with facial and ocular anomalies. Optic nerve anomalies, hypoplasia in particular, are frequently associated with holoprosencephaly.

Between the second and fourth gestational months, the neurones in the ventricular and subventricular zones

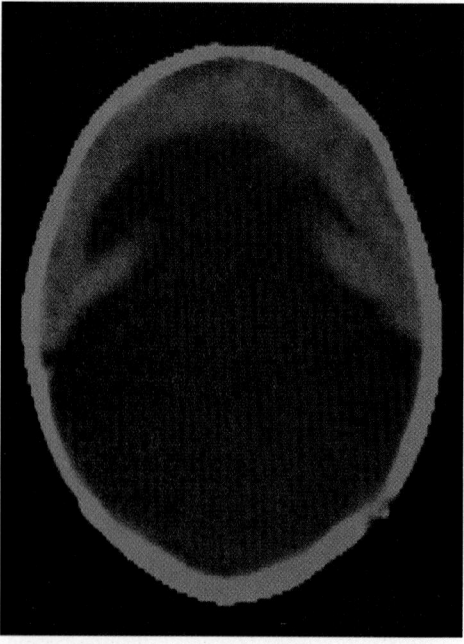

Fig. 54.1 Alobar holoprosencephaly. There is a complete failure to form separate ventricles.

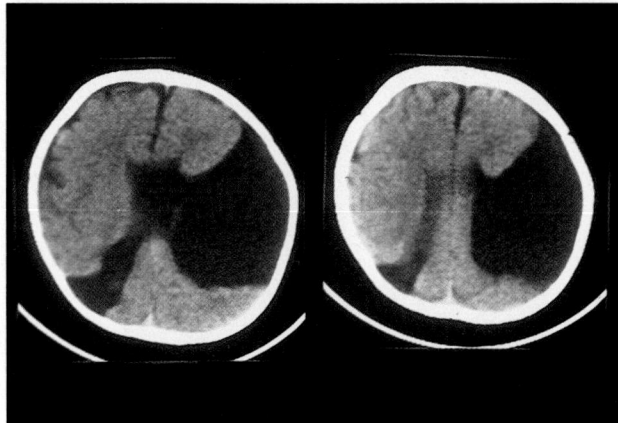

Fig. 54.2 Schizencephaly in a patient with holoprosencephaly.

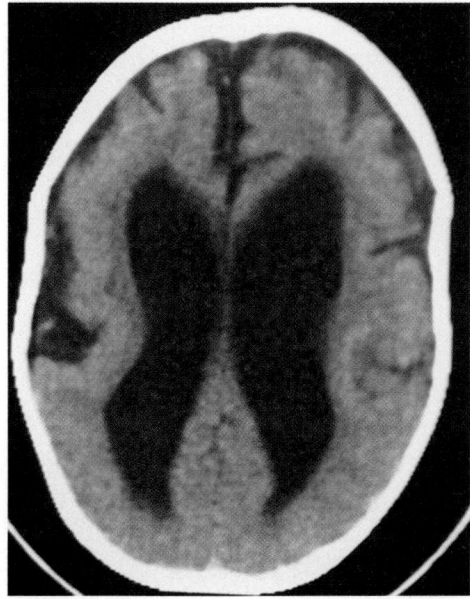

Fig. 54.3 Agyria. Agyria is a severe form of lissencephaly. On this CT scan it can be seen that the surface of the brain posteriorly is smooth. The rest of the brain is atrophic as shown by the large sulci and ventricles.

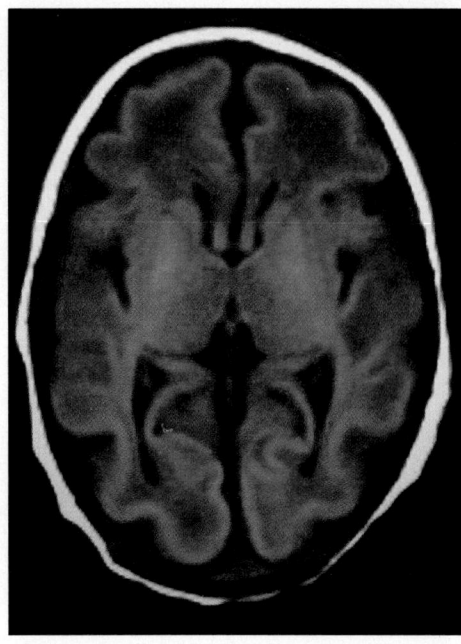

Fig. 54.4 Pachygyria. This disorder is similar to lissencephaly and shows the crude form and smooth surface of the gyri.

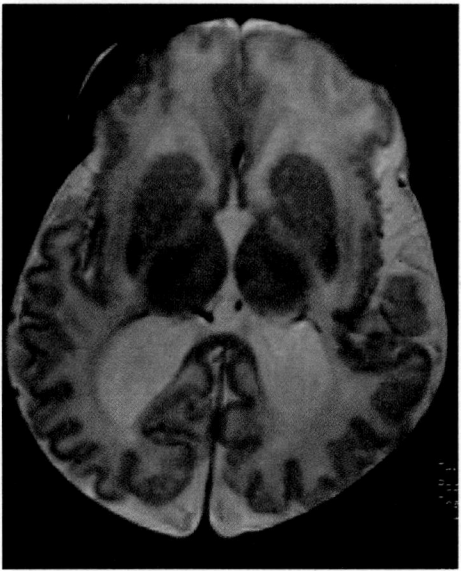

Fig. 54.5 Polymicrogyria. Gyri are variably small and 'bumpy'.

proliferate and then migrate to the cortical plates. While neurones early in embryogenesis migrate relatively short distances, neurones later in development often migrate long distances across the intermediate zones. Their migration may be facilitated by radial glial cells which appear to serve as guidelines (Rakic 1972). The neurones arriving first in the cortical mantle assume the deepest locations, while neurones arriving later assume a more superficial location.

Aberrations in neuronal migration may result in a variety of neural abnormalities. Lissencephaly (smooth brain) occurs when neurones end their migration in the intermediate zone, resulting in an absence of cortical gyri

(Fig. 54.3). Pachygyria (Fig. 54.4) is related to lissencephaly, but develops when neuronal migration is disturbed at a later stage; it is characterized by reduced numbers of gyri, abnormally thick cortex and fewer cortical neurones than normal. Polymicrogyria (Figs 54.5, 54.6) may occur secondary to an even later neuronal migratory disturbance. The gyri are unusually small with a reduced number of cortical layers and a primitive orientation to the neurones. Neuronal heterotopias (ectopic grey matter) are

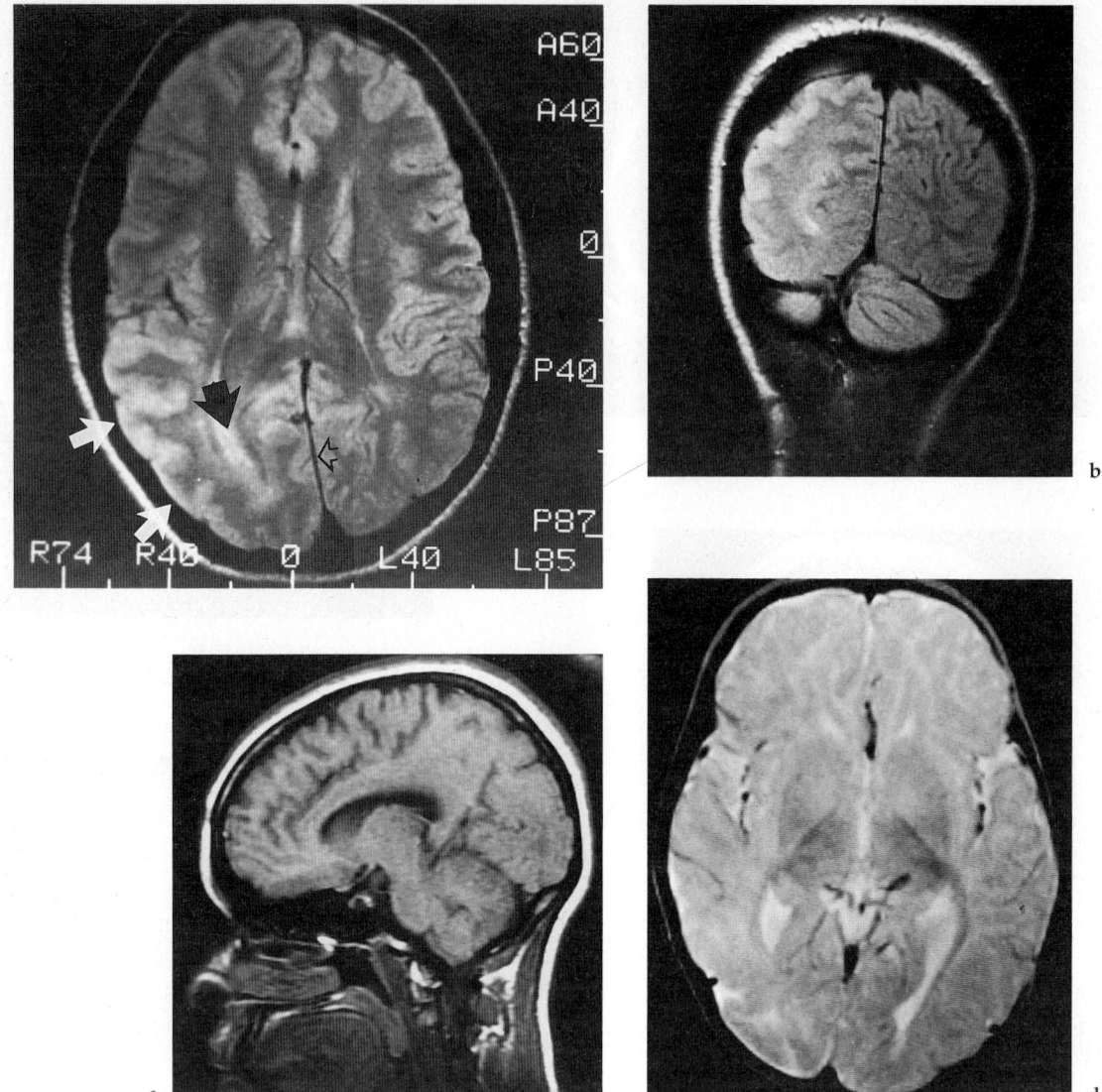

Fig. 54.6 Polymicrogyria. (a) Axial (TE 2000, TR 35) MRI scan of a 23-year-old woman with a seizure disorder and right occipital polymicrogyri. The visual acuity and fields were normal. The polymicrogyri involve the right occipital lobe laterally (white arrows) but spare the visual cortex medially (open arrow). The white matter in the right occipital lobe is also dysplastic (black arrow). (b) Coronal (TR 2000, TE 35) MRI scan of the same patient. There are polymicrogyri in the right occipital lobe laterally and an absence of normal cortical gyri. The visual cortex medially is normal. (c) Sagittal T1-weighted (TR 400, TE 20) MRI scan of the same patient. The polymicrogyri of the right occipital lobe may be clearly distinguished from the normal cortical gyrations and sulci of the frontal lobe. (d) A 9-month-old child noted to have visual inattention to the left at 6 weeks of age by her mother. At 9 months of age the hemianopia was more difficult to detect clinically, but visual evoked potentials recorded from the two hemispheres were grossly asymmetrical. MRI scan shows hypoplasia of the right occipital lobe. The child was the product of a full-term uncomplicated pregnancy and delivery. She is developmentally normal otherwise.

collections of neurones in subcortical white matter (Figs 54.7, 54.8); they are a common accompaniment of severe neuronal migratory disorders and also may be an incidental finding during autopsies. Their significance is unclear in most cases. Infants with lissencephaly and pachygyria frequently die during infancy and have severe neurological abnormalities including seizures and hypotonia. While children with generalized polymicrogyria are frequently neurologically handicapped, those with focal polymicrogyria will often only have seizures or isolated functional abnormalities. Polymicrogyria localized to the striate cortex may result in homonymous hemianopias, often with incongruous margins not honouring the vertical midline (Hoyt 1985). Polymicrogyria, as well as neuronal ectopias and dysplasias, are also frequently found in the inferior frontal and superior temporal regions of the left hemisphere in dyslexic subjects (Galaburda *et al.* 1985; Geschwind & Galaburda 1985). Historically, focal cortical

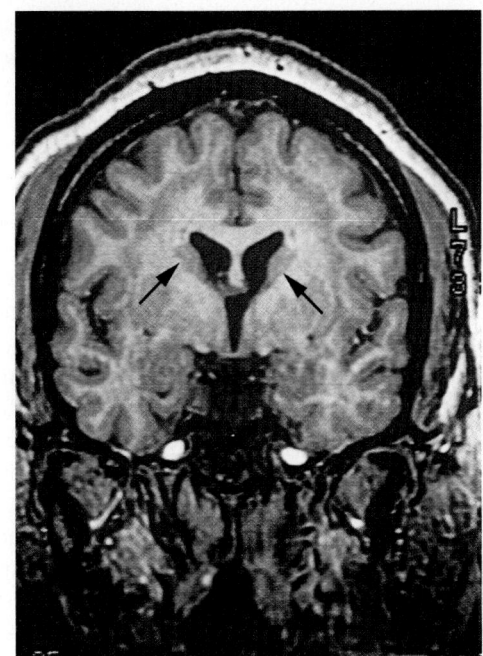

Fig. 54.7 Neuronal heterotopia. Ectopic grey matter (arrows) can be seen impinging on the ventricles in these coronal sections.

gyral anomalies were only identified intraoperatively or at postmortem. In some instances they may now be visualized using magnetic resonance imaging (MRI) (Tychsen & Hoyt 1985).

The fetal brain responds quite differently to injuries compared with the neonatal or adult brain. Injuries to the brain during fetal development cause total dissolution of the affected parenchyma, often with well-circumscribed borders. Insults early in fetal development may result in loss of portions of the brain or schizencephaly, whereas insults later in fetal development result in porencephalic cysts (Fig. 54.9). In contradistinction, full-term infants and children develop encephalomalacia and gliosis after injuries. Schizencephaly and porencephaly may affect large portions of the brain (Fig. 54.10), or only limited regions such as the occipital lobes. The distribution of porencephalic cysts often corresponds to a territory perfused by one of the major cerebral vessels suggesting a vascular aetiology.

Occasionally only the occipital horns of the lateral ventricles are dilated with thinning of the overlying occipital cortex. This condition is known as colpocephaly (Fig. 54.11). The pathogenesis of colpocephaly is unclear (Garg 1982), but may stem from an *in utero* insult or failure of development of the optic radiations. Colpocephaly is commonly associated with optic disc anomalies.

Congenital vascular anomalies may also occur in the occipital lobes resulting in hemianopias or other more subtle field defects. These anomalies may be part of a more widespread vascular disorder such as the Sturge–Weber or Wyburn–Mason syndrome or may occur as isolated arteriovenous malformations. They are often calcified.

Congenital tumours may also occur in the occipital lobes, but are quite uncommon (Fig. 54.12).

Congenital lesions of the geniculostriate pathway may result in trans-synaptic degeneration of the ipsilateral temporal hemiretina which causes thinning of the arcuate

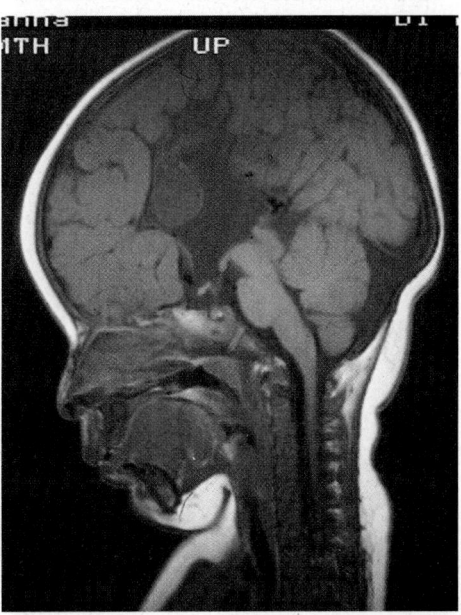

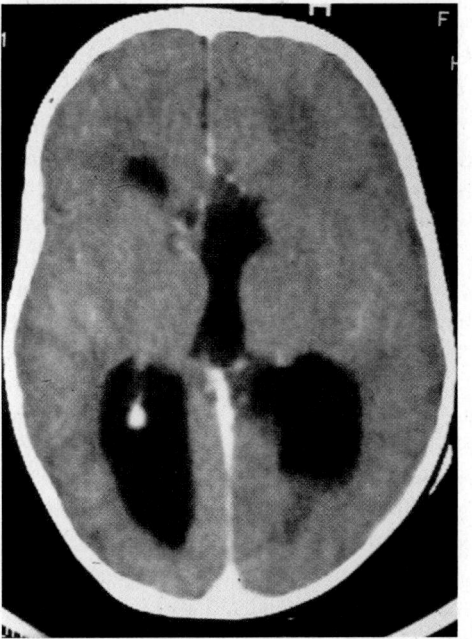

Fig. 54.8 (a) Aicardi's syndrome showing agenesis of the corpus callosum and neuronal heterotopia. (b) Axial section showing cortical heterotopia and abnormal ventricular system.

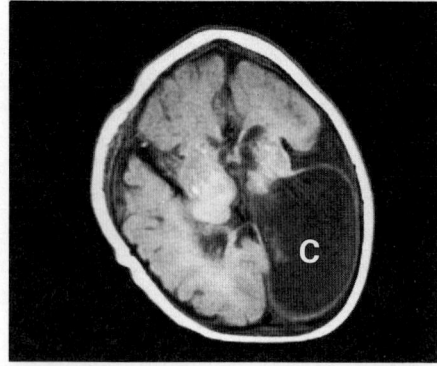
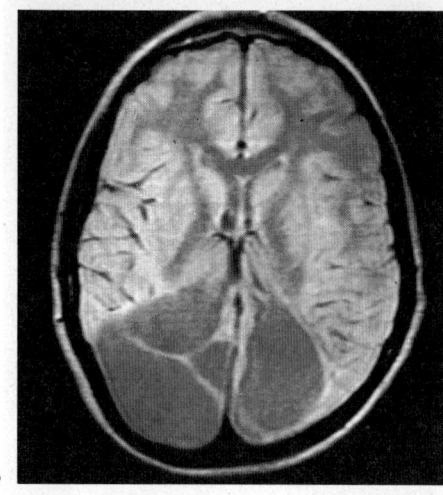

Fig. 54.9 (a) Axial T1-weighted (TR 600, TE 20) MRI scan of a 6-month-old child with a porencephalic cyst in the left occipital lobe **C**; the location of the cyst is suggestive of *in utero* occlusion or maldevelopment of the left posterior cerebral artery. (b) Bilateral porencephalic cysts.

nerve fibre bundles inferiorly and superiorly. Trans-synaptic degeneration of the nasal hemiretina contralateral to the lesion produces a horizontal band of optic disc atrophy (Hoyt 1985). While ablation of the visual cortex results in striking trans-synaptic degeneration of the retinogeniculate pathway even in adolescent non-human primates (Van Buren 1963), the human retinal ganglion cell layer is only known to degenerate after *in utero* insults to the posterior visual pathway (Miller & Newman 1981). Thus an isolated defect of the geniculostriate pathway, associated with either optic nerve atrophy or hypoplasia, implies a prenatal injury.

Congenital homonymous hemianopias often remain undetected until early adulthood (Tychsen & Hoyt 1985; Ragge *et al.* 1991). They frequently occur secondary to periventricular leukomalacia (PVL) but on occasion may occur secondary to lesions of the optic tracts (Bosley *et al.* 1991; Margo *et al.* 1991). Congenital optic tract lesions are also usually associated with congenital nystagmus, which can help to distinguish them from lesions of the geniculo-

striate pathway. Homonymous hemianopias should be suspected in children with lateralized visual evoked potentials (VEPs) (Lambert *et al.* 1990).

Acquired defects

Acquired disorders of the visual cortex may occur secondary to hypoxic, traumatic, infectious or metabolic insults. Hypoxic ischaemic encephalopathy may occur after perinatal asphyxia or later in childhood after cardiorespiratory arrests, intraoperative asphyxia, near-drowning episodes or near-miss cot deaths (Constantinou *et al.* 1989); it is the survival of these critically ill children that has led to the increasing frequency with which the diagnosis is made (Jan & Wong 1991). Although it is often difficult to distinguish the effects of ischaemia (i.e. hypoperfusion) from hypoxaemia (i.e. diminished blood oxygenation), each is associated with specific findings. Generalized ischaemia often results in watershed infarctions of the vulnerable border zones between the areas supplied by the major cerebral arteries. In premature infants, the watershed zone is in the periventricular region between the regions supplied by ventriculopetal and ventriculofugal arteries (DeReuck *et al.* 1972). An ischaemic insult to premature infants most commonly damages the periventricular area resulting first in periventricular cysts and then PVL (Fig. 54.13) several months later (Flodmark *et al.* 1987). Generalized ischaemic insults to full-term infants and adults commonly result in watershed infarctions in the parasagittal and parieto-occipital regions. The trigone area of the lateral ventricles, comprised largely of the optic radiations, is particularly vulnerable to ischaemia since it is a watershed zone for all three major cerebral arteries. Positron emission tomography has demonstrated that the posterior parasagittal region is the most vulnerable region of the brain to hypoxic ischaemic insults in full-term infants (Volpe 1981). Metabolic factors, the distribution of excitatory synapses, and factors affecting myelination are also crucial in determining the long-term sequelae of hypoxic ischaemic insults in neonates (Hill 1991).

Hypoxic ischaemic insults may also produce diffuse cerebral atrophy and ulegyria (Courville 1971). Ulegyria is the loss of neurones and the formation of gliosis in areas of injured cerebral cortex. Biooccipital lobe infarctions may occur after hypoxic insults presumably secondary to compression of the posterior cerebral arteries against the tentorium by oedematous cerebral tissue.

Trauma may damage the visual cortex via a coup or contrecoup mechanism (Griffith & Dodge 1968; Kaye & Heiskowitz 1986). Traumatic injuries to the posterior visual pathway often occur in children secondary to child abuse (see Chapter 62). The injuries may stem from direct trauma as in the battered child syndrome (Kempe *et al.* 1962) or indirect trauma secondary to

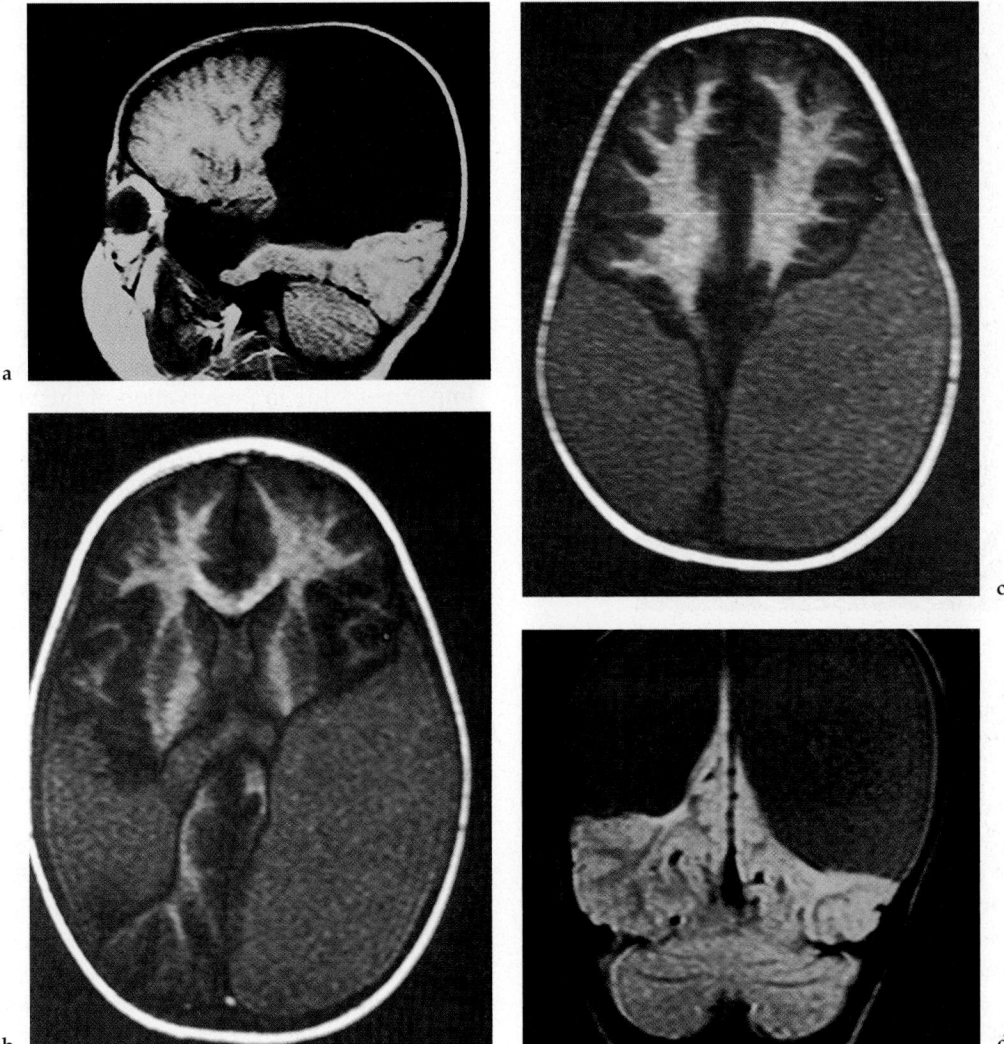

Fig. 54.10 (a–d) Cortical blindness from a prenatal vascular insult: MRI showing loss of large portions of the posteror part of the brain.

vigorous shaking (Frank *et al.* 1985; Lambert *et al.* 1986). Radiographic studies at the time of injury often reveal oedema or haemorrhages in the area of the visual cortex (Fig. 54.14).

Meningitis may affect the visual cortex. *Haemophilus influenzae* meningitis has a predilection for damaging the occipital cortex, often resulting in marked areas of radiolucency in the occipital lobes (Acers & Cooper 1965; DeSousa *et al.* 1978; Ackroyd 1984). Granulomas and parasitic cysts also may cause damage to the visual cortex.

Hydrocephalus frequently damages the anterior and the posterior visual pathways (Smith *et al.* 1966; Arroyo *et al.* 1985). Injuries to the geniculostriate pathway presumably occur by compression of the posterior cerebral arteries against the tentorium (Lindenberg & Walsh 1964) (see Chapter 53).

Metabolic disease

Leigh's disease (see Fig. 54.16), X-linked adrenoleukodystrophy (see Fig. 54.15) and other metabolic diseases (see Chapter 57) may cause cerebral visual defects.

Cortical visual impairment

Cortical visual impairment refers to the loss of vision secondary to injuries to both geniculostriate pathways (Good *et al.* 1994; Brodsky *et al.* 1996). Since injuries to both the optic radiations and the visual cortex affect vision, cerebral visual impairment is perhaps a more accurate term (Granet *et al.* 1993). Cortical visual impairment should be suspected in any child with decreased vision and an otherwise normal ocular examination including normal pupillary light responses. The visual loss may be either transient or permanent (Hoyt & Walsh 1958).

Transient cortical blindness may stem from a number of causes. Hypoxic insults to the posterior visual pathway

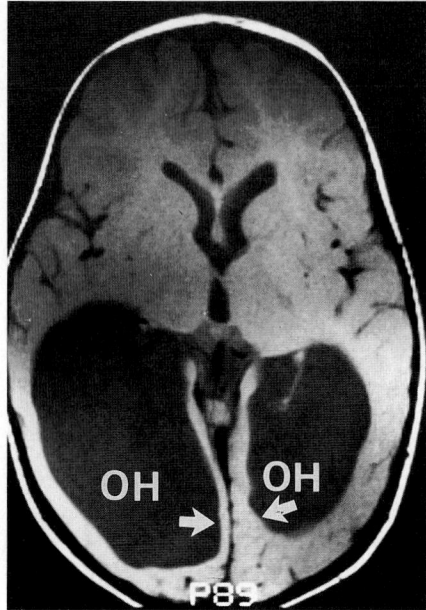

Fig. 54.11 Axial T1-weighted MRI scan of a patient with colpocephaly with dilated occipital horns (OH), but otherwise normal lateral ventricles. There is thinning of the occipital cortex (arrows), but the visual acuity was normal and there were no visual field defects.

may result in episodes of no light perception with a subsequent partial or complete restoration of vision. These episodes may occur as sequelae of generalized hypotension, cardiac surgery, birth asphyxia or metabolic derangements. Hypertensive crises and hydrocephalus may also result in transient episodes of cortical blindness possibly due to occlusion of the posterior cerebral arteries (Tychsen & Hoyt 1984). Cortical visual impairment secondary to trauma is also reversible in certain instances.

A complete restoration of vision is unusual after an episode of cortical visual impairment (Barnet *et al.* 1970); more commonly some residual vision loss persists (Wong 1991). In two large series of children with cortical visual impairment, more than half of the children showed a significant improvement in vision over time (Whiting *et al.* 1985; Lambert *et al.* 1987); however, the visual recovery was slow in many instances lasting months to years. Usually the children had no apparent light perception initially, but then with time regained colour vision and form perception, and finally improved visual acuity. All the children manifested residual perceptual difficulties, even when there was a recovery of good visual acuity. These difficulties included an apparent preference for touching rather than looking at objects, a reliance on peripheral vision, and a 'crowding' phenomenon with acuity levels better with single letters than when looking at groups of letters. While some have obvious homonymous hemianopias or constricted fields, most do not have easily char-

acterized visual defects, perhaps due to the difficulty of assessing the visual fields of children or to the more diffuse nature of their injuries (Scher *et al.* 1989).

VEPs have proved quite helpful in determining the potential for visual recovery in both neonates and older children with the recent onset of cortical visual impairment (McCulloch *et al.* 1991; Taylor & McCulloch 1991; McCulloch & Taylor 1992). Normal VEPs are generally associated with an excellent visual recovery, whereas abnormal or non-recordable VEPs are frequently associated with an unfavourable visual recovery. On rare occasions, VEPs may be normal despite severe cortical visual impairment due to preservation of the visual cortex but loss of the visual association areas (Bodis-Wollner *et al.* 1977). Forced choice preferential looking can also be an effective means of evaluating the visual acuity of children with cortical visual impairment (Scher *et al.* 1989; Granet *et al.* 1993).

Neuroimaging studies of the brain can be helpful in the evaluation of children with cortical visual impairment.

Three neuropathological patterns occur (Martin & Barkovich 1995) and are reflected in MRI.

1 Selective neuronal necrosis, particularly in the hippocampus and the deep grey matter.
2 Periventricular leukomalacia (PVL).
3 Focal or more widespread infarction.

The more premature the infant, the more severe the damage found. Martin and Barkovich (1995) found a good correlation between normal MRIs in the first 24–72 hours and a good neurological outcome, even after severe asphyxia. Extensive brain oedema with effacement of the cortical ribbon, and lesions in the thalami and dorsal striatum are associated with a poor prognosis, irrespective of the birth variables (APGAR, and so on).

In one large series of children with cortical visual

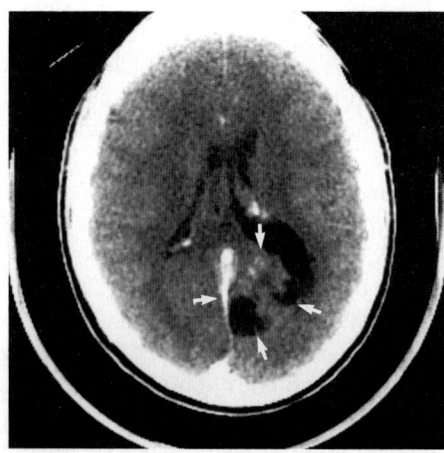

Fig. 54.12 Axial CT scan of a 24-year-old man with a gangliogioma (arrows) of the left occipital lobe. The patient has a congenital right homonymous hemianopia.

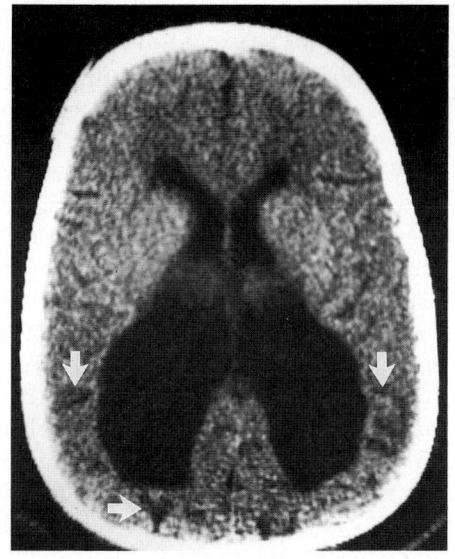

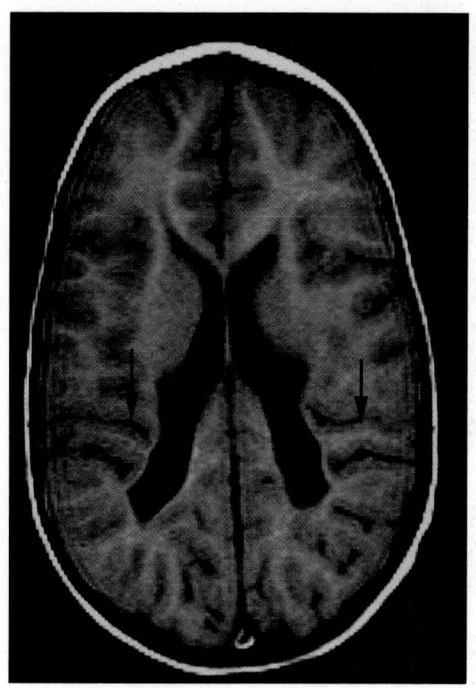

Fig. 54.13 (a) Axial section of a child with severe periventricular leukomalacia who was asphyxiated at birth. The occipital horns of the lateral ventricles are dilated and the cortical sulci impinge directly on the ventricles (arrows).(b) Periventricular leukomalacia in a 3-year-old boy who was substantially premature and had periventricular haemorrhages in the neonatal period. The cortical sulci (arrows) impinge directly on the ventricle.

impairment, normal computed tomographic (CT) or MRI scans were associated with a good prognosis, while changes in the optic radiations were highly associated with a poor visual outcome (Lambert *et al.* 1987). Surprisingly, radiographic changes in the visual cortex were not correlated with the visual outcome. Most children with severe injuries to the optic radiations had PVL. Presumably the optic radiations lack the plasticity of the visual cortex and are less likely to recover from significant injury. While diffuse atrophy is the most common radiographic abnormality seen in children with cortical visual impairment, biooccipital lobe infarctions, PVL and parietooccipital 'watershed' infarctions are also frequently found. Children with cortical visual impairment often have other associated neurological deficits including mental retardation, cerebral palsy, seizure disorders, microcephaly or hydrocephalus. Infantile spasms (Appleton 1993) themselves produce apparent visual impairment and 'add on' to any organic brain defect.

Periventricular and intraventricular haemorrhage

Periventricular and intraventricular haemorrhages occur in many premature infants. The haemorrhages arise from poorly supported small vessels in the subependymal germinal matrix and frequently occur after hypoxic insults or hypertensive episodes. The haemorrhages usually extend into the ventricular system and severe haemorrhages dilate the ventricles and may dissect into the brain substance. The haemorrhages occur a median of 38 hours after birth and may result either in a catastrophic deterioration or in a more clinically silent, 'saltatory' course. Survival is related to the severity and site of the haemorrhage; hydrocephalus, motor and intellectual deficits commonly occur in survivors.

Periventricular intraventricular haemorrhages may result in severe damage to the posterior visual pathway by destroying portions of the optic radiations or visual cortex. Porencephalic cysts commonly develop in areas of the brain into which intracerebral haemorrhages have dissected.

Tamura and Hoyt (1987) reported tonic downward and esotropic deviations in 11 infants after severe intraventricular haemorrhages. The downward deviations improved in all cases after 9–21 months, but remained to a limited degree in three patients. The esotropias were permanent. The deviations may have a similar pathogenesis to the downward and convergent deviations adults experience after thalamic haemorrhages.

Extrageniculostriate visual system

In humans and other primates there is evidence suggesting that there is a second visual pathway bypassing the lateral geniculate body and the visual cortex (Weiskrantz 1963). The pathway extends from the superior colliculus,

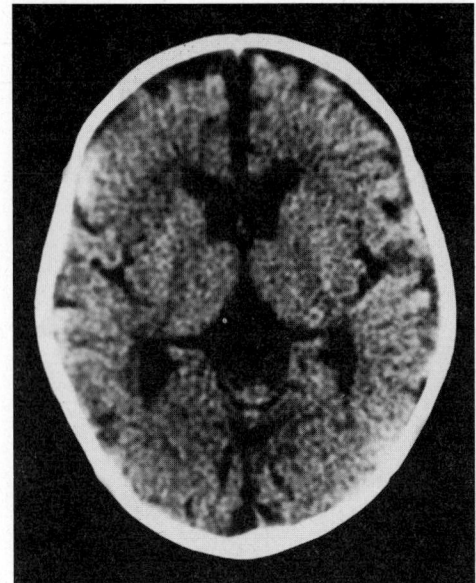

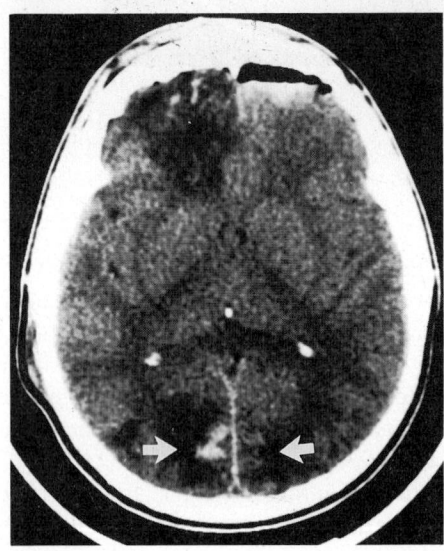

Fig. 54.14 (a) CT scan of non-accidental injury shows extensive cortical atrophy in a 6-month-old infant with retinal haemorrhages. (b) Axial CT scan of a youth who fell off a cliff and landed on his face. There are contracoup contusion injuries to both occipital lobes with oedema and haemorrhage involving the visual cortex (arrows). The patient had no light perception for 1 week, but by 2 weeks his vision had returned to normal.

extrageniculate visual pathways (Humphrey & Weiskrantz 1967; Denny-Brown & Chambers 1976). It has been proposed that humans utilize the extrageniculate pathway after injuries to their geniculostriate pathway (Zihl & Von Cramon 1979; Barbur *et al.* 1980; Bridgeman & Staggs 1982). Most of the evidence in support of these claims has been derived from testing adults with dense homonymous hemianopias perimetrically. Since fixation and light scattering have been inadequately controlled in some of these tests, the significance of these results is unclear (Campion *et al.* 1983). In one of the most convincing studies demonstrating the existence of the extrageniculate pathway, Rafal *et al.* (1990) demonstrated that projecting a light into a 'blind' hemifield slightly before or simultaneously with a light projected into the sighted field acts as a distractor for the initiation of a saccade to the stimulus in the sighted hemifield even though there was no conscious awareness of the stimulus in the 'blind' hemifield.

Children with cortical visual impairment may have a striking dissociation of their visual acuity and function. Jan *et al.* (1986) suggested that the extrageniculate pathway may have been responsible for the good navigational skills of a child with severely impaired vision. The extrageniculate visual pathway may also help to explain how children lacking occipital lobes are still able to perform some visual functions (Summers & MacDonald 1990).

through the pulvinar nucleus to the parastriate cortex (Brodman's areas 18 and 19). The extrageniculate visual pathway seems to mediate the detection of light and movement on a subconscious level (Weiskrantz *et al.* 1974), which has been referred to as 'blindsight'. In neonates some visual responses may be mediated through the extrageniculate system (Dubowitz *et al.* 1986). After the ablation of the striate cortex, non-human primates gradually regain visual function, possibly by using their

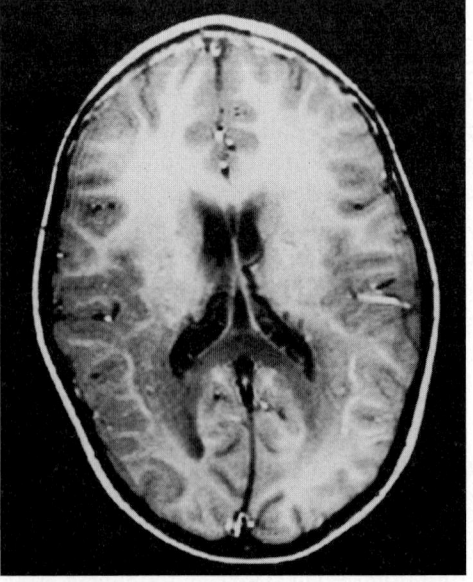

Fig. 54.15 Adrenoleukodystrophy. This 5-year-old boy presented with blindness with normal eyes. The T_1-weighted MRI scan shows posterior periventricular lucency and enhancement.

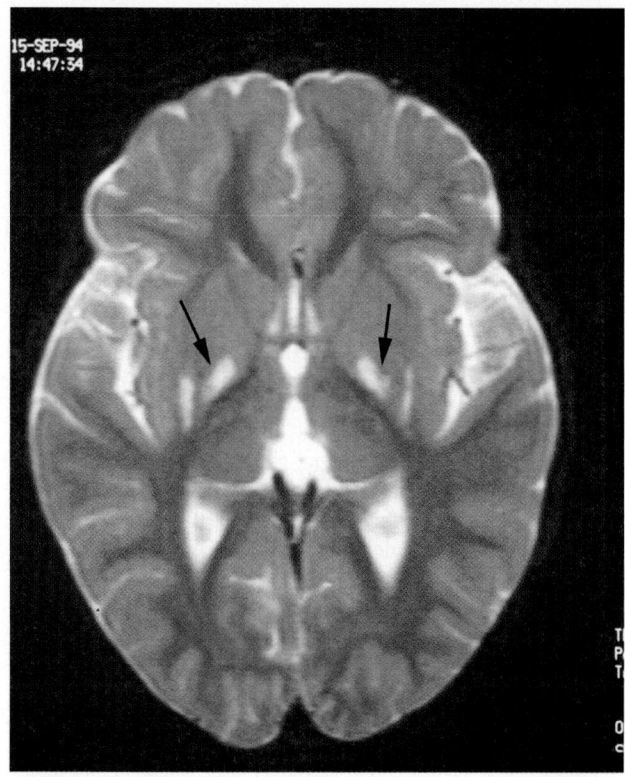

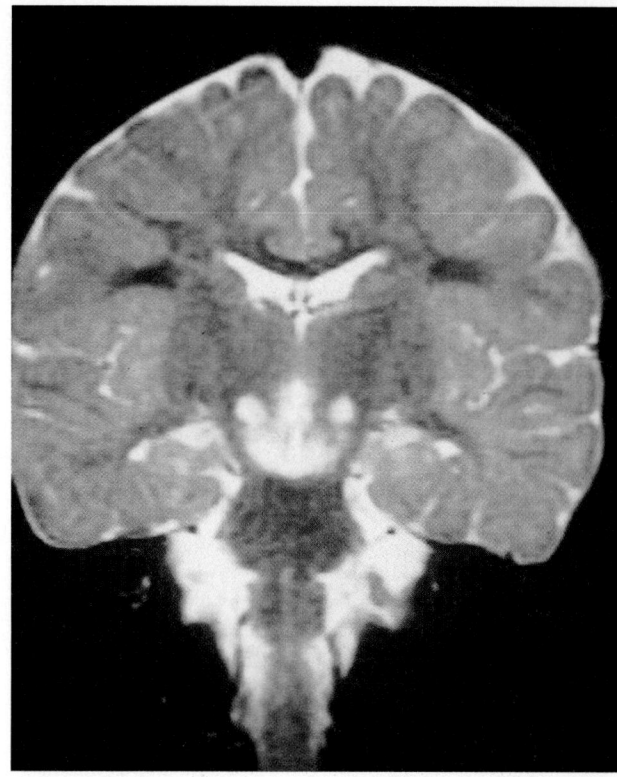

Fig. 54.16 Leigh's disease. (a) The MRI scan shows gliosis in the putamen and globus pallidus (arrow) and (b) the midbrain.

References

Acers TE, Cooper WC. Cortical blindness secondary to bacterial meningitis. *Am J Ophthalmol* 1965; **59**: 226–9.

Ackroyd RS. Cortical blindness following bacterial meningitis: a case report with reassessment of prognosis and aetiology. *Dev Med Child Neurol* 1984; **26**: 227–30.

Appleton R. Infantile spasms. *Arch Dis Child* 1993; **69**: 614–18.

Arroyo HA, Jan JE, McCormick AQ *et al*. Permanent visual loss after shunt malfunction. *Neurology* 1985; **35**: 25–9.

Barbur JL, Ruddock KH, Waterfield VA. Human visual responses in the absence of the geniculo–calcarine projection. *Brain* 1980; **103**: 905–28.

Barnet AB, Manson JI, Wilner E. Acute cerebral blindness in childhood. Six cases studied clinically and electrophysiologically. *Neurology* 1970; **20**: 1147–56.

Bodis-Wollner I, Atkin A, Raab E *et al*. Visual association cortex and vision in man: pattern-evoked occipital potentials in a blind boy. *Science* 1977; **198**: 629–31.

Bosley TM, Kiyosawa M, Moster M *et al*. Neuro-imaging and positron emission tomography of congenital homonymous hemianopsia. *Am J Ophthalmol* 1991; **111**: 413–18.

Bridgeman B, Staggs D. Plasticity in human blindsight. *Vision Res* 1982; **22**: 1199–203.

Brodsky MC, Baker RS, Hamed LM. *Pediatric Neuro-Ophthalmology*. New York: Springer-Verlag, 1996.

Campion J, Latto R, Smith YM. Is blindsight an effect of scattered light, spared cortex and near-threshold vision? *Behav Brain Sci* 1983; **6**: 423–86.

Constantinou J, Gillis J, Ouvrier R, Rahilly P. Hypoxic ischaemic encephalopathy after near-miss sudden infant death syndrome. *Arch Dis Child* 1989; **64**: 703–8.

Courville CB. *Birth and Brain Damage*. Pasadena: Margaret Courville, 1971.

Denny-Brown D, Chambers RA. Physiological aspects of visual perception. Functional aspects of visual cortex. *Arch Neurol* 1976; **33**: 219–27.

DeReuck J, Chattha AS, Richardson EP. Pathogenesis and evolution of periventricular leukomalacia in infancy. *Arch Neurol* 1972; **27**: 229–36.

DeSousa AL, Kleiman MB, Mealey J Jr. Quadriplegia and cortical blindness in *Haemophilis influenzae* meningitis. *J Pediatr* 1978; **93**: 253–4.

Dubowitz LM, Mushin J, De Vries L *et al*. Visual function in the newborn infant: is it cortically mediated? *Lancet* 1986; **i**: 1139–41.

Dutton G. Cognitive visual dysfunction. *Br J Ophthalmol* 1994; **78**: 723–6.

Flodmark O, Roland EH, Hill A *et al*. Periventricular leukomalacia: radiologic diagnosis. *Radiology* 1987; **162**: 119–24.

Frank Y, Zimmerman R, Leeds NM. Neurological manifestations in abused children who have been shaken. *Dev Med Child Neurol* 1985; **27**: 312–16.

Galaburda AM, Sherman GF, Rosen GD *et al*. Developmental dyslexia: four consecutive patients with cortical anomalies. *Ann Neurol* 1985; **18**: 222–33.

Garg BP. Colpocephaly. An error of morphogenesis? *Arch Neurol* 1982; **39**: 243–6.

Geschwind N, Galaburda AM. Cerebral lateralisation: biological mechanisms, associations and pathology I. A hypothesis and a program for research. *Arch Neurol* 1985; **42**(Part 1): 428–59.

Good WV, Jan JE, Desa L, Barkovich J, Groenveld M, Hoyt C. Cortical visual impairment in children. *Surv Ophthalmol* 1994; **38**: 351–64.

Granet DB, Hertle RW, Quinn GE *et al*. The visual-evoked response in infants with central visual impairment. *Am J Ophthalmol* 1993; **116**: 437–43.

Griffith JF, Dodge PR. Transient blindness following head injury in children. *N Engl J Med* 1968; **278**: 648–51.

Hill A. Current concepts of hypoxic ischemic cerebral injury in the term newborn. *Pediatr Neurol* 1991; **7**: 317–25.

Hoyt WF. Congenital occipital hemianopia. *Neuro-Ophthalmol* 1985; **2**: 252–9.

Hoyt WF, Walsh FB. Cortical blindness with partial recovery following acute cerebral anoxia from cardiac arrest. *Arch Ophthalmol* 1958; **60**: 1061–9.

Humphrey NK, Weiskrantz L. Vision in monkeys after removal of the striate cortex. *Nature* 1967; **215**: 595–7.

Jan J, Wong P. The child with cortical visual impairment. *Semin Ophthalmol* 1991; **6**: 194–200.

Jan JE, Wong PK, Groenveld M *et al*. Travel vision: 'collicular visual system'? *Pediatr Neurol* 1986; **2**: 359–62.

Kaye EM, Heiskowitz J. Transient post-traumatic cortical blindness: brief versus prolonged syndromes in childhood. *J Child Neurol* 1986; **1**: 206–10.

Kempe GH, Silverman FN, Steele BF *et al*. The battered child syndrome. *J Am Med Assoc* 1962; **181**: 17–24.

Lambert SR, Hoyt CS, Jan JE *et al*. Visual recovery from hypoxic cortical blindness during childhood: computed tomographic and magnetic resonance imaging predictors. *Arch Ophthalmol* 1987; **105**: 1371–7.

Lambert SR, Johnson TE, Hoyt CS. Optic nerve sheath and retinal hemorrhages associated with the shaken baby syndrome. *Arch Ophthalmol* 1986; **104**: 1509–12.

Lambert SR, Kriss A, Taylor D. Detection of isolated occipital lobe anomalies during early childhood. *Dev Med Child Neurol* 1990; **32**: 451–5.

Lindenberg R, Walsh FB. Vascular compressions involving intracranial visual pathways. *Trans Am Acad Ophthalmol Otolaryngol* 1964; **68**: 677–94.

McCulloch DL, Taylor MJ. Cortical blindness in children: utility of flash VEPs. *Pediatr Neurol* 1992; **8**: 156.

McCulloch DL, Taylor MJ, Whyte HE. Visual evoked potentials and visual prognosis following perinatal asphyxia. *Arch Ophthalmol* 1991; **109**: 229–33.

Margo CE, Hamed LM, McCarty J. Congenital optic tract syndrome. *Arch Ophthalmol* 1991; **109**: 1120–2.

Martin E, Barkovich AJ. Magnetic resonance imaging in perinatal asphyxia. *Arch Dis Child* 1995; **72**: 62–70.

Miller NR, Newman SA. Transsynaptic degeneration (letter). *Arch Ophthalmol* 1981; **99**: 1654.

Rafal R, Smith J, Krantz J *et al*. Extrageniculate vision in hemianopic humans: saccade inhibition by signals in the blind field. *Science* 1990; **250**: 118–20.

Ragge NK, Barkovich AJ, Hoyt WF *et al*. Isolated congenital hemianopia caused by prenatal injury to the optic radiation. *Arch Neurol* 1991; **48**: 1088–91.

Rakic P. Mode of cell migration to the superficial layers of fetal monkey neocortex. *J Comp Neurol* 1972; **145**: 61–83.

Scher MS, Dobson V, Carpenter NA *et al*. Visual and neurological outcome of infants with periventricular leukomalacia. *Dev Med Child Neurol* 1989; **31**: 353–65.

Smith JL, Walsh TJ, Shipley T. Cortical blindness in congenital hydrocephalus. *Am J Ophthalmol* 1966; **62**: 251–7.

Summers CG, MacDonald JT. Vision despite tomographic absence of the occipital cortex. *Surv Ophthalmol* 1990; **35**: 188–90.

Tamura EE, Hoyt CS. Oculomotor consequences of intraventricular haemorrhages in premature infants. *Arch Ophthalmol* 1987; **105**: 533–5.

Taylor MJ, McCulloch DL. Prognostic value of VEPs in young children with acute onset cortical blindness. *Pediatr Neurol* 1991; **7**: 111–15.

Tychsen L, Hoyt WF. Hydrocephalus and transient cortical blindness (letter). *Am J Ophthalmol* 1984; **98**: 819–21.

Tychsen L, Hoyt WF. Occipital lobe dysplasia. Magnetic resonance findings in two cases of isolated congenital hemianopia. *Arch Ophthalmol* 1985; **103**: 680–2.

Van Buren JM. Trans-synaptic retrograde degeneration in the visual system of primates. *J Neurol Neurosurg Psychiatr* 1963; **26**: 402–9.

Volpe JJ. Neonatal intraventricular haemorrhage. *N Engl J Med* 1981; **304**: 886–91.

Weiskrantz L. Contour discrimination in a young monkey with striate cortex ablation. *Neuropsychologia* 1963; **1**: 145–64.

Weiskrantz L, Warrington EK, Sanders MD *et al*. Visual capacity in the hemianopic field following a restricted occipital ablation. *Brain* 1974; **97**: 709–28.

Whiting S, Jan JE, Wong PK *et al*. Permanent cortical visual impairment in children. *Dev Med Child Neurol* 1985; **27**: 730–9.

Wong V. Cortical blindness in children: a study of etiology and prognosis. *Pediatr Neurol* 1991; 178–84.

Zihl J, Von Cramon D. The contribution of the 'second' visual system to directed visual attention in man. *Brain* 1979; **102**: 835–56.

55: Cerebral Palsy

Jean-Pierre Lin

Cerebral palsy (CP) and the epilepsies of childhood account for the bulk of neurological morbidity in children. The child with CP presents with a complex movement disorder which continues to pose challenges in terms of definition, diagnosis, pathogenesis, assessment, treatment and prevention.

Definition

The term CP refers to the motor manifestations of damage to or anomalies of the developing brain. Damage may arise by any means (e.g. genetic defects, migrational defects, cerebral malformation, hypoxic ischaemic encephalopathy, trauma, infection/inflammation, stroke, haemorrhage) but the damaging process is static in contrast to the progressive neurological disorders which continue to damage the brain. In the absence of extremely severe initial damage, the brain continues to grow and develop, often at a slower rate than normal. This contin-ued growth and development, coupled with physical growth, produces a changing clinical picture. In addition to excluding conditions of progressive neurological damage, the term CP usually excludes disorders of the spinal cord, peripheral nerves, neuromuscular junction and muscles. The motor manifestations include both delayed development and abnormal function of the voluntary motor system including gross motor and fine motor function, feeding, speech and eye movements. Epilepsy, behaviour, learning and cognitive disorders, including disorders of vision and hearing, are complications of the same injury which produced the motor disorder of cerebral palsy. Typically, this early brain damage produces abnormalities of muscle tone, reflexes, posture and movement control.

Epidemiology

Modern accounts of CP begin with the attribution of CP to difficult deliveries by William Little (1843), i.e. to perinatal causes. Fifty years later, Freud speculated that CP could represent the effects of 'deeper-lying influences' on the development of the fetus, i.e. antenatal causes, an issue later taken up by Collier (1924) when writing about the pathogenesis of cerebral diplegia. For an up-to-date review of pathogenetic mechanisms see Kuban and Leviton (1994).

The pathophysiology of brain damage in CP remains poorly understood, but for the majority of term infants (born after 37 weeks gestation) who later develop CP, there is no identifiable birth injury or evidence of hypoxic ischaemic insult. Premature babies have 50–70 times the risk of developing CP compared with the term population: they differ both in their pathogenetic associations and in their clinical manifestations.

The determination of the incidence of CP is complicated by the fact that there is a continuously changing relationship between the brain lesion and the functional impairment. The diagnosis may not be clear until the end of the first or second year. In the Collaborative Perinatal Project, two-thirds of the children with 'spastic diplegia' and half of all children with signs of 'CP' at their first birthday outgrew their symptoms by the age of 7 years (Nelson & Ellenberg 1982). As a result it is often several years before data on the incidence of CP in a given birth cohort can be ascertained.

The changing motor patterns and signs within the same child over time reflect underlying neuronal maturation and axonal myelination. A further complication is that some very slowly progressive disorders may mistakenly be taken for CP so that unexpected deteriorations in a child's neurological condition should always lead to a questioning of the original diagnosis.

Incidence and prevalence

The prevalence varies from 1.5 to 2.5 per 1000 live births for moderately or severe CP. Prospective studies, which include mild CP cases, have a higher estimate of prevalence than service registers, which only tend to see severely affected children.

Despite changes in obstetric care practices including the identification of at-risk mothers, and the establishment of neonatal units for the care of the newborn, the prevalence of CP has changed little over the past 30 years, indicating non-obstetrical causes for CP.

Although the premature infant is 50–70 times more at risk of developing CP than his or her term counterpart, there is no doubt that the absolute incidence of CP in the lowest birth weight groups has increased in parallel with the increased survival of such infants: the relative incidence is, however, unchanged since it is also the case that many more low birth weight infants survive without motor disability as well (Forfar *et al.* 1994). This also suggests that neonatal intensive care does not 'produce' brain-damaged infants.

Classification, clinical subtypes and topography

There are many ways of classifying the cerebral palsies.
1 Mode of onset: genetic, malformation, deformation, destruction, infective, infarct, intraventricular haemorrhage, periventricular leucomalacia (PVL).
2 Site of brain injury: cortex, subcortex, basal ganglia, brain stem, global.
3 Topography: monoplegia, diplegia, triplegia, quadriplegia, double hemiplegia.
4 Motor manifestations: spastic, dystonic, dyskinetic (choreoathetoid), hypotonic and/or ataxic.
5 According to severity: mild, moderate, severe or 'impairment', 'disability', 'handicap'.

The correlation between observable brain damage on neuroimaging (computed tomographic (CT) scanning) and functional impairment is not necessarily tight (Wiklund & Uvebrandt, 1991; Lin *et al.* 1993) (Fig. 55.1). Severe CP may be present with normal imaging and vice versa.

But magnetic resonance imaging (MRI) is proving to be more discriminatory.

Complications and associations

Epilepsy accompanies one-third of all cases: 50% in the case of hemiplegic CP and even higher in quadriplegic CP.

The risk of subsequent learning difficulties is much higher if CP is complicated by epilepsy and, conversely, the prognosis for educational development is far higher in the absence of fits. As a distinct group, cases with pure basal ganglia (extrapyramidal) syndromes, though severely motor impaired may nevertheless have normal intelligence. Conversely, mixed forms of CP do worse.

Speech and feeding are particularly difficult in the quadriplegic and extrapyramidal (dyskinetic) groups. The dyskinetic CP children have difficulty in initiating voluntary movements as well as difficulty in suppressing unwanted movements. This produces chaotic voice control and swallowing at every level of motor control, i.e. disorganized chest, airway, laryngeal, pharyngeal, palatal, tongue and lip muscle co-ordination.

Visual impairment ranges from strabismus with failure to develop binocular vision, through field defects and degrees of visual agnosia. The ex-premature infant is also at risk of retrolental fibroplasia (see Chapter 43).

Risk factors

Term infants

It has been customary to look for risk factors of 'birth asphyxia' in children with CP (Table 55.1).

Premature infants

Changes in the white matter of the brain such as PVL correlate better with the risk of CP than do intraventricular haemorrhages (IVH) (Levene 1990; Lin *et al.* 1992). Up to 22–100% of premature babies with PVL grow up to have CP, and this rate increases if there are cysts in the white

Table 55.1 Risk factors for birth asphyxia. It is often overlooked that 95% of infants with these risk factors do not have cerebral palsy. After Cohen and Duffner (1981).

Short or long birth spacing
History of spontaneous abortions or stillbirth
Thyroid hormone or oestrogen replacement in pregnancy
Twin pregnancy
Malpresentation
Postmaturity, i.e. > 42 weeks gestation, 'senile placenta'
Low APGAR scores
Abnormal fetal heart rate during labour
Congenital anomalies

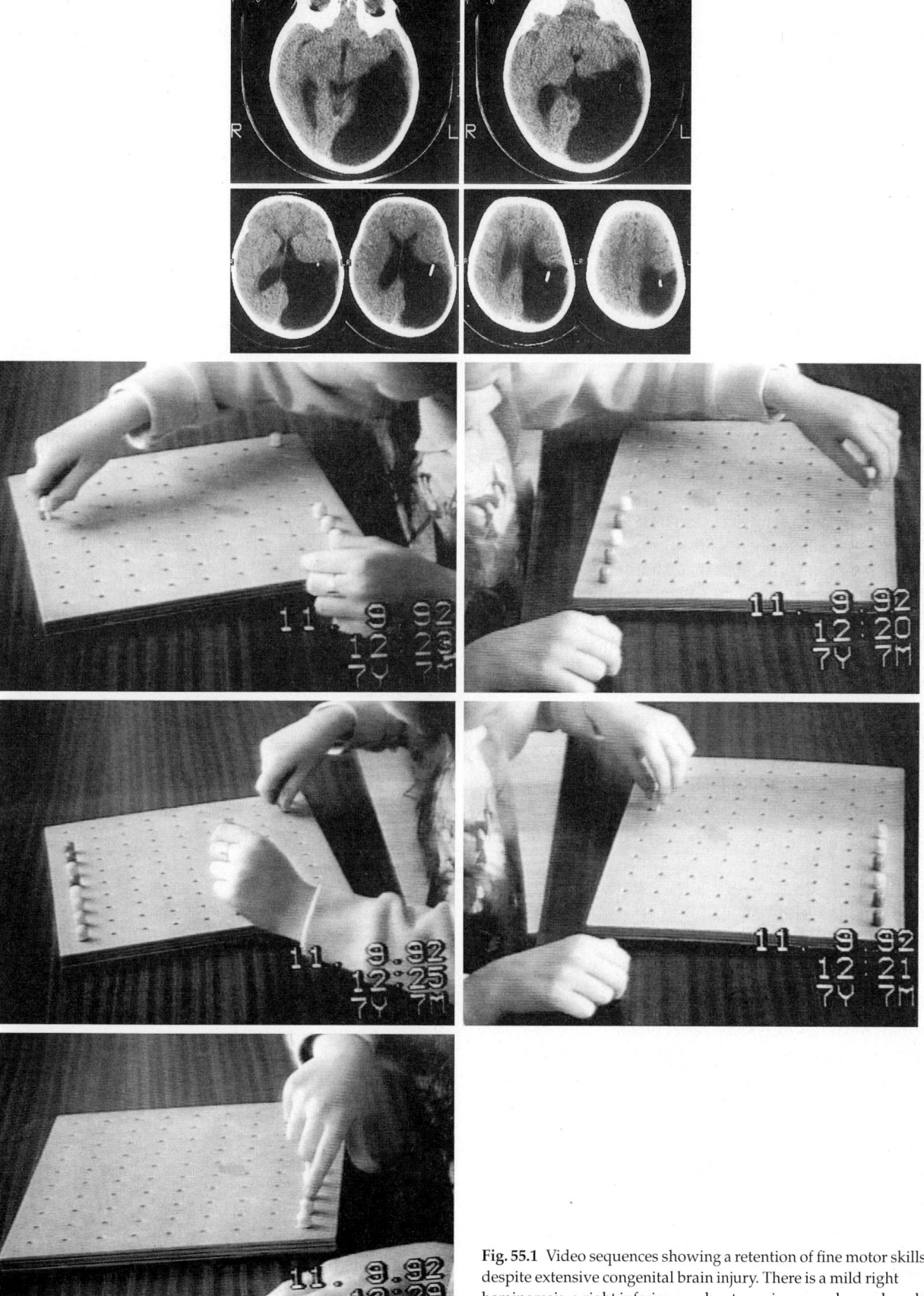

Fig. 55.1 Video sequences showing a retention of fine motor skills despite extensive congenital brain injury. There is a mild right hemiparesis, a right inferior quadrantanopia, normal speech and the child attends a normal school. The right pincer grip is awkward. From Lin *et al.* 1993 with permission from the publisher (courtesy of Dr Robert A. Minns).

Table 55.2 Risk factors for periventricular leucomalacia. After Kuban & Leviton (1994).

Placental vascular anastomoses
Twin gestation
Antepartum haemorrhage and abruption
Inflammation of the umbilical cord or membranes, i.e. amnionitis
Low gestational age
Acidosis, low APGARs or asphyxia
Intracranial haemorrhage
Hypotension
Patent ductus arteriosus
Sepsis
Necrotizing enterocolitis or surgery

matter and especially if these are large, posterior and bilateral. The risk factors for PVL are indicated in Table 55.2.

A relatively new hypothesis is that *in utero* infections such as chorio-amnionitis trigger the onset of premature labour with the release of destructive cytokines, e.g. tumour necrosis factor alpha (Leviton 1993). This is supported by a recent study demonstrating an increased risk of CP associated with maternal chorioamnionitis, prolonged rupture of membranes and maternal infection (Murphy *et al.* 1995). Perhaps surprisingly, the same study demonstrated a reduced risk of CP associated with maternal pregnancy-induced hypertension.

Assessment and objective measurements of 'muscle tone'

A lack of operational definitions limits not only the understanding of the problem of hypertonus, but also the understanding of its role in producing disability and the search for treatments.

Examples of the usefulness of operationally defined measurements include temperature, respiration rate and blood pressure. It is worth considering, by way of analogy, the significance of the discovery of the sphygmomanometer to the definition and management of hypertension, a multifactorial syndrome which may result from cardiovascular, renal, endocrine or psychological diseases. The underlying pathophysiology determines the therapeutic strategy. Serial measurements of arterial blood pressure under prescribed conditions allow evaluation of any given intervention or simple observation of the untreated natural history of the condition. Such measurements allow rational debate regarding the indications, effectiveness and complications of treatment.

Many pitfalls in the treatment of CP arise from the fundamental assumption that the problems of CP are caused by spasticity alone, while failing to understand CP as a comprehensive disorder of the development of movement (Leonard *et al.* 1991), posture (Nashner 1985), 'muscle tone' including dystonia and reflex excitability (Lin &

Brown 1992; Lin *et al.* 1994a, b). This continues to cause much confusion.

Muscle tone can be defined as the product of a number of different physical factors acting in concert but constantly changing. A good analogy is 'the weather' of which the international literature is rich in apt literary, pictorial, musical and scientific descriptions. The meteorologist makes measurements of temperature, wind speed, atmospheric pressure, humidity, sunshine and cloud covering which not only describe the current state of the weather in different parts of the globe, but also attempt to predict changes in the weather based on known patterns of behaviour of combinations in these measurements. Nevertheless, despite the economic importance to fishing, aviation, agriculture and sport, the reliability of weather reports is notoriously questionable.

Clinically, the appreciation of muscle tone is obtained by passively stretching a muscle by rotating a limb about a joint. The factors resisting stretch may be non-electrical (biophysical) and electrical (neural) phenomena (Table 55.3; Lin *et al.* 1994a).

The way the muscle is stretched allows measurement of each of these factors. The measurement of tone encompasses many techniques.

1 Clinical, non-parametric rating (e.g. Ashworth scale 0–4).
2 Length–tension measurements.
3 Work of stretch.
4 Plastic properties of muscle: stress relaxation, creep and moulding.
5 Measurement of muscle stiffness (resonant frequency).
6 Ramp stretching and sinusoidal stretching (velocity-dependent reflexes).
7 Contractile properties of muscle following an ankle jerk.

Table 55.3 Contributing factors to muscle tone. After Lin *et al.* (1994).

Non-electrical (biomechanical) factors
Elasticity (length-dependent)
Viscosity (velocity-dependent)
Inertia (acceleration-dependent)
Plastic (time-dependent)
Contracture (short muscle/short tendon)

Electrical (neural) factors
Myotonia (a slowness to relax)
Reflex excitability (velocity-dependent) and spasticity (low velocity-dependent threshold and high gain)
Dystonia (fluctuations with changes in labyrinthine input, body contacts and non-specific afferent inputs)
Posture (voluntary and involuntary, e.g. hemiposture)
Movement (voluntary and involuntary)

Clinical non-parametric rating

This is an important starting point allowing categorization according to whether tone is normal, raised or depressed. Observation will indicate whether the tone fluctuates (dystonia), is constant (as in physical contracture and parkinsonian rigidity) or is only evident when the limb is rapidly stretched (spasticity). The presence or absence of clonus, and its frequency can be measured (see below).

Length–tension measurements

This can be measured by using incremental torques. As the stretch torque is increased, so the muscle length increases. This increase in muscle length can be gauged by measuring the joint angle and plotting this against stretch torque.

Work of stretch and plastic properties of muscle

There is invariable hysteresis in the angle–torque plot: the joint angle being greater for any given torque as the torque is incrementally decreased. The area of the hysteresis represents the work absorbed by the 'plastic properties' of muscle. It is thought that this represents the work required to break weak chemical bonds between the sliding filaments and possibly also the non-contractile elements in the muscle.

Stress relaxation, creep and moulding

Using a constant torque (applied with a trapezoid wave form to avoid velocity effects), the muscle appears to reach a given length and then to gradually creep to a longer length (Walsh *et al.* 1994). The increase in joint angle can be very considerable. To prevent creep in the joint angle, i.e. to maintain it at a constant angle, it would be necessary to keep reducing the stretch torque over time: this is stretch relaxation. If the stretch torque is removed completely, the muscle only gradually returns to its original length, a process which may take many seconds or minutes: this is moulding. It is probably these phenomena which every parent of a CP child encounters every morning when applying a splint: a prolonged passive stretch is initially required to apply the splint, but thereafter, the limb sits comfortably in the splint all day, i.e. the muscles have been moulded to a different length until the splint is removed. (This must be contrasted with the dystonic limb in which active involuntary muscle contractions often force the limb out of the splint while at the same time causing pressure sores.)

Measurement of muscle stiffness (resonant frequency)

A non-specific measure of muscle stiffness can be obtained by measuring the resonant frequency (RF) of the muscle obtained by sinusoidally oscillating a limb about a joint at gradually increasing frequencies (chirps). The RF is obtained at the moment of maximum displacement when elastic and inertial forces cancel out. (NB. Many vehicles and machines will start to vibrate violently at a certain velocity threshold: this is known as the natural frequency or RF and is unique to that vehicle or machine.) When oscillated at weak driving torques, the RF is high, i.e. the muscle is stiff, but this value will fall to a constant as the torque is increased.

The RF will change depending on whether or not the muscle is voluntarily or involuntarily contracting and so may provide a valuable (but non-specific) tool for assessing tone, and should be measured along with the electromyogram (EMG) to determine if the muscle is 'on' or 'off'. RF measures can be obtained in hypotonic or hypertonic states (Brown *et al.* 1991), i.e. regardless of whether the muscles are myotonic, spastic, dystonic, involuntarily or voluntarily activated. However, the oscillation is usually perceived as quite pleasurable and may actually be therapeutic in its own right. Also the stiffness will be altered by the history of movement of the muscle owing to changes in the thixotropic or plastic properties of muscle (Lakie *et al.* 1984).

Ramp stretching and sinusoidal stretching

Standard pulsed torques can be used to apply stretches at graded velocities which allows measurements of the reflex velocity threshold and velocity gain of the EMG response generated both monosynaptically and polysynaptically. This can be used as a measure of reflex excitability. This technique provides one objective way of measuring spasticity in which the velocity threshold is lowered and the gain for any given velocity of stretch is increased.

Contractile properties of muscle following an ankle jerk

Isometric measurements of the mechanical contraction and relaxation of the muscle in response to a tendon tap can be made. This involves the muscle spindles, afferent nerves, alpha motor neurones in the spinal cord and the voluntary muscles. This allows the non-invasive physiological assessment of the interaction between muscle spindle, spinal cord and voluntary muscle in the short and long term. Slow relaxation times of the soleus muscle in children compared with adults have already been reported (Lin *et al.* 1994c, 1996, in press).

The effects of short- and long-term loading (stretching)

and unloading (releasing) of muscles can be studied in healthy adults and children and in the child with CP. The effects of interventions (short and long term) can be followed and the profound effects on the muscle twitch characteristics and corresponding reflex excitability measured (Lin *et al.* 1996, in press). These studies show that motor neurone excitability and muscle twitch characteristics alter with the length of the muscle which is in turn conditioned by the applied stretch force. The concept of the functional active joint range and optimal joint angle for voluntary dexterity has been explored in detail and shown to be close to the mid range of the muscle's length (Lin *et al.* 1996; Lin *et al.* in press).

A note on the definition and measurement of spasticity in cerebral palsy

The term 'spasticity' today refers to a clinical neurological syndrome characterized by an injury to the central nervous system which produces heightened velocity-dependent stretch reflexes, clonus, an extensor Babinski response as well as distal weakness and loss of fine motor dexterity (Lance 1980; Lin *et al.* 1994a, b), yet the mode of onset and the mechanism(s) of spasticity remain elusive. One of the disappointments of the past 100 years of scientific work on spasticity has been a failure to make the measurement of spasticity relevant to the clinical management of the patient. Animal models have been of limited use in the understanding of the pathophysiology of spasticity. A further difficulty has been the association of specific anatomical sites of damage with the development of spastic states; a 'pyramidal lesion' for example (occurring at any point along the course of a corticospinal fibre) may be flaccid or spastic and the natural history may be to stay flaccid or to become spastic over time.

One obvious shortcoming of many clinical studies has been a failure to grasp that CP syndromes comprise a disorder of movement, posture and muscle tone. The disturbance of tone may be dystonic, spastic or relate to intrinsic biomechanical changes in the properties of the muscles, i.e. both the well-understood visco-elastic and the less well-known plastic properties of muscle.

The ideal theory of spasticity should (i) be capable of describing the phenomenon in clear operational terms; (ii) explain why it takes days or often weeks for spasticity to emerge after spinal or cerebral injury; and (iii) offer clues for the rehabilitation of the patient which are likely to be beneficial.

The ideal measurement(s) should be simple to use and relate to the pathological process as well as predict the likely effects of intervention for planning a course of treatment.

The classical models for spasticity have involved the study of the roles of the muscle spindle (intrafusal fibres), type Ia and type II sensory nerve afferents, alpha motor neurone, gamma motor neurone (fusimotor) and spinal interneurones in the pathophysiology of spasticity. Such studies have established that there is no change in muscle spindle sensitivity to stretch and no evidence for fusimotor overactivity in the production of spasticity. Studies using muscle vibration have established the likelihood of a loss of presynaptic inhibition between the dorsal root afferents and the alpha motor neurone resulting in a lowering in the reflex velocity threshold and an increase in reflex gain to a given velocity of muscle stretch as measured by the EMG response of the muscle.

Recent studies indicate that changes in the contractile properties of the extrafusal fibres, the muscle proper, contribute to the clinical manifestation of reflex excitability in relation to short-term muscle stretches in healthy as well as spastic individuals. Such effects of short-term unloading or loading of muscles has led to a study of the longer term changes induced by tendon lengthening or immobilization in a cast and confirmed that muscle unloading results in fast twitchy muscle and increased reflex excitability and clonus (Lin *et al.* in press), whereas muscle loading produces the opposite effect, i.e. is 'antispastic', and reduces or abolishes clonus. Unloading particularly increases the speed of relaxation of the muscle whereas loading slows the speed of relaxation. These studies provide predictive measurements of the likely effects of muscle loading and unloading and go some way to explaining the natural history of spasticity after acute neurological injury. According to this model, paresis results in muscle unloading and muscular transformation at the level of the sarcoplasmic reticulum and myosin adenosine triphosphatase (ATPase) isoforms to produce fast-twitch muscles, brisk reflexes and clonus over the first few weeks. This phenomenon of muscular change, over both the short and long term, can be measured and altered in a variety of ways both to the benefit and detriment of the patient (see Barry *et al.* 1994 for the effects of unloading on muscle). This model argues strongly in favour of the notion that strengthening and slowing muscles is essentially antispastic. Muscle is designed to move and work. Use and disuse affects the properties of muscle and alters reflex excitability.

Treatment in cerebral palsy

The overall objective of treatment in CP is to improve function and prevent deformity. As seen above, the phenomena which the clinician is attempting to alter are extremely complex. The successful outcome of any intervention depends on a number of factors including the following.
1 Case definition.
2 Understanding of the pathophysiology of the underlying problem.

Table 55.4 Treatment in cerebral palsy.

Physical therapies (Bobath, Voitja, Domen–Delicato, Peto, high
 resistance exercise)
Orthotics (solid and hinged)
Plaster immobilization
Drugs: diazepam, baclofen, (oral and intrathecal), dantrolene, L-
 dopa, nerve blocks
Botulinum toxin (intramuscular injections)
Therapeutic and functional electrical stimulation
Orthopaedic surgery (single and multiple soft tissue releases with or
 without bone surgery)
Selective dorsal rhizotomy (multiple divisions of dorsal sensory
 afferent rootlets)

3 Understanding of the mechanism of action of the proposed treatment.
4 Objective (operationally defined) methods of evaluation.
5 Criteria for the success or failure of the treatment (treatment goals).

A comprehensive review of treatments in CP (Table 55.4) testifies to fundamental gaps in our understanding of the pathophysiology of CP (Lin *et al.* 1994a, b).

The use of physical therapies combined with orthotics with occasional plaster immobilization and surgery remain the pillars of interventional management in CP, although much remains to be learned regarding the effects of such treatments on the muscles and the nervous system (Barry *et al.* 1994; Lin *et al.* 1994a, b, in press). Muscle strengthening as an avowed aim of treatment has still to enter the framework of routine care in contrast to 'tone lowering' by slow passive stretching. Whatever the overall approach, it must not be forgotten that muscles are designed to work and to move. The three treatments which have received most attention in the past 5 years are intrathecal baclofen, selective dorsal rhizotomy and local botulinum toxin injections to the muscles. These will be examined in turn with regard to the following factors.

1 Safety.
2 Efficacy.
3 Complications.
4 Practicality.
5 Repeatability.
6 Cost.

Intrathecal baclofen

Baclofen is a gamma aminobutyric acid beta (GABA-beta) receptor agonist which was first used in the treatment of spasticity in 1970 at the Prince Henry Hospital in Australia in two quadriparetic and four quadriplegic adults over a 3-month period. The study concluded that baclofen reduced the velocity sensitivity to stretch (dynamic sensitivity), reducing muscle spasms in three out of six and

clonus in two out of four cases without causing weakness (Jones *et al.* 1970). Overall, baclofen proved superior to diazepam (a GABA-alpha receptor agonist) in five out of six cases. A further open trial in 115 patients with spinal and cerebral lesions, using larger doses for up to 6 years, demonstrated that baclofen was largely beneficial to those patients with spinal spasticity in whom 87% (69 of 79) had improved and in 52% (41 of 79) spasticity was 'no longer a problem' so that the limiting factors to mobility were the underlying weakness produced by the paraparesis or paraplegia.

Complications included: dreams, hallucinations or visual illusions (eight of 110), drowsiness (eight of 110), depression (two of 110), paranoia (two of 110), headache (two of 110), blurred vision (two of 110), nausea (two of 110) and tremor (two of 110); i.e. cumulative side-effects were noted in 20% of cases receiving treatment. There were no biochemical or haematological side-effects, but one case attempted suicide by taking 1000 mg of baclofen which produced coma requiring ventilation for 6 hours associated with hypotonia and areflexia and flexor plantar responses. All the features of spasticity returned as the baclofen wore off.

This early trial demonstrated potential benefits in the use of baclofen but already indicated its limited usefulness in cerebral motor disorders, potential 'central' side-effects and the risks of overdosage. Further studies confirmed that the GABA-beta receptors are concentrated in the presynaptic endings of afferent fibres entering the dorsal horns of the spinal cord (Price *et al.* 1984; Bowery 1989) which accords with the view that spasticity arises in part as a result of a loss of presynaptic inhibition.

Intrathecal infusions of baclofen emerged as a strategy for overcoming the central effects produced by large doses and chronic use. The first report showed improvements in the Ashworth scale in six adults who had programmable pumps implanted (Penn & Kroin 1985). Technical difficulties included problems of pump implantation, programming, overdosage causing light-headedness, weakness, drowsiness and loss of consciousness requiring ventilation. Catheter blocks and leaks were also reported.

Trials of intrathecal baclofen have been reported by Armstrong *et al.* (1992) in two ventilator-dependent children with chronic post-traumatic mixed cranial and spinal spasticity, spasms and rigidity. Both children had been given trials of oral baclofen but developed symptoms of sedation at attempted increases in the dose (30 mg/day for one case and 100 mg/day in the other). The first case showed evidence of gradual tolerance to intrathecal baclofen which culminated in doubling the daily intrathecal dose from 600 µg/day to 1200 µg/day over a 16-month period. Problems with breakthrough spasms resulted in myelography which demonstrated a spinal block to flow from an arachnoiditis attributed to the original injury 6 years previously. Breakthrough spasms eventually resulted in a selective dorsal rhizotomy at 18 months into intrathecal baclofen therapy. One year after rhizotomy, the upper limb dystonic posturing returned but was again controlled by intrathecal baclofen. The second case died following a bolus infusion of 800 µg of intrathecal baclofen after a partially beneficial trial of intrathecal baclofen which had necessitated many revisions of the infusion pump concentration and infusion rate over an 18-month period. A postmortem in the second case revealed inflammatory changes in the lumbar spinal meninges and in the posterior horns of the spinal cord indicating long-standing inflammation.

Both cases illustrate the complexity surrounding continuous intrathecal baclofen infusions along with the associated morbidity and possible mortality arising from overdosage. These problems cast doubt on the advisability of intrathecal baclofen therapy in CP: in specialist hands it may have a place in severe spinal spasticity. However, the years of baclofen evaluation have shed light on the pathophysiology of spasticity and spurred research into GABA receptor type, distribution and function.

Selective dorsal rhizotomy

Unlike intrathecal baclofen, there have been no reported deaths using selective dorsal rhizotomy (SDR). In common with the baclofen rationale, the use of SDR is aimed at reducing spasticity. However, it has been principally targeted at the child with cerebral diplegia who has already attained walking mobility, is free from cognitive impairments or seizures, has well-motivated parents, access to good physical therapy facilities and shows no evidence of extrapyramidal manifestations (Peacock & Staudt 1990; Park & Owen 1992). The basic assumptions underlying the pathogenesis of the movement disorder in 'spastic diplegia', the case selection for SDR, and the selection of the rootlets for section during the operation have been systematically questioned by Landau and Hunt (1990) and ensuing correspondence (Rhizotomy Correspondence 1991).

One overt aim of rhizotomy is to 'once and for all' treat spasticity while at the same time preventing the need for multiple orthopaedic procedures over many years. Neither aim has been fulfilled as increasing numbers of studies reveal the return of spasticity in as little as a year after SDR and the need for repeated orthopaedic interventions (Bretas & Dias 1991; Thomas *et al.* 1994). Specific complications include: excessive dorsiflexion and valgus requiring orthotic correction (Cahan *et al.* 1990); spondylolisthesis and scoliosis from laminectomy (Peters *et al.* 1990); rapid hip subluxation (Goldberg 1991); and acquired vertical talus (Mooney & Koman 1994).

The prospective follow-up in an observational study of 34 children with 'spastic CP' (24 diplegic, 10 quadriplegic), while showing a reduction in spasticity as judged by the Ashworth scale and deep tendon reflexes, showed 'considerable variability' in outcome (McLaughlin *et al.* 1994). Another randomized control study of 24 children, 12 of whom were randomized to SDR, showed no statistical differences in the gross motor function scores of children undergoing SDR (Wright *et al.* 1994): while improvements in stride length, stride time and velocity were noted, the significance of these findings was weak (Sheil *et al.* 1994).

The popularity of SDR is virtually confined to North America. The surgery, which may last up to 8–10 hours, is costly. The target group is that in whom one would expect the best prognosis for walking, and the aim of preventing repeated orthopaedic interventions or the use of orthotics and aggressive physiotherapy has not been fulfilled. However, the results of clinical trials and comparative studies of the potential benefits of SDR are awaited.

Botulinum toxin

As has been seen, the lack of predictability of a successful outcome after intrathecal baclofen or SDR combined with the medical investment in human resources and equipment required to deliver such services significantly limit their clinical usefulness.

The use of botulinum toxin, which began with the treatment of blepharospasm, laryngospasm and torticollis in patients suffering from dystonia, appears ideal for the management of dynamic deformities and postures.

Botulinum toxin inhibits the release of acetylcholine from the presynaptic nerve ending of the neuromuscular junction. This effect reaches a maximum over a few weeks but lasts several months. It has the potential benefit of being repeatable if and when signs recur.

An additional advantage is that since the muscle is the final common pathway of all motor activity, botulinum toxin abolishes voluntary and involuntary movements, dystonia, spasticity and reflex excitability. It is therefore suitable for the treatment of dynamic hypertonus of any origin. However, by definition, treated muscles will become weak, if not paralysed.

Whether or not botulinum toxin prevents contractures remains to be fully established, though early studies of its use in the lower limb for dynamic equinus (Cosgrove *et al.* 1994; Sutherland *et al.* 1994) and for use in the upper limb (Corry *et al.* 1994) appear promising.

This chronic 'poisoning' of the muscles is a relatively new form of treatment but botulinum does provide the ability to tailor treatments individually at relatively low cost in a way which proves impossible with conventional orthopaedic surgery or rhizotomy.

The risk of systemic poisoning with respiratory failure is small but nonetheless exists, particularly in cases in whom respiratory function is already compromised by poor co-ordination and spinal deformities.

Dilemmas in the clinical management

The needs of a child with CP may range from being indistinguishable from the normal child to total dependency with a developmental age fixed at less than 3 months. Treatment depends on the expectations of the parents, the carers and the child.

The first objective is to retain the trust of the parents and to be open and honest about problems. In infancy, it is essential to avoid the possibility of the child being rejected. Rejection may lead to the child being abandoned to fostering, while denial may lead to unrealistic expectations, anger and frustration. It is all too often the case that the child is too young to be consulted at a time when radical treatments such as orthopaedic surgery are carried out. As the children become adults, their needs are often neglected. It is vital to bear in mind that the 'natural history' of CP may also be acting in the child's favour in terms of slow, but continued development.

Broadly speaking, if a child can sit independently at the age of 2 years, they are likely to progress to standing and walking, though they may need orthotics (splints and crutches) and exercise tolerance may be extremely limited. The onus on carers is to ensure as far as possible that the child can benefit from this slow development.

At present, there is insufficient understanding of the pathophysiology of CP for prescriptive treatment. Current methods of assessment poorly predict the likely effects of any given intervention. Treatments and their evaluation remain crude, often relying on one-off procedures to alter a dynamic and continuous process. It should be remembered that CP is a disorder of motor control, i.e. a movement disorder due to abnormal muscular activation patterns producing abnormal movements (Leonard *et al.* 1991) and postures (Nashner 1985).

The issue of mobility is particularly complex and important for children at several levels, and helps to focus beyond considerations of mere impairment of a given limb or limbs to include vision, a sense of direction, a sense of danger to self and others, of time (arriving early or more usually late), of energy demands and economy and finally the complex fusion of choice and desire. Mobility therefore equates with independence and control over one's surroundings. Often, a distinction must be made between home and community mobility. At home the child may continue to crawl or walk with a rolator or other aids but community mobility may be impossible without the aid of a wheelchair which may need to be powered. The child who learns to walk or to steer a wheelchair is using visual skills as well as demonstrating visual awareness. It is a common experience to see overprotected children who by dint of being passively transported in their chairs behave as passengers in a vehicle: they look about in an undirected fashion and so fail to develop the skills of looking for obstacles which becomes second nature when one is self-mobile.

Prevention of brain damage

This is the challenge of the next 20 years. Mechanisms have been identified which may alter the incidence of CP. Intrauterine growth retardation (IUGR) and premature delivery are two particular major areas of interest. Both are multifactorial and raise interesting biological questions: should premature delivery be prevented or does it reflect a hostile intrauterine environment from which the baby should be rescued? One major cause of premature delivery is maternal infection such as chorioamnionitis and a major multicentre study on prevention of maternal infection with antibiotics is under way.

At a mechanistic level for the cause of brain injury or cerebral malformation, the cerebro-protective role of magnesium sulphate ($MgSO_4$), a natural NMDA receptor blocker, appears promising in animal models in which it can be demonstrated that the effects of the excitotoxic amino acid glutamate (or chemical glutamate agonists), which acts on the *N*-methyl-D-aspartate (NMDA) receptor, can be prevented by an appropriately timed bolus injection of $MgSO_4$. Ulegyrias, porencephalic cysts and cortical–subcortical hypoxic lesions can all be prevented (Marret *et al.* 1995) apparently by the ability of $MgSO_4$ to alter the excitotoxic cascade involving massive calcium influx into the neurones as well as altering calcium channels. The Eclampsia Trial Collaborative Group (1995) were able to demonstrate a dramatic lowering of the risk of recurrent convulsions when $MgSO_4$ was given, compared with the use of either diazepam or phenytoin, and the same women were much less likely to require ventilation or develop pneumonia than when treated with diazepam or phenytoin. This sort of evidence gives support to the use of agents such as $MgSO_4$ in pregnancy, probably after neuronal migration at around 20 weeks when damage to the newly formed cortex can occur. The question is how to target such treatments. From among 155636 births in four Californian counties over the period 1983 and 1985, Nelson and Grether (1995) identified 42 singleton infants weighing less than 1500g (very low birthweight, VLBW) surviving to 3 years with moderate or severe congenital CP. Maternal exposure to $MgSO_4$ of these affected children was compared to that of mothers of 75 randomly selected VLBW control survivors according to whether the mother had received $MgSO_4$ to prevent maternal convulsions or eclampsia or had been used as a tocolytic agent. Their results showed that 36% of the 75 control VLBW infant's mothers had received $MgSO_4$ on admission for delivery compared with only 7.1% of the 42 mothers of the affected children, leading to the conclusion that in utero exposure to $MgSO_4$ may be protective against CP. This suggests the possibility of using $MgSO_4$ antenatally, although in another case control study, (Murphy *et al* 1995) pre-eclampsia itself was associated with a reduced risk of cerebral palsy. A success story such as the prevention of neural tube defects with folate is a possible example of population prevention.

Postnatal birth asphyxia presents another challenge for neonatologists (Bax & Nelson 1993; Blair 1993) and a major MgSO$_4$ trial to reduce the effects of hypoxic ischaemic encephalopathy is currently under way.

References

Armstrong RW, Steinbok P, Farrell K *et al*. Continuous intrathecal baclofen treatment of severe spasms in two children with spinal cord injury. *Dev Med Child Neurol* 1992; **34**: 731–8.

Barry JA, Cotter MA, Cameron NE, Patullo MC. The effect of immobilisation on the recovery of rabbit soleus muscle from tenotomy: modulation by chronic electrical stimulation. *Exp Physiol* 1994; **79**: 515–25.

Bax MCO, Nelson K. Birth asphyxia: a statement. *Dev Med Child Neurol* 1993; **35**: 1022.

Blair E. A research definition of birth asphyxia. *Dev Med Child Neurol* 1993; **35**: 449.

Bowery N. GABA-beta receptors and their significance in mammalian pharmacology. *Trends Pharmacol Sci* 1989; **10**: 401–7.

Bretas CT, Dias LS. Selective dorsal rhizotomy. *Dev Med Child Neurol* 1991; **33**(Suppl. 64): 46.

Brown JK, Rodda J, Walsh EG, Wright GW. Neurophysiology of lower limb function in hemiplegic children. *Dev Med Child Neurol* 1991; **33**: 1037–47.

Cahan LD, Adams JM, Perry J, Beeler LM. Instrumented gait analysis after selective dorsal rhizotomy. *Dev Med Child Neurol* 1990; **32**: 1037–43.

Cohen ME, Duffner PK. Prognostic indicators in hemiparetic cerebral palsy. *Ann Neurol* 1981; **9**: 353–7.

Collier JS. The pathogenesis of cerebral diplegia. *Proc Royal Soc Med* 1924; **17**(neurology section): 1–11.

Corry IS, Cosgrove AP, Walsh EG *et al*. Botulinum A toxin in the hemiplegic upper limb: a double blind trial. *Dev Med Child Neurol* 1994; **36**(Suppl. 70): 11.

Cosgrove AP, Corry IS, Graham K. Botulinum toxin in the management of the lower limb in cerebral palsy. *Dev Med Child Neurol* 1994; **36**: 386–96.

Eclampsia Trial Collaborative Group. Which anticonvulsant for women with eclampsia? Evidence from the Collaborative Eclampsia Trial. *Lancet* 1995; **345**: 1455–63.

Forfar JOF, Hume R, McPhail FM *et al*. Low birthweight: a 10-year outcome study of reproductive casualty. *Dev Med Child Neurol* 1994; **36**: 1037–48.

Goldberg MJ. Rapid progression of hip subluxation in cerebral palsy after selective posterior rhizotomy. *J Paediatr Orthop* 1991; **11**: 494–7.

Jones RF, Burke D, Marosszeky JE, Gillies JD. A new agent for the control of spasticity. *J Neurol Neurosurg Psychiatr* 1970; **33**: 464–8.

Kuban KCK, Leviton AL. Cerebral palsy. *N Engl J Med* 1994; **330**: 188–95.

Lakie M, Walsh EG, Wright GW. Resonance at the wrist demonstrated by the use of a torque motor: an instrumental analysis of muscle tone in man. *J Physiol (Lond)* 1984; **353**: 265–85.

Lance JW. Pathophysiology of spasticity and clinical experience with baclofen. In: Feldman RG, Young RR, Koella WP, eds. *Spasticity:*

Disordered Motor Control. Chicago/London: Year Book Medical Publishers: 1980; 185–203.

Landau WM, Hunt CC. Dorsal rhizotomy: a treatment of unproven efficacy. *J Child Neurol* 1990; **5**: 174–8.

Leonard CT, Hirschfeld H, Forssberg H. The development of independent walking in children with cerebral palsy. *Dev Med Child Neurol* 1991; **33**: 567–77.

Levene MI. Cerebral ultrasound and neurological impairment: telling the future. *Arch Dis Child* 1990; **65**: 469–71.

Leviton A. Preterm birth and cerebral palsy: is tumour necrosis factor the missing link? *Dev Med Child Neurol* 1993; **35**: 553–8.

Lin J-P. Interaction of muscle maturation with movement and postures. In: Forssberg H, Connolly K, eds. *Neurophysiology and Psychology of Motor Development. Clinics in Developmental Medicine Series*. Cambridge: Mac Keith Press, 1997 in press.

Lin J-P, Brown JK. Peripheral and central mechanisms of hindfoot equinus in childhood hemiplegia. *Dev Med Child Neurol* 1992; **34**: 949–65.

Lin J-P, Brown JK, Brotherstone R. Assessment of spasticity in hemiplegic cerebral palsy I. Proximal lower limb reflex excitability and function. *Dev Med Child Neurol* 1994a; **36**: 116–29.

Lin J-P, Brown JK, Brotherstone R. Assessment of spasticity in hemiplegic cerebral palsy II. Distal lower limb reflex excitability and function. *Dev Med Child Neurol* 1994b; **36**: 290–303.

Lin J-P, Goh W, Brown JK, Steers AJ. Heterogeneity of neurological syndromes in survivors of grade 3 and 4 periventricular haemorrhage. *Child Nervous System* 1993; **9**: 205–14.

Lin J-P, Goh W, Brown JK, Steers AJ. Neurological outcome following neonatal posthaemorrhagic hydrocephalus: the effects of maximum raised intracranial pressure and ventriculo-peritoneal shunting. *Child Nervous System* 1992; **8**: 190–7.

Lin J-P, Brown JK, Walsh EG. The maturation of motor dexterity: or why Johnny can't go any faster. *Dev Med Child Neurol* 1996; **38**: 244–54.

Lin J-P, Brown JK, Walsh EG. Soleus muscle length, stretch reflex excitability and the contractile properties of muscle in children and adults: a study of the functional joint angle. *Dev Med Child Neurol* in press.

Lin J-P, Brown JK, Walsh EG. The continuum of reflex excitability in hemiplegia: the influence of muscle length and muscular transformation after heel-cord lengthening and immobilisation on the pathophysiology of spasticity and clonus. *Dev Med Child Neurol* in press.

Lin J-P, Brown JK, Walsh EG. Physiological maturation of muscles in childhood. *Lancet* 1994c; **343**: 1386–9.

Little WJ. Course of lectures on the deformities of the human frame. *Lancet* 1843; **1**: 318–22.

McLaughlin JF, Bjoornson KF, Astley SJ *et al*. The role of selective dorsal rhizotomy in cerebral palsy: critical evaluation of a prospective clinical series. *Dev Med Child Neurol* 1994; **36**: 755–769.

Marret S, Gressens P, Gadisseux J-F, Evrard P. Prevention by magnesium of excitotoxic neuronal death in the developing brain: an animal model for clinical intervention studies. *Dev Med Child Neurol* 1995; **37**: 473–84.

Mooney JF, Koman AL. Acquired vertical talus after selective dorsal rhizotomy. *Dev Med Child Neurol* 1994; **36**(Suppl. 70): 20.

Murphy DJ, Sellars S, MacKenzie IZ, Yudkin PL, Johnson AM. Case-control study of antenatal and intrapartum risk factors for cerebral palsy in very preterm singleton babies. *Lancet* 1995; **346**: 1449–54.

Nashner LM. A functional approach to understanding spasticity. In: Struppler A, Weindl A, eds. *Electromyography and Evoked Potentials*. Berlin: Springer, 1985: 22–9.

Nelson KB, Ellenberg JH. Children who 'outgrew' cerebral palsy.

Pediatrics 1982; **69**: 529–36.

Nelson KB, Grether JK. Can magnesium sulfate reduce the risk of cerebral palsy in very low birthweight infants? *Pediatrics*, 1995; **95**: 263–9.

Park TS, Owen JH. Surgical management of spastic diplegia in cerebral palsy. *N Engl J Med* 1992; **326**: 745–9.

Peacock WJ, Staudt LA. Spasticity in cerebral palsy and the selective dorsal rhizotomy procedure. *J Child Neurol* 1990; **5**: 179–85.

Penn RD, Kroin JS. Continuous intrathecal baclofen for severe spasticity. *Lancet* 1985; **(ii)**: 125–7.

Peters JC, Hoffman EB, Arens LJ, Peacock WJ. Incidence of spinal deformity in children after multiple level laminectomy for selective posterior rhizotomy. *Child Nervous System* 1990; **6**: 30–2.

Price GW, Kelly JS, Bowery NG. The location of GABA–beta receptor binding sites in the mammalian spinal cord. *Synapse* 1987; **1**: 530–8.

Price GW, Wilkin GP, Turnbull MJ, Bowery NG. Are baclofen-sensitive GABA-beta receptors present on primary afferent terminals of the spinal cord? *Nature* 1984; **307**: 71–4.

Rhizotomy Correspondence. *J Child Neurol* 1991; **6**: 173–80.

Shiel EMH, Wright FV, Naumann S *et al*. Randomized control trial of selective dorsal rhizotomy: biomechanical evaluation. *Dev Med Child Neurol* 1994b; **36**(Suppl. **70**): 19–20.

Sutherland DH, Langmann KR, Wyatt MP, Mubarak SJ. Effects of botulinum toxin on gait of patients with cerebral palsy: preliminary results. *Dev Med Child Neurol* 1994; **36**(Suppl. **70**): 11–12.

Thomas SS, Aiona MD, Buckon CE. Does gait continue to improve two years following selective dorsal rhizotomy? *Dev Med Child Neurol* 1994; **36**(Suppl. **70**): 20.

Wiklund LM, Uvebrant P. Hemiplegic cerebral palsy: correlation between CT morphology and clinical findings. *Dev Med Child Neurol* 1991; **33**: 512–23.

Walsh EG. *Muscles Masses, and Motion: Clinics in Developmental Medicine*, No. 125. Oxford: Mac Keith Press, 1992.

Walsh EG, Lin J-P, Brown JK, Dutia MB. Muscular creep in juvenile hemiplegia. *Proc Physiol Soc (Lond)* Bristol Meeting 1994.

Wright FV, Shiel EMH, Naumann S *et al*. Gross motor function following selective dorsal rhizotomy — results of a randomized control trial. *Dev Med Child Neurol* 1994a; **36**(Suppl. **70**): 18.

Section 5
Selected Topics in Paediatric Ophthalmology

56: Non-Organic Visual Disorders

David Taylor

What is it that causes otherwise well children to have symptoms, the reality of which cannot be doubted, without evidence of organic disease and why is the visual system so often chosen as the site for these manifestations?

Association with organic disease

Non-organic symptoms are common amongst children referred to a paediatric ophthalmology service (Schlaegel & Quilala 1955), and their prompt and correct diagnosis, with appropriate management, saves the doctor, the child and the parents much heartache and time and saves the discomfort and risk of unnecessary investigations.

> The fear of missing organic disease means that doctors have become more cautious about diagnosing hysteria. Several conditions previously regarded as hysterical are now thought to have an organic basis including spasmodic torticollis, blepharospasm, and writer's cramp, there may be some more to come. Nevertheless, there is a nucleus of patients for whom no diagnosis, other than hysteria, seems right. (Lloyd 1986)

The concept of hysteria in the eyes of the public has achieved such a distorted and variable meaning that its use has been criticized and the American Pediatric Association's classification now does not use the term. In practice, however, clinicians use the terms 'hysteria', 'functional' and 'psychogenic' rather loosely (Mace & Trimble 1991). But the clinical subdivisions that were included in the catch-all term 'hysteria' are used instead, the most relevant of which to childhood ocular disorders is 'conversion disorder'. Marsden (1986) defines conversion disorder as a loss or distortion of neurological function not fully explained by organic disease. In psychiatry, it is well recognized that the presence of organic disease may be associated with non-organic disease, with the classic situation being the occurrence of pseudoseizures in epileptics (Fenton 1986). The same may well be true of ocular hysterics, but in childhood the symptoms usually occur free of organic disease, or psychiatric disease (Jones & Levy 1983; Catalano *et al.* 1986). In adults, organic disease may be found in a substantial proportion of hysterics (Kathol *et al.* 1983) and a significant proportion may be deliberate deceivers. Thompson (1985) described this type as: 'The Deliberate Malingerer — this patient is a villain who, with malicious intent, deliberately feigns visual loss'.

Patients with self-inflicted injuries, known as the ocular Munchausen's syndrome (Rosenberg *et al.* 1986), and malingerers are rare in childhood. The child who has non-organic ocular symptoms seems to be very different from the adult. He is a normal child, usually not from a very disturbed background (although serious underlying social problems may co-exist), and he does not have any eye or psychiatric disease.

Freud, nurtured by Charcot, developed the forerunner of the conversion theory. He believed that the patient had an internal conflict (usually sexual) of which he was unaware, which became converted into a symptom as a means of expression after a process of dissociation, which is a mental mechanism whereby underlying feelings and the symptoms are separated.

Clinical presentation and symptoms

Mersky (1986) made a useful clinical definition of conversion symptoms.

1 They correspond to an idea in the mind of the patient concerning physical or sensory changes or psychological dysfunction.

2 They are definable, if somatic, in terms of positive evidence and, if psychological, by techniques of clinical examination.

3 They are related to emotional conflict.

Three terms are commonly applied to this situation: one is hysterical visual loss and the others are functional and non-organic visual loss. The latter two are used rather loosely to describe the same phenomenon, implying that the impairment is the result of a disorder of function rather than structure and is therefore restorable (Thompson 1985). Hysterical visual loss is a more specific description of one form of functional visual loss.

Conversion disorders are rare under 6 years old, and the sex ratio is equal up to 10 years, then females outnumber males by 3 : 1. Family disharmony is common and incestuous relationships should be borne in mind as an underlying cause (Editorial 1991).

The child with a non-organic ocular defect is aged between 6 and 16 years, most frequently 10 years old (Jones & Levy 1983), girls are more frequently affected than boys (Yasuna 1951). There may be a family history of illness or of eye disease, such as retinitis pigmentosa (Holden & Duvall-Young 1994). The symptoms seem to come on gradually in most cases, often the first problem being a marginal failure at a school eye test. Subsequent examinations by optometrists or ophthalmologists reveal varying degrees of acuity and visual field loss, often worsening as time goes on, but rarely to the extent that the child becomes bilaterally blind. The remarkable thing is how little most children are inconvenienced by an apparently marked visual loss. Repeated objective examinations and further examinations, including neurophysiology and radiology, are all normal. The condition is usually bilateral (Yasuna 1951), the most common complaints are of 'just not seeing', blurred vision, or distorted or small images; occasionally symptomatic visual field defects are described, such as 'tunnel vision' which is the most common, and hemianopias are occasionally encountered (Keane 1979). Central scotomas are rare and should make one think of associated organic disease. Non-ocular defects occasionally also occur, including spasm of the near reflex, headaches, voluntary nystagmus (Catalano *et al.* 1986), and eye movement tics (Shawkat *et al.* 1992); horizontal gaze paresis has occurred in an adult (Troost & Troost 1979), contraversive eye deviation (Armon 1991) and accommodation paralysis has also been described.

Psychological background

Enquiry into the background, looking for the underlying stress that produces the symptoms, should centre on two main areas: (i) the home and family; and (ii) the school. Conflict between children, sibling rivalry, the child who needs more attention, an unhappy marriage, overcrowd-

ing, sexual abuse or harassment by relatives or others, or conflict with neighbours and their children may all be predisposing factors. In the school it is the slow child who is being overstretched, or the bright child who is being understretched who may produce visual symptoms, but unsympathetic or aggressive teachers, teasing or bullying, sexual or non-sexual harassment are all factors to look for as predisposing to hysterical visual loss. It is of utmost importance to enlist the help of the parents, and to tell them explicitly of the possible underlying problems so that they can best help their own child, because it is by relieving underlying factors that the symptoms are best treated.

Detection of hysterical ocular disorders in children

It is of crucial importance that the diagnosis is made positively, with the clear demonstration of signs that are widely outside the bounds of physiological possibility. Marginal anomalies should be treated with the greatest of caution.

There are certain situations that are particularly suggestive of hysteria.

1 A severe functional defect in the presence of a normal physical examination and especially when there is a severe unilateral defect with normal pupil reactions and no refractive error.

2 The sudden onset of a disorder related to an emotionally significant event or situation.

3 Step-like deterioration, with the patient's acuity becoming one or two lines worse on each examination but with no objective abnormalities.

4 The ability of a patient to achieve a better acuity or better visual fields with coaxing or cajoling.

5 A monotonous and excessively slow reading of all the letters on a letter chart, regardless of whether they are large or small.

6 A single symptom is most frequent in hysterics whereas psychoneurotic patients will tend to have numerous symptoms. Children rarely have substantial ocular complaints.

7 A previous history of hysterical manifestations, ocular or non-ocular, is a recognized predisposing factor to further hysterical disorders.

8 The occurrence of visual problems in other members of the family, especially if serious.

Bilateral total blindness

Although unusual, this severe disturbance is usually easy to detect as being non-organic.

1 Direct threat or throwing a ball on a string at the patient while the eyes are open invariably produces a blink (Fig. 56.1). By asking the patient to close his eyes, the

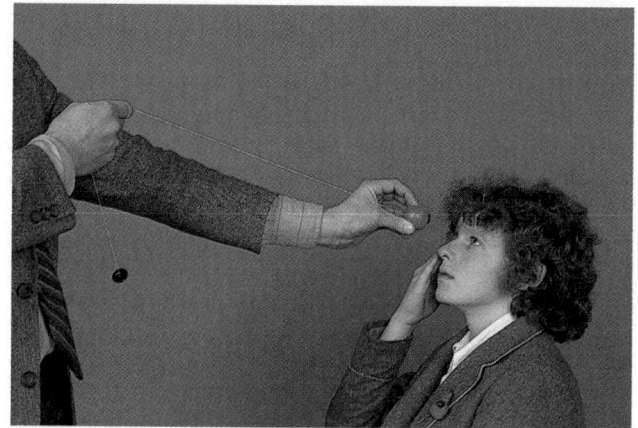

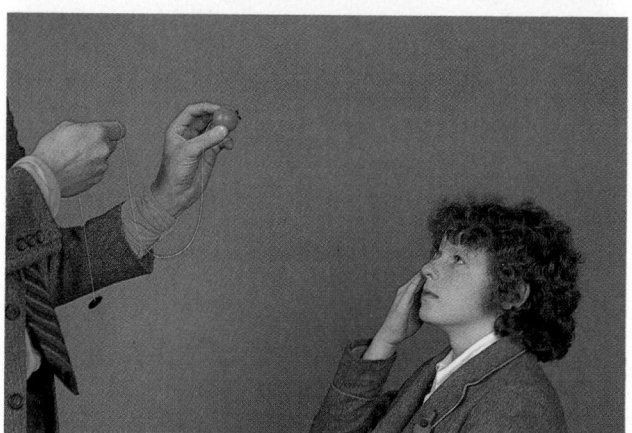

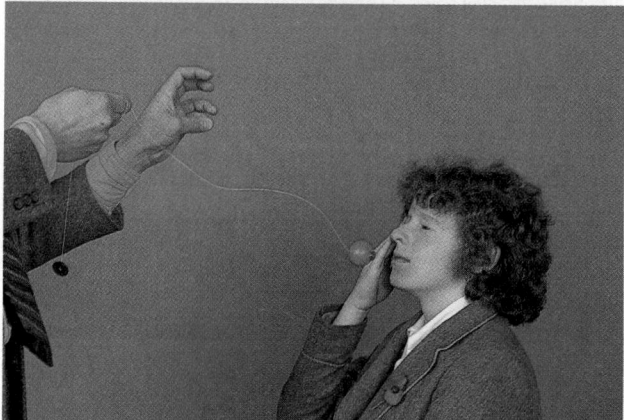

Fig. 56.1 Bilateral non-organic blindness. The ball on a string is measured for distance (a), withdrawn (b) and then thrown at the child, eliciting a blink if she is indeed sighted (c).

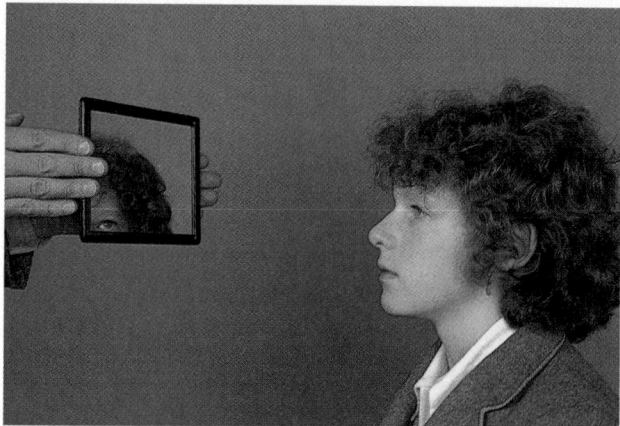

Fig. 56.2 When a blind person looks at a mirror, no movement takes place when the mirror is rotated. The sighted person's eyes will move as the mirror rotates although he feels he is looking straight ahead.

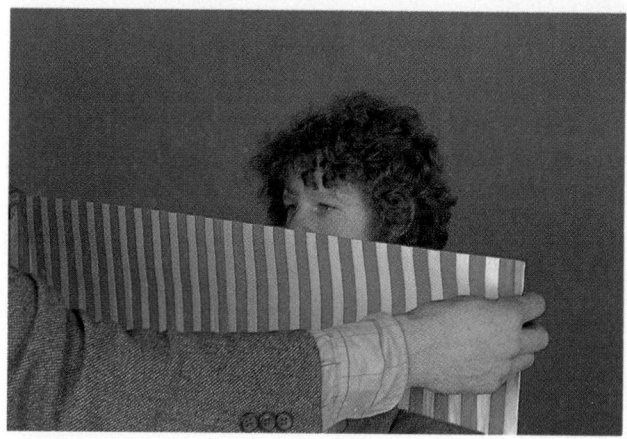

Fig. 56.3 Bilateral non-organic blindness. As long as the patient does not 'look through' the tape, the patient's eyes will move with the OKN tape.

string can be concealed before the ball is thrown, making the test more effective.

2 When facing a mirror a patient will involuntarily move his eyes when the mirror is rotated about a vertical axis running through the centre of the mirror. The velocity of the eye movement is proportional to the velocity of rotation of the mirror and the only way in which the patient can inhibit the eye movement is by 'looking

through' the mirror, usually easily detected by a change in convergence of the eyes and an associated pupil reaction (Fig. 56.2).

3 An optokinetic drum or tape, subtending a large angle at the eye, can be held in front of the patient and the drum rotated to elicit visual evoked movement (Fig. 56.3). It is possible for the patient to look through the tape or drum giving the impression that he is not seeing it. If a large drum, in which the patient sits, is available (some eye movement laboratories have these), this provides whole field stimulation and an irresistible source of visual evoked eye movement. Some workers (Aichnair & Rubi 1976) have found the Catford drum (Catford & Oliver 1971) is a useful test in functional visual loss but this is not a universal experience since it is very easy to avoid fixation of the target of this machine.

4 Another occasionally useful device is to hold up a car-

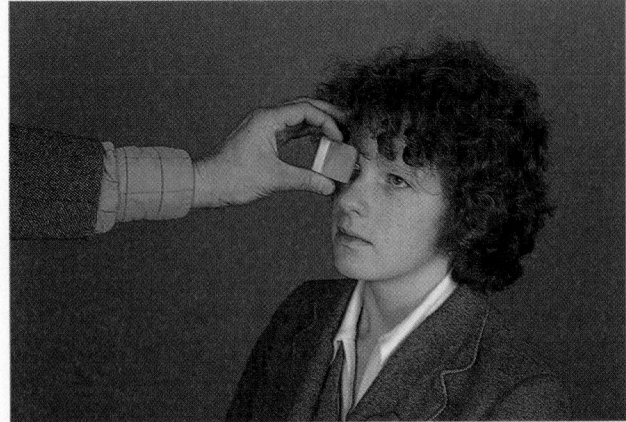

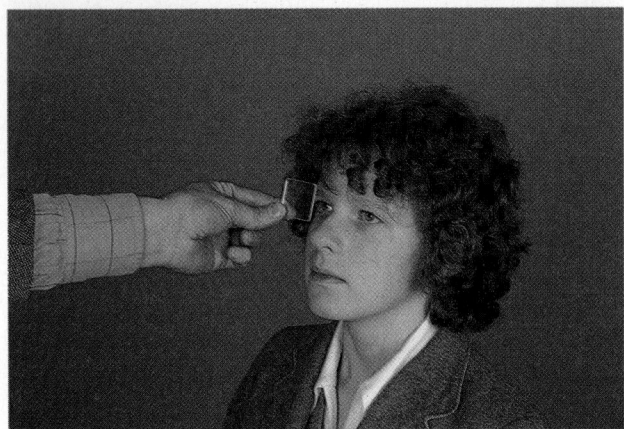

Fig. 56.4 A 25 dioptre prism (a) elicits a movement even with only peripheral vision. A 4 dioptre prism (b) requires central vision to elicit a movement.

toon or joke on a card in order to obtain a reaction. This is considerably less effective than the adult equivalent (holding up a pornographic photograph) but may help if the child's emotional state and the joke are appropriate.

5 A 5 or 25 dioptre prism placed base out in front of a seeing eye will normally induce an appropriate, and totally involuntary, fusional movement (Fig. 56.4). This will not occur in severe visual defect.

Unilateral blindness

The same test as described in the previous section can be used by covering the normal eye. In addition there are several subtle tests that can be applied.

1 A dextrous refractionist can usually manage to confuse the patient into reading with the 'blind' eye while he thinks that he is using his good eye. Putting a high plus lens or rotating two cylinders (Fig. 56.5) from a cancelling to an additive position to occlude the good eye causes the patient to unsuspectingly read down the chart to a normal level. Polaroid lenses or polaroid projection devices can also be used to trick the patient into reading with the affected eye.

2 Worth's dots, in which four illuminated spots, two green, one white and one red, are viewed by the patient wearing a red goggle over the right eye and a green over the left (Fig. 56.6). A normal person will see two spots with the right eye (the red and the white appear red) through the red filter and three with the left eye (two green and one white all appearing green through the green filter). With both eyes open the patient sees four dots if he is able to fuse the two white dots. If there is a latent or manifest strabismus without suppressions he sees five dots. If the patient sees more than three green or two red he must be using both eyes.

3 Various tests of stereoacuity are available but the one most useful for this purpose is the Frisby stereotest (Hinchcliff 1978) since this does not require the use of

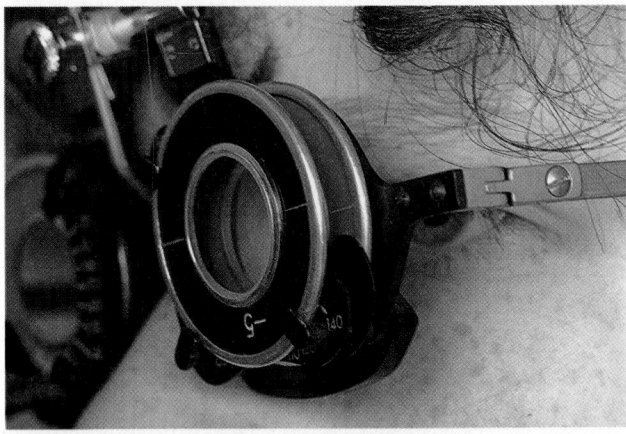

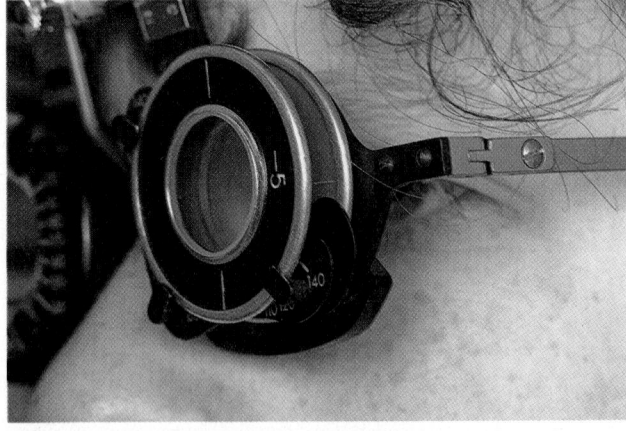

Fig. 56.5 The right eye is suspected of seeing better than the patient indicates; the ophthalmologist puts two cancelling cylinders at the same axis in front of the left eye (a), obscures the patient's view of the test type by moving across him, switches the lenses to add to each other (b) and occlude the left eye and as he moves away from the patient urges him to read quickly. The left eye is obscured by the lens combination and the right is forced to be used, the patient does not usually detect the change to being forced to use the right eye.

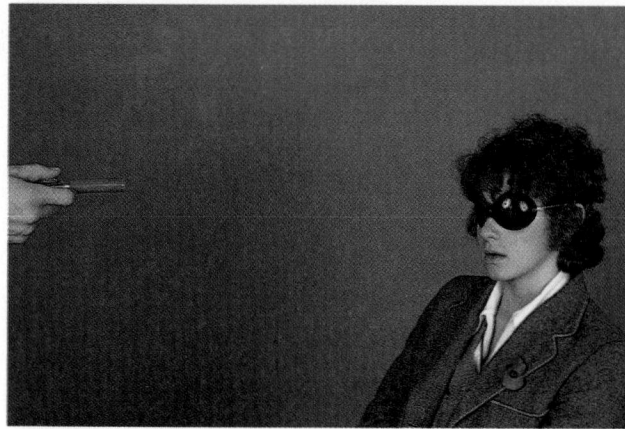

Fig. 56.6 Worth's four dot test being used to detect non-organic unilateral visual defect (see text).

polaroid or red/green glasses to achieve dissociation of the eyes. While the plate shown is held steadily (movement induces parallax and detection of the target) the patient is invited to point out the square containing a circle. It requires quite a high degree of binocular vision to achieve this.

4 Either a horizontal prism, as described in the previous section, or a vertical prism may be placed in front of the apparently defective eye. The vertical prism, if over 5 dioptres in power, usually involves diplopia and the patient may report this or terminate the examination.

5 It is in this group that pupil reactions are most useful; if one eye is blind and the other is normal there is always a relative afferent pupil defect.

6 Bar reading is a commonly used technique in orthoptics. To read with a bar placed in an appropriate position between the reading matter and the patient's eyes requires both eyes to work simultaneously in order to read a complete line.

7 A pseudoscope (Fig. 56.7) is a device in which a system of mirrors in a box is used to confuse the observer as to which eye he is using. When the patient thinks he is covering one eye he is in fact covering the other. The device is fitted with lens holders to enable refraction to be carried out.

Unilateral partial acuity loss

In this group the same tests that are used for unilateral complete visual loss are applicable. The results, however, are often less easy to interpret. Pupil reactions are rarely helpful and since there are no clear norms for the correlation between acuity and stereoacuity, the stereoacuity tests are difficult to interpret. The pseudoscope and the confusion–refraction test are most useful in this situation.

Bilateral partial acuity loss

This group is the most difficult to diagnose as non-organic but they nearly always have associated functional field defects that can establish the diagnosis.

1 The finding of an acuity that greatly varies in terms of the angle subtended, at different distances is an indicator of the hysterical defect. The patient may sometimes, by the use of a second chart with different sized figures or a mirror placed so as to hide the increased distance between the patient and the chart, be induced to read letters of a size that he was not previously able to read. Similarly, near vision testers, using Snellen near equivalent letters, may show a disparity.

2 A severe bilateral loss of acuity due to organic disease is not compatible with a high level of stereoacuity.

3 Similarly it is unusual for a patient to make fusional movement when a 5 dioptre prism is placed base out in front of the other eye, if that eye has organically reduced acuity.

Visual field defects

When having their visual fields tested, even normals may apparently perform in a non-organic manner if the examination is not carefully conducted. Abnormal fields are often associated with an apparently reduced acuity in functional visual loss, or sometimes with other symptoms including reading disability (Leary & Van Selm 1987).

Tunnel vision is the most common of hysterical field defects (Eames 1947; Yasuna 1951). In tunnel vision the size of the field is the same at all distances; usually the field is also small. Purely constricted fields, for instance in retinitis pigmentosa, are conical becoming larger as the patient moves away from the testing screen. The defect is

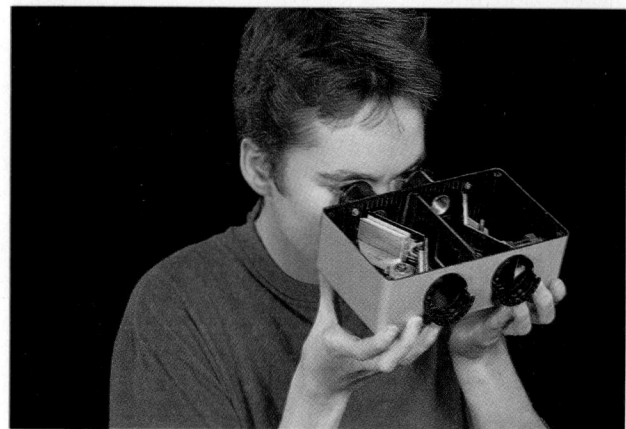

Fig. 56.7 The pseudoscope is a system of mirrors arranged to be used in a device similar to a pair of binoculars. The patient obscures what he or she thinks is (say) the left aperture but is actually obscuring the right eye. The apparatus is seen here with the lid removed.

always gross; there is an apparently dense defect involving the whole visual field only a few degrees away from the fixation point and this is the same size whether tested at 1, 2 or more metres away from the screen.

The defect, characterized by the piling of isoptres, is usually 'sharp edged' so that both large and small targets are perceived at the same point which is often remarkably constant. This 'piling up' of the isoptres may occur even in the face of gross changes in the contrast between the brightness of the background and the target; a distinctly unphysiological effect!

The absolute nature of the defect may make it easier to detect as being hysterical.

1 In a confrontation technique, if the patient alternates fixation between the examiner's eye and a fixation point on a stick held by the examiner, and at a time when he is fixing the examiner's eye, the fixation point is moved (Fig. 56.8). If the patient has organic disease with constricted fields, he will have difficulty in relocating the spot, whereas a hysteric will find it accurately.

2 On parting, the examiner fixes the patient in the eye and, without speaking, raises his hand from the elbow as though to shake hands. Given the variations of social backgrounds, most patients with organically constricted fields do not see the examiner's hand, while the hysteric will.

Using large targets, one may obtain a square visual field, the target when moved inwards from one direction being detected in areas previously blind.

On successive testing the field may become smaller. If the target is moved inwards as though around a clockface the target becomes detectable at an ever decreasing distance from fixation giving rise to 'spiralling'.

A binasal field defect is rare and may be a hysterical phenomenon (Pilley & Thompson 1975). Pilley and Thompson pointed out that with a binasal hemianopia, if the patient fixes the examiner, there is a blind area between the two which is wedge-shaped, with a base between the patient's eyes and the apex at the examiner's nose. In organic disease targets that were not visible in this wedge are visible and the hysteric therefore may see them. Hysterical binasal defects are usually clear-cut, organic ones are not.

In the very rare bitemporal hysterical visual field defect there is a wedge of blindness extending away from the fixation point. Therefore, if the patient fixes the examiner's nose and then fixes a point between the examiner's nose and himself, if the bitemporal hemianopia is complete there will be a loss or blurring of the central features of the examiner's face. Obviously this does not occur in hysterical amblyopia.

De Schweinitz (1906) stressed the importance of inverted colour fields in hysteria. In this, the red targets are detected more peripherally than the blue targets of identical size and brightness, whereas the reverse is normal. This is not a test frequently done today but may be a useful adjunct.

Lastly it must be emphasized that an examiner skilled in testing for hysteria should not let his enthusiasm for testing to allow him either to overlook co-existing organic disease, or to encourage the patient to give apparently hysterical results when none are normally present, and do not forget that Eames (1947) demonstrated tunnel vision in 9% of 193 normal schoolchildren! The visual field testing is best done with a tangent screen but defects can be detected even using automated perimetry (Smith & Baker 1987).

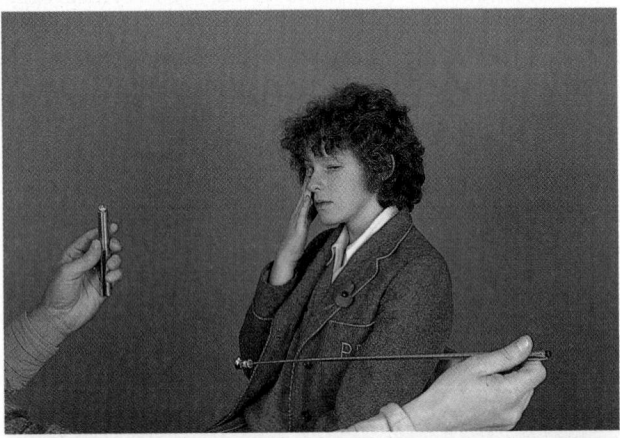

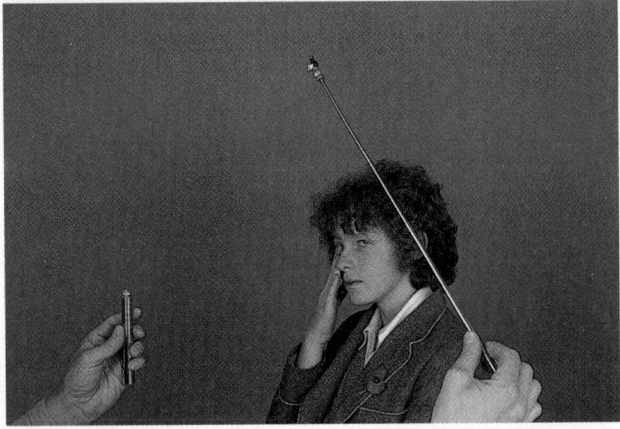

Fig. 56.8 The patient, who has been shown to have very constricted visual fields, looks accurately between the light and the mobile target which moves in the apparently blind part of the visual field.

Confirmatory studies

Once the clinician has made a positive diagnosis of non-organic visual loss and has not found evidence of any disease, there remains little to do from the point of view of diagnosis and one can easily argue that the more one investigates the child the more stress one creates and the more one reinforces his underlying problem. If there is any doubt in the mind of the doctor, parent or the older child, about the possibility of organic disease, detailed neurophysiological studies, including an electroretinogram and pattern visually evoked responses may be very reassuring and may inspire sufficient confidence to base the treatment only on reassurance. Hysterical symptoms may also occur in brain disorders such as Batten's disease or adrenoleukodystrophy, many of which are accompanied by neurophysiological changes. So these are useful confirmatory studies in many cases and are risk-free. Further investigations such as a computed tomography or magnetic resonance imaging are not completely risk-free and are therefore only indicated if the neurophysiological tests are abnormal or if there is real doubt in the doctor's mind.

Management

The most important thing is to try to find the underlying cause and this is possible in most cases; appropriate and sensitive modification of these underlying predisposing factors will abolish the symptom. It is useful to demonstrate the non-organic nature of the defect to the parents and to reassure them strongly that it is such a common problem that it could almost be regarded as a 'normal stress reaction'. There is a very strong need to discuss the condition in full with both child and parents, in language appropriate to both; it is this that makes most paediatric ophthalmologists' hearts fall when they make the diagnosis in the middle of a busy clinic! The contributions of a psychiatrist or psychologist may be helpful in refractory cases but it is probably preferable to avoid involvement with too many professionals, because this may tend to reinforce the problem.

Prognosis

The prognosis is good (Jones & Levy 1983; Catalano *et al.* 1986) and strong reassurance with minimal follow-up is indicated. Psychiatric help may be useful in certain cases and it is likely that 'integrative' and family therapy may improve the prognosis (Turgay 1990). Good prognostic factors are younger age, treatment compliance, early intervention, healthy family functioning, lack of psychopathology, insight and acceptance by the family of the psychological natures of the illness (Turgay 1990). If there is any indication of an underlying psychiatric disorder, or of a more widespread psychoneurosis, for instance if the patient has recurrent episodes especially affecting more than one system, the psychiatrist's expert help is mandatory.

References

Aichner H, Rubi E. Objective Seh Scharf Bentimmung bei Kleinstkmodern. *Klin Mbl Augenheilkd* 1976; **169**: 255–9.

Armon C. The alternating eye deviation sign. *Neurology* 1991; **41**: 1845.

Catalano RA, Simon JW, Krohel GB, Rosenburg PN. Functional visual loss in children. *J Am Acad Ophthalmol* 1986; **93**: 385–91.

Catford GV, Oliver A. A method of visual acuity detection. Proceedings of the Second International Orthoptic Congress, Amsterdam. *Excerpta Med* 1971; 183–20.

De Schweinitz GW. Neuroses and psychoses. In: Posey WC, Spiller WG, eds. *The Eye and the Nervous System*. Lippincott, 1906: 614–96.

Eames TH. A study of tubular and spiral central fields. *Am J Ophthalmol* 1947; **30**: 610–11.

Editorial. Neurological conversion disorders in childhood. *Lancet* 1991; **337**: 889–90.

Fenton GW. Epilepsy and hysteria. *Br J Psychiatr* 1986; **149**: 28–37.

Hinchcliff H. Clinical evaluation of stereopsis. *Br Orthopt J* 1978; **35**: 46–50.

Holden R, Duvall-Young J. Functional visual deficit in children with a family history of retinitis pigmentosa. *J Pediatr Ophthalmol Strabismus* 1994; **31**: 323–4.

Jones JB, Barklage NE. Conversion disorder: camouflage for brain lesions in two cases. *Arch Int Med* 1990; **150**: 1343–5.

Jones RB, Levy IS. Hysterical blindness in pediatric ophthalmology. In: Wybar KC, Taylor DSI, eds. *Pediatric Ophthalmology*. New York: Marcel Dekker, 1983: 399–405.

Kathol RG, Cox TA, Corbett JJ, Thompson HS. Functional visual loss. *Arch Ophthalmol* 1983; **101**: 729–35.

Keane JR. Hysterical hemianopia. *Arch Ophthamol* 1979; **97**: 865–6.

Leary PM, Van Selm JL. Tunnel vision presenting as reading disability. *J Roy Soc Med* 1987; **80**: 585–7.

Lloyd GG. Hysteria: a case for conservation. *Br Med J* 1986; **293**: 1255–6.

Mace CJ, Trimble MR. 'Hysteria', 'functional' or 'psychogenic'? A survey of British neurologist's preferences. *J Roy Soc Med* 1991; **84**: 471–6.

Marsden CD. Hysteria: a neurologist's view. *Psychol Med* 1986; **149**: 28–37.

Mersky H. Disorders of conscious awareness: hysterical phenomena. *Br J Hosp Med* 1986; **19**: 305–9.

Pilley SJH, Thompson HS. Binasal field loss and prefixation blindness. In: Glaser J, Smith JL, eds. *Neuro-ophthalmology*, Vol. 8. St Louis: CV Mosby, 1975: 277–84.

Rosenberg PN, Krohel GB, Webb RM, Hepler RS. Ocular Munchausen's syndrome. *Ophthalmology* 1986; **93**: 1120–4.

Schlaegel TF Jr, Quilala FV. Hysterical amblyopia; statistical analysis of 42 cases found in a survey of 800 unselected eye patients at a state medical center. *Arch Ophthalmol* 1955; **54**: 875–84.

Shawkat F, Harris C, Jacobs M, Taylor D, Brett E. Eye movement tics. *Br J Ophthalmol* 1992; **76**: 697–9.

Smith TJ, Baker RS. Perimetric findings in functional disorders using automated techniques. *J Am Acad Ophthalmol* 1987; **94**: 1562–7.

Thompson SH. Functional visual loss. *Am J Ophthalmol* 1985; **100**: 209–13.

Troost TB, Troost GE. Functional paralysis of horizontal gaze. *Neurology* 1979; **29**: 82–5.

Turgay A. Treatment outcome for children and adolescents with conversion disorder. *Canad J Psychiatr* 1990; **35**: 585–9.

Yasuna ER. Hysterical amblyopia in children and young adults. *Arch Ophthalmol* 1951; **45**: 70–6.

57: Neurometabolic Disease

David Taylor

Gangliosidoses

Amaurotic family idiocy is a term which used to be applied to a variety of neurometabolic diseases. It has outlived its usefulness because it is inappropriately non-specific and often hurtful to parents.

GM2 gangliosidoses

GM stands for ganglioside monosialo and the numbers 1, 2 and 3 for their positions on a thin layer plate.

Tay–Sachs disease (GM2 type I)

Warren Tay, a London ophthalmologist, first described this disease but it was the frequency of the gene in people of Ashkenazi Jewish stock that led to the finding of the disease in New York where it was described as 'amaurotic family idiocy' by Bernard Sachs in 1887. It is an autosomal recessive disorder in which a deficient activity of hexosaminidase A leads to an accumulation of GM2 ganglioside in the neurones of the brain and elsewhere. Children with the disease present early in their first year of life with a loss of skills already acquired, blindness, seizures, spasticity and an exaggerated startle response to sound and light flash stimuli which may be the first abnormality noted by the parents. The head enlarges and the child usually dies by 4 years of age.

Ophthalmoscopy at an early stage reveals the characteristic cherry red spot which is due to ganglioside accumulation in the retinal ganglion cells (Cogan & Kuwabara 1959). The absence of ganglion cells at the fovea gives rise to the red spot surrounded by white diseased cells.

As the ganglion cells die the cherry red spot fades and optic atrophy becomes apparent. The electroretinogram (ERG) is normal or large (Godel *et al.* 1978) but the visual evoked response (VER) extinguished (Honda & Sudo 1976). The injection of placental hexosaminidase A enzyme did not improve these neurophysiological parameters in three patients (Godel *et al.* 1978).

The gene has been mapped to 15q23–q24 (Nakai *et al.* 1987).

Sandhoff's disease (GM2 type II)

These children have a clinical disease similar to that of Tay–Sachs patients, but have a deficient activity of both hexosaminidase A and B. The gene frequency in the Jewish population is one in 1000, but in this case, the disease is more frequent in non-Jews, in whom the frequency is probably one in 600 (Canter & Kabach 1985).The gene for hexosaminidase B has been localized to 5q31–qter (Fox *et al.* 1984).

Juvenile (GM2 type III)

This is a very rare variant with an onset of ataxia between 2 and 6 years with late onset of blindness, which may lead to it being misdiagnosed as Batten's disease. However, the ERG is normal in gangliosidoses. There is a partial defect of hexosaminidase A. A faint cherry red spot sometimes occurs (Brett *et al.* 1973). Patients may have eye movement defects including pursuit and vestibulo-ocular reflex suppression defects and saccadic dysmetria; the ERG and VER are normal (Musarella *et al.* 1982).

GM1 gangliosidoses

Infantile (GM1 type I)

This is a rare autosomal recessive trait with deficient activity of beta-galactosidase leading to the accumulation of GM1 gangliosides. There is no racial predilection.

Children are affected at birth or very early in infancy with the following symptoms.
1 Severe cerebral degeneration and regression with death by 2 years.
2 Seizures in some patients.
3 Visceral involvement of liver, spleen, bone marrow and kidney.
4 Coarse features with a Hurler's syndrome-like appearance.

5 A cherry red spot, retinal haemorrhages, and occasionally corneal clouding (Emery *et al.* 1971).

The diagnosis may be suspected by finding large foamy histiocytes in bone marrow aspirate and vacuolated lymphocytes in peripheral blood but clinicians usually seek confirmation by enzyme analysis as a first procedure.

Late infantile (GM1 type II)

This autosomal recessive disease presents in older children with mental and motor regression and seizures, followed by spasticity and decerebrate rigidity. Their facial features appear normal, but they may have kyphoscoliosis. They have abnormal marrow histiocytes and deficient beta-galactosidase. Neuro-ophthalmological problems are not dominant in the clinical picture.

Prenatal diagnosis in the gangliosidoses

Prenatal diagnosis is available by assaying the enzymes from cultured amniotic cells or chorionic villus biopsy and is applicable to parents with one or more affected children but the gene frequency is not sufficiently high for screening in most populations.

Batten's disease (neuronal ceroid lipofuscinosis)

In childhood, four main forms of Batten's disease occur. All are characterized by visual deterioration with retinal degeneration and a severely abnormal ERG, seizures and mental regression. Because the infantile and late infantile types have a rapid downhill course and are already diagnosed by the neurologist, the paediatric ophthalmologist rarely has a role to play.

Excellent reviews of pathological aspects of Batten's disease are provided by Lake (1984) and Multiple Authors (1993).

Infantile

- Haltia–Santavuori disease.
- Infantile neuronal ceroid lipofuscinosis.

These babies present between 8 and 18 months of age with myoclonus, mental and motor regression, and visual failure (Santavouri *et al.* 1973). There is severe neuronal destruction with phagocytosis by often binucleated cells, and fibrillary astrocytes are found in the cerebral cortex (Haltia *et al.* 1973) which leads to microcephaly. Blindness occurs early in the course of the disease with an absent ERG or a low amplitude ERG which later becomes isoelectric (Pampiglione & Harden 1977). The flash VER is diminished in amplitude. Death occurs by 4 years. First described in children of Finnish/Swedish stock, cases have been recognized around the world in several racial groups. The retinas show narrow blood vessels, some pigment epithelial changes around the macula and later optic atrophy and clumped retinal pigmentation (Raitta & Santavouri 1973; Bateman & Phillipart 1986). Cherry red spots are not seen. Neurones contain granular osmophilic deposits known by the acronym 'GROD' or as 'Finnish snowballs' and the diagnosis can be made on ultrastructural studies of rectal neurones or of peripheral leucocytes (Baumann & Markesbery 1982). It is inherited as an autosomal recessive trait and it occurs in many races. The gene has been localized to chromosome 1.

Late infantile

* Jansky–Bielschowsky disease.
* Late infantile neuronal ceroid lipofuscinosis.

These children present from 2 to 4 years of age with mental deterioration, ataxia, myoclonic jerks and epilepsy with death by 7 years. They become blind early from retinal degeneration, most marked at the macula, but later the whole retina is affected and appears thinned with clumped pigment, narrow arterioles and optic atrophy. The ERG is extinguished early but there is an extraordinarily enlarged VER amplitude, many times the normal. The electroencephalogram (EEG) shows large spikes at low rates of photic stimulation (Pampiglione & Harden 1977).

Diagnosis is established by the finding of characteristic electron microscopic curvilinear bodies in rectal neurones, lymphocytes (Markesbury *et al.* 1976) or in sural nerve (Bolmers *et al.* 1973) (skin and conjunctival biopsies have also been used). It is inherited as an autosomal recessive trait and there is no racial predilection.

Juvenile

* Batten–Mayou disease.
* Vogt–Spielmeyer disease.
* Spielmeyer–Sjögren disease.
* Juvenile neuronal ceroid lipofuscinosis.

Frederick Batten (1903), a pathologist of the National Hospital, Queen Square, and later a physician at the Hospital for Sick Children, Great Ormond Street, London, described two siblings with a maculopathy and progressive mental retardation and he later (Batten 1914) cited another family described by Vogt in 1905. Other cases were described at this time (Mayou 1904; Spielmeyer 1905). Mayou gave a good description of the retinae when he noted granular pigmentation with a reddish-black spot at the macula. In the discussion following the presentation of Mayou's paper, Mr Sidney Stephenson said 'a number of such cases have been recorded in the last few years and it must be a gratification to the Society [the Ophthalmological Society of the UK] that the first case of this kind was shown at the Society by Mr Rayner Batten in 1897'.

R.E. Batten was F.E. Batten's older brother, but he described patients with only a retinal and not a combined retinal and cerebral degeneration. Not just for chauvinistic reasons has the name Batten stuck!

Juvenile Batten's disease is the most common neurodegenerative disease seen by paediatric ophthalmologists today, and it represents a small but important cause of child blindness in the UK. It is still of considerable clinical and academic interest. Perhaps 25–30% of the children each year registered as blind with acquired retinal or macular disease have Batten's disease (Spalton *et al.* 1980). Its incidence in West Germany is 0.7 per 100 000 live births (Claussen *et al.* 1992).

Children with juvenile Batten's disease present with visual failure between 4 and 10 years, with a peak incidence at 6 years (Spalton *et al.* 1980). The earliest change is a bull's eye maculopathy (Fig. 57.1) but the whole retina is affected early as shown by the ERG changes, which are present early in the disease (Pampiglione & Harden 1977; Hussain & Marshall 1993). Attenuation of the b-wave of the ERG, with initial preservation of the EOG, and later involvement of all elements of the ERG suggested to Pinckers and Bolmers (1974) that the retina between the receptors and ganglion cells was primarily affected. Later there is a widespread retinal degeneration with pigment clumping and sparse bone spicule pigmentation in the periphery, the disc becomes atrophic and the arterioles thinned (Fig. 57.2). The whole retina becomes avascular (De Venecia & Shapiro 1984). The children are usually functionally blind within 3 years.

Most affected children were always dull but mental deterioration and behavioural disturbances occur early, often predating the visual deterioration. They are often quite subtle and their occurrence led Harcourt and Hopkins (1962) to believe that behavioural disturbances were frequent in children with idiopathic retinal dystrophies;

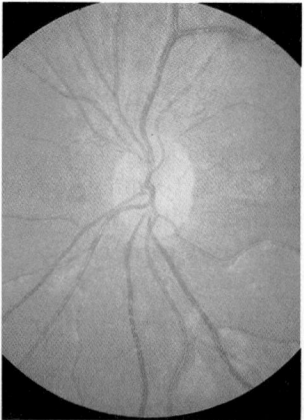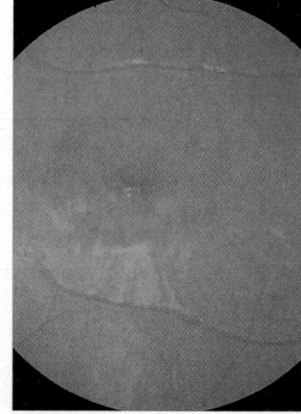

Fig. 57.1 Optic atrophy, arteriolar thinning and bull's eye maculopathy in juvenile Batten's disease.

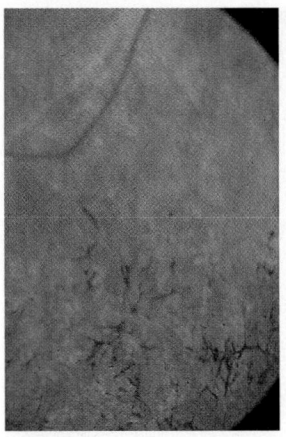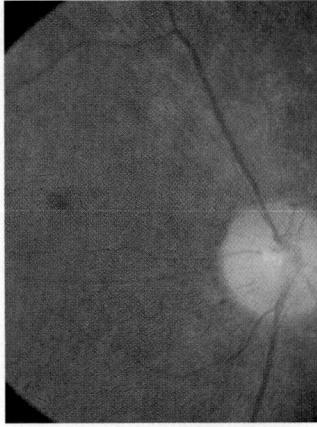

Fig. 57.2 Late retinal changes in juvenile Batten's disease include bone-spicule pigmentation, optic atrophy and extreme arteriolar narrowing.

some of these children subsequently developed Batten's disease.

It is the onset of fits between 7 and 16 years of age that often leads to the diagnosis. The delay in diagnosis is understandably frequent; it was by as much as 9 years in four patients in Spalton *et al.*'s (1980) series. The seizures are not usually difficult to control, and are often infrequent initially. The flash VER may show reduced early components initially, but becomes extinguished and the EEG shows runs of large amplitude and slow wave and spike complexes (Pampiglione & Harden 1977; Westmoreland *et al.* 1979). Computed tomographic (CT) scanning shows diffuse supra- and intratentorial brain atrophy (Valavanis *et al.* 1980; Raininko *et al.* 1990).

One characteristic finding at presentation is of eccentric viewing, with the patient tending to overlook the 'target' (Good 1992) and this may be due to a relative preservation of the upper retina. Affected children tend to rub or poke their eye and this may account for the keratoconus and cataracts seen in some patients. Fluorescein angiography may show leakage in rapidly degenerating retinae, but generally only shows evidence of retinal pigment epithelial degeneration.

The disease follows a depressingly slow downward path with dementia occurring in the teens and death sometimes well into the second or third decade.

Juvenile Batten's disease occurs with equal frequency in both males and females, seems to have no racial predilection and is inherited as an autosomal recessive trait.

Diagnosis is suspected by finding vacuolated lymphocytes (Fig. 57.3) in the peripheral blood smears and is confirmed by the finding of characteristic 'fingerprint' (Fig. 57.4) inclusions in neurones on electron microscopy studies of rectal biopsies (Lake 1976). Other biopsy material can be examined ultrastructurally including skin, conjunctiva and lymphocytes (Baumann & Markesbery 1978;

Jaben *et al.* 1983; Brod *et al.* 1987). 'A spectrum of biochemical defects has been implicated in these disorders, but many of these biochemical changes are no longer regarded as useful in detecting affected but asymptomatic individuals, carriers or even normals in a highly reproducible manner' (Rider *et al.* 1992). Attention was focused on the presence of ceroid and lipofuscin in neurones, hence the name neuronal ceroid lipofuscinosis. It was thought that there was a defect in peroxidation of fatty acids (Den Tandt & Van Martin 1978), and the finding of low levels of docosahexanoic acids in leucocytes was used to support this (Pullarkat *et al.* 1978). Antioxidant treatment, however, failed to influence the disease (Santavuori & Moren 1977). The neuronal deposits are autofluorescent pigments which were thought to be retinoyl complexes (Wolfe *et al.* 1977) but more recently attention has focused on phosphorylated dolichol (Hall & Patrick 1987) and on subunit C of mitochondrial adenosine triphosphate (ATP) synthase complex (Multiple Authors 1992, 1993).

There is no treatment though prenatal diagnosis is pos-

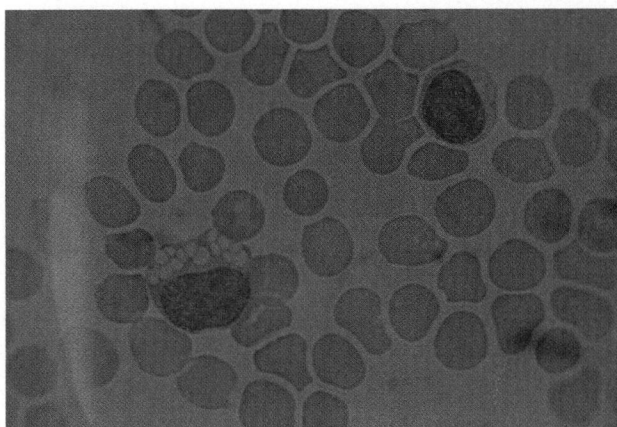

Fig. 57.3 Juvenile Batten's disease—lymphocyte inclusions.

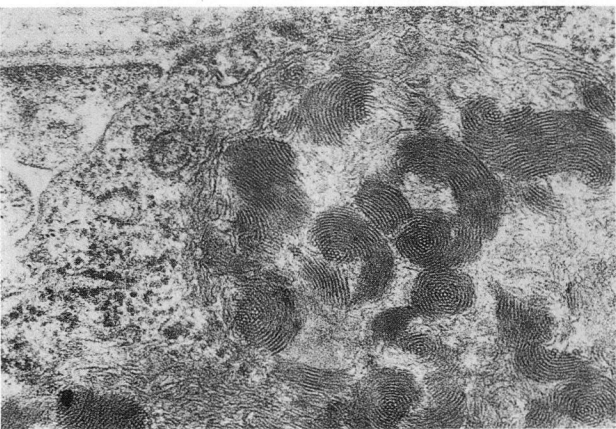

Fig. 57.4 Juvenile Batten's disease—'fingerprint' inclusions in rectal neurones.

sible. Bone marrow transplantation is not promising (Deeg *et al*. 1990). Parents may be offered presymptomatic diagnosis for apparently unaffected siblings but many prefer to await the course of events. The gene is at 16p12.1 (Gardiner *et al*. 1990; Mitchison *et al*. 1993; Batten's Disease Consortium 1995).

Early juvenile Batten's disease

Several patients with presentation around 5 years of age similar to the late infantile form but with a course and histopathology similar to the juvenile form have been described (Lake & Cavanagh 1978; Kohlschütter *et al*. 1993) but there are no vacuolated lymphocytes.

Kufs' disease

Kufs' disease is an adult onset form of Batten's disease with no ophthalmological abnormalities (Martin 1993).

Niemann–Pick disease

As a result of an international symposium Niemann–Pick disease is now classified into two basic groups (Elleder & Jirasek 1983).

Group 1

These patients are sphingomyelinase deficient with a profound lack of lysosomal sphingomyelinase activity, and can be divided into the following types.
- Type A: neurovisceral—infantile, juvenile, adult (rare).
- Type B: visceral only—infantile (rare), juvenile, adult.

The gene for sphingomyelinase has been assigned to chromosome 17 (Konrad & Wilson 1987).

Type A

These children present in the first 6 months of life with hepatosplenomegaly and failure to thrive, intellectual deterioration with death by 3 years. This is the classical form, it is autosomal recessive and most frequently seen in offspring of Ashkenazi Jewish parents. Cherry red spots (Fig. 57.5) lead on to retinal ganglion cell degeneration and optic atrophy (Goldstein & Wexler 1931; Walton *et al*. 1978); there is minimal corneal opacification and a brown discoloration of the anterior lens capsule occurs (Walton *et al*. 1978).

Type B

In this type the onset is later, from 2 years to adulthood. The sphingomyelinase deficiency is less severe than type A. Massive visceral enlargement, pulmonary infiltration, bone changes, and haematological problems with throm-

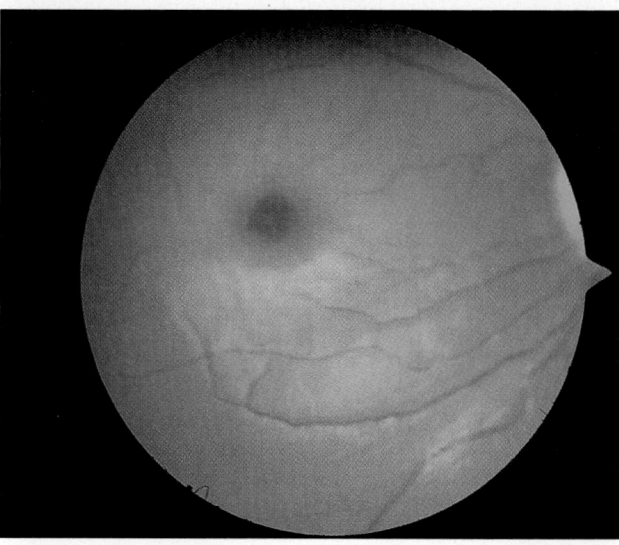

Fig. 57.5 Cherry red spot in Asian patient with Niemann–Pick type A: the spot is red because of dark background pigmentation.

bocytopenia occur. A macular halo has been described (Harzer *et al*. 1978; Matthews *et al*. 1986). It is an autosomal recessive disease and more frequent in Ashkenazi Jews. Some hope for the future is indicated by a successful bone marrow transplant which cleared liver and bone marrow of sphingomyelin (Vellodi *et al*. 1987).

Group 2

These patients are not sphingomyelinase deficient, but the sphingomyelin accumulates in the spleen and a little in the liver (serum cholesterol is raised). Brain sphingomyelin is normal. Sphingomyelinase is normal. There may be a defect in cholesterification in fibroblasts. Group 2 patients can be divided into the following types.
- Type C: neurovisceral with variable sphingomyelin deposition.
- Type D: juvenile variant found in Nova Scotia (possibly the same as C).

Type C

This is also known as ophthalmoplegic lipidosis; juvenile dystonic lipidosis; neurovisceral storage disease with vertical supranuclear ophthalmoplegia; Neville–Lake syndrome; and many others!

There seem to be three phenotypes (Fink *et al*. 1989).

1 Early onset, in infancy, with liver dysfunction, hepatosplenomegaly, severe prolonged jaundice in 60%, and psychomotor dysfunction. Early death may occur. Between 2 and 10 years neurological involvement occurs as in phenotype 2.

2 Between 4 and 6 years there is the onset of mild intellec-

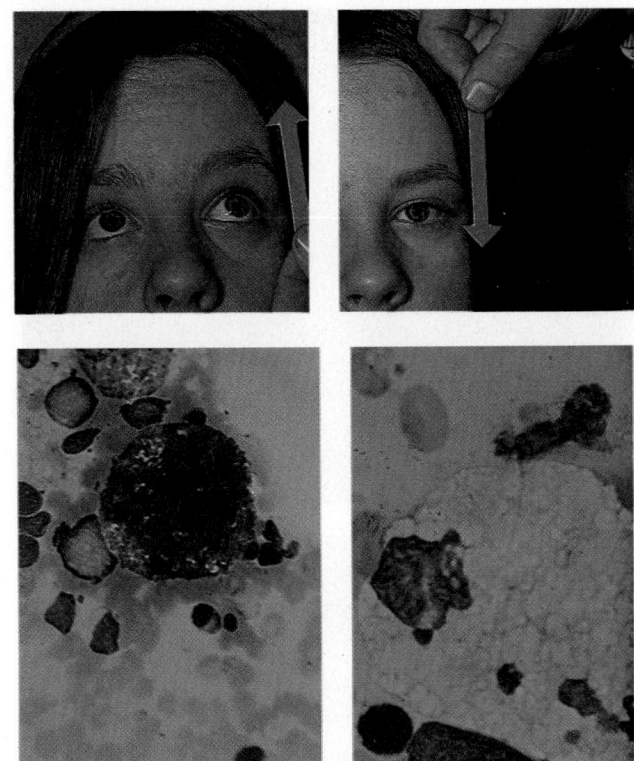

Fig. 57.6 (a) Downgaze palsy in child with Niemann–Pick type C. The arrow denotes the direction that the child is being told to look. Horizontal and upgaze were normal (Mr M.D. Sanders' patient). (b) Niemann–Pick type C showing foamy macrophages (right) and sea-blue histiocytes (left).

tual problems with a supranuclear palsy (Fig. 57.6) and ataxia. Dystonia is quite a frequent finding but it is not consistently present; seizures are common but not usually frequent. The supranuclear palsy, which is so characteristic, was described by Norman *et al.* (1967) and Dunn and Sweeney (1971), but clearly defined by Neville *et al.* (1973). There is loss of voluntary vertical saccades (rapid eye movements), and fast phases of optokinetic nystagmus (OKN), especially downwards; there is preserved doll's eye movements. There may be vertical pursuit and sometimes horizontal supranuclear eye movement defects or a supranuclear disorder of convergence. Head thrusts may be used to compensate for the saccade disorder. A faint cherry red spot, due to opalescence of the perifoveal retina, has been observed in one case (Taylor *et al.* 1981).

3 An adolescent or adult form, slowly progressive with organomegaly and neurological problems.

Phenotypes 1 and 2 can occur in the same family (Fink *et al.* 1989).

Bone marrow aspirate shows numerous foamy macrophages (Fig. 57.6b) with non-uniform vacuoles and ingested red blood cells. They have densely staining nuclear fragments. Older patients have only a few 'sea-blue' histiocytes which stain an intense blue with Giemsa; these cells are principally found in type B disease and it is strictly incorrect to call type C 'the sea-blue histiocyte syndrome', however euphonic the name. Neurones, including those in the retina (Taylor *et al.* 1981), show membrane-bound polymorphous cytoplasmic bodies containing concentric multilamellated bodies. It is an autosomal recessive condition characterized by abnormalities of intracellular translocation of exogenous cholesterol (Vanier *et al.* 1991). Prenatal diagnosis is now possible (Vanier *et al.* 1991).

Type D

This is a rare disease which is very similar to type C but which occurs in a Nova Scotian population; affected patients can be traced to common ancestors. It seems to be biochemically only very subtly different from type C (Butler *et al.* 1987).

Gaucher's disease

In all forms of Gaucher's disease there is a defect in glucocerebrosidase, which is the enzyme that cleaves glucose from glucosyl ceramide. They all have characteristic Gaucher cells in almost all tissues; the cells are large and have a 'crinkly' cytoplasm with the appearance of crumpled tissue paper. They contain no fat or cholesterol. Fibrillar inclusions are seen on electron microscopy.

It results from a variety of mutations but in Ashkenazi Jews four mutations account for 97% of cases. Within each genotype there is considerable phenotypic variation. Bone marrow transplant may be effective, but it is risky. Glucocerebrosidase intravenous infusion is effective but costly (Beutler 1992).

Type I

This is only occasionally seen in childhood and presents with marked hepatosplenomegaly and with hypersplenism. Dark brown–yellow pingueculae occur in the nasal bulbar conjunctivae which are characterized by numerous Gaucher cells on histological examination. Rarely macular and perimacular degeneration has been described (Eyb 1952; Collier 1961; Miller *et al.* 1973; Petrochelos *et al.* 1975; McKeran *et al.* 1985).

Type II

This presents in early infancy with delayed development, fits and spasticity, squint, and a cherry red spot in some patients with later optic atrophy. Death occurs by 1 year old. Retinal haemorrhages have been described (Reich *et al.* 1951).

Type III ('Norrbottnian type')

This subacute disease begins from birth to 14 years with splenomegaly and fever, growth retardation, and bone changes with thinning of the cortices in all cases. Later there is intellectual deterioration and seizures in some. Pingueculae are rare; squint occurred in 13 out of 22 cases studied by Dreborg *et al.* (1980), and perivascular infiltrates were shown in seven out of 210 cases examined. Nearly half the patients had oculomotor apraxia (Tripp *et al.* 1977; Dreborg *et al.* 1980) emphasizing the need for a systemic investigation of children with a supranuclear eye movement disorder. The apraxia includes vertical movements. The apraxia may be congenital (Bolthauser *et al.* 1984) and is probably associated with perivascular infiltration in the brain stem with Gaucher cells (Winkleman *et al.* 1983). Retinal neovascularization and white dots have been described in what may be this form (Jaime & Dalmas 1989; Rodriguez *et al.* 1992).

Neuraminidase deficiency

Sialidosis type I

This is also known as the cherry red spot–myoclonus syndrome. This disease presents in childhood with cherry red spots (Fig. 57.7), a progressive myoclonus, but normal intelligence (Rapin *et al.* 1975; Lowden & O'Brien 1979; Thomas *et al.* 1979).

Insidious visual loss brings these children to the ophthalmologist who discovers the cherry red spot which fades with age and neuronal loss. First, myoclonus develops and becomes debilitating by the late teens; then there follows periodic alternating nystagmus, dementia and cataracts (Swallow *et al.* 1979). The children appear normal but some may have mild bony changes.

The diagnosis is made by the finding of a defect in lysosomal neuraminidase with normal beta-galactosidase. Sialyloligosaccharides are excreted in the urine but not mucopolysaccharides.

Sialidosis type II

These patients have coarse features, similar to a child with Hurler's disease (Fig. 57.8). They have progressive loss of vision from corneal clouding and bilateral cherry red spots (Goldberg *et al.* 1971). They become deaf and mentally retarded, and may have nystagmus. They do not have mucopolysacchariduria but excrete sialyloligosaccharides. Both neuraminidase and beta-galactosidase are abnormal. Histopathological examination has shown lamellated inclusions in retinal ganglion cells, amacrine cells but not in the optic nerve which showed marked demyelination (Usui *et al.* 1991b).

There are some nosological difficulties between neu-

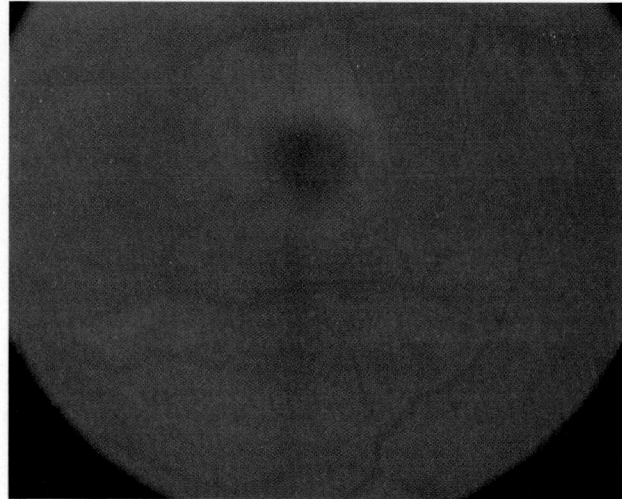
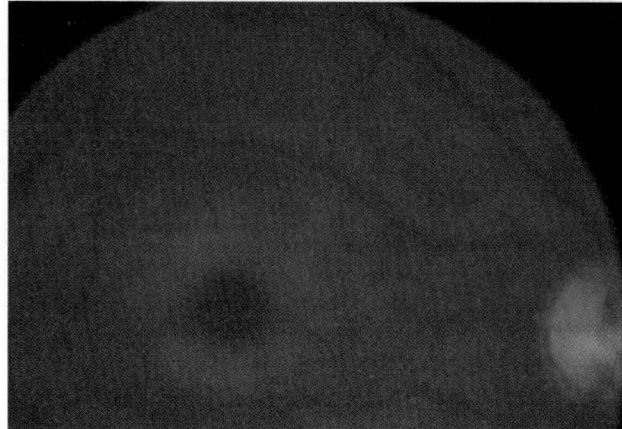

Fig. 57.7 Cherry red spot in a patient with sialidosis type I (Mr M.D. Sanders' patient).

raminidase deficiency and mucolipidoses (McKusick 1986).

Mucopolysaccharidoses

These are a group of diseases characterized by variable combinations of bony changes, mental retardation, corneal clouding, retinal degeneration and mucopolysaccharide in the urine.

Historical associations have caused the eponyms to be retained despite the detailed classification into six main types and at least 16 subtypes on urinary glycosaminoglycan excretion and enzyme analysis. The old term gargoylism is incorrect and too offensive to the patients and their parents to be retained (Table 57.1).

A quick clinical guide to diagnosis for the ophthalmologist can be based on the facial features and the bony and eye changes.

1 Hurler's-like phenotype with cloudy cornea, retinal

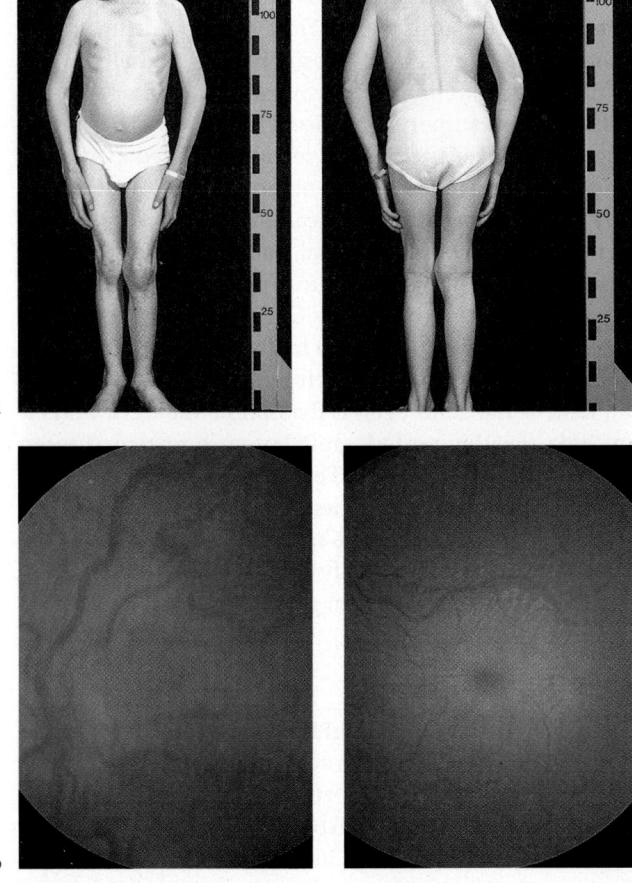

Fig. 57.8 Patient with sialidosis type 2. He has marked bony changes (a) and a cherry red spot (b).

degeneration and optic atrophy. This can be subdivided into:

(a) MPS IH—Hurler's syndrome;

(b) MPS VI — Maroteaux–Lamy syndrome (mentally normal);

(c) MPS VII—beta-glucuronidase deficiency (eye findings not reported).

2 Mild facial changes and cloudy cornea. This can be subdivided into:

(a) MPS IS — Scheie's disease: hand deformity, aortic incompetence, retinal degeneration, normal intelligence;

(b) MPS IV — Morquio's disease: severe skeletal changes and dwarfing, normal intelligence and no retinal degeneration.

3 Mental retardation, facial changes without cloudy cornea.

(a) MPS II Hunter's: occasional mild corneal changes, severe skeletal changes, retinal degeneration, mental retardation;

(b) MPS III Sanfilippo: severe mental retardation, mild facial changes, moderate skeletal changes, and retinal degeneration present.

The above classification is incomplete, but serves as an *aide mémoire*. MPS V is not present; it is MPS IS (Scheie's syndrome).

The gene for MPS IS has been assigned to 22pter–q11(Schuchmann *et al.* 1984) and MPS VI to 5q13–q14 (Litjens *et al.* 1989).

The paediatric ophthalmologist is rarely involved with Hunter's, Hurler's, Sanfilippo or MPS VII because their mental retardation and short lives often preclude treatment for their corneas. Nevertheless, they are not infrequently asked to see patients with Maroteaux–Lamy, Morquio's and Scheie's disease whose pathological and ocular clinical features have many similarities, although they are not identical.

Ocular findings and management

Corneal clouding

When the corneas are affected they take on a 'ground

Table 57.1 A classification of the mucopolysaccharidoses (MPS). After Wraith (1995).

Type	Eponym	Stored material	Enzyme deficiency
MPS IH	Hurler	DS, HS	Iduronidase
MPS IS	Scheie	DS, HS	Iduronidase
MPS IH/S	Hurler–Scheie compound	DS, HS	Iduronidase
MPS II	Hunter	DS, HS	Iduronidase sulphate sulphatase
MPS IIIA	Sanfilippo	HS	Heparan N-sulphatase
MPS IIIB		HS	N-acetylglucosaminidase
MPS IIIC		HS	Acetyl-CoA-glucosaminidase acetyltransferase
MPS IIID		HS	N-acetylglucosamine-6-sulphatase
MPS IVA	Morquio	KS	Galactosamine-6-sulphatase
MPS IVB		KS	Beta-galactosidase
MPS VI	Maroteaux–Lamy	DS	N-acetylgalactosamine-4-sulphatase
MPS VII	Sly	CS, DS, HS	Beta-glucuronidase

DS, dermatan sulphate; HS, heparan sulphate; KS, keratan sulphate; CH, chondroitin sulphate.

glass' appearance that in some instances is better seen with illumination from the side, than on slit-lamp examination (Figs 57.9, 57.10). All layers of the corneas are symmetrically infiltrated, both within cells and in the extracellular space, with acid mucopolysaccharide. In some studies the cells have been involved preferentially (Zabel *et al.* 1989). Although not clinically affected, the conjunctiva (which is readily biopsied) also shows intracellular inclusions on electron microscopy which are mucopolysaccharide-containing lysosomes (Kenyon 1976). The only treatment for the cloudy cornea is by corneal transplantation. Unfortunately, the co-existence of retinal degeneration, optic atrophy, severe mental retardation or a markedly shortened lifespan often contraindi-

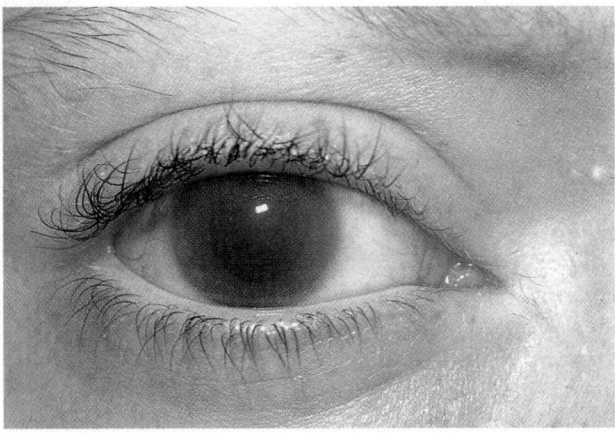

Fig. 57.9 Opaque cornea in Scheie's MPS IS. The acuity was 6/12 at this stage.

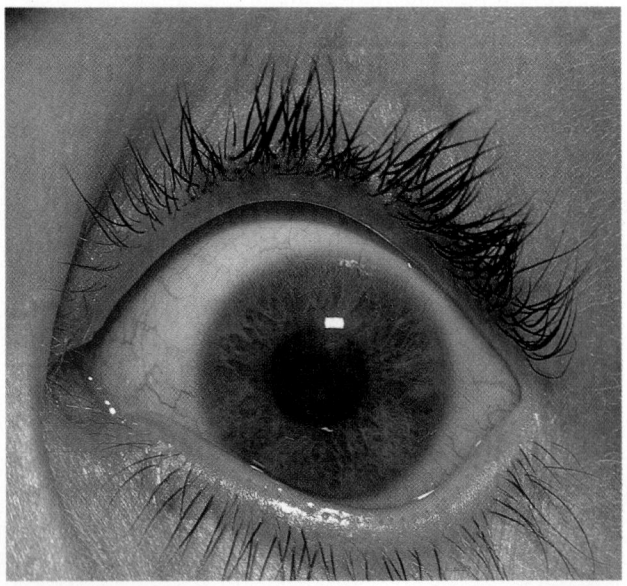

Fig. 57.10 Very mild corneal cloudiness in Morquio's disease MPS IV. Normal vision.

cates treatment. Careful assessment of the patient's needs together with neurophysiological studies and magnetic resonance imaging (MRI) to establish the viability of the retina and postretinal pathways are mandatory before embarking on surgery. The visual improvement is rarely long lived but sometimes gives an extended period of vision to children who would otherwise be blind. Reports vary but we have found corneal grafts may remain clear for months, rejection is unusual, and the graft re-opacifies by involvement with the original process. An interesting phenomenon was reported by Orgül *et al.* (1991): the partial clearing of the host cornea in the post-transplant period. Provided the cases are carefully selected the procedure can benefit the child even if the ophthalmologist finds it tiresome that his perfect graft becomes opacified more quickly than he is used to! They can always be regrafted provided that retinal degeneration or optic atrophy has not supervened. After bone marrow transplantation the clearing of the corneas is only partial, but reaccumulation does not occur in a successful graft.

Retinal degeneration

This is seen in most forms but has not yet been recorded in Morquio's disease. It has a very insidious onset and is usually overshadowed by the corneal opacities. The more intelligent child with MPS IS or MPS VI may note onset of night-blindness or dimness in addition to the blurring of the corneal disease. Histopathologically, most tissues of the eye are affected especially the retinal pigment epithelium (Del Monte *et al.* 1983; Lavery *et al.* 1983, McDonnell *et al.* 1983). Kenyon (1976) found the retinal pigment epithelial cells were filled with mucopolysaccharide but were generally intact. The outer retina is also affected. A macular oedema like change and pseudopapilloedema have been described in a patient with MPS IS who had a retinal degeneration (Usui *et al.* 1991a).

No treatment is available and detection of the retinal degeneration is mandatory before corneal grafting is undertaken.

Optic disc swelling and atrophy

Histopathological studies show that both the ganglion cells and the nerve fibre layer of the retina, and optic nerve itself are severely affected. Kenyon (1976) thought that the optic nerve axons might be compressed or nutritionally compromised by the infiltration of glial cells. Optic disc swelling (Fig. 57.11) occurs in most of the MPS patients and leads frequently to optic atrophy (Collins *et al.* 1990). Optic atrophy can also be caused by glaucoma. Neurophysiological studies help to delineate optic nerve and cortical visual defect.

Beck (1983) and Beck and Cole (1984) published two papers the first of which gave the case report of a man

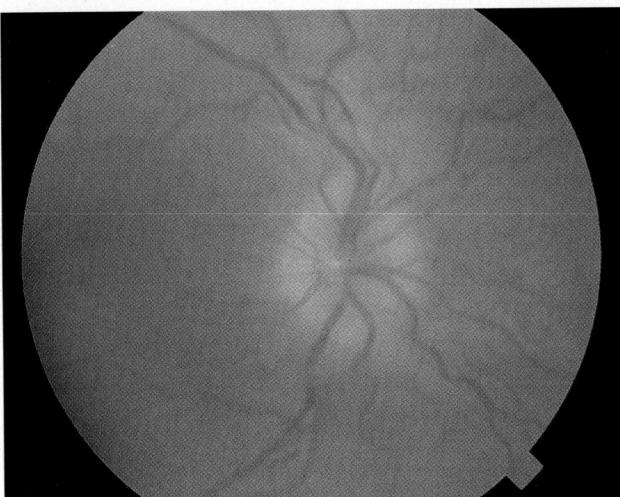

Fig. 57.11 Optic disc swelling in a patient with MPS IV—Maroteaux–Lamy syndrome. The picture is hazy due to corneal clouding.

with Hunter's MPS II who had documented 11 years with gross bilateral papilloedema with no evidence of raised intracranial pressure. They noted in this paper the severity of the systemic disease which led to his death and to his histopathology being reported by Beck and Cole (1984). They found a grossly thickened sclera with MPS deposition that caused compression of the optic nerve in its intrascleral course. The sclera at the posterior pole was 2.9 mm.

Glaucoma

Glaucoma probably occurs in all of the mucopolysaccharidoses and some other metabolic diseases with cloudy corneas. It was clearly described by Spellacy *et al.* (1980) in MPS IH, and it also occurs in MPS IS and MPS IV (Cahane *et al.* 1990; Iwamoto *et al.* 1990), with histopathological studies of a trabeculectomy specimen showing MPS-laden cells in the aqueous draining channels. The cloudy corneas, which often appear large because of the cloudiness alone, make it a diagnosis easily missed. The incidence is probably not high enough to warrant routine examinations under anaesthetic unless there is clinical suspicion of raised intraocular pressure.

Diagnosis

Diagnosis is made by a combination of clinical and radiological studies with analysis of urinary MPS and leucocyte enzymes. Prenatal diagnosis is available by enzyme assay from cultured amniotic fluid cells or by analysis of amniotic fluid MPS derived from the fetal urine.

General management

The general management is best carried out by a paediatrician with appropriate experience and with access to the relevant diagnostic and radiological facilities. Skeletal and respiratory problems, deafness, blindness, hydrocephalus, cardiomyopathy and valvular defect and many other problems provide a great test of the paediatrician's skills. Treatment is symptomatic at present but bone marrow transplantation in infancy offers some hope for future years (Hobbs *et al.* 1981).

Mucolipidoses

These children have a mixture of features of mucopolysaccharidoses and neurolipidoses but without MPS excretion in the urine. As the metabolic basis of subtypes becomes clear they are removed from this classification (Spranger & Wiedemann 1970).

Mucolipidosis I

There are some nosological difficulties to this disease which has some close resemblance to neuraminidase deficiency sialidosis type II. Lake (1984) divides mucolipidosis type I into sialidosis types I and II.

Patients have coarse facies, corneal clouding, cataract (Cibis *et al.* 1983) a cherry red spot and skeletal dysplasia.

Mucolipidosis II

These children are Hurler-like with a chronic course. They have characteristic inclusions in cultured fibroblasts on phase contrast microscopy, giving rise to the name 'I-cell disease'. Conjunctival biopsy is useful in diagnosis (Libert *et al.* 1977b). A retinal degeneration occurs (Newell *et al.* 1975).

Mucolipidosis III

The children have a more chronic course, but are otherwise similar clinically to ML II. Conjunctival biopsy may help in the diagnosis (Libert *et al.* 1977a). Affected children have a progressive stiffening of the joints from the early years, with coarsening of the features and a kyphoscoliosis. Corneal clouding, hypermetropic astigmatism, normal ERG and optic disc oedema of uncertain mechanism were reported by Traboulsi and Maumenee (1986); these authors also noted a diffuse retinal haze which they felt might have resulted from accumulation of storage material in ganglion cells. The retina was also 'wrinkled' in two patients.

Mucolipidosis IV

ML IV is important to the paediatric ophthalmologist because of the ocular features which may form a major defect.

Children with ML IV present with corneal clouding and progressive retardation without skeletal changes (Goutieres *et al.* 1979). Many have Ashkenazi Jewish parents. Mild cases have been described, with the corneal changes being the most prominent problem (Lake *et al.* 1982; Casteels *et al.* 1992). Most patients present with hypotonia, corneal clouding and puffy lids; they often do not progress beyond a developmental age of 15 months and live until their teens or occasionally up to their thirties (Chitayat *et al.* 1991). Mild forms have been reported (Lake *et al.* 1982; Casteels *et al.* 1992), and cases re-reported (Reis *et al.* 1993).

ML IV patients have cloudy corneas from early life but the clouding is mainly epithelial (Fig. 57.12) (Kenyon *et al.* 1979; Lake *et al.* 1982; Riedel *et al.* 1985). The corneal epithelial defect may have a whorl-like form (see Fig. 24.28) (Casteels *et al.* 1992). Rapid regrowth of epithelium makes the clarity of grafts very short lived despite the absence of rejection. Conjunctival transplantation may improve corneal clarity for up to 1 year (Dangel *et al.* 1985). In some instances corneal surface irregularities are associated with episodic pain (Newman *et al.* 1990).

Cataracts form and the presence of a retinal degeneration may make treatment unrewarding (Reidel *et al.* 1985).

Diagnosis is made by the finding of multiple concentrically lamellated bodies in cornea and conjunctiva on ultrastructural studies (Merin *et al.* 1975; Lake *et al.* 1982; Reidel *et al.* 1985).

Mannosidosis

Patients show a variable retardation, skeletal dysplasia, deafness and mental retardation. Macroglossia, deafness and other features make this reminiscent of Hurler's disease. Corneal opacity is not usually marked and cataract, of a 'spoke-like' configuration, is probably more frequent (Arbisser *et al.* 1976; Letson & Desnick 1978; Montgomery *et al.* 1982). The spokes are posterior cortical, composed of multiple discrete clear round vacuoles lying at different depths in the lens, best seen by slit-lamp retroillumination (Murphree *et al.* 1976). MRI findings suggest demyelination and there is cerebellar atrophy and a thick calvarium (Dietmann *et al.* 1990).

Fucosidosis

Fucosidosis exists in two forms which vary mainly in that type I is more severe and occurs in infancy. Both have mental regression, coarse features and bone dysplasia. Type II may have a skin abnormality similar to the angiokeratoma of Fabry's disease (George & Graham-Brown 1994).

Willems *et al.* (1991) found the following results in 77 patients surveyed:

- 95% experienced mental deterioration;
- 87% experienced motor deterioration;
- 79% had coarse facies;
- 78% had growth retardation;
- 78% experienced recurrent infections;
- 58% had dysostosis multiplex;
- 52% had angiokeratoma corposis diffusum;
- 44% had visceromegaly; and
- 38% experienced seizures.

They have conjunctival and retinal vascular tortuosity (Barrone *et al.* 1974; Snodgrass 1976; Snyder *et al.* 1976; Libert & Toussaint 1982). A bull's eye maculopathy was described by Snodgrass (1976) and central and epithelial corneal opacities (Snyder *et al.* 1976) which may be 'lobulated' rather than diffuse.

Diagnosis is by analysis of α-L-fucosidase in cultured fibroblasts or leucocytes (Libert *et al.* 1976b): prenatal diagnosis is possible.

Fabry's disease (angiokeratoma diffusum)

The usual presenting symptom is the presence of clusters of punctate dark-red telangiectases or blobs in the skin in the bathing trunk area and on the mucous membranes. Episodes of burning pain in the limbs occur and are probably due to a peripheral neuropathy (Kocen & Thomas 1970). Diagnosis is often delayed because of the nonspecific symptoms and signs in the early stages, the mean age of diagnosis in one centre being 29 years (Morgan & Crawford 1988).

Renal disease is a frequent cause of death. It is inherited as an X-linked recessive trait with the affected boys having a defect of alpha-galactosidase in leucocytes or cultured fibroblasts and amniotic fluid cells. The gene has been

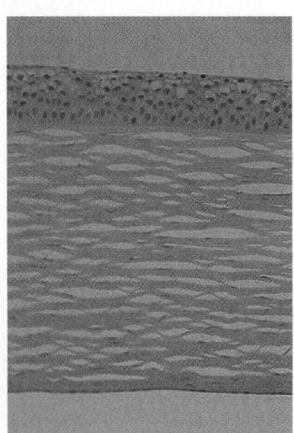
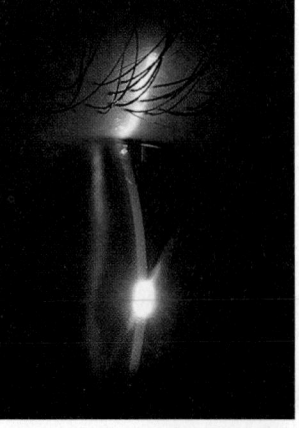

Fig. 57.12 Mucolipidosis IV. The corneal clouding is due mainly to epithelial changes.

linked to Xq22 by *in situ* hybridization (Astrin *et al.* 1989). Sometimes heterozygous females may be symptomatic. Franceschetti (1976) carried out a review of 470 cases, documenting the ocular findings. Earlier reports by Spaeth and Frost (1965), and Weingeist and Blodi (1971) confirmed the earlier observations of corneal abnormality by Weicksel (1925). From Franceschetti (1976) and Sher *et al.* (1979) the ocular findings are as follows.

Conjunctival vessel tortuosity

This occurred in 45% of affected males and 25% of females.

Lid oedema

This occurred in 13 of 470 cases. Angiokeratoma of the lids is rare.

Corneal lesions

Slit-lamp examination shows one or more lines radiating from a point near the centre of the cornea with a whorl-like appearance ('cornea verticillata'; Fig. 57.13a). The opacity is made up of myriads of white to yellow–brown dots in the epithelial or subepithelial layers. It is not distinguishable from drugs causing cornea verticillata, such as chlorpromazine, amiodarone, quinacrine, chloroquine and indomethacin. In young patients the corneal opacities may appear as a diffuse haze (Sher *et al.* 1979). They occur in virtually all hemizygotes and heterozygotes.

Lens opacities

These occur in two ways.
1 A granular white subcapsular cataract, wedge-shaped with the base at the lens equator, especially inferiorly.
2 Opacities seen in retroillumination that are spots radiating from the posterior pole of the lens, along the sutures (Fig. 57.13b).
    These lens opacities are probably unique to Fabry's disease.

Fundus lesions

Retinal vascular tortuosity occurs, especially affecting the veins, in the second decade. The vessels become beaded, have sheathing and may develop arteriovenous anastomoses and thromboses. Affected males are more severely affected than the hemizygotes. Retinal vascular occlusion may be the initial symptom, in one case in a 16-year-old boy (Sher *et al.* 1978). Optic disc oedema may occur, probably secondary to the vascular lesions. Myelinated nerve fibres have been reported twice (Calmettes *et al.* 1967; Sher *et al.* 1978).

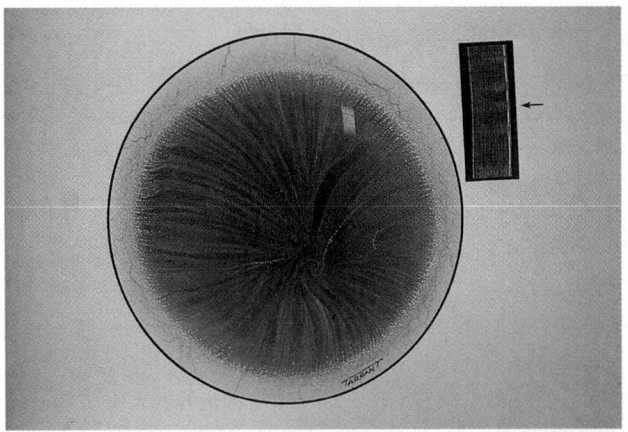

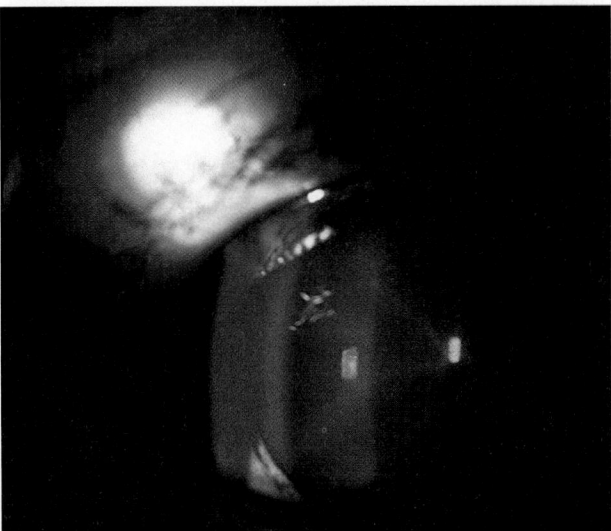

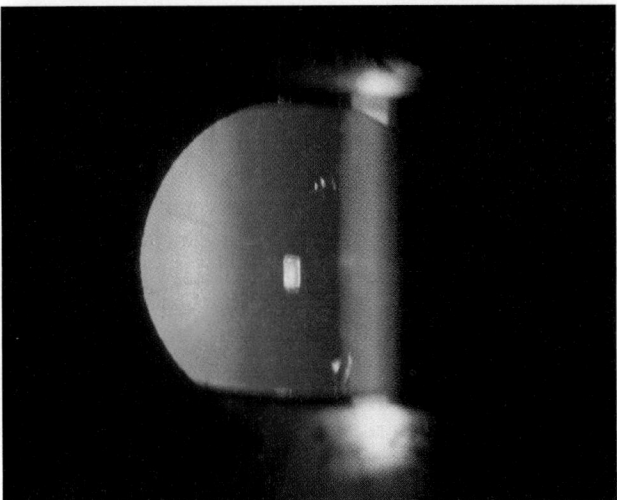

Fig. 57.13 (a) Fabry's disease: a painting of cornea verticillata. Usually the whorled lines are very faint, and cannot be seen without slit-lamp microscopy. (b) Fabry's disease: characteristic spoke-like posterior cortical sutural cataract on direct illumination, (c) on retroillumination.

Neuro-ophthalmological problems

Nystagmus was found in six cases in the literature, third nerve palsy in three cases, and strabismus in nine cases (seven were divergent). Optic atrophy, internuclear ophthalmoplegia, seizures and strokes have all been described, but are rare. Vision defects seem to be unusual.

Diagnosis

The diagnosis can be made by enzyme assay or conjunctival biopsy (Libert *et al.* 1976a); prenatal diagnosis is available.

Whorl-like corneal opacities (differential diagnosis)

1 Well-defined whorls:
   (a) Fabry's disease;
   (b) mucolipidosis IV (Casteels *et al.* 1992);
   (c) drug deposition — indomethacin, chloroquine, hydroxychloroquine, amiodarone, phenothiazines, especially chlorpromazine, and mepacrine.
2 Corneal opacities resembling whorls:
   (a) Tangier disease;
   (b) Melkersson syndrome/amyloidosis V;
   (c) tyrosinaemia.
3 Other names for whorl-like opacities:
   (a) Fleischer's vortex dystrophy;
   (b) cornea verticillata;
   (c) whorl-like corneal dystrophy.

Farber's disease

This autosomal recessive disease is characterized by the onset in infancy of multiple subcutaneous nodules, lymphadenopathy, hoarse cry and variable involvement of lung, heart and liver. The course is variable with death between 1 and 18 years. The more severely affected children may have eye changes including a cherry red spot that consists of a faint grey ring around the fovea (Cogan *et al.* 1966), nodular corneal opacity (Ozaki *et al.* 1978) and a pingueculum-like conjunctival lesion (Zetterstrom 1958). The retinal ganglion cells in a child with cherry red spots were grossly distended with inclusions (Zarbin *et al.* 1985) but most ocular tissues had some involvement.

The diagnosis is made by the assay of ceramidase activity of cultured fibroblasts or by biopsy of the nodules.

Leucodystrophies

The leucodystrophies are a group of conditions characterized by demyelination, or failure to form normal myelin, in the central white matter of the brain.

Clinically, they present with ataxia, paralysis and eye movement disorders whereas 'grey matter' diseases such as the neuronal storage diseases present with seizures, mental retardation, retinal disorders and optic atrophy. Demyelination and primary neuronal disease occur in both groups: it is the proportion that is different.

Metachromatic leucodystrophy

All types of metachromatic leucodystrophy (MLD) are associated with a defect in aryl sulphatase A; there are excess sulphatides in many tissues, especially in the nervous system.

The late infantile form has an onset between 1 and 2 years and patients have progressive motor problems due to central and peripheral nervous system involvement. Mental deterioration occurs later and seizures are unusual. Death usually occurs by 6 years of age.

The juvenile form starts later and has a slower course. In addition to the motor problems, there are often marked behavioural difficulties which often obscure the diagnosis for some time (MacFaul *et al.* 1982).

Most patients with MLD present to paediatricians or psychiatrists with motor or behavioural problems, but ophthalmological disorders may be important, especially in later onset cases (Libert *et al.* 1979). Optic atrophy is found in one-third of cases and blindness from this and cerebral causes is frequent (François 1979). The optic atrophy may be caused by retinal ganglion cell degeneration (Renard *et al.* 1963; Goebel *et al.* 1978), but metachromatic granules have also been found in the optic nerve (Renard *et al.* 1963; Hammami *et al.* 1973). Retinal involvement may also include a cherry red spot (Allen *et al.* 1962; Cogan *et al.* 1970; Hammami *et al.* 1973; Bateman *et al.* 1984). The retina and optic nerve, however, are not invariably involved (Quigley & Green 1972; Bosch & Hart 1978). It is not surprising that the eye is frequently involved; aryl sulphatase A and B are widely distributed in the eye but show highest activities in the retina (Hara *et al.* 1979). Nystagmus is infrequent, possibly related to poor vision (Libert *et al.* 1979). The ERG may be abnormal in some cases (Weiter *et al.* 1980) but it is not a feature of most cases apart from subtle pattern ERG changes; Zlotgora *et al.* (1981) commented that Weiter *et al.*'s case may have not truly been MLD.

The diagnosis is made by examination of the urine for intracellular metachromic substances and assay of aryl sulphatase A in white blood cells. It is autosomal recessive and familial cases tend to run a similar course among family members.

Krabbe's disease (globoid cell leucodystrophy)

Krabbe's disease is associated with deficient activity of galactocerebrosidase. It presents in an early and a more rare late infantile form with central white matter disease in both and a peripheral neuropathy (Baker *et al.* 1990) in the early form. The early infantile cases present in early infancy with failure to thrive, extreme irritability, retardation, an exaggerated startle response and a peripheral neuropathy. The disorder starts so early that a careful history is necessary to differentiate the disease from cerebral palsy. It is autosomal recessive, and the gene locus has been mapped to chromosome 14 (Zlotogora *et al.* 1990).

A visual defect is common and caused by optic atrophy or cortical blindness (François 1975) but is often overshadowed by the rapid neurological deterioration. The optic nerve contains globoid cells (Cogan & Kuwabara 1968; Emery *et al.* 1972; Yunis & Lee 1972; Brownstein *et al.* 1978) and tubular inclusions (Harcourt & Ashton 1973); demyelination is frequent; MRI changes include a bilaterally increased T2 signal in periventricular white matter in occipital, parietal and posterior temporal lobes (Baker *et al.* 1990). The diagnosis is made by enzyme assay of leucocytes or cultured fibroblasts.

Adrenoleucodystrophy (Addison–Schilder disease)

This is a rare X-linked disease that presents usually in the first decade with visual defects (Schaumberg *et al.* 1975; Wray *et al.* 1976a) and regression. The association with hypoadrenalism causes a presentation with skin pigmentation (Hormia 1978) or hypogonadism (Fettes *et al.* 1979) which are associated with Addison's disease. A not infrequent symptom, usually only elicited by direct questioning, is that the patient's summer suntan failed to fade. The visual symptoms are easily dismissed as being hysterical because initially the eye examination is normal and there are quite marked behavioural changes. Boys with hysterical blindness should be suspected of having adrenoleucodystrophy; neurophysiological studies are very helpful (Battaglia *et al.* 1981): the ERG is normal, the VER reduced and the EEG shows irregular slow activity over the posterior parts of the brain. The auditory evoked response can be used to detect carriers (Moloney & Masterson 1982). Somatosensory evoked responses may be more sensitive for carrier detection (Garg *et al.* 1983).

CT or MRI is helpful in making the diagnosis in the early stages (Quisling & Andriola 1979) as it shows low density zones in the periventricular white matter, especially posteriorly (Fig. 57.14; Fig. 57.15). The grey matter is spared and the lesions are remarkably symmetrical and confluent, contiguous over the midline via the splenium.

Optic atrophy occurs later. Ocular histopathology showed inclusions in optic nerve macrophages, retinal neurones and macrophages, and retinal photoreceptor and pigment epithelial degeneration (Cohen *et al.* 1983; Glasgow *et al.* 1987). One of Cohen *et al.*'s (1983) cases had a cataract and cystoid macular oedema. The inclusions in optic nerve macrophages are not invariable (Wray *et al.* 1976a).

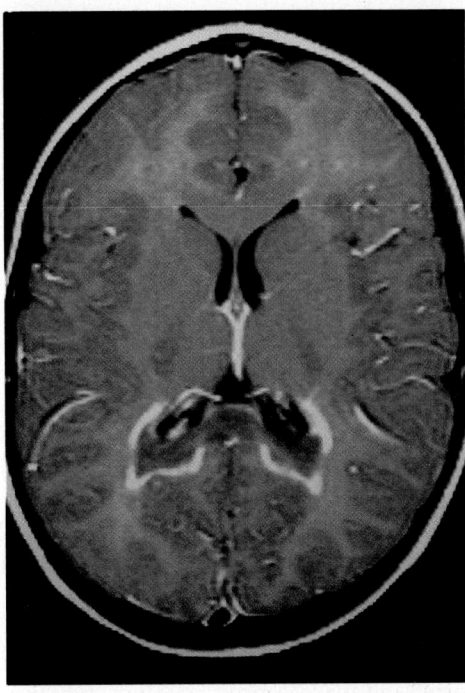

Fig. 57.14 Adrenoleucodystrophy. MRI scan showing characteristically predominant early involvement of the occipital lobes and visual pathway with high signal from the periventricular white matter. See also Fig. 51.21.

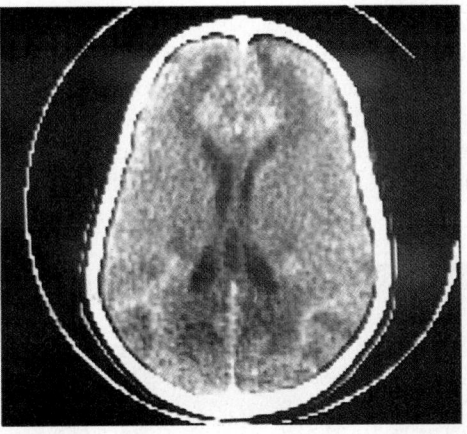

Fig. 57.15 Adrenoleucodystrophy. Periventricular lucency and enhancement on CT.

Progressive neurological deterioration occurs with death within a few years. A milder form, with lateral presentation and slow progress, mainly affecting the spinal cord is known as adrenoleucomyeloneuropathy.

The diagnosis is made by a combination of the clinical, CT, neurophysiological and endocrine studies, and measurement of long chain fatty acids, which may also be abnormal in carriers.

The results of bone marrow transplant or dietary

treatment are as yet uncertain (Green 1991; Moser *et al.* 1992).

Canavan's disease and Alexander's leucodystrophy

These are two rare diseases with progressive neurological deterioration which occur in childhood, with a rapid downhill course. Ophthalmological symptoms are overshadowed by the overwhelming neurological deterioration. Canavan's disease is an autosomal recessive disease associated with aspartoacyclase deficiency; it occurs particularly in Ashkenazi Jewish families.

Cogan (1976) described two cases of Canavan's disease who had flutter-like oscillations of the eyes together with another case without nystagmus. The two cases with nystagmus were blind with optic atrophy.

Prenatal diagnosis, based on amniotic fluid levels of *N*-acetyl-L-aspartate and enzyme assay, is available (Bennett *et al.* 1993).

Alexander's leucodystrophy (Fig. 57.16) presents in infancy with neurological deterioration leading to dementia, seizures and macrocephaly. Hiccups may be an early sign, brain biopsy may be the only way to make the definitive diagnosis of this non-genetic disease (Brett 1991).

Other metabolic diseases

Organic acidaemias

This is a group of disorders, including maple syrup urine disease, propionic acidaemia, glutaric aciduria, methyl malonic aciduria, and multiple acyl coenzyme A (CoA) dehydrogenase deficiency, that are autosomal recessive enzyme disorders of amino acid catabolism. They present in infancy with a severe metabolic acidosis with rapid deterioration and ketosis or as failure to thrive or a variety of neurological problems including seizures, dystonia or as an ataxia in older children. Most of the ophthalmological problems have been recorded in infants with maple syrup urine disease.

A variety of gaze pareses occur, both vertical (Zee *et al.* 1974; McDonald & Sher 1977) and horizontal and vertical mixed gaze pareses (Mainardi 1966; Schwartz & Kolendrianos 1969; Chhabria *et al.* 1979). Ptosis is frequent (Lonsdale *et al.* 1963; Zee *et al.* 1974; Chhabria *et al.* 1979).

Before diagnosis the infant is hypotonic with a divergent squint, poor eye movements and ptosis. As treatment is started, before recovery takes place, there are bursts of wild eye movements and eyelid movements (Dickinson *et al.* 1969). Older children may present with nystagmus (Morris *et al.* 1961).

Rapid diagnosis is essential to reduce the permanent neurological defects, since the outcome becomes worse after the first 24 hours with progressively severe permanent neurological sequelae (Naughten *et al.* 1982).

Diabetes

See Chapter 49.

Urea cycle disorders

This is a group of diseases which may present at any age but occurs particularly severely in the neonatal period when they present with the gradual onset of lethargy, seizures and liver failure. They have abnormal liver enzymes, raised ammonia, and excess urinary orotic acid.

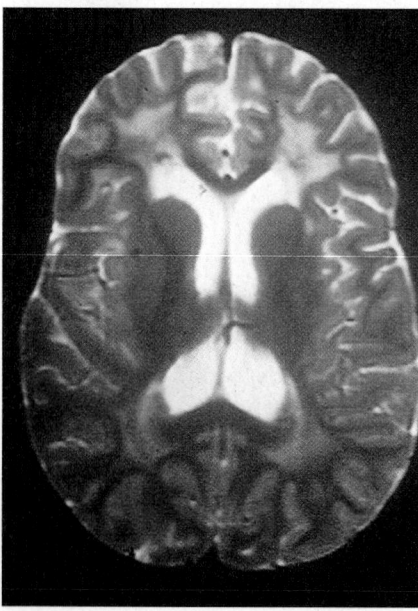 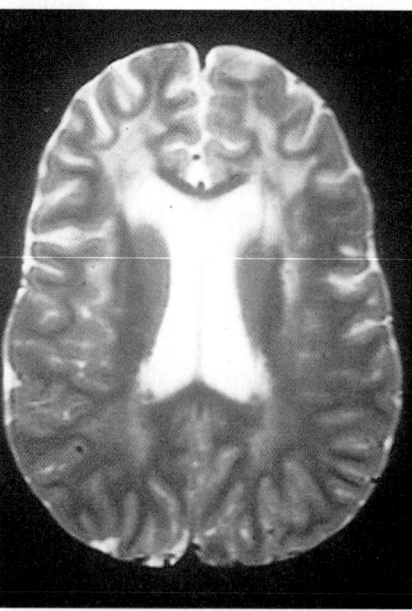

Fig. 57.16 Alexander's leucodystrophy T2-weighted sequence.

Later onset disorders present in a much more chronic fashion; papilloedema has been described in late onset citrullinaemia (Hayasaka *et al.* 1974). Ornithine carbamyl transferase deficiency is inherited as an X-linked dominant condition in which the male infants usually die but the females survive and thrive poorly. One male has been recorded as having survived with marked myopia vitiligo and hyperammonaemia and transient visual disturbances (Snebold *et al.* 1987).

Menkes' disease

- Kinky hair syndrome.
- Steely hair syndrome.
- Tricholipodystrophy.

This is an X-linked recessive disease of copper metabolism. The Menkes mutation probably affects copper transport from the cystosol to organelles (Kodama 1993). Serum copper and caeruloplasmin levels are extremely low. It occurs in one in 254 000 live births in Europe (Tønnensen *et al.* 1991). The Menkes gene is distal to the X inactivation centre and proximal to the phosphoroglycerate kinase locus in Xq13. This can be used for prenatal diagnosis (Tønnensen *et al.* 1991).

The babies are often premature but slow to mature with failure to grow. When the second hair grows it is stubbly, stiff, fractures easily and feels like wire wool. Affected children progressively deteriorate with increasing spasticity and seizures.

The eyebrows are sparse, twisted (pili torti) and white, with the eyelashes better preserved and pigmented than the brows (Horn & Warburg 1976). There is a retinal dystrophy affecting the outer nuclear layer and photoreceptors in the macular area (Toussaint & Davis 1978) or more widespread (Seelenfreund *et al.* 1968; Billings & Degnam 1971; Horn & Warburg 1976; Wray *et al.* 1976b). Tortuous retinal vessels are frequent (Billings & Degnan 1971; Levy *et al.* 1974); the ERG becomes extinguished (Billings & Degnan 1971; Levy *et al.* 1974; Horn & Warburg 1976). The ERG is unaffected by raising the copper levels (Levy *et al.* 1974). Optic atrophy is probably secondary to retinal degeneration.

Demyelination is found in the optic nerve histopathologically (Wray *et al.* 1976b) and diffuse neuronal loss and demyelination on MRI scanning (Johnsen *et al.* 1991).

Amino acid and protein disorders

- Alkaptonuria (see Chapter 22).
- Cystinosis (see Chapter 24).
- Amyloidosis (see Chapter 24).
- Tyrosinaemia type 2, Richner–Hanhart (see Chapter 24).
- Wilson's disease (see Chapter 24).
- Lowe's syndrome (see Chapter 39).
- Homocystinuria (see Chapter 39).
- Phenylketonuria.

Phenylketonuria

Phenylketonuria is a rare autosomal recessive disorder of phenylalanine metabolism due to the lack of the enzyme phenylalanine hydroxylase.

Despite the gene frequency of about one in 510 of the population, untreated cases are rare because of neonatal screening which is universal in the Western world. Sadly a few cases each year have false negative results or are missed for one reason or another and they present with a gradual mental deterioration, sometimes with seizures, and they are often fair haired, blue eyed and with a pale rough skin. Treatment is by a diet low in phenylalanine which should be continued for the first decade of life. Phenylketonuric mothers have a high incidence of congenital anomalies and microcephaly in their children. In late diagnosed cases the eyes have blue irides even in those of dark skinned stock but the hypopigmentation does not seem to have the same associations, i.e. strabismus as in albinos (Zwaan 1983). High refractive errors are common (Cotticelli *et al.* 1985). Cataracts are quite frequent: they may occur in older children or in adult life and may be related to trauma and treatment (Zwaan 1983); they may be congenital (Parks & Schwilk 1963; Cotticelli *et al.* 1985).

Lipid metabolism disorders

Hyperlipoproteinaemias

The hyperlipoproteinaemias may occasionally cause corneal arcus (type IIa, IIb), xanthomas (type I, IIa, IIb), and lipaemia retinalis may very rarely be found in occasional children with type IV.

Lecithin cholesterol acyltransferase deficiency

Homozygotes with this disease, which is autosomal recessive, have central corneal clouding and arcus-like changes. The central corneal changes are grey dots occupying the full thickness of the stroma, mainly centrally, with peripheral condensation to form the arcus-like changes (Vrabec *et al.* 1988). Patients have a haemolytic anaemia which may lead to renal failure.

Tangier disease

This rare autosomal recessive disease may present in childhood with a neuropathy including facial diplegia and orange-coloured tonsils and sometimes a yellowish tinge to the conjunctiva, and stromal corneal clouding (Hoffman & Fredrickson 1965).

Fish eye disease

This very rare disease was described in a man and his three daughters by Carlson and Philipson (1979). They had eyes like those of a boiled fish, normal serum cholesterol, and raised triglycerides, very low density lipoprotein (VLDL), and very high density lipoprotein (VHDL).

Urbach–Wiethe syndrome (lipoid proteinosis)

This autosomal recessive disease is characterized by nodules and plaques in skin and mucous membranes. Laryngeal nodules and thickening give rise to hoarseness and the skin changes consist of the following features.
1 Multiple pigmented varioliform scarring on the face, elbows and knees resulting from vesicular eruptions (Feiler-Ofry *et al.* 1979).
2 Nodules at the margins of the lids (Blodi *et al.* 1960) and mucous membranes of the mouth and pharynx.

The lid nodules rarely give rise to problems but corneal changes (Muirhead & Jackson 1963; Newton *et al.* 1971; Charlin & Fernandez 1978), glaucoma and cataract (François *et al.* 1968; Charlin & Fernandez 1978), and retinal changes including a pigmentary retinopathy (Schilovitz *et al.* 1973) and drusen (Charlin & Fernandez 1978) occur.

Metabolic diseases with ophthalmological presentation

Corneal abnormalities

Those presenting with this include the following.
- Mucopolysaccharidoses (all except MPSII and MPSIII).
- Mucolipidoses.
- Fucosidosis.
- Mannosidosis.
- Farber's disease (one case).
- Sialidosis II.
- LCAT disease 1, Tangier disease 1, fish eye disease.
- Cystinosis.
- Tyrosinaemia.
- Wilson's disease.

Corneal disease and angiokeratoma corporis diffusum

Those presenting with this include the following.
- Fabry's disease (see pp. 782–784).
- Mucolipidosis I.
- Fucosidosis type II.

Visual failure

Those associated with this include the following.

- Juvenile Batten's disease.
- Leucodystrophies.
- Gangliosidoses.
- Abetalipoproteinaemia.

Eye movement disorders

Those associated with this include the following.
- Niemann–Pick type C (vertical gaze palsy).
- Sialidosis type I (periodic alternating nystagmus, myoclonus).
- Gaucher's disease type III (congenital oculomotor apraxia).
- Pelizaeus–Merzbacher disease (see Chapters 63 and 64).
- Organic acidaemias.
- Urea cycle disorders (bursts of chaotic eye movements).
- Sialidosis type II (nystagmus).
- GM2 type III (pursuit + vestibulo-ocular reflex defects).
- Canavan's disease (flutter-like oscillations).

Cherry red spot

This occurs in the following.
- GM2 type I, II and III.
- GM1 type I.
- Niemann–Pick type A.
- Sialidosis type I and II.
A faint or irregular cherry red spot occurs in the following.
- Niemann–Pick type C, type B1 MLD.
- Farber's disease.
- Mucolipidosis III.

References

Allen RJ, McCusker JJ, Tourtelotte WW. Metachromatic leucodystrophy. Clinical, histochemical and cerebrospinal fluid abnormalities. *Pediatrics* 1962; **30**: 629–38.

Arbisser AI, Murphree AL, Garcia CA, Howell RR. Ocular findings in mannosidosis. *Am J Ophthalmol* 1976; **82**: 465–71.

Astrin KH, Falk CT, Vlasak I *et al.* Linkage between alpha-galactosidase A and DXS17, 87, 94, 101, 106 and 287. *Cytogenet Cell Genet* 1989; **51**: 953–7.

Baker RH, Troutmann JC, Younge BR, Nelson KD, Zimmerman D. Late juvenile-onset Krabbe's disease. *Ophthalmology* 1990; **97**: 1176–81.

Barrone R, Gatti R, Trias X, Durnad P. Fucosidosis. *J Pediatr* 1974; **84**: 727–35.

Bateman J, Philippart M. Ocular features of the Hagberg–Santavuori syndrome. *Am J Ophthalmol* 1986; **102**: 262–72.

Bateman J, Philippart M, Isenberg SJ. Ocular features of multiple sulfatase deficiency and a new variant of metachromatic leucodystrophy. *J Pediatr Ophthalmol* 1984; **21**: 133–40.

Battaglia A, Harden A, Pampiglione G, Walsh PJ. Adreno-leucodystrophy: neurophysiological aspects. *J Neurol Neurosurg Psychiatr* 1981; **44**: 781–5.

Batten FE. Cerebral degeneration with symmetrical changes in the maculae in two members of a family. *Trans Ophthalmol Soc UK* 1903;

23: 386–90.

Batten FE. Family cerebral degeneration with macular change (so-called juvenile form of family amaurotic idiocy). *Q J Med* 1914; **7**: 444–54.

Batten's Disease Consortium. Isolation of a gene underlying Batten disease CLN3. *Cell* 1995; **22**: 949–57.

Baumann RJ, Markesbery WR. Juvenile amaurotic idiocy (neuronal ceroid lipofuscinosis) and lymphocyte fingerprint profiles. *Ann Neurol* 1978; **4**: 531–6.

Baumann RJ, Makersbery WR. Santavuori disease: diagnosis by leucocyte ultrastructure. *Neurology* 1982; **32**: 1277–81.

Beck M. Papilloedema in association with Hunter's syndrome. *Br J Ophthalmol* 1983; **67**: 174–7.

Beck M, Cole G. Disc oedema in association with Hunter's syndrome: ocular histopathological findings. *Br J Ophthalmol* 1984; **68**: 590–5.

Bennett MJ, Gibson KM, Sherwood WG *et al.* Reliable prenatal diagnosis of Canavan disease (aspartoacyclase deficiency): comparison of enzymatic and metabolite analysis. *J Inherit Metab Dis* 1993; **16**: 831–36.

Beutler E. Gaucher disease: new molecular approaches to diagnosis and treatment. *Science* 1992; **256**: 794–9.

Billings DM, Degnam M. Kinky hair syndrome: a new case and review. *Am J Dis Child* 1971; **121**: 447–52.

Blodi FC, Whinery RD, Hendricles CA. Lipoid proteinosis (Urbach–Wiethe) involving the lids. *Trans Am Ophthalmol Soc* 1960; **58**: 155–6.

Bolmers DJM, Gabreels FJM, Joosten EMG, Gabreeles–Festen A. Ceroid lipofuscinosis (Batten's disease), first ophthalmological report of cytoplasmic inclusions in Schwann's cell of the sural nerve in two patients with an amaurotic familial idiocy. *Acta Ophthalmol* 1973; **51**: 47–57.

Bolthauser E, Schirmert G, Gitzelmann R, Henn V. *Ocular Apraxia in Gaucher's Disease Type III. Presented at the Vth International Neuro-ophthalmological Society*. Belgium: Elsevier, 1984.

Bosch EP, Hart MN. Late adult-onset metachromatic leucodystrophy. *Arch Neurol* 1978; **35**: 475–81.

Brett EM. *Paediatric Neurology*. London: Churchill Livingstone, 1991: 175.

Brett EM, Ellis RB, Haas L *et al.* Late onset GM2 gangliosidosis. Clinical pathological and biochemical studies in eight patients. *Arch Dis Child* 1973; **48**: 775–85.

Brod RD, Packer AJ, Van Dyk JL. Diagnosis of neuronal ceroid lipofuscinosis by ultrastructural examination of peripheral blood lymphocytes. *Arch Ophthalmol* 1987; **105**: 1388–93.

Brownstein S, Meagher-Villemure K, Polomeno RC, Little JM. Optic nerve in globoid leucodystrophy (Krabbe's disease). *Arch Ophthalmol* 1978; **96**: 864–70.

Butler J De B, Camly M, Kruth H, Vanier M *et al.* Niemann–Pick variant disorders: comparison of errors of cellular cholesterol homeostasis in group D and C fibroblasts. *Proc Natl Acad Sci USA* 1987; **84**: 556–60.

Cahane M, Treister G, Abraham F, Melamed S. Glaucoma in siblings with Morquio syndrome. *Br J Ophthalmol* 1990; **74**: 382–4.

Calmettes L, Deodati F, Dupre A, Bec P. Manifestations oculaires du syndrome de Fabry. *Bull Soc Ophthalmol* 1967; **59**: 513–17.

Canter RM, Kabach MM. Sandhoff disease, heterozygote frequency in North American Jewish and non-Jewish populations: implications for carrier screening. *Am J Hum Genet* 1985; **37**: A48.

Carlson LA, Philipson B. Fish eye disease. *Lancet* 1979; **ii**: 921–3.

Casteels I, Taylor DSI, Lake BD, Spalton DJ, Bach G. Mucolipidosis IV: presentation of a mild variant. *Ophthalmol Paediatr Genet* 1992; **13**: 205–10.

Charlin C, Fernandez FL. The Urbach–Wiethe syndrome. *Arch Oph-*

thalmol (Paris) 1978; **35**: 521–6.

Chhabria S, Tomasi LG, Wong PWK. Ophthalmoplegia and bulbar palsy in variant form of maple syrup urine disease. *Ann Neurol* 1979; **6**: 71–81.

Chitayat D, Meunier CM, Hodgkinson KA *et al.* Mucolipidosis type IV: clinical manifestations and natural history. *Am J Med Genet* 1991; **41**: 313–18.

Cibis GW, Harris DJ, Chapman AL, Tripathi RC. Neurolipidosis I. *Arch Ophthalmol* 1983; **101**: 933–9.

Claussen M, Heim P, Knispel J, Goebel H, Kohlschütter A. Incidence of neuronal ceroid-lipofuscinoses in West Germany. *Am J Med Genet* 1992; **42**: 536–8.

Cogan DG. Ocular manifestations of spongy degeneration. *Birth Defects Orig Article Ser* 1976; **12**: 527–34.

Cogan DG, Kuwabara T. Histochemistry of the retina in Tay–Sachs disease. *Arch Ophthalmol* 1959; **61**: 414–23.

Cogan DG, Kuwabara T. The sphingolipidoses and the eye. *Arch Ophthalmol* 1968; **79**: 437–52.

Cogan DG, Kuwabara T, Moser H. Metachromatic leucodystrophy. *Ophthalmologica* 1970; **180**: 2–17.

Cogan DG, Kuwabara T, Moser H, Hazard GW. Retinopathy in a case of Farber's lipogranulomatosis. *Arch Ophthalmol* 1966: **75**: 752–8.

Cohen SMZ, Green WR, de la Cruz C *et al.* Ocular histopathologic studies of neonatal and childhood adrenoleucodystrophy. *Am J Ophthalmol* 1983; **95**: 82–96.

Collier MM. Dégénéréscence maculaire d'un type special dans un cas de maladie de Gaucher. *Bull Soc Ophthalmol Franc* 1961; **7**: 497–500.

Collins M, Traboulsi E, Maumenee I. Optic nerve head swelling and optic atrophy in the systemic mucopolysaccharidoses. *Ophthalmology* 1990; **97**: 1445–50.

Cotticelli L, Costagliola C, Rinaldi E, DiMeo A *et al.* Ophthalmological findings in phenylketonuria: a survey of 14 cases. *J Pediatr Ophthalmol Strabismus* 1985; **22**: 78–9.

Dangel ME, Bremer DL, Rogers GL. Treatment of corneal opacification in mucolipidosis IV with conjunctival transplantation. *Am J Ophthalmol* 1985; **99**: 137–42.

De Venecia G, Shapiro M. Neuronal ceroid lipofuscinosis—a retinal trypsin digest study. *Ophthalmology* 1984; **91**: 1406–11.

Deeg HJ, Shulman HM, Albrechtsen D, Craham TC, Storb R, Koppang N. Batten's disease: failure of allogenic bone marrow transplantation to arrest disease progression in a canine model. *Clin Genet* 1990; **37**: 264–70.

Del Monte MA, Maumenee IH, Green WR, Kenyon KR. Histopathology of Sanfilippo's syndrome. *Arch Ophthalmol* 1983; **101**: 1255–62.

Den Tandt WR, Van Martin JJ. Peroxidase in ceroid lipofuscinosis. *J Neurol Sci* 1978; **38**: 191–3.

Dickinson JP, Holton JB, Lewis OM *et al.* Maple syrup urine disease: 4 years experience with dietary treatment of a case. *Acta Pediatr Scand* 1969; **58**: 341–3.

Dietmann JL, Filippi de la Palavesa MM, Trauchant C, Kastler B. MR findings in mannosidosis. *Neuroradiology* 1990; **32**: 485–7.

Dreborg S, Erikson A, Hagberg B. Gaucher's disease (Norrbothnian type). I. General clinical description. *Eur J Pediatr* 1980; **133**: 107–18.

Dunn HC, Sweeney VP. Progressive supranuclear palsy, an unusual juvenile variant of Niemann–Pick disease. *Neurology* 1971; **21**: 442–3.

Elleder M, Jirasek A. International symposium on Niemann–Pick disease. *Eur J Pediatr* 1983; **140**: 90–1.

Emery JM, Green WR, Huff DS. Krabbe's disease. *Am J Ophthalmol* 1972; **74**: 400–6.

Emery JM, Green WR, Wyllie RG, Howell RR. GM(I) gangliosidosis, ocular and pathological manifestations. *Arch Ophthalmol* 1971; **85**: 177–87.

Eyb C. Augenhintergrundveranderungen bei der Rindlichen gaucherschen Erkrankurg. *Klin Wochtenschr* 1952; **64**: 38.

Feiler-Ofry V, Lewy A, Regenbogen L *et al.* Lipid proteinosis (Urbach–Wiethe syndrome). *Br J Ophthalmol* 1979; **63**: 694–8.

Fettes I, Killinger D, Volpe R. Adrenoleucodystrophy: report of a familial case. *Clin Endocrinol* 1979; **11**: 151–60.

Fink JK, Filling-Katz MR, Sokol J *et al.* Clinical spectrum of Niemann–Pick disease type C. *Neurology* 1989; **39**: 1040–9.

Fox MF, Du Toit DL, Warnich L, Retief AE. Regional localization of alpha galactosidase (CLS) to Xpter–q22, hexosaminidase B (HEXB) to 5q31–qter, and arylsulfatase B (ARSB) to 5pter–q13. *Cytogenet Cell Genet* 1984; **38**: 45–9.

Franceschetti AT. Fabry disease: ocular manifestations. *Birth Defects Orig Article Ser* 1976; **12**: 195–208.

François J. Ocular manifestations in demyelinating disease. *Adv Ophthalmol* 1979; **39**: 1–36.

François J. Ocular manifestations in inborn errors of carbohydrate and lipid metabolism. In: *Krabbe's Disease*, Part II, Section G. Basel: Karger, 1975: 98–100.

François J, Backulin J, Follmann P. Ocular manifestations of Urbach–Wiethe syndrome. *Ophthalmologica (Basel)* 1968; **155**: 433–48.

Gardiner M, Sandford A, Deadman M *et al.* Batten disease/Spielemeyer–Vogt disease, juvenile onset neuronal ceroid-lipofuscinosis gene (CLN3) maps to human chromosome 16. *Genomics* 1990; **8**: 387–90.

Garg BP, Markand ON, Dellyer WE, Warren C Jr. Evoked response studies in patients with adrenoleucodystrophy and heterozygous relatives. *Arch Neurol* 1983; **40**: 356–59.

George S, Graham-Brown R. Angiokeratoma corporis diffusum in fucosidosis. *J Roy Soc Med* 1994; **87**: 707.

Glasgow BJ, Brown HH, Hannah JB, Foos RY. Ocular pathologic findings in neonatal adrenoleucodystrophy. *J Am Acad Ophthalmol* 1987; **94**: 1054–61.

Godel V, Blumenthal M, Goldman B *et al.* Visual functions in Tay–Sachs disease patients following enzyme replacement therapy. *Metab Ophthalmol* 1978; **2**: 27–32.

Goebel HH, Shimokawa K, Argyrakis A, Pilz H. The ultrastructure of the retina in adult metachromatic leucodystrophy. *Am J Ophthalmol* 1978; **85**: 841–9.

Goldberg MF, Cotlier E, Fichenscher LG *et al.* Macular cherry red spot, corneal clouding and beta galactosidase deficiency. *Arch Int Med* 1971; **138**: 387–9.

Goldstein E, Wexler D. Niemann–Pick disease with cherry red spots in the macula. *Arch Ophthalmol* 1931; **5**: 704–6.

Good W. Overlooking: a sign of bilateral central scotomata in children. *Dev Med Child Neurol* 1992; **34**: 69–73.

Goutieres F, Arsenio-Nunes M-L, Aicardi J. Mucolipidosis IV. *Neuropediatrics* 1979; **10**: 321–31.

Green SH. Adrenoleucodystrophy. *Arch Dis Child* 1991; **66**: 830–3.

Hall NA, Patrick AD. Accumulation of phosphorylated dolichol in several tissues in ceroid-lipofuscinosis (Batten's disease). *Clin Chim Acta* 1987; **170**: 323–36.

Haltia M, Rapola J, Santavuori P, Keranen A. Infantile type of so-called neuronal ceroid lipofuscinosis 2. Morphological and biochemical studies. *J Neurol Sci* 1973; **18**: 269–85.

Hammami H, Daicker B, Streiff E *et al.* Leucodystrophie metachromatique associes au syndrome de Lowe. *Bull Mem Soc Fr Ophthalmol* 1973: **86**: 106–7.

Hara S, Hayasaka S, Mizuno K. Distribution and some properties of lysosomal arylsulfatases in the bovine eye. *Exp Eye Res* 1979; **28**: 641–50.

Harcourt B, Ashton N. Ultrastructure of the optic nerve in Krabbe's leucodystrophy. *Br J Ophthalmol* 1973; **57**: 885–91.

Harcourt B, Hopkins D. Tapeto-retinal degeneration in childhood presenting as a disturbance of behaviour. *Br Med J* 1962; **i**: 202–5.

Harzer K, Ruprecht KW, Seuffer-Schulze D, Jans U. Morbus Niemann–Pick B—enzymatisch giesichert mit unwarteter retinaler Beteiligung. *Graefe's Arch Clin Exp Ophthalmol* 1978; **296**: 79–88.

Hayasaka S, Kiyosawa M, Nomura H, Takase S. Papilledema in late-onset citrullinemia. *Am J Ophthalmol* 1974; **97**: 242–3.

Hobbs JR, Hugh-Jones K, Barrett AJ *et al.* Reversal of clinical features of Hurler's disease and biochemical improvement after treatment by bone marrow transplantation. *Lancet* 1981; **ii**: 709–11.

Hoffmann H, Fredrickson DS. Tangier disease. *Am J Ophthalmol* 1965; **39**: 582–5.

Honda Y, Sudo M. Electroretinogram and visually evoked cortical potential in Tay–Sachs disease; a report of two cases. *J Pediatr Ophthalmol* 1976; **13**: 226–9.

Hormia M. Diffuse cerebral sclerosis, melanoderma and adrenal insufficiency (adreno-leucodystrophy). *Acta Neurol Scand* 1978; **58**: 128–33.

Horn M, Warburg M. Menke's disease. *Birth Defects Orig Article Ser* 1976; **12**: 557–62.

Hussain AA, Marshall J. Nosological significance of retinopathies in neurodegenerative disorders with emphasis on Batten disease. *J Inherit Metab Dis* 1993; **16**: 267–71.

Iwamoto M, Nawa Y, Maumenee IH *et al.* Ocular histopathology and ultrastructure of Morquio syndrome (systemic mucopolysaccharidosis IV). *Graefe's Arch Clin Exp Ophthalmol* 1990; **228**: 342–9.

Jaben SL, Flynn JT, Parker JC. Neuronal ceroid lipofuscinosis: diagnosis from peripheral blood smear. *Ophthalmology* 1983; **90**: 1373–7.

Jaime S, Dalmas MF. Un cas de maladie de Gaucher associé à une ischémie rétinienne peripherique. *J Fr Ophthalmol* 1989; **12**: 461–3.

Johnsen DE, Coleman L, Poe L. MR of progressive neurodegenerative change in treated Menkes' kinky hair disease. *Neuroradiology* 1991; **33**: 181–2.

Kenyon KR. Ocular manifestations and pathology of systemic mucopolysaccharidoses. *Birth Defects Orig Article Ser* 1976; **12**: 133–53.

Kenyon KR, Maumenee IH, Green WR, Libert J, Hiatt RL. Mucolipidosis IV. *Arch Ophthalmol* 1979; **97**: 1106–12.

Kocen RS, Thomas PK. Peripheral nerve involvement in Fabry's disease. *Arch Neurol* 1970; **22**: 81–8.

Kodama H. Recent developments in Menkes disease. *J Inherit Metab Dis* 1993; **16**: 791–9.

Kohlschütter A, Gardiner RM, Goebel HH. Human form of neuronal ceroid-lipofuscinosis (Batten disease). *J Inherit Metab Dis* 1993; **16**: 241–4.

Konrad R, Wilson D. Assignment of the gene for acid lysosomal sphingomyelinase to human chromosome 17. *Cytogenet Cell Genet* 1987; **46**: 641.

Lake BD. The differential diagnosis of the various forms of Batten's disease by rectal biopsy. *Birth Defects Orig Article Ser* 1976; **12**: 455–64.

Lake BD. Lysosomal enzyme deficiencies. In: Adams JH, Corsellis JAN, Duchen LW, eds. *Greenfield's Neuropathology*, 4th edn. London: Edward Arnold, 1984: 491–572.

Lake BD, Cavanagh NPC. Early juvenile Batten's disease. *J Neurol Sci* 1978; **36**: 265–71.

Lake BD, Milla PJ, Taylor DSI, Young EP. A mild variant of ML4. *Birth Defects Orig Article Ser* 1982; **18**: 391–404.

Lavery MA, Green WR, Jabs EW, Luckenbach MW, Cox JL. Ocular histopathology and ultrastructure of Sanfilippo's syndrome, type IIIB. *Arch Ophthalmol* 1983; **101**: 1263–74.

Letson RD, Desnick RJ. Punctate lenticular opacities in type II mannosidosis. *Am J Ophthalmol* 1978; **85**: 218–24.

Levy NS, Dawson WW, Rhodes BJ, Garnica A. Ocular abnormalities in Menke's kinky hair syndrome. *Am J Ophthalmol* 1974; **77**: 319–25.

Libert J, Kenyon KR, Maumenee IH. Mucolipidosis III (pseudo-Hurler polydystrophy) ultrastructure of conjunctival biopsies. *Metab Ophthalmol* 1977a; **1**: 145–8.

Libert J, Tandeur M, Van Hoof F. The use of conjunctival biopsy and enzyme analysis in tears for the diagnosis of homozygotes and heterozygotes with Fabry's disease. *Birth Defects Orig Article Ser* 1976a; **12**: 221–39.

Libert J, Toussaint D. Tortuosities of retinal and conjunctival vessels in lysosomal storage disorders. *Birth Defects Orig Article Ser* 1982; **18**: 347–58.

Libert J, Van Hoof F, Farriaux J-P, Toussaint D. Ocular findings in I cell disease (mucolipidosis type II). *Am J Ophthalmol* 1977b; **83**: 617–28.

Libert J, Van Hoof F, Tandeur M. Fucosidosis: ultrastructural study of conjunctiva and skin and enzyme analysis of tears. *Invest Ophthalmol Vis Sci* 1976b; **15**: 626–39.

Libert J, Van Hoof F, Toussaint D *et al.* Ocular findings in metachromatic leucodystrophy. *Arch Ophthalmol* 1979; **97**: 1495–504.

Litjens T, Baker EG, Backmann KR, Morris CP, Hopwood J, Callen DF. Chromosomal localization of the ARSB, the gene for human *N*-acetylgalactosamine-4-sulphatase. *Hum Genet* 1989; **82**: 67–8.

Lonsdale D, Mercer RD, Faulkner WR. Maple syrup urine disease. *Am J Dis Child* 1963; **106**: 258–66.

Lowden JA, O'Brien JS. Sialidosis: a review of human neuraminidase deficiency. *Am J Hum Genet* 1979; **31**: 18–24.

McDonald JT, Sher PK. Ophthalmoplegia: a sign of metabolic disease in the newborn. *Neurology (Minn)* 1977; **27**: 971–3.

McDonnell J, Green W, Maumenee I. Ocular histopathology of systemic mucopolysaccharidosis, type IIA Hunter syndrome, severe. *Ophthalmology* 1983; **92**: 1772–80.

MacFaul R, Cavanagh N, Lake BD, Stephens R, Whitfield AE. Metachromatic leucodystrophy: review of 38 cases. *Arch Dis Child* 1982; **57**: 168–75.

McKeran RO, Bradbury P, Taylor D, Stern G. Neurological involvement in type I (adult) Gaucher's disease. *J Neurol Neurosurg Psychiatr* 1985; **48**: 172–5.

McKusick VA. *Mendelian Inheritance in Man.* Baltimore: Johns Hopkins University Press, 1986.

Mainardi P. Un caso di malattia dello sciroppo d'acero. *Pediatr Minerva* 1966; **18**: 1969–72.

Markesbery WR, Shield LK, Egel RT, Jameson MD. Late infantile neuronal ceroid-lipofuscinosis: an ultrastructural study of lymphocyte inclusions. *Arch Neurol* 1976; **33**: 630–5.

Martin JJ. Adult type of neuronal ceroid-lipofuscinosis. *J Inherit Metab Dis* 1993; **16**: 237–40.

Matthews JD, Weiter JJ, Kolodry EH. Macular halos associated with Niemann–Pick type B disease. *Ophthalmology* 1986; **93**: 933–8.

Mayou MS. Cerebral degeneration with symmetrical changes in the maculae in three members of a family. *Trans Ophthalmol Soc UK* 1904; **24**: 142–5.

Merin S, Livini N, Berman ER, Yatziv S. Mucolipidosis IV; ocular, systemic, and ultrastructural findings. *Invest Ophthalmol* 1975; **14**: 437–48.

Miller JD, McCliver R, Kanfer J. Gaucher's disease: neurologic disorder in adult siblings. *Ann Int Med* 1973; **78**: 883–7.

Mitchison HM, Williams RE, McKay TR *et al.* Redefined genetic mapping of juvenile onset neuronal ceroid lipofuscinosis on chromosome 16. *J Inherit Metab Dis* 1993; **16**: 339–41.

Moloney J, Masterson JG. Detection of adrenoleucodystrophy carriers by means of evoked potentials. *Lancet* 1982; **i**: 852, vol II,

no 8303.

Montgomery TR, Thomas GH, Valle DL. Mannosidosis in an adult. *Johns Hopkins Med J* 1982; **151**: 113–17.

Morgan SH, Crawford M d'A. Anderson–Fabry disease. *Br Med J* 1988; **297**: 872–3.

Morris MD, Lewis BD, Doolan PD, Harper HA. Clinical and biochemical observations of an apparently non-fatal variant of branched-chain ketoaciduria. *Pediatrics* 1961; **28**: 918–23.

Moser HW, Moser AB, Smith KD *et al.* Adrenoleucodystrophy: phenotypic variability and implications for therapy. *J Inherit Metab Dis* 1992; **15**: 645–64.

Muirhead JF, Jackson P. Urbach Wiethe disease. *Arch Ophthalmol* 1963; **69**: 174–9.

Multiple Authors. NCL Symposium. *J Clin Neuropathol* 1992; **11**: 157–66.

Multiple Authors. NCL Symposium. *J Inherit Metab Dis* 1993; **16**: 225–349.

Murphree AL, Beaudet AL, Palmer EA, Nichols BL. Cataract in mannosidosis. *Birth Defects Orig Article Ser* 1976; **12**: 319–25.

Musarella MA, Raab EI, Rudolph S, Grabowski GA, Desnick RJ. Oculomotor abnormalities in chronic GM2 gangliosidosis. *J Pediatr Ophthalmol Strabismus* 1982; **19**: 80–9.

Nakai H, Byers MG, Shows TB. Mapping HEXA to 15q 23q24. *Cytogenet Cell Genet* 1987; **46**: 667.

Naughten ER, Jenkins J, Francis DEM, Leonard JV. Outcome of maple syrup urine disease. *Arch Dis Child* 1982; **57**: 918–21.

Neville BCR, Lake BD, Stevens R, Sanders MD. A neurovisceral storage disease with vertical supranuclear ophthalmoplegia and its relationship to Niemann–Pick disease — a report of nine patients. *Brain* 1973; **96**: 97–120.

Newell FW, Matalon R, Meyer S. A new mucolipidosis with psychomotor retardation, corneal clouding, and retinal degeneration. *Am J Ophthalmol* 1975; **80**: 4410–49.

Newman NJ, Starck T, Kenyon K, Lessell S, Fish I, Kolodny EH. Corneal surface irregularities and episodic pain in a patient with mucolipidosis IV. *Arch Ophthalmol* 1990; **108**: 251–4.

Newton FH, Rosenberg RN, Laupert PW, O'Brien JS. Neurologic involvement in Urbach–Wiethe's disease (lipid proteinosis). *Neurology* 1971; **21**: 1205–13.

Norman RM, Forrester RM, Tingey AH. The juvenile form of Niemann–Pick disease. *Arch Dis Child* 1967; **42**: 91–6.

Orgül S, Daiker B, Kain H-L. Simultane Hornhaut transplantation bei mucopolysaccharidose. *Klin Mbl Augenheilkd* 1991; **198**: 430–2.

Ozaki H, Mizutani M, Hayashi H. Farber's disease. *Acta Med Okayama* 1978; **32**: 69–79.

Pampiglione G, Harden A. So-called neuronal ceroid lipofuscinosis. Neurophysiological studies in 60 children. *J Neurol Neurosurg Psychiatr* 1977; **40**: 323–30.

Parks MM, Schwilk NF. Bilateral lamellar-type cataracts in a case of phenylketonuria. *Am J Ophthalmol* 1963; **56**: 140–2.

Petrochelos M, Tricoules D, Kotziras T, Vauzoukos A. Ocular manifestations of Gaucher's disease. *Am J Ophthalmol* 1975; **80**: 1006–11.

Pinckers A, Bolmers D. Neuronal ceroid lipofuscinosis (ERG et EOG). *Ann Ocul (Paris)* 1974; **207**: 523–9.

Pullarkat RK, Patel UK, Brokerhoff H. Leucocyte docosahexanoic acid in juvenile form of ceroid lipofuscinosis. *Neuropaediatrics* 1978; **9**: 127–30.

Quigley MA, Green WR. Clinical and ultrastructural ocular histopathologic studies of adult-onset metachromatic leucodystrophy. *Am J Ophthalmol* 1972; **82**: 472–9.

Quisling RG, Andriola MR. Computed tomographic evaluation of the early phase of adrenoleucodystrophy. *Neuroradiology* 1979; **17**: 285–8.

Raininko R, Santavouri P, Heiskala H, Sainio K, Palo J. CT findings in neuronal ceroid-lipofuscinosis. *Neuropaediatrics* 1990; **21**: 95–101.

Raitta C, Santavouri P. Ophthalmological findings in infantile type of so-called neuronal ceroidlipofuscinosis. *Acta Ophthalmol* 1973; **51**: 755–63.

Rapin I, Katzmann R, Engel J Jr. Cherry red spots and myoclonus without dementia: a distinct syndrome with neuronal storage. *Arch Neurol* 1975; **32**: 349–54.

Reich C, Seife M, Kessler B. Gaucher's disease: a review and discussion of 20 cases. *Medicine* 1951; **30**: 1–20.

Reis S, Sheffer RN, Merin S, Luder AS, Bach G. Mucolipidosis IV: a mild form with late onset. *Am J Med Genet* 1993; **4**: 392–4.

Renard G, Bargeton E, Dhermy P, Aran J-J. Etude histologique des deterations de la retine et du nerf optique au cours de la leucodystrophie metachromatique. *Bull Mem Soc Fr Ophthalmol* 1963; **76**: 40–58.

Rider JA, Dawson G, Siakotos AN. Perspective of biochemical research in the neuronal ceroid lipofuscinosis. *Am J Med Genet* 1992; **42**: 519–24.

Riedel KG, Zwaan J, Kenyon KR *et al.* Ocular abnormalities in mucolipidosis IV. *Am J Ophthalmol* 1985; **99**: 125–37.

Rodriguez MJG, Conde HP, Nieto CL, Puerta AC, Carrete PT. La participation rétinienne dans la maladie de Gaucher. *J Fr Ophthalmol* 1992; **15**: 185–90.

Santavouri P, Haltia M, Rapola J, Raitta C. Infantile type of so-called neuronal ceroid lipofuscinosis I. A clinical study of 15 diseases. *J Neurol Sci* 1973; **18**: 257–67.

Santavouri P, Moren R. Experience of antioxidant treatment in neuronal ceroid-lipofuscinosis of Spielmeyer–Sjögren type I. *Neuropediatrics* 1977; **8**: 333–4.

Schaumberg HH, Powers JM, Raine CS, Suzuki K, Richardson JO. Adrenoleucodystrophy: a clinical and pathological study of 17 cases. *Arch Neurol* 1975; **32**: 577–91.

Schilovitz G, Grupper Ch, Payran P. Urbach–Wiethe's disease. Association with retinitis pigmentosa. *Ann Ocul (Paris)* 1973; **206**: 105–14.

Schuchman EH, Astrin KH, Aula P, Desnick RJ. Regional assignment of the structural gene for human alpha-L-iduronidase. *Proc Natl Acad Sci USA* 1984; **81**: 1169–73.

Schwartz JF, Kolendrianos ET. Maple syrup urine disease. A review with a report of an additional case. *Dev Med Child Neurol* 1969; **11**: 460–70.

Seelenfreund MH, Gartner S, Vinger F. The ocular pathology of Menke's disease. *Arch Ophthalmol* 1968; **80**: 718–23.

Sher NA, Letson RD, Desnick RJ. The ocular manifestations in Fabry's disease. *Arch Ophthalmol* 1979; **97**: 671–6.

Sher NA, Reiff W, Letson RD, Desnick RJ. Central retinal artery occlusion complicating Fabry's disease. *Arch Ophthalmol* 1978; **96**: 815–17.

Snebold NG, Rizzo JF, Lessell S, Pruett RC. Transient visual loss in ornithine trans carbamoylase deficiency. *Am J Ophthalmol* 1987; **104**: 407–12.

Snodgrass M. Ocular findings in fucosidosis. *Br J Ophthalmol* 1976; **60**: 508–13.

Snyder RO, Carlow TJ, Ledman J, Wenger DA. Ocular findings in fucosidosis. *Birth Defects* 1976; **12**: 241–6.

Spaeth GK, Frost P. Fabry's disease, its ocular manifestations. *Arch Ophthalmol* 1965; **74**: 760–9.

Spalton DJ, Taylor DSI, Sanders MD. Juvenile Batten's disease; an ophthalmological assessment of 26 patients. *Br J Ophthalmol* 1980; **64**: 726–32.

Spellacy E, Kennerly-Bankes JL, Crow J, Dourmashkin R, Shah D, Watts RWE. Glaucoma in a case of Hurler disease. *Br J Ophthalmol* 1980; **94**: 773–9.

Spielmeyer W. Weitere Mittheilung uber eine besondere form von familiarer amaurotischer idiotie. *Neurol Centralbl* 1905; **24**: 1131–2.

Spranger JW, Wiedemann HR. The genetic mucolipidoses: diagnosis and differential diagnosis. *Hum Genet* 1970; **9**: 113–19.

Swallow DM, Evans L, Stewart G, Thomas PK, Abrahams JD. Sialidosis type I. *Ann Hum Genet* 1979; **43**: 27–35.

Taylor D, Lake BD, Marshall J, Garner A. Retinal abnormalities in ophthalmoplegic lipidosis. *Br J Ophthalmol* 1981; **65**: 484–9.

Third International Conference on the Neuronal Ceroid Lipofuscinosis (Batten disease), Indianapolis, Indiana, USA. *Am J Med Genet* 1992; **42**: 516–18.

Thomas PK, Abrams JD, Swallow D, Stewart G. Sialidosis type I: cherry red spot myoclonus syndrome with sialidase deficiency and altered electrophoretic mobilities of some enzymes known to be glycoproteins. *J Neurol Neurosurg Psychiatr* 1979; **42**: 873–80.

Tønnensen T, Peterson A, Kruse TA, Gerdes A-M, Horn N. Multipoint linkage analysis in Menkes disease. *Am J Hum Genet* 1992; **50**: 1012–17.

Tønnensen T, Kleijer WJ, Horn N. Incidence of Menkes disease. *Hum Genet* 1991; **86**: 408–10.

Toussaint D, Davis P. Dystrophie maculaire dans une maladie de Menkes. Etude histologique oculaire. *J Fr Ophthalmol* 1978; **1**: 457–60.

Traboulsi EI, Maumenee IH. Ophthalmologic findings in mucolipidosis III (pseudo-Hurler polydystrophy). *Am J Ophthalmol* 1986; **102**: 592–7.

Tripp JH, Lake BD, Young E, Ngu J, Brett EM. Juvenile Gaucher's disease with horizontal gaze palsy in three siblings. *J Neurol Neurosurg Psychiatr* 1977; **40**: 470–68.

Usui T, Sawaguchi S, Abe H, Iwata K, Oyanagi K. Late infantile type galactosialidosis: histopathology of the retina and optic nerve. *Arch Ophthalmol* 1991b; **109**: 542–7.

Usui T, Shirakashi M, Takagi M, Abe H, Iwata K. Macular edema-like change and pseudopapilloedema in a case of Scheie syndrome. *J Clin Neuro-ophthalmol* 1991a; **11**: 183–5.

Valavanis A, Friede RL, Schubiger O, Hayek J. Computed tomography in neuronal ceroid lipofuscinosis. *Neuroradiology* 1980; **19**: 35–8.

Vanier MJ, Pentchev P, Rodriguez-Lafrasse C, Rousson R. Niemann–Pick disease type C: an update. *J Inherit Metab Dis* 1991; **14**: 580–95.

Vellodi A, Hobbs JR, O'Donnell NM, Coulter BS, Hugh-Jones K. Treatment of Niemann–Pick disease type B by allogenic bone marrow transplantation. *Br Med J* 1987; **295**: 1375–6.

Vrabec MP, Shapiro MB, Koller E, Wiebe DA, Henricks J, Albers JJ. Ophthalmic observations in lecithin cholesterol acyltransferase deficiency. *Arch Ophthalmol* 1988; **106**: 225–30.

Walton DS, Robb RM, Crocker AC. Ocular manifestations of group A Niemann–Pick disease. *Am J Ophthalmol* 1978; **85**: 174–80.

Weicksel J. Angiomatosis bzw: Angiokeratosis universalis. *Dtsch Med Wochenschr* 1925; **51**: 890–900.

Weingeist TA, Blodi FC. Fabry's disease—ocular findings in a female carrier. A light- and electron-microscopic study. *Arch Ophthalmol* 1971; **85**: 169–76.

Weiter JJ, Feingold M, Kolodny EH, Raghaven SA. Retinal pigment epithelial degeneration associated with leucocytic arylsulfatase A deficiency. *Am J Ophthalmol* 1980; **90**: 768–72.

Westmoreland BF, Groover RV, Sharbrough FW. Electrographic findings in three types of cerebromacular degeneration. *Mayo Clin Proc* 1979; **54**: 12–21.

Willems J, Gatti R, Darby JK, Romeo G, Durand P, Dumon JE, O'Brien JS. Fucosidosis revisited: a review of 77 patients. *Am J Med Genet*

1991; **38**: 111–31.

Winkelman MD, Banber BQ, Victor M, Moser HW. Non–infantile neuronopathic Gaucher's disease: a clinicopathologic study. *Neurology* 1983; **33**: 394–8.

Wolfe LS, Ng Ying Kin NMK, Baker RR, Carpenter S, Anderman F. Identification of retinol complexes as the autofluorescent component of the neuronal storage material in Batten disease. *Science* 1977; **195**: 1360–4.

Wraith JE. The mucopolysaccharidoses: a clinical review and guide to management. *Arch Dis Child* 1995; **72**: 263–7.

Wray SH, Cogan DG, Kuwabara T, Schaumberg HH, Powers JM. Adrenoleucodystrophy with disease of the eye and optic nerve. *Am J Ophthalmol* 1976a; **82**: 480–5.

Wray SH, Kuwabara T, Sanderson P. Menke's kinky hair disease: a light and electron microscopic study of the eye. *Invest Ophthalmol Vis Sci* 1976b; **15**: 128–38.

Yunis EJ, Lee RE. Further observations on the fine structure of globoid leucodystrophy. *Hum Pathol* 1972; **3**: 371–88.

Zabel RW, MacDonald IM, Mintsioulis G, Addison DJ. Scheie's syndrome: an ultrastructural analysis of the cornea. *Ophthalmology* 1989; **96**: 1631–8.

Zarbin MA, Green WR, Moser HW, Morton SJ. Farber's disease. *Arch Ophthalmol* 1985; **103**: 73–80.

Zee DS, Freeman JM, Holtzman NA. Ophthalmoplegia in maple syrup urine disease. *J Pediatr* 1974; **84**: 113–15.

Zetterstrom R. Disseminated lipogranulomatosis (Farber's disease). *Acta Paediatr* 1958; **47**: 501–10.

Zlotgora J, Chakraborty S, Knowlton RG, Wenger DA. Krabbe disease locus mapped to chromosome 14 by genetic linkage. *Am J Hum Genet* 1990; **47**: 137–44.

Zlotgora J, Schaap T, Bach G. Retinal pigment epithelial degeneration and arylsulfatase A deficiency. *Am J Ophthalmol* 1981; **92**: 136–8.

Zwann J. Eye findings in patients with phenylketonuria. *Arch Ophthalmol* 1983; **101**: 1236–7.

58: Specific Learning Disorders (Dyslexia)

Nicholas Cavanagh

Practical aspects

Reasons for academic failure in childhood include mental retardation, a sensory disability such as blindness or deafness, a primary emotional disturbance, or inadequate education. In addition there is a small but significant proportion (perhaps 5%) of children who in the absence of any of the above explanations, show profound difficulties in one or more of listening, thinking, talking, reading, writing, spelling or mathematics. In this book these children will be referred to as having specific learning difficulties, but there is considerable confusion and disagreement about terminology and in another context they might be described as having dyslexia, specific developmental dyslexia, minimal brain dysfunction, the attention deficit syndrome, hyperactive child syndrome, perceptual handicaps, the chronic brain syndrome, developmental dyspraxia, and so on (Wheeler & Watkins 1978). Even the term specific learning disability has its critics (Crystal 1982). What is abundantly clear from this prolifer-ation of terms is that there are many facets to the problem and that the affected children may present in a variety of ways.

Presentation

Usually the difficulties manifest for the first time soon after schooling begins, though sometimes there are overt problems much earlier. Some children are slow to learn to dress, have problems knowing which way round things go, or may be slow to show hand preference (usually this is becoming evident around 18 months to 2 years of age). They have great difficulty using scissors, eat messily, appear clumsy and unable to cope with buttons and laces; they seem to trip over 'nothing', fall frequently, and drop things excessively. These are the children who later may be shown to have a relatively low performance intelligence (IQ) on the Wechsler intelligence scale for children (WISC III) compared with higher verbal abilities. They go on to have problems learning to write smoothly and efficiently. Their writing is slow, untidy and messy. They cannot take down dictation, and fail examinations because they cannot commit their knowledge to paper. They have difficulty in distinguishing left from right, and tend to lose their place on the page. These are dyspraxic children.

A relationship between early speech delay and impaired language development, and subsequent learning difficulties has been suspected for a long time (McCready 1910). By 1979 Vellutino claimed that there was moderately suggestive evidence for this, and both the Dunedin (Silva 1980; Silva *et al.* 1983) and Waltham Forest (Graham *et al.* 1980) longitudinal studies of language delay in children show significant reading and spelling delay compared with controls. However, it is Stevenson's opinion (1984) that it is not possible to establish from the published data why the results represented a specific learning difficulty with reading that is not accounted for by the low intelligence scores of the children. Such children may show a discrepancy between their poor ability to express themselves and their ideas, and their normal or superior understanding of what is said to them. Alternatively, the problems may be the reverse with good expressive language, but inability to receive information and act on it or respond to it appropriately. These children may appear in a dream and forget messages or what they have been asked to do.

Problems of concentration, distractibility or overactivity are often present from an early age. Sometimes as babies they have been noticeably wriggly even when breastfeeding, have required very little sleep, have been very light sleepers, and have been constantly on the go.

It is upon a background of such problems early in life that the children then go on to have difficulties reading and writing, show bizarre spelling, confusion of b and d, saw and was, and more profound problems of syntax and semantics. Difficulties in memorizing may be more for visual input than auditory or vice versa, or sometimes both, manifesting with difficulty in learning by heart. Sometimes short-term memory deficits are paramount, and sometimes the difficulties are more to do with numbers than letters.

Finally all these problems commonly lead to behavioural disturbance. The children may lose confidence in themselves, and feel they are stupid. These feelings may be reinforced by their peers and ignorant teachers. They may become withdrawn and depressed. Aggression is a common consequence. Alternatively they may cease to try and become deliberately inattentive to the teaching of what they find hard to understand.

Diagnosis

The majority of children with specific learning difficulties are undetected until they start school, and even if their parents or preschool teachers have been concerned, it is unlikely that their problems will be investigated earlier. This delay results from a combination of factors: it may not be appreciated that the presenting symptoms portend learning difficulties and instead they may be attributed to immaturity; there may be a fear of making the problem worse by emphasizing it; there may be a belief that the child will compensate for it; and finally it may be asked what could be done anyway at such a young age? This important question is discussed below.

The role of the paediatrician

In most educational systems, even if the parent or teacher decides that a child does have learning difficulties, the sequence of events in establishing the diagnosis is still exceedingly haphazard and there is considerable uncertainty, in the lay, educational and medical spheres, about the ideal course of action. Some of this uncertainty results from the variability of the presenting symptoms, but partly reflects the ambivalence of some professionals about the validity of the concept of specific learning difficulties. This ambivalence is not shared by the British Paediatric

Association or the British Neurological Association (Gordon *et al.* 1983) or in the editorial column of the *Journal of Paediatrics* (Deuel 1981). They contended that the paediatrician is ideally suited to be in overall charge of management, seeking to correlate the essential contributions of educationalist and psychologist and referring when necessary to their ophthalmological, audiological, neurological and psychiatric colleagues. They might also seek the help, when appropriate, of a number of therapists; physiotherapists, occupational therapists, specialists in perceptual problems, speech and language therapists, or remedial teachers, and so on. In many societies a greater problem seems to be to find *anyone* with appropriate skills and interests to care for the child with specific learning difficulties.

The role of the psychologist

Although specific learning difficulties may be suspected by parent, teacher or doctor, the diagnosis of such problems can only be made by the psychologist; a detailed review of the tests needed for this is beyond the scope of this text. Although the age of the child concerned will determine to some extent the tests used, any assessment will need to measure the overall level of intelligence, reading ability (including both accuracy and comprehension), spelling age, mathematical ability, visual, and auditory discrimination, and so on. If over 6 years of age, the WISC III is the most useful test of general intellectual functioning since it provides information about both verbal and performance abilities. On the verbal scale, the subtests assess vocabulary, abstract verbal concepts, general knowledge, verbal reasoning, auditory sequential memory and mental arithmetic. On the performance scale, the subtests assess spatial organization and reasoning, visual perception, conceptual sequencing and visual associative learning and memory.

The role of the ophthalmologist

The attitude of the American Academy of Pediatrics, the American Association for Pediatric Ophthalmology and Strabismus, and the American Academy of Ophthalmology, is unequivocal about this (1992):

> Decoding of retinal images occurs in the brain after visual signals are transmitted from the retina via the visual pathways. Unfortunately, however, it has become common practice among some to attribute reading difficulties to one or more subtle ocular or visual abnormalities. Although the eyes are obviously necessary for vision, the brain interprets visual symbols. Therefore, correcting subtle visual defects cannot alter the brain's processing of visual stimuli. Children with dyslexia or related learning disabilities have the same ocular health statistically

as children without such conditions. There is no peripheral eye defect that produces dyslexia or other learning disabilities, and there is no eye treatment that can cure dyslexia or associated learning disabilities.

The ophthalmological status of dyslexics is probably the same as non-dyslexics (Aasved 1987) but an eye problem may combine to form an additional burden. There may be a higher incidence of convergence insufficiency in dyslexics (Latvala *et al.* 1994) but causality is difficult to prove.

The role of the physician

Ocular defects should be identified as early as possible and when correctable, managed by the ophthalmologist. These treatable conditions include refractive errors, focusing deficiencies, eye muscle imbalances and motor fusion deficiencies. The ophthalmologist may be consulted early, but if no ocular defect is found, the child should be referred to a paediatrician to co-ordinate required multi-disciplinary care.

Controversies

Eye defects, subtle or severe, do not cause reversal of letters, words or numbers. No scientific evidence is available to support claims that the academic abilities of dyslexic or learning disabled children can be improved with treatment based on:
1 visual training, including muscle exercises, ocular pursuit, tracking exercises or 'training' glasses (with or without bifocals or prisms);
2 neurological organizational training (laterality training, crawling, balance board, perceptual training); or
3 tinted or coloured lenses.
Some controversial methods of treatment result in a false sense of security that may delay or even prevent proper instruction or remediation. The expense of these methods is unwarranted and they cannot be substituted for appropriate remedial educational measures. Claims of improved reading and learning after visual training, neurological organization training, or use of tinted or coloured lenses, are typically based upon poorly controlled studies that rely on anecdotal information or testimony. These studies are frequently carried out in combination with traditional educational remedial techniques.

These views do not meet with universal acceptance. For example Dunlop (1972), an orthoptist, points to a higher instance of esophoria in reading disabled children compared with normals and advocates orthoptic intervention. Also, Stein and Fowler (1982) claim that just over 50% of dyslexics show 'unstable ocular motor dominance with possible consequent failure to develop dependable associ-

ation between retinal and ocular motor signals' and recommend treatment with uniocular occlusion.

Audiological assessment

The same uncertainty that exists about the role of the eyes in specific learning difficulties also attends the ears. By definition 'dyslexia' can only be diagnosed in the absence of significant hearing impairment, but this requirement does not refer to the possible role of transient, though significant, auditory difficulties during the early, critical years of life when language is being developed. The findings of Glass (1981) indicated that there is a connection between early conductive hearing loss and several measures of auditory learning (auditory perception, auditory vocal associations and auditory sequential memory). Zinkus *et al.* (1978) point out the language and auditory processing deficits experienced by children aged 6–11 years of age who in the first 3 years of life had chronic severe otitis media; they also found evidence that children with history of severe otitis media experience difficulty in performing tasks that require the integration of visual and auditory processing skills.

The question of which ear is dominant for language has been nearly as much a matter of study as eye dominance and vision. There seems to be unequivocal evidence of right ear dominance (left hemisphere) in right-handed normal people, fairly good evidence that it is established by the age of 5 years, and recent evidence that in children with dyslexia there is a strong left ear dominance (Chasty 1982).

The role of the paediatric neurologist

One of the problems of managing children with specific learning difficulties is that their problems often transcend the conventional speciality boundaries or remain at the periphery of several. An example of this is clumsiness, which is usually a dyspraxia but may be due to a neurological disorder of cerebellar or extrapyramidal pathways or be due to unsuspected hemiplegia. Other examples are children with wide verbal/performance discrepancies and children with the attention deficit syndrome. It would be beneficial for all such children to be referred at least once to a paediatric neurologist for a full neurological history, examination and, if indicated, investigation (e.g. neuroimaging) and treatment, e.g. with methylphenidate or piracetam. Of course, it does not take a neurologist to recognize 'soft' neurological signs, e.g. the fine involuntary movements of the outstretched fingers, right/left confusion, confused laterality, synkinesis, clumsiness with fine manipulative tasks, and so on. Nor does it need a neurologist to confirm that the significance of such findings is uncertain and not specific to children with specific learning difficulties. But in many instances an authoritative analysis of the signs and symptoms and firm advice on their meaning and relevance, and on the role of treatment or necessity for further investigation, makes a neurological consultation helpful to both the parents and the child, and those trying to help them.

Differential diagnosis

Some of the differential diagnoses of specific learning disabilities are mentioned in the first paragraph of this chapter. Distinction between mild to moderate mental retardation and specific learning difficulties depends upon the results of psychological testing. If mental retardation is found it may be present by itself or be part of a recognizable syndrome with genetic and possibly therapeutic implications: these children should always be referred to a paediatric neurologist. There are some dysmorphic features that might alert the ophthalmologist to possible mental handicap, e.g. macrocephaly (large head circumference), large stature as found in Soto's syndrome, cutaneous naevi such as achromic naevi or café-au-lait patches as found in tuberous sclerosis and neurofibromatosis, respectively, coarse features as may be present in mucopolysaccharidosis, short stature as may be found in hypothyroidism, or hypertelorism signifying underlying agenesis of the corpus callosum, and so on. This further emphasizes the role of the ophthalmologist in the detection and management of systemic disease and the fact that the paediatric ophthalmologist needs to have appropriate measuring apparatus and developmental scales readily available.

Progressive degenerative disease of the central nervous system may be so insidious as to masquerade as a static disorder or result in deterioration that is matched in tempo by natural adaptation and therefore be unrecognized in the early stages. Slowing down in acquisition of skills rather than frank loss of them may be the main indication of this but a careful developmental history will alert the physician (Cavanagh & Lobascher 1983).

Finally, it is important not to overlook the gifted child who, if unrecognized, may express his boredom with disturbed behaviour, withdrawal, depression and failing to progress at school (Lobascher & Cavanagh 1977).

Management

General

A significant aspect of the management of a problem is its recognition and delineation. Sometimes this is all that can be done but the beneficial effect in terms of relief by the patient or parents that there is not something more sinister afoot, that the problems are often partly self-limiting, that the child is not 'repeated' or that there are many other children with similar problems, must not be under-rated. Evi-

dence is emerging that there is a stage beyond the diagnosis, and that 'treatment' can be offered, its efficacy monitored and its benefits measured. Such optimism is relatively new. Yule (1976) asked 'does remedial help, help in relation to the school-aged child?' and concluded that there was no good evidence that it did confer any long-term benefits. Six years later a review of the intervening literature led Hewitson (1982) to the same conclusion, but Hicks (1986) pointed out some promising results with the combined strength deficit-orientated approach, i.e. remedial help which both capitalizes on a child's strengths as well as improves weaknesses (Hicks 1980). She refers to the study by Hicks and Spurgeon (1982) which characterized patterns of error in reading and spelling of the child with 'auditory' problems and the child who has difficulty attaching a verbal label to visual stimuli.

There are now widespread efforts to provide perceptual motor training for 'clumsy children', i.e. those with a relatively low performance compared with verbal IQ and showing a motor dyspraxia. The experience of M. Lobascher *et al.* (personal communication, 1990) at Great Ormond Street Hospital, London, with 100 such children, has shown that where there is good verbal function (VIQ greater than 105), expert therapy will lead to a closing of the V/P gap over a 6-month period with the performance IQ coming up to the verbal IQ. This effect, as measured by formal psychological assessment, is mirrored by a marked functional improvement but for this to be maintained the child has to continue to work to a 'recipe' and needs refresher courses in perceptual motor training over several subsequent years.

A variety of treatments are directed at correcting 'scotopic sensitivity', minor eye defects, eye dominance problems and crossed laterality. Whilst the initiators of these treatments may be enthusiastic, the studies refuting them are often not long behind (Bishop 1989; Robinson & Conway 1990; Menacker *et al.* 1993). 'The ophthalmologist must explain to the child and to the parent that dyslexia usually has no ophthalmological or visual cause, but is a disability with a neurophysiological background still unknown in which the only efficient treatment is within the area of pedagogy' (Lennarstrand & Ygge 1992).

Drug treatment

Hyperactivity, impulsiveness and distractibility are behavioural disturbances which are difficult to quantitate and, when attributed to a child, often raise the question of whether the observation is simply in the eye of the beholder. Nevertheless, there are a number of children with specific learning difficulties who appear to their teachers to have a very short attention span and to be unduly susceptible to environmental distractions. Treatment of such children with methylphenidate (Ritalin) may bring about a great improvement in their concentration, which on occasions has meant the difference between the child being accepted at his school as opposed to being expelled for unmanageable behaviour (Ottenbacher & Cooper 1983). There are two important criticisms to the use of this medication: (i) the danger of side-effects; and (ii) there is no proven long-term academic benefit to children so treated.

In the author's 20 years plus experience of using this medication in a dose of 0.6 mg/kg body weight per day in two divided doses (the second dose not being given after 2 o'clock in the afternoon), there have been no extrapyramidal side-effects nor depression of appetite, nor misery. In order to prevent the potential (but not proven) side-effects of growth inhibition, it is recommended that the medication is prescribed only from Monday to Friday and only during the school term. There is not yet any evidence that children treated with Ritalin perform any better academically in the long term, though Sebrecht *et al.* (1986) have shown its effectiveness in producing benefits in the performance of a number of basic cognitive tasks.

The author has no personal experience in the use of piracetam, which is claimed (Chase *et al.* 1984) to improve reading accuracy and comprehension, reading speed and writing accuracy as compared with a placebo-controlled group.

Psychiatric problems

Depression, aggression and behavioural disturbances may be very substantial problems for the child with specific learning disability. Generally they are symptoms secondary to the impact on the child of having specific learning disability, and resolve spontaneously with the benefit of appropriate remedial help for the learning disability. But sometimes the help of a child psychiatrist may be useful.

Theoretical considerations

Conceptual aspects

The questions, 'dyslexia — does it exist? Is it a disease?', have been revisited recently by Rosenberger (1992), provoked by a study from Shaywizt *et al.* (1992). That study showed that reading skills vary along with intelligence in the normal population, and that dyslexic children fall within the normal distribution. Nevertheless, Rosenbergen continues to believe that among the causes of underachievement in reading in relation to general ability, 'are the individual aptitude deficits that we refer to as "dyslexia"'.

Genetic aspects

The belief that there is an inherited basis to specific learn-ing difficulties goes back many years. Hermann's (1959) classic study on twins with dyslexia showed that in 12 monozygotic twins there was 100% concordance and in 33 dizygotic twins, a 33% concordance. An earlier study by Hallgren (1950) had shown a very high familial incidence in 116 cases with parent–sibling or first-degree relative involvement in all but 12 cases and he had concluded that there was an autosomal dominant pattern of inheritance. This is difficult to reconcile with the universal observations that boys are four times more commonly affected than girls.

Other viewpoints have been expressed, for example Rutter *et al.* (1970) who indicates the greater importance of biological rather than hereditary factors, and by Finucci *et al.* (1976) who concluded that there is no single mode of inheritance and urged more accurate subgrouping and categorization. An annotation 'The genetics of dyslexia' (Pennington 1990) is a useful update. That there is familial aggregation (familiarity) in dyslexia seems undoubted. The evidence to date of that familiarity indicating genetic transmission is most convincing in the expression of the view that 'the heritable component in dyslexia at the written language level is in phonological coding and the heritable precursor to that deficit in phonological coding is a deficit in phoneme awareness' (Pennington 1990). The modes of transmission are still not determined (though genetic heterogeneity seems likely), and the finding (Smith *et al.* 1983) of linkage between dyslexia and chromosome 15 heteromorphisms has yet to be confirmed independently.

Neuropathology and neuroimaging findings

Hier *et al.* (1978) performed a computed tomographic (CT) brain scan on 24 patients with dyslexia and found that in 10 there was a reversal in the normal pattern of cerebral asymmetry in that the right temporoparietal-occipital region was larger than the left. Even allowing for the fact that six of the 24 patients were left-handed, this figure was statistically significant. Duara *et al.* (1991), with magnetic resonance imaging (MRI) scans, pinpointed the asymmetry more specifically to the angular gyrus region, and also demonstrated a larger splenium in the corpus callosum of dyslexic compared with non-dyslexic subjects.

The first postmortem report on the brain of a dyslexic child (Drake 1968), indicated excess subcortical white matter neurones. A number of more recent postmortem studies show disorders of neuronal migration in the left cortex, particularly around the sylvian fissure and left planum temporale, foci of ectopic neurones in the subcortical white matter, and bilateral abnormalities of the thalami (Galaburda & Kempner 1979; Galaburda *et al.* 1983). Whilst these studies do not indicate the precise aetiology of the neuronal disturbance, they do indicate an organic rather than purely behavioural explanation for specific learning difficulties, and to a disturbance affecting early brain development. Recent MRI studies, however (Schultz *et al.* 1994), have failed to show differences between dyslexics and non-dyslexics.

Immunology

Geschwind and Behan (1984) reported an association between childhood dyslexia and immune disorders. A further study (Behan *et al.* 1985) has shown the presence of raised anti-Ro antibody titres in the serum of mothers with dyslexic children in a significantly greater proportion than in controls, raising the possibility that the antibody may play a role in the pathogenesis of dyslexia, perhaps synergistically with the male hormone (Geschwind & Behan 1982).

Electroencephalogram

The electroencephalogram (EEG) recorded conventionally in the form of a continuously fluctuating tracing on a polygraph, does not have any significant role in the investigation or management of children with specific learning difficulties. However, re-displaying the EEG in terms of the amount of energy or power occurring at a given moment in time for each of the frequencies of the EEG across the entire spectrum of frequencies (quantitative topographic mapping) and in colour has demonstrated a difference between dyslexia and normal controls that can be used diagnostically and which points to aberrant neurophysiology in dyslexia (Duffy *et al.* 1979, 1980a, b).

Ocular aspects

The literature relating to ocular movements and reading disability is a confusing one, partly because of the difficulty in defining reading disability and partly because of lack of normal controls. These problems of interpretation are discussed by Pavlides and Miles (1981), and Pavlides in his own studies takes great care to define what he means by dyslexia and to include controls. His studies confirmed the observations that dyslexic children show abnormali-

ties of duration of eye fixation, perceptual span, ocular sweeps and increased regressions of the eyes during reading. By comparing dyslexic children with backward readers with the same chronological and reading age, he was able to discount the effect of patient difficulties with textual comprehension. His development of a test to assess a child's ability to follow sequentially illuminated lights, aimed to overcome environmental, psychological and intellectual factors by avoiding the use of a text, and he has shown that dyslexic children demonstrate specific difficulties. The question then posed is whether the difficulties derive from impaired oculomotor control of the eyes or from an inability to sequence. Causality is always difficult to prove, which has been one of the reasons why many ophthalmologists and others have felt that the eye movement and some other problems seen in dyslexic children may be the effect of the reading difficulties rather than the cause. Stein *et al.* (1987, 1988) however, feel that a defect in vergence control is an important cause, but not the only cause of dyslexia. They note that some children make mainly phonological errors and that others do not improve with the occlusion that may help those with vergence defects, and speculate that the underlying cause may exert its effect by a combination of vergence defect and by disturbing phonemic segmentation.

The Dunlop test (Fig. 58.1) is a synoptophore test in which foveal-sized fusion slides are placed in the synoptophore tubes with the controls towards the examiner and they are viewed with each eye separately (a and b). The child is asked to move the tubes to join (fuse) the two slides so that he sees one house and two trees (c).

Whilst the child is concentrating on the door of the house the examiner abducts the synoptophore tubes and asks the child to tell him whether the large or the small tree moves. The tree that moves indicates the non-dominant eye. This is carried out at least six times then repeated with the positioning of the slides reversed.

Stein *et al.* (1986) have shown that 30% of a group of 753 schoolchildren have an unstable reference eye on the Dunlop test, the incidence falling with increasing age. Children with unstable responses were much more likely to be backward readers. One very valid point is that in reading-aged children, a treatment by supervised monocular

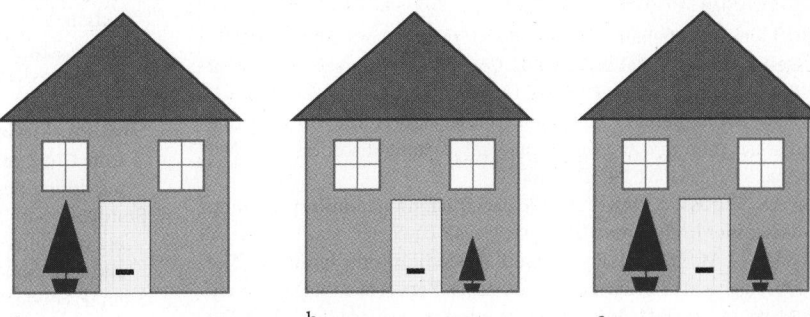

Fig. 58.1 The Dunlop test: see text.   a   b   c

occlusion is very unlikely to do harm, but its worth is not established.

References

Aasved, H. Ophthalmological status of schoolchildren with dyslexia. *Eye* 1987; **1**: 61–8.

American Academy of Paediatrics, American Association for Paediatric Ophthalmology and Strabismus/American Academy of Ophthalmology. A policy statement: learning disabilities, dyslexia and vision. *Paediatrics* 1992; **90**: 124–6.

Behan M, Behan P, Geschwind N. Anti-Ro antibodies in mothers of dyslexic children. *Dev Med Child Neurol* 1985; **27**: 538–42.

Bishop DVM. Unfixed reference, monocular occlusion and developmental dyslexia—a critique. *Br J Ophthalmol* 1989; **73**: 209–16.

Cavanagh N, Lobascher M. Childhood dementia. *Med Int* 1983; **31**: 1682–5.

Chase CH, Schmitt RL, Russell G, Tablal P. A new chemotherapeutic investigation: piracetam effects on dyslexia. *Ann Dyslexia* 1984; **34**: 29–48.

Chasty H. Dichotic listening techniques and brain specialisation. In: *Current Research into Specific Learning Difficulties: Neurological Aspects*. Bath: Better Books, 1982: 50–9.

Crystal D. Linguistic factors in specific learning difficulty. In: *Current Research into Specific Learning Difficulties. Neurological Aspects*. Bath: Better Books, 1982: 1–14.

Deuel R. Minimal brain dysfunction, hyperkinesis, learning difficulties and attention deficit disorder. *J Pediatr* 1981; **98**: 912–15.

Drake WE. Clinical and pathological findings in a child with developmental learning disability. *J Learn Disab* 1968; **1**: 9–25.

Duara R, Kusheh A, Gross-Glenn K. Neuroanatomic differences between dyslexia and normal readers on magnetic resonance imaging scans. *Arch Neurol* 1991; **48**: 410–16.

Duffy F, Burchfield J, Lombroso C. Brain electrical activity mapping (BEAM): a method for extending the clinical utility of EEG and evoked potential data. *Ann Neurol* 1979; **5**: 309–21.

Duffy FH, Denckla MB, Bartels P, Sandini E. Dyslexia: regional differences in brain electrical activity by topographic mapping. *Ann Neurol* 1980a; **7**: 412–20.

Duffy FH, Denckla MB, Bartels P, Sandini G, Kiessling LS. Dyslexia: automated diagnosis by computerised classification of brain electrical activity. *Ann Neurol* 1980b; **7**: 421–8.

Dunlop P. Dyslexia. The orthoptic approach. *Aust Orthop J* 1972; **12**: 16–20.

Finucci JM, Guthrie JT, Childs AL, Abbey H, Childs B. The genetics of specific reading disability. *Ann Hum Genet* 1976; **40**: 1–23.

Galaburda AM, Kempner TL. Cytoarchitectonic abnormalities in developmental dyslexia: a case study. *Ann Neurol* 1979; **6**: 94–100.

Galaburda AM, Sherman GF, Geschwind N. Developmental dyslexia: third consecutive case with cortical anomalies. *Neurosci Abstr* 1983; **9**: 940.

Geschwind N, Behan P. Laterality, hormones and immunity. In: Geschwind N, Galaburda A, eds. *Cerebral Dominance: The Biological Foundations*. Harvard: Harvard University Press, 1984: 211–24.

Geschwind N, Behan P. Left handedness: association with immune disease, migraine and developmental learning disorders. *Proc Nat Acad Sci USA* 1982; **79**: 5097–100.

Glass R. The association of middle-ear effusion and auditory learning difficulties in children. *Rehab Lit* 1981; **42**: 81–5.

Gordon N, McKinlay I, Rosenbloom R. Medical contribution to: The Management of Children with Dyslexia. Report of a Working Party set up by the British Paediatric Neurology Association. *Arch Dis Childhood* 1984; **59**: 588–90.

Graham P, Stevenson J, Richman N. Epidemiology of language delay in childhood. In: Rose FC, ed. *Clinical Neuroepidemiology*. Tunbridge: Pitman Medical, 1980.

Hallgren B. Specific dyslexia: a clinical and genetic study. *Acta Psychiatr Neurol* 1950; **65**(Suppl.): 1–287.

Hermann K. *Reading Disability: A Medical Study of Blindness and Related Handicap*. Springfield, Illinois: CC Thomas, 1959.

Hewitson J. The current status of remedial intervention for children with remedial problems. *Dev Med Child Neurol* 1982; **24**: 183–93.

Hicks C. Modality preference and the teaching of reading and spelling to dyslexic children. *Br Educ Res J* 1980; **6**: 175–87.

Hicks C. Remediating specific reading disabilities: a review of approaches. *J Res Read* 1986; **9**: 39–55.

Hicks C, Spurgeon M. Two-factor analytic studies of dyslexic subtypes. *Br J Ed Psychol* 1982; **52**: 289–300.

Hier DB, Le May M, Rosenberger PB, Perlo VP. Developmental dyslexia. *Arch Neurol* 1978; **35**: 90–2.

Latvala M-L, Korhonen TT, Pentinen M. Ophthalmic findings in dyslexic schoolchildren. *Br J Ophthalmol* 1994; **78**: 339–43.

Lennarstrand G, Ygge J. Dyslexia: ophthalmologic aspects. *Acta Ophthalmol* 1992; **70**: 3–13.

Lobascher M, Cavanagh N. The other handicap: brightness. *Br Med J* 1977; **2**: 1269–71.

McCready EB. Biological variations in the higher cerebral centres causing retardation. *Arch Pediatr* 1910; **27**: 506–13.

Menacker S, Breton M, Radcliffe J, Gole G. Do tinted lenses improve the reading performance of dyslexic children? A cohort study. *Arch Ophthalmol* 1993; **111**: 213–18.

Ottenbacher KJ, Cooper HM. Drug treatment of hyperactivity in children. *Dev Med Child Neurol* 1983; **25**: 358–66.

Pavlides G, Miles TR, eds. *Dyslexic Research and its Application to Education*. Chichester: Wiley, 1981.

Pennington BF. Annotation: the genetics of dyslexia. *J Child Psychol Psychiatr* 1990; **31**: 193–201.

Robinson G, Conway R. The effects of Irlen colored lenses on students' specific reading skills and their perception of ability: a 12-month validity study. *J Learn Dis* 1990; **23**: 589–96.

Rosenberger PB. Dyslexia is it a disease? *N Engl J Med* 1992; **326**: 192–3.

Rutter M, Tizard J, Whitmore K. *Education, Health and Behaviour*. London: Longmans, 1970. (Reprinted Krieler, Huntington, New York, 1981.)

Schultz RJ, Cho NK, Staib LH *et al*. Brain morphology in normal and dyslexic children: the influence of sex and age. *Ann Neurol* 1994; **35**: 732–42.

Sebrecht M, Shaynitz S, Shaynitz B, Jatlan P, Anderav G, Cohen D. Components of attention: methylphenidate dosage and blood levels in children with attention deficit syndrome. *Pediatrics* 1986; **7**: 222–8.

Shaywitz SE, Escobar MD, Shaywitz BA, Fletcher JM, Makuch R. Evidence that dyslexia may represent the lower tail of a normal distribution of reading ability. *N Engl J Med* 1992; **326**: 145–50.

Silva PA. The prevalence, stability and significance of developmental language delay in pre-school children. *Dev Med Child Neurol* 1980; **22**: 768–77.

Silva PA, McGee R, Williams SM. Developmental language delay from 3 to 7 years and its significance for low intelligence and reading difficulties at age 7. *Dev Med Child Neurol* 1983; **25**: 783–93.

Smith SD, Kimberling WJ, Pennington BF, Lubbs HA. Specific reading disability: identification of an inherited form through linkage and analysis. *Science* 1983; **219**: 1345–7.

Stein JF, Fowler S. Diagnosis of dyslexia by means of a new indication of eye dominance. *Br J Ophthalmol* 1982; **66**: 332–6.

Stein JF, Riddell PM, Fowler MS. Disordered vergence control in dyslexic children. *Br J Ophthalmol* 1988; **72**: 162–7.

Stein JF, Riddell PM, Fowler MS. The Dunlop test and reading in primary school children. *Br J Ophthalmol* 1986; **70**: 317–20.

Stein, JF, Riddell PM, Fowler MS. Fine binocular control in dyslexic children. *Eye* 1987; **1**: 433–9.

Stevenson J. Predictive value of speech and language screening. A review article. *Dev Med Child Neurol* 1984; **26**: 528–38.

Vellutino FR. Dyslexia. In: *Theory and Research*. Cambridge, Massachusetts: MIT Press, 1979: 237.

Wheeler TJ, Watkins EJ. Dyslexia: the problem of definition. *Dyslexia Rev* 1978; **1**: 1–4.

Yule W. Issues and problems in remedial education. *Dev Med Child Neurol* 1976; **18**: 674–82.

Zinkus P, Gottlieb M, Schapiro M. Developmental and psychoeducational sequelae of chronic otitis media. *Am J Dis Child* 1978; **132**: 1100–4.

59: Pupil Anomalies and Reactions

Creig S. Hoyt

Whilst an understanding of the anatomy (Fig. 59.1), physiology and pathophysiology of the pupillary pathways is of paramount importance to the paediatric ophthalmologist, they are dealt with so excellently in other books (most

notably by Miller 1985) that only aspects relevant to children will be discussed here.

Development

The pupillary light response is absent in infants of 29 gestational weeks or less, but is usually present by 31 or 32 weeks (Robinson 1966; Isenberg *et al.* 1990). At birth the pupil is small: it enlarges in the first months of life and is probably at its largest at the end of the first decade, before gradually becoming small again in old age. The pupil reactions of term or premature infants are often of small amplitude and because of their small resting size they may be difficult to elicit clinically. Cocaine and hydroxyamphetamine are less potent in infants than in the older children suggesting that the miosis of the newborn is due to decreased sympathetic tone (Korczyn *et al.* 1978). In very premature babies the pupil may not have fully formed; during the seventh month the vascular pupillary membrane atrophies and the pupil appears. Until after 32 weeks of gestation mydriasis should not be taken as necessarily indicating a central nervous system lesion and an unresponsive pupil does not necessarily indicate an afferent defect (Isenberg *et al.* 1990).

Dynamic retinoscopy (Haynes *et al.* 1965) indicates that the infants from 6 days to 1 month of age exhibit no evidence of accommodation but that normal function is achieved by 3–4 months. The effect of this lack of accommodation is defocusing of the higher spatial frequencies, the detection of which requires a greater discrimination than the younger infant is capable of. Braddick *et al.* (1979), however, using photorefraction have demonstrated an ability to accommodate of over 1 dioptre in the neonate, and this increases rapidly in the first month and to a lesser extent in the first few years of life, with high amplitudes from 4 years onwards until presbyopia sets in.

The near synkinesis

When someone looks from a far to a near point, the eyes converge, the pupils constrict and the eyes focus (accommodate); these three components are separate in origin

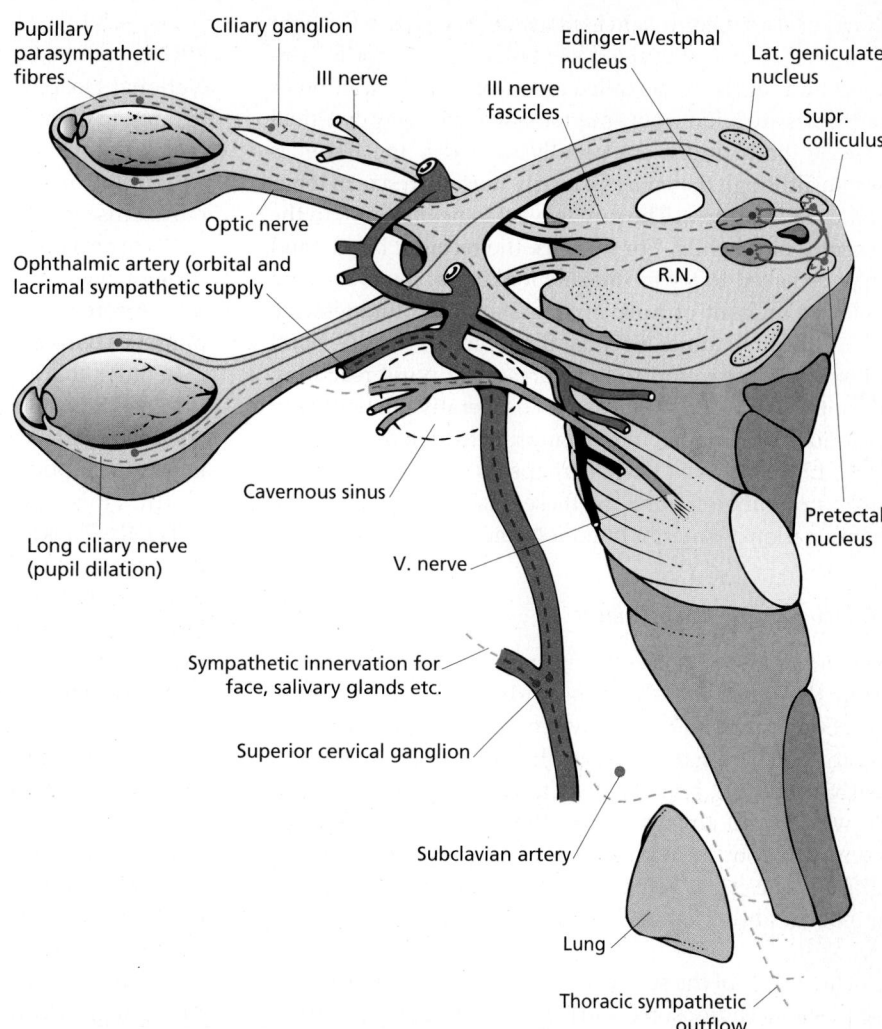

Fig. 59.1 Schematic representation of the efferent and afferent pathways involved in pupillary reactions. Red = blood vessels and parasympathetic. Blue = afferent visual pathways. Green = sympathetic pathway.

but linked together as a common response except in some disease states or by pharmacological manipulation when one or more elements may be selectively impaired. Disturbances in the relationship between the amount of accommodation and convergence are important aspects of most childhood squints and the manipulation of that ratio may be important in management (see Chapters 65, 66 and 67).

In small children the testing of the near pupil response is much more difficult than the pupil response to light. The most important factor in testing is to provide a suitable fixation target, for example, a small internally lit toy for an infant, a mobile toy with sufficient detail to need focusing for a small child and letters or numbers for the literate.

Congenital and structural abnormalities

Congenital, structural and developmental anomalies in the pupil include the following (see also Chapters 38 and 50).

- Aniridia.
- Micropupil (congenital idiopathic microcoria).
- Polycoria and corectopia.
- Coloboma.
- Peninsula pupil: an inherited partial iris sphincter atrophy with dilated oval pupils (Bosanquet & Johnson 1981).
- Persistent pupillary membrane.
- Congenital mydriasis and miosis (see Miller 1985).
- Irregular pupils.
- Abnormalities of iris colour.

Abnormalities of pupil reactivity

Afferent pupil defects

Amaurotic pupils

A totally blind eye resulting from eye or optic nerve disease usually has no pupil reaction to a light shone on it. If the blindness is unilateral the affected eye has no pupil reaction at all when a light is shone on it but when the light is shifted to the unaffected eye both pupils rapidly constrict and this is the so-called amaurotic pupil reaction. If both eyes are blind from anterior visual pathway or retinal disease, both pupils are usually dilated if the lesion is recent although they may be nearly normal in size in long-standing blindness. The pupils react to near stimuli in the recently blind child. For instance the recently blind child may be asked to try to imagine looking at his own hand held up in front of him; in long-standing blindness the child usually cannot do this. Sometimes a totally blind person may be found to have preserved pupil reactions, despite careful technique and a co-operative patient who is genuinely blind and not attempting to look near (Taylor 1982; Lhermitte *et al.* 1984). Perhaps there are a few surviving pupillomotor fibres in these cases, or they have a combination of anterior blindness and cortical disease.

Relative afferent pupil defect

When one optic nerve afferent pathway is more affected than the other there may be a difference in the pupil reactions based on the relative conduction of the pupillomotor fibres from the two eyes. It is very useful in the preverbal child but requires meticulous technique, the basis of which is to always subject the two eyes to the same stimulus, both in intensity and direction. It only distinguishes one eye as being more affected than the other and is not an absolute assessment or measurement of pupil function.

The details of the set-up and performance of the test are important (Thompson & Corbett 1991). In a dimly lit room the observer uses a bright light (hence the alternative name 'the swinging flash light test') which is shone on each eye individually while the child, if possible, has his fixation maintained at one position, preferably in the distance. Any difference in reaction is noted. Then the light is shone on the expected 'better' eye for about 3 seconds and then rapidly moved to the suspected 'worse' eye (Thompson *et al.* 1981). If the second eye is really worse both pupils will dilate by a direct and consensual reaction driven by the pupil afferent system from the worse eye. Similarly if the light is moved from the worse to the better eye the pupils will constrict. In either direction of movement there may be a momentary constriction when the pupil is first stimulated.

Although the clinical test is not a measurement it can be graded, usually I–IV, with IV being an amaurotic pupil. Measurement using graded filters or pupillography (Fison *et al.* 1979; Bell *et al.* 1993) is usually too difficult in a child. If there is also a unilateral efferent defect or ocular defect the test can still be performed because the reactions from one eye are always bilateral and the pupil whose efferent system is intact can be observed for the assessment of both afferent systems.

The relative afferent pupil defect (RAPD) is usually attributed to Marcus Gunn, an ophthalmologist at the National Hospitals for Nervous Diseases, London, at the beginning of this century.

The RAPD is essentially a test of optic nerve function although it may be abnormal in patients with extensive retinal disease. As Miller (1985) points out it *never* occurs with corneal disease, cataract, a moderately sized vitreous haemorrhage, central serous retinopathy or drusen of the disc. Afferent defects may occur with profoundly amblyopic eyes (Greenwald & Folk 1983; Portnoy *et al.* 1983).

In older children a useful subjective addition to the test is to ask the child which eye sees the light brightest. The child may be asked a question, 'if the light in the good eye is worth 1 pound/dollar how much is the other one worth?', this may give a very rough quantification.

The RAPD is a very sensitive test even in children and it is common experience to find normal acuity and colour vision in the presence of an afferent defect, most particularly in children in the recovery phase of an optic neuropathy, but also in posterior lesions involving the afferent pathway in the midbrain (Forman *et al.* 1990).

A technique known as the edge-light pupil cycle time (Miller & Thompson 1978a, b) may help to give information about individual eyes as opposed to the relative information of the RAPD. The technique needs a very co-operative patient because it involves measuring the time between stimulus and response when a light is shone on the pupil margin; this can be done by simple observation with the beam of a slit lamp reduced to 0.5 mm thick and shone at the margin of the pupil in such a way that when the light goes through the pupil it causes it to constrict to a degree that it then blocks completely the admission of light to the eye. At least 10 cycles are timed with a stopwatch and the total time divided by the number of cycles to obtain the time in milliseconds. A normal response is less than 954 milliseconds in either eye and there is normally less than 70 milliseconds difference between the two eyes. The cycle time increases with age (Manor *et al.* 1981).

Chiasmal, optic nerve and tract lesions do not produce by themselves anisocoria and a chiasmal defect, unless it involves the optic nerve, does not have a RAPD. Because of the greater proportion of crossing than uncrossing fibres in the chiasm (Burde 1967) a complete (but not a partial) optic tract lesion may be associated with a contralateral RAPD (Newman & Miller 1983): this is not easy to detect clinically.

Light-near dissociation

When the pupil reacts better to a near than to a light stimulus or vice versa there is said to be light-near dissociation; a relatively poor, rather than an absent light reaction is much more common. It must be remembered that a bright light is necessary to test the pupil's light reaction otherwise the powerful near reflex will always appear better than the light reaction. With the expectation of errors in testing techniques or poor patient co-operation there is no pathological situation where the pupillary light reflex is normal while the near response is defective.

Afferent pupillomotor defects

Any cause of an afferent pupil light reflex will cause the pupil to react less well than to near light than near targets but there are several relatively specific entities.

Damage to the pupillomotor fibres in the dorsal midbrain after they have branched from the optic tract and before they have become associated with the fibres of the near response in the Edinger–Westphal nucleus may cause a relatively poor response to the light with relatively intact pupil response to a near stimulus.

Argyll Robertson pupils

The archetypal light-near pupillary dissociation was described by Douglas Argyll Robertson in 1869. This type of abnormality is usually seen in adults with tabes dorsalis or other forms of tertiary syphilis but is said to be occasionally seen in young persons with congenital syphilis. Typically the pupils are small, irregular and they constrict more fully and more briskly to a near stimulus than to light. They may dilate less well than normal pupils. If the slit lamp is used, a light response may just be detected. Vision is normal unless there is associated visual pathways disease. The iris is often seen to be atrophic on slit-lamp examination. There is still considerable discussion as to the site of the lesion but Miller (1985), after an elegant discussion, concludes that it is due to neuronal damage in the region of the sylvian aqueduct.

Sylvian aqueduct syndrome

Expanding lesions dorsal to the sylvian aqueduct in children include pinealomas, ependymomas, 'trilateral' retinoblastoma, granulomas and cystic lesions. Compression of the dorsal midbrain produces light-near dissociation that may be associated with a vertical gaze palsy, lid retraction, accommodation defects and convergence–retraction nystagmus: the resting size of the pupils is usually larger than normal. Sometimes, probably in more rapidly enlarging tumours, the pupils may be large, and poorly reactive to light or near stimuli.

Others

Adie's pupils (see below) may react better to near than to light stimuli, and in aberrant regeneration of the third nerve the pupil may respond better to near stimuli.

Uneven or sinuous pupil reactions

In some conditions the pupil reactions may appear to be segmental, or 'sinuous', with one part of the iris sphincter reacting better in one segment than another, the pupil is often irregular in shape. The phenomenon may sometimes be seen with the naked eye but it is better seen with magnification by loupe or by slit-lamp examination.

Adie's syndrome (tonic pupil syndrome)

This condition may occur in children (Thompson 1977a) but is more frequently found in young adults, especially women. It is usually unilateral but may be bilateral, sometimes with an asynchronous onset (Dulton & Paul 1992).

Children rarely have symptoms related to the onset but they may fail a school near vision test, or complain of blurred near vision or photophobia. The potential for the development of anisometropic amblyopia must be considered in the hyperopic child with Adie's syndrome. In the author's experience it is the parents noticing an anisocoria that most often brings it to the attention of the doctor. It has been described in association with opsoclonus and neuroblastoma (West & Repka 1992).

The acutely affected pupil is usually a little larger than its (uninvolved) fellow but if viewed in darkness, it may be smaller as the normal pupil is free to dilate widely. It always has a segmental paralysis of the iris sphincter (Thompson 1978) which may be extensive with virtually all of the pupil being paralysed and only reacting sluggishly and in a sinuous fashion (the 'tonic' pupil). There is also a defect in accommodation which is often marked at first (Bell & Thompson 1978) but which gradually improves over 2 or more years (Thompson 1977a). Corneal sensation may be reduced when tested with an aesthesiometer (Purcell *et al.* 1977) or even with a whisp of cotton wool. This is probably due to damage to the sensory fibres which also pass through the ciliary ganglion.

Patients with Adie's syndrome may be hyporeflexic or areflexic in their extremities. Adie's syndrome may be diagnosed by finding an internal ophthalmoplegia, unilateral or asymmetrical with sinuous pupil reactions in a healthy person with normal corrected vision. Denervation hypersensitivity of the pupil may be demonstrated by finding pupillary constriction 20 minutes after instillation of pilocarpine 0.1% (Bourgon *et al.* 1978); methacholine 2.5% is probably a less sensitive and less pharmacologically stable alternative. Pharmacological hypersensitivity (Fig. 59.2) may occur with postciliary ganglionic as well as preciliary ganglionic lesions (Ponsford *et al.* 1982).

Deep tendon reflex abnormalities with an intact vibration sense suggest more widespread neural involvement

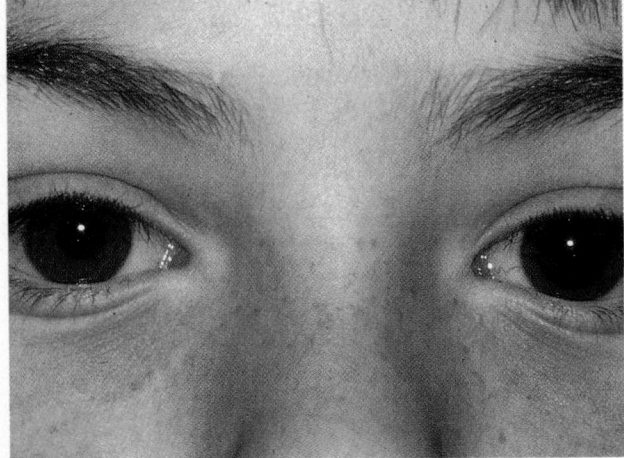

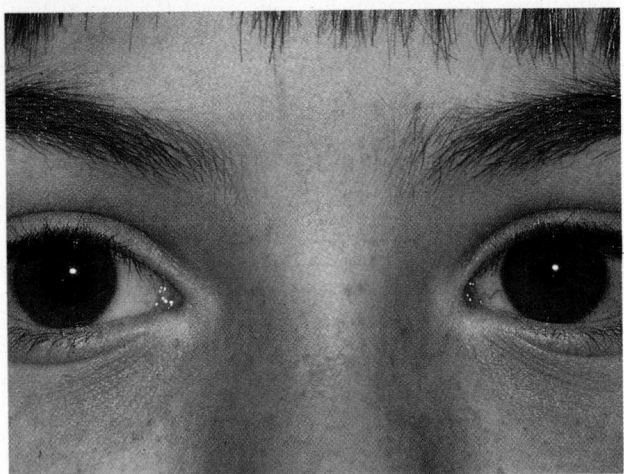

Fig. 59.2 (a) Left Adie's pupil before bilateral instillation of 0.1% pilocarpine. (b) Left Adie's pupil 20 minutes after instillation of 0.1% pilocarpine. The right pupil is unchanged, the left constricts due to denervation hypersensitivity.

and this is supported by Selhorst *et al.*'s findings (Selhorst *et al.* 1984) of dorsal root nerve loss.

In time, Adie's pupils become smaller and the accommodation paresis becomes less but the other features remain.

Loewenfeld and Thompson (1967, 1981) have proposed that the site of the lesion of the tonic pupil is in the ciliary ganglion and that many of its features can be explained by aberrant regeneration. The cause is unknown but it may be due to a neurotropic virus. Most patients do not require treatment but they may be helped with their photophobia and occasionally with symptoms due to accommodation paresis by dilute pilocarpine (0.1% three times daily). Young children with Adie's or other tonic pupils should have the unaffected or better eye occluded for a short period each day to avoid amblyopia.

Iris abnormalities

Damage to the iris by trauma, irradiation, uveitis, ischaemia, previous involvement by leukaemia (Fig. 59.3) or haemorrhage, or involvement with a tumour such as lymphoma, leukaemia, juvenile xanthogranuloma, leiomyoma, or neurofibroma may all give rise to sinuous pupil reactions.

Episodic pupillary dysfunction ('springing pupil')

Episodic unilateral mydriasis lasting minutes to weeks and usually accompanied by blurred vision and headaches has been reported. Accommodation is usually affected but other signs of lid or extraocular muscle dysfunction are absent (Hallett & Cogan 1970).

Midbrain corectopia

Damage to some midbrain pupillary fibres may give rise

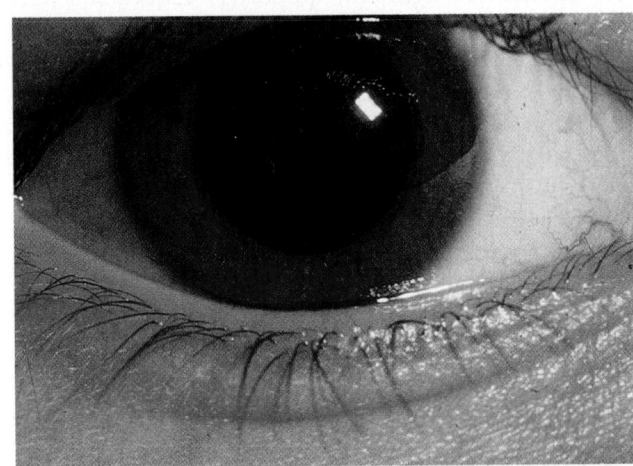

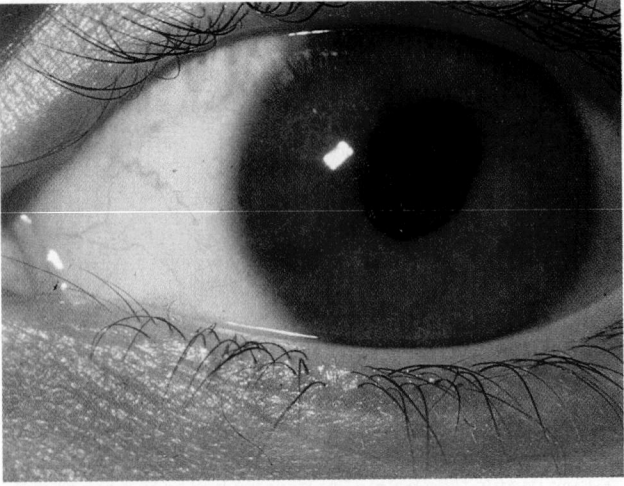

Fig. 59.3 Left iris abnormality with sluggish reactions and small pupil due to leukaemic infiltration.

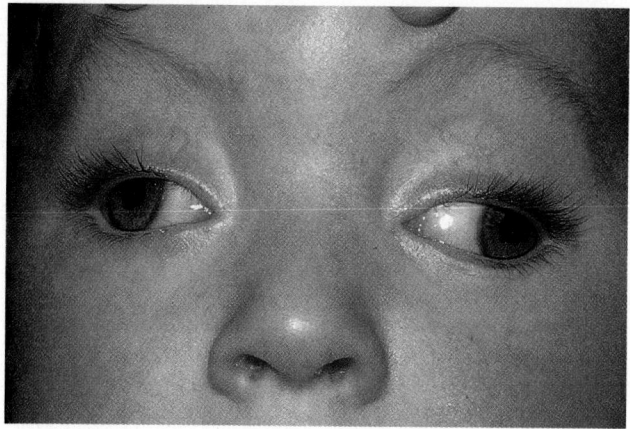

Fig. 59.4 Bilateral congenital third nerve palsy with fixed and unreactive pupils; the pupil made very slow bilateral size changes.

to unequal upward and inward distortion of the pupil (Selhorst *et al.* 1976) and an unequal, sinuous pupil reaction to light and near stimuli. The patients described have often but not always been comatose.

Third nerve palsy

In complete third nerve palsy the pupil is unreactive (Fig. 59.4) but in partial or recovering third nerve palsy the ipsilateral pupil reactions may be sluggish and react in an uneven fashion.

Sometimes the pupil shape may be irregular and the reactions sinuous.

1 In acute partial lesions of the third nerve (Fisher 1980; Marshall *et al.* 1983) presumably due to selective loss of function in some but not all third nerve fibres.

2 In cyclic oculomotor spasm (see Chapters 21 and 66).

3 Sinuous iris movements due to sector contractions of the iris sphincter and abnormal spontaneous pupillary contractions occur in aberrant regeneration (Fig. 59.5) following third nerve palsy (Czarneki & Thompson 1978). The pupil may even be small in long-standing lesions (Fig. 59.6).

Riley–Day syndrome

In the Riley–Day syndrome (familial dysautonomia) there is a hypersensitivity to dilute parasympathomimetic agents (i.e. pilocarpine 0.1%). Although it has been suggested that these children may have a tonic pupil, Korcyzn *et al.* (1981) found no evidence of this on pupillography of 10 patients.

Iris sphincter or dilator muscle spasms

Spasm of the iris dilator (Thompson *et al.* 1983) gives rise to 'tadpole-shaped' pupils which usually occurs in young

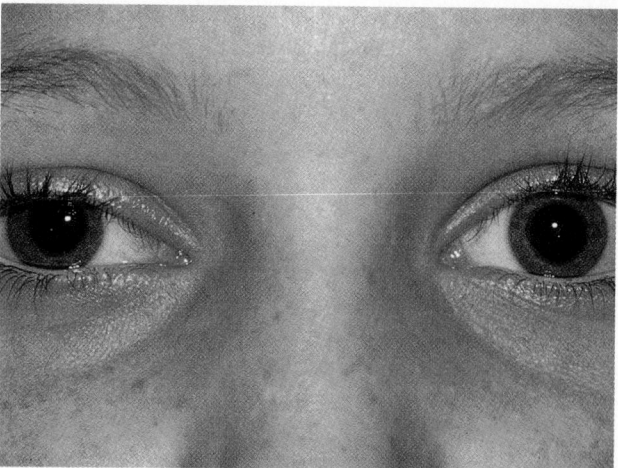

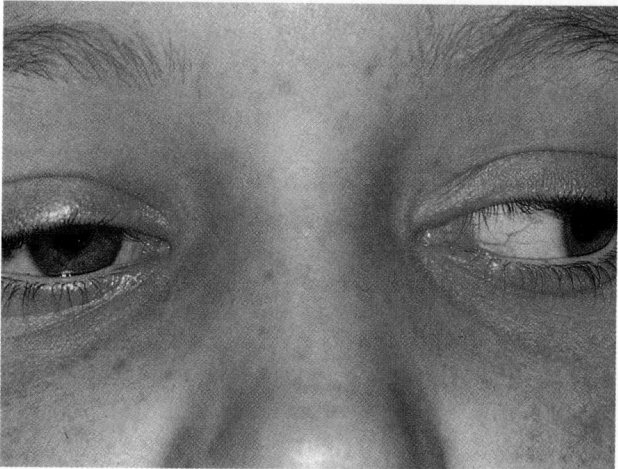

Fig. 59.5 Aberrant regeneration following partial recovery from right traumatic third nerve palsy: the right pupil constricts on attempted adduction.

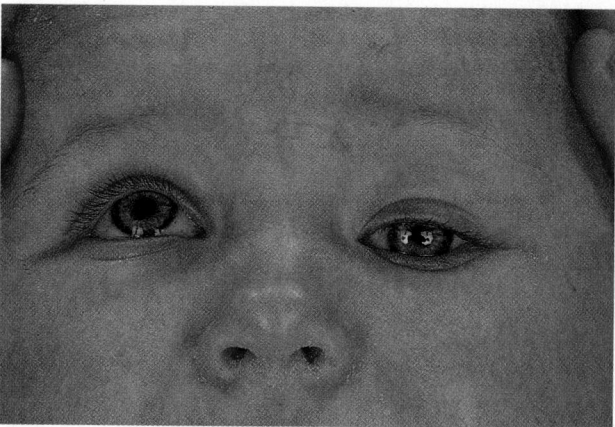

Fig. 59.6 Left congenital third nerve palsy. In long-standing cases the pupil may be small.

adults who are otherwise healthy. The pupils are peaked in one direction for a few minutes and it may occur on several separate occasions. This may represent a subset of patients who carry the diagnosis of springing pupil.

Other causes of tonic pupils

Although Adie's syndrome is the classic tonic pupil, other causes of ciliary ganglion damage give rise to a similar syndrome, confined to the affected eye, unlike Adie's syndrome which may be bilateral and have systemic abnormalities. A tonic pupil has been described in an infant with an orbital glial-neural hamartoma (Brooks-Kayal *et al.* 1995). Traumatic, infectious or inflammatory diseases and a wide variety of exanthemas have been described causing a tonic pupil and they may also occur as part of a variety of widespread neuropathies including: syphilis, diabetes, Guillain–Barré syndrome, Miller–Fisher syndrome, pandysautonomia, hereditary sensory neuropathy (Miller *et al.* 1976), Charcot–Marie–Tooth disease, and trilene poisoning. Autonomic neuropathy and chronic relapsing polyneuropathy due to paraneoplastic disease has been reported to cause tonic pupils (Van Lieshout *et al.* 1986).

Paradoxical pupils

In children and in older people with retinal disease a curious phenomenon may occur in which the pupil size in the light is larger than that in the dark (Barricks *et al.* 1977) despite the other responses being normal. The parents may occasionally remark on this themselves but it is usually a sign that has to be elicited. When clearly present it is extremely helpful as it virtually only occurs in retinal diseases.

The best way to record paradoxical pupils is to take a polaroid photograph of the child in a fully lit room and in a nearly fully darkened room. The photographs may clearly show the difference and can be kept as a record. Simple observation, however, is perfectly adequate. It is important to leave the child for at least a minute in the dark; the pupils can be observed there by using a flashlight for a moment, or with an infrared viewing device or video. Most typically the response is found in patients with cone dysfunction syndromes, achromatopsia, or congenital stationary night-blindness (Price *et al.* 1985) but it also has been described in Leber's amaurosis, dominant optic atrophy, optic neuritis and other retinal disease and even amblyopia. Nevertheless, in the young child with nystagmus the presence of the paradoxical pupil suggests an electroretinogram (ERG) should be obtained.

The mechanism has not been adequately explained (Price *et al.* 1985) but it is interesting that dark-rearing chicks to maturity causes them to have paradoxically constricted pupils in the dark (Yinon *et al.* 1981).

Horner's syndrome

Sympathetic denervation in childhood is not uncommon and may be congenital or acquired.

Clinical characteristics

Miosis

The pupils are unequal with the difference greatest in the dark due to the defect being in a failure of the dilator pupillae muscle. The difference also depends on the completeness of the lesion and the alertness of the child, as a drowsy child is more likely to have a small resting pupillary tone and the inequality will be less obvious. There is also a lag in the dilatation of the affected side (Thompson 1977b); this lag (Fig. 59.7) results in a greater anisocoria at 5 seconds than at 15 seconds after the lights are turned out; it is best measured on polaroid photographs. Pupil reactions to light and near and accommodation are unaffected.

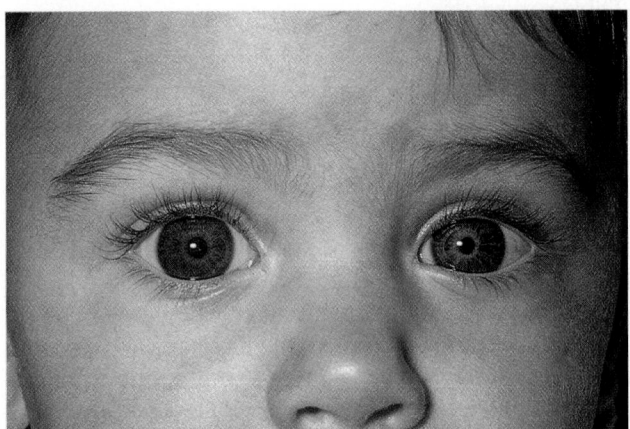

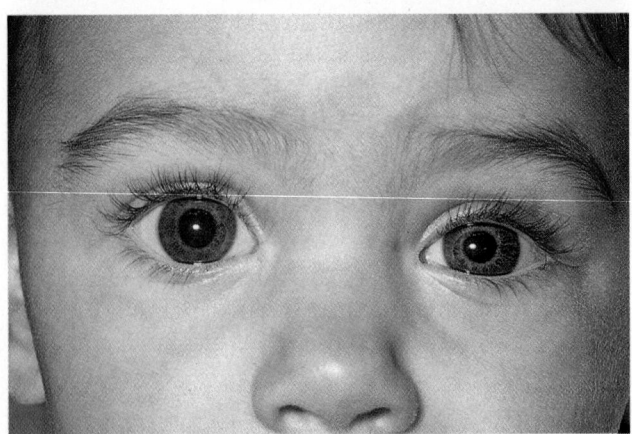

Fig. 59.7 (a) Left Horner's syndrome with mild ptosis. Photograph taken in the light. (b) Same patient 5 seconds after lights turned out showing dilation lag.

Ptosis

A 1–2 mm ptosis of the upper lid is present (Fig. 59.8) but it may be so slight and so variable that it escapes notice. The lower lid may also be affected giving rise to a more obvious narrowing in the palpebral fissure (Nielsen 1983b). This narrowing gives rise to the false appearance of enophthalmos in a few cases.

Ipsilateral anhidrosis

Lesions before the superior cervical ganglion, where the sweat and piloerector fibres split off to go with the external carotid artery, will damage these fibres and cause an ipsilateral flushed face and conjunctiva and nasal stuffi-ness in acute lesions whilst in longer standing lesions there is a defect of sweating with a dry, warm side to the face when the other is cool and sweaty. In chronic lesions the affected side may be pale due to denervation hyper-sensitivity to circulating catecholamines.

Heterochromia

In congenital Horner's syndrome the iris fails to become fully pigmented giving rise to heterochromia with the light iris on the affected side (Fig. 59.9); this is most marked in heavily pigmented irides. Occasionally hete-rochromia has been recorded as happening very gradual-ly following injury or surgery to the carotid in childhood (Miller 1985). However, progressive heterochromia has

Fig. 59.8 (a) Left Horner's syndrome. This child presented with the complaint of a sudden onset ptosis and small pupil. (b) Chest X-ray showing left apical mass. (c) Barium swallow showing constriction of the oesophagus. The cause was a large benign ganglioneuroma.

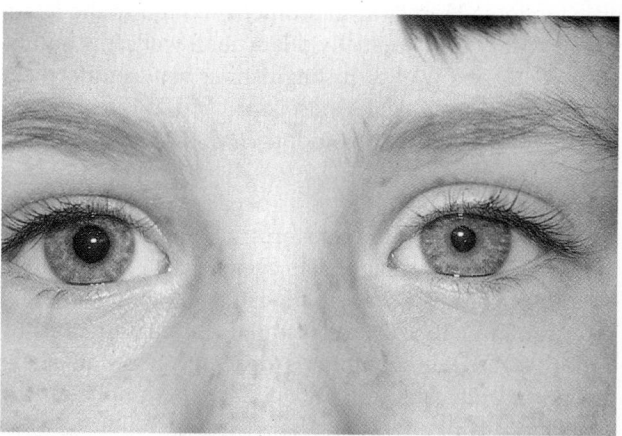

a

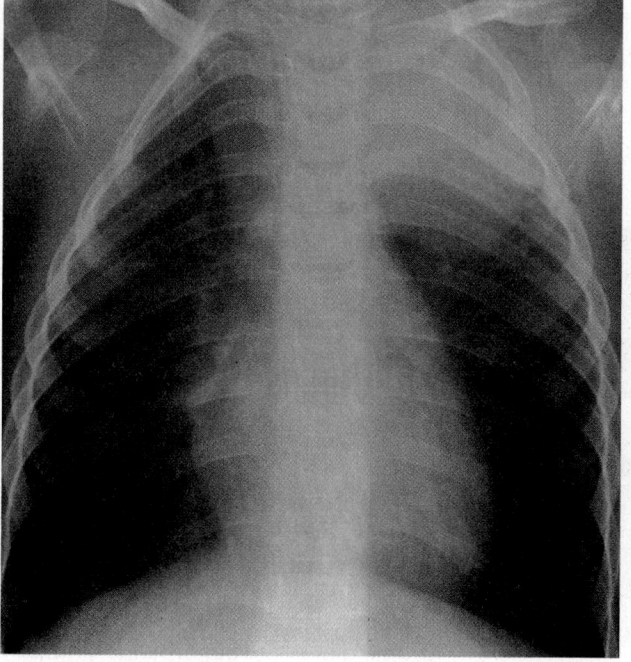

b

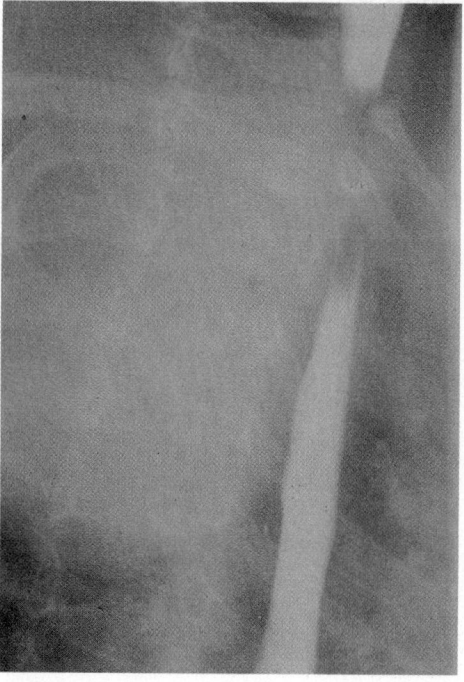

c

been reported following acquired Horner's syndrome even in adults (Makley & Abbott 1965). Heterochromia is not invariably present in congenital Horner's syndrome especially in light coloured irides or if insufficient time has elapsed (Woodruff *et al.* 1988). Histopathologically, in one case (McCartney *et al.* 1992), the iris pigment epithelium was normal, there were no iris sympathetic fibres and the stromal melanocytes were reduced in number, but contained normal melanosomes. The anterior border cells were depleted.

Pharmacological responses

Cocaine 10% blocks re-uptake of noradrenaline by the sympathetic nerve endings. In postganglionic lesions the nerve is dead and contains no noradrenaline (norepinephrine) and since cocaine has no direct effect, the pupil fails to dilate whilst it dilates in normals and in a preganglionic Horner's syndrome, although in the latter situation it does not usually dilate at all well. It is highly effective as one way of distinguishing between normals (even with physiological anisocoria) and anisocoria due to Horner's syndrome (Kardon *et al.* 1990a, b; Moster 1990).

Hydroxyamphetamine 1% releases noradrenaline from presynaptic nerve terminal stores; it should be instilled into the conjunctival sac of both eyes at least 24 hours after the use of cocaine. Where the postganglionic neurone is intact noradrenaline is present and the pupil is dilated but if the postganglionic neurone is 'dead' it contains no noradrenaline and does not dilate. Hydroxyamphetamine takes about 40 minutes to work.

Adrenaline 0.1% (1:1000) does not normally dilate the pupil but in postganglionic Horner's syndrome there is denervation hypersensitivity and the pupil dilates. Adrenaline 0.1% has the advantage of being more readily available and it is not a proscribed drug.

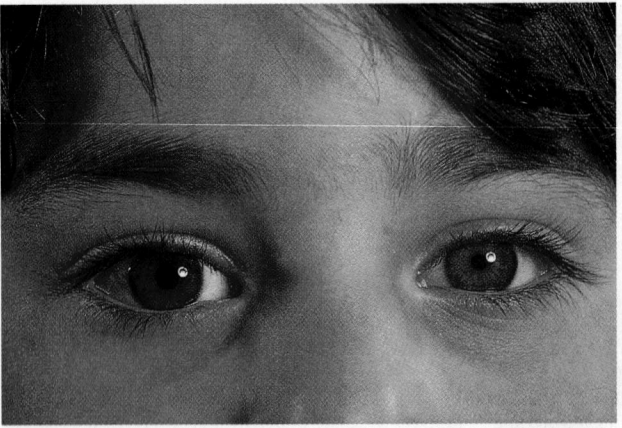

Fig. 59.9 Left congenital Horner's syndrome with heterochromia.

Pharmacological testing is frequently not necessary to establish the diagnosis but because ipsilateral ptosis and miosis co-exist quite frequently due to the frequency of physiological anisocoria with lid and other abnormalities, it may be diagnostic in some instances (Thompson *et al.* 1982). In children, the main problem is measuring the inequality and changes in light and dark; this may be helped by polaroid photographs.

Other characteristics

There have been various reports of ipsilateral accommodative increase or decrease but the difference does not seem to be reliably present or easy to measure in children. The ipsilateral central cornea may be thicker on the affected side (Nielsen 1983a).

Congenital Horner's syndrome

Weinstein *et al.* (1980) divided congenital Horner's syndrome into three causal types.

1 With obstetric trauma to the internal carotid artery and its sympathetic nerve plexus. These children were usually delivered by forceps and they had a postganglionic Horner's syndrome on drug testing, i.e. they did not dilate with 1% hydroxyamphetamine. They had no facial anhidrosis.

2 With surgical or obstetric trauma to the preganglionic sympathetic pathway (the pupil dilates with 1% hydroxyamphetamine). This group includes patients with brachial plexus injury, known traditionally as Klumpke's palsy (Klumpke 1885). Cardiothoracic surgery is a common cause in most children's hospitals.

3 Those without a history of birth trauma but with a Horner's syndrome with evidence of a lesion at, or peripheral to, the superior cervical ganglion. These patients also had anhidrosis (absence of sweating on the ipsilateral face) presumably due to a lesion after the separation of the sweat fibres which pass from the superior cervical ganglion to the external carotid artery. A note of caution was sounded by Woodruff *et al.* (1988) who had two patients with congenital or early onset Horner's with a preganglionic lesion with anhidrosis which were caused by neuroblastoma.

Congenital Horner's syndrome may also be found with hemifacial atrophy (Mobius 1884), cervical vertebral anomalies (Robinson *et al.* 1965), congenital tumours (Jaffe *et al.* 1975; Sauer & Levinsohn 1976; Sayed *et al.* 1983; Stewman 1983; Woodruff *et al.* 1988), arachnoidal cysts and holoprosencephaly (Woodruff *et al.* 1988), and with the congenital varicella syndrome (Borzyskowksi *et al.* 1981). Despite the above list of causes, it must be said that most children with congenital Horner's syndrome have no abnormality found despite extensive investigation.

Postnatally acquired Horner's syndrome

Some authors (Sauer & Levinsohn 1976) have emphasized the seriousness of the causes of acquired Horner's syndrome in childhood. It may occur in the following.

1 As a 'central' lesion. This occurs with brain stem trauma, brain stem tumours and vascular malformations (Guy *et al.* 1989), infarcts and haemorrhages, syringomyelia. Bilateral 'pinpoint' pupils are found particularly in comatose patients with pontine haemorrhages.

2 As a 'preganglionic' lesion, i.e. of the second neurone between the spinal cord and the superior cervical ganglion. This occurs with neck trauma, neuroblastoma (Woodruff *et al.* 1988), and other tumours.

3 As a 'postganglionic' lesion, i.e. of the final neurone after the superior cervical ganglion. Cavernous sinus lesions (tumours, aneurysms, or inflammatory disease), neuroblastoma, and trauma may cause this type of Horner's syndrome.

Management

Congenital

Since birth trauma or early cardiothoracic surgery are the most frequent causes, further investigations are not usually necessary (Giles & Henderson 1958; Leone & Russell 1970). However, the occurrence of tumours in those children with congenital Horner's syndrome of no obvious cause may warrant investigation with a chest X-ray, head and neck tomography and a 24-hour catecholamine assay (Woodruff *et al.* 1988).

Treatment with weak adrenergic substances (Campbell & Hill 1978) is rarely necessary.

Acquired

Where there is no obvious cause, such as trauma or surgery, a child with acquired Horner's syndrome should be investigated by or in conjunction with a neurologist and the further investigations should include a chest X-ray, computed tomography (CT) or magnetic resonance imaging (MRI) scan and 24-hour catecholamine assay.

Pupil changes from high sympathetic 'tone'

Cases have been described in which an intermittent dilated pupil, with or without widening of the palpebral fissure, occurs associated with a cervicomedullary syrinx (Lowenstein & Levine 1944), post spinal cord injury (Kline & McCluer 1984), lung tumours, seizures (Gadoth *et al.* 1981) or migraine. In seizures and migraine (Pant *et al.* 1966) there may well be a lowering of parasympathetic tone at the same time, but sympathetic induced spasm is suggested by pallor and sweating (Jammes 1980).

Pupil changes from damage to the parasympathetic system

Internal ophthalmoplegia (paralysis of the sphincter pupillae and accommodation) is occasionally seen without external ophthalmoplegia from nuclear lesions. It is bilateral and often associated with other oculomotor palsies (Daroff 1971).

Damage to the third nerve in the interpeduncular fossa, where the pupillomotor fibres are confined to the superomedial aspect of the nerve, may occur from aneurysm or tumour when it is usually associated with external ophthalmoplegia, but meningitic lesions can cause an isolated internal ophthalmoplegia.

In uncal herniation the comatose patient develops a dilated pupil on the side of the herniation, together with an asymmetrically sluggish reaction to light. The pupil signs may be the only abnormality other than coma for a period of some hours. Flexion of the neck, by stretching the brain stem, may worsen the dilation or even cause both pupils to dilate but this is not a recommended procedure! Later ipsilateral external ophthalmoplegia and hemiplegia develop, contralateral ophthalmoplegia and then more profound brain stem signs. The syndrome is caused by the uncus of the temporal lobe herniating under the tentorial edge to compress the posterior cerebral artery, third nerve and the midbrain with the opposite tentorial edge cutting into the cerebral peduncle. Midbrain compression occludes the Sylvian aqueduct worsening the already raised supratentorial pressure.

Pharmacological agents

Numerous pharmacological agents affect pupil size and reactivity. Systemic agents usually affect the pupils symmetrically whilst topical agents are often only instilled into one eye and may be asymmetrical.

Pupil-dilating agents

Parasympatholytic agents

Atropine 0.5–1%, homatropine 2%, cyclopentolate 0.5–1% and tropicamide 1% are all commonly used agents to dilate the pupil and cause cycloplegia. Homatropine and atropine have a prolonged action and are not often indicated diagnostically or therapeutically unless their long action is desirable. Hyoscine 0.5% has an action similar to atropine but is less long lived. They may cause respiratory failure in children with congenital central hypoventilation (Oren *et al.* 1987).

Sympathomimetics

Adrenaline 0.1–1% or phenylephrine 2.5–10% may be

used to dilate the pupil in association with a parasympatholytic. They have no action on accommodation but are not sufficient by themselves to produce good dilation. They must be used with great care, and at lowest dilution, if at all, in premature babies, those with cardiac or vascular disease or with hypertension.

Pupil-constricting agents

Cholinergic drugs

Pilocarpine 1–4% is commonly used to constrict the pupil and as treatment for glaucoma. It has little effect on infantile glaucoma.

Anticholinesterases

Phospholine iodide (ecothiopate) 0.03–0.125%, eserine 0.5% and isofluorophate 0.025% are occasionally used for treatment of glaucoma. Isoflurophate is used in the USA and phospholine iodide was used in Europe to cause peripheral accommodation and 'unlink' the association between accommodative convergence and accommodation in some high AC : A ratio squints (see Chapters 65 and 66).

Sympatholytic agents

Guanethidine 5% (ismelin) can be used to counter lid retraction in hyperthyroidism. Thymoxamine 1% may also cause pupil construction.

Systemic agents

Atropine, scopolamine and benztropine can cause pupil dilatation and paralysis of accommodation in sufficient quantities. The seeds of jimson weed, the berries of deadly nightshade and henbane have all been known to cause a serious or fatal poisoning. The symptoms have been described as 'hot as a hare, blind as a bat, dry as a bone, red as a beet, mad as a hen'. When proof of atropine poisoning is needed in the absence of facilities for assay it is said that a few drops of the child's urine put into one eye of a cat may suggest the diagnosis. Mydriasis from topical atropine or atropine-like drugs is not counteracted by pilocarpine 1% but in systemic poisoning it may be.

Antihistamines and some antidepressants produce a mydriasis.

Heroin, morphine and other opiates, marijuana and some other psychotropic drugs cause bilateral pupil constriction.

Abnormalities of the near reflex

Congenital absence

Children may be born with a defect in the near reflex. They have absent accommodation and poor convergence and the pupil fails to constrict to a near stimulus, but it constricts to light (Chrousos *et al.* 1985).

Familial cases of accommodation defect occur (Karseras *et al.* 1974; Hibbert *et al.* 1975). The cause is unknown but it may be peripheral in origin (Hibbert *et al.* 1975), in the ciliary body or lens.

Acquired defects

Psychogenic

Children in the second decade may present with symptoms of difficulty with reading due to non-organic causes. They can usually be cajoled into a normal near response or tricked by prisms and minus lenses; the synoptophore is particularly useful here. In older persons, malingering may be suspected especially when compensation for injury is a possibility.

Sylvian aqueduct (Parinaud's) syndrome

Premature presbyopia is one of the signs of tumours encroaching on the dorsal midbrain together with the more classic signs of convergence, i.e. retraction nystagmus, vertical gaze defects, eyelid retraction, convergence defect, and pupil light-near dissociation.

Systemic disease

Botulism, diphtheria, diabetes, and head and neck trauma may all give rise to accommodation defects either isolated or associated with eye movement and vergence defects. Wilson's disease has been shown to be associated with a defect in the near response in some cases. It is not yet clear but the cause may be central rather than in the eye (Curran *et al.* 1982).

Pharmacological agents

See above.

Eye disease

Defective accommodation occurs in children with severe iridocyclitis, dislocated lenses, large colobomas, buphthalmos, very high myopia, and direct eye trauma including retinal detachment surgery.

Other neurological causes

Adie's tonic pupil syndrome and third nerve paralysis may cause defective accommodation. Sinus disease, presumably by affecting the short ciliary nerves, may cause cycloplegia and accommodation defect (Hein 1961).

Accommodation in schoolchildren

One expects a school-aged child to have a high amplitude of accommodation irrespective of refractive error (Donders 1864). Low amplitudes of accommodation have been reported in children who specialize in music as opposed to sport (Mantyjarvi 1988). It has been suggested that there is a causal relationship between a defective near response and some cases of dyslexia (Hammerberg & Norn 1974).

It is important, however, to distinguish clearly between reading difficulties due to a defective near response, which can be improved by exercises, and dyslexia which is a specific defect in the perceptual process involved with reading and writing and which cannot be remedied by simple exercises. Stein *et al.* (1987) have suggested that because they found that 67% of dyslexics had electro-oculographic evidence of poor or 'unstable' vergence control in response to a small fusion stimulus, associated with low stereoacuity, whilst most good readers had good vergence control, there may be a causal link. It was difficult for them to show a direct causal link but 51% of the dyslexics with unstable vergence movements improved after monocular occlusion as opposed to 24% who had no occlusion. Occlusion is, if nothing else, a harmless treatment in the older child.

Spasm of the near reflex

Spasm of the near reflex consists of episodes of a combination of:
1 accommodation-induced myopia;
2 convergence of the eyes; and
3 miosis.

The symptoms are usually of blurred, double vision, and ocular pain or headache. These cases are rarely due to organic disease and a truly causal relationship with organic pathology is often not easy to establish. Safran *et al.* (1982) described three cases with pre-existing eye movement defects, and a small number of other associations have been described including neurosyphilis, myasthenia gravis, and multiple sclerosis. Upper brain stem pathology is often suspected but rarely found.

In most cases it is not possible to demonstrate any organic disease and the phenomenon is assumed to be psychogenic. The episodes have a sudden onset and can last many hours and may be very variable. There is blurred vision and photophobia. The eyes are crossed and

may mimic a bilateral sixth nerve paresis but the essential finding is of the pupils constricting increasingly as the deviation increases. Pupils that become constricted on attempted lateral gaze are also a clue to the functional nature of the complaint. It is unusual in childhood but may occur. Occasionally symptoms may be recurrent over several years.

The treatment is to reassure the patient and parents and sometimes they are helped by miotics but more usually by a combination of cycloplegia with bifocal glasses. Unless there are any neurological signs no investigations are required and the prognosis is good.

Anisocoria

Anisocoria (unequal pupils), occurs when there is a local abnormality in the iris, or its musculature, or when there is an asymmetrical abnormality in the efferent pathways that drive pupil constriction or dilatation. Afferent (visual) defects never cause anisocoria, even if they are highly asymmetrical, unless they are associated with an efferent defect. Apart from the size abnormality there is usually a change in reactivity which is usually the clue to the diagnosis.

Physiological anisocoria

This is also known as simple anisocoria or occasionally as central anisocoria. Lam *et al.* (1987) determined pupil size in 128 normal individuals: 41% showed anisocoria of 0.4 mm or greater; 80% showed 0.2 mm or greater. The difference is rarely more than 1 mm between the two sides and may vary from time to time (see also Chapter 6). The size difference is usually apparent in light and dark and the pupil reactions are normal. Direct clinical measurements are often difficult in children and this may be avoided by making measurements from polaroid photographs.

Anisocoria during reflex responses to unilateral light stimulation, with the direct light reaction exceeding the consensual, can be shown by pupillometry in a significant number of normals (Smith *et al.* 1979). This 'contraction anisocoria' was repeatable and the difference was about 6%.

Diagnosis

The diagnosis of anisocoria can be difficult. It is frequently found that the patient and the doctor mistake which is the abnormal pupil, especially in Horner's syndrome in which there are no associated visual or ocular motor symptoms.

The abnormality is usually sorted out in three simple stages:
1 The reactions to light and accommodation. If they are

abnormal, whether unilateral or bilateral, the diagnosis is of an efferent, parasympathetic or local cause.

2 Slit-lamp examination will show sinuous pupil reactions and iris anomalies, uveitis, and so on.

3 The size difference in light and dark will help to diagnose sympathetic and parasympathetic lesions. In Horner's syndrome the anisocoria is greater in the dark because the dilator pupillae fails to function. In a parasympathetic lesion the difference is greatest in the light because of the failure of the sphincter pupillae.

In nearly all situations the pupil abnormality can be diagnosed by looking at the pupil and by looking for accompanying clinical grounds. It is usually difficult even with the aid of drug testing, especially in small wriggling children who never seem to want to be still at the time you want to measure. The flow chart in Chapter P.21 summarizes a clinical approach and has some notes on drug testing for completeness. It is not meant to be absolutely complete or totally foolproof but acts as a guide to diagnosis and is not helpful when both pupils are abnormal.

References

Barricks ME, Flynn JT, Kushner BJ. Paradoxical pupillary responses in congenital stationary night blindness. *Arch Ophthalmol* 1977; **95**: 1800.

Bell RA, Thompson SA. Ciliary muscle dysfunction in Adie's syndrome. *Arch Ophthalmol* 1978; **96**: 638–42.

Bell R, Waggoner P, Boyd W, Akers R, Yee C. Clinical grading of relative afferent pupillary defects. *Arch Ophthalmol* 1993; **111**: 938–42.

Borzyskowski M, Harris R, Jones R. The congenital varicella syndrome. *Eur J Pediatr* 1981; **137**: 335–8.

Bosanquet RC, Johnson GJ. Peninsula pupil: anomaly unique to Newfoundland and Labrador? *Arch Ophthalmol* 1981; **99**: 1824–6.

Bourgon P, Pilley SFJ, Thompson SH. Cholinergic supersensitivity of the iris sphincter in Adie's tonic pupil. *Am J Ophthalmol* 1978; **85**: 373–7.

Braddick O, Atkinson J, French J, Howland H. A photorefractive study of infant accommodation. *Vision Res* 1979; **19**: 1319–30.

Brooks-Kayal AR, Liu GT, Menacker SJ, Heher KL, Katowitz JA, Bilaniuk LT. Tonic pupil and orbital glial-neural hamartoma in infancy. *Am J Ophthalmol* 1995; **119**: 809–11.

Burde RM. The pupil. *Int Ophthalmol Clin* 1967; **7**: 839–55.

Campbell WW, Hill TA. A good treatment for Horner's syndrome. *N Engl J Med* 1978; **299**: 835–37.

Chrousos GA, O'Neill JF, Cogan DG. Absence of the near reflex in a healthy adolescent. *J Pediatr Ophthalmol Strabismus* 1985; **22**: 76–7.

Curran RE, Hedges TR III, Boger WP III. Loss of accommodation and the near response in Wilson's disease. *J Pediatr Ophthalmol Strabismus* 1982; **19**: 157–60.

Czarneki JSC, Thompson HS. The iris sphincter in aberrant regeneration of the third nerve. *Arch Ophthalmol* 1978; **96**: 1606–10.

Daroff RB. Ocular motor manifestations of brainstem and cerebellar dysfunction. In: Smith JL, ed. *Neuroophthalmology*, Vol. 5. St Louis: CV Mosby, 1971: 104–18.

Donders FC. *Accommodation and Refraction of the Eye*. London: New Sydenham Society, 1864.

Dulton G, Paul R. Adie syndrome in a child: a case report. *J Pediatr Ophthalmol Strabismus* 1992; **29**: 126.

Fisher CM. Oval pupils. *Arch Neurol* 1980; **37**: 502–3.

Fison PN, Garlick DJ, Smith SE. Assessment of unilateral afferent pupillary defects by pupillography. *Br J Ophthalmol* 1979; **63**: 195–9.

Forman S, Behrens M, Odel J, Spector R, Hilal S. Relative afferent pupillary defect with normal visual function. *Arch Ophthalmol* 1990; **108**: 1073–5.

Gadoth N, Margalith D, Bechar M. Unilateral pupillary dilatation during focal seizures. *J Neurol* 1981; **225**: 227–30.

Giles CL, Henderson DA. Horner's syndrome, an analysis of 216 cases. *Am J Ophthalmol* 1958; **46**: 289–301.

Greenwald MJ, Folk ER. Afferent pupillary defects in amblyopia. *J Pediatr Ophthalmol Strabismus* 1983; **20**: 63–7.

Guy J, Day AL, Mickle JP, Selatz NJ. Contralateral trochlear nerve paresis and ipsilateral Horner's syndrome. *Am J Ophthalmol* 1989; **107**: 73–7.

Hallett M, Cogan DG. Episodic unilateral mydriasis in otherwise normal patients. *Arch Ophthalmol* 1970; **84**: 130–9.

Hammerberg E, Norm MS. Defective dissociation of accommodation and convergence in dyslexic children. *Br Orthopic J* 1974; **31**: 96–8.

Haynes H, White BL, Held R. Visual accommodation in human infants. *Science* 1965; **148**: 528–30.

Hein PA. Unilateral paralysis of accommodation. *Am J Ophthalmol* 1961; **52**: 711–12.

Hibbert FG, Goldstein V, Osborne SM. Defective accommodation in members of one family. *Tr Ophthalmol Soc UK* 1975; **95**: 455–61.

Isenberg S, Molarte A, Vazquez M. The fixed and dilated pupils of premature neonates. *Am J Ophthalmol* 1990; **110**: 168–72.

Jaffe H, Cassady JR, Filler RM, Petersen R, Traggis D. Heterochromia and Horner's syndrome associated with cervical and mediastinal neuroblastoma. *J Pediatr* 1975; **87**: 75–7.

Jammes JL. Fixed dilated pupils in petit mal attacks. *Neuro-ophthalmol* 1980; **1**: 155–9.

Kardon RH, Dennison CE, Brown CK, Thompson HS. Cortical enucleation of the cocaine test in the diagnosis of Horner's syndrome. *Arch Ophthalmol* 1990a; **108**: 384–7.

Kardon RH, Dennison CE, Brown CK, Thompson HS. Reply to: the cocaine test and Horner's syndrome (letter). *Arch Ophthalmol* 1990b; **108**: 1667–8.

Karseras A, Unwin B, Wybar KC. Defective accommodation in young people. *Br Orthoptic J* 1974; **31**: 91–5.

Kline LB, McCluer SM. Oculosympathetic spasm with cervical spinal cord injury. *Arch Neurol* 1984; **41**: 61–4.

Klumpmke A. Contribution a l'etude des paralyses du plexus brachial. *Rev Med (Paris)* 1885; **5**: 591–616.

Korczyn AD, Laor N, Nemet P. Autonomic pupillary activity in infants. *Metab Ophthalmol* 1978; **2**: 391–4.

Korczyn AD, Rubenstein AE, Yahr MD, Axelrod FB. The pupil in familial dysautonomia. *Neurology* 1981; **31**: 628–9.

Lam BL, Thompson HS, Corbett JJ. The prevalence of simple anisocoria. *Am J Ophthalmol* 1987; **104**: 69–73.

Leone CR, Russell DA. Congenital Horner's syndrome. *J Pediatr Ophthalmol Strabismus* 1970; **7**: 152–6.

Lhermitte F, Guillaumat L, Lyon-Caen O. Monocular blindness with preserved direct and consensual pupillary reflex in multiple sclerosis. *Arch Neurol* 1984; **41**: 993–4.

Loewenfeld IE, Thompson HS. Mechanism of tonic pupil. *Ann Neurol* 1981; **10**: 275–6.

Loewenfeld IE, Thompson HS. The tonic pupil: a re-evaluation. *Am J Ophthalmol* 1967; **63**: 46–87.

Lowenstein O, Levine AS. Periodic sympathetic spasm and relaxation and role of sympathetic system in pupillary innervation. *Arch Ophthalmol* 1944; **31**: 74–94.

McCartney A, Riordan-Eva P, Howes R, Spalton D. Horner's syndrome: an electron microscopic study of human iris. *Br J Ophthalmol* 1992; **76**: 746–9.

Makley LB, Abbott K. Neurogenic heterochromia: A report of an interesting case. *Am J Ophthalmol* 1965; **59**: 297–9.

Manor RS, Yassur Y, Siegal R, Ben-Sira L. The pupil cycle time test: age variations in normal subjects. *Br J Ophthalmol* 1981; **65**: 750–3.

Mantyjarvi MI. Accommodation in school children with music or sports activities. *Pediatr J Ophthalmol Strabismus* 1988; **25**: 3–7.

Marshall LF, Barba D, Toole BM, Bowers SA. The oval pupil. *J Neurosurg* 1983; **58**: 566–8.

Miller NR. *Walsh and Hoyt's Clinical Neuro-ophthalmology*, 4th edn, Vol. 2. Baltimore: Williams & Wilkins, 1985: 385–469.

Miller RG, Nielson SL, Sumner AJ. Hereditary sensory neuropathy and tonic pupils. *Neurology* 1976; **26**: 931–3.

Miller SD, Thompson HS. Edge light pupil cycle time. *Br J Ophthalmol* 1978a; **62**: 495–500.

Miller SD, Thompson HS. Pupil cycle time. *Am J Ophthalmol* 1978b; **83**: 635–42.

Mobius PJ. Zur Pathologie des Halssympathikus. *Klin Wochenschr* 1884; 15–18.

Moster ML. The cocaine test and Horner's syndrome. *Arch Ophthalmol* 1990; **108**: 1667.

Newman SA, Miller NR. The optic tract syndrome: neuro-ophthalmic considerations. *Arch Ophthalmol* 1983; **101**: 1241–50.

Nielson PJ. The corneal thickness and Horner's syndrome. *Acta Ophthalmol* 1983a; **61**: 467–73.

Nielson PJ. Upside down ptosis in Horner's syndrome. *Acta Ophthalmol* 1983b; **61**: 952–8.

Oren J, Kelly DH, Shannon DC. Long-term follow-up of children with congenital central hypoventilation syndrome. *Pediatrics* 1987; **80**: 375–80.

Pant SS, Benton JW, Dodge PR. Unilateral pupillary dilation during and immediately following seizures. *Neurology* 1966; **16**: 837–40.

Ponsford JR, Bannister R, Paul EA. Methacholine pupillary responses in third nerve palsy and Adie's syndrome. *Brain* 1982; **105**: 583–7.

Portnoy JZ, Thompson HS, Lennarson L, Corbett JJ. Pupillary defects in amblyopia. *Am J Ophthalmol* 1983; **96**: 609–14.

Price MJ, Thompson HS, Judisch F, Corbett JJ. Pupillary constriction to darkness. *Br J Ophthalmol* 1985; **69**: 205–12.

Purcell JJ, Krachmer JH, Thompson HS. Corneal sensation in Adie's syndrome. *Am J Ophthalmol* 1977; **84**: 496–500.

Robinson GC, Dikrainian DA, Roseborough GF. Congenital Horner's syndrome and heterochromia iridium: their association with congenital foregut and vertebral anomalies. *Pediatrics* 1965; **35**: 103–7.

Robinson RJ. Assessment of gestational age by neurological examination. *Arch Dis Child* 1966; **41**: 437–41.

Safran AB, Roth A, Gauthier G. Le syndrome des spasmes de convergence 'plus'. *Klin Monatsbl Augenheilkd* 1982; **180**: 471–3.

Sauer C, Levinsohn MN. Horner's syndrome in childhood. *Neurology* 1976; **26**: 216–21.

Sayed AK, Miller BA, Lack EE, Sallan SE, Levey RH. Heterochromia iridis and Horner's syndrome due to para-vertebral neurilemmoma. *J Surg Oncol* 1983; **22**: 15–16.

Selhorst JB, Hoyt WF, Feinsod M, Hosobuchi Y. Midbrain corectopia. *Arch Neurol* 1976; **33**: 193–5.

Selhorst JB, Madge G, Ghatak N. The neuropathology of the Holmes–Adie syndrome. *Ann Neurol* 1984; **16**: 138–9.

Smith SA, Ellis CJK, Smith SE. Inequality of the direct and consensual light reflexes in normal subjects. *Br J Ophthalmol* 1979; **63**: 523–7.

Stein JF, Riddell PM, Fowler MS. Fine binocular control in dyslexic children. *Eye* 1987; **1**: 433–9.

Stewman DA. Unilateral straight hair in congenital Horner's syndrome due to stellate ganglion tumor. *Ann Neurol* 1983; **13**: 345–6.

Taylor D. Congenital tumors of the anterior visual system with dysplasia of the optic discs. *Br J Ophthalmol* 1982; **66**: 455–63.

Thompson HS. Adie's syndrome: some new observations. *Trans Am Ophthalmol Soc* 1977a; **75**: 587–626.

Thompson HS. Diagnosing Horner's syndrome. *Trans Am Ophthalmol Soc* 1977b; **83**: 840–2.

Thompson HS. Segmental palsy of the iris sphincter in Adie's syndrome. *Arch Ophthalmol* 1978; **96**: 1615–20.

Thompson HS, Bell RA, Bourgon P. The natural history of Adie's syndrome. In: Thompson HS, Daroff R, Frisen L, Glaser JS, Sanders MD, eds. *Topics in Neuro-ophthalmology*. Baltimore: Williams & Wilkins, 1979: 96–9.

Thompson HS, Corbett J. Asymmetry of pupillomotor input. *Eye* 1991; **5**: 36–40.

Thompson HS, Corbett JJ, Cox TA. How to measure the relative afferent pupillary defect. *Surv Ophthalmol* 1981; **26**: 39–42.

Thompson BM, Corbett JJ, Kline LB, Thompson HS. Pseudo-Horner's syndrome. *Arch Neurol* 1982; **39**: 108–11.

Thompson HS, Zackon J, Czarnecki SC. Tadpole-shaped pupils caused by segmental spasm of the iris dilator muscle. *Am J Ophthalmol* 1983; **96**: 467–76.

Van Lieshout JJ, Wieling W, Van Montfrans GA *et al*. Acute dysautonomia associated with Hodgkin's disease. *J Neurol Neurosurg Psychiatr* 1986; **49**: 830–2.

Weinstein J, Zweifel TJ, Thompson HS. Congenital Horner's syndrome. *Arch Ophthalmol* 1980; **98**: 1074–8.

West C, Repka M. Tonic pupils associated with neuroblastoma. *J Pediatr Ophthalmol Strabismus* 1992; **29**: 382–3.

Woodruff G, Buncic JR, Morin JD. Horner's syndrome in children. *J Pediatr Ophthalmol Strabismus* 1988; **25**: 40–4.

Yinon U, Urinowsky E, Barishak Y-TR. Paradoxical pupillary constriction in dark reared chicks. *Vision Res* 1981; **21**: 1319–22.

60: Leukaemia

David Taylor

Incidence

Although the ophthalmic manifestations of leukaemia in childhood may be memorably dramatic, a prospective study by Hoover *et al.* (1988) showed that serious eye involvement is rather unusual. Only one of their 82 patients had reduced vision due to the leukaemia from bilateral retinal detachments and vitritis and although half of their surviving patients had cataracts these were of little visual significance. Others have reported a higher incidence (Schachat *et al.* 1989).

Nonetheless, ocular involvement when it occurs is important and demands prompt diagnosis and treatment. Now that survival rates of 50–70% are usual (Niemeyer *et al.* 1985) and even children with non-lymphocytic leukaemia who receive treatment now have survival rates of up to 40% (Stiller & Eatock 1994), the eye complications of the disease and its treatment become more significant. Children dying of leukaemia have a high incidence of eye involvement (Allen & Straatsma 1961; Leonardy *et al.*

1990) and eye involvement may carry a poor prognosis (Ohkoshi & Tsiaras 1992).

Eye involvement in leukaemia is particularly interesting because it is the only site where the leukaemic involvement of nerves and blood vessels can be directly observed, because the eye may act as a 'sanctuary' for leukaemic cells against chemotherapy, and because in the occasional patient the eye complications may be the major residual disability (Taylor & Day 1982).

Acute lymphoblastic leukaemia is the most common leukaemia in childhood. Over the last two decades mortality during remission induction fell from 3.5 to 1% whilst death during remission remained at 5–6%. Increased risk factors included young age, high white cell count, the need for bone marrow transplant and Down's syndrome (Atra *et al.* 1993). Deaths in remission due to herpes and measles virus decreased whilst deaths associated with intensification of treatment and gut toxicity increased. Avoidance of chemotherapy-related late effects remains a very important aim for the oncologist (Pinkerton 1992).

Orbit

Oakhill *et al.* (1981) found that of 27 children presenting with unilateral proptosis over an 8.5-year period, three had leukaemia. The incidence in other series, i.e. Porterfield (1962), has varied probably mainly because of varying referral patterns, but leukaemia is probably a small, but significant cause of proptosis in children. In Kincaid and Green's (1983) postmortem study of patients of all ages orbital involvement was found in 14% of eyes with chronic leukaemia and 7.3% in acute leukaemia. It was more common in lymphatic leukaemia (12%) than in myeloid leukaemia (8%).

Children presenting with proptosis caused by leukaemic infiltration may cause considerable diagnostic problems. When the biopsy is reported as 'benign' (Humayun *et al.* 1992) or inflammatory the cautious clinician will first make sure that the biopsy was from the centre of the abnormal area, not on the periphery where secondary inflammatory signs may occur. Collaboration with an oncologist colleague ensures that there is no systemic or bone marrow evidence of leukaemia.

Orbital involvement may be due to bone (Fig. 60.1) or soft tissue infiltration, tumour formation or haemorrhage. Orbital presentation may occur without ocular involvement and it may be the only manifestation, especially in myeloid leukaemia (Zimmerman & Font 1975).

In orbital involvement with some forms of myeloid leukaemia in childhood the tumour takes on a greenish tinge, which has given rise to the name chloroma; the colour is said to be due to the enzyme myeloperoxidase, but probably also results from the presence of altered blood products. Children with orbital involvement present with proptosis, chemosis and, rarely, with muscle involvement and these may occur early in the course of the disease (MacManaway & Neely 1994). Because it may be difficult to differentiate between primary leukaemia infiltration and complications such as haemorrhage or opportunistic infection a biopsy may be necessary (Rubinfield *et al.* 1988).

Lids

The lids are usually only involved as a part of orbital infiltration, but Kincaid and Green (1983) saw a 4-year-old girl who relapsed with lid swelling due to leukaemic infiltration.

Conjunctiva

The conjunctival vessels may be involved by haemorrhage (Fig. 60.2), infiltration (Allen & Straatsma 1961) or by hyperviscosity when the vessels are tortuous or comma-shaped (Swartz & Jampol 1975). Conjunctival mass formation is rare, but can be the presenting sign in acute leukaemia (Kincaid & Green 1983).

Cornea and sclera

Being avascular, the cornea is not often involved in the

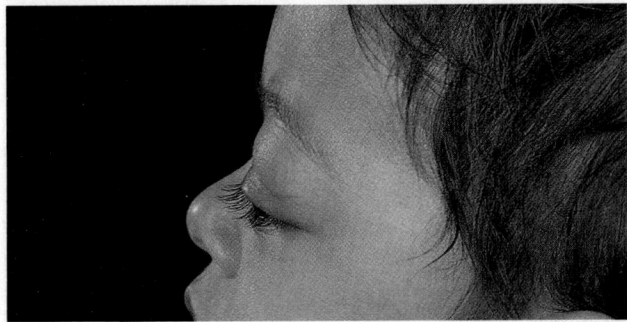

Fig. 60.1 Myeloid leukaemia presenting as proptosis and orbital mass.

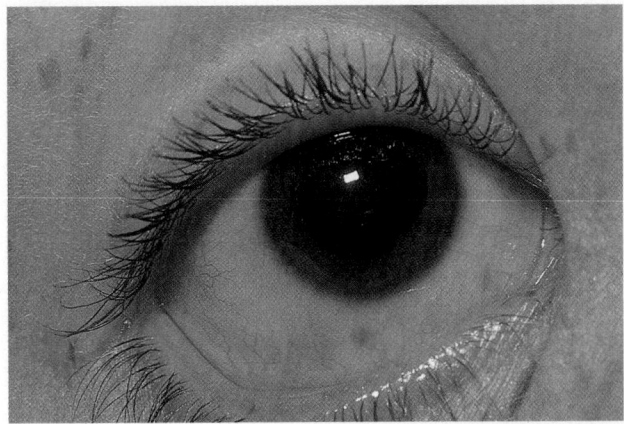

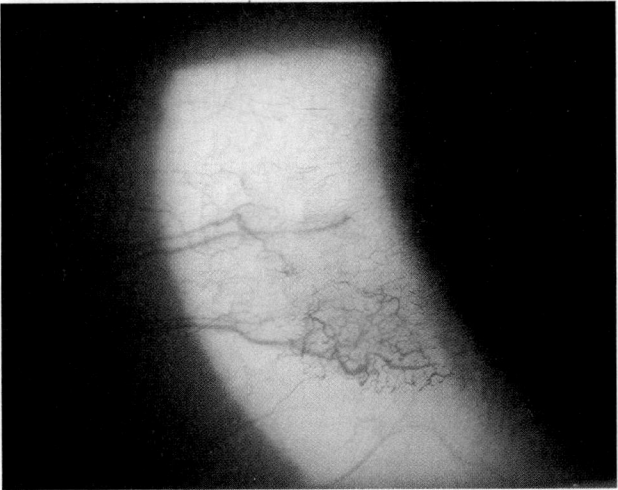

Fig. 60.2 (a) Conjunctival haemorrhages and infiltration in acute lymphoblastic leukaemia. (b) Conjunctival infiltration with leukaemic cells.

leukaemias (Fig. 60.3), but it may be involved by herpes simplex or zoster in the immunocompromised child or by other inflammatory disease. Conjunctival staining with fluorescein may be exacerbated by bone marrow transplantation and total body irradiation (Bray *et al.* 1991), due to dry eye and decreased epithelial viability.

Corneal ring ulcers may be the presenting sign in acute leukaemia (Bhadresa 1971; Wood & Nicholson 1973) or in chronic leukaemia in adults (Eiferman *et al.* 1988). They may respond to topical antibiotics and steroids. Perilimbal infiltrates have been described in a young adult with acute monocytic leukaemia (Font *et al.* 1985). Scleral involvement has mainly been an autopsy finding (Kincaid & Green 1983).

Lens

Cataracts occur frequently in patients who have had total body irradiation, related not only to the total dose but also to the rate and fractionation of administration (Livesey *et*

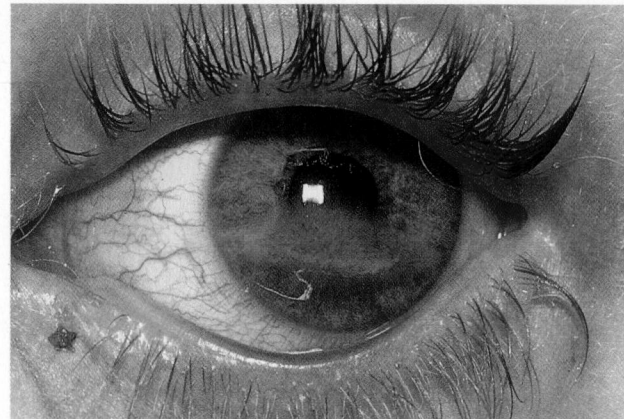

a

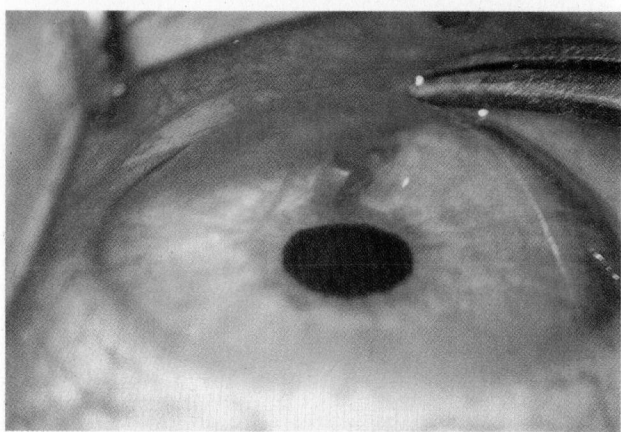

b

Fig. 60.3 (a) Corneal inflammatory infiltrate in a patient with acute lymphoblastic leukaemia who had a bone marrow transplant. The infiltrate started with symptoms and signs similar to a recurrent erosion. (b) After 2 years the same patient had an infiltrated cornea fed by an iris vessel.

al. 1989; Bray *et al.* 1991). The use of steroids to treat graft-versus-host disease may exacerbate the cataracts (Livesey *et al.* 1989).

The treatment of the cataracts, when visually significant, is usually by lens aspiration or phacoemulsification with lens implantation – the prognosis is good.

Anterior chamber, iris and intraocular pressure

The anterior segment is an uncommon site of extramedullary relapse accounting for between 0.5 and 2.6% of all relapses (Allen & Straatsma 1961; Kincaid & Green 1983; Bunin *et al.* 1987); it is seen most frequently in lymphoblastic leukaemia, but occasionally occurs in other forms of leukaemia (Perry & Mallen 1979; Tabbara & Beckstead 1980; Novakovic *et al.* 1989). Most reported cases have been in acute lymphoblastic leukaemia in relapse, but rarely children may present with a leukaemic hyphaema or hypopyon (Tabbara & Beckstead 1980).

The pathogenesis of anterior segment disease is unknown, but the relative infrequency of concurrent central nervous system relapse suggests that seeding from the central nervous system is not an important mechanism (Novakovic *et al.* 1989). The infiltration is most likely to be blood-borne and the relatively frequent occurrence of isolated anterior segment relapse supports Ninane *et al.*'s (1980) concept of the eye as a 'sanctuary' site. Because of the blood–eye barrier, chemotherapeutic agents do not penetrate the eye as well as many other sites and this, together with the avoidance of the eye in cranial irradiation, allows the survival of leukaemia cells which most frequently cause symptoms after chemotherapy has been stopped.

Symptoms include redness, watering, photophobia and the parents may notice changes in the shape or reactions of the pupil or in the colour and appearance of the iris. Pain and visual loss may occasionally occur.

Clinical findings are variable (Figs 60.4–60.7) with iritis and hypopyon being the most common. Ciliary injection,

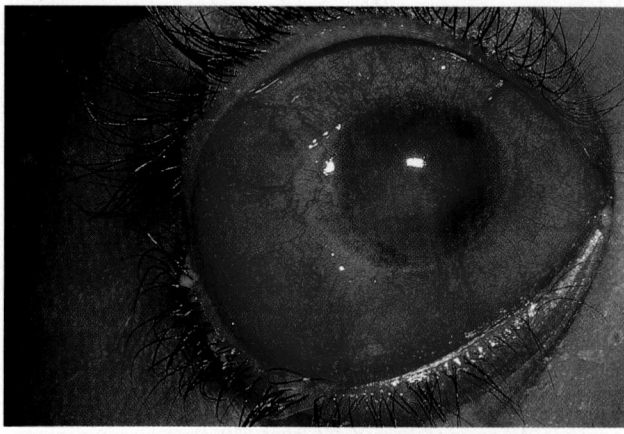

Fig. 60.4 Acute lymphoblastic leukaemia in relapse with iris, subconjunctival and scleral invasion, with glaucoma.

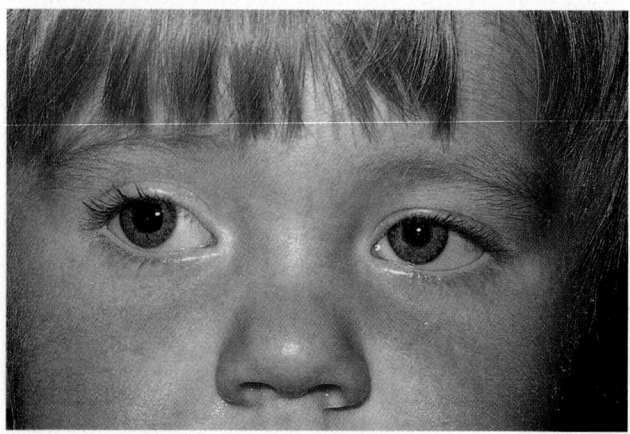

Fig. 60.5 Heterochromia iridis due to iris relapse in the left eye.

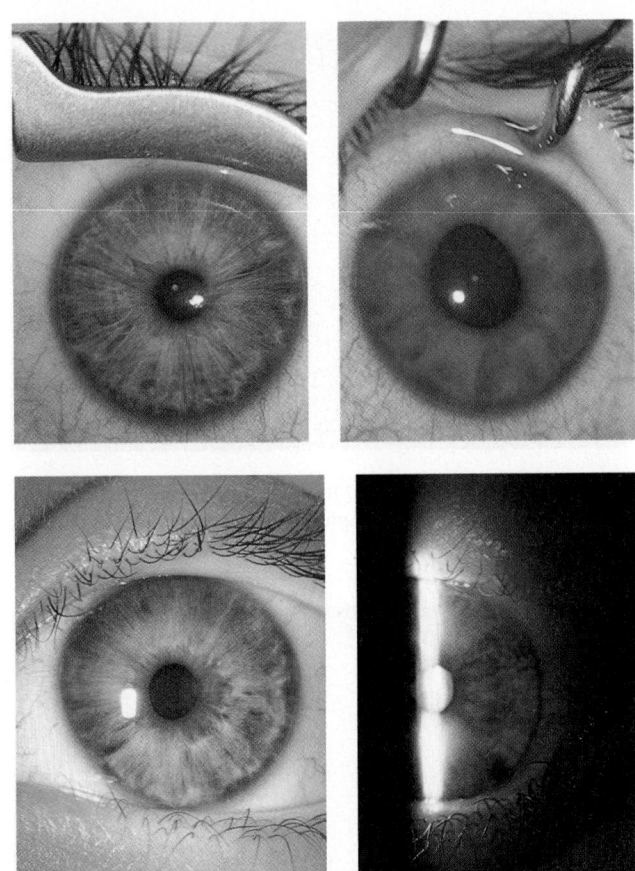

Fig. 60.6 (a) Iris relapse with heterochromia, infiltrated left iris and sluggish pupil reactions. (b) After treatment with 2500 cGy there is iris transilluminance. The right eye had become affected.

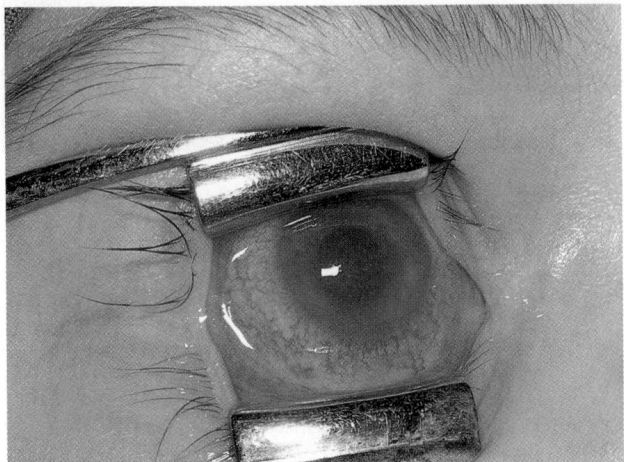

Fig. 60.7 Iris relapse with glaucoma in acute lymphoblastic leukaemia.

keratic precipitates (KP), anterior chamber cells and flare (Zakka *et al.* 1980) are frequant. Posterior synechiae are unusual, but a greyish hypopyon which may be streaked with blood (Hinzpeter *et al.* 1978) is common.

Other causes of hyphaema include juvenile xanthogranuloma, retinoblastoma, retrolental fibroplasia, persistent hyperplastic primary vitreous, iridoschisis, unsuspected trauma, iris vascular malformations, rubeosis iridis and other blood dyscrasias.

Secondary glaucoma is common and is associated with corneal oedema, pain and redness (Tabbara & Beckstead 1980).

The iris may be thickened either diffusely or in the form of one or more nodules or a mass of variable size; the iris may also be thinned with loss of pigment. This iris colour may be changed, usually by a brownish discoloration, and the thickening of the iris obliterates the iris crypts and may give a rather featureless iris. Rubeosis may occur. It is often the failure of standard uveitis treatment that draws the ophthalmologist's attention to the underlying leukaemia. It should not, however, be assumed because a child has leukaemia any uveitis is leukaemic. This is not necessarily the case and histological confirmation must be obtained. The diagnosis is best established by a combination of an anterior chamber paracentesis and an iridectomy. Novakovic *et al.* (1989) pointed out that a paracentesis alone may not be sufficient to give an accurate diagnosis. Pathological studies show leukaemic infiltration of the iris and trabecular meshwork (Kincaid & Green 1983; Jankovic *et al.* 1986) and the hypopyon consists of leukaemic cells, necrotic tissue and proteinaceous exudate. Leukaemic cells may be difficult to find. Patients with glaucoma have histological evidence of leukaemic obstruction of the outflow channels and episcleral vessels (Glaser & Smith 1966). The latter case was an adult, reported by J. Lawton Smith and Dr B. Glaser (the father of Dr Joel Glaser), who presented with limbal injection and raised intraocular pressure which failed to respond to acetazolamide. The leukaemia was discovered on routine investigation after admission and the glaucoma responded well to low-dose radiotherapy.

Treatment of anterior segment relapse usually consists of reinduction of chemotherapy, substantial ocular radiotherapy (usually 3000 cGy) and topical steroid treatment.

Choroid

The choroid is the part of the eye most frequently involved in all types of leukaemia (Allen & Straatsma 1961; Kincaid & Green 1983; Leonardy *et al.* 1990), but it only rarely becomes clinically apparent. The clinical manifestations are the result of serous retinal detachment (Burns *et al.* 1965) or retinal detachment associated with a subretinal mass (MacManaway & Neely 1994). Retinal infarction occurs with ophthalmic artery occlusion, and chronic or focal ischaemia results in retinal pigment epithelial defects and clumping (Clayman *et al.* 1972). Fluorescein angiography demonstrates myriads of diffuse leakage points at the level of the retinal pigment epithelium (Kincaid *et al.* 1979). Similar fluorescein patterns are seen in serous detachments with melanoma, metastatic tumour, Vogt–Koyanagi–Harada disease and posterior scleritis. Leukaemic choroidopathy can be detected by ultrasound even when there is no abnormality on clinical examination (Abramson *et al.* 1983).

Retina and vitreous

The retina, because of its ready visibility, is the part of the eye most frequently found to be involved clinically, and fundoscopy is part of the routine follow-up examination of leukaemic patients.

Hyperviscosity changes

Hyperviscosity of the blood occurs at some stage in most cases of leukaemia, but reaches its most pronounced manifestations in the chronic leukaemias, which are more common in adults.

Vascular tortuosity and dilatation with irregularity or even 'beading' of the veins, sheathing and haemorrhages are probably the earliest manifestations (Fig. 60.8).

Fluorescein angiography (Jampol *et al.* 1975) and trypsin digests (Duke *et al.* 1968; Kincaid & Green 1983) show capillary saccular and fusiform microaneurysms, and neovascularization has also been observed in some cases of chronic myeloid leukaemia in adults; it seems to be more closely related to the longevity of the disease and the increased amounts of blood cells giving rise to a prolonged hyperviscosity, reduced flow with capillary closure, microaneurysm formation and neovascularization (Rosenthal 1983). Microaneurysms do not occur in acute leukaemia (Duke *et al.* 1968).

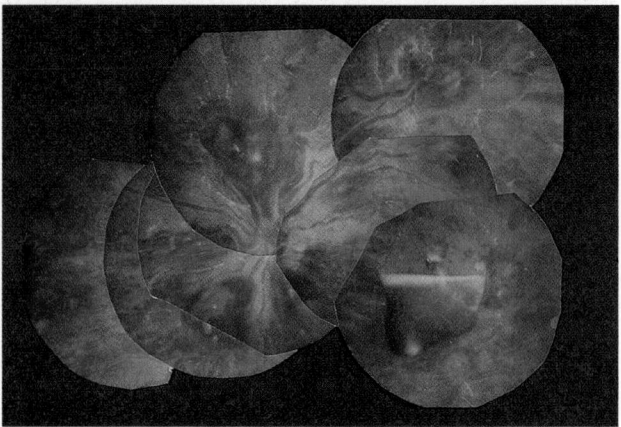

Fig. 60.9 Widespread retinal infiltrates and haemorrhages in all layers of the retina in acute lymphoblastic leukaemia.

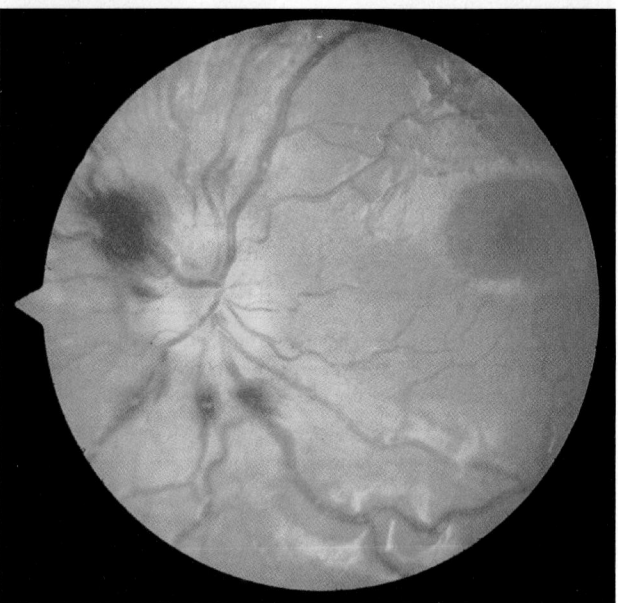

Fig. 60.10 Retinal nerve fibre layer haemorrhages in acute lymphoblastic leukaemia. The tiny white centres to the haemorrhages are light reflexes.

Retinal haemorrhages

Haemorrhages occur as a result of a combination of hyperviscosity, coagulation, infiltration and defective damage to retinal vessel walls and vessel occlusion (Kaur & Taylor 1991).

Haemorrhages occur throughout the retina (Figs 60.9–60.12) and may involve the vitreous. They may be massive and involve the whole eye.

Nerve fibre layer haemorrhages are seen as bright red haemorrhages with at least one margin being 'flame-shaped'. Deeper haemorrhages are not quite so red and usually more rounded. Subhyaloid haemorrhages have

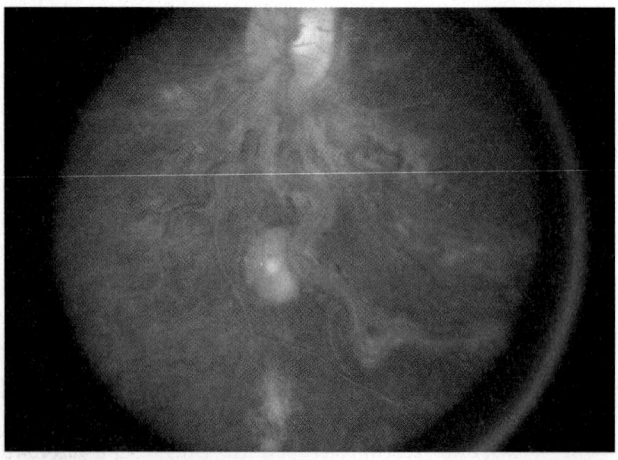

Fig. 60.8 Hyperviscosity changes in chronic myeloid leukaemia in a 20-year-old (Dr S. Day's patient).

sharply defined margins and can form a fluid level in which there may be a layer of white cells.

Some haemorrhages are white centred; this should not be confused with the pinpoint white light reflex from the apex of a haemorrhage, or with haemorrhage around a leukaemic deposit. The white area consists of platelet and fibrin deposits which occlude the vessel, or septic emboli

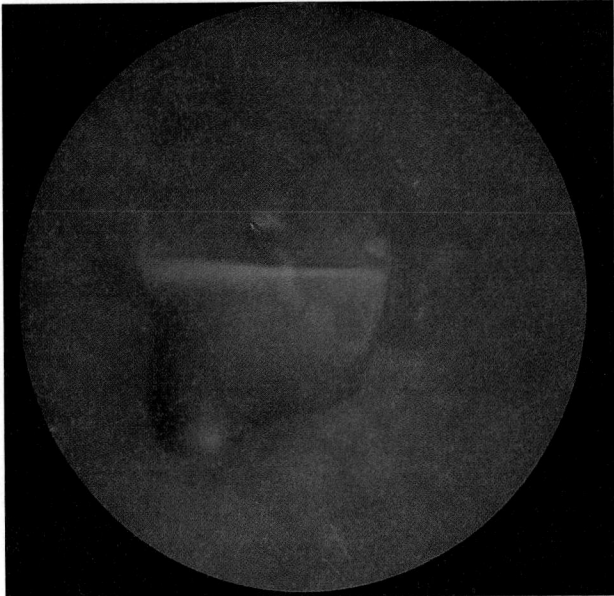

Fig. 60.13 Subhyaloid haemorrhage with a gross leukaemic cell content.

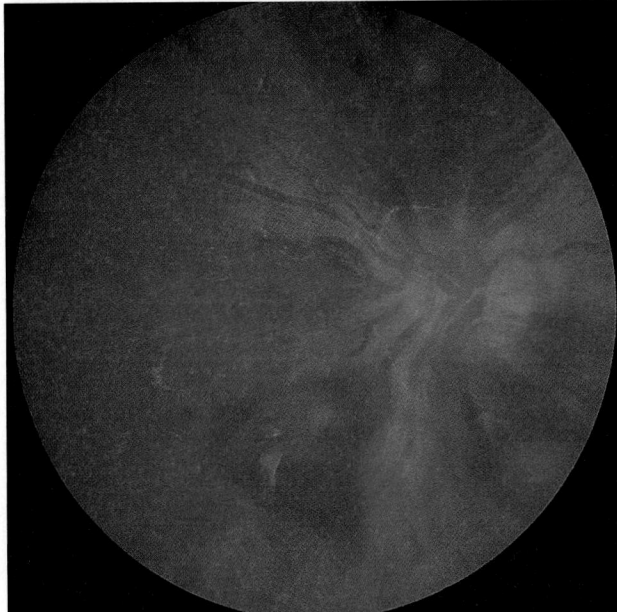

Fig. 60.11 White centred and nerve fibre retinal haemorrhages in acute lymphoblastic leukaemia.

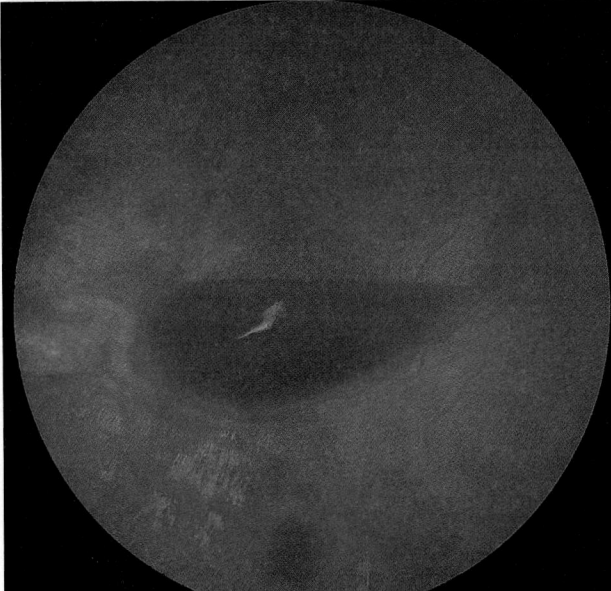

Fig. 60.12 Subhyaloid haemorrhages with acute lymphoblastic leukaemia, profound anaemia and thrombocytopenia.

(Duane *et al.* 1980). The haemorrhage occurs because of infarction and weakening of the vessel wall, which can also be damaged by leukaemic deposits.

White patches

White areas in the retinas of leukaemic children may be caused by the following.
1 Vessel sheathing (Kim *et al.* 1994).
2 Retinal infiltrates — these are nodular deposits which before the era of modern chemotherapy were commonly seen. They are unusual in acute leukaemia today. They are often associated with haemorrhage (Figs 60.13, 60.14). Similar changes have been recorded in B-cell lymphoma (Wender *et al.* 1994).
3 Cotton-wool spots — these are retinal nerve fibre layer infarcts and occur frequently in acute leukaemia (Kincaid & Green 1983) and transiently after bone marrow transplantation (Fig. 60.15). They presumably occur because of retinal vascular occlusion in patients who have recently received bone marrow transplants whether or not they have been treated with cyclosporin. They can recover spontaneously and have been shown to be associated with retinal vascular endotheliopathy (Webster *et al.* 1995).
4 Hard exudates. These small yellowish lesions are seen in relation to vessels that are chronically leaking non-cellular blood elements and are most frequently seen in chronic leukaemias with hyperviscosity.
5 Opportunistic infections with cytomegalovirus or fungus may occur in the immunosuppressed patient.

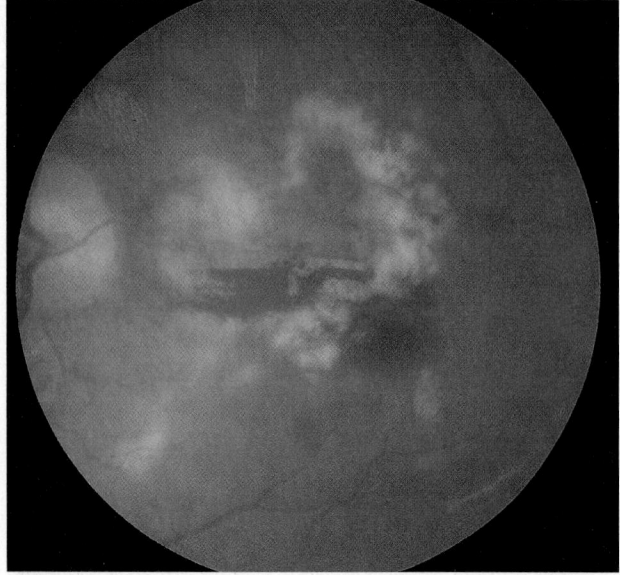

Fig. 60.14 Retinal infiltrates in acute lymphoblastic leukaemia.

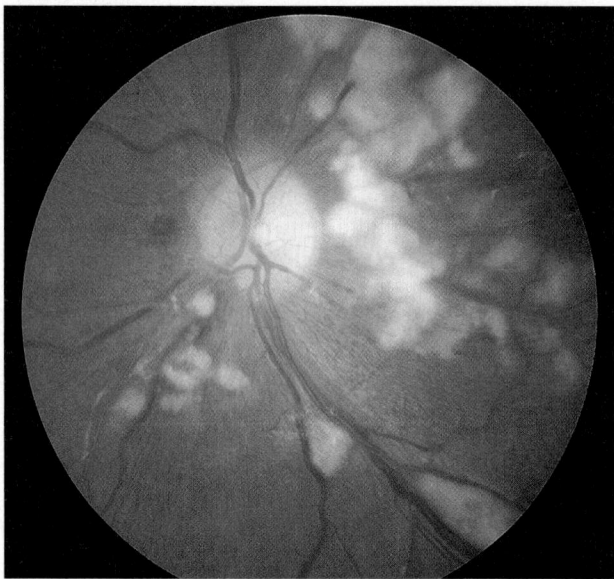

Fig. 60.15 Transient multiple cotton-wool spots after bone marrow transplant.

6 Retinal infarction, in the acute stage gives rise to large areas of cloudy swelling of the retinal nerve fibres and ganglion cell layer.

Retinal infarction

Occlusion of larger retinal arterioles or of the ophthalmic artery occasionally occurs as a preterminal event (Taylor & Day 1982) (Fig. 60.16).

Vitreous cells

Vitreous involvement with leukaemic or blood cells is usually secondary to retinal infiltration or haemorrhage (Kincaid & Green 1983), but may occur without obvious involvement of the retina (Reese & Guy 1933). Occasionally vitreous aspiration may be needed to confirm the diagnosis (Swartz & Schumann 1980) especially if the patient is apparently in remission and there is a possibility of an opportunistic infection. Vitreous organization (Fig. 60.17) is an unusual but serious sequel to widespread retinal or optic nerve infiltration.

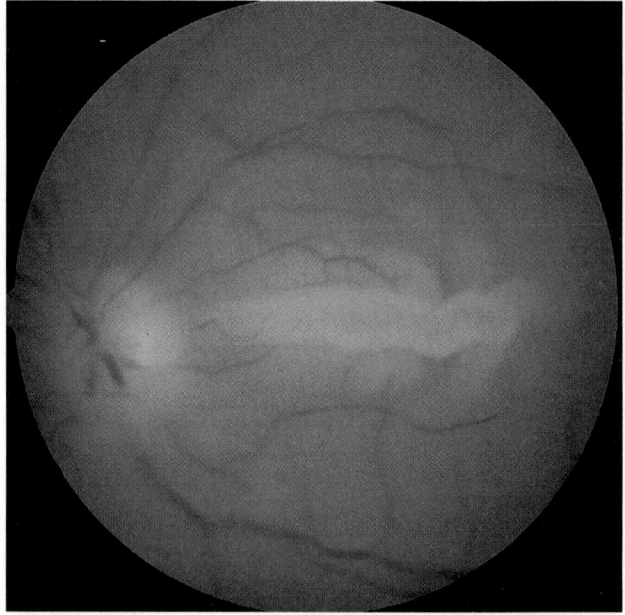

Fig. 60.16 Ophthalmic artery occlusion as a preterminal event.

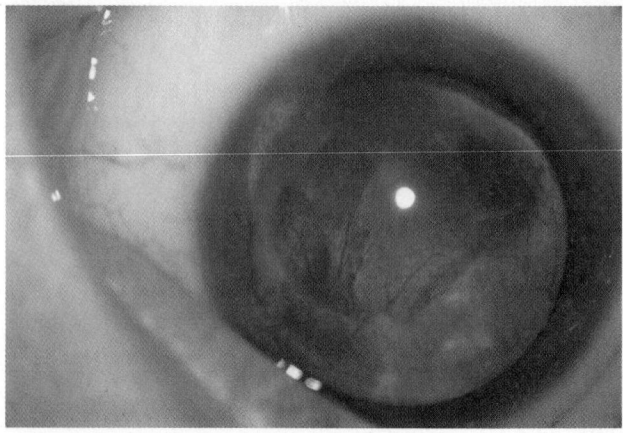

Fig. 60.17 Vitreous organization in acute lymphoblastic leukaemia following leukaemic retinopathy and choroidopathy.

Other retinal manifestations

Serous retinopathy (Burns *et al.* 1965; Kincaid *et al.* 1979) and retinal pigment clumping (Clayman *et al.* 1972) occur as manifestations of choroidal involvement.

Optic nerve

Optic nerve involvement in postmortem cases occurs in nearly one-fifth of acute or chronic leukaemias (Kincaid & Green 1983), although in clinical series it is more frequently seen in acute lymphatic leukaemia (Ellis & Little 1973; Rosenthal *et al.* 1975; Brown *et al.* 1981). Optic nerve involvement, which used to presage death, is now less frequently seen presumably due to aggressive chemotherapy (Rosenthal 1983).

Leukaemic optic neuropathy may have only minimal visual symptoms despite even massive involvement, but often marked loss of central vision is observed (Fig. 60.18), especially with infiltration behind the lamina cribrosa (Rosenthal 1983). With prelaminar infiltration there is ophthalmoscopically visible fluffy white infiltration with haemorrhage, but on occasion, especially if the infiltration is bilateral, the differentiation from papilloedema may be difficult and a lumbar puncture may be necessary.

The response to irradiation with 2000 cGy of radiotherapy may be dramatic (Rosenthal *et al.* 1975); whatever the treatment optic atrophy is a frequent sequel (Nikaido *et al.* 1988).

An optic neuropathy may also be caused by vincristine treatment (Sanderson *et al.* 1976) or by radiotherapy.

Other neuro-ophthalmic involvement

Neurological complications of leukaemia and its treatment are common. Campbell *et al.* (1977) found that 61 of 438 children had significant complications including haemorrhage, which occurred in 1% of children with lymphoblastic leukaemia, and 7% of children with myeloblastic leukaemia. Infection by measles, varicella or mumps occurred in 11 patients and left permanent defects in many. Bacterial infections were less frequent. Methotrexate, vincristine and other drugs may cause significant problems – methotrexate may be given intrathecally or in high doses systemically (Hann 1992).

Central nervous system involvement manifests as meningeal irritation, with headaches and vomiting, fits and cranial nerve involvement. Vessel occlusion gives rise to various defects from transient deafness to a hypoxic encephalopathy (Lilleyman 1993). In addition to the disease, many of the drugs and radiotherapy used may have central nervous system side-effects, both short and long term, including fits and a variable handicap.

Communicating hydrocephalus (De Reuck *et al.* 1979), chiasmal infiltration (Zimmerman & Thorenson 1964) and

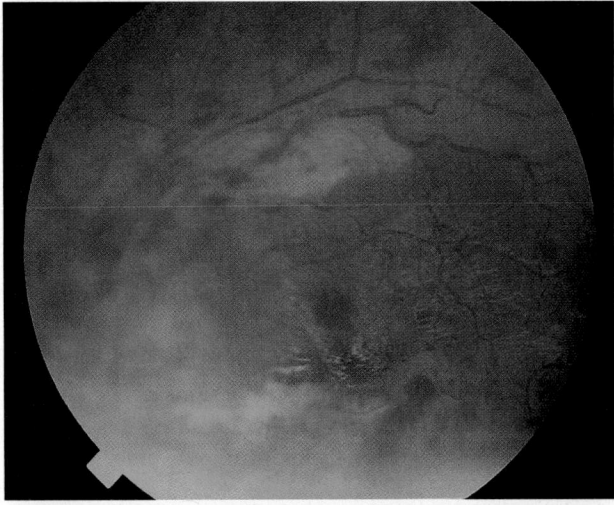

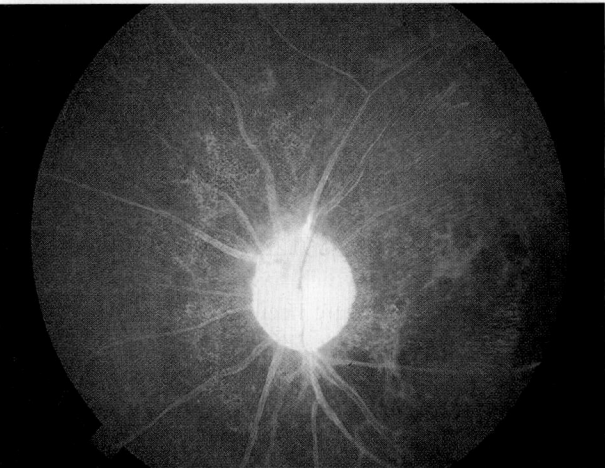

Fig. 60.18 (a) Gross optic nerve head and retinal involvement in acute lymphoblastic leukaemia. (b) Profound optic atrophy and vascular attenuation following treatment with radiotherapy (same patient).

sixth nerve palsies (Abbassidum 1979) have also been described.

Complications of treatment

Drugs

Vincristine and other vinca alkaloids may cause corneal hypoaesthesia, ptosis, third, sixth and seventh nerve palsies (Albert *et al.* 1967), and optic neuropathy (Sanderson *et al.* 1976) which may be reversible if the treatment is stopped early. The neuropathy is dose related (Sandler *et al.* 1969) and is most frequently seen initially as a peripheral neuropathy with abnormal deep tendon reflexes. Fits also occur (Campbell *et al.* 1977).

L-Asparaginase may occasionally and idiosyncratically

be associated with a severe encephalopathy which may be fatal (Gerrard *et al.* 1986).

Cytarabine may cause blurred vision from conjunctivitis, corneal epithelial opacities and microcysts (Hopen *et al.* 1981).

Methotrexate is a significant cause of neurological problems including arachnoiditis from intrathecal administration, fits, depression, ataxia and dementia (Campbell *et al.* 1977).

Steroids may cause posterior subcapsular cataracts. Elliott *et al.* (1985) found cataracts in 32% of 37 children who had been treated with steroids and cranial irradiation, but they were not of great visual significance.

Rapid withdrawal of steroid therapy may cause benign intracranial hypertension (pseudotumour cerebri).

Immunosuppression

Anti-leukaemia chemotherapy, steroids and radiotherapy all contribute to the immunosuppression which allows infection by opportunistic bacteria, viruses (Fig. 60.19, 60.20), fungi or protozoa some of which do not usually cause significant infection in humans.

Herpes simplex and zoster affect the cornea (Fig. 60.21), conjunctiva and lids (Figs 60.22, 60.23). Herpes simplex and cytomegalovirus, which have an affinity for neural tissue, may cause a severe necrotizing retinochoroiditis which may be difficult to differentiate from leukaemic infiltrates, a distinction which can be helped by chorioretinal biopsy (Taylor *et al.* 1981), but can usually be made by culture of urine or saliva.

Yeast and fungus infections are rare, but important complications of immunosuppression (Michaelson *et al.* 1971; Greene & Wiernick 1972; Avenda *et al.* 1978) and, if

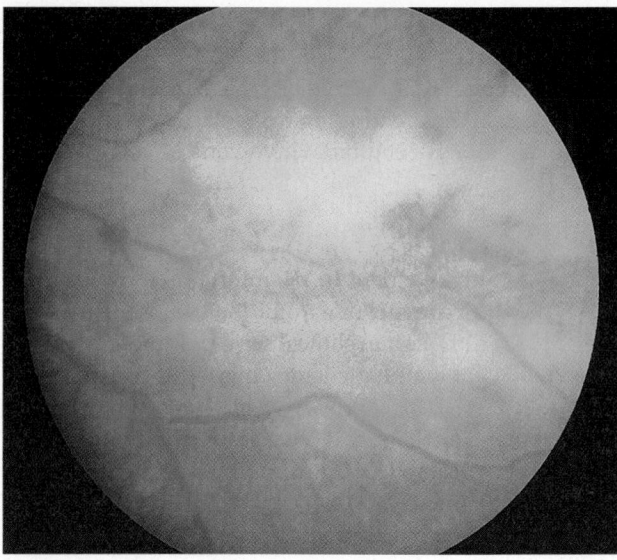

Fig. 60.20 Cytomegalovirus retinitis in acute lymphoblastic leukaemia in relapse.

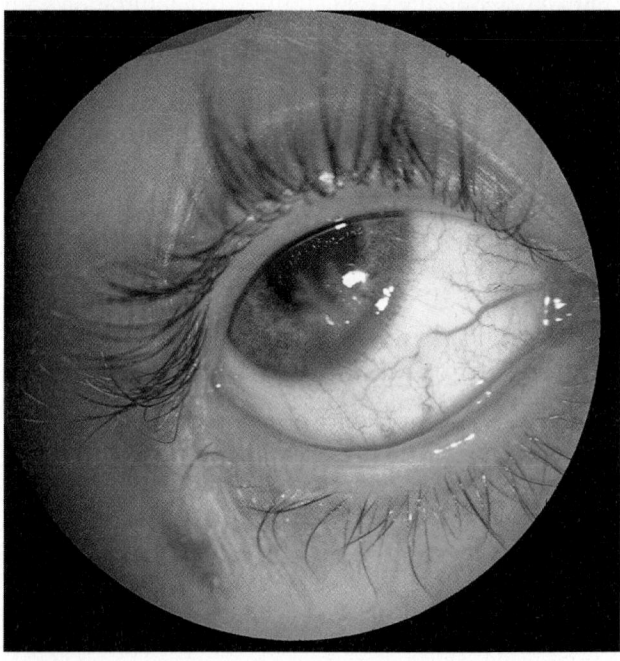

Fig. 60.21 Herpes simplex keratitis in a patient with acute lymphoblastic leukaemia on chemotherapy.

possible, biopsy is necessary to establish the diagnosis and to plan appropriate treatment. Other infections include mucormycosis, toxoplasmosis and aspergillosis (Cogan 1977).

Graft-versus-host disease

In some children with leukaemia in relapse, and in some aplastic anaemias, following total body irradiation and

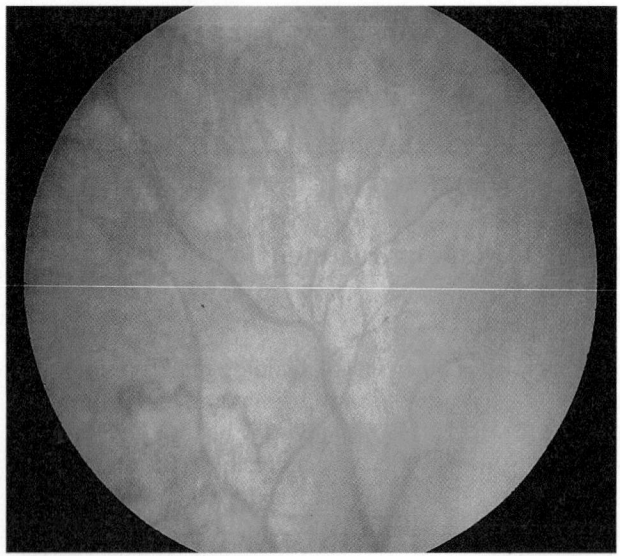

Fig. 60.19 Cytomegalovirus retinitis in acute lymphoblastic leukaemia in relapse.

chemotherapy to destroy the existing marrow, a bone marrow transplant is performed (Chessells 1988) to give a new population of bone marrow cells. There are two types of bone marrow transplant.

1 Allogenic, when donor marrow, matched by HLA typing or from a close relative, is infused.

2 Autologous, when the patient's own stored marrow is used.

Because of failure to recognize the transplant recipient as 'self', the transplanted lymphocytes may attack the recipient and cause graft-versus-host disease.

Acute graft-versus-host disease is characterized by the occurrence within 4 months of the transplant of weight loss, fever, rash, liver dysfunction and a dry mouth.

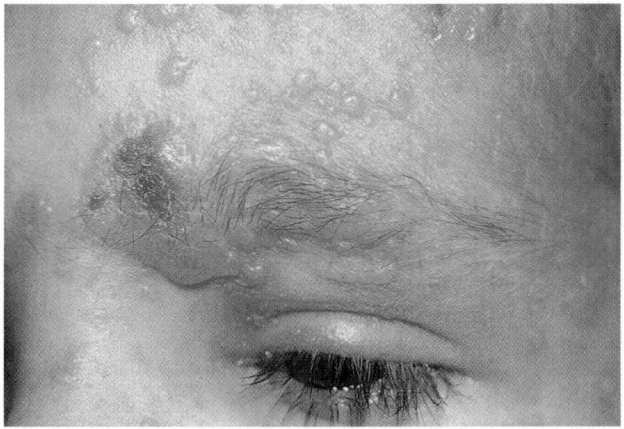

Fig. 60.22 Confluent varicella in a patient with acute lymphoblastic leukaemia in relapse.

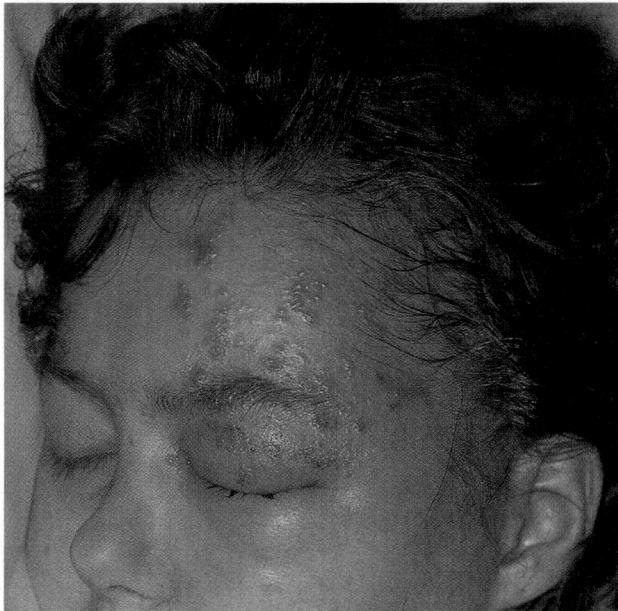

Fig. 60.23 Herpes zoster in a patient with acute lymphoblastic leukaemia on chemotherapy.

Ocular manifestations are common in chronic graft-versus-host disease (Franklin *et al.* 1983; Jack *et al.* 1983) and include dry eye, cicatricial lagophthalmos, sterile conjunctivitis and uveitis. The eye problems are frequently severe and test the ophthalmologist's management of the dry eye. There is a high incidence of visually significant cataract.

About half of patients undergoing bone marrow treatment develop keratoconjunctivitis sicca (Hirst *et al.* 1983) with a pseudomembranous conjunctivitis in some patients. At autopsy the whole eye is affected including the lacrimal gland (Jabs *et al.* 1983). About 10% of patients undergoing bone marrow transplant develop conjunctival involvement with graft-versus-host disease (Jabs *et al.* 1989). Pseudomembranous conjunctivitis was the most frequent manifestation of conjunctival graft-versus-host disease and carried a poor prognosis for life.

An interesting occurrence is the transient appearance of multiple white cotton-wool spots in bone marrow transplant recipients (Gratwahl *et al.* 1983). Coskuncan *et al.* (1994) found retinal complications in 12.8% of 397 patients with bone marrow transplant including retinal or vitreous haemorrhage, cotton-wool spots, optic disc oedema, retinitis, lymphoma, and serous retinal detachments.

The ophthalmologist's role

Since ocular complications are rare (Hoover *et al.* 1988) there is probably no need for routine ophthalmological surveillance in these children and the ophthalmologist usually only becomes involved by the referring oncologist or paediatrician, from whom most ophthalmologists can learn a lot about communication and patient management!

References

Abbassidum K. Headaches, vomiting and diplopia in a 16-year-old child. *Clin Pediatr* 1979; **18**: 191–2.

Abramson DH, Jereb B, Wollner N, Murphy L, Ellsworth RM. Leukemia ophthalmopathy detected by ultrasound. *J Pediatr Ophthalmol Strabismus* 1983; **20**: 92–7.

Albert DM, Wong VG, Henderson ES. Ocular complications of vincristine therapy. *Arch Ophthalmol* 1967; **78**: 709–13.

Allen RA, Straatsma BR. Ocular involvement in leukaemia and allied disorders. *Arch Ophthalmol* 1961; **66**: 490–509.

Atra A, Richards S, Chessells J. Remission death in acute lymphoblastic leukaemia: a changing pattern. *Arch Dis Child* 1993; **59**: 550–4.

Avenda NJ, Tanishima T, Kuwabara T. Ocular cryptococcosis. *Am J Ophthalmol* 1978; **86**: 110–13.

Bhadresa GN. Changes in the anterior segment as a presenting feature in leukaemia. *Br J Ophthalmol* 1971; **55**: 133–5.

Bray LC, Carey PJ, Proctor SJ, Evans RG, Hamilton PJ. Ocular complications of bone marrow transplantation. *Br J Ophthalmol* 1991; **75**: 611–14.

Brown GC, Shields JA, Augsburger JJ, Serota FT, Koch P. Leukaemic optic neuropathy. *Int Ophthalmol* 1981; **3**: 111–16.

Bunin N, Rivera G, Goode F, Hustu HO. Ocular relapse in the anterior chamber in childhood acute lymphoblastic leukaemia. *J Clin Oncol* 1987; **5**: 299–303.

Burns CA, Blodi FC, Williamsen BK. Acute lymphocytic leukaemia and central serous retinopathy. *Trans Am Acad Ophthalmol Otol* 1965; **69**: 307–9.

Campbell RHA, Marshall WC, Chessels JM. Neurological complications of childhood leukaemia. *Arch Dis Child* 1977; **52**: 850–8.

Chessels JMS. Bone marrow transplantation for leukaemia. *Arch Dis Child* 1988; **63**: 879–82.

Clayman HM, Flynn JT, Koch K, Israel C. Retinal pigment epithelial abnormalities in leukemic disease. *Am J Ophthalmol* 1972; **74**: 416–19.

Cogan DG. Immunosuppression and eye disease. *Am J Ophthalmol* 1977; **83**: 777–88.

Coskuncan N, Jabs D, Dunn J *et al*. The eye in bone marrow transplantation VI. Retinal complications. *Arch Ophthalmol* 1994; **112**: 372–9.

De Reuck J, De Coster W, Vander Eecken H. Communicating hydrocephalus in treated leukaemic patients. *Eur Neurol* 1979; **18**: 8–14.

Duane TD, Osher RH, Green WR. White centered haemorrhages: their significance. *Ophthalmology* 1980; **87**: 66–9.

Duke JR, Wilkinson CP, Sigelman S. Retinal microaneurysms in leukaemia. *Br J Ophthalmol* 1968; **52**: 368–74.

Eiferman RA, Levartovsky S, Schulz JC. Leukemic corneal infiltrates. *Am J Ophthalmol* 1988; **105**: 318–19.

Ellis W, Little HL. Leukaemic infiltration of the optic nerve head. *Am J Ophthalmol* 1973; **75**: 867–71.

Elliott AJ, Oakhill A, Goodman S. Cataracts in childhood leukaemia. *Br J Ophthalmol* 1985; **69**: 459–61.

Font R, Mackay B, Tang R. Acute monocytic leukaemia recurring as bilateral perilimbal infiltrates: immunohistochemical and ultrastructural confirmation. *Ophthalmology* 1985; **92**: 1681–6.

Franklin RM, Kenneth R, Kenyon PS *et al*. Ocular manifestations of graft-vs-host disease. *J Am Acad Ophthalmol* 1983; **90**: 4–13.

Gerrard MP, Eden OB, Lilleyman JS. Acute encephalopathy induction therapy for acute lymphoblastic leukaemia. *Paediatr Haematol Oncol* 1986; **3**: 49–58.

Glaser B, Smith JL. Leukaemic glaucoma. *Br J Ophthalmol* 1966; **50**: 92–4.

Gloor B, Gratwahl A, Hahn H *et al*. Multiple cotton wool spots following bone marrow transplantation for treatment of acute lymphotic leukaemia. *Br J Ophthalmol* 1985; **69**: 320–5.

Gratwahl A, Gloor D, Hann H, Speck B. Retinal cotton-wool patches in bone-marrow transplant recipients. *N Engl J Med* 1983; **308**: 110–11.

Greene WH, Wiernick PH. *Candida* endophthalmitis. Successful treatment in a patient with acute leukaemia. *Am J Ophthalmol* 1972; **74**: 1100–4.

Hann IM. CNS directed therapy in childhood acute lymphoblastic leukaemia. *Br J Haematol* 1992; **82**: 2–5.

Hinzpeter EN, Knoeber H, Freund J. Spontaneous haemophthalmos in leukaemia. *Ophthalmologica* 1978; **177**: 224–8.

Hirst LW, Jabs DA, Tutschka PJ, Green WR, Santos GW. The eye in bone marrow transplantation I. Clinical study. *Arch Ophthalmol* 1983; **101**: 580–90.

Hoover DL, Smith LEH, Turner SJ, Gelber RD, Sallan SE. Ophthalmic evaluation of survivors of acute lymphoblastic leukaemia. *Ophthalmology* 1988; **95**: 151–5.

Hopen G, Mondino BJ, Johnson BL. Corneal toxicity with systemic cytarabine. *Am J Ophthalmol* 1981; **95**: 500–5.

Humayun M, Bernstein S, Gould H, Charis R. Orbital childhood acute lymphoblastic leukaemia as the initial presentation. *J Pediatr Ophthalmol Strabismus* 1992; **29**: 252–4.

Jabs DA, Hirst LW, Green WR, Tutschka PJ, Santos GW, Beschorner WE. The eye in bone marrow transplantation II. Histopathology. *Arch Ophthalmol* 1983; **101**: 585–90.

Jabs DA, Wingard J, Green R, Farmer ER, Vogelsang G, Sarah R. The eye in bone marrow transplantation III. Conjunctival graft-vs-host disease. *Arch Ophthalmol* 1989; **107**: 1343–9.

Jack MK, Jack GM, Sale GE, Shulman HM, Sullivan KM. Ocular manifestations of graft-v-host disease. *Arch Ophthalmol* 1983; **101**: 1080–4.

Jampol LM, Goldberg MF, Busse B. Peripheral retinal microaneurysms in chronic leukaemia. *Am J Ophthalmol* 1975; **80**: 242–8.

Jankovic M, Masera G, Uderzo C. Recurrences of isolated leukaemic hypopyon in a child with acute lymphoblastic leukaemia. *Cancer* 1986; **57**: 380–4.

Kaur B, Taylor D. Fundus hemorrhages in infancy. *Surv Ophthalmol* 1991; **37**: 1–19.

Kim T, Duker J, Hedges T. Retinal angiopathy resembling unilateral frosted branch angiitis in a patient with relapsing acute lymphoblastic leukemia. *Am J Ophthalmol* 1994; **117**: 806–8.

Kincaid MC, Green WR. Ocular and orbital involvement in leukaemia. *Surv Ophthalmol* 1983; **27**: 211–32.

Kincaid MC, Green WR, Kelley JS. Acute ocular leukaemia. *Am J Ophthalmol* 1979; **87**: 698–702.

Leonardy NJ, Rupani M, Dent G, Klintworth GK. Analysis of 135 autopsy eyes for ocular involvement in leukaemia. *Am J Ophthalmol* 1990; **109**: 436–45.

Lilleyman J. Neurological complications of acute childhood leukaemia. *J Roy Soc Med* 1993; **86**: 252–3.

Livesey SJ, Holmes JA, Whittaker JA. Ocular complications of bone marrow transplantation. *Eye* 1989; **3**: 271–6.

MacManaway J, Neely J. Choroidal and orbital leukaemic infiltrate mimicking advanced retinoblastoma. *J Pediatr Ophthalmol Strabismus* 1994; **31**: 394–6.

Michelson PE, Stark W, Reeser F *et al*. Endogenous *Candida* endophthalmitis. *Int Ophthalmol Clin* 1971; **11**: 125–47.

Niemeyer CM, Hitchcock-Bryan S, Sallan SE. Comparative analysis of treatment programs for childhood acute lymphoblastic leukaemia. *Semin Oncol* 1985; **12**: 122–30.

Nikaido H, Mishima H, Ono H, Choshi K, Dohy H. Leukemic involvement of the optic nerve. *Am J Ophthalmol* 1988; **105**: 294–9.

Ninane J, Taylor D, Day S. The eye as a sanctuary in acute lymphoblastic leukaemia. *Lancet* 1980; **i**: 452–3.

Novakovic P, Kellie S, Taylor D. Childhood leukaemia: relapse in the anterior segment of the eye. *Br J Ophthalmol* 1989; **73**: 354–9.

Oakhill A, Willshard H, Mann JR. Unilateral proptosis. *Arch Dis Child* 1981; **56**: 549–51.

Ohkoshi K, Tsiaras W. Prognostic importance of ophthalmic manifestations in childhood leukaemia. *Br J Ophthalmol* 1992; **76**: 651–5.

Perry HD, Mallen FJ. Iris involvement in granulocytic sarcoma. *Am J Ophthalmol* 1979; **87**: 530–2.

Pinkerton C. Avoiding chemotherapy related late effects in children with curable tumours. *Arch Dis Child* 1992; **67**: 1116–19.

Porterfield JF. Orbital tumours in children: a report of 214 cases. *Int Ophthalmol Clin* 1962; **2**: 319–35.

Reese AB, Guy L. Exophthalmos in leukaemia. *Am J Ophthalmol* 1933; **16**: 476–8.

Rosenthal AR. Ocular manifestations of leukaemia: a review. *Ophthalmology* 1983; **90**: 899–905.

Rosenthal AR, Egbert PR, Wilbur JR, Probert JC. Leukaemic involvement of the optic nerve. *J Pediatr Ophthalmol* 1975; **12**: 84–93.

Rubinfeld RS, Gootenberg JE, Charis RM, Zimmerman LE. Early onset acute orbital involvement in childhood acute lymphoblastic leukaemia. *J Am Acad Ophthalmol* 1988; **95**: 116–21.

Sanderson PA, Kuwabara T, Cogan DG. Optic neuropathy presumably caused by vincristine therapy. *Am J Ophthalmol* 1976; **81**: 146–50.

Sandler SG, Tobin W, Henderson ES. Vincristine-induced neuropathy. *Neurology* 1960; **19**: 367–74.

Schachat AP, Markowitz JA, Guyer DR, Burke PJ, Karp JE, Graham ML. Ophthalmic manifestations of leukaemia. *Arch Ophthalmol* 1989; **107**: 697–701.

Stiller CA, Eatock EM. Survival from acute non-lymphocytic leukaemia, 1971–88: a population-based study. *Arch Dis Child* 1994; **70**: 219–23.

Swartz M, Jampol LM. Comma-shaped venular segments of conjunctiva in chronic granulocytic leukaemia. *Canad J Ophthalmol* 1975; **10**: 458–61.

Swartz M, Schumann OB. Acute leukaemic infiltration of the vitreous diagnosed by pars plana aspiration. *Am J Ophthalmol* 1980; **90**: 326–30.

Tabbara KF, Beckstead JH. Acute promonocytic leukaemia with ocular involvement. *Arch Ophthalmol* 1980; **98**: 1055–9.

Taylor DSI, Day SH. Neuroophthalmologic aspects of childhood leukaemia. In: Smith JL, ed. *Neuroophthalmology Focus*. New York: Massan, 1982: 281–90.

Taylor D, Day S, Constable I, Marshall W, Tiedemann K. Chorioretinal biopsy in a patient with leukaemia. *Br J Ophthalmol* 1981; **65**: 489–93.

Webster AR, Anderson JR, Richards EM, Moore AT. Ischaemic retinopathy occurring in patients receiving bone-marrow allografts and campath-IG: a clinicopathological study. *Br J Ophthalmol* 1995; **9**: 687–91.

Wender A, Adar A, Maor E, Yassur Y. Primary B-cell lymphoma of the eyes and brain in a 3-year-old boy. *Arch Ophthalmol* 1994; **112**: 450–1.

Wood WJ, Nicholson DH. Corneal ring ulcer as the presenting manifestation of acute monocytic leukaemia. *Am J Ophthalmol* 1973; **76**: 69–72.

Zakka KA, Yee RD, Shorr N *et al.* Leukaemic iris infiltration. *Am J Ophthalmol* 1980; **89**: 204–9.

Zimmerman LE, Font RL. Ophthalmologic manifestations of granulocytic sarcoma (myeloid sarcoma or chloroma). *Am J Ophthalmol* 1975; **80**: 975–90.

Zimmerman LE, Thoreson HT. Sudden loss of vision in acute leukaemia. *Surv Ophthalmol* 1964; **9**: 467–73.

61: Phakomatoses

Creig S. Hoyt

A hamartoma is a tumour mass arising as an anomaly of tissue formation. It is composed of tissue elements normally present in the involved organ or site. Several important syndromes with clinical manifestations in children, involving the neurological, ocular and cutaneous tissues, are characterized by the presence of hamartomas. These hamartomas are frequently also referred to as phakomatoses (Font & Ferry 1972). The most important of them in the practice of paediatric ophthalmology are neurofibromatosis, tuberous sclerosis, Sturge–Weber syndrome, and von Hippel–Lindau syndrome, although others sometimes included in this group are Klippel–Trenaunay–Weber and, previously, ataxia telangiectasia.

Neurofibromatosis

See Chapter 28.

Tuberous sclerosis

In 1908 Vogt presented the classic triad of epilepsy, mental retardation and specific skin lesions in tuberous sclerosis. Skin lesions are an early manifestation of the disease and most diagnostic are angiofibromas (Fig. 61.1) occurring in a 'butterfly' distribution of the nose and cheeks (Nichol & Reed 1962). However, these cutaneous manifestations are rarely seen in the first 2 years of life and, for that reason, careful ophthalmic evaluation of suspected patients may be essential in establishing the diagnosis (Williams & Taylor 1985).

Tuberous sclerosis may be more common than initially realized, affecting as many as one in 12 000 children under 10 years (Sampson *et al.* 1989). The disorder may be inherited in an autosomal dominant fashion; however, as most patients with tuberous sclerosis do not reproduce because of premature death or mental retardation, 75% of cases are spontaneous mutations. The complete syndrome has never been reported in two consecutive generations (Alper & Holmes 1983). Recent evidence suggests there is considerable heterogeneity in tuberous sclerosis. There is evidence for at least two responsible genes, one on chromosome 9 (9q34) in the UK (Fryer *et al.* 1987) and one on chromosome 11 (11q14–q23) in the USA (Smith *et al.* 1990). More recently, a loss of heterozygosity on chromosome 16 (16p13) in hamartomas from tuberous sclerosis patients has suggested that there may be a further gene implicated (Green *et al.* 1994).

Diagnostic criteria

When tuberous sclerosis is classical, the diagnosis is straightforward. However, patients can be mildly affected, and many of the classical signs may not develop in early infancy, only becoming apparent later in childhood. For this reason, Gomez (1979) laid down primary and secondary features to aid in diagnosis which have evolved more recently (Webb & Osbourne 1992, 1995).

Primary features

Only one of the following primary features is necessary to make the diagnosis.
- Ungual fibroma (Fig. 61.2).
- Retinal hamartomas (more than one).
- Facial angiofibromas.
- Subependymal glial nodules on computed tomography (CT) or magnetic resonance imaging (MRI) (Fig. 61.3).
- Multiple cortical tubers (Fig. 61.4).
- Bilateral renal angiomyolipomas.

Primary features with family history

In an individual with an affected first-degree relative, tuberous sclerosis can be diagnosed if one of the following features is present.

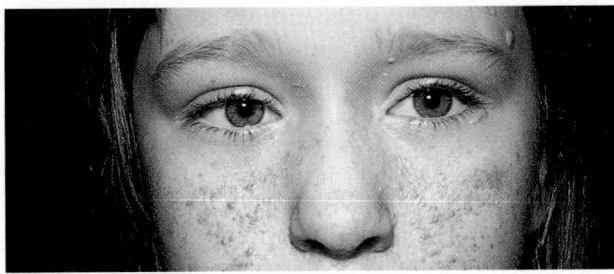

Fig. 61.1 Tuberous sclerosis, angiofibromas of the face—most characteristically seen, as here, over the malar region.

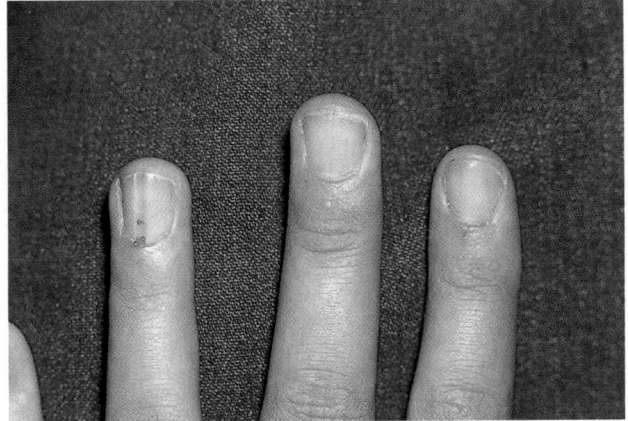

Fig. 61.2 Peri-ungual fibromas.

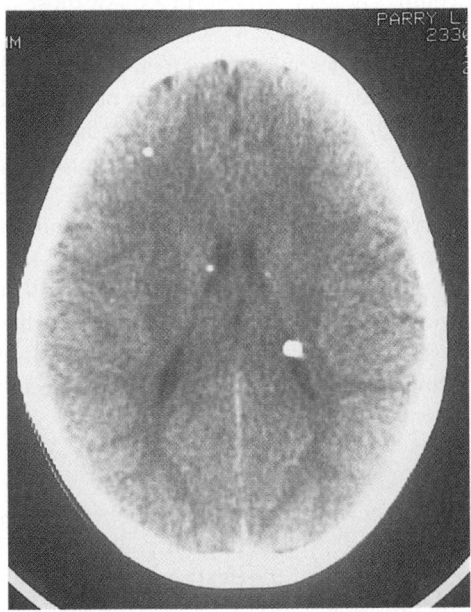

Fig. 61.3 Periventricular calcification in tuberous sclerosis.

- Shagreen patch (Fig. 61.5).
- Forehead fibrous plaque.
- Multiple cardiac rhabdomyomas.
- Giant cell astrocytoma.
- Isolated retinal phakoma.
- Isolated cortical tuber.

Secondary features

If no first-degree relative is affected, the above features are highly suggestive of tuberous sclerosis but not diagnostic. Two of the following features in an individual are diagnostic of the condition.

- Hypomelanic macules (Fig. 61.6).
- Bilateral polycystic kidneys.

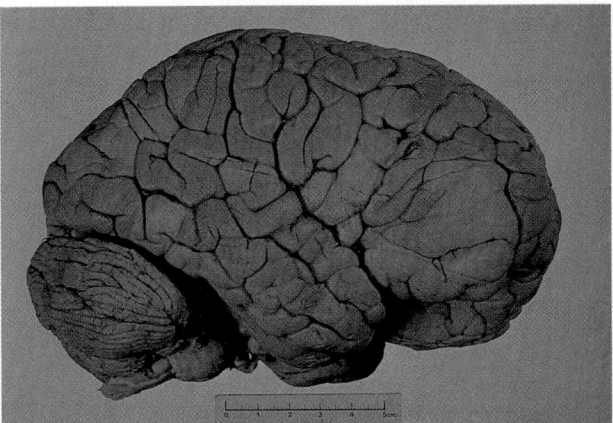

a

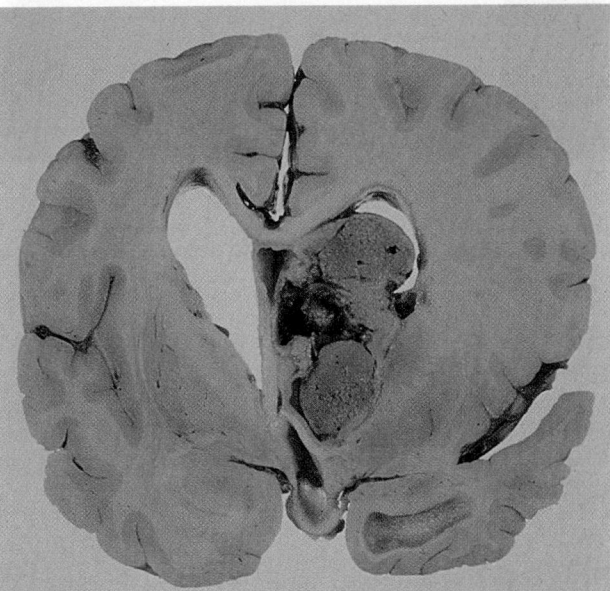

b

Fig. 61.4 (a) Tuberous sclerosis. Brain hamartomas show first as smooth firm pale areas on the gyri. These superficial foci of cortical gliomas (cortical tubers) may appear on the ventricular surfaces as linear lumpy strands or 'candle guttering'. (b) Tuberous sclerosis. Benign astrocytoma with hydrocephalus.

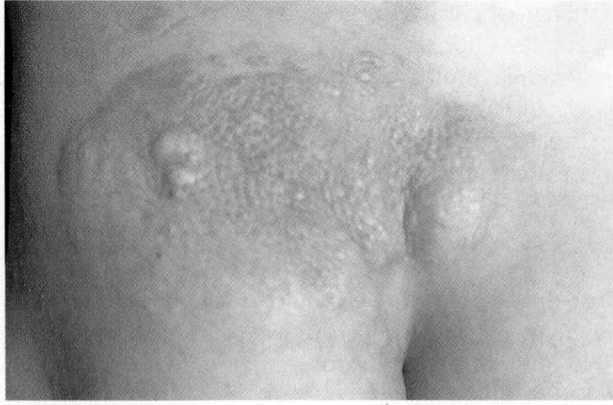

Fig. 61.5 Tuberous sclerosis. Shagreen patch on the skin of the lower back. Shagreen is the name used for a rough form of untanned leather or shark skin.

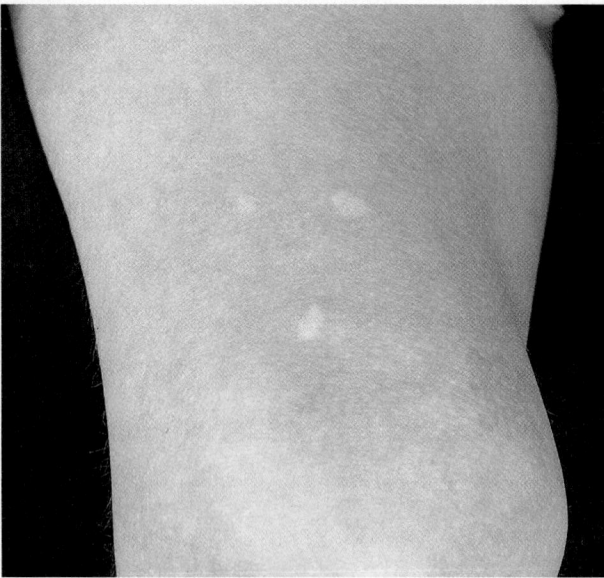

Fig. 61.6 Tuberous sclerosis. Ash-leaf spots are small flat depigmented areas on the skin which occur anywhere on the body, are usually lanceolate in shape and are best seen with a Woods ultraviolet light.

- Isolated cardiac rhabdomyoma.
- Isolated renal angiomyolipoma.
- Pulmonary lymphangiomyomatosis.
- Multiple cortical or subcortical hypomyelinated lesions.

Neurological features

By far the most common manifestation of this disorder is seizures. In infancy, the seizure disorder often takes on the picture of infantile spasms known as 'salaam spasms' (named after the Arabic greeting). These may occur several hundred times a day and quite typically involve flexion and extension movements of the arms and legs. As the child develops, these are replaced by grand mal seizures in 90% of those affected (Lagos & Gomez 1969). The major neurological signs and symptoms in tuberous sclerosis are related to cortical and subependymal astrocystic hamartomas. The cortical 'tubers' occur on the surface of the brain distorting the gyri, whereas the deep subependymal nodules occur most commonly in the region of the basal ganglia and protrude into the lateral and third ventricles (see Fig. 61.4). These may be seen on CT or MRI scanning; visible intracranial calcification can be identified in 50% of patients with tuberous sclerosis. However, calcification is much less frequently seen in infancy. Central nervous system neoplasias occur occasionally in tuberous sclerosis but with much less frequency than in neurofibromatosis. Most commonly, these are subependymal giant cell astrocytomas which, although usually benign, account for 25% of premature death in tuberous sclerosis (Shepherd *et al.* 1991). Mental retardation, although one of the original triad of features, only occurs in 60% of cases.

Cutaneous manifestations

The characteristic cutaneous lesions of tuberous sclerosis include angiofibromas, shagreen patches usually seen on the trunk, forehead fibrous plaques, periungual fibromas, and white depigmented areas known as ash leaf spots. Angiofibromas occur typically in a butterfly distribution over the nose and cheeks and used to be known as adenoma sebaceum. They are present in 85% of those affected, but are rare before the age of 2 years and may not be present until late adolescence. Shagreen patches (Fig. 61.5) are thickened areas of discolored skin occurring usually over the lumbar area in 40% of cases. Forehead fibrous plaques only occur in 25% of cases, but are often present at birth and so are a useful diagnostic feature. Periungual fibromas may grow around the nails of the hands or feet in 50% of cases of tuberous sclerosis. Gum fibromas are much less common. Depigmented 'ash-leaf patches' (see Fig. 61.6) occur in 80% of cases and are the most likely feature of tuberous sclerosis to occur in the first year of life. A Woods ultraviolet light is often required to detect them.

Visceral features

Visceral involvement in tuberous sclerosis is most commonly seen as renal cysts or angiomyolipomas of the kidney. Rhabdomyomas of the heart and cystic lesion of the lung and bone may also occur.

Ocular features

Ocular involvement occurs in at least 50% of patients, although this may not be evident in infancy. The most common ocular manifestations of tuberous scle-

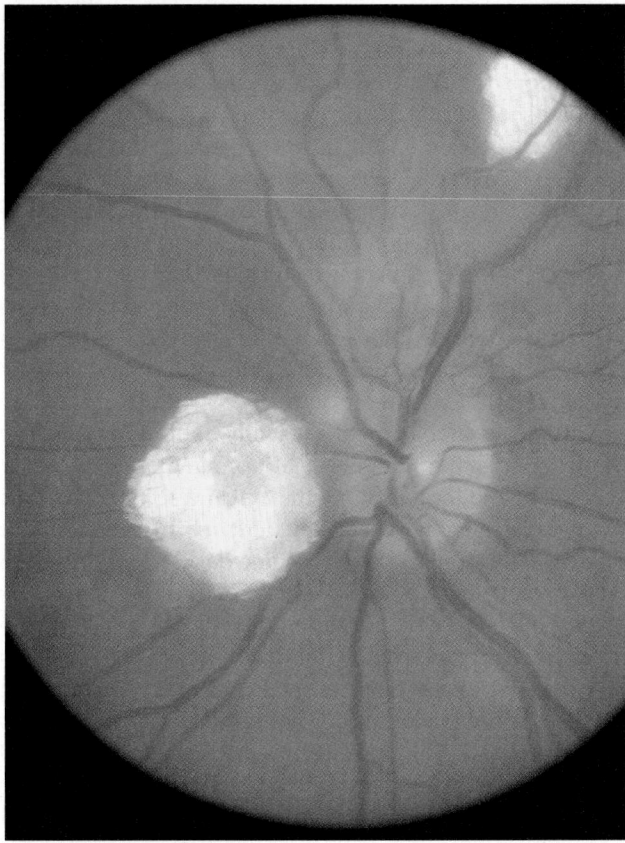

Fig. 61.7 Tuberous sclerosis. 'Mulberry tumours'—these white elevated refractive hamartomas probably evolved from flat translucent lesions.

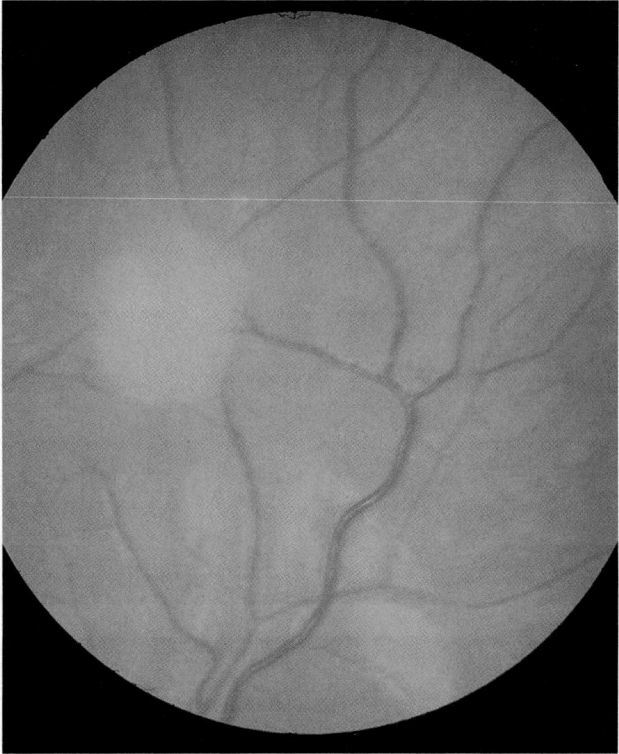

Fig. 61.8 Tuberous sclerosis. Almost flat translucent retinal lesions overlying blood vessels.

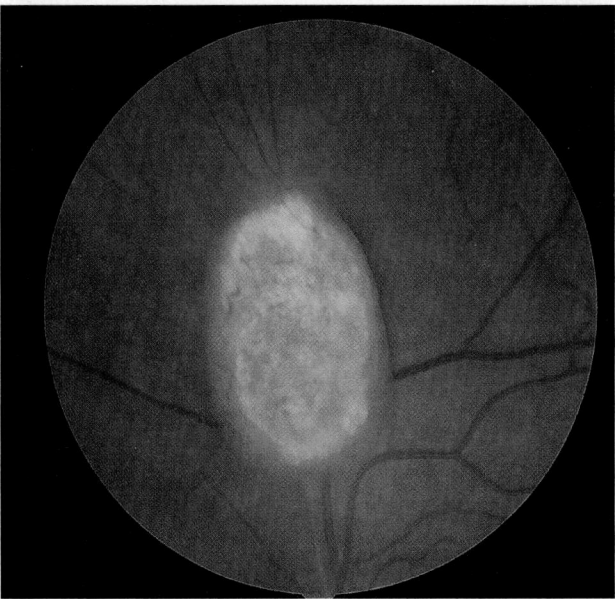

Fig. 61.9 Tuberous sclerosis. Fundus lesions transitional between a flat lesion (Fig. 61.8) and a mulberry tumour (Fig. 61.7).

rosis are hamartomas of the retina and optic nerve (Figs 61.7–61.12). Although these lesions are typically described as being elevated, highly refractile, yellowish, multinodular or cystic masses resembling mulberries (see Fig. 61.7) or clumps of tapioca, this may not be the most predominant type of lesion. Often, the hamartomas are flat, smooth surfaced, semitransparent lesions which are difficult to see and may only manifest as an abnormal light reflex (see Fig. 61.8). Although there is one photographically substantiated report of a lesion evolving from the flat type to the mulberry type over 20 years, in general the lesions remain static, and both types of lesion can be seen in adults and children (Robertson 1988). Retinal hamartomas are not calcified in infancy but become so later in life (see Fig. 61.9) (Zimmer-Galler & Robertson 1995). There may be single or multiple lesions occurring throughout the fundus, although typically they appear clustered around the optic nerve (see Fig. 61.10) or around blood vessels (see Fig. 61.11). These ocular hamartomas rarely interfere with visual function; their presence is of great diagnostic importance, particularly in the evaluation of a child with seizures and evidence of retardation. Rarely, vitreous haemorrhages (see Fig. 61.12) have been reported presumably as the result of bleeding from the abnormal blood vessels involved in the tumour (Atkinson *et al.* 1973). Papilloedema and/or optic atrophy may occur in these patients as signs of asso-

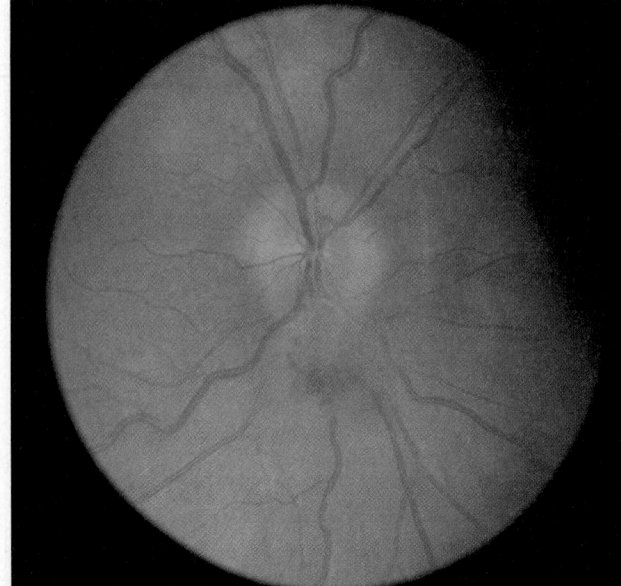

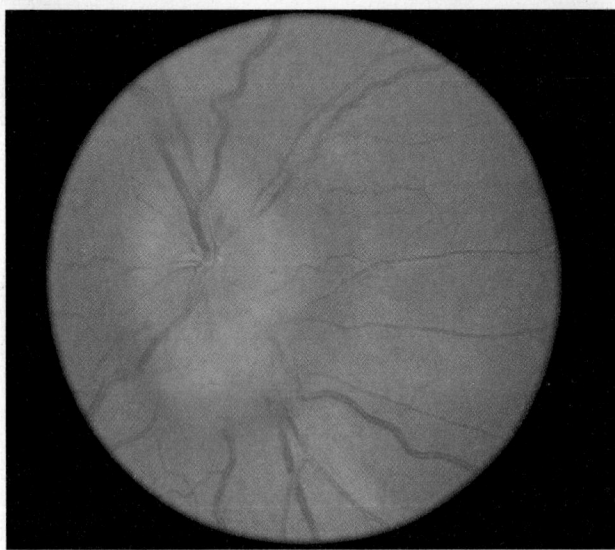

Fig. 61.10 (a) Tuberous sclerosis. Small haemorrhagic flat hamartoma at the disc. Vitreous haemorrhage may occur from these lesions. (b) Tuberous sclerosis. Same patient as (a) but during a period of raised intracranial pressure showing papilloedema and the hamartoma (Williams & Taylor 1985).

ciated intracranial lesions, especially if hydrocephalus has developed. Other ocular lesions include pseudocolobomas of the lens (see Fig. 61.13) and iris (see Fig. 61.14) (Williams & Taylor 1985), and depigmented fundus lesions (see Fig. 61.15).

Sturge–Weber syndrome

The Sturge–Weber syndrome is a neuro-oculocutaneous disorder. Clinically the neurological component manifests

as epilepsy, mental retardation and hemiplegia. The ocular component manifests as glaucoma and vascular malformations of the conjunctiva, episclera, choroid and retina. The dermal involvement is the familiar naevus flammeus (see Fig. 61.16) or port-wine stain (Sullivan *et al.* 1992). The Sturge–Weber syndrome is not familial and generally affects both sexes equally. The clinical manifestations have a common embryological basis. The primary defect is a developmental insult affecting tissues which originate in the pro- and mesencephalic neural crests (Couly & Dourain 1987). These affected precursors then give rise to vascular and other tissue malformations in the meninges, the eye and the dermis.

Cutaneous involvement is usually noticed at birth. The typical port-wine stain or facial haemangioma is usually unilateral and located along the first and second divisions of the trigeminal nerve. It is evident at birth and does not increase in extent but does become darker in colour with age. Hypertrophy of the face may occur on the same side as the haemangioma and the globe on the affected side may be enlarged even without glaucoma. The process may extend to the gingiva and may involve palate and tongue. The cutaneous lesion consists of large dilated capillaries in the dermis and subcutaneous tissues. It does not undergo malignant change or degeneration. Central nervous system involvement is manifest usually as ipsilateral leptomeningeal haemangiomas (although it may be contralateral or bilateral) present over the occipital and/or temporal lobes. Because venous drainage is poor, the metabolic activity of the underlying cortex becomes increasingly dysfunctional. The cerebral tissue becomes atrophic and frequently calcifies, which can be seen on CT scan (Figs 61.17, 61.18). Seizures occur commonly in these

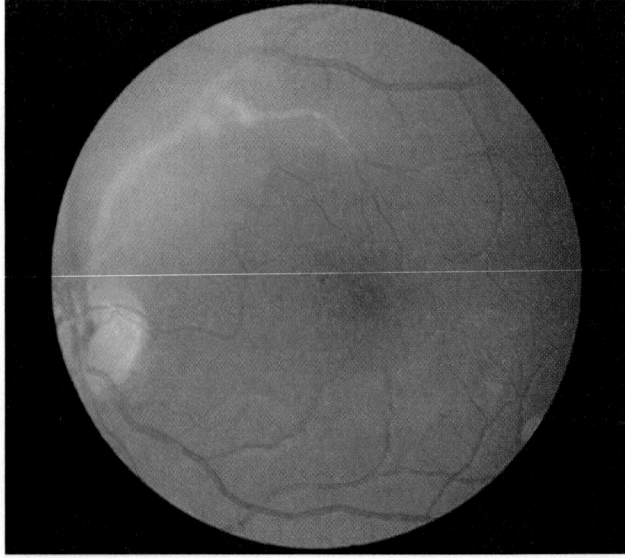

Fig. 61.11 Tuberous sclerosis. Large slightly raised translucent lesion with 'pseudosheathing' (Williams & Taylor 1985).

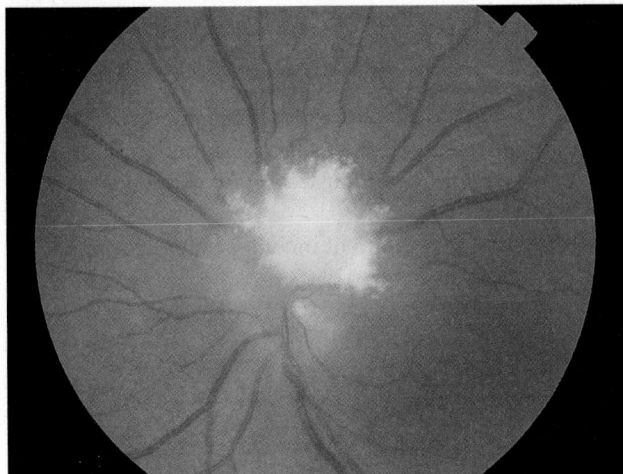

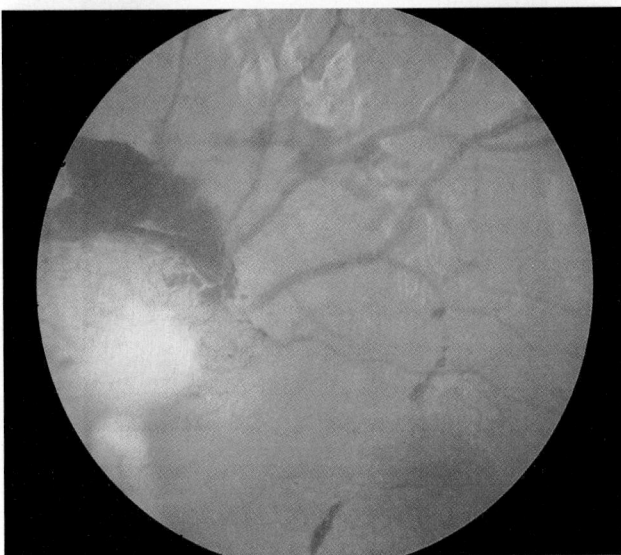

Fig. 61.12 (a) Tuberous sclerosis. Retinal hamartoma at the disc with normal vision. (b) Tuberous sclerosis. Same patient as (a) showing vitreous haemorrhage associated with the hamartoma.

coma before the age of 2 years, and 20% developing glaucoma after the age of 4. This may relate to the pathophysiology of the glaucoma, trabeculodysgenesis playing an important role in infantile onset glaucoma, and raised episcleral venous pressure being more important in late onset glaucoma (Sullivan *et al.* 1992).

Glaucoma associated with Sturge–Weber syndrome has always proved a therapeutic challenge and still remains one of the most difficult causes of raised intraocular pressure to control. Starting from the time of diagnosis, the intraocular pressure, the discs and the corneal diameter need to be measured intermittently, even if an occasional examination under anaesthetic is needed in the first years. The patients are at risk of developing glaucoma at any time in their life and so need long-term follow-up. Iwach *et al.* (1990) looked at the success of goniotomy, trabeculotomy, trabeculectomy, laser trabeculoplasty and medica-

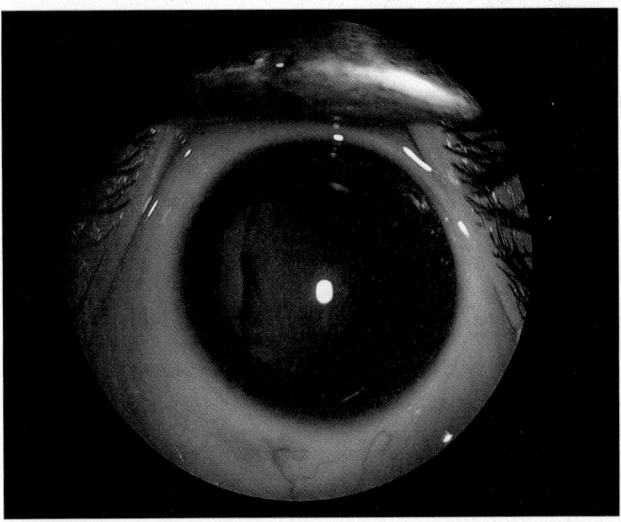

Fig. 61.13 Tuberous sclerosis. Lens pseudocoloboma.

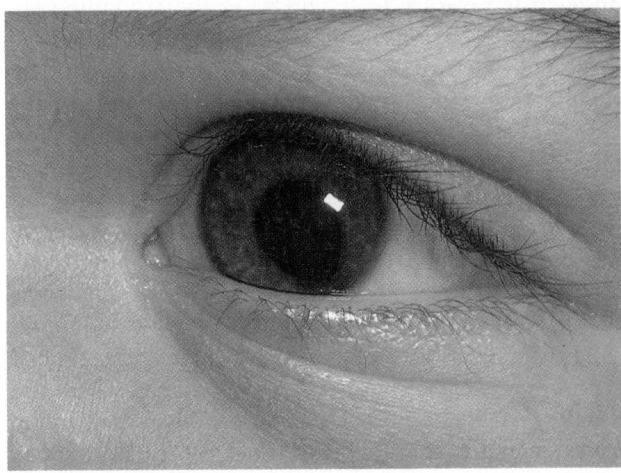

Fig. 61.14 Tuberous sclerosis. Iris pseudocoloboma.

patients. In addition, up to 60% of patients show some degree of mental retardation. Visceral involvement is less common than in other phakomatoses but tumours of the lung, gastrointestinal tract, pituitary, ovaries and pancreas have been reported.

The two primary ocular complications of this syndrome are glaucoma and choroidal haemangiomas. Glaucoma (see Chapter 40) occurs almost exclusively in those patients with ipsilateral eyelid and conjunctival involvement (Phelps 1978). One-third of patients with the Sturge–Weber syndrome develop glaucoma at some time, but of those with episcleral involvement, virtually all develop raised intraocular pressure (Sullivan *et al.* 1992). Infrequently this may be contralateral to the cutaneous lesions. There tends to be a bimodal age of onset of glaucoma in Sturge–Weber syndrome, 50% developing glau-

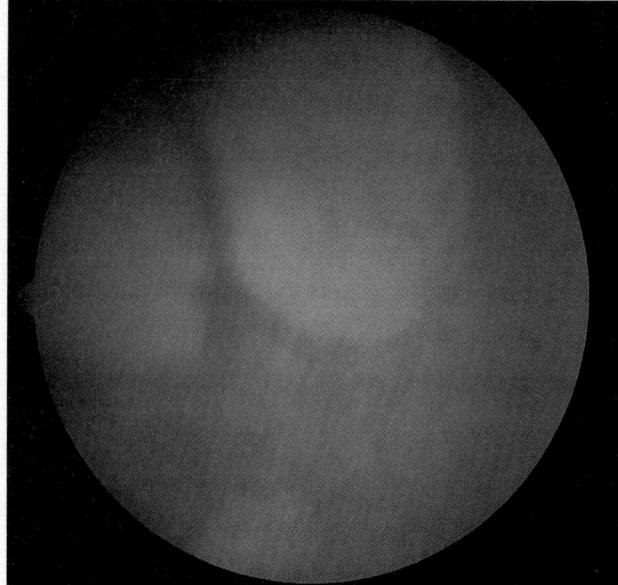

Fig. 61.15 Tuberous sclerosis. Peripheral fundus lesion showing depigmentation. In a girl with seizures the main differential diagnosis was with Aicardi's syndrome.

tion in the management of glaucoma in Sturge–Weber syndrome. They reported two groups of patients, early onset (<4 years) and late onset. The early onset group underwent goniotomy, but the median stable interval after one procedure was only 8 months. With multiple goniotomies and the addition of medical treatment, however, the median stable interval was increased to 9 years. The authors suggest that goniotomy is the primary treatment of choice in early onset glaucoma associated with Sturge–Weber syndrome. Sullivan *et al.* (1992) reported that 28 of their 36 patients with Sturge–Weber syndrome required surgical treatment of glaucoma, and 103 operations were performed. Only 47% of eyes had controlled intraocular pressure (<21 mmHg) at the last follow-up visit, and all but one required the addition of medical treatment. Cyclocryotherapy and cyclodiathermy in combination with surgical treatment may improve the outcome slightly (Wagner *et al.* 1988; Koraszewska-Matuszewska & Samochowiec-Donocik 1989) but glaucoma associated with Sturge–Weber syndrome remains difficult to control and is a significant cause of morbidity in this disorder. The prognosis in a newly diagnosed case of glaucoma associated with Sturge–Weber syndrome should be guarded.

Approximately 40% of patients with the Sturge–Weber syndrome develop choroidal haemangiomas. These are usually seen as flat choroidal lesions lacking pigmentation and showing poorly defined borders. In those cases in which the haemangioma is diffuse, a deep red colour (Fig. 61.19) may appear and has been described as the

'tomato ketchup' fundus (Susac *et al.* 1974). These haemangiomas grow slowly and may lead to degenerative changes of the overlying retina with serous retinal detachment. Ultimately neovascular glaucoma may ensue. Radiotherapy using lens-sparing techniques (Fig. 61.20) may have some role in their treatment (Plowman & Harnett 1988).

Other ocular involvement includes heterochromia with

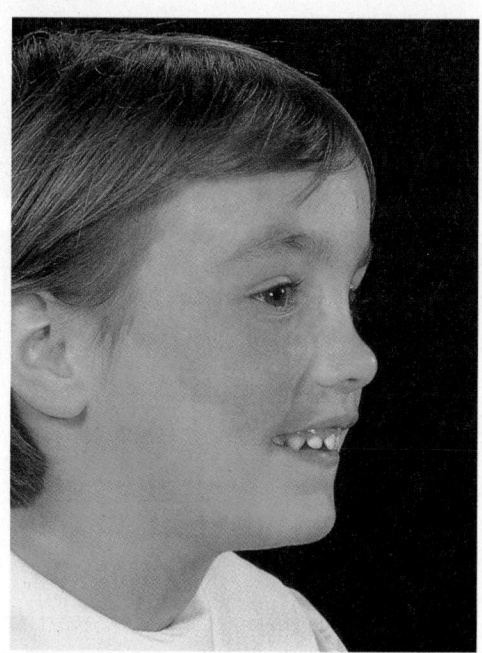

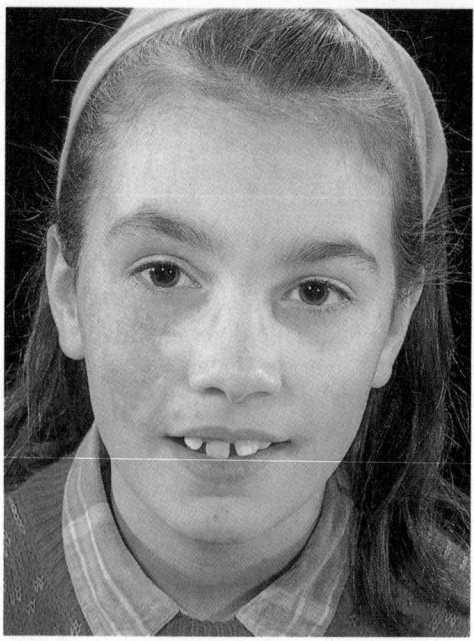

Fig. 61.16 Unilateral facial port-wine stain. In this case it was associated with an ipsilateral choroidal haemangioma (see Fig. 61.20). (a) As a small child the port-wine stain is deep red. (b) The same patient is in the early stages of having laser treatment for the port-wine stain.

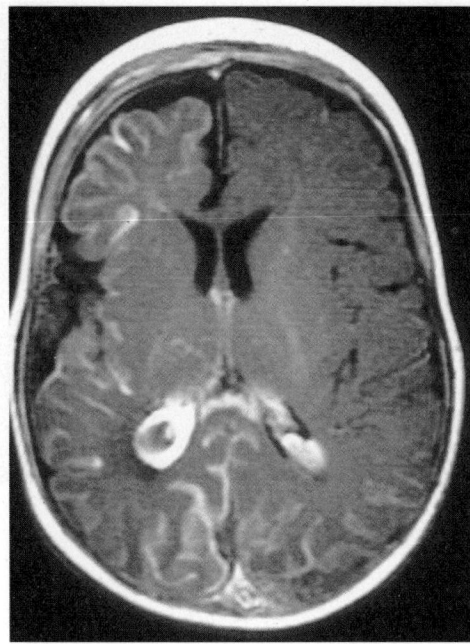

Fig. 61.17 Sturge–Weber syndrome showing hemicerebral atrophy and calcification.

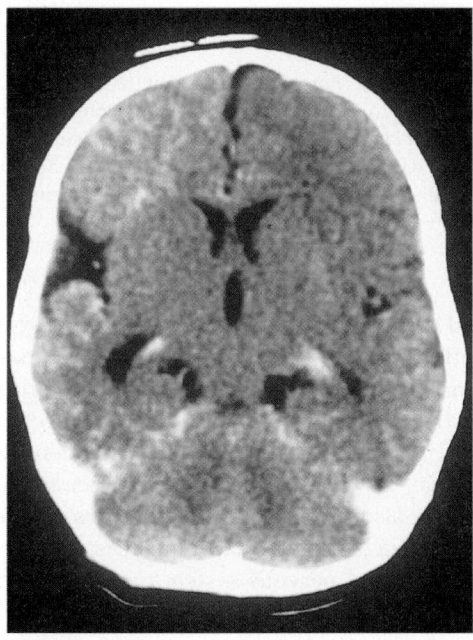

Fig. 61.18 Sturge–Weber syndrome showing diffuse hemicerebral calcification.

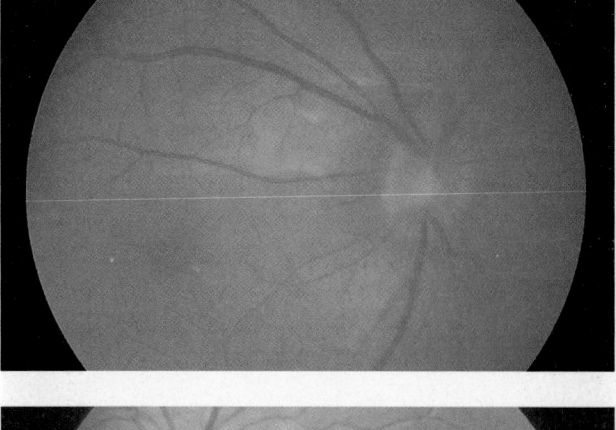

a

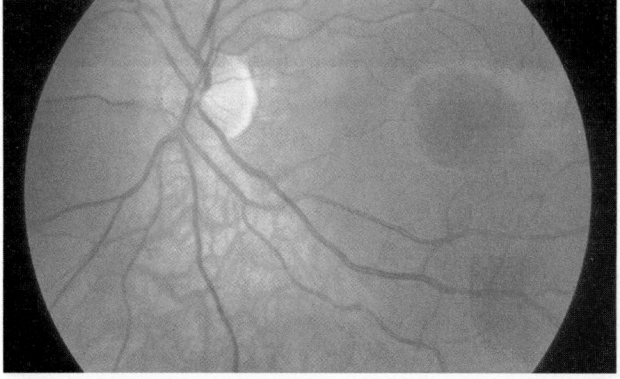

b

Fig. 61.19 (a) Sturge–Weber syndrome with a port-wine stain on the right side of the face: a diffuse choroidal haemangioma ('tomato ketchup fundus') showing the diffuse redness of the right posterior pole. (b) Sturge–Weber syndrome. Same patient showing a normal left fundus.

the darker iris being ipsilateral to the cutaneous lesions, as well as colobomas and ectopia lentis.

For illustrations see Chapter 40.

Von Hippel–Lindau syndrome

The major features of this disorder include retinal angiomatosis, cerebellar, medullary and spinal cord hae-mangioblastomas, renal cell carcinoma and phaeo-chromocytoma. The disorder may be inherited in an autosomal dominant fashion but most cases are sporadic. The gene has been identified on the short arm of chromo-some 3 (3p25–p26) and codes for a tumour suppressor protein (Latif *et al.* 1993). No racial or sexual predilections are known. The incidence of von Hippel–Lindau is about one in 36 000 live births (Maher *et al.* 1991b). Although patients may present at any age, most present in the sec-ond or third decade. Retinal angiomatosis is the most fre-quent complication in patients with von Hippel–Lindau and occurs earlier than other major manifestations, so the ophthalmologist plays a key role in diagnosis and man-agement of the condition. Clinical variability is common in von Hippel–Lindau and patients rarely manifest all fea-tures of the disorder.

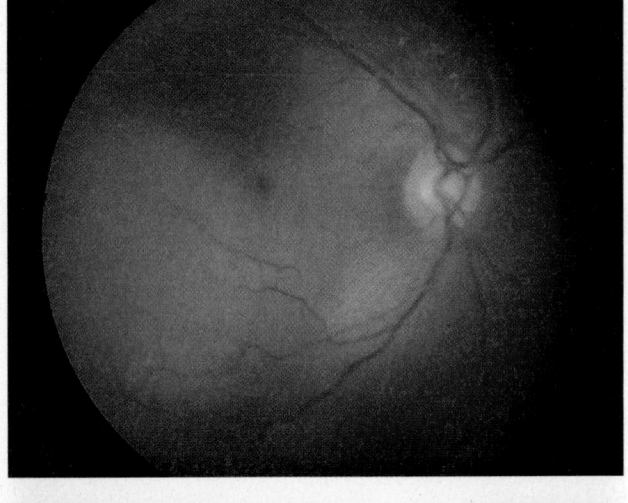

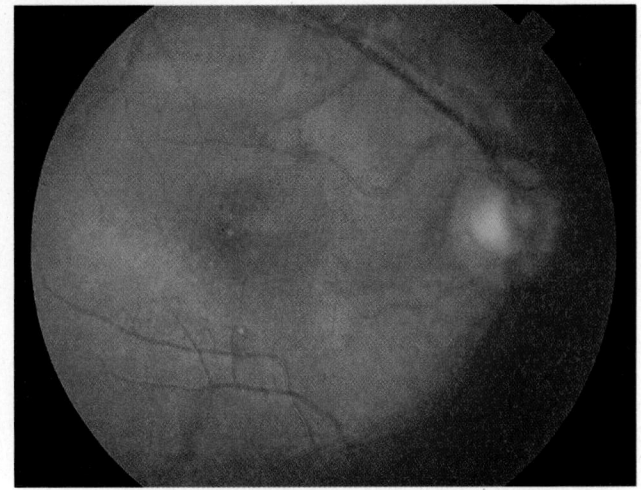

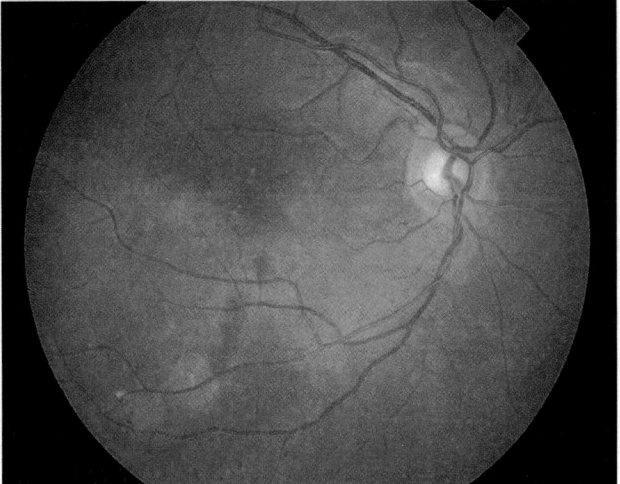

Fig. 61.20 (a) Discrete choroidal angioma abutting the macula giving an acuity reduced to 6/36. (b) Same patient following radiotherapy (see Plowman & Harnett 1988). There had been substantial visual improvement with the acuity at 6/9 after radiotherapy. (c) Same patient 10 years later, after prolonged occlusion treatment the acuity is still 6/9.

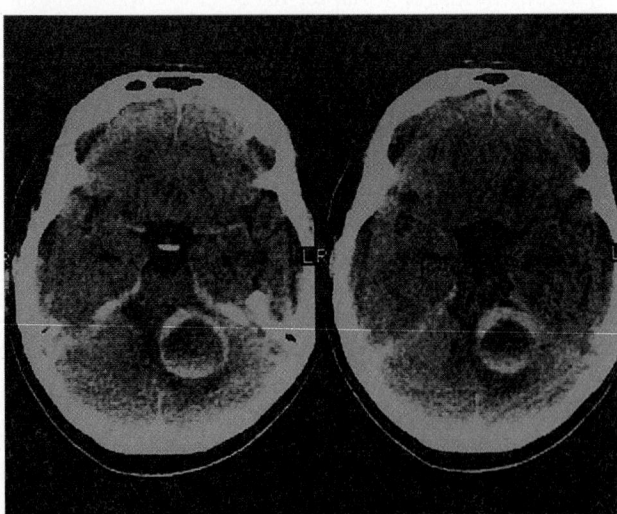

Fig. 61.21 Von Hippel–Lindau syndrome showing cerebellar haemangioblastoma.

Central nervous system involvement in this syndrome is seen primarily as cerebellar haemangioblastomas (Bech & Jensen 1961). These space-occupying posterior fossa tumours (Fig. 61.21) present with typical cerebellar signs or raised intracranial pressure. Less frequently, these tumours may involve the medulla or upper spinal cord. Patients may also present with classic signs of cerebellar dysfunction, including ataxia, clumsiness, and nystagmus. These central nervous system tumours are usually amenable to surgical treatment.

Other visceral manifestations occur not infrequently in this syndrome. Some of these are life-threatening and account for the premature death of these patients. These include angiomas of the kidney, pancreas, liver and spleen, as well as cystic involvement of bone, omentum, ovary and epididymis. The life-threatening lesions associated with this syndrome include hypernephromas, phaeochromocytomas, and cystadenomas of abdominal organs.

The typical ocular lesions of the von Hippel–Lindau syndrome are haemangioblastomas (Welch 1970). These

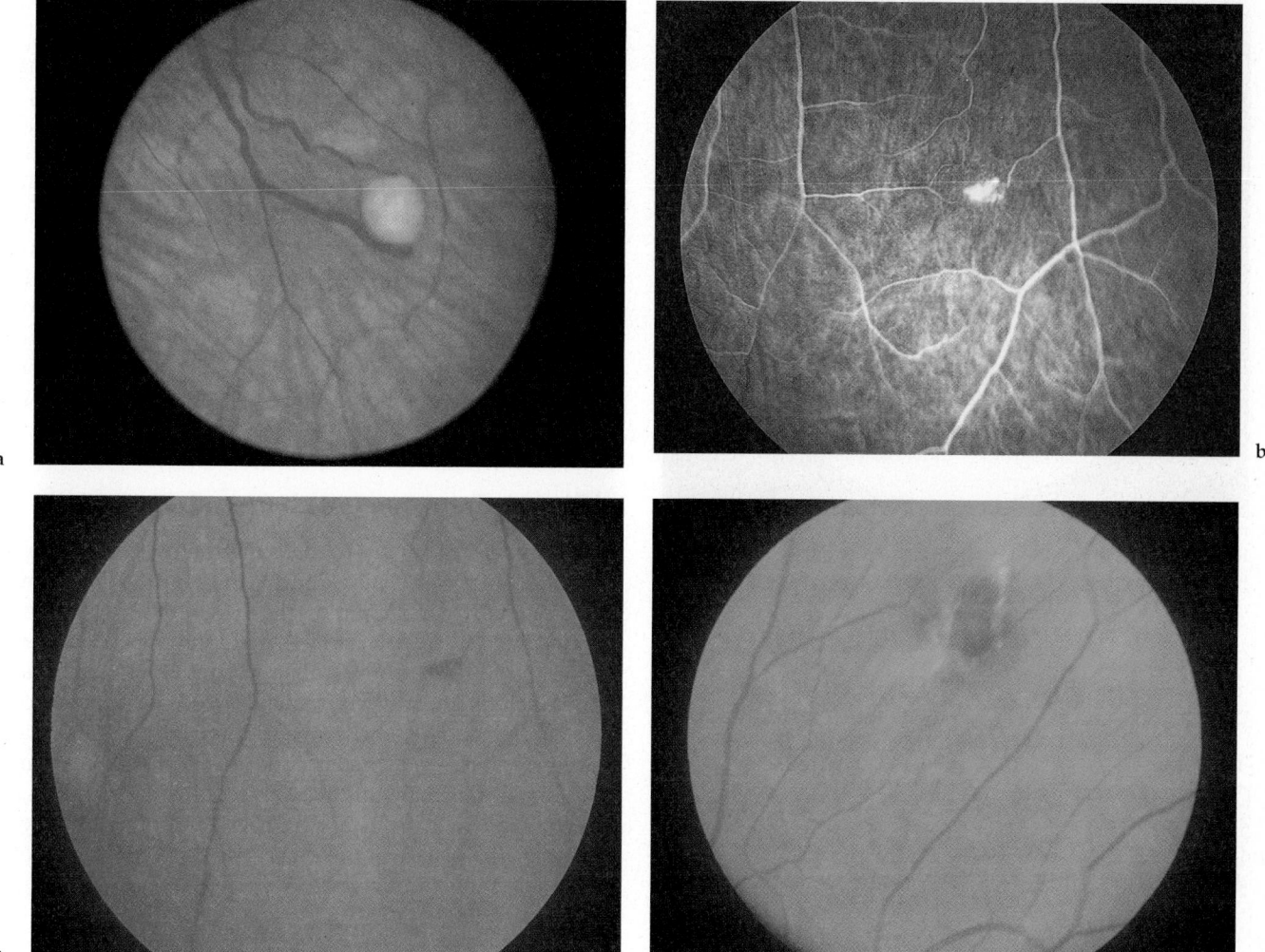

Fig. 61.22 (a) Von Hippel–Lindau syndrome. Haemangioblastoma with large feeding and draining vessel. (b, c) Patient of Mr Tony Moore showing a small, peripheral haemangioblastoma. (d) Patient of Mr Tony Moore showing a treated lesion.

tumours are composed of thin-walled capillaries and solid masses of endothelial cells often showing cystic degeneration (Jesberg *et al.* 1968). These tumours are often multiple with both eyes involved in more than 50% of cases. Patients rarely present with ocular complaints in the first two decades of life although retinal angiomas have been reported in infants and young children (Green *et al.* 1986). Retinal angiomas in von Hippel–Lindau are usually in the midperiphery (Fig. 61.22). Peripapillary angiomas (Fig. 61.23) are much less common and tend to be deep retinal tumours associated with exudation. The natural history of the retinal lesions has not been well determined, but five stages are described (Hardwig & Robertson 1984).

• Stage I, pre-classical: small capillary clusters, initially only the size of a diabetic microaneurysm, often difficult to see ophthalmoscopically but revealed on fluorescein angiography.

• Stage II, classical: typical retinal angiomas.

• Stage III, exudation: from leaking vessels of tumours usually larger than 1 disc diameter.

• Stage IV, retinal detachment: exudative or tractional.

• Stage V, end stage: retinal detachment, uveitis, glaucoma, phthisis.

The classical retinal angioma extends into the vitreous cavity, and is a nodule of capillaries with one feeding artery and vein. As the tumour enlarges, the vein becomes arterialized. Many tumours are progressive (although there are some reports of regression) and may grow as large as 3 disc diameters. Treatment of the early ocular lesions with cryotherapy and/or photocoagulation is frequently successful, especially in small lesions (Annesley *et al.* 1977). In the late stages of this disease these are largely unsuccessful (Annesley *et al.* 1977). When a patient is discovered to have a retinal angioma, all mem-

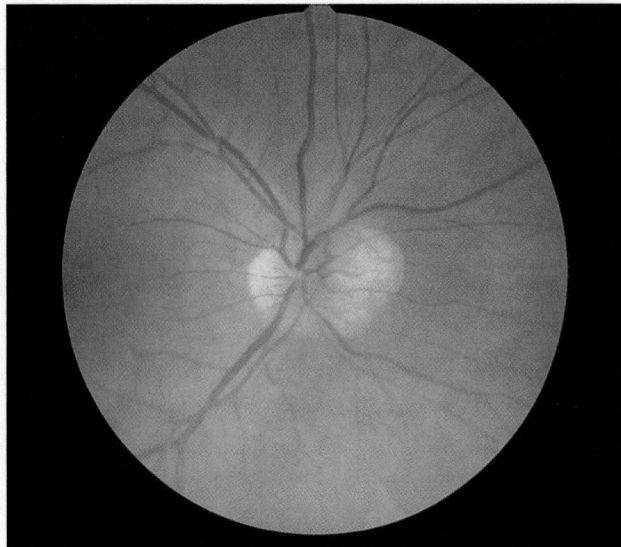

Fig. 61.23 Von Hippel–Lindau syndrome. Peripapillary haemangioma.

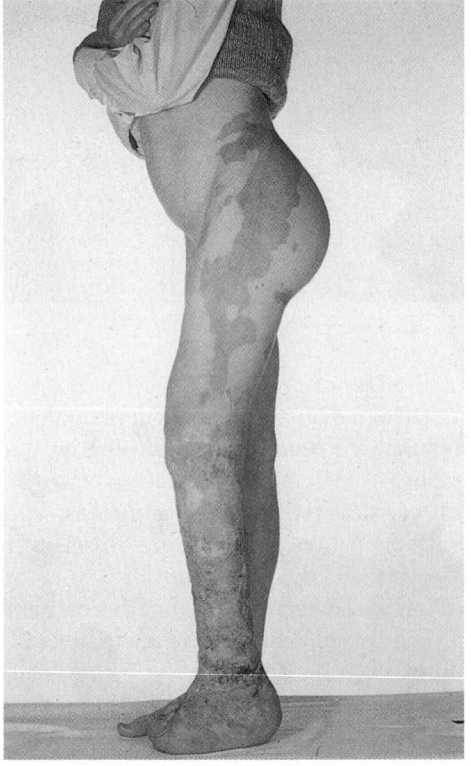

Fig. 61.24 Klippel–Trenaunay–Weber syndrome showing limb hypertrophy and vascular malformation.

bers of the family should be carefully studied for the presence of additional ocular lesions so that early treatment may be initiated if necessary (Welch 1970; Moore *et al.* 1991).

Screening

Patients with von Hippel–Lindau are at risk of developing multiple tumours and the cumulative risk of developing retinal angioma, cerebellar haemangioblastoma and renal cell carcinoma by the age of 60 is 84, 70 and 69%, respectively (Maher *et al.* 1990). Renal cell carcinoma is the most common cause of death. Thus all patients require at least annual follow-up. Screening of relatives at risk of developing von Hippel–Lindau is also worthwhile. Moore *et al.* (1991) detected subclinical disease in 30% of asymptomatic at-risk relatives and they suggest annual screening for these relatives. Now the gene has been isolated, presymptomatic diagnosis of gene carriers is possible.

Klippel–Trenaunay–Weber syndrome

The Klippel–Trenaunay–Weber syndrome has been recognized as a separate clinical entity (Troost *et al.* 1975). It consists of a port-wine lesion on the extremities, varicosities on the affected side (Fig. 61.24), and local hypertrophy of bone and soft tissue on the affected part. Ophthalmic features include orbital varix, retinal varicosities, angioma of the choroid and heterochromia iridium. It is said by some authorities that glaucoma occurs much less commonly in this syndrome; many of the cases reported have features in common with the Sturge–Weber syndrome. Enlargement of the ipsilateral optic nerve and other features of regional giantism have been reported in this syndrome (Good *et al.* 1989).

References

Alper JC, Holmes LB. The incidence and significance of birthmarks in a cohort of 4641 newborns. *Pediatr Dermatol* 1983; **1**: 58–68.

Annesley WH, Leonard BC, Shields JA, Tasman WS. Fifteen year review of treated cases of retinal angiomatosis. *Ophthalmology* 1977; **83**: 446–51.

Atkinson A, Sanders MS, Wong V. Vitreous hemorrhage in tuberous sclerosis. *Br J Ophthalmol* 1973; **57**: 773–9.

Bech J, Jenson OA. On the frequency of coexisting racemose hemangioma of the retina and brain. *Acta Psychiatr Scand* 1961; **36**: 47–50.

Couly GF, Dourain NML. Mapping of the early primordium in quail-chick chimeras II. The prosencephalic neural plate and neural folds: implications for the genesis of cephalic human congenital abnormalities. *Dev Biol* 1987; **120**: 198–214.

Font RL, Ferry AP. The phakomatoses. *Int Ophthalmol Clin* 1972; **36**: 47–50.

Fryer AE, Chalmers AH, Connor JM *et al*. Evidence that the gene for tuberous sclerosis is on chromosome 9. *Lancet* 1987; **i**: 659–60.

Gomez MR, ed. *Tuberous Sclerosis*. New York: Raven Press, 1979.

Good WV, Hoyt CS. Optic nerve shadow enlargement in the Klippel–Trenaunay–Weber syndrome. *J Pediatr Ophthalmol Strabismus* 1989; **26**: 288–9.

Green A, Smith M, Yates J. Loss of heterozygosity on chromosome 16p 13.3 in hamartomas from tuberous sclerosis patients. *Nature Genet* 1994; **6**: 193–6.

Green IS, Bowmer MI, Johnson GI. Von Hippel–Lindau disease in a Newfoundland kindred. *Canad Med Assoc J* 1986; **1**: 134–46.

Hardwig P, Robertson DM. von Hippel–Lindau disease: a familial, often lethal, multisystem phakomatosis. *Ophthalmology* 1984; **91**: 263–9.

Iwach AG, Hoskins HD, Hetherington J, Shaffer RN. Analysis of surgical and medical management of glaucoma in Sturge–Weber syndrome. *Ophthalmology* 1990; **97**: 904–9.

Jesberg DO, Spencer WH, Hoyt WF. Incipient lesion of von Hippel–Lindau disease. *Arch Ophthlamol* 1968; **80**: 632–6.

Koraszewska-Matuszewska B, Samochowiec-Donocik E. Treatment of glaucoma in children in congenital pathologic syndromes. *Klin Oczna* 1989; **91**: 141–3.

Lagos JC, Gomez NR. Tuberous sclerosis: reappraisal of a clinical entity. *Mayo Clin Proc* 1969; **42**: 26–49.

Latif F, Tory K, Gnarra J *et al*. Identification of the von Hippel–Lindau disease tumour suppressor gene. *Science* 1993; **260**: 1317–20.

MacDonald P, Miller NR. Chiasmatic and hypopthalmic extension of nerve glioma. *Arch Ophthalmol* 1968; **101**: 1412–14.

Maher ER, Bentley E, Yates TRW. Localization of the gene for von Hippel–Lindau disease to a small region of chromosome 3 confirmed by genetic linkage analysis. *Genomics* 1991a; **10**: 957–60.

Maher ER, Iselius L, Yates JRW *et al*. von Hippel–Lindau disease: a genetic study. *J Med Genet* 1991b; **28**: 443–7.

Maher ER, Yates JR, Harries R *et al*. Clinical features and natural history of von Hippel–Lindau disease. *Q J Med* 1990; **77**: 1151–63.

Mellman K, Rosen SW. Lindau's disease: review of the literature and a study of a large kindred. *Am J Med* 1964; **36**: 595–8.

Moore AT, Maher ER, Rosen P, Gregor Z, Bird AC. Ophthalmological screening for von Hippel–Lindau disease. *Eye* 1991; **5**: 723–8.

Nichol WR, Reed WB. Tuberous sclerosis: special reference to the microscopic alterations in cutaneous hamartomas. *Arch Dermatol* 1962; **85**: 209–13.

Phelps CD. The pathogenesis of glaucoma in Sturge–Weber syndrome. *Ophthalmology* 1978; **85**: 256–81.

Plowman PN, Harnett AN. Radiotherapy in benign orbital disease 1. Complicated ocular angiomas. *Br J Ophthalmol* 1988; **72**: 286–8.

Robertson DM. Ophthalmological findings. In: Gomez MR, ed. *Tuberous Sclerosis*. New York: Raven Press, 1988: 89–109.

Sampson JR, Scahill SJ, Stephenson JBF, Mann L, Connor JM. Genetic aspects of tuberous sclerosis in the west of Scotland. *J Med Genet* 1989; **26**: 28–31.

Shepherd CW, Gomez MR, Lie JT, Crowson CS. Causes of death in patients with tuberous sclerosis. *Mayo Clin Proc* 1991; **66**: 792–6.

Smith M, Smalley S, Cantor R, Pandolfo M, Gomez M, Baumann R. Mapping of a gene determining tuberous sclerosis to human chromosome 11q14–11q23. *Genomics* 1990; **6**: 105–14.

Sullivan TJ, Clarke MP, Morin JD. The ocular manifestations of the Sturge–Weber syndrome. *J Pediatr Ophthalmol Strabismus* 1992; **29**: 349–56.

Susac JO, Smith JL, Scello PJ. The tomato ketchup fundus in Sturge–Weber syndrome. *Arch Ophthalmol* 1974; **92**: 69–70.

Troost BT, Savino PJ, Lozito JC. Tuberous sclerosis and the Klippel–Trenaunay–Weber syndrome. *J Neurol Neurosurg Psych* 1975; **38**: 500–3.

Van dorp DB, Kwee ML. Tuberous sclerosis: diagnostic problems in a family. *Ophthalmic Paediatr Genet* 1990; **11**: 95–101.

Wagner RS, Caputo AR, Del Negro RG, Niegel J. Trabeculectomy with cryotherapy for infantile glaucoma in the Sturge–Weber syndrome. *Ann Ophthalmol* 1988; **20**: 289–91

Webb DW, Osborne JP. New research in tuberous sclerosis. *Br Med J* 1992; **304**: 1647–8.

Webb DW, Osborne JP. Tuberous sclerosis. *Arch Dis Child* 1995; **72**: 471–4.

Welch RB. von Hippel–Lindau disease. *Trans Am Ophthalmol Soc* 1970; **68**: 367–71.

Williams R, Taylor D. Tuberous sclerosis. *Surv Ophthlamol* 1985; **30**: 143–54.

Zimmer-Galler IE, Robertson DM. Long-term observation of retinal lesions in tuberous sclerosis. *Am J Ophthalmol* 1995; **119**: 318–24.

62: Accidental and Non-Accidental Trauma

William V. Good

Epidemiology of childhood eye trauma

The number of serious eye injuries in children has been estimated at 11.8 per 100 000 per year (Morris *et al.* 1993). At least 35% of serious eye injuries occur in children, and the majority of these eye injuries occur in children under the age of 12 (LaRoche *et al.* 1988; Rapoport *et al.* 1990). These epidemiological data hold constant in many coun-tries, including Israel (Rapoport *et al.* 1990), Ireland (Cana-van *et al.* 1980), Malawi (Ilsar *et al.* 1982) and Brazil (Mor-eira *et al.* 1988). Eye trauma is the most common cause of unilateral blindness in children (National Society for the Prevention of Blindness 1980; Alfaro *et al.* 1994). Despite the significance and scope of eye trauma in children, the amount of research and effort at prevention and treatment has been less than in other areas of ophthalmic research activity.

Aside from the obvious ramifications of vision loss, sig-nificant problems also arise as a consequence of cosmetic problems associated with the disfigurement that often accompanies a serious eye injury. It is difficult to place an objective value or significance on this factor, but studies on the psychosocial consequences of strabismus would suggest that these could be very severe (Satterfield *et al.* 1993).

Several factors can place a child at particular risk for a serious accidental eye injury (Scharf & Zonis 1975; Niiranen & Raivio 1981; Moreira *et al.* 1988; Rapoport *et al.* 1990). The first risk factor is youth: children aged between 0 and 5 years of age are probably at greater risk for serious eye injury than children between the ages of 5 and 18. Second, boys are affected far more frequently than girls, particularly in the age group older than 6 years. Third, a lack of parental supervision is a definite and obvious risk factor for serious eye injury. Younger children are more often injured by a fall or being struck with a sharp projectile. Eye injuries in older children are more likely to be related to a sporting event (e.g. ice hockey or baseball).

The prognosis for recovery of vision after accidental eye trauma is also affected by psychosocial factors. Baxter *et al.* (1994) showed that non-compliance with optical cor-rection and patching was an important factor after child-hood perforating anterior eye injury. These authors emphasized the importance of parental education. In some cases, the use of social services, home nurses and other ancillary personnel may be helpful in improving the visual prognosis. Amblyopia may limit recovery of vi-sion in children under 7 years of age, even in serious eye injuries that would carry a good prognosis in older individuals.

Non-accidental trauma (child abuse)

Epidemiology

Child abuse is defined as endangerment of a child at the hands of a parent or guardian. Endangerment may be physical abuse, sexual abuse or neglect or other forms of maltreatment. Child abuse results in at least 1100 known deaths annually in the USA, and 15% of children who are abused will have permanent physical abnormality as a result (Sedlak 1987). Virtually all abused children have permanent emotional problems.

It is remarkable that laws to protect animals came before description, definition and legal mechanisms for dealing with child abuse in North America and elsewhere. Not until 1946 was child abuse first described in the medical literature. Caffey (1946, 1972) noted that a history of deliberate trauma could be elicited in children who had a combination of subdural haematomas and fractures of the long bones. Henry Kempe *et al.* (1962), at the University of Colorado, are generally credited with having brought the problem of child abuse to national recognition in the USA in 1962. Even so, there was a tendency to discount stories of abuse by children as 'imaginative'. There also was fear among health workers about legal problems if they accused parents of abuse.

Most abused children are under the age of 3 years (Marcus & Albert 1992). Shaking injuries to children will occur in babies but usually not in older children. Very young babies are far more likely to suffer a blow to the head, while older children will show a pattern of recurrent and habitual abuse which may result in various injuries in different stages of healing (Kempe *et al.* 1962). About 40% of abused children have some ophthalmic problem as a result of the abuse (Friendly 1971). Three to four per cent of children who present to an ophthalmology emergency room in the UK have been mistreated (Olver & Hague 1989) and the ophthalmologist is often the doctor who could be responsible for first recognizing the abuse (Marcus & Albert 1992).

Virtually any of the ocular traumatic conditions discussed in this chapter can occur as a result of child abuse, so it must be emphasized that any unexplained periocular or ocular trauma requires investigation for possible abuse. This is particularly the case when the injury cannot be explained by the parent's history, or the history is inconsistent amongst the child's caregivers. The diagnosis of abuse is evident when a parent or guardian admits to it, but often the health-care provider must search for clues. These clues may be categorized as psychological or physical.

The psychological clues that a child has been abused are listed in Table 62.1. The parents' history may show the potential for child abuse if a parent was abused or neglected as a child, or has a history of mental illness, spouse

Table 62.1 Psychological profile of an abusing parent.

History of having been abused
Serious mental illness
Spouse abuse perpetrator or victim
Drug abuse
Criminal record
Young age (< 17 years old)
Single
Socially isolated
Other impulsive behaviours

abuse, drug abuse, a criminal record, or a history of previously abusing other children (Aycub & Pfeifer 1977; Gray *et al.* 1979; Soumenkoff *et al.* 1981). Abusive caregivers also tend to be young (< 17 years of age), and single, to lack financial resources, and to live in chaotic environments. The abuser may be socially isolated (e.g. no telephone, friends, contact with relatives), impulsive and overly identified with the child (Aycub & Pfeifer 1977; Gray *et al.* 1977; Soumenkoff *et al.* 1981). This latter point of identification is an important element to child abuse, as abusive parents will often have unrealistic, lofty goals for their small children. The child's failure to meet these goals translates into parental disappointment. If the parent himself was abused as a child, he may consider that his own child should be treated in the same manner.

In the last 30 years the child abuse syndrome has been further characterized and it now is clear that it may take several physical forms. The first of these is intraocular or periocular trauma, which occurs in approximately 40% of abused children (Friendly 1971). Retinal haemorrhages are the most common ocular injury in non-accidental trauma (Kiffney 1964) and are found in a surprisingly large percentage of children with eye injury, anywhere from 65 to 89% (Aron *et al.* 1970; Billmire & Myers 1985). The relationship of retinal haemorrhage to child abuse is an important one.

Retinal haemorrhages

Accidental trauma is not usually a cause of retinal haemorrhages (Elder *et al.* 1991; Buys *et al.* 1992) and the finding of retinal haemorrhages must raise suspicions of non-accidental injury.

One of two mechanisms may be involved in causing retinal haemorrhages in the setting of child abuse (Kaur & Taylor 1992). The first of these is a rise in intraocular venous pressure, which can be caused either by a rise in intracranial pressure or by an increase in the central venous pressure.

A rapid increase in intracranial pressure will often cause optic nerve sheath haemorrhage. As Kaur and Taylor noted (1992), these haemorrhages may occur as a result of the extension of haemorrhage in the subarachnoid space into a comparable space in the optic nerve sheath (Lambert *et al.* 1986).

Alternatively, vessels within the subarachnoid space of the optic nerve sheath could also be ruptured. No matter which of these two mechanisms is invoked, the result is that pressure is placed on the central retinal vein, and intraocular venous pressure may increase (Muller & Deck 1974). Intraocular haemorrhages do not always occur in the setting of optic nerve sheath haemorrhage (Muller & Deck 1974). When children cry (as when injured and in pain), they force air out of their lungs against resistance. This has the effect of increasing venous pressure via the valsalva manoeuvre, and can also increase central venous pressure. The result can be intraretinal haemorrhages, or even massive haemorrhages, as occurs with Purtscher's retinopathy (discussed below) (Tomasi & Rosman 1975).

An alternative, but not necessarily exclusive, mechanism for an aetiology for retinal haemorrhage is one which invokes shaking and its resultant acceleration and deceleration of the child's head (Lyle *et al.* 1957). The baby's head may be particularly vulnerable to shaking injuries because it is relatively larger than the body, compared to adults, and because head control is not as good in infancy and early childhood (Caffey 1972). Shaking will often cause brain injury as well. And the haemorrhages with shaking injury are particularly severe, often extending out into the vitreous (Fig. 62.1) (Mushin & Morgan 1971).

Clinical characteristics of retinal haemorrhage include intraretinal haemorrhage in mild cases of abuse, and haemorrhages in all of the retinal layers and in the vitreous in more severe cases (Fig. 62.2). As noted above, shaking is particularly likely to cause these severe retinal

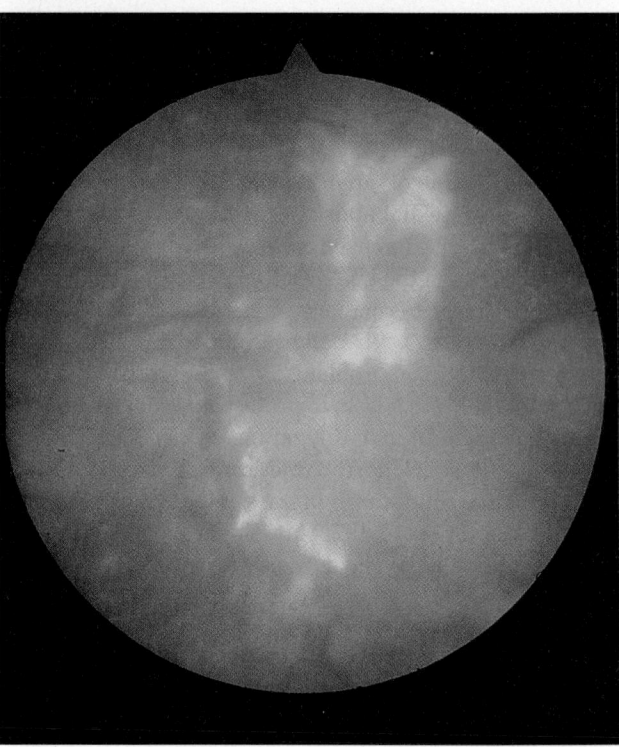

Fig. 62.2 Retinal and vitreous haemorrhages in non-accidental injury. The white areas represent partially organized haemorrhage and the greenish background is caused by altered blood products.

haemorrhages. The haemorrhages do not resolve rapidly (as they do when the aetiology is parturition) and they are known to last even for many months (Jensen *et al.* 1971). Shaking may cause retinal cysts filled with blood. As the blood is absorbed, retinoschisis may develop (Elder *et al.* 1991) and result in a particularly poor visual prognosis (Greenwald *et al.* 1986). Retinal folds (Fig. 62.3), which actually are concentric and outside the vascular arcade which surrounds the macula, may also develop as a result of shaking and vitreous traction (Gaynon *et al.* 1988; Massicotte *et al.* 1991). Perimacular folds cannot be taken as pathognomonic of non-accidental injury as they have been described in Terson's syndrome (Keithahn *et al.* 1993).

The prognosis for retinal haemorrhage in the setting of non-accidental trauma depends on the severity of the haemorrhage and associated neurological damage. When optic atrophy occurs from intra-sheath haemorrhage or other mechanisms, the prognosis is also poor. Retinal haemorrhage in the process of resolving may cause pigment migration into the macula, and this can also impair vision.

Pathological studies show haemorrhages predominantly in the bipolar and nerve fibre layers (Riffenburgh & Sathyavagiswarand 1991). The presence of haemosiderin may be helpful in dating haemorrhages and in particular

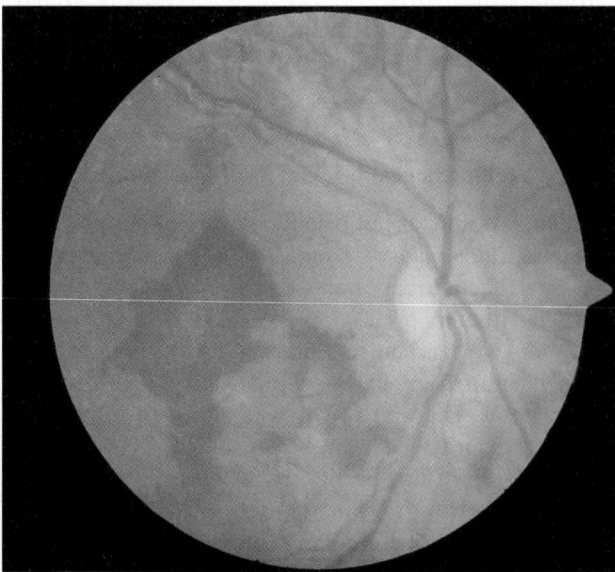

Fig. 62.1 Intraretinal and subhyaloid haemorrhages in non-accidental injury.

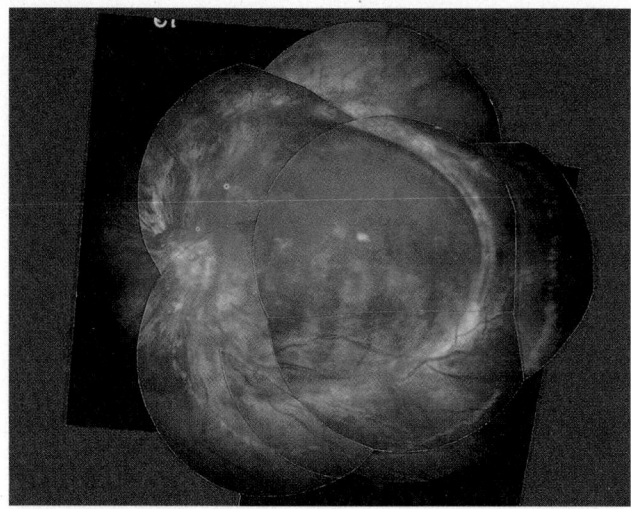

Fig. 62.3 Perimacular folds. The raised nature of the fold can be seen by the shadow created by the fold above. Perimacular folds are suggestive, but cannot be said to be pathognomonic, of non-accidental injury (Yih and Taylor 1996).

in documenting different ages of haemorrhages (Elner *et al.* 1990). The presence of haemosiderin alone does not indicate non-accidental injury (Gilliland *et al.* 1991).

The differential diagnosis of retinal haemorrhages in non-accidental trauma often includes haemorrhages caused by cardiopulmonary resuscitation (CPR). This is particularly the case when a child has rib fractures as a result of presumed resuscitative effort. Spevak *et al.* (1994) studied the question of rib fractures in infants who had been resuscitated and found that none showed rib fractures. Rib fractures would appear to be highly specific for non-accidental trauma.

Conversely, retinal haemorrhages may be the result of chest compression, either on the basis of resuscitative effort or non-accidental trauma (Kirschner & Stein 1985; Goetting & Sowa 1990). Retinal haemorrhages therefore can occur on the basis of CPR. The other items in the differential diagnosis for retinal haemorrhages in children are listed under that topic below.

Central nervous system injury

Ophthalmologists are often called upon to evaluate retinal haemorrhages in the setting of brain injury. Typically, a young child is admitted to the intensive care unit comatose, and non-accidental trauma is suspected. Fifty-one per cent of babies who have intracranial haemorrhages also show retinal haemorrhages (Hollenhorst & Stein 1958). Optic nerve sheath haemorrhages may occur with or without retinal haemorrhages. Retinal haemorrhages occur in 27% of cases of optic nerve sheath haemorrhages (Muller & Deck 1974). The clinician should remember that the absence of retinal haemorrhages does not exclude the possibility of child abuse. Overall, perhaps 80% of babies with interhemispheric haemorrhage caused by non-accidental injury will show retinal haemorrhage (Zimmerman *et al.* 1979). The severity of the retinal haemorrhages may predict the severity of the neurological injury (Wilkinson *et al.* 1989).

The type of central nervous system injury in abuse may take several forms. Generalized brain contusion can occur (Fig. 62.4), as can bilateral subdural haematomas (Newton 1989) (Fig. 62.5). Posterior interhemispheric subdural haematoma is particularly characteristic of a shaking injury, and non-accidental trauma.

Systemic manifestations of child abuse

Child abuse also results in injuries to the child's body at various stages of healing, implying a chronicity to the abuse. When a child is seen with a hand print bruise, human bite marks or cigarette burns, child abuse is usually the cause. Some children have their hair pulled by parents or guardians, and this can cause subgaleal haematomas. Genital injuries are also part of the child abuse syndrome. Additional features include tears in the floor of the mouth and to the frenulum, abdominal injuries, and dehydration or anxiety, which may occur as a consequence of chronic neglect or abuse. An inflammatory orbital tumour occurred in a child who was subsequently shown to have been injured by a parent (Waterhouse *et al.* 1992). Some babies are shaken, and this may cause intracranial and intraocular bleeding without showing any actual external signs of bone fracture, head trauma or bruising (Caffey 1946, 1972).

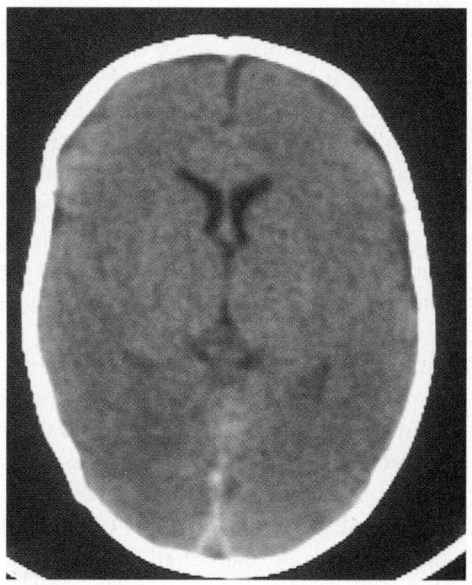

Fig. 62.4 Para-falcine oedema shown on this CT scan.

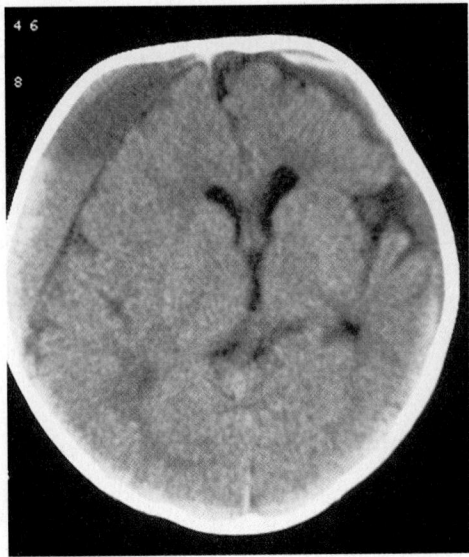

Fig. 62.5 Bilateral subdural haemorrhages in child abuse.

Investigations

X-rays

A full skeletal survey is indicated in all infants under 1 year of age suspected of being injured by any means. Between the ages of 1 and 3 years, a skeletal survey is probably indicated only if there is suspicion of physical abuse, and in the older child a skeletal survey must be performed selectively (Merton *et al.* 1983). Fractures are most commonly present in the under 3 age group (particularly under the age of 1), in boys, and involving extremities, skull and ribs. Bony injuries which characteristically are produced by abuse include epiphyseal-diaphyseal fractures, both spiral and transverse, metaphyseal injuries resulting from shaking or jerking, posterior rib fractures from blunt injuries, occult (often in infants) or occult multiple, or multiple fractures at various stages of healing (Merton *et al.* 1983). Ninety per cent of skull fractures in non-accidental injuries occur in children under the age of 2 and intent to injure is suggested by one or more of the following features: (i) multiple or complex fractures; (ii) depressed fracture; (iii) a fracture with a maximum width of greater than 3 mm; (iv) a growing fracture; (v) involvement of more than one cranial bone; or (vi) non-parietal fracture, or all fractures associated with intracranial injury (Hobbs 1984). Linear fractures of the calvarium are best seen on plain X-ray of the skull. Fractures of the skull-base or depressed fractures are visualized best by computed tomographic (CT) scan (Hershey & Zimmerman 1985).

CT or MRI scanning

In addition to showing skull-base or depressed fractures, CT or magnetic resonance imaging (MRI) may reveal evidence of cerebral swelling and/or intracranial haemorrhage. Cerebral swelling occurs acutely due both to increased cerebral blood flow and oedema, and shows with evidence of absence or compression of the ventricles and increased density in brain substance. Vasogenic oedema may be focal or multifocal and is seen in haemorrhagic contusion and intracerebral haematoma and extends along axon pathways into white matter. It may be evident for as long as 2 months after injury.

Brain contusion may result directly from the injury or from contre coup, and shows as a non-homogeneous area of high density (haemorrhage) and low density (necrosis) areas.

Intracranial bleeding may be of several kinds. Intracerebral haemorrhage occurs at the site of contusion or from blood vessels torn by shearing forces. Often this kind of bleeding occurs at juncture points between cortex and white matter and shows as little areas of focal haemorrhage.

Extracerebral haemorrhage may be epidural, when it can be associated with skull fracture, e.g. in the temporoparietal regions when the bleeding does not then cross skull suture lines. Alternatively, the bleeding may be subdural, which often is associated with underlying brain damage. Bilateral subdurals strongly suggest whiplash injury leading to shearing of bridging veins at fixed sites of attachment to the walls of the sagittal sutures. Shaking may lead to parieto-occipital interhemispheric subdural haematoma. Infants under the age of 6 months with subdurals often present with coma, but in the older age group the signs are less specific, such as lethargy, vomiting, crying, and so on. Concomitant subdural hygroma and atrophy may be indicative of earlier traumatic episodes.

Subarachnoid haemorrhage often occurs in association with other kinds of bleeding mentioned above and shows as an increased density in the region of the falx. Communicating hydrocephalus may be a sequel to this.

Bleeding and clotting studies

The types of bruising and the manner in which they are said to occur may be very similar in non-accidental injury and bleeding disorders (Schwer *et al.* 1982). The tests which must be done to exclude a bleeding disorder (O'Hare & Eden 1984) are: (i) full blood count and film; (ii) platelet count size and shape; (iii) partial thromboplastin time; (iv) prothrombin time; (v) thrombin time; and (vi) fibrinogen and bleeding time. It is, of course, possible that a bleeding diathesis and non-accidental injury may co-exist.

Drug history

It is important to enquire about salicylate and other drug ingestion both around the time that bruises are thought to have occurred and when bleeding and clotting studies are being performed, since they may affect test results. It is also important to be aware of circulating antibodies after minor viral infections in children (O'Hare & Eden 1984).

Radionuclide bone scanning

This may be a useful addition to plain radiography and increase the detection rate of hairline fractures. It should, perhaps, be reserved for occasions where plain X-rays are negative and there is a strong suspicion of non-accidental injury. It should be noted that bone scans and plain X-rays may give false-negative results.

Differential diagnosis

Osteogenesis imperfecta

This condition has to be actively considered in any child suspected of non-accidental injury, since very mild forms may present with fractures in the toddler age group up to adolescence. The clinical features include blue sclera, large fontanelle, excess joint laxity, small stature and poor dentition. The distinguishing radiological features of osteogenesis imperfecta that help to distinguish fractures caused in the condition from non-accidental injuries include the following: the fractures are mainly in the diaphyses of long bones and are rare in the metaphyses. Wormian bones are usually present, and generally there are radiological signs of osteoporosis (Carty 1988).

Copper deficiency

Copper deficiency most commonly has to be considered in the under 2 age group. The clinical features include a predisposing cause (low birth weight, dietary deficiency, malnutrition) and anaemia, neutropenia, pallor, hypotonia, hyperpigmentation, prominent scalp veins, and finally, plasma copper concentrations, usually below 40 mg/dl and caeruloplasmin less than 13 mg/dl. The radiological features include osteoporosis, fraying and cupping of the metaphyses, spur formation, periosteal reactions and fractures. These findings are in contrast to the non-accidentally injured child where the bone texture is normal and there is no cupping or fraying of the metaphysis where a fracture has occurred (Shaw 1988).

Scurvy

In this condition, too, spur formation and corner fractures may occur, but there is no fraying of the metaphyses to distinguish this from copper deficiency and the epiphyses have distinctive etched appearances to distinguish them from both copper deficiency and the bones of the non-accidentally injured child (Carty 1988).

Accidental trauma and natural disease processes

Often, the most difficult aspect of management in suspected child abuse is to be absolutely sure that the cause is not due to a natural disease process or accidental trauma. Since there is no absolutely pathognomonic sign, the diagnosis rests on careful clinical history and examination. The dangers of relying on suspicious circumstances, or unusual emotional reactions of the parents, is that these are so variable that they are only useful as secondary information. Weissgold *et al.* (1995) published details of such a case, in which the parents of a child with a sudden cerebral haemorrhage (without retinal haemorrhages) were unusually stoic about their baby's fatal illness, to the extent that they went on a vacation cruise immediately after the funeral: autopsy revealed a subarachnoid vascular malformation.

Management

Although details of management of suspected non-accidental injury will vary in different parts of the world according to specific legal requirements, there are a number of guiding principles of universal application. These include the following.

1 That all professionals involved must actively guard themselves against feelings of vindictiveness, moral superiority, sexism and any personal crusade.

2 That the aims are correctly to recognize non-accidental injury, help the child and the family in the immediate and long term, and prevent recurrence.

3 That any system designed to achieve these aims will have to strike a balance between extremes. On the one hand, it must not result in the false accusation of innocent people and the disruption of innocent families. On the other hand, it should not miss actual cases.

In practice, a case of suspected non-accidental injury might be managed as follows.

1 Admit the child to hospital under the care of a paediatrician. It is necessary at that stage to express to the parents what your concerns are. Only resort to legal placement of the child in hospital if the parents refuse their consent.

2 Take a full history including details of the pregnancy, delivery, newborn period, developmental milestones, previous illnesses, family history, social history, educational history, drug ingestion, as well as details of the circumstances of the particular injury/injuries in question.

3 Examine the child fully, paying particular attention to the physical injuries, nutritional state, intellectual and developmental progress and growth. Record all findings, make drawings where possible and photograph external injuries.

4 Obtain a social services report.

5 The paediatrican should keep in frequent contact with parents.

6 The paediatrician should decide on the basis of all the information received whether non-accidental injury has occurred. It would be the policy of some doctors to hold a case conference of all the parties involved with the child, perhaps including the police. Some other doctors would not hold a case conference because of concerns expressed by James and Ward (1988).

7 It would be hoped that good liaison with the police would allow for as little punitive intervention on their part as possible.

8 Full liaison should be maintained with the Social Services department which has a statutory duty to promote the welfare of the child, and to appoint a 'key worker' (Department of Health and Social Security 1988).

9 The aim, whenever possible, would be to maintain the family together, and support them in such a way as to prevent re-occurrence. This might involve (i) various agencies, e.g. the family doctor, the National Society for the Prevention of Cruelty to Children, the Local Education Authority, the health visitor or the Housing Department, and so on; (ii) regular outpatient review; and (iii) the offer of respite care from time to time.

10 On-going liaison at all levels between all the parties involved.

11 Particular attention has to be paid to enable the family to provide the environment that prevents the emotional disturbances which so often persist long after the accidental injury (Oates 1984).

Guidelines for physicians who are involved in court cases concerning child abuse have been prepared by Williams (1993).

Munchausen's syndrome by proxy

Munchausen's syndrome by proxy is a peculiar variation of child abuse, whereby caregivers intentionally harm their children but attempt to fool doctors into believing that the results of the abuse are a natural illness (Fig. 62.6). In Munchausen's syndrome, the infliction of self-abuse leads to an illness, which is used by the sufferer to gain access to medical care under the guise of a naturally occurring disease.

The classic cases of Munchausen's syndrome involve people who are usually male, pathological liars, and who travel or wander a great deal (American Psychiatric Association 1980; Folks *et al.* 1990). But the most common profile of the abusive parent in Munchausen's by proxy is that

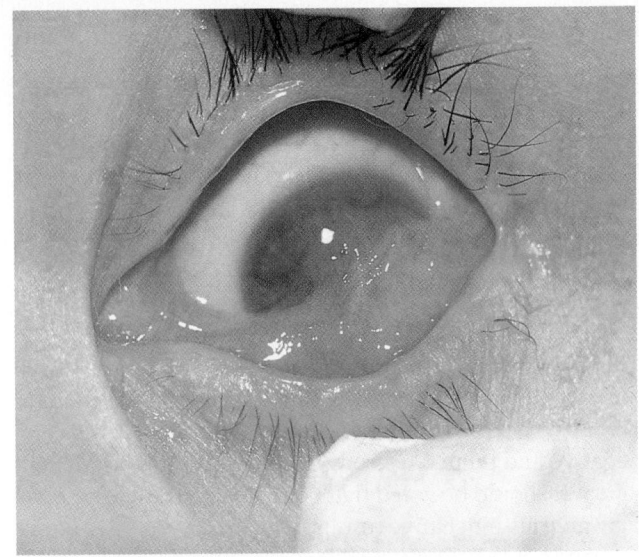

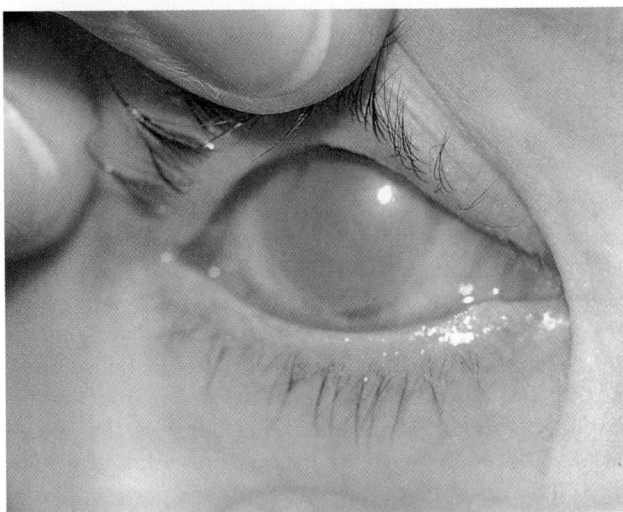

Fig. 62.6 (a) This child had recurrent attacks of keratoconjunctivitis in the left eye which, in the early stages, resolved on admission to hospital but later resulted in an axial pseudopterygium. (b) The right eye became suddenly inflamed 2 years after the left eye had started to develop keratitis. This picture shows the eye 4 days after the onset of the abnormality which was when it was reported. Both injuries were later found to be caused by the mother.

of an intelligent, educated woman, who may be employed in a health-related field. In some cases, Munchausen's by proxy occurs as a result of complex family interactions. A woman who may have a tendency towards somatization joins an authoritarian family (e.g. husband) that is prone to physically abuse children. She is dominated by her husband and displaces her own mental illness (self-abuse, somatization) onto her child (Folks & Houck 1993). There has been some discussion as to the appropriateness of the title and the specificity of the criteria (Fisher & Mitchell 1995; Morley 1995). The American Psychiatric Association DSM IV prefers the term 'factitious disorder by proxy', which should be applied to a perpetrator whose actions fulfil the following criteria.

1 Intentional production or feigning of physical or psychological signs or symptoms in another person who is under the individual's care.

2 The motivation for the perpetrator's behaviour is to assume the sick role by proxy.

3 External incentives for the behaviour (such as economic gain) are absent.

4 The behaviour is not better accounted for by another mental disorder.

Meadow (1995), who described the syndrome, has addressed the nosological difficulties.

Munchausen's by proxy takes several physical manifestations. Parents poisoning a child is common (Lorber *et al.* 1980). The nature of the poisoning may elude detection until or unless the physician suspects that it could occur at the hands of the child's mother. Chemical eye injuries can be inflicted by siblings as well (Taylor & Bentovim 1979). Factitious fevers, rashes and lacerations also occur. Ocular manifestations may include recurrent eye irritation, chemical injury and eyelid oedema/rash.

It is usual to involve expert child psychologists or psychiatrists in the management of these difficult cases (Eminson & Postlewaite 1992) but even with well-managed cases 50% have an unacceptable outcome (Bools *et al.* 1993).

Other forms of non-accidental injury or child abuse

See Chapter P29.

Neglect

This consists of the persistent or severe neglect of a child which results in serious impairment of that child's health or development; it includes exposure to danger, and repeated failure to attend to the physical or developmental needs of a child.

Emotional abuse

This is characterized as the persistent emotional ill-treatment of a child which has an effect on that child's behaviour and development.

Sexual abuse

Sexual abuse may be defined as the involvement of dependant or immature children in sexual activities which they do not really comprehend, and to which they are unable to give informed consent, which violate social taboos of family life and are knowingly not prevented by the carer.

Self-inflicted injury

Self-inflicted injury occurs predominantly in young adults with psychiatric disease. Burning, chemicals or cutting (Yang *et al.* 1981) are frequent methods and autoenucleation is also practised by schizophrenics (Trevor Roper 1980). There is usually evidence of secondary gain from the injury (Taylor & Hyler 1993). Keratoconjunctivitis artefacta, caused by thermal, chemical or mechanical injury, is suggested by sharply demarcated lesions in the inferior and nasal areas of the bulbar conjunctiva and cornea and the skin below the eye (Fig. 62.7) in a patient who shows little concern and has other evidence of psychopathy (Jay *et al.* 1982).

In all children with suspected self-induced injury the possibility of underlying metabolic or psychiatric diseases must be entertained. It is also important to look into the possibility of the self-inflicted injury being the manifestation of stress caused by sexual or other abuse.

In children, severe self-mutilation occurs in the Smith–Magenis syndrome (Finucane *et al.* 1993a, b), the Lesch–Nyhan syndrome, Joubert's syndrome, and possibly in the Gilles de la Tourette syndrome.

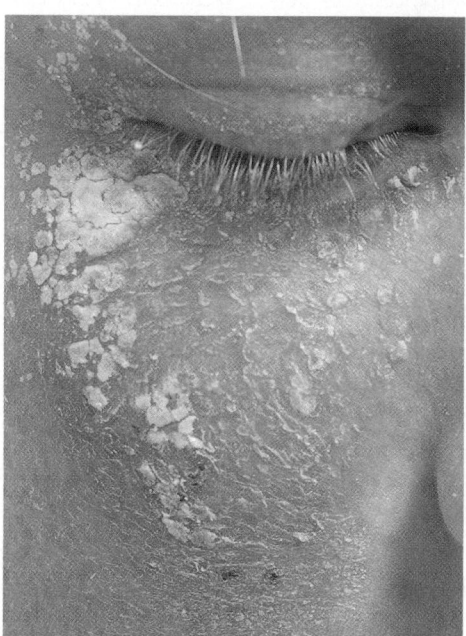

Fig. 62.7 Self-inflicted injury in a teenager. This patient had recurrent attacks of conjunctivitis artefacta and a desquamating skin lesion adjacent to that eye.

Ophthalmic trauma caused by amniocentesis and birth injury

A spectrum of eye injuries can occur in association with amniocentesis. Normally, amniocentesis is performed in the second trimester, with very little risk of fetal loss (Milunsky 1975; Finnegan *et al.* 1985). However, ocular injuries have been the subject of a variety of reports, and clinicians should be aware of the nature of these injuries.

Non-pigmented epithelial iris cysts have been reported after amniocentesis (Rummelt *et al.* 1993). Presumably, these cysts occur as a result of penetrating injury with the amniocentesis needle. The cysts are located anteriorly and have an adherence to the posterior corneal surface. Peripheral anterior synechiae occur.

Naylor *et al.* (1990) reported five cases of presumed ophthalmic amniocentesis injury. One child had a hemianopia and gaze palsy. Two of the cases had presumed needle perforation of the eye resulting in a peaked pupil in one case and chorioretinal scar in the other. In the remaining two of the five cases one showed a small leucoma, and one a limbal corneal scar.

There have been additional reported cases of injury due to amniocentesis including leucocoria (Admoni & Ben-Ezra 1988), third nerve palsy (Patel *et al.* 1993) (Fig. 62.8) and even congenital blindness (Merin & Beyth 1980). Clearly, abnormalities of the anterior segment of the eye or of the retina (Isenberg & Heckenlively 1985) which could have been caused by trauma should be evaluated in the context of whether a baby or young child was exposed to amniocentesis *in utero*. Real-time ultrasound monitoring of the amniocentesis needle may help avoid this injury (Hershey 1993).

Ocular adnexal injuries occur rarely after episiotomy. Upper eyelid laceration (Sachs *et al.* 1986) and lower eyelid laceration (Dorfman & Benson 1993) have been reported. The instrumentation occasionally used in childbirth may also cause other external trauma, including bruising and subconjunctival haemorrhage (Jain *et al.* 1980). The possibility of ruptured globe as caused by childbirth is discussed below.

Orbital injury due to forceps resulting in inferior rectus fibrosis has been described (Hamed & Fang 1992). Forceps should be suspected as the cause of a congenital corneal abnormality in which vertical ruptures in Descemet's membrane (Fig. 62.9) occur with a contralesional occipital depression caused by the other arm of the forceps (McDonald & Burgess 1992).

Eyelid and lacrimal system trauma

Many eyelid injuries result in superficial lacerations which can be closed with fine silk or nylon suture. Clinicians must be aware of two particular types of injuries which require special attention. The first of these is eyelid margin laceration, and the second is injury to the lacrimal drainage system.

In eyelid margin laceration, attention must be directed towards careful reapproximation of the margins of the eyelid. The usual aetiology is sharp or blunt trauma to the lid margin, although other unusual aetiologies are known, for example, dog bite or rat bite (Myers & Christmann 1991) injuries.

Injuries to the canalicular system will occur if the medial eyelid margin is injured, either of the upper or lower lid. Such injuries usually require intubation with silastic tubing material passed through both ends of the canaliculus and into the nose. With deeper injuries, it is important to close deep edges of the wound with fine grade absorbable suture and close the more superficial edges of the wound with fine suture. Once again, if the eyelid margin is cut, failure to reapproximate the margin precisely may result in the formation of a cosmetically undesirable notch.

Dog bite injuries may affect the eyelid margin and the lacrimal system (Jameson *et al.* 1992). In addition, either an inferior oblique palsy or restrictive type of ocular motor problem may occur. Management consists of closure of the laceration, as described above, and strabismus management as required.

Anterior segment trauma

Subconjunctival haemorrhage

Subconjunctival haemorrhages can occur spontaneously or as a result of trauma. Despite their dramatic appearance, subconjunctival haemorrhages are of virtually no significance except in a situation where enough swelling occurs near the limbus so as to interfere with normal corneal protection by the eyelids and tear film. In this case a dellen may occur. A dellen is an excavation of the cornea with or without epithelial defect which occurs adjacent to a mass or bump near the corneal scleral limbus. It is probably caused by localized drying.

Subconjunctival haemorrhages associated with trauma indicate the need for a thorough search for a more serious eye injury (Fig. 62.10). The haemorrhage may mask a penetrating injury, so the examiner should look carefully for other signs of penetrating injury (e.g. uvea in a laceration, distorted pupil, lower intraocular pressure).

Corneal abrasion

Corneal abrasions occur when the corneal epithelium is traumatically removed from its underlying basement membrane. Abrasions can occur in the context of blunt or sharp trauma, and are noteworthy for the significant pain that they cause. Abrasions are diagnosed with a fluorescein test. Fluorescein instilled into an eye with a corneal

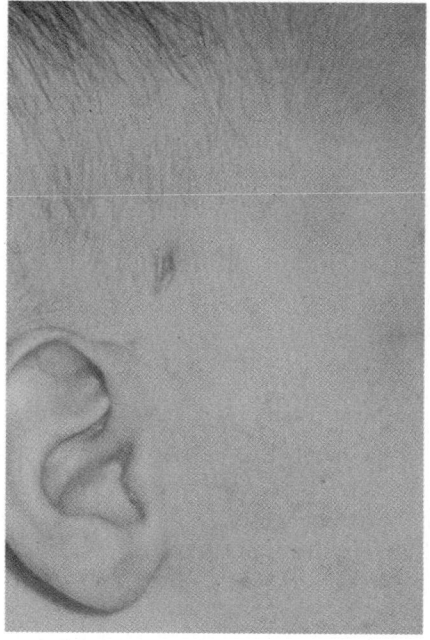

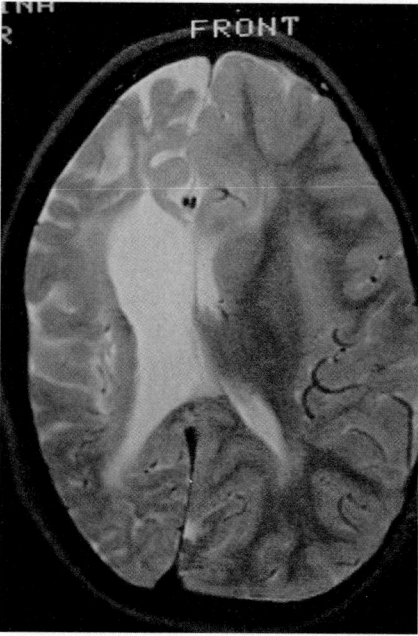

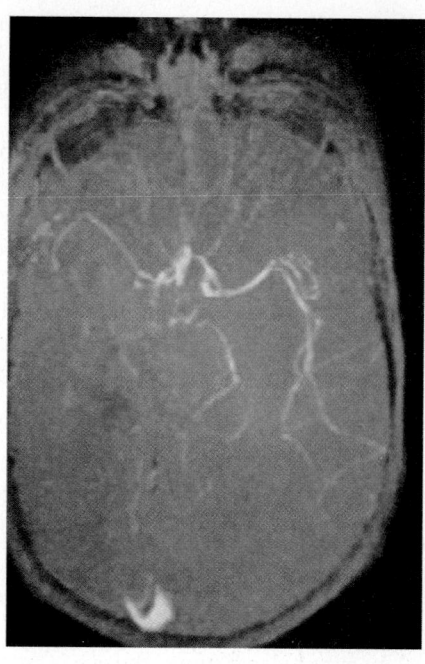

a   b   c

Fig. 62.8 (a) Amniocentesis injury with needle marks on the right temple. (b) Same patient. MRI scan showing right cerebral hemiatrophy. (c) MRI angiography showing occlusion of the right middle cerebral artery.

abrasion will transiently stain the underlying basement membrane and will fluoresce when exposed to a blue light.

The differential diagnosis for corneal abrasion includes viral illness (e.g. herpes simplex keratitis) and corneal basement membrane disease. Herpes infection is usually suggested by a dendritic appearance, while basement membrane disease occurs in older children and adults and is recurrent, with no history of trauma.

Management of corneal abrasions involves prophylaxis against infection, since the epithelial lining of the cornea is a protective barrier against organisms. Most authorities recommend placing an antibiotic ointment into the eye (broad spectrum, accompanied by cycloplegia in order to reduce pain from iridospasm), and with patching over closed lids. The question of patching and its effectiveness is debated. However, most patients will find the patching to be more comfortable than leaving the eyelids open.

Corneal foreign body

A small foreign body may stick on the cornea if it succeeds in penetrating the corneal epithelium. Patients will

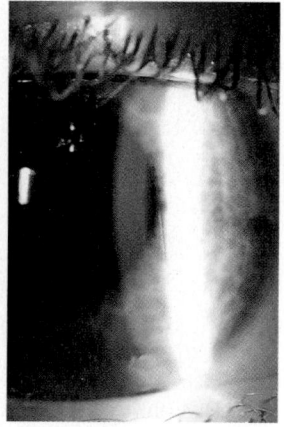

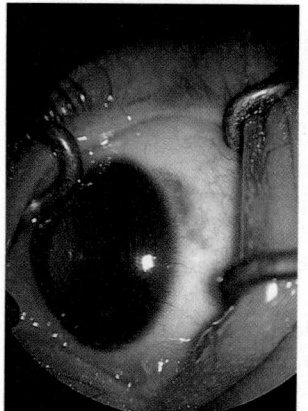

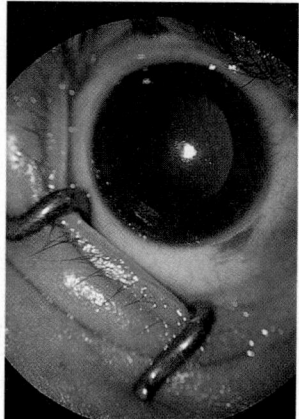

Fig. 62.9 Forceps injury to cornea. The vertically orientated rupture in Descemet's membrane can just be seen to one side of the pupil.

Fig. 62.10 Subconjunctival haemorrhage. In this instance associated with shaking, there were severe intraocular injuries.

complain of pain and foreign body sensation on the eye. There may be a history of injury to the eye, but many patients will not recall anything in particular happening to them.

The foreign body should be removed, usually with irrigation, a rotating 'burr', or simply and carefully with a sharp needle brought towards the eye tangentially and used to flick the foreign body away from the surface of the eye.

The eye should be examined carefully for the possibility of a penetrating eye injury and then managed as a corneal abrasion, once the foreign body is gone.

Eye wall injuries

Aetiology

Eye wall lacerations can be categorized according to two dichotomies: simple laceration versus rupture; and anterior laceration versus posterior.

In simple lacerations, the eye is cut with a sharp object. Virtually any object imaginable has been responsible at one time or another for an eye wall laceration (Figs 62.11–62.14). Very young children usually suffer injury when they fall on a sharp object, such as a pencil, nail or toothpick. Older children, though, may suffer eye wall lacerations from glass (particularly when they wear spectacles), and projectiles. BB or air guns are notorious for causing ocular penetrating injuries and eye wall lacerations (Schein *et al.* 1994). Bottle rockets and knives are other common causes. Unusual causes include the peck of a chicken, which carries the risk of endophthalmitis caused by unusual bacterial species from the bird's beak. Amniocentesis is also a potential cause of eye wall laceration or other type of injury (see above) (Isenberg & Heckenlively 1985).

Predisposition ('brittle corneas')

Certain eyes may be more likely to rupture with relatively minor trauma. In Ehlers–Danlos syndrome, defective collagen cross-linkage (Pinnel *et al.* 1972) leads to scleral and corneal weakness (Fig. 62.15). Patients with Ehlers–Danlos show blue sclera (due to scleral thinning), hyperextensible skin, and hypermobile joints. Spontaneous corneal rupture can occur (Biglan *et al.* 1977; Cameron 1993).

In the brittle cornea, blue sclera and joint hyperextensibility syndrome (Ticho *et al.* 1980; Zlotogora *et al.* 1990), spontaneous rupture of the globe may occur; patients may have red hair and develop keratoglobus, and, unlike Ehlers–Danlos syndrome, they have normal levels of lysyl hydroxylase.

Osteogenesis imperfecta consists of blue sclera, deafness and bone fractures (Ruedemann 1953; Chan *et al.*

1982). Children with this syndrome may also be more prone to corneal rupture in the setting of minor trauma.

Rupture

When a globe is ruptured, it is pushed or squeezed so hard that the eye wall breaks under pressure. The results usually are devastating, with partial or complete expulsion of intraocular contents. Expulsion is facilitated due to the increase in intraocular pressure followed by sudden decompression through a hole in the wall of the eye. Events that can cause ruptured globes include encounters with large, usually blunt, objects. A fist fight can result in a ruptured globe, as can injury from the force of a small projectile, such as a handball, squash ball, racquetball or baseball. For example, in North America, hockey puck injuries were most often responsible for ruptured globes among children prior to the advent of protective eye-wear (Pashby 1985). In the USA, baseball injuries are

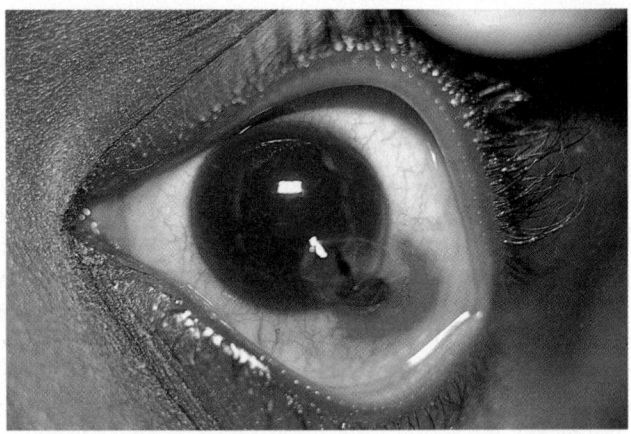

Fig. 62.11 Penetrating injury with iris prolapse and subconjunctival haemorrhage (Dr William Good's patient).

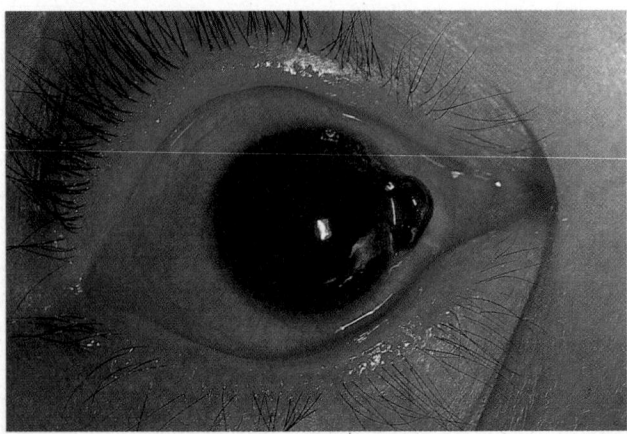

Fig. 62.12 Limbal penetrating injury with iris prolapse. Photograph by courtesy of Dr William Good.

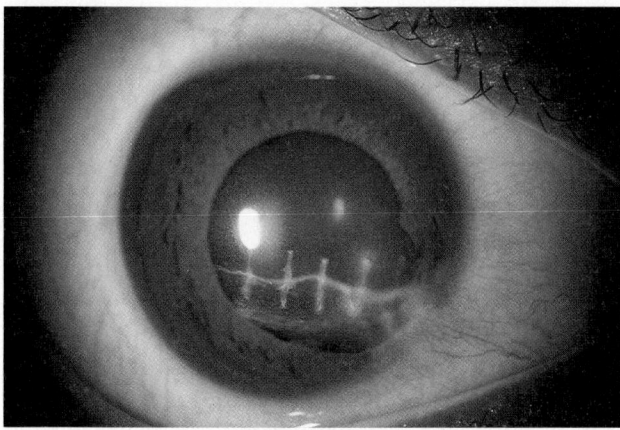

Fig. 62.13 After removal of the corneal sutures a scar persists. Failure to remove suture promptly may cause blood vessel migration and corneal opacification. Note the vessels at the corneoscleral limbus. Photograph by courtesy of Dr William Good.

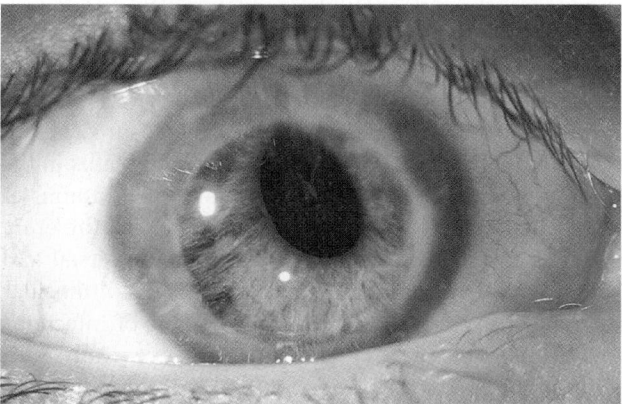

Fig. 62.14 This 5-year-old child had accidental corneal trauma as an infant. Prompt corneal grafting and amblyopia treatment resulted in an acuity of 6/12.

now most likely to result in serious eye injuries in older children.

Globe rupture is more common in boys than girls, reflecting the nature of the causal events. When the intraocular contents are affected the prognosis is poor (Cascairo *et al.* 1994; Rudd *et al.* 1994).

A ruptured globe has even been reported following parturition, and it is assumed that an increase in intraocular pressure could have been caused by force on the globe by a pelvic bone or some other obstacle (Bachynski *et al.* 1986). Eyes are more likely to be ruptured or lacerated in areas where the sclera or cornea are thinnest. The areas under the insertions of the rectus and superior oblique muscles and also the corneoscleral limbus are thin and more likely to give way under pressure.

Anterior versus posterior laceration

A second important dichotomy in the diagnosis of globe lacerations is anterior versus posterior positioning. There is no doubt that anterior locations of injuries carry a better prognosis, so long as the inciting agent does not also cut the retina. Injuries anterior to the pars plana (located approximately 5 mm posterior to the corneal scleral limbus) will not cut the retina, and therefore carry a better prognosis (Eagling 1976; Baxter *et al.* 1994). If a cataract occurs in conjunction with an anterior laceration, the prognosis for recovery of vision is not as good (Eagling 1976). Posterior injuries cut the retina and often result in a complicated retinal detachment. Although these retinal detachments may be amenable to treatment, they carry a far worse prognosis than if the laceration were anterior.

One last set of definitions should be mentioned. Penetrating eye injuries are those in which the causative agent enters the eye but does not pass all the way through. Per-

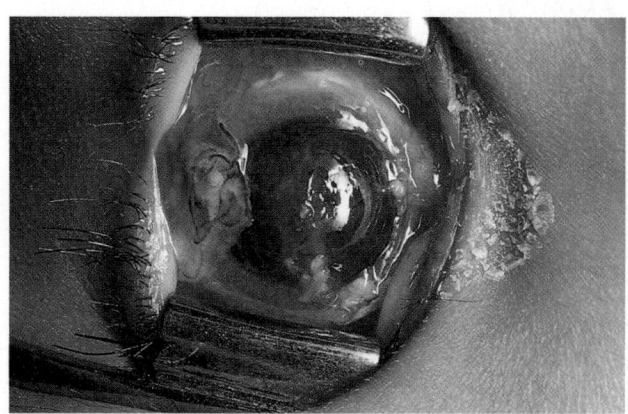

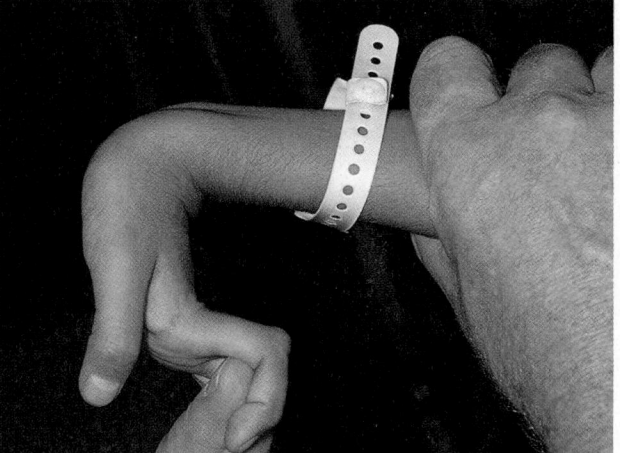

Fig. 62.15 (a) Ehlers–Danlos syndrome with spontaneous rupture of the cornea. This is an autosomal recessive disease. One of this child's siblings, also affected, had a bilateral corneal rupture at the same time during fisticuffs. (b) Ehlers–Danlos syndrome. Hyperflexible joints.

forating eye injuries are those that pass through two walls of the eye. The same definition holds true when referring to different parts of the eye. For example, a penetrating corneal injury is one that penetrates the cornea but does not pass all the way through it. A perforating injury passes all the way through the cornea into the anterior chamber or further into the eye.

Diagnosis

The diagnosis of penetrating eye injury is obvious when a laceration is apparent. Clues to occult penetration include subconjunctival haemorrhage, distorted pupil, wrinkled lens capsule, and lowered intraocular pressure, particularly compared to pressure in the fellow, uninjured eye (see Fig. 62.7). The child's or family's history may or may not corroborate the physical findings.

Management

Prevention

The best form of management for eyeball lacerations is prevention (Vinger 1981). Education to prevent injuries includes the following.
1 The encouragement of the wearing of suitable safety glasses or goggles by players who participate in games involving a small ball.
2 The encouragement of parents and teachers to supervise play and sport when sharp objects (fencing, archery, etc.) are used and teaching young people to respect the use of handguns, even 'low power' or BB or airguns.
3 The use of safety glasses in monocular children is controversial. Although it seems logical to encourage their use, and although compliance may be good (Drack *et al.* 1993) there are many children who will not wear them and it seems to some that their enforcement may be inappropriate except at times of particular risk.
4 A knowledge of when the injuries occur helps (Luff *et al.* 1993): most occur in the home and therefore parental education must be a priority.

Treatment

Once the eye laceration or globe rupture is diagnosed, a protective shield should be placed over the eye. Emergency surgery is indicated, but the patient's overall health status should not be ignored. The eye laceration may accompany head trauma or other head injury. We have had the experience of caring for adolescent patients with multiple gunshot wounds, some of which were nearly ignored due to the focus of attention being placed on the eye injury itself.

Imaging

The role of imaging of the eye in order to determine an intraocular foreign body is an important one. In many cases, a CT scan of the orbits (Figs 62.20, 62.21) will help to identify the location of expected or unexpected intraocular foreign bodies, and ultrasonography also can be very helpful.

Anaesthesia

The anaesthetic induction of the patient is debated. Some would advocate avoiding a depolarizing agent for fear that the contraction of extraocular muscles (which initially occurs) could press on the eye and express intraocular contents. However, there has been no study that actually documents this, and there is a report (Wang *et al.* 1992) which showed no difference in prognosis whether or not a depolarizing agent is used.

Surgery

The main goal of surgery is closure of the eye wall laceration. With anterior lacerations, prompt closure and re-evaluation of the patient's vision and ocular status in the ensuing several days is advisable. We do not administer intraocular antibiotics prophylactically unless there are signs of an infection; but this issue is controversial and some would recommend the use of an intraocular regimen that covers against a broad range of infectious organisms. The prompt closure of an eye wall laceration would seem to be adequate to greatly reduce the incidence of traumatic endophthalmitis. A concurrent traumatic cataract should be removed at the same time as closure of the laceration in young children. Delay in traumatic cataract extraction runs the risk of inducing amblyopia. In older children (>7 years of age), a second operation could be performed and could include intraocular lens implant, so long as the posterior capsule remains intact.

Posterior lacerations almost always cut through the retina. Even so, the initial goal of surgery is wound closure. Most authorities do not use cryosurgery or scleral buckling at initial surgery. The trauma alone is enough to cause a retinal scar around a break, and cryosurgery releases intraocular factors which may increase the likelihood of posterior vitreoretinopathy (PVR). A posterior vitreous detachment occurs 7–10 days after trauma; after this detachment has taken place, the retinal surgery can be undertaken.

Management continues even after successful closure and repair of the wound. Children under the age of 7 years are at risk for amblyopia (Vaegan & Taylor 1979). Prompt refractive management in the form of a contact lens over a corneal laceration (or spectacles if appropriate), and patching should be started as soon as possible (Epstein *et al.* 1988). Additionally, corneal sutures in children attract blood vessels and scarring much more quickly than in adults. Sutures may need to be removed in a matter of weeks in young children. Failure to remove sutures may result in a completely vascularized cornea, which impedes vision.

Prognosis

Prognosis in eye wall lacerations and ruptures in children is debated (Sternberg *et al.* 1984a, b). Without doubt, anterior lacerations carry a better prognosis than posterior lacerations. But in young children, with the risk of amblyopia, the prognosis may not be so good, even with anterior lacerations. When anterior lacerations are combined with cataract, the prognosis worsens (Baxter *et al.* 1994). The prognosis also is highly dependent upon success in the management of amblyopia or the potential for amblyopia.

Traumatic cataracts

Traumatic cataracts can occur either as a result of a sharp penetrating injury to the lens capsule and/or lens, or a blunt concussive force (Angra *et al.* 1991). Traumatic cataracts may occur immediately after the injury, or may occur days to even years after a concussive blow. Cataracts may be partial or complete; trauma may produce a posterior subcapsular cataract which then progresses to a total cataract.

The diagnosis of traumatic cataracts is based on an abnormality in the red reflex. The cataract problem can be confirmed by examining the lens under magnification, either with loupes or a slit lamp. In some cases, a Vossius ring may occur, i.e. a ring of pigment forms on the anterior lens capsule as a result of the posterior (pigmented) aspect of the iris striking the capsule. Examination should establish that there are no other ocular injuries. An effort should be made to search for a rupture in the lens capsule as well, since this usually indicates that the lens opacity will not clear spontaneously, and the lens will need to be removed.

In partial cataracts, an additional important aspect to the examination is an effort at measuring visual function in the involved eye. In older children, of course, this can be done with Snellen acuity. In younger children, an estimate must be made based upon experience with lens clarity and visual functioning under monocular and binocular conditions. Attempts can be made to measure acuity with forced choice preferential looking techniques, but these may be misleading and probably should not be used as the sole determinant to undertaking surgery (Hoyt 1993; Kushner 1994).

If there is doubt as to the value of removing a lens with a cataract, then it should be observed. This is true if the cataract occurs as a result of blunt or penetrating trauma. So long as the child is beyond the age when amblyopia can develop, the initial repair of a corneal or scleral laceration can be followed at a later date with removal of the lens. This 'wait-and-see' strategy has no deleterious effects on the child other than the necessity for a second general anaesthetic.

Surgical management consists of removal of the lens with or without preservation of the posterior capsule. If a lens is removed at the same time that an eye wall laceration is closed, it may be safer to avoid simultaneous lens implant but simultaneous corneal repair, lens aspiration, and posterior chamber lens implantation has its advocates (Anwar *et al.* 1994). The reason for caution is that the implant could conceivably foster survival of bacterial organisms which penetrated the eye as a result of the trauma. Decisions regarding subsequent implants depend on surgeon preference and the presence or absence of corneal refractive problems. If a child has a significant amount of astigmatism and will require contact lens rehabilitation anyway, then any increased risk of a lens implant can be avoided, since the implant would not avert the need for contact lenses. Contact lenses can be successful in post-traumatic aphakia (Riise *et al.* 1977; Jain *et al.* 1985). Amblyopia must also be managed carefully in order to maximize visual potential. Combined keratoplasty and lens implantation may have a role in some cases (Vajpayee *et al.* 1994).

A special type of cataract can occur as the result of electrical injury (Shapiro 1984). A characteristic opacity in the posterior aspect of the lens forms as the result of the transmission of electricity to the eye (Fig. 62.16) itself. If this type of cataract becomes visually significant it can be cared for in the same fashion as cataracts from other causes.

Hyphaema

A hyphaema is a collection of blood in the anterior chamber of the eye. In the setting of trauma, hyphaema occurs as a result of avulsion of blood vessels, usually at the base of the iris. Bleeding occurs and then ceases after clot formation or an increase in intraocular pressure. A hyphaema may be small enough that it can be identified only with a slit-lamp examination, or it can be so extensive as to fill the entire anterior chamber with blood, the so-called '8-ball hyphaema'. In most instances, a superiorly located meniscus develops due to the effects of gravity (Fig. 62.17).

Knowledge of the various other aetiologies of hyphaema is important, particularly since children may not reveal that they fell or were hit by a friend or some other object. Herpes zoster iritis can occasionally cause a hyphaemia. Spontaneous hyphaemas also occur with

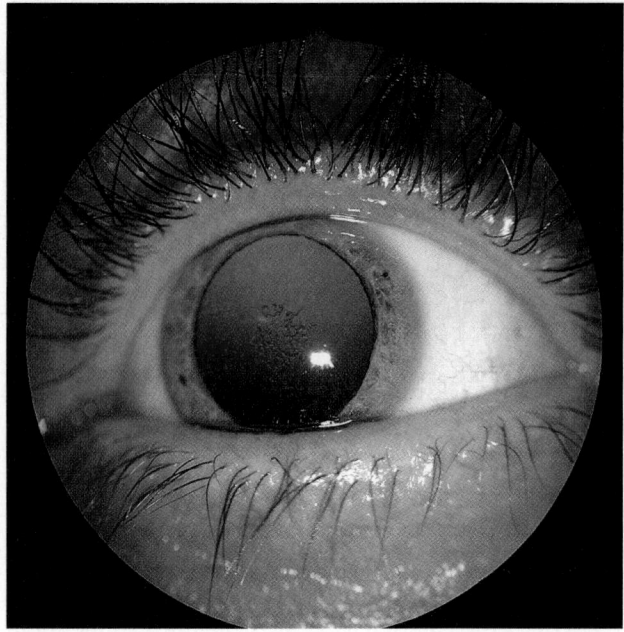

Fig. 62.16 After an electric shock this young man slowly developed a monocular cataract. Photograph by courtesy of Dr William Good.

juvenile xanthogranulomatosis. Most of these cases occur in very young children (< 1 year of age), and may or may not be associated with cutaneous lesions. Hyphaemas may also occur rarely in association with tumours of the eye, particularly retinoblastoma, but also with iris vascular abnormalities or rubeosis.

The management of hyphaemas is debated (Little & Aylward 1993). The natural history of the hyphaema is such that the clot usually retracts between the third and fifth post-traumatic day, at which point the hyphaema may recur. There is a general agreement that very small 'trickle' hyphaemas are less likely to rebleed than larger ones. However, rebleeding cannot be predicted solely on the basis of the size of the hyphaema if it is visible without magnification. For this reason, most advocate some sort of rest regimen for the child. Whether a child should be hospitalized in order to facilitate resting will certainly depend at least on the child's activity level, the family's ability to supervise the child, and perhaps also on the size of the hyphaema. Other efforts at enforcing rest include using light sedation. Antiemetics may prevent vomiting (and transient increases in intraocular pressure and eye movement), and should be considered. A quick, substantial rise in intraocular pressure (a complication of hyphaema) can cause nausea and vomiting.

The use of eye drops is also of unproven benefit. Many would choose to use a long-acting cycloplegic agent in order to put the iris and pupil 'at rest'. Short-acting cycloplegics probably are not worthwhile because movement of the iris could potentially lead to disruption of clot and further bleeding. Topical steroids may be

useful if an inflammatory component (iritis) occurs.

Systemic steroids have been advocated by Rynne and Romano (1980). The use of epsilon aminocaproic acid has been advocated by some, but its value in children has not been proven conclusively (Palmer *et al.* 1986; Kraft *et al.* 1987). Epsilon aminocaproic acid blocks fibrinolysis. Presumably, it can retard or inhibit the dissolution of the clot, and thereby reduce the risk of rebleeding.

Complications of hyphaema are increased intraocular pressure and glaucoma. How much pressure and for how long pressure can be tolerated safely is very individually determined and has not been worked out for children. High pressure runs the risk of causing corneal blood staining and optic nerve damage. To prevent these complications, many would treat pressure and attempt to maintain it below 30 mmHg. Persistent elevation of intraocular pressure may be an indication for surgical evacuation of the hyphaema. In many cases, elevated pressure can be managed with eye drops such as beta-blockers (acetylcholine agents are probably ill advised because they constrict the pupil and may have an effect on the fragile blood vessels). Systemic pressure-lowering agents such as acetazolamide may also be useful.

When a child has sickle cell anaemia, the management of glaucoma caused by hyphaema is more problematic. The only agent available to the physician is a topical beta-blocker, since other agents may either exacerbate the hyphaema (e.g. pilocarpine) or lead to sickle cell crisis. Children with sickle cell with a hyphaema may be candidates for early surgical intervention. Surgical intervention consists of a clot evacuation through a corneal scleral incision. In children who do not have sickle cell, but in whom glaucoma remains a refractory problem, such surgical evacuation may also be advisable.

Blood staining occurs when erythrocytes cross the corneal endothelial membrane and stain the cornea. This

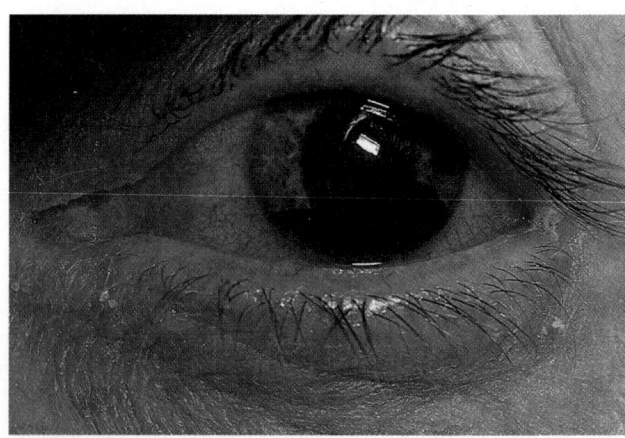

Fig. 62.17 A long-standing hyphaema shown by the dark colour of the blood in this young man. Photograph by courtesy of Dr William Good.

occurs when the intraocular pressure is elevated, and also in situations where the corneal endothelium is damaged. Corneal blood staining is reversible, but takes several years. Corneal blood staining is particularly problematic in children due to the potential for development of amblyopia.

Months and years later, if the angle of the eye has been traumatized and 'recessed', the child may develop a type of open angle glaucoma referred to as 'angle recession glaucoma'. For that reason, any patient who has had a hyphaema probably should have yearly ophthalmology examinations, with intraocular pressure measurements determined. The risk of angle recession glaucoma may be as high as 10% following hyphaema, at least in adult patients (Wolff & Zimmerman 1962; Blanton 1964).

Posterior segment trauma

Commotio retinae

Commotio retinae, also known as Berlin's oedema, can occur after blunt trauma to the front part of the eye. The oedema, which occurs in the outer retinal areas, has a funduscopic appearance that is white or grey–white. The macula may be involved, in which case central vision will be at least temporarily diminished (Blight & Hart 1977; Sipperly *et al.* 1978). But Berlin's oedema can also involve extramacular areas and may actually not be noticed by the patient.

In most cases, the oedema resolves, but there are some cases where pigment migration in the macula might result in loss of central vision. Also, a full-thickness macular hole can follow the formation of this type of oedema (Gass 1987). The differential diagnosis consists of retinal infarction, cotton-wool spot and shallow retinal detachment. No particular treatment is available for commotio retinae.

Purtscher's retinopathy

Severe trauma to the torso or the head itself can cause a type of retinopathy called Purtscher's retinopathy. Purtscher's disease can also be caused by a fat or air embolism (Urbanek 1934; Burton 1980).

Purtscher's retinopathy has the appearance of massive whitening around the optic nerve head associated with haemorrhage. The whitening may represent ischaemic areas or exudate. There is no specific treatment for this problem, which may resolve leaving anything from mild to profound vision loss.

Whiplash injury

A macular hole sometimes occurs as a consequence of a severe whiplash injury (Grey 1978; Kelley *et al.* 1978). Presumably, the head thrusting induces a vitreoretinal inter-face shearing force which tugs at the fovea and creates a partial or full-thickness hole. The hole resembles solar maculopathy, but this latter problem has an altogether different aetiology.

Choroidal rupture

Another potential complication of blunt injury to the front part of the eye is choroidal rupture; it is often associated with widespread damage and vitreous haemorrhage (Fig. 62.18). The choroid may be broken (ruptured) at the level of the inner choroid and retinal pigment epithelium, and often in the most visually sensitive area of the retina, the macula (Gass 1987). The mechanism is mechanical disruption and refraction of tissue (Martin *et al.* 1994). Sometimes the rupture is associated with a serous or haemorrhagic retinal detachment which obscures the nature of the injury. Once the detachment resolves, the patient may be left with diminished vision if there has been scarring or retinal pigment epithelial migration into the area of the macula. Later, choroidal rupture can predispose to a choroidal neovascularization process, which can lead to exudate and haemorrhage under the macula, also diminishing vision. Patients with choroidal rupture should be apprised of this potential consequence, and should monitor their vision on a regular basis, since laser treatment to the choroidal neovascularization may, in some cases, help eliminate the problem.

Retinal haemorrhages

Retinal haemorrhages can be caused by direct head or ocular trauma, or by indirect trauma, as with a shaking injury in non-accidental trauma (Caffey 1972). Haemorrhages occur in normal infants in the perinatal period (Fig. 62.19) in a large percentage of cases, and may also be caused by trauma. Evidence for the traumatic nature of retinal haemorrhages is found in the fact that occipital presentation at birth, the use of obstetrical procedures, labour induction, and prolonged labour are all associated with an increased incidence in retinal haemorrhages (Kauffman 1958). Retinal haemorrhages are uncommon in children born by caesarean section.

A diagnosis of retinal haemorrhages is made by fundoscopic examination. In older children, retinal haemorrhage may be suspected by complaints of altered or decreased vision. In younger children, haemorrhage will be diagnosed in an incidental examination, or when an examination is performed due to suspected non-accidental trauma.

Haemorrhages may occur in any of several layers in the retina or vitreous (Kaur & Taylor 1992). Subretinal pigment epithelial haemorrhages appear dark with an amorphous boundary. Intraretinal haemorrhages are red in appearance, usually small and round. Superficial retinal

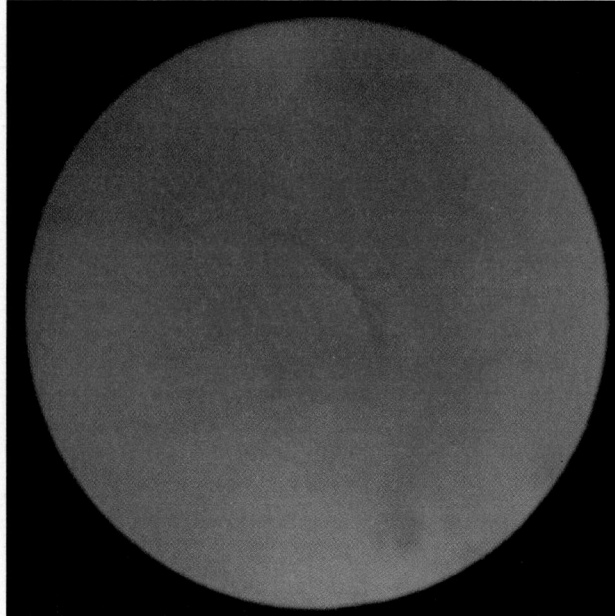

Fig. 62.18 Choroidal rupture. There is a marked vitreous haemorrhage largely obscuring a view of the fundus where a pale organizing clot can barely be made out.

haemorrhages have a splinter appearance because they often occur in the nerve fibre layer. Subhyaloid haemorrhages have a characteristic appearance where blood forms a meniscus in a large cystic filled cavity. Finally, vitreous haemorrhages may also occur in the setting of trauma, and may be localized or diffuse depending on their severity.

Any of these haemorrhages may occur with trauma, but pre-retinal haemorrhages are particularly common in children with subdural or subarachnoid haemorrhages (Hollenhorst & Stein 1958). Since central nervous system haemorrhage is frequently caused by trauma in children, a traumatic aetiology for pre-retinal haemorrhages should be suspected. The relationship of shaken baby to trauma is discussed above.

Other, non-traumatic causes of retinal haemorrhages include Coats' disease (Quinn 1989); persistent hyperplastic primary vitreous (Karr & Scott 1986); retinal dysplastic syndrome, including Norrie's disease and incontinentia pigmenta (Kaur & Taylor 1992); blood dyscrasias (Baum & Bulpitt 1970); hyperviscosity syndromes; infections of the retina, including cytomegalovirus, rickettsia (Giraud 1959); endocarditis; protein C deficiency (Pulido *et al.* 1987), and retinal tumours such as retinoblastoma. In all of these cases the aetiology is usually obvious, but should be searched for prior to diagnosing a traumatic aetiology of retinal haemorrhages for reasons discussed under non-accidental trauma.

There seldom is any particular management for retinal haemorrhages, but the exception would be the baby or young child with a prolonged vitreous haemorrhage. Kaur and Taylor (1992) have commented on the fact that vitreous haemorrhages in children may take longer to absorb because the vitreous gel is more solid in this age group. Prolonged obscuration of vision due to vitreous haemorrhage could cause deprivation amblyopia, and is a reason for early vitrectomy (Ferrone & de Juan 1994), particularly in the first 3–6 months of life. We have encountered children with prolonged vitreous haemorrhage in the setting of profound perinatal hypoxic ischaemia and vigorous resuscitation efforts (Good *et al.* 1994). The children we saw required vitrectomy due to slow absorption of a vitreous haemorrhage.

Traumatic retinal detachment

Blunt trauma to the eye can cause a retinal detachment even if the globe is not cut or ruptured (Cox *et al.* 1966; Weidenthal & Schepens 1966). Typically, the detachment occurs as the result of an avulsion of the vitreous base, often in the superonasal quadrant of the eye. Presumably this location is most vulnerable because a blunt blow to the eye arises from 180° away, in the inferotemporal segment. There have been cases where a blunt object strikes the eye and causes a small or large retinal tear which, days, weeks or even months later leads to a delayed retinal detachment. This is known to occur in boxing injuries, for example.

The clinician should be aware of the vulnerability of the vitreous base and should, to the extent possible, inspect this peripheral area of the retina in order to exclude this possible post-traumatic problem. Retinal detachments

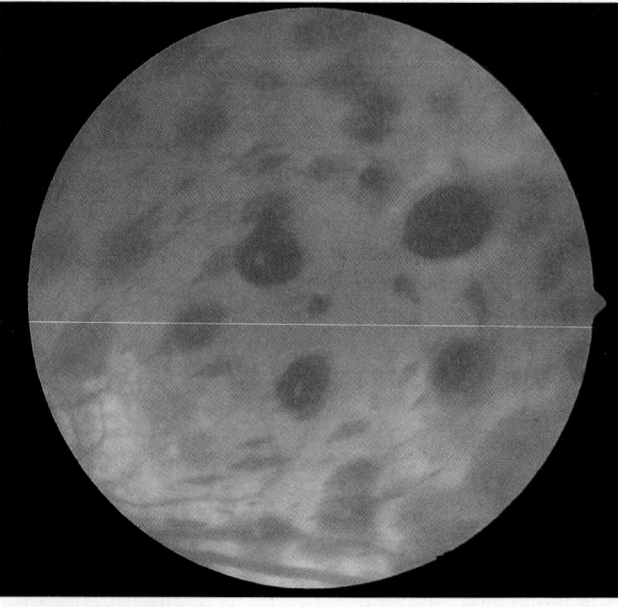

Fig. 62.19 Neonatal retinal haemorrhages in a normal child. Photograph by courtesy of Dr Andrew Q. McCormick, Vancouver.

should be managed promptly, usually with a scleral buckling procedure.

Self-abuse in severely mentally retarded children can also cause retinal detachments by aetiologies mentioned above (Robertson *et al.* 1990; Jan *et al.* 1994). In atopy, constant rubbing to relieve itching increases the risk of retinal detachment (Balyeat 1937; Oka *et al.* 1994).

Orbit trauma

Orbital bone fractures

General

Fractures of the bony orbit are mainly the province of the neurosurgeons and craniofacial team but the high frequency with which the eye is involved (p. 850) demands the involvement of an ophthalmologist in most cases.

Blow-out fratures

The term 'blow-out fractures' was probably first used by Smith and Regan (1957). Blow-out fracture refers to the caving in of one of the orbital bones that surround the eye. In most cases the floor of the orbit is fractured (Fig. 62.20), but the medial wall of the orbit can also be damaged. Blow-out fractures of the superior orbital wall are uncommon and the term 'blow-in' fracture is preferable in such cases because most such fractures involve a caving in of the bones in this area into the orbit (McLachlan *et al.* 1982). Blow-out fractures are unusual in young children, before the sinuses have formed.

Aetiology

Blow-out fractures can occur by one or both of two mechanisms. In the first situation, the eye may be compressed into the orbit, thereby increasing the pressure on the orbital contents. This expansion of tissue in the orbit may cause a dramatic increase of pressure on orbital bones. Since the orbital floor appears to be the weakest, it is the most likely to be fractured (Pfeiffer 1943; Converse & Smith 1960). This first theory is termed the 'hydraulic theory'. A second mechanism of blow-out fracture involves direct transmission of the force of a blow to the orbital rim to the bones of the floor or medial wall of the orbit. Experimental injuries to the orbital rim have demonstrated that a posterior orbital floor blow-out fracture can be induced in this fashion (Fujino 1974; Kersten 1987).

Enophthalmos

Generally speaking, there are three types of problems that can result from a blow-out fracture. Enophthalmos can

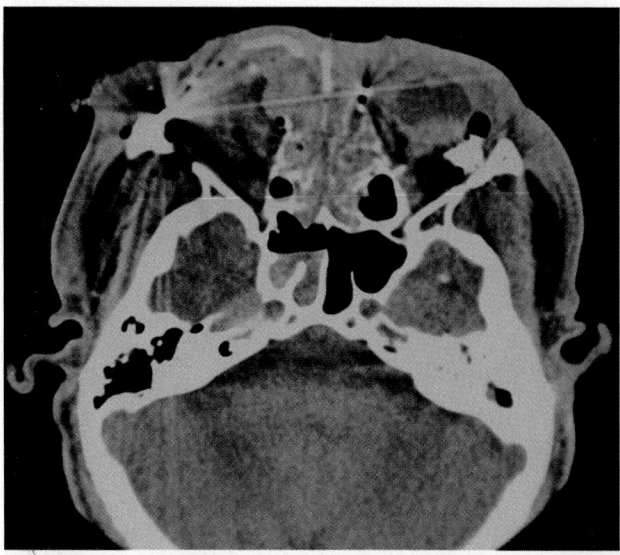

Fig. 62.20 CT scan showing disrupted right globe following a gunshot wound. The left eye was also injured from the concussive effect. Note the vitreous haemorrhage. Photograph by courtesy of Dr William Good.

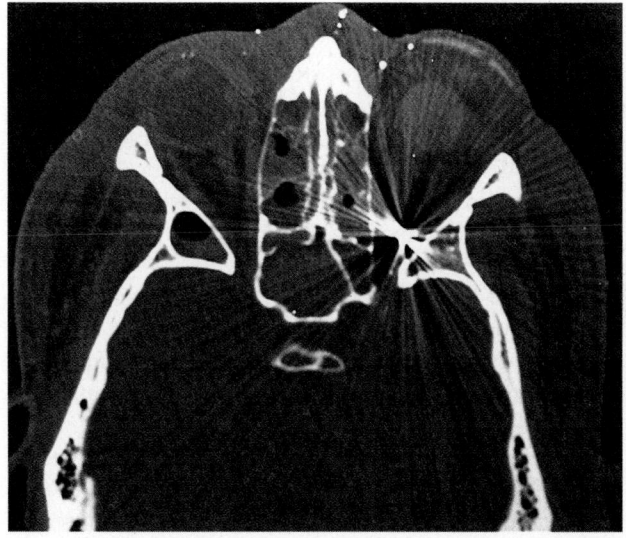

Fig. 62.21 CT scanning is particularly helpful in delineating the presence and location of ocular and orbital foreign bodies: this adolescent was shot in the face with a shotgun.

occur as a result of shifting of intraorbital contents into fractures of the floor or medial wall of the orbit. Enophthalmos may not be apparent in the first few days after trauma due to oedema and swelling in the injured area. Enophthalmos becomes apparent by 5–7 days after injury and should be evaluated at that point. Its management, if cosmetically significant, requires repair of the fracture and replacement of orbital contents in order to reconstitute the orbit to its original volume.

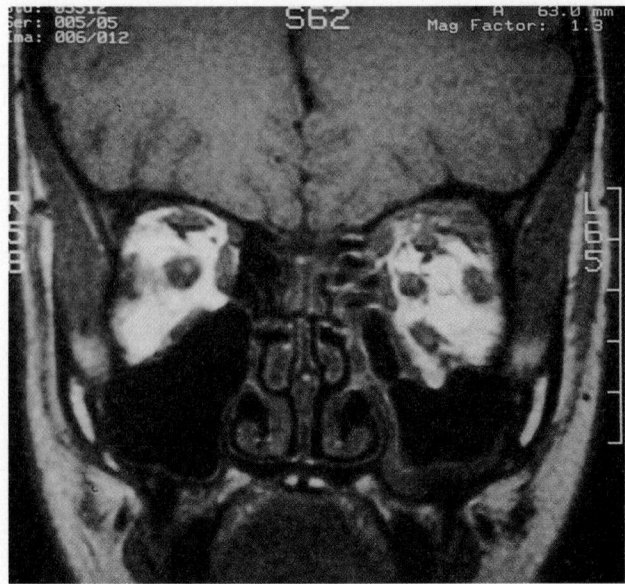

Fig. 62.22 Blow-out fracture showing entrapment of the tissues associated with the inferior rectus in the left orbit.

Strabismus

A second problem is that of strabismus. A variety of strabismus problems can occur after blow-out fracture, including entrapped extraocular muscle, paralysed muscle, actual displacement of the globe in a vertical direction, Brown syndrome, and even cranial nerve injury if the force of the blow damages any of the cranial nerves which innervate the extraocular muscles.

A trapped inferior rectus muscle is the most common cause of strabismus associated with blow-out fracture. The muscle becomes incarcerated in the inferior floor fracture and tethers the eye in a hypotropic position. Most patients experience vertical diplopia, worsening in upgaze. Patients may be able to use their eyes together (fuse) in downgaze. The results of forced duction testing indicate that traction in the upward direction is more difficult in the involved eye than in the uninvolved eye. Treatment usually consists of freeing of an entrapped extraocular muscle, or recession of the inferior rectus muscle of the involved eye.

In some cases, the inferior rectus muscle may be traumatically paralysed or rendered inefficient. In this case, a hypertropia may exist on the involved side, and the problem worsens in downgaze due to inefficiency of the paralysed inferior rectus muscle. Treatment may consist of recession of the contralateral inferior rectus muscle to alleviate the primary gaze problem, and possibly the use of a posterior fixation suture in the contralateral muscle in order to 'match' the downgaze defect in the involved eye.

Occasional cases involve entrapment or tethering of the medial rectus muscle. These cases may emulate a Duane's syndrome because abduction is insufficient and enophthalmos may occur on abduction. Forced duction testing plus radiological evaluation should secure the diagnosis. Treatment consists of freeing the medial rectus muscle and recessing it if the eye is esotropic in primary gaze.

Brown syndrome (limited elevation of the eye in adduction) occurs when damage to the superior oblique trochlea or the superior oblique tendon has occurred. Interestingly, Brown syndrome associated with blow-out fracture or orbital trauma can occur with trauma in any location of the orbit. Therefore, Brown syndrome is not diagnostic of superior orbital damage. Treatment may consist of injection of steroid into the area of the superior oblique tendon, or superior oblique weakening procedures, often accompanied by an inferior oblique weakening procedure in order to alleviate the defect caused by iatrogenic superior oblique palsy.

Large orbital floor fractures may allow periorbital pressure to be transmitted to the orbit, for instance on jaw movement (Brodsky & James 1993).

The third treatment issue with regard to blow-out fractures is whether large fractures should be repaired where there is no functional or cosmetic deficit. Although there is debate, most authorities would not render treatment if there is no functional or cosmetic deficit.

Traumatic optic neuropathy

Aetiology

Traumatic optic neuropathy occurs when head or facial trauma causes direct or indirect injury to the optic nerve. The result is unilateral or bilateral loss of vision, and the vision loss may be partial or complete. Perhaps 5% of all head trauma cases result in damage to the visual axis. Even facial fractures have a high degree of association with optic nerve injury (Gjerris 1976). In a very large series of patients, Turner (1943) demonstrated that 1% of cases of facial fractures result in an optic nerve injury. Frontal bone trauma is most likely to result in optic nerve injury. Even subtle and apparently insignificant frontal head trauma will occasionally involve an optic nerve lesion. The reports of incidence of traumatic optic neuropathy above involve large numbers of adult patients. The exact incidence and risk of optic neuropathy in children is unknown. There is no doubt, however, that children also are susceptible to traumatic optic neuropathy.

There are several possible mechanisms for traumatic optic neuropathy. The first is optic nerve avulsion where the optic nerve is severed or partially severed near its junction with the globe. The usual source of optic nerve avulsion is severe trauma, although mild cases of trauma also have been reported to cause optic nerve avulsion (Hillman *et al.* 1975; Chow *et al.* 1984; Heine 1990). If the fundus can be visualized ophthalmoscopically through clear media, a hole appears in the previous location of the optic nerve head. Sometimes the avulsion can be visualized with a CT scan (Christ *et al.* 1985; Pillai *et al.* 1987). The ultrasonic B scan can also be helpful in demonstrating an avulsed optic nerve and will show a kind of split in the optic nerve head (Talwar *et al.* 1991).

One special circumstance bears mentioning. Patients with severe psychiatric disturbances may attempt to enucleate their own eye and in the process sever the optic nerve at some point in its approach to the globe. If the severance is posterior near the chiasm, a unilateral blindness may be accompanied by a temporal hemianopia in the fellow eye due to chiasmal damage (Krauss *et al.* 1984; Middleton & Smith 1987). Patients who attempt to remove their own eye often experience temporary relief of their psychiatric symptoms if successful; a resurgence of symptoms may lead them to attempt to enucleate their other eye. Such patients should be guarded very closely and their psychotic symptoms should be managed aggressively.

A second mechanism of vision loss is traumatic anterior ischaemic optic neuropathy. The presumed aetiology is closure of one or more posterior ciliary arteries (Hayreh 1975). Thrombosis or transient vasospasm caused by the trauma could play a role in the aetiology.

In some cases an optic sheath haemorrhage results from trauma and causes an optic neuropathy (Hupp *et al.* 1984; Guy *et al.* 1989). In these cases, orbital CT scan or ultrasonography will usually demonstrate enlargement of the optic nerve sheath (Byrne & Glaser 1983). Elucidation of this problem is important because optic nerve sheath fenestration may be helpful in restoring vision or preventing further visual loss (Hupp *et al.* 1984; Mauriello *et al.* 1992).

The most common aetiology of traumatic optic neuropathy is arguably also the most elusive. A posterior traumatic optic neuropathy must be inferred from other aspects of the physical examination, because there are no initial ophthalmoscopic findings.

There are many possible mechanisms for posterior traumatic neuropathy. These include an actual laceration caused by bone fracture, ischaemia, contusion and even haemorrhage (Kline *et al.* 1984). Injuries to the posterior optic nerve can also cause cerebrospinal fluid rhinorrhoea and even disturbances of cerebral or cortical function (McDaniel & McDaniel 1991).

Diagnosis and treatment

The examiner often must rely on signs of unilateral afferent visual dysfunction (afferent pupil defect, diminished colour vision, decreased visual acuity). Unfortunately, many patients who experience such trauma are also neurologically damaged and may not be able to co-operate with a physical examination. The pupillary examination then becomes paramount in establishing the diagnosis.

Treatment of traumatic optic neuropathy can take one of at least three approaches. Although there is increasing evidence that intervention may be useful, in some cases withholding treatment is most sensible, particularly where avulsion is suspected, or where a patient is otherwise so severely injured that surgical or medical intervention is dangerous.

High-dose steroids using methylprednisolone at a dose of 30 mg/kg as an intravenous bolus has been shown to be better than placebo in healing acute spinal cord trauma (Braughler & Hall 1985; Brachen *et al.* 1990). These exceptionally high doses of methylprednisolone may also be efficacious in the treatment of traumatic optic neuropathy (Anderson 1982; Seiff *et al.* 1990; Spoor *et al.* 1990). In the case of traumatic optic neuropathy, doses are 1 mg/kg per day for 72 hours followed by a rapid taper.

A second option involves surgical intervention. Indications include optic sheath haemorrhage, orbital haemorrhage (focal, diffuse or subperiosteal) and an optic canal fracture causing compression of the optic nerve. The role of optic canal decompression or optic nerve defenestration in 'generic' cases of traumatic optic neuropathy is unclear and studies are under way to determine whether surgical intervention is effective in these situations (Seiff 1990; Spoor *et al.* 1990). Transethmoidal decompression may be effective, particularly in younger patients (Levin *et al.* 1994).

Traumatic retrobulbar haemorrhage

Trauma to the eye or orbit will occasionally cause haemorrhage behind the eye. Haemorrhage may be the result of blunt trauma, in which case shearing forces on retrobulbar veins or arteries are suspected. Sharp objects can also penetrate behind the eye without actually injuring the globe itself, and may lacerate blood vessels.

The affected person will have pain with signs of a rapidly increasing mass behind the globe. These signs include proptosis, an increase in intraocular pressure, chemosis and diminished ocular motility.

Trauma is not the only cause of these retro-orbital signs. The clinician should keep in mind that slowly progressive signs may indicate Graves' disease, and that conditions such as orbital cellulitis and traumatic carotid-cavernous fistula can also present in the above-mentioned fashion. Cellulitis may be diagnosed when other signs of infection are present (redness, heat in the area, considerable pain). CT scan usually demonstrates a sinusitis extending into the retro-orbital space, and the patient may have fever and leucocytosis. Carotid-cavernous fistula is suspected when there is pulsating exophthalmos and vessels which appear arterialized in the conjunctiva and retina.

Traumatic retrobulbar haemorrhage occasionally is an

ophthalmic emergency. When the intraocular pressure is elevated and affecting optic nerve function (as demonstrated by decreased visual acuity, decreased colour vision or by an afferent pupil defect) the pressure must be lowered immediately. If there is no visual dysfunction, the pressure can be lowered urgently with medications that may have a more delayed onset of action.

Intraocular pressure can be lowered rapidly (within 1 hour) with carbonic anhydrase inhibitors (acetazolamide) and hyperosmotic agents. A lateral canthotomy can relieve retrobulbar pressure almost immediately. The lateral canthus is excised aggressively to allow orbital contents to shift anteriorly.

Although aqueous paracentesis occasionally is recommended as another method for lowering intraocular pressure, it probably has only a short-term benefit and exposes the patient to the risk of cataract or intraocular infection.

Central nervous system trauma

Prolonged cortical visual impairment following trauma

Many possible mechanisms can account for prolonged cortical visual impairment after head trauma. Trauma that would cause a seizure could then lead to impaired vision on a cortical basis. In addition, a cerebral contusion could result in generalized cerebral oedema and this could cause both transient or prolonged cortical visual impairment (Courville 1953; Browder *et al.* 1961). Increased cerebral oedema could cause the compression of the posterior cerebral arteries which in turn could lead to vascular insufficiency to the visual cortex (Lindenberg 1955; Hoyt 1960). One last possible mechanism invokes the watershed zones between the three major cerebral arteries (anterior, middle and posterior). These zones are most vulnerable to severe hypoxia and/or ischaemia, and damage there may result in cortical visual impairment. Central nervous system hypoxic ischaemia could be a sequel to either generalized trauma with blood loss or even central nervous system vasospasm resulting from more localized trauma. The occipital region is quite susceptible to hypoxia (Courville 1958). Thus, the occipital region of the brain may be selectively involved in events that result in hypoxia and ischaemia.

The shaken baby syndrome may also result in cortical visual impairment. In the situation where the shaken baby syndrome is suspected, the baby's eyes should be examined very carefully for the concurrent finding of retinal haemorrhages (Han & Wilkinson 1990).

Cortical visual impairment following cardiac surgery

Cortical blindness or visual impairment is a well-recognized complication of cardiac surgery. The cause

is not known, although embolism by air or fat has been suspected. The prognosis is usually good.

Post-traumatic transient cortical visual impairment

Cortical visual impairment can be defined as complete, or nearly complete, loss of vision with normal pupillary reflexes, and a normal fundus examination (Whiting *et al.* 1985; Good *et al.* 1994). Cortical visual impairment in children may differ in its manifestations from cortical blindness in adults (Good *et al.* 1994). Children show fluctuating vision, a preference for observing colour (versus black and white), light gazing and, occasionally, photophobia.

A relatively minor blow to the head can cause transient cortical blindness (Rodriguez *et al.* 1993). The type of injury that can cause transient cortical blindness is usually a blow to the parieto-occipital region (Griffith & Dodge 1968; Hass *et al.* 1975). Alpha rhythm may be suppressed for transient periods after a head trauma.

The clinical picture accompanying transient visual loss is diffuse, and usually nearly complete, visual field loss, with visual acuity loss, along with signs and symptoms of migraine. For example, many children will show headache, irritability, nausea and even vomiting (Mitchel & Troost 1980). In fact, the similarities between transient cortical visual impairment and migraine in children have been commented upon by many authorities (Hass *et al.* 1975; Hass & Sovner 1969; Kaye & Herskowitz 1986).

Traumatic cranial neuropathy

Non-fatal head injuries result in cranial neuropathy as much as 13% of the time (Baker & Epstein 1991). The sixth cranial nerve is most commonly traumatized, with the third cranial nerve next in incidence, followed by the fourth cranial nerve (Rush & Younge 1981). Most cases of traumatic cranial neuropathy occur between the ages of 16 and 25 years, but a wide age range can be involved, including even very young children (Kowal 1992).

Diagnosis

In sixth nerve palsy, difficulty or inability to abduct the involved eye is noted. The patient demonstrates a large angle esotropia (usually greater than 30 prism dioptres) in primary gaze. Bilateral sixth nerve palsies can occur, and should be searched for.

Complete third nerve palsies cause dilated pupil, complete ptosis and inability to abduct, depress or elevate the eye. The resulting eye position is one of exotropia and slight hypotropia. Partial third nerve palsies may occur, and affect the individual oculomotor nerve.

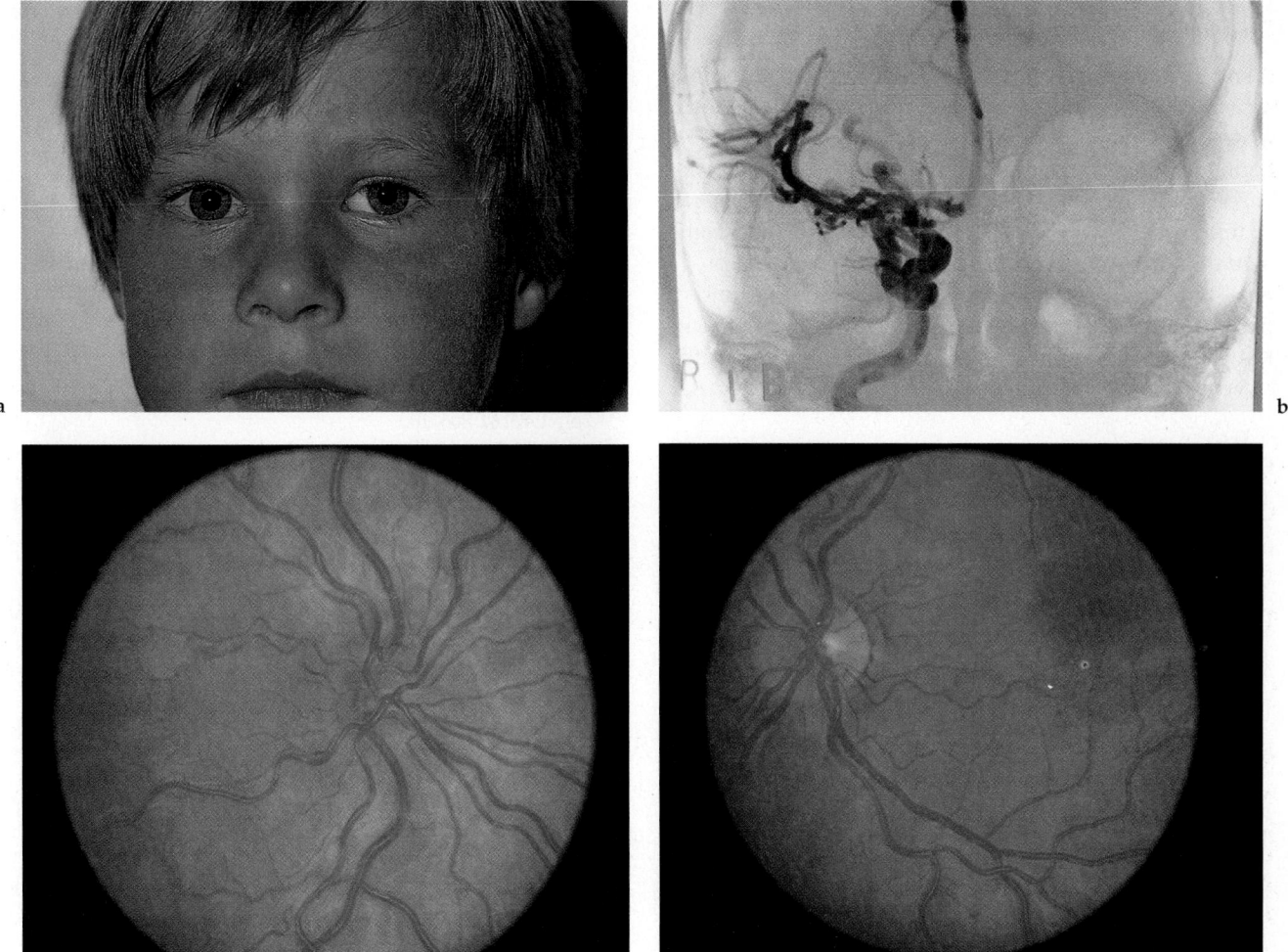

Fig. 62.23 (a) This 5.5-year-old boy developed right proptosis and a squeaky bruit a week after a severe road traffic accident. (b) Carotid angiogram showing the shunt which was later closed with a balloon catheter. Dilated episcleral veins can be seen on the right. Retinal venous congestion and tortuosity with optic disc oedema on the right (c, d).

Traumatic fourth nerve palsies may be unilateral or bilateral. Unilateral cases typically show a hypertropia in primary gaze with inferior oblique overaction. Patients may demonstrate excyclotorsion of the eye, and cyclotorsional double vision up to 8°. Bilateral fourth nerve palsies occur in as many as 30% of cases (Snydor *et al.* 1982). Bilaterality is suggested by the following physical findings: (i) a 'V' pattern esotropia greater than 25 prism dioptres; (ii) alternating hyperdeviation (right hypertropia on right head tilt, and left hypertropia on left head tilt) (Jampolsky 1986); and (iii) an excyclotorsion which exceeds 15° (Ellis & Helveston 1976).

Management

Recovery of cranial nerve function occurs in about 40% of cases when all cases are pooled (Rush & Younge 1981). The prognosis for recovery of a traumatic fourth nerve palsy is a little better (47%), with sixth nerve palsy at 38.6% or third nerve palsy at 36.2% (Rush & Younge 1981).

Neuroimaging is often indicated when a cranial neuropathy is present. MRI is probably more sensitive in detecting subtle intraparenchymal lesions or haemorrhages. The CT scan could be more helpful in discerning skull fractures, which could contribute to the development of the cranial neuropathy.

Management of double vision includes monocular patching and the use of prisms. Most authorities would choose to wait 6 months before considering surgical management. The use of botulism neurotoxin may alleviate symptoms of double vision, at least in primary gaze, in the most acute traumatic period of sixth nerve palsy.

Disorders of accommodation following head trauma

A surprising number of patients will complain of trouble focusing their eyes following head trauma (Kowal 1992). In Kowal's study of referrals to an oculomotility service in Melbourne, Australia, the most common abnormality was paresis of accommodation with no other ocular signs or symptoms. Half of the patients who had trouble accommodating improved within a year. After a year, the prognosis for recovery dropped considerably, and many patients required prolonged reading add treatment. Kowal also noted the occurrence of convergence insufficiency in some of his patients.

Carotid-cavernous fistula

Carotid-cavernous fistulas are rare in children but may occur following severe trauma (Fig. 62.23).

References

Admoni MM, Ben-Ezra D. Ocular trauma following amniocentesis as the cause of leukocoria. *J Pediatr Ophthalmol Strabismus* 1988; **25**: 196–7.

Alfaro DV, Chaudhry NA, Walonker AF, Runyan T, Saito Y, Liggett PPE. Penetrating eye injuries in young children. *Retina* 1994; **14**: 201–5.

American Psychiatric Association. *Diagnostic and Statistical Manual of Mental Disorders*, 3rd edn. Washington DC: American Psychiatric Association, 1980: 288–90.

Anderson RL, Panje WR, Gross CE. Optic nerve blindness following blunt forehead trauma. *Ophthalmology* 1982; **89**: 445–55.

Angra SK, Vajpayee RV, Titayal JS *et al.* Types of posterior capsule breaks and their surgical management. *Ophthalmic Surg* 1991; **22**: 388–91.

Anwar M, Bleik J, von Noorden G, El-Maghraby A, Attia F. Posterior chamber lens implantationfor primary repair of corneal lacerations and traumatic cataracts in children. *J Pediatr Ophthalmol Strabismus* 1994; **31**: 157–61.

Aron JJ, Marx P, Blanck MF *et al.* Ocular symptoms observed in Silverman's syndrome. *Ann Ocul* 1970; **203**: 533–46.

Aycub C, Pfeifer D. The prophylaxis of child abuse and neglect. *Child Abuse Negl* 1977; **1**: 71–5.

Bachynski BN, Andreu R, Flynn JR. Spontaneous corneal perforation and extrusion of intraocular contents in premature infants. *J Pediatr Ophthalmol Strabismus* 1986; **23**: 25–8.

Baker RS, Epstein AD. Ocular motor abnormalities from head trauma. *Surv Ophthalmol* 1991; **35**: 245–67.

Balyeat RM. Complete retinal detachment (both eyes): with special reference to allergy as a possible primary etiologic factor. *Am J Ophthalmol* 1937; **20**: 580–2.

Baum JD, Bulpitt CJ. Retinal and conjunctival hemorrhage in the newborn. *Arch Dis Child* 1970; **45**: 344–9.

Baxter RJ, Hodgkins PR, Calder I, Morrell AJ, Vardy S, Elkington AR. Visual outcome of childhood anterior perforating eye injuries: prognostic indicators. *Eye* 1994; **8**: 349–52.

Biglan AW, Brown SI, Johnson BL. Keratoglobus and blue sclera. *Am J Ophthalmol* 1977; **83**: 225–33.

Billmire ME, Myers PA. Serious head injury in infants: accidental abuse? *Pediatrics* 1985; **75**: 340–2.

Blanton FM. Anterior chamber angle recession and secondary glaucoma, a study of the after-effects of traumatic hyphemas. *Arch Ophthalmol* 1964; **72**: 39–42.

Blight R, Hart JCD. Structural changes in the outer retinal layers following blunt, mechanical, non-perforating trauma to the globe: an experimental study. *Br J Ophthalmol* 1977; **61**: 573.

Bools CN, Neale BA, Meadow SR. Follow-up of victims of fabricated illness (Munchausen syndrome by proxy). *Arch Dis Child* 1993; **69**: 625–30.

Brachen MB, Shepard MJ, Collins WF *et al.* A randomized, controlled trial of methylprednisolone or naloxone in the treatment of acute spinal-cord injury. Results of the Second National Acute Spinal Cord Injury Study. *N Engl J Med* 1990; **322**: 1405–11.

Braughler JM, Hall ED. Current application of 'high-dose' steroid therapy for CNS injury. A pharmacological perspective. *J Neurosurg* 1985; **62**: 806–10.

Brodsky M, James C. Ocular protrusion with contralateral jaw movement. *Arch Ophthalmol* 1993; **111**: 1028–9.

Browder EJ, Kaplan HA, Baldwin M *et al.* Cerebral concussion and its sequelae. *NY State J Med* 1961; **61**: 1864–1903.

Burton TC. Unilateral Purtscher's retinopathy. *Ophthalmology* 1980; **87**: 1096.

Buys Y, Levin A, Enzenaver R *et al.* Retinal findings after head trauma in infants and young children. *Ophthalmology* 1992; **99**: 1718–23.

Byrne SF, Glaser JS. Orbital tissue differentiation with standardized echography. *Ophthalmology* 1983; **90**: 1071–90.

Caffey J. Multiple fractures in the long bones of infants suffering from chronic subdural hematoma. *Am J Roentgenol Radiat Ther* 1946; **56**: 163–73.

Caffey J. On the theory and practice of shaking infants: its potential residual effects of permanent brain damage and mental retardation. *Am J Dis Child* 1972; **124**: 161–9.

Cameron JA. Corneal abnormalities of the Ehlers–Danlos syndrome type VI. *Cornea* 1993; **12**: 54–9.

Canavan VM, O'Flaherty MJ, Archer DB, Elwood JH. A 10-year survey of eye injuries in northern Ireland, 1967–76. *Br J Ophthalmol* 1980; **64**: 618–25.

Carty H. Brittle or battered? *Arch Dis Child* 1988; **63**: 350–2.

Cascairo M, Mazow M, Prager T. Pediatric ocular trauma: a retrospective survey. *J Pediatr Ophthalmol Strabismus* 1994; **31**: 312–17.

Chan CC, Green WR, de la Cruz ZC, Hillis A. Ocular findings in osteogenesis imperfecta congenita. *Arch Ophthalmol* 1982; **100**: 1459–63.

Chow AY, Goldberg MF, Frenkel M. Evulsion of the optic nerve in association with basketball injuries. *Ann Ophthalmol* 1984; **16**: 35–47.

Christ T, Pillunat L, Wagner P. Computerized tomography in partial avulsion of the optic nerve. *Klin Monatsbl Augenheilkd* 1985; **187**: 531–3.

Converse JM, Smith B. Blow-out fracture of the floor of the orbit. *Trans Am Acad Ophthalmol Otolaryngol* 1960; **64**: 676–88.

Courville CB. *Commotio Cerebri*. Los Angeles: San Lucas Press, 1953: 63.

Courville CB. Etiology and pathogenesis of laminar cortical necrosis. *Arch Neurol Psych* 1958; **70**: 7–30.

Cox MS, Schepens CL, Freeman HM. Retinal detachment due to ocular contusion. *Arch Ophthalmol* 1966; **76**: 678–85.

Department of Health and Social Security (DHSS) and Welsh Office. *Working Together: A Guide to Arrangements for Inter-agency Co-operation for the Protection of Children from Abuse.* London: Her Majesty's Stationery Office, 1988.

Dorfman MS, Benson WH. Marginal eyelid laceration after episiotomy. *Am J Ophthalmol* 1993; **116**: 778.

Drack A, Kutschke P, Stair S, Scott W. Compliance with safety glasses wear in monocular children. *J Pediatr Ophthalmol Strabismus* 1993; **30**: 249–52.

Eagling EM. Perforating injuries of the eye. *Br J Ophthalmol* 1976; **60**: 732–6.

Elder JE, Taylor RG, Klug GL. Retinal haemorrhage in accidental head trauma in childhood. *J Paediatr Child Health* 1991; **27**: 286–9.

Ellis FD, Helveston EM. Superior oblique palsy: diagnosis and classification. In: *Strabismus Surgery*. Boston: Little, Brown, 1976: 127–35.

Elner SG, Elner VM, Arnall M, Albert DM. Ocular and associated systemic findings in suspected child abuse: a necropsy study. *Arch Ophthalmol* 1990; **108**: 1094–102.

Eminson D, Postlewaite R. Factitious illness: recognition and management. *Arch Dis Child* 1992; **67**: 1510–16.

Epstein RJ, Fernandez A, Gammon JA. The correction of aphakia in infants with hydrogel extended wear contact lenses. *Ophthalmology* 1988; **95**: 1102–6.

Ferrone P, de Juan E. Vitreous hemorrhage in infants. *Arch Ophthalmol* 1994; **112**: 1185–9.

Finnegan JA, Quarrington BJ, Hughes HE *et al.* Infant outcome following mid-trimester amniocentesis: development and physical status at age six months. *Br J Obstet Gynaecol* 1985; **92**: 1015–23.

Finucane BM, Jaeger ER, Kurtz MB, Weinstein M, Scott CI Jr. Eye abnormalities in the Smith–Magenis contiguous gene deletion syndrome. *Am J Med Genet* 1993a; **45**: 443–6.

Finucane BM, Kurtz MB, Babu VR, Scott CI Jr. Mosaicism for deletion 17p11.2 in a boy with the Smith–Magenis syndrome. *Am J Med Genet* 1993b; **45**: 447–9.

Fisher GC, Mitchell I. Is Munchausen syndrome by proxy really a syndrome? *Arch Dis Child* 1995; **72**: 530–4.

Folks DG, Ford CV, Houck CA. Somatoform disorders, factitious disorders and malingering. In: Stoudemire A, ed. *Clinical Psychiatry for Medical Students*. Philadelphia: JB Lippincott, 1990.

Folks DG, Houck CA. Somatoform disorders, factitious disorders, and malingering. In: Stoudemire A, Fogel BS, eds. *Psychiatric Care of the Medical Patient*. Toronto: Oxford University Press, 1993.

Friendly DS. Ocular manifestations of physical child abuse. *Trans Am Acad Ophthalmol Otolaryngol* 1971; **75**: 318–32.

Fujino T. Experimental 'blow-out' fracture of the orbit. *Plast Reconstr Surg* 1974; **56**: 81.

Gass JDM. 'Berlin's edema'. In: *Stereoscopic Atlas of Macular Diseases: Diagnosis and Treatment*, 3rd edn. St Louis: CV Mosby, 1987: 552.

Gaynon MW, Koh K, Marmor MF *et al.* Retinal folds in the shaken baby syndrome. *Am J Ophthalmol* 1988; **106**: 432–5.

Gilliland MG, Luckenbach MW, Massicotte SJ *et al.* The medicolegal implications of detecting hemosiderin in the eyes of children who are suspected of being abused. *Arch Ophthalmol* 1991; **109**: 321–3.

Giraud P. Alternations vasculaires retineinnes d'origine riskettsienne. *Bull Soc Fr Ophtalmol* 1959; **72**: 621–31.

Gjerris F. Traumatic lesions of the visual pathways. In: Vinken PJ, Bruyn CW, eds. *Handbook of Clinical Neurology*, Vol. 24. Amsterdam: North Holland, 1976: 27–57.

Goetting MG, Sowa B. Retinal hemorrhage after cardiopulmonary resuscitation in children: an etiologic reevaluation. *Pediatrics* 1990; **85**: 585–8.

Good WV. Monocular nystagmus caused by unilateral vision loss. *Dev Med Child Neurol* 1993; **35**: 1100–6.

Good WV, Jan JE, DeSa L, Barkovich AJ, Groenveld M, Hoyt CS. Cortical visual impairment in children. *Surv Ophthalmol* 1994; **38**: 351–64.

Gray JD, Cutler C, Dean J *et al.* Prediction and prevention of child abuse and neglect. *J Soc Issues* 1979; **35**: 127–39.

Greenwald MJ, Weiss A, Oesterle CS *et al.* Traumatic retinoschisis in

battered babies. *Ophthalmology* 1986; **93**: 618–25.

Grey RHB. Foveo-macular retinitis, solar retinopathy, and trauma. *Br J Ophthalmol* 1978; **62**: 543.

Griffith JF, Dodge PR. Transient blindness following head injury in children. *N Engl J Med* 1968; **278**: 648–51.

Guy J, Sherwood M, Day AL. Surgical treatment of progressive visual loss in traumatic optic neuropathy. *J Neurosurg* 1989; **70**: 799–801.

Hamed LM, Fang EN. Inferior rectus muscle contracture resulting from perinatal orbital trauma. *J Pediatr Ophthalmol Strabismus* 1992; **29**: 387–9.

Han DP, Wilkinson WS. Late ophthalmic manifestations of the shaken baby syndrome. *J Pediatr Ophthalmol Strabismus* 1990; **27**: 299–303.

Hass DC, Pineda GS, Lourie H. Juvenile head trauma syndromes and their relationship to migraine. *Arch Neurol* 1975; **32**: 727–30.

Hass DC, Sovner RD. Migraine attacks triggered by mild head trauma and their relation to certain post-traumatic disorders of childhood. *J Neurol Neurosurg Psych* 1969; **32**: 548–54.

Hayreh SS. *Anterior Ischemic Optic Neuropathy*. Berlin: Springer-Verlag, 1975: 12–23.

Heine J. Optic nerve evulsion. *Klin Monatsbl Augeheilkd* 1990; **196**: 484–5.

Hershey D. Ocular injury from amniocentesis. *Ophthalmology* 1993; **100**: 1601–2.

Hershey BL, Zimmerman RA. Pediatric brain computed tomography. *Pediatr Clin North Am* 1985; **32**: 1477–508.

Hillman JS, Myska V, Nissim S. Complete avulsion of the optic nerve. A clinical, angiographic, and electrodiagnostic study. *Br J Ophthalmol* 1975; **59**: 503–9.

Hobbs CJ. Skull fracture and the diagnosis of abuse. *Arch Dis Child* 1984; **56**: 246–52.

Hollenhorst RW, Stein HA. Ocular signs and prognosis in subdural and subarachnoid bleeding in young children. *Arch Ophthalmol* 1958; **60**: 187–92.

Hoyt CS. Cryotherapy for retinopathy of prematurity: 3.5 year outcome for both structure and function. *Arch Ophthalmol* 1993; **111**: 319–20.

Hoyt WF. Vascular lesions of the visual cortex with brain herniation through the tentorial incisura. *Arch Ophthalmol* 1960; **64**: 44–57.

Hupp SL, Buckley EG, Burne SF, Tenzel RR, Glaser JS, Schatz NS. Post-traumatic venous obstructive retinopathy associated with enlarged optic nerve sheath. *Arch Ophthalmol* 1984; **102**: 254–6.

Ilsar M, Chirambo M, Belkin M. Ocular injuries in Malawi. *Br J Ophthalmol* 1982; **66**: 145–8.

Isenberg SJ, Heckenlively JR. Traumatized eye with retinal damage from amniocentesis. *J Pediatr Ophthalmol Strabismus* 1985; **22**: 65–7.

Jain IS, Mohan K, Gupta A. Unilateral traumatic aphakia in children: role of corneal contact lenses. *J Pediatr Ophthalmol Strabismus* 1985; **22**: 137–9.

Jain IS, Singh YP, Gupta SL, Gupta A. Ocular hazards during birth. *J Pediatr Ophthalmol Strabismus* 1980; **17**: 14.

James D, Ward K. Child abuse registers (letter). *Lancet* 1988; **i**: 1398.

Jameson N, Good WV, Hoyt CS. Fat adherence simulating inferior oblique palsy after blepharoplasty. *Arch Ophthalmol* 1992; **110**: 1369.

Jampolsky A. Management of vertical strabismus. In: Crawford JS, Flynn JT, Haik BG *et al.* eds. *Pediatric Ophthalmology and Strabismus. Transactions of the New Orleans Academy of Ophthalmology*. New York: Raven Press, 1986: 141–71.

Jan JE, Good WF, Freeman RD, Espezel H. Eye-poking. *Dev Med Child Neurol* 1994; **36**: 321–5.

Jay J, Grant S, Murray S. Keratoconjunctivitis artefacta. *Br J Ophthalmol* 1982; **66**: 781–5.

Jensen AD, Smith RE, Olson MI. Ocular clues to child abuse. *J Pediatr*

Ophthalmol Strabismus 1971; **8**: 270–2.

Karr DJ, Scott WE. Visual acuity results following treatment of persistent hyperplastic primary vitreous. *Arch Ophthalmol* 1986; **104**: 662–7.

Kauffman ML. Retinal hemorrhages in the newborn. *Am J Ophthalmol* 1958; **46**: 658–60.

Kaur B, Taylor D. Fundus hemorrhages in infancy. *Surv Ophthalmol* 1992; **37**: 1–17.

Kaye EM, Herskowitz J. Transient post-traumatic cortical blindness: brief versus prolonged syndromes in childhood. *J Child Neurol* 1986; **1**: 206–10.

Keithahn M, Bennett S, Cameron D, Mieler W. Retinal folds in Terson syndrome. *Ophthalmology* 1993; **100**: 1187–90.

Kelley JS, Hoover RE, George T. Whiplash maculopathy. *Arch Ophthalmol* 1978; **92**: 834.

Kempe CH, Silverman RN, Steele BF, Droegemueller W, Silver HK. The battered child syndrome. *J Am Med Assoc* 1962; **181**: 17–24.

Kersten RC. Blow-out fracture of the orbital floor with entrapment caused by isolated trauma to the orbital rim. *Am J Ophthalmol* 1987; **103**: 215–20.

Kiffney GT. The eye of the 'battered child'. *Arch Ophthalmol* 1964; **72**: 231–3.

Kirschner RH, Stein RJ. The mistaken diagnosis of child abuse. A form of medical abuse? *Am J Dis Child* 1985; **139**: 873–5.

Kline LB, Morawetz RB, Swaid SN. Indirect injury of the optic nerve. *Neurosurgery* 1984; **14**: 756–64.

Kowal L. Ophthalmic manifestations of head injury. *Aust NZ J Ophthalmol* 1992; **20**: 35–40.

Kraft SP *et al.* Traumatic hyphema in children: treatment with epsilon-amino caproic acid. *Ophthalmology* 1987; **94**: 1232–7.

Krauss HR, Yee RD, Foos RY. Autoenucleation. *Surv Ophthalmol* 1984; **29**: 179–87.

Kushner BJ. Grating acuity tests should not be used for social service purposes in preliterate children (editorial). *Arch Ophthalmol* 1994; **112**: 1030–1.

Lambert SR, Johnson TE, Hoyt CS. Optic nerve sheath and retinal hemorrhages associated with the shaken baby syndrome. *Arch Ophthalmol* 1986; **104**: 1509–12.

LaRoche GR, McIntyre L, Schertzer RN. Epidemiology of severe eye injuries in childhood. *Ophthalmology* 1988; **95**: 1603–7.

Lavin PJM, Troost BT. Traumatic fourth nerve palsy: clinicoanatomic correlations with computed tomographic scan. *Arch Neurol* 1984; **41**: 52–60.

Levin L, Joseph M, Rizzo J, Lessell S. Optic canal decompression in indirect optic nerve trauma. *Ophthalmology* 1994; **101**: 566–9.

Lindenberg R. Compression of brain arteries as pathogenetic factor for tissue necrosis and their area of predilection. *J Neuropathol Exp Neurol* 1955; **14**: 223–43.

Little B, Aylward G. The medical management of traumatic hyphaema: a survey of opinion among ophthalmologists in the UK. *J Roy Soc Med* 1993; **86**: 458–9.

Lorber J, Reckless JP, Watson JB. Non-accidental poisoning, the elusive diagnosis. *Arch Dis Child* 1980; **55**: 643–7.

Luff A, Hodgkins P, Baxter R, Morrell A, Calder I. Aetiology of perforating eye injury. *Arch Dis Child* 1993; **68**: 682–3.

Lyle DJ, Stapp JP, Button RR. Ophthalmologic hydrostatic pressure syndrome. *Am J Ophthalmol* 1957; **44**: 652–6.

McDaniel KD, McDaniel LD. Anton's syndrome in a patient with post-traumatic optic neuropathy and bifrontal contusions. *Arch Neurol* 1991; **48**: 101–5.

McDonald M, Burgess S. Contralateral occipital depression related to obstetric forceps injury to the eye. *Am J Ophthalmol* 1992; **114**: 318–21.

McLachlan DL, Flanagan JC, Shannon GM. Complications of orbital roof fractures. *Ophthalmology* 1982; **89**: 1274–8.

Marcus DM, Albert DM. Recognizing child abuse. *Arch Ophthalmol* 1992; **110**: 766–8.

Martin D, Awh C, McCven B, Jaffe G, Scott J, Machemer R. Treatment and pathogenesis of traumatic chorioretinal rupture (sclopetaria). *Am J Ophthalmol* 1994; **117**: 190–200.

Massicotte SJ, Folberg R, Torczynski E, Gilliland MGF, Luckenbach MW. Vitreoretinal traction and perimacular folds in the eyes of deliberately traumatised children. *Ophthalmology* 1991; **98**: 1124–7.

Mauriello JA, DeLuca J, Krieger A, Schulder M, Frohman L. Management of traumatic optic neuropathy—a study of 23 patients. *Br J Ophthalmol* 1992; **76**: 349–52.

Meadow R. What is, and what is not 'Munchausen syndrome by proxy'? *Arch Dis Child* 1995; **72**: 534–8.

Merin S, Beyth Y. Uniocular congenital blindness as a complication of midtrimester amniocentesis. *Am J Ophthalmol* 1980; **89**: 299–301.

Merton DF, Radkowski MA, Leonidas JC. The abused child, a radiological reappraisal. *Radiology* 1983; **146**: 377–82.

Middleton TH III, Smith RR. Optic nerve avulsion secondary to traumatic enucleation. *Neurosurgery* 1987; **21**: 89–91.

Milunsky A. Risk of amniocentesis for prenatal diagnosis (editorial). *N Engl J Med* 1975; **293**: 932–3.

Mitchel EM, Troost BT. Palinopsia: cerebral localization with computed tomography. *Neurology* 1980; **30**: 887–9.

Moreira CA, Debert-Ribeiro M, Belfort R. Epidemiological study of eye injuries in Brazilian children. *Arch Ophthalmol* 1988; **106**: 781–4.

Morley CJ. Practical concerns about the diagnosis of Munchausen syndrome by proxy. *Arch Dis Child* 1995; **72**: 528–30.

Morris R, Witherspoon CD, Kuhn F, Brown S. *Epidemiology of Pediatric Injuries from the Injury Registry of Alabama (ERA). Presented at the First International Symposium of Ophthalmology.* Bordeaux, France, 9–11 September, 1993.

Muller PJ, Deck JHN. Intraocular and optic nerve sheath hemorrhage in cases of sudden intracranial hypertension. *J Neurosurg* 1974; **41**: 160–6.

Mushin A, Morgan G. Ocular injury in the battered baby syndrome. *Br J Ophthalmol* 1971; **55**: 343–7.

Myers C, Christmann L. Rat bite—an unusual cause of direct trauma to the globe. *J Pediatr Ophthalmol Strabismus* 1991; **28**: 356–8.

National Society for the Prevention of Blindness. *Vision Problems in the United States. National Society for the Prevention of Blindness.* New York: National Society for the Prevention of Blindness, 1980.

Naylor G, Roper JP, Willshaw HE. Ophthalmic complications of amniocentesis. *Eye* 1990; **4**: 845–9.

Newton RW. Intracranial haemorrhage and non-accidental injury. *Arch Dis Child* 1989; **64**: 188–90.

Niiranen M, Raivio I. Eye injuries in children. *Br J Ophthalmol* 1981; **65**: 436–8.

Oates RK. Personality development and physical abuse. *Arch Dis Child* 1984; **59**: 147–50.

O'Hare AE, Eden OB. Bleeding disorders and non-accidental injury. *Arch Dis Child* 1984; **59**: 860–4.

Oka C, Ideta H, Nagasaki H, Watanabe K, Shinagawa K. Retinal detachment with atopic dermatitis similar to traumatic retinal detachment. *Ophthalmology* 1994; **101**: 1050–4.

Olver JM, Hague S. Children presenting to an ophthalmic casualty department. *Eye* 1989; **3**: 415–19.

Palmer DJ *et al.* A comparison of two dose regimens of epsilon-amino caproic acid in the prevention and management of secondary traumatic hyphemas. *Ophthalmology* 1986; **93**: 102–8.

Pashby T. Eye injuries in Canadian amateur hockey. *Can J Ophthalmol* 1985; **20**: 2–4.

Patel CK, Taylor DSI, Russell-Eggitt IM, Kriss A, Demaerel P. Congenital third nerve palsy associated with mid-trimester amniocentesis. *Br J Ophthalmol* 1993; **77**: 530–3.

Pfeiffer RL. Traumatic enophthalmos. *Arch Ophthalmol* 1943; **30**: 718–26.

Pillai S, Mahmood MA, Limaye SR. Complete avulsion of the globe and optic nerve. *Br J Ophthalmol* 1987; **71**: 69–72.

Pinnel SR, Krane SM, Kenzora JE, Glimcher MJ. A heritable disorder of connective tissue: hydroxylysine-deficient collagen disease. *N Engl J Med* 1972; **286**: 1013–20.

Pulido JS, Lingua RW, Cristol S, Byrne SF. Protein C deficiency associated with vitreous hemorrhage in a neonate. *Am J Ophthalmol* 1987; **104**: 546–7.

Quinn G. Vitreous and retina. In: Isenberg SJ, ed. *The Eye in Infancy*. Chicago: Yearbook Medical Publishers, 1989: 350–1.

Rapoport I, Romen M, Kinek M *et al*. Eye injuries in children in Israel: a national collaborative study. *Arch Ophthalmol* 1990; **108**: 376–9.

Riffenburgh R, Sathyavagiswaran L. Ocular findings at autopsy of child abuse victims. *Ophthalmology* 1991; **98**: 1519–24.

Riise R, Kolstad A, Brum S, Espeland A. The use of contact lenses in children with unilateral traumatic aphakia. *Acta Ophthalmol* 1977; **55**: 386–94.

Robertson M, Doran M, Trimble M, Lees AJ. The treatment of Gilles de la Tourette syndrome by limbic leucotomy. *J Neurol Neurosurg Psych* 1990; **53**: 691–4.

Rodriguez A, Lozanoa JA, DelPozo D, Paez JH. Post-traumatic transient cortical visual blindness. *Int Ophthalmol* 1993; **17**: 277–83.

Rudd J, Jaeger E, Freitag S, Jeffers J. Traumatically ruptured globes in children. *J Pediatr Ophthalmol Strabismus* 1994; **31**: 307–11.

Ruedemann AD Jr. Osteogenesis imperfecta congenita and blue sclerotics. *Arch Ophthalmol* 1953; **49**: 6–16.

Rummelt B, Rummelt C, Gottfried O, Naumann H. Congenital nonpigmented epithelial iris cyst after amniocentesis. *Ophthalmology* 1993; **100**: 776–81.

Rush JA, Younge BR. Paralysis of cranial nerves III, IV, and VI. Cause and prognosis in 1000 cases. *Arch Ophthalmol* 1981; **99**: 76–9.

Rynne MD, Romano PE. Systemic corticosteroids and the treatment of traumatic hyphema. *J Pediatr Ophthalmol Strabismus* 1980; **17**: 141–3.

Sachs D, Levin PS, Dooley K. Marginal eyelid laceration at birth. *Am J Ophthalmol* 1986; **102**: 539.

Satterfield D, Keltner JL, Morrison TL. Psychosocial aspects of strabismus study. *Arch Ophthalmol* 1993; **111**: 1100–4.

Scharf J, Zonis S. Perforating injuries of the eye in childhood. *J Pediatr Ophthalmol* 1975; **13**: 326–8.

Schein OD, Enger C, Tielsch JM. The context and consequences of ocular injuries from air guns. *Am J Ophthalmol* 1994; **117**: 501–6.

Schwer W, Brueschke EE, Dent T. Hemophilia. *J Fam Pract* 1982; **14**: 661–4.

Sedlak A. *A Study of National Incidence and Prevalence of Childhood Abuse and Neglect*. Bethesda, MD: Westat, 1987.

Seiff SR. High dose corticosteroids for treatment of vision loss due to indirect injury to the optic nerve. *Ophthalmic Surg* 1990; **21**: 389–95.

Shapiro MB. Lightning cataracts. *Wis Med J* 1984; **83**: 23–4.

Shaw JC. Copper deficiency and non-accidental injury. *Arch Dis Child* 1988; **63**: 448–55.

Sipperly JO, Quigley HA, Gass JDM. Traumatic retinopathy in primates: the explanation of comotio retinae. *Arch Ophthalmol* 1978; **96**: 2267–70.

Smith B, Regan WF Jr. Blow-out fracture of the orbit; mechanism and correction of internal orbital fracture. *Am J Ophthalmol* 1957; **44**: 733–9.

Snydor CF, Seaber BA, Buckley EG. Traumatic superior oblique

palsies. *Ophthalmology* 1982; **89**: 134–8.

Soumenkoff G, Marnefe C, Gerard M *et al*. A coordinated attempt for prevention of child abuse at the antenatal care level. *Child Abuse Negl* 1981; **6**: 87–94.

Spevak MR, Kleinman PK, Belanger PL, Primack C, Richmond JM. Cardiopulmonary resuscitation and rib fractures in infants: A postmortem radiologic-pathologic study. *J Am Med Assoc* 1994; **272**: 617–18.

Spoor TC, Hartel WC, Lensink DB, Wilkinson MJ. Treatment of traumatic optic neuropathy with corticosteroids. *Am J Ophthalmol* 1990; **110**: 665–9.

Sternberg P *et al*. Multivariate analysis of prognostic factors in penetrating ocular injuries. *Am J Ophthalmol* 1984a; **98**: 467–72.

Sternberg P *et al*. Penetrating ocular injuries in young patients. Initial injuries and visual results. *Retina* 1984b; **4**: 5–8.

Talwar D, Kumar A, Verma L, Tewari HK, Khosia PK. Ultrasonography in optic nerve head avulsion. *Acta Ophthalmol (Copenh)* 1991; **69**: 121–3.

Taylor D, Bentovim A. Recurrent non-accidentally inflicted chemical eye injuries to siblings. *J Pediatr Ophthalmol* 1979; **13**: 238–42.

Taylor S, Hyler S. Update on factitious disorders. *Int J Psych Med* 1993; **23**: 81–94.

Ticho U, Ivry M, Merin S. Brittle cornea, blue sclera, and red hair syndrome (the brittle cornea syndrome). *Br J Med* 1980; **64**: 175–7

Tomasi LG, Rosman NP. Purtscher's retinopathy in the battered child syndrome. *Am J Dis Child* 1975; **129**: 1335–7.

Trevor Roper P. The psychopathic eye. *Br J Hosp Med* 1980; **Feb 23**: 137–43.

Turner JWA. Indirect injury of the optic nerves. *Brain* 1943; **66**: 140–5.

Urbanek J. Uber fettemoblie des Auges. *Albrecht Graefe's Arch Ophthalmol* 1934; **131**: 147.

Vaegan, Taylor D. Critical period for deprivation amblyopia in children. *Trans Ophthalmol Soc UK* 1979; **99**: 432–9.

Vajpayee RB, Angra SK, Honavour SG. Combined keratoplasty, cataract extraction, and intraocular lens implantation after corneolenticular laceration in children. *Am J Ophthalmol* 1994; **117**: 507–11.

Vinger PF. Ocular sports injuries. Principles of protection. *Int Ophthalmol Clin* 1981; **21**: 149–61.

Wang ML, Seiff SR, Drasner K. A comparison of visual outcome in open-globe repair: succinylcholine with D-tubocurarine versus non-depolarizing agents. *Ophthalmic Surg* 1992; **23**: 746–51.

Waterhouse W, Enzenauer R, Parmley V. Inflammatory orbital tumor as an ocular sign of a battered child. *Am J Ophthalmol* 1992; **114**: 509–10.

Weidenthal DT, Schepens CL. Peripheral fundus changes associated with ocular contusion. *Am J Ophthalmol* 1966; **62**: 465–77.

Weissgold DJ, Budenz DL, Hood I, Rorke LB. Ruptured vascular malformation masquerading as battered/shaken baby syndrome: a nearly tragic mistake. *Surv Ophthalmol* 1995; **39**: 509–12.

Whiting S, Jan JE, Wong PK *et al*. Permanent cortical visual impairment in children. *Dev Med Child Neurol* 1985; **27**: 730–9.

Wilkinson WS, Arbor A, Han DP, Rappley MD, Owings CL. Retinal haemorrhage predicts neurologic injury in the shaken baby syndrome. *Arch Ophthalmol* 1989; **107**: 1472–5.

Williams C. Expert evidence on cases of child abuse. *Arch Dis Child* 1993; **68**: 712–14.

Wolff SM, Zimmerman L. Chronic secondary glaucoma associated with retro displacement of iris root and deepening of the anterior chamber and angle secondary to contusion. *Am J Ophthalmol* 1962; **54**: 547–63.

Yang SK, Brown GC, Magargal LE. Self-inflicted ocular mutilation. *Am J Ophthalmol* 1981; **91**: 658–63.

Yih J-P, Taylor D. Retinol signs in non-accidental injury. *Asia Pacific J*

Ophthalmol 1996; **8**: 32–3.

Zimmerman RW, Bilaniuk LT, Bruce D *et al.* Computed tomography of craniocerebral injury in the abused child. *Radiology* 1979; **130**: 687–90.

Zlotogera J, Ben-Ezra D, Cohen J, Cohen L. Syndrome of the brittle cornea, blue sclera and joint hyperextensibility. *Am J Med Genet* 1990; **36**: 269–72.

Section 6
Eye Movements and Strabismus

63: Nystagmus and Eye Movement Disorders

Christopher Harris

Nystagmus is a rhythmic oscillation of one or both eyes about one or more axes. There are many kinds of nystagmus. Some can be induced physiologically, others occur spontaneously and are usually pathological. Collectively, spontaneous nystagmus can be associated with conditions ranging from the relatively benign to the life-threatening. Some eye oscillations are really saccadic oscillations, rather than nystagmus, and are discussed in Chapter 64. However, voluntary nystagmus and convergence retraction nystagmus will be discussed here because of common clinical usage. Some cyclic phenomena will also be discussed in this chapter alongside periodic alternating nystagmus.

The correct identification of nystagmus seldom leads to a specific diagnosis, but the differential diagnoses can be narrowed to refine and reduce further investigations. Most nystagmus can be broadly divided into three categories.

1 Nystagmus secondary to a visual deficit.

2 Nystagmus secondary to intracranial lesions and drug toxicities.

3 Congenital benign idiopathic nystagmus.

Often, the child with nystagmus is investigated on the presumption of a sinister intracranial lesion, only to find an unsuspected infantile visual deficit. By far the majority of nystagmus in childhood is either secondary to a visual problem or is congenital idiopathic. The latter group can sometimes only be diagnosed by exclusion, but the most common idiopathic nystagmus, congenital idiopathic nystagmus, can usually be positively identified by eye movement recording, which can save the child from unnecessary neuroimaging.

Conversely, a nystagmus that presages serious neurological disease may not be properly identified until the child presents with more obvious neurological signs.

The mechanisms that give rise to nystagmus are not well understood, but it is worth recognizing that not only must there be a reason for the spontaneous oscillations (healthy children do not have nystagmus even in the dark), but there must also be a reason for the lack of suppression of the nystagmus in the light. There are three possibilities.

1 The nystagmus intensity is too high, or vision is too poor for complete suppression. This occurs in peripheral vestibular disease and in some forms of nystagmus that occur with visual loss.

2 There is a concomitant disorder of the smooth pursuit system. This occurs with central lesions. For example, lesions of the vestibular cerebellum give rise to gaze-paretic nystagmus as well as damaging the smooth pursuit system.

3 The fixation and smooth pursuit systems are themselves at fault and cause the nystagmus. This argument has been used in attempts to explain congenital nystagmus (Tusa *et al.* 1992; Harris 1995).

Terminology and classification

The objective recording of eye movements has transformed our understanding of eye movements and their pathology and has rendered obsolete some older ideas about nystagmus. It continues, nevertheless, to be contentious whether to classify nystagmus on the basis of:

• its clinical appearance, which is pragmatic but frequently in error;

• the waveform as revealed by electronystagmography, which is usually accurate but not without problems and currently unavailable to most clinicians;

• aetiological grounds, which would be ideal, but is inherently retrospective.

None is perfect and the various terminologies have left the clinician with a confusing classification that has been exacerbated by changing definitions of labels already in widespread use. Therefore, for the sake of clarity, all specific types of nystagmus will be abbreviated to distinguish them from the everyday meaning of their constituent words. It is hoped that this will clarify one of the most confusing aspects of nystagmus. To emphasize this point with an analogy: various birds (e.g. crows, rooks, etc.) are examples of black birds, but they are not blackbirds, which are a specific type of bird that happens also to be black. Analogously, some types of nystagmus (e.g. Latent Nystagmus) are examples of congenital nystagmus, but they are not Congenital Nystagmus, which is a specific kind of nystagmus that is also congenital.

Ultimately, the choice of labels is arbitrary, but clinicians need to be aware of the different meanings of terms so that the communication of findings is unambiguous. Above all, the unqualified term 'nystagmus' should be used with extreme care. Some of the confusing terminology is now described.

Congenital, acquired and idiopathic nystagmus

The term 'congenital nystagmus' is used by some to denote any nystagmus with an onset in infancy. For others, it denotes specifically Congenital Idiopathic Nystagmus (CIN) (sometimes called 'motor nystagmus'). For oculomotorists it describes a specific type of nystagmus, Congenital Nystagmus (CN), which may be idiopathic or associated with an infantile sensory defect, such as albinism. In the published literature the usage of the term 'congenital nystagmus' is inconsistent. Whichever use is adopted, 'congenital' nystagmus usually has an onset in the first 3 months of life, but does not typically occur at birth, and so to add to the confusion, it is not strictly congenital. Since some nystagmus due to neurological disease can occur in infancy, Casteels *et al.* (1992) have recommended that the term 'congenital nystagmus' be avoided. They classified nystagmus with an onset before and after 6 months as early and late onset nystagmus. They subdivided early onset nystagmus into three types.

1 Sensory Defect Nystagmus (SDN) and Latent Nystagmus (LN).

2 Congenital Idiopathic Nystagmus (CIN), in which no sensory defect can be established.

3 Neurological Nystagmus (NN), which is usually associated with a neurological disease.

A more general scheme based on Casteel *et al.*'s (1992) is shown in Fig. 63.1.

SDN is associated with an early onset sensory problem (albinism, cataract, etc.). This nystagmus usually has features that distinguish it from any other type of nystagmus, including nystagmus secondary to a late onset visual defect. By ophthalmological investigations and electronystagmography, SDN can be positively identified so that neurological investigations are not usually needed. Other types of nystagmus (NN) (vertical, see-saw, acquired pendular, etc.) are usually associated with neurological disease or, rarely, a late onset visual deficit, and require full investigation usually involving computed tomography (CT) and magnetic resonance imaging (MRI).

Idiopathic nystagmus is more problematic, but usually breaks down into two groups.

1 An early onset idiopathic nystagmus has the same features as SDN, and cannot be distinguished from SDN on the basis of the nystagmus. We call it CIN; it only differs from SDN in that no sensory defect can be established. However, because of the distinct features of this nystagmus, in most cases it can be positively identified, thus saving the child from unnecessary sedation for neuroimaging.

2 Other types of idiopathic nystagmus are not like SDN

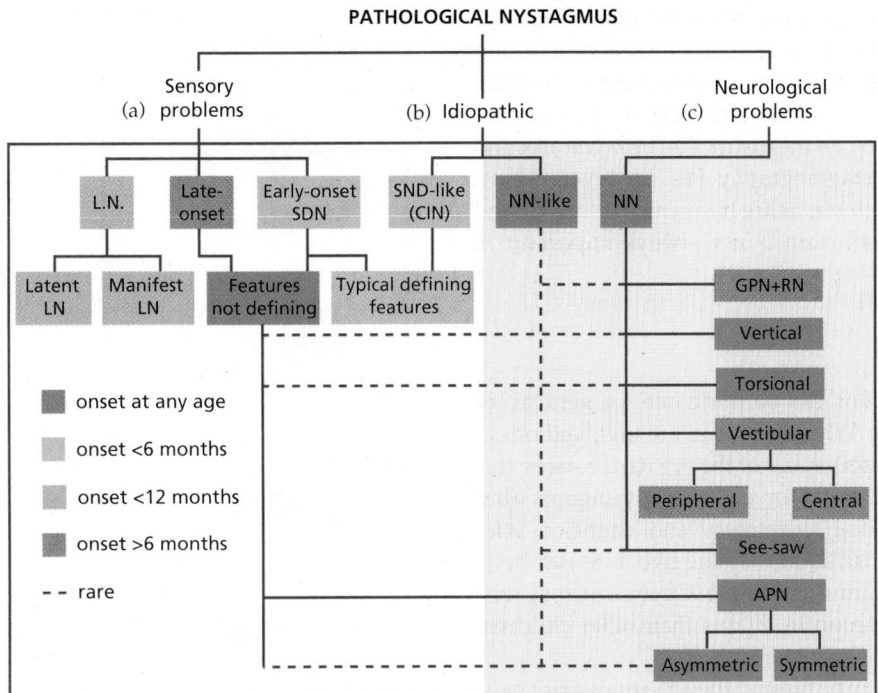

Fig. 63.1 An organizational guide to childhood nystagmus. (a) Sensory nystagmus. A primary visual sensory abnormality (including optic nerve disease), which is usually due to (i) infantile uni-ocular defects (strabismus, anisometropia, cataract, etc.) that lead to LN; (ii) infantile bi-ocular defects (due to foveal hypoplasia, cone dysfunction, etc.) that lead to nystagmus with the defining feature of accelerating slow-phases; (iii) a conjugate or asymmetrical pendular nystagmus due to late onset visual loss (e.g. amblyopia), or occasionally an infantile bi-ocular defect; this nystagmus has no defining features and cannot usually be differentiated from nystagmus secondary to intracranial disease (see red line). (b) Idiopathic nystagmus. No detectable sensory or neurological abnormality. The most common early onset idiopathic nystagmus (CIN) may have the same defining features (accelerating slow-phases) as nystagmus secondary to early onset sensory defect. Idiopathic early onset or late onset nystagmus may not have defining features and is similar to nystagmus with a primary neurological insult. (c) Neurological nystagmus. A primary neurological disorder that gives rise to a specific type of nystagmus (see text).

but are similar to NN (e.g. congenital idiopathic see-saw nystagmus), but these cannot be positively identified from the nystagmus and so full neurological investigations are usually needed.

Since SDN and CIN cannot be distinguished on the basis of their waveforms, we shall denote this nystagmus explicitly by SDN/CIN for the sake of clarity. (This is equivalent to the oculomotorists' definition of CN but without the confusion that surrounds that term.)

It is crucial to note that nystagmus co-existing with a sensory defect is not automatically labelled as SDN. There are many progressive neuro-ophthalmological disorders with optic atrophy or a retinal dystrophy with a nystagmus that do not have the features of SDN, and almost certainly have a neurological origin, regardless of age of onset (including early infancy).

No scheme is perfect, and it is not wise to take a dogmatic approach to the classification or investigation of patients with nystagmus. With or without eye movement recordings, there are inevitably difficult cases. One problem is that some cases of small amplitude pendular SDN do not have any features that distinguish it from acquired pendular nystagmus (which may also have an onset in infancy). Unfortunately, this nystagmus has a predilection for being associated with subtle retinal disorders (congenital stationary night-blindness, cone dysfunction) which may require electrophysiological investigations that are not universally available. Fortunately, this is a small group of patients, and the uncertainty in such cases is clearly identifiable so that they can always be fully investigated.

The cut-off age of 6 months is rather arbitrary, and some cases of LN (which is usually thought of as a type of early onset nystagmus) appear to have an onset after 6 months. However, identification of this nystagmus is seldom a problem.

Jerk and pendular nystagmus

Each cycle of the nystagmus oscillation may have a slow-phase and a fast (saccadic) component called a quick-phase, in which case it is called jerk nystagmus. Oscillations without a quick-phase are called pendular, although the waveform may not be sinusoidal. In some types of nystagmus the waveform may change spontaneously or with different gaze directions. Both jerk and pendular nystagmus may occur simultaneously in compound nystagmus. Historically, the classification of nystagmus had depended on the distinction between jerk and pendular. Electronystagmography has, however, shown that such clinical distinctions are frequently incorrect, and in any case, the distinction is not always important in some early onset nystagmus.

Axes of oscillations

Nystagmus oscillations can be horizontal or vertical, or both simultaneously. When both axes are involved out of phase, the anteroposterior axis of the eye itself rotates: this is circumrotatory, circular or elliptical nystagmus (but sometimes abbreviated to rotatory and confused with rotary). Rarely, the oscillations of the two axes can be in phase and the nystagmus is oblique. Circumrotatory nystagmus is more common in infants than older children, and is not necessarily a sinister sign.

The oscillations may be around the anteroposterior axis. This is torsional (or cyclotorsional) nystagmus, but is sometimes called rotary nystagmus (sometimes confused with rotatory nystagmus). Conventionally intorsion corresponds to the rotation when the top (upper pole) of the eye moves towards the nose and the bottom of the eye moves away. Extorsion is the reverse (Fig. 63.2). More recently conjugate torsional eye movements have been described as 'clockwise' when the upper poles of the eyes rotate towards the patient's right (anti- or counter-clockwise from the observer's viewpoint).

The axis of oscillation may change with gaze position (e.g. circumrotatory in upgaze, horizontal in primary or lateral gaze, etc.).

Direction

The direction of the nystagmus is conventionally described by the direction of the fast phases or beats. However, it is the slow-phase that reflects the pathology (except for some cases of Epileptic Nystagmus, EN). The fast phase is a reflexive compensatory movement to recentre or refixate the eyes. The direction often depends on gaze direction. By definition, pendular nystagmus does not have a direction. Note that the direction is described relative to the head, rather than to the direction of gravity.

Amplitude, frequency and intensity

The amplitude of nystagmus is the excursion of the slow- or quick-phase (measured in degrees). Clinically, it is often classed as being fine, medium or coarse; however, these are subjective descriptions. The frequency (measured in

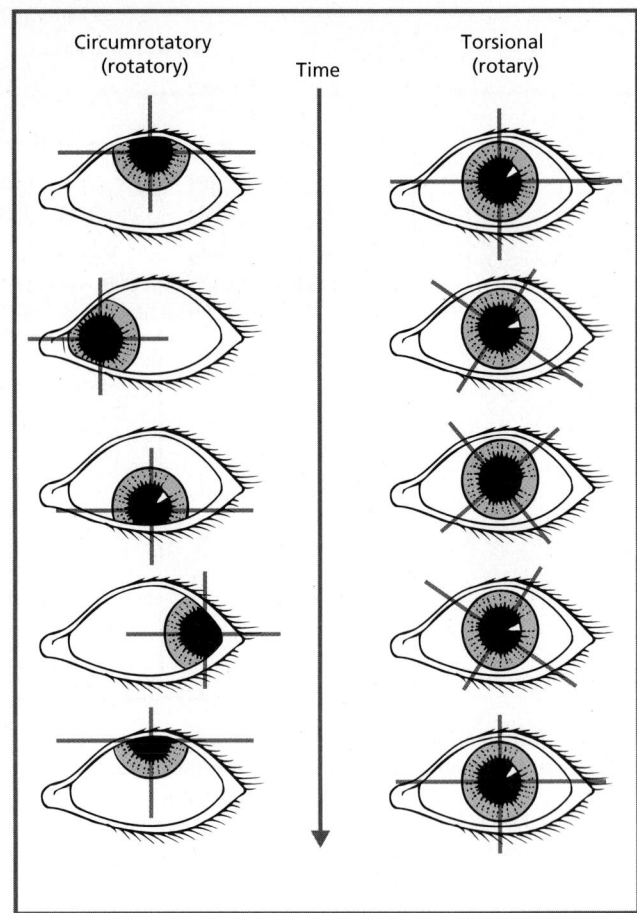

Fig. 63.2 The difference between torsional (rotary) nystagmus and circumrotatory (rotatory, circular, elliptical) nystagmus, shown for left eye only. In torsional nystagmus (right column), the eye rotates around the anteroposterior axis, here shown as extorsion for the left eye or left or anti-clockwise torsion. In circumrotatory nystagmus (left column), the anteroposterior axis itself rotates.

cycles or beats per second) is the number of oscillations per second. The intensity is the product of amplitude and frequency and is approximately equal to the average speed of the slow-phases for jerk nystagmus in degrees per second.

For jerk nystagmus, the amplitude and intensity both depend not only on slow-phase velocity but also on how rapidly quick-phases are triggered, which in turn also depend on slow-phase velocity. Whether the jerk nystagmus is physiological or pathological, there is a gradual developmental trend of increasing frequency and decreasing amplitude over the first few years, but this may take longer with developmental delay or a saccade failure.

Conversely, pendular nystagmus is frequently of small amplitude and high frequency. Presumably, if it were otherwise, quick-phases would be triggered and the nystagmus would become jerk. In early infancy some types of congenital pendular nystagmus may have a very high amplitude, but very low frequency.

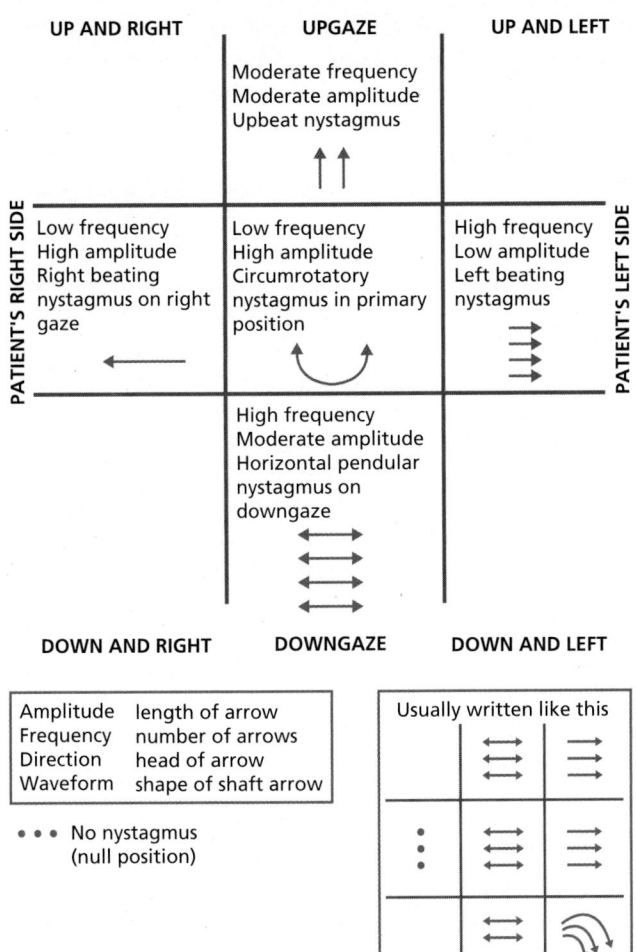

UP AND RIGHT   **UPGAZE**   **UP AND LEFT**

Moderate frequency
Moderate amplitude
Upbeat nystagmus

↑ ↑

PATIENT'S RIGHT SIDE

Low frequency
High amplitude
Right beating
nystagmus on right
gaze

←

Low frequency
High amplitude
Circumrotatory
nystagmus in primary
position

High frequency
Low amplitude
Left beating
nystagmus

→
→
→
→

PATIENT'S LEFT SIDE

High frequency
Moderate amplitude
Horizontal pendular
nystagmus on
downgaze

↔
↔
↔
↔

DOWN AND RIGHT   **DOWNGAZE**   **DOWN AND LEFT**

Amplitude length of arrow	Usually written like this
Frequency number of arrows	
Direction head of arrow	
Waveform shape of shaft arrow	

• • • No nystagmus
(null position)

Fig. 63.3 A descriptive way of documenting nystagmus.

Nystagmus can be descriptively documented clinically by various graphical schemes (Fig. 63.3), where confusion between circumrotatory and torsional nystagmus can be avoided by explicitly stating the presence of Torsional Nystagmus.

The degree of visual loss attributable to the nystagmus is difficult to predict clinically and in the preverbal child caution is needed: only time will tell the final acuity. Visual acuity does not correlate well with nystagmus intensity, but is better predicted by the waveform of the nystagmus, and by the ability of the child to fixate.

One feature of SDN/CIN is a range of possibly eccentric eye positions where the nystagmus is at a minimum (but not necessarily absent). This is called the null zone or null region. Conventionally the null zone corresponds with the region of least intensity, which may not correspond to the region of least amplitude or to the region of least frequency. Amplitude, frequency and intensity do not correspond to any specific waveform. In addition, the position of the null zone may change in time, or depend on movement of the visual scene, or change depending on

previous eye position. All these factors can be important considerations in evaluating a patient for head posture surgery (Abadi & Whittle 1991).

Manifest, latent and latent component nystagmus

Nystagmus that appears only when one eye is occluded is called latent, whereas nystagmus that appears when both eyes are open is called manifest, regardless of the quality of vision in each eye. This distinction is not so simple as it seems. First, LN is a specific type of nystagmus that is usually associated with an early onset strabismus or monocular visual disorder. Because of early onset monocular visual loss or suppression, even with both eyes open, the patient may be effectively monocular, so that the LN is unmasked, i.e. manifest; hence the apparently contradictory, but logical, terms manifest LN (MLN) and latent LN (LLN) have arisen (Dell'Osso *et al.* 1979). Therefore, the term 'manifest' does not help identify the nystagmus, because any type of nystagmus can occur with both eyes open. Also, SDN and CIN often intensify on monocular occlusion, and so exhibit a latent component. Since SDN and CIN may have a null region in primary position, SDN with a latent component may be mistaken for LN.

Gaze-evoked, gaze-paretic and gaze-dependent nystagmus

These terms have been used inconsistently. We use the term gaze-evoked to describe any nystagmus that appears on eccentric gaze but is absent in primary position. For example, SDN/CIN and manifest LN may sometimes appear on lateral gaze but not in primary position, and hence are gaze-evoked. We use the term Gaze-Paretic Nystagmus (GPN) to refer to a specific nystagmus caused by a mismatch between the gaze-holding circuitry and the viscoelastic forces of the extraocular muscles. Thus GPN is another example of a gaze-evoked nystagmus, but not vice versa. The nystagmus may be present in primary position but intensify significantly or change its waveform in eccentric gaze. We call this gaze-dependent nystagmus. Most types of nystagmus are gaze-dependent in some way, with nystagmus usually intensifying in the direction of the beats (Alexander's law). So common is gaze-dependence, that its absence can be significant, possibly indicating Acquired Pendular Nystagmus (APN) (even in early infancy).

Asymmetric and dissociated nystagmus

When the nystagmus is different in each eye, the nystagmus is called asymmetric or dissociated. The nystagmus may be completely absent in one eye, but more often there is just a marked difference between the eyes. Some authors have reserved the term asymmetrical to describe a nystagmus that is dissociated in eccentric gaze (e.g. abduction nystagmus).

Compound nystagmus

Occasionally a patient can exhibit two types of nystagmus simultaneously, often involving a high-frequency pendular nystagmus and a jerk nystagmus (but not always). For example, LN, which is not uncommon in the general population, may be present with APN in a child with intracranial disease and a history of strabismus. In cerebellar or brain stem disorders APN may co-exist with GPN, which clinically may be quite similar to some cases of SDN. It is important not to dismiss one nystagmus merely because the other has been recognized. Compound nystagmus is best examined with eye movement recordings.

Examination of nystagmus

History

Obtaining a reliable history is important in examining the child with nystagmus. Essential questions include the following.

1 Is there any family history of nystagmus or other neuro-ophthalmological problems? The focus should be on conditions associated with nystagmus rather than the presence of nystagmus itself, because the nystagmus may have not been noticed in relatives. The history of the maternal grandfather in particular should also be investigated for the possibility of X-linked recessive associations. Parental consanguinity should be broached since many retinal and macular diseases are autosomal recessive. Many neurodegenerative conditions are inherited. A positive family history of idiopathic nystagmus does not render unnecessary a thorough ophthalmological, and if necessary, neurological investigation of a child with nystagmus.

2 The time of onset, progression, variations in intensity with age, and any changes with lighting conditions. History of an only child or firstborn can be remarkably unreliable. An onset of predominantly horizontal nystagmus in the first 6 months usually indicates SDN/CIN/LN, and only rarely APN. The amplitude of nystagmus typically declines with age particularly during the first year. However, SDN/CIN is notoriously variable and may be exacerbated when the child is tired or stressed at any time in life.

A firmly established onset after 6 months should be presumed to be NN. However, the presence of SDN/CIN/LN may have gone unnoticed from early infancy even by experienced and observant parents, particularly if there is a broad null region around primary position. The nystagmus may only come to light when the child is examined closely for unrelated reasons (school check-ups,

etc.). There are a few well-documented cases of apparently late onset SDN/CIN (Gresty *et al.* 1991), in which the nystagmus may have been precipitated by an illness. In such cases the SDN/CIN must be positively identified, preferably with eye movement studies.

3 Intermittent problems can be difficult to diagnose, especially if an event does not occur during the examination. Are there aspects of intermittency in the nystagmus or symptoms? Is there any family history of seizures? Are there periods of dizziness, vertigo, fainting, and so on, which may be mistakenly identified as seizures or 'attacks'? Are symptoms worse when the head moves or is in a particular position, such as lying supine or prone, looking up or behind? Do visual symptoms worsen during the day? Does diet have any effect?

4 The parents' opinion of the child's vision, of any photophobia, or night vision problems. Asking how the child watches his or her favourite television programme can also be useful: many children with SDN/CIN will watch very close to or with a head turn.

5 The effect of any previous treatments including surgery and previous and current medication. Some types of nystagmus can occur secondary to prescribed and non-prescribed drugs.

Ocular examination

The clinician needs to carry out a full ocular examination including slit-lamp examination for iris transillumination, fundoscopy for retinal or optic disc disease. Colour vision should be tested if the child is old enough. Cycloplegic refraction is important because of the high incidence of astigmatism in young children with nystagmus, which needs correction with spectacles. The best corrected acuity should also be measured with and without abnormal head posture, for distance and for near, and uni-ocularly and with both eyes open.

Electroretinogram and pattern evoked potentials

The diagnosis of CIN should not be made without exclusion of an abnormal electroretinogram (ERG) and pattern visual evoked potential (pVEP). Electrodiagnostics can be useful in establishing a diagnosis of conditions such as congenital stationary night-blindness, cone dysfunction, ocular albinism and optic nerve disease.

ERG and pVEPs are also very useful in the investigation of the child with pendular nystagmus. One of the limitations of nystagmography and clinical examination is distinguishing between a fine horizontal or circumrotatory pendular gaze-independent nystagmus that can be very occasionally SDN or more often APN. This difficulty is further exacerbated by the frequent association of fine pendular SDN with subtle retinal disease.

NN is usually associated with subcortical lesions. Thus,

delayed pVEPs with NN may indicate a disseminated disorder involving white matter. Abnormal ERG and NN are characteristic of some syndromes including Joubert's syndrome, Refsum's disease, Senior's syndrome, Batten's disease, peroxisomal disorders and many others (see Chapters 9, 44, 57).

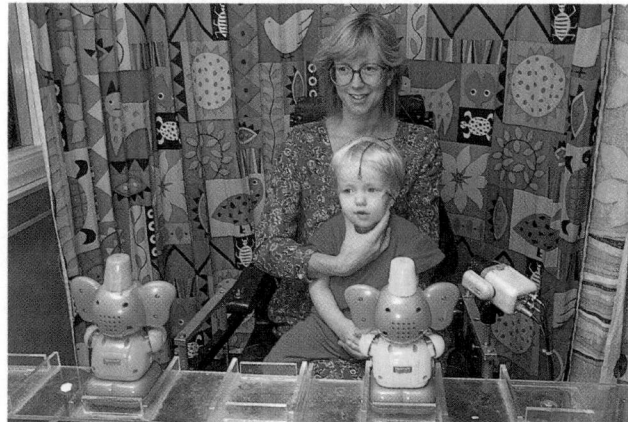

a

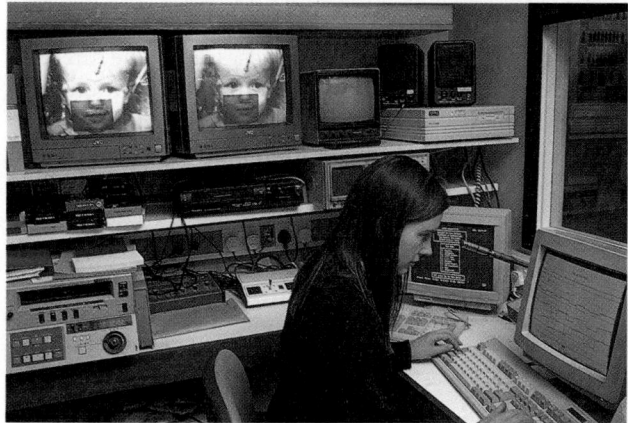

b

Fig. 63.4 The eye movement laboratory at Great Ormond Street Hospital, London. (a) Horizontal eye movements are measured by electrodes placed at the outer canthus of each eye and a ground electrode at the mid-forehead position; a monocular recording can be made with an electrode on the inner canthus, and vertical eye movements can be measured by placing electrodes above and below an eye. The infant sits on a parent's lap with the head held still and any nystagmus is examined in the cardinal gaze positions. Each eye is patched in turn and the viewing eye is abducted and adducted to reveal any latent nystagmus or latent component. Full-field binocular and monocular optokinetic testing is achieved with a brightly coloured attractive curtain that completely encircles the patient and is rotated at various speeds. Saccades are readily elicited by large noisy toys from the very young, or by small lights from the older child. Vestibular nystagmus is induced by completely darkening the room and rotating the chair at constant speed in each direction. The patient is monitored at all times by an infrared camera. (b) The video image and electro-oculographic signals are relayed to the adjacent room for recording and superimposed allowing the eye movement trace and the visual appearance of the eyes to be examined simultaneously (see Jacobs *et al.* 1992; Harris *et al.* 1992).

Oculomotor examination

Axis

Purely vertical or torsional nystagmus, whether it is upbeat, downbeat or pendular, should be presumed to be NN at any age: only rarely is SDN/CIN purely vertical or torsional. Late onset circumrotatory nystagmus should also be presumed to be NN. Early onset circumrotatory nystagmus is ambiguous but it is more likely to be SDN than CIN. Purely horizontal nystagmus, jerk or pendular, in all gaze directions with an early onset usually indicates SDN/CIN or manifest LN, but can be APN or Periodic Alternating Nystagmus (PAN).

Asymmetry

Most nystagmus is conjugate. Asymmetrical nystagmus in primary position, which can have any axis, usually occurs in one of three settings.
1 Secondary to an intracranial lesion, usually involving the chiasm or midbrain.
2 Secondary to monocular visual loss.
3 As part of the spasmus nutans triad. Only very rarely is SDN asymmetrical.

Asymmetric nystagmus in lateral gaze usually occurs in the abducting eye, and is called abduction, dissociated or ataxic nystagmus, and is classically associated with internuclear ophthalmoplegia, but may be mimicked in myasthenia gravis.

Gaze-dependencies and monocular viewing

It is very important to observe the nystagmus for gaze-dependence, a change in its characteristics in different positions of gaze: a fine pendular or jerk nystagmus may become a very intense jerk nystagmus on lateral gaze, which is typical of SDN/CIN. A fine pendular nystagmus that does not change appreciably in horizontal gaze direction should be presumed to be a NN, until proven otherwise.

Examine the nystagmus monocularly for a latent component, especially in the horizontal cardinal positions. In LN the nystagmus often has a null position in far adduction of the fixing eye, whereas GPN usually has a null in primary position and is unaffected by monocular occlusion.

It has sometimes been said that a nystagmus which remains horizontal in all gaze directions is always SDN or CIN. This is not strictly true, since MLN, APN and PAN can also be purely horizontal, but it forms a rough and ready clinical guide.

Fine nystagmus and torsional nystagmus can sometimes be best detected by ophthalmoscopy. Note that the fundus is behind the centre of eye rotation, so it moves in the opposite direction to the front of the eye. In indirect ophthalmoscopy there is an additional inversion from the objective lens!

Electronystagmography (Fig. 63.4)

The waveform of the nystagmus in different gaze-directions is important in identifying nystagmus, and can positively identify SDN/CIN but it cannot distinguish between the various sensory defects or define whether it is idiopathic. Clinical observation of waveforms is unreliable. If eye movement equipment is not available, it is worth noting that most ERG/VEP equipment is quite capable of demonstrating nystagmus waveforms by electro-oculography. For conjugate eye movements, an electrode is attached to each outer canthus, with a reference electrode usually on the mid-forehead. Monocular recordings can be made by placing the electrodes on the inner and outer canthi. Averaging must be turned off. DC coupling is ideal, but for AC coupling, the low cut-on frequency should be set as low as possible so that the decay rate of the AC coupling cannot be confused with a nystagmus slow-phase. From an electrophysiological viewpoint, the signals are large, being about $10\,\mu V$ per degree of eye movement for a 1-month-old infant, and $20\,\mu V$ per degree for an adult (Harris *et al.* 1993a). It should be noted that these signals may be substantially reduced or absent in disorders affecting the retina and retinal pigment epithelium.

There are many different nystagmus waveforms, but it is useful to consider four basic types (Fig. 63.5): jerk nystagmus with an accelerating slow-phase (ASP), with a decelerating slow-phase (DSP), with a constant velocity or linear slow-phase, and pendular nystagmus. Note that the term 'pendular' refers to a lack of quick-phases rather than the shape of the wave form.

Horizontal accelerating slow-phases are considered to be definitive, but not invariable in SDN/CIN (this does not apply to vertical ASP). Therefore, an important goal in examining a patient with horizontal nystagmus is to try to find a direction of gaze in which ASP can be induced. DSP nystagmus is typical of LN and GPN, but can also occur in SDN/CIN. Linear slow-phases are equivocal, since they can occur in jerk nystagmus if the amplitude is small.

Physiological nystagmus

Optokinetic nystagmus

Optokinetic Nystagmus (OKN) is a normal response to a moving visual scene. The slow-phases are in the direction of stimulus motion. Healthy children will, from the time of birth, demonstrate brisk optokinetic nystagmus when viewing binocularly, but will show poor or absent OKN if

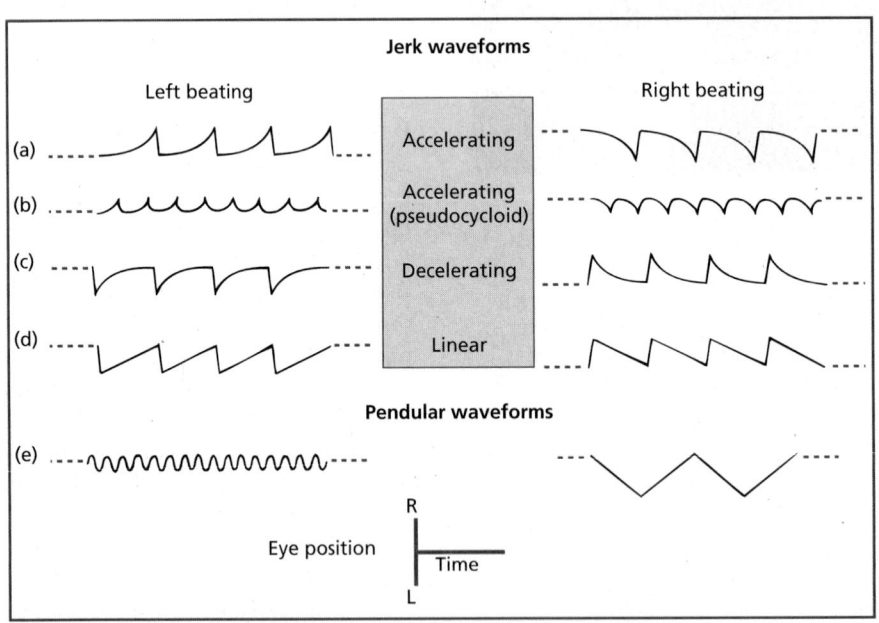

Fig. 63.5 Stylized wave form types seen in horizontal nystagmus for left beating (left column) and right beating (right column). By convention up means right, and down means left. (a) Accelerating slow-phases (ASP) (increasing velocity slow-phases), where the speed of the eye increases with time during the slow phase. (b) A common variant of the ASP waveform, called 'pseudocycloid', which may appear pendular to the naked eye. (c) Decelerating (decreasing velocity slow-phases) DSP. (d) Linear or constant velocity slow-phases where the speed does not change during the slow-phase. (e) Pendular nystagmus (i.e. no quick-phases), with sinusoidal wave form (left) and triangular wave form (right).

viewing monocularly and the stimulus moves in the nasotemporal direction of the viewing eye. Optokinetic nystagmus can normally be suppressed by fixation of a stationary object. The abnormalities of OKN are discussed in Chapter 64.

Induced Vestibular Nystagmus

Vestibular Nystagmus (VN) is a normal response to rotation of the head in the light or dark, and is the type of nystagmus induced by manually spinning an infant. During rotation, the slow-phases are in the opposite direction to rotation, and reverse on sudden cessation of rotation. VN can also be induced by rotation in the light provided the patient has no fixation target or does not have the ability to fix, but the rotation may also induce an optokinetic response. VN is discussed in Chapter 64.

VN can also be induced by caloric irrigation of the ears. By cooling or heating the semi-circular canals on one side of the head, a temporary vestibular imbalance is created, which leads to VN.

End-Point Nystagmus

Many healthy individuals exhibit a jerk nystagmus in far lateral gaze, which beats in the direction of gaze. This End-Point Nystagmus (EPN) usually disappears when the eccentricity is reduced by a few degrees. However, in some children EPN may be quite marked and the question of whether the nystagmus is really GPN may arise. However, the lack of any neurological signs and the lack of any other eye movement abnormality, particularly saccadic pursuit, indicates EPN. Normals with EPN may even show some Rebound Nystagmus (RN) (see below), which in this instance is also physiological (Shallo-Hoffmann *et al.* 1990).

Voluntary nystagmus

About 5% of the population are able to initiate nystagmus at will (Yee *et al.* 1994). The frequency range is 3–42 Hz, and the amplitude range is 0.5–35°. Voluntary nystagmus is usually horizontal, but vertical and circumrotatory nystagmus may occur. It is often associated with convergence effort (Hotson 1984) and facial grimacing, and cannot be sustained. Voluntary nystagmus consists of back-to-back saccades.

Occasionally voluntary nystagmus may occur as a non-organic problem in the schoolchild, in which case its voluntary nature can be difficult to establish. It has been described as a tic (Shawkat *et al.* 1992). The abnormal oscillations must be distinguished from pathological saccadic oscillations, particularly opsoclonus. In opsoclonus the saccades are chaotic, multidirectional and dysmetric (see Chapter 64).

Very rarely a true spontaneous nystagmus may be completely suppressed or released at will. This nystagmus can be released indefinitely giving the appearance of voluntary nystagmus. Facial grimacing is not present. Such patients should be investigated for the cause of their underlying nystagmus.

Latent Nystagmus

Latent Nystagmus (LN) is always a conjugate horizontal jerk nystagmus and usually has an onset before 6 months, but it may start later (onset is difficult to define unless it is manifest). It is probably the most common type of nystagmus due to its association with infantile strabismus, and it is neurologically benign.

Despite the label 'latent', LN may be truly latent (LLN) or manifest (MLN). LLN becomes manifest only on monocular occlusion. However, if there is low vision in one eye the nystagmus may be manifested in both eyes, thereby leading to degraded vision in the normal eye.

Whether manifest or latent, LN beats in the direction of the fixing eye (away from the nose) and becomes more intense when the fixing eye abducts. The direction of LN actually depends on the eye the patient thinks he or she is fixing with, not the actual eye (van Vliet 1973). We have come across a boy who could reverse his LN by trying to fix with his totally blind eye!

LN is always jerk with decelerating or linear slow-phases (see LN versus SDN/CIN below). With monocular viewing, the nystagmus may become manifest in primary position or may appear only on abduction of the fixing eye. In either case, on far adduction of the fixing eye, the nystagmus markedly dampens or even disappears (in a very few cases the nystagmus may show a very slight reversal). A head turn in the direction of the fixing eye may be adopted to capitalize on the better vision in adduction.

When viewing with both eyes open, the nystagmus may be clinically absent in primary position, but may become manifest on lateral gaze with beats in the direction of gaze. This is probably due to partial occlusion of the adducting eye by the nasal bridge. The appearance is strikingly similar to GPN. However, if the abducting eye is occluded the nystagmus will greatly dampen if it is LN, but remain virtually unchanged if it is GPN (Harris *et al.* 1993c).

LN, whether manifest or latent, is usually secondary to early onset interruption of binocular vision. By far the most common aetiology is infantile esotropia, but LN may also occur with unilateral cataract and other uni-ocular defects. A puzzling feature of LN is that not all patients with uni-ocular defects develop LN (Gresty *et al.* 1992; Shawkat *et al.* 1995), and it has been suggested that there may be a genetic predisposition for early onset strabismus and hence LN, which becomes manifest in patients with monocular vision (Kushner 1995).

Latent Nystagmus versus Sensory Defect Nystagmus/Congenital Idiopathic Nystagmus

Eye movement recording reveals that the slow-phases of LN (LLN or MLN) are typically decelerating, but if the amplitude is small, the slow-phases may appear to be linear. With practice, this waveform can sometimes be visualized by the naked eye, but in most cases the waveform can only be resolved by eye movement recording. There is confusion between MLN and SDN/CIN with a latent component because both types are manifest with both eyes open, and the nystagmus direction reverses with alternate occlusion. Since the management and aetiology of MLN and SDN/CIN are different, it is important to make the correct identification.

One area of difficulty, even with eye movement recordings, is that the slow-phases in some patients with what appears to be LLN have an accelerating waveform identical to that seen in SDN/CIN: Gresty *et al.* (1992) have considered this to be a *forme fruste* of SDN/CIN, although these patients do not seem to have a bilateral sensory defect. Clearly this type of nystagmus, which perhaps should be called 'latent SDN/CIN', blurs the distinction between LN and SDN/CIN. In our experience, this type of latent nystagmus is not common, and clinically it should probably be treated as LN rather than SDN/CIN.

Management

LN should be correctly identified and, particularly when manifest, distinguished from SDN/CIN using eye movement recordings if available. Any underlying visual defect or strabismus requires appropriate treatment. Asymptomatic LN requires no treatment.

Although it has long been known that LN (and most other eye movements) can be abolished with barbiturates (Bender 1946), this is not a realistic treatment.

Surgery for symptomatic LN consists of a medial rectus recession, with or without a Faden (posterior fixation suture) or a recess-resect procedure, depending on the presence of strabismus. Surgery should only be contemplated if a tangible benefit to the patient can be reasonably expected, such as a significant improvement in vision or the reduction of a prominent head turn.

It has been reported that MLN may be converted to LLN by either optical or surgical alignment of the optic axes. This has been achieved in patients with long-standing MLN, and Zubcov *et al.* (1990) believe that this is due to the introduction of equal visual input on corresponding retinal loci.

Liu *et al.* (1993) have proposed that the potential value of surgery for LN can be evaluated by injection of botulinum toxin into the medial rectus. With temporary paralysis of the medial rectus more adduction innervation is needed to maintain primary position with dampening of the LN, as normally occurs in adduction. This allows vision to be tested in the absence of manifest nystagmus, and any diplopia to be tested prior to surgery.

Sensory Defect Nystagmus and Congenital Idiopathic Nystagmus

Early onset SDN has an onset in the first few months and can be associated with a wide range of congenital sensory abnormalities including: albinism, cataract, aniridia, coloboma, congenital stationary night-blindness, cone dysfunction, achromatopsia, and many others. It can be 'acquired' neonatally as in keratitis (Ohm 1958; Kommerel & Mehdorn 1982) or cataract. SDN does not usually occur secondary to cortical defects. In some children no sensory defect can be detected, and the nystagmus is labelled as CIN. In the past, many cases of subtle sensory defects have been incorrectly diagnosed as CIN; the best example of this is albinism, subtle examples of which were often not examined for iris transillumination. A full clinical examination, including slit-lamp biomicroscopy, ERG and a pVEP are needed before sensory defects can be excluded. The incidence of SDN to CIN in our experience is about 9:1, but this is determined largely by the nature of our referrals.

SDN/CIN is usually conjugate and horizontal in all gaze directions. However, in infancy the nystagmus may be circumrotatory. There is often a null zone in which the nystagmus is minimal or absent. This null is often around primary position but may be eccentric in one-third of cases (Forsmann 1964), in which case the child may adopt a head posture. The nystagmus often dampens on convergence, but not always (Ukwade & Bedell 1992). The nystagmus usually persists in the dark, but may dampen or disappear with eyelids closed (whether or not in the dark). The nystagmus usually intensifies with fixation effort, or when the child is stressed or tired, and nystagmus intensity decreases with relaxation. However, anomalous instances can arise in which the nystagmus only appears in the dark or in dim illumination, or only during horizontal pursuit (Kelly *et al.* 1989), or vertical pursuit (personal observation), or only on convergence, or can be released and suppressed at will (Tusa *et al.* 1992).

The nystagmus is absent in stage 1 sleep, but is present in rapid eye movement (REM) sleep (Abadi & Dickinson 1986).

Inheritance

CIN may be inherited as an autosomal dominant trait; other modes of inheritance occur, but are less common. The inheritance of SDN depends entirely on the underlying condition; for example, congenital stationary night-blindness is usually inherited as an X-linked recessive trait, but other modes occur.

Optokinetic response

It is claimed that 'inverted' or 'reversed' OKN is a hall-mark of SDN/CIN. The idea arose because, when presented with an optokinetic stimulus, some patients with SDN/CIN respond with beats in the opposite direction expected from normal optokinetic nystagmus (Halmagyi *et al.* 1980a; Abadi & Dickinson 1985). However, this should not be taken literally because it is the slow-phases that determine the optokinetic response, and the terms 'inverted' or 'reversed' OKN are really misnomers. The vast majority of children with SDN/CIN do not have any recognizable OKN, and the response to an OKN stimulus is really their own nystagmus in which sometimes the null has shifted.

To describe the shift in the null, consider a typical adult sufferer of SDN/CIN with a null in primary position: in left gaze the nystagmus will beat towards the left, and in right gaze, towards the right. Now, for an unknown reason, if the patient is presented with an optokinetic or smooth pursuit stimulus moving to the right, the null region moves in the opposite direction, i.e. to the left. Looking straight ahead during this stimulation is now equivalent to looking to the right of the null region, which causes the nystagmus to beat towards the right and thus in the opposite direction to OKN. If reversed, the stimulus induces left beating nystagmus.

Nevertheless, with or without null shifting, the abnormal OKN response can be very useful as an identifying feature SDN/CIN in cases where the waveform is ambiguous. It should be noted that the horizontal OKN response is normal in those rare cases of vertical or torsional SDN/CIN (Abadi & Dickinson 1985).

Waveforms

A feature of jerk SDN/CIN is the distinctive waveforms of the nystagmus. In childhood, accelerating horizontal slow-phases, when present, are virtually unique to SDN/CIN (Dell'Osso & Daroff 1975; Yee *et al.* 1976; Abadi & Dickinson 1986) (although an acquired horizontal ASP nystagmus has been reported secondary to a lumbar puncture in a single adult case of type 1 Arnold–Chiari malformation; Barton & Sharp 1993).

Although the SDN/CIN may be pendular or even absent in primary position, it usually converts to a jerk nystagmus with accelerating slow-phases in lateral gaze.

The waveforms of SDN/CIN do not distinguish among the various sensory defects underlying SDN or between SDN and CIN (Dell'Osso & Daroff 1975; Yee *et al.* 1976; Abadi & Dickinson 1986). Thus, the diagnosis of CIN must be made by the exclusion of any sensory defect by ophthalmological and electrophysiological means. There may, however, be some relationship between waveform and aetiology: cone dysfunction and congenital stationary night-blindness seem to have a predilection for being associated with a fine pendular nystagmus, even in infancy, in our experience.

The presence of horizontal accelerating slow-phases does, however, distinguish SDN/CIN from NN, and this allows CIN to be positively identified when no sensory defect can be found, thus avoiding further investigations.

Accelerating slow-phases are not universally present, and so positive identification by waveform cannot always be made. In the young infant the nystagmus may be large amplitude low frequency and pendular with a sinusoidal or triangular waveform (Reinecke *et al.* 1988). We have seen this waveform in albinos and idiopaths, so it does not distinguish between SDN and CIN. The waveform may not change on lateral gaze (assuming the infant can be persuaded to attempt lateral gaze), and occasionally an ASP nystagmus can be elicited by monocular occlusion if there is a latent component. In any case, with full-field OKN stimulation the nystagmus continues unabated or it may be suppressed, but normal OKN (as expected at this age) cannot be elicited (Fig. 63.6).

More problematic is the presence of a high frequency low amplitude pendular nystagmus that is not gaze-dependent. Such nystagmus cannot be distinguished from APN, which can present in early infancy and be purely horizontal, and can be associated with intracranial disease (see below). SDN may be associated with subtle visual defects such as cone dysfunction and CSNB, which may be detected only by detailed ERG studies (see Chap-

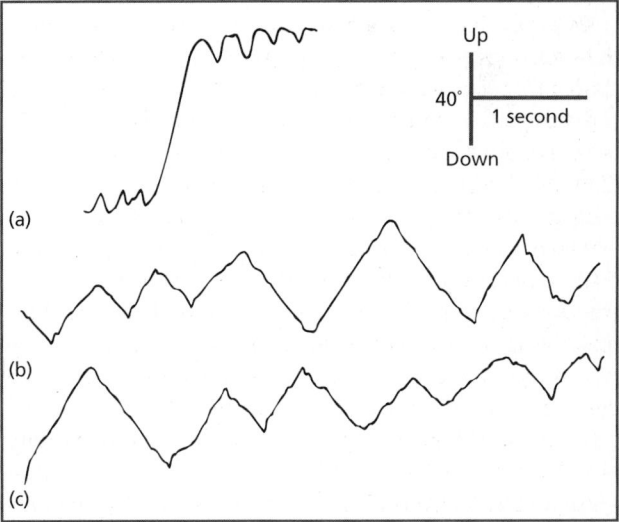

Fig. 63.6 Actual waveforms recorded by electro-oculography. (a) Typical accelerating slow-phase nystagmus recorded from 3-year-old with CIN, showing leftward beats in left gaze and rightward beats in right gaze. (b) Large amplitude low frequency triangular pendular nystagmus recorded from an albino infant aged 3 months. (c) Same infant as (b) but recorded during full-field optokinetic stimulation. Nystagmus remains essentially unaltered (calibration approximate).

ter 9). In most of these cases there is no optokinetic response although the child can track a moving toy. In contrast the child with APN usually shows an optokinetic nystagmus with the nystagmus superimposed on the slow-phases. A few cases of SDN/CIN with gaze-independent pendular nystagmus show an optokinetic response: these must be presumed to be APN until proven otherwise.

A third problem that arises without eye movement recording is that an APN may be compounded with MLN or GPN, and so appears to be pendular in primary position but jerk in lateral gaze. This combination occurs occasionally in neurological disease, and should not be mistaken for SDN/CIN.

Visual performance and Sensory Defect Nystagmus/Congenital Idiopathic Nystagmus

Apart from an underlying early-onset sensory defect in SDN, vision can be degraded in patients because of the nystagmus itself.

A hallmark of SDN/CIN is the enormous variability in the features of the nystagmus (waveform, null zone, sometimes head posture) that can change within minutes, and depend ineffably on such factors as stress, tiredness, fixation effort, distance of visual target, and even whether the patient was looking in lateral gaze in the last few seconds. The combination of these factors is difficult to control, and should always be borne in mind when assessing the visual performance of the patient with SDN/CIN.

When the retinal image moves across the retina at more than a few degrees per second, contrast sensitivity at high spatial frequencies is reduced. Since slow-phase velocities can reach more than 100° per second (Collewijn *et al.* 1985), it is not surprising to find that contrast sensitivity in SDN/CIN depends on the type of waveform, with visual performance being better if there are longer periods of low eye velocity during a cycle of nystagmus ('foveation periods', 'dwell times') (Abadi & Worfolk 1989). This is also true even if there is an underlying visual defect; thus, depending on the waveform, the best performance of an albino can be comparable to the worst performance of a patient with CIN. Pendular waveforms afford short or no foveation periods and tend to reduce contrast sensitivity more than jerk waveforms, all other factors being equal.

An abnormal head posture is often adopted in patients with an eccentric null zone. Although this may reasonably be thought to be an adaptation to optimize contrast sensitivity by allowing the eyes to align with the null, Abadi and Whittle (1991) have found that the head posture does not always correspond to the eye deviation of minimum nystagmus intensity, or minimum nystagmus amplitude, or minimum nystagmus frequency. Moreover, even though the duration of foveation periods is a better indica-

tor of contrast sensitivity than nystagmus intensity (Dickinson & Abadi 1985), Abadi and Whittle found that the duration of foveation periods with eye velocity below 10° per second was actually not a better predictor of head posture either. Thus, although the position of the null is a useful rule of thumb for predicting head posture, it is by no means perfect for as yet unknown reasons.

Contrast sensitivity also depends on the ability to align the visual target with the fovea during foveation periods. Abadi *et al.* (1991) have shown that even with a well-differentiated fovea in patients with CIN, only half of them consistently used the fovea during foveation periods. Surprisingly, about half of their albino patients also used a good 'foveation' strategy in spite of being afoveate.

A higher incidence of with-the-rule corneal astigmatism has been frequently reported in SDN and CIN, and it would seem to be secondary to mechanical deformation or some growth response to anisotropic contrast sensitivity, but the mechanism is obscure (Dickinson & Abadi 1984). Using tachistoscopic presented stimuli, Abadi and King-Smith (1979) have shown lower sensitivity to lines orthogonal to the nystagmus, and this may reflect a meridional amblyopia secondary to longstanding anisotropic visual deprivation (Daroff *et al.* 1973).

Oscillopsia

Oscillopsia is an illusory perception that the world is moving. Under normal lighting conditions most patients with early onset nystagmus do not complain of oscillopsia when gaze is in its habitual position, but oscillopsia may or may not occur in gaze directions eccentric from a null position. Information concerning disturbances of vision, whether from the child or parent, should be considered cautiously since it can be difficult for the young child to understand the difference between diplopia, blurred vision and oscillopsia.

Mechanism

The underlying mechanism of SDN/CIN is unknown; most of the oculomotor systems have been implicated at one time or another and there is little to guide the clinician.

Some have argued that the SDN/CIN is secondary to a congenital malformation, which has been prompted by the association of SDN with albinism and its attendant anomalous visual pathways (Optican & Zee 1984). However, there is little to support this. Patients with CIN or other sensory defects do not show the albinoid crossed VEP asymmetries (see Chapter 9), even in those remarkable families that have inherited both albinism and CIN (Apkarian & Shallo-Hoffmann 1991). Moreover, rarely a patient with the other typical features of albinism may not have nystagmus (Kriss *et al.* 1992a). It has also been claimed that CIN may be due to a chiasmal abnormality (McCarty *et al.* 1992), but as pointed out by Kriss *et al.* (1992a), the available data do not support this. A genuine crossed asymmetry has been reported in extremely rare cases of achiasmic children (Apkarian *et al.* 1993), who exhibited nystagmus described as see-saw. We have also seen a child with achiasmia and other midline defects who had crossed VEP asymmetry and pure see-saw nystagmus (no SDN/CIN). Congenital See-Saw Nystagmus (SSN) is quite distinct from SDN/CIN, and although it is conceivable that in those rare cases of so-called 'congenital idiopathic' SSN there may be anomalous pathways, there is no evidence that patients with CIN have anomalous visual pathways.

Because SDN occurs in association with such a wide range of genetically unrelated congenital and even neonatally acquired visual disorders, its seems most likely that the nystagmus results from an abnormal neurodevelopmental process induced by a visual defect at birth or in early infancy. However, why a few albinos with foveal hypoplasia do not develop nystagmus (Kriss *et al.* 1992b), and why a child with CSNB with a very subtle retinal defect and normal visual acuity does develop SDN remains unknown. And, by definition, the origins of CIN are unknown; whether future technical developments will reveal subtle visual defects in CIN remains to be seen.

Tusa *et al.* (1992) and Harris (1995) have produced rigorous models of the nystagmus based on an abnormality of the fixation or the smooth pursuit systems. Yet, why these putative abnormalities arise from a sensory defect have not been explained, especially since macula defects occurring later in life do not result in this type of nystagmus. One is left with the strong suspicion that the nystagmus results from abnormal visual experience during a critical period of visual development (Harris 1995).

Management

There is no cure for the nystagmus, and the management goals are as follows.
1 To maximize useful vision in the context of the underlying sensory defect (with limited effective treatment options).
2 To provide genetic counselling.
3 To explain the various visual, educational and social problems encountered by patients with SDN/CIN.

These can only be achieved after the nystagmus has been properly identified (using eye movement recordings if necessary), and after the correct diagnosis of the underlying visual deficit has been made. The 'diagnosis' of CIN can only be made by exclusion of any sensory deficit using electrophysiology.

All patients should be refracted. Most treatment of SDN/CIN has been aimed at improving vision by shifting the null to primary position to obviate a head turn (surgery, prisms), or inducing convergence to dampen the nystagmus (prisms, minus lenses).

Treatment

Prisms

Prismatic spectacles will shift the visual scene laterally thereby allowing the child with an eccentric null region to view objects straight ahead without a head turn. The base of the prisms should be away from the null position in the same direction for both eyes. Additional minus lenses will induce excess convergence that may also help to dampen the nystagmus. Prisms are only practical for small head turns. For large head turns they are too thick and unwieldy, and Fresnel lenses introduce distortion and chromatic aberration.

Base-out prisms to induce convergence or minus lens correction to induce accommodation and convergence have limited value, especially in patients with esotropia, which is a common accompaniment to SDN/CIN.

Surgery for nystagmus

Treatment directed at the nystagmus itself to improve visual acuity was first described by Bietti and Bagolini (1960). They performed a large recession of the four horizontal muscles. This technique has enjoyed a recent revival (Helveston *et al.* 1991; von Noorden & Sprunger 1991) but is not yet fully evaluated (Flynn 1991).

Surgery for head posture

Surgery for unacceptable head position has been performed in young children for many years. Kestenbaum (1953) performed equal recessions and resections of all horizontal recti with shifting of the eyes in the direction of the rapid phase of the nystagmus, away from the null point. Anderson (1953) recessed the muscles responsible for the slow component of the nystagmus, and Goto (1954) resected the appropriate muscles without a corresponding recession. Pratt-Johnson (1971) recommended symmetrical surgery on all four horizontal recti when there was no associated strabismus.

Parks (1973) suggested recession of one medial rectus 5 mm and a resection of the lateral rectus 8 mm with the opposite eye receiving a recession of the lateral rectus 7 mm and resection of the medial rectus muscle 6 mm (Fig. 63.7). Because of the high rate of recurrence using this technique, Calhoun and Harley (1973) recommended no surgery in a 15° head turn and increased the amount of the 'classic Parks' surgery by 40%, resulting in surgery of 7, 8.4, 9.8 and 11.2 mm for a 30° head turn and a classic plus 60% for a 45° head turn.

Taylor (1973) recommended an 8–9 mm recession of the

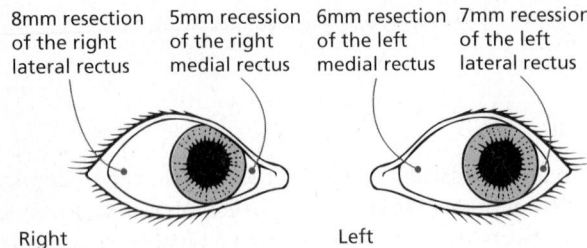

8mm resection of the right lateral rectus   5mm recession of the right medial rectus   6mm resection of the left medial rectus   7mm recession of the left lateral rectus

Right   Left

Fig. 63.7 Head posture surgery to shift null in SDN/CIN illustrated for a head turn to the right (null in left gaze). Arrows show resection of the right lateral and left medial recti and recession of the right medial and left lateral recti. Numbers (mm) show the classic Parks surgery.

lateral rectus muscle on the side of the slow-phase of the nystagmus and a 6 mm recession of the medial rectus muscle of the antagonists. The recommended surgery reported by Scott and Kraft (1984) is as follows.

1 A classic Parks maximum for 20° turn.

2 Classic plus 10–40% for 24–45° turn.

3 Classic plus 40% for 45° or more.

4 Turns over 50° required augmentation of 50–60% to obtain an excellent result.

Mitchell *et al.* (1987) reviewed the records of 48 patients with nystagmus and head turn. They were subdivided into six groups receiving different types of surgery. The results of this series are comparable to the series reported by Scott and Kraft (1984), and by Nelson *et al.* (1984).

It does not require excessive cynicism (Casteels *et al.* 1992) to wonder why, when each report claims success, that successive publications recommend ever more surgery, even to the point, in effect, of creating a gazy palsy (Calhoun & Harley 1973; Scott & Kraft 1984). Null point surgery should be reserved for those with genuine and significant symptoms.

Adelstein and Cüppers (1966) introduced the term 'nystagmus blockage syndrome' to describe a large angle (> 50 prism dioptres) early onset esotropia that was thought to be secondary to sustained convergence effort to block SDN/CIN. Although this became a popular label, it was probably over-used and now many believe it to be rare. The syndrome requires the initial presence of SDN/CIN. The clinical significance of Nystagmus Blockage Syndrome is that surgical outcome is more variable than in essential infantile esotropia.

Drugs

Baclofen has been described as having some success in adults with SDN/CIN by Yee *et al.* (1982) but not by Halmagyi *et al.* (1980b). 5-Hydroxytryptophan has been reported to be successful (Larmande & Pautrizel 1981).

Feedback

Over recent years a number of potential unproven 'therapies' have been proposed to improve vision in SDN/CIN. Their mechanisms are unclear but may function by providing some feedback about the eye oscillations that is otherwise absent due to the lack of oscillopsia in SDN/CIN.

1 Auditory feedback coupled to the intensity of the nystagmus has had some moderate success (Abadi *et al.* 1980; Ciuffreda *et al.* 1980; Kirschen 1983; Mezawa *et al.* 1990).

2 Contact lenses (Abadi 1979; Allen & Davies 1983; Dell'Osso *et al.* 1988) appear to dampen the nystagmus through their provision of tactile feedback via the eyelids.

3 After-image treatment (Stohler 1973) and possibly intermittent photic stimulation (Mallett 1983) may provide visual feedback.

Although these techniques are claimed to improve vision in some patients, their long-term benefit has not been properly assessed with controlled clinical trials. An inherent difficulty is that SDN/CIN is extraordinarily susceptible to changes in mental state. Patients entering a study are likely to be initially anxious, but increasing familiarity with experimental procedures during a clinical trial is likely to reduce stress and thereby improve visual performance, regardless of any treatment effects. Blind studies with placebo controls are therefore essential.

The possibility of providing additional feedback during early infancy, when the nystagmus first appears and when the visual system is most plastic, has not been explored to our knowledge.

Counselling

Genetic counselling should be provided based on the correct diagnosis of the underlying visual deficit (if present). It should be recognized that currently there are numerous adults who have been incorrectly labelled as idiopathic, because a subtle sensory defect (ocular albinism, cone dysfuction, CSNB) has not been detected, or the nystagmus has been incorrectly identified (e.g. MLN). Without thorough ophthalmological, electrophysiological and oculomotor investigations when needed, it is not possible to provide sensible genetic counselling for these patients and their offspring.

SDN/CIN can be a life-long visual and social handicap, and parents should be counselled on the problems their child may encounter later in life.

The nystagmus usually decreases in intensity with age, particularly in the first year, but almost always persists throughout life. It is important to clarify that in most cases the nystagmus is secondary to an underlying visual problem; it is not unusual to meet affected individuals who believe that the nystagmus is the real reason for their poor vision, and who may go to great lengths to obtain a 'cure' or operation for their nystagmus. 'Dizziness' may occur from time to time, especially in unfamiliar surroundings.

Nystagmus never leads to blindness. Spectacles do not correct for nystagmus. An often overlooked point is that the child does not experience oscillopsia; parents often find this a relief. The degree of nystagmus does not correlate well with the degree of the underlying visual deficit.

Problems at school can arise because of poor vision, misinterpretation of abnormal head posture, head-shaking and close-up viewing. A visual problem may not arise until small print is introduced into the classroom, or a low contrast whiteboard is used. Some children with nystagmus may not perform well in moving ball games, but they can be encouraged in other sports that do not require fine vision, such as swimming, and so on. Inevitably, teasing may occur. Some prospective careers should not be encouraged (e.g. military, aircrew, police, etc.).

Eligibility to hold a driving licence depends on visual acuity at some specified distance (not the presence of nystagmus). Most patients with SDN/CIN do not meet the minimum vision requirements. One should also consider the problem of the possible drop in acuity when the SDN/CIN waveform changes during periods of stress, which are not uncommon in driving situations.

Neurological and neuromuscular nystagmus

All NN requires neurological investigation, which usually includes CT and/or MRI. Rarely, forms of nystagmus that are identical to NN can be congenital and idiopathic, but this can only be established by exclusion (see Fig. 63.1). An onset in infancy does not preclude intracranial disease. The various types of NN have been extensively investigated in adults, but much less in children. In describing NN we shall draw heavily from the adult literature, but in the young child the distribution of causes will be biased towards inherited degenerative conditions and structural malformations rather than the acquired lesions that dominate the adult literature.

It is also essential to realize that the presence of a sensory defect (e.g. optic atrophy, progressive retinal dystrophy) does not mean that the nystagmus is SDN, regardless of the age of onset.

Gaze-Paretic and Rebound Nystagmus

Gaze-Paretic Nystagmus (GPN), often called gaze-evoked nystagmus, is a jerk nystagmus that appears on eccentric gaze and beats in the direction of gaze. On lateral gaze, it is horizontal, but there may also be an upbeat GPN in upgaze although the intensity is usually much less than that in lateral gaze. In oblique gaze the nystagmus may be oblique, but it may also be purely horizontal if the vertical gaze-holding apparatus is spared. Downbeat GPN in downgaze is much less common (but horizontal GPN often accompanies primary position downbeat nystagmus). In primary position there is no GPN, but unsteady fixation may occur or there may be a compounding APN. GPN is unaffected by monocular occlusion, which distinguishes it from MLN.

Pathological GPN is rare in early infancy, but at any other age it is probably the most common NN. It is due to a mismatch between the gaze-holding circuitry of the brain stem or cerebellum and the dynamics of the extraocular muscles. It can be experimentally induced in animals by lesions of the cerebellar flocculus (Zee *et al.* 1981) and the perihypoglossal region of the brain stem (Cannon & Robinson 1987).

Other horizontal abnormal eye movements are usually present with GPN, which together form the 'vestibulocerebellar' or 'flocculus' oculomotor syndrome, which consists of low gain or saccadic pursuit, poor or absent suppression of the vestibulo-ocular reflex (VOR), poor or absent OKN, and a hyperactive VOR. In severe cases, the eyes drift so rapidly back to primary position that the child may adopt head thrusts to shift gaze, which can be confused with head thrusts due to a saccade failure (Harris *et al.* 1993b).

GPN is associated with a very wide variety of cerebellar disorders. In children, GPN is often bilateral, but when unilateral it beats towards the side of the lesion. It is usually associated with other cerebellar signs such as truncal or gait ataxia, dysarthria, intention tremor, and so on. (Note that ataxic nystagmus actually refers to abduction nystagmus, not GPN!) GPN may be associated with intermittent saccade failure, as in ataxia telangiectasia.

The possibility of an external cause for GPN should always be considered because GPN can be a side-effect of many drugs, including sedatives, anticonvulsants, alcohol, barbiturates, chloral hydrate, diazepam and marijuana.

GPN may also occur as an inter-ictal phenomenon in episodic/paroxysmal ataxia, which may be mistaken for epilepsy. The inter-ictal GPN does not usually respond to acetazolamide therapy (Baloh & Winder 1991).

GPN has also been reported in various non-progressive familial vestibulocerebellar disorders (Theunissen *et al.* 1989; Harris *et al.* 1993c).

GPN may also occur in myasthenia gravis. In this case the gaze-holding mismatch is peripheral, rather than central, as a result of fatigue of the neuromuscular junction.

Rebound nystagmus

Sometimes GPN exhibits a rebound phenomenon, called

Rebound Nystagmus (RN). When the patient attempts sustained eccentric fixation, the intensity of the GPN may wane or even reverse (Hood *et al.* 1973). Upon returning gaze rapidly to primary position a rebound nystagmus occurs transiently for a few seconds, and beats in the opposite direction to the side of the previous eccentric fixation. RN occurs in the dark and is not dependent on a visual input. Pathological RN is associated with the typical vestibulocerebellar eye movement abnormalities seen with GPN.

As with GPN, RN is associated with a wide range of disorders involving the cerebellum. It is probably a more definite sign of cerebellar disease than GPN, and has been associated with a tumour confined to the flocculus (Yamazaki & Zee 1979). RN is not a constant feature of GPN, and may disappear in progressive disease; we have seen a case where the RN was unilateral with bilateral GPN. RN is said to be associated with more chronic disorders, but this may reflect a lack of rapid progression.

RN has been variably associated with episodic vertigo and ataxia (Theunissen *et al.* 1989; Baloh & Winder 1991) and with a dominantly inherited benign familial vestibulocerebellar disorder (Harris *et al.* 1993c).

Toluene (Baba *et al.* 1988), and epanutin and barbiturate intoxication (Hood *et al.* 1973) may lead to RN.

Normal individuals with End-Point Nystagmus may also exhibit physiological RN (Shallo-Hoffmann *et al.* 1990), but they do not show any other oculomotor abnormality such as low-gain pursuit. RN should not be confused with Periodic Alternating Nystagmus.

'Acquired' Pendular Nystagmus

Acquired Pendular Nystagmus (APN) is usually a high frequency low amplitude nystagmus. It may be purely horizontal, purely vertical, circular or elliptical. It may be completely monocular or more exaggerated in one eye.

APN typically remains pendular in all gaze directions with usually only small changes in amplitude, but a horizontal APN may become circumrotatory on elevation. This gaze-independence is in contrast to pendular SDN/CIN which remains horizontal in elevation and usually becomes jerk on lateral gaze. In most cases of APN there is an optokinetic response with the APN superimposed on the OKN slow-phases. This is in contrast to SDN/CIN, in which there is usually no recognizable OKN response. However, if APN is compounded with GPN, the nystagmus will become jerk on lateral gaze due to the GPN, and there may be no optokinetic response. Eye movement recordings are particularly useful in distinguishing among these different types of nystagmus.

APN is probably the second most common neurological nystagmus in childhood and can occur at any age, and although classified as 'acquired', APN can have an onset in the first few months, at the same time that SDN/CIN may occur (Fig. 63.8). It is therefore important to distinguish horizontal and circumrotatory APN from SDN/CIN in infancy.

APN can be associated with a wide range of brainstem and cerebellar disease, including:

1 Dysmyelinating disease, particularly Pelizaeus–Merzbacher disease (PMD). In some cases of PMD, the nystagmus may be very subtle and compounded with upbeat nystagmus (Trobe *et al.* 1991). In others, the APN may be compounded with GPN and other vestibulocerebellar eye movement abnormalities (Mallinson *et al.* 1983). It has been reported that PMD carriers may also have mildly abnormal eye movements (Huygen *et al.* 1992).

2 APN may be associated with synchronous oscillations of the palate, pharynx and head. This oculopalatal myoclonus (Gresty *et al.* 1982; Nakada & Kwee 1986) does not occur with SDN/CIN. It is thought to be due to a lesion in the dentato-mesencephalic-olivary system with defective VOR adaptation (Nakada & Kwee 1986).

3 APN has also been reported secondary to drug toxicities, including glue-sniffing (Maas *et al.* 1991).

4 Demyelinating disease (Gresty *et al.* 1982).

Asymmetric nystagmus

Asymmetrical or even monocular APN may be secondary to late onset visual loss and has been reported in amblyopia. This is rare in children. In some cases of APN caused by a neurodegenerative disease there may be progressive visual loss due to an associated retinal dystrophy or optic atrophy; the APN in these cases may be complicated by the increasing visual sensory defect.

In children, APN is often associated with intrinsic or extrinsic lesions of the optic chiasm, usually gliomas or craniopharyngiomas. The APN may be asymmetric and accompanied by head nodding or head shaking. A similar clinical picture is presented by the child with a self-limiting benign condition called spasmus nutans. Neuroimaging is essential in all cases of APN.

APN is sometimes associated with a saccade failure ('ocular motor apraxia'), as in Cockayne's syndrome (Coker *et al.* 1979), PMD, Joubert's syndrome, Dandy–Walker malformation, Cornelia de Lange syndrome and perinatal hypoxia (Harris *et al.* 1996). Head thrusting may not be present.

See-Saw Nystagmus

See-Saw Nystagmus (SSN) is a rare nystagmus in which one eye elevates and usually intorts as the other eye depresses and extorts, and it may be associated with a bitemporal hemianopia (Maddox 1914). The vertical components are disjunctive and the torsional components are conjugate. SSN may be congenital idiopathic or acquired.

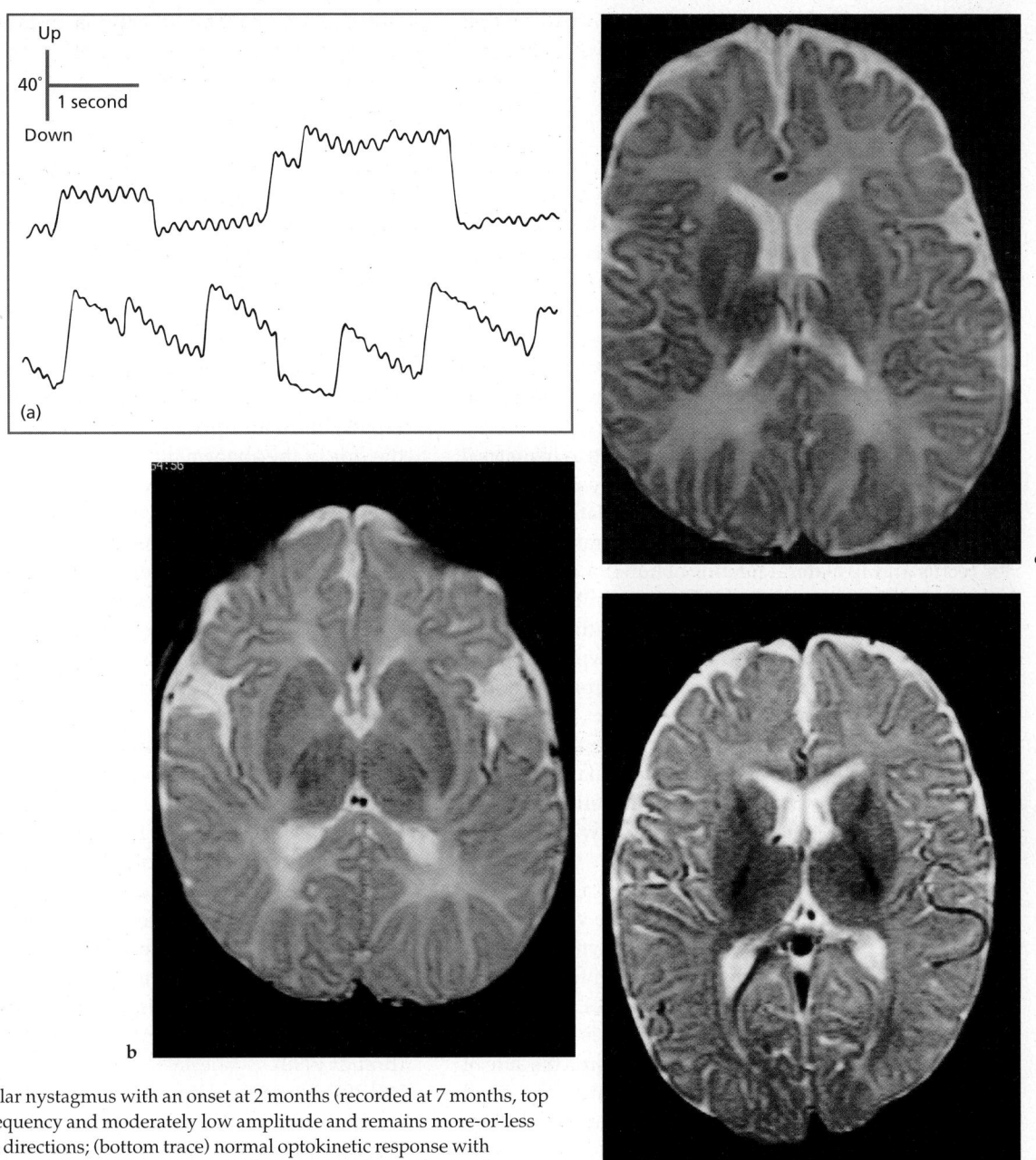

Fig. 63.8 (a) Pendular nystagmus with an onset at 2 months (recorded at 7 months, top trace) has a high frequency and moderately low amplitude and remains more-or-less constant in all gaze directions; (bottom trace) normal optokinetic response with spontaneous nystagmus superimposed. In spite of early onset, this nystagmus has no defining features of early onset Sensory Defect or Congenital Idiopathic Nystagmus. (b, c) MRI showed severe dysmyelination and a diagnosis of Pelizaeus–Merzbacher disease was eventually made. (d) Age-matched MRI (at that time 6 months old) with myelination clearly seen in the internal capsule.

In congenital idiopathic SSN the elevating eye may extort, but intorsion has also been described in association with retinitis pigmentosa (Bergin & Halpern 1986). Full-blown SSN is very distinctive, but sometimes the vertical component may be barely discernible and it may be confused with pure torsional nystagmus.

SSN is usually associated with parasellar or chiasmal lesions, and is thought to be the result of bilateral pressure on the midbrain, rather than a visual deficit (Miller 1985).

The nystagmus is usually pendular, but a jerk see-saw has been associated with unilateral lesion of the mesodiencephalic junction (Halmagyi *et al.* 1994).

Recently SSN has been recorded in children with optic chiasmal dysplasia, in which there is no decussation at the chiasm (Apkarian *et al.* 1993). This raises the question as to whether SSN may, after all, be of visual origin, or whether there is also a subtle malfomation of the midbrain. In a case we have seen there were other midline malformations, although no midbrain lesion could be discerned. It should also be noted that in our case, each eye intorted on elevation.

Vestibular Nystagmus

Spontaneous Vestibular Nystagmus (VN) is due to vestibular disease, either peripheral (labyrinths and vestibular nerve) or central. It is usually accompanied by symptoms of dizziness, vertigo and oscillopsia.

Acute peripheral disease usually gives rise to a mixed nystagmus reflecting a static unbalanced excess of tone from the remaining intact semi-circular canals. For single canal involvement the nystagmus occurs in the plane of that canal.

For example, the posterior canal gives rise to ipsilateral intorsion and depression through excitatory pathways to the ipsilateral superior oblique and contralateral inferior rectus (and inhibitory pathways to the contralateral superior rectus and ipsilateral inferior oblique). Loss of tonus from the left anterior canal will leave an imbalance that causes torsional slow-phases to the left (beats to the opposite side of the lesion), and with downward slow-phases (upbeating), due to the excess tone from the unopposed right posterior canal. If gaze is directed to the right, the torsional component will increase because the torsional axis becomes more perpendicular to the posterior canal plane. If gaze is to the left, the vertical component will increase as the vertical axis aligns with the canal plane (see Fig. 64.4).

Acute unilateral labyrinthine loss leads to a mixed horizontal/torsional nystagmus. In this case the vertical components from the intact posterior (downward) and anterior (upward) canals cancel, but their intorsion components add and cause torsional slow-phases towards the side of the lesion. The intact lateral canal is unopposed and so there is a horizontal slow-phase towards the side of lesion as well. Because of the arrangement of the canal planes, pure vertical or pure torsional nystagmus seldom occurs with peripheral disease. The direction of slow-phases due to excitation of each canal are summarized in Table 64.2.

An important aspect of the vestibular system is its ability to adapt and compensate centrally for tone imbalances. Thus, after an acute lesion, over some days peripheral VN subsides. If the acute attacks are intermittent and remit (as in Menière's disease), the central adaptation will cause a temporary Recovery Nystagmus that beats towards the side of the lesion. Static imbalance can sometimes be detected by observing a transient nystagmus after vigorous head shaking or nodding.

In peripheral disease the nystagmus becomes more prominent when fixation is broken, as in the dark or with Frenzel lenses. This is in contrast to the central lesions which commonly affect smooth pursuit.

In children acute peripheral VN and vertigo is often due to vestibular neuritis.

Positional nystagmus

Positional nystagmus is a pathological form of vestibular nystagmus that occurs when the head is moved. In the majority of cases this is due to a peripheral disorder and is usually associated with benign paroxysmal positional vertigo (BPPV), in which patients complain of episodes of vertigo, which is usually rotational, on certain head movements. The condition is usually benign but may be protracted over years.

The nystagmus is induced by moving the patient rapidly from an upright into the head-down position to the side of the abnormality (Hallpike manoeuvre). After a few seconds, nystagmus occurs and then gradually wanes in less than 40 seconds. It is mixed with a torsional component consisting of beats extorting relative to the lower eye, and a vertical component with upward beats. The nystagmus may be asymmetrical, being more torsional in the lower eye, and more vertical in the upper. The nystagmus also becomes more torsional when viewing laterally (i.e. down) and more vertical in the opposite direction (up).

A reversed but weaker nystagmus occurs upon sitting. The positional nystagmus wanes with repeated manoeuvres.

It is believed that BPPV is due to detachment of degenerated otoliths from the utricle, which then deposit on, or interfere with, the cupula of the posterior canal (cupulolithiasis). The increased mass of the cupula then gives rise to abnormally excitatory signals during head motion, which are relayed to the ipsilateral superior oblique and contralateral inferior rectus, so causing intorsion ipsilateral to the canal and downward slow-phases (Brandt 1990).

BPPV is unusual in childhood and rarely occurs in the first decade. BPPV can be secondary to viral neurolabyrinthitis or trauma, although it is not always clear which came first. BPPV may occur after migraine attacks, and may also be a permanent side-effect of aminoglycoside toxicity (Baloh *et al.* 1987). Among children presenting with vertigo and dizziness, BPPV is also uncommon.

BPPV must be differentiated from intermittent pure DBN.

Vertical nystagmus

The child with vertical nystagmus should always be investigated on the suspicion of an intracranial disorder. Rarely, vertical nystagmus can be congenital and inherited (Forsythe 1955; Sogg & Hoyt 1962; Bixenman 1983) or transient in a normal infant (Hoyt 1987; Weissman *et al.*

1988). Vertical nystagmus is usually divided into three—pendular, downbeat and upbeat—but these may co-exist in some patients depending on gaze direction, head position and degree of convergence. In children, vertical nystagmus is often intermittent and may be mislabelled as opsoclonus. Vertical nystagmus, particularly upbeat, may depend on head position, and it has been argued that it is really a central positional nystagmus involving the otolithic centres (Fisher *et al.* 1983). Whether these various features of vertical nystagmus cluster into different aetiological categories is not yet known. We recommend that a child with an apparently intermittent vertical nystagmus be examined in different positions, particularly supine.

Upbeat nystagmus appearing only in elevation is a common associate of horizontal GPN, which is discussed above. Vertical pendular nystagmus is a common variant of APN, which is also discussed above.

Downbeat Nystagmus

Downbeat Nystagmus (DBN) usually occurs in the primary position and often with a distinctive increase in vertical amplitude on lateral gaze (Yee 1990). In lateral gaze there is also often a horizontal component (GPN) causing the nystagmus to become oblique. However, in primary position the nystagmus may be a small amplitude vertical pendular or may even be clinically absent (Baloh & Yee 1989). In elevation the nystagmus diminishes and may convert to upbeat, but sometimes the DBN may actually intensify (Baloh & Yee 1989). The nystagmus may appear or intensify with convergence (Cox *et al.* 1981; Baloh & Yee 1989). DBN may also change with head position (Halmagyi *et al.* 1983). DBN is often associated with horizontal deficits of smooth pursuit, OKN and suppression of the VOR, and other cerebellar signs are usually present.

DBN is classically associated with abnormalities of the craniocervical junction, which require imaging with MRI, and include: Arnold–Chiari malformation, basilar invagination, syringobulbia, medullary glioma, as well as deformation of the cervical spine at C5–6, and the Klippel–Feil syndrome.

DBN may occur in cerebellar degenerative conditions. The increase in vertical amplitude in lateral gaze is not obligatory but is more common with cerebellar involvement (Yee 1990).

DBN may also occur with raised intracranial pressure due to remote supratentorial causes (Phadke *et al.* 1981; Lavin & Bahntge 1983).

DBN can be secondary to anticonvulsant therapy and sedatives (Miller 1985), and in adults DBN has also been reported in magnesium and thiamine deficiency secondary to chronic alcoholism (Saul & Selhorst 1981). In alcoholic DBN the distinctive enhancement on lateral gaze is not usually present.

DBN has been reported as a transient phenomenon in the healthy infant (Hoyt 1987; Weissman *et al.* 1988). In infantile 'paroxysmal tonic upgaze', there is usually DBN (see Chapter 64).

It should be noted that DBN may have accelerating upward slow-phases, but this feature does not imply SDN/CIN (Fig. 63.9).

Upbeat Nystagmus

Upbeat Nystagmus (UBN) in primary position is much less common than DBN. The vertical component of UBN does not increase on lateral gaze, but may become oblique due to a compounding horizontal GPN. UBN usually increases on elevation and decreases on depression, but the reverse may occur. In some cases UBN nystagmus changes to DBN on downgaze, and may stop or become downbeat with convergence. UBN may be enhanced or diminished in a supine position or with a head tilt (Fisher *et al.* 1983; Baloh & Yee 1989; Hirose *et al.* 1991). UBN can be associated with APN and poor horizontal pursuit, GPN and RN (Kattah *et al.* 1983).

UBN has been associated with acquired lesions of the pontomedullary tegmentum, the brachium conjunctivum, the midbrain and the vermis. The nystagmus is thought to be due to an imbalance of the vertical VOR and the otoliths.

UBN, with or without APN, has been associated with cerebellar degeneration, including olivopontocerebellar atrophy (Baloh & Yee 1989), atrophy of the anterior vermis (Kattah *et al.* 1983), and dysmyelination as in Pelizaeus–Merzbacher disease (Mallinson *et al.* 1983). UBN can be an early sign of cerebellar astrocytoma (Traccis *et al.* 1989). UBN can also be a long-term phenomenon in survivors of medulloblastoma: in such cases it does not necessarily indicate active disease (Elliot *et al.* 1989). UBN is not always due to central disturbances and has been reported in chronic middle ear disease (Gresty *et al.* 1988). UBN is not usually associated with Arnold–Chiari or other craniocervical malformations.

Congenital intermittent UBN has been reported in a non-progressive, probably autosomal dominant, familial disorder (Sogg & Hoyt 1962). Furman *et al.* (1985) also reported a probably dominantly inherited infantile condition with UBN and typical horizontal vestibulocerebellar eye movement abnormalities, which were associated with anterior vermis atrophy. UBN may also be a transient phenomenon in the healthy infant (Hoyt 1987; see also Chapter 64).

UBN has been reported secondary to organophosphate poisoning (Jay *et al.* 1982).

Torsional Nystagmus

Torsional Nystagmus (TN) is a nystagmus in which the

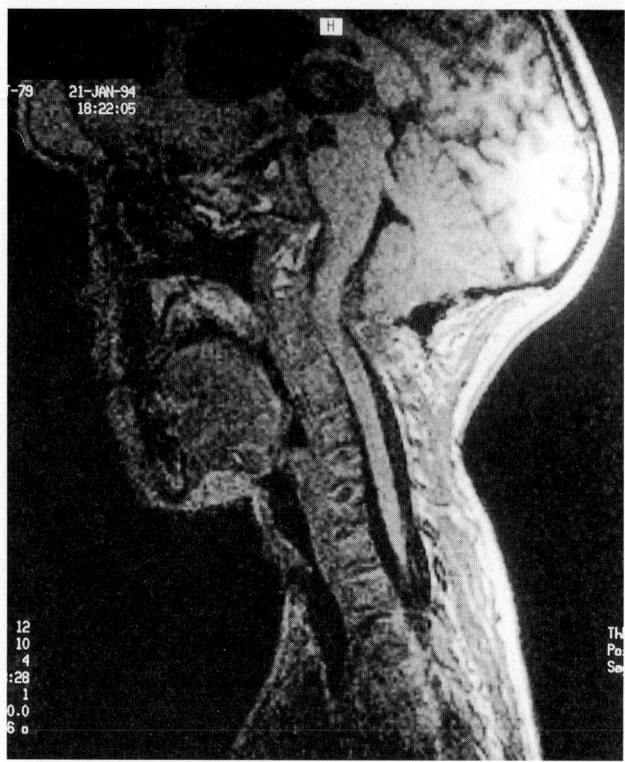

a

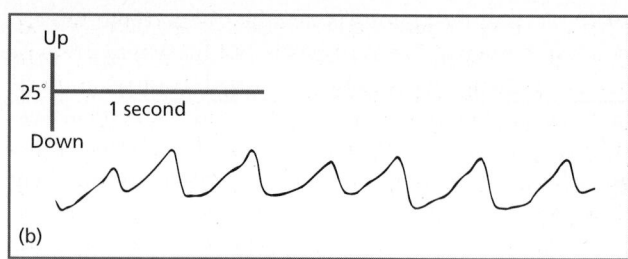

(b)

Fig. 63.9 (a) Cervicomedullary malformation. Downbeat nystagmus was acquired at 13 years following accidental brain stem compression during intubation. (b) Note that in vertical nystagmus accelerating upward slow phases do not indicate sensory defect or congenital idiopathic nystagmus.

oscillations are around the anteroposterior axis of the eye (see Fig. 63.2). Although the angle of torsion may be quite large, TN can be difficult to detect without ophthalmoscopy or specialized equipment (electro-oculography or infrared limbus eye tracker cannot detect torsion), and consequently TN may be under-reported.

Torsional eye movements occur as part of SSN or as part of peripheral vestibular nystagmus (see above). Small torsional movements may also occur in conjunction with early onset nystagmus (SDN/CIN or LN), but do not indicate additional pathology.

Pure TN is rare but usually indicates central pathology, and has been associated with midpontine lesions (possibly affecting central vestibular connections) (Noseworthy *et al.* 1988).

Very rarely CIN may be purely torsional, and may have accelerating slow-phases in the torsional axis (M.A. Gresty, personal communication), but as with vertical nystagmus, accelerating slow-phases in this axis do not necessarily indicate SDN/CIN (Noseworthy *et al.* 1988).

Abduction Nystagmus

Abduction Nystagmus is an asymmetrical ('dissociated') nystagmus that occurs predominantly in the abducting eye in lateral gaze. The nystagmus beats towards the abducting eye, and a less intense nystagmus may also occur in the adducting eye. It is most often associated with internuclear ophthalmoplegia. There has been no consensus on the pathophysiology of this nystagmus. Confusingly, abduction nystagmus has sometimes been labelled as 'ataxic nystagmus'.

Abduction Nystagmus as a part of a 'pseudo-internuclear ophthalmoplegia' has also been reported in association with myasthenia gravis (Jay *et al.* 1987).

Various mixtures of abduction and adduction nystagmus may occur following strabismus surgery.

Periodic Alternating Nystagmus and other cyclic phenomena

Periodic Alternating Nystagmus (nystagmus alternans)

Periodic Alternating Nystagmus (PAN) is a horizontal jerk nystagmus that spontaneously reverses direction every few minutes. In adults PAN is usually acquired, but it is more commonly associated with SDN/CIN in children as congenital PAN.

During a PAN cycle the intensity gradually increases for a minute or so, then decreases and becomes minimal during the neutral phase, which usually lasts a few tens of seconds. The intensity then increases once more in the opposite direction. Typically a reversal takes about 90 seconds to 2 minutes (period = 3–4 minutes) and consequently PAN can easily be overlooked. Shorter reversals of 10–20 seconds have been reported and are said to be more common in congenital PAN (Keane 1993). Even shorter reversals have been reported in PAN associated with infectious mononucleosis (Reis *et al.* 1989). Sometimes the PAN may be directionally asymmetric, with longer phases in one direction. Even an aperiodic alternating nystagmus has been reported (Nuti *et al.* 1986). PAN should not be confused with Rebound Nystagmus, although some have argued for a common underlying mechanism.

Acquired PAN is associated with lesions of the cerebellum or lower brain stem including: multiple sclerosis, brain stem encephalitis, syphilis, tumours of the fourth ventricle or cerebellum, aqueductal stenosis, vertebrobasilar artery insufficiency, cysticercosis, ataxia telangiectasia, Friedreich's ataxia, Arnold–Chiari malformation, and syringobulbia. PAN has also been reported secondary to otitis media. It has been said that acquired PAN is usually associated with chronic rather than acute disorders (Daroff & Dell'Osso 1974). Acquired PAN is thought to arise from brain stem disinhibition by the cerebellar vermis, both nodulus and uvula (Leigh *et al.* 1981).

PAN as a drug side-effect is unclear: in one report, PAN was related to phenytoin intoxication in a chronic alcoholic (Campbell 1980); in another, PAN was thought to be due to primidone/phenobarbitone intoxication in an epileptic patient on constant phenytoin medication (Schwankhaus *et al.* 1989). Both patients were adults.

PAN has been reported to occur in the dark or secondary to cataract and vitreal haemorrhage: the PAN was suppressed on restoration of vision (Cross *et al.* 1982; Jay *et al.* 1985).

Acquired PAN is rare in childhood. It is usually associated with other oculomotor abnormalities including DBN (Keane 1974), GPN, RN (Baloh *et al.* 1976), oculopalatal myoclonus, saccadic smooth pursuit, and saccadic dysmetria which can be best detected during the neutral phase of the PAN. Patients complain of oscillopsia, particularly during the maximal phases, and they may present with other cerebellar signs.

There have been many reports of a congenital PAN (cPAN) associated with SDN/CIN (Robb 1972). In cPAN the slow-phases are typically accelerative (but not always, see Fig. 63.10) with the direction reversing spontaneously every few minutes. In a recent study of 32 albinos, Abadi and Pascal (1994) reported PAN in 37%! PAN with SDN/CIN represents a spontaneous shift in the null region. This may also induce a spontaneous change in an associated abnormal head posture, and therefore it is important to observe candidates for head posture surgery for some minutes. The period of the reversal may be longer if the patient relaxes, and oscillopsia may be reported during the maximal phases.

For acquired PAN, some success with baclofen treatment has been reported (Halmagyi *et al.* 1980b; Nuti *et al.* 1986; Troost *et al.* 1990), but this is variable (Uemura *et al.* 1988).

Periodic Alternating Gaze deviation

Periodic Alternating Gaze (PAG) deviation is an alternating conjugate deviation, thought to be PAN with a co-existing saccade failure, and has been reported in the late stages of neurodegeneration (Grant *et al.* 1993). PAG, although rare, tends to be more common in children. PAG should be differentiated from ping-pong gaze.

Periodic Alternating Esotropia

Periodic Alternating Esotropia (PAE) is very rare and is usually associated with a compensatory head turn (Staudenmaier & Buncic 1983). Hamed and Silbiger (1992) reported a 9-month-old girl with PAE, neonatal apnoea, developmental delay, and no spontaneous nystagmus. MRI revealed a marked hypoplastic vermis, small brain stem, and large fourth ventricle. This case has many similarities to Joubert's syndrome (see Chapter 44).

Ping-pong gaze (short-cycle periodic alternating gaze)

In ping-pong gaze the eyes change direction immediately or after a few seconds (less than 10). The deviations may be extreme or restricted to one side (Ishikawa *et al.* 1993). It is seen in comatose or stuporous patients. Ping-pong gaze is usually associated with bilateral acute cerebral lesions (Stewart *et al.* 1979) in which case the prognosis is usually

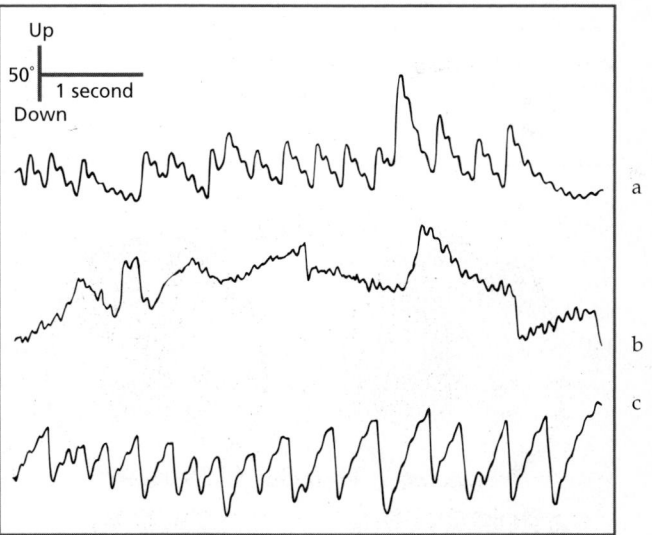

Fig. 63.10 Congenital PAN recorded from a 9-year-old albino: (a) (top trace) nystagmus just before the null period; (b) during the null period; and (c) after the null period showing reversed direction of beats. This unusual compound waveform shows: (i) a jerk nystagmus with predominantly linear slow-phases, which reversed direction spontaneously about every 100 seconds (traces are not contiguous); (ii) a superimposed constant low amplitude high frequency pendular nystagmus. Note that neither waveform is definitive of early onset sensory defect nystagmus.

very poor, but it may occur with severe, widespread developmental disorders. Recovery is possible when secondary to toxic encephalopathy.

Epileptic Nystagmus

Epileptic Nystagmus (EN) is a rare type of nystagmus that occurs only during seizures, and is absent between seizures. EN may be the only clinical sign, but is usually accompanied by other clonic phenomena including lid twitching. Associated pupillary oscillations have also been reported (Lavin 1986). It has been described mostly in adults, but EN can occur in early childhood (Beun *et al.* 1984). EN is confirmed by its consistent correlation with abnormal EEG activity and must not be confused with other types of intermittent nystagmus or a nystagmus that may develop secondary to anticonvulsant therapy.

The conscious patient may complain of a variety of ictal

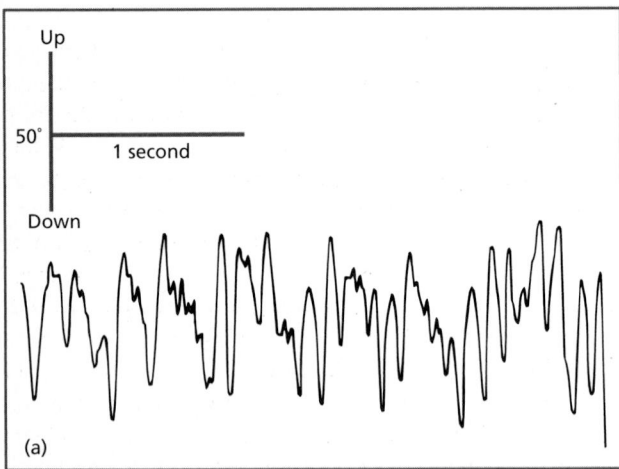

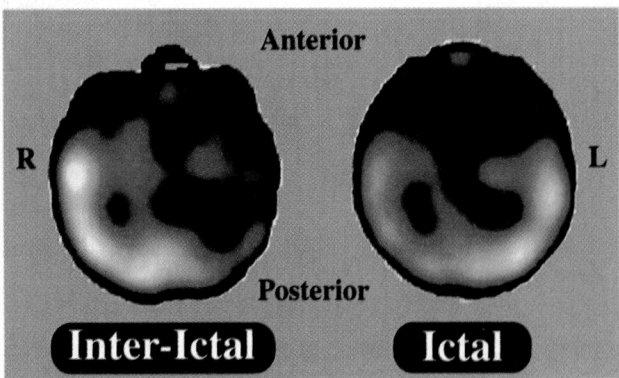

Fig. 63.11 Epileptic nystagmus recorded during a seizure from a 9-month-old girl with cortical dysplasia of the left temporal/occipital/parietal region. (a) The erratic right beating nystagmus, which crossed the midline, had rapid slow-phases and a very large amplitude. (b) Inter-ictal SPECT showed relative hypofusion in left temporal area. Ictal SPECT (radiolabel injected at onset of nystagmus) showed hyperfusion during seizure. Seizures and nystagmus completely resolved following left cortical resection.

visual phenomena including oscillopsia, blurred vision, blindness, and simple or complex hallucinations. Seizures may occur spontaneously or be induced by flashing lights, image blurring, eccentric gaze deviations, changes in light intensity, eyeball pressure, stress or fatigue (Stolz *et al.* 1991).

EN is usually horizontal and conjugate, but rarely it may be vertical, pendular, or even monocular (Jacome & FitzGerald 1982). In most cases the nystagmus beats contraversive to the side of the focus; however, the direction may reverse if the focus alternates (Stolz *et al.* 1991). The eyes may also show intermittent contraversive tonic deviations (i.e. in the same direction as the beats), but these deviations may sometimes be ipsiversive (in the direction of the slow-phases) (Tusa *et al.* 1990). We have seen contraversive and ipsiversive deviations on different days in the same infant.

Two types of horizontal EN are recognized. In one, the slow-phases are large amplitude and cross the midline. It has been argued that seizures activate the ipsilateral smooth pursuit and optokinetic cortical centres in the temporo-occipito-parietal area, which cause ipsiversive slow-phases across the midline, and are supposedly reset by normal reflexive contraversive quick-phase (Tusa *et al.* 1990). In the second, the slow-phases do not cross the midline and the nystagmus stays contralateral to the focus. It is thought that the focus stimulates contraversive saccades which are followed by decelerating slow-phases back to the midline due to poor gaze-holding ability. The focus is also usually in the contralateral temporo-occipitoparietal region. A requirement for this type of EN is poor gaze-holding (leaky integrator), which may be secondary to sedatives and anticonvulsants (Kaplan & Tusa 1993). Thus this is a unique type of nystagmus since it is the quick-phases that are pathological.

Vertical EN is rare and probably results from bilateral frontal foci (Kaplan & Lesser 1989).

Lid nystagmus

Oscillations of the lids are usually associated with vertical nystagmus, being most prominent with upbeat nystagmus. Lid twitching may also occur as an ictal phenomenon in EN. Isolated lid oscillations are, however, very rare and have been described as being induced bilaterally with convergence (Pick's) nystagmus (Sanders *et al.* 1968; Safran *et al.* 1982; Howard 1988). This has been associated with posterior fossa lesions, including the cerebellum, medulla and midbrain.

Convergence–Retraction Nystagmus

In Convergence–Retraction Nystagmus (CRN), attempts to make upward saccades or quick-phases cause the eyes to make rapid movements with saccadic-like velocities and may also cause the globes to retract due to an abnormal innervation of all rectus muscles. CRN may also occur with horizontal saccades. CRN may be brought out with a downward optokinetic stimulus, which induces convergence retraction instead of normal upward quick-phases. It may be quite uncomfortable. This may be the only oculomotor abnormality.

CRN is due to opposed saccades and is not a true nystagmus. It has been induced in monkeys with lesions of the posterior commissure. Clinically CRN is associated with lesions in or near the dorsal midbrain, and may be part of the full dorsal midbrain syndrome (Parinaud's syndrome). Such lesions may be intrinsic to the midbrain or extrinsic, including hydrocephalus.

CRN should be distinguished from a true nystagmus induced by convergence, which may occur in Voluntary Nystagmus (CRN is uncomfortable and also causes facial grimacing), or may rarely be a DBN appearing with convergence.

Head oscillations

Abnormal head movements can occur in a number of clinical contexts in the young child. Head shaking or nodding is often intermittent and should not be confused with the head movements used to shift gaze in a child with a gaze or saccade palsy. The hypermetric head thrusts seen in saccade palsy can appear oscillatory if the child attempts to shift gaze frequently between two targets. The terms head shaking and head nodding have been used interchangeably and do not indicate horizontal and vertical head oscillations, respectively.

It is important to establish the presence or absence of spontaneous nystagmus by examining the child with the head still, and in various positions, and when looking at different distances:

1 In the normal child, head shaking induces a compensating VOR which tends to keep the eyes pointing straight ahead, and could be mistaken for nystagmus as the head oscillates.

2 In some cases the nystagmus disappears during head shaking, perhaps suppressed by the VOR (Gresty & Halmagyi 1981).

3 The nystagmus may be dampened if the child is allowed to adopt an extreme head turn (Chrousos *et al.* 1985).

4 The nystagmus and head shaking may only occur at near distances (Chrousos *et al.* 1986), or only at far distances if convergence dampens the nystagmus.

5 The head shaking may only occur under strong fixation effort, or when the child is tired or stressed due to other factors.

6 Other children may only exhibit head shaking when they believe they are not being watched!

The question of whether head oscillations help to stabilize retinal images or are a concomitant abnormality has frequently been asked, but there is no consensus and there may be different reasons for head shaking (Gresty & Halmagyi 1981). It is difficult to judge any compensatory role of head shaking clinically but a patient who head shakes when concentrating on an object of interest is perhaps more likely to have a head shake that improves his vision, and therefore a better prognosis than one with a head shake that occurs even when not concentrating.

Head shaking and sensory defect nystagmus/congenital idiopathic nystagmus

By far, the most common association of head shaking is with SDN/CIN.

Spasmus nutans

Spasmus nutans (Latin for nodding spasm) is a self-limiting, benign triad of asymmetric APN, head nodding, and a head turn or tilt. Some cases may not have an abnormal head posture. The nystagmus often has a phase difference between the eyes. The pathogenesis is unknown. First described in the nineteenth century, this condition was thought to be prevalent in children from poor families and raised in dark surroundings. It is now a rare condition, but it is more prevalent in some centres than others.

The onset is typically between 4 and 12 months, but up to 2 years is not uncommon. The nystagmus precedes the head nodding, and both are usually horizontal, but may be vertical, oblique or torsional. The head nodding is intermittent and usually has a lower frequency than the nystagmus (Gottlob *et al.* 1992). Head nodding may suppress the nystagmus (Gresty *et al.* 1976) or compensate for the nystagmus by altering the nystagmus frequency (Gottlob *et al.* 1992). Chrousos *et al.* (1985) have also argued for suppression of the nystagmus by head movement.

The condition resolves before 5 years, although in some cases the nystagmus may persist intermittently at a subclinical level (Weissman *et al.* 1987).

Although many children with spasmus nutans are healthy, some have a history of prematurity, strabismus, developmental delay or other systemic disease. Chiasmal glioma is an association (Arnoldi & Tychsen 1995) and patients with spasmus nutans should have a neurophysiological assessment (see Chapter 9) and if this is abnormal, neuroimaging should also be done.

The diagnosis of spasmus nutans cannot be made on clinical signs. There are no reliable diagnostic clues to differentiate this self-limiting condition from APN due to intracranial lesions (Gottlob *et al.* 1990). In addition the diagnosis of spasmus nutans cannot be made without excluding subtle retinal disorders such as congenital stationary night-blindness (Lambert & Newman 1993).

Even Leigh's subacute necrotizing encephalomyelopathy has been mistaken for spasmus nutans (Sedwick *et al.* 1984).

Spasmus nutans should properly only be regarded as a retrospective diagnosis.

Bobble-headed doll syndrome

The bobble-headed doll syndrome (BHDS) is a rare rhythmic bobbing or nodding of the head, sometimes involving the trunk, associated with hydrocephalus and a third ventricle cyst or suprasellar mass. However, BHDS may be acquired acutely with ventricular shunt obstruction (Dell 1981).

According to Benton *et al.* (1966) 'The movement is reminiscent of that seen in dolls with weighted heads resting on a coiled spring'. The head oscillation is usually vertical but may be horizontal, or both. It usually disappears during volitional movements such as reaching, and during sleep (Russo & Kindt 1974). Accompanying oscillatory eye movements are the normal VOR to the head bobbing and so BHDS is not really an oculomotor abnormality. The bobbing usually has an onset in early childhood but may be mistaken for a 'tic' and go undiagnosed for years. The bobbing may or may not remit after apparently successful intervention

The bobbing may be variably associated with truncal and peripheral extrapyramidal signs, seizures, obesity, diabetes insipidus, precocious puberty, thermoregulatory abnormalities, sleep disorders and enuresis, behavioural problems, aggressiveness, bulimia, memory loss, mental dullness or retardation, optic atrophy and strabismus. These are presumably due to associated involvement of the hypothalamus, limbic system, and visual pathways.

The pathophysiology of the head bobbing is unclear but dilatation of the third ventricle may compress adjacent thalamic structures and interfere with the basal ganglio-thalamocortical loops (Russo & Kindt 1974).

Ocular bobbing

Over the years, the term 'ocular bobbing' has come to indicate a tetrad of distinctive unusual abnormal spontaneous vertical, usually conjugate eye movements: ocular bobbing (*per se*), reverse ocular bobbing, ocular dipping and reverse ocular dipping. These movements tend to be irregular and are not strictly nystagmus. They are usually seen in coma or in the locked-in syndrome.

In ocular bobbing *per se*, there is an initial rapid downward eye movement, with a brief period of maintained tonic downgaze, followed by a slow drift upward to the midline. Other reflex eye movements are usually absent. Ocular bobbing is typically associated with intrinsic pontine lesions (haemorrhage, tumour, infarct), but may also occur with extra-axial compressive pontine lesions,

encephalitis, and metabolic/toxic encephalopathies. Prognosis is usually very poor, but survival has been reported in a case of subarachnoid haemorrhage from a pontine arteriovenous malformation, although the oculomotor abnormalities persisted (Clarke & Stern 1976).

In reverse ocular bobbing the initial rapid phase is upward followed by a downward slow-phase. It is less localizing and has been described in comatose patients with metabolic encephalopathy. It has also been described in patients with combined phenothiazine/benzodiazapine overdose, and may be a *form fruste* of the oculogyric crisis (Lennox 1993).

In ocular dipping ('inverse bobbing'), the initial phase is slow and downward followed by a rapid upward phase. Roving horizontal conjugate or dysconjugate eye movements may occur, and reflex eye movements may be present. Ocular dipping has been associated with anoxic coma, or after prolonged status epilepticus. The pathology is unclear, but cortical depression may be responsible (Mehler 1988). Pontine dysfunction is unusual, but has been reported (Herishanu *et al.* 1991).

In reverse ocular dipping ('converse bobbing') the initial phase is slow but upward, followed by a downward rapid phase. This is the rarest of the tetrad and has been reported in the awake patient (Mehler 1988). It has been associated with metabolic or viral encephalopathy and pontine infarction.

Acknowledgements

I thank the charities Help a Child to See and Iris Fund for their support. I also thank Peter West, Fatima Shawkat, Christine Timms and Laura Mezey for their help in preparing this chapter, and I thank the Nystagmus Action Group (UK) for many informative discussions.

References

Abadi RV. Visual performance with contact lenses and congenital idiopathic nystagmus. *Br J Ophthalmol* 1979; **33**: 32–7.

Abadi RV, Carden D, Simpson JA. New treatment for congenital nystagmus. *Br J Ophthalmol* 1980; **64**: 2–6.

Abadi RV, Dickinson CM. The influence of pre-existing oscillations on the binocular optokinetic response. *Ann Neurol* 1985; **17**: 578–86.

Abadi RV, Dickinson CM. Waveform characteristics in congenital nystagmus. *Doc Ophthalmol* 1986; **64**: 153–67.

Abadi RV, Dickinson CM, Pascal E. Sensory and motor aspects of congenital nystagmus. In: Schmid R, Zambarbieri, eds. *Oculomotor Control and Cognitive Processes.* Elsevier: North Holland, 1991: 249–62.

Abadi RV, King-Smith PE. Congenital nystagmus modifies orientational detection. *Vis Res* 1979; **19**: 1409–11.

Abadi RV, Pascal E. Periodic alternating nystagmus in humans with albinism. *Invest Ophthalmol Vis Sci* 1994; **35**: 4080–6.

Abadi RV, Wittle J. Nature of head postures in congenital nystagmus. *Arch Ophthalmol* 1991; **109**: 216–20.

Abadi RV, Worfolk R. Retinal slip velocities in congenital nystagmus.

Vis Res 1989; **29**: 195–205.

Adelstein FE, Cüppers C. Zum Problem der echten und der scheinbaren Abducenslähmung (Das sogenannte 'Blockierungssyndrom'). *Augenmuskell Büch Augenarzt* 1966; **46**: 371.

Allen ED, Davies PD. Role of contact lenses in the management of congenital nystagmus. *Br J Ophthalmol* 1983; **67**: 834–6

Anderson JR. Causes and treatment of congenital eccentric nystagmus. *Br J Ophthalmol* 1953; **37**: 267–81.

Apkarian P, Bour L, Barth PG. A unique achiasmatic anomaly detected in non-albinos with misrouted retino-fugal projections. *Eur J Neurosci* 1993; **6**: 501–7.

Apkarian P, Shallo-Hoffmann J. VEP projections in congenital nystagmus: VEP asymmetry in albinism: a comparison study. *Invest Ophthalmol Vis Sci* 1991; **32**: 2653–61.

Arnoldi KA, Tychsen L. Prevalence of intracranial lesions in children initially diagnosed with disconjugate nystagmus (spasmus nutans). *J Pediatr Ophthalmol Strabismus* 1995; **32**: 296–301.

Baba K, Sakata E, Inoue I. Complete gaze nystagmus and rebound nystagmus in all directions. A case with chronic toluene intoxication. *Equilib Res* 1988; **47**: 339–44.

Baloh RW, Honrubia V, Jacobson BA. Benign positional vertigo: clinical and oculographic features in 240 cases. *Neurology* 1987; **37**: 371–8.

Baloh RW, Honrubia V, Konrad HR. Periodic alternating nystagmus. *Brain* 1976; **99**: 11–26.

Baloh RW, Winder A. Acetazolamide-responsive vestibulocerebellar syndrome: clinical and oculographic features. *Neurology* 1991; **41**: 429–33.

Baloh RW, Yee RD. Spontaneous vertical nystagmus. *Rev Neurol (Paris)* 1989; **145**: 527–32.

Barton JJS, Sharpe JA. Oscillopsia and horizontal nystagmus with accelerating slow phases following lumbar puncture in the Arnold–Chiari malformation. *Ann Neurol* 1993; **33**: 418–21.

Bender MB. Effects of barbiturates on ocular movements (nystagmus). *Confinia Neurol* 1946; **7**: 144–7.

Benton JW, Nellhaus G, Huttenlocher PR, Ojemann RG, Dodge PR. The bobble-head doll syndrome. *Neurology* 1966; **16**: 725–9.

Bergin DJ, Halpern J. Congenital see-saw nystagmus associated with retinitis pigmentosa. *Ann Ophthalmol* 1986; **18**: 346–9.

Beun AAM, Beintema CD, Binnie CD *et al.* Epileptic nystagmus. *Epilepsia* 1984; **25**: 609–14.

Bietti GB, Bagolini B. Traitement medicochirugical du nystagmus. *L'Anee Ther Clin Ophthalmol* 1960; **11**: 268–93.

Bixenman WW. Congenital hereditary downbeat nystagmus. *Can J Ophthalmol* 1983; **18**: 344–8.

Brandt T. Positional and positioning vertigo and nystagmus. *J Neurol Sci* 1990; **95**: 3–28.

Calhoun JH, Harley RD. Surgery for abnormal head position in nystagmus. *Trans Am Ophthalmol Soc* 1973; **71**: 70–87.

Campbell WW. Periodic alternating nystagmus in phenytoin intoxication. *Arch Neurol* 1980; **37**: 178–80.

Cannon SC, Robinson DA. Loss of the neural integrator of the oculomotor system from brain stem lesions in monkey. *J Neurophysiol* 1987; **57**: 1383–409.

Casteels I, Harris CM, Shawkat F, Taylor D. Nystagmus in infancy. *Br J Ophthalmol* 1992; **76**: 434–7.

Chrousos GA, Matsuo V, Ballen AE, Cogan DG. Near-evoked nystagmus in spasmus nutans. *J Pediatr Ophthalmol Strabismus* 1986; **23**: 141–3.

Chrousos GA, Reingold DR, Chu FC, Cogan DG. Habitual head turning in spasmus nutans: an oculographic study. *J Pediatr Ophthalmol Strabismus* 1985; **22**: 113–16.

Ciuffreda KJ, Goldrich SG, Neary C. Auditory biofeedback as a potentially important new tool in the treatment of nystagmus. *J Am Optom Assoc* 1980; **51**: 615–17.

Clarke C, Stern R. Ocular bobbing with survival. *J Neurol Neurosurg Psychiatr* 1976; **39**: 58–60.

Coker S, Susac JI, Sharpe J, Smallridge R. Cockayne's syndrome. Neuro-ophthalmic CAT scan and endocrine observations. In: Smith JL, ed. *Neuro-ophthalmology Focus*. New York: Mason, 1979: 379–85.

Collewijn H, Apkarian P, Spekreijse H. The oculomotor behaviour of human albinos. *Brain* 1985; **108**: 1–28.

Cox TA, Corbett JJ, Thompson HS, Lennarson L. Upbeating nystagmus changing to downbeat nystagmus with convergence. *Neurology* 1981; **31**: 891–2.

Cross SA, Smith JL, Newton EWD. Periodic alternating nystagmus clearing after vitrectomy. *J Clin Neuro-ophthalmol* 1982; **2**: 5–11.

Daroff RB, Dell'Osso LF. Periodic alternating nystagmus and the shifting null. *Can J Otolaryngol* 1974; **3**: 367–71.

Daroff RB, Hoyt WF, Bettman JW, Lessel S. Suppression and facilitation of congenital nystagmus by vertical lines. *Neurology* 1973; **23**: 530–3.

Dell S. Further observations on the 'bobble-headed doll syndrome'. *J Neurol Neurosurg Psychiatr* 1981; **44**: 1046–9.

Dell'Osso LF, Daroff RB. Congenital nystagmus waveforms and foveation strategy. *Doc Ophthalmol* 1975; **39**: 155–82.

Dell'Osso LF, Schmidt D, Daroff RB. Latent, manifest latent and manifest nystagmus. *Arch Ophthalmol* 1979; **97**: 1877–85.

Dell'Osso LF, Traccis S, Abel LA, Erzurum SI. Contact lenses and congenital nystagmus. *Clin Vis Sci* 1988; **3**: 229–32.

Dickinson CM, Abadi RV. Corneal topography of humans with congenital nystagmus. *Ophthal Physiol Opt* 1984; **4**: 3–13.

Dickinson CM, Abadi RV. The influence of nystagmoid oscillation on contrast sensitivity in normal observers. *Vis Res* 1985; **25**: 1089–96.

Elliot AJ, Simpson EM, Oakhill A, Decock R. Nystagmus after medulloblastoma. *Dev Med Child Neurol* 1989; **31**: 43–6.

Fisher A, Gresty M, Chambers B, Rudge P. Primary position upbeating nystagmus: a variety of central positional nystagmus. *Brain* 1983; **106**: 949–64.

Flynn JT, Scott WE, Kushner BJ *et al.* Large rectus muscle recessions for the treatment of congenital nystagmus. *Arch Ophthalmol* 1991; **109**: 1636–7.

Forssman B. A study of congenital nystagmus. *Acta Otolaryngol* 1964; **57**: 427–9.

Forsythe WI. Congenital hereditary vertical nystagmus. *J Neurol Neurosurg Psych* 1955; **18**: 196–8.

Furman JM, Baloh RW, Chugani H, Waluch V, Bradley WG. Infantile cerebellar atrophy. *Ann Neurol* 1985; **17**: 399–402.

Goto N. A study of optic nystagmus by electro-oculogram. *Acta Soc Ophthalmol Jap* 1954; **58**: 851–965 (abstracted in *Ophthal Lit London* 1954; **8**: 1493).

Gottlob I, Zubcov A, Catalano RA *et al.* Signs distinguishing spasmus nutans (with and without central nervous system lesions) from infantile nystagmus. *Ophthalmology* 1990; **97**: 1166–75.

Gottlob I, Zubcov AA, Wizow SS, Reinecke RD. Head nodding is compensatory in spasmus nutans. *Ophthalmology* 1992; **99**: 1024–31.

Grant MP, Cohen M, Petersen RB *et al.* Abnormal eye movements in Creutzfeldt–Jakob disease. *Ann Neurol* 1993; **34**: 192–7.

Gresty M, Halmagyi GM. Head nodding associated with idiopathic childhood nystagmus. *Ann NY Acad Sci* 1981; **374**: 614–18.

Gresty M, Leech J, Sanders M, Eggars H. A study of head and eye movement in spasmus nutans. *Br J Ophthalmol* 1976; **60**: 652–4.

Gresty MA, Bronstein AM, Brookes GB, Rudge P. Primary position upbeating nystagmus associated with middle ear disease. *Neuro-ophthalmology* 1988; **8**: 321–8.

Gresty MA, Bronstein AM, Page NG. Congenital type nystagmus emerging later in life. *Neurology* 1991; **41**: 653–6.

Gresty MA, Ell JJ, Findley LJ. Acquired pendular nystagmus: its characteristics, localising value and pathophysiology. *J Neurol Neurosurg Psychiatr* 1982; **45**: 431–9.

Gresty MA, Metcalfe T, Timms C, Elston J, Lee J, Liu C. Neurology of latent nystagmus. *Brain* 1992; **115**: 1303–21.

Halmagyi GM, Aw ST, Dehaene I, Curthoys IS, Todd MJ. Jerk-waveform see-saw nystagmus due to unilateral meso-diencephalic lesion. *Brain* 1994; **117**: 789–803.

Halmagyi GM, Gresty MA, Leech J. Reversed optokinetic nystagmus (OKN): mechanism and clinical significance. *Ann Neurol* 1980a; **7**: 429–35.

Halmagyi GM, Rudge P, Gresty MA *et al.* Treatment of periodic alternating nystagmus. *Ann Neurol* 1980b; **8**: 609–12.

Halmagyi GM, Rudge P, Gresty MA, Sanders MD. Downbeating nystagmus, a review of 62 cases. *Arch Neurol* 1983; **40**: 777–84.

Hamed LM, Silbiger J. Periodic alternating esotropia. *J Pediatr Ophthalmol Strabismus* 1992; **29**: 240–2.

Harris CM. Problems in modelling congenital nystagmus: towards a new model. In: Findlay JM, Walker R, Kentridge RW, eds. *Eye Movement Research: Processes, Mechanisms and Applications.* Amsterdam: Elsevier, 1995: 239–53.

Harris CM, Jacobs M, Shawkat F, Taylor D. The development of saccadic accuracy in the first 7 months. *Clin Vis Sci* 1993a; **8**: 85–96.

Harris CM, Jacobs M, Shawkat F, Taylor D. Human ocular motor neural integrator failure. *Neuro-ophthalmology* 1993b; **13**: 25–34.

Harris CM, Kriss A, Shawkat F, Taylor D. The use of video in assessing and illustrating abnormal eye movements in young children. *J Audiovis Media Med* 1992; **5**: 113–16.

Harris CM, Shawkat F, Russell-Eggitt I, Wilson J, Taylor D. Intermittent horizontal saccade failure ('ocular motor apraxia') in children. *Br J Ophthalmol* 1996; **80**: 151–8.

Harris CM, Walker J, Wilson J, Russell-Eggitt I. Eye movements in a familial vestibulocerebellar disorder. *Neuropediatrics* 1993c; **24**: 117–22.

Helveston EM, Ellis FD, Plager DA. Large recession of the horizontal recti for treatment of nystagmus. *Ophthalmology* 1991; **98**: 1302–5.

Herishanu YO, Abarbanel JM, Frisher S, Farkash P, Berginer J, Amir-Schechter D. Spontaneous vertical movements associated with pontine lesions. *Isr J Med Sci* 1991; **27**: 320–4.

Hirose G, Kawada J, Tsukada K, Yoshioka A, Sharpe JA. Upbeat nystagmus: clinicopathological and pathophysiological considerations. *J Neurol Sci* 1991; **105**: 159–67.

Hood JD, Kayan A, Leech J. Rebound nystagmus. *Brain* 1973; **96**: 507–26.

Hotson J. Convergence-initiated voluntary flutter: a normal intrinsic capability in man. *Brain Res* 1984; **294**: 299–304.

Howard RS. A case of convergence-evoked eyelid nystagmus. *J Clin Neuro-ophthalmol* 1988; **74**: 386–93.

Hoyt CS. Nystagmus and other abnormal ocular movements in children. *Pediatr Clin North Am* 1987; **34**: 1415–23.

Huygen PL, Verhagen WI, Renier WO. Oculomotor and vestibular anomalies in Pelizaeus–Merzbacher disease: a study on a kindred with two affected and three normal males, three obligate and eight possible carriers. *J Neurol Sci* 1992; **113**: 17–25.

Ishikawa H, Ishikawa S, Mukuno K. Short-cycle periodic alternating (ping-pong) gaze. *Neurology* 1993; **43**: 1067–70.

Jacobs M, Harris CM, Shawkat F, Taylor D. The objective assessment of abnormal eye movements in infants and young children *Austral NZ J Ophthalmol* 1992; **20**: 185–95.

Jacome DE, FitzGerald R. Monocular ictal nystagmus. *Arch Neurol* 1982; **39**: 653–6.

Jay WM, Marcus RW, Jay MS. Primary position upbeat nystagmus with organophosphate poisoning. *J Pediatr Ophthalmol Strabismus* 1982; **19**: 318–19.

Jay WM, Nazrian SM, Underwood DW. Pseudointernuclear ophthalmoplegia with downshoot in myasthenia gravis. *J Clin Neuro-ophthalmol* 1987; **7**: 74–6.

Jay WM, Williams BB, De Chicchis A. Periodic alternating nystagmus clearing after cataract surgery. *J Clin Neuro-ophthalmol* 1985; **5**: 149–52.

Kaplan PW, Lesser RP. Vertical and horizontal epileptic gaze deviations and nystagmus. *Neurology* 1989; **39**: 1391–3.

Kaplan PW, Tusa RJ. Neurophysiologic and clinical correlations of epileptic nystagmus. *Neurology* 1993; **43**: 2508–14.

Kattah JC, Kolsky MP, Guy J, O'Doherty D. Primary position vertical nystagmus and cerebellar ataxia. *Arch Neurol* 1983; **40**: 310–14.

Keane JR. Cysticercosis: unusual neuro-ophthalmologic signs. *J Clin Neuro-ophthalmol* 1993; **13**: 194–9.

Keane JR. Periodic alternating nystagmus with downbeat nystagmus. *Arch Neurol* 1974; **30**: 399–402.

Kelly BJ, Rosenberg ML, Zee DS, Optican LM. Unilateral pursuit-induced congenital nystagmus. *Neurology* 1989; **39**: 414–16.

Kestenbaum A. A nystagmus operation. *Proc XVII Council Ophthalmol* 1953; **2**: 1071–8.

Kirschen DG. Auditory feedback in the control of congenital nystagmus. *Am J Optom Physiol Opt* 1983; **60**: 364–8.

Kommerel G, Mehdorn E. Is an optokinetic defect the cause of congenital and latent nystagmus? In: Lennerstrand G, Zee DS, Keller EL, eds. *Functional Basis of Ocular Motility Disorders.* New York: Pergamon Press, 1982: 159–67.

Kriss A, Harris C, Lambert SR. Ocular motility anomalies in developmental misdirection of the optic chiasm. *Am J Ophthalmol* 1992a; **113**: 601–2.

Kriss A, Russell-Eggitt I, Harris CM, Lloyd IC, Taylor D. Aspects of albinism. *Ophthalmic Paediat Genet* 1992b; **13**: 89–100.

Kushner BJ. Infantile uniocular blindness with bilateral nystagmus. *Arch Ophthalmol* 1995; **113**: 1298–300.

Lambert SR, Newman NJ. Retinal disease masquerading as spasmus nutans. *Neurology* 1993; **43**: 1607–9.

Larmande P, Pautrizel B. Traitement du nystagmus congenital par 1-5-hydroxytryptophane. *Nouv Presse Med* 1981; **10**: 3166.

Lavin PJM. Pupillary oscillations synchronous with ictal nystagmus. *Neuro-ophthalmology* 1986; **6**: 113–16.

Lavin PJM, Bahntge MF. Downbeat nystagmus with supra-tentorial disease. *Neuro-ophthalmology* 1983; **3**: 235–7.

Leigh RJ, Robinson DA, Zee DA. A hypothetical explanation for periodic alternating nystagmus: instability in the optokinetic-vestibular system. *Ann NY Acad Sci* 1981; **374**: 619–35.

Lennox G. Reverse ocular bobbing due to combined phenothiazine and benzodiazepine poisoning. *J Neurol Neurosurg Psychiatr* 1993; **56**: 136–7.

Liu C, Gresty M, Lee J. Management of symptomatic latent nystagmus. *Eye* 1993; **7**: 550–3.

McCarty JW, Demer JL, Hovis LA, Nuwer MR. Ocular motility anomalies in developmental misdirection of the optic chiasm. *Am J Ophthalmol* 1992; **113**: 86–95.

Maddox EE. See-saw nystagmus with bitemporal hemianopia. *Proc Roy Soc Med* 1914; **7**: 12–13.

Mallett RFJ. The treatment of congenital idiopathic nystagmus by intermittent photic stimulation. *Ophthalmic Physiol Opt* 1983; **3**:

341–56.

Mallinson AI, Longridge NS, Dunn HG, McCormick AQ. Vestibular studies in Pelizaeus–Merzbacher disease. *J Otolaryngol* 1983; **12**: 361–4.

Mass EF, Ashe J, Spiegel P, Zee DS, Leigh RJ. Acquired pendular nystagmus in toluene addiction. *Neurology* 1991; **41**: 282–5.

Mehler MF. The clinical spectrum of ocular bobbing and ocular dipping. *J Neurol Neurosurg Psychiatr* 1988; **51**: 725–7.

Mezawa M, Ishikawa S, Ukai K. Changes in waveform of congenital nystagmus associated with biofeedback treatment. *Br J Ophthalmol* 1990; **74**: 472–6.

Miller NR. *Walsh Hoyt's Clinical Neuro-ophthalmology.* Baltimore: Williams & Wilkins, 1985: 753–61.

Mitchell PR, Wheeler MB, Parks MM. Kestenbaum surgical procedure for torticollis secondary to congenital nystagmus. *J Pediatr Ophthalmol Strabismus* 1987; **24**: 87–92.

Nakada T, Kwee IL. Oculopalatal myoclous. *Brain* 1986; **109**: 31–41.

Nelson LB, Ervin-Mulvey LD, Calhoun JH *et al.* Surgical management for abnormal head position in nystagmus: the augmented modified Kestenbaum procedure. *Br J Ophthalmol* 1984; **68**: 796–800.

Noseworthy JH, Ebers GC, Leigh RJ, Dell'Osso LF. Torsional nystagmus: quantitative features and possible pathogenesis. *Neurology* 1988; **38**: 992–4.

Nuti D, Ciacci G, Giannini F, Rossi A, Federico A. Aperiodic alternating nystagmus: report of two cases and treatment by baclofen. *Ital J Neurol Sci* 1986; **7**: 453–9.

Ohm J. *Nystagmus und Schielen bei Sehschwachen und Blinden.* Stuttgart: Enke, 1958.

Optican LM, Zee DS. A hypothetical explanation of congenital nystagmus. *Biol Cybern* 1984; **50**: 119–34.

Parks MM. Congenital nystagmus surgery. *Am Orthop J* 1973; **23**: 35–9.

Phadke JG, Hern JEC, Blaiklock CT. Downbeat nystagmus — a false localising sign due to communicating hydrocephalus. *J Neurol Neurosurg Psychiatry* 1981; **44**: 459.

Pratt-Johnson JA. The surgery of congenital nystagmus. *Can J Ophthalmol* 1971; **6**: 628–77.

Reinecke RD, Guo S, Goldstein H. Waveform evolution in infantile nystagmus: an electro-oculographic study of 35 cases. *Binoc Vis* 1988; **3**: 191–202.

Reis J, Ebner AM, Warter JM, Gut JP, Collard M, Bataillard M. Alternating nystagmus and infectious mononucleosis. *Neuro-ophthalmology* 1989; **9**: 289–92.

Robb RM. Periodic alternation of null point in congenital nystagmus. *Arch Ophthal* 1972; **87**: 167–201.

Russo RK, Kindt GW. A neuroanatomical basis for the bobble-head doll syndrome. *J Neurosurg* 1974; **41**: 720–3.

Safran AB, Berney J, Safran E. Convergence-evoked eyelid nystagmus. *Am J Ophthalmol* 1982; **93**: 48–51.

Sanders MD, Hoyt WF, Daroff RB. Lid nystagmus evoked by ocular convergence. *J Neurol Neurosurg Psychiatr* 1968; **31**: 368–71.

Saul RF, Selhorst JB. Downbeat nystagmus with magnesium depletion. *Arch Neurol* 1981; **38**: 650–2.

Schwankhaus JD, Kattah JC, Lux WE, Masucci EF, Kurtzke JF. Primidone/phenobarbital-induced periodic alternating nystagmus. *Ann Ophthalmol* 1989; **21**: 230–2.

Scott WE, Kraft SP. Surgical treatment of compensatory head position in congenital nystagmus. *J Pediatr Ophthalmol Strabismus* 1984; **21**: 85–95.

Sedwick LA, Burde RM, Hodges FJ. Leigh's subacute necrotizing encephalomyelopathy manifesting as spasmus nutans. *Arch Ophthalmol* 1984; **102**: 1046–8.

Shallo-Hoffmann J, Schwarze H, Simonsz H, Muhlendyck H. A re-examination of endpoint nystagmus in normals. *Invest Ophthalmol Vis Sci* 1990; **31**: 388–92.

Shawkat F, Harris CM, Jacobs M, Taylor D, Brett E. Eye movement tics. *Br J Ophthalmol* 1992; **76**: 697–9.

Shawkat FS, Harris CM, Taylor DSI, Thompson DA, Russell-Eggitt I, Kriss A. The optokinetic response differences between congenital profound and non-profound unilateral visual deprivation. *Ophthalmology* 1995; **102**: 1615–22.

Sogg RL, Hoyt WF. Intermittent vertical nystagmus in a father and son. *Arch Ophthalmol* 1962; **68**: 515–17.

Staudenmaier C, Buncic JR. Periodic alternating gaze deviation with dissociated secondary face turn. *Arch Ophthalmol* 1983; **102**: 202–5.

Stewart JD, Kirkham TH, Mathieson G. Periodic alternating gaze. *Neurology* 1979; **29**: 222–4.

Stohler T. After image treatment in nystagmus. *Am Orthopt J* 1973; **23**: 65–7.

Stolz SE, Chatrian G-E, Spence AM. Epileptic nystagmus. *Epilepsia* 1991; **32**: 910–18.

Taylor JN. Surgery for horizontal nystagmus: Anderson–Kestenbaum operation. *Aus J Ophthalmol* 1973; **1**: 114–16.

Theunissen EJJM, Huygen PLM, Verhagen WIM. Familial vestibulo-cerebellar dysfunction: a new syndrome? *J Neurol Sci* 1989; **89**: 149–55.

Traccis S, Rosati G, Aiello I *et al.* Upbeat nystagmus as an early sign of cerebellar astrocytoma. *J Neurol* 1989; **236**: 359–60.

Trobe JD, Sharpe JA, Hirsh DK, Gebarski SS. Nystagmus of Pelizaeus–Merzbacher disease. A magnetic search coil study. *Arch Neurol* 1991; **48**: 87–91.

Troost BT, Janton F, Weaver R. Periodic alternating oscillopsia: a symptom of alternating nystagmus abolished by baclofen. *J Clin Neuro-ophthalmol* 1990; **10**: 273–7.

Tusa RJ, Kaplan PW, Hain TC, Naidu S. Ipsiversive eye deviation and epileptic nystagmus. *Neurology* 1990; **40**: 662–5.

Tusa RJ, Zee DS, Hain TC, Simonsz H. Voluntary control of congenital nystagmus. *Clin Vis Sci* 1992; **7**: 195–210.

Uemura T, Inoue H, Hirano T. The effects of baclofen on periodic alternating nystagmus and experimentally induced nystagmus. *Adv Oto-Rhino Laryngol* 1988; **42**: 254–9.

Ukwade MT, Bedell HE. Variation of congenital nystagmus with viewing distance. *Optom Vis Sci* 1992; **69**: 976–85.

Van Vliet AGM. On the central mechanism of latent nystagmus. *Acta Ophthalmol* 1973; **66**: 772–81.

von Noorden GK, Sprunger DT. Large rectus muscle recession for the treatment of congenital nystagmus. *Arch Ophthalmol* 1991; **109**: 221–4.

Weissman BM, Dell'Osso LF, Abel LA, Leigh RJ. Spasmus nutans. A quantitative prospective study. *Arch Ophthalmol* 1987; **105**: 525–8.

Weissman BM, Dell'Osso LF, DiScenna A. Downbeat nystagmus in an infant. Spontaneous resolution during infancy. *Neuro-ophthalmology* 1988; **8**: 317–19.

Yamazaki A, Zee DS. Rebound nystagmus: EOG analysis of a case with floccular tumour. *Br J Ophthalmol* 1979; **63**: 782–6.

Yee RD. Downbeat nystagmus: characteristics and localization of lesions. *Trans Am Ophthalmol Soc* 1990; **87**: 984–1032.

Yee RD, Baloh RW, Honrubia V. Effect of baclofen on congenital nystagmus. In: Lennerstrand G, Zee DS, Keller EL, eds. *Functional Basis of Ocular Motility Disorders.* Oxford: Pergamon, 1982: 151–7.

Yee RD, Spiegel PH, Yamada T, Aabel LA, Suzuki DA, Zee DS. Voluntary saccadic oscillations, resembling ocular flutter and opsoclonus. *J Neuro-ophthalmol* 1994; **14**: 95–101.

Yee RD, Wong EK, Baloh MD, Honrubia V. A study of congenital nystagmus: waveforms. *Neurology (Minn)* 1976; **26**: 326–33.

Zee DS, Yamazaki A, Butler P, Gucer G. Effects of ablation of flocculus and paraflocculus on eye movements in primates. *J Neurophysiol* 1981; **46**: 878–99.

Zubcov AA, Reinecke RD, Gottlob I, Manley DR, Calhoun JH. Treatment of manifest latent nystagmus. *Am J Ophthalmol* 1990; **110**: 160–7.

64: Other Eye Movement Disorders

Christopher Harris

Abnormal eye movements in children may be associated with a wide range of neuro-ophthalmological disorders resulting from muscle conditions, intracranial disease or neurodegenerative conditions, and abnormal visual experience in early infancy

A special problem encountered in the assessment of the non-verbal patient is the interdependence between eye movements and vision. First, in order for the child to make an appropriate oculomotor response to a visual target, the target must be visible. Second, vision in infants and older children is often assessed by the eye and head movement response to a visual target. It is not uncommon to discover that a 'blind baby', as determined by fixation patterns, really has normal sensory function but is unable to generate the appropriate orienting reflex (such as in ocular motor apraxia). As another example, the ability to follow a moving stimulus requires a different motor response than orienting towards a static target. Informal assessment with moving toys can give a completely false impression of vision; it pays to be constantly aware of what behaviour the child is expected to produce for visual assessment.

This chapter considers dynamic eye movements in general, without specific reference to nystagmus. For more in-depth (non-paediatric) treatments see Miller (1985), Carpenter (1988), Kennard and Rose (1988) and Leigh and Zee (1991). Eye movements will be divided into subsystems: the neural integrator (NI), saccades, vestibulo-ocular reflex (VOR), optokinesis, smooth pursuit (SP) and vergence. This systematizes the oculomotor investigation of the patient, but it should be recognized that clinical abnormalities are seldom confined to one system.

Eye movement systems

The neural integrator

A fundamental oculomotor function is the so-called eye position neural integrator (NI), which is needed for all conjugate eye movements.

When the eye rotates away from its natural resting position, there is an imbalance in tensions between agonist and antagonist muscles. This imbalance induces a mechanical force that restores eye position back to its resting position, much like in a stretched elastic band. This force is considerable: it moves the eyes back towards primary position with a speed of about 5° per second for every degree of eccentricity. For example, for 20° eccentricity, eye velocity would initially be 100° per second, but as the eyes get closer to primary position the restoring force decreases, so eye velocity also decreases, theoretically reaching 0° per second when resting position is reached. Thus, the eyes are forced back towards resting position with a decreasing velocity, or decelerating, profile.

In healthy individuals (including infants over a few weeks of age) the eyes do not fall back to the resting position when eccentric fixation is attempted, even in the dark, due to a tonic signal innervating the muscles keeping the eyes in their desired eccentric position; this tonic signal must be more intense for greater eccentricities. If the tonic signal were insufficient for the desired eccentricity, the eyes would slip back to some intermediate eccentricity where the restoring force and the tonic force were in equilibrium. This slippage would cause the image of the desired visual target to fall off the fovea, so that a saccade would be required to refoveate the target, which would then be followed inevitably by drift again back towards primary position, and so on.

To move the eyes at a given speed, for example when tracking a moving target, two signal components are needed to drive the muscles. One represents the desired speed (phasic component) and the other is the tonic component that precisely counterbalances the elastic restoring force that depends on eye position. When the eyes move away from resting position, the tonic component must increase at just the right rate, and when the eyes move towards their resting position the tonic must decrease by just the right rate. The greater the speed, the faster must be the tonic change.

Robinson (1973) realized that this changing tonic component could be precisely generated by a premotor neural circuit which computed the mathematical integration of the velocity signal; hence the term 'neural integrator'. If the phasic and tonic components are applied in the correct proportion, the restoring force of the globe is always exactly counterbalanced, whatever the desired direction and speed of the eyes.

The role of the NI and its dysfunction are most clearly seen in the saccadic system. In order to fixate a visual target, a pulse (a velocity signal) is sent to the muscles which causes the eyes to move rapidly to the desired eccentricity. This pulse is integrated by the NI (in the mathematical sense) to yield the tonic signal which is also applied to the muscles and holds the eyes in their new desired position. Once the saccade is over, there is no longer any velocity signal, so the NI has no more signal to integrate, and its output (the tonic signal) would remain constant holding the eyes at the desired position in perpetuity (Fig. 64.1).

However, as in all biological systems, the NI is not perfect and the tonic signal slowly decays or 'leaks' away, hence the term 'leaky integrator'. This decay is not normally seen in the light because the smooth pursuit/fixation system holds steady gaze using visual feedback. However, in the dark the eyes do drift back with a time-constant of about 25 seconds in healthy adults (Becker & Klein 1973).

When the NI time-constant is low, the eyes drift back more rapidly to their resting position. The NI is excessively leaky, which we call NI dysfunction (NID); the lower the time-constant, the more severe the disorder, and the faster the eyes drift back to primary position. If there were no NI function, the time-constant would be at its lowest limit set by the dynamics of the muscles, which is about one-fifth of a second, but some residual NI function is usually present. When the time-constant is t seconds, and the eyes are at $e°$ eccentricity, the eyes will drift back towards the resting position with a speed of:

$v = e/t$ degrees per second.

So, at the limit of gaze (~50°), and with a normal NI time-

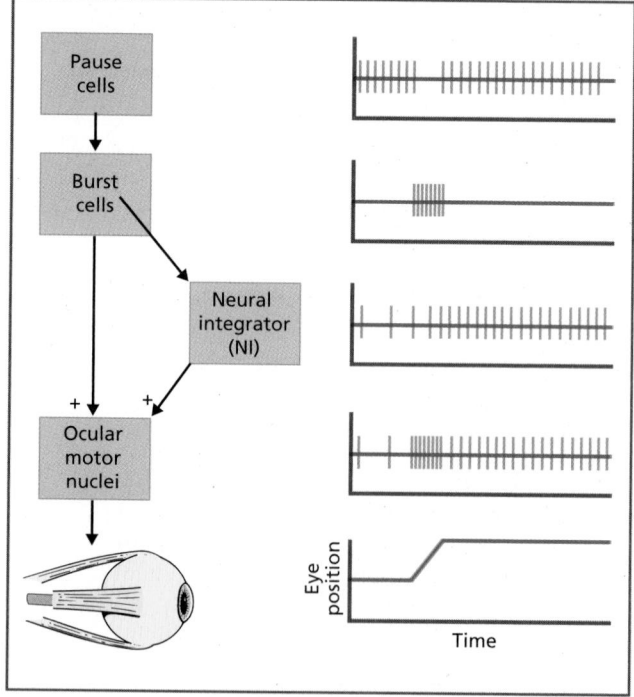

Fig. 64.1 The role of the NI in the generation of saccades. Tonic pause neurones are inhibited by a high-level triggering signal. This disinhibits burst units, which then fire rapidly to yield an intense phasic signal that is transmitted via the appropriate ocular motor nuclei to the agonist extra-ocular muscle, while the antagonist muscle is inhibited. Simultaneously the burst signal is passed to the NI which counts the spikes in the burst (integrates) and generates a new tonic signal that is appropriate for the new eye position. This tonic signal is also relayed to the extraocular muscles via the oculomotor nuclei and holds the eyes steady at the end of a saccade.

constant of 25 seconds, the eyes will drift back at a maximum speed of $50/25 = 2$ degrees per second, which is sufficient to maintain normal visual acuity.

Little is known about the development of the NI. It is difficult for the very young infant to maintain eccentric gaze. Informal abrupt rotations of the young infant and watching for maintenance of eccentric gaze suggests that NI starts out leaky. By 1 month of age, at the latest, we have seen no post-saccadic drifts that suggest a leaky integrator, and gaze-paretic nystagmus (GPN) is rare in infancy.

Testing

The simplest way to measure the NI time-constant is to ask the patient to maintain far eccentric gaze in the dark and observe (with an infrared camera) or record stability of gaze. With NID the eyes will quickly drift back towards primary position necessitating saccades to maintain eccentric gaze. This test is possible in the young schoolchild although it is usually necessary to employ some means of head restraint.

In most cases of NID there is a concomitant failure of the SP system, so that in eccentric gaze-holding in the light the eyes drift back to primary position.

Neural substrate

Both clinically and experimentally the cerebellum is intimately involved in this integration because lesions of the flocculus and paraflocculus lead to poor eccentric gaze-holding (Zee *et al.* 1976, 1981). However, NI function is not completely abolished, and there is a residual NI time-constant of about 1–2 seconds. Experimental work undertaken in the mid-1980s led to the discovery that the mammalian prepositus hypoglossus and medial vestibular nucleus were also involved (Cheron *et al.* 1986a, b; Cannon & Robinson 1987). There seem to be two components to the NI:

1 A brain stem component with a time-constant of about 1.5 seconds.
2 A cerebellar circuit that augments this to its normal value of about 25 seconds.

Neural integrator dysfunction

The most common clinical manifestation of NID is GPN (Fig. 64.2h) and low gain SP, which are signs of acquired cerebellar disease. It is not clear why these two abnormalities frequently co-exist, but it may be because SP and NI depend on similar circuitry in the cerebellar flocculus/paraflocculus. Because SP is dysfunctional, suppression of VOR and the optokinetic response are also abnormal. Fixation in primary position may also be quite unsteady. Thus, NID is a part of the 'flocculus' or vestibulocerebellar

oculomotor syndrome: GPN, poor SP, VOR suppression (VORS), low gain or absent optokinetic nystagmus (OKN), and unsteady fixation (Leigh & Zee 1991).

NID also affects induced vestibular nystagmus (VN) by causing the slow phases to decelerate as the eyes move

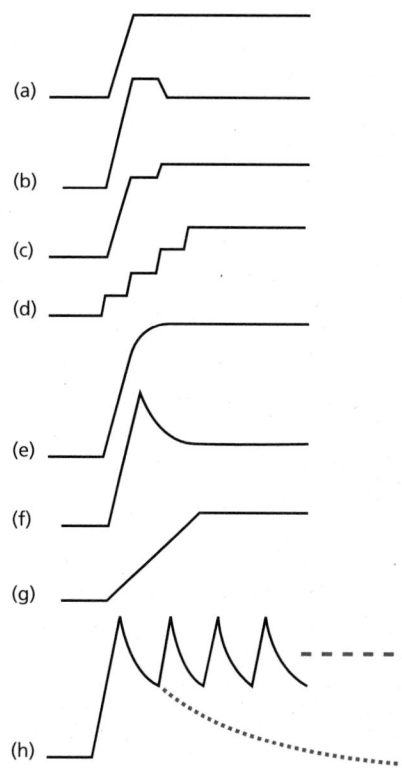

Fig. 64.2 Some common types of saccade abnormalities. (a) Target reached in a single accurate saccade (normal). (b) Saccade overshoots target and requires a secondary corrective in the opposite direction; gain hypermetria is often secondary to cerebellar disease. (c) Saccade undershoots target requiring secondary corrective in the same direction; some gain hypometria is normal in children and adults. Pathological hypometria occurs in cerebellar disease and is often associated with saccade failure ('ocular motor apraxia'); (d) when the hypometria is severe, many saccades are needed to reach the target. This is physiological in the first 3 months of life, but otherwise is pathological and may occur with saccades into a hemianopic visual field, as well as in cerebellar disease and severe saccade failure. (e) When the pulse is too small for the desired target eccentricity, the end of the saccade is slow because the eyes are driven only by the tonic signal (pulse–step mismatch). Pulse hypometria is uncommon in children. (f) When the pulse is too large for the target the eyes overshoot and decay back to the desired position without an intersaccadic interval. In children pulse hypermetria is most often seen during the resolution of opsoclonus–myoclonus. (g) Slow saccades can be caused by brain stem disease, myopathies and neuromuscular disease. (h) Although not strictly a saccadic disorder, failure of the NI is most easily detected from saccades made away from primary position. The tonic signal cannot be maintained allowing the eyes to drift back towards primary position (dotted line). In the attentive patient this is prevented by subsequent saccades that attempt to re-foveate the target, giving rise to GPN.

away from resting position. Eventually the eyes will become stationary when the restoring force balances the vestibular driving force. Using the formula above, consider the head to be rotated at 10° per second with a perfectly compensatory VOR. If the NI time-constant was 2 seconds (not uncommon in cerebellar disease), in primary position the eyes would initially move at 10° per second, but they would become ever slower as they became more eccentric and would come to a rest with a tonic deviation at $10 \times 2 = 20°$ from resting position. This tonic deviation would gradually decay as the vestibular command decayed (see below). This eye movement behaviour is somewhat more complicated because of the quick-phases, but if the NI time-constant is extremely short, then even quick-phases do not occur, and rotation simply causes a tonic deviation. This really occurs, not only in experimental animals, but also in children with severe NID (Harris *et al.* 1993b).

With a pefect NI, any eye velocity command would move the eyes at the desired speed at all eccentricities. It follows that any pathological nystagmus that changes its intensity or waveform with eccentricity along the axis of the nystagmus, probably involves a leaky NI. Most types of jerk nystagmus intensify when gaze is directed in the direction of quick-phases (Alexander's law), and for VN, Robinson *et al.* (1984) have shown that Alexander's law is due to a leaky NI that has physiologically adapted in response to the vestibular imbalance. A similar argument has also been proposed to account for the null in sensory defect nystagmus/congenital idiopathic nystagmus (SDN/CID) and possibly even in latent nystagmus (LN) (Harris 1995).

Saccades

Saccades are fast conjugate eye movements that are used to shift gaze from one visual object to another. The quick (fast) phases of induced and spontaneous jerk nystagmus are also saccadic. Circuitry for saccadic control is widespread throughout the brain, so abnormalities of saccades occur frequently, but by the same token they are difficult to localize. Because of their fleeting nature, saccadic abnormalities can be overlooked or misinterpreted as nystagmus.

The brain stem horizontal saccadic centres are ipsilateral and consist of a variety of units in the pontine tegmentum that have saccade-related burst activity. Horizontal saccades are generated by excitatory and inhibitory burst units (EBNs and IBNs) and pause units. Pause neurones fire tonically and inhibit EBNs and their activity inhibits the triggering of saccades: their role in disorders of saccadic triggering is not clear since experimental lesions of pause neurones lead to slow saccades rather than saccadic oscillations (Kaneko & Fuchs 1987). The EBNs project directly to the ipsilateral sixth nucleus, and to interneu-

rones that relay the premotor signal via the contralateral medial longitudinal fasciculus (MLF) to the contralateral third nucleus. EBNs also drive IBNs which inhibit the contralateral sixth motorneurones and interneurones.

Premotor circuitry for vertical saccades resides in the mesencephalon, particularly the rostral interstitial nucleus of the MLF (riMLF), where upward and downward control are separated (upward control is more medial than downward control). The posterior commissure is an important link in the generation of upward saccades. Vertical circuitry does not have its own pause neurones, and depends to some extent on the integrity of the lower brain stem horizontal saccade structures. However, the vertical system appears to be more independent of the horizontal saccade system in humans than in the monkey.

The superior colliculus (SC) is thought be an important centre for computing the correct amplitude and meridian of saccades, but the brain stem also receives a direct connection from the frontal eye fields (FEFs) in the frontal cortex (Schiller *et al.* 1980). The SC receives saccade-related signals from a variety of sources including the posterior parietal cortex, the frontal cortex directly (Fries 1984) and indirectly via the caudate nucleus and substantia nigra (pars reticulata) (Hikosaka 1989). There are also intercortical saccade related pathways (Cavada & Goldman-Rakic 1989). In addition the saccadic system is under continual adaptive control by the cerebellum, particularly the flocculus and the posterior cerebellar vermis (Optican & Robinson 1980).

Thus, the saccadic pathways are widespread and complex, and the relative roles of each pathway in generating and suppressing various types of saccades (e.g. reflexive, voluntary, etc.) is unclear.

Testing

The main way of testing saccades is to suddenly present a target at a known eccentricity to the patient whose head is held. For most clinical purposes large targets are as effective as small targets with the advantage of being readily seen by the child who has a visual disorder. The addition of sound to a visual target eases the elicitation of saccades from small infants (Jacobs *et al.* 1992). Abnormalities are better visualized in larger amplitude saccades. For children with alternating esotropia it is necessary to occlude one eye since the peripheral target may be foveated by cross-fixation.

Abnormalities of saccades

A common phenomenon in normal or abnormal saccades is some degree of 'dysmetria'. In 'gain dysmetria', the saccade is executed with a normal profile but it misses the target and corrective saccades are needed for foveation. In 'pulse-step mismatch' ('pulse-step dysmetria'), the saccade has an abnormal profile where the pulse component is too large or too small for the desired target eccentricity. The difference is difficult to disentangle without objective eye movement recordings (Leigh & Zee 1991).

Gain dysmetria

The accuracy of saccades is usually classified in one of the following three categories:

1 Orthometria: the target is fixated in a single accurate saccade.

2 Hypometria: the first saccade falls short of the target and one or more secondary saccades are needed.

3 Hypermetria: the first saccade goes past the target and one or more secondary saccades are needed.

In healthy adults and children aged over about 1 year, saccades are typically slightly hypometric reaching about 90–100% of the target distance, followed by secondary saccades. This normal hypometria is properly called normometria, which, strictly speaking, is not quite the same as orthometria.

Primary saccades made by young healthy infants can be hypometric requiring as many as four or five secondary saccades (Aslin & Salapatek 1975). If the head is held still, this hypometria can be seen clinically under about 3 months of age especially for large saccades. The progression towards normometria lasts at least for the first 7 months (Harris *et al.* 1993a). Consistent marked hypometria below 90% after 7 months of age should be considered suspicious of neurological disease; however, even healthy adults will make the occasional grossly hypometric saccade.

Hypermetria is more easily detected and appears flutter-like (but should not be mistaken for ocular flutter). Hypermetria is abnormal at any age, and when conjugate it is almost always associated with cerebellar disease (Selhorst *et al.* 1976a), although saccadic overshoot can also occur in Wallenberg's syndrome (see below).

If the hypermetria is severe, the corrective saccade may be as large as the primary saccade thus causing the eyes to oscillate back and forth with saccades. This has been called macrosaccadic oscillations (Selhorst *et al.* 1976b). Hypometria is also usually associated with cerebellar disease, and mixed hypometria and hypermetria may also occur.

Hypometria (but not hypermetria) is also associated with 'ocular motor apraxia' (Harris *et al.* 1996) (see below).

In homonymous hemianopia, saccades into the blind field are often multiple hypometric, 'staircase' or 'searching'. Hemianopic hypermetria as a strategy to bring the target into the functioning visual field (Meienberg *et al.* 1981) is rare in childhood in our experience, although the child may make surprisingly accurate saccades to the remembered location of a target in the blind field. If the ipsilateral parietal cortex is also involved it will reduce SP and optokinetic responses for stimulus motion towards the side of the lesion. Informal visual assessment using moving targets may therefore give a different impression than using stationary targets.

Gain dysmetria can be secondary to changes in visual magnification. The removal of aphakic spectacles may lead to a temporary gain dysmetria until adaptation takes place.

In basal ganglia disease, voluntary saccades may be hypometric with more or less normal reflexive saccades.

During the resolving stage of isolated (type 1) delayed visual maturation (DVM) in infants, saccades may be transiently hypometric for age (Harris *et al.* 1995), but if the hypometria is prolonged, a neurological explanation should be sought since this may indicate DVM type 2.

Pulse-step mismatch

Another saccadic abnormality occurs when the proportions of the pulse and step components are not properly matched. When the pulse is too large the eyes overshoot the target and drift back to a steady position, which may appear as a flicker or twitch at the end of a saccade. This may be mislabelled as ocular flutter or even nystagmus unless eye movements are recorded. When the pulse is too small, the eyes slow down too early and creep more slowly towards the target. This is more difficult to see clinically but may appear as a slow saccade (Fig. 64.2).

Pulse-step mismatch may occur bilaterally (conjugately) or monocularly, and with central or peripheral pathology. Central pulse-step mismatch is usually a cerebellar sign.

Pulse-step mismatch may occur asymmetrically if one eye is paretic. If the paretic eye is the preferred eye, the other eye may show overshoot due to central adaptation to augment the signals for the paretic eye. Conversely, if the non-paretic eye is preferred, the paretic eye may show dynamic undershoot. This disorder is uncommon in children, but it may be found secondary to strabismus surgery.

Slow saccades

Slow saccades are difficult to detect clinically unless severe. Slow saccades may be a brain stem sign indicating involvement of the ipsilateral paramedian pontine reticular formation; they also occur in progressive external ophthalmoplegia, myasthenia gravis, basal ganglia disease (Kirkham & Kamin 1974), and in Duane's syndrome, presumably due to co-contraction of antagonist muscles.

In adults, slow saccades have been reported secondary to therapeutic and toxic levels of certain sedative hypnotics.

When saccades are very slow they may be mistaken for an SP response, but SP cannot usually be generated without a moving target.

Fast saccades

Excessively fast saccades are rare in clinical practice. However, they have been associated with opsoclonus (Bergenius 1986).

Saccade initiation failure ('ocular motor apraxia')

The term 'congenital ocular motor apraxia' was coined by Cogan (1952) to describe an inability from birth to make horizontal saccades.

Strictly, the term 'ocular motor apraxia' indicates a difficulty in generating voluntary saccades, and is usually acquired in adulthood following bilateral parietal lesions secondary to stroke, metastases, Alzheimer's disease or trauma. It is associated with other high-level disorders such as optic ataxia, and various visual agnosias as in Balint's syndrome (Pierrot-Deseilligny *et al.* 1986). We are not aware of any reported case of Balint's syndrome in childhood, and it is inappropriate to equate the adult acquired condition with the childhood congenital or acquired condition by using the term 'apraxia'. Moreover, in childhood so-called ocular motor apraxia always involves missed reflexive nystagmus quick-phases (Cogan 1972; Harris *et al.* 1996) (Fig. 64.3). The term saccade palsy would be more appropriate, but this term is also used by some to describe slow saccades. We will use the term 'saccadic initiation failure' (SIF) to describe the intermittent or total failure of saccades and quick-phases, regardless of their speed.

SIF may be congenital or acquired and may affect only horizontal, or only vertical saccades, or in progressive disease it may eventually affect both. For horizontal defects, it is important to distinguish between SIF (the inability to trigger a saccade) and a gaze palsy (an inability to move the eyes beyond the midline). SIF is always supranuclear.

SIF is intermittent (Harris *et al.* 1996), often being more noticeable when the child is under stress, is suffering from tiredness or is trying very hard to look at an object. Total SIF has been reported in advanced stages of Gaucher's disease (Vivian *et al.* 1993). In congenital SIF the saccades, when they occur, usually have normal speeds (Zee *et al.* 1977).

Adaptive strategies. Whether their SIF is congenital or acquired, affected children often adopt various compensating strategies in order to shift gaze.

In head thrusting, the head is abruptly turned towards the peripheral target. This induces a VOR causing the eyes to deviate fully in the opposite direction so that they are brought around towards the target by the head movement. The child must bring the head past the target to fixate it with the fully deviated eyes. Once the target is fixated the head is brought back to the straight-ahead position whilst the VOR keeps the target fixated. These hypermetric head thrusts are quite distinct from head shaking/nodding and distinct from the head movements in external ophthalmoplegia, although close examination is sometimes needed.

Head thrusting is not a constant feature of SIF, and may not develop until 2–3 months of age in the otherwise healthy child (Rosenberg & Wilson 1987), or may develop much later, or not at all in the severely retarded child, as in some cases of Joubert's syndrome. Shifting gaze with the head may also compensate for a gaze palsy, hemianopia, slow saccades, or even poor eccentric gaze holding (Harris *et al.* 1993b).

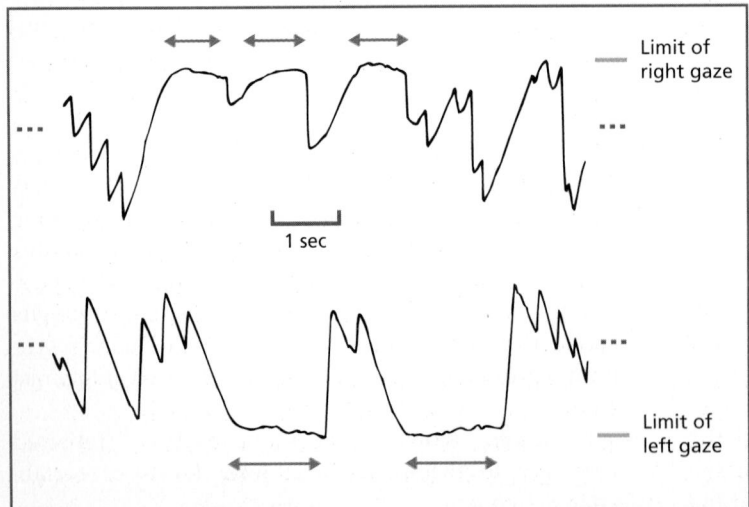

Fig. 64.3 Saccade initiation failure revealed by 'locking up' during OKN with full-field curtain rotating at 50° per second to the right (upper panel) and to the left (lower panel). Note intermittent periods of missed quick-phases allowing the eyes to deviate to the mechanical limit of gaze (shown by arrows), followed by resumption of normal OKN. Patient was a 17-month-old with microcephaly and a history of neonatal septicaemia, hyperbilirubinaemia and hypoglycaemia.

Older children facilitate the triggering of saccades by blinking synkinetically. These blinks are difficult to detect, and may give the appearance that the condition has undergone some improvement although head thrusting may still emerge when the child is feeling tired or under stress.

In most children with SIF, vertical saccades appear to be normal and some children may tilt the head to shift horizontal gaze with vertical saccades. Rarely, other strategies may be seen; we have seen a child who would read by moving the book rather than scanning with the eyes or head.

Detection. The most reliable means of detection is to examine the quick-phases of induced OKN and VN. All affected children will show an intermittent failure of quick-phases which intermittently allows the eyes to become deviated to the mechanical limit of gaze ('locking-up'). Ideally, testing is carried out in an eye movement laboratory. However, if one is not available testing may be accomplised by manual spinning.

Associations. SIF is not a diagnosis; whether congenital or acquired it is associated with a wide range of conditions (Table 64.1), although a large minority are eventually found to be idiopathic. Careful attention must be paid to clinical history, assessment of vision, examination for any neurological signs, and any other malformation (dysmorphic facies, polydactyly, etc.).

SIF has been reported in twins and in families (Moe 1971; Narbona *et al.* 1980; Borchert *et al.* 1987; Prasad & Nair 1994).

Vision is usually found to be normal in idiopaths who also demonstrate normal electroretinograms (ERGs) and visual evoked potentials (VEPs) (Gittinger & Sokol 1982; Shawkat *et al.* 1996), but in others the vision depends on the underlying condition. A poor VEP or ERG and SIF is suggestive of associated disease. Shawkat *et al.* (1996) found that head thrusting was less likely to be present if VEPs were abnormal, presumably reflecting neurological disease.

Strabismus is common. Nystagmus is uncommon and usually indicates a neurological association.

Apart from the association of SIF with agenesis of the corpus callosum most structural abnormalities occur in and around the fourth ventricle or posterior cerebellum (vermis). Magnetic resonance imaging (MRI) is the preferred imaging technique.

Regardless of aetiology (including idiopaths), some infants with SIF tend to be hypotonic, sometimes with mild developmental delay manifest by late sitting and walking. Such children tend to be clumsy with a wide-based gait, although frank cerebellar signs are uncommon. Speech development is slow, and reading difficulties are common. There is evidence to suggest that SIF may be part of a wider developmental syndrome (Rappaport *et al.* 1987).

There is no treatment for SIF. In spite of a usually good visual and clinical outcome, delayed speech development and poor reading as well as clumsiness can lead to educational problems in later childhood.

Whether the condition improves with age is still unknown. The development of adaptive strategies improves the ability of the child to shift gaze rapidly. However, such strategies may belie the fact that the underlying condition has not have changed.

Pathophysiology. The pathophysiology of SIF is unknown. Early reports proposed a cerebral origin (Alfano 1955) and there was some OKN locking-up in a hemispherectomized infant (Braddick *et al.* 1992). The association of agenesis of the corpus callosum with SIF probably reflects concomitant midline defects in the cerebellum or brain stem (Eda *et al.* 1984). In many congenital and in acquired cases (Joubert's syndrome, ataxia telangiectasia) there is evidence of a cerebellar origin. The autopsy of an idiopath showed cerebellar abnormalities but a normal cerebrum and brain stem (Fielder *et al.* 1986). In others with neurometabolic disease, there is probably brain stem degeneration that progresses to involve other eye movement centres. This is consistent with a report of an autopsy showing brain stem gliosis in a child with 'congenital ocular motor apraxia' and juvenile Gaucher's disease (Büttner-Ennever *et al.* 1988). Yet, in other cases, the involvement of the basal ganglia seems likely, as in Wilson's and Huntingdon's diseases.

Structural abnormalities seldom occur in isolation, which makes localization very difficult. In a recent neuroradiological study of 62 children, 61% had abnormal scans with abnormalities in the cerebellum and brain stem being most correlated with SIF, but abnormalities of the cerebral cortex/basal ganglia were also important (Shawkat *et al.* 1995b).

In summary, the pathophysiology of SIF seems to be related to more than one site, but there is overwhelming evidence that SIF in childhood can be caused by subtentorial disorders.

Vertical saccade failure

Vertical SIF, whether congenital or acquired, is much less common. Compensatory behaviours include vertical head thrusting or synkinetic blinks. An upward saccade failure may sometimes be compensated by the Bell's phenomenon.

Vertical SIF usually involves bilateral lesions of the midbrain, particularly the riMLF, which are believed to be the site of vertical burst units (Büttner-Ennever & Büttner 1978). Congenital non-progressive cases have been reported (Ro *et al.* 1989), with bilateral riMLF lesions confirmed

Table 64.1 Clinical associations of horizontal saccade initiation failure (SIF) in childhood.

Idiopathic	*Perinatal problems* Hypoxia Hydrocephalus Cerebral palsy Seizures

Congenital malformations
Agenesis corpus callosum
Dilatation of the fourth ventricle and vermis hypoplasia
Joubert's syndrome (Moore & Taylor 1984; Lambert *et al.* 1989a;
    Harris *et al.* 1996)
Dandy–Walker malformation (Harris *et al.* 1996)
Immature development of putamen (Steinlin *et al.* 1990)
Heterotopia of grey matter (Steinlin *et al.* 1990)
Porencephalic cyst (Harris *et al.* 1996; Walsh & Hoyt 1969)
Hamartoma near foramen of Monro (Walsh & Hoyt 1969)
Macrocephaly (Orrison & Robertson 1979; Harris *et al.* 1996)
Microcephaly (Eustace *et al.* 1994; Harris *et al.* 1996)
Posterior fossa cysts (Pebenito & Cracco 1988)
Chondrodystrophic dwarfism and hydrocephalus (Cogan 1966)
Encephalocoele (Pebenito & Cracco 1988)
Occipital meningocoele (Alfano 1955)
	Acquired disease
	Post-immunization encephalopathy (possible) (Morimoto *et al.* 1985;
	    Harris *et al.* 1996)
	Herpes encephalitis (Harris *et al.* 1996)
	Posterior fossa tumours (Lyle 1961; Wybar 1971; Zaret *et al.* 1980;
	    Summers *et al.* 1987; Harris *et al.* 1996)
	Bilateral frontoparietal lesions (Balint's syndrome) (reported only in
	    adults, see text)

Neurodegenerative conditions with an infantile onset of SIF
Infantile Gaucher's disease (type 1) (Cogan *et al.* 1981; Catalano *et al.*
    1988; Vivian *et al.* 1993)
Pelizaeus–Merzbacher disease (Harris *et al.* 1996)
Krabbe's leukodystrophy (Harris *et al.* 1996)
Propionic acidaemia (Harris *et al.* 1996)
GM1 gangliosidosis (Harris *et al.* 1996)
Infantile Refsum's disease (Harris *et al.* 1996)
4-hydroxybutyric aciduria (Rating *et al.* 1984; Eustace *et al.* 1994)
	Other associations
	Alagille's syndrome (Alvarez *et al.* 1983)
	Bardet–Biedl syndrome (Lavy *et al.* 1995/6)
	Carotid fibromuscular hypoplasia (Harris *et al.* 1996)
	Cockayne's syndrome (Eustace *et al.* 1994)
	Cornelia de Lange syndrome (Harris *et al.* 1996)
	Juvenile nephronophthisis (Donaldson *et al.* 1985)
	Lowe's syndrome (Gresty & Ell 1982)
	Neurofibromatosis type 1 (Glover & Powe 1985)
	Orofacial digital syndrome (Manson 1973)
	X-linked muscle atrophy with congenital contractures (Wieacker
	    et al. 1985)

Neurodegenerative conditions usually with a later onset of SIF
Ataxia telangiectasia (Stell *et al.* 1989; Woods & Taylor 1992)
Spinocerebellar degenerations (various) (Aicardi *et al.* 1988; Awaya
    et al. 1986; Araie *et al.* 1977; Koeppen 1976; Ozawa *et al.* 1974;
    Wadia & Swami 1971; Inoue *et al.* 1971)
Juvenile Gaucher's disease (type 3)
Huntington's disease (Starr 1967; Avanzini *et al.* 1979)
Hallervorden–Spatz disease (Angelini *et al.* 1992)
Wilson's disease (Kirkham & Kamin 1974)	

in one case (Ebner *et al.* 1990). Adult acquired vertical SIF has been reported in bilateral thalamic lesions, but the thalamosubthalamic territory may have been involved (Mills & Swanson 1978).

Vertical SIF is a cardinal sign of Niemann–Pick type C disease (Sanders & Wybar 1969; Neville *et al.* 1973), and it may also be a presenting sign (Shawkat *et al.* 1994). Progressive involvement of vertical smooth pursuit, horizontal saccades and convergence may occur. Vertical SIF, particularly for downward saccades, may also occur in Gaucher's disease (types 2 and 3), although the horizontal SIF is more prominent (Vivian *et al.* 1993). Vertical SIF has also been reported in association with kernicterus and hydrocephalus. Transient tonic 'paroxysmal' upward and downward deviations of infancy may result from a vertical jerk nystagmus with an intermittent failure of quick-phases (see below).

Disorders of latency

The latency of a saccade is the time between the stimulus onset and the beginning of the appropriate saccade. In adults, latencies are typically about one-fifth of a second, but this depends to some extent on the visual target and whether the fixation target is extinguished or not at the same time as the peripheral target onset. Latency also depends on arousal state.

Saccade latency for infants is normally much longer than in adults, up to about 1 second (Aslin & Salapatek 1975). Latencies of secondary saccades are also long, about 400 milliseconds (140–200 in adults), and slowly decrease with age (Harris *et al.* 1993a). In OKN and VN, quick phases occur less frequently in infants and toddlers than in adults (Ornitz *et al.* 1979; Hainline *et al.* 1984).

In childhood, prolonged saccade latencies usually occur

in association with SIF. It is important to distinguish between a saccade that is slow to be initiated and a saccade that is slow during its execution.

Opsoclonus and ocular flutter

Opsoclonus is a striking saccadic disorder characterized by intermittent bursts of wild conjugate oscillations of the eyes in all directions. 'Ocular flutter' describes such oscillations when they occur only in the horizontal direction. During resolution of the condition opsoclonus may be followed by ocular flutter and then saccade dysmetria.

Typically, opsoclonus has a very high frequency of 5–13 oscillations per second, and the amplitude can be tens of degrees. The number of bursts can vary enormously, being almost incessant in acute cases, or sometimes every few minutes. Other eye movements are usually normal, although Shawkat *et al.* (1993) reported prolonged post-rotatory VN. A burst of opsoclonus usually occurs at the time of saccades or nystagmus quick-phases. Opsoclonus bursts can be evoked by upgaze or by OKN or VN; these tests may not be possible as the distraught child may become completely unco-operative. Bursts may appear spontaneously during fixation; these may be triggered by small saccades, when they are sometimes known as 'flutter dysmetria'.

Opsoclonus may be mistaken for nystagmus and vice versa (Allarakhia & Trobe 1995). Eye movement recordings reveal that opsoclonus is a burst of back-to-back saccades with no intersaccadic intervals (Vignaendra 1977), without the rhythm of nystagmus and without slow phases. Rarely, there may also be a constant fine high frequency acquired pendular nystagmus (APN).

Non-organic ('voluntary') nystagmus can be superficially similar to opsoclonus (Shawkat *et al.* 1992), but other abnormalities such as saccadic dysmetria are absent. In difficult cases, eye movement recordings are definitive.

Acquired opsoclonus is usually associated with myoclonus and has been described variously as: opsoclonus–myoclonus, dancing eye syndrome, dancing eye–dancing feet, myoclonic encephalopathy of infants and infantile polymyoclonia. There is usually an acute or subacute onset. Ataxia, vomiting and irritability are common. It usually occurs as a post-infectious encephalopathy, or as a paraneoplastic phenomenon of occult neuroblastoma/ganglioneuroma. In the latter group, the presence of opsoclonus confers a favourable survival rate. A history of prodromal disease does not preclude occult neuroblastoma. The opsoclonus may have an onset after treatment for neuroblastoma, but this may also herald a recurrent neuroblastoma (Basco *et al.* 1995).

In children, opsoclonus has also been associated with hydrocephalus, sepsis, poliovirus vaccine or infection and thallium intoxication. In adults, opsoclonus has also been reported with tricyclic antidepressant overdose, haloperidol and lithium toxicity, and exposure to chlorinated insecticide (Digre 1986).

Opsoclonus–myoclonus may be self-limiting, but adrenocorticotrophic hormone (ACTH) or steroid therapy can have a dramatic short-term effect on reducing the symptoms in some children. Unfortunately, not all children respond so well, and the opsoclonus and other cerebellar signs may become steroid-dependent and re-emerge on attempts to taper the treatment, or during an intercurrent illness. Regardless of the short-term response, children with opsoclonus usually have long-term developmental problems, including motor and cognitive handicaps (Koh *et al.* 1994). Alternative therapies have been sought (Cher *et al.* 1995; Petruzzi & de Alarcon 1995).

Opsoclonus may also be congenital. Opsoclonus occurred in 8 of 242 healthy neonates in the first 3 days of life: it resolved by 6 months (Hoyt *et al.* 1980). However, neonatal opsoclonus is not always benign, and may be associated with intrauterine anoxia, intracranial haemorrhage, microcephaly, epilepsy, truncal ataxia, mental retardation and congenitally poor vision (Walsh 1947; Bienfang 1974).

Although acquired opsoclonus probably involves an immune mechanism, its neural substrate remains a mystery. Zee and Robinson (1979) suggested that saccadic oscillations could result from a defect in the brain stem saccadic pause neurones, but this seems unlikely since experimental and clinical lesions of pause neurones lead to slow saccades rather than fast oscillations (Kaneko & Fuchs 1987; Bronstein *et al.* 1990), and autopsies have shown the pontine region of the pause neurones to be normal in opsoclonus (Ridley *et al.* 1987). Because of the associated ataxia, tremor and saccadic dysmetria, many have proposed a cerebellar origin but there is also some evidence for a midbrain origin (Keane & Devereaux 1974) or a neurotransmitter imbalance (Pranzatelli *et al.* 1995).

Antisaccades and intrusive saccades

In the antisaccade test, the patient is instructed to make a saccade in the opposite direction to an abruptly appearing peripheral visual target (Hallett & Adams 1980). This requires the patient to suppress the reflexive saccade to the visual target while generating a voluntary saccade in the opposite direction: it is largely untried on young children, but it can sometimes be used in the first decade though normative data are lacking.

It is thought that the antisaccade task taps into the higher level control of saccadic eye movements, and in adults, failure has been reported in patients with frontal lesions (Guitton *et al.* 1985) or basal ganglia disorders (Lasker *et al.* 1987).

Failure of antisaccades is associated with distractibility and intrusive saccades, which reflect the general inability of the patient with basal ganglia disease to suppress unwanted saccades. The presence of saccadic intrusions may be so severe as to make the smooth pursuit task virtually impossible.

Other types of intrusive saccades are small saccades away from the current fixation followed after a delay by another saccade back to the target. If the amplitude is less than about 5°, these are called 'microsquare wave jerks', and occur in some healthy adults, but in our experience much less frequently in children. When the amplitude is large, they are called 'macrosquare wave jerks', which are pathological, and usually associated with cerebellar disease; but these are also rare in childhood. These rather stereotyped intrusions appear similar to flutter and are distinct from the involuntary shifts of gaze seen in the distractible child with or without pathology.

Macrosaccadic oscillations are large amplitude oscillations of the eye about the fixation point with an intersaccadic interval of about 200 milliseconds. They are seen in acute cerebellar disease.

The vestibulo-ocular reflex

VOR refers to the conjugate eye movements that are induced reflexively by head movements. VOR is driven by head motion signals derived from the semi-circular canals. It is not visually mediated and can be elicited in the dark; it is present at birth. VOR is a useful means of generating eye movements in infants and unco-operative children.

When the head is suddenly rotated, the walls of the semi-circular canal move relative to the endolymph fluid within the canal. This relative motion bends hair cells which are embedded in a gelatinous cupula in the ampulla of each canal. The net effect is that the vestibular ganglia relay signals that are mostly proportional to head velocity over the physiological range of natural head movements (Carpenter 1988). The velocity signals are then distributed by the vestibular nuclei to the various ocular motor nuclei,

thus forming a classic three-neurone arc: vestibular ganglion–vestibular nucleus–ocular motor nucleus.

There are six semi-circular canals, three on each side, arranged as pairs at approximate right angles to each other, and they are maximally stimulated by head rotation in the planes of the canal pairs. The right lateral and left lateral canals are maximally stimulated with horizontal head movements (with the head pointing down a few degrees). The left posterior and right anterior (superior) canals are maximally stimulated by moving the head up and to the left, and down and to the right, respectively. The right posterior and left anterior canals are stimulated maximally by the head moving up and to the right, and down and to the left, respectively. Since the VOR is compensatory, excited canals cause the eyes to move towards the side opposite the canal (Table 64.2).

The canal planes are roughly similar to the planes of action of the extraocular muscle pairs, and each canal is excitatorily connected to a pair of agonist muscles and inhibitorily to a pair of antagonist muscles. Thus, if the head rotates backwards and to the right, the right posterior canal is maximally excited which activates the right superior oblique and left inferior rectus. This causes the eyes to predominantly depress with gaze to the left, or predominantly left tort with gaze to the right, thereby compensating for the head movement in all gaze directions (Fig. 64.4) (for further details see Leigh & Zee 1991). Most head movements involve all canals, but with this elegant arrangement, the appropriate combination of agonist and antagonist muscles are always activated to compensate for the head movement in any direction. It should be noted, however, that this arrangement is only approximate and all muscles are recruited for all canals to some extent.

By itself, the three-neurone arc or 'direct' vestibular pathway is not sufficient to drive the eyes with the correct velocity in all gaze positions because of the strong restoring force of the muscles towards primary position. To overcome the viscous and elastic tensions of the muscles,

Table 64.2 Effect of stimulating a single semi-circular canal. Based on Leigh & Zee (1991).

Canal	Head movement	Eye movement in		Agonist		Antagonist	
		R gaze	L gaze	R	L	R	L
R Post	R and up	L Tors	Down	SO	IR	IO	SR
R Ant	R and down	Up	L Tors	SR	IO	IR	SO
R Lat	R	L	L	MR	LR	LR	MR
L Post	L and up	Down	R Tors	IR	SO	SR	IO
L Ant	L and down	L Tors	Up	IO	SR	SO	IR
L Lat	L	R	R	LR	MR	MR	LR

Post, posterior; Ant, anterior; Lat, lateral (horizontal) canal; R/L Tors, cyclotorsion with upper poles of eyes moving to patient's right/left; SO/IO, superior/inferior oblique; SR/IR/LR/MR, superior/inferior/lateral/medial rectus.

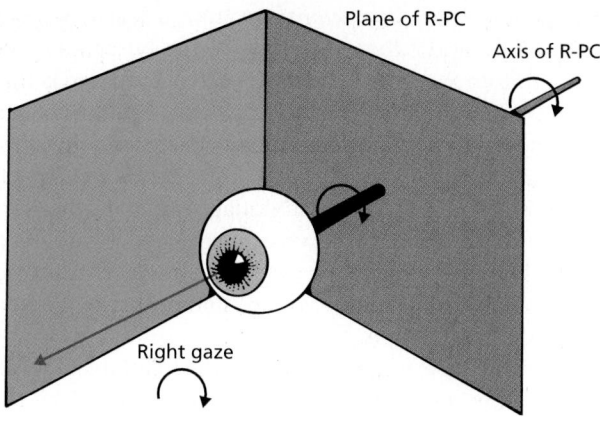

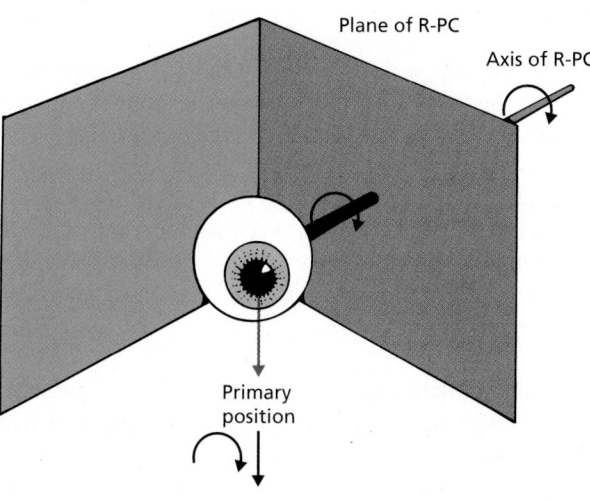

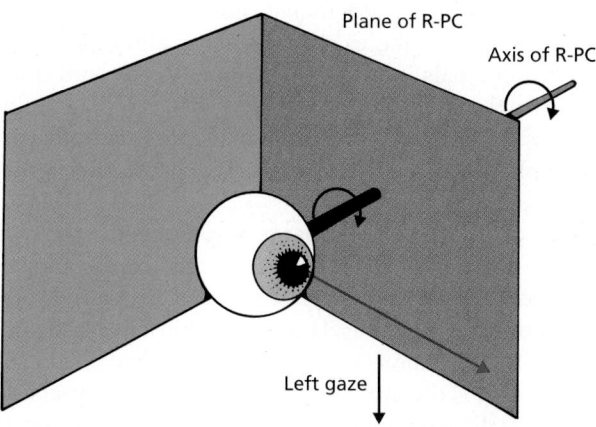

Fig. 64.4 Stimulating the right posterior semi-circular canal causes the eyes to rotate in the plane of the canal regardless of the position of the eyes. In right gaze this induces a predominantly left torsion of the eyes (upper poles of eyes rotate to patient's left). In left gaze the eyes predominantly depress. In primary position left torsion and depression occur.

the eye position NI provides an additional tonic signal. An abnormal NI can distort the VOR leading to some interpretative difficulties.

Gain. The gain of the VOR is the ratio of the angle of eye rotation to the angle of head rotation. Thus perfect compensation would require a gain of 1. In adults the gain is lower than 1, typically 0.6–0.9, which increases to 1 for rotation in the light. In newborns, however, the gain is near unity in the dark (Finochio *et al.* 1991) and gradually decreases over the preschool years. The reason for this high gain is not clear since high gain full-field OKN is present from birth (Roy *et al.* 1989). However, SP is very poor in the young infant, and perhaps the unity VOR gain helps stabilize images of small visual targets. Conversely, because neither the canals nor the eyes are on the axis of head rotation, higher gains are needed to stabilize images of near targets than far targets. So perhaps infant resting VOR gain is more attuned to nearer targets than adults (Reisman & Anderson 1989).

Vestibular nystagmus and time-constant. When there is a constant imbalance in tonus from the canals, the eyes will be driven in a direction determined by the net imbalance at a more-or-less constant (linear) velocity with quick-phases that 'reset' eye position (VN). An imbalance can be caused pathologically by over-excitability of a canal (as in benign paroxysmal positional vertigo, see Chapter 63), or by under-excitability of a canal, for example due to infection. For example, loss of left anterior canal function would result in excess tonus from the right posterior canal leading to VN with downward and left-torting slow phases, depending on gaze direction (see Chapter 63).

A physiological VN can also be induced by sustained rotation of the head in the dark (per-rotatory VN). Although this does not happen naturally, the VN has some useful properties that make it of clinical value. With constant rotation in the dark, the springy cupula will gradually regain its original resting position (the endolymph 'catches up' with the canal), and no longer generates an excitatory signal. So the VN will gradually decay, with ever slower slow-phases, until it disappears. If all other cues of motion could be eliminated, the patient would have no sensation of motion and believe himself to be stationary. If the rotation is then suddenly stopped, the endolymph will move relative to the canal wall in the opposite direction causing a reverse (post-rotatory) nystagmus, with a sensation of self-rotation (circularvection) in the opposite direction to the previous actual rotation. Eventually the cupula will restore and the nystagmus and circularvection will disappear.

Measurements on animals have shown that the time-constant[1] of this decay of per- or post-rotatory nystagmus as measured at the vestibular ganglion is about 5–6 seconds. However, the actual nystagmus takes much longer to decay, with a time-constant of 12 seconds or so in humans. This augmentation of the cupula time-constant has been labelled the velocity storage mechanism (VSM). It is a neural function, which probably involves reverberatory local commissural connections between opposite vestibular nuclei in the brain stem. However, it is also under adaptive control by the nodulus and uvula in the cerebellar vermis and experimental lesions lead to an excessively long VSM time-constant (Waespe *et al.* 1985). The VSM is also thought to be responsible for the time-constant of the delayed OKN system.

VN can be elicited from the full-term and premature infant. As with OKN, the amplitude of a typical slow phase is much higher, and the beat frequency much lower than in adults (Ornitz *et al.* 1979; Cordero *et al.* 1983). The time-constant is on average short in the infant (about 7 seconds), which is roughly expected from the cupula alone, and matures over the first 5 years. This trend most likely reflects neural development of the VSM rather than physical growth of canals.

If rotation is maintained in the dark after per-rotatory VN has decayed, a weaker secondary nystagmus will occur in the opposite direction to the immediately preceding nystagmus. A secondary post-rotatory (post-post-rotatory) nystagmus also occurs. The relative intensity of this secondary nystagmus is higher in infants than in adults (Ornitz *et al.* 1979) and has a shorter time-constant with protracted development. Secondary VN is thought to be a central adaptive neural mechanism for compensating for imbalances within the vestibular system. It has been implicated in the timing of pathological periodic alternating nystagmus (PAN) (Leigh *et al.* 1981) (see Chapter 63), and the relatively shorter reversal rates of childhood PAN could be a manifestation of the short time-constant of this adaptive mechanism.

Testing

In eye movement laboratories, VOR is usually tested in complete darkness to avoid any confounding visual input. The patient is either oscillated back and forth sinusoidally at different frequencies, or is rotated at a constant speed for a minute or so (step rotation). Sinusoidal rotation yields relatively reliable measures of gain and phase, but a number of different frequencies need to be tested, which can be time-consuming for the young sick child. It is also difficult to distinguish between abnormalities of eye velocity control (VSM) from abnormalities of eye position control (NI).

Step rotation allows the VSM time-constant to be easily

---

[1] The time-constant is measured as the time taken for eye velocity to fall to 37% of its initial value. As a rule of thumb, the nystagmus will persist for a total time of about 3×the time-constant.

examined without contamination from a leaky NI, and some information about the state of the NI can also be gleaned from the slow phases. Another advantage is that quick-phase failure can also be detected. Spurious head movements do not interfere much with the ongoing nystagmus, although excessive head tilting can dampen post-rotatory nystagmus. The disadvantage is that the measure of gain (peak slow phase velocity divided by rotation speed) is not as reliable. Nevertheless, given the limited time available for testing a young child or infant, we routinely use step rotation.

Clinically, VOR must be tested in the light; fixation can be broken by Frenzel lenses if they are tolerated by the child. The following two techniques are generally employed.

The oculocephalic or doll's head manoeuvre. Passive or active turns of the head are a quick test for vestibular function, and can be used to test vertical as well as horizontal VOR. The movements should be rapid. Head movements also stimulate proprioceptors in the neck muscles and joints, which can give rise to the cervico-ocular reflex (COR) which may be more active in infants (Reisman & Anderson 1989) and in patients with no functioning labyrinths (Bronstein & Hood 1986).

Spinning. Manual spinning of an infant is not a pure rotational vestibular test; it is in the light and there is head translation as well as rotation. Nevertheless it is particularly informative as part of a routine clinical examination.

In the light, the examiner holds the infant at arm's length face-to-face and rotates himself and the infant clockwise (i.e. to the examiner's right) through several revolutions. This induces a per-rotatory VN with quick phases to the infant's right (examiner's left). If the rotation is abruptly stopped, a post-rotatory VN is induced with quick-phases to the infant's left. The procedure is then reversed.

Because infant VN has a large amplitude, the per-rotatory nystagmus is clearly visible with large conjugate excursions. Since the test is carried out in the light, the post-rotatory nystagmus dampens within a few beats due to visual stabilization (VOR suppression). Sustained post-rotatory VN is therefore a sign of poor VOR suppression, which in the young infant indicates low vision or an abnormality of the early optokinetic pathway. This test can also sometimes help to distinguish between a questionable esotropia and a sixth nerve palsy since the eyes are usually driven well beyond the midline; patching the fellow eye for a few minutes prior to spinning may help. During manual spinning, infants with SIF will demonstrate a complete or intermittent failure of quick-phases, so that the eyes stay fully deviated (locked up) in the mechanical limit of gaze. The same phenomenon can be elicited by rotating the child in a swivel chair. To test for vertical VOR place the child on his side (on a parent's lap if needed) and rotate.

Abnormalities of the vestibulo-ocular reflex

Abnormal gain. Abnormally high gain has been reported in lesions of the cerebellar flocculus and possibly the inferior olive (Zee *et al.* 1976; Baloh *et al.* 1981; Thurston *et al.* 1987). The flocculus, and therefore its climbing fibre input from the inferior olive, are widely regarded as important in adaptive control of VOR gain (Lisberger *et al.* 1984). Mildly high gains have also been reported in familial vestibulocerebellar disorders (Theunissen *et al.* 1989; Harris *et al.* 1993c).

Abnormally low gain is more difficult to interpret due to the wide variations of gain in the dark. In the young child, very low gain may indicate involvement of the vestibular nerve, and is sometimes seen in meningitis and the CHARGE syndrome.

Asymmetrical gain is a more reliable indicator of acquired vestibular disease, but needs to be assessed in the context of other oculomotor and possibly auditory abnormalities, to distinguish among peripheral, brainstem, cerebellar, and cortical causes.

Abnormal time-constant. The VSM time-constant can be abnormally short due to disease of the end organ, the vestibular nerve or central disease (Baloh *et al.* 1988). There is considerable variability among normal individuals, especially infants, which leads to difficulty in interpretation.

Ultra low time-constants have been reported in Arnold–Chiari type I malformation, olivopontocerebellar degeneration (Baloh *et al.* 1988), demyelinating disease (Huygen *et al.* 1990), congenital and acquired blindness (Sherman & Keller 1986), and bilateral vestibulopathy secondary to ototoxic drugs (Baloh *et al.* 1984). It is important not to confuse the VSM and its time-constant with the eye position NI and its time-constant in gaze-holding. The two functions are clinically distinct (Baloh *et al.* 1988; Harris *et al.* 1993b), but VN can be distorted by an abnormal NI, which is a problem with sinusoidal stimulation for testing VOR, where both short VSM and short NI timeconstants may occur, as in healthy young infants (Weissman *et al.* 1989), and in disease of the brain stem and cerebellum. Even with step rotation, a very leaky NI prevents normal VN (Harris *et al.* 1993b).

An abnormally long time-constant is rare. Shawkat *et al.* (1993) recorded prolonged post-rotatory VN from a child in the acute stage of opsoclonus–myoclonus.

Absent quick-phases. Absent quick-phases may be an indication of SIF; most affected children will show a similar failure during OKN, but in a few cases, only VN shows the failure. This probably indicates a very subtle form of saccade failure, and by itself is probably of little clinical significance.

When the NI has an ultra short time-constant (i.e. effectively absent), rotation in the dark causes a tonic deviation of the eyes rather than a nystagmus. The angle of tonic deviation increases with the speed of rotation, and may reach the limit of gaze, appearing similar to saccade failure.

Some healthy infants may show lock-up during VN in the first 2–3 weeks, which may be prolonged in the infant with delayed visual maturation (Hoyt *et al.* 1985). Whether this is due to a genuine immaturity of the saccadic system or an immaturity of the NI is not yet clear.

Vestibular Nystagmus and Sensory Defect Nystagmus/ Congenital Idiopathic Nystagmus (see Chapter 63). VOR is usually absent or very erratic in children with SDN/CIN, whether elicited by calorics, constant rotation, or sinusoidal oscillation. Demer and Zee (1984) were able to elicit a response with sinusoidal oscillation at high frequencies. They proposed that this indicated either an ultra low VSM time-constant or an ultra low NI time-constant (see Harris *et al.* 1993b; Harris 1995).

In those few children who do have a vestibular response to constant rotation in the dark, we have occasionally observed quick-phase failure (locking up). The reason for this is obscure, but it should not be confused with saccade failure and a neurological nystagmus.

Optokinesis

Optokinesis refers to reflexive conjugate slow following of the eyes to movement of large areas of the visual scene. It is most readily elicited by full-field motion, which is encountered naturally during head and eye movements, or unnaturally by looking out of the window of a moving vehicle. Optokinesis may also be elicited by small-field motion induced by a moving drum, tape or television picture. In some circumstances, such as in delayed visual maturation (DVM), a full-field smooth response can be elicited in the absence of a small-field response.

OKN (optokinetic nystagmus) is a physiological nystagmus where the slow-phase optokinetic pursuit response is reset by quick-phases (saccades). The direction of OKN is conventionally described by the direction of the quick-phases but the optokinetic response actually refers to the slow phases, and here we shall refer to the direction of OKN by the direction of the stimulus or slow phases.

OKN is measured by the velocity of the eyes during the slow phases, or gain (the speed of the slow phases divided by stimulus speed). However, beat frequency has been used as a more convenient measure in the very young. Beat frequency is typically about 0.5–1 beats per second, which is about half that of adults (Hainline *et al.* 1984), and there is a more or less linear relationship between beat frequency and slow phase velocity (Harris *et al.* 1994).

Early versus delayed optokinetic nystagmus. Because it is reflexive, OKN is a clinically useful test in the preverbal or neurologically impaired child. In primates, OKN is a remarkably complicated response. In the developmental literature there has been much debate about the cortical and subcortical neural substrate for the development of OKN.

In primates OKN has at least two distinct components.
1 Delayed (indirect, slow) OKN (OKNd). OKNd is closely linked to the VOR and VSM. It has a slow build-up (tens of seconds) and gives rise to optokinetic after-nystagmus (OKAN), which is a gradual decay of nystagmus when the lights are switched off. OKNd is driven by visual motion signals in the visual cortex via the nucleus of the optic tract in the pretectum and the vestibular nuclei.
2 Early (direct, fast) OKN (OKNe). OKNe has a fast build-up (<1 second) (Abadi *et al.* 1994) and ceases promptly in the dark. The OKNe pathway is similar to the SP pathway, which is mediated by a cortico-ponto-cerebellar route, and it is doubtful that the pretectum has a direct role in the OKNe/SP pathway, although it may be important for adaptive control of OKNe/SP.
Each has different neural pathways that are mostly parallel (Fuchs & Mustari 1993).

During optokinetic stimulation of healthy human adults, both OKNe and OKNd are activated, but OKNe is completely dominant in the light. The presence of OKNd can only be detected by looking for OKAN after the lights are switched off. However, the OKNd system may be uncovered in patients in whom the OKNe/SP system has been lesioned; this can occur with parietal lesions (Baloh *et al.* 1982), in vestibulocerebellar disorders (Zee *et al.* 1976; Harris *et al.* 1993c), and possibly in brain stem disease (Pierrot-Deseilligny *et al.* 1984). Many authors have not distinguished between OKNd and OKNe, thus giving a false impression of absent SP in the presence of OKN, where probably OKNd was really being measured.

Although OKNe is dominant in primates, it is only rudimentary in the cat (Evinger & Fuchs 1978). Thus the kitten is not a homologue of the human infant, since the kitten will not develop human-like OKNe/SP when it matures. Probably OKN has a fast build-up in infants from at least as young as 1 month (Hainline *et al.* 1984; Harris *et al.* 1994), indicating OKNe rather than OKNd function. This implies cortical function from an early age, which is consistent with the OKN deficit caused by cortical lesions (Braddick *et al.* 1992; Jacobs *et al.* 1993).

Stare versus look optokinetic nystagmus. Adult OKN is sensitive to attentional state (Ter Braak 1936). In look or 'active' OKN, the subject attends specific features of the moving stimulus and the OKN has high gain, large amplitude, and low beat frequency. With stare or 'passive' OKN, individual stimulus features are not attended, the OKN has a lower gain (particularly at high stimulus speeds), low amplitude and high frequency. It is unlikely that stare versus look OKN is related in any way to OKNd or OKNe (Pola & Wyatt 1993), but rather they are both aspects of OKNe.

In the preverbal child it is not possible to be sure which type of OKN is elicited. Infants produce a fast build-up, large amplitude, low frequency OKN similar to that seen in adult look OKN. However, infants also produce large amplitude VN in the dark. In the early visually unresponsive stage of isolated DVM, OKN has a similar high amplitude and low frequency as in normal age-matched infants (Harris *et al.* 1995). Thus, it seems probable that most infant OKN is actually stare OKN, where the low beat frequency reflects an immaturely long latency to generate quick-phases.

Testing

Optokinetic responses can often be obtained by inducing the child to look at a drum or tape which traditionally has black and white stripes which can be rotated horizontally or vertically; in fact, any interesting or patterned target can be used. These bedside clinical tests do not generate a large-field motion stimulus.

There is no clear demarcation between a full- and small-field. For some investigators the sensation of self-motion is an indication of a true OKN response; this takes about 5 seconds or so to build up, and cannot be ascertained in the pre/non-verbal child. The sensation of self-motion is called circularvection when viewing a rotating optokinetic curtain, and linearvection for the sensation of self-translation when viewing a flat-projected or TV moving stimulus.

The failure to elicit OKN with a hand-held drum or tape does not preclude a normal full-field optokinetic response.

Abnormalities of optokinetic nystagmus

Bilateral absence of optokinetic nystagmus

There are four principal reasons for absent OKN.
1 Poor vision. The response to a full-field OKN stimulus is difficult to suppress, so the presence of OKN demonstrates sight in the visually unresponsive child. The degree of vision needed for an optokinetic response depends on stimulus speed, direction, distance, size, pattern, whether the child is monocular, the presence of spontaneous nystagmus, underlying neurological disease, and alertness. Thus OKN is a poor way to quantify visual acuity (Mackie & McCulloch 1995). We use a full-field brightly patterned curtain containing many spatial frequencies

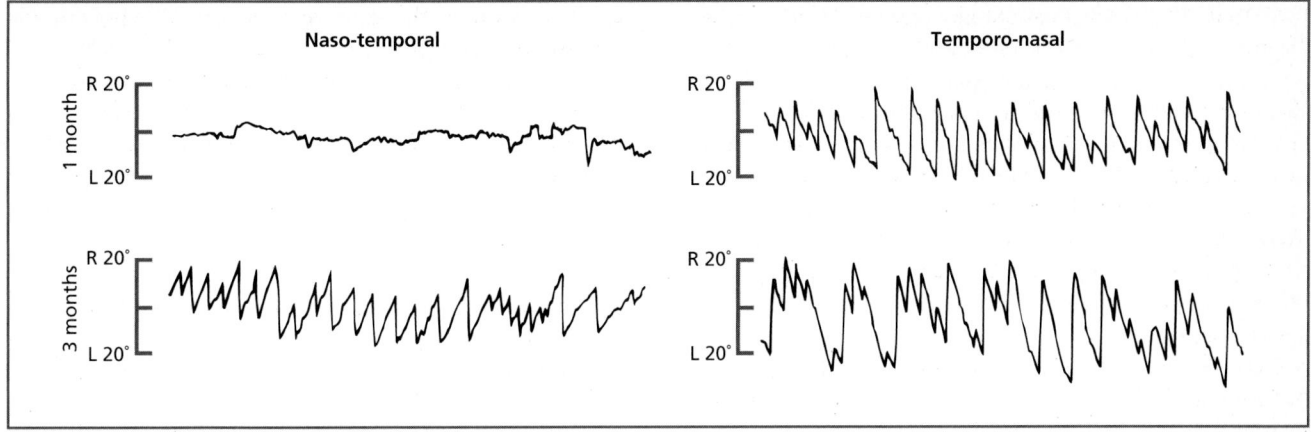

Fig. 64.5 OKN elicited by a full-field curtain from a healthy infant viewing monocularly with the right eye. At 1 month of age a normal OKN can be elicited with slow phases in the temporonasal direction of the viewing eye (i.e. to the left), but there is no response in the nasotemporal direction. By 3 months, the nasotemporal OKN has much improved.

which is attractive to young children while yielding OKN even with extremely poor vision.

2 Early onset nystagmus (SDN/CIN). This is usually associated with a failure of OKN. During testing, the nystagmus persists unabated, but the waveform may change (null shifting), or occasionally the SDN/CIN may become completely quiescent, still without OKN. The presence of optokinetic slow phases with superimposed pendular nystagmus may indicate APN associated with neurological disease at any age (including early infancy). Absent OKN and GPN occur in association with vestibulocerebellar disorders, so that the presence of spontaneous nystagmus without OKN does not automatically indicate SDN/CIN.

3 Intracranial lesions. Bilateral lesions of the optokinetic pathway may abolish all horizontal OKN and SP. This can occur with lesions of the brain stem, cerebellum or cortex. Some OKN may be present with a slow build-up of tens of seconds if the delayed OKN pathway is intact. With posterior fossa lesions, other cerebellar or brain stem signs are usually present. Children or adults with GPN and no OKN may appear to have an optokinetic response or 'pseudo-OKN' (Harris *et al.* 1993c). Here, the patient looks in the opposite direction to stimulus motion, thereby inducing his own GPN with slow phases in the same direction as stimulus motion. Upon reversal of stimulus motion, gaze is shifted to the opposite side thereby inducing GPN in the other direction. To test for an OKN response, the patient should look straight ahead at the stimulus. In unco-operative children, the VOR suppression test may be more fruitful.

4 SIF. Delay or failure of the triggering of quick-phases is a feature of SIF and is easily detected with full-field OKN since the eyes lock-up. This does not occur in healthy infants over 1 month of age. With a hand-held drum quick-phase failure can be mistaken for absent OKN if the eyes are not driven to the limit of gaze.

Binocular asymmetry of optokinetic nystagmus

Asymmetrical abnormalities of binocular OKN and SP can be caused by unilateral lesions anywhere in the optokinetic pathway, including brain stem, cerebellum and parietal lobe (Yee *et al.* 1982). There are other clinical or oculomotor signs that may distinguish these sites. Isolated binocular OKN asymmetry suggests a parietal lesion, and has been reported in infants as young as 4–5 months (Braddick *et al.* 1992; Jacobs *et al.* 1993).

Lesions of the posterior cortex often involve both the occipital and parietal lobes with a contralateral homonymous hemianopia and an ipsilateral SP deficit: unilateral lesions restricted to the occipital lobe lead to hemianopia but symmetrical OKN (Smith 1962) or there may be an OKN asymmetry with normal fields.

Children often do not demonstrate hemi-neglect, so OKN testing can often detect parietal lesions.

Monocular asymmetry of optokinetic nystagmus

Healthy neonates demonstrate an optokinetic response that is symmetrical when both eyes are open but asymmetrical if one eye is occluded (Fig. 64.5). In this asymmetry of monocular OKN (mOKN), the speed of the slow phases and the beat frequency are lower for stimulus motion in the nasotemporal (NT) direction of the viewing eye, than in the temporonasal (TN) direction (Atkinson 1979). This normal asymmetry declines over the first 6 months for moderate stimulus speeds (about 30° per second) but it persists beyond 6 months at high stimulus speeds (Roy *et al.* 1989; Harris *et al.* 1994).

With early disturbances of binocular vision due to strabismus, anisometropia or unilateral cataract, the mOKN asymmetry usually becomes permanent and usually in both eyes. Whereas with an onset after about 1–2 years mOKN symmetry remains (Schor & Levi 1980; Maurer *et al.* 1983; Westall & Shute 1992).

Although persistent mOKN asymmetry has been related to the lack of binocular development (van Hof-van Duin & Mohn 1986), it seems that the development of mOKN symmetry and binocularity may be separate processes because:

1 In individual subjects there is only a weak correlation between the development of mOKN symmetry and binocularity (Wattam-Bell *et al.* 1987).

2 At high stimulus speeds, the normal development of symmetry is protracted well beyond the time of normal development of stereopsis: there is no special age at which mOKN symmetry develops (Roy *et al.* 1989; Harris *et al.* 1994).

3 Stereodeficient subjects show a wide range of OKN asymmetries, with some being nearly symmetrical (Westall *et al.* 1989).

4 Infants with no possible binocularity due to profound congenital monocular visual loss can exhibit symmetrical monocular OKN in their functioning eye (Shawkat *et al.* 1995a).

5 Some stereoblind non-amblyopic esotropes with an onset before 2 months demonstrate symmetrical monocular OKN for stimulus speeds as high as 75° per second in each eye (Timms *et al.* 1995).

6 Three infants with early onset esotropia gained high-grade stereopsis after surgical alignment before 5 months, but did not develop symmetrical mOKN (Aiello *et al.* 1994).

These studies seem to suggest that mOKN asymmetry may be particularly sensitive to very early abnormal and probably rivalrous vision from both eyes.

Occasionally a schoolchild may present with strabismus and an unknown history, and clinically it would be reassuring to be able to date the true onset of the strabismus by looking for asymmetrical mOKN. However, persistent mOKN asymmetry is not a constant feature of early onset strabismus. In two large studies of esotropes, a large percentage with an onset before 6 months demonstrated symmetrical mOKN (Bourron-Madignier *et al.* 1987; Demer & von Noorden 1988). These studies were based on subjective estimation, but using electro-oculography (EOG) in a small sample, Timms *et al.* (1995) found definite mOKN symmetry in non-amblyopic stereoblind esotropes. Thus, symmetrical OKN does not preclude an early onset esotropia. Asymmetrical mOKN is, however, strong presumptive evidence for an esotropia with an onset in the first year (Bourron-Madignier *et al.* 1987; Demer & von Noorden 1988; Schor *et al.* 1995). Asymmetry in only one eye (affected or normal eye) has been described as more likely when there is a later onset of strabismus (Westall *et al.* 1989).

Thus, although asymmetrical mOKN is more likely in early onset strabismus, the correlation is not perfect, and the ability to date the onset of strabismus later in childhood is not precise.

'Manifest' monocular asymmetry of optokinetic nystagmus

Existing mOKN asymmetry may appear with both eyes viewing if vision in one eye is very poor or is suppressed. OKN testing with both eyes open will then appear like binocular OKN asymmetry. Even when there is neurological impairment in a child, the possibility of a manifest mOKN asymmetry must be considered because early onset strabismus is not an uncommon association of neurological disease (Table 64.3).

Smooth pursuit and vestibulo-ocular reflex suppression

Smooth pursuit (SP) is when the eyes smoothly follow a small smoothly moving visual target across a visual background. SP is not synonymous with 'following' or 'tracking' since those terms usually imply any ability to follow a moving target including SP, saccades or head movements.

When the head moves there is a reflexive vestibulo-ocular reflex (VOR) that moves the eyes in the opposite direction, which would normally prevent fixation of any visual target that moved at the same speed as the head. VORS is the ability to suppress this VOR. SP and VORS are probably manifestations of the same oculomotor function (Barnes 1993).

Although OKNe and SP probably share an extracortical pathway, they are not exactly the same and are partially dissociated in early infancy. SP is volitional and requires attention to a small moving region of the visual field with suppression of the stationary visual background. The young infant has difficulty in following small moving targets and tracking is often saccadic, but full-field OKN can be easily elicited. The reason for this dissociation is not clear. Obviously the infant conjugate eye movement system is quite capable of generating slow movements, and the targets in most studies should be resolvable by the afferent visual pathways. One hypothesis is that there is an immaturity in driving the OKNe pathway with small regions of moving visual field, so that SP response improves with larger targets. This would account for the different experimental results where some have reported no SP until 2–3 months (Aslin *et al.* 1981), while others, using larger targets, have found a response at younger ages including the neonatal period (Kremenitzer *et al.* 1979).

For children over 1 year, the clinical difference between SP and OKNe deficits are minor (see also Büttner 1988).

Table 64.3 Clinical guide to the horizontal optokinetic nystagmus (OKN) asymmetries without spontaneous nystagmus.

	Both eyes open		Right eye viewing		Left eye viewing		
	R	L	R (n-t)	L (t-n)	R (t-n)	L (n-t)	Typical aetiology
(1)	+	+	+	+	+	+	> 6 month normal
(2)	+	+	−	+	+	−	< 6 month normal
							> 6 month DVM; early onset uniocular problems
(3)	+	+	+	+	−	−	Low vision in *left* eye without (2)
	+	+	−	−	+	+	Low vision in *right* eye without (2)
(4)	+	−	+	−	+	−	Lesion of *left* occipitoparietal cortex
	−	+	−	+	−	+	Lesion of *right* occipitoparietal cortex
(5)	−	+	−	+	−	−	Low vision in *left* eye with (2) *or* lesion of *right* occipitoparietal cortex with (2)
	+	−	−	−	+	−	Low vision in *right* eye with (2) *or* lesion of *left* occipitoparietal cortex with (2)
(6)	−	−	−	−	−	−	Bilateral low vision *or* bilateral lesions of occipitoparietal cortex

DVM, delayed visual maturation; R/L, stimulus motion to patient's right/left; n-t, nasotemporal; t-n, temporonasal. +, OKN normal; −, OKN absent/poor.

Testing

SP is tested by getting the patient to follow a relatively slowly (10–40° per second) moving target horizontally and vertically without head movements. As with saccades, this is not a test of visual acuity, so an easily resolvable target is needed. In normal children over 6 months the eye movements should be smooth and conjugate.

In VORS the patient is rotated or oscillated back and forth in a swivel chair while fixating a target that is fixed to the chair. Alternatively, the patient may hold with his teeth a wooden tongue depressor to which is attached a pin; he shakes his head slowly while looking at the pin. If the patient is attending the target, the VOR response is suppressed resulting in no movements of the eyes relative to the head. Failure of VORS results in an incompletely cancelled VOR which appears as a nystagmus with beats in the direction of rotation. In unilateral disorders, VORS and SP failures are in the same direction of stimulus motion.

SP or VORS testing requires attention. Saccadic pursuit implies that the child is at least attending the target because he can be seen to follow the target, whereas in VORS testing, failure to fixate the target may reflect either poor SP or simply poor attention to the target. Another advantage of SP testing is that catch-up saccades are readily detected, but nystagmus due to poor VORS may be subtle.

The advantage of VORS testing is that the eyes do not have to deviate from primary position. LN becomes manifest frequently on lateral gaze with both eyes open and can appear strikingly similar to GPN, even to the point that both yield saccadic SP. VORS is usually normal in LN but abnormal in GPN.

Neural substrate

The geniculostriate visual pathway relays visual information to extra-striate cortex in the parieto-occipito-temporal areas, which are essential for SP and OKNe function. SP signals descend directly to the pons, to the ipsilateral dorsolateral pontine nuclei (DLPN), which relay SP signals to the cerebellar flocculus and posterior vermis, and then to the oculomotor centres in the brain stem (Büttner 1988).

Unilateral lesions in the cortex and cerebellum lead to deficits in SP towards the side of the lesion. Brain stem lesions are seldom so circumscribed, but a pure SP deficit has also been reported with a lesion in the ipsilateral basal pons (Thier *et al.* 1991).

Abnormalities of smooth pursuit

SP failure is not localizing by itself. Intracranial lesions of the cortex and cerebellum affecting SP usually have a similar affect on OKN (see above), although a dissociation has been reported in acquired thalamic lesions in an adult (Ohtsuka *et al.* 1991). As with OKN, persistent monocular SP asymmetries may persist in patients with early onset strabismus but not with late onset strabismus (Tychsen *et al.* 1985; Sokol *et al.* 1991).

There is a complete dissociation in the initial unresponsive stage of DVM, where no following can be elicited to any hand-held stimulus, but binocular OKN is usually normal (Harris *et al.* 1995). It is unlikely that this dissociation is due to immature acuity, since the pattern VEPs are normal. It may reflect a delayed development of extra-striate cortical function (Tressider *et al.* 1990).

Vergence

Vergence is the ability to change the angle between the two visual axes to permit both near and far foveation, to maintain single vision and stereopsis; it is driven by retinal image disparity and accommodative blur. Fixation of a near target induces accommodation and pupillary constriction as well as convergence.

Cells in the mesencephalic reticular formation dorsal to the oculomotor nucleus fire in relation to both vergence angle and vergence velocity (Zee & Levi 1989).

Little is known about the development of human vergence because of the difficulties in measuring relatively small eye movements simultaneously in both eyes in infants. The absolute measurement of static vergence angle in the infant is hampered by two problems.
1 The angle between the line of sight and the pupillary axis changes in early infancy (Slater & Findlay 1975).
2 An inconsistent retinal locus may be used for fixation in the immature macula (Hainline *et al.* 1990).

Accommodation-driven vergence can be detected at 2 months, and disparity-driven vergence at about 4 months, which is similar to the age when both fusion and stereopsis develop (see Aslin 1993).

Abnormalities of vergence

The major abnormality of vergence in childhood is in association with strabismus; other vergence abnormalities are rare in childhood.

Spasm of the near-reflex

Convergence spasm associated with accommodation and pupillary constriction is most commonly a non-organic problem, although the spasm can hardly be considered 'voluntary'. Blurred vision and diplopia occur, and the patient may complain of eye-ache. Attempts to abduct an eye may lead to abduction nystagmus. The spasms may last from seconds to minutes.

Organic problems are rare but include midbrain lesions, encephalitis, posterior fossa lesions, metabolic problems, anticonvulsant toxicities, myasthenia gravis and cyclic oculomotor palsy (see Miller 1985; Leigh & Zee 1991). It must be distinguished from bilateral sixth nerve palsies.

Treatment with cycloplegics may relieve the accommodative component and the pain whereas miotics may reduce the central drive by causing a genuine miosis and accommodation.

Divergence paralysis

Divergence paralysis appears as a convergent strabismus when looking at distance but with normal convergence. It is usually associated with a partial sixth nerve palsy (unilateral or bilateral).

Convergence insufficiency

Convergence insufficiency usually appears in adolescence and gives rise to symptoms of eye strain following close work. A poorly controlled exophoria on near fixation is found with the cover test. Eye movements and reading acuity are normal, and there should be no neurological abnormalities. The child and parents should be reassured that there is no disease, and reading at a further distance with a bright light and for shorter periods should be encouraged. There may occasionally be underlying psychological problems. Convergence insufficiency should be distinguished from dorsal midbrain problems.

Midbrain lesions

Organic vergence abnormalities occur in midbrain disease. Convergence may be paralysed, or it may be excessive causing reading difficulties, and giving the appearance of a sixth nerve palsy. Excessive convergence may lead to convergence spasm. Convergent retraction nystagmus may occur on attempted upgaze or with a downward optokinetic stimulus (which elicits upward quick-phases), and may become more exaggerated on extension of the neck (Mossman *et al.* 1990). Other abnormalities are associated with organic vergence abnormalities including limitations of upgaze, lid retraction, skew deviation (SD) and downbeat nystagmus. Pupillary responses may be abnormal and may react better to accommodation than light (light-near dissociation).

Lesions may be intrinsic to the midbrain, or due to extrinsic pineal tumours or secondary to aqueductal stenosis bringing pressure to bear on the posterior commissure.

Oculomotor defects in localized brain disease

Brain stem

Medulla

Medullary malformations have been associated with a wide range of oculomotor abnormalities including Downbeat Nystagmus, PAN, Torsional Nystagmus, GPN and Rebound Nystagmus, positional nystagmus, internuclear ophthalmoplegia, skew deviation and alternating skew deviation, saccade dysmetria, poor SP, abnormal VOR gain and time-constants (Leigh & Zee 1991). Some of these abnormalities are secondary to the cerebellar rather than medullary involvement. Convergence nystagmus has also been associated with Arnold–Chiari malformation, but this may have been caused by distortion of the midbrain and aqueduct (Mossman *et al.* 1990).

Wallenberg's lateral medullary syndrome results from medullary ischaemia in the territory of the posterior inferior cerebellar artery. Symptoms include vertigo, facial and corneal insensitivity and a compelling sensation of being pulled to one side (lateropulsion). The main oculomotor abnormality is saccade dysmetria with overshoot towards the side of the lesion and contralateral undershoot. Wallenberg's syndrome is extremely rare in childhood (Klein *et al.* 1976).

Pons

Lesions of the pons are not common in childhood but can cause a range of complex oculomotor abnormalities depending on involvement of supranuclear, nuclear, or infranuclear structures. The precise localization of gaze abnormalities is poorly understood. Sixth nerves pareses are discussed in Chapter 66.

A horizontal gaze palsy describes a difficulty in moving both eyes across the midline: it may affect one or more types of eye movement. If all movements are affected it implies that the final gaze pathway is affected; if single eye movement subtypes are affected it implies that the palsy is supranuclear.

Lesions of the paramedian pontine reticular formation (PPRF) lead to slow ipsiversive saccades and an ipsilateral gaze palsy, but pursuit and VOR may be preserved. A very circumscribed lesion of the basal pons may lead to an ipsiversive SP deficit with preserved saccades (Thier *et al.* 1991). Convergence is usually spared. Acute pontine lesions are rare in childhood, but a progression from intermittent saccade failure, to slow saccades, and then to a gaze palsy with idiosyncratic sparing of pursuit or VOR may occur in Niemann–Pick type C.

Internuclear ophthalmoplegia. In internuclear ophthalmoplegia (INO), a unilateral lesion of the MLF interrupts abducens relay signals from reaching the contralateral oculomotor nucleus, impairing adduction. In demyelinating disease the lesion is usually rostral to the abducens, above the decussation where abducens axons enter the contralateral fasciculus (Bronstein *et al.* 1990).

The degree of deficit may range from a complete lack of adduction of the ipsilateral eye to slow adducting saccades with full range. In bilateral INO there is impaired adduction of both eyes, although the severity may be asymmetrical. In some cases, vergence may also be affected and there may be a vertical nystagmus, or skew deviation, presumably due to collateral damage at the midbrain level. In INO there is usually a dissociated abduction nystagmus in the contralateral eye (see Chapter 63).

In the 'one-and-a-half' syndrome, there is an additional gaze palsy (i.e. limiting both eyes) towards the side of the lesion due to additional lesions or an extended lesion affecting the PPRF or the abducens. In the full-blown condition only abduction of the contralateral eye is spared.

In childhood, INO is unusual, and unlike adults, demyelinating disease is rare (Steinlin *et al.* 1995). More common causes of childhood INO are posterior fossa tumours, in which INO may be a presenting sign (Cogan & Wray 1970), and Arnold–Chiari malformations (Arnold *et al.* 1990). Other associations include parainfectious vasculitis, head trauma (Mueller *et al.* 1993), polyarteritis nodosa (Kirkali *et al.* 1991), sickle cell disease (Leavitt & Butrus 1994), and rarely progressive neurodegenerative disease (Sloane *et al.* 1994).

Skew deviation. Skew deviation (SD) is a supranuclear disorder of vertical eye alignment. The vertical deviation may be comitant or non-comitant. It is usually acquired with an acute onset secondary to brain stem lesions (Keane 1975). SD diminishes with time and is said to be rare in progressive disease.

Brandt and Dieterich (1993) reported torsion in all of their 56 adult unilateral cases, with intorsion of the elevated eye or extorsion of the depressed eye, or both occurring in 50% of cases. They found pontomesencephalic lesions on the same side as the elevated eye or pontomedullary lesions on the opposite side of the elevated eye.

SD is often associated with other brain stem oculomotor abnormalities such as INO, Wallenberg's syndrome, and gaze limitations. Acquired SD is rare in childhood, but must be carefully distinguished from trochlear palsies and vertical strabismus.

In alternating SD, the deviation reverses on changing lateral gaze, with the adducting eye being lower, or higher, or either. This has most commonly been attributed to midbrain lesions and has been associated with vertical gaze palsies, pupillary abnormalities and convergence-retraction nystagmus (Keane 1985). The association with downbeat nystagmus has implicated cervicomedullary involvement.

In a study of 242 neonates, Hoyt *et al.* (1980) detected congenital SD in 22, five of whom later developed a large angle esotropia.

Midbrain

The midbrain is involved in the control of vertical eye movements and vergence. The proximity of the posterior commissure, the nuclei of the riMLF, and the interstitial nuclei of Cajal (INC), the nucleus of the posterior commissure, the periaqueductal grey matter, and the third nucleus leads to a variety of vertical and vergence abnormalities, which may be supranuclear, nuclear or infranuclear.

Each riMLF contains burst units for upward, downward, and torsional saccades/quick-phases, where the torsional component is ipsiversive: the right riMLF causes right-torsion, i.e. the upper poles of the eyes tort to the patient's right, and are connected by the posterior commissure. Bilateral lesions (or a unilateral lesion that also involves the posterior commissure) are needed to create a pure vertical saccade deficit.

In neurodegeneration due to Niemann–Pick type C disease, there is a predilection for vertical saccade involvement, presumably involving the riMLFs (Shawkat *et al.* 1994), which may eventually involve horizontal saccades.

The INCs are involved in vertical gaze holding (the vertical NI), and relay downward control via ipsilateral pathways to their third subnucleus: they relay upward control by contralateral pathways via the posterior commissure to their third subnucleus (Leigh & Zee 1991).

The setting-sun sign

Intrinsic posterior commissure lesions, or extrinsic pressure on the posterior commissure, may cause an upward saccade failure as well as an upgaze palsy, which probably accounts for the tonic downgaze, 'setting-sun', as seen in acute hydrocephalus.

The dorsal midbrain syndrome

This is also known as Parinaud's syndrome, pretectal syndrome, Sylvian aqueduct syndrome and Koerber–Salus–Elschnig syndrome. The dorsal midbrain syndrome consists of the following.
1 Impairment of upgaze (with downgaze involvement sometimes).
2 Disturbance of vergence eye movements (convergence-retraction nystagmus).
3 Lid retraction (Collier's sign).
4 SD.
5 Near-reflex dissociation.
Ptosis may also occur, presumably due to third nucleus involvement.

Transient vertical gaze abnormalities of infancy

Paroxysmal tonic upgaze may occur in infancy (Ouvrier & Billson 1988; Ahn *et al.* 1989; Echenne & Rivier 1992; Campistol *et al.* 1993). The onset ranges from 4 to 19 months, typically starting at 9 months. The attacks may be less frequent in the mornings and more frequent during an intercurrent illness (Deonna & Meyer 1990), but decrease over the first year and usually disappear by 1–4 years. A chin-down posture may be adopted. Early development is characterized by hypotonia, late walking and ataxia. MRI is usually normal, although periventricular leukomalacia and poor myelination has been reported in one case (Sugie *et al.* 1995). The EEG is normal. Horizontal SP has been reported to be abnormal in one case (Deonna

& Meyer 1990). A common feature is intermittent downbeat nystagmus, often being more intense in downgaze. Antiepileptic, corticosteroid and acetazolamide therapies have had no clinical benefit, although levodopa has been helpful in some cases (Ouvrier & Billson 1988; Campistol *et al.* 1993), but not in all (Gieron & Korthals 1993). A normal outcome is usual. The underlying pathology is unknown.

Spontaneous downgaze has been reported as a benign transient phenomenon occurring in neonates that spontaneously remits in the first year (Hoyt *et al.* 1980). It has been described in preterm infants with an onset at 36–38 weeks gestation (Kleinman *et al.* 1994). Vertical eye movements are full, usually without lid retraction. In a similar benign condition, neonatal downward deviations have been associated with upbeat nystagmus (Goldblum & Effron 1994). Thus there may be a range of abnormality depending on the ability of the infant to generate upward quick-phases. Except for the different time of onset and reversed direction, there is a similarity to the paroxysmal tonic upgaze.

This must be distinguished from tonic downgaze, in which there is difficulty in eliciting upgaze and lid retraction since this can indicate hydrocephalus (Cernerud 1975).

A paroxysmal downgaze with upper eyelid closure has been described as a transient phenomenon in retarded spastic infants with white matter disease (Yokochi 1991).

Cerebellum

The cerebellum either modulates or mediates all eye movement systems. Abnormal eye movements most frequently result from cerebellar disease.

The SP and fast optokinetic response are mediated via the flocculus/paraflocculus and vermis. The flocculus/paraflocculus is also important in the augmentation of the brain stem NI.

The nodulus and uvula are important for controlling the VSM, which is needed for the VOR and optokinetic after-nystagmus.

The posterior vermis is intimately involved in controlling the accuracy of saccades as well as being involved in the SP system.

The cerebellum may also be involved in the timing of saccades and quick-phases, and may be implicated in some cases of SIF.

Cerebellar disorders also give rise to a wide variety of nystagmus including: downbeat nystagmus, upbeat nystagmus, APN, GPN, rebound nystagmus and PAN.

Thalamus

Vertical eye movement disorders have often been associated with thalamic lesions, but they are more likely due to collateral damage to nearby rostral mesencephalic structures.

MRI is necessary to demonstrate midbrain involvement since CT can be inadequate (Siatkowski *et al.* 1993).

Horizontal deficits including tonic deviations and saccadic hypometria have been attributed to thalamic lesions, although it is not clear whether this is due to the destruction of thalamic oculomotor centres or descending fibres.

Basal ganglia

The basal ganglia are important in the higher control of eye movements, particularly saccades (Kennard & Lueck 1989), and they are involved in a variety of childhood neurodegenerative conditions.

The basal ganglia link the frontal eye fields with tectal and cerebellar saccadic centres. Basal ganglia eye movement abnormalities are virtually impossible to distinguish from those due to frontal disease (distractibility of gaze, intrusive saccades, antisaccade failure). Basal ganglia saccade abnormalities can also be similar to cerebellar/brain stem eye movement disorders (hypometria, lock-up during nystagmus, slow saccades).

Involuntary movements, dystonia, psychiatric disturbances, and a positive family history are common. It is doubtful that disorders of the basal ganglia alone can give rise to nystagmus, although gaze-evoked nystagmus has been reported in a pedigree of striatonigral degeneration (Rosenberg *et al.* 1976).

Parkinson's disease is rare in childhood except as a post-encephalitic phenomenon, but a number of Parkinsonian syndromes occur. Huntington's disease is an autosomal dominant disorder characterized by an inexorable degeneration of the caudate nucleus and the putamen followed by atrophy of the whole brain. Six per cent of cases have an onset before 21 years and 3% before 15 (Caviness 1985). The earliest reported onset is 2 years. There are slow long-latency saccades (Avanzini *et al.* 1979; Lasker *et al.* 1988), difficulty in suppressing reflexive saccades (Tian *et al.* 1991); horizontal and vertical saccade failure including quick-phase failure during OKN and VN (Starr 1967) and saccadic pursuit without GPN (Beenen *et al.* 1986).

Eye tics, blepharospasm and involuntary eye deviations have been described in Gilles de la Tourette syndrome (Frankel & Cummings 1984). One study revealed normal eye movements (Bollen *et al.* 1988), but we have observed intrusive saccades and poor antisaccades in a 13-year-old boy. 'Tourettism' has also been associated with Huntington's disease (Jankovic & Ashizawa 1995).

In Sydenham's chorea, Schieken *et al.* (1973) reported diplopia and involuntary rapid jerky random 'choreiform' eye movements only in the right eye in two children with right hemichorea.

Hallervorden–Spatz disease is a rare disorder and it is

characterized by a progressive dystonia particularly in the jaw, retinal degeneration and dementia. Onset is after early childhood and death usually occurs in the second or third decade. There is degeneration of the globus pallidus and the substantia nigra, with a characteristic 'eye-of-the-tiger' appearance of T2-weighted MRI of the pallidum (Sethi *et al.* 1988). Slow or absent horizontal saccades with compensating head turns have been reported (Angelini *et al.* 1992).

In Wilson's disease there may be an upgaze palsy with slow horizontal voluntary saccades and with horizontal saccade failure during OKN and VN (Kirkham & Kamin 1974), and loss of accommodation and the near response (Curran *et al.* 1983). There may be midbrain involvement in addition to basal ganglia disease.

Leigh's disease (subacute necrotizing encephalomyelopathy) typically has an onset in the first 2 years with rapid progression leading to death by 6, although longer survival occurs. Optic atrophy is frequent and the basal ganglia (putamen, globus pallidus, caudate nucleus), upper and lower brain stem, thalamus, cerebellum, and anterior visual pathways (Montpetit *et al.* 1971) are frequently involved. Nystagmus is more common with onset in the second year (Pincus 1972) and is either secondary to cerebellar/brain stem disease or visual loss due to optic atrophy.

Cerebral cortex

Frontal lobe

Oculomotor manifestations of diseases of the frontal cortex are difficult to delineate and to differentiate from basal ganglia disease in children, although it is possible to elicit predictive, anti- and voluntary saccades late in the first decade.

Temporal lobe

The 'vestibular cortex' lies in the temporo-parietal junction, and is thought to be the centre for the sense of circularvection. This is a compelling sensation of self-rotation which is induced by large-field optokinetic stimulation, and it is impossible to distinguish from real self-rotation without other cues. Circularvection is a remarkably resilient sensation which is readily elicited in patients with SDN/CIN who have no normal OKN response. Lesions may abolish this sensation (Straube & Brandt 1987).

Hemispherectomized patients exhibit an asymmetrical vestibular response with slower compensatory (slow) eye movements towards the side of the lesion (the same as OKN/SP) (Estanol *et al.* 1980; Sharpe & Lo 1981). Jacobs *et al.* (1993) reported a similar deficit in a 5-month infant with a large parietal cyst. It is plausible that these asymmetries were due to ipsilateral temporal lobe involvement. In any case, it is important to recognize that VOR asymmetries do not always have their origin in the hindbrain.

Occipital and parietal lobes

Unilateral occipitoparietal lesions lead to a homonymous hemianopia in the contralateral field and poor pursuit/OKN for stimulus motion to the side of the lesion (see above).

Oculomotor 'syndromes'

Single eye movement abnormalities seldom occur in isolation and it is worth recognizing some common patterns or 'syndromes'. These are summarized below.

Eye movements in the healthy infant

Normal in early infancy: hypometric saccades, dissociation of binocular pursuit and OKN with low gain pursuit and normal OKN; monocular asymmetries of SP and OKN; slightly high VOR gain and short VOR time-constant; no nystagmus. This constellation does not occur in acquired disease but may be prolonged in the developmentally delayed infant.

Delayed visual maturation

No fixing or following. VOR present but some locking up may occur during manual spinning. Full-field OKN usually present, with no small-field response.

Infantile esotropia

* Early onset monocular visual deprivation (esotropia, cataract, etc.).
* Possible LN.
* Possible dissociated vertical deviation.
* Normal binocular SP and OKN (if no nystagmus, otherwise variable).
* Possible permanent monocular asymmetries of OKN and variable SP.
* Normal VOR.

Sensory defect/congenital idiopathic nystagmus

* Usually typical nystagmus waveforms.
* No OKN response (with rare exceptions).
* Erratic or absent VOR.

Cerebellar 'flocculus/paraflocculus syndrome'

* GPN (which must be distinguished from manifest LN),

and poor eccentric gaze-holding in the dark.
* Other types of nystagmus may be present including rebound nystagmus, upbeat nystagmus in upgaze; downbeat nystagmus in primary position, APN in all gaze directions, and rarely PAN.
* Saccadic pulse-step mismatch but normal saccadic gain.
* Low gain or saccadic SP.
* Slow build-up or absent OKN when viewing straight ahead. Pseudo-OKN may occur if eyes are deviated towards the opposite direction of stimulus motion.
* VOR may have moderately high gain and VN slow phases may be decelerating.
* Other cerebellar signs.

Cerebellar dorsal vermis syndrome

* Hypometric or hypermetric saccades.
* Intermittent saccade failure may occur.
* Other cerebellar signs.

Saccade initiation failure ('oculomotor apraxia')

See above.

Unilateral occipitoparietal lesion

* Multiple hypometric (searching) saccades to the opposite side of the lesion, due to hemianopia in contralateral field.
* Poor or absent SP towards the side of the lesion.
* Poor or absent OKN for stimulus motion towards the side of the lesion.
Note: if monocular OKN asymmetry is present (e.g. due to age, DVM or early onset esotropia) then the eye contralateral to the lesion may show no smooth following behaviour in either direction (thus appearing to be a blind eye), and the ipsilateral eye will only show smooth following towards the side opposite the lesion.

Two special presentations

Visual unresponsiveness in infancy

Infant vision is often assessed by an eye and/or head movement response to a moving or suddenly appearing visual object, eye contact or by smiling to a silent smile. Failure to detect a response gives the impression of a blind infant and may be due to sensory, motor or cortical problems.

Full ophthalmological investigations are needed including slit-lamp examination. Nystagmus should be identified and distinguished from the aimless horizontal and vertical roving eye movements of the blind. The majority of infants with nystagmus have a defect of the eye or anterior visual pathways. If the nystagmus has a very large amplitude, as is often the case in SDN/CIN in early infancy, it may not be possible to elicit any convincing horizontal ocular orienting response. For small amplitude nystagmus most infants will shift average gaze towards a visual target. However, in dysmyelinating disease there may be an APN concurrent with a saccade failure, as in Pelizaeus–Merzbacher disease.

When there is no nystagmus and no detectable visual defect, an absent visual motor response indicates one of three possibilities.

1 Cortical blindness (see Chapters 9 and 54).

2 SIF.

3 DVM (see Chapter 3).

Tests that depend on an orienting response, such as preferential looking, are not helpful and pattern VEPs are the investigation of choice provided age-matched normative data are available (Lambert *et al.* 1989b).

DVM cannot be distinguished from SIF by electrophysiology since pattern VEPs may be normal in both (Lambert *et al.* 1989b; Shawkat *et al.* 1996). In SIF head thrusts may not develop until later or not at all in the delayed child, and although vertical saccades are usually spared it is often difficult to obtain a convincing vertical tracking response in the young infant. We recommend testing with full-field horizontal OKN. In isolated DVM, the infant may be completely visually unresponsive to a hand-held drum or tape, but has a normal full-field bi-ocular OKN response (Harris *et al.* 1995). Unlike the infant with a saccade failure, quick-phases are not intermittently missed and lock-up does not occur. Monocular OKN in the NT direction is significantly reduced for age, and may be absent.

Manual spinning induces a vestibular rather than an optokinetic response. Normal quick-phases indicate DVM rather than a saccade failure. However, missed quick-phases (locking up) may not distinguish between these two conditions on the initial visit because VN quick-phases may be intermittently absent as a transient phenomenon in the healthy infant up to about 2–3 weeks, and possibly up to about 3 months in the DVM infant (Hoyt *et al.* 1985).

If nystagmus does not develop, the visual outcome in infants with DVM or saccade failure is usually very good, but the possibility of neurological problems cannot be ruled out, and the child needs to be followed up.

Children with reading difficulties

Ophthalmologists sometimes become involved in the assessment of the schoolchild with reading difficulties. For the most part, this takes the form of excluding any underlying visual or oculomotor problem. Reading, however, is little affected by oculomotor abnormalities, but when it is these children are not dyslexic. The question of

whether a particular child has a reading difficulty because of an oculomotor problem is not the same as asking whether dyslexic children as a group have oculomotor abnormalities (Evans & Drasdo 1990; Olson *et al.* 1991; Fischer & Biscaldi 1996).

Reading is a highly complex process that consists of an alternating sequence of fixations and saccades scanning across the text, with occasional regressions (saccades back to previously fixated words), and with a large saccade from the end of the current line to the beginning of the next line. Inwardly, reading is a process of acquiring lexical information in the specific sequence laid down by the text.

Monitoring eye movements during reading is not very revealing for the following reasons:

1 It is practically difficult to record the small reading eye movements from the child who has difficulty or does not want to read.

2 Frequently there is no obvious abnormality.

3 When abnormalities do occur (such as excessive regressive saccades), it is not clear whether they are the cause or the result of the reading difficulty.

A general oculomotor examination (including SP and OKN) is often more fruitful.

Reading can be hampered by sensory deficits, such as low contrast sensitivity or oscillopsia, which can be caused by early or late onset nystagmus, or by diplopia. Larger print size and higher contrast can be of some help. However, reading can be completely devastated by relatively subtle saccade abnormalities, such as abnormalities of saccadic timing or triggering.

It is important to distinguish between developmental rather than acquired reading difficulties, since the latter may be a sign of a serious neurological or ophthalmological disease.

Some of the rare oculomotor causes of reading difficulties that we have encountered include the following:

1 Gaze-evoked nystagmus may reduce contrast sensitivity or lead to oscillopsia when the eyes are not in primary position or in the accustomed null region, such as when a child is admonished for adopting a head posture. An LN may become intermittently manifest if the child suppresses one eye during attempted reading. Occasionally reading problems may be the presenting symptom of nystagmus.

Reading difficulties may emerge with a change in classroom practice, such as the introduction of small print, or the use of a blackboard. Poor contrast sensitivity at moderate spatial frequencies is more deleterious to reading than low acuity' levels, *per se*. We are reminded of a recent case of an articulate bright 7-year-old girl with congenital idiopathic nystagmus, who was having noticeable reading difficulties. Upon questioning, it was soon discovered that she had been moved towards the back of the classroom, and that the new 'blackboard' consisted of light-green marker on a white board. Reflections of sunlight further reduced this already unacceptably low contrast.

In early onset nystagmus, stress and tiredness can affect reading ability.

2 Saccadic inaccuracy disturbs reading, particularly large saccades to the beginning of a new line. Narrower columns of text can sometimes be easier to read. Slow saccades can make reading virtually impossible.

3 A failure to initiate saccades is a cause of reading difficulty but it is often not recognized. Since many affected children may also have delayed expressive speech development, the reading difficulty may be mistakenly ascribed to a more general language problem. Saccade failure can be difficult to detect since by reading age the tell-tale head thrusting will usually have been supplanted by subtle synkinetic blinks. Locking up during OKN or VN is a more reliable indicator of saccade failure.

Intrusive saccades can devastate reading, as was recently exemplified in our laboratory by an intelligent 13-year-old boy with a long history of Tourette syndrome who was no longer able to read. Eye movement recording demonstrated abundant intrusive saccades and a complete failure of anti-saccades.

The ophthalmologist has no magic remedies for reading difficulties, but he or she can be a support to the child and parents by (i) explaining the underlying cause of the reading problem, when known; (ii) by providing common-sense advice to parents and teachers about the need for suitable and practical visual aids in the classroom and at home; and (iii) by explaining some of the adaptive but effective strategies that some children may adopt.

Acknowledgements

I thank the charities Help a Child to See and Iris Fund for their support. I also thank Peter West, Fatima Shawkat, Christine Timms and Laura Mezey for their help in preparing this chapter, and I thank the Nystagmus Action Group (UK) for many informative discussions.

References

Abadi RV, Howard IP, Ohmi M, Howard T, Lee EE, Wright MJ. The rise time and steady-state gain of the human optokinetic response (OKR). *Invest Ophthalmol Vis Sci* 1994; **35** (Suppl.): 2035.

Ahn JC, Hoyt WF, Hoyt CS. Tonic upgaze in infancy. *Arch Ophthalmol* 1989; **107**: 57–8.

Aicardi J, Barbosa C, Andermann E *et al.* Ataxia–ocular motor apraxia: a syndrome mimicking ataxia–telangiectasia. *Ann Neurol* 1988; **24**: 497–502.

Aiello A, Wright KW, Borchert M. Independence of optokinetic nystagmus asymmetry and binocularity in infantile esotropia. *Arch Ophthalmol* 1994; **112**: 1580–3.

Alarakhia IN, Trobe JD. Opsoclonus–myoclonus presenting with features of spasmus nutans. *J Child Neurol* 1995; **10**: 67–8.

Alfano JE. Spasm of fixation. *Am J Ophthalmol* 1955; **40**: 724.

Alvarez F, Landrieu P, Laget P, Lemonnier F, Odievre M, Alagille D. Nervous and ocular disorders in children with cholestasis and vitamin A and E deficiencies. *Hepatology* 1983; **3**: 410–14.

Angelini L, Nardocci N, Runi V, Zorzi C, Strada L, Savoiardo M. Hallervorden–Spatz disease: clinical and MRI study of 11 cases diagnosed in life. *J Neurol* 1992; **239**:417–25.

Araie M, Ozawa T, Awaya Y. A case of congenital ocular motor apraxia with cerebellospinal degeneration. *Jpn J Ophthalmol* 1977; **21**: 355–65.

Arnold AC, Baloh RW, Yee RD, Hepler RS. Internuclear ophthalmoplegia in the Chiari type II malformation. *Neurology* 1990; **40**: 1850–4.

Aslin RN. Development of smooth pursuit in human infants. In: Fisher DF, Monty RA, Senders JW, eds. *Eye Movements: Cognition and Visual Perception*. Hillsdale, New Jersey: Erlbaum, 1981: 31–51.

Aslin RN. Infant accommodation and convergence. In: Simons K, ed. *Early Visual Development, Normal and Abnormal*. Oxford: Oxford University Press, 1993: 30–8.

Aslin R, Salapatek P. Saccadic localization of visual targets by the very young human infant. *Percept Psychophys* 1975; **17**: 293–302.

Atkinson, J. Development of optokinetic nystagmus in the human infant and monkey infant. An analogue to development in kittens. In: Freeman RD, ed. *Developmental Neurobiology of Vision*. New York: Plenum Press, 1979: 227–87.

Avanzini G, Girotti F, Caraceni T, Spreafico R. Oculomotor disorders in Huntington's chorea. *J Neurol Neursurg Psychiatr* 1979; **42**: 581–9.

Awaya Y, Sugie H, Fukuyama Y. A hereditary variant of spinocerebellar degeneration associated with choreoathetosis and ocular motor apraxia of early onset. *Acta Paediatr Jpn* 1986; **28**: 271.

Baloh RW, Beykirch K, Tauchi P, Yee RD, Honrubia V. Ultralow vestibulo-ocular reflex time constants. *Ann Neurol* 1988; **23**: 32–7.

Baloh RW, Honrubia V, Yee RD, Hess K. Changes in the human vestibulo-ocular reflex after loss of peripheral sensitivity. *Ann Neurol* 1984; **16**: 222–8.

Baloh RW, Yee RD, Honrubia V. Clinical abnormalities of optokinetic nystagmus. In: Lennerstrand G, Zee DS, Keller EL, eds. *Functional Basis of Ocular Motility Disorders*. New York: Pergamon, 1982: 311–20.

Baloh RW, Yee RD, Kimm J, Honrubia V. Vestibulo-ocular reflex in patients with lesions involving the vestibulocerebellum. *Exp Neurol* 1981; **72**: 141–52.

Barnes GR. Visual-vestibular interaction in the control of head and eye movement: the role of visual feedback and predictive mechanisms. *Prog Neurobiol* 1993; **41**: 435–72.

Basco WT, Abboud M, Holden KR. Opsoclonus–myoclonus and recurrent neuroblastoma. *J Pediatr* 1995; **126**: 847–8.

Becker W, Klein HM. Accuracy of saccadic eye movements and maintenance of eccentric eye positions in the dark. *Vision Res* 1973; **13**: 1021–34.

Beenen N, Buttner U, Lange HW. The diagnostic value of eye movement recordings in patients with Huntington's disease and their offspring. *Electroencephalogr Clin Neurophysiol* 1986; **63**: 119–27.

Bergenius J. Saccade abnormalities in patients with ocular flutter. *Acta Otolaryngol (Stockh)* 1986; **102**: 228–33.

Bienfang DC. Opsoclonus in infancy. *Arch Ophthalmol* 1974; **91**: 203–5.

Bollen EL, Roos RAC, Cohen AP *et al.* Oculomotor control in Gilles de la Tourette syndrome. *J Neurol Neurosurg Psychiatr* 1988; **51**: 1081–3.

Borchet MS, Sadun AA, Sommers JD, Wright KW. Congenital ocular motor apraxia in twins. *J Clin Neuro Ophthalmol* 1987; **7**: 104–7.

Bourron-Madignier M, Ardoin ML, Cypres C, Vettard S. Study of optokinetic nystagmus in children. In: Lenk-Schafer M, ed. *Transactions of the Sixth International Orthoptics Congress*. Harrogate: International Orthoptics Congress, 1987: 134–9.

65: Concomitant Strabismus

John Elston

Concomitant strabismus denotes a misalignment of the visual axes in which the angle of deviation is constant, irrespective of the direction of gaze, and the range of movement of each eye is full. In most cases, the misalignment is horizontal (eso- or exotropia) but a vertical deviation is often also present on lateral gaze. A secondary change in horizontal alignment on up- and downgaze will then usually be found.

Concomitant strabismus in childhood is relatively common. There is a spectrum of abnormality ranging from large manifest strabismus through stable microtropia with reduced binocular functions, to intermittent deviations.

The epidemiological data must be interpreted with caution as they depend on the diagnostic criteria used as well as the sampling methods, tests employed and age at examination. Graham (1974) examined 4784 children, 99% of all those born in Cardiff (UK) during 1 year, at the age of 4–5 years. The cover test was in some way abnormal in

7.1% and these children were referred for more detailed examination, a manifest strabismus being confirmed in 5.3% of the total. Other prevalence estimates range from 5% (Simons & Reinecke 1978) to 3.8% of children (Freidman *et al.* 1980). Most recent studies of epidemiology have concerned subgroups of strabismus and not the whole range of abnormality.

Binocular visual development

The presence of childhood strabismus is a physical sign of a disturbance of normal binocular visual development. At birth, afferent visual function is poorly developed. The eyes are usually exotropic, and sensory and motor interactions between the two eyes are absent or rudimentary (Nixon *et al.* 1985). Motion processing is immature, i.e. there is a pursuit eye movement response to visible objects moving in the temporal to nasal direction in front of each eye, but not to nasal to temporal movement. The postnatal development of high visual acuity depends on differentiation, myelination and the establishment of synaptic connections in the eye, visual pathways and primary visual cortex (V1). The substrate for sensory binocular interaction is the development of horizontal synaptic connections between the ocular dominance columns of the two eyes in V1 (Tychsen & Burkhalt 1995). These connections are largely excitatory, summating the slight disparity between what is seen by each eye to achieve stereopsis. There are also inhibitory connections which may have a role in physiological suppression (i.e. eliminating physiological diplopia) and in binocular rivalry. Both facilitation and suppression are normal features of the function of the primary visual cortex. At the same time as sensory interactions between the two eyes are developing, motion processing is maturing to achieve temporonasal and nasotemporal symmetry. Motion processing appears to be a function of the adjacent extrastriate visual cortex, and it is likely that these developments are co-ordinated (Atkinson 1992) and mediated by magnocellular pathways. As these processes occur, the neonatal exodeviation reduces, orthotropia is achieved and motor fusion develops (Sondhi *et al.* 1988).

The susceptibility of visual development to disruption by extrinsic factors progressively decreases as, with increasing age, the anatomical and physiological substrate develops. The nature and timing of a disturbance to developing binocular vision determine the consequences. In the first weeks of life there is a latent period during which motor abnormalities such as unilateral lateral rectus palsy or sensory deficits (e.g. due to retinal haemorrhage) are unimportant (Elston & Timms 1992). Also during this period, transient supranuclear disturbances of gaze, for example upbeating nystagmus, may be observed in healthy neonates but do not compromise normal binocular development (Hoyt *et al.* 1980). After the age of approximately 6 weeks, sensitivity to disruption rises quickly to a peak, probably early in the first year of life, then slowly declines over the next 5 or 6 years. If the disruption to developing binocularity is not too severe or for too long, structure and function are partly preserved or may recover. The capacity to develop normal binocular function is robust and can be achieved despite disorders of extraocular movement. In congenital superior oblique underaction for example, the resulting vertical squint is compensated for by a head posture, and full binocularity usually develops with a large vertical fusion range (Reynolds *et al.* 1984). In Duane's retraction syndrome, despite evidence of paradoxical innervation of the lateral rectus dependent on the position of gaze, good quality binocular function frequently develops often with an abnormal head posture in unilateral cases. The development of normal binocular functions has also been described in a case of isolated total unilateral horizontal gaze palsy of presumed pontine origin (Hoyt *et al.* 1977).

Aetiology of childhood strabismus

The cause of most cases of childhood strabismus cannot be determined. In many cases, the history and physical signs will give some indication of the chronological timing of the disturbance of normal binocularity but not its nature. The following should be considered in the assessment of the individual case.

Anatomy

Unilateral or asymmetric bilateral developmental abnormalities of the eye or optic nerve will lead to strabismus, usually convergent. Examples are optic nerve hypoplasia and coloboma. Visual pathway abnormalities, for example the near total decussation of the chiasm in albinism, will mean that the anatomical substrate for binocularity is absent (Coleman *et al.* 1979). Visual cortical maldevelopment will also prevent binocular development.

Structural factors involving the overall size, depth and relative disposition of the orbits may produce strabismus, particularly exotropia. Note that in hypertelorism, the wide lateral displacement of the orbits may simulate an exodeviation. In some craniofacial dysostoses, maxillary hypoplasia is associated with shallow laterally directed orbits and an exotropia (Fig. 65.1). Abnormalities of the number and insertions of the extraocular muscles may contribute as well as abnormal patterns of reciprocal innervation and inhibition caused by excyclorotation of the orbits (Diamond *et al.* 1980; Cheng *et al.* 1993).

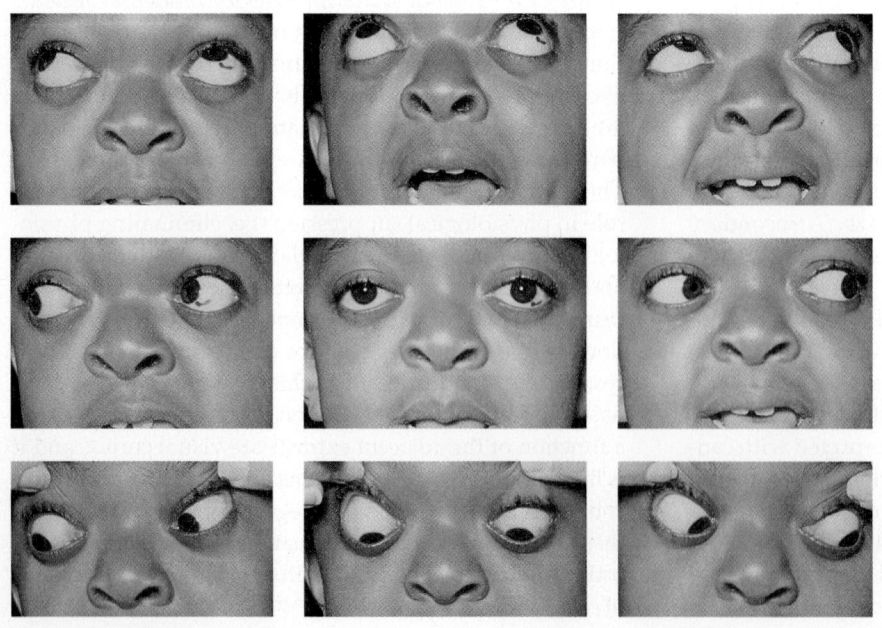

Fig. 65.1 Apert's syndrome with shallow orbit, a V pattern exotropia with overacting inferior obliques.

Genetics

Genetic factors contribute to some extent to the development of infantile esotropia. Twenty-five per cent of children with childhood onset strabismus have either a parent or a sibling with strabismus (Graham 1974). Twin and genealogical data suggest that multiple modifying factors are involved (Francois 1961; McKussick 1978). High refractive error is known to be associated with strabismus and is to a large extent genetically determined with evidence for both autosomal dominant and recessive pedigrees for high myopia, high hypermetropia and anisometropia. Anisometropia is a potent cause of amblyopia and therefore strabismus. The degree and axis of astigmatism may be inherited (Sorsby *et al.* 1962). Moreover the broad categories of esotropia and exotropia seem to be under some genetic control and strabismus may appear at the same age in identical twins (Chimonidou *et al.* 1977). Reduced divergence fusional amplitudes may be found in families of patients with accommodative convergent squint (Nash *et al.* 1975).

The development of the normal relationship between accommodative convergence and accommodation (AC : A ratio) is also to some extent under genetic control and in families with an esotropic propositus it is on average significantly higher in unaffected family members than in normals (Franceschetti & Burian 1970).

Neurological dysfunction

Between 20 and 40% of cases of cerebral palsy have an esotropia (Breakey 1995). Strabismus is also very common in hydrocephalus and in children with multiple handicaps, including a number of specific syndromes with neurological involvement such as Down's (Harcourt 1974).

Some neurotropic viral infections (e.g. varicella) may cause strabismus by specifically damaging developing binocular functional circuitry. Anecdotal reports of strabismus occurring during an infectious disease in childhood are probably due to a phoria decompensating to a tropia. Rarely, closed head injury seems to disrupt fusional amplitudes and cause a manifest strabismus (Pratt-Johnson 1973; Stanworth 1974).

Prematurity

Very low birth weight is associated with an increased incidence of strabismus, particularly if there is evidence of peri- or intraventricular haemorrhage (Palmer *et al.* 1982; Fawer *et al.* 1985). Children who have had retinopathy of prematurity have a high incidence of abnormal refraction including high myopia, astigmatism and anisometropia. Strabismus is common in this group (Kushner 1982). Perinatal hypoxia predisposes to infantile esotropia, possibly

because the motion processing areas in the extrastriate visual cortex are vulnerable.

Functional deficits in concomitant strabismus

Amblyopia

Amblyopia is commonly found in strabismus but the relationship between the two is complex and they are only partly interdependent. Amblyopia is relatively uncommon in primary exodeviations. It rarely occurs in infantile esotropia unless the condition is treated surgically. It is common in childhood esotropia but normal vision in each eye does not exclude small angle strabismus. Anisometropic amblyopia may not be associated with strabismus, and these 'straight-eyed amblyopes' may escape detection until vision is tested in each eye separately at school entry. In these cases, binocular functions usually develop indicating facilitatory overlap of receptive fields in V1. However, treatment of the amblyopia may precipitate strabismus.

Stereopsis

Sensory stereopsis may be normal in intermittent exotropia, even with very large deviations. Motor fusion is defective. Sensory stereopsis is always reduced in manifest esotropia but motor fusion may be relatively well maintained.

Parents often ask about the value of stereoscopic vision and its importance in education, sports and career choice. It is evident that providing one eye has reasonable visual acuity, the absence of stereopsis does not interfere in any way with education. Sporting prowess is multifactorial and stereoscopic vision is probably only important in the judgement of speed and angle in small ball games such as squash. Good visual acuity in each eye is a requirement for a number of jobs and the holding of a heavy goods vehicle licence in the UK; stereoscopic vision is required in some jobs in the Armed Forces and medicine, including ophthalmic surgery.

Oblique muscle dysfunction

From the parents' perspective, oblique muscle dysfunction may be the most obvious feature of their child's strabismus. Inferior oblique overaction with elevation of the eye on adduction greater in the amblyopic or non-fixing eye is the most common abnormality (Weakley *et al.* 1992). This is associated with a V pattern of eye movement (Fig. 65.2). Superior oblique overaction, again often asymmetric with downshoot of the eye in adduction, produces an A pattern (Fig. 65.3). Combinations of oblique muscle dysfunction may give an X, Y or inverted Y pattern.

The cause is not known, but there is evidence for an

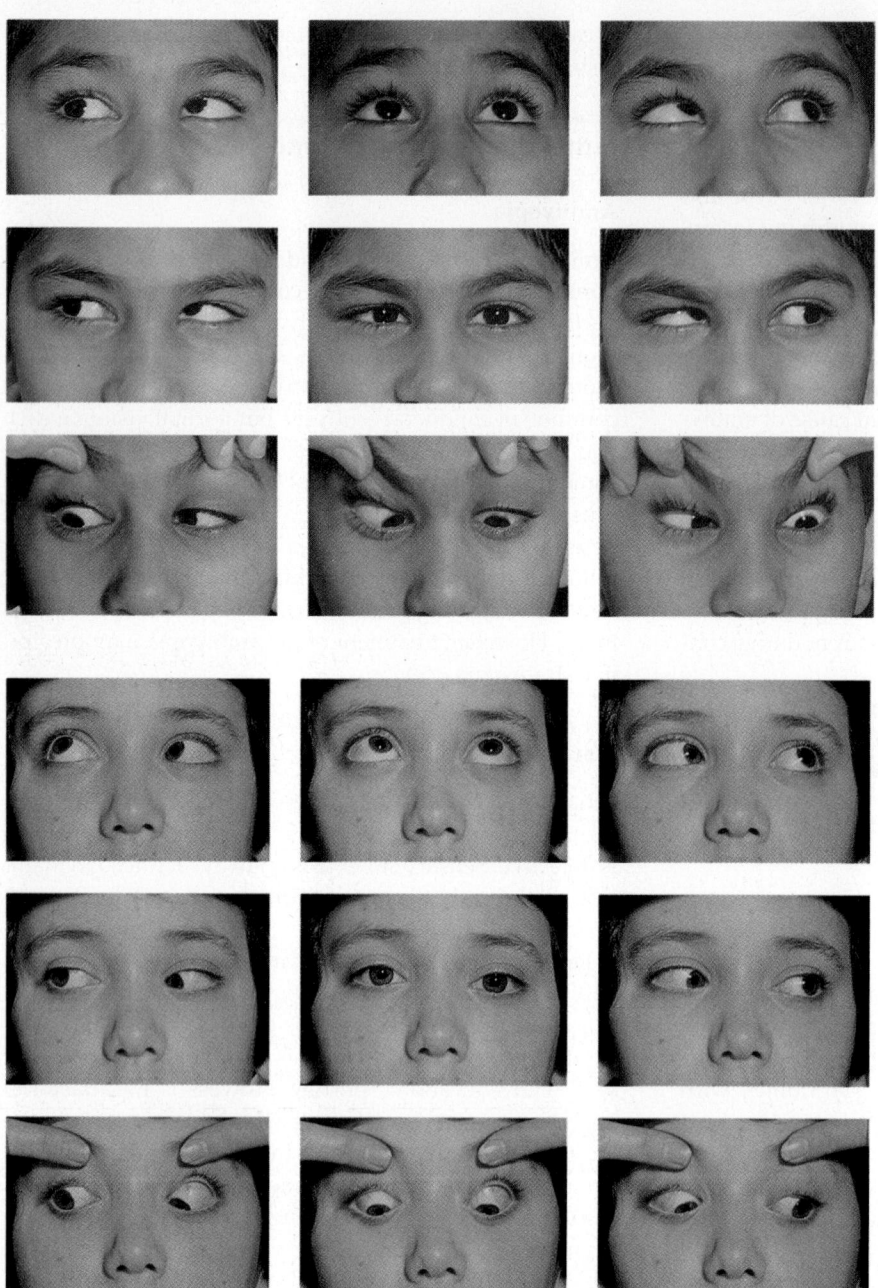

Fig. 65.2 'V' pattern esotropia showing both eyes on upgaze, marked convergent squint on downgaze, overacting inferior obliques and underacting superior obliques.

Fig. 65.3 'A' pattern esotropia on upgaze and overacting superior obliques.

underlying instability of cyclovertical muscle balance. Physiological elevation of each eye in adduction has been described and a 12–24-hour period of uniocular occlusion in visually mature adults, may result in measurable ipsilateral (or bilateral) inferior oblique overaction with a V pattern (Slavin *et al.* 1988). Complete dissociation of the visual axis in strabismus may therefore exacerbate this tendency. Superior oblique overaction may result in other individuals by decompensation of the opposite minor cyclovertical instability. Once established, the oblique muscle dysfunction will tend to progressively increase.

Excyclorotation of the non-fixing eye is a recognized feature of essential infantile esotropia and may be the pri-

mary factor in disrupting the cyclovertical muscle balance in these cases (Kushner 1985). Some authors have argued that the primary abnormality in many cases of childhood strabismus is oblique muscle dysfunction, with the disturbance of the balance between the vertically acting components of the superior and inferior oblique muscles — sagittalization of one or other oblique muscle axis (Gobin 1968). It is argued that the horizontal deviation (convergent or divergent) develops secondarily from a phoria due to the oblique muscle imbalance disrupting developing binocular functions. It is true that an A or V pattern with appropriate oblique muscle dysfunction may rarely occur without manifest horizontal strabismus in the primary position. Alternatively, in these cases binocularity may be maintained with an abnormal head posture. These cases may be explained by orbital anatomical factors but in the vast majority of cases of childhood strabismus, the horizontal deviation precedes the cyclovertical one.

An A pattern with superior oblique overaction is a frequent finding in hydrocephalus (see Fig. 53.8). It is due to forward displacement of the trochlea due to differential bone growth altering the cyclovertical muscle balance on adduction in favour of the depressor fibres of the superior oblique.

Attempts to implicate a central disturbance of ocular motor control as the cause of the A and V patterns in childhood strabismus are unconvincing (Hamed *et al.* 1993). It should be noted, however, that a V pattern with inferior oblique overaction is a feature of bilateral fourth nerve palsy and that elevation of each eye in adduction occurs in alternating skew deviation.

An A pattern occurs when there is isolated bilateral inferior rectus underaction (e.g. in ocular myasthenia gravis) and can also be produced by stereotactic pretectal lesions (Nashold & Seaber 1972). However, it is unlikely that a central disturbance of ocular motor control is responsible for the A and V patterns seen in childhood strabismus. Likewise, orbital anatomical factors such as sagittalization of the oblique muscle axis seem inadequate to explain such a stereotyped and frequently observed abnormality.

Dissociated deviations

Dissociated vertical deviation (DVD) consists of elevation of the eye when retinal illumination is reduced ipsilaterally either by an occluder or a neutral density filter. Occasionally it may be manifest spontaneously, for example when day-dreaming. It is always accompanied by extorsion of the eye and a horizontal deviation, usually a divergence (Harcourt *et al.* 1980). An A pattern of eye movement with superior oblique overaction is usually seen but note that dissociated deviations are often manifest on lateral gaze, simulating inferior oblique overaction. Dissociated deviations may be found in all categories of childhood strabismus but are most common in infantile esotropia and early onset primary exodeviations (Helvesten 1969). In general terms, the later the onset of the strabismus the less frequently a dissociated deviation will occur and the less marked it will be. It is a bilateral abnormality, often asymmetric with the larger deviation in the amblyopic or non-fixing eye. It is always associated with latent nystagmus occurring in the fixing eye with the fast phase directed towards that side (Gresty *et al.* 1992). The esotropic drift of the fixing eye in latent nystagmus may be a motor manifestation of the failure of maturation of motion processing as both dissociated deviations and latent nystagmus are frequently accompanied by direc-

tional asymmetry of the optokinetic responses (Kommerel & Mehdorn 1982).

The suggestion that dissociated deviations are accompanied or caused by abnormal visual pathway projections (Fitzgerald & Billson 1984) has not been confirmed (Kriss *et al.* 1989).

Cosmetic

The cosmetic defect associated with childhood strabismus is determined by the size and nature of the deviation and the facial features of the individual. From the parents' point of view, it is often an aspect of major importance. It is important that parents are given the opportunity to discuss these concerns but they must also be educated in the importance of other aspects, particularly amblyopia.

Diagnosis and assessment

The history is important in the diagnosis since many deviations are initially intermittent. A child's mother is very rarely wrong if she says that she has definitely seen an inward or outward turn of the eye at times. Strabismus may initially occur only during an intercurrent illness or when the child is overtired. A family history of strabismus, amblyopia, hypermetropia or anisometropia should be sought.

Examination

Visual acuity should be tested in each eye separately using methods appropriate for the age of the child. The cover test is the most important determinant of the presence or absence of strabismus in clinical practice. The gross appearance of ocular alignment is an unreliable guide. Variations in the shape and form of the palpebral apertures, orbital and ocular factors may either mask or simulate strabismus. The cover test must be performed both without accommodation (distance fixation) and with accommodation maximally stimulated (appropriate near target, not a light). The test should also be performed at far distance (infinity) in children with exodeviations. Apart from the presence or absence of strabismus and the steadiness of fixation with each eye, performing a cover test will allow latent nystagmus and dissociated deviations to be analysed. The alternate cover test progressively increases dissociation between the eyes allowing the maximum size of a deviation (particularly a latent one) to be assessed and fusional vergence to be observed.

The range of eye movements should be tested, with a light as target to eliminate accommodation. Limitations and oblique dysfunction should be noted. Accommodative vergence should also be controlled in the head tilt test. Elevation of the eye on ipsilateral tilt indicates ipsilateral superior oblique underaction or superior rectus contracture. Elevation on contralateral tilt is seen in dissociated deviations.

The sensory binocular status will be investigated using random dot stereo presentations and on the synoptophore. Information about the motor fusion range may be helpful both diagnostically and in planning surgery. The prism adaptation test may provide information on the response to surgery (Prism Adaptation Research Group 1990).

All children with strabismus or suspected strabismus should have a cycloplegic refraction at first examination. Retinoscopy must be performed along the visual axis to avoid cylindrical errors. It is important to treat any anisometropia since it destabilizes normal binocular development. Pupil dilatation will enable anatomical abnormalities in the posterior segment to be identified. Children with intracranial pathology may present with concomitant strabismus and whilst most of these 'strabismus masquerade syndromes' will be identified by an examination such as the above, it is important to keep an open mind, particularly if unusual or inconsistent features are seen.

Classification

Esodeviations

Essential infantile esotropia

Formerly known as congenital esotropia, this condition usually develops around the second or third month of life as the neonatal exotropia resolves.

Initially the angle of esotropia may be variable but characteristically becomes large with good vision in each eye and cross-fixation (Fig. 65.4). Oblique muscle dysfunction develops in over two-thirds of patients, with an A pattern more common than a V. About half develop dissociated deviations (Von Noorden 1988).

Variants of infantile esotropia include the nystagmus blockage syndrome in which a jerk nystagmus with a quick phase towards the side of the fixing eye is present in abduction. Each eye is held in extreme adduction and the torticollis necessary for fixation is prominent (Von Noorden 1976).

Genetic factors appear to play a small part in the development of infantile esotropia. Environmental influences can be identified in approximately half of the affected children. Prematurity and dysmaturity predispose to the development of the condition, as does perinatal hypoxia. Maternal smoking and/or alcohol consumption during pregnancy have also been incriminated. High refractive error (myopia or hypermetropia) may also cause the syndrome, emphasizing the importance of a full examination on presentation (see above). Accommodative esotropia (see below) may very rarely present in the first 6 months of life.

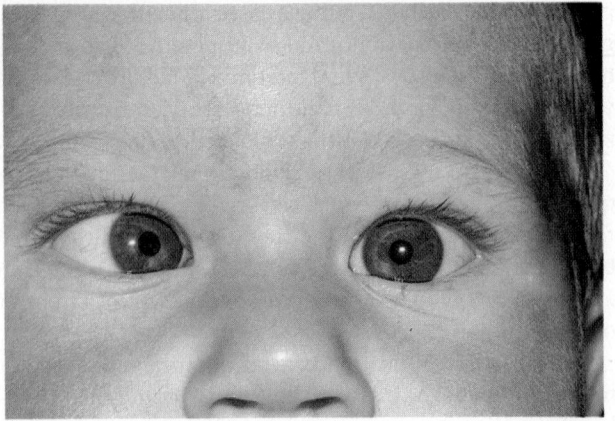

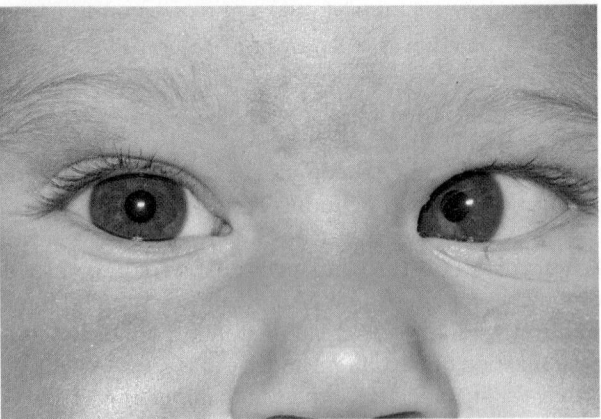

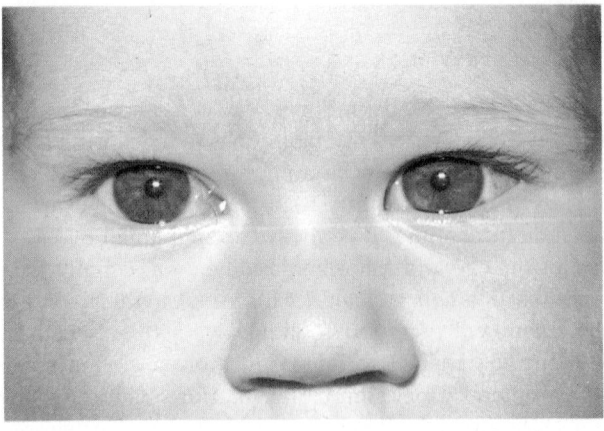

Fig. 65.4 (a, b) Infantile esotropia showing alternating fixation and (c) same patient immediately following surgery, showing small residual esotropia.

The majority of children with infantile esotropia are neurologically and developmentally normal. The esotropia is presumed to develop because of a failure of maturation of motion processing, possibly in relation to the function of the extrastriate visual cortex, specifically area MT, the middle temporal visual area. The other features of the syndrome apart from the esotropia, for example latent nystagmus, dissociated deviation, oblique muscle dysfunction and lack of binocular connectivity in the primary visual cortex, are secondary to the failure to develop symmetric motion processing (Helvesten 1993). Alternatively, there may be delayed development or a congenital defect of retinal disparity sensitivity in V1.

Principles of management

Untreated, infantile esotropes will develop excellent vision in each eye but a persistent esodeviation usually associated with oblique dysfunction. The underlying asymmetry of motion processing as tested by optokinetic responses persists (Aiello *et al.* 1994). Because of this and the speed at which the visual system develops in the first months of life, it is unlikely that infantile esotropia is functionally curable. Despite increasingly early surgery, bifoveal fixation with full binocular function has not been convincingly demonstrated in a typical infantile esotrope (Archer *et al.* 1986; Charles & Moore 1992). In most cases, combined orthoptic and surgical management can achieve satisfactory alignment of the eyes with peripheral sensory fusion but no stereopsis.

High hypermetropia or myopia will require appropriate spectacle (or rarely contact lens) correction. Theoretically, relatively early surgical alignment (within the first 2 years of life) may result in better quality binocular function although this hypothesis has never been rigorously tested. From the cosmetic point of view, and possibly that of the developing parent–child relationship, early surgery is also preferable. However, there are disadvantages in operating too early. The surgery is technically more difficult and since the posterior segment of the eye in infancy is relatively underdeveloped, a standard medial rectus recession in the first few months of life could result in reduced eye movement later on. In most cases, oblique dysfunction is difficult to assess in the first year of life and may not develop until later. Cross-fixating infantile esotropes usually become amblyopic in one eye after surgery and this may be difficult to detect and treat. The results of early surgery (at mean age 15 months) are the same in normal and neurologically impaired esotropes (Charles & Moore 1992).

A balance between the theoretical requirements of early ocular alignment and the practical difficulties has to be struck. The diagnosis of infantile esotropia will be made in the first few months of life. At this stage, a full explanation of the condition to the parents is required. Emphasis should be placed on the inevitability of repeated visits to the clinic, the likelihood of patching for amblyopia at some stage and the necessity for at least one operation, probably on both eyes. The number of children requiring a second operation at some stage varies between 15 and 30%.

Botulinum toxin treatment in infantile esotropia is attractive in that it avoids incisional surgery and its com-

plications. It can also be used to test the hypothesis that the condition is functionally curable if treated early enough. If both medial rectus muscles are injected and an exotropia produced in the first months of life, orthophoria should be achieved as the muscles recover function. However, the results are no better than standard surgery (Ing 1993) and probably not as good as those reported with larger amounts of muscle surgery very early in infancy (Ing 1991; Shauly *et al.* 1994).

Simultaneous horizontal and cyclovertical (oblique) muscle surgery is usually advocated. Asymmetric oblique muscle dysfunction should be treated with appropriately graded weakening procedures. Inferior oblique myotomy usually produces a larger correction than recession and may lead to superior oblique overaction, i.e. overcorrection. Dissociated deviations may be addressed surgically as a secondary procedure. It is important that parents appreciate that it is not possible to eliminate the abnormality completely but it can usually be substantially reduced. It is often asymmetric (affecting the amblyopic or non-fixing eye more) and asymmetric hangback of the superior rectus is the simplest effective procedure.

Nystagmus blockage syndrome as defined above, should be identified as the surgical treatment is different. There is evidence that large bimedial recessions with posterior fixation give the best functional and cosmetic results (Hoyt 1977).

Infantile esotropia secondary to structural abnormalities

A full ocular examination will identify cases due to uniocular or asymmetric structural abnormalities of the eye. The visual defect in the non-fixing eye may be partly due to amblyopia and consideration should be given to patching of the fixing eye. In most cases, cosmetic surgical alignment of the eyes is best left until the child is of school age.

Later onset (childhood) esotropia

Esotropia developing from the age of 6 months onwards, with a peak at between 3 and 4 years, differs from infantile esotropia in several respects. Associated amblyopia increases as the age of presentation rises, as do refractive errors especially anisometropia and high hypermetropia.

Refractive error is to a large extent genetically determined and a family history of esotropia is commonly found. Whereas in infantile esotropia a normal relationship between accommodative convergence and accommodation is usually found, in childhood esotropia over half the cases have an abnormal ratio, in most cases very high. Dependent on the age of onset and the factors that have led to a disruption of normal binocular visual development, variable degrees of amblyopia and variable binocular potential will be present.

Principles of management

At the initial consultation, the diagnosis will be established and the parents and child given an explanation of the disorder and an outline of the treatment proposed. This is usually spectacle correction of full refractive error with or without patching for amblyopia. There is frequently an accommodative element in childhood esotropia, which will be controlled by a hypermetropic spectacle correction. In many cases, surgery may well be required subsequently. Preoperative prism adaptation can be used to see if correction of the angle of strabismus induces further convergence. In those cases with a larger prism adapted angle of deviation, appropriately augmented surgery is indicated (Prism Adaptation Research Group 1990).

Parents often do not appreciate that spectacles and patching are the mainstay of treatment and not something that is tried before surgery. However, particularly if there is more than one child in the family with esotropia, the amounts of time, energy and expense that are required by the parents in supervising these treatments are considerable. This is apart from visits to the orthoptic department which should be kept to the minimum necessary to monitor and encourage the child.

Accommodative esotropia

Fully accommodative esotropia

The eyes are normally aligned for distance fixation but on accommodation, an esotropia develops. By definition this is completely controlled by wearing the full hypermetropic spectacle correction (Fig. 65.5), and this is the preferred treatment in the UK and USA. Some authors have postulated that accommodative esotropia develops because of minor degrees of cyclovertical muscle incomitance acting as a barrier to fusion for near. Simultaneous medial rectus recession and repositioning (or desagittalization) of the oblique muscles is advised, and the accommodative component of the deviation is said to resolve postoperatively (Gobin 1991). Dissociated deviation may be a prominent feature of accommodative esotropia and require appropriate surgery.

Convergence excess esotropia

In contrast to a fully accommodative esotropia, the convergence of the visual axes on accommodation is not controlled by the full spectacle correction (Fig. 65.6). The AC:A ratio is high or very high (Ludwig *et al.* 1988). The convergence excess may be controlled by the addition of the full near correction (+3). The near addition may be gradually eliminated over months with control maintained. However, most cases will require a full bimedial

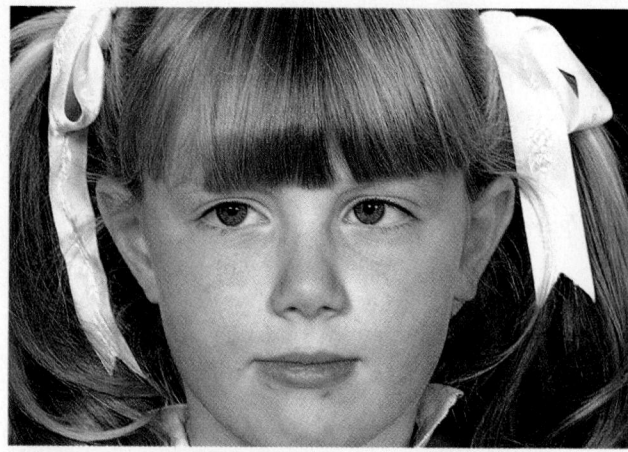

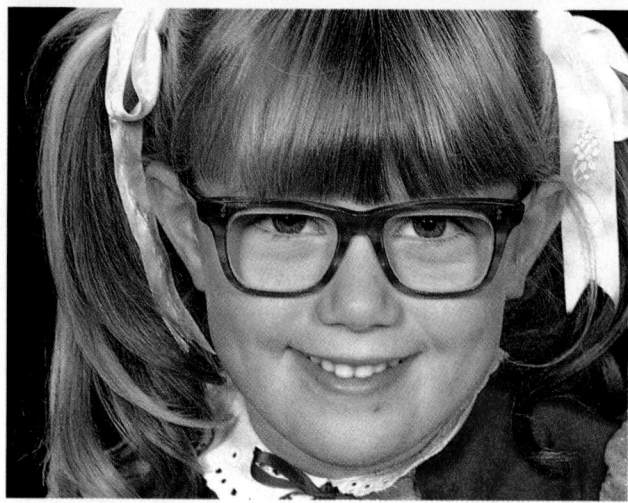

Fig. 65.5 Accommodative esotropia showing (top) left esotropia without glasses, and (bottom) straight eyes and good binocular vision with hypermetropic spectacles on.

recession. The AC:A ratio reduces postoperatively, particularly if it is very high preoperatively and there is a risk of consecutive exotropia which increases in the absence of fusion (Lucas *et al.* 1994).

Microesotropia

Microesotropia is best considered as a small (less than 5°), stable, cosmetically insignificant convergent strabismus that is usually associated with mild amblyopia and reduced binocular functions (Helvesten & Von Noorden 1967). It may occur primarily or secondary to surgical or optical treatment of a larger esotropia. If primary, there is a risk of decompensation to a larger esotropia. The fundamental abnormality in primary cases is usually mild anisometropia producing amblyopia and sensory adaptations resulting in the development of abnormal retinal correspondence but with good stereopsis maintained by binocular motor responses. At the smallest angle of esodeviation, the cover test may be negative if the amblyopic

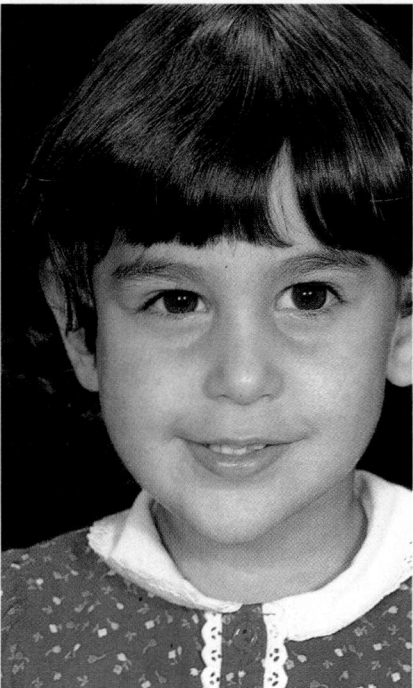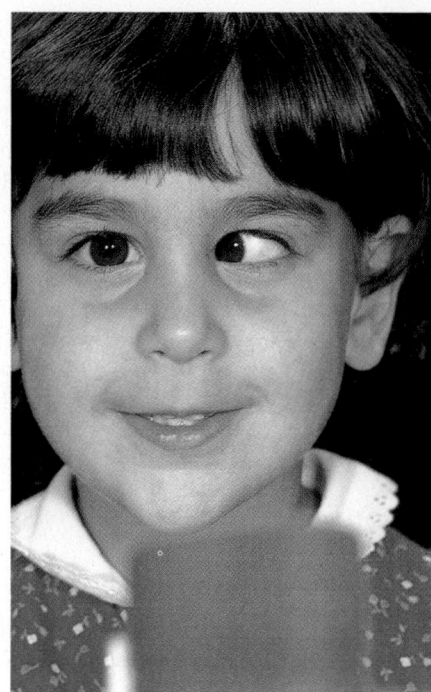

Fig. 65.6 This child, who has no refractive error, has an esotropia only when fixing an accommodative target. On the left the eyes can be seen to be straight when the child is fixing a light. On fixing a solid detailed target a left esotropia rapidly develops. Her AC : A ratio is high.

eye fixes with a high acuity extrafoveal point. In most cases, however, a small abducting movement is seen when the eye with better vision is covered (Lang 1969). Primary microesotropia may be genetically determined (Cantolino & Von Noorden 1969).

Primary microesotropia is treated with spectacle correction of any anisometropia or refractive errror. Patching for amblyopia may also be required. There is a risk that patching will lead to decompensation to a larger esotropia, and this needs to be explained to the parents. A secondary microesotropia denotes an excellent surgical result of the treatment of a larger deviation.

Late onset normosensorial esotropia

This is an unusual form of esotropia with onset after early childhood, usually between 8 and 12 years, after visual maturity has been achieved. The esotropia may be initially intermittent, most often observed in the morning on waking but tending to become constant. Alternate day esotropia is a variant, but has very rarely been described with central nervous system disease (Pillae & Duand 1987). Double vision is present but there are no signs of lateral rectus palsy. Refraction is usually normal. Normal potential binocularity can usually be demonstrated.

The cause is not understood. The onset may follow systemic illness or even be related to stress. The prognosis for restoration of full binocularity, or sometimes a stable microesotropia, is good. Management options include prisms in the short term, botulinum toxin injection to one medial rectus muscle or surgery (Ohtsuki *et al.* 1994).

Exodeviations

The term exodeviation encompasses both divergent strabismus (exotropia) and latent divergence (exophoria). Exodeviations are relatively unusual and in Graham's series, of the 339 children with an abnormal cover test, 20% had an exodeviation (80% an esodeviation). Nearly half of the exodeviations were phorias. Fifty per cent of exodeviations occur in the first year of life and all studies show a consistent sex difference with between 65 and 70% occurring in girls. The control of an intermittent exodeviation may either spontaneously improve or decline during childhood (Hiles *et al.* 1968). The disturbance of the normal development of binocular vision associated with an exodeviation differs from that seen in esodeviations and children often do not show any fixation preference. Significant amblyopia is uncommon. Sensory aspects of binocularity are usually well developed whilst there are reduced or absent divergence fusional amplitudes. Double vision does not occur when the deviation is manifest implying that suppression of vision in the deviating eye is complete, occurring over the whole temporal hemi-retina. Exodeviations characteristically worsen in bright sunlight and children often shut one eye under these conditions, which may be a useful diagnostic clue.

Aetiology

In primary exodeviations, genetic factors do not seem to be important. The range of refraction in a group of children with exodeviations is the same as that in controls. An abnormality of the AC : A ratio is not of aetiological significance but the ratio is frequently high as a secondary response to achieve binocularity for near.

Orbital anatomical development may predispose to an exotropia. The birth and general medical history is usually unremarkable with no over-representation of prematurity or neurological dysfunction. The underlying pathophysiology is presumed to be a disturbance of normal binocular development resulting in disordered motor fusion with secondary temporal hemi-retinal suppression, on a cortical basis. Oblique muscle function may also occur secondarily producing A and V patterns. Children often seem to find it more difficult to control an exophoria on upgaze so that a V pattern may be present without oblique dysfunction.

Classification

Congenital exotropia

Most children have an exotropia or intermittent divergence of the visual axes in the first weeks of life. An exotropia that persists into infancy is designated congenital exotropia (Fig. 65.7) and neurological defects are more frequently found in these children than in congenital or infantile esotropes. The angle of divergence is usually large and in the more severely neurologically impaired children, afferent visual development may be poor with or without delayed visual maturation.

The management of a child with congenital exotropia would usually be in the hands of a paediatric neurologist or a paediatrician. The ophthalmologist should ensure that amblyopia does not develop and offer surgery for cosmetic improvement when appropriate.

Primary exodeviations

The generally agreed classification is dependent on cor-

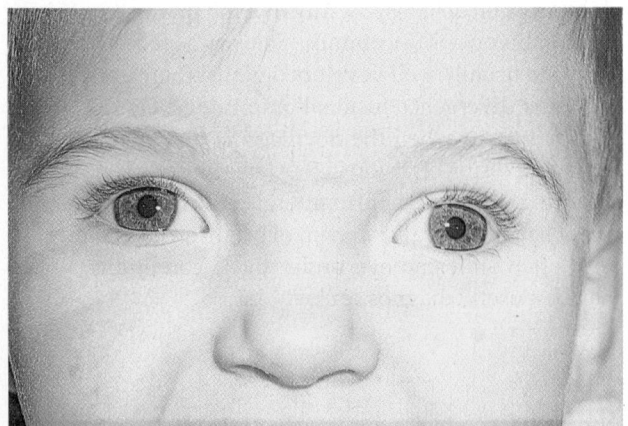

Fig. 65.7 Congenital exotropia. Neurological defects are more frequently found in congenital exotropia than in congenital esotropia.

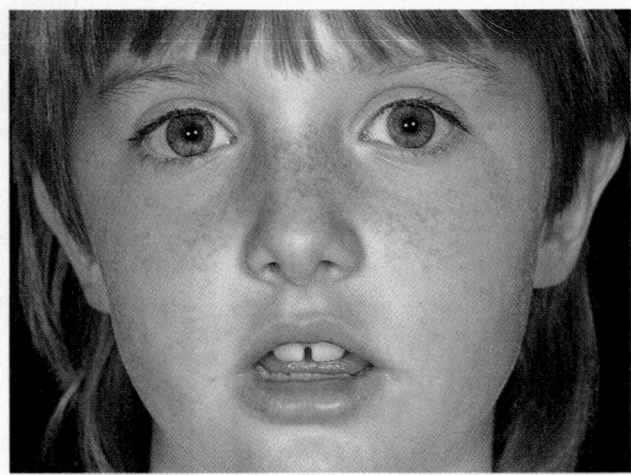

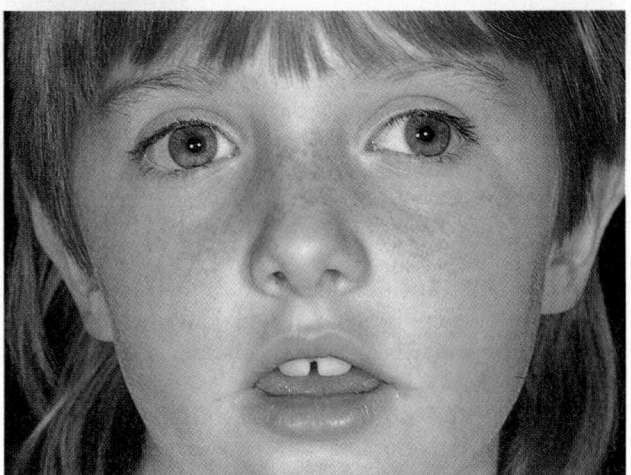

Fig. 65.8 Intermittent exotropia. This child, who has no refractive error, was noted by her parents to have an eye which drifted when she was day-dreaming or tired, especially when she looked in the distance. The top figure shows her fixing a near target and the bottom shows her fixing a distance target.

rect examination and should provide information that is useful in selecting treatment options in individual cases. Three categories are recognized: (i) basic; (ii) divergence excess (real or simulated); and (iii) convergence insufficiency (Burian & Franceschetti 1970).

In basic exodeviation, the size of the strabismus is the same for near and distance fixation. About 50% of cases are in this category. In divergence excess (17%), the deviation is greater at distance than near (Fig. 65.8). This difference may be real or simulated by accommodative convergence which reduces the near measurement. The two can be differentiated by eliminating accommodation with a + 3 lens for the near measurement. Simulated divergence excess revealed by this test should be managed as a basic exodeviation.

In convergence insufficiency, the near deviation is greater than that at distance (33%).

In order to ensure correct classification, assessment

should include measurement of the exodeviation at far distance fixation (30 m or 100 ft), with +3 lenses in divergence excess and sometimes after prolonged (several hours) patching of the deviating eye to disrupt binocularity maintained by convergence (Burian & Smith 1971).

Management. The first step is the correction of refractive error. If the child is myopic with divergence excess, this may be all that is needed to control the strabismus. Also, some children with hypermetropia and exotropia respond completely to spectacle correction (Iacobucci *et al.* 1993). If this is not the case, provided there is no amblyopia, symmetric low hypermetropia need not be treated unless there is significant astigmatism. It is possible to control an emetrope with divergence excess by prescribing low myopic spectacles. Amblyopia should be managed conventionally.

Orthoptic treatment is particularly valuable in divergence excess where the recognition of pathological diplopia (i.e. double vision occurring when the visual axes diverge) may sometimes be achieved by alternate eye patching. Convergence insufficiency usually responds reasonably well to convergence exercises in the short term but is often recurrent. The surgical treatment of intermittent exotropia can be difficult. There is a strong tendency for the exodeviation to recur weeks, months or years postoperatively. Conversely, in visually immature children a consecutive esotropia may be followed by the development of amblyopia and loss of binocular functions. The margin between benefit and potential permanent damage to the developing visual system is narrow. The best results appear to follow a small esotropia in the immediate postoperative period but amblyopia may result in up to 10% of cases. Traditionally, surgery has been carried out later in exodeviation than in esodeviation but some authors have suggested that better results are obtained with early surgery (median age 2.5 years) (Pratt-Johnson *et al.* 1977).

Logically, divergence excess exodeviations should be treated with bilateral lateral rectus recessions, convergence insufficiency with bilateral medial rectus resections and the basic deviation with a recess-resect operation. Appropriate oblique muscle surgery will also be required. Many surgeons achieve good results with a recess-resect procedure in all cases.

Secondary (sensory) exotropia

This may occur in unilateral or asymmetric ocular developmental disorders such as unilateral high myopia. It can also occur with sensory deprivation, particularly following trauma. It may be the presenting sign of optic nerve or retinal pathology including retinoblastoma. The management will obviously be directed primarily towards the underlying abnormality with cosmetic strabismus surgery considered as necessary.

Consecutive exotropia

There is a considerable element of unpredictability in the response to strabismus surgery for esotropia (Bradbury & Doran 1993). Parents should always be warned of the possibility of a second operation being necessary either for recurrent esotropia or consecutive exotropia. Provided a surgical misadventure such as loss of the sutures from the medial rectus during surgery or apparent 'slipping' of the medial rectus in the immediate postoperative period has not occurred, a consecutive exotropia in the first days after esotropia surgery should be managed conservatively. If it persists, particularly in cases with pre-existing binocular functions, early intervention is indicated. If there is no limitation of adduction and the exodeviation is small to moderate, botulinum toxin injection to the lateral rectus may be indicated. Otherwise, re-operation will be needed.

References

Aiello A, Wright KW, Borchert M. Independence of optokinetic nystagmus asymmetry and binocularity in infantile esotropia. *Arch Ophthalmol* 1994; **12**: 1580–3.

Archer SM, Helvesten EM, Miller KK, Ellis FD. Stereopsis in normal infants and infants with congenital esotropia. *Am J Ophthalmol* 1986; **101**: 591–6.

Atkinson J. Early visual development: differential functioning of parvocellular and magnocellular pathways. *Eye* 1992; **6**: 129–35.

Bradbury JA, Doran RML. Secondary exotropia: a retrospective analysis of matched cases. *J Pediatr Ophthalmol Strabismus* 1993; **30**: 163–6.

Breakey AS. Ocular findings in cerebral palsy. *Arch Ophthalmol* 1995; **52**: 852–6.

Burian HM, Franceschetti AT. Evaluation of diagnostic methods for the classification of exodeviations. *Trans Am Ophthalmol Soc* 1970; **68**: 56–71.

Burian HM, Smith DR. Comparative measurement of exodeviations at 30 and 100 feet. *Trans Am Ophthalmol Soc* 1971; **69**: 188–99.

Cantolino SJ, Von Noorden GK. Heredity in microtropia. *Arch Ophthalmol* 1969; **81**: 753–7.

Charles SJ, Moore AT. Results of early surgery for infantile esotropia in normal and neurologically impaired infants. *Eye* 1992; **6**: 603–6.

Cheng H, Burdon MA, Shun-Shin GA, Czypionka S. Dissociated eye movements in cranio-synostosis: a hypothesis re-visited. *Br J Ophthalmol* 1993; **77**: 563–8.

Chimonidou E, Palimeris G, Koliopoulos J, Velissaropoulos Z. Family distribution of concomitant squint in Greece. *Br J Ophthalmol* 1977; **61**: 27–9.

Coleman J, Sydnar CF, Wolbarsht ML, Creel DJ. Abnormal visual pathways in human albinos studied with visually evoked potentials. *Exp Neurol* 1979; **65**: 667–79.

Diamond GR, Katowitz JA, Whitaker LA, Quinn GE, Schaffer DB. Variations in extra-ocular muscle number and structure in craniofacial dysostosis. *Am J Ophthalmol* 1980; **90**: 416–18.

Elston JS, Timms C. Clinical evidence for the onset of the sensitive period in man. *Br J Ophthalmol* 1992; **76**: 327–8.

Fawer C-L, Calarne A, Furrer M-T. Neurodevelopmental outcome at 12 months of age related to cerebral ultrasound appearances of high-risk preterm infants. *Early Hum Dev* 1985; **11**: 123–32.

Fitzgerald BA, Billson FA. Dissociated vertical deviation: evidence for abnormal visual pathway projection. *Br J Ophthalmol* 1984; **68**: 801–6.

Franceschetti AT, Burian HM. Gradient accommodative convergence accommodation ratio in families with and without esotropia. *Am J Ophthalmol* 1970; **70**: 558–62.

Francois J. *Heredity in Ophthalmology.* St Louis: CV Mosby, 1961: 255–69.

Friedman L, Biedner B, David R, Sachs V. Screening for refractive errors, strabismus and other ocular anomalies from ages 6 months to 3 years. *J Pediatr Ophthalmol Strabismus* 1980; **17**: 315–17.

Gobin MH. Sagittalisation of the oblique muscles as a possible cause for the A, V and X phenomena. *Br J Ophthalmol* 1968; **52**: 13–18.

Gobin MH. The surgical correction of accommodative esotropia. In: Tilson G, ed. *Advances in Amblyopia and Strabismus, Transactions of the VIIth International Orthoptic Congress.* Lauf-Fahner: Verlag, 1991: 105–9.

Graham PA. Epidemiology of strabismus. *Br J Ophthalmol* 1974; **58**: 224–31.

Gresty MA, Metcalfe T, Timms C, Elston JS, Liu C. Neurology of latent nystagmus. *Brain* 1992; **115**: 1303–22.

Hamed LM, Fang EN, Fanous MM *et al.* The prevalence of neurologic dysfunction in children with strabismus who have superior oblique overaction. *Ophthalmology* 1993; **100**: 1483–7.

Harcourt B. Strabismus affecting children with multiple handicaps. *Br J Ophthalmol* 1974; **58**: 272–9.

Harcourt B, Mein J, Johnson F. Natural history and associations of dissociated vertical divergence. *Trans Ophthalmol Soc UK* 1980; **100**: 495–7.

Helvesten EM. Exotropia, alternating sursumduction and superior oblique overaction. *Am J Ophthalmol* 1969; **67**: 3772–80.

Helvesten EM. The origins of congenital esotropia. *J Pediatr Ophthalmol Strabismus* 1993; **30**: 215–32.

Helvesten EM, Von Noorden GK. Microtropia: a newly defined entity. *Arch Ophthalmol* 1967; **78**: 272–81.

Hiles DA, Davies GT, Costenbader FD. Long-term observations on unoperated intermittent exotropia. *Arch Ophthalmol* 1968; **80**: 436–42.

Hoyt CS. Nystagmus compensation (blockage) syndrome. *Am J Ophthalmol* 1977; **83**: 423–4.

Hoyt CS, Billson FA, Taylor H. Isolated unilateral gaze palsy. *J Pediatr Ophthalmol* 1977; **154**: 343–5.

Hoyt CS, Mousel DK, Weber AA. Transient supranuclear disturbances of gaze in healthy neonates. *Am J Ophthalmol* 1980; **89**: 708–12.

Iacobucci I, Archer S, Giles C. Children with exotropia responsive to spectacle correction of hyperopia. *Am J Ophthalmol* 1993; **116**: 79–83.

Ing M. Botulinum alignment for congenital esotropia. *Ophthalmology* 1993; **100**: 318–32.

Ing MR. Early surgical alignment for congenital esotropia. *Trans Am Ophthalmol Soc* 1991; **79**: 625–63.

Kommerel G, Mehdorn E. Is an optokinetic defect the cause of congenital and latent nystagmus? In: Lennerstrand G, Zee DS, Keller EL, eds. *Functional Basis of Oculomotility Disorders.* Oxford: Pergamon Press, 1982: 159–67.

Kriss A, Timms C, Elston J, Taylor D, Gresty M. Visual evoked potentials in dissociated vertical deviation—a re-appraisal. *Br J Ophthalmol* 1989; **73**: 265–70.

Kushner BJ. The role of ocular torsion on the aetiology of A and V patterns. *J Pediatr Ophthalmol Strabismus* 1985; **22**: 171–9.

Kushner BJ. Strabismus and amblyopia associated with regressed retinopathy of prematurity. *Arch Ophthalmol* 1982; **100**: 256–61.

Lang J. Microtropia. *Arch Ophthalmol* 1969; **81**: 758–62.

Lucas E, Bentley CR, Aclimandos WA. The effect of surgery on the AC/A ratio. *Eye* 1994; **8**: 109–14.

Ludwig IH, Parks MM, Getson PR, Kammerman LA. Rate of deterioration in accommodative esotropia correlated to the AC/A relationship. *J Pediatr Ophthalmol Strabismus* 1988; **25**: 8–13.

McKusick VA. *Mendelian Inheritance in Man.* Baltimore and London: Johns Hopkins University Press, 1978: 359–60.

Nash AJ, Hegmann JP, Spivey BE. Genetic analysis of vergence measurements in populations with varying incidence of strabismus. *Am J Ophthalmol* 1975; **79**: 978–84.

Nashold BS, Seaber JH. Defects of ocular motility after stereotactic midbrain lesions in man. *Arch Ophthalmol* 1972; **88**: 245–8.

Nixon RB, Helveston EM, Miller K, Archer SM, Ellis FD. Incidence of strabismus in neonates. *Am J Ophthalmol* 1985; **100**: 798–801.

Ohtsuki H, Hasebe S, Kobashi R, Okano M, Furese T. Critical period for restoration of normal stereo acuity in acute onset comitant esotropia. *Am J Ophthalmol* 1994; **118**: 502–8.

Palmer P, Dubowitz LMS, Levene MI, Dubowitz V. Developmental and neurological progression of preterm infants with intraventricular haemorrhage and ventricular dilation. *Arch Dis Child* 1982; **57**: 748–53.

Pillae P, Duand VK. Cyclic esotropia with central nervous system disease, report of two cases. *J Pediatr Ophthalmol Strabismus* 1987; **24**: 237–41.

Pratt-Johnson JA. Central disruption of fusional amplitude. *Br J Ophthalmol* 1973; **57**: 347–50.

Pratt-Johnson JA, Barlow JM, Tilson G. Early surgery in intermittent exotropia. *Am J Ophthalmol* 1977; **84**: 689–94.

Prism Adaptation Research Group. Efficacy of prism adaptation in the surgical management of acquired esotropia. *Arch Ophthalmol* 1990; **108**: 1248–56.

Reynolds JD, Biglan AW, Hiles DA. Congenital superior oblique palsy in infants. *Arch Ophthalmol* 1984; **102**: 1503–5.

Shauly Y, Prager TC, Mazow ML. Clinical characteristics and long-term post-operative results of infantile esotropia. *Am J Ophthalmol* 1994; **117**: 183–9.

Simons K, Reinecke RD. Amblyopia screening and stereopsis. Symposium on Strabismus In: *Transactions of the New Orleans Academy of Ophthalmology.* St Louis: CV Mosby, 1978: 15–50.

Slavin ML, Potash SD, Rubin SE. Asymptomatic physiological hyperdeviation in peripheral gaze. *Ophthalmology* 1988; **95**: 778–81.

Sondhi N, Archer SM, Helveston HM. Development of normal ocular alignment. *J Pediatr Ophthalmol Strabismus* 1988; **25**: 210–11.

Sorsby A, Sheridan M, Leary GA. Refraction and its components in twins. Medical Research Council's special reports. Series no. 303. London 1962; 1–43.

Stanworth A. Defects of ocular movement and fusion after head injury. *Br J Ophthalmol* 1974; **58**: 266–71.

Tychsen L, Burkhalt ERA. Neuro-anatomic abnormalities of visual cortex in infantile esotropia. In: Lennerstrand G, ed. *Update on Strabismus and Pediatric Ophthalmology.* Florida: CRC Press, 1995: 73–6.

Von Noorden GK. Current concepts of infantile esotropia. *Eye* 1988; **2**: 343–58.

Von Noorden GK. The nystagmus compensation (blockage) syndrome. *Am J Ophthalmol* 1976; **82**: 283–90.

Weakley DR, Urso RG, Dias EL. Asymmetric inferior oblique overaction and its association with amblyopia in esotropia. *Ophthalmology* 1992; **99**: 590–3.

66: Incomitant Strabismus and Cranial Nerve Palsies

John Elston

Incomitant strabismus in childhood is rare: no precise epidemiology is available, but it is notable that amongst 149 000 new patients presenting with strabismus (adults and children) to an eye hospital, only 126 (0.84%) had one of the most common varieties of incomitant strabismus, Duane's syndrome (Kirkham 1970). Incomitant strabismus may also present to paediatricians, neurologists and neurosurgeons, making data collection difficult.

In infancy, diagnosis may be difficult because of problems with the limited range of eye movement, particularly up- and downgaze, that can readily be elicited. Eye movement testing may be augmented in two ways. First, an infant can be held face to face with the examiner with the head supported and rotated on the vertical and horizontal axes to elicit vestibulo-ocular reflexes and assess the integrity of movement in each eye. Second, the infant is held as above, facing the examiner who spins around the vertical axis (for example on a rotating chair). The eyes deviate against the direction of spinning and saccade back to refixate. Provided the infant has a normal afferent visual and central nervous system, the integrity of the infranuclear oculomotor system can be assessed clinically by comparing the speed and extent of the refixation saccades in each eye. With these methods, a lateral rectus palsy, for example, can usually be differentiated from a concomitant convergent squint.

The most frequent observations by parents of affected children are of abnormal eye alignment, abnormal eye movement (with or without abnormal eyelid and/or pupil movement) or a head posture. The common ocular motility causes of a compensatory head posture (CHP) are superior oblique palsy (unilateral or bilateral), unilateral lateral rectus palsy, Duane's and Brown's syndrome and idiopathic congenital nystagmus (Kraft *et al.* 1992).

Occasionally associated features such as facial diplegia in Möbius' syndrome or epibulbar dermoid in Goldenhar's syndrome may be the presenting problem. Children who do not move their eyes normally, for example due to a gaze palsy, may also be referred because of a suspected sensory visual defect.

Incomitant strabismus is caused by two broad groups of disorders: (i) developmental abnormalities (principally Duane's, Möbius' and Brown's syndromes); and (ii) ocular motor palsies.

Developmental abnormalities

Duane's syndrome

Although originally described in the European literature at the end of the nineteenth century by Stilling and Türk, the disorder is properly named after Duane who described 54 cases in 1905, detailing the consistent ocular features. In the most typical form, there is a congenital deficiency of abduction of the eye with widening of the palpebral aperture on attempted abduction. This is combined with variable impairment of adduction with retraction of the globe and narrowing of the palpebral aperture

(Figs. 66.1, 66.2) and abnormal vertical movements (Duane 1905).

The vertical movements (upshoots or downshoots, rarely both) occur when the eye turns away from the field of action of the primarily involved muscle—for example on adduction in a typical (type 1) case (Figs. 66.3, 66.4). The movement may be very marked so that only sclera is visible. It has been attributed to the leash or banding effect of a tight horizontal muscle, in this example a lateral rectus, which slips upwards or downwards around the globe rotating it on its anteroposterior axis and converting the ipsilateral antagonist into an elevator or depressor. This hypothesis has some support from the observation that a

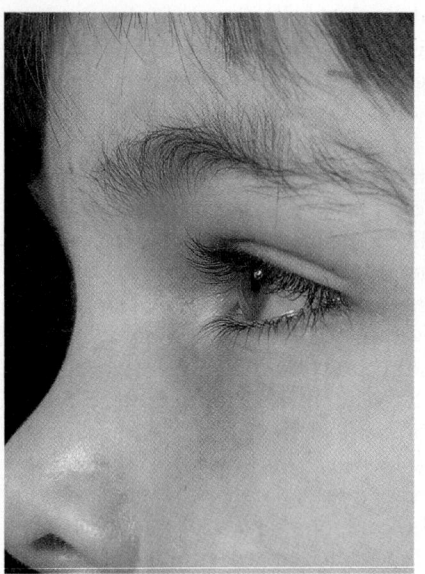
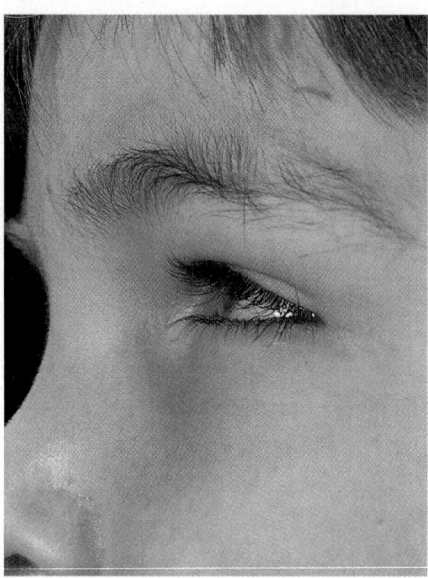

Fig. 66.1 Duane's syndrome. The left-hand picture shows the left eye in straight ahead gaze. The right-hand picture shows the left eye in right gaze showing marked retraction.

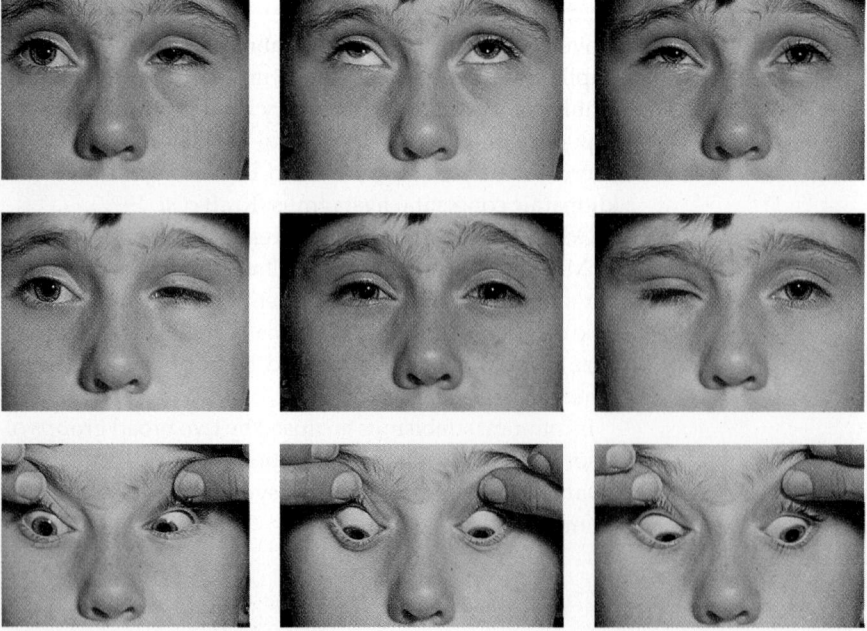

Fig. 66.2 Bilateral typical Duane's syndrome. There is no deviation in the straight ahead position, narrowing of the palpebral fissure in the adducting eye and weak abduction.

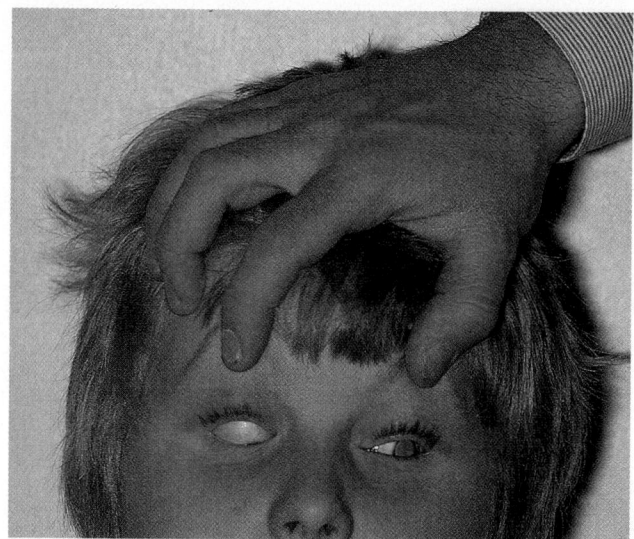

Fig. 66.3 Duane's syndrome showing gross downshoot of the right eye on adduction.

traction (forced duction) test is positive in most cases of Duane's. However, dynamic (multi-sequence) magnetic resonance imaging (MRI) does not show any muscle slip (Bloom *et al.* 1991) suggesting the abnormal vertical movements are primarily innervational in origin.

Duane's syndrome is usually unilateral and more common on the left side (Pfaffenbach *et al.* 1972) but may be bilateral in 15–20% of cases (Cross & Pfaffenbach 1972; Isenberg & Urist 1977). Bilaterality is probably more common than reported—careful inspection in many unilateral cases shows subtle abnormalities of contralateral lid and eye movement. This clinical suspicion may be supported by eye movement recordings (Gourdeao *et al.* 1981) and autopsy findings in one case (Mulhern *et al.* 1994). It is more common in females than males (Pfaffenbach *et al.* 1972) and may be familial (Kirkham 1970) (Fig. 66.5). There is a spectrum of abnormality of eye movement, and some authors have classified the condition into types I, II and III, dependent on the relative limitations of abduction and adduction.

1 Type I patients have normal adduction and reduced abduction.

2 Type II patients have normal abduction and reduced adduction.

3 Type III patients have reduced abduction and adduction.

Although there is some electrophysiological (electromyographic, EMG) support for this classification (Huber 1974) it is not very useful clinically since most cases of Duane's syndrome are explicable on a single pathology (see below). The syndrome may perhaps be best regarded as typical as described by Duane, or atypical (having other features such as marked reduction of adduction).

One of the notable features of the condition is the frequently normal development of sensory and motor binocular function despite profoundly abnormal eye movements. Binocularity may only be maintained with an abnormal head posture, usually of head turn towards the side of the lesion. Amblyopia, usually due to anisometropia or astigmatism, occurs in 10% of cases, 25% if the condition is bilateral. If a manifest strabismus is present, it is characteristically less than 25 dioptres. However, three patients with large angle infantile esotropia and limited abduction were shown to have Duane's syndrome after bilateral medial rectus recessions (Elsas 1991).

Numerous ocular associations of Duane's syndrome have been described (Table 66.1). The most common are ptosis (palpebral aperture less than the normal side by greater than 1 mm), cataracts, heterochromia, coloboma of iris choroid and optic disc, optic nerve hypoplasia, Morning Glory optic disc, epibulbar dermoid (see below) and oculocutaneous albinism. Other systemic developmental abnormalities are present in between 30 to 50% of cases.

Table 66.1 Duane's syndrome.

Isolated
Typical
Type I
  normal adduction
  reduced abduction

Atypical
Type II
  normal abduction
  reduced adduction
Type III
  reduced adduction
  reduced abduction

Associations
Deafness
Wildervanck's syndrome
Others
  Goldenhar's syndrome
  Hemivertebra
  Syndactyly
  Other limb malformation
  Okihiro syndrome
  Urogenital abnormalities
  Marcus Gunn jaw–winking
  Crocodile tears

Causes
Thalidomide
Fetal alcohol

Acquired Duane's syndrome
Orbital myositis
Orbital fractures and metastasis

Vertical Duane's syndrome

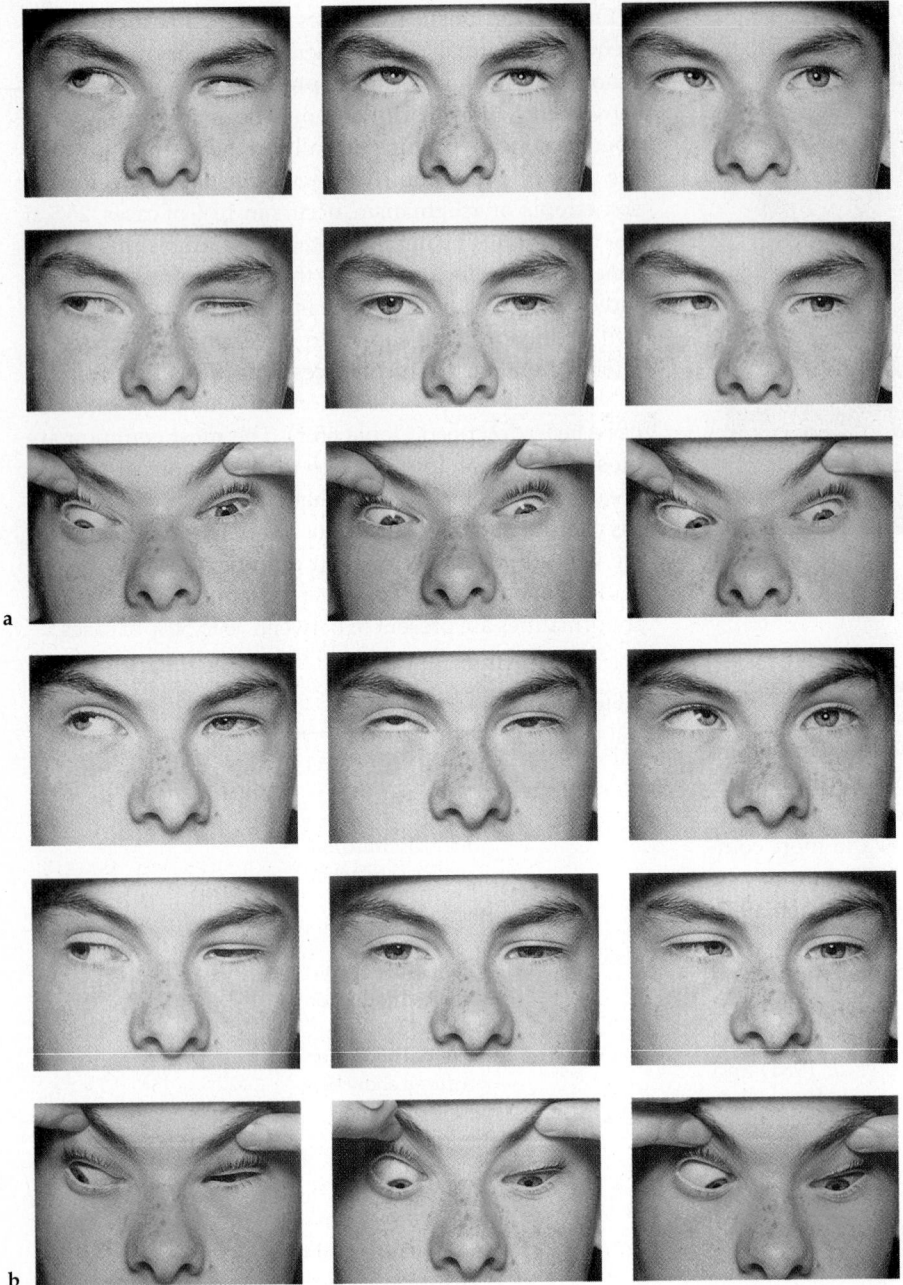

a

b

Fig. 66.4 (a) Left Duane's with gross upshoot of the left eye on adduction. (b) Same patient following splitting and recession of the left lateral rectus.

1 Deafness. The most important is perceptive deafness (10.7%, Kirkham 1970; 9.6%, Shauly *et al.* 1993) which may be severe in infancy and lead to a speech defect. Missing or hypoplastic auricle and facial palsy may occur.

2 Wildervanck's syndrome. The triad of Duane's, deafness and Klippel–Feil anomaly (an abnormality of the cervical spine leading to a short neck with reduced movements and a low posterior hairline) may be inherited as an autosomal dominant condition known as Wildervanck's syndrome. There is variable penetrance and different features in affected family members (Kirkham 1970).

3 Others. Other developmental anomalies include the following.

(a) Goldenhar's syndrome. It is evident that Wildervanck's (cervico-oculo–acoustic) syndrome is closely related to Goldenhar's (oculo-auriculo–vertebral) syndrome and the two may represent a continuum of abnormality (Baum 1992; Coyle 1992).

(b) Hemivertebra.

(c) Syndactyly.

(d) Other (usually terminal) limb malformations (Pfaffenbach *et al.* 1972).

(e) Okihiro's syndrome consists of autosomal domi-

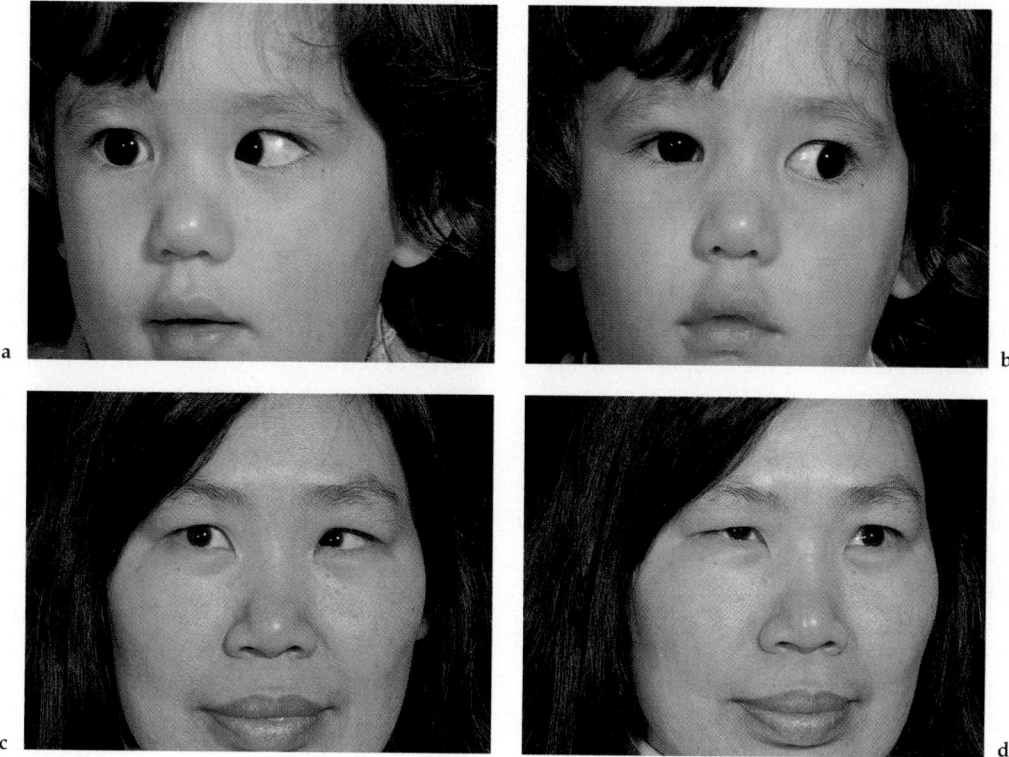

Fig. 66.5 Atypical right Duane's syndrome in a child (a, b) with a similar abnormality in her mother (c, d).

nant Duane's syndrome with radial ray deformity, thenar hypoplasia (or absence) and deafness (Collins *et al.* 1993; Hayes *et al.* 1985; MacDermott & Winter 1987). Again some similarity with Goldenhar's and Wildervanck's syndromes is evident from the clinical descriptions.

(f) Familial Duane's has also been reported with urogenital abnormalities and an abnormality of chromosome 22 (Cullen *et al.* 1993), and a case associated with bilateral ptosis and mental retardation had a 4q27–31 deletion (Chew *et al.* 1995).

(g) Marcus Gunn jaw–winking and 'crocodile tears' (Ramsay & Taylor 1980) are also recognized associations.

The pathophysiology of the condition was a matter of speculation until the development of the technique of extraocular muscle EMG. A study in 1972 showed normal innervation of the medial rectus, but a wide variation of lateral rectus innervational abnormalities, with co-firing on adduction, reduced activity on attempted abduction, and inappropriate activity on up- and downgaze (Scott & Wong 1972). It became clear that retraction (and secondary palpebral aperture narrowing) on adduction was due to co-contraction often in the superior and inferior as well as the lateral rectus, and the abnormal vertical movements (upshoots and downshoots) may in some cases be due to a

primary innervational anomaly. The results were taken to indicate an absent sixth nerve, with the peripheral third nerve supplying all the extraocular muscles in an abnormal way; a primary brain stem origin for the abnormality was thought likely. This conclusion had been reached earlier, principally on clinical grounds, by Hoyt and Nachtigaler (1965). Confirmation of the EMG findings was provided by Strachan and Brown (1972), who showed paradoxical innervation of the lateral rectus, and Huber (1974) who was able to distinguish the clinical subtypes of Duane's with EMG and suggest that the features depended on the relative contribution and pattern of third nerve supply to the lateral rectus, and fibrosis in the muscle. More recently, Saad and Lee's (1993) EMG work has shown regional abnormalities in the medial rectus in four cases (two each with types I and II) who showed medial rectus activity on attempted abduction. The authors speculated on a possible abnormal supranuclear input to the medial rectus motoneurones. Eye movement recordings showing slow horizontal saccadic movements in both the affected and unaffected eyes of patients with unilateral Duane's, also suggest that the premotor horizontal gaze system is abnormal (Gourdeao *et al.* 1981).

The first comprehensive report of the postmortem findings, both intracranial and orbital, in a case of bilateral Duane's syndrome appeared in 1980 (Hotchkiss *et al.* 1980). Both abducens nuclei and nerves were absent from the brain stem, and the lateral rectus muscles were partly innervated by branches from the oculomotor nerves.

Abducens interneurones must be present but may be abnormally innervated. An autopsy in a case of unilateral (left) Duane's confirmed these findings, and firmly established the disorder as a developmental neurological abnormality (Miller *et al.* 1982). This finding has been confirmed (Mulhern *et al.* 1994). Innervation of the lateral rectus may be patchy with histological evidence of fibrosis in non-innervated parts of the muscle. There may be a more extensive brain stem abnormality in some cases. Nine out of 14 patients with Duane's showed increased latency in wave III of the brain stem auditory evoked potential (Jay & Hoyt 1980) which is generated by the superior olivary complex in the pons. Seventeen out of 18 cases of congenital crocodile tears in the literature also had Duane's syndrome, suggesting more extensive pontine dysgenesis in these cases (Ramsay & Taylor 1980).

It will be evident from the above that there is a very extensive literature on the phenomenology of Duane's and good evidence for the underlying pathology. However, the cause in most cases remains a mystery. Some insight may be gained from the observation that Duane's is commonly seen in thalidomide embryopathy (Stromland & Miller 1993). Thalidomide is a hypnotic and antiemetic, widely prescribed in Western Europe (especially in western Germany) from 1957 to 1962. It caused a characteristic embryopathy and 54% of survivors have ocular abnormalities, 30% having Duane's, 10% bilateral horizontal gaze palsies. Other notable associations, also seen in idiopathic Duane's are deafness, facial palsy, Goldenhar's and Wildervanck's syndromes and crocodile tears (Miller & Stromland 1991). Exposure to thalidomide between postconception days 20 and 24 is a consistent feature and the damage must therefore be to cells destined to form the respective brain stem nuclei. Duane's syndrome may be a stereotypical or predictable reparative process to a non-specific insult to these cells at this stage in development (Miller 1992). Duane's has also been reported in the fetal alcohol syndrome (Holzman *et al.* 1990) suggesting other environmental agents might be responsible in some cases.

A syndrome exactly mimicking Duane's syndrome occurs in orbital myositis (Timms *et al.* 1989). Pain and pain on eye movements are prominent features and the involved extraocular muscles may be clinically enlarged and inflamed (Fig. 66.6). Retraction on gaze away from the involved muscle is prominent, presumably due to failure of elongation or active muscle spasm. The diagnosis can be confirmed on ultrasound, computed tomography (CT) or MRI (Moorman & Elston 1995).

The differential diagnosis of acquired Duane's also includes orbital trauma—usually a medial wall blow-out fracture—or damage to the lateral rectus and adjacent lateral orbital wall. Metastasis may also present this way.

A vertical retraction syndrome has been described and suggested to be related to Duane's. The features are con-

genital limitation of up- or downgaze, with retraction and narrowing of the palpebral aperture on attempting the opposite movement. The superior rectus is more often involved than the inferior rectus and there is a variable esotropia or exotropia. The literature is sparse, however, and there are no reports of pathology: some cases described (Pruksacholawit & Ishikawa 1976) may well be partly recovered congenital third nerve palsies. Other unusual patterns that may be related include an adduction deficit with bilateral abduction on attempted lateral gaze into the field of action of the apparently paretic muscle (synergistic divergence) (Wilcox *et al.* 1981; Wagner *et al.* 1987). Of the 14 cases recorded in the literature, two were bilateral and in one of these the Marcus Gunn phenomenon was also evident. EMG has suggested neural mis-wiring is responsible (Thomas *et al.* 1993).

Management

The parents of a child with Duane's syndrome need an explanation of the underlying developmental problem, emphasizing that although the condition is not progressive, it will not resolve, and it is not possible to create normal eye movements surgically. The developmentally significant associations (see above), particularly deafness, should be excluded. An accurate refraction is required, and ametropia or anisometropia and amblyopia treated.

The overall plan depends on the primary position alignment, the presence of an abnormal head posture, the severity of the retraction and the pattern of upshoot and downshoot, and accompanying A, V or X pattern (Kraft 1988).

The indications for surgical treatment are the presence of a tropia, compensatory head posture, upshoots or downshoots or marked globe retraction. The surgical options are outlined in Table 66.2.

If the child is binocular with the head held straight, no surgical treatment is necessary; if binocular with a noticeable head posture (turn towards the side of the lesion) then surgery to move the eye in the direction of the head turn may be helpful. Specialized surgical techniques are required, however, since resection of the affected muscle will have an excessive effect and increase retraction: recession should be avoided. A temporal transfer of the superior and inferior rectus to produce some abduction, combined with a small medial rectus recession may be required (Gobin 1974). In cases where retraction on adduction is the chief cosmetic abnormality, it can be reduced by recessing the medial and lateral rectus equally on the affected eye. Similarly up- and downshoots of the eye may be amenable to mechanical stabilization of the position of the extraocular muscles on the globe by splitting and recessing the lateral rectus; recessing it alone or recessing both medial and lateral (von Noorden 1992) (Fig. 66.4). In

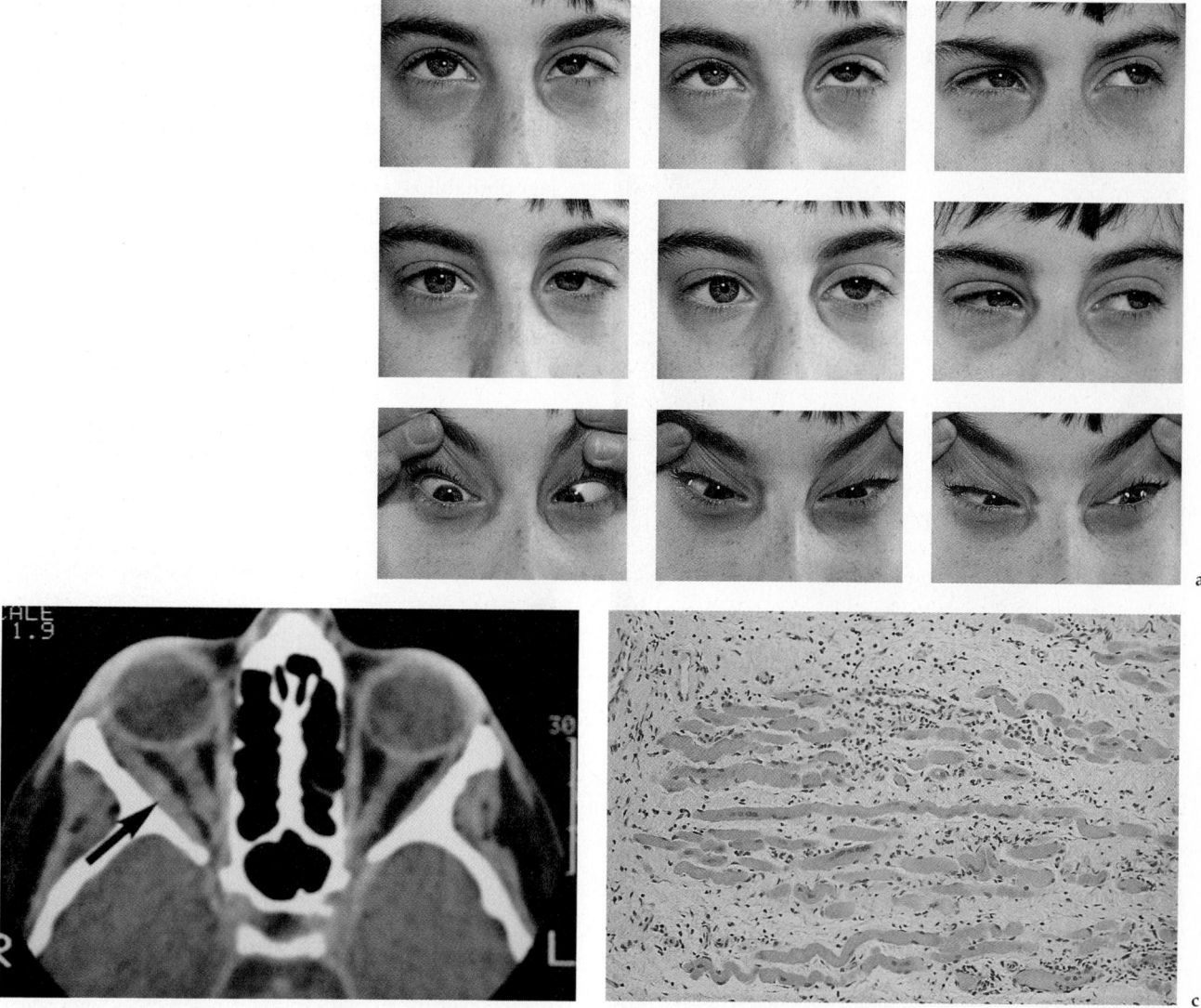

Fig. 66.6 (a) This 10-year-old patient presented with double vision and swollen lids. He had a typical Duane's syndrome, more marked on the right than the left. (b) CT scan showing 'shaggy' and enlarged lateral recti, particularly on the right. (c) Biopsy of the lateral rectus muscle shows the muscle fibres infiltrated with inflammatory cells. The symptoms and signs were completely abolished by a short course of steroids.

cases with a constant strabismus (usually convergent) surgery will also be required.

Möbius' syndrome

The syndrome of congenital facial diplegia with failure of abduction was first described by Von Graefe in 1880, more completely by Möbius in 1888 (Van Allen & Blodi 1960). The facial palsies are often incomplete (sparing the lower

Table 66.2 Surgical options in Duane's syndrome.

Esotropia/ compensatory head posture	Unilateral	Medial rectus recession or if deviation > 20 dioptres bimedial recession or superior and inferior rectus temporal transfer + later medial rectus recession
	Bilateral	Bimedial recession or as above (NB, if retraction is prominent, recess ipsilateral lateral rectus as well)
Exotropia/ compensatory head posture	Unilateral	Lateral rectus recession or if deviation > 30 dioptres bilateral lateral rectus recession
	Bilateral	Bilateral lateral rectus recession
Upshoot/ downshoot		Consider splitting and recession or recession and posterior fixation of horizontal muscles

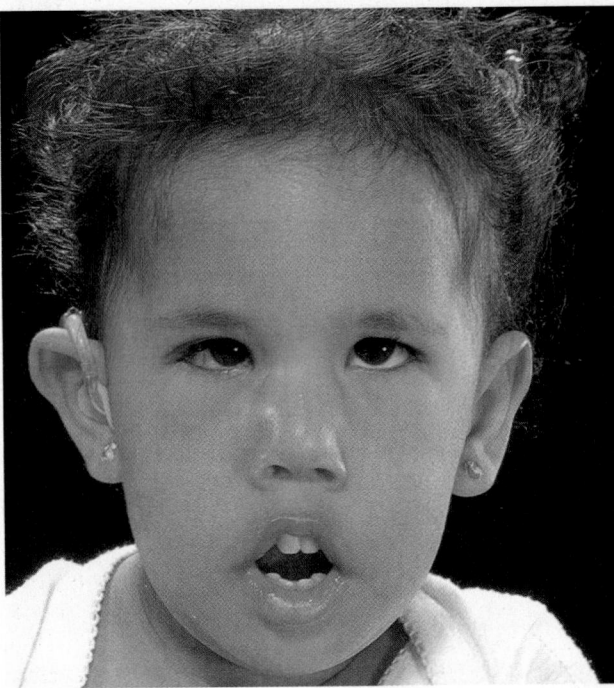

Fig. 66.7 Möbius' syndrome. This child has only a minimal strabismus in the primary position, a bilateral seventh nerve palsy and deafness.

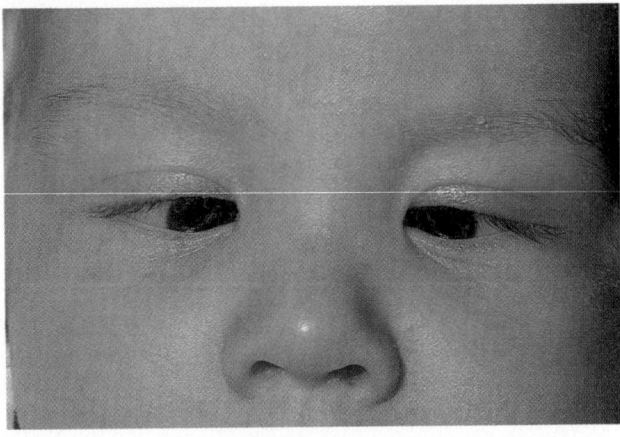

Fig. 66.8 Möbius' syndrome. Marked convergence with bilateral sixth nerve palsy and a seventh nerve palsy evidenced by rather 'expressionless' eyes. Many parents of infants with Möbius' syndrome find their child's apparent (but false) lack of response, due to the facial palsy, difficult to accept.

face) and asymmetrical but are an invariable feature. The eyes, which do not close normally but are protected by Bell's phenomenon, are often straight, not convergent (Figs. 66.7, 66.8, 66.9), indicating bilateral horizontal gaze palsies. Forty-five out of 61 cases reviewed by Henderson (1939) showed both these signs, whilst 15 had in addition bilateral partial third nerve palsies. Three of 18 cases studied by Amaya *et al.* (1990) had limitation of elevation. The

vertical eye movements are otherwise normal, as are the pupils, the vision, and the optic nerves and fundus.

Ametropia is common and primary position strabismus almost invariable (16 out of 18, Amaya *et al.* 1990). Crocodile tears occurred in three of 18 of Amaya's cases and excessive tearing was otherwise common, probably due to lagophthalmos and reduced blinks. Corneal sensation (Fig. 66.10) may also be defective (Miller *et al.* 1989). Eighteen of Henderson's cases had partial atrophy of the tongue, which characteristically shows longitudinal furrowing (Fig. 66.11). There may also be paralysis of the soft palate.

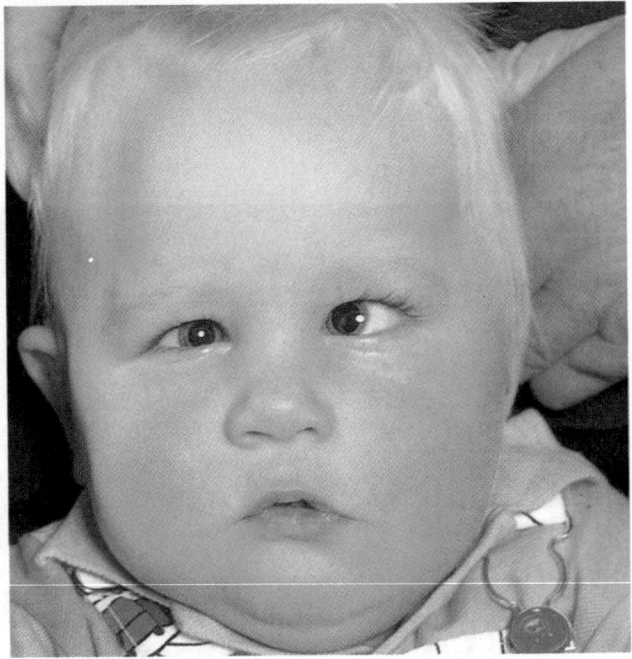

Fig. 66.9 Möbius' syndrome showing 'expressionless' face and a marked left esotropia. There is a bilateral sixth nerve palsy.

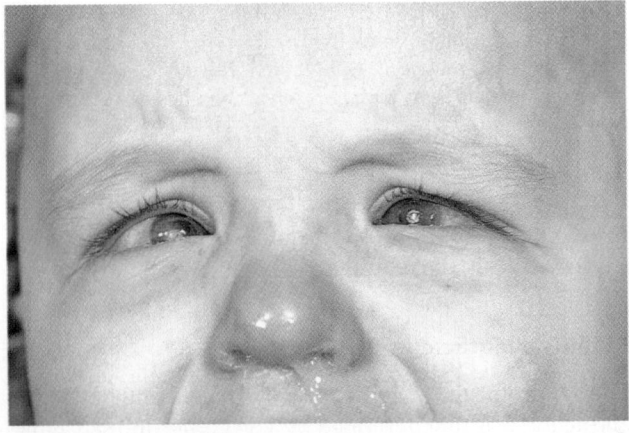

Fig. 66.10 Möbius-like syndrome with anaesthetic corneas from fifth nerve palsy and exposure due to seventh nerve palsy.

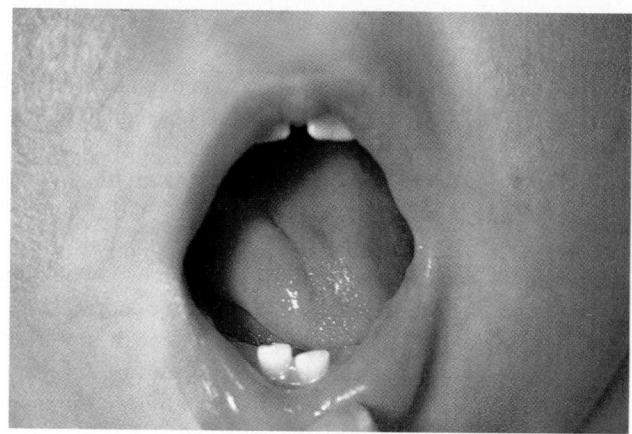

Fig. 66.11 Hypoplasia of the tongue with longitudinal furrowing in Möbius' syndrome.

Other associated developmental anomalies include skeletal malformations—agenesis or dysgenesis of limbs, or terminal limb defects such as syndactyly or polydactyly (Rogers *et al.* 1977). Dental anomalies (malocclusion and crowding exacerbated by micrognathia) may occur and other described associations include cerebral and cerebellar malformations, endocrine disturbances (e.g. hypogonadism, diabetes insipidus) and cardiovascular abnormalities (e.g. patent ductus or ventricular septal defect).

There appears to be a distinct syndrome of Möbius' sequence, peripheral neuropathy, and hypogonadotrophic hypogonadism (Kawai *et al.* 1990). Psychological problems are common (Amaya *et al.* 1990). Physical factors such as lack of facial and tongue movements may make communication difficult. Peer group and even parental rejection may occur. Mental deficiency, however, is relatively unusual (10% of Henderson's cases), belying the external appearance.

The combination of Möbius' syndrome and terminal limb hypogenesis is designated terminal transverse defect with orofacial malformation (TTV-OFM).

In some cases, this spectrum of abnormality may be accompanied by the Poland anomaly—unilateral absence of the sternocostal head of pectoralis major and the breast (Fig. 66.12) and synbrachydactyly of the ipsilateral hand. The Sprengel anomaly in which one or both scapulae are hypoplastic and the Klippel–Feil anomaly can also occur in combination with TTV-OFM defects.

Möbius' syndrome may be familial (Merz & Wojtowicz 1967) but Baraitser (1977) has suggested, from a study of the siblings and parents of 15 children, that if primary skeletal defects, agenesis of limbs, syndactyly, and so on, are included as obligatory in the diagnosis, the risk to subsequent offspring is very low (2%). A number of other conditions, however, may present with Möbius-like facies in infancy. These include disorders of the anterior horn cell

such as hypoplasia of the involved cranial nerve nuclei (Towfighi *et al.* 1979), brain stem tegmental necrosis (Thakkar *et al.* 1977) and myopathy, for example facioscapulo–humeral dystrophy (Hanson & Rowland 1971).

In Möbius' syndrome, the facial muscles show no EMG potentials on attempted activity (Merz & Wojtowicz 1967): the lateral rectus may, however, show some evidence of co-contraction with the medial rectus on attempted abduction, i.e. similar to Duane's syndrome (Van Allen & Blodi 1960; Merz & Wojtowicz 1967). Postmortem evidence shows that the underlying problem is agenesis of the sixth, seventh and twelfth cranial nerve nuclei (Towfighi *et al.* 1979). The extraocular muscles themselves are normal, but a traction test is often strongly positive, probably due to secondary fibrotic changes.

Möbius' syndrome and the spectrum of abnormality encompassed by TTV-OFM may be the result of an ischaemic insult in early pregnancy causing primary cranial nuclear hypoplasia and limb reduction defects (Bouwes Bavink & Weaver 1986; St Charles *et al.* 1994). Possible mechanisms interrupting blood vessel development include extrinsic factors such as amniotic bands or environmental influences, for example infections or drugs. Severe limb reduction defects may occur after chorionic villus sampling (CVS) at 56–66 days gestation (Firth *et al.* 1991) and some affected children also have orofacial malformations including Möbius' syndrome. Of 75 published cases of limb reduction defects in babies exposed to CVS *in utero*, 19 had Möbius' or Möbius-like syndromes (Firth *et al.* 1994).

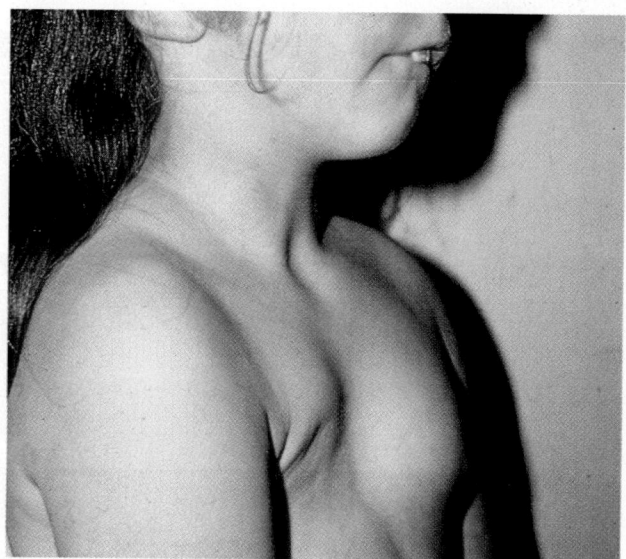

Fig. 66.12 Möbius' syndrome showing seventh nerve palsy and a unilateral Poland's anomaly (absence of pectoralis major and minor on the right side and the absence of the right breast).

Management

These children benefit from a multidisciplinary management approach. There may be serious feeding problems in infancy (Amaya *et al.* 1990). Surgery may be required for cardiovascular abnormalities. The psychological problems need attention. The ophthalmologist will need to identify and treat ametropia, amblyopia and primary position nystagmus. Medial rectus recession is the most appropriate surgical procedure. Lateral tarsorrhaphy may be necessary to protect the corneas, especially if they are anaesthetized (Miller *et al.* 1989).

Brown's syndrome

Brown's syndrome denotes a series of clinical findings that may have a variety of causes. There is a failure of elevation of the affected eye, which is complete when the eye is adducted, and reduces progressively with abduction (Fig. 66.13) (Brown 1973). The traction test is positive on attempted passive elevation of the eye in adduction, which distinguishes Brown's syndrome from isolated inferior oblique palsy or idiopathic superior oblique overaction. A V pattern of eye movement with exotropia in upgaze is usual. Although overaction of the ipsilateral superior oblique is classically absent, it may be present in one-fifth of patients (Sato *et al.* 1987). The palpebral aperture usually widens on adduction. Ten per cent of all cases are bilateral (Brown 1973), and the condition may be familial, when it is always bilateral (Moore *et al.* 1988; Hamed 1991b). Mirror image Brown's syndrome has been described in twins (Wortham & Crawford 1988). It has been described with congenital con-tralateral superior oblique palsy (Castanera de Molina & Munos 1991).

Most cases of Brown's syndrome seen in childhood are congenital and due to developmental anomalies of the superior oblique tendon. The trochlear and superior oblique tendon are derived from the same mesenchymal tissue, and develop into separate entities by differential growth (Sevel 1981). In the embryo, septae extend from the tendon to the trochlea, and the syndrome may be due to persistence of these septae or restriction of normal tendon movement through the sheath. In others, the anterior (reflected) part of the tendon is short preventing elevation in adduction. A cyst or focal expansion of the tendon may also be responsible.

Brown's syndrome may occasionally be acquired in childhood. Focal trauma or surgery in the region of the trochlea is the usual cause (Dobler *et al.* 1993), but cases due to inflammatory disease (Herman 1978; Moore & Morin 1985; Wang *et al.* 1984; Bradshaw *et al.* 1993), a metastasis (Booth-Mason *et al.* 1985; Slavin & Goldstein 1987), and trochlear involvement by tumour (Biedner *et al.* 1988) have been described in the Hurler–Scheie syndrome (Bradbury *et al.* 1989) and morphoea (Olver & Laidler 1988). It has been described as a transient phenomenon after an uncomplicated delivery (Christiansen & Thomas 1994).

Children with Brown's syndrome usually present with an abnormal head posture, turning their heads to move the affected eye into abduction, sometimes combined with elevation of the chin, in order to achieve binocularity. Sometimes binocularity has been lost by the time of presentation, in which case the parents notice a vertical strabismus, with over-elevation of the normal eye the most prominent feature.

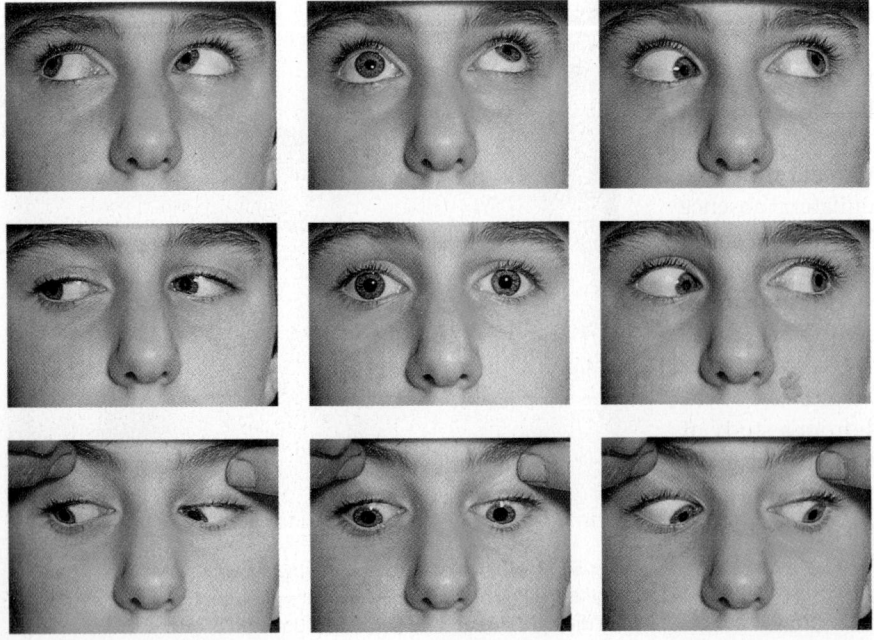

Fig. 66.13 Right Brown's syndrome with poor elevation of the eye in adduction but no residual hypotropia in the primary position.

Management

There is an overall tendency for spontaneous improvement (Waddell 1982) and complete resolution may occur, preceded by a period of intermittency between the ages of 7 and 10 often characterized by an audible and palpable 'click' as the tendon passes through the trochlea. The improvement may be due to progressive atrophy or disruption of abnormal septa (see above). In children who are binocular, with no deviation in the primary position and no gross head posture, management can therefore be expectant.

The indications for surgical treatment are a CHP, a vertical deviation in the primary position or deteriorating binocularity. The diagnosis is confirmed at surgery by a positive traction test. The most effective operation is a superior oblique tenectomy (Sprunger *et al.* 1991). Secondary operations are common with an average of more than two procedures per patient. A repeat tenectomy, ipsilateral inferior oblique recession or contralateral inferior rectus recession may be needed. Simultaneous superior oblique tenectomy and inferior oblique recession is no longer recommended.

Extraocular muscle fibrosis syndromes

Congenital fibrosis of the extraocular muscles

This is an autosomal dominant disorder with high penetrance (Harley *et al.* 1978; Hiatt & Halle 1983; Houtman *et al.* 1986; Lawford 1988). It has been described in patients from many races. Concordance within affected families is high and the phenotype is homogeneous between families. Occasionally it has been reported as being sporadic (Crawford 1970), presumably a new mutation.

It is usually isolated, but similar conditions have been described in association with amyloidosis (Sharma *et al.* 1991), Joubert's syndrome (Appleton *et al.* 1989), and oculocutaneous albinism (Brodsky *et al.* 1989). One family has been described with congenital fibrosis, internal ophthalmoplegia and iris transillumination due to a posterior pigment epithelial defect: it is notable that the ciliary and extraocular muscles and the posterior pigmented epithelium of the iris are all of neural crest origin (Cibis *et al.* 1992). A family was described (Fig. 66.14) in which one patient had a chromosome defect (Catford 1966). The gene has been mapped to the centromeric region of chromosome 12 (Engle *et al.* 1994).

Congenital fibrosis of the extraocular muscles (CFEOM) is characterized by a congenital, stationary, bilateral ptosis and external ophthalmoplegia, usually with a chin-up abnormal head posture. The forced duction test is markedly abnormal. Some abnormal, jerky, limited movement may remain, but mostly gaze is transferred by head movements.

Myopia, astigmatism and amblyopia are common (Catford 1966; Crawford 1970; Fells *et al.* 1984).

The pathophysiology is unclear: its congenital and stationary nature is against a myopathy, and although 'miswiring' has been suggested as a prenatal underlying cause (Brodsky *et al.* 1989), there are some cases with a marked convergence at birth whose only residual movement is a convergence jerk on attempted gaze in any direction (Figs. 66.15, 66.16). This 'convergence-only' defect may be associated with a deterioration in the forced duction test, it being better at attempts earlier in the child's life suggests that the early defect may be a 'mis-wiring' defect with secondary fibrous changes; these cases are very rare and are sometimes associated with more widespread neurological abnormalities and it is likely that most cases are a primary developmental muscle disorder (Engle *et al.* 1994).

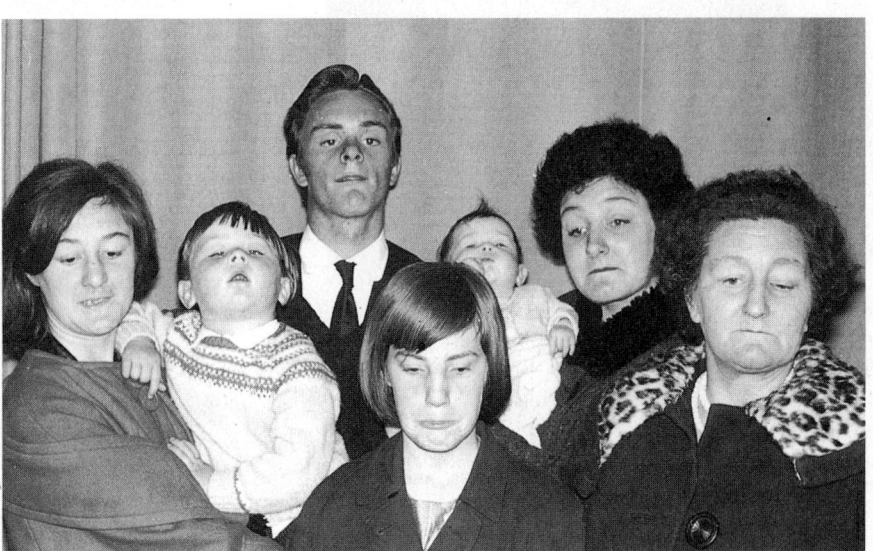

Fig. 66.14 Familial generalized fibrosis of the ocular muscles showing a similar phenotype in all generations (see Catford 1966). Courtesy of Mr Gordon Catford.

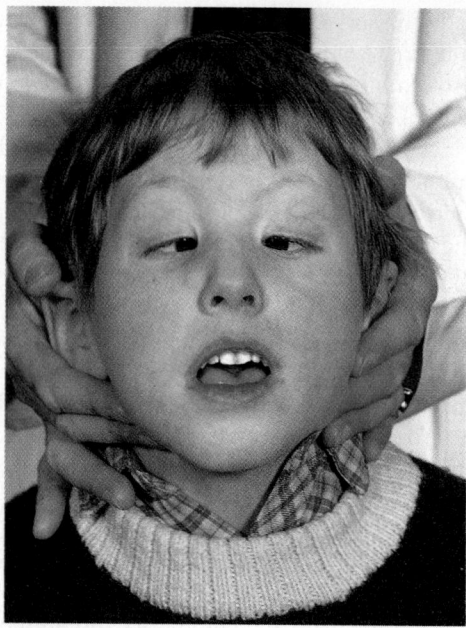

Fig. 66.15 Convergence-only defect. This patient was born with absence of any movement of the eyes except convergent movements which occurred on attempting gaze in any direction. There is a bilateral ptosis. A brain stem aetiology is suggested by the freeness of movement on a forced duction test. Intelligence is normal.

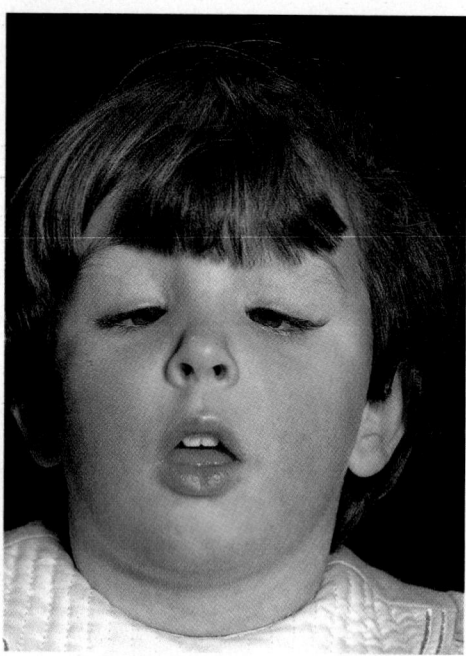

Fig. 66.16 Convergence-only defect.

Management

Refractive error and amblyopia must be identified and treated conventionally. To reduce or overcome the abnormal head posture, a very large recession or a free tenoto-my of the affected muscles, possibly combined with postoperative traction may be carried out.

Asymmetrical fibrosis

Unilateral globe displacement with ptosis, enophthalmos and limited eye movements can occur congenitally without a family history. Imaging suggests the presence of fibrous tissue in the orbit, confirmed on biopsy (Hertle *et al*. 1992). The extraocular muscles, orbital fat, Tenon's capsule and conjunctiva are involved. There is often a history of neonatal periorbital swelling and bruising, and the condition may be secondary to cranial haemorrhage. The other eye is normal.

Fibrosis of individual muscles

1 Medial rectus (strabismus fixus convergens). This is a congenital condition with gross fibrosis of the medial recti, a gross convergent strabismus, no ptosis and variable vertical muscles.
2 Lateral rectus (strabismus fixus divergens). In this, the lateral recti are primarily affected. In strabismus fixus treatment is only for cosmesis, the prognosis should be guarded: extra large recessions or clearance of fibrous tissue and free tenotomy of the muscle may be of benefit.
3 Inferior rectus fibrosis (IRF). This is very similar in its clinical appearance to a double elevator palsy (DEP): upward movements are variably limited, equally in adduction and abduction; there is a pseudoptosis (Fig. 66.17) and, if the defect is still present in downgaze, a chin-up abnormal head posture may be present. The difference between the two, clinically, is that in IRF the forced duction test is abnormal; in DEP it is normal. It may well be that IRF results from fibrosis following long-standing DEP. Refractive errors need to be corrected and amblyopia treated. Indications for surgery are a significant cosmetic defect, or inability of the eye to reach the primary position. In IRF a large recession of the inferior rectus alone may allow the eye to reach primary position. In DEP a vertical transposition of the horizontal muscles is the operation of choice in most cases.
4 Superior rectus. A congenitally 'tight' superior rectus (Weiss & Manley 1985).
5 Congenital fibrosis of the vertically acting muscles (Gillies *et al*. 1995).

Others

Goldenhar's syndrome

Goldenhar's syndrome (oculo-auriculovertebral dysplasia with hemifacial microsomia) may be accompanied by congenital ophthalmoplegia or Duane's syndrome. A

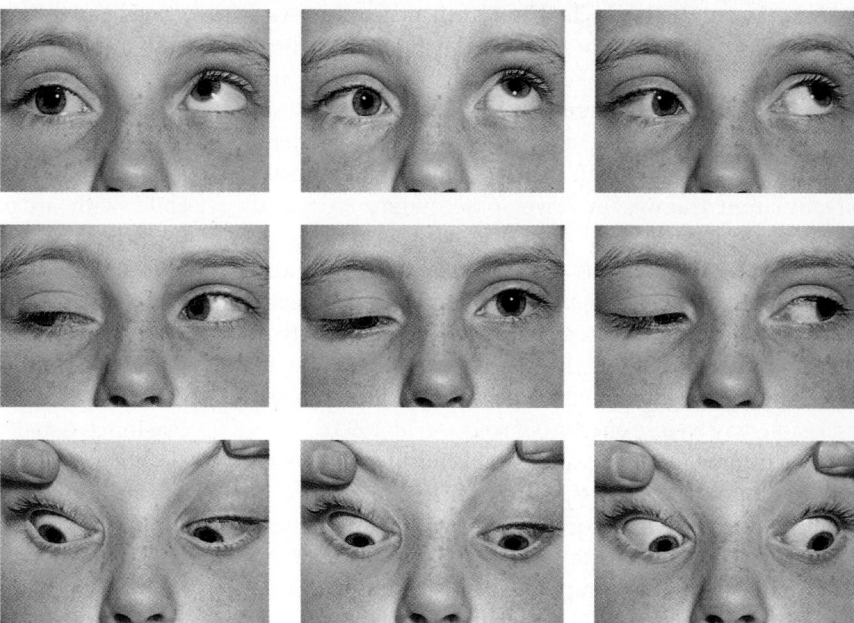

Fig. 66.17 Right inferior rectus fibrosis with right hypotropia especially in upgaze. There is a right pseudoptosis.

postmortem study in one case showed agenesis of the fourth and sixth nerve nuclei (Aleksic *et al.* 1976).

Craniosynostoses

Incomitant strabismus is a feature of the craniosynostosis syndromes. Exotropia with a vertical deviation and V pattern is seen in Crouzon's and Pfeiffer's syndromes whilst esotropia is more common in Apert's syndrome. Maldevelopment of the orbits with anomalous extraocular muscle insertions is a factor in determining the abnormal eye movements emphasized by the occurrence of specific muscle underactions or overactions in limited syndromes such as frontonasal dysplasia. Extraocular muscles may also be absent or poorly developed (Robb & Boger 1983). Cheng and colleagues have drawn attention to the excyclorotation of the eye (visible on ophthalmoscopy) and muscle cone in these patients. The dissociated eye movements, for example elevation in adduction, result from Hering's law as the abducting muscles become the lateral rectus and superior rectus with contralateral adduction achieved by the medial rectus and superior rectus (Cheng *et al.* 1993).

Anomalous insertions

Rarely, an anomalous muscle insertion may be an isolated abnormality not associated with other orbital pathology (Rosenbaum & Jampolsky 1975; Mather & Saunders 1987).

Acquired oculomotor nerve dysfunction

The oculomotor system consists of supranuclear, internu-

clear, nuclear and infranuclear components; only the latter will be considered in this section. Infranuclear oculomotor disorders in childhood may be isolated, or associated with other symptoms (for example pain or headache) or signs (for example other cranial nerve palsies). Isolated individual ocular motor (third, fourth or sixth cranial nerve) disorders will be discussed first.

Children with third, fourth or sixth cranial nerve palsies may present to ophthalmologists, neurologists, neurosurgeons or paediatricians, so that it is difficult to collect data from a representative group of patients, and the epidemiology is sparse. In an unselected, retrospective study of 1000 cases of all ages (all with acquired palsies), Rush and Younge (1981) found that 90% of the patients were over 19 years at presentation. This figure was confirmed in a later study of 4278 cases of both congenital and acquired oculomotor palsies (Richards *et al.* 1992). Of 160 palsies in children, over half were sixth nerve palsy, a quarter were third nerve palsy and the remainder were either multiple or fourth nerve palsies (Kodsi & Younge 1992). For all palsies, trauma was the most common cause, accounting for 42.5% of paediatric cases but only 15% in adults. Children are injured in road traffic accidents both as pedestrians and as unrestrained passengers; they may be injured at play (e.g. falling from a tree or climbing frame) or occasionally, deliberately, by a parent or other person responsible for their care.

Closed head injury with or without skull fracture may cause a complete third nerve palsy; the injury is usually severe, and may be associated with prolonged loss of consciousness and other neurological signs (Elston 1984). Bilateral fourth nerve palsies follow less severe head injuries often without loss of consciousness, when the head is flexed on the neck. The fourth nerve roots are avulsed from the superior medullary velum. The diagnosis is difficult to make on eye movement testing and may be missed; measurements of ocular torsion are necessary to distinguish a unilateral from a bilateral fourth nerve palsy. Sixth nerve damage may result directly from trauma, or develop secondary to raised intracranial pressure.

Concomitant strabismus (usually esotropia) may also be precipitated by closed head trauma; any case, however, in which there is an inconsistency between the severity of the reported trauma and the subsequent physical signs should be investigated neuroradiologically. A predisposing lesion may be responsible (Chrousos *et al.* 1993).

Facial trauma may also cause strabismus. In a blow-out fracture, anterior orbital trauma results in a fracture of either the medial wall or orbital floor, with displacement of orbital contents. There is enophthalmos and limitation of eye movement due to trapping of either the extraocular muscles or their associated fascia in the fracture. Extraocular muscle dysfunction may also be due to intramuscular haemorrhage, in which case spontaneous recovery may be expected, or traumatic denervation. Whereas in adults spontaneous improvement is the rule, in children this is not the case, and early surgery to free trapped tissue is advised, but may not be successful (McGarry & Fells 1984).

The most common tumour causing oculomotor palsies in childhood is probably a brain stem glioma (17% of Kodsi & Younge's cases). The presentation is in the first decade, most commonly with a sixth, occasionally a fourth and rarely a third nerve palsy.

Presentation

Isolated ocular motor nerve palsies in infancy usually present with the parents' observation of an abnormality of eye or eyelid movement, or pupil size. Older children may complain of double vision, and although this symptom can be the result of the recognition of physiological diplopia, it should always be taken seriously. The distance esotropia of a mild lateral rectus palsy, for example, may be minimal, but early diagnosis is important. Other presentations in childhood include the shutting of one eye and adoption of an abnormal head posture.

A full history is important; recent infections including exposure to neurotropic viruses, may be of aetiological importance. General symptoms such as headache and fever should be sought, and may determine the urgency of investigation. The drug history may be relevant, for example, tetracycline (Maroon & Mealy 1971) and nalidixic acid (Cohen 1973) may cause intracranial hypertension.

The differential diagnoses include concomitant strabismus, neuromuscular disease, orbital disease and supranuclear and internuclear ophthalmoplegias. Myasthenia gravis may present in infancy and childhood with ptosis and ophthalmoplegia (Berkovitz *et al.* 1977). Juvenile myasthenia resembles the adult type, and may be associated with thyroid dysfunction. Lid signs (twitches and 'hops') are often prominent and should be specifically looked for. Forceful eye closure should be tested in any child with an ophthalmoplegia. Neonatal myasthenia, due to cross-placental transfer of anti-acetylcholine receptor antibodies from a mother with the disease, is usually transient. Mitochondrial cytopathy may present in childhood with symmetrical ophthalmoplegia and ptosis (Land *et al.* 1981).

Orbital disease in childhood, such as metastatic neuroblastoma, usually presents as a mass lesion with proptosis, but may also mechanically restrict the eye movements, as may orbital trauma.

Supranuclear and internuclear ophthalmoplegia must be excluded before the diagnosis of peripheral ocular motor palsy is made. For example, skew deviation of any aetiology may mimic a vertical muscle palsy. Monocular elevation paresis (double elevator palsy) may be caused by a unilateral pretectal lesion (Jampel & Fells 1968); in this condition there is no ocular deviation in the primary position or downgaze, no ptosis and normal pupils, but defective upgaze in both adduction and abduction (Metz 1981). Divergence paralysis with raised intracranial pressure produces the signs of a mild bilateral sixth nerve palsy and may be the same condition (Kirkham *et al.* 1972).

Third nerve

Congenital palsy

This is a rare condition (Victor 1976). The vast majority of cases are unilateral. The clinical features are ptosis (Fig. 66.18) and exotropia with variable involvement of third nerve innervated extraocular muscles producing

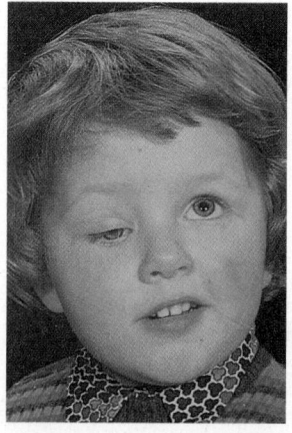
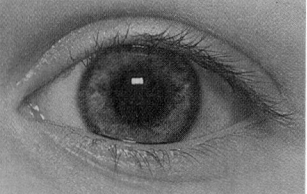
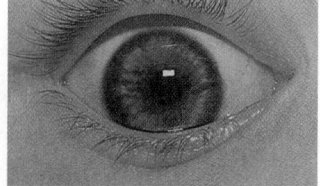

Fig. 66.18 Congenital third nerve palsy with smaller pupil on the affected side (see text).

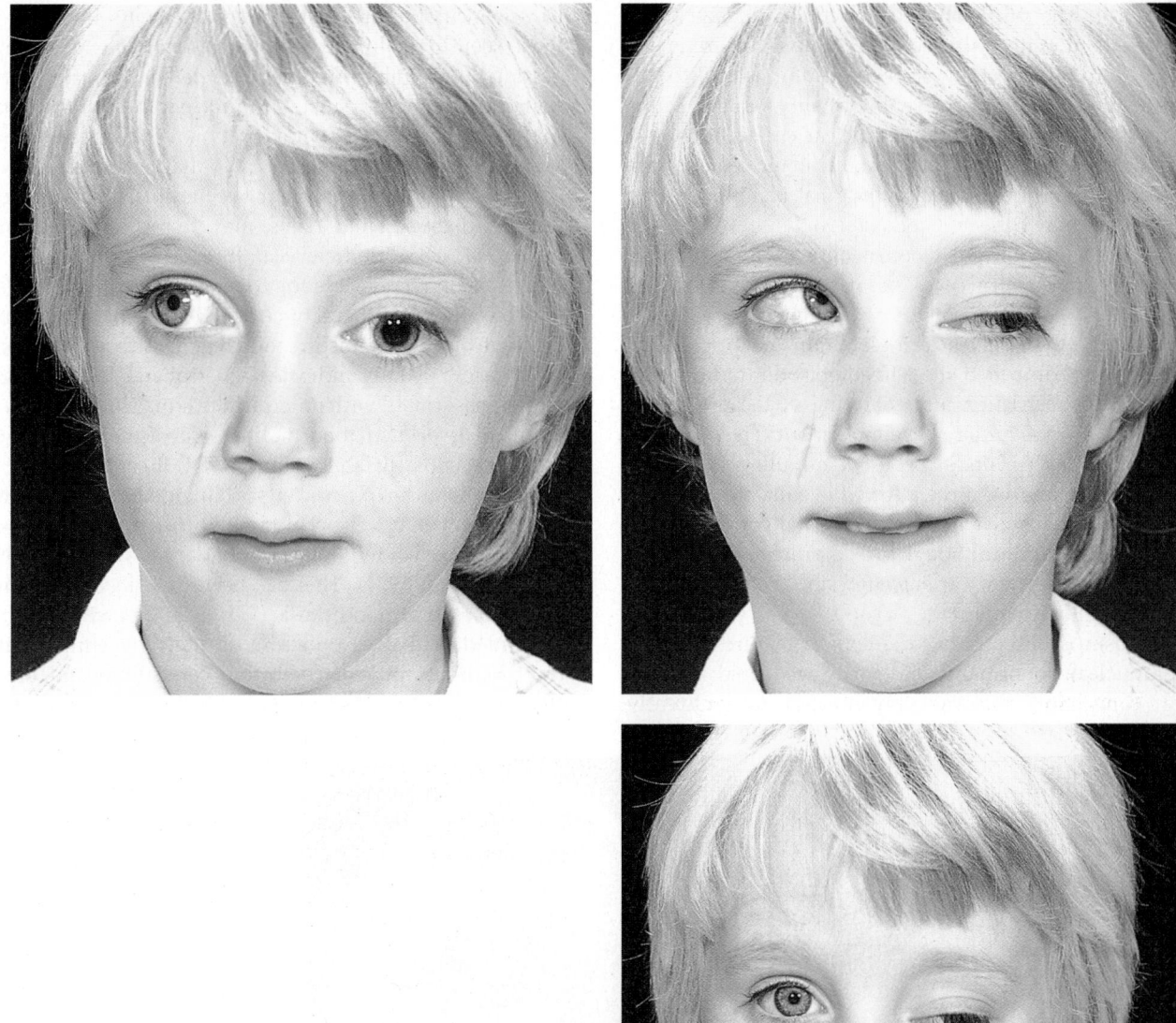

Fig. 66.19 Third nerve palsy with aberrant regeneration, causing relative lid elevation on adduction. The cause was 'ophthalmoplegic migraine' and after a further episode the aberrant regeneration was abolished.

reduced adduction, elevation and depression (Victor 1976; Miller 1977). The pupil although usually large may be smaller than the normal size, although the smallness has never satisfactorily been explained (Lotufo *et al.* 1983), and was present in only two out of 12 cases in Victor's series, seven having larger pupils (Victor 1976). However, the pupil may be dilated at birth and subsequently become miosed (Hamed 1991a). Amblyopia on the affected side is very common, but four out of 12 of Hamed's cases had

better vision in the affected eye due to contralateral nystagmus.

Many cases develop signs of abnormal re-innervation (Fig. 66.19) which may be superimposed on limited normal innervation. Two patterns are recognized: (i) oculomotor synkinesis ('misdirection regeneration'), which is common; and (ii) cyclic spasms of oculomotor function, which is uncommon. In oculomotor synkinesis, the upper lid elevates and the pupil contracts on adduction and downgaze. The pupil often contracts on upgaze when globe retraction may also be seen. Although there is evidence that misdirection of regenerating axons to the 'wrong' muscle underlies the abnormality, central synaptic reorganization altering internuclear connections may be partly responsible. The synkinetic movements are stereotyped and occasionally abnormal contralateral lid movements may be seen (Guy *et al.* 1989).

Cyclic oculomotor palsy occurs only after a congenital third nerve palsy or one acquired in the first 2 years of life (Loewenfeld & Thompson 1975). The child presents the features of a more or less complete third nerve palsy on which is superimposed short-lived episodes of lid elevation, pupil constriction and centering of the eye in the orbit with a small range of eye movement. The oculomotor spasms last seconds to half a minute and can be induced by fixing with the affected eye or attempting to adduct it. They may also occur spontaneously and in sleep. The condition, although rare, is probably more common than was formerly appreciated since Fells and Collin (1979) diagnosed nine cases over a 4-year period. The mechanism is obscure, but the clinical features imply a supranuclear abnormality, i.e. partly recovered infranuclear connections that can only function intermittently.

During oculomotor spasms lid movements identical to those seen in oculomotor synkinesis can be elicited suggesting the two abnormalities are related, the latter being sustained by more robust supranuclear and internuclear inputs. Other authors, however, have suggested that peripheral mechanisms such as ephaptic transmissions (cross talk) or intermittent nerve impulse transmission through demyelinated axons, may be responsible (Kommerel *et al.* 1988; Friedman *et al.* 1989).

The lesion responsible for congenital third nerve palsy may be either peripheral or central. An isolated palsy and the development of misdirection regeneration (the majority of cases) usually indicates a peripheral lesion which may be associated with mild birth trauma (Victor 1976). If there are associated abnormalities such as hemiparesis or hydrocephalus (Balkan & Hoyt 1984) a central origin is likely. The third nerve nucleus is damaged and little or no function develops. The underlying cause may be primary nuclear aplasia or hypoplasia secondary to vascular occlusion (Norman 1974). This has been described following mid-trimester amniocentesis (Fig. 66.20) in a child with a presumed fetal skull puncture on the right temple with right hemi-atrophy of cerebrum, cerebellum and brain stem (Patel *et al.* 1993). Severe birth trauma may also

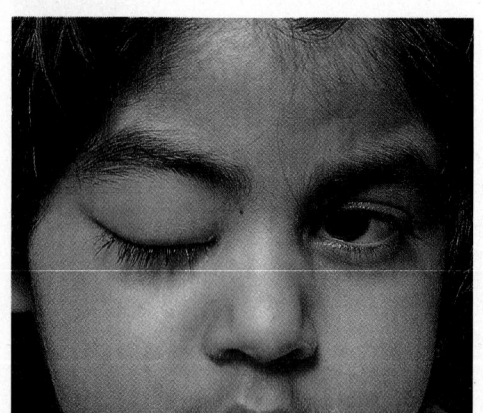
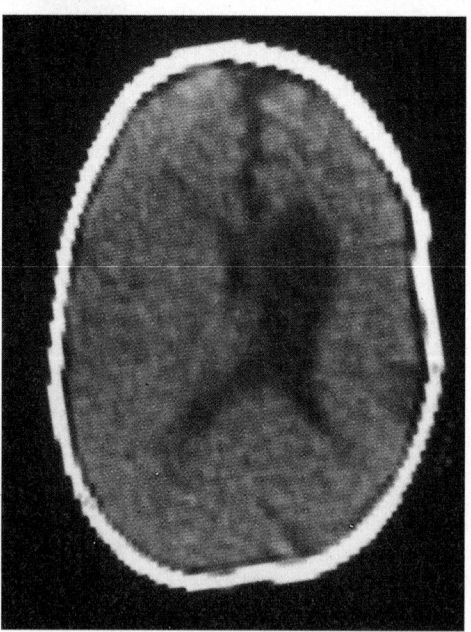
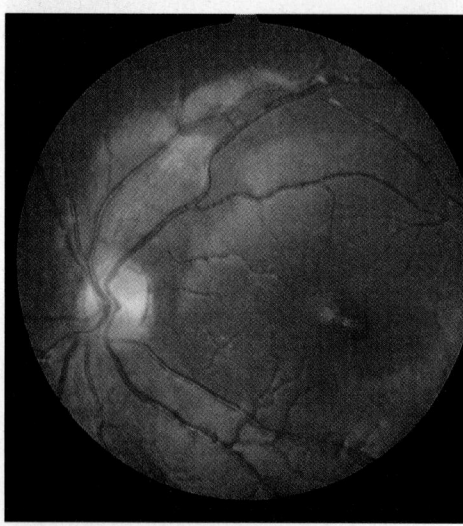

Fig. 66.20 (a) Right third nerve palsy, associated with (b) a porencephalic cyst. The left optic disc (c) shows band atrophy reflecting the left homonymous hemianopia from right optic tract involvement.

be responsible (Hamed 1991a). The clinical distinction between peripheral and central cases is not necessarily reliable and MRI in apparently isolated cases may reveal other abnormalities.

Two cases of congenital oculomotor palsy, cerebellar hypoplasia and facial capillary haemangioma have been described (White *et al.* 1992). The mechanism is not known. Bilateral congenital third nerve palsy is usually associated with substantial brain abnormalities (Good *et al.* 1991).

Congenital palsy of individual third nerve innervated muscles is occasionally found. The most common involve the inferior rectus (Von Noorden & Hansel 1991) and inferior oblique (Pollard 1993).

Management

Because of the associated neurological abnormalities, all cases should be assessed by a paediatric neurologist. If a central origin is suspected, neuroimaging is required. Amblyopia must be treated from the onset with vigorous patching, which may be combined with the use of low concentration (0.1%) pilocarpine, which, by mediating accommodation, will bring the child into focus for near objects. Surgical treatment may be needed, and if the eye is markedly exotropic, should be carried out early (e.g. during the second year) to allow it to be used during occlusion treatment without a gross head turn. The surgical technique will depend on the amount of third nerve function. At least two operations are usually required (for the horizontal and vertical components). Nasal transfer of the vertical rectus muscles is not helpful for the exotropia. The superior oblique tendon can be used to adduct the eye. It is important for the parents to appreciate that normal eye movements can never be achieved, but it is usually possible to centre the eye in the orbit in the primary position. The ptosis is not usually severe enough to require early treatment to enable patching to be effective. If it does require treatment at a late stage, the lid should be raised cautiously, as Bell's phenomenon may be defective, and corneal exposure may become a problem.

Acquired palsy

The important consideration in this group is the aetiology; the clinical features vary according to the extent of third nerve involvement, and the associated symptoms according to the underlying cause. The differential diagnoses, if the pupil is not involved, include myasthenia gravis which may present in infancy or childhood (Berkovitz *et al.* 1977).

Trauma is the most common cause accounting for 31 out of 43 cases in one series and six out of 17 in another (Miller 1977; Ing *et al.* 1992). Most occur in road traffic accidents, and some are due to penetrating trauma (Keane 1993).

Trauma alone may not be a sufficient explanation, however, and if a third nerve palsy follows minor head injury without loss of consciousness, neuroradiological investigation is indicated. Three patients with parasellar or clivus tumours presented with a third nerve palsy in such circumstances, the nerve being stretched over the tumours (Eyster *et al.* 1972).

Infection is the next most common cause. Thirteen of 147 cases of bacterial meningitis caused by *Haemophilus influenzae*, *Neisseria meningitidis* and *Streptococcus pneumoniae* had third nerve palsies (a different 13 had sixth nerve palsies), all of which recovered fully on treatment, unlike nerve deafness in meningitis (Dodge & Swartz 1965). Other infectious agents described include varicella (Sharf & Hyams 1972) in which the pupil may be in-volved, infectious mononucleosis (Nellhaus 1966) and tuberculosis.

Tumours may present as an isolated third nerve palsy; this has been described in brain stem glioma, which accounts for 10% of all central nervous system tumours in childhood. Other tumours presenting with the third nerve palsy include craniopharyngioma (Hoff & Patterson 1972), leptomeningeal sarcoma (Miller 1976) and as a complication of enlargement of the third ventricle associated with intracranial tumour (Osher *et al.* 1978). Although intracranial aneurysms can occur in early childhood (Matson 1965; Patel & Richardson 1971), the earliest published age at which posterior communicating artery aneurysm (Fig. 66.21) has caused isolated, pupil involved, third nerve palsies is 14 years. Angiography to exclude aneurysm is not justified below the age of 10. Sphenoid sinus mucocoele (Fig. 66.22a) and orbital tumours (Fig. 66.2b,c) are rare causes.

Charcot coined the phrase 'ophthalmoplegic migraine' in 1890, and large numbers of cases were described by Möbius and Ehlers (Alpers & Yaskin 1951). These early cases were diagnosed clinically, however, and it is now clear that the symptoms and signs can result from many causes, so that full examination and neuroimaging is mandatory. The condition presents with pain in or above the eye, sometimes with vomiting, for 24–48 hours; as the pain lessens, a third nerve palsy develops over the next 24–48 hours. The palsy recovers over the next 3 days to 1 month (Bickerstaff 1964). The condition may be recurrent, either on the same or opposite side; the first attack almost always occurs before the age of 12, and it is more common in boys than girls. It may persist into adult life. There may be a family history of migraine and it has also been described in siblings (Van Pelt & Andermann 1964). The first attack may be in infancy (see Fig. 66.19).

The aetiology is uncertain; carotid angiography following the onset of the palsy has been described as normal (Alpers & Yaskin 1951) or showing narrowing of the intracavernous carotid artery (Walsh & O'Doherty 1960). It has been suggested that the intracavernous vasa nervorum to

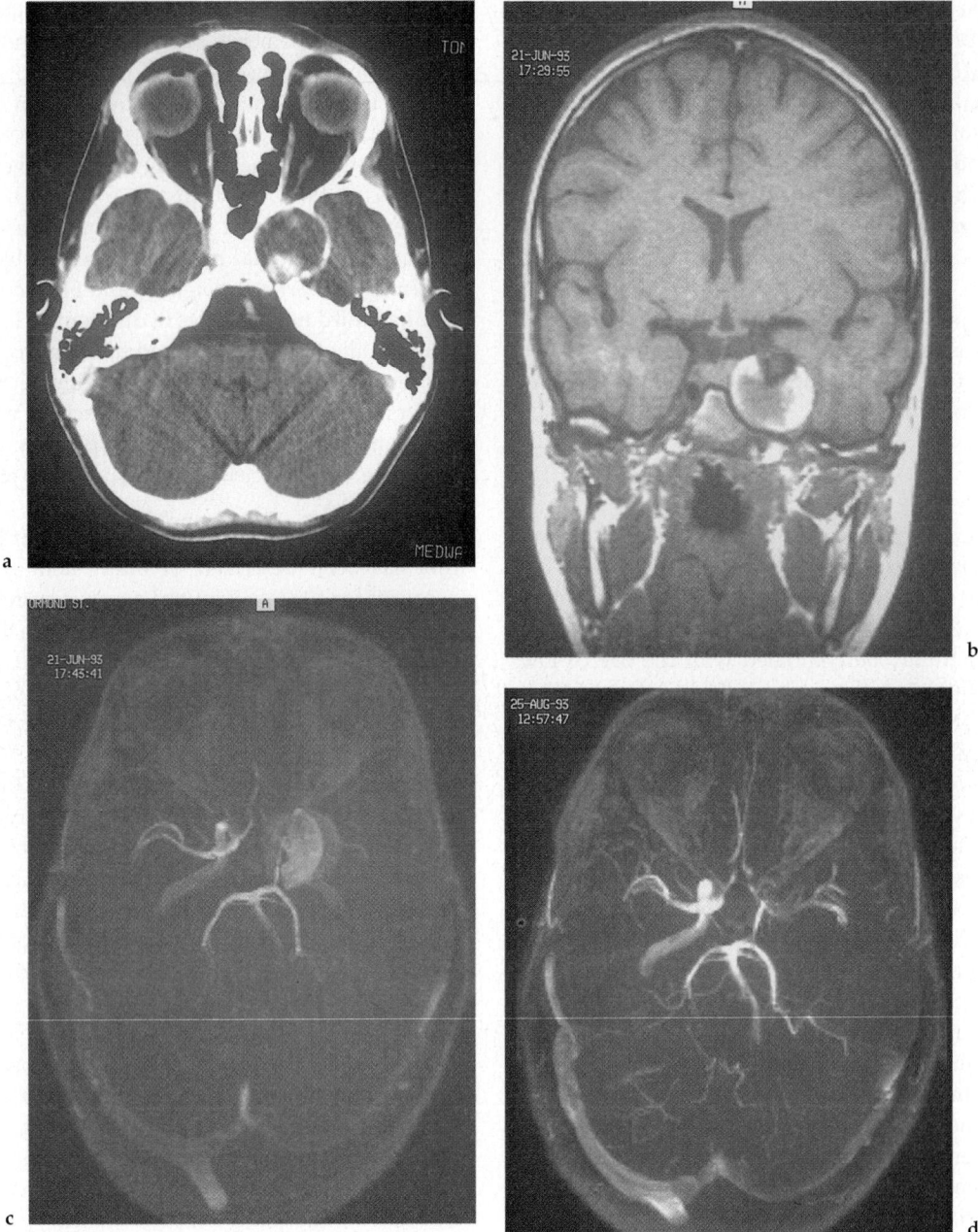

Fig. 66.21 (a, b) Right third nerve palsy associated with a large anterior communicating artery aneurysm in a 7-year-old child. (c) MRI angiography of the same case. (d) MRI angiography following balloon occlusion.

the third nerve are in spasm or blocked, that the nerve is compressed by oedema of the intracavernous carotid, or that the increased cerebral volume that may accompany migraine compresses the nerve (Harrington & Flocks 1953). The recognition of the development of oculomotor synkinesis after migrainous ophthalmoplegia (O'Day *et al.* 1980) supports the suggestion of a peripheral (probably microvascular) aetiology. Gadolinium-enhanced MRI in

one case showed a lesion of the third nerve at its point of exit from the brain stem (Strommel *et al.* 1993).

Despite extensive investigation including arteriography and CT scanning, some cases of acquired third nerve palsy in childhood remain unexplained (Mizen *et al.* 1985). Characteristically, there is no recovery of function in these cases. Repeat MRI at approximately 2-yearly intervals is recommended in these cases. In five patients a mass (schwannoma or meningioma) was subsequently demonstrated after initial investigations were negative (Abdul-Rahim *et al.* 1989).

The pattern of recovery in acquired third nerve palsy depends largely on the cause, and varies from complete,

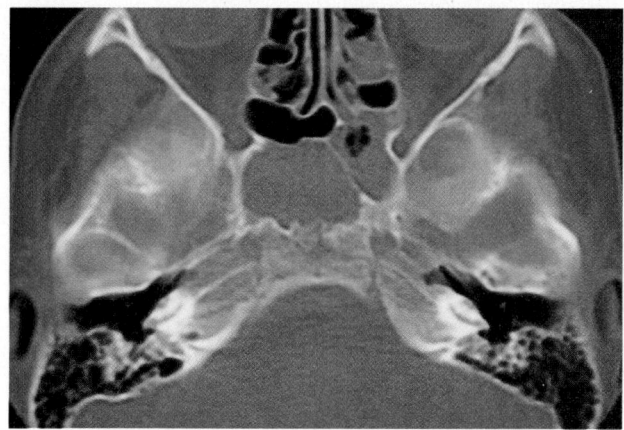

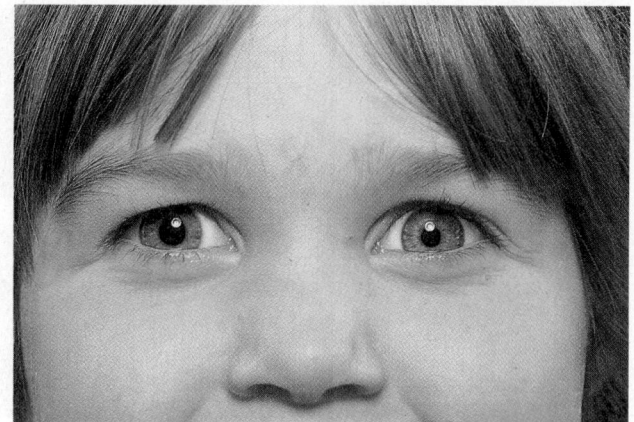

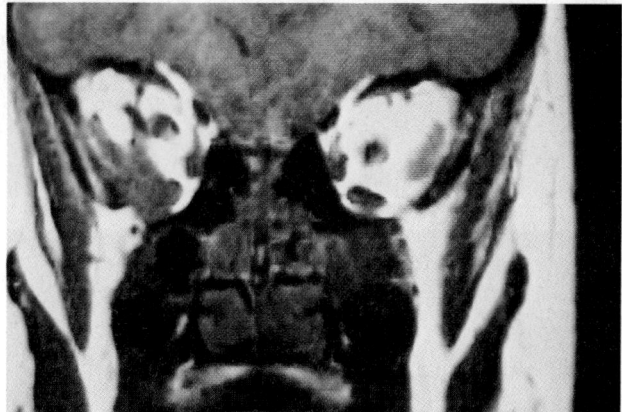

Fig. 66.22 (a) Sphenoid sinus mucocoele associated with third nerve palsy. (b) Congenital right third nerve palsy associated with an inferior orbital tumour probably a neuroma. (c) CT scan showing inferior orbital tumour on the right. The condition remained unchanged over 12 years.

to incomplete with or without oculomotor synkinesis or, if the onset was in infancy, cyclic spasm. Isolated bilateral third nerve palsy has been described due to a mesencephalic haematoma from a cavernous angioma (Getenet *et al.* 1994).

Management

The management is primarily that of the underlying cause. Occlusion treatment may be necessary to prevent or treat amblyopia. Spontaneous recovery must be allowed for before surgery is contemplated, and stable orthoptic measurements for at least 6 months must be obtained. The operation needed will depend on the extent of recovery, and whether or not there is a vertical as well as horizontal component. In cases with oculomotor synkinesis and lid elevation in adduction, the abnormal lid movements can be used to advantage, by recessing the lateral and resecting the medial rectus of the contralateral (normal) eye. This effectively treats both the horizontal strabismus and the ptosis on the affected side. Unusually large recessions and resections are usually required when surgery is on the affected eye.

Fourth nerve

Congenital palsy

Congenital superior oblique underaction may be due to a variety of causes. Some cases are undoubtedly innervational in origin (congenital fourth nerve palsy) but Helveston has drawn attention to the importance of anatomical factors in many cases (Helveston *et al.* 1992). The superior oblique tendon may be found at operation to be redundant, misdirected, inserted into posterior Tenon's capsule or even absent. Orbital anatomical variations may also cause superior oblique underaction by altering the balance of the vertically acting muscles in adduction, for example in plagiocephaly. Patients with Goldenhar's syndrome may have a congenital fourth nerve palsy due to agenesis of the nucleus (Aleksic *et al.* 1976).

Congenital superior oblique underaction or fourth nerve palsy becomes apparent when the infant is old enough to have developed head control (2–4 months). It is usually unilateral. The characteristic turn and tilt of the head away from the side of the lesion is then adopted in the interests of binocularity. The demonstration of a vertical strabismus when the head is straightened, and elevation of the affected eye when the head is tilted to that side

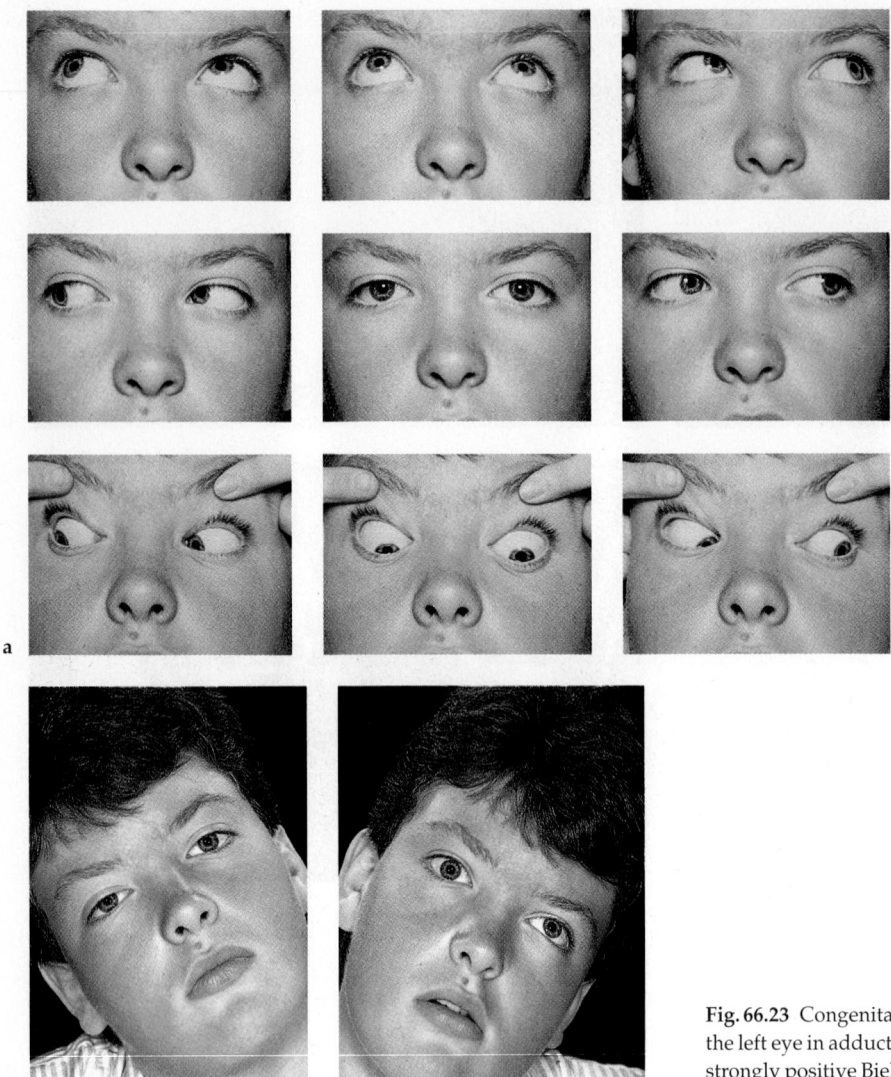

a

b

Fig. 66.23 Congenital fourth nerve palsy showing (a) elevation of the left eye in adduction and weak depression in adduction and (b) a strongly positive Bielschowsky head tilt test. (c, d) The improvement following a 14 mm recession of the left inferior oblique.

in the Beilschowsky head tilt test (Fig. 66.23) are possible by the age of 6 months (Reynolds *et al.* 1984). The differential diagnoses of upshoot of the eye in adduction include inferior oblique overaction, dissociated vertical deviation, Duane's syndrome and contralateral superior rectus underaction when fixing with the paretic eye.

Adults with congenital unilateral superior oblique palsy commonly have facial asymmetry due to hypodevelopment on the contralateral side (Wilson & Hoxie 1993); it may be that the facial asymmetry develops as a consequence of the palsy, rather than the two developing as the result of a common developmental abnormality (Paysee *et al.* 1995). It is possible that eye muscle surgery in childhood to correct an abnormal head posture may prevent or reduce facial asymmetry. Congenital superior oblique palsy 'plus' consists of the palsy with facial asymmetry, ptosis, amblyopia and horizontal strabismus (Helveston *et al.* 1992). Congenital absence of the superior oblique tendon is suggested by a large hypertropia in the primary position with amblyopia and horizontal strabismus (Wallace & Von Noorden 1994).

The differential diagnosis of torticollis in infancy includes disorders of the sternomastoid and cervical spine, hemianopias and other eye movement disorders such as nystagmus, oculomotor apraxia, and Brown's and Duane's syndromes.

When the child is old enough to allow full eye movement testing, the underaction of the superior oblique and overaction of ipsilateral inferior oblique and contralateral inferior rectus become evident. A large vertical fusion range will be demonstrable.

Some apparently unilateral cases are in fact bilateral (Reynolds *et al.* 1984). Scott and Kraft (1986) found that a third of their cases were bilateral, but often highly asymmetric, with the lesser affected eye masked by the contralateral hypertropia. The greater the degree of excyclotorsion, the greater the likelihood of it being bilateral (Kraft *et al.* 1993).

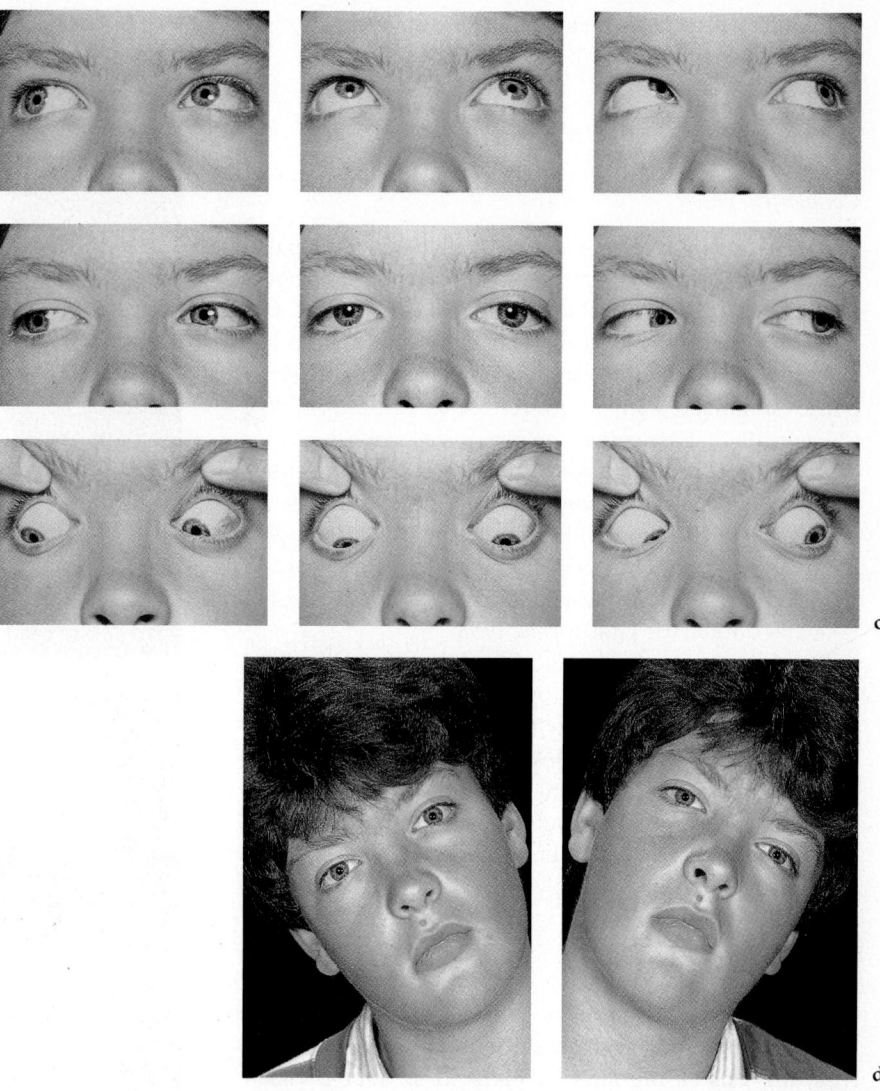

Fig. 66.23 *Continued.*

Management

Provided the child remains binocular and does not have a gross head posture, surgical treatment can be delayed until it is possible to assess the visual system fully orthoptically. There may, however, be a case for early surgery to prevent secondary facial asymmetry (Goodman *et al.* 1995). The indications for surgery are an anomalous head posture, asthenopia or vertical/torsional diplopia. If the tendon is found to be redundant or lax at operation, a superior oblique tuck should be carried out (Morris *et al.* 1992). Otherwise an ipsilateral inferior oblique recession is the best treatment. Sometimes contralateral inferior rectus recession is required. Bilateral cases need to be detected and treated with bilateral surgery in the first instance (Kushner 1988).

Acquired palsy

Acquired fourth nerve palsy may be unilateral or bilateral;

the physical signs, apart from underaction of the superior oblique muscles, consist of a V pattern of eye movement with esotropia, and increasing excyclotorsion in downgaze. Patients therefore adopt a head posture of chin depression to achieve binocularity. The differential diagnoses include alternating skew deviation, in which a vertical strabismus, with the adducting eye higher, develops on lateral gaze, and the V pattern due to bilateral inferior oblique 'overaction' seen in concomitant strabismus (see above). A positive Bielschowsky head tilt test to right and left and a large cyclotropia are indicators of bilaterality.

The most common cause is closed head trauma; if there is no history of trauma, full neurological examination and investigation is indicated, since posterior fossa tumours may present this way. Surgical treatment must be deferred until spontaneous recovery has stopped; bilateral advancement of the anterior half of the superior oblique tendons corrects the excyclotorsion and increases depression in adduction, reducing the V pattern. A bilateral palsy is frequently asymmetric.

An inferior rectus recession on the less severely affected side may be required.

Sixth nerve

Congenital palsy

The most common form of congenital lateral rectus palsy is Duane's syndrome, considered in more detail above. Diagnostic features include familial occurrence and increased frequency in girls than boys, and on the left rather than right side. Transient unilateral lateral rectus palsies in newborn infants were first recognized in 1962 (Benson 1962). Subsequent reports have established that the condition is benign and not associated with either other neurological or developmental abnormalities, or strabismus in childhood (Elston & Timms 1992). It may be relatively common, but not often detected (Reisner *et al.* 1971) with figures of one in 182 and one in 124 normal neonates quoted (de Grauw *et al.* 1983).

Typically the pregnancy is normal, but the delivery is more likely to have been by forceps than in normal neonates. The full recovery with normal binocularity suggests that it is a peripheral lesion. Normal neonates who show this abnormality should have a full medical and neurological examination, but if this is normal, they may not need further investigation, and should be treated expectantly.

Acquired palsy

Dependent on the age of the child, acquired abduction deficit in childhood will present with a head turn away from the palsied muscle (if unilateral) or double vision (unilateral or bilateral palsies), worse for distance fixation. The child may not complain of double vision, but be seen to shut one eye, for example when watching television. Alternatively, parents may notice the sudden onset of a convergent strabismus. Associated symptoms such as headache, drowsiness or earache may give important aetiological clues.

The majority of acquired sixth nerve palsies in childhood are due to trauma (42%) and with basal skull fracture there may be associated signs such as facial palsy (Fig. 66.24) or deafness. The next most common single cause is neoplasm (16%) but only exceptionally rarely is an isolated sixth nerve palsy the presenting sign. In Kodski and Younge's series of 18 cases due to neoplasm, 15 had other neurological signs whilst two of the three others were known to have metastatic malignant disease. However, two cases of isolated sixth nerve palsy in girls aged 7 and 13, spontaneously resolving then recurring, were found subsequently to be due to clivus chordoma (Volpe & Lessel 1993). Pontine glioma is the most common neoplasm (Fig. 66.25) and lateral rectus palsy (with other

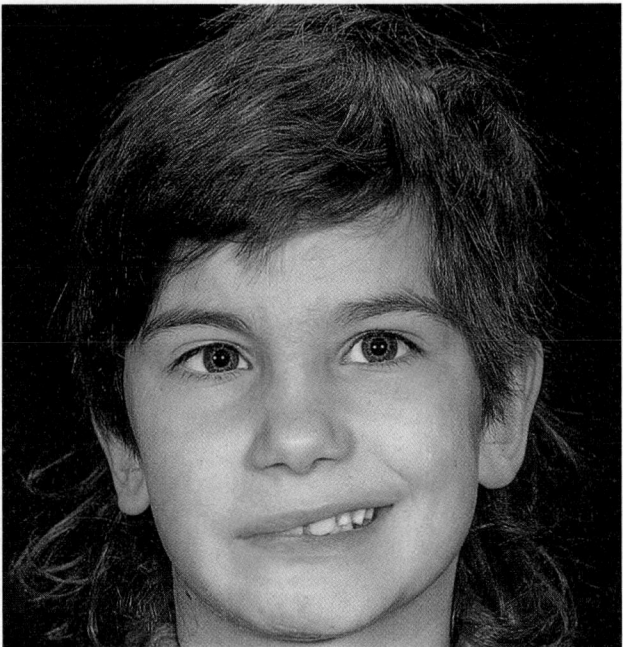

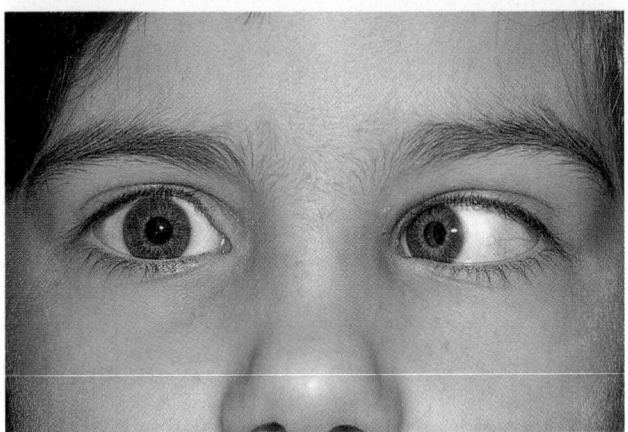

Fig. 66.24 Traumatic right sixth and seventh nerve palsy.

signs) is the most common presentation of this tumour, which occurs at an average age of 6.5 years. Brain stem gliomas are amongst the most common central nervous system tumours of childhood and adolescence (Panitch & Berg 1970) and may produce unilateral or bilateral sixth nerve palsy, rarely a third nerve palsy. Benedikt's syndrome (third nerve palsy with contralateral ataxia and tremor due to destruction of the cerebello-rubrothalamic tract) or Weber's syndrome (third nerve palsy with contralateral hemiparesis) may develop. The abduction deficit is usually progressive, and may evolve into a gaze palsy (Bucy & Keplinger 1959). Pyramidal signs and other cranial nerve palsies, most frequently facial palsy, develop thereafter (Bray *et al.* 1958). Thirty-five per cent of cases develop papilloedema at some stage. By contrast, metastatic neuroblastoma, which may cause an isolated lateral rectus palsy in its early stages, presents in children

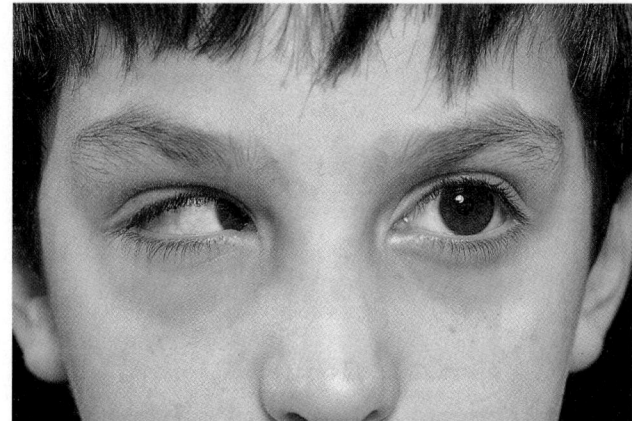

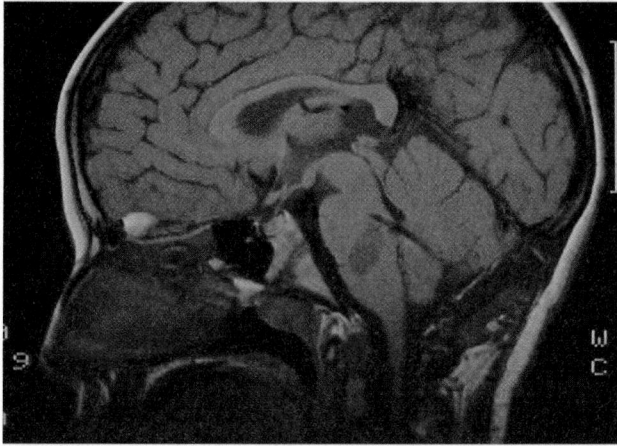

Fig. 66.25 (a) This 10-year-old boy had had strabismus surgery as an infant and was well controlled for many years but the squint deteriorated and it became evident that he had a sixth nerve palsy on the left. This was associated with a brain stem glioma (b).

under the age of 3 years. Other primary intracranial tumours, in the posterior fossa particularly, may present with raised intracranial pressure which produces papilloedema and bilateral abduction deficit (Fig. 66.26). In these cases, as with third nerve palsy, minor head trauma may precipitate the palsy (Robertson *et al.* 1970; Chrousos *et al.* 1993). A lateral rectus palsy has been described as the presenting sign in orbital rhabdomyosarcoma (Sananman & Weintraub 1971).

Raised intracranial pressure is a well-recognized cause of sixth nerve palsy. Benign intracranial hypertension (BIH) can present in childhood, either in its idiopathic form, or secondary to middle ear disease and cerebral venous sinus thrombosis or drugs. Those incriminated include tetracycline (Maroon & Mealy 1971), nalidixic acid (Cohen 1973) and steroids (Cohen 1973). Contrary to previous assumptions, severe permanent visual loss can occur in childhood BIH and treatment should be aggressive (Lessell & Rosman 1986).

'Benign' recurrent sixth nerve palsy

Infection is another relatively common cause of lateral rectus palsy. It occurs in bacterial meningitis (Dodge & Swartz 1965) and has been described in varicella (Nemet *et al.* 1974) and Lyme borreliosis (Packner & Steere 1985). Vascular causes are unusual in the paediatric age group, although an arteriovenous malformation has been incriminated (Robertson *et al.* 1970) and microvascular disease in the second decade (Moster *et al.* 1984).

In some cases, no cause may be established, yet full recovery occurs. Such benign sixth nerve palsies in childhood were first recognized in 1967 (Knox *et al.* 1967) when 12 cases, aged 18 months to 15 years at presentation, were described. The features are now well established: the palsy is isolated, painless and resolves spontaneously within 8–12 weeks. Investigation, including CT and MRI scanning and cerebrospinal fluid examination, is normal. The original cases were described as following a viral illness with fever and upper respiratory tract infection, and accompanying peripheral blood lymphocytosis. Infectious diseases implicated include Epstein–Barr virus, cytomegalovirus and Q fever (Straussberg *et al.* 1993). The condition has also been described following immunization, for example for rubella, rubeola and mumps (Werner *et al.* 1983), or occurring without an identifiable precipitant (Boger *et al.* 1984). It may be recurrent (Bixenman & Von Noorden 1981), usually ipsilaterally (Boger *et al.* 1984), and occur in infants as young as 2.5 months. Episodes may continue into adult life. Recovery may be incomplete especially after multiple recurrences, and extraocular muscle surgery may be necessary (Bixenman & Von Noorden 1981). Amblyopia may develop during the period of palsy, and prophylactic patching is advisable (Scharf & Zonis 1975).

The aetiology is obscure, and both microvascular (arteritic) and primary demyelinating pathologies have been proposed (Werner *et al.* 1983). It is a diagnosis of exclusion that is made retrospectively and after a period of close observation: full neurological examination and investigation are mandatory, as is emphasized by the cases of remitting sixth nerve palsy in skull base tumours noted above.

Amongst other causes of sixth nerve palsy in childhood are those that follow lumbar puncture, and in the older age group, those associated with multiple sclerosis and posterior fossa developmental abnormalities (Bixenman & Laguna 1987).

Management

The management depends on the underlying cause; once this is established by neuroimaging (Bloom *et al.* 1993) and other studies, the natural history becomes clearer, and the extent of spontaneous recovery more predictable.

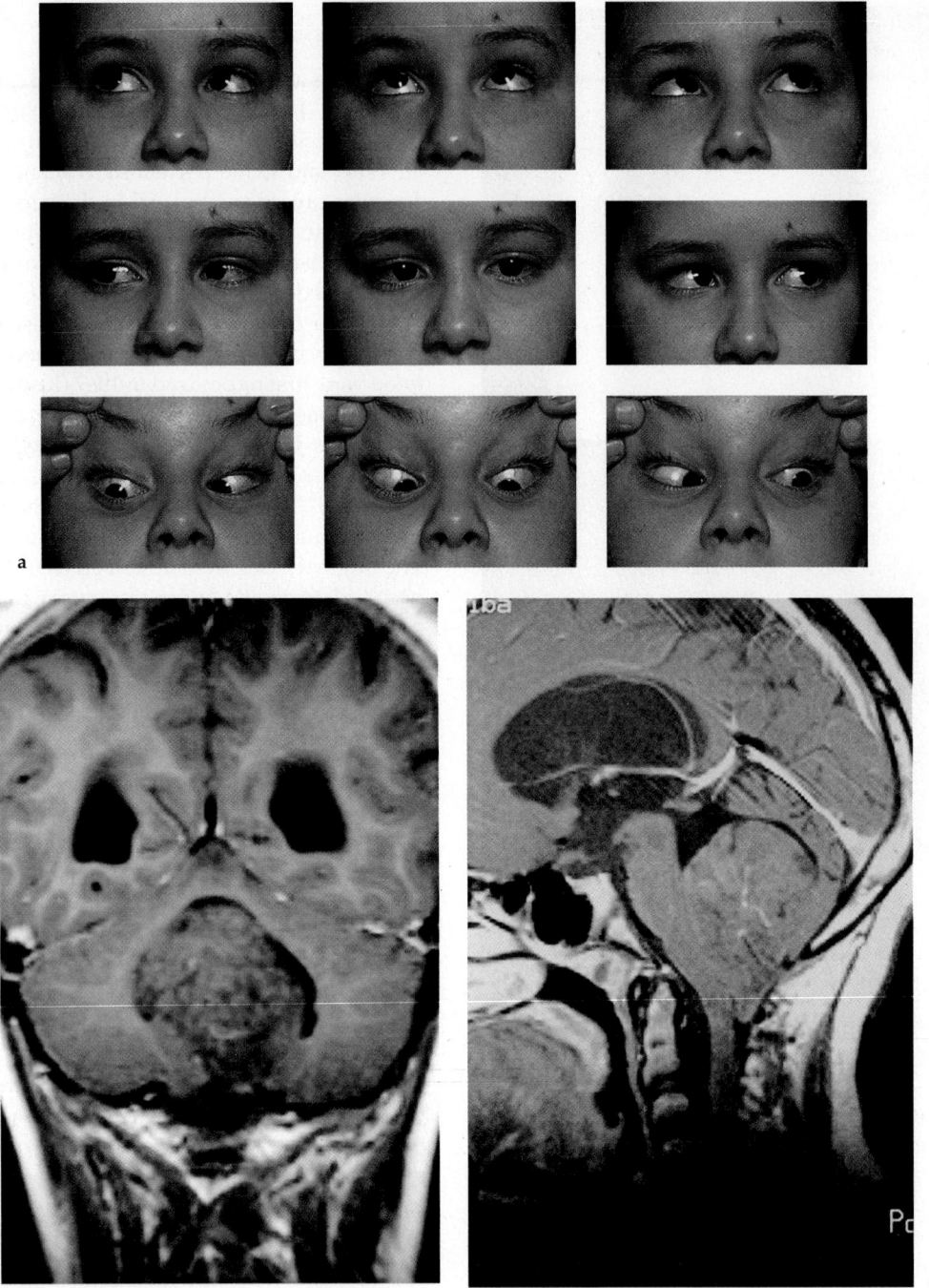

Fig. 66.26 This teenage girl developed intermittent double vision. There was minimal reduction of abduction of the right eye (a) and an esophoria that was greater in the distance than for near. It was associated with hydrocephalus caused by a brain stem ependymoma (b,c).

Patching to prevent amblyopia, or the teaching of a head posture to maintain binocularity may be all that is necessary. In visually immature children, treatment of the ipsilateral medial rectus with botulinum toxin may enable binocularity to be maintained during the period of palsy.

It may also prevent medial rectus contracture and may therefore improve the prospects for full spontaneous recovery. If full recovery does not occur, surgery is necessary; if near full abduction returns, with a normal abducting saccadic velocity but a persistent esotropia, binocularity can be regained either by recession of the medial and resection of the lateral rectus, or by an injection of botulinum toxin into the medial rectus. If an injection is used, a short period of exotropia must be expected (Elston & Lee 1985).

In unrecovered lateral rectus palsy, because of the

secondary overaction of both the ipsilateral and contralateral medial rectus muscles, a large esotropia is produced, and the treatment objective becomes more limited — the re-establishment of binocularity in the primary position and downgaze. It is necessary to redistribute the forces generated by the extraocular muscles on the affected side, and to provide an abducting vector by a full vertical muscle temporal transfer preceded by botulinum injection of the medial rectus. Again a period of exotropia is produced but the eyes may reconverge. If so, one or both medial rectus muscles will need recessing (Fitzsimmons *et al.* 1988).

Combinations of third, fourth and sixth nerve palsies

If isolated ocular motor nerve palsies are rare in childhood, a review of the available literature suggests that combinations of palsies are extremely unusual. Of Kodski and Younge's 160 patients, 18 had multiple oculomotor palsies mostly due to trauma. The differential diagnoses include conditions discussed above and considered in more detail below such as myasthenia gravis and mitochondrial cytopathy.

Miller–Fisher syndrome

The Miller–Fisher variant of Guillain–Barré syndrome consists of ophthalmoplegia, ataxia and areflexia. It may occur in childhood, with the youngest reported case at 22 months (Marks *et al.* 1977). Six of the eight cases of less than 18 years discussed by these authors had internal as well as external ophthalmoplegia, but relative sparing of the levator is characteristic. Increased cerebrospinal fluid protein without cells is characteristic, and in children the condition appears to have a benign course with complete recovery. A specific antiganglioside antibody (GQ1b) is found in the serum of patients with Miller–Fisher syndrome and causes the physical signs. Plasmapheresis to remove the antibody is very helpful in reducing the time course of the disease.

Sphenocavernous sinus syndromes

Combinations of oculomotor palsies are otherwise most commonly due to lesions in the cavernous sinus or superior orbital fissure. Clinical differentiation between these two sites is difficult, and they are best regarded together as the sphenocavernous syndrome. This consists of a third, fourth and sixth nerve palsy with involvement of the first and, in the cavernous sinus, second division of the fifth (trigeminal) nerve. There may also be involvement of the oculosympathetic nerve, and sometimes an optic neuropathy; proptosis may develop. Apart from double vision, pain is often a prominent symptom. Subtle pupillary signs including sinuous pupil reactions and super-sensitivity to 0.1% pilocarpine occur (Slamovits *et al.* 1987).

The sphenocavernous syndrome has been described in childhood most frequently due to rhabdomyosarcoma (Sananaman & Weintraub 1971; Takahashi *et al.* 1982). Other causes include a primary intrasellar germinoma that evolved into a choriocarcinoma (Guiffre & Lorenzo 1975) and histiocytosis-X (Beller & Kornbleuth 1951). The rarity of ocular motor nerve involvement in this condition, however, has been emphasized (Moore *et al.* 1985). Burkitt's lymphoma, which is rare in developed countries, presents at an average age of 11.5 years with abdominal involvement; it has, however, been described as causing bilateral total external ophthalmoplegia by extension from the ethmoid sinus (Trese *et al.* 1980). A craniopharyngioma can rarely invade the cavernous sinus and produce ocular motor palsies (Neetens & Selosse 1977).

Orbital apex syndrome

The orbital apex syndrome differs from the above in presenting with proptosis, optic neuropathy, and (at least initially) mechanical limitation of eye movement. Other signs, such as ocular sympathetic involvement and conjunctival oedema, frequently develop. Secondary neuroblastoma and other metastatic disease (e.g. leukaemia) are the most common causes in childhood.

Neuromuscular disease and incomitant strabismus in infancy and childhood

A number of neuromuscular disorders, including myopathies, muscular dystrophies, mitochondrial cytopathy and myasthenia gravis, may involve the extraocular muscles and levator in infancy and childhood. The differential diagnoses, which may also include the fibrosis syndrome and combinations of third, fourth and sixth nerve palsies, may be difficult and depends on the clinical features and family history as well as muscle enzyme studies, EMG and muscle biopsy.

Congenital and juvenile myopathies

Amongst congenital myopathies, which produce muscle weakness and hypotonia, congenital fibre type disproportion (CFTD) may rarely be associated with exotropia, ophthalmoplegia and ptosis from birth (Owen *et al.* 1981). Centronuclear myopathy, a familial cause of generalized muscle weakness, is consistently associated with ptosis and external ophthalmoplegia in the survivors to the second decade (Bradley *et al.* 1970). Visually insignificant mid-cortical cataracts have also been reported in this condition (Hawkes & Absolon 1975).

The eye movements are normal in both congenital and Duchenne muscular dystrophy, although there may be orbicularis oculi weakness in both (Honda & Yoshioka 1978). Myotonic dystrophy, however, may present in infancy or childhood with either ptosis (including eyelid myotonia) or more often reduced eye movements (Dodge *et al.* 1965). Such cases have been misdiagnosed as Möbius' syndrome; the family history and examination of relatives may be important in making the correct diagnosis.

Freeman–Sheldon syndrome

In the whistling face, or Freeman–Sheldon syndrome, there is a high incidence of strabismus and ptosis; the extraocular muscles are stiff on forced duction testing (O'Keefe *et al.* 1986). The children have many other features attributable to increased muscle tone including a small mouth which may make anaesthesia hazardous.

They are usually of normal intelligence and the inheritance is autosomal dominant.

Mitochondrial cytopathy

Mitochondrial cytopathy has diverse neuromuscular and central nervous system manifestations (Fig. 66.27). The onset is in the first or second decade in the majority of cases, characteristically with progressive external ophthalmoplegia and limb weakness on exertion. Ptosis is also a common presenting symptom (Petty *et al.* 1986). A pigmentary retinopathy is not usually prominent in childhood, but electrodiagnostic studies may be abnormal.

The younger the age at presentation, the more likely the patient is to develop systemic abnormalities such as cardiac conduction defects, generalized hypotonia, cerebel-

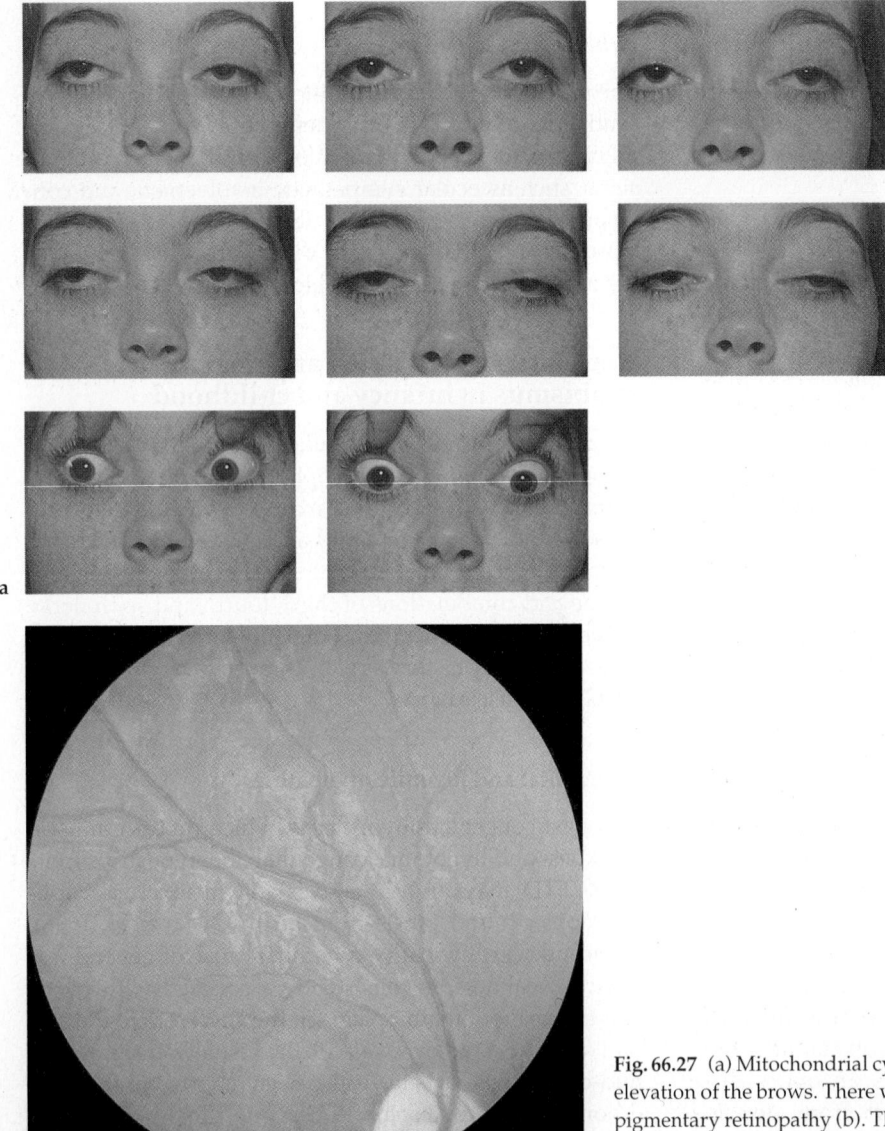

Fig. 66.27 (a) Mitochondrial cytopathy. Bilateral symmetrical ptosis with elevation of the brows. There was poor vision associated with a bilateral pigmentary retinopathy (b). The pigmentary retinopathy in children with this condition is not similar to retinitis pigmentosa but it is usually a granular retinal pigment epithelial disturbance, optic atrophy and vessel thinning.

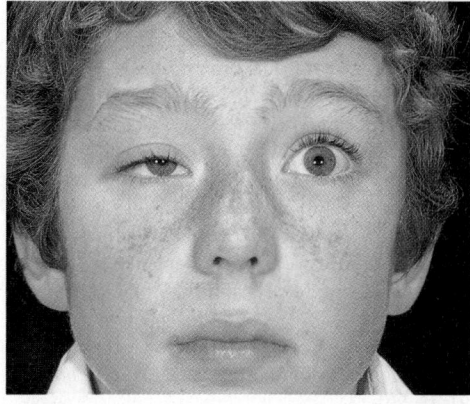

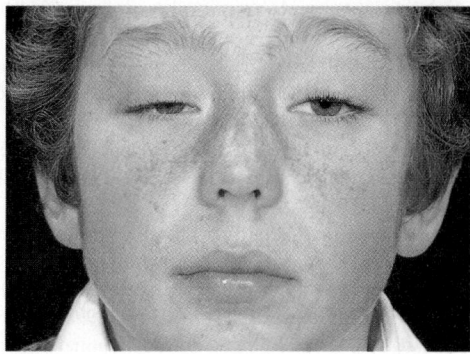

Fig. 66.28 Myasthenia with variable ptosis, squint and orbicularis weakness. Photographs taken 10 minutes apart.

lar ataxia, endocrine abnormalities (e.g. diabetes mellitus) and retinal pigmentation (Mitsumoto *et al.* 1983). A family history suggesting mitochondrial inheritance may be helpful in making the diagnosis. Muscle biopsy (including extraocular muscle biopsy) will show ragged red fibres (Ringel *et al.* 1979).

Myasthenia gravis

Myasthenia gravis is rare in the first decade; neonatal myasthenia, due to cross-placental transfer of anti-acetylcholine receptor antibodies, occurs in approximately one in seven children of myasthenic mothers, and recovers spontaneously in 1–12 weeks. Congenital myasthenia has the same clinical characteristics, but occurs in the absence of antibodies and is more common in boys than girls. It may be inherited as an autosomal recessive trait in some cases. Unlike the juvenile variant (see below) it shows no tendency to remit, and may be due to a different disease process (Simpson 1981).

Juvenile myasthenia, with onset before 17 years (Fig. 66.28), occurs nearly five times more commonly in girls than boys; the spontaneous remission rate is high (30% by 15 years of follow-up) and higher after thymectomy (Rodrigues *et al.* 1983). Diagnosis may be difficult and the initial presentation may suggest concomitant strabis-

mus. A number of children have had extraocular muscle surgery before the diagnosis is made. A battery of diagnostic tests including single fibre EMG, anti-acetylcholine receptor antibodies and Tensilon tests may be required. Rarely, other diseases may produce an ophthalmoplegia; in abetalipoproteinaemia, for example, mild ptosis, and exotropia may be the presenting signs (Yee *et al.* 1976).

Other unusual causes

Thyroid ophthalmopathy

Graves' ophthalmopathy, usually with hyperthyroidism, may present in the second decade with double vision. The management principles are the same as in adults and in general the prognosis is good. Graves' ophthalmopathy and ocular myasthenia gravis may co-exist.

Ocular neuromyotonia

Ocular neuromyotonia consists of short-lived episodes of involuntary ocular muscle contraction usually in third nerve innervated muscles. Most cases follow a period of chronic compressive neuropathy (e.g. by an extending pituitary-based tumour) followed by decompression with variable recovery, then radiotherapy treatment. Neuromyotonia affecting the lateral rectus producing an exotropia with reduced adduction and retraction of the globe has been described in a 7-year-old boy after radiation therapy for a thalamic glioma (Barroso & Hoyt 1993).

Botulism

A variety of combinations of eye muscle and bulbar palsies may occur in botulism (Simcock *et al.* 1994).

Idiopathic congenital eye muscle enlargement

A single case report by Dickson *et al.* (1994) described unilateral congenitally large muscles in a child with a vertical and horizontal strabismus.

Synergistic divergence

This is a congenital defect of adduction with abduction movements of both eyes on attempted gaze into the field of action of the involved side. It may be bilateral (Hamed *et al.* 1992; Thomas *et al.* 1993). It is probably a 'mis-wiring' phenomenon.

References

Abdul-Rahin A, Savino PJ, Zimmerman RA, Sergott RC, Bosley TM. Cryptogenic oculomotor nerve palsy. *Arch Ophthalmol* 1989; **107**: 387–90.

Aleksic S, Budzilovich G, Choy A *et al*. Congenital ophthalmoplegia in oculoauriculo vertebral dysplasia — hemifacial microsomia (Goldenhar–Gorbin syndrome). *Neurology* 1976; **26**: 638–44.

Alpers BJ, Yaskin EH. Pathogenesis of ophthalmoplegic migraine. *Arch Ophthalmol* 1951; **45**: 555–66.

Amaya LG, Walker J, Taylor D. Möbius syndrome: a study and report of 18 cases. *Binocular Vis* 1990; **5**: 119–32.

Appleton RE, Chitayat D, Jan JE, Kennedy R, Hall JG. Joubert's syndrome associated with congenital ocular fibrosis and histidinaemia. *Arch Neurol* 1989; **46**: 579–82.

Apt L, Axelrod RN. Extra-ocular muscle fibrosis. *Am J Ophthalmol* 1978; **85**: 822–9.

Balkan R, Hoyt CS. Associated neurologic abnormalities in congenital third nerve palsies. *Am J Ophthalmol* 1984; **97**: 315–19.

Baraitser M. Genetics of Möbius' syndrome. *J Med Genet* 1977; **14**: 415–17.

Barroso L, Hoyt WF. Episodic exotropia from lateral rectus neuromyotonia — appearance and remission after radiation therapy for a thalamic glioma. *J Ped Ophthalmol Strabismus* 1993; **30**: 56–7.

Baum J. Goldenhar's syndrome. *Arch Ophthalmol* 1992; **110**: 750.

Beller AJ, Kornbleuth W. Eosinophilic granuloma of the orbit. *Br J Ophthalmol* 1951; **35**: 220–5.

Benson PF. Transient unilateral external rectus muscle palsy in newborn infants. *Br Med J* 1962; **1**: 1054–5.

Berkovitz S, Beklin M, Tenenbaum A. Childhood myasthenia gravis. *J Pediatr Ophthalmol* 1977; **14**: 269–73.

Bickerstaff ER. Ophthalmoplegic migraine. *Rev Neurol* 1964; **110**: 582–7.

Biedner B, Monos T, Frilling F, Mozeo M, Yassur Y. Acquired Brown's syndrome caused by frontal sinus osteoma. *J Pediatr Ophthalmol Strabismus* 1988; **25**: 226–30.

Bixenman WW, Laguna JF. Acquired esotropia as initial manifestation of Arnold–Chiari malformation. *J Pediatr Ophthalmol Strabismus* 1987; **24**: 83–6.

Bixenman WW, Von Noorden GK. Benign recurrent sixth nerve palsy in childhood. *J Pediatr Ophthalmol Strabismus* 1981; **18**: 29–34.

Bloom J, Cadera W, Heiberg E, Karlik S. A magnetic resonance imaging study of horizontal rectus muscle palsies. *J Pediatr Ophthalmol Strabismus* 1993; **30**: 296–300.

Bloom JN, Gravis ER, Mardelli PG. A magnetic resonance imaging study of the upshoot–downshoot phenomenon of Duane's retraction syndrome. *Am J Ophthalmol* 1991; **111**: 548–54.

Boger WP, Puliafito CA, Magoon EH, Syndnor CF, Knupp JA, Buckley EG. Recurrent isolated sixth nerve palsy in children. *Ann Ophthalmol* 1984; **16**: 237–44.

Booth-Mason S, Kyle GM, Rossor R, Bradbury P. Acquired Brown's syndrome: an unusual cause. *Br J Ophthalmol* 1985; **69**: 791–4.

Bouwes Bavinck JN, Weaver JD. Subclavian artery supply disruption sequence: hypothesis of a vascular aetiology for Poland, Klippel–Feil and Möbius' anomalies. *Am J Med Genet* 1986; **23**: 903–18.

Bradbury JA, Martin L, Strachan IM. Acquired Brown's syndrome associated with Hurler–Scheie's syndrome. *Br J Ophthalmol* 1989; **73**: 305–9.

Bradley WG, Price DL, Watanabe CK. Familial centronuclear myopathy. *J Neurol Neurosurg Psych* 1970; **33**: 687–93.

Bradshaw DJ, Bray VJ, Enzenaver RW, Enzenaver RJ, Truwit CL, Damiano TR. Acquired Brown syndrome associated with enteropathic arthropathy: a case report. *J Pediatr Ophthalmol Strabismus* 1993; **31**: 118–19.

Bray PF, Carter S, Taveras JM. Brainstem tumours in children. *Neurology* 1958; **8**: 1–7.

Brodsky MC, Fritz KJ, Carney SH. Iatrogenic inferior rectus palsy. *J Pediatr Ophthalmol Strabismus* 1992; **29**: 113–15.

Brodsky MC, Pollok SC, Buckley EG. Neural misdirection in congenital ocular fibrosis syndrome: implications and pathogenesis. *J Pediatr Ophthalmol Strabismus* 1989; **26**: 159–61.

Brown HW. True and simulated superior oblique tendon sheath syndromes. *Doc Ophthalmol* 1973; **34**: 123–36.

Bucy PC, Keplinger JE. Tumours of the brain stem with special reference to ocular manifestations. *Arch Ophthalmol* 1959; **62**: 541–54.

Burke JP, Ruben JB, Scott WE. Vertical transposition of the horizontal recti (Knapp procedure) for the treatment of double elevator palsy: effectiveness and long-term stability. *Br J Ophthalmol* 1992; **76**: 734–7.

Castanera de Molina A, Munos LG. Brown syndrome associated with contralateral superior oblique palsy. *J Pediatr Ophthalmol Strabismus* 1991; **28**: 310–13.

Catford GV. A familial musculo-fascial anomaly. *Trans Ophthalmol Soc UK* 1966; **86**: 19–36.

Cheng H, Burdon MA, Shun-Shin GA, Czypionka S. Dissociated eye movements in craniosynostosis: a hypothesis revised. *Br J Ophthalmol* 1993; **77**: 563–8.

Chew CKS, Foster P, Hurst JA, Salmon JF. Duane's retraction syndrome associated with chromosome 4q27–31 segment deletion. *Am J Ophthalmol* 1995; **119**: 807–9.

Christiansen S, Thomas A. Postpartum Brown's syndrome. *Arch Ophthalmol* 1994; **112**: 23–5.

Chrousos G, Dipaolo F, Kattah J, Laws E. Paresis of the abducens nerve after trivial head injury. *Am J Ophthalmol* 1993; **116**: 387–8.

Cibis GW, Tripathi RC, Tripathi BJ, Seidel FG. Familial total ophthalmoplegia with iris transillumination. *Am J Ophthalmol* 1992; **113**: 443–6.

Cohen DN. Intracranial hypertension and papilloedema associated with nalidixic acid therapy. *Am J Ophthalmol* 1973; **76**: 680–2.

Cohn GA. Pseudotumour cerebri in children secondary to administration of adrenal steroids. *J Neurosurg* 1963; **20**: 784–6.

Colins A, Baraitser M, Pembrey M. Okihiro syndrome: thenar hypoplasia and Duane anomaly in three generations. *Clin Dysmorphol* 1993; **2**: 237–40.

Coyle TJ. In reply: Goldenhar's syndrome. *Arch Ophthalmol* 1992; **110**: 750.

Crawford JS. Congenital fibrosis syndrome. *Can J Ophthalmol* 1970; **5**: 331–6.

Cross HE, Pfaffenback DD. Duane's retraction syndrome and associated congenital abnormalities. *Am J Ophthalmol* 1972; **73**: 442–50.

Cullen P, Rodgers CS, Callen DF *et al*. Association of familial Duane anomaly and urogenital abnormality in bi-satellited marker derived from chromosome 22. *Am J Med Genet* 1993; **47**: 925–30.

de Grauw AJC, Rotteveel JJ, Cruysberg JRM. Transient sixth cranial nerve paralysis in the newborn infant. *Neuropediatrics* 1983; **14**: 164–5.

De Respinis PA, Caputo AR, Wagner RS, Guo S. Duane's retraction syndrome. *Surv Ophthalmol* 1993; **38**: 257–88.

Dickson J, Kraft S, Jay V, Blaser S. A case of unilateral congenitally enlarged extraocular muscles. *Ophthalmology* 1994; **101**: 1902–7.

Dobler A, Sondhi N, Cantor L, Ku S. Acquired Brown's syndrome after a double-plate Molteno implant. *Am J Ophthalmol* 1993; **116**: 641–2.

Dodge PK, Gamsford I, Byers RK, Russell P. Myotonic dystrophy in infancy and childhood. *Paediatrics* 1965; **35**: 3–19.

Dodge PK, Swartz MN. Bacterial meningitis — a review of selected aspects. *N Engl J Med* 1965; **272**: 954–60.

Duane A. Congenital deficiency of abduction, associated with impairment of adduction, retraction movements, contraction of the palpebral fissure and oblique movements of the eye. *Arch Oph-*

thalmol 1905; **34**: 133–59.

Dulley B, Fells P. Long-term follow-up of orbital blow-out fractures with and without surgery. In: Ravault AP, Lenz M, eds. *Orbital Disorder, Proceedings of the Second International Symposium*, Vol. 14. Basel: Karger, 1975: 467–70.

Elsas FJ. Occult Duane's syndrome: co-contraction revealed following strabismus surgery. *J Pediatr Ophthalmol Strabismus* 1991; **28**: 328–32.

Elston JS. Traumatic third nerve palsy. *Br J Ophthalmol* 1984; **68**: 538–43.

Elston JS, Lee JP. Paralytic strabismus: the role of botulinium toxin. *Br J Ophthalmol* 1985; **69**: 891–6.

Elston JS, Timms C. Clinical evidence for the onset of the sensitive period in man. *Br J Ophthalmol* 1992; **76**: 327–8.

Engle EC, Kunkel LM, Specht LA, Beggs AH. Mapping a gene for congenital fibrosis of the extraocular muscles to the centromeric region of chromosome 12. *Nature Genet* 1994; **7**: 69–73.

Eyster EP, Hoyt WF, Wilson CB. Oculomotor palsy from minor head trauma. *J Am Med Assoc* 1972; **220**: 1982–6.

Fells P, Collin JRO. Cyclic oculomotor palsy. *Trans Ophthalmol Soc UK* 1979; **99**: 192–6.

Fells P, Waddell E, Alvarez M. Progressive, exaggerated A pattern strabismus with presumed fibrosis of extraocular muscles. In: Reinecke RD, ed. *Strabismus II: Proceedings of the Fourth Meeting of the International Strabismological Association.* Orlando: Grune & Stratton, 1984: 335–43.

Firth HV, Boyd PA, Chamberlain P, MacKenzie IZ, Lindenbaum RH, Huson SM. Severe limb abnormalities after chorion villus sampling at 56–66 days gestation. *Lancet* 1991; **337**: 762–3.

Firth HV, Boyd PA, Chamberlain PF, MacKenzie IZ, Morris-Kay GM, Huson SM. Analysis of limb reduction defects in babies exposed to chorion villus sampling. *Lancet* 1994; **343**: 1069–71.

Fitzsimmons R, Lee JP, Elston JS. Treatment of unrecovered sixth nerve palsy with combined botulinium toxin chemodenervation and surgery. *Ophthalmology* 1988; **95**: 1535–42.

Friedman DI, Wright KW, Sadun AH. Oculomotor palsy with cyclic spasms. *Neurology* 1989; **39**: 1263–4.

Getenet J-C, Vignetto A, Nighoghossian N, Trouillas P. Isolated bilateral third nerve palsy caused by a mesencephalic hematoma. *Neurology* 1994; **44**: 981–2.

Gillies WE, Harris AJ, Brooks AMV, Rivers MR, Wolfe RJB. Congenital fibrosis of the vertically acting extraocular muscles: a new group of dominantly inherited ocular fibrosis with radiologic findings. *Ophthalmology* 1995; **102**: 607–12.

Gobin MH. Surgical management of Duane's syndrome. *Br J Ophthalmol* 1974; **58**: 301–6.

Good WV, Barkovich AJ, Nickel BL, Hoyt CS. Bilateral congenital oculomotor nerve palsy in a child with brain abnormalities. *Am J Ophthalmol* 1991; **111**: 555–8.

Goodman CR, Chabner E, Guyton DL. Should early strabismus surgery be performed for ocular torticollis to prevent facial asymmetry? *J Pediatr Ophthalmol Strabismus* 1995; **32**: 162–6.

Gottlob I, Catalano RA, Reinecke RD. Surgical management of oculomotor nerve palsy. *Am J Ophthalmol* 1991; **111**: 71–6.

Gourdeao A, Miller N, Zee D, Morris J. Central oculomotor abnormalities in Duane's retraction syndrome. *Arch Ophthalmol* 1981; **99**: 1809–10.

Guiffre R, Lorenzo ND. Evolution of a primary intrasellar germinomatous teratoma into a choriocarcinoma. *J Neurosurg* 1975; **42**: 602–4.

Guy J, Engel HM, Lessner AM. Acquired contralateral oculomotor synkinesis. *Arch Neurol* 1989; **46**: 1021–3.

Hamed LM. Associated neurologic and ophthalmologic findings in congenital oculomotor palsy. *Ophthalmology* 1991a; **98**: 708–14.

Hamed LM. Bilateral Brown syndrome in three siblings. *J Pediatr Ophthalmol Strabismus* 1991b; **28**: 306–9.

Hamed LM, Lingua RW, Farous MM, Saunders TG, Lusby FW. Synergistic divergence: saccadic velocity analysis and surgical results. *J Pediatr Ophthalmol Strabismus* 1992; **29**: 30–7.

Hanson PA, Rowland LP. Möbius' syndrome and facio–scapulohumeral dystrophy. *Arch Neurol* 1971; **24**: 31–9.

Harley RD, Rodrigues MM, Crawford JS. Congenital fibrosis of the extraocular muscles. *J Pediatr Ophthalmol Strabismus* 1978; **15**: 346–58.

Harrington DO, Flocks M. Ophthalmoplegic migraine. *Arch Ophthalmol* 1953; **40**: 643–55.

Hawkes CH, Absolon MJ. Myotubular myopathy associated with cataract and electrical myotonia. *J Neurol Neurosurg Psych* 1975; **38**: 761–4.

Hayes A, Costa T, Polomeno RC. The Okihiro syndrome of Duane anomaly, radial ray abnormalities and deafness. *Am J Med Genet* 1985; **22**: 273–80.

Helveston EM, Krach D, Plager DA, Ellis FD. A new classification of superior oblique palsy based on congenital variations in the tendon. *Ophthalmology* 1992; **99**: 1609–15.

Henderson JL. The congenital facial diplegia syndrome: clinical features, pathology and aetiology. *Brain* 1939; **62**: 381–403.

Herman JS. Acquired Brown's syndrome of inflammatory origin. *Arch Ophthalmol* 1978; **96**: 1228–9.

Hertle RW, Katowitz JA, Young TL, Quinn GE, Forbes MG. Congenital unilateral fibrosis, blepharoptosis and enophthalmos syndrome. *Ophthalmology* 1992; **99**: 347–55.

Hiatt RL, Halle AA. General fibrosis syndrome. *Ann Ophthalmol* 1983; **15**: 1103–10.

Hoff JT, Patterson RH. Craniopharyngiomas in children and adults. *J Neurosurg* 1972; **36**: 299–302.

Holzman AE, Chrousos GA, Kozma C, Traboulsi EI. Duane's retraction syndrome in the fetal alcohol syndrome. *Am J Ophthalmol* 1990; **110**: 564–5.

Honda Y, Yoshioka M. Ophthalmological findings in muscular dystrophies: a survey of 53 cases. *J Pediatr Ophthalmol Strabismus* 1978; **15**: 236–8.

Hotchkiss MD, Miller NR, Clark AW, Green WR. Bilateral Duane's retraction syndrome: a clinicopathologic case report. *Arch Ophthalmol* 1980; **98**: 870–4.

Houtman WA, van Weeden TW, Robinson PH, de Vries B, Hoogenraad TU. Hereditary congenital external ophthalmoplegia. *Ophthalmologica* 1986; **193**: 207–18.

Hoyt WF, Nachtigaler H. Anomalies of ocular motor nerves. *Am J Ophthalmol* 1965; **70**: 443–8.

Huber A. Electrophysiology of the retraction syndromes. *Br J Ophthalmol* 1974; **58**: 293–300.

Ing EB, Sullivan TJ, Clarke MP, Buncic JR. Oculomotor nerve palsies in children. *J Pediatr Ophthalmol Strabismus* 1992; **29**: 331–6.

Isenberg S, Urist MJ. Clinical observations in 101 consecutive patients with Duane's retraction syndrome. *Am J Ophthalmol* 1977; **84**: 419–25.

Jamal GA, Ballantyne JP. The localization of the lesion in patients with acute ophthalmoplegia, ataxia and areflexia (Miller–Fisher syndrome). *Brain* 1988; **111**: 95–114.

Jampel RS, Fells P. Monocular elevation palsy caused by a central nervous system lesion. *Arch Ophthalmol* 1968; **80**: 45–57.

Jay W, Hoyt CS. Abnormal brain stem auditory evoked potentials in Stilling–Turk–Duane's retraction syndrome. *Am J Ophthalmol* 1980; **89**: 814–18.

Kaban T, Smith K, Orton R, Noel L, Clarke W, Candera W. Natural history of presumed congenital Brown syndrome. *Arch Ophthalmol* 1993; **111**: 943–6.

Kalpakian B, Bateman BJ, Sparkes RS, Wood GK. Congenital ocular fibrosis syndrome associated with the Prader–Willi syndrome. *J Pediatr Ophthalmol Strabismus* 1986; **23**: 170–3.

Kawai M, Momoi T, Fuji T, Nakano S, Itagaki Y, Mikawa H. The syndrome of Möbius' sequence, peripheral neuropathy, and hypogonadotrophic hypogonadism. *Am J Med Genet* 1990; **37**: 578–82.

Keane JR. Third nerve palsy due to penetrating trauma. *Neurology* 1993; **43**: 1523–7.

Kirkham TH. Duane's syndrome and familial perceptive deafness. *Br J Ophthalmol* 1969; **53**: 335–9.

Kirkham TH. Inheritance of Duane's syndrome. *Br J Ophthalmol* 1970; **54**: 323–9.

Kirkham TH, Bird AC, Sanders MD. Divergence paralysis with raised intracranial pressure. *Br J Ophthalmol* 1972; **56**: 776–82.

Kishore K, Kumar H. Congenital ocular fibrosis with musculoskeletal abnormality: a new association. *J Pediatr Ophthalmol Strabismus* 1991; **28**: 283–6.

Knox DL, Clark DB, Schuster FF. Benign sixth nerve palsies in children. *Pediatrics* 1967; **40**: 560–4.

Kodsi S, Younge B. Acquired oculomotor trochlea and abducent cranial nerve palsies in pediatric patients. *Am J Ophthalmol* 1992; **114**: 568–74.

Kommerell G, Mehdorn E, Ketelsen UP, Vollrath-Junger CH. Oculomotor palsy with cyclic spasms. *Neuro-ophthalmology* 1988; **8**: 9–22.

Kraft SP. A surgical approach for Duane's syndrome. *J Pediatr Ophthalmol Strabismus* 1988; **25**: 119–31.

Kraft SP, O'Donoghue EP, Roarty JD. Improvement of compensatory head postures after strabismus surgery. *Ophthalmology* 1992; **99**: 1301–8.

Kraft S, O'Reilly C, Quigley P, Allan K, Eustis H. Cyclotorsion in unilateral and bilateral superior oblique paresis. *J Pediatr Ophthalmol Strabismus* 1993; **30**: 361–7.

Kushner BJ. The diagnosis and treatment of bilateral masked superior oblique palsy. *Am J Ophthalmol* 1988; **105**: 186–95.

Land JM, Hockaday JM, Hughes JT, Ross BD. Childhood mitochondrial myopathy with ophthalmoplegia. *J Neurol Sci* 1981; **51**: 371–82.

Lawford JB. Congenital hereditary defect of ocular movements. *Trans Ophthalmol Soc UK* 1988; **8**: 262–74.

Lee JP. Congenital extra-ocular muscular defects. *Eye* 1992; **6**: 181–3.

Lessell S, Rosman P. Permanent visual impairment in childhood pseudotumour cerebri. *Arch Neurol* 1986; **43**: 801–4.

Loewenfeld IE, Thompson HS. Oculomotor palsy with cyclic spasms. A critical review of the literature and a new case. *Surv Ophthalmol* 1975; **20**: 81–124.

Lotufo DG, Smith JL, Hopen GR, Pollard F. The pupil in congenital third nerve misdirection syndrome. *J Clin Neuro-ophthalmol* 1983; **3**: 193–5.

MacDermot KD, Winter RM. Radial ray defect and Duane anomaly: report of a family with autosomal dominant transmission. *Am J Med Genet* 1987; **27**: 313–19.

McGarry B, Fells P. Difficulties in the management of orbital blow-out fractures in patients under 20 years old. In: Ravalt AP, Lenk M, eds. *Transactions of the Vth International Orthoptic Congress*. Lyon: Lips, 1984: 283–7.

Marks HG, Augustyn P, Allen RJ. Fisher's syndrome in children. *Pediatrics* 1977; **60**: 726–9.

Maroon JC, Mealy J. Benign intracranial hypertension. *J Am Med Assoc* 1971; **216**: 1479–80.

Matson DD. Intracranial aneurysms in childhood. *J Neurosurg* 1965; **23**: 578–83.

Mather TR, Saunders RA. Congenital absence of the superior rectus muscle: a case report. *J Pediatr Ophthalmol Strabismus* 1987; **24**: 291–6.

Merz M, Wojtowicz S. The Möbius' syndrome. *Am J Ophthalmol* 1967; **63**: 837–40.

Metz HS. Double elevator palsy. *J Pediatr Ophthalmol Strabismus* 1981; **18**: 31–5.

Miller MT. Ocular teratology. Observations, speculations, questions, principles re-affirmed. *Eye* 1992; **6**: 177–80.

Miller MT, Ray V, Owens P, Cheu F. Möbius' and Möbius-like syndromes. *J Pediatr Ophthalmol Strabismus* 1989; **26**: 176–89.

Miller MT, Stromland K. Ocular motility in thalidomide embryopathy. *J Pediatr Ophthalmol Strabismus* 1991; **28**: 47–55.

Miller NR. Isolated oculomotor nerve palsy in childhood from leptomeningeal polymorphic sarcoma. *J Pediatr Ophthalmol* 1976; **13**: 211–14.

Miller NR. Solitary oculomotor nerve palsy in childhood. *Am J Ophthalmol* 1977; **83**: 106–11.

Miller NR, Kiel SM, Green WR, Clark AW. Unilateral Duane's retraction syndrome (type I). *Arch Ophthalmol* 1982; **100**: 1468–72.

Mitsumoto H, Aprille JR, Wray SH, Nemni R, Bradley WG. Chronic progressive external ophthalmoplegic (CPEO) clinical morphological and biochemical studies. *Neurology (Cleve)* 1983; **33**: 452–61.

Mizen TR, Burde RM, Klingele TG. Cryptogenic oculomotor nerve palsies in children. *Am J Ophthalmol* 1985; **100**: 65–7.

Molarte AB, Rosenbaum AL. Vertical rectus muscle transposition surgery for Duane's syndrome. *J Pediatr Ophthalmol Strabismus* 1990; **27**: 171–7.

Moore AT, Morin JD. Bilateral acquired inflammatory Brown's syndrome. *J Pediatr Ophthalmol Strabismus* 1985; **22**: 26–31.

Moore AT, Pritchard J, Taylor D. Histiocytosis X: an ophthalmological review. *Br J Ophthalmol* 1985; **69**: 7–14.

Moore AT, Walker J, Taylor D. Familial Brown's syndrome. *J Pediatr Ophthalmol Strabismus* 1988; **25**: 202–4.

Moorman C, Elston JS. Acute orbital myositis. *Eye* 1995; **9**: 96–101.

Morris RJ, Scott WE, Keech RV. Superior oblique tuck surgery in the management of superior oblique palsies. *J Pediatr Ophthalmol Strabismus* 1992; **29**: 337–46.

Moster ML, Savino PJ, Sergott RC, Bosley TM, Schatz NJ. Isolated sixth-nerve palsies in younger adults. *Arch Ophthalmol* 1984; **102**: 1328–30.

Mulhern M, Keohane C, O'Connor G. Bilateral abducens nerve lesions in unilateral type 3 Duane's retraction syndrome. *Br J Ophthalmol* 1994; **78**: 588–91.

Neetens A, Selosse P. Oculomotor anomalies in sellar and parasellar pathology. *Ophthalmologica (Basel)* 1977; **175**: 80–104.

Nellhaus G. Isolated oculomotor nerve palsy in infectious mononucleosis. *Neurology* 1966; **16**: 221–4.

Nemet P, Ehlich D, Lazar M. Benign abducens palsy in varicella. *Am J Ophthalmol* 1974; **78**: 859.

Norman MG. Unilateral encephalomalacia in cranial nerve nuclei in neonates: report of two cases. *Neurology* 1974; **24**: 424–7.

O'Day J, Burston F, King J. Ophthalmoplegic migraine and aberrant regeneration of the oculomotor nerve. *Br J Ophthalmol* 1980; **64**: 534–6.

O'Keefe M, Crawford JS, Young JDH, Macrae WG. Ocular abnormalities in the Freeman–Sheldon syndrome. *Am J Ophthalmol* 1986; **102**: 346–9.

Olver J, Laidler P. Acquired Brown's syndrome in a patient with combined lichen sclerosis et atrophicus and morphoea. *Br J Ophthalmol* 1988; **72**: 552–8.

Osher RH, Corbett JJ, Schatz NJ, Savino PJ, Orr LS. Neuro-ophthalmological complications of enlargement of the third ventricle. *Br J*

Ophthalmol 1978; **62**: 536–42.

Owen JS, Kline LB, Oh SJ, Miles NE, Benton JW. Ophthalmoplegia and ptosis in congenital fiber type disproportion. *J Pediatr Ophthalmol Strabismus* 1981; **8**: 55–60.

Packner AR, Steere AL. The triad of neurological manifestations of Lyme disease, meningitis, cranial neuritis and radiculoneuritis. *Neurology* 1985; **35**: 47–53.

Panitch HS, Berg BD. Brain stem tumour of childhood and adolescence. *Am J Dis Child* 1970; **119**: 465–72.

Parks MM, Sprague EH. Simultaneous superior oblique tenotomy and inferior oblique recession in Brown's syndrome. *J Am Acad Ophthalmol* 1987; **94**: 1043–7.

Patel AN, Richardson AG. Ruptured intracranial aneurysms in the first two decades of life. *J Neurosurg* 1971; **35**: 571–3.

Patel CK, Taylor, DSI, Russell-Eggitt IM, Kriss A, Demaerel P. Congenital third nerve palsy associated with mid-trimester amniocentesis. *Br J Ophthalmol* 1993; **77**: 530–3.

Paysee EA, Coats DK, Plager DA. Facial asymmetry and tendon laxity in superior oblique palsy. *J Pediatr Ophthalmol Strabismus* 1995; **32**: 158–61.

Petty RKH, Harding AE, Morgan-Hughes JA. The clinical features of mitochondrial myopathy. *Brain* 1986; **109**: 915–38.

Pfaffenbach DD, Cross HE, Kearns TP. Congenital anomalies in Duane's retraction syndrome. *Arch Ophthalmol* 1972; **88**: 635–9.

Pollard ZF. Diagnosis and management of inferior oblique palsy. *J Pediatr Ophthalmol Strabismus* 1993; **30**: 15–18.

Pruksacholawit K, Ishikawa A. A typical vertical retraction syndrome: a case study. *J Pediatr Ophthalmol* 1976; **13**: 215–20.

Ramsay J, Taylor D. Congenital crocodile tears: a key to the aetiology of Duane's syndrome. *Br J Ophthalmol* 1980; **64**: 518–22.

Reisner SH, Perlman M, Ben-Tovim N, Dubrawski C. Transient lateral rectus muscle paresis in the newborn infant. *J Pediatr* 1971; **78**: 461–5.

Reynolds JD, Biglan AW, Hiles DA. Congenital superior oblique palsy in infants. *Arch Ophthalmol* 1984; **102**: 1503–5.

Richards B, Jones F, Younge B. Causes and prognosis in 4278 cases of paralysis of the oculomotor, trochlear and abducens cranial nerves. *Am J Ophthalmol* 1992; **113**: 489–96.

Ringel SP, Wilson WB, Barden MT. Extra-ocular muscle biopsy in chronic progressive external ophthalmoplegia. *Ann Neurol* 1979; **6**: 326–39.

Robb RM. Idiopathic superior oblique palsies in children. *J Pediatr Ophthalmol Strabismus* 1990; **27**: 66–70.

Robb RM, Boger WP. Vertical strabismus associated with plagiocephaly. *J Pediatr Ophthalmol Strabismus* 1983; **20**: 58–62.

Robertson DM, Hines JD, Rucker CW. Acquired sixth-nerve palsy in children. *Arch Ophthalmol* 1970; **83**: 574–9.

Rodriguez M, Gomez MR, Howard FM, Taylor WF. Myasthenia gravis in children: long-term follow-up. *Ann Neurol* 1983; **13**: 504–10.

Rogers GL, Hatch GF, Gray I. Möbius' syndrome and limb abnormalities. *J Pediatr Ophthalmol* 1977; **14**: 134–8.

Rosenbaum AL, Jampolsky A. Pseudoparalysis caused by anomalous insertion of superior rectus muscle. *Arch Ophthalmol* 1975; **93**: 535–7.

Rush JA, Younge BR. Paralysis of cranial nerves III, IV and VI. Cause and prognosis in 1000 cases. *Arch Ophthalmol* 1981; **99**: 76–9.

Saad N, Lee JP. Medial rectus electromyographic abnormalities in Duane's syndrome. *J Pediatr Ophthalmol Strabismus* 1993; **30**: 88–91.

Sananman ML, Weintraub MI. Remitting ophthalmoplegia due to rhabdomyosarcoma. *Arch Ophthalmol* 1971; **86**: 459–61.

Sato SE, Ellis FD, Pinchoff BS, Helveston EM, Rummel JH. Superior oblique overaction in patients with true Brown's syndrome. *J Pediatr Ophthalmol Strabismus* 1987; **24**: 282–7.

Scharf J, Zonis S. Benign abducens nerve palsy in childhood. *J Pediatr Ophthalmol* 1975; **12**: 165.

Scott AB, Knapp P. Surgical treatment of the superior oblique tendon sheath syndrome. *Arch Ophthalmol* 1972; **88**: 282–6.

Scott AB, Wong GM. Duane's syndrome: an electromyographic study. *Arch Ophthalmol* 1972; **87**: 140–7.

Scott WE, Kraft SP. Classification and treatment of superior oblique palsy. *J Pediatr Ophthalmol Strabismus* 1986; **23**: 265–75.

Sevel D. Brown's syndrome — a possible etiology explained embryologically. *J Pediatr Ophthalmol Strabismus* 1981; **18**: 26–31.

Sharf B, Hyams S. Oculomotor palsy following varicella. *J Pediatr Ophthalmol* 1972; **9**: 245–7.

Sharma P, Gupta NK, Arora R, Prakash P. Strabismus fixus convergens secondary to amyloidosis. *J Pediatr Ophthalmol Strabismus* 1991; **28**: 236–7.

Shauly Y, Weissman A, Meyer E. Ocular and systemic characteristics of Duane's syndrome. *J Pediatr Ophthalmol Strabismus* 1993; **30**: 178–83.

Simcock P, Kelleher S, Dunne J. Neuro-ophthalmic findings in botulism type B. *Eye* 1994; **8**: 646–8.

Simpson JA. Myasthenia gravis and myasthenic syndromes. In: Walton J, ed. *Disorders of Voluntary Muscle*. Edinburgh: Churchill Livingstone, 1981: 585–624.

Slamovits TL, Miller NR, Burde RM. Intracranial oculomotor nerve paresis with anisocoria and pupillary parasympathetic hypersensitivity. *Am J Ophthalmol* 1987; **104**: 401–7.

Slavin ML, Goodstein S. Acquired Brown's syndrome caused by focal metastasis to the superior oblique muscle. *Am J Ophthalmol* 1987; **103**: 598–9.

Sprunger DT, Von Noorden GK, Helveston EM. Surgical results in Brown's syndrome. *J Pediatr Ophthalmol Strabismus* 1991; **28**: 164–8.

St Charles S, Di Mario FJ Jr, Grunnet ML. Möbius sequence: further *in vivo* support for the subclavian artery supply disruption sequence. *Am J Med Genet* 1994; **47**: 289–93.

Stommel EW, Ward TN, Harris RD. MRI findings in ophthalmoplegic migraine. *Headache* 1993; **33**: 234–7.

Strachan IM, Brown BH. Electromyography of extraocular muscles in Duane's syndrome. *Br J Ophthalmol* 1972; **56**: 594–9.

Straussberg R, Cohen AH, Amir J, Varsano I. Benign abducens palsy associated with EBV infection. *J Pediatr Ophthalmol Strabismus* 1993; **30**: 60.

Stromland K, Miller MT. Thalidomide embryopathy revisited 27 years later. *Acta Ophthalmol* 1993; **71**: 238–45.

Takahashi T, Murase TT, Isayama Y, Tamaki N, Fujiwara K, Matsumoto S. Rhabdomyosarcoma presenting as Garcia's syndrome. *Surg Neurol* 1982; **17**: 269–72.

Thakkar N, O'Neil W, Duvally J, Liv C, Ambler M. Möbius' syndrome due to brain stem tegmental necrosis. *Arch Neurol* 1977; **34**: 124–6.

Thomas R, Mathai A, Gieser S, Ratnammal J. Bilateral synergistic divergence. *J Pediatr Ophthalmol Strabismus* 1993; **30**: 122–3.

Timms C, Russell-Eggitt I, Taylor D. Acquired Duane's syndrome. *Binocular Vis* 1989; **4**: 109–12.

Towfighi J, Marks K, Palmer E, Vannucci R. Möbius' syndrome: neuropathological observations. *Acta Neuropathol (Berl)* 1979; **48**: 11–17.

Trese MT, Krohel GB, Hepler RS, Naeim F. Burkitt's lymphoma with cranial nerve involvement. *Arch Ophthalmol* 1980; **98**: 2015–17.

Van Allen MW, Blodi FC. Neurological aspects of the Möbius' syndrome. *Neurology* 1960; **10**: 249–59.

Van Pelt W, Andermann F. On the early onset of ophthalmoplegic migraine. *Am J Dis Child* 1964; **107**: 628–31.

Victor DI. The diagnosis of congenital unilateral third-nerve palsy.

Brain 1976; **99**: 711–18.

Volpe NJ, Lessell S. Remitting sixth nerve palsy in skull base tumours. *Arch Ophthalmol* 1993; **111**: 1391–5.

Von Noorden GK. Congenital hereditary ptosis with inferior rectus fibrosis. *Arch Ophthalmol* 1970; **83**: 378–80.

Von Noorden GK. Recession of both horizontal recti muscles in Duane's retraction syndrome with elevation and depression of the adducted eye. *Am J Ophthalmol* 1992; **114**: 311–13.

Von Noorden GK, Hansell R. Clinical characteristics and treatment of isolated inferior rectus paralysis. *Ophthalmology* 1991; **98**: 253–7.

Waddell E. Brown's syndrome revisited. *Br Orthop J* 1982; **39**: 17–21.

Wagner RS, Caputo AR, Frohman LP. Congenital unilateral adduction deficit with simultaneous abduction: A variant of Duane's retraction syndrome. *Ophthalmology* 1987; **94**: 1049–54.

Wallace DK, Von Noorden GK. Clinical characteristics and surgical management of congenital absence of the superior oblique tendon. *Am J Ophthalmol* 1994; **118**: 63–9.

Walsh JP, O'Doherty DS. A possible explanation of the mechanism of ophthalmoplegic migraine. *Neurology* 1960; **10**: 1079–84.

Wang FM, Wertenbaker C, Behrens MM, Jacobs JC. Acquired Brown's syndrome in children with juvenile rheumatoid arthritis. *Ophthalmology* 1984; **91**: 23–7.

Weiss A, Manley D. Congenital tight superior rectus muscle. *J Pediatr Ophthalmol Strabismus* 1985; **22**: 51–3.

Werner DB, Savino PJ, Schatz NJ. Benign recurrent sixth nerve palsies in childhood. *Arch Ophthalmol* 1983; **101**: 6073–8.

White WL, Mumma JV, Tomasovic JJ. Congenital oculomotor nerve palsy, cerebellar hypoplasia and facial capillary hemangioma. *Am J Ophthalmol* 1992; **113**: 497–500.

Wilcox LM, Gittinger JW, Breinin GM. Congenital adduction palsy and synergistic divergence. *Am J Ophthalmol* 1981; **91**: 1–7.

Wilson EM, Hoxie J. Facial asymmetry in superior oblique muscle palsy. *J Pediatr Ophthalmol Strabismus* 1993; **30**: 315–18.

Wortham E, Crawford JS. Brown's syndrome in twins. *Am J Ophthalmol* 1988; **105**: 562–3.

Yee RD, Cogan DG, Zee DS. Ophthalmoplegia and disassociated nystagmus in abetalipoproteinaemia. *Arch Ophthalmol* 1976; **94**: 571–5.

Ziffer AJ, Rosenbaum AL, Demer JL, Yee RD. Congenital double elevator palsy: vertical saccadic velocity utilising the scleral search coil technique. *J Pediatr Ophthalmol Strabismus* 1992; **29**: 142–9.

67: Strabismus Surgery

Robert Morris

The management of strabismus involves careful assessment of patients, treatment of amblyopia and refractive errors, and in certain cases surgical correction of the strabismus. Amblyopia should be treated prior to surgery and the different stages in the management of the strabismus should be made clear to parents. As a general rule, refractive errors should be fully corrected and any surgery based on the residual angle in spectacles. Following surgery children need continued follow-up until at least the age of visual maturity to monitor their vision and refraction, as well as the stability of the strabismus. Surgery may be functional or cosmetic and the indications for each differ.

The assessment of strabismus should include measurement and recording of the deviation, with the appropriate refractive error, at near and distance in primary position and at distance in nine positions of gaze where possible (Jampolsky 1971; Vivian & Morris 1993; O'Flynn 1994). Sensory assessment of the strabismus is essential to determine the binocular potential or function. All children with strabismus require at least one cycloplegic refraction. Where appropriate other investigations such as Hess charts, active forced generation tests and forced duction tests may be necessary. Only with this information can an informed decision regarding surgery be made.

Parents typically expect surgery to be carried out on the squinting eye but in general it is advantageous to perform symmetrical surgery. Uniocular surgery is, however, indicated if one eye has poor vision, there has been previous surgery on the other eye or in cases of complex strabismus with restriction or limitation of ocular movement.

Surgical anatomy

It is a common misconception that the challenge of strabismus surgery is the decision of which muscles to operate on. Poor surgery will compromise even the best decisions and a good knowledge of the surgical anatomy is essential.

Conjunctiva

The conjunctiva is a key structure in strabismus surgery and poor surgical technique can lead to scarring and redness. The plica semilunaris is a particularly important structure as if it is inadvertently advanced towards the limbus it leaves unsightly scarring. The conjunctiva is fused to Tenon's capsule anteriorly, and both are fused to the sclera at the limbus. The rectus muscles and their anterior ciliary arteries are often visible through the conjunctiva, although this may be impossible in young patients when both conjunctiva and Tenon's capsule are thick.

Tenon's capsule and intermuscular septum

Tenon's capsule is the fascial layer that extends from the limbus fusing posteriorly to the optic nerve. It is a dense white structure (Fig. 67.1) in children but becomes atrophic in adults. Divided into anterior and posterior parts at the point at which the extraocular muscles penetrate it posterior to the equator, it separates the globe and extraocular muscles from the orbital fat. Strabismus surgery is carried out within Tenon's capsule, which if pierced can lead to orbital fat prolapse and resultant scarring with restriction of ocular movements. From its undersurface check ligaments extend to the surface of the capsule of the rectus muscles. The intermuscular septum (Fig. 67.2), a thin fascial plane, connects the rectus muscles from the point at which they pierce Tenon's capsule and anteriorly fuses with it and the conjunctiva at the limbus. During strabismus surgery both Tenon's capsule and the intermuscular septum need to be divided to hook and dissect a rectus muscle. From the outer surface of Tenon's capsule septae run through the orbital fat to the orbital periosteum (Koornneef 1977). The orbital fat extends anteriorly to within 10 mm of the limbus and can be clearly seen through the conjunctiva in the inferior fornix.

Rectus muscles

The rectus muscles originate at the orbital apex, are all approximately 40 mm long and insert onto the sclera anteriorly. They insert along the spiral of Tillaux at varying distances from the limbus (Table 67.1). Apt (1980, 1982) has studied their relationship to the limbus in detail. He found a wide variation in the distance between the limbus and insertion, and also demonstrated that clinically the width of the limbus can vary from 0.4 to 1.6 mm, being thinnest medially and widest superiorly. He emphasized that the distance from the muscle to the insertion is least in the centre of the insertion and greatest at the poles. During strabismus surgery the insertion may become displaced towards the limbus making measurements from the insertion inaccurate, and the distance from the limbus to the insertion should therefore always be measured before manipulation of the muscle (Keech *et al.* 1990). This displacement is thought to be a combination of shortening of the sclera anterior to the insertion as well as in some cases lamellar tearing of the sclera. V-shaped deformities of the insertion stump have also been described by Kushner *et al.* (1987). Although careful surgical technique may minimize these artefacts they are difficult to eliminate.

Superior oblique muscles

The superior oblique muscle, the longest and thinnest of the extraocular muscles, arises from the orbital apex, passes through the trochlea as a cord-like tendon and then

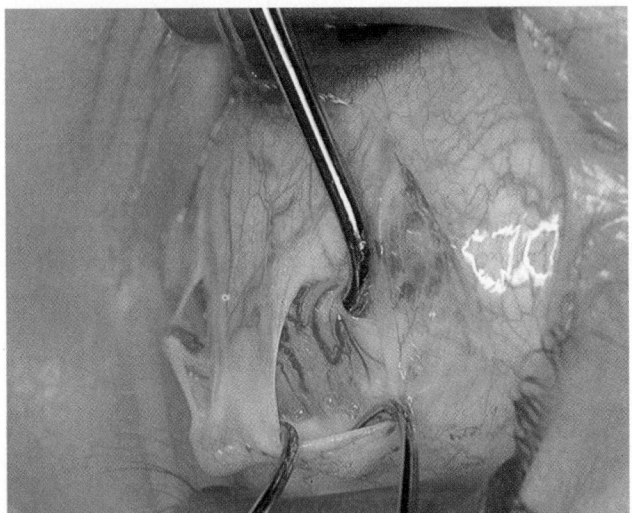

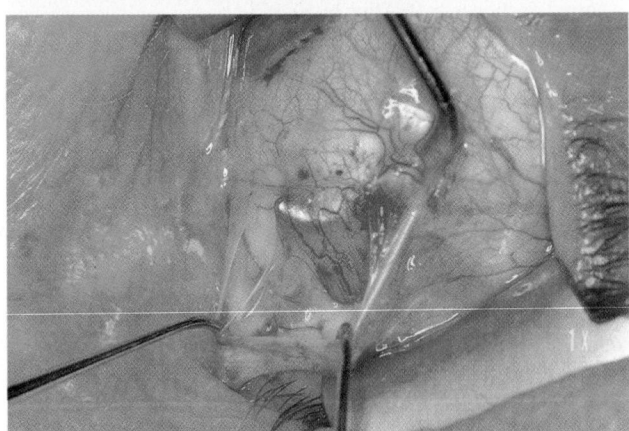

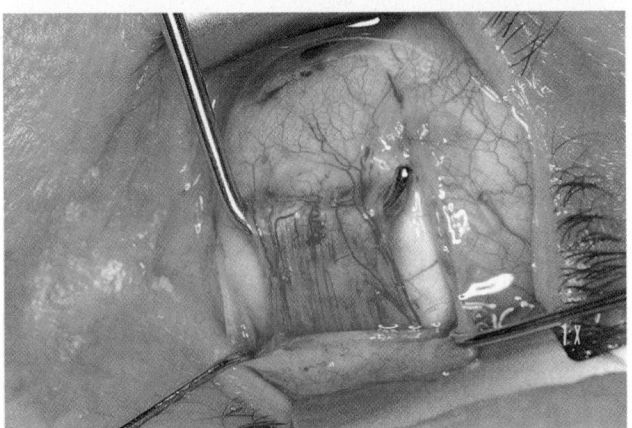

Fig. 67.1 (a) Tenon's capsule overlying the superior rectus. (b) Intermuscular septum and check ligaments displayed with tenotomy hooks. (c) Muscle after dissection. Note anterior ciliary arteries.

Table 67.1 Rectus muscle dimensions.

	Distance from cornea to midpoint of insertion (mm)	Length of muscle (mm)	Width at insertion (mm)	Length of tendon (mm)
Medial rectus	5.5	40	10.3	3.7
Inferior rectus	6.5	40	9.8	5.5
Lateral rectus	6.9	48	9.2	8.8
Superior rectus	7.7	42	10.8	5.8

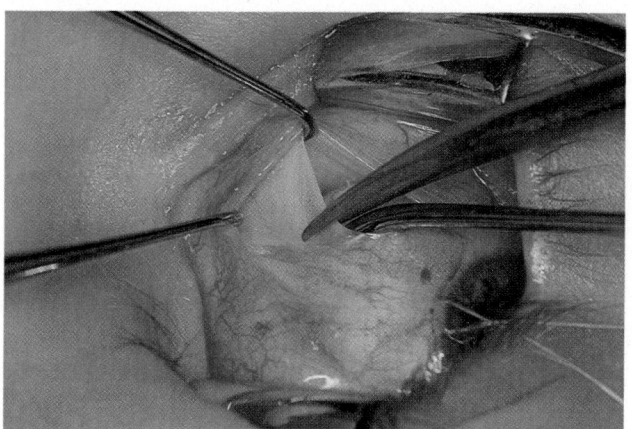

Fig. 67.2 Intermuscular septum and check ligaments overlying medial rectus being incised with scissors.

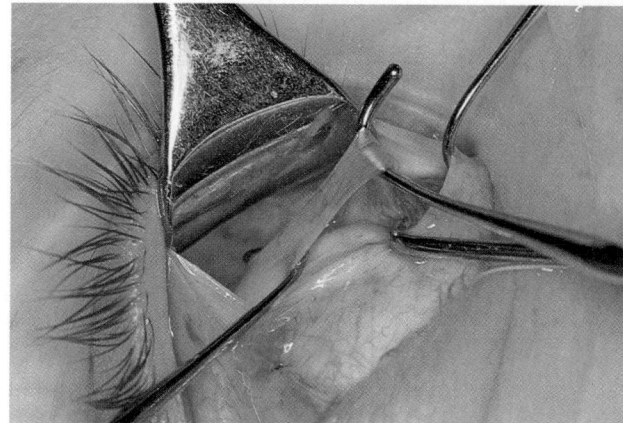

Fig. 67.4 Strabismus hooks beneath superior oblique tendon demonstrating tendon laxity in a patient with a lax superior oblique tendon.

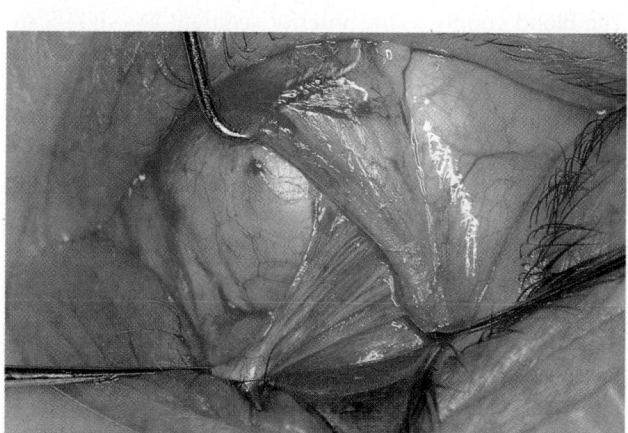

Fig. 67.3 Superior oblique tendon inserting beneath the superior rectus (right eye viewed from above).

runs posterolateral at an angle of approximately 54°, before fanning out and passing under the superior rectus inserting on the superotemporal quadrant of the globe (Fig. 67.3). The anterior end of the insertion lies about 4 mm from the lateral insertion of the superior rectus muscle; the width of the insertion is about 11 mm, but varies considerably (Fink 1951, 1962).

Functionally the trochlea acts as the insertion of the superior oblique muscle. The main action of the muscle in

adduction is depression. In abduction its main actions are intorsion and abduction.

The anatomy of the superior oblique tendon is often anomalous. In one study 87% of patients undergoing surgery for congenital superior palsies had an anomalous tendon (Helveston *et al.* 1992). The tendon may be redundant or lax (Fig. 67.4), misdirected, have an anomalous insertion nasal to the superior rectus or into Tenon's capsule, and the trochlea or the tendon may even be absent (Helveston *et al.* 1992). Wallace and von Noorden (1994) have described the clinical signs indicative of absence of the superior oblique tendon in nine patients. Intraoperative exaggerated forced duction testing can demonstrate laxity of the superior oblique tendon indicating an anomaly of the tendon (Plager 1990). The nasal superior oblique tendon has fascial relationships with the superior nasal intermuscular septum which envelopes the superior oblique tendon to form the superior oblique capsule. If the nasal intermuscular tendon is removed while performing a nasal tenotomy the cut tendon ends have no support, will freely separate and a palsy may result. There is also a frenulum between the undersurface of the superior rectus and the superior oblique (Fig. 67.5), which must be divided for effective recession of either of these muscles (Jampolsky 1986).

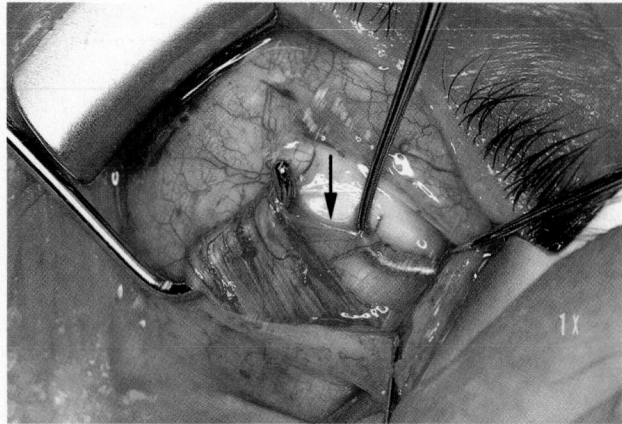

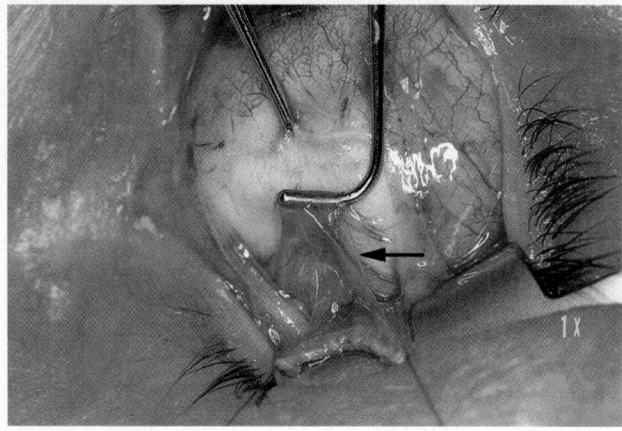

Fig. 67.5 Right eye. (a) Chavasse hook beneath superior rectus and Stevens hook beneath the superior oblique showing the fascial attachment between them. (b) Undersurface of disinserted superior rectus showing fascial attachment between it and the superior oblique tendon.

Inferior oblique muscles

The inferior oblique muscle is the shortest of the extraocular muscles (37 mm), with a short tendon of only 1–2 mm. It passes posteriorly, laterally and upwards, from its origin adjacent to the lacrimal sac, to its insertion 8–10 mm posterior to the inferior border of the lateral rectus insertion. It runs at an angle of approximately 51° to the vertical plane of the globe. As the muscle passes the inferior temporal quadrant it overlies the vortex vein. The width of the insertion is about 9 mm long, but varies considerably, and the posterior aspect of it overlies the macula (Fink 1962). The neurovascular bundle enters the muscle as it passes beneath the nasal border of the inferior rectus muscle.

The main action of the muscle in adduction is elevation, and in abduction cyclotorsion and abduction. Inferior oblique overaction is a common occurrence and is seen most frequently in association in patients with horizontal strabismus, usually congenital esotropia and intermittent exotropia, and superior oblique palsies. Overactions can be graded on a scale of I–IV (Jampolsky 1971; Vivian &

Morris 1993; O'Flynn 1994). Inferior oblique overaction must be distinguished from dissociated vertical deviation, and the two conditions may co-exist (Scott & Morris 1990). Inferior oblique underactions are less common and usually secondary to superior oblique overactions; although inferior oblique palsies have been described they are rare. Inferior oblique underaction can be distinguished from Brown's syndrome by the presence of a normal forced duction test (Pollard 1993).

Globe dimensions

The adult globe measures 24 mm in length. The neonatal globe is only 17 mm (Swan & Wilkins 1984), although the anterior portion of the globe is proportionately larger, the distance from the muscle insertions to the limbus being 80% of that in a normal adult eye, and at 6 months equal to it (Swan & Wilkins 1984). The clinical relevance of this is that the equator of the globe is only a small distance behind the muscle insertion, and therefore surgery in infants should be undertaken with caution. During the first 2 years of life there is rapid growth of the eye, the average length being 20.3 mm at 6 months and 22.8 mm at 20 months of age (Swan & Wilkins 1984).

Blood supply

The blood supply to the anterior segment has significant practical importance as certain types of strabismus surgery can lead to anterior segment ischaemia. From an understanding of the functional blood supply those procedures likely to cause ischaemia can be predicted. In humans there is a three-layered collateral blood supply to the anterior segment consisting of an anterior episcleral arterial circle, an incomplete intramuscular arterial circle and a major arterial circle. The major contribution to this arterial circulation comes from the anterior ciliary arteries – each rectus muscle has two except the lateral which has one. The contribution of the two long posterior ciliary arteries is less significant (Olver & Lee 1989; Olver & McCartney 1989a, b; Lee & Olver 1990).

General principles of surgery

Anaesthetic

In children a general anaesthetic is always used. Most children are induced for anaesthesia either intravenously or by gaseous induction and are paralysed and ventilated. The advent of laryngeal masks and avoidance of premedication enables rapid recovery from anaesthesia (Luff *et al.* 1993). Topical local anaesthesia (Habib *et al.* 1993), locally injected bupivicaine (El Kasaby *et al.* 1993) and nonsteroidal anti-inflammatory agents (Morrison & Repka 1994) have all been advocated for reduction of postoperative pain. Postoperative pain is worse with multiple muscle surgery, and reoperations and resections are more painful then recessions; relief may require strong analgesia although opiates are rarely required.

Instruments

Each surgeon has their own preference for the type of instruments used, but certain principles apply. A selection of strabismus hooks is invaluable (Fig. 67.6), including a Chavasse, Jameson or Green muscle hook; these spread the rectus muscles evenly and prevent bunching of the muscle (Fig. 67.7). Stevens tenotomy hooks are useful for retracting conjunctiva and sclera, and essential for oblique muscle surgery. In some cases Desmarres or Fison retractors are necessary for adequate exposure. 6–0 Vicryl (polyglactin-910) is the most commonly used suture material for muscle reattachment (Schwartz & Koller 1981). It has the advantages of causing minimal tissue reaction, a high tensile strength, good knot-holding ability and absorbs in 2–3 months (Bladyes 1975). Its main disadvantages are that it snags tissues and in rare instances can produce an allergic reaction (Bladyes 1975). When reattaching a muscle to the globe the needle should be placed in through the superficial third to half of the sclera with the tip visible at all times. Spatulate needles which cut the tissues at the sides and tip are preferable, and provided the needle is held parallel to the sclera during its intrascleral course the risk of globe perforation is low (Morris *et al.* 1990). In most circumstances a three-eighths needle is preferable, but a half-circle needle can be advantageous where suture placement is difficult because of poor access and allows a shorter scleral bite of the same depth. A reverse cutting needle with a cutting edge on its convex surface can be used, but has a theoretically greater risk of scleral perforation. Its advantage, however, is that it does

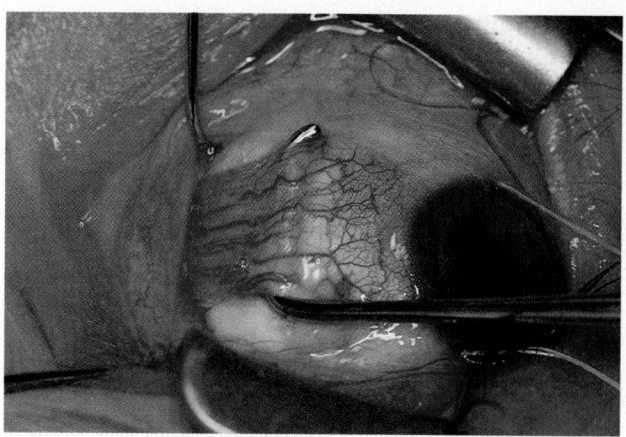

Fig. 67.7 A Chavasse muscle hook under medial rectus. Note the even spreading of the muscle tendon on the hook and anterior ciliary arteries

not have to be placed exactly parallel to the scleral surface during its intrascleral course. My preference for conjunctival closure is 8–0 virgin silk or 8–0 Vicryl.

All strabismus surgery should be performed with magnification. Most surgeons use spectacle-mounted loupes, but others advocate using the operating microscope which has the advantage of good lighting and magnification, but the disadvantages of reducing the field size and depth of focus, and restricting the surgeon's mobility.

Forced duction tests (traction tests)

Forced duction tests, the passive movement of a patient's eye in a particular direction to test for mechanical restriction, should be conducted routinely before any strabismus operation. They can help distinguish mechanical restriction from muscle weakness. Interpretation of the test requires experience in the technique and even then it is difficult to detect subtle restrictions. In the presence of restriction the test is positive, a negative test indicates free passive movement of the globe. If positive the test should be repeated throughout surgery, particularly when the muscle thought to be responsible for the restriction has been disinserted. In adults it can be conducted in the clinical setting using topical local anaesthesia, but in children is usually performed under general anaesthetic. If succinylcholine has been used in the induction of anaesthesia, muscle tone is increased and this may have an influence on the test.

The assessment of the rectus and oblique muscles requires different techniques. To assess the rectus muscles the globe should be held at the limbus with fixation forceps moved in the opposite direction. For example, to assess restriction due to the inferior rectus the eye is held at 6 o'clock and the globe fully elevated. The important point is that the globe should be pulled forwards, rather

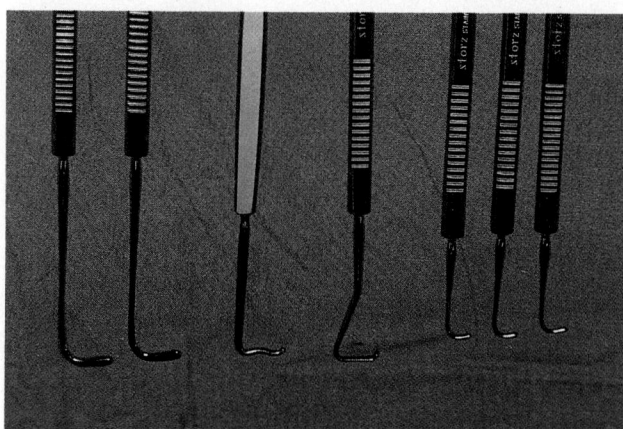

Fig. 67.6 Strabismus hooks from right to left: three Stevens tenotomy hooks, a Green muscle hook, a Chavasse hook and two von Graefe hooks.

than pushed backwards, to put the rectus muscles on the stretch. If the globe can be fully rotated then no mechanical restriction is present. Guyton (1981) has described an exaggerated forced duction test to assess the tightness of the oblique muscles. It aids in the diagnosis of congenital superior oblique palsy as well as in Brown's syndrome. The eye is held with toothed forceps at 3 and 9 o'clock and retropulsed into the orbit thereby stretching the oblique muscles. The eye is then excyclotorted and elevated in adduction. In Brown's syndrome there is restriction to elevation. In congenital superior oblique palsy there is absence of the normal resistance felt (Plager 1990). The technique is also useful to assess the efficacy of superior oblique weakening procedures for Brown's syndrome and in assessing the tightness of the tendon after a superior oblique tuck. A similar technique can be used to assess the tightness of the inferior oblique, primarily to assess the tightness of the muscle when it is overacting having been previously weakened.

Conjunctival incisions

There are three main types of conjunctival incision, the limbal, cul-de-sac and Swan. My preference is to use a limbal incision (Fig. 67.8) for rectus muscle surgery as it is easy to perform, gives good exposure, induces little scarring or adhesion formation and can be combined with conjunctival recession where indicated (von Noorden 1968, 1969). This type of incision is particularly advantageous for reoperations or when muscle transposition is performed because of the exposure it provides. The major disadvantage of the technique is that an unsightly conjunctival ridge can develop if there is poor reapposition of the conjunctiva. Although many surgeons use only one relaxing incision with this technique this can result in irregular tearing of the conjunctiva and two should be employed.

The cul-de-sac incision (Fig. 67.9), pioneered by Parks (1968), is quick, produces minimal scarring, leaves the limbal conjunctiva intact and in skilled hands does not need a conjunctival suture. The other advantage of this technique is that adjacent rectus muscles can be approached through the same incision. There is also animal evidence to suggest that fornix conjunctival incisions cause less severe anterior segment ischaemia than limbal incisions (Fishman *et al.* 1990), but this has not been shown to be the case clinically (Saunders *et al.* 1994). The incision is placed on the bulbar conjunctiva 8 mm from the limbus and not actually in the fornix, but rather 1–2 mm limbal to it. The conjunctival incision is pulled over the muscle to

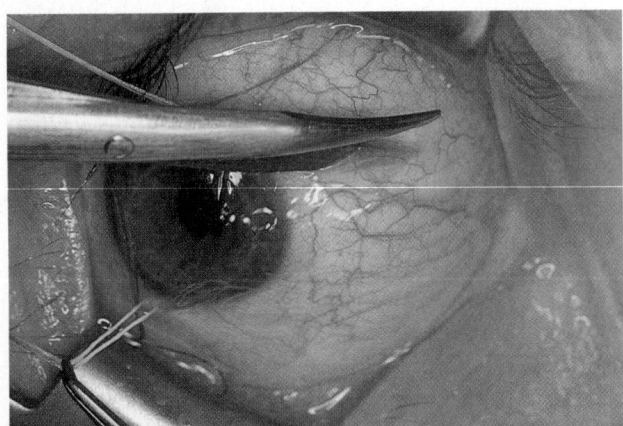

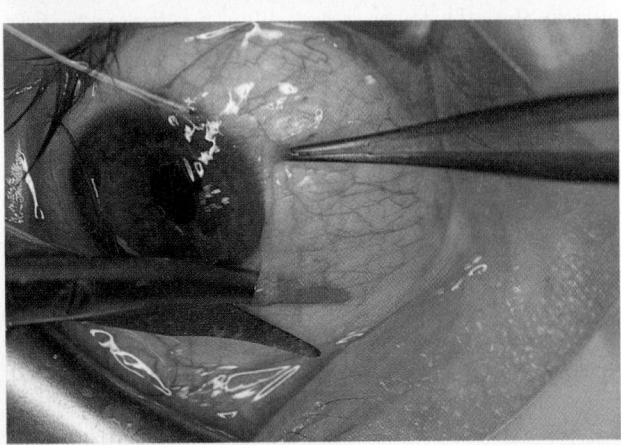

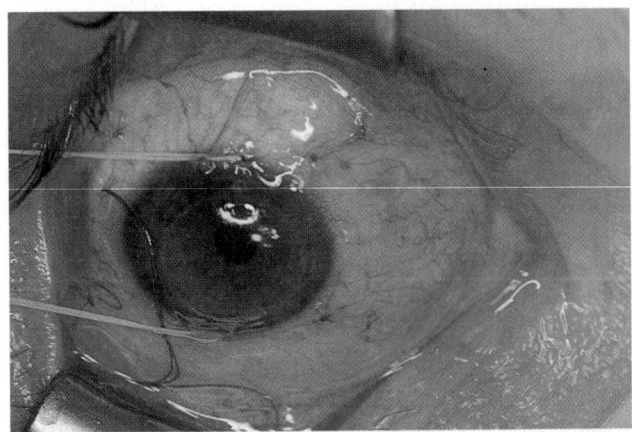

Fig. 67.8 Limbal conjunctival incision. (a) Superior conjunctival relaxing incision; this is followed by the limbal incision. (b) Inferior conjunctival relaxing incision parallel to superior conjunctival incision following completion of peritomy. (c) Accurate apposition of conjunctiva following rectus muscle surgery.

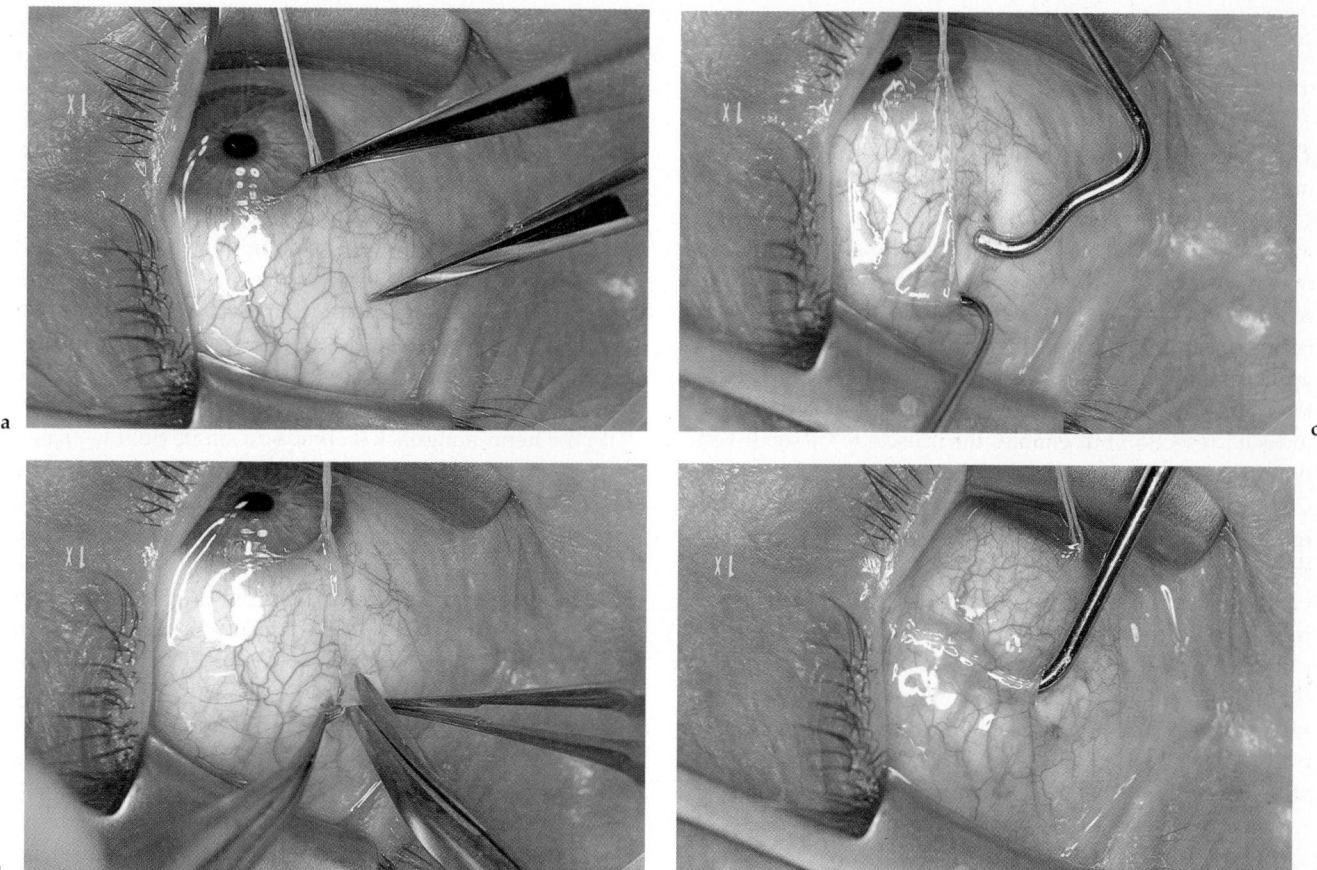

Fig. 67.9 Cul-de-sac conjunctival incision. (a) Conjunctival incision 8 mm from the limbus. (b) Intact Tenon's capsule being incised after incision of the conjunctiva. (c, d) Placement of strabismus hook under the rectus muscle following division of Tenon's capsule.

allow it to be exposed. It is, however, technically more demanding for rectus muscle surgery, particularly for reoperations, and a skilled assistant is essential. In adults with thin conjunctiva there is a risk of large conjunctival tears occurring. Although widely used for oblique muscle surgery it is less popular for rectus muscle surgery.

The Swan incision (Swan & Talbot 1954) is made over the muscle insertion but is now rarely used. The main disadvantage of this technique is haemorrhage resulting from inadvertent trauma to the anterior ciliary vessels or muscle itself when exposing the muscle.

Extraocular muscle surgery

Principles

Meticulous attention to detail is essential for successful surgery. Surgery is easier, outcomes more predictable and complications reduced. Careful dissection should enable

good exposure of the extraocular muscles, will limit formation of adhesions and minimize inadvertent muscle and vessel trauma, as well as fat prolapse. Good haemostasis makes surgery easier and reduces postoperative inflammation and adhesions. Any bleeding should be avoided if possible but when present bleeding points should be identified and cauterized. Saline solution can be used to facilitate identification of bleeding points and also help prevent the charring and shrinkage of conjunctiva sclera and muscle tissue which occurs when dry tissue is cauterized.

Rectus muscle surgery

Once a rectus muscle has been exposed, excessive Tenon's should be removed from the surface of the muscle to allow accurate placement of sutures and reduce the risk of tissues snagging on the suture. The anterior ciliary vessels should then be cauterized before being cut to prevent bleeding. Cauterizing the vessels after suture placement runs the risk of burning through the suture. Whether using a single or double suture technique careful placement of the suture in the muscle with accurate knots reduces the risk of sutures looping and muscle slippage (Mimms 1992).

Weakening procedures

Recessions

The easiest and most effective technique for weakening a horizontal or vertical rectus muscle is a recession. Its effect is maximal in the field of action of the muscle but there is also a significant effect in primary position. Recessions are faster, easier, more predictable and produce less inflammation and conjunctival scarring than resections. For a recession suture placement prior to disinsertion should be approximately 0.5–1 mm from the insertion with secure lock bites at both poles. This minimizes the amount of induced resection but enables the muscle to be secure on the suture and be disinserted without exposing the suture. Care must be taken not to drag muscle capsule or Tenon's into the knot as this will make it less secure and may predispose to retention cysts.

Surgeons vary in their preference of whether to measure recessions from the limbus or the original insertion of the muscle. The advantage of measuring from the limbus is that it is a fixed anatomical point whereas the insertion of the muscles, particularly the medial rectus, varies (Apt & Call 1982). If measurements are made from the insertion it should be measured before the muscle is disinserted as it can creep forwards towards the limbus following its disinsertion (Kushner *et al.* 1987; Keech *et al.* 1990). One practical difficulty of limbal measurements is that its precise location may be difficult to locate clinically as it can be up to 1.5 mm wide (Apt 1980; Apt & Call 1982).

Most surgeons perform fixed recessions using either a single or double suture technique (Fig. 67.10a, b). The advantage of fixed recessions is that the muscle is sutured directly at the site of the desired placement of the recessed muscle, and the muscle can be readily supra- or infraplaced if needed. However, the disadvantages of this method are that needle passes through the thinnest sclera, increasing the potential risk of globe perforation, particularly for large recessions where needle placement can be technically difficult. In addition the suture knot is tied where Tenon's is thick and can readily become incorporated into the knot.

Rectus muscles can also be recessed using the 'hangback' or less commonly the 'hemi-hangback' technique. The hangback technique allows the rectus muscle to be suspended on a single 6–0 vicryl suture from its original insertion (Fig. 67.10c). It is easier and quicker and has the theoretical advantage of reducing the risk of scleral perforation as the needle is passed through the thick sclera anterior to the insertion of the muscle, although this has not been proven. The disadvantages of the technique are that the muscle width is contracted with central sagging, there is a risk the muscle might migrate anteriorly and it is not possible to infra- or supraplace the muscle using this technique. Large recessions of the superior rectus used for the treatment of dissociated vertical deviation are effectively hangback recessions. I prefer to use an anchored hangback suture technique with superficial scleral passes at the desired point of recession, with deeper scleral bites at or just anterior to the insertion where the sclera is thickest (Figs 67.10d, 67.11). This has several advantages: the muscle is placed in the desired position preventing central muscle sag and the muscle creeping forwards, and small superficial scleral needle passes in the thin sclera minimize the risk of globe perforation. Before the knot is tied the position of the muscle can be checked and the sutures replaced if necessary. The knot is tied anteriorly so that the risk of dragging Tenon's capsule into the knot is reduced.

In the hemi-hangback technique a single double-armed suture is used and the needles are placed posterior to the insertion (Fig. 67.10e). The muscle is then allowed to 'hangback' on the suture. It has been advocated for large recessions where exposure can be difficult. The technique has the disadvantage that the suture is passed through thin sclera. This technique should not be confused with the loop recession described by Gobin (1968). In this technique a non-absorbable suture is placed through each pole of the muscle, which is then sutured to the sclera behind the insertion suspended on a 1.5–2.0 mm loop of the suture (Fig. 67.10f).

The amount of recession required to correct a deviation (Tables 67.2, 67.3) depends on many factors, but correlates most significantly with the preoperative deviation, and the influence of axial length and refractive error are not clinically important (Kushner *et al.* 1993). As a general rule recession of previously unoperated muscles produces more predictable effect than recession of previously operated muscles, which produce a greater effect per millimetre of recession, as does recession of tight muscles associated with mechanical restriction.

Table 67.2 Esotropia. These guidelines vary depending on the surgeon, the surgical technique, the age of the patient, presence of lateral incomitance, previous strabismus surgery, and presence of oblique muscle dysfunction or cerebral palsy.

Deviation	BMRc	MRc and LRs	BLRs
10–15	3.0	3.0/3.5	5.0
15–20	3.5	3.5/4.5	5.5
20–25	4.0	4.0/5.5	6.0
25–30	4.5	4.5/6.5	6.5
30–35	5.0	5.0/7.0	7.0
35–40	5.5	5.5/7.5	7.5
45–50	6.0	6.0/8.0	8.0
50–60	6.5	6.5/8.0	
60–70	7.0		

BMRc, bilateral medial rectus recessions; MRc and LRs, medial rectus recession and lateral rectus resection; BLRs, bilateral lateral rectus resections.

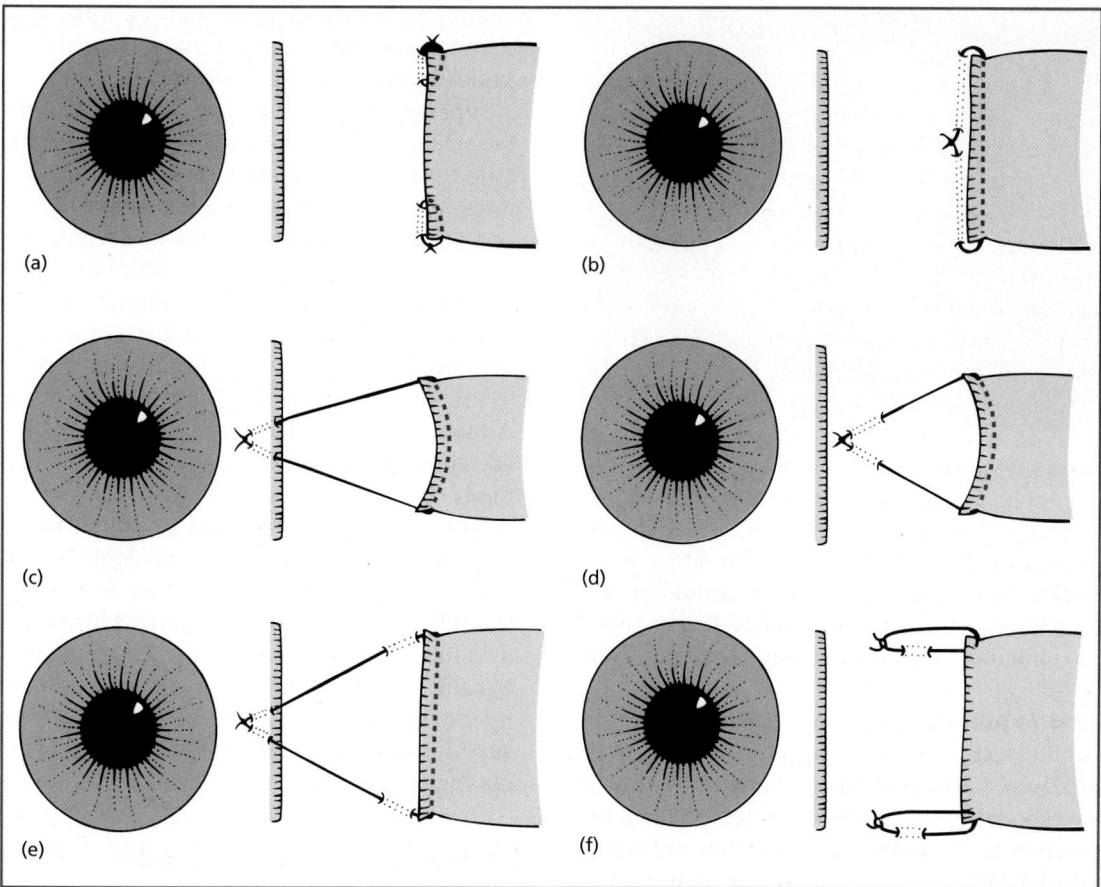

Fig. 67.10 Rectus muscle recession. (a) Fixed recession (two single sutures). (b) Fixed recession double-armed suture. (c) Hangback recession (note central bowing). (d) Hemi-hangback recession. (e) Anchored hangback suture. (f) Gobin's loop recession.

Table 67.3 Exotropia. These guidelines vary depending on the surgeon, the surgical technique, the age of the patient, presence of lateral incomitance, previous strabismus surgery, and presence of oblique muscle dysfunction and cerebral palsy.

Deviaton	BLRc	MRs	BMRs	MRs and LRc
15	4.0		4.0	3.0/4.0
20	5.0		5.0	4.0/5.0
25	6.0		6.0	5.0/6.0
30	7.0			6.0/7.0
35	8.0			6.0/8.0
40	7.0	+4.0		7.0/8.0
45	7.0	+5.0		7.5/8.5
50	7.0	+6.0		7.0/9.0
60	7.0		+5.0	8.0/10.0
70	7.0		+7.0	9.0/10.0
80	8.0		+7.0	10.0/10.0

BLRc, bilateral lateral rectus recessions; MRs, medial rectus resection; BMRs, bilateral medial rectus resections; MRs and LRc, medial rectus resection and lateral rectus recession; +, medial rectus surgery in addition to bilateral lateral rectus recession.

Horizontal muscle recession

The medial rectus can be recessed to 11.5 mm from the limbus without compromising adduction. There has, however, been an increasing trend for large bilateral medial rectus recessions in the management of large angle infantile esotropia, because of the high incidence of undercorrection in these patients with conventional recession (Ing *et al.* 1966). Medial rectus recessions of 6–8 mm have been reported to correct large infantile esotropias successfully (Nelson *et al.* 1987; Weakley & Parks 1990; Damanakis *et al.* 1994), but a high incidence of consecutive exodeviation (nearly 40% of 88 patients) has been reported (Stager *et al.* 1994). Calhoun has suggested that late overcorrection occurs not from medial rectus underaction, but from the development of lateral rectus overaction or the absence of binocularity (Calhoun 1994). Recessions of up to 1.5 mm behind the equator, determined ultrasonographically, do not give underactions nor do bilateral medial rectus recessions of 11 mm from the limbus cause late progressive overcorrection (Kushner *et al.* 1994). Other authors suggest three or four muscle surgery to correct large angle congenital esotropia (Lee & Dyer 1983; Scott *et al.* 1986). Kushner *et al.* (1994) have suggested that a prospective trial of large bilateral medial rectus recessions versus three

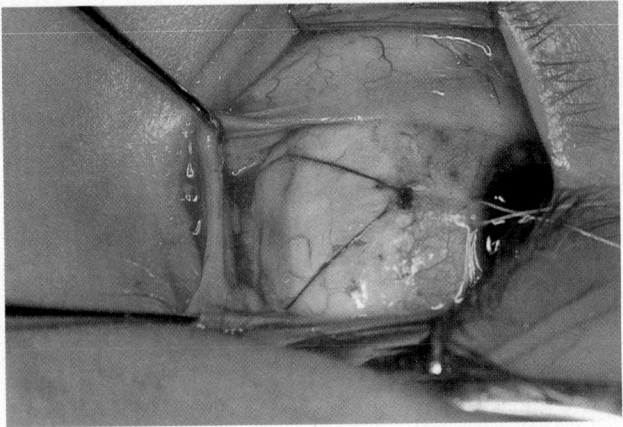

Fig. 67.11 Anchored hangback suture.

to four muscle surgery in patients with large angle esotropia be carried out. Large recessions should be performed with caution if combined with a lateral rectus resection as limitation of adduction may develop postoperatively.

The lateral rectus has a longer arc of contact with the globe than other rectus muscles and large recessions, up to 10 or even 12 mm, can be performed without limitation of movement, especially in patients with large axial lengths. As the insertion of the lateral rectus is more consistent than the medial rectus most surgeons measure recessions of this muscle from the insertion rather than the limbus.

Vertical muscle recession

Inferior rectus recession is associated with retraction of the lower lid in many cases, and the degree of retraction increases with increasing amounts of inferior rectus recession (Pacheco *et al.* 1992). For this reason recessions of more than 5 mm should not be performed. The muscle should be carefully freed from the intermuscular septum, from check ligaments as far back as the vortex veins, and particularly from its attachment to Lockwood's ligament to reduce the risk of this complication (Helveston 1986). Various techniques have been described to limit this complication including suturing the capsulopalpebral head to the recessed inferior rectus muscle and adjustable lower lid retractor surgery (Jampolsky 1986; Kushner 1992b; Pacheco *et al.* 1992).

Overcorrection of the deviation in downgaze from excessive recession of the muscle should be avoided, as downgaze is such a functionally important position of gaze. Late overcorrections following inferior rectus recession due to the muscle slipping have also been reported and patients should, initially, be slightly undercorrected with an inferior rectus recession (Sprunger & Helveston 1993). The reason for this late slippage is thought to be related to its attachment to Lockwood's ligament and the

inferior rectus exerting a downward force on the muscle; contracture of the ipsilateral superior rectus may also play a role (Sprunger & Helveston 1993).

Superior rectus recessions are an effective procedure in the management of true vertical deviations and also dissociated vertical deviation. In order to achieve an effective recession of the muscle, the fascial attachments between it and the superior oblique must be divided. Recession of 1 mm corrects approximately 3 prism dioptres of vertical deviation. Recessions of greater than 5 mm are best avoided except in the special case of dissociated vertical deviation (Scott *et al.* 1982) when hangback recessions of up to 9 mm are indicated for large deviations (Fig. 67.12). Although surgery on the superior rectus does cause upper lid retraction, in contrast to inferior rectus surgery, this is rarely clinically significant (Pacheco *et al.* 1992).

As a general rule, because of the potential complications of inferior rectus recessions, if a comitant vertical deviation of less than 15 prism dioptres is corrected, surgery should be confined to a superior rectus recession. If the deviation is larger than this, then surgery should be split equally between the superior rectus and the contralateral inferior rectus. If the deviation increases on upgaze a superior rectus recession is indicated and if it increases in downgaze an inferior rectus recession is indicated.

The Faden or posterior fixation operation

This is a technique which weakens a muscle by placing a non-absorbable suture (5–0 mersilene or 5–0 Dacron) through the belly of the muscle behind the equator, usually 12–16 mm from the insertion, and in practice as posterior as possible (Fig. 67.13) (Cuppers 1976). A semi-circular needle makes suture placement easier. Its main advantage is that it weakens the muscle in its field of action with little or no effect on the deviation in primary position. For it to be effective it must produce an underaction of the muscle. The mechanism by which it produces its effect is thought

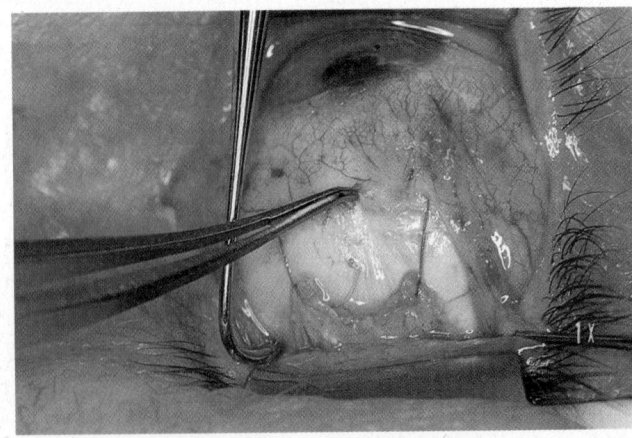

Fig. 67.12 Superior rectus hangback recession.

effect on the lateral rectus. The technique may be combined with a recession of the muscle (Kushner 1983).

The best indication for a Faden suture is in the management of incomitant strabismus, when there is little or no deviation in primary position and an incomitant deviation in the field of action of a single underacting muscle (von Noorden 1978). The suture is placed on the contralateral overacting yoke muscle. A good example is seen in patients with inferior rectus underaction following a blow-out fracture, who have no deviation in primary position but an increasing hyperdeviation on downgaze. The Faden suture is placed on the contralateral inferior rectus. Other indications for posterior fixation sutures include nystagmus blockage syndrome, convergence excess esotropia, dissociated vertical deviation, nystagmus with a face turn, residual strabismus after recession of a muscle, and Duane's syndrome where troublesome upshoots and downshoots might be reduced with placement of the suture on the lateral rectus (von Noorden 1978; Guyton 1985).

Technically the Faden procedure is difficult to perform, although suture placement is easier when the technique is combined with a recession. The vortex veins are close to the site of suture placement and the insertion of the superior oblique makes placement of the lateral suture on superior rectus difficult. There is a higher risk of scleral perforation than with conventional recession (Lyons *et al.* 1989). The biggest problem with the procedure, however, is that it produces an unpredictable effect.

Marginal myotomy

Marginal myotomy of the rectus muscles is an unpredictable and irreversible procedure. The superior and inferior borders of the muscle are cut 75% of the width of the muscle, about 5 mm apart, so that all fibres of the muscle are cut as the procedure is otherwise ineffective (Helveston 1993). There are few indications for the procedure, but it can be useful if a fully recessed muscle requires further weakening or if recession is contraindicated because of thin sclera, such as occurs in high myopia.

Strengthening procedures

Resections

Resection of a muscle enhances its action particularly when combined with a recession of the antagonist muscle in the same eye. Resections are, however, more difficult to perform than recessions, and produce more conjunctival tissue reaction and redness particularly if excess conjunctival tissue is hooded over the cornea. Large resections may produce limitation of ocular movement in the opposite direction of gaze, by a mechanical leash effect. This

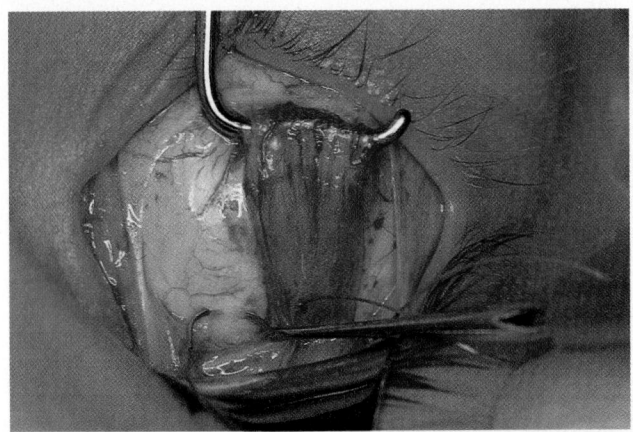

a

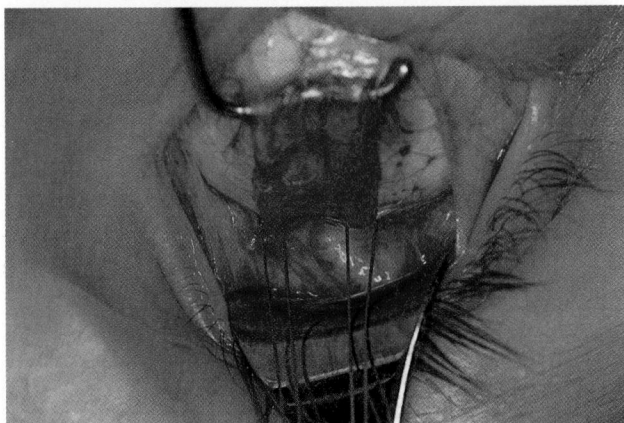

b

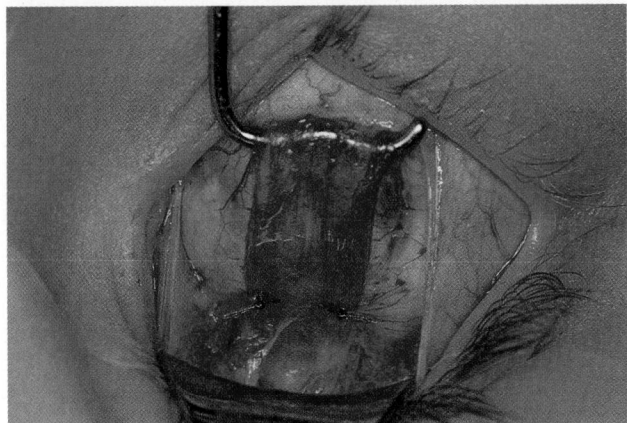

c

Fig. 67.13 Superior rectus posterior fixation suture. (a) Scleral placement of suture at medial border of superior rectus, lateral suture already placed through sclera and muscle. Surgeon's view from above. (b) Sutures prior to tying. View from in front. (c) Completed procedure. Surgeon's view.

to be the result of the effective insertion being moved to the point of the Faden suture, increasing the arc of contact of the muscle with the globe and reducing the lever arm, thereby weakening the muscle in its field of action (Scott 1977). It is most effective on the medial rectus, equally effective on the superior and inferior recti, but has little

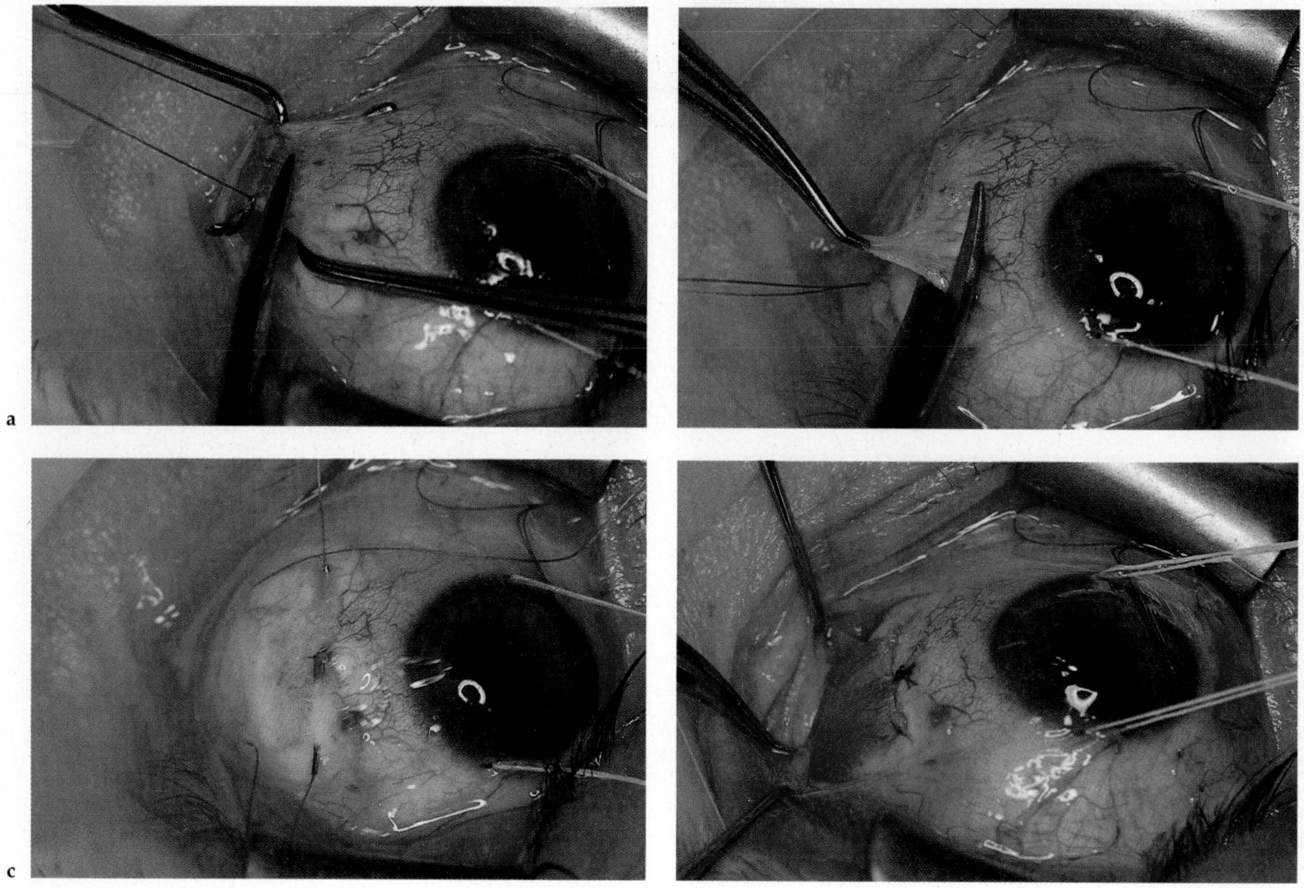

Fig. 67.14 A 4 mm single double-armed suture rectus muscle resection. (a) Suture placed 4 mm from muscle insertion. Muscle being cut anterior to the suture. (b) Removal of redundant muscle tissue. (c) Scleral placement of sutures anterior to insertion. Note the needle point exits near to each other. (d) Final position of muscle following suture tying. Note absence of central sagging of resected

lock bites taken at either end (Fig. 67.14a). A muscle clamp is then placed in front of the suture line and the muscle disinserted from the sclera. The redundant tissue is then removed, the end cauterized and the clamp removed (Fig. 67.14b). Many surgeons advocate leaving a stump of tissue at the insertion site to attach the resected muscle to. My own preference is not to leave this stump but to remove it and place the sutures in the sclera just anterior to the insertion, rather than just behind the insertion in thin sclera, providing a more secure scleral attachment.

The guidelines for the amount a muscle can be resected for a given deviation vary depending on the exact surgical technique. A consistent surgical technique is essential for predictable surgical results. The maximum amount a rectus muscle can be resected depends on the muscle. A horizontal muscle can be resected 10 mm or more, but at the expense of limitation of ocular movements in the opposite field. This may be appropriate in correcting a large deviation in a densely amblyopic eye. Large resections should, however, be avoided in most cases as they lead to restricted movement away from the muscle which leads to incomitant deviations. Resections greater than 5 mm of the superior and inferior recti should be avoided as they will be associated with advancement of the lid and narrowing of the palpebral fissure.

effect is maximal during the initial postoperative period and tends to diminish with time.

Resection of a muscle requires more complete dissection of the intermuscular septum and check ligaments than recession, ideally 5 mm beyond the extent of the resection. This ensures that Tenon's is not advanced as the muscle is resected. Particular care must be taken when resecting a lateral rectus to free the inferior oblique from its lower border to prevent it being included in the resection. Once the muscle has been dissected free from its attachments two hooks are placed under it. There are several suture techniques for rectus muscle resection, the most common being a single double-armed suture, two double-armed sutures, and two single-ended sutures. The aim of the resection should be to shorten the muscle and maintain its width without any central sagging. I prefer a single suture technique, the suture being placed through the muscle at the required distance from the insertion and

In cases where the resected muscle is tight or a muscle is being advanced from a previously recessed position, I prefer to use two double-armed sutures — the technique is similar to the single suture technique but each suture passes through only half the width of the muscle (Parks 1983a). Advancement of a slipped or previously recessed muscle is a powerful way of enhancing the effect of a rectus muscle, which has a greater effect per millimetre of advancement than resection. The precise effect varies depending on the degree of underaction of the muscle, previous surgery and the findings at surgery. If the muscle is advanced 2 mm anterior to the original insertion rather than to its original insertion then a greater effect is achieved. In consecutive exotropia medial rectus advancement anterior to the insertion or bilateral surgery should be considered for deviations greater than 25 prism dioptres (Biender *et al.* 1991; Ohtsuki *et al.* 1993). Muscle advancement is associated with the same difficulties as resection, but the problems are more pronounced, particularly if dissection near the orbital fat is required. For consecutive exotropia a simple advancement of the muscle to the original insertion (Ohtsuki *et al.* 1993) may suffice, although it is usually preferable to combine the advancement with a recession, ideally placing the recessed muscle on an adjustable suture.

A rectus muscle can also be strengthened using a tuck or plication. The only indication for these procedures is if there is concern about the risk of anterior segment ischaemia as it is possible to leave the anterior ciliary vessels intact.

Inferior oblique surgery

Indications

The indications for weakening procedures of the inferior oblique relate principally to overactions of the muscle, either primary or secondary. Weakening procedures are most commonly indicated for inferior oblique overaction associated with V pattern strabismus and overaction secondary to superior oblique underaction. Strengthening procedures first described by Wheeler in 1935 are rarely performed as, in contrast to superior oblique tucks, they are ineffective (Wheeler 1935).

In V pattern strabismus, inferior oblique surgery is likely to be most effective in those cases where the amount of V pattern is greatest between primary gaze and upgaze, as the main inferior oblique abducting effect occurs in upgaze. Bilateral inferior oblique weakening will correct up to 20 prism dioptres horizontal deviation in upgaze, having little or no effect on the horizontal deviation in primary position or downgaze (Stager & Parks 1973). In cases of symptomatic unilateral superior oblique palsy inferior oblique surgery is indicated if there is an incomitant hyperdeviation increasing in the field of action of the inferior oblique and associated with inferior oblique overaction. If the size of the deviation is less than 15 prism dioptres then inferior oblique surgery alone may suffice, but if greater then surgery on other muscles should be considered (Scott & Kraft 1986).

Surgical procedures

Inferior oblique surgery is based on weakening or changing the action of the muscle, which is easily approached through an inferotemporal conjunctival fornix incision 8 mm from the limbus. Direct visualization of the muscle is required and good lighting, if necessary with a headlight, is essential if the posterior fibres of the muscle are to be adequately seen. The assistant places a strabismus hook under the inferior and lateral rectus muscles to help exposure and protect these muscles from inadvertent dissection. The surgeon should use a large strabismus hook to retract conjunctiva, Tenon's and the orbital fat and a small hook to secure the inferior oblique once its posterior border has been visualized. Posterior fibres of the muscle can easily be missed but identified, in the V formed by the hook holding the anterior fibres, as a strand of muscular tissue running in the direction of the original line of the muscle.

Once isolated, a variety of weakening procedures are practised, the most common being myectomy (Fig. 67.15), disinsertion and recession (Fig. 67.16) (Dyer 1962; Parks 1972; Apt & Call 1978). All are effective in correcting inferior oblique overaction. Although myectomy of the muscle, involving removal of a segment of 5–8 mm of muscle, is an effective procedure, myotomy and Z-plasty are less effective. One of the advantages of a recession is that it can be graded allowing small recessions to be performed when there is little inferior oblique overaction. In a standard recession the muscle is placed 2 mm lateral and 3 mm posterior to the lateral border of the inferior rectus, equivalent to approximately a 10 mm recession of the muscle (Parks 1972). The more medial and anterior the muscle is placed the greater the weakening effect.

Anterior transposition of the inferior oblique is achieved by placing the muscle just anterior and parallel to the inferior rectus insertion, producing a J-shaped deformity of the muscle (Elliott & Nankin 1981; Mimms & Wood 1989). In this position, anterior to the equator of the globe, the inferior oblique becomes a functional depressor and in addition there may also be some mechanical restriction to elevation (Bremer *et al.* 1986; Kratz *et al.* 1989; Stager *et al.* 1992; Ziffer *et al.* 1993). The more anterior the muscle is placed, particularly the posterior fibres, the greater this effect (Kratz *et al.* 1989); this may be further enhanced by combining it with a myectomy of the muscle (Gonzalez & Klein 1993). The exact mechanism is uncertain but it is proposed that the effective origin of the muscle is changed either to the neurovascular bundle or

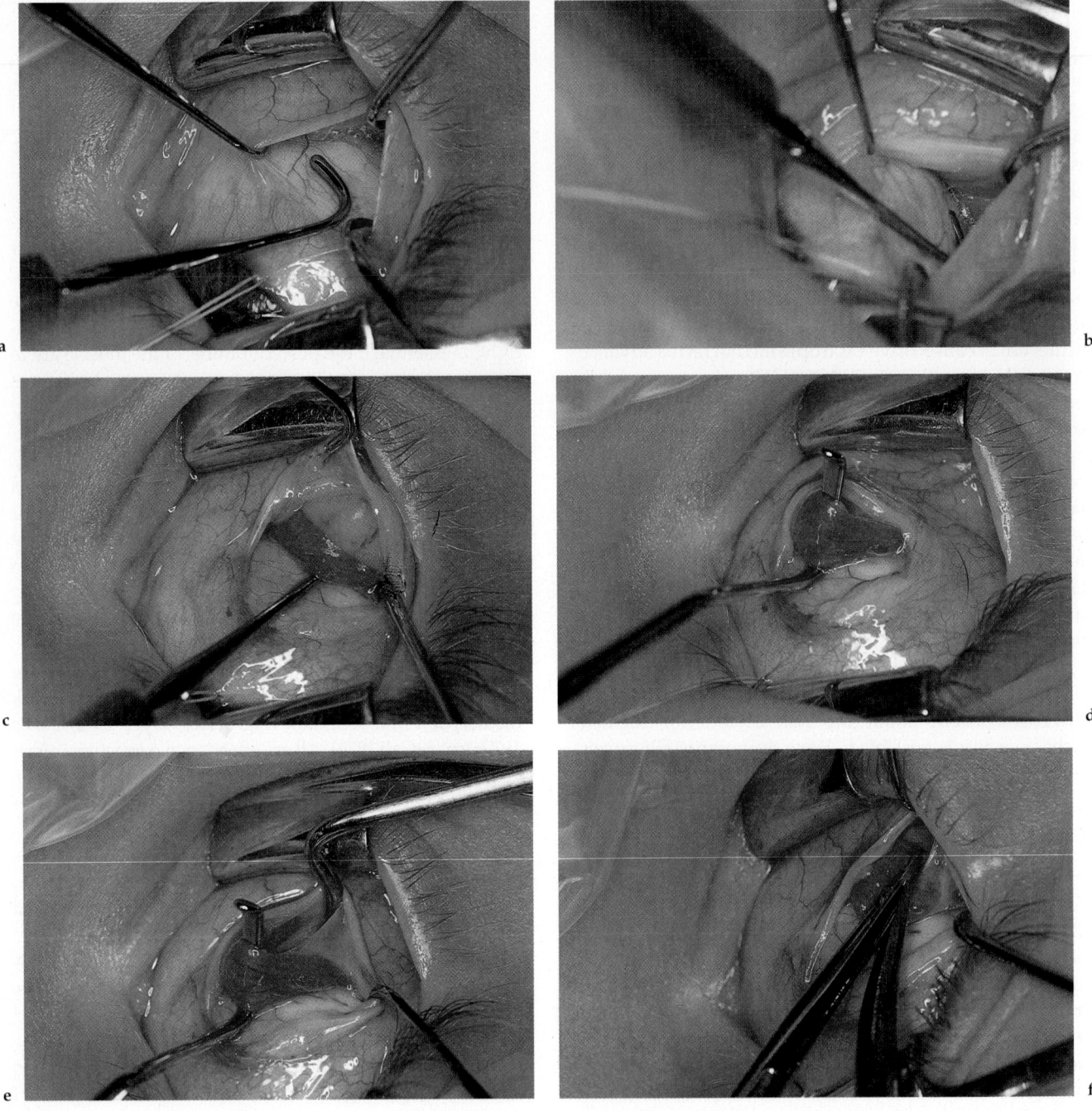

Fig. 67.15 Inferior oblique myectomy; surgeon's view from above. (a) Inferolateral conjunctival fornix incision. (b) Visualization of posterior border of inferior oblique. (c) Stevens tenotomy hook under both inferior oblique muscle and orbital fat. (d) Hook under inferior oblique, the orbital fat having been freed. (e) Intermuscular septum between inferior oblique and Tenon's capsule. (f) Inferior oblique being disinserted from the globe, a straight artery clamp having been placed along its insertion.

Lockwood's ligament and therefore when the muscle contracts the globe is pulled downwards (Bremer *et al.* 1986; Kratz *et al.* 1989; Stager *et al.* 1992). It is a useful technique for marked inferior oblique overaction, and when inferior oblique overaction and dissociated vertical deviation coincide then it is most effective in eyes with preoperative deviations of less than 15 prism dioptres in primary position (Kratz *et al.* 1989; Burke *et al.* 1993). It may also be used when superior rectus surgery has proved ineffective for dissociated vertical deviation. It is best performed bilaterally as unilateral surgery produces a postoperative hypotropia and this effect is exacerbated by inadvertent

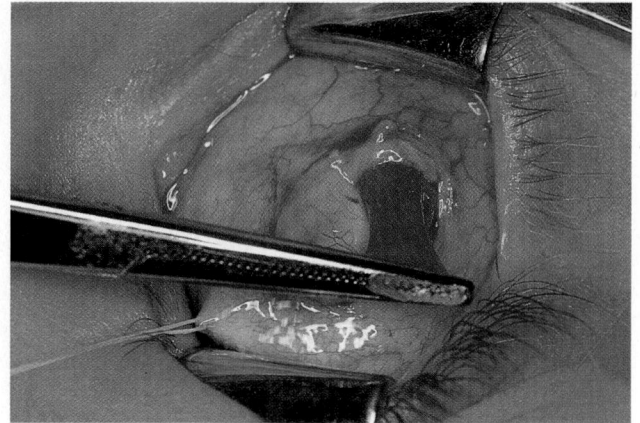

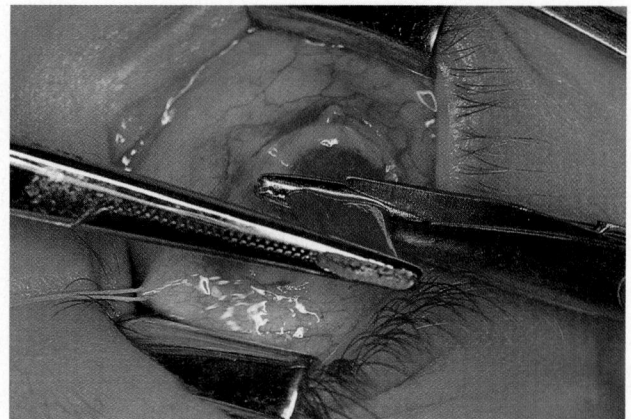

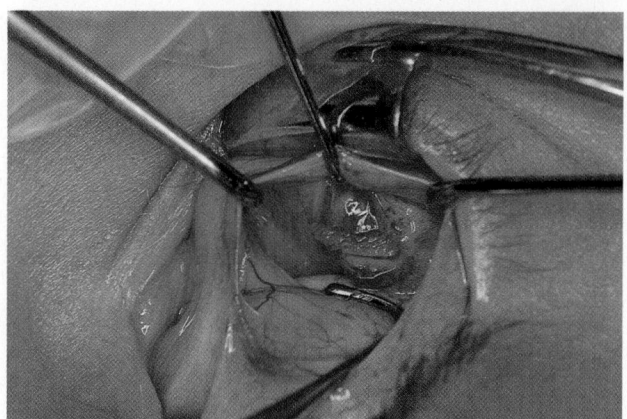

Fig. 67.15 *Continued.* (g) Inferior oblique muscle having been disinserted. (h) A segment of muscle being removed. (i) Cut border of inferior oblique visible, retracting into Tenon's capsule.

resection of the muscle, which should be avoided (Bremer *et al.* 1986).

Denervation and extirpation may be indicated if other procedures have been ineffective in resolving marked inferior oblique overaction, but should not be used as a primary procedure. The nerve to the inferior oblique is cauterized as it enters the muscle at the lateral border of the inferior rectus, but the muscle function can recover as the nerve regrows. To overcome this Gonzales (1976) suggested removing as much of the inferior oblique as technically possible, tracing it as far back within Tenon's capsule as possible. Del Monte and Parks (1983) have reported good results with this procedure finding it superior to large recessions.

Specific complications

The key factor in the success of inferior oblique weakening procedures is identification of the posterior border of the muscle by direct visualization, as the most common cause of persistent inferior oblique overaction is incomplete division of these fibres (Fig. 67.17). It is, however, important to distinguish such overaction from dissociated vertical deviation, particularly in patients with congenital strabismus (Scott & Morris 1990). Inferior oblique fat

adherence syndrome is a less common but important complication resulting in hypotropia and restriction of elevation of the eye in adduction following surgery (Parks 1972). It is associated with rupture of posterior Tenon's capsule and prolapse of the orbital fat with associated haemorrhage which leads to dense scarring at the site of surgery. Both these complications can be minimized with meticulous surgical technique. Other complications include inadvertent disinsertion of the lateral or inferior rectus muscle, pupillary dilation and haemorrhage from either the cut end of the muscle or damage to the inferior temporal vortex vein.

Superior oblique surgery

Weakening procedures

The main indications for superior oblique weakening are in Brown's syndrome and superior oblique overaction in the presence of a vertical or an A pattern strabismus which is affecting fusion or causing a significant compensatory head posture. Several different types of procedure have been described, all are difficult to quantify and none entirely satisfactory. Most are non-selective and produce global weakening of torsion, depression and abduction.

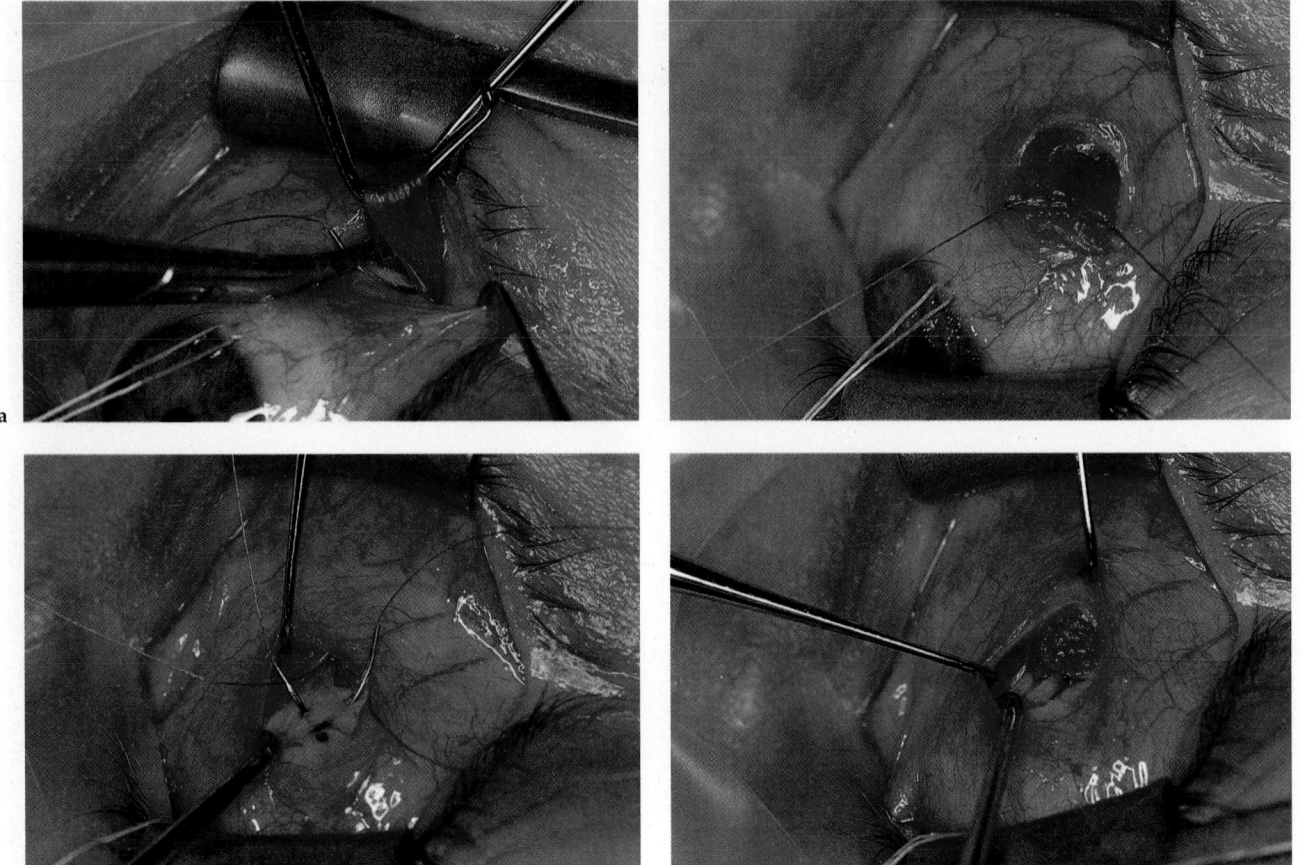

Fig. 67.16 Inferior oblique recession; surgeon's view from above. (a) Suture being placed at the insertion of the inferior oblique using a double-armed vicryl suture. (b) Double-armed vicryl suture through inferior oblique muscle. (c) Needles placed lateral and posterior to the lateral border of the inferior rectus (the strabismus hook in the bottom left of the picture is under the insertion of the inferior rectus). (d) Muscle in recessed position.

Superior oblique tenotomies and tenectomies can be performed nasal or temporal to the superior rectus insertion. The closer the tenotomy is to the trochlea the greater the weakening effect of the procedure. Temporal tenotomies tend to have little effect, partly due to the fascial attachment between the superior oblique and the undersurface of the superior rectus which does not allow retraction of the oblique tendon.

Surgically the nasal portion of the superior oblique tendon can be approached via a nasal (Fig. 67.18) (Berke 1946; Parks & Helveston 1970) or a superotemporal conjunctival fornix incision (Parks 1983b). The former is easier technically but the latter leaves the nasal intermuscular tendon intact and Parks (1983b) has suggested that this reduces the incidence of postoperative superior oblique palsy, as the cut ends of the tendon are supported by the septum. With either technique direct visualization of the tendon is

essential to reduce the complications induced by blind hooking, particularly incomplete tenotomy and inadvertent transection of the superior rectus (McNeer 1972; Raymond & Parks 1995). However, with any of these techniques there is a significant incidence of consecutive superior oblique underaction. In patients with Brown's syndrome, tenotomy leads to consecutive underaction of the superior oblique in 66–85% of cases (Crawford *et al.* 1980; von Noorden & Olivier 1982). To avoid this complication Z-tenotomy of the superior oblique has been advocated. The tendon is lengthened by partial width marginal tenotomies, but in practice it is difficult to perform and produces unpredictable weakening of superior oblique function (Souza Dias & Uesugui 1986).

Superior oblique recession has the advantage of being a graded weakening procedure, but it can result in bunching of the tendon fibres anterior to the equator, which changes the function from depression and abduction to elevation and adduction (Caldeira 1975). Although recession is more predictable than tenotomy, it tends to result in undercorrection and has similar complications to tenotomy with no clear advantage over it (Buckley & Flynn 1983).

Disinsertion of the tendon produces mild weakening of muscle action. As with recession, in order for it to be

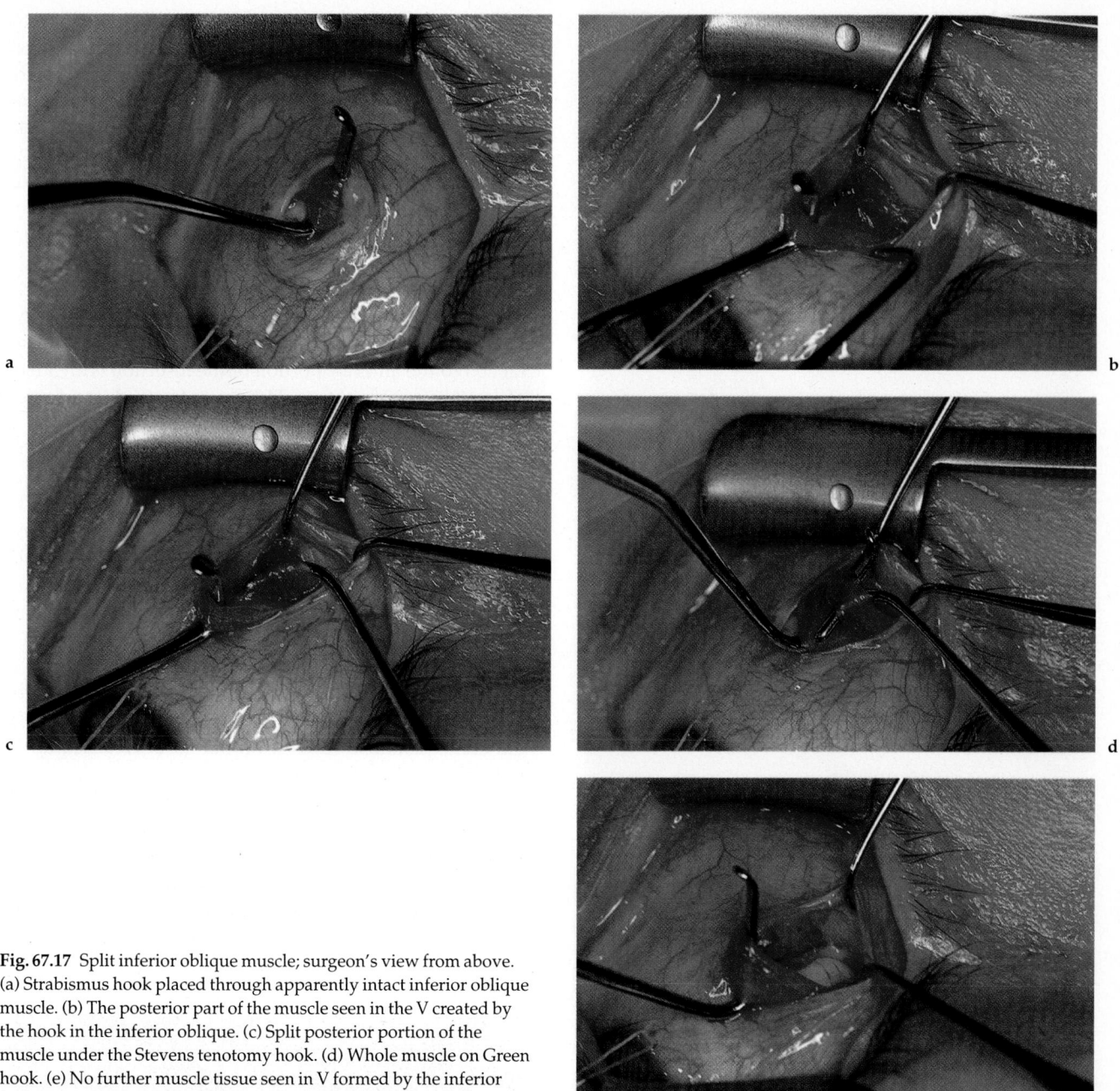

Fig. 67.17 Split inferior oblique muscle; surgeon's view from above. (a) Strabismus hook placed through apparently intact inferior oblique muscle. (b) The posterior part of the muscle seen in the V created by the hook in the inferior oblique. (c) Split posterior portion of the muscle under the Stevens tenotomy hook. (d) Whole muscle on Green hook. (e) No further muscle tissue seen in V formed by the inferior oblique. This illustration emphasises how important meticulous technique is in avoiding unnecessary complications.

effective the fascial attachments between it and the superior rectus above need to be divided. Disinsertion of the posterior fibres selectively weakens depression (Wheeler 1935).

The use of a superior oblique silicone tendon expander is advocated by Wright (1991) as a method of weakening the muscle. A segment of 240 silicone retinal band is inserted between cut ends of the nasal portion of the tendon (Fig. 67.19). Although producing global weakening of superior oblique function, the procedure can be quantified using different lengths of tendon. It is suitable for both

Brown's syndrome and superior oblique overaction (Manners *et al.* 1994), and a low incidence of secondary superior oblique underaction is reported.

Posterior tenectomy has been advocated for mild A pattern esotropia to weaken the abducting and depressor functions selectively yet maintaining the incyclotorsion function. A wedge resection of the posterior and medial fibres is performed preserving the anterior intorting fibres (Prieto-Diaz 1988; Shin *et al.* 1996).

Scott and Kraft (1988) have suggested that careful preoperative selection criteria minimize the risks of bilateral

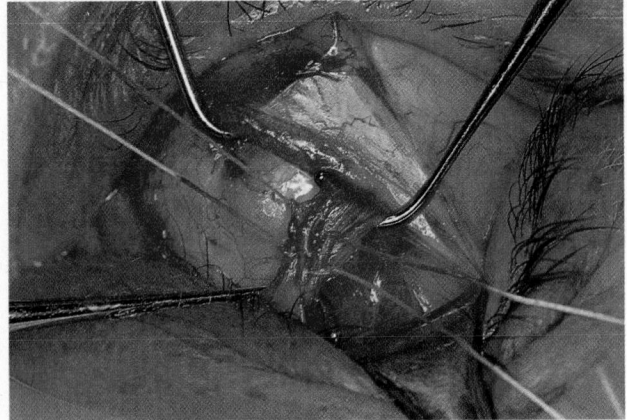

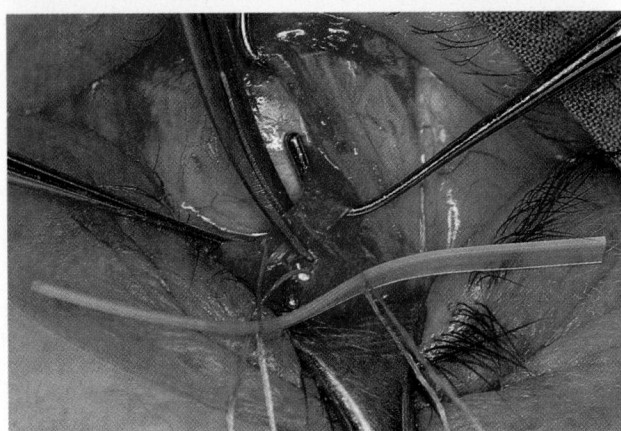

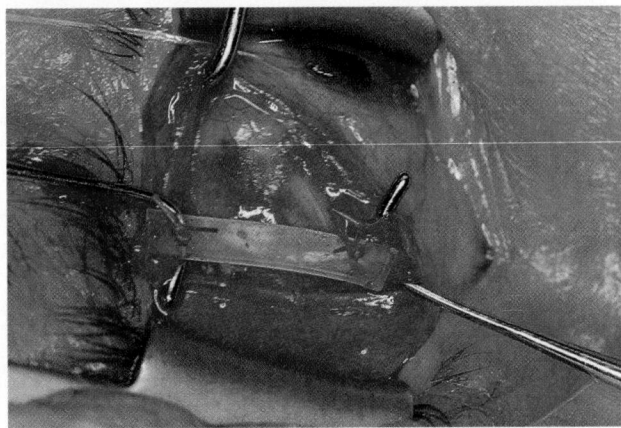

Fig. 67.18 Superior oblique tendon expander; surgeon's view from above. (a) Non-absorbable double-armed sutures closed through superior oblique tendon. (b) Segment of silicone band inserted and tendon being divided. (c) Tendon following division and insertion of silicone band.

superior oblique tenotomies and did not find that fusion was adversely affected in their series. They suggest it should only be carried out in the presence of a 45 prism dioptre A pattern with moderate to marked superior oblique overaction and no inferior oblique overaction. In this study up to 12 prism dioptres of exodeviation was

corrected in primary position and up to 45 prism dioptres in downgaze. Bilateral posterior tenectomies can be used to correct up to 15 prism dioptres of A pattern and scleral disinsertion up to 25 prism dioptres. For larger A patterns superior oblique tenotomy may be combined with horizontal muscle surgery. The magnitude of reduction of the A pattern corresponds to the size of the preoperative A pattern and the correction in primary position is greater in patients with exodeviations than esodeviations (Shuey *et al.* 1992).

Gobin (1982) has described desagittalization of the superior oblique by anteropositioning the tendon with a loop. The tendon is disinserted and the anterior tip reattached to the anterior portion of the insertion with a loop of non-absorbable suture. This procedure reduces depression in adduction (Gobin 1982).

The most frequent complication of superior oblique weakening procedures is secondary superior oblique underaction. In most instances this can be dealt with by ipsilateral inferior oblique weakening, but in patients with fusion superior oblique surgery can induce torsional and/or vertical diplopia. Bilateral superior oblique weakening procedures can lead to the development of a postoperative V pattern and torsion. Poor surgical technique and blind hooking of the tendon can lead to posterior fibres not being identified at surgery and left intact causing persistent overaction of the muscle. Fat adherence can also result if orbital fat is breached at the time of surgery.

Another technique for weakening the function of the superior oblique involves subluxating the tendon out of the trochlea through an anterior orbitotomy approach, or alternatively dislocating the trochlea from the bony orbit using a periosteal approach (Mombaerts *et al.* 1995). The authors report good results with both techniques, but

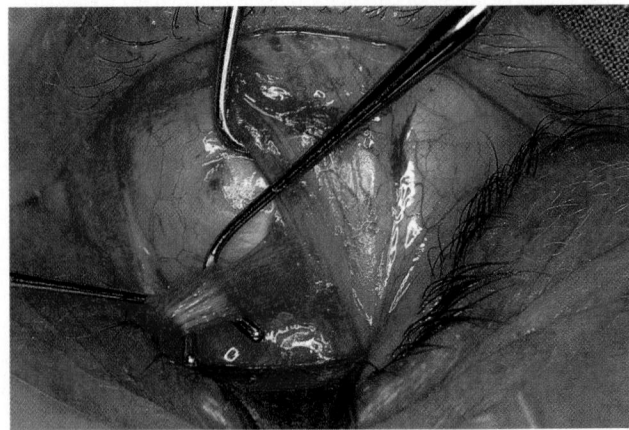

Fig. 67.19 Superior oblique tenotomy. The superior oblique tendon is identified via the nasal approach with two Stevens tenotomy hooks beneath it. The muscle is divided between the hooks for a superior oblique tenotomy.

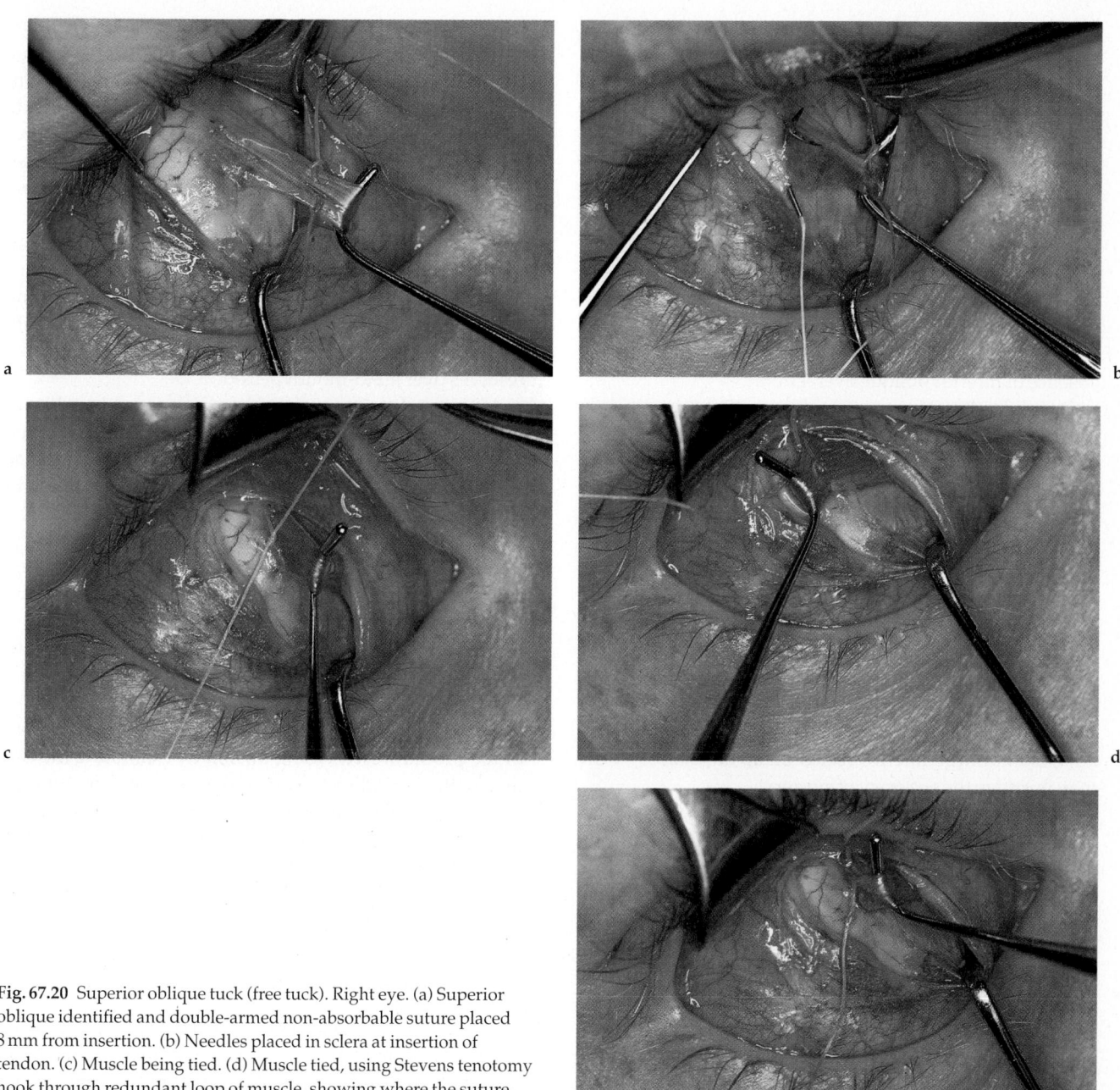

Fig. 67.20 Superior oblique tuck (free tuck). Right eye. (a) Superior oblique identified and double-armed non-absorbable suture placed 8 mm from insertion. (b) Needles placed in sclera at insertion of tendon. (c) Muscle being tied. (d) Muscle tied, using Stevens tenotomy hook through redundant loop of muscle, showing where the suture has been passed through the tendon. (e) Final position of muscle after tuck. Note Stevens tenotomy hook through redundant loop of muscle.

favour the latter as there is less risk of damage to the supratrochlear neurovascular bundle, the technique can be graded and it is technically easier.

Strengthening procedures

Superior oblique tuck

Non-selective enhancement of the function of the superior oblique muscle can be achieved by tucking the superior oblique tendon. McGuire (1947) recognized that in most cases of superior oblique palsy the muscle was rarely completely paralysed and suggested that the most logical surgical approach in these cases was a strengthening procedure of the superior oblique tendon. McLean (1948) first described a temporal approach to the tendon thereby avoiding disinsertion of the superior rectus muscle (McGuire 1969). Tuck surgery is helpful in the management of selected patients with both unilateral and bilateral superior oblique palsies. A tuck can be performed using a tendon tucker, or a free tuck (Fig. 67.20) can be performed (Scott & Kraft 1988).

Despite reports of the efficacy of superior oblique tuck surgery, there is no consensus in the literature on the role of this procedure – many authors feel that the complications outweigh the advantages (Khawam *et al.* 1967; Johnson 1971; Anderson *et al.* 1974; Mittleman & Folk 1976; Helveston & Ellis 1983; Saunders & Tomlinson 1985; Saunders 1986). However, a study by Morris *et al.* (1992) of 45 patients showed that many cases of superior oblique palsy can be effectively treated with superior oblique tucks. They suggest that the procedure is indicated in those patients with an incomitant vertical deviation which is greatest in the field of action of the superior oblique, with associated superior oblique underaction and in the absence of inferior oblique overaction.

Quantification of superior oblique tucks is difficult. Morris *et al.* (1992) found that the effect of an isolated tuck ranged from no effect to 11 prism dioptres in primary position (mean 3.6 prism dioptres) and from 0 to 40 prism dioptres (mean 14.3 prism dioptres) in the field of maximum deviation and did not find any correlation between the size of the tuck and the amount of deviation corrected. This is likely to be due to the fact that it is not just the size of the tuck which determines the amount of correction obtained. Other important factors include the laxity of the superior oblique tendon and the size of the preoperative deviation. In patients undergoing contralateral inferior rectus recessions in conjunction with a tuck, postoperative adjustment of the inferior rectus on an adjustable suture may improve the accuracy of surgery.

Intraoperative adjustment of the tuck by forced ductions is essential to prevent development of a significant postoperative iatrogenic Brown's syndrome (Saunders & Tomlinson 1985; Saunders 1986) although it does not help determine the amount of vertical deviation corrected. Using this technique the incidence of clinically significant Brown's syndrome is small (Morris *et al.* 1992).

Bilateral superior oblique tucks are indicated in patients with bilateral superior oblique palsies in whom there is a significant esodeviation on downgaze and alternating hyperdeviations on sidegazes. In the absence of these features bilateral modified Harada–Ito procedures to correct symptomatic torsion are indicated.

An alternative to a superior oblique tuck is a resection or advancement of the muscle, but both have the disadvantage of disinserting the muscle from its insertion and therefore altering its function.

The Harada–Ito procedure

The intorting action of the superior oblique muscle can be enhanced by selectively strengthening the anterior portion of the muscle. This procedure was first reported by Harada and Ito (1964) who described anterior and lateral positioning of the anterior fibres of the superior oblique, without disinsertion, for the correction of excylotorsion in bilateral superior oblique palsies. Fells (1974) subsequently described a modification of the technique, suggesting disinserting the anterior fibres and advancing them anteriorly and temporally 8 mm posterior to the superior border of the lateral rectus muscle insertion (Fig. 67.21). The anterior third of the tendon is transposed in this technique. This modification of the procedure is effective in reducing excyclotorsion and is indicated in patients with bilateral superior oblique palsies in whom torsion is the main finding (Price *et al.* 1987). The procedure corrects about 11° of excyclotorsion without inducing a vertical deviation (Mitchell & Parks 1982). Typically an initial postoperative overcorrection is produced, which resolves over a 2–3-month period.

A greater abducting effect in downgaze can be achieved if the anterior fibres are placed more posteriorly than 8 mm from the insertion of the superior border of the lateral rectus, and this should be considered in patients with significant esotropic deviations in downgaze (Mitchell & Parks 1982). Conversely, it is important to avoid placing the tendon closer than 8 mm to the lateral rectus insertion, as this anteroplaces the muscle and may produce an undesirable esotropic deviation. If some posterior fibres are included in the transposition this produces a greater depressor effect and may be useful in correcting small hypertropias.

Guyton (1984) has suggested intraoperative adjustment of the procedure, assessing torsion by examining the fundus with the indirect ophthalmoscope, and monitoring the change in the position of the fovea in relationship to the optic disc. Metz and Lerner (1981) have described an adjustable suture technique for this procedure, but it has not gained popularity, as it is technically difficult to perform the adjustment.

Superior oblique tendon transposition

Transposition of the superior oblique tendon, combined with a large medial rectus recession and lateral rectus resection, is useful in some cases of complete third nerve palsy (Helveston 1993). The superior oblique tendon is cut at the medial border of the superior rectus, the tendon is then resected and sutured to the globe just above the insertion of the medial rectus (Fig. 67.22a). The transposed tendon adducts the globe both mechanically and by exerting some functional rotational action. This effect can be enhanced by combining the procedure with dislocation of the trochlea allowing the muscle to lie parallel to the medial rectus. Pratt-Johnson and Tillson (1995) suggest that this dislocation of the trochlea should be reserved for cases with a hypotropia, in primary position, of less than 15 prism dioptres, but in cases with greater superior oblique function and hypotropias of 20 prism dioptres or more this step is not required. Postoperatively traction sutures should be used to hold the eye in adduction to prevent

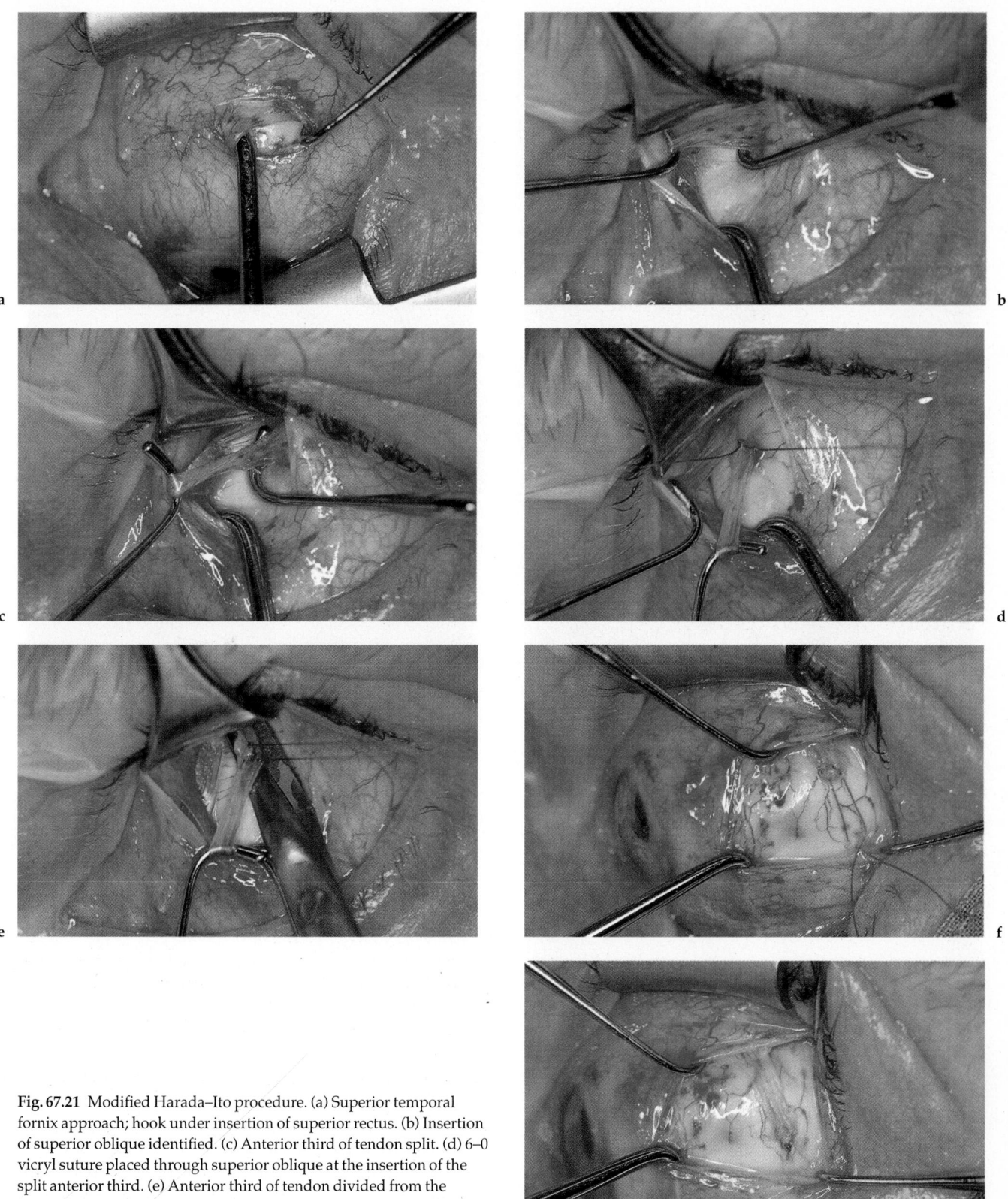

Fig. 67.21 Modified Harada–Ito procedure. (a) Superior temporal fornix approach; hook under insertion of superior rectus. (b) Insertion of superior oblique identified. (c) Anterior third of tendon split. (d) 6–0 vicryl suture placed through superior oblique at the insertion of the split anterior third. (e) Anterior third of tendon divided from the globe. (f) Double-armed suture placed above superior border of lateral rectus 8 mm from insertion; hook in lower left of picture is under insertion of lateral rectus. (g) Final position of tendon.

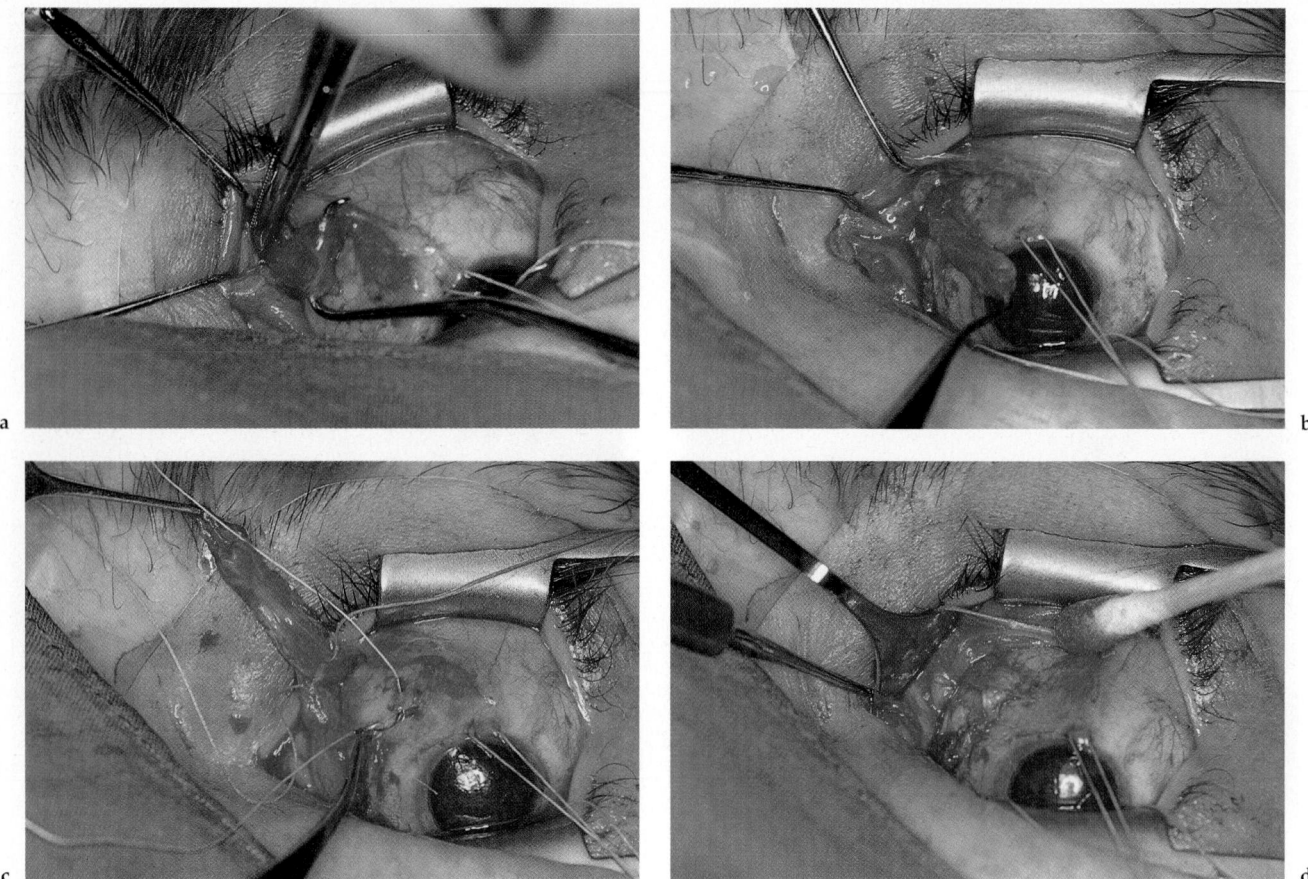

Fig. 67.22 Superior oblique tendon transposition. (a) Tendon under Green hook, artery forceps being used to fracture trochlea. (b) Tendon disinserted and moved nasally. (c) Suture placed through tendon and sutured above the insertion of the medial rectus. (d) Tendon sutured to sclera (redundant tendon tissue having been excised). Note the medial rectus has also been resected.

the insertion of the lateral rectus muscle creeping forwards.

Transposition procedures

Muscle transposition procedures move the muscle out of the normal line of action changing their function.

Vertical transposition of the horizontal rectus muscles

Probably the most common transposition procedure performed in strabismus surgery is a vertical transposition of the horizontal rectus muscles in the management of A and V patterns (Knapp 1959). This type of procedure should only be considered if there is no demonstrable inferior oblique overaction in a V pattern, and no superior oblique overaction in an A pattern. V patterns are considered clinically significant if there is a difference of 15 prism dioptres

between upgaze of 25° and downgaze of 25°. A 10 prism dioptre difference is considered significant for A patterns. Surgical correction of the pattern should be considered in the presence of a chin-up or chin-down head position, or if the pattern is precluding fusion. Surgery on A and V patterns is rarely indicated for cosmetic strabismus surgery (Miller 1960; Tamler 1961; Scott *et al.* 1989).

The simple rule for vertical displacement of the horizontal recti is that in V patterns the medial rectus is always moved inferiorly towards the apex of the V (Fig. 67.23). This applies for both resections and recessions of the muscle. The lateral recti are moved in the opposite direction. In A patterns the medial recti are moved towards the apex of the A, that is superiorly, and the lateral recti inferiorly (Fig. 67.23). The principle of the procedure is that a horizontal rectus muscle is recessed and transposed in the direction in which the greatest weakening effect is required (Knapp 1959). Therefore in a V pattern esotropia, recession and inferior displacement of the medial recti weakens them more in downgaze than upgaze. Resection and superior displacement of the lateral recti produces less abducting effect in upgaze than in downgaze.

The amount of effect produced depends on how much the muscle is displaced and the size of the preoperative pattern, but there is no consistent correlation (Ribeiro *et al.*

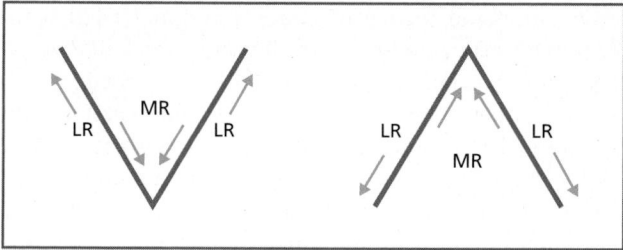

Fig. 67.23 Direction which medial and lateral recti moved in A and V patterns.

1995). A half tendon width displacement produces a reduction in the pattern of approximately 10–20 prism dioptres, and a full tendon width 25–30 prism dioptres (Scott *et al.* 1989; Metz 1993). The amount of horizontal surgery performed should be based on the deviation in primary position as transposing the muscles has little effect on the deviation in this position. Unilateral surgery moving the medial rectus and lateral rectus in opposite directions combined with recession and resection can be

performed and should be considered if surgery needs to be confined to one eye (Goldstein 1967; Metz 1977). Surgery is equally effective in collapsing the pattern if bilateral symmetrical surgery or unilateral surgery is performed (Scott *et al.* 1989).

Technically the important points to remember when performing this procedure include a conjunctival incision with a larger relaxing incision in the direction in which the muscle is to be displaced. As with resections, the intermuscular septum and check ligaments should be dissected far enough back to allow the muscle to be moved freely. Finally, the displaced muscle, when reattached, should remain concentric with the limbus (Fig. 67.24).

An alternative to vertical transposition of the muscle in the management of A or V patterns is to slant the muscle insertion (Biender & Rothkoff 1995). In V pattern esotropia the inferior pole of the medial rectus is recessed more than the upper pole, weakening the muscle more in downgaze. In A pattern esotropia the converse applies.

Horizontal muscle transposition procedures can also be used to correct a small comitant vertical deviation associ-

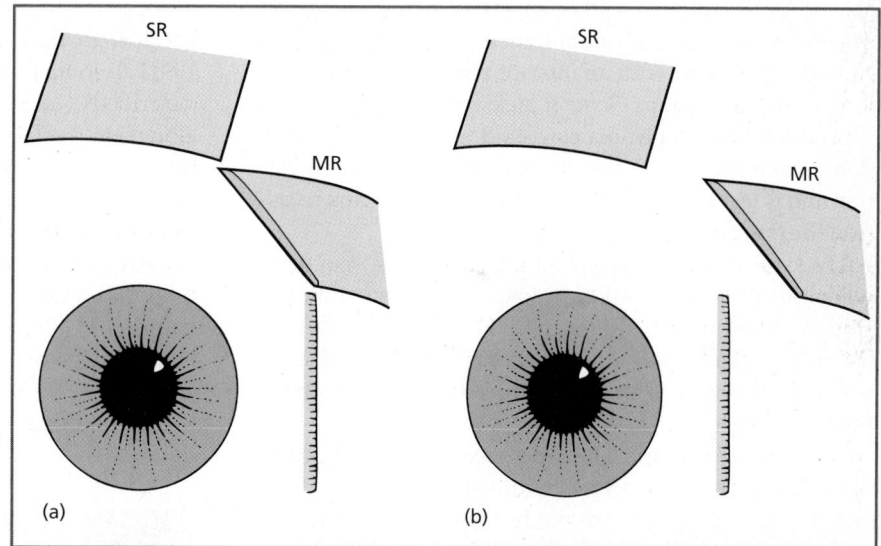

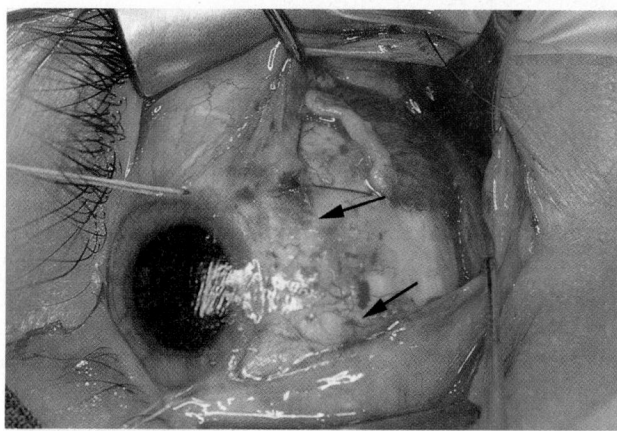

Fig. 67.24 For an A pattern, the medial rectus may be raised by up to one tendon width (a). For an A esodeviation, the medial rectus is recessed and supraplaced (anchored hangback technique) (b, c). Original insertion indicated by arrows (c).

ated with a horizontal strabismus. This technique can be applied with uniocular surgery, moving the rectus muscle in the opposite direction of the vertical deviation; for example, in the presence of a hypertropia both medial and lateral recti should be lowered (O'Neill 1978; Metz 1988). As a rule of thumb 1 mm of vertical displacement will correct 1 prism dioptre of vertical deviation (O'Neill 1978; Metz 1988). The same principle can be used to correct a small horizontal deviation when performing vertical rectus muscle surgery for vertical deviations (Metz 1988).

Horizontal muscle transposition procedures are useful in vertical deviations resulting from underaction or paresis of vertical rectus muscles. Superior vertical transposition of the horizontal recti is carried out to correct elevator palsies (Knapp procedure) or inferior transposition to correct depressor palsies (Dunlap procedure) (Knapp 1969; Dunlap 1971). Knapp described transposing both medial and lateral recti alongside the superior rectus, and reported correcting an average of 38 prism dioptres of hypotropia with this technique. The best indication for the procedure is a double elevator palsy with a hypotropia in primary position and a chin-up head posture, in the absence of a positive forced duction test. A positive forced duction test indicates inferior rectus restriction, which should be released with an inferior rectus recession prior to a Knapp procedure (Scott & Jackson 1977; Metz 1988). The amount of hypotropia corrected increases over time, does not correlate with the size of the preoperative deviation and is less predictable after prior inferior rectus recession (Burke *et al.* 1992).

The same principles apply for inferior rectus weakness, when the horizontal recti are transposed inferiorly alongside the inferior rectus (Dunlap 1971). This procedure is useful in patients with inferior rectus paresis such as may occur following a blow-out fracture (Lipton *et al.* 1990; Burke & Keech 1995).

Both the Knapp and Dunlap procedures can be combined with a recess resect procedure of the medial and lateral recti if there is a co-existent horizontal deviation (Lee *et al.* 1986; Scott *et al.* 1989; Buckley & Townsend 1991).

Horizontal transposition of the vertical rectus muscles

Horizontal transposition of the vertical recti is indicated in some cases of complete sixth nerve palsy. The first procedure was described by Hummelsheim (1907) for the correction of sixth nerve palsy, who advocated transposition of the temporal half of the superior and inferior recti alongside the lateral rectus, suturing the muscles to the lateral rectus. O'Connor (1921) modified the technique, transposing the whole of the superior and inferior recti by suturing them to the sclera adjacent to the lateral rectus. Because of the risk of anterior segment ischaemia associated with these techniques, when combined with medial

rectus recession, these procedures were superseded by the Jensen (1964) procedure. This carries less risk of anterior segment ischaemia as the rectus muscles are not disinserted. The superior and inferior recti are split in half and the temporal halves sutured with a non-absorbable suture (5–0 Dacron or 4–0 mersilene) to the superior and inferior halves of a split lateral rectus. The suture around the muscle should be loose to minimize the risk of anterior segment ischaemia from direct constriction of the anterior ciliary arteries; the sutured muscles are fixed to the globe 12–15 mm from the limbus. The procedure is combined with a 5–6 mm medial rectus recession, ideally with preservation of the anterior ciliary arteries, or alternatively botulinum toxin to the medial rectus. The Jensen procedure is an effective technique, but does produce mechanical restriction to adduction although this contributes to stabilizing the surgical outcome and preventing recurrence of the esotropia (Scott *et al.* 1979; Rosenbaum *et al.* 1984; Metz 1993).

An alternative to the Jensen procedure is full temporal transposition of the superior and inferior recti combined with a medial rectus botulinum toxin injection. The timing of the toxin injection is not critical and may be up to a week prior to surgery or even postoperatively (Rosenbaum *et al.* 1984; Fitzsimons *et al.* 1988; Rosenbaum *et al.* 1991). Two methods of temporal transposition have been described. The insertion of the vertical recti can be either alongside the lateral rectus, between their original insertion and the lateral rectus (Fitzsimons *et al.* 1988), or they can be placed parallel with the upper and lower borders of the lateral rectus, the superior rectus 3 mm above the superior border and the inferior rectus 1 mm below the inferior border of the lateral rectus (Fig. 67.25) (Rosenbaum *et al.* 1984). These procedures reduce but do not eliminate the risk of anterior segment ischaemia (Keech *et al.* 1990; Lee & Olver 1991).

Vertical deviations can be induced with all these tech-

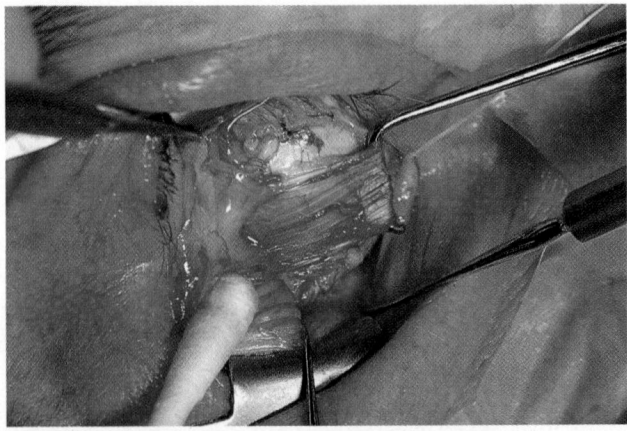

Fig. 67.25 Temporal transposition of superior and inferior recti parallel to the upper and lower borders of the lateral rectus.

niques, most commonly hyperdeviations. To overcome this an adjustable suture modification of the full temporal transposition has been described (Laby & Rosenbaum 1994).

Horizontal transposition procedures can be effective in some cases of type 1 Duane's syndrome (Gobin 1974; Molatre & Rosenbaum 1990) and also in cases of lost medial or lateral rectus muscles. The Jensen procedure is contraindicated in Duane's syndrome because of the mechanical restriction it produces.

Adjustable suture techniques

The concept of adjustable sutures was first described in the 1930s, but it is only since the mid-1970s that the technique has become popular. Although adjustable suture surgery can be carried out under local anaesthesia with on table adjustment, most surgeons prefer a two-staged approach, initial surgery being carried out under general anaesthesia with postoperative adjustment under topical anaesthesia. Most adjustable suture surgery is done on the rectus muscles, but an adjustable Harada–Ito procedure has been described (Metz & Lerner 1981).

The indications for adjustable sutures are varied: some surgeons use them in all patients who they feel will tolerate the procedure (Table 67.4). They are most useful in cases where conventional surgery is likely to be unpredictable, particularly in strabismus reoperations when scarring, tethering or contracture of extraocular muscles is present (Morris & Luff 1992). They should be considered in any patient undergoing vertical or horizontal rectus muscle surgery where the indication for surgery is diplopia, as their use facilitates achieving the maximal field of binocular single vision.

Although adjustable sutures require the co-operation of the patient they can be performed in children as young as 8 years, and it is my experience that girls tend to be more co-operative than boys. Careful preoperative assessment will give an indication of the suitability of a patient for adjustment. A patient who can tolerate a cotton bud manipulating the bulbar conjunctiva, anaesthetized with topical anaesthetic, or alternatively applanation tonometry, is likely to tolerate the procedure.

The key to the two-stage approach is general anaesthesia planned so that the patient is alert and co-operative with minimal nausea in the postoperative period. Intra-

Table 67.4 Indications for adjustable suture surgery.

Previous strabismus surgery
Large angle squints
Thyroid eye disease
Strabismus following retinal detachment surgery
Combined horizontal and vertical muscle procedures

venous anaesthetic agents can facilitate this (Luff *et al.* 1993). Ideally the adjustment should be performed within 6 hours; leaving it longer than 24 hours may lead to difficulty as the tissues are beginning to adhere to the globe (Holmes & Townshend 1995).

Any type of conjunctival incision can be used, but the limbal technique is easiest, the main disadvantage being that it can be difficult to cover the suture knot with conjunctiva after the adjustment. 6–0 vicryl is currently the best suture material as it has a high tensile strength and little tendency to snag. A dyed suture facilitates identification of the suture for adjustment, a white suture being difficult to see. There are two main methods for muscle reattachment, the bow tie and the sliding, or cinch knot. In the bow tie technique the sutures are placed just anterior to the insertion through scleral tunnels emerging 1.5 mm apart to facilitate tying a bow (Fig. 67.26). At adjustment the bow is undone and the muscle can be advanced or recessed, and when in the desired position the knot is tied. Fells has described a modification of this using two scleral passes for each suture so that the suture forms a Z configuration (Fells 1988) (Fig. 67.27). The alternative technique is the cinch method in which a second suture is tied tightly around the two arms of the muscle suture; this knot can be slid up or down the muscle sutures to enable adjustment, but this technique produces a larger knot and more conjunctival tissue reaction postoperatively (Eustis & Hesse 1993). At the end of surgery the long suture ends of the adjustable suture can be taped to the lid and tucked into the inferior fornix.

Most adjustable sutures are put on recessed muscles, and more than one muscle can be placed on an adjustable suture. Some surgeons prefer to deliberately over-recess a muscle as it is easier to advance than recess a muscle at the time of adjustment. Although resected muscles can be placed on adjustable sutures, they are more difficult to adjust and there is a greater risk of muscle slippage.

At adjustment the patient's deviation should be measured and the ocular movements assessed with the patient wearing the appropriate spectacle correction. Depending on the findings, muscles can be advanced or recessed as needed, although it is important not to recess a muscle so far that it would lead to underaction of the muscle. For patients with large deviations, especially vertical deviations, it is better to place more than one muscle on an adjustable suture rather than try to achieve the whole effect with one muscle. Post-adjustment drift occurs in the first 12 months, horizontal deviations tending to undercorrection and vertical deviations to overcorrection (Rosen *et al.* 1991).

Adjustable sutures do have advantages over conventional surgery and are associated with a lower reoperation rate, with most authors reporting an adjustment rate of about 40%. Specific complications are rare. Nausea induced by the adjustment is the most common. Bradycardia, suture breakage and inability to adjust the suture can all occur.

Botulinum toxin therapy

Botulinum neurotoxin therapy for strabismus has been advocated for many types of strabismus in adults, but has fewer indications in children. Botulinum toxin is a large protein molecule, produced by *Clostridium botulinum*, which binds with the motor nerve terminals at the neuromuscular junction and causes paralysis by blocking acetylcholine release. Injection of the drug into an extraocular muscle produces a local paralytic effect, which is maximal at 4–7 days, with no scarring and little risk of complications. Recovery of function occurs over a period of 4–16 weeks, and as antibodies rarely form to the toxin repeated injections can be given.

Botulinum toxin is injected transconjunctivally using an electromyographic (EMG) recording to ensure accurate placement of the needle tip in the muscle (Fig. 67.28). The needle is insulated except at its tip which acts as a monopolar electrode and is connected to an EMG amplifier, which monitors the signal from the muscle audibly or visually. As the needle is advanced into the muscle the signal increases and is maximal when the direction of gaze is towards the muscle. The signal diminishes when the drug is injected. In adults topical anaesthesia is adequate for anaesthesia but in young children ketamine anaesthesia is used, as the EMG signal is preserved whereas other anaesthetics diminish the signal.

There are few clear indications for the use of botulinum toxin in strabismus (Lee 1995). It is best reserved for horizontal strabismus with angles less than 40 prism dioptres, for residual postoperative under- and overcorrections, and cases of strabismus after multiple strabismus or retinal detachment procedures. The best indication is in the management of chronic sixth nerve palsies. Some cases of persistent esotropia due to medial rectus contracture may be cured. Toxin chemodenervation of the medial rectus as adjunct to vertical muscle transposition surgery in unrecovered sixth nerve palsy is now the treatment of choice in these patients. It is also widely used in acute sixth nerve palsies, where spontaneous improvement is likely. The rationale for treatment, in this situation, is that it will prevent contracture of the medial rectus and limit any residual esotropia which may result. However, there are conflicting reports in the literature as to whether there is any long-term benefit of this treatment (Metz & Mazow 1988; Lee *et al.* 1994). Other indications for its use in strabismus are listed in Table 67.5. The best results are seen in patients with small angle deviations and good fusion.

Specific complications of botulinum toxin injection are common but serious complications are rare. The most common complications result from local spread of the drug to adjacent muscles, the levator being particularly susceptible. Ptosis has been reported in 40% of cases, most commonly after medial rectus injection, but is usually mild. Induced vertical deviations are also common. Subconjunctival haemorrhage is common but orbital haemor-

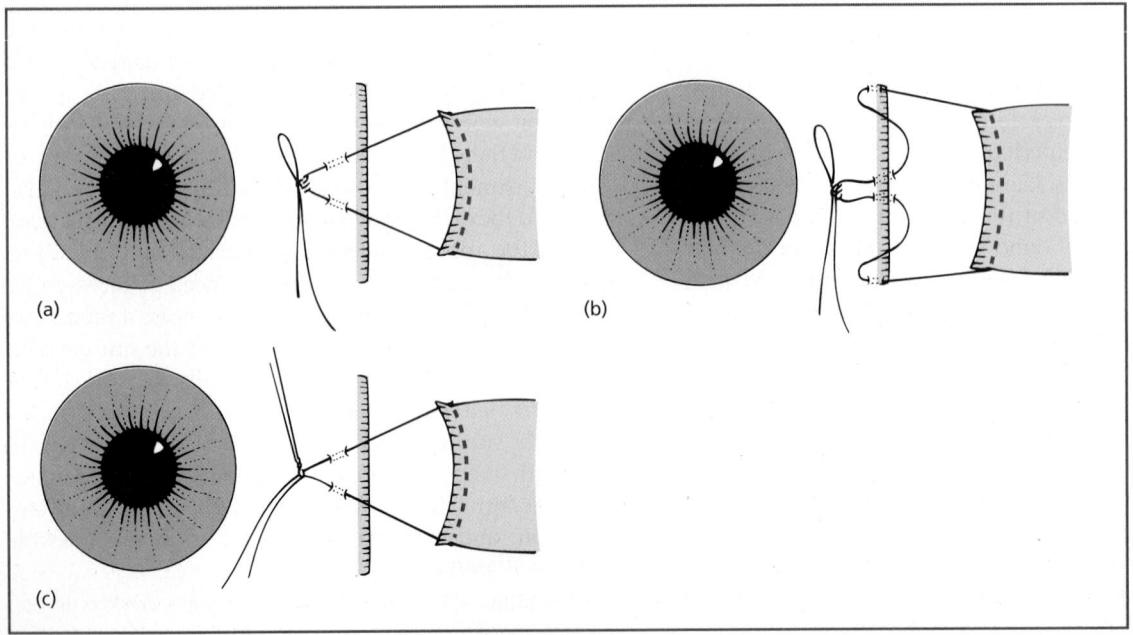

Fig. 67.26 (a–c) Adjustable suture techniques. (a) Bow-tie technique. (b) Fells' technique. (c) Cinch technique. (d–h) Bow-tie adjustable suture technique using limbal conjunctival approach.

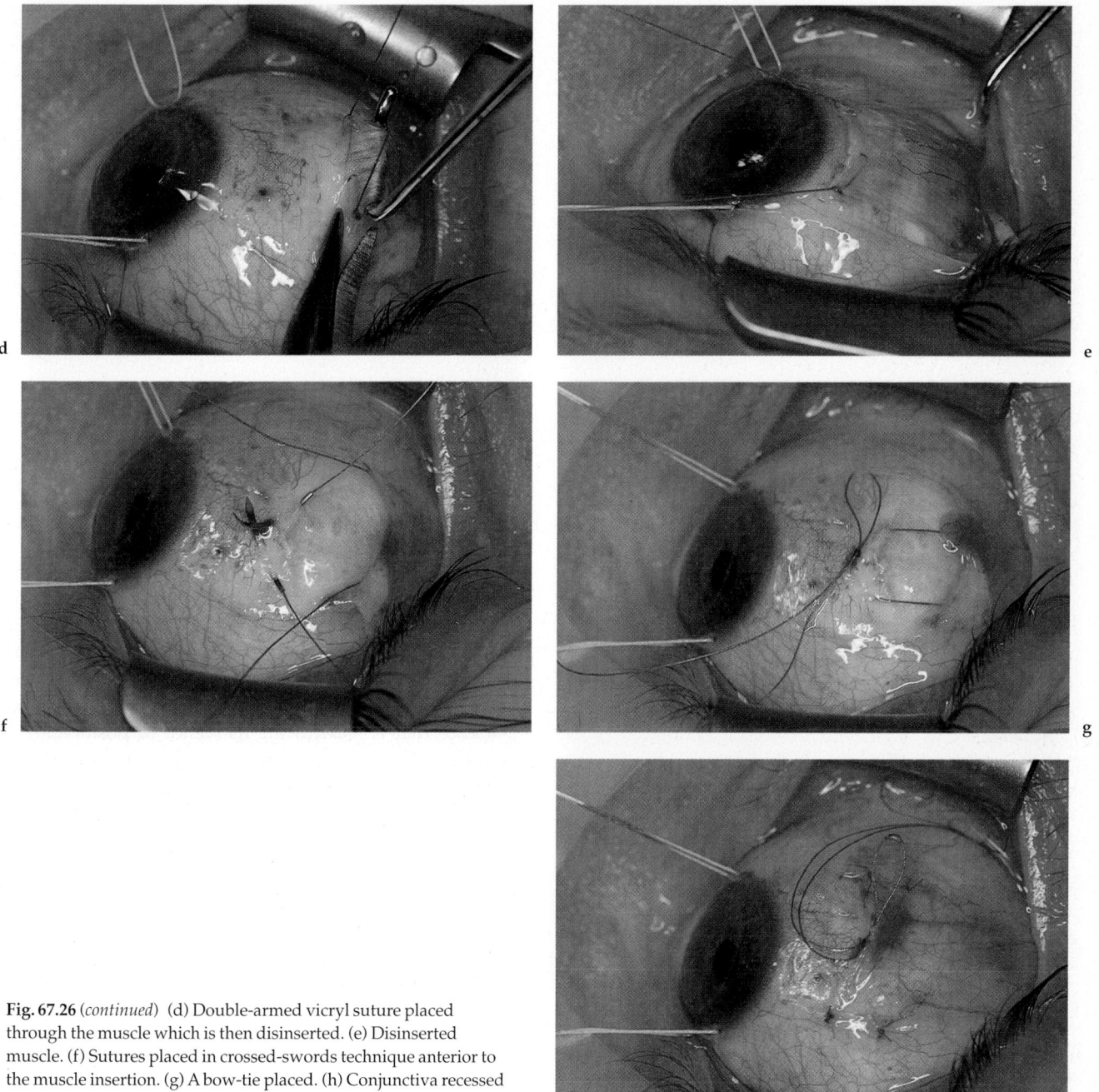

Fig. 67.26 (*continued*) (d) Double-armed vicryl suture placed through the muscle which is then disinserted. (e) Disinserted muscle. (f) Sutures placed in crossed-swords technique anterior to the muscle insertion. (g) A bow-tie placed. (h) Conjunctiva recessed to the level of the knot to facilitate adjustment of the suture.

rhage rare. The incidence of scleral perforation is 0.11%, Scott (1989) and Scott *et al.* (1990) reporting perforation in nine out of 8300 cases. Pupillary dilatation has been reported.

The use of botulinum toxin in children is not universally accepted. One of the concerns about treating children is the risk of amblyopia if ptosis or small vertical deviation is induced by the injection. It has been advocated mainly for the treatment of congenital esotropia and sixth nerve palsies. In congenital esotropia the rationale of treatment is to induce an exodeviation and, in some children treated under the age of 1 year, a face turn will develop to allow alignment of the eyes with fusion. In Magoon and Scott's (1987) series of 82 children, 85% required more than one injection to achieve alignment within 10 prism dioptres of orthotropia. In a larger series, 356 children were investigated and 223 were aligned within 10 prism dioptres of orthotropia, and on average 1.6 injections were required (Scott *et al.* 1990). Despite a 33% incidence of transient ptosis none of the patients developed amblyopia (Scott *et al.*

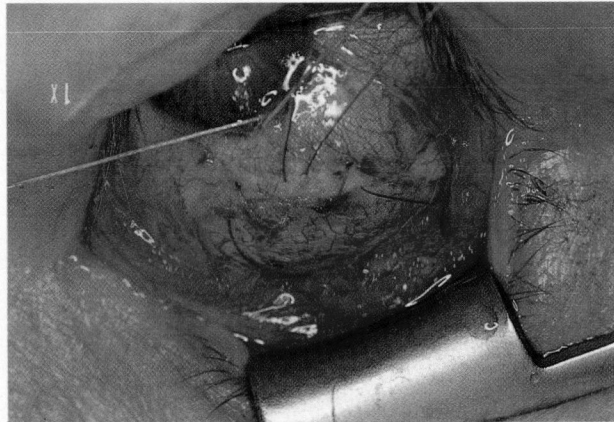

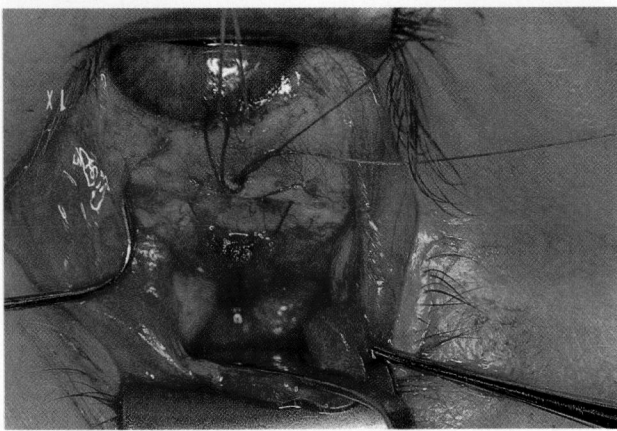

Fig. 67.27 Fells' adjustable suture (placed on a slipped inferior rectus which is being advanced). (a) Suture through sclera. (b) Adjustable bow tied.

1990). Other possible indications for botulinum toxin in children are strabismus following temporary ocular occlusion and cases of acute late onset esotropia.

Complications

Complications are an inevitable result of any surgery and strabismus surgery is no exception; however, they can be minimized by careful surgical technique

Anaesthetic

All general anaesthetics carry a small risk to the patient but there are some complications of specific interest to the strabismus surgeon. The risks are often stated as being that one in 10 000 anaesthetics in a healthy child are complicated by cardiac or respiratory arrest, and that one in ten of these cases will die or be left with a permanent disability.

• Manipulation of the extraocular muscles, especially the medial rectus, may induce cardiac arrhythmias, most commonly bradycardia. This effect of the oculocardiac

Table 67.5 Potential indications for botulinum toxin.

Esotropia
Congenital esotropia
Surgically overcorrected intermittent exotropia
Postoperative residual esotropia

Exotropia
Consecutive exotropia
Surgically overcorrected esotropia
Postoperative residual exotropia

Restrictive strabismus
Thyroid eye disease (acute phase only)
Strabismus following retinal detachment surgery

Paralytic strabismus
Sixth nerve palsy
Third nerve palsy

reflex during surgery can be prevented using intravenous atropine.

• Postoperative nausea and vomiting is said to be more common after strabismus surgery than many other surgical procedures, particularly in children. Its incidence is partly related to the use of opiates and opiate-related drugs for premedication. Droperidol has been advocated as premedication for strabismus patients as there is some evidence that it reduces the incidence of postoperative vomiting. The use of modern intravenous anaesthetic agents such as propofol also seems to reduce the incidence of postoperative vomiting. Although many children do experience nausea and vomiting postoperatively it is rare that this prevents them being managed as day cases.

• Patients using phospholine iodide drops are at risk of prolonged apnoea if succinylcholine is used during induction of anaesthesia. The drug should therefore be stopped some weeks before the time of any planned strabismus surgery.

Haemorrhage

Bleeding during strabismus surgery relates principally to surgical technique, the muscle being operated on and the extent of scarring present in reoperations. It can always be controlled by careful surgical technique using wet field cautery. Delayed haemorrhage following strabismus surgery is rare, but orbital haemorrhage has been described.

Globe perforation

Scleral perforation during surgery typically occurs during placement of scleral sutures to reattach recessed muscles, but can also occur during muscle resection and the placement of stay sutures leading to shallowing of the anterior

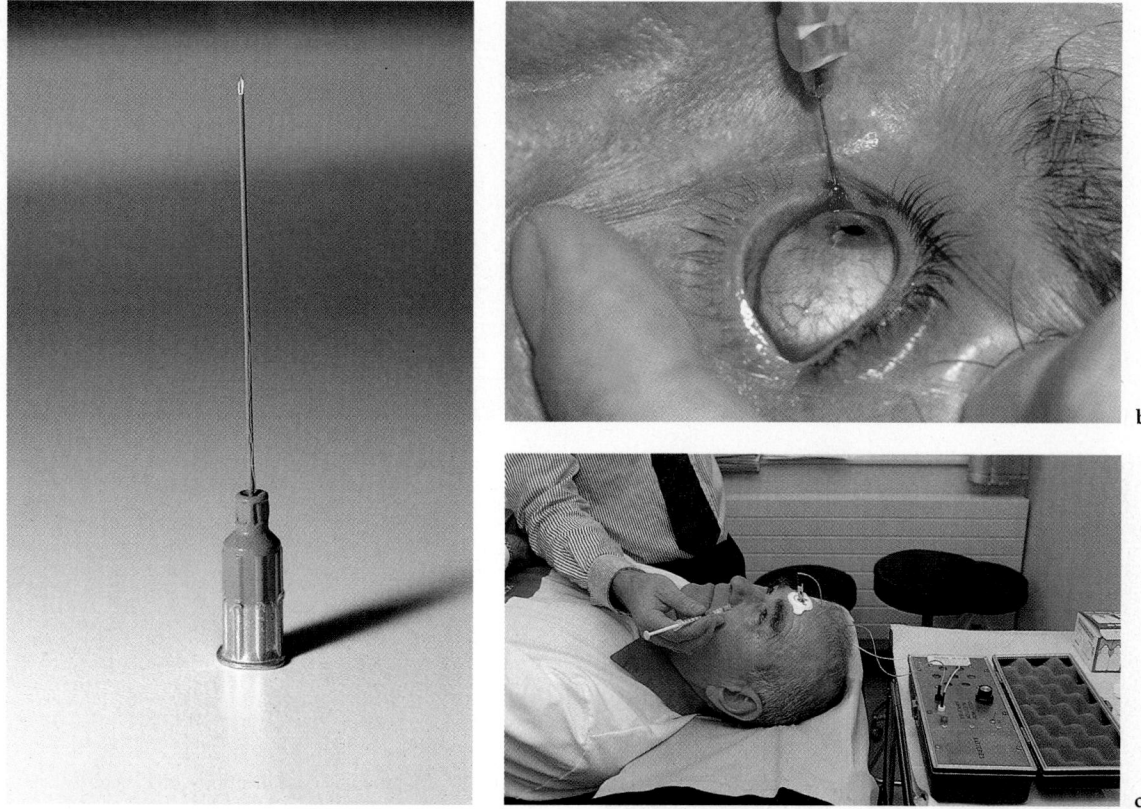

Fig. 67.28 Botulinum toxin injection. (a) Insulated needle. (b) Needle placed in medial rectus. (c) EMG unit (Oculinum Inc.).

chamber or a hyphaema. Rarely globe perforation may occur during disinsertion of rectus muscles, particularly in reoperations, placement of traction sutures beneath the lateral rectus and preplacement of muscle sutures (Simon *et al.* 1992). A recent prospective study on inadvertent perforation of the globe reported an incidence of less than 1% (Morris *et al.* 1990). This contrasts with the previous retrospective reports of between 9.2 and 10.2%, although these authors did not study consecutive patients and so this may not reflect the true incidence (Gottleib & Castro 1970; Kalunzny *et al.* 1977). This decline is the result of the introduction of fine spatulate needles for strabismus surgery, as well as improved techniques of illumination and magnification. The incidence is higher for Faden sutures as these are placed through thin posterior sclera (Lyons *et al.* 1989).

Scleral perforation can lead to localized retinal haemorrhage, vitreous haemorrhage, retinal detachment and endophthalmitis. However, these complications are rare and in most cases a localized chorioretinal scar develops (Fig. 67.29) (Simon *et al.* 1992). If a scleral perforation is suspected at surgery the retina should be inspected, and antibiotics administered, but the use of cryotherapy

is controversial (Gottleib & Castro 1970; Basmadjian *et al.* 1975). Most surgeons feel it is not indicated, a view supported by the rare reports of retinal detachment following strabismus surgery, and there is animal evidence to suggest cryotherapy may have a detrimental effect (Basmadjian *et al.* 1975; Mittleman & Bakos 1984).

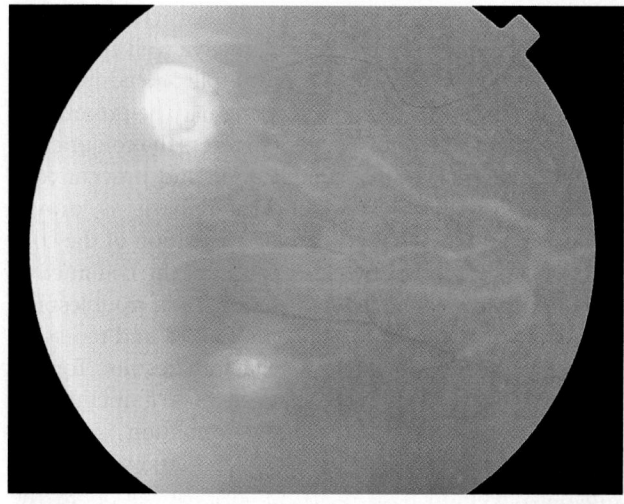

Fig. 67.29 Localized chorioretinal scars following scleral perforation at strabismus surgery.

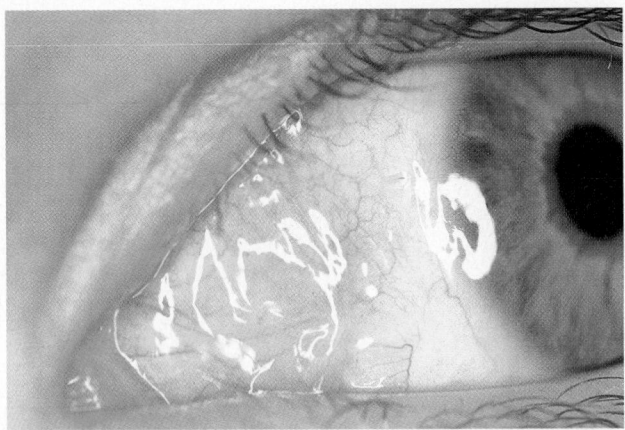

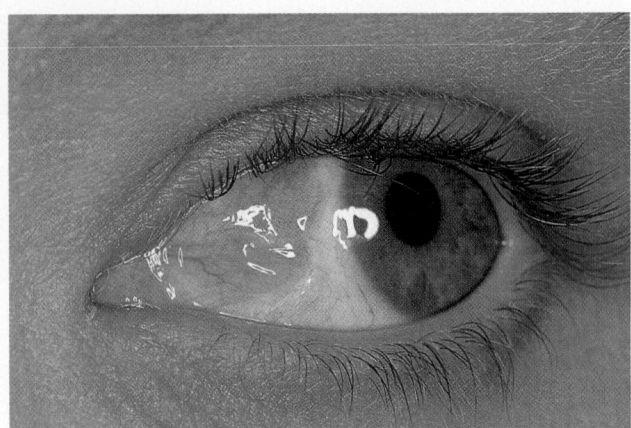

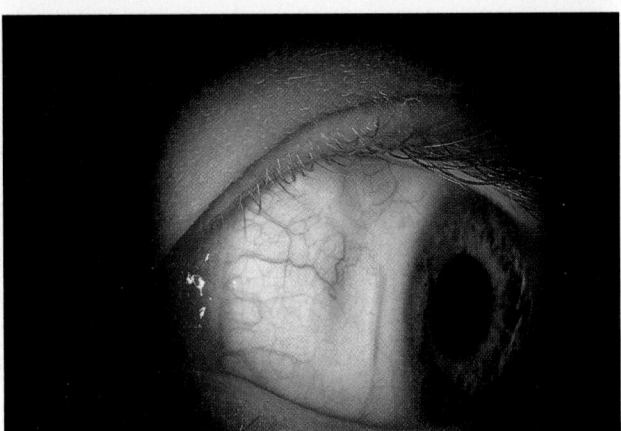

Fig. 67.30 Conjunctival complications. (a) Unsightly conjunctival scarring over medial rectus. (b) Plica semilunaris drawn towards limbus following medial rectus surgery. (c) Raised conjunctiva at the limbus due to early postoperative slippage.

Conjunctival-related complications

Most conjunctival-related complications are the result of poor surgical technique. Meticulous handling of conjunctival tissues during surgery and their accurate apposition will reduce the incidence of complications.

A conjunctival scar is inevitable, but provided surgery is performed carefully and the conjunctiva well apposed it is not clinically significant. After multiple procedures conjunctival vascularization and scarring may be prominent. In reoperations it is often prudent to recess the conjunctiva to reduce the risk of this complication and prevent conjunctival restriction. The plica semilunaris is drawn towards the limbus either by poor apposition of the conjunctiva at surgery, or by cicatrization of the conjunctiva following multiple procedures (Fig. 67.30). If troublesome the conjunctiva and plica can be mobilized and recessed, but it is difficult to achieve satisfactory results. Topical antimetabolites have been suggested as a method of reducing hypertrophic scar tissue formation in at-risk patients (Urban *et al.* 1993; Cruz & Matkovich 1995). Unsightly conjunctival scarring also develops if the orbital fat is penetrated at surgery and is advanced subconjunctivally lending a pink fleshy appearance to the conjunctiva. Patients with conjunctival scarring frequently complain of irritable red eyes especially in dry environments or after swimming.

Prolapse of Tenon's capsule through the conjunctival wound, usually the result of incomplete conjunctival closure, produces a dense white appearance contrasting with the pinker conjunctiva. It usually shrinks spontaneously within a few weeks, but can be excised if excessively bulky.

Conjunctival epithelial inclusion cysts (Fig. 67.31) are uncommon, and may develop many years after surgery (Kushner 1992a). They arise from small fragments of conjunctival epithelium within the wound, are usually small but may enlarge progressively. If small they can be left, but larger cysts need to be excised intact to prevent recurrence.

Dellen, areas of corneal thinning secondary to drying usually adjacent to the limbus, may form following strabismus surgery. They are not usually clinically significant and if patients are symptomatic treatment is with artificial tear substitutes. Resection or advancement of a medial rectus muscle is the most common cause of dellen formation as the conjunctiva is more frequently folded or chemotic after this procedure.

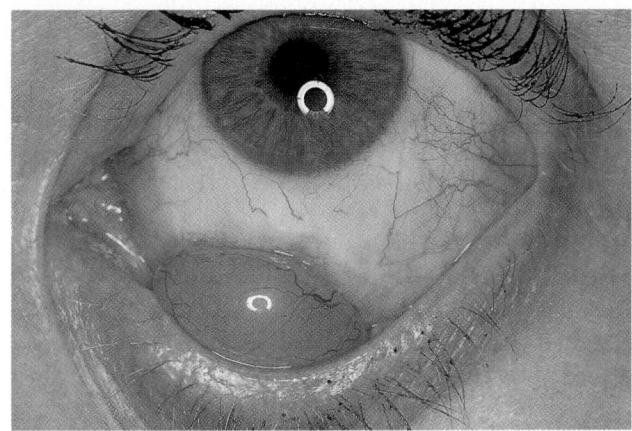

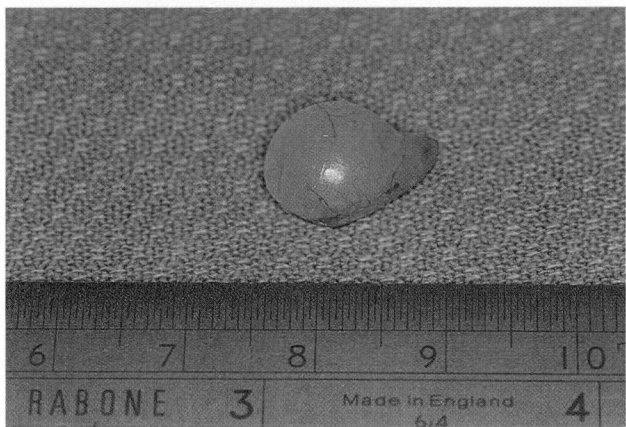

Fig. 67.31 (a) Conjunctival epithelial inclusion cyst over inferior rectus. (b) Conjunctival epithelial inclusion cyst following excision.

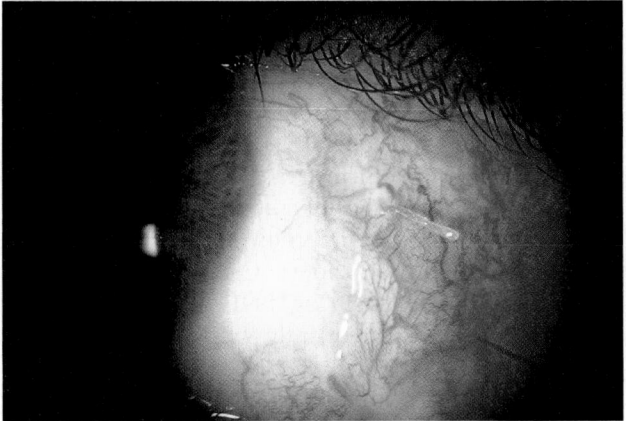

Fig. 67.32 Vicryl suture reaction.

Suture-related complications

Allergic reactions to suture material used in strabismus surgery are now uncommon since the advent of synthetic absorbable sutures (Fig. 67.32). Such reactions were much more commonly seen when the use of organic suture material was widespread. They usually present as a prolonged inflammatory reaction over the site of the sutures, and respond to treatment with topical steroids. Suture granulomas occur in less than 0.5% of patients (Helveston 1993), usually over the site of the knot (Fig. 67.33). In most cases they are small and resolve spontaneously, but large granulomas can require excision. Stitch abscesses are rare (Fig. 67.34).

Lid changes

Vertical muscle surgery can lead to changes in the palpebral aperture. In practice this is only seen with inferior rectus recession because of its attachments to the lower lid retractors (Pacheco *et al.* 1992). Large recessions of the inferior rectus are commonly associated with lower lid retraction and several techniques have been described to overcome this complication (Jampolsky 1986; Kushner 1992; Pacheco *et al.* 1992). An upper lid ptosis can occur

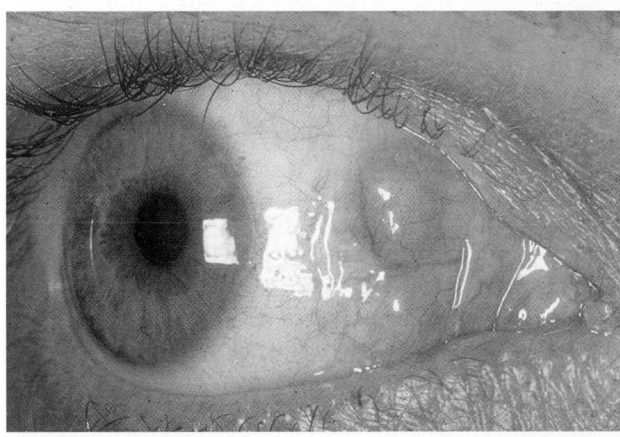

Fig. 67.33 Suture granuloma.

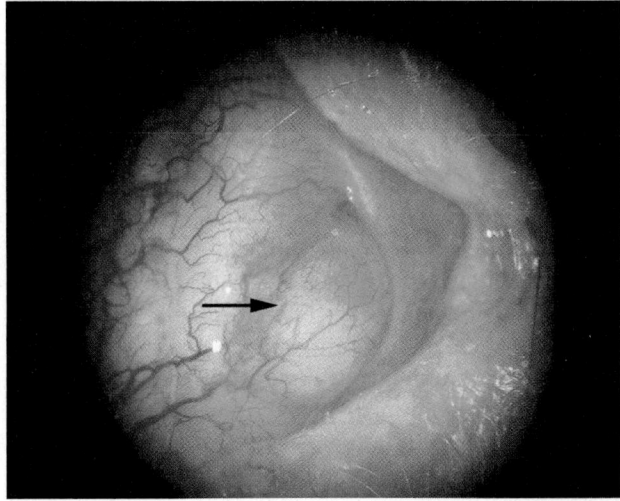

Fig. 67.34 Localized stitch abscess. Note fluid level in abscess (arrow).

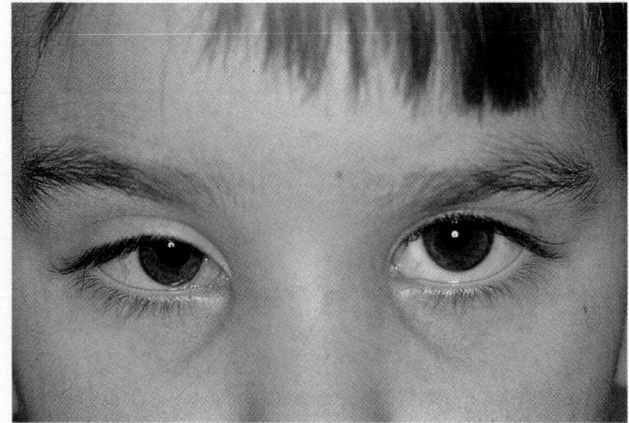

Fig. 67.35 Narrowing of right palpebral fissure following right medial rectus readvancement.

following large superior rectus resections but upper lid retraction is rarely seen even with larger recessions of the superior rectus. Horizontal rectus muscle surgery can cause narrowing of the palpebral fissure if large recess-resect procedures induce some retraction of the globe (Fig. 67.35). This may follow advancement and resection of a previously recessed or 'lost' muscle.

Anterior segment ischaemia

Severe anterior segment ischaemia following strabismus surgery is rare, occurring in 30 of 400 000 strabismus cases, 16 of which were associated with transposition procedures (Simon *et al.* 1984; France & Simon 1986). Mild cases are common, and clinically not significant. In severe cases the signs include conjunctival chemosis, corneal oedema, anterior chamber cellular activity, lens opacities, hypotony and late iris atrophy. Lee and Olver (1990), studying adults with anterior segment fluorescein angiography, found iris sector perfusion defects in six out of 35 cases. Surgery on the vertical rectus muscles produced iris sector hypoperfusion more readily then horizontal muscle surgery, and further surgery on the same muscle did not typically cause further hypoperfusion, as restoration of blood flow was largely the result of remodelling of the deep collateral circulation rather than recanalization of the anterior ciliary vessels. Recovery of the iris circulation occurred in most patients within 4 weeks and in all patients by 12 weeks (Olver & Lee 1992). In children there is almost complete absence of sector infarction (Olver & Lee 1989). These findings are similar to those found in primates where simultaneous removal of all four recti produced severe anterior segment ischaemia, but staged removal of the recti did not, suggesting a remodelling of the circulation (Virdi & Hayreh 1987). The type of conjunctival incision has been said to influence anterior segment ischaemia by an effect on the anterior episcleral arterial circle (Fishman *et al.* 1990), limbal incisions predisposing

to more severe ischaemia than the fornix approach. However, Olver suggests that as the anterior episcleral arterial circle lies in the deepest episcleral layer, it is unlikely to be damaged by the reflection of the conjunctiva that occurs with a limbal incision (Olver 1989).

Two-muscle rectus surgery rarely causes anterior segment ischaemia, unless there is a predisposing risk factor. Horizontal rectus muscle surgery combined with one vertical muscle is safe in children, but surgery of both vertical recti together with a horizontal rectus muscle, especially the medial rectus, is likely to lead to anterior segment ischaemia (Olver & Lee 1989, 1992). However, staged surgery does not produce a cumulative effect and three or even four rectus muscles can be safely detached after a 3–4-month interval. Remodelling of the collateral circulation and an increased contribution from the long posterior ciliary arteries is the likely mechanism for this (Virdi & Hayreh 1987; Olver & Lee 1989).

Risk factors for anterior segment ischaemia include microvascular disease, sickle cell disease, chronic lymphocytic leukaemia, thyroid eye disease, high myopia and previous scleral buckling or strabismus surgery (Olver & Lee 1989; Lee & Olver 1990). Microvascular dissection of the anterior ciliary arteries has been advocated as a method of preserving the anterior ciliary artery circulation in strabismus surgery in high-risk cases, but its clinical applications and benefits are not yet clearly defined (McKeown *et al.* 1989).

Infection

Postoperative infection is rare after strabismus surgery. Preoperative instillation of povidone iodine into the conjunctival sac and preoperative use of topical antibiotics reduce the bacterial load (Apt 1984), but their role in reducing the incidence of infection is not proven. Although most surgeons routinely use antibiotics alone or with steroid drops postoperatively, many patients comply poorly with this treatment and it is of doubtful benefit (Wortham *et al.* 1990). Postoperative conjunctivitis is the most common type of infection and usually resolves rapidly with topical antibiotics. Orbital cellulitis is rare (one in 1000–1900 cases) (Ing 1991) and Gram-positive cocci are the most frequently implicated organisms (Kilvin & Wilson 1995). It presents with pain, lid swelling, chemosis, limitation of ocular movement and proptosis, together with systemic signs of infection (von Noorden 1972). It requires hospital admission and parenteral antibiotic therapy. Endophthalmitis is rare (one in 30000 cases) (Ing 1991) and occurs only if the globe has been perforated at surgery. Full-thickness perforation may be followed by early and rapid endophthalmitis, whereas endophthalmitis associated with partial-thickness perforation is more likely to occur after a few days.

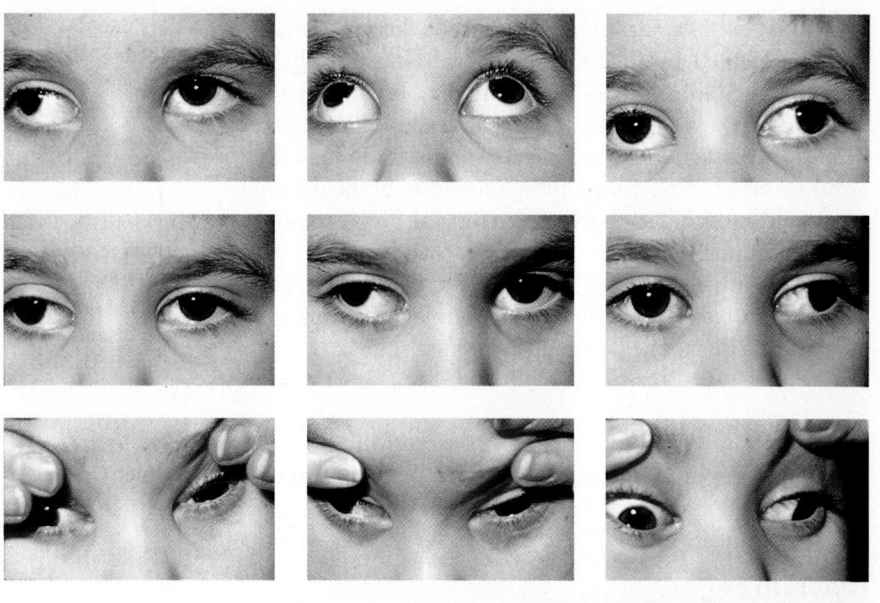

Fig. 67.36 (a) Patient with slipped medial rectus muscle. Note large exodeviation and underaction of medial rectus. (b) Findings at surgery. Strabismus hook under pseudotendon of medial rectus 11 mm from limbus. Forceps indicating anterior end of medial rectus muscle. Note the change in colour between muscle tissue and pseudotendon.

Motility and diplopia

The most common complication in strabismus surgery is over- and undercorrection: experience is that about 80% of patients have the desired postoperative outcome, although initially good postoperative alignment may change with time. Patients with poor or no fusion, amblyopia or those who have had multiple surgical procedures are most likely to have unstable ocular alignment. Limitation of extraocular movements may occur after inferior oblique surgery as described above, but also after multiple surgery and excessive resections or recessions.

Diplopia may occur postoperatively for a variety of reasons, but is usually transient in children, who suppress the diplopic image. Scott reported a 39% incidence of diplopia in adults 6 weeks postoperatively, but only 1.4% were left with residual diplopia (Scott *et al.* 1994).

Extraocular muscle complications

Rupture of a rectus muscle at the time of surgery can occur, typically during reoperations when excessive force from a muscle hook is applied to a thin muscle, the rupture occurring at the junction of the tendon and muscle. A 'lost' muscle can occur at the time of surgery if a disinserted muscle retracts into Tenon's capsule (MacEwan *et al.* 1992). Apart from the medial rectus, which in contrast to the other rectus muscles does not have attachments to the obliques, the muscle can usually be readily identified. The medial rectus can, however, be difficult to identify and it is important not to look for it on the surface of the globe but within Tenon's capsule.

A 'lost' or slipped muscle can develop postoperatively, either immediately or some weeks later (Plager & Parks 1990; MacEwan *et al.* 1992). It is seen more commonly after resections and advancements of previously recessed muscles. Its occurrence can be reduced with meticulous surgical technique particularly in the placement of muscle and scleral sutures. Patients present with a large deviation and marked underaction of the muscle (Fig. 67.36a). At surgery the muscle is usually attached to the sclera by a pseudotendon, which in some cases is extremely flimsy.

Care must be taken to leave this intact as the muscle can often be located by following this strand posteriorly. A subtle change in colour of the tissue may be seen at the junction of the pseudotendon and muscle (Fig. 67.36b). Posterior dissection to locate the muscle is usually required and haemorrhage and penetration of the orbital fat should be avoided to minimize the risk of postoperative restrictions.

Postoperatively muscle action may be temporarily reduced, probably because of pain, trauma, inflammation and relative ischaemia (Arnold 1992).

Refractive changes

Minor changes in astigmatism may occur in the postoperative period (Preslan *et al.* 1992).

References

Anderson L, Gorman C, Luton J. Superior oblique strengthening procedures in hypertropia I and II. *J Pediatr Ophthalmol Strabismus* 1974; **16**: 43–8.

Apt L. An anatomical re-evaluation of rectus muscle insertions. *Trans Am Ophthalmol Soc* 1980; **78**: 365–75.

Apt L, Call NB. An anatomical re-evaluation of rectus muscle insertions. *Ophthalmic Surg* 1982; **13**: 108–12.

Apt L, Call NB. Inferior oblique muscle recession. *Am J Ophthlmol* 1978; **95**: 95–100.

Apt L, Isenberg S, Yoshimori R, Paez J. Chemical preparation of the eye in ophthalmic surgery III. Effect of povidone-iodine on the conjunctiva. *Arch Ophthalmol* 1984; **102**: 728.

Arnold R. Pseudo-slipped muscle due to perioperative inflammatory palsy. *J Pediatr Ophthalmol Strabismus* 1992; **29**: 189–90.

Basmadjian G, Labelle P, Dumas J. Retinal detachment after strabismus surgery. *Am J Ophthalmol* 1975; **79**: 305–9.

Berke R. Tenectomy of the superior oblique for hypertropia. *Trans Am Ophthalmol Soc* 1946; **44**: 304–42.

Biender B, Rothkoff L. Treatment for 'A' or 'V' pattern esotropia by slanting muscle insertion. *Br J Ophthalmol* 1995; **79**: 807–8.

Biender B, Yassur Y, David R. Advancement and insertion of one medial rectus muscle as treatment for surgically overcorrected esotropia. *Binocular Vis* 1991; **6**: 197–200.

Bladyes J. The use of polyglactin-910 in muscle surgery. *Ophthalmic Surg* 1975; **6**: 39–41.

Bremer D, Roger G, Quick D. Primary position hypotropia after anterior transposition of the inferior oblique. *Arch Ophthalmol* 1986; **104**: 229–32.

Buckley EG, Flynn JT. Superior oblique recession versus tenotomy: a comparison of surgical results. *J Pediatr Ophthalmol Strabismus* 1983; **20**: 112–17.

Buckley EG, Townsend LM. A simple transposition procedure for complicated strabismus. *Am J Ophthalmol* 1991; **111**: 302–6.

Burke J, Keech RV. Effectiveness of inferior rectus transposition of the horizontal rectus muscles for acquired inferior rectus paresis. *J Pediatr Ophthalmol Strabismus* 1995; **32**: 172–7.

Burke J, Ruben J, Scott WE. Vertical transposition of the horzontal recti (Knapp procedure) for the treatment of double elevator palsy. *Br J Ophthalmol* 1992; **76**: 734–7.

Burke J, Scott WE, Kutshke P. Anterior transposition of the inferior oblique muscle for dissociated vertical deviation. *Ophthalmology* 1993; **100**: 245–50.

Caldeira JAF. Graduated recession of the superior oblique muscle. *Br J Ophthalmol* 1975; **59**: 553–9.

Calhoun JH. Discussion on how far a medial rectus can be safely recessed and delayed consecutive exotropia following 7-millimetre bilateral medial rectus recession for congenital esotropia. *J Pediatr Ophthalmol Strabismus* 1994; **31**: 151–2.

Crawford JS, Orton RB, Labow-Daily L. Late results of superior oblique tenotomy in true Brown's syndrome. *Am J Ophthalmol* 1980; **89**: 824–9.

Cruz OA, Matkovich L. Effects of intraoperative mitomycin-C on strabismus surgery in the rabbit: a preliminary study. *Ophthalmic Surg* 1995; **26**: 237–40.

Cuppers C. The so-called 'faden operation' (surgical correction by well-defined changes in the arc of contact). In: Fells P, ed. *Second Congress of the International Strabismus Association*. Marseilles: Diffusion Generale de Librairie, 1976: 395–400.

Damanakis A, Arvanitis P, Laddas I, Theodossiadis G. 8-mm bimedial rectus recession in infantile esotropia of 80–90 prism dioptres. *Br J Ophthalmol* 1994; **78**: 842–4.

Del Monte M, Parks M. Denervation and extirpation of the inferior oblique. An improved weakening procedure for marked overaction. *Ophthalmology* 1983; **90**: 1178–85.

Dunlap E. Vertical displacement of the horizontal recti. In: Burian H, Dunlap E, Dyer J, eds. *Symposium on Strabismus*. St Louis: CV Mosby, 1971: 307–29.

Dyer J. Tenotomy of the inferior oblique muscle at its scleral insertion. *Arch Ophthalmol* 1962; **68**: 176–81.

Elliott L, Nankin J. Anterior transposition of the inferior oblique. *J Pediatr Ophthalmol Strabismus* 1981; **18**: 35–8.

El-Kasaby HT, Habib NE, Marczak AM. Subconjunctival bupivacaine in strabismus surgery. *Eye* 1993; **7**: 346–9.

Eustis H, Hesse R. Conjunctival reaction using adjustable sutures: a comparison of the cinch and bow knot methods. *J Pediatr Ophthalmol Strabismus* 1993; **30**: 149–53.

Fells P. Adjustable sutures. *Eye* 1988; **2**: 33–5.

Fells P. Management of paralytic strabismus. *Br J Ophthalmol* 1974; **58**: 255–65.

Fink WH. *Surgery of the Oblique Muscles of the Eye*. St Louis: CV Mosby, 1951.

Fink WH. *Surgery of the Vertical Muscles of the Eye*, 2nd edn. Springfield, Illinois: Charles C. Thomas, 1962.

Fishman PH, Repka MX, Green WR, D'Anna S, Guyton D. A primate model of anterior segment ischaemia after strabismus surgery. The role of the conjunctival circulation. *Ophthalmology* 1990; **97**: 456–61.

Fitzsimons R, Lee J, Elston J. Treatment of sixth nerve palsy in adults with combined botulinum toxin chemodenervation and surgery. *Ophthalmology* 1988; **95**: 1535–42.

France T, Simon J. Anterior segment ischaemia following muscle surgery: the AAPOS experience. *J Pediatr Ophthalmol Strabismus* 1986; **23**: 87–91.

Gobin MH. Recession of the medial rectus muscle with a loop. *Ophthalmologica* 1968; **12**: 102–7.

Gobin MH. Surgical management of Duane's syndrome. *Br J Ophthalmol* 1974; **58**: 301–6.

Goldstein J. Monocular displacement of the horizontal rectus muscles in the A and V pattern. *Am J Ophthalmol* 1967; **64**: 265–7.

Gobin MH. Desagittalisation of the oblique muscles as a surgical treatment for strabismus. In: Boschi MC, Frosini R. (eds) *Proc Int Strab Symp*. Florence June 21–23 1982.

Goldstein J, Prepas S, Conrad S. The effect of needle characteristics in strabismus surgery. *Arch Ophthalmol* 1982; **100**: 617–18.

Gonzalez C. Denervation of the inferior oblique, current status and long-term results. *Trans Am Acad Ophthalmol* 1976; **81**: 899–901.

Gonzalez C, Klein B. Myectomy and anterior transposition of the inferior oblique muscle: a new surgical procedure and its results in 49 operations. *Binocular Vis* 1993; **8**: 249–58.

Gottlieb F, Castro J. Perforation of the globe during strabismus surgery. *Arch Ophthalmol* 1970; **84**: 151–7.

Guyton D. An exaggerated forced duction test for the oblique muscles. *Ophthalmology* 1981; **88**: 1035–9.

Guyton D. The posterior fixation procedure: mechanism and indications. *Int Ophthalmol Clin* 1985; **25**: 79–88.

Guyton D. Torsion and elevation under general anaesthesia and during voluntary eye closure (Bell phenomenon): discussion. *J Pediatr Ophthalmol Strabismus* 1984; **21**: 78.

Habib N, El-Kasaby H, Marczak A, Hsuan J. Subconjunctival bupivacaine versus topical amethocaine in strabismus surgery. *Eye* 1993; **7**: 757–9.

Harada M, Ito Y. Surgical correction of cyclotropia. *Jpn J Ophthalmol* 1964; **8**: 88.

Helveston E. Complications of strabismus surgery. In: *Pediatric Ophthalmology Strabismus. Transactions of the New Orleans Academy of Ophthalmology.* New York: Raven Press, 1986: 61–70.

Helveston E. *Surgical Management of Strabismus. An Atlas of Strabismus Surgery.* St Louis: Mosby Year Book, 1993.

Helveston EM, Ellis FD. Superior oblique tuck for superior oblique palsy. *Aust NZ J Ophthalmol* 1983; **11**: 215–20.

Helveston E, Ellis F, Plager D. A new classification for superior oblique palsy based on congenital variations in the tendon. *Ophthalmology* 1992; **99**: 1609–15.

Holmes JM, Townshend AM. Optimum timing of postoperative adjustment in a rabbit model of adjustable suture surgery. *Ophthalmic Surg* 1995; **26**: 241–3.

Hummelsheim E. Weitene Erfahrungen mit partieller Schnenuberpflanzung an den Augenmuskeln. *Arch Augenheilk* 1907; **62**: 71–4.

Ing MR. Infection following strabismus surgery. *Ophthalmic Surg* 1991; **22**: 41–3.

Ing MR, Costenbader FD, Parks MM, Albert D. Early surgery for congenital esotropia. *Am J Ophthalmol* 1966; **61**: 1419–27.

Jampolsky A. Management of vertical strabismus. In: *Pediatric Ophthalmological Strabismus. Transactions of the New Orleans Academy of Ophthalmology.* New York: Raven Press, 1986: 154–7.

Jampolsky A. A simplified approach to strabismus diagnosis. In: *Symposium on Strabismus. Transactions of the New Orleans Academy of Ophthalmology.* St Louis: CV Mosby, 1971: 34–92.

Jensen C. Rectus muscle union: a new operation for paralysis of rectus muscles. *Trans Pacific Coast Oto–Ophthalmol Soc* 1964; **45**: 359–84.

Johnson J. A review of superior oblique tuck. *South Med J* 1971; **64**: 941–3.

Kaluzny J, Ralcewicz H, Perlikiewicz-Kikielowa A. Eye fundus periphery after operation for squint. *Klin Oczna* 1977; **47**: 557–8.

Keech R, Morris R, Ruben J, Scott W. Anterior segment ischaemia following vertical muscle transposition and botulinum toxin injection. *Arch Ophthalmol* 1991; **108**: 176.

Keech R, Scott W, Baker J. The medial rectus insertion site in infantile esotropia. *Am J Ophthalmol* 1990; **109**: 79–84.

Khawam E, Scott A, Jampolsky A. Acquired superior oblique palsy. *Arch Ophthalmol* 1967; **77**: 761–8.

Kilvin JD, Wilson ME and the Periocular Infection Study Group. Periocular infection after strabismus surgery. *J Pediatr Opthalmol Strabismus* 1995; **32**: 42–9.

Knapp P. The surgical treatment of double elevator paralysis. *Trans Am Acad Opthalmol* 1969; **67**: 304.

Knapp P. Vertically incomitant horizontal strabismus: the so-called

'A' and 'V' pattern syndromes. *Trans Am Ophthalmol Soc* 1959; **57**: 666–9.

Koorneef L. New insights in the human orbital connective tissue. *Arch Ophthalmol* 1977; **95**: 1269–73.

Kratz R, Roher G, Bremer D, LeGuire L. Anterior displacement of the inferior oblique for DVD. *J Pediatr Ophthalmol Strabismus* 1989; **26**: 212–17.

Kushner B. Evaluation of the posterior fixation suture plus recession with saccadic velocities. *J Pediatr Ophthalmol Strabismus* 1983; **20**: 202.

Kushner B. Subconjunctival cysts as a complication of strabismus surgery. *Arch Ophthalmol* 1992a; **110**: 1243–5.

Kushner B. A surgical procedure to minimize lower lid retraction with inferior rectus recession. *Arch Ophthalmol* 1992b; **110**: 1011–14.

Kushner B, Fisher M, Lucchese N, Morton G. Factors influencing response in strabismus surgery. *Arch Ophthalmol* 1993; **111**: 75–9.

Kushner B, Fisher M, Lucchese N, Morton G. How far can a medial rectus safely be recessed? *J Pediatr Ophthalmol Strabismus* 1994; **31**: 138–46.

Kushner B, Preslan M, Vrabec M. Artifacts of measurement during strabismus surgery. *J Pediatr Ophthalmol Strabismus* 1987; **24**: 159–64.

Laby D, Rosenbaum A. Adjustable vertical rectus muscle transposition surgery. *J Pediatr Ophthalmol Strabismus* 1994; **31**: 75–8.

Lee DA, Dyer LA. Bilateral medial rectus muscle recession and lateral rectus muscle resection in the treatment of congenital esotropia. *Am J Ophthalmol* 1983; **96**: 218–28.

Lee J. Botulinum toxin in the management of ocular muscle disorders. *Am Orthop J* 1995; **45**: 115–25.

Lee J, Collin J, Timms C. Elevating the hypotropic globe. *Br J Ophthalmol* 1986; **70**: 26–32.

Lee J, Harris S, Cohen J, Cooper K, MacEwan C, Jones S. Results of a prospective randomised trial of botulinum toxin therapy in acute unilateral sixth nerve palsy. *J Pediatr Ophthalmol Strabismus* 1994; **31**: 283–6.

Lee J, Olver J. Anterior segment ischaemia. *Eye* 1990; **4**: 1–6.

Lee J, Olver J. Anterior segment ischaemia following vertical muscle transposition and botulinum toxin injection. *Arch Ophthalmol* 1991; **109**: 174.

Lipton J, Page A, Lee J. Management of diplopia in downgaze following orbital trauma. *Eye* 1990; **4**: 535–7.

Luff A, Morris R, Wainwright A. Day case management in adjustable suture strabismus surgery. *Eye* 1993; **7**: 694–6.

Lyons C, Fells P, Lee J, MacIntyre A. Chorioretinal scarring after the Faden operation. *Eye* 1989; **3**: 401–3.

MacEwan C, Lee J, Fells P. Aetiology and management of the 'detached' rectus muscle. *Br J Ophthalmol* 1992; **76**: 131–6.

McGuire W. Paresis of the superior oblique. Surgical correction: recess or tuck? *South Med J* 1969; **62**: 941–3.

McGuire W. The surgical correction of paresis of the superior oblique. *Trans Am Ophthalmol Soc* 1947; **44**: 527–49.

McKeown C, Lambert H, Usaf M, Shore J. Preservation of the anterior vessels during extraocular muscle surgery. *Ophthalmology* 1989; **96**: 499–507.

McLean J. Direct surgery of underacting superior oblique muscles. *Trans Am Ophthalmol Soc* 1948; **46**: 633–51.

McNeer KW. Untoward effects of superior oblique tenotomy. *Ann Ophthalmol* 1972; **4**: 747–50.

Magoon E, Scott A. Botulinum toxin chemodenervation in infants and children. An alternative to incisional strabismus surgery. *J Pediatr* 1987; **110**: 719–22.

Manners R, O'Flynn E, Morris RJ. Superior oblique tendon lengthening for acquired superior oblique overactions. *Br J Ophthalmol* 1994;

78: 280–4.

Metz H. The use of vertical muscle offsets with horizontal strabismus surgery. *Ophthalmology* 1988; **95**: 1094–7.

Metz H. XXth Annual Frank Costenbader Lecture. Muscle transposition surgery. *J Pediatr Ophthalmol Strabismus* 1993; **30**: 346–53.

Metz H, Lerner H. The adjustable Harada–Ito procedure. *Arch Ophthalmol* 1981; **99**: 624–6.

Metz H, Mazow M. Botulinum toxin treatment of acute sixth and third nerve palsies. *Graefe's Arch Klin Exp Ophthalmol* 1988; **226**: 141–4.

Metz H, Schwartz L. The treatment of A and V patterns by monocular surgery. *Arch Ophthalmol* 1977; **95**: 251–3.

Miller J. Vertical recti transplantation in the A and V syndromes. *Arch Ophthalmol* 1960; **64**: 175–9.

Mimms J. Forming and teaching true knots in strabismus surgery. *Ophthalmic Surg* 1992; **23**: 477–81.

Mimms J, Wood R. Bilateral anterior transposition of the inferior obliques. *Arch Ophthalmol* 1989; **107**: 41–4.

Mitchell P, Parks M. Surgery for bilateral superior oblique palsy. *Ophthalmology* 1982; **89**: 484–8.

Mittleman D, Bakos I. The role of retinal cryopexy in the management of experimental perforation of the eye during strabismus surgery. *J Pediatr Ophthalmol Strabismus* 1984; **21**: 186–9.

Mittleman D, Folk E. The evaluation and treatment of superior oblique muscle palsy. *Trans Am Acad Ophthalmol Otolaryngol* 1976; **81**: 893–8.

Molarte A, Rosenbaum A. Vertical muscle rectus transposition surgery for Duane's syndrome. *J Pediatr Ophthalmol Strabismus* 1990; **27**: 171–7.

Mombaerts I, Koornneff L, Everhard YS, Hughes DS, Maillette de Buy Wenniger-Prick LJJ. Superior oblique luxation and trochlear luxation as new concepts in superior oblique muscle weakening surgery. *Am J Ophthalmol* 1995; **120**: 83–91.

Morris RJ, Luff A. Adjustable sutures in squint surgery. *Br J Ophthalmol* 1992; **76**: 560–2.

Morris RJ, Rosen P, Fells P. Incidence of inadvertent globe perforation during strabismus surgery. *Br J Ophthalmol* 1990; **74**: 490–3.

Morris RJ, Scott WE, Keech R. Superior oblique tuck surgery in the management of superior oblique palsies. *J Pediatr Ophthalmol Strabismus* 1992; **29**: 337–46.

Morrison N, Repka M. Ketorolec versus acetaminophen or ibuprofen in controlling postoperative pain in patients with strabismus. *Ophthalmology* 1994; **101**: 915–18.

Nelson LB, Calhoun JH, Simon JW, Wilson T, Harley RD. Surgical management of large angle congenital esotropia. *Br J Ophthalmol* 1987; **71**: 380–3.

O'Connor R. Transplantation of ocular muscles. *Am J Ophthalmol* 1921; **4**: 838–41.

O'Flynn E. Strabismus documentation: an alternative approach. *Br Orthop J* 1994; **51**: 10–14.

O'Neill J. Surgical management of small angle hypertropia by vertical muscle offsets. *Am Orthop J* 1978; **28**: 32–43.

Ohtsuki H, Hasebe S, Tadokoro Y, Kobashe R, Watanabe S, Okano M. Advancement of medial rectus muscle to the original insertion for consecutive exotropia. *J Pediatr Ophthalmol Strabismus* 1993; **30**: 301–5.

Olver JM, Lee JP. The effects of strabismus surgery on the anterior segment circulation. *Eye* 1989; **3**: 318–26.

Olver JM, Lee JP. Recovery of the anterior segment circulation after strabismus surgery. *Ophthalmology* 1992; **99**: 305–15.

Olver JM, McCartney AC. Anterior segment vascular casting. *Eye* 1989a; **3**: 302–7.

Olver JM, McCartney AC. Orbital and ocular micro-vascular corrosion casting in man. *Eye* 1989b; **3**: 588–96.

Pacheco E, Guyton D, Repka M. Changes in eyelid position accompanying vertical rectus muscle surgery and prevention of lower lid retraction with adjustable surgery. *J Pediatr Ophthalmol Strabismus* 1992; **29**: 265–72.

Parks M. Fornix incisions for horizontal rectus muscle surgery. *Am J Ophthalmol* 1968; **65**: 907–15.

Parks MM. *Atlas of Strabismus Surgery*. Philadelphia: Harper & Row, 1983a: 116–31.

Parks MM. Superior oblique tendon surgery. In: *Atlas of Strabismus Surgery*. Philadelphia: Harper & Row, 1983b: 189–209.

Parks MM. Weakening surgical procedures for eliminating overaction of the inferior oblique muscle. *Am J Ophthalmol* 1972; **73**: 107–22.

Parks MM, Helveston E. Direct visualization of the superior oblique tendon. *Arch Ophthalmol* 1970; **84**: 491–4.

Plager D. Traction testing in superior oblique palsy. *J Pediatr Ophthalmol Strabismus* 1990; **27**: 136–40.

Plager D, Parks M. Repair and recognition of the 'lost' rectus muscle. *Ophthalmology* 1990; **97**: 131–6.

Pollard Z. Diagnosis and treatment of inferior oblique palsy. *J Pediatr Ophthalmol Strabismus* 1993; **30**: 15–18.

Pratt-Johnson JA, Tillson G. *Management of Strabismus and Amblyopia. A Practical Guide*. New York: Thieme Medical, 1995: 175–6.

Preslan M, Ciofffi G, Min Y. Refractive error changes following strabismus surgery. *J Pediatr Ophthalmol Strabismus* 1992; **29**: 300–4.

Price N, Vickers S, Lee J, Fells P. The diagnosis and surgical management of acquired bilateral superior oblique palsy. *Eye* 1987; **1**: 78–85.

Prieto-Diaz J. Management of superior overaction in A-pattern deviations. *Graefe's Arch Ophthalmol* 1988; **226**: 126–31.

Raymond WR, Parks MM. Transection of the superior oblique rectus muscle during intended superior oblique tenotomy: a report of three cases. *Ophthalmic Surg* 1995; **26**: 244–9.

Ribeiro G, Brooks S, Archer S, Del Monte M. Vertical shift of the medial rectus muscles in the treatment of A-pattern esotropia: analysis of outcome. *J Pediatr Ophthalmol Strabismus* 1995; **32**: 167–71.

Rosen P, Morris R, McCarry B, Fells P, Lee J. Variability following adjustable suture strabismus surgery. In: Tilson G, ed. *Advances in Amblyopia and Strabismus. Transactions of the VIIth International Orthoptic Congress*. Germany: Fahner Verlag, 1991: 89–93.

Rosenbaum A, Foster R, Ballard E, Resales T, Gruenberg P, Choy A. Complete superior and inferior rectus transposition for abducens palsy. In: Reinecke R, ed. *Strabismus II: Proceedings of the IVth Meeting of the International Strabismological Association*. Florida: Grune & Stratton, 1984: 599–605.

Rosenbaum A, Kushner B, Kirschen D. Vertical rectus muscle transposition and botulinum toxin (oculinum) to medial rectus for abducens palsy. *Arch Ophthalmol* 1991; **109**: 1345–6.

Saunders RA. Treatment of superior oblique palsy with tendon tuck and inferior oblique muscle myectomy. *Ophthalmology* 1986; **93**: 1023–7.

Saunders RA, Bluestein EC, Wilson ME, Berland JE. Anterior segment ischaemia after strabismus surgery. *Surv Ophthalmol* 1994; **38**: 456–66.

Saunders RA, Tomlinson E. Quantitated superior oblique tendon tuck in the treatment of superior oblique muscle palsy. *Am Orthop J* 1985; **35**: 81–9.

Schwartz R, Koller H. Survey of sutures used in strabismus surgery. *J Pediatr Ophthalmol Strabismus* 1981; **18**: 39–41.

Scott AB. Botulinum toxin in the treatment of strabismus. Focal points. *Clin Mod Ophthalmol* 1989; **7**: 1–11.

Scott AB. The Faden operation: mechanical effects. *Am Orthop J* 1977;

27: 44–7.

Scott AB, Magoon E, McNerr K *et al*. Botulinum toxin treatment of strabismus in children. *Trans Am Ophthalmol Soc* 1990; **87**: 174–80.

Scott WE, Drummond G, Keech R. Vertical offsets of the horizontal recti in the management of A and V pattern strabismus. *Aust NZ J Ophthalmol* 1989; **17**: 281–8.

Scott WE, Jackson O. Double elevator palsy: the significance of inferior rectus restriction. *Am Orthop J* 1977; **27**: 5–10.

Scott WE, Kraft SP. Classification and surgical treatment of superior oblique palsies I. Unilateral superior oblique palsies. In: *Symposium on Pediatric Ophthalmology and Strabismus: Transactions of the New Orleans Academy of Ophthalmology*. New York: Raven Press, 1986: 15–38.

Scott WE, Kraft SP. Surgery of the superior oblique. In: Waltman S, Keates R, Hoyt C, Frueh B, Herschler J, Carroll D, eds. *Surgery of the Eye*. New York: Churchill Livingstone, 1988: 789–801.

Scott WE, Kutschke P, Lee W. Diplopia in adult strabismus. *Am Orthop J* 1994; **44**: 66–9.

Scott WE, Morris RJ. Dissociated vertical deviation and inferior oblique overaction in infantile esotropia. *Arch Ophthalmol* 1990; **108**: 1081.

Scott WE, Reese PD, Hirsch CR, Flabetich C. Surgery for large angle congenital esotropia. *Arch Ophthalmol* 1986; **104**: 374–7.

Scott WE, Sutton V, Thalaker J. Superior rectus recession for dissociated vertical deviation. *Ophthalmology* 1982; **89**: 317–22.

Scott WE, Werner D, Lennarson L. Evaluation of Jensen procedures by saccades and diplopic fields. *Arch Ophthalmol* 1979; **97**: 1886–9.

Shin GS, Elliott RL, Rosenbaum AL. Posterior superior oblique tenotomy at the scleral insertion for collapse of A-pattern strabismus. *J Pediatr Ophthalmol Strabismus* 1996; **33**: 211–18.

Shuey T, Parks M, Friendly D. Results of combined surgery on the superior oblique and horizontal rectus muscles for A pattern horizontal strabismus. *J Pediatr Ophthalmol Strabismus* 1992; **29**: 199–201.

Simon J, Lininger L, Scherage J. Recognised scleral perforation during eye muscle surgery: incidence and sequelae. *J Pediatr Ophthalmol Strabismus* 1992; **29**: 273–5.

Simon J, Price EC, Krohel G, Poulin R, Reinecke R. Anterior segment ischaemia following strabismus surgery. *J Pediatr Ophthalmol Strabismus* 1984; **21**: 179–84.

Souza-Dias C, Uesugui CF. Efficacy of different techniques of superior oblique weakening in the correction of the A anisotropia. *J Pediatr Ophthalmol Strabismus* 1986; **23**: 82.

Sprunger D, Helveston E. Progressive overcorrection after inferior rectus recession. *J Pediatr Ophthalmol Strabismus* 1993; **30**: 145–8.

Stager D, Parks M. Inferior oblique weakening procedures: effect on primary position horizontal alignment. *Arch Ophthalmol* 1973; **90**: 15–16.

Stager D, Weakley D, Everett M, Birch E. Delayed consecutive exotropia following 7-millimetre bilateral medial rectus recession for congenital esotropia. *J Pediatr Ophthalmol Strabismus* 1994; **31**: 147–52.

Stager DR, Weakley D, Stager D. Anterior transposition of the inferior oblique: anatomic assessment of the neurovascular bundle. *Arch Ophthalmol* 1992; **110**: 360–2.

Swan K, Talbot T. Recession over Tenon's capsule. *Arch Ophthalmol* 1954; **51**: 32–41.

Swan K, Wilkins J. Extraocular muscle surgery in early infancy. *J Pediatr Ophthalmol Strabismus* 1984; **21**: 44–9.

Tamler E. Pure and impure AV syndromes. *Arch Ophthalmol* 1961; **66**: 524–7.

Urban RJ, Kaufman L. Mitomycin in the treatment of hypertrophic conjunctival scars after strabismus surgery. *J Pediatr Ophthalmol Strabismus* 1993; **30**: 96–8.

Virdi P, Hayreh S. Anterior segment ischaemia after recession of various recti. An experimental study. *Ophthalmology* 1987; **94**: 1258–67.

Vivian A, Morris R.J. Diagrammatic representation of strabismus. *Eye* 1993; **7**: 565–71.

von Noorden G. Indications of the posterior fixation operation in strabismus. *Ophthalmology* 1978; **85**: 512–20.

von Noorden G. The limbal approach to surgery of the rectus muscle. *Arch Ophthalmol* 1968; **80**: 94–7.

von Noorden G. Modification of the limbal approach to surgery of the rectus muscle. *Arch Ophthalmol* 1969; **82**: 349–50.

von Noorden G. Orbital cellulitis following extraocular muscle surgery. *Am J Ophthalmol* 1972; **74**: 627–9.

von Noorden G, Olivier P. Superior oblique tenectomy in true Brown's syndrome. *Ophthalmology* 1982; **89**: 303–9.

Wallace DK, Von Noorden GK. Clinical characteristics and surgical management of congenital absence of the superior oblique tendon. *Am J Ophthalmol* 1994; **118**: 63–9.

Weakley DR, Parks MM. Results from 7-mm bilateral recessions of the medial rectus muscles for congenital esotropia. *Ophthalmic Surg* 1990; **21**: 827–30.

Wheeler J. Advancement of the superior oblique and inferior oblique muscles. *Am J Ophthalmol* 1935; **18**: 1–5.

Wortham E, Anandkrishnan I, Kraft S, Smith D, Morin J. Are antibiotic steroid drops necessary following strabismus surgery? A prospective, randomised, masked trial. *J Pediatr Ophthalmol Strabismus* 1990; **27**: 205–7.

Wright K. Superior oblique silicone expander for Brown syndrome and superior oblique overaction. *J Pediatr Ophthalmol Strabismus* 1991; **28**: 101–7.

Ziffer A, Isenberg S, Elliott R, Apt L. The effect of anterior transposition of the inferior oblique muscle. *Am J Ophthalmol* 1993; **116**: 224–7.

Appendix—Problems

P1: Clinical Investigations of Bilateral Poor Vision from Birth

David Taylor

In most cases the cause of apparently poor vision from birth is obvious to the ophthalmologist, for clinical examination (Fig. P1.1) will show anterior or posterior segment abnormalities; management of these cases depends on the cause.

When the eyes are found to be normal (Table P1.1) it is important to exclude 'pseudo-blindness' as in delayed visual development or saccade palsies (the absence of rapid eye movements makes the baby appear blind). Babies with normal fundi can still be blind from such conditions as Leber's amaurosis, cone dysfunction syndromes, cerebral blindness (perinatal anoxia, meningitis, developmental anomalies or hydrocephalus), or high ametropia. The nystagmus may be primary, not due to eye disease, and this itself will give rise to poor vision.

When the fundus is thought to be normal it is most important to exclude the presence of optic nerve hypoplasia by a combination of direct and indirect ophthalmoscopy.

Abnormalities of the pupil reactions are useful in the clinical investigations of bilateral poor vision from birth. A paradoxical pupil (in which the pupil is larger in the light than in the dark) is indicative of retinal disease, whereas sluggishly reacting pupils indicate anterior visual pathway disease. A relative afferent pupil defect suggests there is asymmetrical anterior visual pathway disease.

A paediatric neurological consultation and further investigations such as visually evoked responses, electroretinogram, computed tomography (CT) scanning, and biochemistry are carried out where indicated. Invasive tests such as CT scanning need not be used unless positive information likely to influence management is to be gained.

The history of the child's prenatal, perinatal and postnatal development, and the history of the onset of the poor vision or of the age at which it was detected are vital in the clinical investigation of suspected poor vision from birth. A family history, including the presence of consanguinity and some general questions into the child's general developmental milestones, as well as the presence of any systemic abnormalities such as seizures and the medications

that the child may be on for these is most important. The parents should both be examined clinically and in some cases (i.e. Best's disease) neurophysiological studies may be indicated.

The visual assessment of the child is carried out in the usual way (see Chapter 8).

Examination of the external eyes will reveal the presence of nystagmus or squint and the anterior segment of the eye can be inspected both by the naked eye and the slit lamp to exclude such conditions as albinism, cataract, corneal abnormalities, and so on.

It is vital that every patient of any age is refracted since high ametropia can give rise to poor vision from early in life, and may be a clue to the underlying diagnosis: high hypermetropia, for instance, is common in Leber's amaurosis (see Chapter 7).

The vitreous should be examined with the ophthalmoscope, direct or indirect, and with the slit lamp and such abnormalities as haemorrhage from non-accidental injury or bleeding disorders as in the leukaemic patient can be excluded. Retinopathy of prematurity, retinal dysplasia, persistent hyperplastic primary vitreous, hyaloid abnormalities and retinoblastoma seedlings may be found on examination.

The fundus should be examined with the pupil dilated with both the direct and indirect ophthalmoscope. Optic disc abnormalities such as coloboma, hypoplasia, anomalous optic disc, optic atrophy or swollen optic discs may reveal the cause of the poor vision. Similarly, retinal abnormalities including coloboma, retinopathy of prematurity, maculopathy, retinal dystrophy, retinal folds, retinoblastoma, retinitis, haemorrhages, albinism, or metabolic disease (for instance cherry red spot) may be diagnosed.

The diagnosis can be made in most cases by clinical examination alone as outlined in Fig. P1.1, or with the help of neurophysiological studies (see Chapter 9), neuroradiology or occasionally metabolic studies. There are, however, some clinical clues in the *apparently* blind infant which can direct the clinician to the diagnosis *when there are no obvious abnormalities on examination*.

1 High hypermetropia is suggestive of a congenital reti-

Table P1.1 Common causes of poor vision in infancy with reportedly normal eyes.

	Ophthalmoscopy	Pupils	EEG	Flash ERG	Flash VEP	Pattern VEP	CT/MRI scan	Slit lamp	Refraction
DVM	Normal	Normal	Normal	Normal	Normal	Normal	Normal	Normal	Normal
Optic nerve hypoplasia (Chapter 50)	Abnormal but direct ophthalmoscopy essential	Afferent defect	Normal or enhanced	Normal	Abnormal	Abnormal	Normal or abnormal	Normal	Normal
Optic atrophy (Chapter P16)	Abnormal	Afferent defect	Normal unless associated brain diseases	Normal	Abnormal	Abnormal	Depends on cause	Normal	Normal
Cortical blindness (Chapter 54)	Normal	Normal	Often abnormal	Normal	Usually abnormal	Usually abnormal	Usually abnormal	Normal	Normal
Albinism (Chapter 38)	Abnormal	Normal	Normal	Normal or enhanced	Cross-over defect	Cross-over defect	Not usually indicated	Iris transillumination	Myopia or astigmatism frequent
Cone dystrophy (Chapter 45)	Normal or abnormal	Normal or paradoxical	Normal	Abnormal	Abnormal	Abnormal	Not usually indicated	Normal	Hypermetropia or myopia
Retinal dystrophy (Chapter 44)	Usually abnormal	Normal	Normal	Abnormal	Usually normal	Usually normal	Normal	Normal	Usually normal
Leber's amaurosis (Chapter 44)	Usually normal	Paradoxical or sluggish	Normal	Very abnormal or absent	Abnormal	Absent	Normal often not indicated	Normal	High hypermetropia

nal dystrophy, especially Leber's congenital amaurosis (see Chapter 44).

2 Myopia may suggest prematurity (with brain problems as the cause of the visual defect) or certain retinal diseases (see Chapter 7).

3 An asymmetrical (i.e. relative) afferent pupil defect suggests anterior visual pathway disease, often compressive.

4 A bilateral symmetrical afferent pupil defect with apparently normal eyes suggests severe bilateral retinal disease, i.e. Leber's congenital amaurosis or severe anterior visual pathway, particularly chiasmal, disease.

5 A high frequency low amplitude pendular nystagmus is seen in cone dystrophies: it is not pathognomonic but with otherwise normal eyes it is highly suggestive.

6 The association of seizures, developmental delay, mid-line facial defects, and a wide variety of other dysmorphic features suggests a brain problem.

7 A positive family history, or a history of consanguinity makes certain diseases more likely. For instance, a child with first cousin normal parents and hypermetropia, who is blind with normal eyes is likely to have a congenital retinal dystrophy. A myopic baby with nystagmus and a partially sighted maternal grandfather is likely to have congenital stationary night-blindness.

8 A history of a problematic pregnancy may be helpful: bleeding, fetal distress and perinatal difficulty suggests brain problems, whilst maternal diabetes, drug ingestion, or significant alcohol intake indicate optic nerve hypoplasia.

9 A detailed history of the postnatal problems of premature infants will help to grade their risk of having brain,

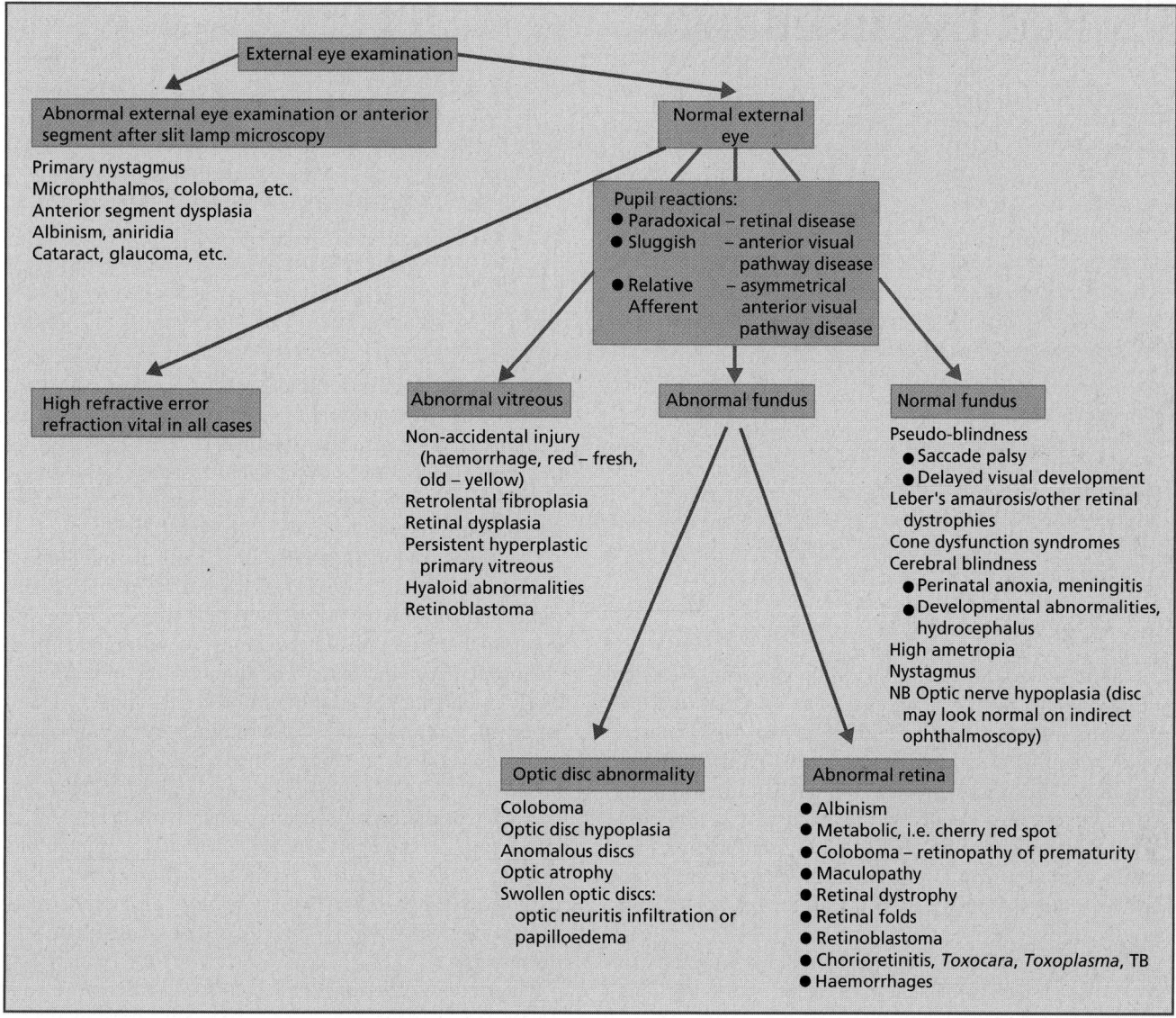

Fig. P1.1 The clinical investigation of bilateral poor vision from birth.

retinal (which should be obvious on examination) or optic nerve problems.

10 Paradoxical pupils are found in congenital stationary night-blindness, Leber's amaurosis and cone dystrophies.

11 A baby that doesn't fix and whose eyes deviate on being spun around, without developing the fast phases of nystagmus, may have congenital oculomotor apraxia, especially if vertical rapid fixation movements can be demonstrated (see Chapter 64).

P2: Red Eye in Infancy

Creig S. Hoyt

The taking of a detailed history, when a patient presents with the complaint of a red eye, is as important as the eye examination, and as important as any further tests, however sophisticated. Any experienced clinician, however busy his or her practice, would confirm that an extra few minutes spent on the history will not only give the diagnosis (to be confirmed by examination and further tests), but will also provide the time necessary to start to build a 'bond' between the doctor, parent and child.

Infants most commonly develop a red eye secondary to an ocular infection, haemorrhage or non-infectious inflammatory disorders. Infections during infancy can be both life-threatening and vision-threatening. They therefore demand urgent investigation and should be treated promptly.

Causes

Conjunctivitis

See also Chapters 15, 17 and 18. The most common cause of red eye during infancy is conjunctivitis. Conjunctivitis during the first 48 hours may be a toxic reaction to silver nitrate prophylaxis. This develops rapidly in up to 90% of infants so treated. It is usually self-limited and resolves in 24–48 hours.

A purulent discharge during the first week of life is suggestive of gonococcal conjunctivitis. It has been reported that 42% of neonates exposed to *Neisseria gonorrhoeae* during delivery will develop conjunctivitis (Laga *et al.* 1986). A Gram stain should be immediately performed and if Gram-negative diplococci are seen in the neutrophils, a third-generation cephalosporin should be administered systemically (Holmes *et al.* 1987). Although the prevalence rate of penicillin-resistant gonococcal neonatal conjunctivitides varies between centres, this is a concern throughout the world (Jarvis *et al.* 1987).

Chlamydia conjunctivitis usually occurs during the first 3 weeks of life and is typically bilateral. Prophylaxis with topical erythromycin or tetracycline may prolong the interval before a child becomes symptomatic from chlamydial conjunctivitis. The diagnosis may be definitively established by immunofluorescent staining of conjunctival scrapings or by identifying intracytoplasmic inclusion bodies in conjunctival epithelial cells. The possibility of *Neisseria gonorrhoeae* and *Chlamydia trachomatis* coexisting as causative agents must be kept in mind since in a recent study of neonatal conjunctivitis in Kenya 50% of the patients demonstrated both pathogens (Laga *et al.* 1986). Chlamydial conjunctivitis should be treated with a 2-week course of systemic erythromycin.

A variety of other bacterial agents may also cause conjunctivitis in neonates, most especially staphylococcal species followed by culture-negative (normal) flora (Jarvis *et al.* 1987). The bacteria found in the conjunctiva of the newborn reflect the mode of delivery. Infants delivered vaginally exhibit organisms of the female genital tract, whereas in babies born by caesarean section the contamination of the conjunctival flora is a function of time elapsed between membrane rupture and delivery (Isenberg *et al.* 1988). Conjunctival cultures should be performed and antibiotic treatment initiated based on the results of these cultures.

Discharge is the hallmark of bacterial conjunctivitis. Red eyes are a feature of infective conjunctivitis, whereas the eye is rarely red in nasolacrimal duct obstruction.

Virus conjunctivitis

See also Chapter 18. Adenovirus conjunctivitis may also occur during infancy. It is usually bilateral and associated with periorbital oedema, a mucoserous discharge and conjunctival chemosis and hyperaemia. Follicles do not develop in the conjunctiva of infants. The diagnosis should be made only after carefully excluding other more serious infections. No specific therapy is usually required.

Keratitis

See Chapter 18. Keratitis may also cause a red eye in infancy. Keratitis is usually caused by a viral infection in infants, but on occasion can be bacterial. Herpes simplex and adenovirus are the most common causes of viral keratitis during infancy. Approximately 70% of neonatal herpes simplex virus infections are type II. Interestingly in cases of herpes simplex infection with ocular involvement in which the virus was subtyped, 40% were type I. All cases of neonatal chorioretinitis, however, involve type II (Grosskreutz & Smith 1987). Vesicles are usually present on the eyelids or in the periorbital region in infants with a primary herpes simplex infection. Corneal involvement may consist of a punctate or a dendritic keratopathy. Vesicles on the skin may be cultured for herpes simplex. Infants suspected of having an ocular herpes simplex infection should be treated with systemic acyclovir because of their high risk of developing a disseminated herpes simplex infection (Nahmias & Hagler 1972). Topical antiviral therapy is also recommended.

Adenovirus conjunctivitis

Adenovirus conjunctivitis may also occur during infancy. It is usually bilateral and associated with periorbital oedema, a mucoserous discharge, conjunctival chemosis and hyperaemia. Follicles do not develop in the conjunctiva of infants. The diagnosis should be made only after carefully excluding other more serious infections.

Endophthalmitis

See also Chapter 17. Endophthalmitis may also occur in infants. It is usually endogenous and requires immediate systemic antibiotics. It should also be suspected in the infant who has had recent eye surgery or periorbital or facial trauma or if there is evidence of *Meningococcus* infection in the child or family members. It may follow surgery for congenital heart defects or result from a systemic infection with an agent such as group B beta *Streptococcus* acquired at birth. Meningitis frequently occurs concurrently. It should be recalled that nearly 50% of cases of metastatic or endogenous endophthalmitis are unilateral. Although an intraocular tap may be necessary, the responsible pathogen can sometimes be identified by culturing blood, cerebrospinal fluid, urine or an infected wound (Greenwald *et al.* 1986).

Chorioretinitis

See also Chapter 38. An active toxoplasmosis chorioretinitis may also on occasion be associated with a red eye during infancy. An accompanying vitritis and iridocyclitis is usually present which may obscure the underlying chorioretinitis. Active toxoplasmosis chorioretinitis should be treated with a course of systemic antibiotics (Feldman & Remington 1987) (see Chapter 13).

Haemorrhage

A periocular haemorrhage may also cause a red eye during infancy. Subconjunctival haemorrhages may occur spontaneously, or secondary to trauma or conjunctivitis. If a red eye exists after trauma, a ruptured or perforated globe should be suspected. If necessary an examination under anaesthesia should be performed to determine the intraocular pressure and to inspect the globe carefully. Subconjunctival haemorrhages may also occur spontaneously or secondary to a Valsalva manoeuvre, as in coughing during pertussis infection. Subconjunctival haemorrhages are frequent in the neonate due to birth trauma. In the older child non-accidental injury should be considered as a cause.

Other causes

There are several other causes of red eye in infancy.

1 Uveitis. This can be either primary or secondary to an intraocular tumour or infiltration (see Chapter 38).

2 Glaucoma. Red eye occurs sometimes when the intraocular pressure elevation is sudden and severe. The eye may be red, as well as photophobic, the cornea is usually cloudy and the infant usually fractious.

3 Vascular malformations and shunts. A red eye may be associated with conjunctival vascular malformations or arteriovenous shunts which involve the orbital venous system.

4 Episcleritis and scleritis. This is very rare in infancy but may occur in autoimmune disease, dry eye and graft-versus-host disease.

5 Foreign bodies. These should be suspected if there is a localized area of redness and especially if there is localized fluorescein staining. Slit-lamp examination may be required and it is important to look under the upper lid.

References

Feldman HA, Remington JS. Toxoplasmosis. In: Behrman RE, Vaughan VC (eds) *Nelson's Textbook of Pediatrics*, 13th edn. Philadelphia: WB Saunders, 1987; 736–8.

Greenwald MJ, Wohl LG, Sell CH. Metastatic bacterial endophthalmitis: a contemporary reappraisal. *Surv Ophthalmol* 1986; **2**: 81–101.

Grosskreuz ZC, Smith LBH. Neonatal conjunctivitis. *Int Ophthalmol*

1987; **2**: 81–101.

Holmes KK, Hook EW, Judson FN *et al*. Policy guidelines for the detection, management and control of antibiotic-resistant strains of *Neisseria gonorrhoeae*. *Morbid Mortal Rep* 1987; **36**: 13–14.

Isenberg SJ, Apt L, Yoshimori R. Source of the conjunctival bacterial flora at birth and neonatorum prophylaxis. *Am J Ophthalmol* 1988; **106**: 458–62.

Jarvis BM, Levine R, Asbell PA. Ophthalmia neonatorum: study of a decade of experience at Mt Sinai Hospital. *Br J Ophthalmol* 1987; **71**: 295–300.

Laga M, Plummer FA, Nzanze H. Epidemiology of ophthalmia neonatorum in Kenya. *Lancet* 1986; **ii**: 1145–9.

Nahmias AJ, Hagler AJ. Ocular manifestations of herpes simplex in the newborn. *Int Ophthalmol Clin* 1972; **12**: 191–213.

P3: Sticky Eye in Infancy

Creig S. Hoyt

Nasal lacrimal duct obstruction

A sticky eye in infancy is usually indicative of congenital dacryostenosis or blepharoconjunctivitis. Tests of patency carried out on newborns suggest that 50% of nasal lacrimal ducts are still not patent at birth; however, the persistent membranous obstruction at the nasal end breaks down quickly in most newborns and as a result only a few infants become symptomatic (Korchmarof *et al.* 1976). Mild congenital dacryostenosis may only be associated with epiphora, but a moderate or severe obstruction is generally associated with dacryocystitis and a mucopurulent discharge, often intermittently. The diagnosis can be confirmed by expressing mucopus from the lacrimal sac. Massaging, effectively increasing the hydrostatic pressure of the lacrimal sac by applying digital pressure over the lacrimal sac, may hasten the resolution of nasal lacrimal duct obstruction (Kushner 1982). Most nasolacrimal duct obstructions resolve spontaneously by 6 months of age (Peterson & Robb 1978). If dacryocystitis persists beyond 6–9 months of age the lacrimal system should be probed (Katowitz & Welsh 1987). This treatment strategy has recently been challenged by Paul and Shepherd (1994) who have suggested that the most costeffective strategy involves probing at 4 months of age in the office.

Conjunctivitis

Conjunctivitis may be bacterial, viral or allergic in aetiology. Bacterial conjunctivitis is usually associated with conjunctival papillae and a purulent discharge. When bacterial conjunctivitis is suspected a Gram stain and culture should be obtained to include *Neisseria gonorrhoea* or *N. meningococcus* injection and to direct the antibiotic therapy specifically. Gonococcal conjunctivitis is typically associated with a copious purulent discharge and lid oedema. Gonococcal conjunctivitis should be treated promptly with systemic steroids. Untreated gonococcal conjunctivitis can rapidly progress to corneal perforation. *Neisseria meningococcus* conjunctivitis is also associated with purulent discharge and places a child at increased risk of meningitis and should be treated promptly with systemic antibiotics (Al-Mutalaq *et al.* 1987).

A conjunctival infection with a variety of other bacterial agents, including *Streptococcus*, *Pneumococcus* and *Haemophilus influenzae*, may also result in purulent ocular discharge. A conjunctival infection with *Staphylococcus aureus* is usually accompanied by a mucopurulent discharge and crusting along the margins of the lids.

Viral conjunctivitis is most commonly caused by an adenovirus, is usually bilateral and associated with mucoserous discharge with a preauricular and occasionally submandibular adenopathy. A punctate keratopathy may also develop which occasionally progresses to subepithelial opacities that may reduce visual acuity. Antibiotics are ineffective against an adenovirus. A herpes simplex blepharoconjunctivitis (type I or II) can also be associated with a sticky eye. A primary infection is usually accompanied by vesicles on the eyelids. A keratitis may or may not be present. Infants with an ocular herpes simplex infection should be treated with systemic acyclovir. Topical antiviral agents should be used to treat neonates with herpes simplex, keratitis or blepharoconjunctivitis.

Allergic conjunctivitis

Allergic conjunctivitis is rare in infancy but it may occur and be associated with a mucopurulent discharge, lid oedema, and conjunctival chemosis and hyperaemia. Affected patients usually have intense pruritus as well. Gram staining of a conjunctival scraping typically reveals eosinophils. If the allergic reaction is to a topically applied ocular preparation the adjacent skin will frequently have an eczematoid dermatitis. Treatment should be initiated with cold compresses and/or topical mast cell inhibitors applied four to six times a day topically. Short courses of topical steroids may also be administered but are to be discouraged in chronic usage.

Parinaud's oculoglandular syndrome

A sticky eye may also be caused by Parinaud's oculoglandular conjunctivitis. Affected children typically have a unilateral conjunctival hyperaemia with a watery discharge, a conjunctival granuloma and regional lymphadenopathy. A Gram-negative bacillus transmitted by cats has been implicated as the causative agent for the condition known as cat-scratch disease (Wear *et al.* 1985).

Vernal conjunctivitis

Vernal conjunctivitis may also be associated with a mucoserous discharge but it is rare in infancy. In addition, affected patients usually have severe photophobia. Giant papillae are typically present on the upper tarsal conjunctiva or along the limbus. A punctate epithelial keratitis or corneal plaque may develop (Buckley 1981). The condition most commonly afflicts children in warm climates and is associated with seasonal exacerbations.

A diagnosis can be established by identifying eosinophils from conjunctival scraping of a child with giant papillary conjunctivitis. Mast cell inhibitors and occasionally steroids may be used to treat acute exacerbations. A superficial keratectomy may be necessary if a corneal plaque fails to resolve after treatment with topical mast cell inhibitors and steroids (Buckley 1981).

Other causes

1 Dry eye. A dry eye may be found in dysautonomia (Riley–Day syndrome), or other causes of deficient tear production. It is especially serious in graft-versus-host disease. The discharge is usually not mucopurulent. It is due to the accumulation of mucus in response to the dryness.

2 Foreign bodies that do not excite an acute reaction may cause stickiness by reactive mucus production.

References

Al-Mutalaq F, Byorne-Rhodes KA, Tabbara KF. *Neisseria meningitides* conjunctivitis in children. *Am J Ophthalmol* 1987; **104**: 280–2.

Buckley RJ. Vernal keratopathy and its management. *Trans Ophthal Soc UK* 1981; **101**: 234–8.

Katowitz ZA, Welsh MG. Timing of initial probing and irrigation in congenital nasolacrimal duct obstruction. *Ophthalmology* 1987; **94**: 698–705.

Korchmarof I, Szalavy E, Fodor M, Jablonsky E. Rate of spontaneous opening of congenitally blocked lacrimal pathways. ICRS J Med Science: Anatomy and Human Biology in Medicine: The Eye 1976; **4**: 541–5.

Kuschner BJ. Congenital nasolacrimal duct obstruction. *Arch Ophthalmol* 1982; **100**: 597–600.

Paul TO, Shepherd R. Congenital nasolacrimal duct obstruction: natural history and the timing of optimal intervention. *J Pediatr Ophthalmol Strabismus* 1994; **31**: 362–7.

Peterson RA, Robb RM. The natural course of congenital obstruction of the nasolacrimal duct. *J Pediatr Ophthalmol Strabismus* 1978; **15**: 246–50.

Wear DJ, Nelpy RH, Zimmerman LE *et al.* Cat scratch disease bacilli in the conjunctiva of patients with Parinaud's oculoglandular syndrome. *Ophthalmology* 1985; **92**: 1282–90.

P4: The Unusual Appearing Eye

John Elston

Many parents cannot put into words what they see with their eyes. Nowhere is this more true than with leukocoria when they may be at a loss to describe the glinting reflex they see in certain gaze directions.

The first step is to establish with the parent, and if possible the child, the exact complaint. 'Odd-looking eye' may be used to refer to abnormalities of the eyelids (e.g. a lump) or eye movements (e.g. incomitant strabismus) as

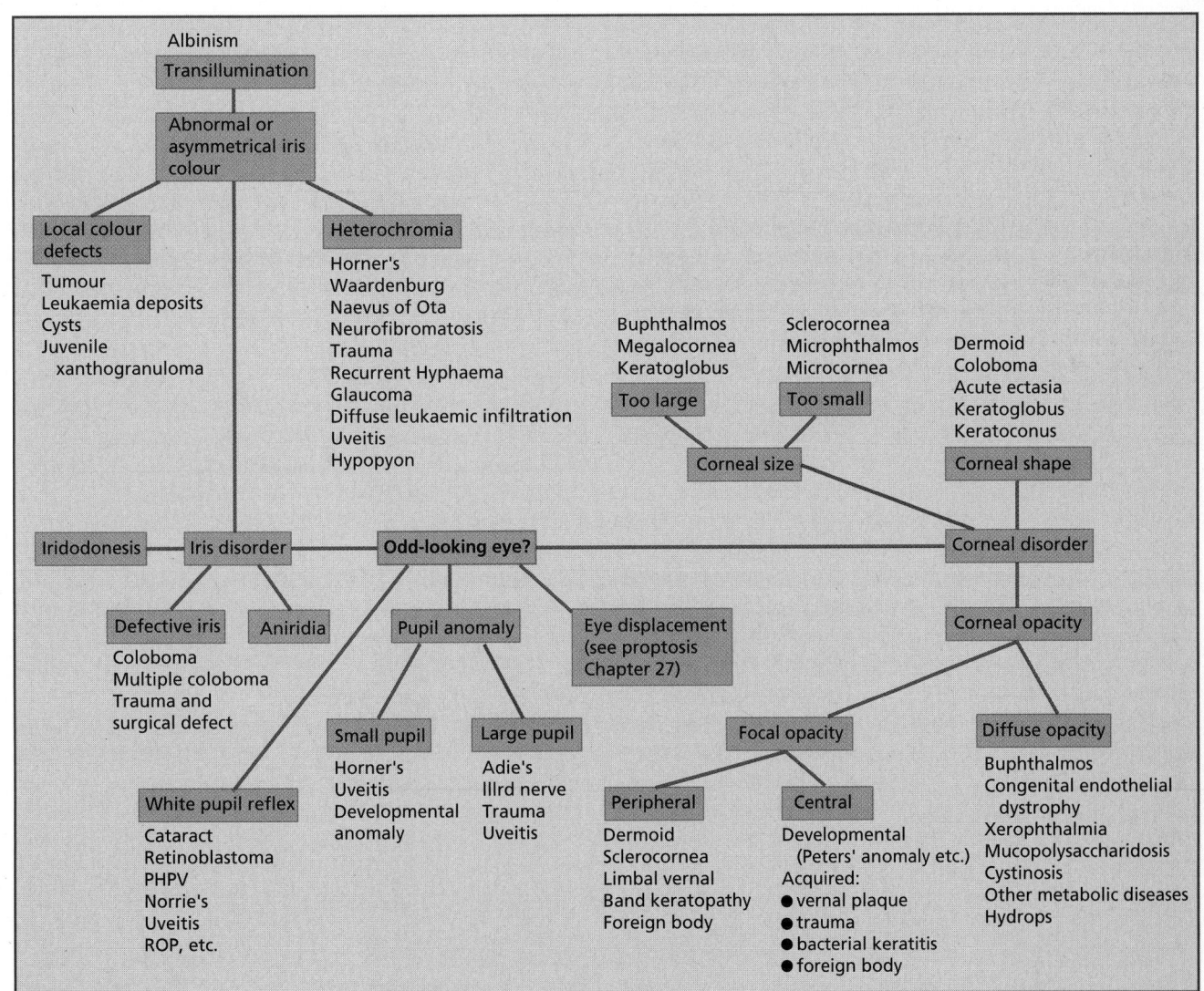

Fig. P4.1 Causes of an odd-looking eye.

well as the eye itself. The problem is best approached anatomically. The unusual appearing eye may have an abnormal colour, iris or pupil; this is determined by investigation including the slit-lamp examination.

Trauma is always worth bearing in mind as a cause of an unusual appearing eye; it may be responsible for traumatic mydriasis, iris prolapse, iris root dialysis or hyphaema.

P5: The Lump in the Lid

Creig S. Hoyt

Although a variety of disorders can cause lumps in the lids of children, most can be distinguished clinically by their pattern of growth and clinical appearance.

Rhabdomyosarcoma

The most serious disorder which needs to be considered when evaluating a lump in the lid is a rhabdomyosarcoma. It most commonly occurs in children between the ages of 5 and 8 years (Shields *et al*. 1987). It may begin as a discrete mass or as a diffuse swelling of the upper eyelid associated with ptosis. Proptosis usually develops soon thereafter as the mass often rapidly grows. More advanced cases produce severe conjunctival chemosis. If a rhabdomyosarcoma is suspected, a computed tomography (CT) and/or a magnetic resonance imaging (MRI) scan of the orbit should be performed to look for bony destruction and a non-encapsulated irregular mass. A biopsy is necessary to confirm the diagnosis. Combined radiation therapy and chemotherapy has resulted in a high cure rate for orbital rhabdomyosarcomas (Abrahamson *et al*. 1979) (see Chapter 30).

Other than rhabdomyosarcomas, most other lumps in the lids of children are benign. A careful clinical examination will usually allow these lesions to be distinguished from one another.

Capillary haemangiomas

Capillary haemangiomas frequently involve the eyelids (see Chapters 21 and 37). At birth they are usually clinically insignificant, but during the first 6 months of life they may enlarge. Superficial capillary haemangiomas are often referred to as 'strawberry naevi' and have a reddish colour. Subcutaneous capillary haemangiomas are manifested clinically as soft, bluish lumps. Capillary haemangiomas should be treated if they cause form-deprivation, strabismic or anisometropic amblyopia. They may be treated with an intralesional injection of depot steroids or systemic steroids (Kushner 1982). While both are quite effective in hastening the involution of capillary haemangiomas if performed during infancy, rebound growth may occur after discontinuing systemic steroids. Laser therapy, while effective in treating the skin discoloration, has thus far not been as effective in reducing the mass effect of these lesions. If a capillary haemangioma is not causing amblyopia, treatment is not necessary. Most capillary haemangiomas spontaneously involute later in childhood.

Dermoids

Dermoids are choristomas which primarily arise along the upper orbital rim in the margin of the eyebrow (see Chapter 35). They are manifested clinically as slow growing, painless, well-encapsulated nodules which may or may not be mobile. They may rupture spontaneously or as a result of trauma, causing cellulitis. On occasion, dermoids have 'stalks' extending through bony canals to the underlying orbital dura. Although their clinical appearance is usually diagnostic, a CT scan of the orbit is helpful in identifying dermoids with intraorbital extensions prior to surgery; mobile, clinically classical dermoids probably do not require scanning. Dermoids should be treated surgically by complete excision, usually through a skin incision.

Chalazion

See also Chapter 21. A chalazion is a lipogranuloma of the eyelids which is manifested clinically as a painless hard nodule. They are uncommon during infancy but occur frequently in older children. *Staphylococcus aureus* blepharitis often occurs concurrently. Warm compresses, cleaning of the lid margins with bland solutions, massage and topical antibiotics frequently hasten their resolution. If conservative therapy proves ineffective, they may also be treated by surgical drainage or with intralesional depot steroids (Kushner 1982).

Orbital cysts

Orbital cysts may occur in association with microphthalmia (Weiss *et al.* 1985) (see Chapter 35). The cysts may often be palpated. Both the orbital cyst and the deformed microphthalmic globe may be excised and replaced with a prosthesis for improved cosmesis.

Styes

Styes are commonly treated by the child's paediatrician or general practitioner, so they are not often seen by ophthalmologists. They are painful abscesses of the sebaceous glands at the root of the lashes. They can be cured simply by removing the lash and allowing the abscess to drain. Antibiotic ointment may sometimes be necessary.

Other causes

1 Naevi, basal cell carcinomas, and metastatic tumours are all rare in infancy.

2 Molluscum contagiosum, verrucae and simple papilloma.

3 Inflammatory lesions due to sarcoidosis, fungal infections (especially in immunocompromised infants) or foreign bodies.

4 Juvenile xanthogranuloma.

5 Squamous cell carcinoma is rare except in patients with xeroderma pigmentosa.

6 Cysts are usually developmental, occurring in the upper outer or inner quadrant away from the lid. If they are small and mobile they may be found in the lid itself. Traumatic implantation cysts are rare.

7 Calcifying epithelioma of Malherbe is a pink hard lump arising in a lid hair follicle.

References

Abrahamson DH, Ellsworth RM, Trelter P. The treatment of orbital rhabdomyosarcoma with irradiation and chemotherapy. *Ophthalmology* 1979; **86**: 1330–5.

Kushner BJ. Intralesional corticosteroids injection for infantile adnexal hemangioma. *Ophthalmology* 1982; **93**: 496–506.

Shields JA, Shields CL, Eagle RC, Nowinski T. Orbital rhabdomyosarcoma. *Arch Ophthalmol* 1987; **105**: 700–6.

Weiss A, Martinez C, Greenwald M. Microphthalmos with cyst: clinical presentation and computed tomographic findings. *J Pediatr Ophthalmol Strabismus* 1985; **22**: 6–12.

P6: Abnormal Blinking and Eye Closure

John Elston

Eye opening and closure are determined by reciprocal activity in the levator palpebrae (third nerve, nucleus in mid-brain) and orbicularis oculi (seventh nerve, nuclei in pons) (van Allen & Blodi 1962). Although the levator motor nucleus is an unpaired midline structure, premotor control is in part lateralized, allowing eye winking, i.e. unilateral levator inhibition and orbicularis activation as well as bilateral blinking (Schmidtke & Buttner-Ennever 1992). A typical blink lasts 80 milliseconds and the upper lid movement both up and down is fast and due to active muscle contraction (Doane 1980). In periodic blinking and gentle eye closure, the pretarsal and preseptal portions of orbicularis oculi are involved whilst in forceful eye closure the orbital part is also recruited (Gordon 1951).

The fundamental purpose of blinking is the maintenance of the anatomical and optical integrity of the corneal epithelium by the precorneal tear film. Infants and children up to 18 months have a low periodic blink rate (2–5 per minute), progressively increasing thereafter to achieve the adult rate (14–20 per minute) in the second decade (Zametkin *et al.* 1979). This rate is greater than that required for visual purposes. Many blinks are incomplete but if the pupil is covered, vision is suppressed by a neural mechanism as it is during saccadic eye movements (Riggs *et al.* 1981). Periodic blinks are accompanied by an eye movement — usually downwards and inwards, with or without globe retraction — and followed by a re-fixation saccade with or without a vergence movement. Bell's phenomenon of (usually) upwards and outwards eye move-ment accompanies forceful eye closure (Collewijn *et al.* 1985).

Voluntary blinking and forceful eye closure are controlled by the pyramidal system. Threshold stimulation of the precentral motor gyrus produces contralateral eye closure, whilst with suprathreshold stimuli the response is bilateral (Penfield & Rasmussen 1968). The extrapyramidal system is the initiator of periodic blinking. Pathways connect the thalamus, basal ganglia, supplementary motor area and brain stem. Lesions that interfere with emotional or periodic blinking may not affect voluntary movement and vice versa (Miller 1985).

The periodic blink rate is relatively constant in an individual under fixed conditions (Carney & Hill 1982). It is modestly increased by intellectual activity including reading, and by anxiety, and can be markedly elevated in thyrotoxicosis, schizophrenia, Tourette's syndrome and to a lesser extent in depression. It decreases with alertness, a function of the reticular activating system, and is reduced in myxoedema and in diseases involving the basal ganglia.

Reflex blinking occurs in response to corneal touch, irritation or drying, eyelid margin or conjunctival stimulation, bright light or loud noise. Reflex blinks in response to electrical stimulation of the supratrochlear nerve can be recorded by surface electrodes when two components are recognized. R_1 is a short latency (9–10 milliseconds) oligosynaptic ipsilateral response and R_2 is a long latency (30 milliseconds) polysynaptic bilateral response (Trontelj & Trontelj 1978). Habituation occurs to the late response but is not seen in infancy, when R_1 is also prolonged. The blink reflex to bright light is a long latency brain stem reflex via the pretectum persisting in the absence of the visual cortex and superior colliculi (Tavy *et al.* 1984). Thus cortically blind infants may shut their eyes in response to a sudden increase in illumination. Both corticobulbar and extrapyramidal inputs to the blink reflex arc appear to be facilitatory, although there is pyramidal inhibition of facial motor neurones (Berardelli *et al.* 1985).

Absolute eyelid position is constantly changing in response to eye movements; the levator and lower lid retractors receive a 'copy' of the neuronal input to the vertically acting extraocular muscles, probably via the rostral interstitial nucleus of the medial longitudinal fasciculus (riMLF). Some widening of the palpebral aperture on abduction is normal (Schmidtke & Buttner-Ennever 1992).

Modification of the periodic blink rate

Excessive blinking

Excessive blinking occurs in a miscellaneous group of disorders in some of which the explanation is obvious, in others less so. Any cause of excessive tear production or poor tear drainage, even if not accompanied by actual watering of the eye, may be associated with an increased blink rate. This activates the 'tear pump' function of the orbicularis oculi. Excessive blinking may also be seen in children with large phorias who use blinks to control the ocular deviation; narrowing or squinting the palpebral apertures to overcome a refractive error may also be accompanied by intermittent excessive blinking. Intermittent or persistent unilateral eye closure may be used to overcome double vision rather than complain of the symptom. Children with an exodeviation often shut one eye in bright sunlight although the reason is unclear. Blinks may be used to initiate saccadic eye movements (the blink–saccade synkinesis). Blinks are used partly to break fixation and partly to inhibit pause cells to enable a fast eye movement to be generated (Zee *et al.* 1983). For example, this may be seen in oculomotor apraxia when excessive blinking rather than head thrusts may be the prominent feature. Photophobia with excessive blinking or blepharospasm also occur as a consistent feature of photoreceptor dystrophies.

Infrequent blinking

The low periodic blink rate of infancy may persist into late childhood. Diseases of the basal ganglia are associated with a low spontaneous blink rate and may occur, for example, after hypoxic damage in childhood (Karson 1983). In Tourette's syndrome forced staring may be seen.

Specific disorders of blinking and eye closure

These occur in three circumstances: an abnormality of the sensory input, the motor response or the central control mechanism.

Abnormal sensory input

Photophobia, lacrimation, excessive blinking and blepharospasm are features of irritative disorders of the eyelids, conjunctiva and cornea including abrasions and foreign bodies. This response is reduced or abolished by topical anaesthesia. Childhood onset corneal dystrophies involving the epithelium, e.g. Reis Buckler's, or corneal crystals, e.g. cystinosis, may present this way.

Inflammatory eye disease (acute anterior uveitis) may produce similar symptoms. The chronic uveitis of juvenile rheumatoid arthritis is notably asymptomatic.

Normal sensation is important in the maintenance of corneal integrity and an anaesthetic cornea is vulnerable to exposure. It may become opaque and vascularized leading to severe visual handicap. This is seen, for example, in the Riley–Day syndrome.

The combination of corneal anaesthesia and facial palsy which may occur after posterior fossa surgery is particularly damaging. Children on ventilators in the intensive care unit are vulnerable to corneal exposure since lid and orbital oedema are common and eye closure may be incomplete. The high ambient temperature leads to rapid drying. Permanent scarring can result unless appropriate protective measures are taken.

Abnormal motor response

Lower motor neurone facial palsy, unless accompanied by corneal anaesthesia, rarely causes corneal exposure problems in childhood, provided the vertical eye movements are intact. Sometimes the eye may have to be taped shut at night. In post-facial palsy synkinesis (misdirection–regeneration of the facial nerve) there is usually mild persistent weakness of orbicularis oculi and periodic blinks are asymmetrical. On attempted forced lid closure synkinetic movements are seen in the mid and lower face.

Eyelid myokymia

Eyelid myokymia is a repetitive muscle contraction usually seen on the lower lid laterally. It is common and self-limiting and may be seen particularly in children under stress, for example when coming up to examinations. If myokymia is extensive and persistent a lesion in the dorsal pons should be suspected. Appropriate neuroimaging (magnetic resonance imaging, MRI) should be undertaken and glioma and tuberculoma are the usual pathologies (Boghen *et al.* 1970; Tenser & Corbett 1974). Extensive bilateral facial myokymia has also been described in the Guillain–Barré syndrome (GBS) (Mateer *et al.* 1983) and demyelination (Tenser 1976).

Eye blinking tic

This is a common cause of abnormal blinking in childhood and it is usually possible to make the diagnosis by history alone. Tics — purposeless, stereotyped, repetitive movements — are common in childhood (a prevalence of up to 13% between the ages of 6 and 12 years) and are most frequently facial, the most common being eye winking or

Table P6.1 Diagnostic steps.

Take a careful history from the parents—most cases of tic will be identifiable.

Examine the face and eyelids looking for
   myokymia
   facial weakness ± misdirection–regeneration
   hemifacial spasm
   blepharospasm

Examine the eyes to identify
   any cause of watering eye (e.g. punctal stenosis)
   ocular surface disorders
   inflammatory eye disease
   photoreceptor dystrophy

Examine the eye movements to identify
   phoria
   exodeviation
   ocular motor palsy
   blink: saccade synkinesis
   myasthenia gravis
   misdirection–regeneration (third nerve)
   dorsal midbrain syndrome

---

blinking tics (Lees 1985). Boys are three times as commonly affected as girls. There are rapid exaggerated contractions of the orbicularis oculi which increase with boredom, tiredness and anxiety. In contrast to other movement disorders, tics are temporarily suppressible. There is often a family history of tic. Mild focal trauma, for example a foreign body or lash in the eye, may trigger the tic. They have also been described after closed head trauma in individuals with a family history of tics. The prognosis is good and the parents and child should be strongly reassured and told to expect complete spontaneous resolution without specific treatment. Psychiatric referral is inappropriate.

Some children with eye winking or blinking tics have other facial tics such as grimacing, nostril flaring or head shaking. Eye movement tics — usually oblique conjugate saccadic movements — may also be seen (Shawkat *et al.* 1992). These also usually resolve spontaneously (Binyon & Prendergast 1991).

In Gilles de la Tourette's syndrome eye blinking and facial tics are combined with more widespread motor tics such as head twisting and gesticulation and vocal or phonic tics. These include throat clearing, sniffs, shouts, barks and clicks, and complex vocal tics especially echolalia (repetition of someone else's words or phrases), palilalia (repetition of one's own words or phrases) and coprolalia (shouting of profanities or obscenities) (Kurlan 1989). 'Sensory tics' — brief episodes of objective sensory disturbance, often in the face or around the eyes—are common. Some children exhibit self-injurious behaviour and

serious bilateral eye damage has been reported. In florid cases the diagnosis is obvious but there is a wide spectrum of abnormality. The condition has an autosomal dominant inheritance with the expression of the gene being in part determined by sex, manifesting as Tourette's syndrome in males, obsessive–compulsive disorder in females (Lees 1985). It often responds to dopamine receptor antagonist drugs. Intelligence is normal and the prognosis is quite good with most interference from the tics occurring in adolescence and 60–70% of adults having only mild tics. Other neuro-ophthalmic manifestations include sustained blepharospasm, forced staring, involuntary gaze deviation, oculogyric crisis and an eye movement tic (Frankel & Cummings 1984). Paracentral kinetic visual field defects have been described (Enoch *et al.* 1988).

Hemifacial spasm

In hemifacial spasm there is episodic co-contraction of facial nerve innervated muscles on one side; eye closure, brow elevation, lateral movement of the corner of the mouth and platysma contraction are typical. Bursts of hemifacial spasm occur and may be triggered by talking, eating or tight eye closure. Sometimes more sustained clonic contraction is seen. Hemifacial spasm in adults is usually due to microvascular compression of the facial nerve in the root exit zone and surgical decompression is usually curative (Tash *et al.* 1991). In infancy, hemifacial spasm may be the presenting sign of a posterior fossa tumour (Langston & Tharp 1976; Bills & Hanich 1991) or vascular anomaly (Flueler *et al.* 1990). In childhood, it may be due to an intrinsic pontine lesion (e.g. glioma) involving the facial nerve fascicles or extra-axial compression of the facial nerve by an abnormal blood vessel or tumour (Tenser & Corbett 1974). All infantile and childhood cases require neuroimaging (MRI) (Figs P6.1–P6.3). Very rarely hemifacial spasm may be familial (due to a familial vascular anomaly) and such cases may start in childhood (Carter *et al.* 1990).

Idiopathic blepharospasm

Primary or idiopathic blepharospasm is usually a disorder of adults not children; it consists of repeated forceful bilateral eye closure, often accompanied by photophobia and not due to an underlying eye or eyelid disorder. Synchronous mid and lower facial muscle contractions are often seen (Grandas *et al.* 1988). Blink reflex studies characteristically show hyperexcitability of the facial nuclei (Berardelli *et al.* 1985). The cause is not known but there is often a family history of idiopathic blepharospasm, focal dystonia or tic, and it seems likely that the facial nuclear hypersensitivity is secondary to extrapyramidal dysfunction. Some cases are associated with rostral brain-stem lesions (Jankovic & Patel 1983).

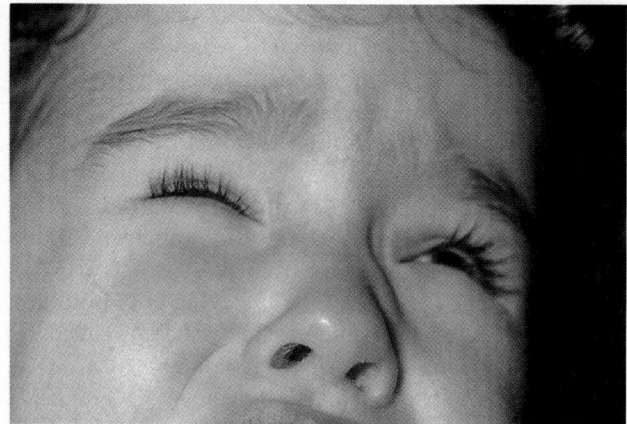

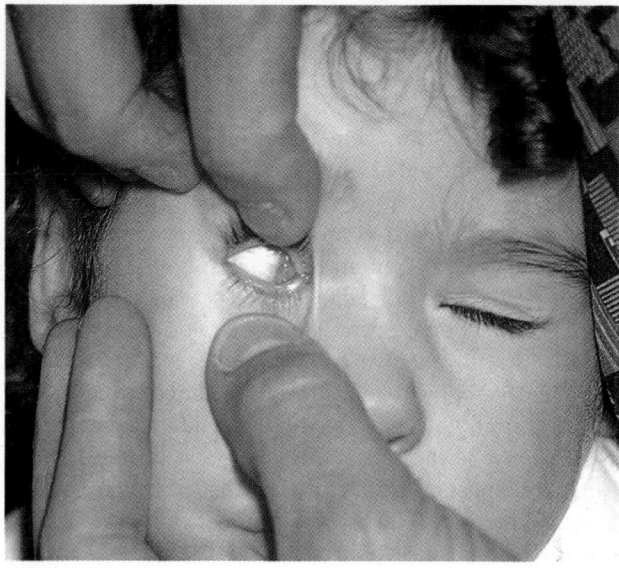

Fig. P6.1 Two-year-old child with intermittent right hemifacial spasm from 1 year of age. The attacks occurred about 20 times a day, were painful and caused the whole right half of the face to go into spasm (a). The attacks resolved spontaneously after 13 months and never recurred over 6 years. There were no abnormalities on CT scanning. The eye movements were normal, the Bell's phenomenon (a) was present during the attack and there were no cranial nerve defects during the intervals between attacks.

There is often a prodrome of increased periodic blinking, photophobia and intermittent blepharospasm which may begin in the second decade. Some affected adults have had an eye blinking tic in childhood (Elston *et al.* 1989). Neuroleptic drug administration may precipitate idiopathic blepharospasm.

Reflex blepharospasm in response to bright lights or other stimuli can occur without ocular disorders as a congenital familial characteristic (Irvine *et al.* 1968). It has also been described as an acquired disorder due to bilateral basal ganglia lesions (Larumbe *et al.* 1993). Lateral gaze-evoked blepharoclonus may occur in multiple sclerosis (Keane 1978).

In a variant of idiopathic blepharospasm, the eyes appear to be passively shut and the brows elevated but attempts on the part of the patient or examiner to open the eyes lead to spasm in the lids. This is pretarsal blepharospasm or involuntary levator palpebrae inhibition, formerly known as apraxia of eyelid opening (Elston 1992). The differential diagnoses include myasthenia gravis, orbicularis oculi myotonia and central bilateral ptosis due to a lesion in the caudal nucleus of the third nerve.

A number of cortical disorders affecting eye opening or closure are described. Right hemisphere lesions have

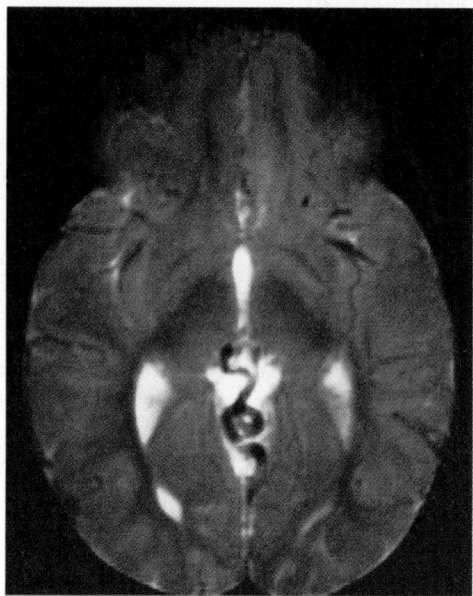

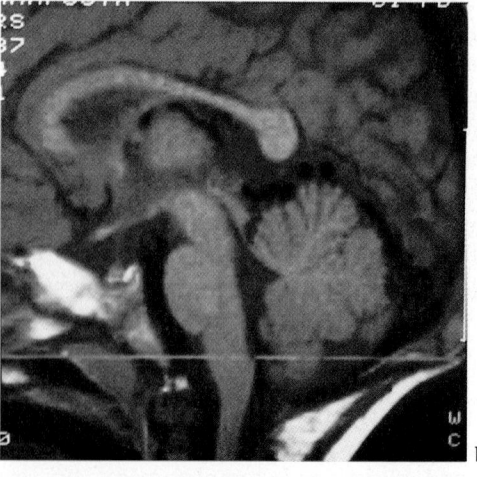

Fig. P6.2 Right-sided facial spasm occurred about every 10 minutes in this 3-year-old who had anomalous shunt vessels secondary to an occluded sigmoid sinus demonstrated by angiography and MRI scanning (a, b). The child had become severely dehydrated at age 1 year and was 'off-colour' for 6 months afterwards when the blepharospasm started. The abnormal vessels lie in the cerebellar, cerebellomedullary and pontine cisterns.

eye on the command to gently close both eyes (Onkawa *et al.* 1993). Supranuclear paralysis of voluntary lid closure has been described in bilateral frontal cortical lesions (Lessell 1972).

Miscellaneous disorders affecting eyelid position and movement

Other disorders which may present in childhood with abnormal eyelid movements are myasthenia gravis, partly recovered third nerve palsy and the Marcus Gunn phenomenon. Overshooting, hyperdynamic upper eyelid movements may be a prominent feature in myasthenia gravis and can dominate the physical signs. Lid hops on horizontal eye movements and lid twitches (Cogan's sign) on vertical eye movement are described. Fatiguability and variability of both eye and eyelid movement will also be present. The abnormal lid movements accompanying misdirection–regeneration of a third nerve palsy are stereotyped; partial ptosis with lid elevation on attempted adduction and downgaze (pseudo-von Graefe sign). The variable lid movements of cyclic oculomotor palsy may also cause confusion. In the plus–minus lid syndrome, due to a paramedian mesencephalic lesion contiguous with the third nerve nucleus, a third nerve palsy with ptosis is accompanied by contralateral lid retraction (Gaymard *et al.* 1992).

In the Marcus Gunn phenomenon, there is a synkinesis between the pterygoid muscles (lateral or medial) and the levator. A partial ptosis may be present and the condition usually presents in infancy with abnormal upper lid movements noted when feeding.

Bilateral upper lid retraction may occasionally be seen in the normal neonate; it is usually intermittent, symmetrical and resolves spontaneously. Pathological upper lid retraction is part of the dorsal midbrain syndrome indicating that the lesion involves the posterior commissure. Sympathetic overactivity in hyperthyroidism may also be responsible for this syndrome.

References

Berardelli A, Accornero N, Grucci G *et al.* The orbicularis oculi response after hemispheral damage. *J Neurol Neurosurg Psychiatr* 1983; **46**: 837–43.

Berardelli A, Rothwell J, Day BL, Marsden CD. Pathophysiology of blepharospasm and oromandibular dystonia. *Brain* 1985; **108**: 593–608.

Berlin L. Compulsive eye opening and associated phenomena. *Arch Neurol Psychiatr* 1955; **73**: 597–601.

Bills DC, Hanich A. Hemifacial spasm in an infant due to fourth ventricular ganglioglioma. *J Neurosurg* 1991; **75**: 134–7.

Binyon S, Prendergast M. Eye movement tics in children. *Dev Med Child Neurol* 1991; **33**: 352–5.

Boghen D, Filistrault R, Descarnes L. Myokymia and facial contraction in brain stem tuberculoma. *Neurology* 1970; **27**: 270–2.

Carney LG, Hill RM. The nature of normal blinking patterns. *Acta*

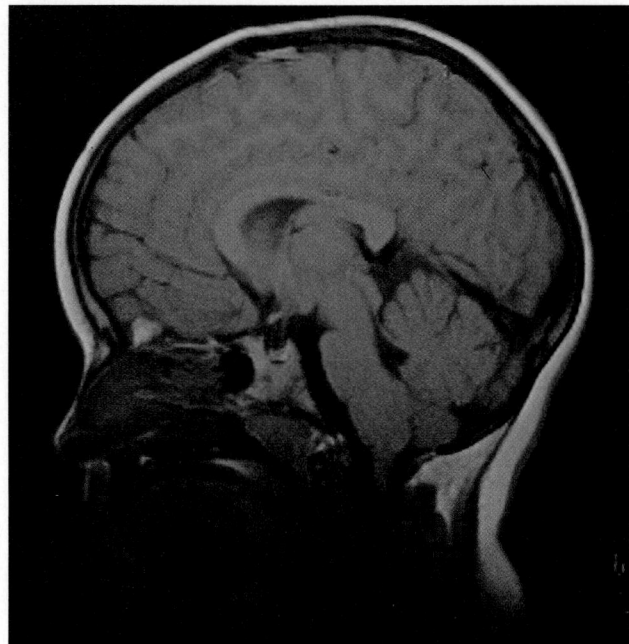

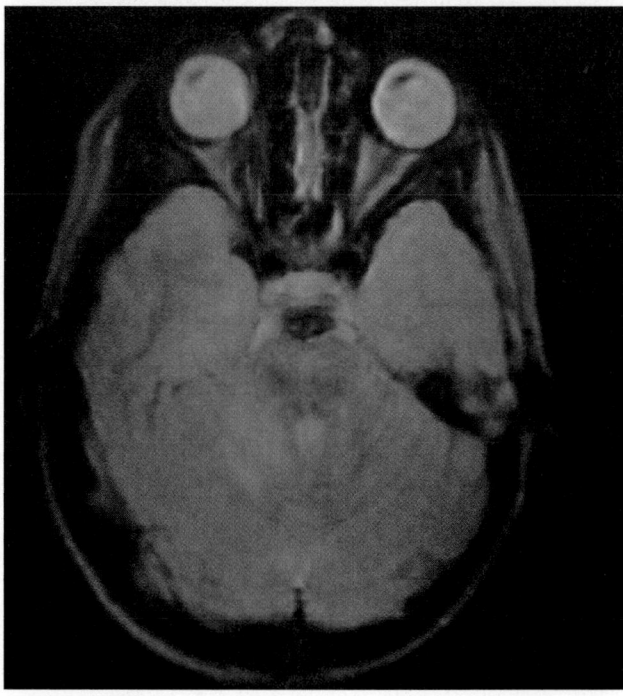

Fig. P6.3 Presumed pontine glioma presenting with unilateral blepharospasm. She presented with attacks of right-sided blepharospasm occurring every few minutes and accompanied by discomfort. CT scans carried out on two occasions were normal and MRI scan (a, b) done 2 years after the onset demonstrated the tumour. This scan carried out 4 years after the onset showed no change in the size of the tumour.

been associated with compulsive eye opening (Berlin 1955) and also bilateral ptosis with apraxia of eyelid opening (Nutt 1977). Acute infarcts in the right middle cerebral artery territory may lead to excessive closure of the right

Ophthalmol 1982; **60**: 427–33.

Carter JB, Patrinely JR, Jankovic J, McCrary JA, Boniuck M. Familial hemifacial spasm. *Arch Ophthalmol* 1990; **108**: 249–50.

Collewijn H, Van Der Steenjp Stinman RM. Human eye movements associated with blinks and prolonged eye closure. *J Neurophysiol* 1985; **54**: 11–27.

Doane NG. Interaction of eyelids and tears in corneal wetting and dynamics of the normal human eye blink. *Am J Ophthalmol* 1980; **89**: 507–16.

Elston JS. A new variant of blepharospasm. *J Neurol Neurosurg Psychiatr* 1992; **55**: 369–71.

Elston JS, Cas Granje F, Lees AJ. The relationship between eye-winking tics, frequent eye blinking and blepharospasm. *J Neurol Neurosurg Psychiatr* 1989; **52**: 477–80.

Enoch JM, Itzhaki A, Lakshminarayanan V, Comerford JP, Liebeman M, Lowe T. Gilles de la Tourette syndrome: visual effects. *Neuro-ophthalmology* 1988; **8**: 251–7.

Flueler U, Taylor D, Hing S, Kendall B, Finn JP, Brett E. Hemifacial spasm in infancy. *Arch Ophthalmol* 1990; **108**: 812–15.

Frankel M, Cummings JL. Neuro-ophthalmic abnormalities in Tourette's syndrome — functional and anatomical implications. *Neurology (Cleveland)* 1984; **34**: 359–61.

Gaymard B, Lafitte C, Gelot A, De Toffol B. Plus–minus lid syndrome. *J Neurol Neurosurg Psychiatr* 1992; **55**: 846–8.

Gordon G. Observations upon the movements of the eyelids. *Br J Ophthalmol* 1951; **35**: 339–51.

Grandas F, Elston J, Quinn N, Marsden RD. Blepharospasm — a review of 264 patients. *J Neurol Neurosurg Psychiatr* 1988; **51**: 767–72.

Irvine AR, Daroff RB, Sanders MD, Hoyt WF. Familial reflex blepharospasm. *Am J Ophthalmol* 1968; **65**: 889–90.

Jankovic J, Patel SC. Blepharospasm associated with brain stem lesions. *Neurology (Cleveland)* 1983; **33**: 1237–40.

Karson CN. Spontaneous eye blink rates and dopaminergic systems. *Brain* 1983; **106**: 643–53.

Keane JR. Gaze-evoked blepharoclonus. *Ann Neurol* 1978; **3**: 243–5.

Kurlan R. Tourette's syndrome; current concepts. *Neurology* 1989; **39**: 1625–30.

Langston JW, Tharp BR. Infantile hemifacial spasm. *Arch Neurol* 1976; **33**: 302–3.

Larumbe R, Vaamonde J, Artieda J, Zubieta JL, Obeso JA. Reflex blepharospasm associated with bilateral basal ganglia lesions. *Move Dis* 1993; **8**: 198–200.

Lees AJ. *Tics and Related Disorders*. Edinburgh: Churchill Livingstone, 1985; 12–14.

Lessell S. Supranuclear paralysis of voluntary lid closure. *Arch Ophthalmol* 1972; **88**: 241–4.

Mateer JE, Gutmann L, McComas CF. Myokymia in Guillain–Barré syndrome. *Neurology (Cleveland)* 1983; **33**: 374–6.

Miller NR. In: *Walsh and Hoyt's Clinical Neuro-Ophthalmology*, Vol. 2. Baltimore/London: Williams & Wilkins, 1985: 961.

Nutt JG. Lid abnormalities secondary to cerebral hemisphere lesions. *Ann Neurol* 1977; **1**: 149–51.

Onkawa S, Yamadori A, Maeda K *et al*. Excessive closure of the right eye; a new sign of infarction in the territory of the ipsilateral right middle cerebral artery. *J Neurol Neurosurg Psychiatr* 1993; **56**: 894–6.

Penfield W, Rasmussen T. *The Cerebral Cortex of Man*, 2nd edn. New York: Hasner, 1968; 51–2, 67–76.

Riggs LA, Volkmann FC, More RK. Suppression of the blackout that would otherwise be caused by blinks. *Vis Res* 1981; **21**: 1077–9.

Schmidtke K, Buttner-Ennever JA. Nervous control of eyelid function—a review of clinical experimental and pathological data. *Brain* 1992; **115**: 227–47.

Shawkat F, Harris CM, Jacobs M, Taylor D, Brett EM. Eye movement tics. *Br J Ophthalmol* 1992; **76**: 679–89.

Tash R, De Merritt J, Sze G, Leslie D. Hemifacial spasm; MRI features. *Am J Neuroradiol* 1991; **12**: 839–42.

Tavy DLJ, Van Woerkorn CAM, Botf GTAM, Endtz LJ. Persistence of blink reflex to sudden illumination in a comatose patient. *Arch Neurol* 1984; **41**: 323–4.

Tenser RB. Myokymia and facial contractions in multiple sclerosis. *Arch Intern Med* 1976; **136**: 81–3.

Tenser RB, Corbett JJ. Myokymia and facial contraction in brain stem glioma. *Arch Neurol* 1974; **30**: 45–7.

Trontelj MA, Trontelj JV. The reflex arc of the first component of the human blink reflex: a single motoneuron study. *J Neurol Neurosurg Psychiatr* 1978; **41**: 538–47.

Van Allen NW, Blodi F. Electromyographic study of reciprocal innervation in blinking. *Neurology* 1962; **12**: 371–7.

Zametkin AJ, Stevens JR, Pitman R. Ontogeny of spontaneous blinking and habituation of the blink reflex. *Ann Neurol* 1979; **5**: 453–7.

Zee DS, Chew FC, Leigh RJ *et al*. Blink–saccade synkinesis. *Neurology (Cleveland)* 1983; **33**: 1233–6.

P7: The Child who Closes One Eye

David Taylor

The complaint by the parent that their child closes one eye is not infrequent. The typical case is a child of about 3–8 years old and it is unusual for the child to present to the ophthalmologist with a history shorter than 2 weeks unless the underlying cause is inflammatory or associated with glaucoma. Associated symptoms are very important, for example:

- watering indicates underlying glaucoma, keratitis or uveitis;
- discharge indicates conjunctivitis or keratitis;
- pain indicates uveitis, keratitis or glaucoma; and
- redness indicates uveitis, conjunctivitis and keratitis.

Most cases can be diagnosed by simple eye examination. However, a few cases defy diagnosis. Mostly these are psychogenic and will improve with time but unless the diagnosis is clear it is appropriate to keep the child under observation.

The following conditions need to be excluded:

1 Intermittent divergent squint. The child in this instance will tend to close one eye, nearly always the same eye, and especially in sunlight. Occasionally double vision can be described (see Chapter 65).

2 Eye blinking tic. This is often unilateral or predominantly unilateral but there are usually other associated features, such as grimacing, and the tic may occur at particular times of stress or in certain social situations (see Chapter P6).

3 Unilateral corneal disease. Keratitis, trauma, or foreign body abrasion, i.e. subtarsal foreign body, may be the underlying cause, and slit-lamp microscopy with fluorescein staining is often helpful.

4 Unilateral conjunctivitis. This is usually accompanied by a discharge and watering together with redness of the eye.

5 Uveitis. Uveitis can present with photophobia and watering, usually with redness, and may be unilateral.

6 Abnormal motor response i.e. eyelid myokymia, eye blinking tic, hemifacial spasm and idiopathic blepharospasm (see Chapter P6).

7 Abnormalities of the lid. These include chalazia, or styes, and may present with the child intermittently closing one eye.

P8: Dry Eye and Inappropriate Tearing

David Taylor

Signs and symptoms

The child with a dry eye rarely complains that it is 'dry'. He says that it is 'burning'. It may also be irritable, somewhat red, gritty and with a small to moderate amount of discharge. The symptoms are often worse in dry atmospheres such as in a hot department store or in dry weather, and they may first present when the central heating is turned on. Sometimes the parents or the child's doctor will have tried a variety of drops. One clue to the underlying cause being a dry eye is that many different drops make the eye feel better, but only momentarily. The parents should be asked whether he sleeps with his eyes even

a little open at night, and if so, whether the cornea is exposed; this is most important in lid or orbital abnormalities and when corneal abnormalities are found along areas that are likely to be exposed. Excessive blinking or screwing up the eyes is another frequent symptom. An enquiry should be made into the presence of joint, skin, gut and respiratory disease, any previous eye disease or local treatment, especially radiotherapy. Rarely the child may complain of photophobia or itching; blurred vision is sometimes complained about.

Diagnosis

Dry eye in a child is relatively uncommon and this is one of the main reasons why it is underdiagnosed. Having suspected it, diagnosis depends on three main procedures.

External inspection

This includes blink rate and blink effectiveness (is the cornea completely covered by the blink?), and the presence of Bell's phenomenon; also, lid abnormalities, skin lesions and scars around the eyes and elsewhere should be looked for.

Slit-lamp examination

This should include looking at the lids for blepharitis and meibomitis, at the tear film for mucus and debris, signs of instability of the film and focal drying, and for punctate keratitis shown with rose bengal or fluorescein stain, scarring of the lids and conjunctiva, and conjunctival thickening or wrinkling. Mucus filaments and plaques may also be seen.

Slit-lamp observations of the tear film may include the tear film break-up time (BUT) (Norn 1969; Baum 1985): if a dry spot appears within 10 seconds of a blink this is considered abnormal. A variety of entities other than dry eye may reduce BUT (Baum 1985).

Slit-lamp examination may also show the presence of a narrower than normal tear meniscus alongside the lid or the presence of a dellen, which is a localized area of thinning of the cornea at a persistent dry spot.

Schirmer's test

The Schirmer's tear test may be difficult to perform in children but where it is possible it may give useful confirmation of a clinical impression of dryness.

After carefully and reassuringly explaining the procedure to the child, a filter paper strip is placed in the lower fornix laterally, and the length of the filter paper that has been wetted is noted after 5 minutes. Less than 5 mm is definitely abnormal and most children will wet 15 mm or more. Anaesthetic drops may be needed but this will reduce the tear production by lessening reflex tearing from corneal stimulation. Some ophthalmologists use this as a test of reflex tearing.

Other tests

Impression cytology (Petroutsos *et al.* 1992; Rivas *et al.* 1992) may reveal changes in older children or under anaesthetic.

Causes of dry eyes

Tear mucin deficiency

The very innermost layer of tears is formed from mucin produced in goblet cells of the conjunctiva and is important in its ability to stabilize the tear film. Its importance in dry eye is not as obvious as it may seem (Thoft 1985), nonetheless in conjunctival and corneal surface disease mucus abnormalities seem to be important (Holly & Lemp 1977). Vitamin A deficiency and trachoma are the most common causes worldwide but in the Western world the Stevens–Johnson syndrome, toxic epidermal necrolysis, burns and pemphigoid (occasionally seen in older children) are the main causes.

Tear lipid-layer deficiency

The meibomian glands produce a thin oily layer on the surface of the tears which reduces evaporation, and deposits of meibomian secretion at the lid margins prevent entry of skin fatty acids which could disrupt the integrity of the film (Tiffany 1985). Loss of meibomian glands causes increased tear evaporation and dry eye (Mathers 1993). Blepharitis, meibomitis and damage to these glands by irradiation may be a contributory factor to dry eye symptoms, and meibomitis and blepharitis should be treated vigorously by massage and cleaning of the lid margins using bland isotonic solutions or dilute baby shampoo (one teaspoon in a cup of water) on a cotton-wool ball or bud gently but firmly at least twice a day.

A short course of an antibiotic/corticosteroid combination ointment, applied in small quantities to the very margin of the lid, may help at the beginning of the treatment.

Aqueous tear deficiency—keratoconjunctivitis sicca

The aqueous middle layer of the tear is produced in the lacrimal glands and this is deficient in most dry eye states.

Keratoconjunctivitis sicca (KCS) is classically a disease of middle age, usually developing in the absence of systemic disease. When it occurs with rheumatoid arthritis, systemic lupus erythematosus, sarcoidosis, coeliac disease, Hashimoto's thyroiditis, systemic sclerosis or other autoimmune disease it is known as Sjögren's syndrome. Defective aqueous tear production also occurs in a variety of other diseases in childhood.

Congenital alacrima

Traditionally, it was thought that neonates produce no tears but Patrick (1974) showed that tears are present from the first day of life and he proposed that the absence of tearing and crying was accounted for by an efficient tear pump.

It is common experience that the parents of some children note that he does not tear when he cries when upset. This, when not accompanied by any external eye abnormality or other symptoms, is of no concern and is presumably due to an abnormality of reflex tear secretion to emotional stimuli. A congenital absence of the lacrimal gland has been proposed but this is difficult to prove. Treatment, in the absence of symptoms or signs other than the absence of emotional tearing itself, is never required. Since damage to the cornea may follow in a minority of these children (Sjögren & Erikson 1950), they might be seen from time to time and especially frequently if there are symptoms (O'Driscoll 1975).

Unilateral cases with corneal dessication and blindness (Morton 1884; Smith *et al.* 1968) are rare.

A bilateral, hereditary alacrima due to hypoplasia of the lacrimal gland suggested by pharmacological testing and by lacrimal gland biopsy, has been described as an autosomal dominant trait (Mondino & Brown 1976).

Defective reflex tearing

In children with congenital insensitivity to pain or with fifth nerve damage from tumour or trauma, there is, in addition to the neuropathic effects of the anaesthesia, also a defect in reflex tearing which further jeopardizes corneal integrity.

Localized drying

To achieve a healthily wetted cornea, a moderate wettable

area is necessary; this is usually reflected in the width of the palpebral fissure. Reduction of the palpebral fissure width by tarsorraphy is a mainstay of treatment in severe cases. Blink rate is also important (Tsubota & Nakamori 1995); a 'trick', commonly used to increase the blink rate in infants wearing contact lenses, is to induce one or more blinks by blowing on the eyelids.

Localized drying can occur because of lagophthalmos, due to lid abnormalities following excessive ptosis surgery, proptosis or facial palsy. Following squint surgery where small pieces of conjunctiva may be left standing above the rest, or in conjunctival tumours, around dermoids, and so on, small dellen (localized tiny dimples caused by dessication) may form and, although they are not a problem by themselves, they weaken the cornea's resistance to infection and keratitis may result.

Infective keratitis from drying can be very difficult to treat and needs vigorous treatment directed both toward the infection and the drying.

Familial glucocorticoid deficiency with achalasia of the cardia

In early childhood these children develop hypoglycaemia and changes in skin pigmentation, dysphagia due to achalasia of the cardia, and symptomatic dry eyes (Allgrove *et al.* 1978).

Ectodermal dysplasia

The ectodermal dysplasias are a group of conditions resulting from a morphological alteration of ectodermal-derived organs (Masse 1994) and characterized by dry skin with (in the hypohydrotic forms), absence of sweat glands and sebaceous glands, poor hair formation, and nail and dental abnormalities. A decrease in tear formation is present in ectodermal dysplasia (Wilson *et al.* 1973) and also in the related syndrome associated with ectrodactyly and cleft palate (EEC syndrome) (Baum & Bull 1974). Eyelid cysts, palmoplantar keratosis, hypodontia and hypotrichosis occur as a possible autosomal recessive trait (Font *et al.* 1986).

Other ocular abnormalities including lacrimal drainage anomalies (Beckerman 1973) and a macular dystrophy (Ohdo *et al.* 1983) also occur in association with ectodermal dysplasia. Although they are usually autosomal reces-sive, the genetics are complicated and require the help of a geneticist experienced in dermatological problems.

Cranial and facial malformations

Dry eyes have been described with Goldenhar's syndrome (Sugar 1967; Baum & Feingold 1973; Mohandessan & Romano 1978) or with craniosynostosis (Schroder & Dietze 1973). They have also been noted in Duane's syndrome (Pfaffenbach *et al.* 1972; Ramsay & Taylor 1980) and Möbius syndrome.

Multiple endocrine neoplasia type IIb

Along with their Marfan-like appearance and characteristic facies with large lips, multiple mucosal neuromas and café-au-lait spots, thickened peripheral and corneal nerves and an increased tendency to thyroid, adrenal and parathyroid tumours, these young people may have lid neuromas, thick lids, nasal displacement of the lacrimal puncta and decreased tear formation (Spector *et al.* 1981).The gene for multiple endocrine neoplasia type IIa and IIb may be on chromosome 10 (Jackson *et al.* 1988).

Familial dysautonomia (Riley–Day syndrome)

The Riley–Day syndrome is an autosomal recessive condition almost exclusively occurring in children of Ashkenazi Jewish parentage. The underlying defect is unknown but may involve the gene concerned with nerve growth factor.

Systemic features include emotional lability, paroxysmal hypertension, sweating, cold hands and feet, and a blotchy skin. They tend to drool and have difficulty in swallowing and they lack fungiform papillae on the tongue (Riley *et al.* 1949; Brunt & McKusick 1970).

As well as a progressive sensory neuropathy (Axelrod *et al.* 1981) which gives rise to absent deep tendon reflexes, a profound corneal hypoaesthesia (Fig. P8.1) together with lack of tears combine to make corneal ulceration prominent amongst the problems of these children. They also have an increased incidence of myopia, exodeviations, anisocoria, ptosis and retinal vascular tortuosity (Dunnington 1954; Goldberg *et al.* 1968).

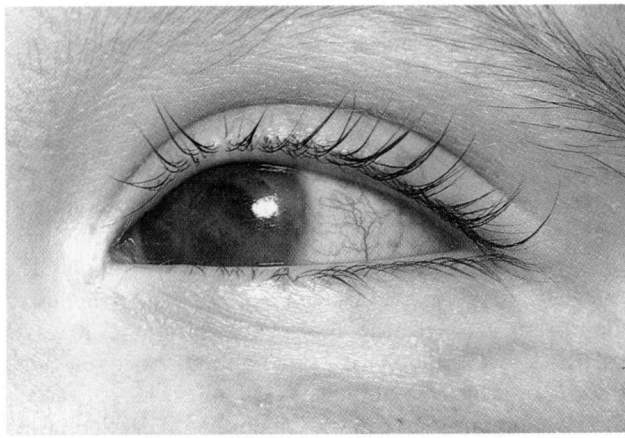

Fig. P8.1 Corneal drying, ulceration, scarring, and vascularization in familial dysautonomia. The combination of anaesthesia and dryness makes keratitis a significant problem for many of these children.

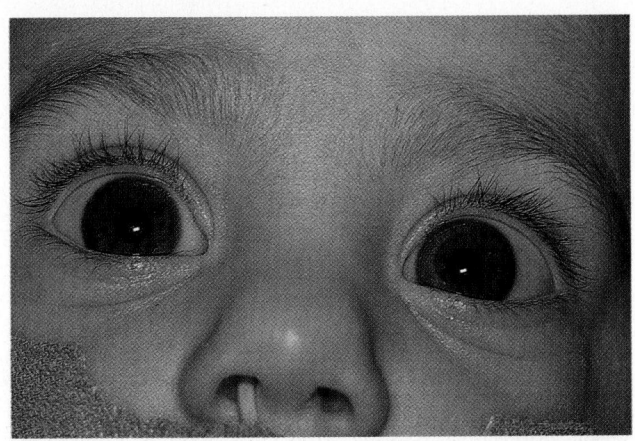

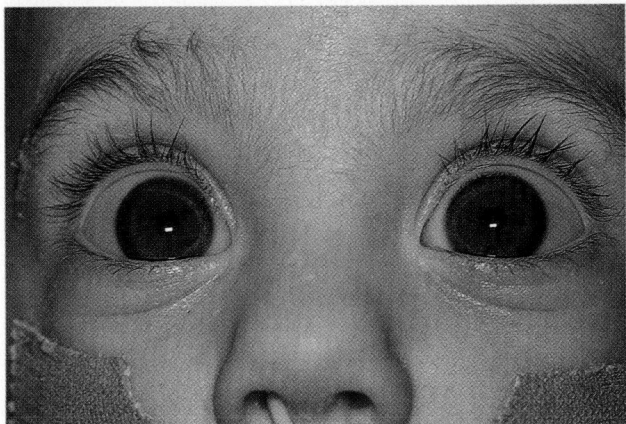

Fig. P8.2 (a) Familial dysautonomia at the time of instillation of pilocarpine 0.1%. There is no change in pupil size in normal children. (b) Same patient, same lighting conditions, 20 minutes later. The denervation hypersensitivity is indicated by the pupil constriction.

There are several syndromes which closely resemble the Riley–Day syndrome; probably the most certain way to establish the diagnosis is by the histopathological changes on sural nerve biopsy (Pearson *et al.* 1975), but this procedure is not often necessary. Other confirmatory findings include the induction of miosis by 0.1% pilocarpine or 2.5% methacholine (Fig. P8.2), which indicates denervation hypersensitivity, and the absence of flare after intradermal injection of histamine.

The management of the child as a whole requires conscientious symptomatic and supportive therapy which is the only way to prolong their lives (Axelrod *et al.* 1976), but it is unusual for them to survive beyond 30 years. The care of their eyes requires an unusual degree of dedication by the parents and the ophthalmologist, the main treatment being directed towards the dryness.

Sjögren's syndrome

This syndrome is not common in childhood, occurring mainly in adults who have rheumatoid arthritis or other autoimmune disease, together with dryness of the mouth and other mucous membranes, and with dry eye. They may also have bronchitis, pneumonia or pulmonary disease together with the other manifestations of autoimmune disease. It is occasionally seen in children with polyarteritis nodosa, Wegener's granulomatosis, the Churg–Strauss syndrome (asthma, eosinophilia and fever), Crohn's disease, acquired immunodeficiency syndrome (AIDS), and graft-versus-host disease after bone marrow transplantation.

Other syndromes and conditions with alacrima

Alacrima has also been described in patients with congenital absence of the lacrimal puncta and aptyalism (Caccamise & Townes 1980), in craniosynostosis (Schroder & Dietze 1973) and in Goldenhar's syndrome (Romano 1978), where it was also associated with a neuroparalytic keratitis. Alacrima has also been noted after craniofacial surgery in oral dysostoses. It has been recorded in 100% of patients with 'benign' botulism (Konig *et al.* 1975).

Treatment of dry eyes

Treatment of dry eyes is frequently unrewarding for both doctor and patient. The doctor's treatment is helped by the occurrence of spontaneous relative remissions but the patient is only actively helped by his own or his parents' compliance with what is often a demanding but successful regime (Lemp 1987).

Treatment of the cause

Treatment of the cause is only possible in drug-induced dry eyes and in xerophthalmia. Biannual vitamin A administration prevents xerophthalmia (Djunaedi *et al.* 1988).

Reduction of tear loss

Avoidance of dry atmospheres, of excessive central heating, the active use of humidification of the main living and sleeping rooms, and of locally increasing humidity by the use of glasses with side arms or of goggles (even swimming goggles) are important methods to reduce the loss of tears by evaporation. The parents' lives may be radically altered even to the extent of having to choose holidays in humid climates. Hydrophilic contact lenses, frequently wetted with preservative-free isotonic drops, may help but are prone to infection (Mackie 1985).

Conservation of tears, first by punctal occlusion with collagen, gelatin or silicone rods and later permanently by punctal thermocautery, may be helpful (Wright 1985).

Stimulation of tear production, enhancement of the

lipid layer of the tear film, osmotic systems, methyl cellulose inserts, and constant infusion apparatuses have all been used with varying success (Wright 1985).

Simple punctal cautery is usually adequate and laser 'punctoplasty' is no more effective and is thus unnecessary (American Academy 1992). It is surprising (when you want the punctae to scar and close) how difficult it is to achieve the desired result. Excision of the punctae, ligature of the ducts and skin closure may be necessary—this usually works!

Reduction of the wetted area

Although strongly resisted by parents, a lateral third or half tarsorrhaphy, which can easily be reduced later, is an essential part of treatment of severe dry eye states where there is associated corneal hypoaesthesia; it should preferably be performed before irretrievable corneal damage has occurred.

Treatment of excess mucus

It is debatable whether mucus is a help or a hindrance to the vitality and comfort of the cornea in patients with dry eye. Acetylcysteine drops (10 or 20%) may be tried four times daily for those children in whom tacky mucus may be causing corneal epithelial defects.

Treatment of dry exposed corneas

Taping or padding the lid, unless expertly done can be more harmful than helpful and is best avoided unless it can be carefully controlled. A temporary tarsorrhaphy with butyl-cyanoacrylate glue or suture may help and the use of simple eye ointment (ointment without antibiotic) or if infected, antibiotic eye ointment, is a good temporary solution.

Artificial tears

Artificial tears are the mainstay for symptomatic dry eyes. A variety are available, including simple saline solution, polyethylene glycol, polyvinyl alcohol, methyl cellulose and dextrans. An expensive alternative suggestion for severe, acute problems is Healonid. The advantage of the water-soluble polymers over saline is mainly that they have a longer action. It may be that hypo-osmolar solutions are more effective (Gilbard 1985). Although there is probably little to choose between the various forms, most ophthalmologists have their favourite preparations, but it is probably better not to use preparations that have the preservative benzalkonium, which unstabilizes the tear film. If used frequently, preservative-free drops are to be preferred.

Salivary gland and duct transfer may be appropriate for

very severe, sight-threatening cases (MacLeod & Robbins 1992).

Inappropriate tearing

Eye irritation including subtarsal foreign body

The symptom of a watering eye calls for a thorough search for a subtarsal foreign body, for uveitis, external eye disease and for a misplaced lash. The most common source of a persistent watering eye with a foreign body sensation is a subtarsal foreign body. It may be transparent so it can be prudent to sweep the tarsal conjunctiva with a cotton-wool bud; one newly appointed British consultant acquired instant fame and fortune in so diagnosing one of our previous Queens who had previously fruitlessly consulted several greybeards!

Crocodile tears

The gastrolacrimal reflex, also known as 'crocodile tears' from the legend that crocodiles weep before eating their victims, is usually found in patients following traumatic or inflammatory conditions of the facial nerve, or the greater superficial petrosal nerve, presumably by misdirection of the regrowing secretomotor fibres that subserve salivation. In adults, facial synkinesis is often associated (Golding-Wood 1963).

Congenital crocodile tears are often associated with Duane's syndrome or what has been described as a sixth nerve palsy (Ramsay & Taylor 1980) and these patients also have other deformities including oxycephaly, facial asymmetry, syndactyly and other limb deformities, deafness and abnormal auricles. This association between Duane's syndrome and crocodile tears is thought to be due to a discrete lesion in the vicinity of the abducens nucleus with innervation of both the lateral rectus and the salivary gland by oculomotor fibres, the latter abnormally carrying fibres from the salivatory areas in the brain stem (Ramsay & Taylor 1980).

References

Allgrove J, Clayden GS, Grant DB, MaCaulay JC. Familial glucocorticoid deficiency with achalasia of the cardia and deficient tear production. *Lancet* 1978; **8077**: 1284–6.

American Academy. Information statement. Punctal occlusion for the dry eye. *Ophthalmology* 1992; **99**: 639–40.

Axelrod FB, Lyer K, Fish I, Pearson J, Sein ME, Speilholz N. Progressive sensory loss in familial dysautonomia. *Pediatrics* 1981; **67**: 517–22.

Axelrod F, Mittag TW, Green JP. Familial dysautonomia. *Nature* 1976; **262**: 742.

Baum J. Clinical manifestation of dry eye states. *Trans Ophthalmol Soc UK* 1985; **104**: 415–23.

Baum J, Bull MJ. Ocular manifestation of the ectrodactyly, ectodermal dysplasia, cleft-palate syndrome. *Am J Ophthalmol* 1974; **78**: 211–16.

Baum JL, Feingold M. Ocular aspects of Goldenhar syndrome. *Am J Ophthalmol* 1973; **75**: 250–3.

Beckerman BL. Lacrimal anomalies in anhidrotic ectodermal dysplasia. *Am J Ophthalmol* 1973; **75**: 728–80.

Brunt PW, McKusick VA. Familial dysautonomia. *Medicine* 1970; **49**: 343–74.

Caccamise WC, Townes PL. Congenital absence of the lacrimal punctae associated with alacrima and aptyalism. *Am J Ophthalmol* 1980; **89**: 62–5.

Djunaedi E, Sommer A, Pandji A, Taylor HR. Impact of vitamin A supplementation on xerophthalmia. *Arch Ophthalmol* 1988; **106**: 218–23.

Dunnington JH. Congenital alacrima in familial autonomic dysfunction. *Arch Ophthalmol* 1954; **52**: 925–31.

Font RL, Seabury-Stone M, Schanzor MC, Lewis RA. Apocrine hidrocystomas of the lids, hypodontia, palmar plantar hyperkeratosis, and onychodystrophy. A new variant of ectodermal dysplasia. *Arch Ophthalmol* 1986; **104**: 1811–13.

Gilbard JP. Topical therapy for dry eye. *Trans Ophthalmol Soc UK* 1985; **104**: 484–98.

Goldberg MF, Payne JW, Brunt PW. Ophthalmologic studies of familial dysautonomia. *Arch Ophthalmol* 1968; **80**: 732–43.

Golding-Wood P. Crocodile tears. *Br Med J* 1963; June 8: 1518–21.

Holly FJ, Lemp MA. Tear physiology and dry eyes. *Surv Ophthalmol* 1977; **22**: 69–82.

Jackson IE, Norum RA, O'Neal LW, Nikolai TF, Delaney JP. Linkage between MEN IIb and chromosome 10 markers linked to MEN IIa. *Am J Hum Genet* 1988; **43**: A147.

Konig H, Gassman HB, Jenzer G. Ocular involvement in benign botulism B. *Am J Ophthalmol* 1975; **80**: 430–2.

Lemp MA. Recent developments in dry eye management. *Ophthalmology* 1987; **94**: 1299–305.

Mackie IA. Contact lenses for dry eyes. *Trans Ophthalmol Soc UK* 1985; **104**: 477–83.

MacLeod A, Robbins S. Submandibular gland transfer in the correction of dry eye. *Austr NZ J Ophth* 1992; **20**: 99–103.

Masse JF, Perusse R. Ectodermal dysplasia. *Arch Dis Child* 1994; **71**: 1–2.

Mathers WD. Ocular evaporation in meibomian gland dysfunction and dry eye. *Ophthalmology* 1993; **100**: 347–51.

Mohandessan MH, Romano PL. Neuroparalytic keratitis in Goldenhar–Gorlin syndrome. *Am J Ophthalmol* 1978; **85**: 111.

Mondino BJ, Brown SI. Hereditary congenital alacrima. *Arch Ophthalmol* 1976; **94**: 1478–80.

Morton AS. Congenital, unilateral absence of lacrimation. *Trans Ophthalmol Soc UK* 1884; **4**: 350–1.

Norn MS. Dessication of the precorneal tear film. I. Corneal wetting time. *Acta Ophthalmol* 1969; **47**: 865–80.

O'Driscoll TG. Alacrima. *Trans Ophthalmol Soc UK* 1975; **95**: 13–14.

Ohdo S, Hirayama K, Terawaki T. Association of ectodermal dysplasia, ectrodactyly and macular dystrophy. *J Med Genet* 1983; **20**: 52–7.

Patrick RK. Lacrimal secretions in full-term and premature babies. *Trans Ophthal Soc UK* 1974; **94**: 283–90.

Pearson J, Dancis J, Axelrod F, Grover N. The sural nerve in familial dysautonomia. *J Neuropathol Exp Neurol* 1975; **34**: 413–24.

Petroutsos G, Paschides CA, Karakostos KX, Psitas K. Diagnostic tests for dry eye disease in normals and dry eye patients with and without Sjögren's syndrome. *Ophthalmic Res* 1992; **24**: 326–31.

Pfaffenbach DD, Cross HE, Kearns TP. Congenital anomalies in Duane's syndrome. *Arch Ophthalmol* 1972; **88**: 635–9.

Ramsey J, Taylor D. Congenital crocodile tears: a clue to the aetiology of Duane's syndrome? *Br J Ophthalmol* 1980; **64**: 518–22.

Riley CM, Day RL, Greeley DMcL, Langford WS. Central autonomic dysfunction with defective lacrimation. *Pediatrics* 1949; **3**: 468–72.

Rivas L, Oroza MA, Perez-Esteban A, Murube-del-Castillo J. Morphological changes in ocular surface in dry eyes and other disorders by impression cytology. *Graefe's Arch Clin Exp Ophthalmol* 1992; **230**: 329–34.

Romano P. Neuroparalytic keratitis in Goldenhar syndrome. *Am J Ophthalmol* 1978; **85**: 111–13.

Schroder D, Dietze U. Bilateral congenital absence of tears, keratitis sicca and premature synostosis of all cranial sutures. *Klin Monatsbl Augenheilk* 1973; **163**: 239–41.

Sjögren H, Erikson A. Alacrima congenita. *Br J Ophthalmol* 1950; **34**: 691–4.

Smith RS, Maddox SF, Collins BE. Congenital alacrima. *Arch Ophthalmol* 1968; **79**: 45–8.

Spector B, Klintworth GK, Wells SA. Histologic study of the ocular lesions in multiple endocrine neoplasia syndrome type IIB. *Am J Ophthalmol* 1981; **91**: 201–14.

Sugar HS. An unusual example of the oculo-auriculo-vertebral dysplasia syndrome of Goldenhar. *J Pediatr Ophthalmol* 1967; **4**: 9–11.

Thoft RA. Relationship of the dry eye to primary ocular surface disease. *Trans Ophthalmol Soc UK* 1985; **104**: 452–7.

Tiffany JM. The role of meibomian secretion in the tears. *Trans Ophthalmol Soc UK* 1985; **104**: 396–401.

Tsubota K, Nakamori K. Effects of ocular surface area and blink rate on tear dynamics. *Arch Ophthalmol* 1995; **113**: 155–8.

Wilson FM, Grayson M, Pieroni D. Corneal changes in ectodermal dysplasia. *Am J Ophthalmol* 1973; **75**: 17–27.

Wright P. Other forms of treatment of dry eyes. *Trans Ophthalmol Soc UK* 1985; **104**: 407–8.

P9: Photophobia

Susan Day

Definition

Photophobia is light sensitivity in normal lighting conditions which makes the child uncomfortable. A child may be unable to describe his symptom, and parents may interpret slight closing of the eyes in bright sunlight as light sensitivity. True photophobia, in which the child is uncomfortable, is an uncommon symptom in infants and children.

Causes

Corneal

Most causes of true photophobia are of corneal origin. Photophobia may be caused either by epithelial disruption, as with a foreign body, or by intrastromal changes, such as with corneal oedema.

The most important cause of corneal photophobia is buphthalmos. Buphthalmos is the hallmark of congenital glaucoma. The corneas are enlarged due to breaks in Descemet's membrane which allow stretching of the cornea in the infantile eye. The cornea further thickens as a result of abnormal Descemet's function, and with this thickening haziness may occur. With extensive changes, actual scar formation may develop which ultimately may limit clarity of the media.

The baby with congenital glaucoma may be extremely photophobic. Mothers report that their babies keep their eyes closed at all times in outdoor lighting and that only with dim illumination will the eyes open. The child may be erroneously treated for possible nasolacrimal duct obstruction since the photophobia also results in epiphora. The accurate diagnosis, however, must be expediently made, as early treatment can prevent blindness in these infants.

Corneal dystrophies may also create photophobia in infancy. Congenital hereditary endothelial dystrophy, a rare autosomal recessive condition, may result in corneal clouding in the first few months of life. The photophobia is less striking than with buphthalmos, perhaps since the epithelium is not as disturbed.

Aniridia is a familiar cause of photophobia as a consequence of the abnormal irides and may include a corneal epithelial component of photophobia particularly in the older child. With aniridia, epithelial disruption with pannus formation occurs peripherally in many individuals.

Another cause of corneal photophobia is scarring. This most commonly occurs after trauma in which a corneal or corneal–scleral wound involves the optical axis. Iatrogenic scarring from refractive procedures can also create glare; hopefully this would not be found in children.

Another major cause of corneal photophobia is with disruption of the corneal epithelium, as with keratitis or corneal foreign body. Keratitis commonly occurs in conjunction with common childhood diseases such as chickenpox and measles. It is important to exclude concurrent uveitis in such patients. Herpetic keratitis may occur in children highlighting the need to perform a careful fluorescein assessment in any child with keratitis. Congenital herpetic keratitis is particularly important to diagnose as its treatment warrants systemic antiviral agents to prevent significant central nervous system sequelae. Corneal foreign bodies occur commonly in children, and may be particularly difficult to diagnose due to examination constraints and the lack of a clear-cut history.

Other epithelial disruptions, as caused by trauma, such as by children's fingernails, may be the cause of photophobia. Cystinosis, a systemic metabolic disorder, results in crystalline-like deposits in the corneal stroma. This tends to be a progressive condition and photophobia may become a feature of the child's symptoms. Several forms of cystinosis occur, with one presenting within the first few years of life and another remaining clinically silent until the mid-teens. The diagnosis is particularly important to make, as renal malfunction is another hallmark feature of this condition.

In the Richner–Hanhart syndrome (tyrosinaemia type II) photophobia occurs with skin lesions on the pressure points of the palms and soles (see Chapter 24).

Uvea

Abnormalities of the uvea can result in photophobia. Two mechanisms are present for this. First, the uveal pigment acts as a filter to incoming light. If the uveal pigment is missing, as with albinism, photophobia may be present. Another uveal abnormality, aniridia, may cause photophobia since the pupillary aperture is large and constant. Uveitis includes photophobia in its triad of symptoms: pain, redness, photophobia. Childhood acute iritis is most commonly either infectious in aetiology (such as with chickenpox) or traumatic in origin, perhaps in association with corneal abnormalities. One of the more significant forms of iritis is that associated with juvenile rheumatoid arthritis (JRA), which unfortunately does not usually have associated photophobia. This form of childhood iritis must be found in its early stages by routine slit-lamp examination of the child with diagnosis of JRA.

Lens

A partial cataract can result in photophobia. This symptom is uncommon in infants with complete cataracts, but may be present in children with partial cataracts. The photophobia usually reduces or disappears when the cataract is removed.

The symptoms of photophobia are important to discuss in patients undergoing chemotherapy, since posterior subcapsular cataracts may occur in association with dry eye in this treatment and since posterior subcapsular cataracts are particularly prone to create photophobia. Subluxed and dislocated lenses can also induce photophobia. The diagnosis of Marfan's syndrome, homocystinuria, previous trauma, and Weill–Marchesani syndrome must be considered.

Optic nerve

Although visual loss is by far the most important symptom of optic neuritis, photophobia may be a concurrent symptom. The photophobia is almost paradoxical, as vision may be extremely poor, yet light may be particularly aggravating. Some patients report that fluorescent bulb illumination is particularly bothersome with optic neuritis.

Vitreous

Vitritis, as an isolated finding, is not common in infants and children. There is usually an associated chorioretinitis or endophthalmitis. Nevertheless, in children on chemotherapy, possible *Candida* vitritis may be present. Metastatic endophthalmitis may result in a difficult-to-define photophobia. This diagnosis must be entertained in any child who has had previous trauma, including manipulations such as dental work.

Retina

Congenital cone dystrophies may result in a presentation of photophobia in an infant. The infant appears not to have photophobia indoors, but will immediately close the eyes when taken outside. The key feature which distinguishes this condition from other causes of photophobia in infancy is relatively poor vision which is associated with a high frequency, low amplitude nystagmus. The nystagmus may consequently be very difficult for the parents to notice, and even primary care clinicians may have difficulty discerning any abnormality. As the child grows older, vision difficulties become more apparent in addition to the light sensitivity.

Macular oedema may also result in photophobia. This condition may cause light sensitivity in the postoperative aphakic infant and child. These children must have a complete examination, as secondary glaucoma could also cause photophobia.

Central nervous system

The central nervous system can account for photophobia. Children with meningitis and encephalitis may be extremely light sensitive. Such symptoms are common with less serious conditions such as childhood measles. The mechanism for the photophobia is rather curious; the fifth cranial nerve, responsible for much of the sensation in the periorbital region, is also responsible for meningeal innervation. It is possible that the photophobia is a referred symptom. Such children nevertheless must be examined to exclude the possibility of concurrent keratitis or iritis (Huber 1976; Safran *et al.* 1980; Cummings & Gittinger 1981). Marmor *et al.* (1990) have described three children in which photophobia, epiphora, and torticollis were the presenting features of posterior fossa tumours.

Strabismus

The apparent light sensitivity associated with strabismus is far different than the child with a corneal foreign body.

Nevertheless, the child with an intermittent exotropia will consistently close one or the other eye when going from indoors to outdoors. This may be interpreted as photophobia by the parents. The squinting is felt by some to eliminate diplopia in such a child (Wang & Chryssanthou 1988). It is thought that fusion control is more difficult in brightly illuminated situations; thus an exophoria becomes a manifest tropia.

Other causes

Other causes of photophobia are perhaps more difficult to define. They are important, however, as apparent light sensitivity is a rather common complaint. Children who are very fair skinned seem to be photophobic. Although a complete examination is in order, normal findings provide reassurance to the parent that this will most likely be outgrown. Another interpretation of photophobia is in the child, typically 5–7 years old, who suddenly begins to blink in furious spurts. Very often, no anticipated conjunctivitis, foreign body, allergy or other pathology is found. It is important to observe during the examination for an apparent on/off switch for the blinking. One can be reassured that this is a benign condition when the blinking seems to be an attention-seeking device.

Examination

The examination must be tailored to the degree of co-operation, yet should be complete to exclude all possible conditions. It is best to consider what the most likely diagnoses are given the child's age. In an infant, congenital glaucoma must be the primary diagnosis of exclusion. In the toddler, trauma and possible corneal foreign body must be sought, since a specific history is often lacking. Another cause in this age group is keratitis associated with a childhood illness. In the preschool child, conditions which are also associated with reduced vision must be considered. At this age, objects of interest become smaller and greater demands are placed on vision than those required by a 2-year-old to stack blocks. Monochromatism, albinism and aniridia may often first come to an ophthalmologist's attention at this time. In the school-age child, the attention-getting form of photophobia seems prevalent. A further common cause at this age is manifestation of intermittent exotropia.

All aspects of the examination are important, even when the ophthalmologist is accustomed to not performing systematically a complete examination in young age groups. Visual acuity, slit-lamp examination, ocular motility and fundus examination are essential. When all appears to be normal, then electroretinography and visual evoked responses should be requested. When the symptoms justify it, an examination under anaesthetic may be useful in the unco-operative child, especially to carry out biomicroscopy, fundus examination, and on the rare occasion that it cannot be carried out without anaesthesia, neurophysiological studies (see Chapter 9).

Management

The management of a child with photophobia is highly dependent on the underlying cause. Buphthalmos, of course, requires immediate steps to lower the intraocular pressure. Iritis may need cycloplegic agents and steroids. Herpetic keratitis requires antiviral agents.

Management of the specific symptom of photophobia is rather practical, consisting of the use of tinted glasses, hats which shade the sunlight, change of residence and avoidance of brighter outdoors illumination. In children with monochromatism, special brown-tinted glasses may enhance vision as much as possible, and children with albinism often respond favourably to rose-tinted spectacles. Management of children who blink excessively is predominantly one of parental education, although occasionally 'magic drops' consisting of artificial tears will help the child. The management of such children certainly requires discussion with the parents, emphasizing the normal aspects of the examination and the high probability that the symptoms will be outgrown.

References

Cummings JL, Gittinger JW. Central dazzle: a thalamic syndrome? *Arch Neurol* 1981; **38**: 372–4.

Huber A. *Eye Signs in Brain Tumours*, 3rd edn. St Louis: CV Mosby, 1976.

Marmor MA, Beauchamp G, Maddox S. Photophobia, epiphora, and torticollis: a masquerade syndrome. *J Pediatr Ophthalmol Strabismus* 1990; **27**: 202–5.

Safran AB, Kline LB, Glaser JS. Positive visual phenomena in optic nerve disease. In: JS Glaser (ed.) *Neuro-ophthalmology*. St Louis: CV Mosby, 1980; **10**: 225–31.

Wang M, Chryssanthou G. Monocular eye closure in intermittent exotropia. *Arch Ophthalmol* 1988; **106**: 941–2.

P10: The Watering Eye

Susan Day

Signs and symptoms

Tearing in childhood is a common clinical problem, especially within the first year of life.

A child with excessive tearing causes great frustration for the parent. Whilst shopping, strangers will ask why the baby is 'crying', the skin becomes excoriated from frequent wiping and rubbing, and parents avoid taking the child to windy or dusty places, where the tearing is aggravated. The paediatrician's reassuring words that the child will 'outgrow' the condition often lose their credibility.

Associated symptoms must be elicited to focus on the appropriate diagnosis. Presence of a scratchy sensation will lead the examiner to suspect a foreign body; morning discharge may indicate keratitis or exposure keratopathy. Photophobia is an ominous associated symptom since congenital glaucoma may present with it. More than one excellent physician has misdiagnosed nasolacrimal duct obstruction or external infection for infantile glaucoma simply by failing to register the complaint of watering and photophobia.

Diagnosis

External inspection

The epiphora may be obvious, with a watery appearance just as if the child had been crying. The skin may be shiny, roughened or erythematous. More subtle tearing problems may be represented by a larger-than-usual tear meniscus above the lower lid. Secondary bacterial infection may occur with a non-patent nasolacrimal system; dacryocystitis and, more commonly, conjunctivitis with purulent discharge may then be the presenting symptom.

Slit-lamp examination

The slit-lamp examination will help assess for the presence or absence of the nasolacrimal punctae. If congenital abnormalities of the punctae are present, involvement of the upper and lower punctae must usually co-exist in order for epiphora to be apparent but the lower punctae are probably also a cause of epiphora when involved alone. An unsuspected foreign body or corneal abrasion may also be detected with the slit lamp. Other evidence of keratitis or corneal abnormality must be sought.

Fluorescein testing

Fluorescein is a valuable method of diagnosing causes of epiphora. Corneal abrasions, keratitis and other superficial irregularities may be detected because of the bright-green staining of epithelial defects when viewed in blue light. Fluorescein can also be used to judge patency of the nasolacrimal system: 5 minutes after instillation, it should be visible either in the nasal cavity or the oropharynx by inspection with a cobalt blue light.

Intraocular pressure

In the baby with excess tearing who also has photophobia, the physician must ensure that glaucoma is not present. Any corneal enlargement, clouding or breaks in

Descemet's membrane (Haab's striae) visible on slit-lamp examination suggest this diagnosis. The intraocular pressure must be assessed by an applanation technique, such as with the Perkins hand-held tonometer. Tactile measurements are notoriously inaccurate. Chloral hydrate sedation will allow accurate measurement of the intraocular pressure (Jaafar 1988). If the diagnosis is obvious, then an examination under anaesthesia proceeding to surgery is appropriate even though the anaesthesia will have to be modified to measure intraocular pressure (Walton 1979; Quigley 1982; De Luise & Anderson 1983) (see Chapter 40).

Causes and treatment

Non-patent nasolacrimal system

Epiphora first apparent between 3 and 6 weeks after birth affects approximately 6% of all neonates (Calhoun 1987). In large part, management is by the primary care doctor and includes antibiotics to prevent secondary infection and massage to encourage establishment of patency (Peterson & Robb 1978; Nelson *et al.* 1985; Paul 1985). The ophthalmologist may be consulted if there is no resolution by 6–9 months, if there is recurrent infection or anxious parents.

Treatment by the ophthalmologist must include proper medical management including massage and antibiotics where there is clinical infection (Kushner 1982). With persistent epiphora, probing of the nasolacrimal system is indicated. Some ophthalmologists advocate probing as young as 3 months, citing high success rate and ability to perform as an outpatient procedure as its advantages (Baker 1985), whereas others prefer to delay probing, hoping for natural resolution of the problem and opting for general anaesthesia and a more controlled environment to encourage better success (Kushner 1982). The technique of probing as well as indications for more extensive surgery are discussed elsewhere (see Chapter 26).

Foreign body

The history of recent trauma accompanied by excess tearing and foreign body sensation usually leads to an obvious suspicion of a corneal or conjunctival foreign body. In preverbal children, the history may be more difficult to obtain. The diagnosis must usually be made with the aid of magnification with either the slit lamp or, in instances of less co-operation, loupes or a +20 lens. When the foreign body is not immediately apparent, the upper lid should always be everted for closer inspection. Often, suspicions of a subtarsal foreign body are founded on the pattern of fluorescein staining of the cornea. Multiple, irregular tracks, particularly in the upper half of the cornea, are created by blinking.

Removal of a foreign body requires sufficient co-operation from the patient. If the foreign body is not embedded, removal with an applicator moistened with topical anaesthetic may be possible. If not easily dislodged, a dental burr drill or needle must be used. General anaesthesia or systemic ketamine and topical anaesthesia with appropriate monitoring is required when co-operation is in doubt, as chloral hydrate or other sedation will not usually allow the necessary manipulation.

Keratitis and conjunctivitis

A watery eye is a common symptom in keratitis. The child often has a history of upper respiratory infection. Eye involvement is usually bilateral but may be asymmetrical in its onset or severity. Epidemic keratoconjunctivitis must be accurately diagnosed so that further transmission to schoolmates, neighbours and family members can be kept at a minimum with proper hygiene. Keratitis related to chickenpox (Marsh 1973), measles (Fedukowicz & Stenson 1985), and mumps (Riffenburgh 1961) must be carefully examined for associated uveitis or optic neuritis. Rarely, watery irritated eyes may be the earliest symptom related to Stevens–Johnson syndrome although the severity of the associated systemic findings pre-empts the eye findings. Such children deserve early assessment and careful following by an ophthalmologist.

Allergic conjunctivitis

Although itching represents the primary symptom of this condition, excess tearing is a prominent feature. The diagnosis is usually easy to make on the basis of seasonal exacerbations, known allergic associations such as asthma, hay fever or eczema, and a family history (see Chapter 18).

Contact lens-related epiphora

In the older child or the aphakic infant with contact lenses epiphora may result from numerous causes. Improper fitting, change in corneal curvature, build-up of deposits, chips or tears at the edge of the contact lens can all create watery eyes from epithelial irregularities. The upper tarsal plate must be assessed for giant papillary conjunctivitis (GPC) in the long-term contact lens wearer (Allansmith 1977). Treatment may include refitting of lenses, obtaining new lenses, and disodium cromoglycate for patients with GPC (Allansmith & Abelson 1983). In all such patients, especially infant aphakes, care must be taken that no corneal ulcer is present, and parents of contact lens wearing infants are warned to be sure to have the lens removed within a few hours in the event of a red, sticky, watery or photophobic eye.

Congenital glaucoma

As previously mentioned, epiphora in conjunction with photophobia may herald congenital glaucoma. Buphthalmos and corneal clouding are also usually present. The diagnosis must be made on the basis of clinical findings including documentation of elevated intraocular pressure, and treatment, usually surgical, instituted promptly to prevent optic nerve damage (see Chapter 40).

Crocodile tears

One peculiar form of tearing occurs only when the patient salivates, most typically when eating, but also possible when the patient is thinking of a good meal (Golding-Wood 1963). The lesion may be at the level of the geniculate ganglion of the seventh cranial nerve but central mechanisms have been postulated. In this region, the preganglion parasympathetic fibres to the lacrimal gland are coursing with similar fibres to the submandibular gland. Presumably, 'miswiring' is present in this region, resulting in the anomalous tearing with salivation. Most typically this phenomenon occurs after injury or surgery on the ear (Axelsson & Laage-Hellman 1962) or as a sequel to Bell's palsy (McGovern 1940). Congenital crocodile tears has been reported in association with another 'miswiring' phenomenon, Duane's syndrome (Ramsay & Taylor 1980).

References

Allansmith MR, Abelson MB. Ocular allergies. In: Smolin G, Thoft R (eds) *The Cornea*. Boston/Toronto: Little, Brown, 1983; 231–43.

Allansmith MR, Greiner JV, Henriquez AS *et al.* Giant papillary conjunctivitis in contact lens wearers. *Am J Ophthalmol* 1977; **83**: 697–708.

Axelsson A, Laage-Hellman JE. The gusto-lacrimal reflex: the syndrome of crocodile tears. *Acta Otolaryngol* 1962; **54**: 239–42.

Baker JD. Treatment of congenital nasolacrimal system obstruction. *J Pediatr Ophthalmol Strabismus* 1985; **22**: 34–5.

Calhoun J. Problems of the lacrimal system in children. *Pediatr Clin N Am* 1987; **34**: 1457–65.

De Luise VP, Anderson DR. Primary infantile glaucoma. *Surv Ophthalmol* 1983; **28**: 1–19.

Fedukowicz HB, Stenson S. *External Infections of the Eye*, 3rd edn. Connecticut: Appleton-Century-Crofts, 1985.

Golding-Wood PH. Crocodile tears. *Br Med J* 1963; **i**: 1518.

Jaafar MS. Care of the infantile glaucoma patient. In: RD Reinecke (ed.) *Ophthalmology Annual*. New York: Raven Press, 1988; 15–37.

Kushner BJ. Congenital nasolacrimal system obstruction. *Arch Ophthalmol* 1982; **100**: 597–600.

McGovern FH. Paroxysmal lacrimation during eating following recovery from facial palsy. *Am J Ophthalmol* 1940; **23**: 1388–42.

Marsh RJ. Herpes zoster keratitis. *Trans Ophthalmol Soc UK* 1973; **93**: 181–90.

Nelson LB, Calhoun JH, Menduke H. Medical management of congenital nasolacrimal duct obstruction. *Ophthalmology* 1985; **92**: 1187–90.

Paul TO. Medical management of congenital nasolacrimal duct obstruction. *J Pediatr Ophthalmol Strabismus* 1985; **22**: 68–70.

Peterson RA, Robb RM. The natural course of congenital obstruction of the nasolacrimal duct. *J Pediatr Ophthalmol Strabismus* 1978; **15**: 246–50.

Quigley HA. Childhood glaucoma, results with trabeculotomy and study of reversible cupping. *Ophthalmology* 1982; **89**: 119–26.

Ramsay J, Taylor DSI. Congenital crocodile tears: a clue to the aetiology of Duane's syndrome. *Br J Ophthalmol* 1980; **64**: 518–22.

Riffenburgh RD. Ocular manifestations of mumps. Special reviews. *Arch Ophthalmol* 1961; **66**: 739–42.

Walton DS. Diagnosis and treatment of glaucoma in childhood. In: Chandler PA, Grant WM (eds). *Glaucoma*. Philadelphia: Lea & Febiger, 1979; 319–20.

P11: Proptosis

Christopher Lyons and Jack Rootman

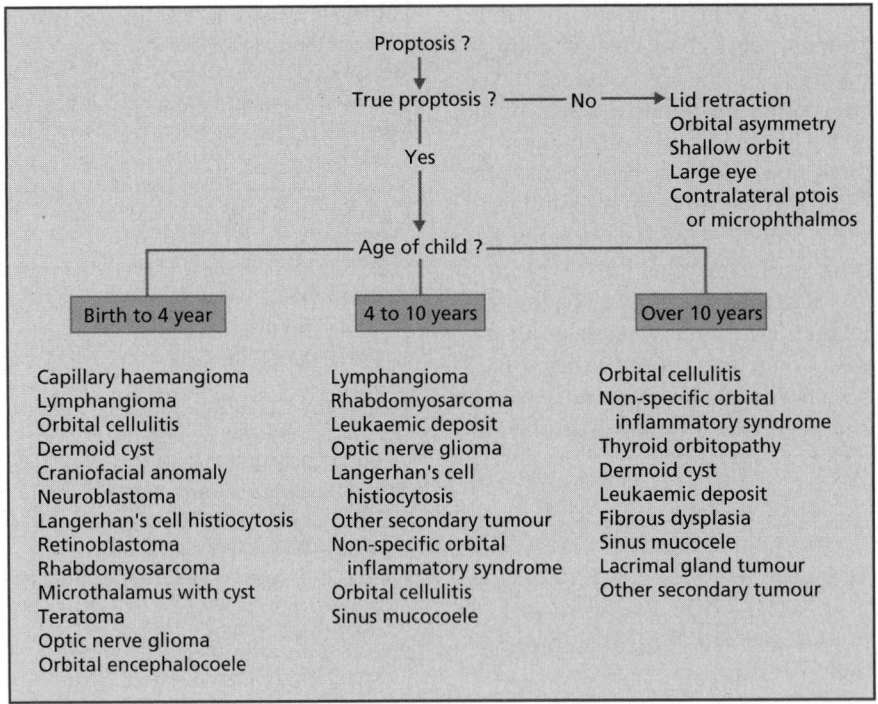

Fig. P11.1 The causes of proptosis vary with the age of the child and there is considerable overlap between both the age groups and the various centres. This figure lists causes in approximate order of frequency. Details of each condition should be sought in the text. In making a clinical diagnosis, the history and progression of the condition as well as the clinical findings are of vital importance. See Chapter 27 for a more detailed and different approach.

P12: Eye Pain

Susan Day

Definition and anatomy

'My eye hurts' is about as simple a definition of this symptom as can be found. Eye pain is a highly subjective complaint, and one which does not always match the physical findings. In a preverbal child, eye rubbing, light sensitivity, excessive blinking, irritability with a red eye may be viewed by the parent as being associated with pain. The older child may complain of eye pain when the underlying cause is anything from a foreign body to an attention-seeking device.

In general, the aetiology for eye pain can be better defined on the basis of the quality of the pain. A superficial foreign body sensation implies epithelial irregularities or foreign bodies on the cornea or conjunctiva. A deeper aching pain is more characteristic of severe intraocular pressure elevation or uveitis. Eye pain more specifically characterized by burning or itching leads one toward concerns about dry eye, allergy and chemical irritation. Pain induced by bright light classically implies uveitis although photophobia can also occur in patients with retinal and optic nerve disease as well as glaucoma.

Eye pain occurs when pain receptors are stimulated. Over-stimulation of other types of sensory fibres does not cause pain; thus another explanation, such as induced ciliary body spasm, must be found for the statement that 'light hurts my eyes'. Two fibre systems, myelinated and unmyelinated, transmit pain fibres; the former appears to transmit sharp transient pain sensations, the latter transmits dull aching sensations.

Pain fibres innervating the eye and periorbital structures arise from the trigeminal, or fifth cranial nerve. The first (ophthalmic) division is the most important division responsible for eye pain (Miller 1985). It innervates the globe, forehead, lacrimal gland, canaliculi and lacrimal sac, as well as the frontal sinus, upper lid and side of the nose. Its intracranial source is the Gasserian ganglion, from which it extends through the cavernous sinus. Branching just behind the superior orbital fissure into the lacrimal, frontal and nasociliary nerves, it then enters the superior orbital fissure. An important intracranial branch of the ophthalmic division supplies the meninges. The second major branch (V2), the maxillary nerve, supplies the cheek, lower eyelid, sometimes a small lower segment of the cornea, upper lip, side of the nose, maxillary sinus, roof of the mouth and temporal region; it too arises from the Gasserian ganglion and courses either within or just lateral to the cavernous sinus. It then passes through the inferior orbital fissure after giving rise to dural branches. Although coursing within the orbit, its terminal branches do not include intraorbital structures. The third (V3) division, or mandibular nerve, supplies sensation to other regions of the cheek as well as sensation within the mouth and preauricular area. After rising from the Gasserian ganglion, it passes through the foramen ovale to the infratemporal fossa. Although pain is most commonly generated at the site of the insult, referred pain may occur if the sensory pathway is stimulated in other regions. This phenomenon is particularly important when discussing eye pain, as intracranial stimulation of the dura may result in a sensation of retrobulbar pain.

The cornea represents one of the areas of greatest density of pain nerve endings in the body, with the greatest concentration occurring in the central cornea. There are more fibres horizontally than vertically, corresponding to the exposed area of the interpalpebral fissures.

Non-corneal structures show, in descending order, less sensitivity: eyelids, caruncle and conjunctiva (Norn 1973). Other ocular structures can be associated with pain including the uvea, sclera and optic nerve sheaths. Although the precise mechanism for the pain is poorly understood, its amelioration, either natural or in response to treatment, has led to commonly accepted explanations. The aggravating pain of ciliary body spasm is often relieved with cycloplegic agents. Anti-inflammatory agents can abate pain associated with episcleritis and, less commonly, scleritis. Pain of retrobulbar optic neuritis has been interpreted as nerve sheath inflammation. The retina and optic nerve have no pain fibres in and of themselves.

Eye pain in any given individual may include several components which require therapeutic attention. The child with a corneal foreign body will have a corneal cause for pain as well as possible reflex ciliary body spasm. Therapeutically, the epithelium must be restored by removal of the irritating cause and pressure patching if the epithelial defect is sufficiently large, and cycloplegic agents will help alleviate the ciliary spasm.

Causes

Cornea

The majority of eye pain in children is associated with underlying corneal pathology. Beware the 2-year-old child who arrives in your office with one eye tightly held shut; this child has a corneal or conjunctival foreign body until proven otherwise! Trauma can result in either a corneal abrasion or in a corneal foreign body. The older child may report that the eye feels like it has sand in it, or feels scratchy. Commonly, a child's cornea may be scratched by fingernails; this usually occurs rather innocuously, since a toddler's eye is at the height where an adult's hand rests.

Cat scratches to the eye are a particular worry due to the abundance of aerobic and anaerobic bacteria under the claws. The presence of a localized granuloma, preauricular adenopathy and a positive response to cat antigen gives rise to the cat-scratch disease or preauricular syndrome of Parinaud (Carithers 1970, 1978; Golnik et al. 1994). Corneal injury may also be non-accidental, and children's eyes have been burned with cigarettes. Foreign bodies most often occur as a child is playing with toys which can break and become splintered. The symptoms are identical to that of an abrasion. Corneal abrasions and foreign bodies often result in severe photophobia as well as pain. With time a red eye may develop or a corneal infiltrate may ensue.

Infection represents the second most common cause of cornea-induced eye pain. Keratitis typically occurs with epidemic keratoconjunctivitis but can also be present with other viral causes. Herpetic keratitis, although uncommon in children, must be clearly differentiated from these other causes. Keratitis is a common association of allergic conjunctivitis; a scratchy foreign body symptom thus may accompany this condition. Keratitis may occur in children who wear contact lenses, either acutely due to badly fitting contact lenses, or chronically due to the changing dimension of the child's cornea or deposit build-up on the lens. A sterile or bacterial ulcer must be ruled out in contact lens wearers. Exposure keratopathy can occur in children with especially prominent eyes and shallow orbits, such as occur with craniofacial abnormalities. Children with Down's syndrome may fail to close their eyes sufficiently when sleeping, thus resulting in chronic keratopathy. Their symptoms may be aggravated by chronic blepharitis (Shapiro & France 1985). Most corneal dystrophies do not result in pain although some epithelial dystrophies may cause painful photophobia.

Conjunctiva

Isolated conjunctivitis does not cause pain unless there is an associated keratitis or iritis. If pain is present, then episcleritis must be considered as an alternative or associated diagnosis.

One common circumstance in which the conjunctiva is apparently responsible for eye discomfort is in the postoperative strabismus patient. The conjunctival suture often causes a foreign body sensation probably by corneal stimulation. One argument for the cul-de-sac incision is to provide better postoperative comfort since the suture position is away from the immediate perilimbal position.

Episclera and sclera

Inflammation of the episclera can be either nodular, as in the chickenpox lesion, or diffuse. Episcleritis is associated with subconjunctival injection and may involve the overlying conjunctiva as well. It also may be accompanied by a relatively mild ache in the eye.

Scleritis is rare in children; it is characterized by deep eye pain, pain on movement, deep redness and mild proptosis, and the vision may be reduced by a serous retinal detachment (Wald et al. 1992). It may be associated with Wegener's granulomatosis (Sacks et al. 1991).

Lacrimal gland

Pain secondary to dry eyes is an uncommon occurrence in children. Dry eyes may occur as a side-effect of cancer chemotherapy; these children are often given artificial tears prophylactically. Absent tear production associated with Riley–Day syndrome, although a cause of dry eyes and recurrent corneal ulceration, is devoid of any eye pain since corneal sensation is absent. Lacrimal gland swelling is rare in children though it may occur with parotid gland swelling in mumps. Dacryoadenitis occurs rarely in association with a childhood viraemia and produces vague discomfort around the eyes. Lacrimal gland infarction associated with sickle cell disease can result in rapid swelling of the gland and mimic acute bacterial cellulitis. Childhood inflammatory orbital disease, with signs and symptoms compatible with orbital pseudotumour, is often associated with pain (Mottow & Jakobiec 1978).

Lacrimal sac

Acute dacryocystitis may occur in infants with a non-patent nasolacrimal system. The pain is accompanied by swelling in the region of the nasolacrimal sac as well as other signs of acute infection.

Glaucoma

The eye pain of congenital glaucoma is also associated with photophobia. Both result from corneal abnormalities as the neonate's cornea is stretched by the high pressure. With breaks in Descemet's membrane, stromal oedema and epithelial irregularities develop, leading to pain and photophobia. The child whose pressure is brought under control may continue to have light sensitivity as a consequence of corneal scarring.

Uvea

Since the iris is supplied with pain fibres, iritis is associated with pain, which may be augmented by ciliary spasm. The symptom of pain may be difficult to distinguish from photophobia: the combination results in an extremely uncomfortable eye. Childhood iritis may occur in association with infection (measles, chickenpox), often in conjunction with keratitis. The iritis of juvenile rheumatoid arthritis is only occasionally painful. Iritis may occur in conjunction with hyphaema, which is usually traumatic. If not associated with trauma, infiltrative processes such as childhood leukaemia or juvenile xanthogranuloma must be considered.

More posterior forms of childhood uveitis include pars planitis and *Toxocara* lesions. These inflammations usually present as visual loss rather than with eye pain. Because the iris and uvea include many pain fibres, this must be considered when doing laser procedures on co-operative children. A laser peripheral iridectomy or retinal photocoagulation may be uncomfortable without appropriate anaesthesia.

Optic nerve

The retina and optic nerves do not contain pain fibres but the optic nerve sheath does. Eye pain may occur with childhood optic neuritis. As with adult optic neuritis, the pain most commonly is initiated by looking from side to side; this puts the inflamed nerve sheath on stretch, eliciting pain. More chronic distention of the nerve sheath, such as occurs with optic nerve sheath glioma in children, does not elicit pain.

Lids

Acute distention of all or part of the lids results in vague pain. A child with a stye (hordeolum) complains of pain much more consistently than those with chalazion. Preseptal cellulitis results in tremendous stretching of the lid tissue, and pain is one of the hallmark symptoms.

Lids of children with chronic allergy may itch rather than cause true pain. Their skin becomes scaly with the eczematous reaction.

Orbit and central nervous system

Orbital pain may result from local irritation of pain fibres. Such pain usually implies an acute event, such as a rapidly expanding mass or pseudotumour (Mottow & Jakobiec 1978). The pain, however, may be referred pain from intracranial irritation of the dura. Cavernous sinus inflammation, such as occurs in individuals with Tolosa–Hunt syndrome, causes pain within the orbit, but does not often occur in children (Kline 1982). Rarely brain stem glioma may present with episodic pain, sometimes with facial spasm.

Painful third nerve palsy

Adults with posterior communicating artery aneurysms may complain that for years before their acute painful third nerve palsy they had had intermittent eye or orbital pain, but unless they complain of diplopia or have physical signs when they are examined they usually go undiagnosed for years. Ophthalmoplegic migraine, although its name implies an associated headache, is often pain free.

Painful sixth nerve palsy

In childhood the sudden onset of a sixth nerve palsy, the sudden worsening of an existing concomitant squint with the appearance of features of incomitance or the onset of a convergent squint worse in the distance, together with facial pain should make one think of petrous apex osteitis secondary to mastoiditis or suppurative otitis media (Gradenigo's syndrome). This was common in pre-antibiotic days but now painful sixth nerve palsy is probably more frequently seen with orbital or retro-orbital disease.

Herpes zoster ophthalmicus

Although relatively unusual in children this condition does occur and it may give rise to severe discomfort in the acute phase. Post-herpetic neuralgia, however, seems to be exceptionally unusual in children. As opposed to adults with herpes zoster ophthalmicus, children with this condition have a significant incidence of systemic disease, including immune deficiency and leukaemia. Treatment with antiviral agents and steroids may reduce the incidence of post-herpetic neuralgia.

Trigeminal neuralgia

Trigeminal neuralgia is predominantly a disease of old age (Poser 1975) but cases have been described in early childhood (Harris 1943). It may be secondary to pontine tumours or tumours including vascular anomalies which press on the fifth nerve. It has been associated with multiple sclerosis (Harris 1950) but, especially in childhood, this is probably not significant. The pain is severe and paroxysmal lasting seconds but leaving the child shaking and upset for a while afterwards. The fact that it is facial pain causing the problem is not obvious in the smaller child who may not be able to communicate his problem so well. Detailed neuroradiology of the course of the fifth nerve is indicated.

Headache

A child may occasionally talk about eye pain when in fact the complaint is a more generalized headache. The interpretation as 'eye pain' may be an important localizing symptom for a further discussion of childhood headache (see Chapter P17).

Functional eye pain

The child between 5 and 8 years has learned that complaining about pain leads to parental attention. Occasionally, this complaint may centre around his eyes. The child may really be asking for glasses, as further questioning may reveal this motive. Siblings of children with bona fide eye problems may have observed the extra commotion and attention given the sibling and hope for equal treatment by complaining of eye pain. Nevertheless, a diagnosis of a functional disorder is purely one of exclusion in any child which usually can be made with ease after listening to and observing the child.

Diagnostic techniques

Since the majority of underlying pathology is either corneal or conjunctival in origin, these structures must be carefully examined under magnification.

The slit-lamp examination can be performed on children of all ages. Staining the cornea with fluorescein or rose bengal should only be performed after corneal sensation has been assessed. In children who cannot co-operate for a slit lamp, the cobalt blue Wood's light, which is normally used for assessing fit of hard contact lenses, can be used or a +20 dioptre lens with the cobalt blue filter fitted over the indirect ophthalmoscope.

In the unco-operative child, the +20 lens or operating loupes may provide adequate magnification. If one decides that a lid speculum must be used, a topical anaesthetic drop must be used. Application of the drops to the fellow eye may suppress the blink reflex reducing squeezing of the lids. If a lid speculum is not available, a paper clip with the round end bent over will provide lid retraction. When a foreign body is suspected but not seen, double lid eversion must be performed. When metallic foreign bodies are suspected in the setting of a metal-on-metal, e.g. hammer and nail injury, one must consider radiological studies to exclude foreign bodies situated more deeply in the eyes. It is also important to document the absence of foreign bodies after treatment if any doubt is present.

The slit lamp or magnification with loupes also provides information about the adnexal structures and is particularly important in cases of chronic keratoconjunctivitis.

The diagnosis of congenital glaucoma includes accurate measurement of intraocular pressure. The Perkins tonometer is particularly helpful, as the pneumotonometer appears to be more affected by corneal scarring and other factors. Examinations under sedation may be necessary for accurate intraocular pressure assessment since the pressure is liable to be altered under anaesthesia.

The assessment of possible preseptal cellulitis is aimed at excluding the diagnosis of orbital cellulitis or primary ocular infection. The globe itself must be seen, as lid swelling can occur secondary to endophthalmitis, and as signs of orbital cellulitis are found by examining the globe. A lid speculum is usually required.

The diagnosis of iritis may be particularly difficult to make in children because the slit lamp must be used in every case—not an easy task in many children. Miosis as well as irregularity of the pupil due to synechiae may support the diagnosis of iritis when examination with the slit lamp is difficult. Many direct ophthalmoscopes include a slit aperture which can be used in lieu of a slit lamp if the situation demands.

Neuroradiological studies are required whenever orbital swelling persists or when the quality of retro-orbital pain and presence of associated symptoms suggests intracranial pathology. Orbital abscesses, optic nerve sheath pathology, and lacrimal gland swelling are all usually detectable with these studies. A bone scan is rarely indicated when concern about a lacrimal gland infarct in association with sickle cell disease is present. Debate often occurs as to when a neuroradiological study should be performed in cases of presumed periorbital cellulitis. If the child fails to respond to intravenous antibiotics after 36–48 hours, then computed tomography or magnetic resonance imaging should be performed to exclude the possibility of orbital mass (such as retinoblastoma, rhabdomyosarcoma or abscess).

Treatment

The treatment of eye pain depends upon the underlying cause. Smaller corneal abrasions are often left unpatched in children, since the patch itself may be uncomfortable. If the symptoms have persisted for 2 days, then a pressure patch is indicated. The addition of a cycloplegic agent to prevent ciliary spasm may make the patient more comfortable. If the cause of the abrasion is potentially infectious (such as a cat scratch) then the patient must be followed very carefully to ensure that a corneal ulcer does not develop.

Foreign bodies must be removed. Start simply, as if you were removing an eyelash, pulling the lower lid down and instructing the patient to look around. Then try a cotton bud moistened with topical anaesthetic. If these simple techniques do not work, then the examiner must judge if the child is sufficiently co-operative to have the foreign body removed with more traditional techniques of dental burrs or small gauge needles. When in doubt, sedate the child or arrange anaesthesia, as the risk of a more significant scar is not worth the pride of doing it 'the adult way'. Many children can co-operate, however, and it is up to the examiner to set the stage for co-operation.

Folk remedies in some Middle-Eastern countries have relied upon women who remove the foreign body with their tongue; although this treatment has apparently withstood the test of time, its mention here should not be taken as an endorsement!

References

Carithers HA. Cat-scratch disease. *Am J Dis Child* 1970; **119**: 200–3.

Carithers HA. Oculoglandular disease of Parinaud. *Am J Dis Child* 1978; **132**: 1195–200.

Golnik K, Maretto M, Farous M *et al.* Ophthalmic manifestations of Rachadimaea species. *Am J Ophthalmol* 1994; **118**: 145–51.

Harris W. Rare forms of trigeminal neuralgia and their relation to disseminated sclerosis. *Br Med J* 1950; **ii**: 1015–19.

Harris W. Trigeminal neuralgia at an exceptionally early age. *Br Med J* 1943; **ii**: 39.

Kline L. The Tolosa–Hunt syndrome. *Surv Ophthalmol* 1982; **27**: 79–95.

Miller N. Anatomy and physiology of the trigeminal nerve. In: *Walsh and Hoyt's Clinical Neuro-ophthalmology*, 4th edn. Baltimore: Williams & Wilkins, 1985; 999–1043.

Mottow LS, Jakobiec FA. Idiopathic inflammatory orbital pseudotumor in childhood. I. Clinical characteristics. *Arch Ophthalmol* 1978; **96**: 1410–17.

Norn M. Conjunctival sensitivity in normal eyes. *Acta Ophthalmol* 1973; **51**: 58–66.

Poser CM. Facial pain: diagnostic dilemma, therapeutic challenge. *Geriatrics* 1975; **30**: 110–15.

Sacks R, Stock E, Crawford S, Greenwald M, O'Grady R. Scleritis and Wegener's granulomatosis in children. *Am J Ophthalmol* 1991; **111**: 430–4.

Shapiro MB, France TD. The ocular features of Down's syndrome. *Am J Ophthalmol* 1985; **99**: 659–63.

Wald K, Spaide R, Patalano V, Sugin S, Yanuzzi L. Posterior scleritis in children. *Am J Ophthalmol* 1992; **113**: 281–6.

P13: Blurred and Weak Vision

Susan Day

Signs and symptoms

A young child rarely complains that he is unable to see unless the visual loss is acute and bilateral. Poor vision is usually suspected by the parents, other relatives, or school teachers on the basis of the child's behaviour or performance at a school screening examination. Parents may relate that the child sits close to the television, seems disinterested in all objects except those in his hand, or holds a book close to one eye. They may note a turn of the head or squeezing of the eyelids when an effort to see is being made. School teachers may sense a child's difficulty in seeing the blackboard or in reading a book. Difficulty with vision is often perceived as an underlying cause for a child's slow learning or poor reading abilities.

A clear distinction needs to be made between blurred and weak or dim vision: an older child can tell the difference between a defocused image and one that is dimmer than normal (or compared to the other eye) or is just not as good as expected. Blurred vision implies an optical problem, i.e. one involving the refractive media; other symptoms direct attention to the retina and beyond.

Acute bilateral vision loss is rare. A change in behaviour is noted, such as a child's stumbling around a familiar room. He may complain that the lights should be turned on or, paradoxically, complain bitterly of photophobia.

The observant child may even say that colours have become faded.

Associated symptoms, both ocular and systemic, usually indicate causes of visual loss other than refractive error. Eye pain or redness, photophobia and leukocoria may be observed by those close to the child. Headache, failure to thrive, seizure disorders, delayed or premature puberty, all may accompany visual loss in the child. The ophthalmologist needs to inquire about systemic health in every child who presents with visual loss.

Monocular visual loss or 'blurred' vision presents in an entirely different fashion. For chronic underlying causes, strabismus may occur, since there is no fusional drive to 'keep the eyes straight'. A non-seeing eye will usually turn inward if the defect is present from an early age and will turn outward in older individuals, but there are very many exceptions to this classic teaching. When strabismus is associated with poor vision in one eye, the visual loss cannot be attributed to simple amblyopia until other more ominous causes of visual loss have been excluded.

Monocular visual loss is often first detected at a school screening examination. These tests usually assess vision monocularly and may include other tests of binocular function.

Finally, concern about possible blurred vision may be raised in the context of a family history of eye problems.

Diagnosis

Visual acuity

This must be assessed at both distance and near since a discrepancy between the two will possibly suggest a refractive error. When blurred vision is the presenting complaint or when the recorded acuity is less than expected, the ophthalmologist must check the visual acuity himself. Hesitation on the child's part, adopting an abnormal head position, squeezing the eyes shut, all can be seen only by observing not only what the child sees but how the child sees. Record this behaviour in the patient's notes: this provides much more information than a simple fractional notation.

Refraction

See Chapter 7.

Optic nerve function

This includes assessment for pupillary responses, colour vision and visual fields as well as clinical evaluation of the optic nerve appearance. These functions should be checked carefully whenever systemic symptoms demand or whenever acuity cannot be improved to an expected level despite appropriate optical correction. For details of specific examination techniques, see Chapter 8.

Media examination

This includes a search for any preretinal abnormality interfering with vision. The retinoscope provides the quickest way to assess media clarity and should be used before the pupils are dilated. In this way, the impact of ptosis, corneal irregularities, anterior segment abnormalities, lens opacities and vitreous opacities can be ascertained in the normal non-dilated state. Although the retinoscope will not always pinpoint the location of the abnormality, it will highlight the amount of interference with the optical axis.

Whenever the retinoscopy defines a problem with media clarity other than ptosis a slit-lamp examination is mandatory. This will define whether the alteration is corneal, anterior segment, lenticular or in the vitreous (see Chapter 8). The direct and indirect ophthalmoscope may aid in further definition of posterior media abnormalities.

Fundoscopy

Both the direct and indirect ophthalmoscope should be used whenever the cause for blurred vision remains a puzzle. Details, such as changes in the retinal nerve fibre layer and foveal pigment irregularities, are best appreciated with the direct ophthalmoscope, whereas the panoramic view is gained from indirect ophthalmoscopy; both are necessary.

Neurological testing

When the history suggests a neurological cause for blurred vision, simple neurological examination such as finger-to-nose testing of cerebellar function or observation of tandem-walking skills is a helpful aid to diagnosis and assessment. Other testing of cranial nerves, motor function and cognitive tasks may be undertaken when appropriate.

Causes and treatment

Refractive error

Blurred vision in association with refractive error reflects not only the type of refractive error but also the accommodation. It is uncommon for children to present with refractive-error blurred vision before 9–12 years old because of the prevalence of low to moderate hyperopia with excellent accommodation. Change in refractive error toward myopia typically occurs between 10 and 14 years (Brown 1938; Slataper 1950). The increase in myopia is more pronounced before than after puberty and changes are more pronounced in a myopic child than a hyperopic child (Mantyjarvi 1985).

Children with hyperopia in general do not have reduced vision unless the refractive error exceeds 5–6 dioptres. Uncommonly, however, bilateral isoametropic amblyopia may be found with hyperopia as low as 4 dioptres. The most common form of presentation of moderate hyperopic refractive errors is as accommodative esotropia rather than blurred vision.

Myopic children typically have blurred distance vision with difficulty seeing the school blackboard, habitual television viewing at a close distance, and peering in an attempt to see. Such a child may try on someone's glasses and note the dramatic improvement in vision. Extremely high myopic refractive errors capable of inducing isoametropic amblyopia may present early as parents become concerned about the child's vision.

Purely astigmatic refractive errors are unusual causes for blurred vision despite the high incidence of astigmatism in the first years of life (Mohindra & Held 1981; Dobson *et al.* 1984). Gwiazda *et al.* (1985) were unable to find any differences in visual development in astigmatic infants who were given correction and those who were not given optical correction. Nevertheless, true meridional amblyopia has been demonstrated (Mitchell *et al.* 1973) in adults.

Refractive errors are rarely responsible for poor school performance. Print in school books is usually large, and refractive errors which are significant usually present as difficulty with distance vision (Tongue 1987).

'Failed school examination'

The parents often bring a child for further examination with a note from school expressing concern about a failed vision screening examination. Often the parent will volunteer that there is no problem with the child's visual behaviour. Occasionally, the parent will be afraid that the child is going blind, has a brain tumour or has been medically neglected.

Although a child who has failed a screening examination deserves thorough examination to exclude pathology, the 'yield' is very low. Most commonly, the child's co-operation or understanding of the test may have been limited, and a simple thorough recheck may reveal normal acuity. Also, the content of the screening examination may include areas such as 'visual motor integration', 'accommodative facility' and other measurements not in general regarded as important by ophthalmologists. It helps if the ophthalmologist is acquainted with the local screening techniques and participates in their establishment and review (Simon & Metz 1985).

Media opacities

Anything which interferes with a clear image being focused on the retina may be regarded as a media opacity and the closer it is to the nodal point of the eye, the more significant it is. Thus, a posterior capsular cataract usually has a more devastating effect on vision than an anteriorly placed lens opacity.

The most anterior of 'media opacities' is lid anomalies. Ptosis can occlude the visual axis or induce astigmatism which creates a 'blur'. It most commonly induces amblyopia with unilateral involvement although refractive errors are frequently also present. Capillary haemangiomas also warrant early intervention whenever their presence interferes with the visual axis or induces astigmatism (Nelson *et al.* 1984; Pasyk *et al.* 1984).

Acquired corneal clouding or inflammation can induce visual blurring. Keratitis from any cause may reduce acuity in association with irritation and watery discharge. Symptoms due to keratoconus usually present during the second decade as slowly progressive visual loss, perhaps with multiple attempts at correction with glasses or contact lenses (Leibowitz 1984).

Dystrophies presenting within the early years of life can result in recurrent epithelial defects or reduced vision (Waring *et al.* 1984).

Blurred vision as a consequence of anterior segment inflammation is usually associated with pain, redness, and photophobia. However, in Still's disease (juvenile rheumatoid arthritis, JRA) vision may become impaired without any associated symptoms. Iridocyclitis is most commonly found in the pauciarticular form, seronegative for rheumatoid factor, and positive antinuclear antibody testing. The ocular involvement may even precede arthritic involvement.

In the older child with cataract a blurring of vision may occur, such as with an acquired metabolic or traumatic cataract or in a child who has been on long-term systemic or topical steroids. A unilateral or sometimes bilateral congenital cataract may cause symptoms and present in older children. The child may also report glare when a partial cataract is present.

Vitreous opacities including haemorrhage, vitritis, retinoblastoma seedlings or vitreous cysts are uncommon causes of blurred vision. When the vitreous is too opacified to allow visualization, other diagnostic tests must be performed such as ultrasound and/or computed tomography (CT) scanning of the eyes and orbits.

Retinal and vitreous causes

Retinoblastoma

Approximately 5% of children with retinoblastoma have visual difficulties as a presenting feature (Ellsworth 1987). More slowly growing and unilateral tumours may present at a later age and retinoblastoma must be excluded in any child presenting with poor vision or strabismus.

Persistent hyperplastic primary vitreous

Mild persistent hyperplastic primary vitreous (PHPV) may rarely cause blurred vision if there is not complete suppression and amblyopia and if the refractive error differs significantly from the fellow eye, or if there is progression of the opacity or secondary glaucoma.

Retinopathy of prematurity

Retinopathy of prematurity (ROP) can create various levels of reduced vision, but fortunately resolves spontaneously in the vast majority of cases. Nevertheless, ROP represents a significant cause of visual loss amongst children (Phelps 1981), and since these children are prone to myopia and retinal detachment, any complaint about vision should be taken seriously.

When they are older, premature infants may have blurred vision from myopia (Nissenkorn *et al.* 1983; Gordon & Donzis 1986), or as a consequence of isoametropic amblyopia or of vitreous or retinal detachment.

Coats' disease

Coats' disease is characterized by poor vision, usually unilateral, affecting males more than females, usually within the first decade of life (Ridley *et al.* 1982) (see Chapter 46).

Retinal dystrophies

The visual disturbances with retinal dystrophies are variable. Family history of early visual loss may be present, and bilaterality is the rule. There may be associated systemic findings. Blurred vision is rarely a complaint in retinitis pigmentosa in the early stages; rather, night-blindness and loss of peripheral visual field occur. These children also tend to have high myopic or hypermetropic refractive errors (see Chapters 7 and 44).

P15: The Deaf–Blind Child

Isabelle Russell-Eggitt

It is important that sensory impairment is diagnosed early particularly in young children and especially if the defect is dual. An awareness of syndromes and associations will encourage screening for occult defect and clarify diagnosis so that prognosis and genetic counselling can be given.

It is also important to remember that there is a high incidence of visual defects in deaf children (Armitage *et al.* 1995), and hearing impairment is frequent in children with visual defects.

As in the field of vision assessment, there have been recent major advances in the non-invasive assessment of hearing loss in infants and young children. These range from the simple distraction tests similar to those used to assess field of vision to transient evoked otoacoustic emission recording (Norton 1993). History taking is vital; often there have been family concerns considerably preceding medical diagnosis.

The infant with congenital vision and hearing impairment

Intrauterine infection

Rubella

Rubella may be transmitted to a fetus during primary infection of the mother and extremely rarely during a subsequent exposure to virus. If the fetus survives an infection before 12 weeks gestation then the vascular lens may be infected resulting in cataract and microphthalmos.

Involvement of the lens may be unilateral. At birth the lens is milky white (there may be a clear cortical zone), and the corneal stroma is often hazy and there may be signs of intraocular inflammation or of glaucoma. The iris may become atrophic. Unless screened for, an associated hearing or cardiac defect may not be apparent. Hearing may be affected without major ocular defect especially where exposure is between 12 and 20 weeks gestation. The associated rubella retinopathy usually only mildly reduces acuity, but there is a high incidence of strabismus and of refractive error. Rarely macular subretinal neovascularization may lead to legal blindness late in childhood.

Cytomegalovirus

Cytomegalovirus primary maternal infection during pregnancy may be associated with severe sequelae of congenital infection, mostly due to neurological damage. In one study sensorineural hearing loss was found in 15% of a primary infected group and in 8% the loss was bilateral (Fowler 1992). In the same study seven of 112 children had chorioretinitis, in three causing vision impairment. These children may be asymptomatic at birth.

Toxoplasma gondii

Toxoplasma gondii infection in adults is often asymptomatic. There is evidence that the fetus may be infected both by primary and by recurrent infection of the mother. In the congenitally infected infant the organism may become widely disseminated with encephalitis and hepatosplenomegaly. There is often microcephaly and there may be intracranial calcification. Hydrocephalus can coexist with microcephaly and porencephaly leading to difficulty in diagnosis of raised intracranial pressure. Long-term problems in survivors are seizures, developmental delay, microcephaly, deafness and visual loss. The most severe disease seems to occur in those infected during the first trimester. The most common ocular manifestation of congenital infection is chorioretinitis.

The typical chorioretinal scars have a circumscribed

hyperpigmented border with a pale centre. The scars have a predilection for the macular region, but are often unilateral and the infant may only present later when a squint develops or when poor acuity is detected. Chorioretinitis may be severe, presenting at birth with leukocoria, a dense yellow retrolental mass with overlying white dots and blood vessels. The anterior segment shows signs of chronic inflammation (keratitis and posterior synechiae). The eye may be small, with persistent pupillary membrane and hyaloid artery, suggesting arrested ocular development.

Premature birth

Premature birth may be associated with visual handicap due to cortical as well as retinal damage and deafness (Bowen *et al.* 1993; Cooke 1993; Litt *et al.* 1993; Whyte *et al.* 1993; Enns-Dokkum *et al.* 1994). Cooke (1993) analysed the outcome at 3 years of age for 1499 infants of less than 1500 g birth weight. Whilst 3.5% had severe vision impairment, 1.3% had severe sensorineural deafness. It was not stated how many individuals were in both groups.

Genetic

Cockayne's syndrome

Cockayne's syndrome is a rare disorder of RNA and DNA repair inherited as an autosomal recessive trait. There is a great variation in severity (Nance & Berry 1992). The typical dysmorphic features of disproportionate cachectic and progeric dwarfism may not be apparent until the age of about 2 years. More than half have mild to severe sensorineural deafness, which may be congenital or not become manifest until the teens. The eyes appear sunken due to fat atrophy. In severe disease cataracts may be present from birth and survival is poor. However, in milder cases the lens may be clear and central vision may be good until about the third decade when symptoms of a progressive rod–cone dystrophy may present (Traboulsi *et al.* 1992). Other features include a photodermatitis and corneal opacities, which may be due to a recurrent erosion syndrome or anhidrosis with reduced blink.

Syndromes of unknown aetiology

CHARGE syndrome

CHARGE syndrome usually occurs sporadically. It is likely that individuals with this phenotype may have a variety of aetiologies. There is evidence for abnormalities of chromosome 22 in some cases and others may be the result of a teratogenic insult. CHARGE is an acronym for coloboma, heart defects, atresia choanae, retardation of growth and of development, genitourinary anomalies and ear abnormalities, both external and internal. Hearing loss is often severe and congenital due to structural abnormality within the temporal bone as well as external ear malformation. The main causes of ocular morbidity are coloboma of the optic nerve, often combined with coloboma of the choroid and retina, and colobomatous microphthalmos.

Rare syndromes

Rare syndromes which include early hearing and vision defect in their manifestations include the following.
1 Trisomy 13.
2 KIDS (keratitis, ichthyosis and deafness) (de Berker *et al.* 1993).
3 X-linked ataxia, posterior column demyelination deafness and optic atrophy (Arts *et al.* 1993).
4 Yemenite deaf–blind hypopigmentation syndrome (Warburg *et al.* 1990).
5 A report of ocular albinism in a three-generation kindred with both females and males affected and associated sensorineural congenital deafness, vestibular abnormalities and macromelanosomes on skin biopsy (Lewis 1978).
6 Wisniewski *et al.* (1985) reported the association of infantile neuroaxonal dystrophy, deafness and oculocutaneous albinism in a 5-year-old black girl.
7 A congenital cone–rod dystrophy may rarely be associated with infantile cardiomyopathy and sensorineural deafness (Russell-Eggitt *et al.* 1989). This is now known to be the early presentation of Alström's syndrome.
8 Osteopetrosis.

Congenital or infantile vision loss with subsequent hearing impairment

Norrie's disease

Norrie's disease is a severe neurodevelopmental disorder with an X-linked inheritance pattern for which a candidate gene has been identified (Berger *et al.* 1992; LaRussa & Wesson 1992; Parsons *et al.* 1992; Chen 1993b). A mutation in the same gene has been reported in a pedigree with the familial exudative vitreoretinopathy (FEVR) phenotype (Chen 1993a). The gene product may regulate neural cell differentiation and proliferation. Males with Norrie's disease have leucocoria and congenitally detached retinas with persistent hyperplastic primary vitreous and retinal dysplasia at birth. The eye may be small, normal sized or even enlarged. Secondary corneal opacity, posterior synechiae, ectropion uveae and cataract develop. Phthisis occurs by the age of 10 years (Warburg 1961). More than one-third develop severe sensorineural deafness, one-third are severely mentally retarded and one-third moderately retarded. As yet audiometric testing has not proven to be helpful in identifying carriers of Norrie's disease (Parving & Schwartz 1991); however, genetic tests may be helpful in some families. There is still difficulty in diagnosis and genetic counselling in single cases.

Peroxisome disorders

Peroxisome disorders may manifest in infancy as dysmorphism, hypotonia, hepatomegaly, rod–cone dystrophy and sometimes fits. One of these disorders is Zellweger's syndrome: very long chain fatty acids accumulate in the serum, but phytanic acid may not be raised (Ek *et al.* 1986). Affected infants may be initially diagnosed as having Leber's amaurosis, but also fail to thrive and are dysmorphic. Neonatal adrenoleukodystrophy should be considered as a differential diagnosis. Another disorder of peroxisomal enzymes is infantile Refsum's disease, which is distinct from the later onset classic Refsum's disease, but serum phytanic acid is raised in both conditions and both result in progressive sensorineural deafness (Weleber *et al.* 1984; Naidu & Moser 1991). There is a wide variation in the presentation of infantile Refsum's syndrome, with one end of the spectrum presenting as Leber's amaurosis with hypotonia and dysmorphic features, and the other as a delayed toddler with sensorineural hearing loss, mildly reduced vision, abnormal fundus pigmentation and reduced electroretinogram.

Alström's syndrome

Alström's syndrome is probably inherited as an autosomal recessive trait (Charles *et al.* 1990). Affected individuals are obese with profound sensorineural deafness, blindness due to retinal dystrophy and insulin-dependent diabetes mellitus. Other features include acanthosis nigricans (particularly in flexures at puberty), male hypogenitalism, hyperuricaemia, hypertriglyceridaemia, baldness, kyphosis, renal dysfunction and hypothyroidism (Charles *et al.* 1990). There is a severe early onset cone dystrophy, with an initially normal rod electroretinogram. However, the rod function also rapidly deteriorates during early childhood and may be undetectable by the age of 5 years (Tremblay *et al.* 1993). Hearing loss may not be evident until school age and diabetes mellitus until the teens or twenties; by this stage the electroretinogram is usually undetectable. Although Alström *et al.* (1959) reported that carriers may be detected on glucose tolerance or hearing testing, Charles *et al.* (1990) found no carrier signs.

X-linked ocular albinism

X-linked ocular albinism is very rarely associated with a progressive middle-age onset sensorineural deafness (Winship *et al.* 1984).

Juvenile vision loss with subsequent hearing loss

Refsum's syndrome

Refsum's syndrome most commonly presents to the ophthalmologist and commonly there is a delay in making the diagnosis until other signs develop; these include: sensorineural hearing loss, mixed motor-sensory polyneuropathy, ataxia and ichthyosis. Night-blindness is the first symptom in the majority and usually presents in teenage but can occur as young as 6 years of age (Claridge *et al.* 1992). There is a progressive salt and pepper retinopathy with deterioration in acuity and visual field constriction. Both the electro-oculogram and electroretinogram are reduced or absent. Diagnosis is made on the finding of raised serum phytanic acid and treatment is dietary. The retinal dystrophy is progressive with legal blindness usually by middle age. Lipid deposition within the iris may cause pupil miosis and the majority develop posterior subcapsular cataracts.

Wolfram's (DIDMOAD) syndrome

Presenting symptoms of Wolfram's syndrome are usually of diabetes mellitus in the first decade. However, the diabetes is of variable severity and presentation may be with visual or hearing loss. By the second decade visual acuity is reduced and the optic discs are pale. More than half develop moderate to severe hearing loss without vestibular abnormality (Higashi 1991). There is evidence that inheritance may be either autosomal recessive or mitochondrial (Bu & Rotter 1993). There may be an associated neurodegenerative disorder with ataxia and fits (Kinsley & Firth 1992).

Early sensorineural hearing loss with subsequent vision impairment

Rubella

Macular changes in children congenitally deaf as a result of congenital rubella may rarely cause visual loss (see above).

Cockayne's syndrome

In patients without early onset cataract in Cockayne's syndrome deafness may precede visual loss due to rod–cone retinal dystrophy (see above).

Usher's syndrome

Usher's syndromes, type I and II, are genetically distinct autosomal recessive conditions, but have a similar phenotype (Smith *et al.* 1994). Together they account for about 4% of all congenital deafness (Fraser 1976). The gene for Usher's syndrome type I maps to the short arm of chromosome 11 (Keats *et al.* 1994). The gene for type I may be homologous to the defective gene on mouse chromosome 7 which causes the shaker-1 deaf mutant (Evans *et al.* 1993). Usher type I is characterized by a profound congenital deafness with vestibular dysfunction and a later onset progressive retinal dystrophy with retinal pigment changes. Night-blindness is the first retinal symptom in more than 90% of cases and will be evident before the age of 10 years (Nuutila 1970). The electroretinogram will be abnormal by the time that there are symptoms. At the end of the second decade more than half will have reduced visual acuity, but less than 10% will be legally blind at this age. However, visual loss and constriction of the visual field is progressive. Early adult onset of posterior subcapsular cataracts may be due to free radical damage of the lens as postulated in other pigmentary retinopathies.

A gene for Usher's syndrome type II has been localized to the long arm of chromosome 1 (1q32); however, there is evidence for genetic heterogeneity amongst the Usher type II phenotype (Pieke Dahl *et al.* 1993); affected patients have an early onset pigmentary retinopathy, high frequency deafness with intact vestibular reflexes.

Beighton *et al.* (1993) described an autosomal recessive deafness with a progressive rod–cone retinal dystrophy and Fanconi's syndrome which is distinct but can be confused with Usher's syndrome.

Deafness–choroideraemia deletion syndrome

Choroideraemia is a rare X-linked progressive degenerative disease of the retina and choroid. The abnormal gene that causes choroideraemia is contiguous with a gene causing a stapedial anomaly and a mixed profound congenital deafness (Merry *et al.* 1989). Affected males with a deletion in the region Xq13–q21 are mentally retarded and suffer from progressive night-blindness and central blindness by the third to fourth decade of life.

Stickler's, Kniest's and Marshall's syndromes

These syndromes are now thought to be allelic expressions of the same dominant gene locus (Stratton *et al.* 1991). Abnormalities within the procollagen gene COL2A1 on chromosome 12 have been identified in Stickler and Kniest phenotypes as well as in other more rare disorders also with abnormalities of cartilage and vitreous (Spranger *et al.* 1994). Prenatal diagnosis may be possible (Zlotogora *et al.* 1994). Congenital high myopia with vitreoretinal degeneration and risk of early retinal detachment and sensorineural hearing loss occur in these conditions. As well as classic peripheral lattice degeneration typically there is radial 'lattice' extending far posteriorly, making these difficult retinas to treat. Glaucoma, which may present as buphthalmos or later in life, is an uncommon feature. The dysmorphic and skeletal features distinguish the phenotypes. There is a high incidence of lens opacity in the Stickler phenotype, with cortical wedge and fleck opacities in children, but not usually sufficient to warrant surgery until adult years (Seery *et al.* 1990).

Refsum's disease

Rarely young children with a peroxisomal enzyme disorder such as infantile Refsum's disease may present initially with generalized delay and hearing loss, only later being found to have defective vision (Weleber *et al.* 1984).

Acquired hearing and vision loss during childhood

Meningitis

This is still the most common cause of acquired deafness due to damage to both the auditory and vestibular parts of the inner ear. Children who survive bacterial meningitis may develop cerebral palsy with damage to the higher visual pathways and severe sensorineural deafness. A recent report from Australia showed *Haemophilus influenzae* to be the major pathogen and advocated an immunization programme (Hanna & Wild 1991).

Craniostenosis syndromes

The reported incidence of hearing loss in the craniostenosis syndromes varies from about 10% (Bertelsen 1951) to about 33% in Crouzon's syndrome (Konigsmark & Gorlin 1976). This may be as a result of stenosis of the external auditory canal, eighth cranial nerve compression in the auditory canal or changes in the middle ear, especially in oxycephaly and Crouzon's syndrome. Congenital fixation of the stapedial footplate has been described in Apert's syndrome. The causes of ocular morbidity include: corneal exposure with scarring, deprivational and strabismic amblyopia, optic atrophy due to raised intracranial pressure or direct compression in the optic canal and cortical visual loss. Up to 80% incidence of optic nerve damage has been reported in the Crouzon's syndrome (Bertelsen 1958).

Mitochondrial cytopathy

There is a wide phenotypic variation in mitochondrial cytopathy due to deletion of mitochondrial DNA. The typical features of Kearns–Sayre — ptosis, progressive external ophthalmoplegia and pigmentary retinopathy—may be present with sensorineural hearing loss. Vision may be well preserved into the fourth decade or beyond with a salt and pepper fundus appearance, and the electroretinogram may be normal or show reduced cone-mediated responses. However, there may be a severe receptor dystrophy progressing to blindness, with evolution of either a retinitis pigmentosa fundus appearance or a severe retinal pigment epithelial atrophy (which may mimic choroideraemia) and an unrecordable electroretinogram (Mullie 1985). Other features of the MELAS complex (mitochondrial encephalopathy, stroke-like episodes and lactic acidosis) may be present in the same individual or in siblings (Zupanc *et al.* 1991).

Biotinidase deficiency

This is an autosomal recessively inherited biochemical disorder which may present in infancy (Salbert *et al.* 1993) or at any stage during the first decade. Keratoconjunctivitis, skin rash and hair loss are common presentations, but there may be acute visual loss. Without treatment with biotin optic neuropathy and sensorineural hearing loss occur and may even progress on therapy.

Cockayne's syndrome

Milder cases of Cockayne's syndrome may not present with sensorineural hearing loss and progressive rod–cone dystrophy until the teens, when the diagnosis will already be evident due to severe dysmorphism (see above).

Mucopolysaccharidoses

Visual loss in the mucopolysaccharidoses occurs because of the development of corneal opacity, glaucoma, optic atrophy (Collins *et al.* 1990), macular epiretinal membranes and retinal dystrophy. Sensorineural deafness may be another complication.

Friedreich's ataxia

This usually presents with progressive ataxia and cerebellar eye signs about the age of 10 years, but may have an onset from 3 years or as late as the teens (Harding 1981). Cardiac symptoms from progressive cardiomyopathy usually occur later and the child becomes kyphoscoliotic with pes cavus. Optic atrophy is an occasional feature and often occurs in association with deafness and diabetes mellitus. Deafness and optic atrophy (which may be secondary to a retinal degeneration) may be features of other spinocerebellar degenerations.

Congenital hearing loss with eye signs

Waardenburg's syndrome

Waardenburg's syndrome is the most common deafness–depigmentation disorder, present in 2.7% of deaf scholars in a South African study. There is a wide variation in phenotype and there is evidence for genetic heterogeneity. Features include dystopia canthorum, true hypertelorism, laterally displaced punctum, dacryocystitis, heterochromia iridis, heterochromia of the fundus (Goldberg 1966), poliosis (white forelock), congenital deafness (partial to profound) and cleft lip and palate.

Types I and III are due to a mutation in the PAX3 gene on the long arm of chromosome 2 (Tassabehji *et al.* 1992). Type III is similar to type I but also has musculoskeletal abnormalities. Type II is a heterogeneous group with no dystopia canthorum. About 20% of families have a mutation in the MITF (microphthalmia) gene on the short arm of chromosome 3 (Tassabehji *et al.* 1995). Type IV, the Shah–Waardenburg syndrome, has associated Hirschsprung disease and is thought to be autosomal recessive, whilst types I, II, and III are autosomal dominant. A defect in endothelin receptor B or endothelin 3 genes may cause this disorder (Edery *et al.* 1996).

The Möbius complex

The Möbius complex is a cluster of features not now thought to be due to a single cause. The phenotype has been associated with various teratogens during pregnancy as well as vascular insult and there also appears to be a group of truly genetic conditions with various inheritance patterns exhibiting the same spectrum of features (Kumar 1990). Mobius complex may present as congenital strabismus. Deafness occurs in about 15% of individuals with this syndrome due to external, middle and inner ear abnormalities (Saito *et al.* 1981). The associated facial diplegia and sixth nerve paresis or horizontal gaze palsy should alert the ophthalmologist to the diagnosis. Affected individuals are often at risk of corneal scarring due to facial weakness, reduced blink, poor eyelid closure and corneal hypoaesthesia.

Wildervanck's syndrome

Wildervanck's syndrome may present with congenital esotropia due to bilateral Duane's syndrome. The neck appears very short due to Klippel–Feil abnormality and there is sensorineural or conductive deafness. There is overlap with Goldenhar's syndrome with some cases having an epibulbar dermoid.

Juvenile hearing loss with eye signs

Alport's syndrome

Alport's syndrome (Flinter 1990) is the eponym used for a variety of hereditary nephritides. Presentation is with haematuria and renal failure, which is more severe in males. Eye signs are rarely detected until the late teens and usually cause only mild visual loss. Anterior lenticonus develops bilaterally and occasionally is associated with an anterior polar cataract. Posterior lenticonus is less common. There may be a gradual increase in axial myopia. Retinal flecks in the macula and coalescing in the retinal periphery are more common in males. A macular degeneration resembling cone dystrophy has been reported. Corneal changes similar to posterior polymorphous dystrophy have been described.

Neurofibromatosis type 2

Neurofibromatosis type 2 is inherited as an autosomal dominant condition with a defect on a gene on chromosome 22 (Wertelecki *et al.* 1988). It is characterized by bilateral acoustic neuromas with hearing loss and intracranial or intraspinal tumours. The acoustic neuromas rarely present in the first decade, but rather more usually in the third. A rare presenting sign (reported as young as 4 years of age) is an epiretinal membrane of the macula associated with a retinal hamartoma (Tonsgard & Oesterle 1993). Presenile posterior subcapsular cataracts occur in more than half of the cases of neurofibromatosis type 2, but are usually only apparent after the systemic diagnosis has already been made.

Management of the deaf–blind child

Many children have useful residual sight or hearing or even both. However, a small group have profound dual handicap often also with other disabilities. It may be very difficult for a deaf–blind child, especially if both handicaps are profound, to acquire very basic skills such as spatial awareness and self/non-self differentiation. The early relationship between parents, especially the mother, and the infant is important for the child to achieve his or her full potential and not to develop frustrated, inturned and often self-injurious behaviour. There are several excellent books detailing care programmes such as *The Deaf/Blind Baby* written by the mother of a multisensorially handicapped girl (Freeman 1985). Other useful texts include: Wyman (1986), McInnes and Treffry (1982) and Best (1987). The family unit when first faced with a devastating diagnosis needs more than just information from the ophthalmologist. Support groups such as SENSE will need to be involved at an early stage.

Education may be as basic as teaching self-feeding skills (Luiselli 1993). There is a goal of developing a sign system so that the child may communicate and acquire some control over his or her environment (Watkins & Clark 1991). Video tapes illustrating an American 'easy to feel, easy to relate to the referent and easy to make' sign system are available to teachers and families (Watkins & Clark 1991). Many children have some potentially useful residual sight and hearing and early sensory training may improve outcome (Michael & Paul 1990).

Psychosocial support

Both deaf and blind children may have difficulty in coming to terms with their handicap and difficulty with social and communication skills (Abolfotouh & Telmesani 1993). A dual sensory defect can be even more disabling and in severe early onset disorders as yet only a partial communication system can be achieved (Downing 1993).

Cochlear implantation

Cochlear implantation(Ramsden *et al.* 1993; Hinderlink *et al.* 1994) may now be feasible in some severely hearing impaired children.

Visual function in children with congenital sensorineural hearing loss

There is an increased incidence of ocular problems in children with hearing impairment apart from the conditions which lead to severe visual loss which are noted above (Prickett *et al.* 1992; Siatkowski *et al.* 1993). Paramount amongst these are refractive errors. Obtaining the clearest possible vision is especially important to the hearing impaired child, for signing and reading.

Useful addresses

SENSE (The National Deaf/Blind and Rubella Association), 11–13 Clifton Terrace, Finsbury Park, London N4 3SR, UK (tel. 0171 272 7774; fax: 0171–272–6012).

The Anne Sullivan Foundation for Deaf–Blind, 40 Lower Drumcondra Road, Dublin 9, Ireland (tel. 0001 300 562).

Toys for the visually handicapped: Playring Limited, 53 Westbere Road, West Hampstead, London NW2, UK.

See also P30.

References

Abolfotouh MA, Telmesani A. A study of some psycho-social characteristics of blind and deaf male students in Abha City, Asir region, Saudi Arabia. *Public Health* 1993; **107**: 261–9.

Alström CH, Hallgren B, Nilsson LB, Asander H. Retinal degeneration combined with obesity, diabetes mellitus and neurogenous deafness. *Acta Psychiatr Neurol Scand* 1959; **34** (Suppl. 129): 1–35.

Armitage IM, Burke JP, Buffin JT. Visual impairment in severe and profound sensorineural deafness. *Arch Dis Childhood* 1995; **73**(1): 53–6.

Arts WF, Loonen MC, Sengers RC, Slooff JL. X-linked ataxia, weakness, deafness and loss of vision in early childhood with a fatal course. *Ann Neurol* 1993; **33**: 535–9.

Beighton P, Bartmann L, Bingham G, Sellars S. Rod–cone dystrophy, sensorineural deafness, and renal dysfunction: an autosomal recessive syndrome. *Am J Med Genet* 1993; **47**: 832–6.

Berger W, Meindl A, Van de Pol TJR *et al*. Isolation of a candidate gene for Norrie disease by positional cloning. *Nature Genet* 1992; **1**: 199–203.

Bertelsen TI. The etiology of the premature synostosis of the cranial sutures. *Acta Ophthalmol* 1958; **36** (Suppl. 51): 1–176.

Bertelsen TI. The premature synostosis of the cranial sutures. *Acta Ophthalmol* 1951; **51**: 87–117.

Best AB. *Steps to Independence: Practical Guide on Teaching People with Mental and Sensory Handicaps*. Kidderminster: British Institute of Mental Handicap Publications, 1987.

Bowen JR, Starte DR, Arnold JD, Simmons JL, Ma PJ, Leslie GI. Extremely low birthweight infants at 3 years: a developmental profile. *J Paediatr Child Health* 1993; **29**: 276–81.

Bu X, Rotter JI. Wolfram syndrome: a mitochondrial disorder? *Lancet* 1993; **342**: 598–600.

Charles SJ, Moore AT, Yates JR, Green T, Clark P. Alström's syndrome: further evidence of autosomal recessive inheritance and endocrinological dysfunction. *J Med Genet* 1990; **27**: 590–2.

Chen ZY, Battinelli EM, Fielder A *et al*. A mutation in the Norrie disease gene (NDP) associated with X-linked familial vitreoretinopathy. *Nature Genet* 1993a; **5**: 180–3.

Chen ZY, Battinelli EM, Hendriks RW *et al*. Norrie disease gene: characterization of deletions and possible function. *Genomics* 1993b; **16**: 533–5.

Claridge KG, Gibberd FB, Sidey MC. Refsum disease: the presentation and ophthalmic aspects of Refsum disease in a series of 23 patients. *Eye* 1992; **6**: 371–5.

Collins MLZ, Traboulsi EI, Maumenee IH. Optic nerve head swelling and optic atrophy in the systemic mucopolysaccharidoses. *Ophthalmology* 1990; **97**: 1445–9.

Cooke RW. Annual audit of the 3-year outcome in very low birthweight infants. *Arch Dis Child* 1993; **69**: 295–8.

de Berker D, Branford WA, Soucek S, Michaels L. Fatal keratitis, ichthyosis and deafness syndrome (KIDS). *Am J Dermatopathol* 1993; **15**: 64–9.

Downing JE. Communication intervention for individuals with dual sensory and intellectual impairments (review). *Clin Comm Dis* 1993; **3**: 31–42.

Edery P, Attie T, Amiel J *et al*. Mutation of the endothelin-3 gene in the Waardenburg–Hirschsprung disease (Shah–Waardenburg syndrome). *Nat Genet* 1996; **12**(4): 442–4.

Ek J, Kase BF, Reith A, Bjorkhem I, Pedersen JI. Peroxisomal dysfunction in a boy with neurologic symptoms and amaurosis (Leber disease): clinical and biochemical findings similar to those observed in Zellweger syndrome. *J Pediatr* 1986; **108**: 19–24.

Enns-Dokkum MH, Johnson A, Schreder AM *et al*. Comparison of mortality and rates of cerebral palsy in two populations of very low birthweight infants. *Arch Dis Child* 1994; **70**: F96–100.

Evans KL, Fantes J, Simpson C *et al*. Human olfactory marker protein maps close to tyrosinase and is candidate gene for Usher type 1. *Hum Mol Genet* 1993; **2**: 115–18.

Flinter F. Alport's syndrome. A clinical and genetic study (review). *Contrib Nephrol* 1990; **80**: 9–16.

Fowler KB, Stagno S, Pass RF, Britt WJ, Boll TJ, Alford CA. The outcome of congenital cytomegalovirus infection in relation to maternal antibody status. *N Engl J Med* 1992; **326**: 663–7.

Fraser GR. *The Causes of Profound Deafness in Childhood*. Baltimore: Johns Hopkins University Press, 1976.

Freeman P. *The Deaf/Blind Baby: A Programme of Care*. London: Heinemann, 1985.

Goldberg MF. Waardenburg's syndrome with fundus and other anomalies. *Arch Ophthalmol* 1966; **76**: 797.

Hanna JN, Wild BE. Bacterial meningitis in children under 5 years of age in Western Australia. *Med J Aust* 1991; **155**: 160–4.

Harding AE. Friedreich's ataxia: a clinical and genetic study of 90 families with an analysis of early diagnostic criteria and intrafamilial clustering of clinical features. *Brain* 1981; **104**: 589–620.

Higashi K. Otologic findings of DIDMOAD syndrome. *Am J Otol* 1991; **12**: 57–60.

Hinderlink JB, Brokx JP, Mens LH, van den Broek P. Results from four cochlear implant patients with Usher's syndrome. *Ann Otorhinolaryngol* 1994; **103**: 285–93.

Keats BJ, Nouri N, Pelias NZ, Deininger PL, Litt M. Tightly linked flanking microsatellite markers for the Usher type 1 locus on the short arm of chromosome 11. *Am J Hum Genet* 1994; **54**: 681–6.

Kinsley BT, Firth RG. The Wolfram syndrome: a primary neurodegenerative disorder with lethal potential (review). *Irish Med J* 1992; **85**: 34–6.

Konigsmark W, Gorlin RJ. *Genetic and Metabolic Deafness*. Philadelphia: WB Saunders, 1976.

Kumar D. Moebius syndrome. *J Med Genet* 1990; **27**: 122–6.

LaRussa F, Wesson MD. Norrie's disease versus PHPV: one family's dilemma. *J Am Optom Assoc* 1992; **63**: 404–8.

Lewis RA. Ocular albinism and deafness. *Am J Hum Genet* 1978; **30**: 57A.

Litt R, Armon Y, Seidman DS, Yafe H, Gale R. The effect of mode of delivery on long-term outcome of very low birthweight infants. *Eur J Obstet Gynecol Repro Biol* 1993; **52**: 5–10.

Luiselli JK. Training self-feeding skills in children who are deaf and blind. *Behav Mod* 1993; **17**: 457–73.

McInnes JM, Treffry JA. *Deaf–Blind Infants and Children: A Developmental Guide*. Toronto: University of Toronto Press, 1982.

Merry DE, Lesko JG, Sosnoski DM *et al*. Choroideremia and deafness with stapes fixation: a contiguous gene deletion syndrome in Xq21. *Am J Hum Genet* 1989; **45**: 530–40.

Michael MG, Paul PV. Early intervention for infants with deaf–blindness (review). *Exceptional Children* 1990; **57**: 200–10.

Mullie MA. The retinal manifestations of mitochondrial myopathy. A study of 22 cases. *Arch Ophthalmol* 1985; **103**: 1825–30.

Naidu SB, Moser H. Infantile Refsum disease. *Am J Neuroradiol* 1991; **12**: 1161–2.

Nance MA, Berry S. Cockayne syndrome: review of 140 cases. *Am J Med Genet* 1992; **42**: 68–84.

Norton SJ. Application of transient evoked otoacoustic emissions to pediatric populations (review). *Ear Hearing* 1993; **14**: 64–73.

Nuutila A. Dystrophia retinae pigmentosa–dysacusis syndrome (DRD). A study of the Usher or Hallgren syndrome. *J Genet Hum* 1970; **18**: 57.

Parsons MA, Curtis D, Blank CE, Hughes HN, McCartney AC. The ocular pathology of Norrie disease in a fetus of 11 weeks gestational age. *Graefe's Arch Clin Exp Ophthalmol* 1992; **230**: 248–51.

Parving A, Schwartz M. Audiometric tests in gene carriers of Norrie's disease. *Int J Pediatr Otorhinolaryngol* 1991; **21**: 103–11.

Pieke Dahl S, Kimberling WJ, Gorin MB *et al*. Genetic heterogeneity of Usher syndrome type II. *J Med Genet* 1993; **30**: 843–8.

Prickett HT, Prickett JG. Vision problems among students in schools and programs for deaf children. A survey of teachers of deaf students. *Am Ann Deaf* 1992; **137**: 56–60.

Ramsden RT, Boyd P, Giles E, Aplin Y, Das V. Cochlear implantation in the deaf blind. *Adv Otorhinolaryngol* 1993; **48**: 177–81.

Russell-Eggitt IM, Taylor DSI, Clayton PT, Garner A, Kriss A, Taylor JFN. Leber's congenital amaurosis. A new syndrome with cardiomyopathy. *Br J Ophthalmol* 1989; **73**: 250–4.

Saito H, Kishimoto S, Furuta M. Temporal bone findings in a patient with Mobius syndrome. *Ann Otol Rhinol* 1981; **90**: 80.

Salbert BA, Astrue J, Wolf B. Ophthalmic findings in biotinidase deficiency. *Ophthalmologica* 1993; **206**: 177–81.

Seery CM, Pruett RC, Liberfarb RM, Cohen BZ. Distinctive cataract in the Stickler syndrome. *Am J Ophthalmol* 1990; **110**: 143–8.

Siatkowski RM, Flynn JT, Hodges AV, Balkany TJ. Visual function in children with congenital sensorineural deafness. *Trans Am Ophthalmol Soc* 1993; **91**: 309–18; discussion 318–23.

Smith RJ, Berlin CI, Hejtmancik JF *et al*. Clinical diagnosis of the Usher syndromes. Usher Syndrome Consortium. *Am J Med Genet* 1994; **50**: 32–8.

Spranger J, Winterpacht A, Zabel B. The type II collagenopathies: a spectrum of chondrodysplasias (review). *Eur J Pediatr* 1994; **153**: 56–65.

Stratton RF, Lee B, Ramirez F. Marshall syndrome. *Am J Med Genet* 1991; **41**: 35–8.

Tassabehji M, Read AP, Newton VE *et al*. Waardenburg syndrome patients have mutations in the human homologue of the Pax-3 paired box gene. *Nature* 1992; **355**: 635–6.

Tassabehji M, Newton VE, Liu XZ *et al*. The mutational spectrum in Waardenburg syndrome. *Hum Mol Genet* 1995; **4**(11): 2131–7.

Tonsgard JH, Oesterle CS. The ophthalmologic presentation of NF-2 in childhood. *J Pediatr Ophthalmol Strabismus* 1993; **30**: 327–30.

Traboulsi EI, De Becker I, Maumenee IH. Ocular findings in Cockayne syndrome. *Am J Ophthalmol* 1992; **114**: 579–83.

Tremblay F, LaRoche RG, Shea SE, Ludman MD. Longitudinal study of the early electroretinographic changes in Alström's syndrome. *Am J Ophthalmol* 1993; **115**: 657–65.

Warburg M. Norrie's disease. *Acta Ophthalmol* 1961; **39**: 757–72.

Warburg M, Tommerup N, Vestermark S *et al*. The Yemenite deaf–blind hypopigmentation syndrome. A new oculo-dermato-auditory syndrome. *Ophthalmol Paediatr Genet* 1990; **11**: 201–7.

Watkins S, Clark TC. A coactive sign system for children who are dual-sensory impaired. *Am Ann Deaf* 1991; **136**: 321–4.

Weleber RG, Tongue AC, Kennaway NG, Budden SS, Buist NRM. Ophthalmic manifestations of infantile phytanic acid storage disease. *Arch Ophthalmol* 1984; **102**: 1317–21.

Wertelecki W, Rouleau GA, Superneau DW *et al*. Neurofibromatosis 2: clinical and DNA linkage studies of a large kindred. *N Engl J Med* 1988; **319**: 278–83.

Whyte HE, Fitzhardinge PM, Shennan AT, Lennox K, Smith L, Lacy J. Extreme immaturity: outcome of 568 pregnancies of 23–26 weeks gestation. *Obstet Gynecol* 1993; **82**: 1–7.

Winship I, Gericke G, Beighton P. X-linked inheritance of ocular albinism with late-onset sensorineural deafness. *Am J Med Genet* 1984; **19**: 797–803.

Wisniewski KE, Laure-Kamionowska M, Sher J, Pitter J. Infantile neuroaxonal dystrophy in an albino girl. A cliniconeuropathologic study. *Acta Neuropathol* 1985; **66**: 68–71 .

Wyman R. *Multiply Handicapped Children*. London: Souvenir Press, 1986.

Zlotogora J, Granat M, Knowlton RG. Prenatal exclusion of Stickler syndrome. *Prenatal Diag* 1994; **14**: 145–7.

Zupanc ML, Moraes CT, Shanske S, Langman CB, Ciafaloni E, DiMauro S. Deletion of mitochondrial DNA in patients with combined features of Kearns–Sayre and MELAS syndromes. *Ann Neurol* 1991; **29**: 680–3.

P16: Optic Atrophy in Infancy and the Child with Optic Atrophy and Neurological Disease

Creig S. Hoyt

Presentation and diagnosis

Small children with optic atrophy do not have a pathognomonic mode of presentation connected with the optic atrophy itself. Rather, they present with either the general behavioural characteristics of visual loss or the ocular motor consequences thereof. The history is vital and particular attention should be paid to any family history of poor vision, consanguinity of the parents, the progress of the pregnancy and suspicion of the lack of weight gain as well as any immediate prenatal problem. The most important time in a child's life for acquiring non-refractive visual defects is in the perinatal period, particularly if the baby is premature or of low birth weight. The parents of these children should be questioned in detail about their baby's early life: whether the child had to be in the incubator, have added oxygen, be ventilated, or had any difficulty in breathing. Episodes of bradycardia or apnoea must be noted; also whether the child had to be resuscitated, or the parents warned by the neonatologist that survival was in jeopardy.

If the onset was in postnatal life the mode of onset and the progression of any visual field defect should be detailed as well as possible, including the child's visual behaviour. Many observant parents will make relevant observations about the vision and even about the state of the pupils, presence of nystagmus, squint or structural abnormalities of the eye. Their observations should be noted because they will be useful in determining progression, especially in the preverbal child who cannot perform standard subjective visual acuity tests.

An assessment of a child's visual function should be made together with the state of the pupil reactions, which if reacting sluggishly to light or showing a relatively afferent pupillary defect, will suggest anterior visual pathway disease. In older children, an acquired defect of colour (usually red/green) vision may help in identifying optic nerve disease, especially if asymmetrical.

A careful examination of the fundus with both direct and indirect ophthalmoscopy is mandatory in order to establish the diagnosis of optic atrophy. The optic disc itself will appear pale with fewer than normal vessels on the surface. The pallor may be diffuse or segmental, and it is most important to pay attention to the presence of the nerve fibre layer atrophy which will show as an enhancement of the normal reflex from the retinal vessels, which normally do not stand up greatly against the internal limiting membrane: in optic atrophy where the nerve fibre layer has atrophied, the vessels stand out. If the optic atrophy is severe the vessels stand out like cords seen in the light reflected in parallax from the internal limiting membrane as it passes over the vessels.

The differential diagnosis on fundoscopy is between optic atrophy and optic disc hypoplasia or other congenital disc anomalies or even glaucoma. Here it is most important that the optic disc be examined by direct ophthalmoscopy. Structural anomalies of the optic disc may also be mistaken if the outline of the disc is not grossly abnormal and similarly glaucoma may be missed if the cup of the disc is not noticed during a hasty examination without adequate magnification. It is most important to pay very close attention to the state of the optic disc in order to be certain that it is either abnormal or entirely normal and that the visual defect may be attributed appropriately to either an optic disc problem or to some other cause, for instance, delayed visual development.

It is not possible to establish a cause in every case (Repka & Miller 1988) and in published series the cause varies enormously between centres; the tertiary referral teaching centre will see cases biased by a close association with neurology, neurosurgery or metabolic departments while developmental centres will see mainly cases associated with cerebral palsy.

Causes

Figure P16.1 provides guidelines for diagnosis (see text for details).

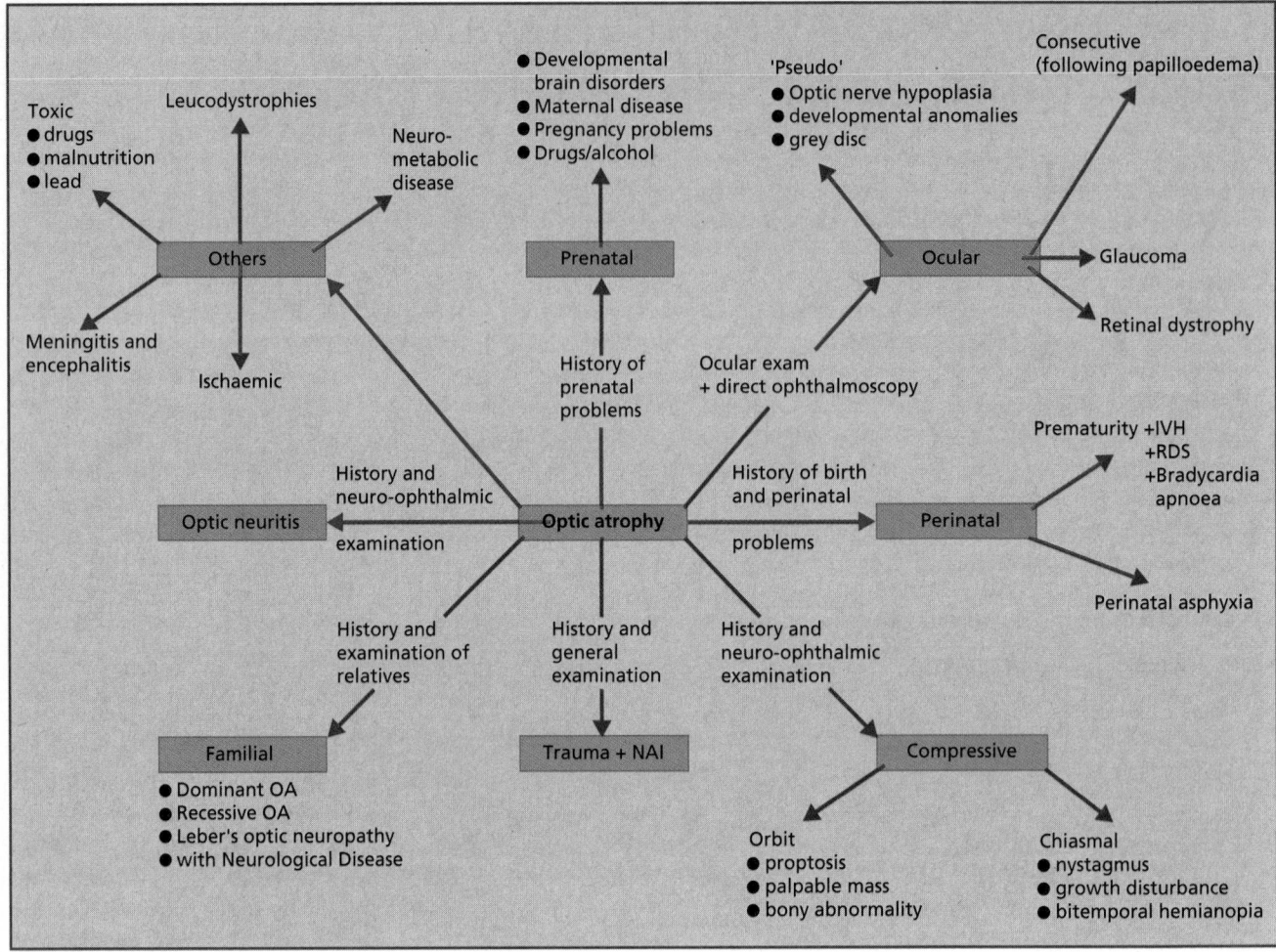

Fig. P16.1 Guidelines for diagnosis of optic atrophy in infancy.

Optic atrophy occurs in late prenatal or early postnatal life (Hoyt & Good 1992). Early prenatal onset damage to the anterior visual system results in a hypoplastic or anomalous optic disc. In postnatal life optic atrophy is an indication that the damage is anterior to the lateral geniculate. When the optic atrophy is definitely unilateral, the cause is anterior to the chiasm and when it is definitely bilateral it is either due to bilateral disease or disease involving pathways posterior to the chiasm. It is possible that late prenatal brain damage may, by trans-synaptic degeneration, give rise to optic atrophy without hypoplasia, but there is little clear evidence for this in human studies. Prenatal causes of optic atrophy include the hereditary optic neuropathies and metabolic causes. If there is a history of pre- or perinatal problems they may well be the cause, especially if there is a history of significant perinatal hypoxia.

Conversely, one should be cautious about attributing optic atrophy to a relatively mild perinatal insult and it is rare for optic atrophy caused by perinatal problems to not be associated with other obvious central nervous system damage. Postnatal causes include tumours invading or encroaching on the visual pathways. Clues to this in the diagnosis may be in the history of progression of the visual defect and associated eye movement disorders or the presence of systemic diseases such as neurofibromatosis. There may be a clear history of trauma or meningitis and a careful history should be taken of any drug ingestion.

Hydrocephalus may also result in optic atrophy but it is an entirely unusual presenting symptom of this disorder. The child with repeated shunt failures or infections is particularly prone to develop optic atrophy. Optic atrophy in hydrocephalus may be difficult to assess even in later life as acuity may be preserved much later than other aspects of vision. Babies with lactic acidosis (i.e. Leigh's disease, mitochondrial cytopathy, pyruvate decarboxylase or cytochrome oxidase deficiency) have a high incidence of optic atrophy, sometimes profound (Hayasaka *et al.* 1986). Other optic neuropathies in many of the hereditary optic neuropathies present later in childhood or the teens.

Investigation

Structural eye disease must be excluded, especially retinal disorders, even if the retina appears normal. An electroretinogram is important in establishing that optic atrophy is not associated with a primary retinal disorder. The integrity of the visual pathways may also be assessed by visually evoked responses. A CT or MRI scan may also be indicated. Systemic investigations are carried out where appropriate.

Prognosis

The prognosis depends on the diagnosis and the natural history of the condition. Much caution should be used in giving a prognosis to parents whose child has recently suffered optic atrophy from an acute cause such as tumour or hydrocephalus, since very dramatic recovery can take place up to 2 or occasionally more years after the onset of the visual loss. As a general rule it is better to be optimistic rather than pessimistic and this should especially be so if there is still some response to a flash stimulus on the visual evoked responses. Every paediatric ophthalmologist has seen examples of remarkable late recovery in vision with optic atrophy or cerebral disorders in infancy.

The uncertainty about prognosis, however, should not inhibit the ophthalmologist from registering the visual handicap with the appropriate authority, although reassessment should be suggested periodically.

References

Hayasaka S, Yamaguschio K, Misuro K, Miyabayashi S, Narasawa K, Tada K. Ocular findings in childhood lactic acidosis. *Arch Ophthalmol* 1986; **104**: 1656–8.

Hoyt CS, Good WV. Do we understand the difference between optic nerve hypoplasia and atrophy? *Eye* 1992; **6**: 201–4.

Repka M, Miller NR. Optic atrophy in children. *Am J Ophthalmol* 1988; **106**: 191–4.

P17: Headaches

David Taylor

Headache in childhood is common (Hockaday 1983) and by the time young adulthood is reached they are almost universal (Blau 1990). The incidence varies but in all studies headache occurs in over half of all children but is not necessarily reported to their doctor (Hockaday 1983). Certain principles are important.

1 The shorter the history the greater the reason for concern.

2 The younger the child the more likely it is that the headache is organic (Hockaday 1983).

3 The history is usually the clue to the diagnosis: most cases are diagnosed on history alone.

4 Important historical detail (i.e. trauma) may be missing.

5 Every headache that interferes with the child's ordinary activity must be regarded seriously unless it is shown to follow a pattern acceptable as migraine. It is possible to subdivide most headaches into one of four groups (Lance 1978; Rothner 1983; Silberstein 1990).

1 Acute single episodes (minutes or hours):
(a) intracranial disease: meningitis; encephalitis; subarachnoid haemorrhage; and trauma;
(b) arterial hypertension;
(c) systemic infections with fever;
(d) sinusitis and mastoiditis;
(e) uveitis, optic neuritis or glaucoma; and
(f) the first attack of migraine.

2 Acute recurrent episodes:
(a) migraine and migraine-like syndromes;
(b) raised intracranial pressure — intermittent hydrocephalus;
(c) subarachnoid haemorrhage; and
(d) tic doloureux and cluster headache (Ryan & Ryan 1989) are rare in childhood.

3 Subacute (days or weeks):
(a) intracranial tumour, abscess or subdural haematoma; and
(b) benign intracranial hypertension (pseudotumour cerebri).

4 Chronic:
(a) stress;
(b) eye strain;
(c) temporomandibular joint and dental problems;
(d) psychological or psychiatric states; and
(e) analgesic abuse.

There are numerous areas where the above guidelines overlap. For instance, intracranial tumour may present as a chronic headache, or stress headaches may present to the doctor with only a short history, but the important point is that a detailed history will correctly classify virtually all headaches.

Stress headaches

Stress headaches are probably the most common of childhood headaches, and as modern treatments for stomach ulcer pain decimate the role models for stomach ache among children's relatives, the symptom of headache becomes a more frequent excuse for missing days at school.

The mechanism producing the pain may be increased muscle tension, hence the term 'tension' headache, and this is borne out by the occurrence of ache and pain in groups of muscles that are made to contract in a sustained manner. Tension was thought to induce relative ischaemia by vasoconstriction (Wolff 1963).

The headaches have usually occurred for some months

by the time the child is seen by an ophthalmologist and they are usually bifrontal or bitemporal; only rarely are they occipital in childhood. They are unusual below 6 years of age. Headaches are frequent in other family members, in particular in the mother. They do not have the migraine accompaniments of visual or other prodromal symptoms and vomiting, although affected individuals may feel ill at ease or unwell enough to want to lie down.

The headaches occur daily or a few times a week but they are not often clearly related to any particular factor (such as school, working, exercise, etc.). Occasionally they are clearly related to the 'causative' factor, for example they only occur at school, in church or at the weekly scout meeting.

Environmental factors are important in childhood headaches but the underlying stress factors which give rise to the tension are often much more difficult to identify than in hysterical visual defects. The parents should be asked to search for appropriate factors such as teasing at school, poor performance or being 'understretched' at school, or sibling rivalry. Attempts need to be made to modify the life of those affected to get around the stress. Analgesics such as paracetamol are helpful but should only be used occasionally. Only rarely is further treatment such as relaxation therapy or psychiatric or psychological help needed. Probably the most important treatment, after exclusion of organic disease, is explanation and reassurance of parent and child.

Hypertension

Although rare in childhood, hypertension is a significant cause of serious disability, e.g. blindness and neurological complications (Hulse *et al.* 1979; Trompeter *et al.* 1982).

One of the main problems is failure of doctors who see a child with neurological problems in the early stages (e.g. facial palsy, convulsions and altered levels of consciousness), to take the blood pressure. Many hospitals do not even have paediatric sphigmomanometer cuffs! The delay in diagnosis significantly increases the permanent sequelae of the hypertension. The cause is usually renal or renovascular disease, with reflux nephropathy and chronic glomerulonephritis being the most common.

Although headache is rarely caused by hypertension, it is the most common symptom of childhood hypertension: it is usually severe and generalized, it may wake the child or be present on waking and be made worse by stooping or lifting heavy objects. Hypertensive retinopathy or papilloedema is often present on the first examination (Trompeter *et al.* 1982).

The visual defect may occur from hypertensive damage to the retina, optic nerve and choroid (Hayreh 1986d) and from cortical blindness. Optic nerve infarction occurs as a sudden event when the systemic blood pressure has dropped in a patient in whom ophthalmic and cerebral arterial blood vessels have constricted by autoregulation to compensate for the high blood pressure. The sudden drop in blood pressure causes flow in the constricted vessels to cease, even though the blood pressure may be 'normal' (Hulse *et al.* 1979; Hayreh *et al.* 1986a).

Retinal (Hayreh 1986b) and, more commonly, choroidal (Hayreh 1986c) damage are less frequent causes of permanent visual sequelae, but may cause focal defects.

Hemianopias (Hulse *et al.* 1979) and cortical blindness may result from hypertensive encephalopathy and stroke.

Altered intracranial pressure

Raised intracranial pressure

Headache is very frequent in patients with raised intracranial pressure (ICP) and increases in severity and frequency as the ICP rises. Headache occurs in over half of children with brain tumours, particularly infratentorial tumours (Childhood Brain Tumour Consortium 1991).

Rossi and Vassella (1989) compared the headaches of 67 children with brain tumour with 600 migraineurs. In brain tumours the headaches were characteristically:
1 nocturnal;
2 on waking;
3 associated with vomiting; and
4 increasing in frequency.
Neurological signs appeared 2–6 months after the headaches.

Intermittent at first if the ICP rise is transient, the headaches may become constant and be exacerbated from time to time presumably as the ICP varies. The older child is often manifestly distressed by the pain and may describe it as 'bursting' or 'blowing up'. With sudden rises in ICP, as in posterior fossa tumours, there may be vomiting, sometimes 'projectile'. For example, he vomits with a suddenness and force that is disastrous for the house furnishings and his parents' clothes. The vomiting often improves the headache. Younger children just go 'off-colour' or babies become disgruntled and unhappy. Raised ICP in infants can be felt by tenseness of the open fontanelle and the 'expert parent' (perhaps of a child with hydrocephalus) may know how to recognize the association between tense fontanelle and the child going off-colour.

A major difficulty in paediatric neuro-ophthalmology is headaches which occur in children with treated hydrocephalus. Papilloedema is an inconstant and late sign in children with raised ICP and optic atrophy and cannot be relied on. Many of these cases resolve themselves simply into those caused by raised ICP from a blocked shunt or other obvious headache syndrome but there remains a group in whom no cause is found; the shunt is functioning, the scan shows no changes suggestive of currently raised ICP, there is no intellectual deterioration and no papilloedema. Undoubtedly a number of these have stress headaches, perhaps exacerbated by parental worries about the child, but in some there is no stress factor identifiable and they can only be managed by reassurance, analgesics and close monitoring. Occasionally ICP monitoring may help (Minns 1977), but with so few signs to go on, and with significant risks in shunt management, a 'watch and wait' policy is often the safest option: it is inevitable that some cases will have (especially in retrospect!) a less than optimal outcome.

The headache is usually generalized but in some instances overlies an area of an abscess or tumour. Pituitary tumours may have a point headache at the vertex; it is instructive to ask the child to point with one finger to where the ache is.

Classic observations on the localization and significance of headache were made by Northfield (1938) and Wolff (1963): the localization of the headache is probably less significant than the other aspects.

Benign intracranial hypertension (pseudotumour cerebri)

Benign intracranial hypertension (BIH, pseudotumour cerebri) is not uncommon in childhood; it has been reviewed by Lessell (1992). It can occur without obvious precipitating cause (Grant 1971). Causes may include: withdrawal of steroids (Liu *et al.* 1994); vitamin A intoxication; tetracycline or ciprofloxacin (Winrow & Supramanian 1990) ingestion; dural sinus thrombosis (after dehydration in infancy); head trauma or surgery (Lam *et al.* 1992); even minor; protein S and fibrinogen abnormalities (Pasquale *et al.* 1990); hyperviscosity, as in polycythaemia and thrombocytosis; and systemic lupus erythematosus (Grant 1971; Carlow & Glasser 1974; Weisberg & Chutorian 1977; Orcutt *et al.* 1984). Probably the most common cause is withdrawal of the steroids used in the treatment of leukaemia, eczema or autoimmune disease. Grant (1971) found an equal sex incidence in children.

The headaches are often frontal and severe but often not associated with vomiting. The children are often unwell during an attack. Transient visual loss, lasting never more than 2 or 3 seconds, may occur in severe papilloedema of any cause. These episodes are known as obscurations and are often posture-related—most frequently the child loses vision on standing up. Many children, perhaps because the vision loss is so transient, do not describe 'loss of vision' but 'blurriness, blacking, mistiness' or other terms.

The papilloedema is usually bilateral and roughly symmetrical. It may be highly asymmetrical or even unilateral when there is an anomaly of the optic nerve or its dural sheath (Sedgwick & Burde 1983), when there is direct involvement of one optic nerve or when there is profound unilateral optic atrophy with insufficient nerve fibres remaining to form papilloedema.

Visual loss is not often associated with BIH in childhood, but Baker *et al.* (1985) made it quite clear that severe visual loss can occur especially when the papilloedema is severe, when dural venous sinus thrombosis is the cause, and when there are retinal nerve fibre layer haemorrhages.

Diagnosis is essentially one of exclusion, made much easier by computed tomography (CT) or magnetic resonance imaging (MRI). Middle ear disease, drug ingestion, previous dehydration, trauma and hyperviscosity of the blood can be excluded by appropriate historical questions and examination.

Treatment of the headache of BIH is treatment of the condition. The number of different modes of treatment implies that none is clearly superior. These include Diamox, steroids, repeated lumbar punctures, glycerol ingestion and of course withdrawal of any precipitating factor. Most cases show spontaneous improvement but for those in whom the headaches do not improve and are disabling, if there is a consequent or threatened neurological deficit or threatened visual loss, a variety of surgical procedures may be indicated including ventriculoperitoneal shunting, bitemporal decompression and optic nerve sheath decompression.

Optic nerve sheath decompression

In this procedure (Galbraith & Sullivan 1973) a hole or slit is made in the optic nerve sheath usually from the nasal side; it has a reasonably low morbidity in adults (Plotnik & Kosmorsky 1993) and children (Billson & Hudson 1975; Tompkins & Spalton 1984; Hupp *et al.* 1987). Various techniques have been used including multiple slits (Sergott *et al.* 1988) and fenestration via a lateral orbitotomy (Corbett *et al.* 1988). The procedure is much safer and easier if the sheath can be seen to be expanded on neuroimaging (Fig. P17.1). The procedure may improve vision even after patients have failed to improve following one or more lumbar–peritoneal shunting procedures (Sergott *et al.* 1987). Although most cases are stable postoperatively, nearly one-third have further visual deterioration and long-term follow-up is appropriate in most cases (Spoor & McHenry 1993). The optic nerve subarachnoid space is patent postoperatively (Brourman *et al.* 1988) and although there are alternative hypotheses, the mechanism of its action is probably by causing decompression of the optic nerve and the intracranial contents by filtration of cerebrospinal fluid through the slit or fenestration (Keltner 1988; Hamed *et al.* 1992). The haemodynamics of the optic disc improve significantly which may emphasize the role of ischaemia in visual loss with papilloedema (Mittra *et al.* 1993).

Adjunctive treatment such as the use of filtration tubes

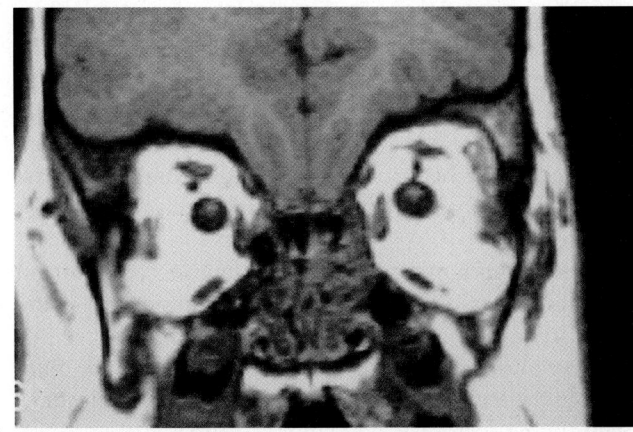

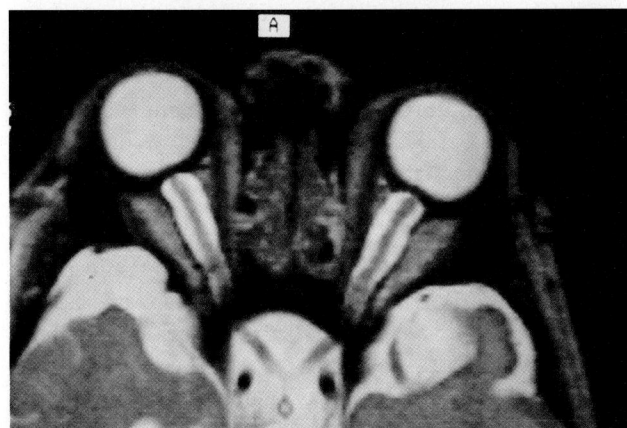

Fig. P17.1 MRI scan showing widely dilated optic nerve sheaths. (a) T1-weighted coronal image. (b) T2-weighted axial image.

and antimetabolites may enhance the results (Spoor *et al.* 1994).

Low intracranial pressure

Lumbar puncture headaches seem to be much less frequent in children, who do not suffer the days of severe bursting headache of some adults who have had lumbar punctures. Some, however, complain of headache and may be 'grizzly' for a few hours.

Eye and oculomotor disease

Eye disease, especially uveitis, glaucoma and corneal disease, gives rise to eye pain; chronic eye pain is often also referred to areas around the eye and may result in symptoms of headache.

Parents, teachers and others frequently suspect that refractive error or eye muscle 'imbalance' cause headache, but only occasionally are they right.

The headaches usually are related to school or reading and are very rarely present on waking. They are most often frontal or around the eyes and they are present almost every day, often not being present on weekends or holidays.

The causes can be divided into those from refractive errors, latent strabismus, convergence insufficiency and accommodation defects. Refractive errors usually cause headaches or 'eye strain' by making the child peer at objects through narrow palpebral fissures in a pin-hole effect. It is probably the prolonged muscular contraction that causes the symptoms.

Latent strabismus usually does not cause headache or eye strain, even with large angle deviations; occasionally, however, when the latent deviation is barely controlled, symptoms may develop.

Eye strain is more frequent when there is convergence insufficiency. The symptoms are usually directly related to reading and the child complains that he cannot read or that concentration is difficult. Diagnosis is simply made by getting the child to look at a near detailed (accommodative) target and observing the eye position or asking him to tell you when he sees double; considerable exhortation should be used after the initial test to see how hard he is trying! Treatment is by near-point exercises.

Accommodation defects result in reading difficulty similar to presbyopia. Nearly all are psychogenic and respond well to reassurance, relief of stress factors when these can be identified, and near-point exercises. Organic causes of accommodation defects include Adie's pupil, pharmacological blockade by atropine-like drugs, and incipient nerve palsies. Not many clinicians will correctly diagnose at the first visit the child or young person who presents with symptoms of defective accommodation secondary to a Sylvian aqueduct syndrome—but they do occur!

Bone and sinus disease

Sinus disease and related osteomyelitis is not uncommon in older children but the severity and frequency are less since the advent of antibiotics. The pain is usually localized over the affected sinus, or in the case of the ethmoids it is usually felt 'between the eyes'. It is often severe and intermittent, worse on bending or coughing and often better on lying down. There may be tenderness on pressing or tapping on the affected area. The diagnosis can be confirmed by radiology but often the help of an otorhinolaryngologist is required.

Headache with intracranial disease

Meningism

Irritation of the meninges (meningism) causes headache and a stiff neck which increases and becomes painful on flexing. The cause can be infectious meningitis, when fever is also present, or blood in the cerebrospinal fluid following subarachnoid haemorrhage from aneurysm, arteriovenous malformation or trauma. Local tenderness or ache may occur if the meningeal disease is localized. Minor trauma giving rise to meningism from subarachnoid haemorrhage should make one suspicious of an arteriovenous malformation.

Subarachnoid haemorrhage

Cerebral aneurysms occasionally occur in childhood, associated with food or generalized neurological signs. The 'sentinel' headache is due to rapid expansion of the aneurysm or a small bleed and occurs before the main bleed. It is immediate, severe, unique for that patient ('like a thunderclap in a clear sky') and may, if diagnosed correctly, lead to early and satisfactory treatment of the aneurysm (Hughes 1992).

Trauma

The headaches that occur soon after head trauma are usually related to meningism, sinus diseases or direct skull or muscle trauma. Headaches frequently continue for several months after the trauma. This post-traumatic headache is less frequent in children than in adults and usually has a better prognosis, but is more frequently associated with temper tantrums, lack of concentration and behavioural disorder (Dillon & Leopold 1961).

Posterior fossa tumours

Posterior fossa tumours most often give a headache due to the raised ICP but some patients with Arnold–Chiari malformations may have a more or less specific headache which is protracted, suboccipital or occipital, and aggravated by the Valsalva manoeuvre, effort or cough (Pascual *et al.* 1992).

Migraine

Migraine is an important cause of headache in children and is frequently associated with visual or ocular symptoms (Bille 1962).

Migraine is paroxysmal, occurring in attacks lasting hours or days, every few weeks or months. The child is free of symptoms in the intervals between attacks.

A variety of premonitory symptoms precede the attacks by a matter of hours and include dizziness, nausea, excitability and depression; children, however, are often unaware of them until asked directly. Classically, visual symptoms occur next but are not often of the typical 'fortification spectrum' type complained of by adults. Scotomas, scintillating spots or haemianopias are frequent and transient and they may be followed by a 'free interval' with mood changes, speech or thought disturbance or somatic symptoms (Blau 1992) but usually the headache

follows within the hour. Usually the headache is very severe, unilateral and of a boring quality. There may be associated symptoms of sensory or motor disturbances in the head or limbs and dysphasia. Photophobia is severe in some children and many like to lie down in a darkened quiet room. The headache passes off in hours but can last days and leaves many patients feeling weak and shaky for a while.

Some authors make a distinction between classic and common migraine (Spector 1984); the classic form being associated with premonitory visual symptoms.

Many cases have typical or partial attacks and the diagnosis in these cases in particular rests on the history alone. Scintillating scotomas, hemianopia, central scotoma, altitudinal hemianopia, diplopia and the other symptoms may occur without headache (Wiley 1979; O'Connor & Tredici 1981).

Migraine is probably related to calibre changes in meningeal vessels that penetrate the outer cortex (Blau 1978) and although it has been reported to resolve after the removal of brain arteriovenous malformation (Troost *et al.* 1979) this is distinctly unusual. If the history is typical and if there is a family history, further investigations are not usually necessary. That the visual symptoms are usually cortical is attested to by their occurrence in people without eyes (Peatfield & Rose 1981).

Episodic mydriasis may occur in childhood migraine during the headache (Woods *et al.* 1984).

Complicated migraine

Hemiplegic

In this form the migraine attacks are accompanied by a hemiplegia or hemisensory attack. The attacks may alternate from side to side (Hosking *et al.* 1978), and the condition may be familial (Zifkin *et al.* 1980).

Ophthalmoplegic

This condition usually has its onset in childhood with the sudden onset of a unilateral third nerve palsy usually involving the pupil (Friedman *et al.* 1962). Pain or headache is not always present (Durkan *et al.* 1971). The third nerve palsy usually resolves at least partially, only to recur after an interval of up to a few years. The mechanism is obscure, but is probably peripheral. Anomalous re-innervation may occur and then be obliterated by a further attack. The diagnosis should only be made after careful exclusion of other causes by scanning and arteriography: as the resolution of scanning improves the diagnosis of ophthalmoplegic migraine will surely become more rare. There may be a family history of migraine.

Fourth and sixth nerve pareses are even less frequent.

Basilar

This is presumed to be due to transient abnormalities of the vertebrobasilar vascular system (Bickerstaff 1961). Symptoms include vertigo, hemianopias, ataxia and occipital headache. It is important to establish the absence of hypertension and neurological signs or symptoms between attacks.

Retinal, choroidal and optic nerve

These are diagnosed by the history of the visual defects. They are monocular transient visual defects including altitudinal hemianopias, central or arcuate scotomas or total visual loss. Permanent visual loss has occurred in some cases, attributed to a variety of mechanisms (Spector 1984). It is usually diagnosed in adults only.

Cluster headaches

These include Raeder's syndrome, Horton's cephalalgia, migrainous neuralgia, and so on. These excruciating, recurrent facial headaches, sometimes with sympathetic nervous system signs, are found in middle-aged adults, but occasionally can be dated back to late childhood (Ryan & Ryan 1989).

Other causes of headache

Hypoglycaemia causes irritability and headache in some children (Hockaday 1983). Fever of any cause may be associated with headache and many of the exanthemas, especially measles, cause eye pain on lateral gaze.

Patients with posterior fossa tumours or vascular malformations (Epstein *et al.* 1990) may present with atypical facial and head pain.

Nerve entrapment may occur in children with bone disorders such as fibrous dysplasia, craniometaphyseal dysplasia, mucopolysaccharidoses or histiocytosis-X.

Arthritis of the temporomandibular joint or at the craniocervical junction is rare but may occur in children predisposed to 'wear and tear' arthritis by injury, developmental defects or metabolic disease, e.g. ochronosis.

Investigation

The diagnosis is made by the history — the examination either confirms it or excludes any associated abnormalities such as hypertension or central nervous system signs. A small proportion of patients will require further investigation by plain X-rays, CT or MRI scanning, especially those in whom raised ICP, intracranial tumour or sinus disease is suspected. Careful selection by history and examination is appropriate otherwise neuroimaging is likely to be unrewarding (Chu & Shinnar 1992).

References

Baker RS, Carter D, Hendrick EB, Buncic JR. Visual loss in pseudotumour cerebri of childhood. *Arch Ophthamol* 1985; **103**: 1681–6.

Bickerstaff ER. Basilar artery migraine. *Lancet* 1961; **i**: 15–17.

Bille B. Migraine in schoolchildren. *Acta Paediatr Scand* 1962; **51**(Suppl.).

Billson FA, Hudson FA. Surgical treatment of chronic papilloedema in children. *Br J Ophthalmol* 1975; **59**: 92–5.

Blau JN. Classical migraine: symptoms between the visual aura and headache onset. *Lancet* 1992; **340**: 355–6.

Blau JN. Common headaches: types, duration, frequency and implications. *Headache* 1990; **30**: 701–4.

Blau JN. Migraine: a vasomotor instability of the meningeal circulation. *Lancet* 1978; **ii**: 1136–9.

Brourman ND, Spoor TC, Ramocki JM. Optic nerve sheath decompression for pseudotumor cerebri. *Arch Ophthalmol* 1988; **106**: 1378–83.

Budd KS, Kedsady JH. Investigation of environmental factors in pediatric headache. *Headache* 1989; **29**: 569–73.

Carlow TJ, Glaser JS. Pseudotumor cerebri syndrome in systemic lupus erythematosus. *J Am Med Assoc* 1974; **228**: 197–200.

Childhood Brain Tumour Consortium. The epidemiology of headache among children with brain tumour. *J Neuro-oncol* 1991; **10**: 31–46.

Chu ML, Shinnar S. Headaches in children younger than 7 years of age. *Arch Neurol* 1992; **49**: 79–82.

Corbett JJ, Nerad JA, Tse DT, Anderson RL. Results of optic nerve sheath fenestration for pseudotumor cerebri. *Arch Ophthalmol* 1988; **106**: 1391–7.

Dillon H, Leopold RL. Children and the postconcussion syndrome. *J Am Med Assoc* 1961; **175**: 86–91.

Durkan GP, Troost BT, Slamovits S, Spoor TC, Kennerdell JS. Recurrent painless oculomotor palsy in children. A variant of ophthalmoplegic migraine? *Headache* 1971; **21**: 281–4.

Epstein MA, Berman PH, Schut L. Cavernous angioma presenting as atypical facial and head pain. *J Child Neurol* 1990; **5**: 27–30.

Friedman AP, Harter DH, Meritt HH. Ophthalmoplegic migraine. *Arch Neurol* 1962; **7**: 320–31.

Galbraith JEK, Sullivan JH. Decompression of the perioptic meninges for relief of papilledema. *Am J Ophthalmol* 1973; **76**: 687–92.

Grant DN. Benign intracranial hypertension: a review of 79 cases in infancy and childhood. *Arch Dis Child* 1971; **46**: 651–5.

Hamed L, Tse D, Glaser J, Byrne S, Schtaz N. Neuroimaging of the optic nerve after fenestration for management of pseudotumor cerebri. *Arch Ophthalmol* 1992; **110**: 636–40.

Hayreh SS, Servais GE, Virdi PS. Fundus lesions in malignant hypertension IV. Focal intraretinal periarteriolar transudates. *Ophthalmology* 1986a; **93**: 60–74.

Hayreh SS, Servais GE, Virdi PS. Fundus lesions in malignant hypertension V. Hypertensive optic neuropathy. *Ophthalmology* 1986b; **93**: 74–8.

Hayreh SS, Servais GE, Virdi PS. Fundus lesions in malignant hypertension VI. Hypertensive choroidopathy. *J Am Acad Ophthalmol* 1986c; **93**: 1383–400.

Hayreh SS, Servais GE, Virdi PS, Marcus ML, Rojas P, Woolson RF. Fundus lesions in malignant hypertension III. Arterial blood pressure, biochemical and fundus changes. *Ophthalmology* 1986d; **93**: 45–60.

Hockaday JM. Headache in children. *Br J Hosp Med* 1983; **27**: 383–92.

Hosking GP, Cavanagh NPC, Wilson J. Alternating hemiplegia: complicated migraine of infancy. *Arch Dis Child* 1978; **53**: 656–60.

Hughes RL. Identification and treatment of cerebral aneurysms after sentinel headache. *Neurology* 1992; **42**: 1118–19.

Hulse JA, Taylor DSI, Dillon MJ. Blindness and paraplegia in severe childhood hypertension. *Lancet* 1979; **ii**: 553–6.

Hupp SL, Glaser JS, Frazier-Byrne S. Optic nerve sheath decompression. Review of 17 cases. *Arch Ophthalmol* 1987; **105**: 386–9.

Keltner J. Optic nerve sheath decompression. *Arch Ophthalmol* 1988; **106**: 1365–9.

Lam BL, Schatz NJ, Glaser J, Bowen B. Pseudotumor cerebri from cranial venous obstruction. *Ophthalmology* 1992; **99**: 706–12.

Lance JW. Outpatient problems: headache. *Br J Hosp Med* 1978; **19**: 377–9.

Lessell S. Pediatric pseudotumor cerebri (idiopathic intracranial hypertension). *Surv Ophthalmol* 1992; **37**: 155–66.

Liu G, Kay M, Bienfung D, Schatz N. Pseudotumor cerebri associated with corticosteroid withdrawal in inflammatory bowel disease. *Am J Ophthalmol* 1994; **117**: 352–7.

Minns RA. Clinical application of ventricular pressure monitoring in children. *Z Kinderchir* 1977; **22**: 4310–43.

Mittra R, Sergott R, Flaharty P *et al*. Optic nerve decompression improves hemodynamic parameters in papilledema. *Ophthalmology* 1993; **100**: 987–97.

Northfield DW. Some observations on headache. *Brain* 1938; **61**: 133–62.

O'Connor PS, Tredici TJ. Acephalgic migraine, 15 years experience. *Am Acad Ophthalmol* 1981; **88**: 999–1002.

Orcutt J, Page NGR, Sanders MD. Factors affecting visual loss in benign intracranial hypertension. *Ophthalmology* 1984; **91**: 1303–13.

Pascual J, Oterino A, Berciano J. Headache in type 1 Chiari malformation. *Neurology* 1992; **42**: 1519–21.

Pasquale LR, Moster ML, Schmaier A. Dural sinus thrombosis with abnormalities of protein S and fibrinogen. *Arch Ophthalmol* 1990; **108**: 644–9.

Peatfield RC, Rose FC. Migrainous visual symptoms in a woman without eyes. *Arch Neurol* 1981; **38**: 466–8.

Plotnik J, Kosmorsky G. Operative complications of optic nerve sheath decompression. *Ophthalmology* 1993; **100**: 683–90.

Rossi LN, Vassella F. Headache in children with brain tumour. *Child's Nerv Syst* 1989; **5**: 307–9.

Rothner RD. Diagnosis and management of headache in children and adolescents. *Neurol Clin* 1983; **1**: 511–26.

Ryan RE Jr, Ryan RE Sr. Cluster headache. *Otolaryngol Clin N Am* 1989; **22**: 1131–44.

Sedwick LA, Burde RM. Unilateral and asymmetric optic disc swelling with intracranial abnormalities. *Am J Ophthalmol* 1983; **6**: 484–7.

Sergott RC, Savino PJ, Bosley TM. Modified optic nerve sheath decompression provides long-term visual improvement for pseudotumor cerebri. *Arch Ophthalmol* 1988; **106**: 1384–90.

Silberstein SD. Twenty questions about headaches in children and adolescents. *Headache* 1990; **30**: 716–24.

Spector RH. Migraine. *Surv Ophthalmol* 1984; **29**: 193–207.

Spoor T, McHenry J. Long-term effectiveness of optic nerve sheath decompression for pseudotumor cerebri. *Arch Ophthalmol* 1993; **111**: 632–5.

Spoor T, McHenry J, Shin D. Optic nerve sheath decompression with adjunctive mitomycin and Molteno device implantation *Arch Ophthalmol* 1994; **112**: 25–6.

Tomkins CM, Spalton DJ. Benign intracranial hypertension treated by optic nerve sheath decompression. *J R Soc Med* 1984; **77**: 141–3.

Trompeter RS, Smith RL, Hoare RD, Neville BGR, Chandler C. Neurological complications of arterial hypertension. *Arch Dis Child* 1982; **57**: 913–17.

Troost BT, Mark LE, Maroon JC. Resolution of classic migraine after removal of an occipital lobe arteriovenous malformation. *Ann Neurol* 1979; **5**: 199–201.

Weisberg LA, Chutorian AM. Pseudotumor cerebri of childhood. *Am J Dis Child* 1977; **131**: 1243–8.

Wiley RG. The scintillating scotoma without headache. *Ann Ophthalmol* 1979; **11**: 581–5.

Winrow AP, Supramaniam G. Benign intracranial hypertension after ciprofloxacin administration. *Arch Dis Child* 1990; **65**: 1165–6.

Wolff HG. *Headache, and Other Related Pain*. New York: Oxford University Press, 1963.

Woods D, O'Connor PO, Fleming R. Episodic unilateral mydriasis and migraine. *Am J Ophthalmol* 1984; **98**: 229–35.

Zifkin B, Andermann E, Andermann F, Kirkham T. An autosomal dominant syndrome of hemiplegic migraine, nystagmus, and tremor. *Ann Neurol* 1980; **8**: 329–31.

P18: Peculiar Visual Images

David Taylor

Children probably have visual experiences that are not 'usual' much more frequently than is realized. They have difficulty in describing them, preferring to call their vision blurred or fuzzy or just 'funny' to giving a more accurate description which they have difficulty in expressing. Their parents, quite understandably, often do not report the symptoms because they have difficulty in understanding them. Ophthalmologists rarely ask children whether they have odd visual images because of a mistaken fear of being misunderstood.

Dysmetropsia

Changes in the size or shape of an object.

Micropsia

A sensation that objects are smaller than they should be is a common experience in childhood and it is usually not based on any organic disease unless associated with other symptoms. Micropsia with metamorphopsia, hallucinations or visual defects is always organic.

Most of the children I have seen with this condition have been between 7 and 15 years, of either sex, and it has been an isolated complaint. Often they have been reading in bed in the evening and have noticed a progressive diminution in the size of their book; looking up they see familiar surroundings clearly but greatly diminished in size; if they walk around they have a peculiar sensation that they are in a Lilliputian land. The sensation frightens only the most timid. It lasts a few minutes and usually goes more quickly than it comes. Sometimes the disappearance is instantaneous whereas the onset is so gradual that it is difficult to say when it began. There is no adequate explanation of the cause but it could be related to a 'mismatch' between accommodation and convergence because when divergence is induced by mirrors or prisms in the absence of a change in accommodation or change in image size, an increase in the perceived size of the image is experienced. The reverse occurs when convergence is induced. The symptoms usually disappear in a few months and reassurance is the only treatment.

Micropsia also occurs with retinal macular disease, particularly with macular oedema or any disease in which the retinal elements are abnormally separated including dystrophies and neuroretinitis. In retinal micropsia there is usually an uncorrectable acuity defect, only a minimal colour defect and the child notices blurred or distorted central vision especially if the disorder is bilateral (Fig. P18.1).

Micropsia may be noticed at the first wearing of myopic spectacles or contact lenses for hypermetropia, and it may be prolonged if the lenses are too strong.

Cerebral abnormalities have been reported as causing micropsia, including migraine, cortical defects and a chiasmal tumour (Bender & Savitsky 1943) which gave rise to a nasotemporal field size difference. Hallucinations also occurred with Lilliputian images (Savitsky & Tarachov 1941) in a child with scarlet fever.

The key to the diagnosis therefore is the history and examination of the child: with isolated micropsia and no abnormality on examination there is no need for further investigation.

Macropsia

Macropsia is much rarer than micropsia. It may occur with

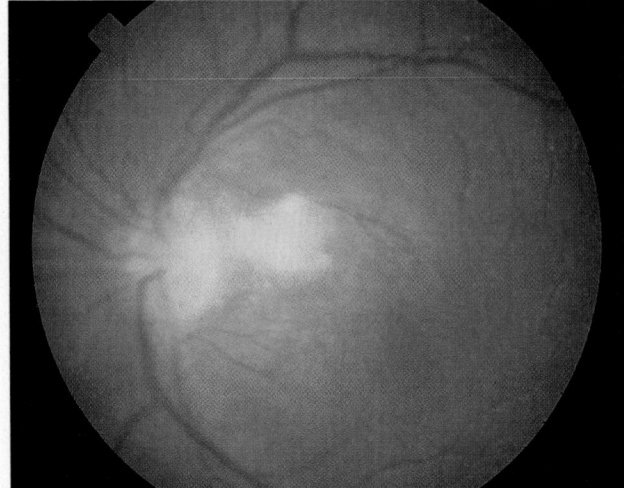

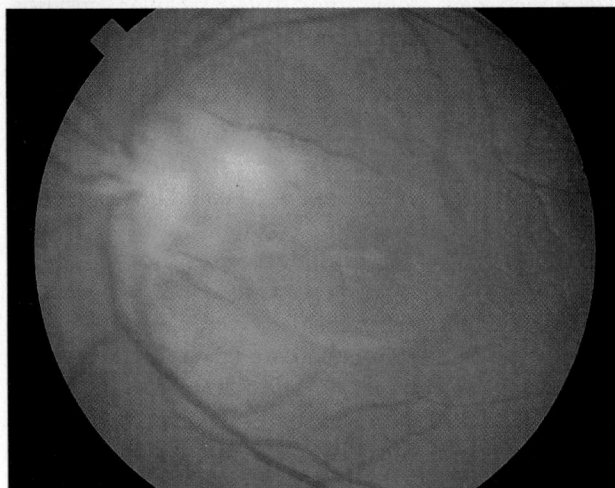

Fig. P18.1 (a) Neuroretinitis with micropsia. This 9-year-old girl complained of dullness of the vision in both eyes, and smallness of objects with distortion on the right. The white area temporal to the optic disc represents retinal nerve fibre swelling and vascular leakage. The retinal oedema extends to the fovea. (b) As the retinal oedema increased and extended across the macula the acuity dropped to 6/36 and the micropsia disappeared.

retinal diseases where the foveal cones are pushed together or with cortical disease. Rarely it is found as a non-organic or benign disorder in the same way that micropsia occurs.

Metamorphopsia

Distortion of central vision — which the child reports as 'lines are bent', 'objects appear broken up' or, in younger children, that things are blurred or that they just cannot see properly—occurs only with organic disease, usually of the anterior visual system. It is accompanied by clinical or neurophysiological evidence of central visual disorders. Metamorphopsia also occurs with brain abnormalities but

it is usually accompanied by hallucinations or with visual field defects or both. A variety of dysmetropias, erythropsia and metamorphopsia has been reported in the course of infectious mononucleosis (Epstein–Barr virus infection). The bizarre images of the body and external objects have prompted the term 'Alice in Wonderland syndrome' (Copperman 1977; Cinbis & Aysun 1992).

Erythropsia and 'coloured clouds'

A sensation that everything is red (erythropsia) is sometimes noted by patients, including children, for a few days or weeks after cataract surgery. It does not seem to have any significance and usually does not trouble the child very much.

'Coloured clouds' are a sensation reported by some children and adults when lying in a sleepy state in oblique sunlight or bright light. They see whorls of multicoloured lights, predominantly red and blue, which swirl in their vision when the lids are closed; it is normal and is probably an entoptic phenomenon.

Entoptic phenomena

Entoptic phenomena are visual observations of normal phenomena within the eye that are made in unusual viewing conditions. Examples include the viewing of retinal vessels by rubbing the eye with a light through closed lids, or seeing spots moving when looking at a bright clear blue sky or an open field of snow (Scheerer's phenomenon).

Phosphenes and photopsias

Phosphenes are transient tiny spots of light seen in an otherwise intact field of vision which usually occur because of retinal stimulation. There are many examples of phosphenes including the following.
1 The bright lights seen when the eye is rubbed through closed lids.
2 Bright lights may occur as a result of retinal traction in vitreous disease. When associated with seeing spots these are an indication for careful ophthalmoscopy since they are the cardinal symptoms of a retinal tear.
3 'Moore's lightning streaks' are larger blue or white lights that meander in the vision for a second or so especially when the lights are dimmed. Their origin is unknown and they seem to be harmless.
4 Flick phosphenes are the eye movement-related spots of light caused by retinal traction.
5 Transient flashes of light may be seen in retinal embolic disease.

Photopsias are larger, longer lasting visual phenomena that may also be related to movement. Davis *et al.* (1976) described their occurrence in patients with optic neuropathies, the relationship to movement presumably being due to traction on the optic nerve. Rarely a patient with an optic neuropathy may complain of seeing a bright light or a flash of light when stimulated by sound (Page *et al.* 1982; Jacobs *et al.* 1987). Thus many of the transient flashes of light seen by children can be of serious significance and should not necessarily be dismissed as being 'invented'.

Complaints about poor vision in special lighting conditions should never be dismissed. They may be a form of photophobia (see P9), due to an optic neuropathy causing altered visual perception, or due to a cerebral defect.

Monocular diplopia

Monocular diplopia in children requires especially careful questioning to determine its true nature. It is most often due to small axial cataracts or corneal disease, cataracts where one part of the lens has a higher refractive index than another, or occasionally due to retinal disease or simple refractive errors (Coffeen & Guyton 1988). Careful questioning may also reveal more than two images, each of varying sharpness.

An interesting example of monocular diplopia occurs when, in a child who has anomalous retinal correspondence associated with squint, the eyes are realigned surgically; he sees two images with the eye that was squinting before surgery. It fades gradually over weeks or months as one or other image predominates depending on the success of the realignment. With both eyes open there can be a binocular triplopia. Diplopia may occur with brain disease (Safran *et al.* 1981) when either eye is viewing but is very rare. In many cases no cause can be found and the underlying problem may be hysterical (see Chapter 56) or stress-related.

Hallucinations

Hallucinations, being entirely personal subjective phenomena, are impossible for the clinician to verify, so their definition by Esquirol as 'false sensory impressions not due to disease of the sense organs' makes a positive diagnosis impossible. There is no totally satisfactory definition of these images, which the patient thinks are real but which arise within the mind in the absence of sense organ stimulation.

Pseudohallucinations are described as hallucinations where the subject realizes they are not 'real' images. Illusions are misinterpretations of actual images.

Social deprivation

Children deprived, intentionally or otherwise, of social contact may develop elaborate visual and auditory images of imaginary friends or animals that can last hours and are usually enjoyed by the child, who is preoccupied by them (Bender 1954). They are probably extensions of the normal imaginary companions that many children have (Bender & Vogel 1941).

Sensory deprivation and visual loss

People who have been isolated for prolonged periods, especially in conditions of total sensory deprivation, may develop elaborate visual and other sensory hallucinations which are often quite pleasant.

Hallucinations occur quite frequently in visual loss; this is a common experience in age-related macular degeneration or senile cataract and the phenomenon is enhanced by the patient's nervousness and exposure to drugs, especially alcohol (and its withdrawal) and premedication drugs.

Patients with sudden cortical visual loss have formed hallucinations that usually, but not always, occur in the area of defective visual field (Lance 1976). These hallucinations are 'irritative' phenomena that are similar to those that occur after encephalitis (Mize 1980) or with epilepsy. However, they occur in any part of the visual field. Patients with eye disease may develop hallucinations that diminish in their clarity, frequency and duration as the blindness progresses (White 1980). When vivid, pleasant hallucinations occur in the elderly with preserved intellectual functions and eye disease, they are known as the Charles Bonnet syndrome (Damas-Mora *et al.* 1982; Siatkowski *et al.* 1990; Brown & Murphy 1992). I have seen a child with adrenoleukodystrophy with cortical blindness and optic atrophy who had vivid and pleasant hallucinations of animals. White and Jan (1992) described a fascinating case in a child who was blind after surgery for optic glioma; the child's mental state was normal and he was initially frightened by the vivid images of familiar objects.

Visual phenomena with localized brain disease

Hallucinations should not be thought of as arising from disease of any particular part of the brain, but some phenomena are more common with disease of certain areas of the brain (Gittinger *et al.* 1982). Disease of the posterior visual pathways and particularly the occipital cortex usually gives rise to unformed, crude, repetitive hallucinations. These are usually 'irritative', i.e. due to an epileptic form of discharge as opposed to the hallucinating due to anterior visual pathways disease which 'releases' the brain from vision, which normally suppresses unwanted discharges (Cogan 1973).

Temporal lobe lesions are said to give rise to formed and detailed visual and olfactory hallucinations. In one case, that of an elderly man with a stroke, the hallucinations were exclusively provoked by watching television (Safran *et al.* 1981).

The evidence for midbrain disorders giving rise to hallucinations is less clear. L'Hermitte (1922) and Van Bogaert (1927) described cases with pathological confirmation. Van Bogaert coined the term peduncular hallucinosis because he believed that involvement of the cerebral peduncles was a vital feature. The name is so euphonic that it has remained. The hallucinations are remarkably vivid (Geller & Bellur 1987; Kölmel 1991; Serra Catafu *et al.* 1992), like a film in many cases, coloured and occasionally accompanied by unformed sound.

Hypnagogic and hypnopompic hallucination

Hallucinations on going to sleep (hypnagogic) or waking (hypnopompic) are quite common in adults. They are often pleasant and have the frustrating quality that when they are concentrated upon they disappear. Although said to be common, occurring in perhaps one-fifth of a population of doctors (Lessell 1975), I have found them so rarely in children that I am reluctant to ask.

Drug-induced hallucination

Barbiturates, valium and alcohol withdrawal after chronic intoxication may all be associated with hallucinations. Chronic abuse is very rare in childhood, but must be remembered with the withdrawal of barbiturates in epileptic children.

Atropine, cyclopentolate and some other cycloplegic drugs are potent causes of visual hallucinations, which occur as part of an organic psychosis with confusion and signs of intoxication (hot, red-faced, dilated pupils, tachycardia).

Ketamine, widely used for examinations under anaesthesia, produces visual and frightening hallucinations especially if the child is wakened roughly.

LSD and mescalin cause hallucinations that may occur long after the taking of the drug but usually within the first 6 hours, starting shortly after ingestion. Micropsia, macropsia, palinopsia and remarkable formed visual hallucinations that are not stereotyped also occur (Lessell 1975).

Psychoneuroses and psychiatric disease

Hallucinations, particularly auditory, occur in about 15% of children with behavioural problems (Bender 1954). Powerful auditory and visual hallucinations, often religious or persecutory and frightening, are characteristic of schizophrenia, which may have its onset in later childhood. They are true hallucinations, believed by the patient. In adolescent psychoses, hallucinations occur in 75% of children and are most fre-quently auditory or auditory and visual (Garralda & Ainsworth 1987).

Children with conduct or emotional disorders who also suffered from hallucinations were older than similar children without hallucinations. They also had lower IQs and were more frequently admitted to hospital for the disorder. The hallucinating children were more likely to be depressed, to have a family history of mood changes and to have more symptoms suggestive of cognitive perceptual disorder (Garralda 1984a). When followed to adulthood the association with hallucinations did not carry an increased risk for psychoses, depressive illness, organic brain disease or other psychiatric disorder (Garralda 1984b).

Palinopsia (visual perseveration in time)

Palinopsia is when there is a 'flashback' of part of a visual scene that was experienced seconds, minutes or hours previously. Part or whole of the visual field may be affected by the palinopsic image and there may also be auditory perseveration (Lessell 1975). It occurs in evolving lesions of different types, usually in defective areas of the visual fields. There is almost invariably a visual field defect and the right parietal lobe is most frequently affected (Bender *et al.* 1968).

Occipital epilepsy

Benign occipital epilepsy of childhood is a condition which may be familial (Nagendran *et al.* 1989) and gives rise to unformed visual experiences of transient loss of vision that occur in brief attacks up to several times a day. Electroencephalography shows epileptiform discharges over the occipital region that are abolished by eye opening. Symptoms may be improved by antiepileptic drugs (Nagendran *et al.* 1989).

Occipital epilepsy also occurs as a condition with very serious implications; Lortie *et al.* (1993) reported 12 neonates with often generalized seizures who had severe visual and general developmental abnormalities.

References

Bender L. Hallucinations in children. In: *A Dynamic Psychopathology of Childhood*. Illinois: CC Thomas, 1954.

Bender L, Vogel BF. Imaginary companions of children. *Am J Orthopsychiatr* 1941; **11**: 56–65.

Bender MB, Feldman M, Sobin AJ. Palinopsia. *Brain* 1968: **91**: 321–38.

Bender MB, Savitsky N. Micropsia and teleopsia limited to the temporal fields of vision. *Arch Ophthalmol* 1943; **29**: 904–8.

Brown GC, Murphy RP. Visual symptoms associated with choroidal neovascularisation: photopsias and the Charles Bonnet syndrome. *Arch Ophthalmol* 1992; **110**: 1251–6.

Cinbis M, Aysun S. Alice in Wonderland syndrome as an initial manifestation of Epstein–Barr virus infection. *Br J Ophthalmol* 1992; **76**: 316.

Cogan DG. Visual hallucinations as release phenomena. *Graefe's Arch Klin Exp Ophthalmol* 1973; **188**: 139–50.

Coffeen O, Guyton DL. Monocular diplopia accompanying ordinary refractive errors. *Am J Ophthalmol* 1988; **105**: 451.

Copperman SM. Alice in Wonderland syndrome as a presenting sign of infectious mononucleosis. *Clin Pediatr* 1977; **16**: 143–6.

Damas-Mora J, Skelton-Robinson M, Jenner FA. The Charles Bonnet syndrome in perspecive. *Psychol Med* 1982; **12**: 251–61.

Davis FA, Bergen D, Schauf C, McDonald WI, Deutsch W. Movement phosphenes in optic neuritis: a new clinical sign. *Neurology* 1976; **26**: 1100–4.

Garralda ME. Hallucinations in children with conduct and emotional disorders. The clinical phenomenon. *Psychol Med* 1984a: **14**: 589–96.

Garralda ME. Hallucinations in children with conduct and emotional disorders. The follow-up study. *Psychol Med* 1984b; **14**: 597–604.

Garralda ME, Ainsworth P. Psychoses in adolescence. In: Coleman J (ed.) *Working with Troubled Adolescents*. London: Academic Press, 1987; 169–86.

Geller T, Bellur SN. MRI confirmation of mesencephalic infarction during life. *Ann Neurol* 1987; **21**: 602–3.

Gittinger WW, Miller NR, Keltner JL, Burde RM. Sugar plum fairies. Visual hallucinations. *Surv Ophthalmol* 1982; **27**: 42–8.

Jacobs L, Karpic A, Bozian D, Gothgen S. Auditory–visual synesthesia. *Arch Neurol* 1987; **38**: 211–16.

Kölmel HW. Peduncular hallucination. *J Neurol* 1991; **238**: 457–9.

Lance JW. Simple formed hallucinations confined to the area of a specific visual field defect. *Brain* 1976; **99**: 719–34.

Lessell S. Higher disorders of visual function: positive phenomena. In: Glaser JS, Smith JL (eds) *Neuro-ophthalmology*, Vol. 8. St Louis: CV Mosby, 1975; 27.

L'Hermitte J. Syndrome de la calotte du pédoncule cérébral. Les troubles psycho-sensoric dans les lésions du mésocephale. *Rev Neurol* 1922; **2**: 1359–65.

Lortie A, Plouin P, Pinard J-M, Dulac O. Occipital epilepsy in neonates and infants. In: Occipital seisures and epilepsies in children. In: Andermann A, Beaumanoir A, Mira L, Roger J, Tassinari CA (eds) *Occipital Seizures and Epilepsies in Children*. John Libbey, 1993; 121–32.

Mize K. Visual hallucinations following viral encephalitis; a self report. *Neuropsychologica* 1980; **18**: 193–202.

Nagendran K, Prior PF, Rossiter M. Benign occipital epilepsy of childhood: a family study. *J R Soc Med* 1989; **82**: 684–5.

Page NGR, Bolger JP, Sanders MD. Auditory evoked phosphenes in optic nerve disease. *J Neurol Neurosurg Psychiatr* 1982; **45**: 7–12.

Safran AB, Kline LB, Glaser JS, Daroff RB. Television-induced formed visual hallucinations and cerebral diplopia. *Br J Ophthalmol* 1981; **65**: 707–11.

Savitsky N, Tarachov S. Lilliputian hallucinations during convalescence from scarlet fever in a child. *J Nerv Ment Dis* 1941; **93**: 310–12.

Serra Catafu J, Rubio F, Peres Serrra J. Peduncular hallucinosis associated with posterior thalamic infarction. *J Neurol* 1992; **239**: 89–90.

Siatkowski RM, Zimmer B, Rosenberg PR. The Charles Bonnet syndrome. *J Clin Neuro-ophthalmol* 1990; **10**: 215–18.

Van Bogaert L. L'hallucinose pédonculaire. *Rev Neurol* 1927; **47**: 608–17.

White C, Jan J. Visual hallucinations after acute visual loss in a young child. *Dev Med Neurol* 1992; **34**: 252–65.

White NJ. Complex visual hallucinations in partial blindness due to eye disease. *Br J Psychiatr* 1980; **136**: 284–6.

P19: The Child who Fails at School

Nicholas Cavanagh

The ophthalmologist is usually unwillingly dragged into a child's educational problems but nonetheless it is important that he understands the variety of reasons why a child may have come to see him. The educational psychologist is the expert in this area and all children with significant learning problems will need assessment by one as early as possible, with full, detailed, and careful psychometry.

Some indication of the extent and nature of the problem will have been provided by the school with comments and reports. These will need to be supplemented by a history from the parents and child, and sometimes it is helpful to see them separately. The history should cover early development, social circumstances, behaviour of the child and the family's perception of the problems (Fig. P19.1).

Causes of failure

Intellectual

The most common reason is that the child has moderate or severe learning difficulties. Alternatively, the child may have been normal mentally and then regressed with time because of a degenerative disease of the brain. Unrecognized frequent fitting, or minor motor status epilepticus should be considered.

Conditions causing regression are often associated with visual failure.

Specific learning disability

A child may be of normal intelligence but have a specific disability. One such example is dyslexia, but another might be dyspraxia or a specific problem of memory whether of long- or short-term memory or of auditory or visual memory. Other examples include perceptual problems or specific language disabilities. Many specific disabilities are compounded by attention deficits or behavioural problems.

Social and emotional

Social and/or emotional causes of school failure may be mainly due to the child and his family, or in part due to an adverse interaction between the child and his teacher in

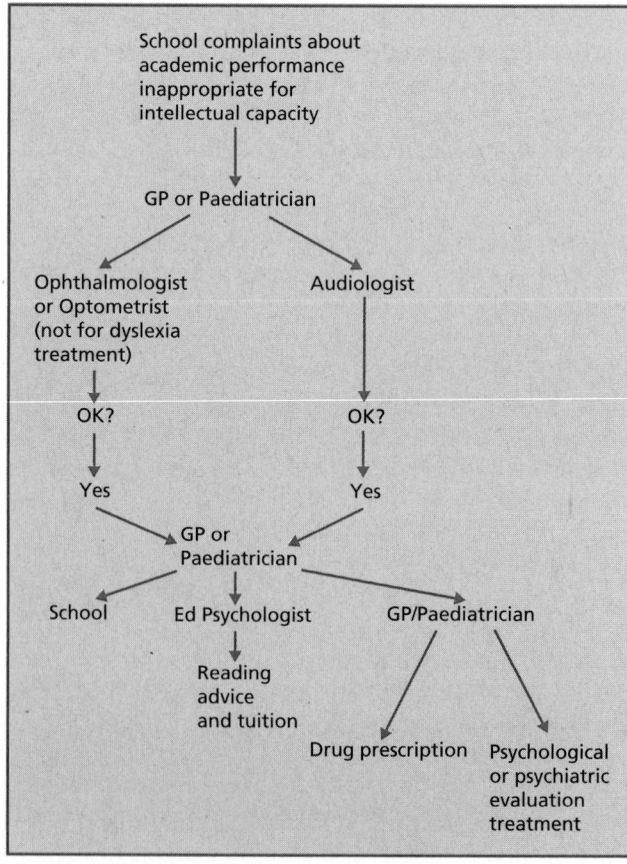

Fig. P19.1 Guidelines to evaluate the child who fails at school.

school. Causes in the former category include the child having a 'difficult' personality, poverty, poor parenting, abuse, bereavement, mixing with the 'wrong' crowd, drug taking, truancy, and so on. Examples in the latter category might include child–teacher personality conflict or poor social integration of the child with his peers due to cultural or racial differences.

Educational reasons

The school or its teachers may be at fault or the syllabus inappropriate, boring or too advanced for the child. Not all children respond well to all teaching methods and school-based factors in educational failure should be sought.

Hearing defects

Clearly serious hearing defects will have significant implications for learning. Less severe defects may go unrecognized longer and have deteriorating effects for that reason. Hearing loss may fluctuate and therefore underlie erratic achievements. Hearing impairment during the sensitive years of speech acquisition may have lasting repercussions upon language abilities.

Sight and oculomotor defects

Although there is a significant proportion of dyslexics who have a variety of minor visual and oculomotor anomalies, it is not proven that these are the cause of the problem. Therefore reading exercises and so on, without remedial teaching, are unlikely to cause significant improvement. Uncorrected refractive errors, convergence insufficiency, poor vision from any cause and some oculomotor disturbances may occasionally be implicated in educational failure.

The ophthalmologist's role

The ophthalmologist has a simple role. He has to exclude significant eye disease, refractive error or oculomotor dysfunction. Some ophthalmologists may take a greater interest in dyslexia and become involved in various forms of special 'treatment'. Their role as wise counsel and guide to the appropriate investigation and management of the child who fails at school is, we believe, more important.

P20: Abnormal Pupil Appearance in Infancy

David Taylor

Parents often have difficulty in expressing their observations regarding abnormalities of their child's pupils. They may be encouraged to be specific as to whether the pupil is large, small, or abnormally shaped or sited, but when the abnormality is actually due to the iris or the appearance of the pupil reflex it may be more difficult for the parent to find the appropriate words.

Their vagueness should not be dismissed, because it is rarely a symptom without foundation. Examination, including slit-lamp microscopy and fundoscopy, usually reveals the cause. Figure P20.1 provides guidelines on the causes.

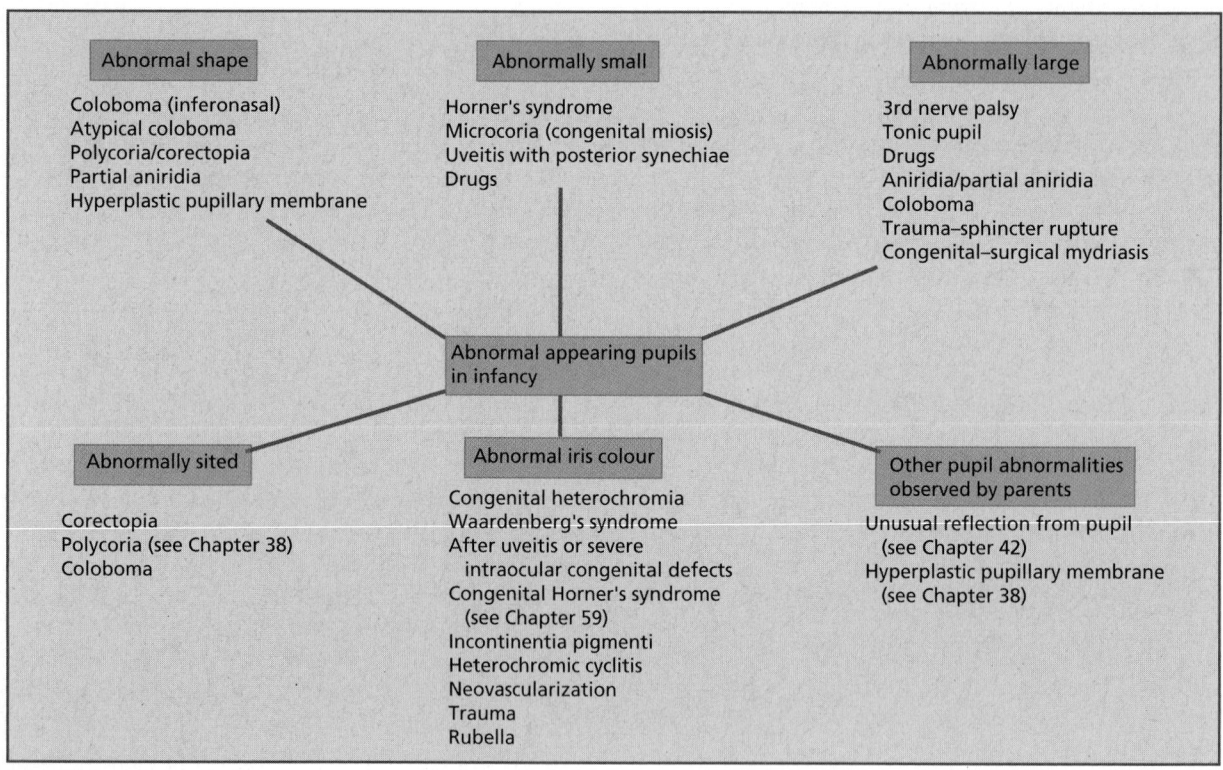

Fig. P20.1 Guidelines on the causes of abnormal pupils in infancy.

P21: Clinical Investigation of Anisocoria

David Taylor

When anisocoria is found in a child a simple stage-by-stage routine can be followed as outlined in Fig. P21.1. This is designed to be a guide only.

Pharmacological testing may occasionally be helpful, but most cases can be diagnosed clinically by their size in different lighting conditions and by their neurological accompaniments.

Slit-lamp examination will reveal developmental abnormalities and sinuous reactions.

The pupil reactions to a bright light and to a near stimulus are noted. The pupil sizes in the dark and in bright light are recorded and preferably photographed. Physiological anisocoria is common in minor degrees; it is usually equal in light and dark and the reactions are normal.

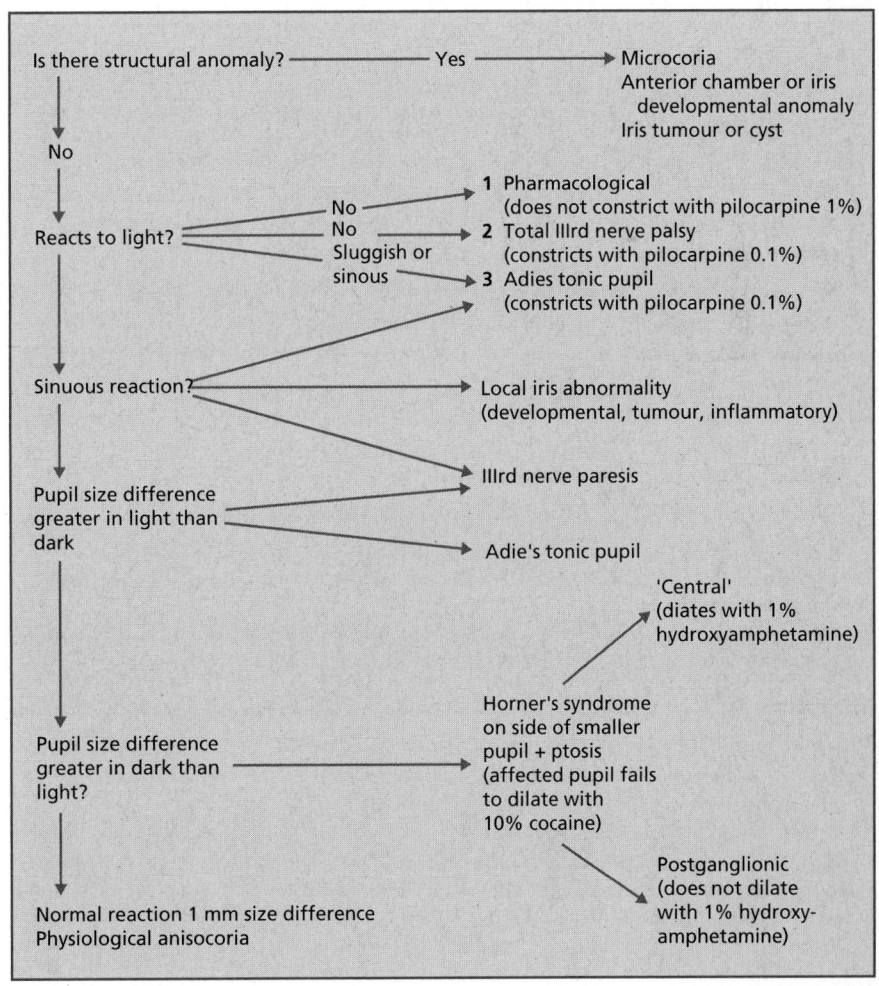

Fig. P21.1 A guide to the routine investigation of anisocoria.

P22: Wobbly Eyes in Infancy

David Taylor

It is surprising how few parents notice nystagmus. Their attention is more frequently drawn to the associated squint or poor vision. The history of the nystagmus is important: both prenatal factors such as drug ingestion or a difficult delivery, and postnatal factors such as the mode of onset, associated systemic and ocular illnesses, drugs and the history of the vision itself.

Some information can be gleaned from the directional characteristics of nystagmus. Nystagmus may be purely vertical, horizontal or rotary, which are characteristics of certain disorders, or it may have specific characteristics (i.e. monocular, see-saw, etc.) which have anatomical or pathogenetic significance (Fig. P22.1).

If the nystagmus is not specific in its characteristics it may help to follow the guidelines in Fig. P22.1. They are not complete but may be helpful in systematically reaching a diagnosis. See also Chapters 63 and 64.

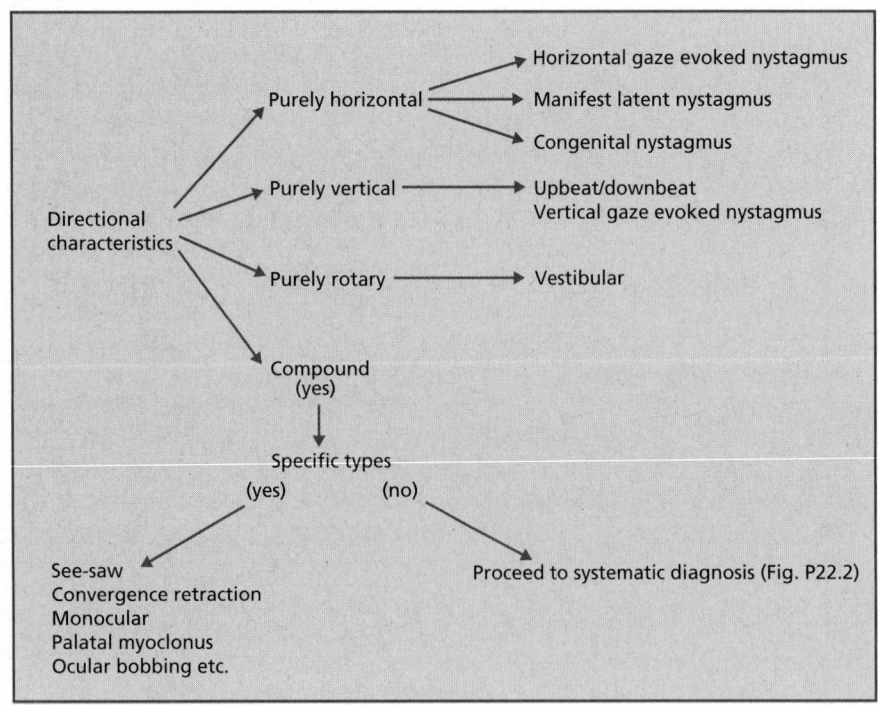

Fig. P22.1 Directional characteristics of wobbly eyes in infancy.

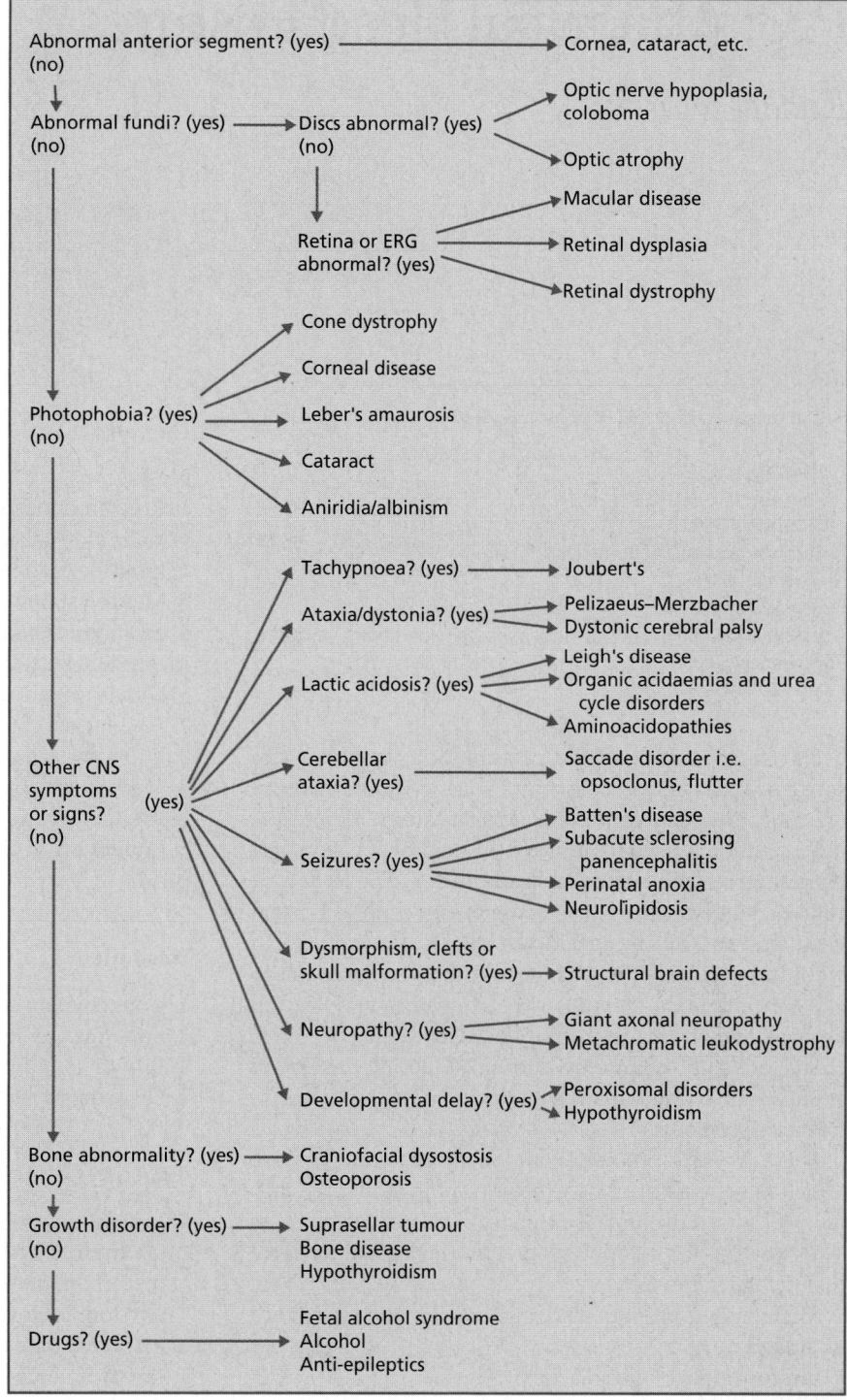

Fig. P22.2 Systematic diagnosis of wobbly eyes in infancy.

P23: Abnormal Head Postures

Robert Morris

Children may adopt a head posture for a variety of reasons, most frequently defects in the cervical musculature or spine, and, less commonly, ocular causes. Where the head position is used to improve the quality of vision, it is usually termed an abnormal head posture. The term torti collis is sometimes used synonymously with abnormal head posture, but is generally reserved for patients in whom the head position includes a component of head tilt.

A long-standing anomalous head posture may lead to facial asymmetry (Horton *et al.* 1967; Goodman *et al.* 1995) characterized by a flattened shortened face on the side of the head tilt, changes in neck muscle tone and rarely cervical spine problems.

There are three potential components to a head posture which may be present alone or in combination: (a) a face turn; (b) a head tilt; and (c) a chin up or chin down posture. The reasons for adopting an abnormal head posture include the following.

1 Maintenance of binocular single vision and avoidance of diplopia.

2 Improvement of visual acuity.

3 To enable fixation when eye movement is restricted.

4 Centralization of a limited field of vision.

Ocular causes of abnormal head posture

There are a large number of causes of an abnormal head posture (Kushner 1979), but the most common causes are superior oblique underaction, lateral rectus paresis, Duane's syndrome, Brown's syndrome and congenital nystagmus (Kraft *et al.* 1992).

Face turn

Nystagmus.

1 Congenital idiopathic or other nystagmus with a null point in side gaze.

2 Infantile esotropia with manifest latent nystagmus.

3 Micronystagmus associated with a congenital squint.

4 Nystagmus blockage syndrome.

Incomitant strabismus.

1 Duane's syndrome.

2 Sixth nerve paresis.

3 Third nerve paresis.

4 Mechanical limitation of abduction, e.g. medial wall blow-out fracture.

5 Limitation of adduction, e.g. internuclear ophthalmoplegia.

Head tilt

1 Congenital nystagmus.

2 Superior oblique underaction.

3 Brown's syndrome.

4 Dissociated vertical deviation.

Chin up

1 Limitation of elevation of ocular movement:
    (a) thyroid eye disease;
    (b) orbital floor fractures;
    (c) double elevator palsy;
    (d) congenital ocular fibrosis;
    (e) supranuclear eye movement disorders.

2 A pattern esotropia.

3 V pattern exotropia.

4 Congenital nystagmus with null point in down gaze.

5 Congenital ptosis.

Chin down

1 A pattern exotropia.

2 V or Y pattern esotropia.

3 Inferior rectus paresis.

4 Bilateral superior oblique palsies.
5 Congenital nystagmus with null point in upgaze.

Non-ocular causes of abnormal head posture
(Boutros & Al-Mateen 1995)

1 Muscular torticollis:
  (a) congenital muscular torticollis
  (b) acquired non-traumatic inflammatory torticollis.
2 Neurological
  (a) Arnold–Chiari malformation
  (b) extrapyramidal dystonias.
3 Skeletal torticollis:
  (a) Klippel–Feil syndrome
  (b) cervical spine abnormalities.
4 Neoplasia of the cervical cord or vertebra.
5 Traumatic torticollis.
6 Miscellaneous:
  (a) unilateral deafness;
  (b) idiopathic;
  (c) benign paroxysmal torticollis of infancy
  (d) habitual.
  (e) hemianopias

Assessment

History

Parents of children with ocular torticollis often report that the head was tilted from birth, when the baby was lying down. Review of family photographs of the child may be helpful in establishing the onset of the head posture.

Examination

Facial asymmetry should be assessed first. An abnormal head posture can usually be readily seen on casual observation of a child, but to assess it in detail the child should be standing up or sitting straight in a chair and asked to view a detailed target; reading down the Snellen chart is ideal. Infants should be seated so that the parent is not supporting the head, once head control has been established. The most accurate method of recording is to photograph the patient. Assessment of the head position should be made with the patient fixing for near and distance. The head posture should be assessed under monocular and binocular viewing. If patching an eye eliminates a head posture this confirms it is binocular in origin and also provides a clue as to possible improvement that might occur if the underlying cause were treated surgically. Non-ocular and monocular head postures do not improve with monocular occlusion.

Patients with nystagmus who adopt an abnormal head posture to maintain the null point, should achieve better visual acuity with the head in their preferred position than can be achieved with the head straightened. A head posture is usually more apparent on distance testing as the convergence associated with near vision may dampen the amplitude of the nystagmus. Assessment for micronystagmus not apparent on ordinary observation may be the cause of an abnormal head posture, particularly in cases of infantile esotropia, and is best seen on ophthalmoscopic examination with the patient looking away from the preferred position.

A cover test should be performed with the head posture present, and then repeated with the head straightened. A manifest squint or nystagmus which is present with the head straight may be eliminated or reduced when the patient holds the head in their preferred position. Ocular movements may demonstrate a limitation or under-action of eye movement or an increase in nystagmus, when the patient is forced to direct the eyes into the position of gaze that is avoided by the abnormal head posture. In cases where the patient uses the head posture to control a manifest strabismus, the examiner should try to confirm the presence of binocular vision when the head is held in the preferred position.

Visual field assessment should be considered in patients with a face turn, in whom there is a possibility of a field defect, for example in children with a hemiplegia. Patients with non-ocular causes of head postures will typically have a reduced range of neck movement, whilst those with ocular head postures should have full neck movement. This may be a useful distinguishing feature in the early stages, but is not diagnostic (Williams *et al.* 1996).

Management

The first step is to prove that the abnormal head posture is secondary to ocular pathology and to diagnose the ocular defect. Treatment involves treating the underlying ocular cause, and may include surgery to improve the range of eye movement in patients with incomitant strabismus, or surgery to centralize the null position in patients with nystagmus. In cases where the head posture is small, cosmetically good and comfortable, treatment is not indicated.

The timing of extraocular muscle surgery to improve an abnormal head posture will depend on the severity of the head posture, and the natural history of the underlying condition. The possibility of development of secondary neck changes if the abnormal head position persists must also be considered, although there are no data available on the time span for the development of irreversible changes. As a general guide, in cases of relatively straightforward incomitant strabismus with significant head postures, treatment should be undertaken as soon as accurate assessment can be made, the condition is shown to be stable, significant refractive errors have been corrected and amblyopia has been treated. Early intervention is particularly important if the patient stops adopting a head posture and starts to squint. Goodman *et al.* (1995) suggest that early strabismus surgery may help to correct facial asymmetry associated with a head tilt, but feel that alternating head positions during sleep may be more important.

The success of surgery in eliminating an abnormal head posture depends on the underlying cause. Kraft *et al.* (1992) have quoted success rates of 75.6% for superior oblique palsies, 87.2% with Duane's syndrome, and all five patients with Brown's syndrome. In cases of congenital nystagmus with a null point the aim of surgery is to eliminate or reduce the head posture without inducing strabismus in fusing patients. In this group surgery should be delayed until at least age 5 years but ideally until 10 years, because of the variability of congenital nystagmus in the early years of life, and the tendency for some improvement. As the head position seems to vary considerably with visual attention in young children with nystagmus, secondary neck changes are rarely a problem. Kestenbaum (1953) and Anderson (1953) suggested that surgery for congenital nystagmus could improve the posture if the eyes were shifted away from the null point in the direction of the rapid phase of the nystagmus. Since their original reports other authors have suggested increased amounts of surgery because of the high incidence of undercorrections (Pratt-Johnson 1971; Parks 1973; Calhoun & Harley 1973; Mitchell *et al.* 1987). It is generally accepted that to be effective surgery must limit ductions, and even then there is a significant tendency for the head posture to return some years after surgery. See Chapter 63.

References

Anderson JR. Causes and treatment of congenital eccentric nystagmus. *Br J Ophthalmol* 1953; **37**: 267–81.

Boutrous GS, Al-Mateen M. Symposium: abnormal head posture of ophthalmic and non-ophthalmic origin. Non-ophthalmic causes of torticollis. *Am Orthoptic J* 1995; **45**: 68–73.

Calhoun JH, Harley RD. Surgery for abnormal head position in congenital nystagmus. *Trans Am Ophthalmol Soc* 1973; **71**: 70–87.

Goodman CR, Chabner E, Guyton DL. Should early strabismus surgery be performed for ocular torticollis to prevent facial asymmetry. *J Pediatr Ophthalmol Strabismus* 1995; **3**: 162–6.

Horton CE, Crawford HH, Adamson JE, Ashbell TS. Torticollis. *South Med J* 1967; **60**: 953–8.

Kestenbaum A. Nouvelle operation de nystagmus. *Bull Soc Ophthalmol Fr* 1954; **2**: 1071–8.

Kraft SP, O'Donoghue EP, Roarty JD. Improvement of compensatory head postures after strabismus surgery. *Ophthalmology* 1992; **8**: 1301–8.

Kushner BJ. Ocular causes of abnormal head postures. *Ophthalmology* 1979; **86**: 2115–25.

Mitchell PR, Wheeler MB, Parks MM. Kestenbaum surgical procedure for torticollis secondary to congenital nystagmus. *J Pediatr Ophthalmol Strabismus* 1987; **24**: 87–93.

Parks MM. Congenital nystagmus surgery. *Am Orthoptic J* 1973; **23**: 35–9.

Pratt-Johnson JA. The surgery of congenital nystagmus. *Can J Ophthalmol* 1971; **64**: 268–72.

Williams CRP, O'Flynn E, Clarke NMP, Morris RJ. Torticollis secondary to ocular pathology. *J Bone Joint Surg* 1996; **78**: 620–4.

P24: The Uncooperative or Difficult Parent

Susan Day

Uncooperative parents are few and far between. Most parents would do anything to help a child with a visual problem. Many have great fears about what an eye examination may reveal: Will my baby see? Are glasses necessary? Will my child have blue eyes? The significance of the parents' questions and concerns may not be the same as the ophthalmologist's concerns, but to properly care for the child, the parents' worries, regardless of how trivial, must be addressed.

The doctor's interactions with the parents must be initiated at the time of the initial visit. Even though the child is your medical charge, the information must go through the parents, particularly when treatment is indicated; thus it is appropriate for your staff to strongly recommend or indeed to have a policy at the time an appointment is made that at least one parent attend the appointment, rather than a more distant relative, nanny or friend. Such a policy ensures that a better history can be taken, that the parent understands what has happened during the appointment, and that the parent has communicated in a face-to-face fashion. A telephone call hours later from someone the doctor has never met simply does not come close to an appropriate personal interaction.

Parental attitudes towards doctors vary from culture to culture. Some groups are very demanding, expecting almost encyclopedic explanations. Other groups may demand nothing but perfection from their children and the doctors caring for them. Yet others would not think to question any doctor about anything, nor to admit that treatment goals have fallen short of instructions. When language barriers exist, communication which enhances understanding and trust in the doctor is compromised, and an experienced interpreter, who is able to give both good and distressing news, is invaluable.

The doctor's role in bringing out the worst of uncooperative parents deserves attention as well. Often, a pure and simple communication problem is at the root of the dissonance. Communication takes time to listen and respond. If the interaction with parent and child is hurried, the chances are much greater that the parent will be 'uncooperative'.

Finally, nobody is perfect for every type of patient. When an uncooperative atmosphere cannot be remedied, it is best for all, particularly the patient, that referral be made elsewhere.

How is the parent uncooperative?

Non-compliance with treatment or failure to keep return appointments

Non-compliance with treatment typically takes the form of failure to enforce patching or the wearing of spectacles. Each of these treatments is a tall order for some children and some parents. When treatment is recommended, it is critical to explain the purpose of the treatment, what might happen if treatment is not given, and what common pitfalls there may be. Such an explanation should be as free as possible from parental distraction toward other siblings, dirty diapers or nappies, feeding responsibilities, and so on. Any noise outside the consulting room should be minimized by closing the door. We are all accustomed to providing informed consent for surgical procedures, and might do well to think of medical treatments in a similar format. Distribution of pamphlets or other educational material intended for the public may assist in promoting compliance by reiterating what was discussed at the appointment; be familiar with any such material, however, and address areas which particularly apply to the specific patient.

When treatment has not been given appropriately, find out why. Did a skin rash develop? Was there teasing by peers or siblings? Were the parents frustrated or embarrassed in some way? Address any issue such as these, offering positive solutions while reinforcing why treatment is needed. Keep a reference list of parents who have been through similar circumstances—another parent may be better than you in offering suggestions.

1085

If treatment at home is not successful and you feel that an absence of discipline is part of the issue, be firm in reviewing the consequences of non-treatment. Emphasize vision development and the transient nature of the plasticity of the visual system. For a child who is 4 or 5 years or older, include the child in the discussion and in the choices in a way that the child will 'buy into' the need for treatment. Suggest rewards which may add to the treatment success.

When appointments are not kept, the ophthalmologist must be aware, since a measure of responsibility still rests with the doctor despite the non-compliance of the family. Note any missed appointments in the chart, and develop a follow-up protocol with your staff. When the patient has a potentially serious consequence of failing an appointment (such as a retinopathy of prematurity follow-up during acute stages) consider a call from yourself or a call to the primary care clinician.

One of the most extreme examples of parental non-compliance relates to refusal of treatment on grounds of religious belief. When the withholding of medical treatment is potentially life-threatening (such as the refusal of treatment for a retinoblastoma), most cultures have instituted legal mechanisms for court-ordered treatment. Since such circumstances arise so rarely within ophthalmology, it is appropriate to remind the ophthalmologist of his or her responsibility to pursue such intervention if required. Usually, hospitals with paediatric wards have staff members who are familiar with the legal requirements and their initiation; these individuals serve as a valuable resource to the ophthalmologist faced with such decisions.

Hostility towards the doctor

Remember that any family coming to you has usually been to many doctors before you. Their attitude towards you may be a consequence of these previous experiences. Perhaps these experiences have resulted in a generalized mistrust of doctors, or a resentment towards perceived high income, or a suspicion about the effectiveness of health care. Your ability to negate these attitudes will have potential great repercussions, not only towards the parents' interactions with future doctors, but also towards the child's developing attitudes towards the medical profession. The diffusion of such hostility, in addition to helping a specific patient to receive better care, is part of our responsibility to our profession.

Hostility can develop after treatment is initiated. Often, it is initiated by a relative who did not attend the earlier appointment. Recently, this author overheard a returning 4-year-old boy exclaim to my receptionist 'Where is that doctor that broke my eyes?' Shortly thereafter, an entourage of relatives with less than pleasant facial expressions were in my room: they had not attended the initial consultation. Ultimately, the cause for the hostility was found to be that the grandfather had tried on the patient's newly obtained glasses and found his vision to be blurred. Even he could not see with these glasses, therefore they must have been wrong!

As difficult as it is to understand this perspective, we nevertheless must be prepared to respond so that the child can be helped. If hostility is sensed by the doctor, the air must be cleared. It is essential that the doctor keep his or her emotions in check, difficult though this may be. Try your best not to be defensive, and to put yourself in the parent's spot. Resist accusations towards the parents. If a shouting match develops, remember that the young patient is observing this, and address the child to reassure the child that he or she has done nothing wrong. Consider excusing yourself from the room in order to check your own emotions.

Finally, examine your role in the perceived hostility. Perhaps the wait in your office was excessive. Perhaps you failed to listen to or answer questions. Interruptions during the appointment or even a defensive or uncaring posture might have induced a negative change in the parents. Examine your staff's telephone and reception etiquette and manner. Make changes in any of these areas which can reduce the likelihood of a hostile parental attitude.

Family dynamics

Every child has two parents, and four grandparents, and so forth! Add a few siblings, well-meaning (or otherwise!) more distant relatives, and a bevy of educational specialists, and the possibility of any dysfunctional component is magnified. Often, the more distant advisor can compare the perceived medical problem of the child to another individual. When your treatment differs from that given to the other person, then free advice is often given in a well-intended fashion to the parent. Especially if the patient is the first child of a parent, there may be a big component of insecurity which will make this parent particularly troubled by such advice; it is important to ask a parent if this has occurred if you sense an altered trust in you.

Family dynamics become strained simply as a consequence of the existing responsibilities. The young couple may be overwhelmed by their various schedules, financial pressures and worries about the future. There simply is not much left-over energy to deal with an unanticipated illness or medical problem. It is therefore easy to understand that the doctor may become an inappropriate recipient of the frustration and exhaustion felt by the parents. Sometimes, shift the focus to the parent, and ask simply, 'And how are *you* doing?'

When the nuclear family's integrity is not present, family dynamics may lead to an even more painful warring over a child's health care. So often, there is a distrust of anything that the other spouse has done. The child becomes an accidental pawn in such dynamics. One parent may insist that glasses be worn, and the other encourage that the glasses not be worn. Tackle these issues as they arise, not in a judgemental fashion, but in a way in which you take no side except that of the child.

Complex medical problems

Every ophthalmologist has experienced the disbelief or the anger which parents display when confronted with a dismal prognosis. The rapid evolution of the parent's reactions often parallels those found in a dying patient: denial, anger, depression and, ultimately, acceptance. Particularly when a new diagnosis is given, the parents must be given extra time, the freedom to discuss with you over the days that follow, and the benefit of a second opinion.

The ophthalmologist must remember that these intense experiences also reflect upon the ophthalmologist's own fragilities—the inability to cure every situation, the uncertainty of the unusual diagnosis, the sad drama observed as the parents cope with their grief. The less experienced clinician should discuss such a situation with a consultant who has perhaps been through similar circumstances before.

It is good practice to suggest a second opinion in these circumstances and provide a list of skilled colleagues or even make an appointment yourself.

Unusual dynamics towards the child

Sometimes the clinician views the attitude of the parent towards the child as being a roadblock to the examination. The most extreme of examples is the child who has sustained a non-accidental injury. Usually, such a child is already in a hospital when the ophthalmologist is consulted; in this circumstance, the ophthalmologist rarely is in a position to interact with the parent. If an extraordinary circumstance occurs where the suspicion for non-accidental injury is first raised in the ophthalmologist's office, protection of the child must remain the ophthalmologist's role, however this must be accomplished.

At the opposite end of this spectrum is the parent who overly pampers and hovers over his or her child. The child may even have been 'warned' about going to a doctor, or, worse still, led to believe that the child was being taken to a toy store, or that the appointment was for the parent. This bed of dishonesty must be set straight by the ophthalmologist in a forthright, positive manner.

The parent who coaches the child on various aspects of the examination (such as visual acuity measurements) must also be requested to withdraw from the testing process. At times, the parent may even be encouraged to leave the examination room in order to gain more accurate testing of the child.

It must always be remembered that the ophthalmologist's vocation is to care for the patient's particular problem. Even if there is a temptation on the doctor's part to judge what he or she deems to be inappropriate parent–child interaction, it is not the doctor's business unless the child's health is at risk. We must understand that our glimpses of such family dynamics are but fractions of time, and we must remain focused on our vocational responsibilities.

What can the doctor do in a positive manner?

Communication

Communication is a two-way street. It requires listening by both parties, and appropriate discussion. In recent patient surveys by the American Academy of Ophthalmology, listening and discussing a patient's condition was a far more valued trait than efficiency, cost or geographic convenience.

Listening is probably the more difficult half of this equation for clinicians. Traditional medical training spends little time in developing this skill. Listening is particularly complex when the patient is a child, since both the child and the parent deserve to tell the story. Listening takes time, which is a precious commodity for most doctors. A counter argument would be that getting the story straight from the start may ultimately save time.

Communication to the parent and child from the doctor is by more than just words. Is eye contact made? Does the doctor remain standing or get level with the parent and child? What does the doctor's posture or body language communicate? Is the room quiet or chaotic? How often is the doctor interrupted during the examination? What contribution, either negative or positive, is made by the office staff? Words spoken by the ophthalmologist must be directed at the level of the recipient. A canned speech about amblyopia or accommodative esotropia will fall on deaf ears. Simplify to the level of the recipient; even the child can be told what is happening fairly accurately.

At the conclusion of an examination, it is appropriate always to ask if the parent and child have any further questions; give them the final opportunity to have issues clarified.

When the medical news is bad, or difficult for the parents, find something positive to express about the child and the parents; it is extremely rare that bad news cannot be tempered with good. Address the possibility of parental guilt if this has not been raised, for otherwise the parents are erroneously likely to dwell on some action of theirs as the cause for their child's diagnosis.

Tactful challenge

An alert doctor can sense when the doctor–patient/parent relationship is awry. Often, it is appropriate to call attention to this stress, but this must be done with care and tact. The parent should not feel attacked by the clinician. Place the child's interest at the centre of such comments: few parents would be offended by this. Ask the parent if there is anything which the doctor has failed to notice, or if the parent is anxious about something in particular. If you sense that the parent's response might be an explosive one, excuse the child to the toy room after explaining that you need to talk directly with the parents.

In one circumstance, challenge may not be appropriate. When previous actions or history have revealed a particularly violent behaviour, antagonism in any form may precipitate unfortunate events. Everyone is sadly familiar with the irate ex-employee or former customer returning for a shooting spree as an act of revenge. If a doctor ever senses that a similar circumstance is developing, attention must be given immediately for the sake of the patient, other patients, office staff and innocent bystanders. Know where security guards are at your institution and know how they can be reached.

Keep the focus on the child

Much of the problems associated with the uncooperative parent dissipate if the clinician maintains attention on the child. Once the parent sees that his or her child is happy, their own feelings become less important. One cannot appear to ignore the parent, but rather regard the parent as an assistant to your helping the child. In conversations with the parent, remember the child's world, not primarily the parent's expectations.

Insist on parental attendance at the appointments

The importance of attendance at the child's eye appointment must be made clear at the time the appointment is made. The parent needs to know who you are, and establish a level of trust that cannot be made with a telephone conversation afterwards. The parent provides important historical data that cannot be provided by others. The parent acts as the child's surrogate as the clinician administers medicines and performs procedures; without his or her attendance, the ophthalmologist must be very cautious in such actions from a medicolegal standpoint. The parent's attendance should also be important from the child's perspective as a new territory is explored.

When all else fails

Discussion with referring doctor

Most children are sent to an ophthalmologist by a paediatrician or primary care clinician who has identified a possible problem. When an uncooperative parent cannot be dealt with effectively, this doctor may be able to provide some insight into the problem, since presumably he or she has seen the child on many other occasions in the past.

It is appropriate to be forthright with your colleague. Tell this person if there was a particular triggering event (such as a long wait), since this parent will quite likely raise a complaint to him or her about you. Suggest to the referring doctor that another ophthalmologist might be more effective in helping the child if you feel this is the case.

Proper referral and notification

The ophthalmologist does not wish to be placed in the uncomfortable position of abandonment of a patient. Remember that your and the patient's family's definition of this term may vary. Nevertheless, the ophthalmologist does carry a responsibility for the medical care of an individual until confirmation of a change in care has been made.

Always be co-operative with any ophthalmologist that assumes the care of one of your patients. Send previous records, as well as a summary note when indicated. Offer to further discuss if this is ever desired.

When treatment goes badly: the courage to admit failure

Most ophthalmological treatment and surgery carries a good prognosis, but occasionally the results are worse than the doctor hoped for, complications occur, or the results are not up to the parent's expectations. Every ophthalmologist has experienced stony-faced or angry parents who feel the treatment has failed and suspect the doctor is to blame.

There are certain points that may help in this situation.
1 A detailed and frank preoperative discussion of the risks, likely outcomes including any problems that may be transient (such as diplopia, pain, swelling, redness, etc.), and benefits and costs is a vital way of preventing postoperative worry and disappointment. A parent that has been warned before a strabismus operation that a slipped muscle is a recognized complication, should not be angry if his child suffers that problem. Even disastrous complications, such as endophthalmitis, do not necessarily lead to destruction of trust in the doctor if appropriately managed, before and after the operation. Proper informed con-

sent rests on communication with the family, not a form provided by the hospital.

2 A face-to-face preoperative discussion is infinitely preferable to any number of pamphlets or videos. Many parents may perceive the latter as a commercial way of reducing patient–doctor contact time but these methods, in addition to discussion, may help the parent.

3 If the outcome really is bad, it is better to agree than disagree with the parents; then steps can be taken to remedy the situation, and the parents are less likely to be antagonized. All doctors, understandably, have difficulty in handling this situation, but most parents prefer a frank approach.

4 Encourage a second opinion early. Offer names of reputable specialists to the family and indicate your willingness to co-operate fully with other consultants.

5 If a wrong decision has been made, a wrong operation performed (which is not exceptionally rare in strabismus surgery) or an incorrect treatment given, it is vital to be absolutely honest with the parents. Many lawsuits are initiated by the combination of a bad result and suspicion of a cover-up.

6 Do not alter previous medical records in any fashion as this raises suspicion of dishonesty and cover-up. It may be appropriate to add a dated note to the records outlining your immediate thoughts about a case which has not gone well.

Suggested reading

Francis V, Korsch B, Morris M. Gaps in doctor–patient communication. *N Engl J Med* 1969; **280**: 535–40.

Groves JE. Care of the hateful patient. *N Engl J Med* 1978; **298**: 883–7.

Kitchen L. Taking care of the hateful patient. *N Engl J Med* 1978; **299**: 366–7.

Like R, Zyzanski SJ. Patient satisfaction with the clinical encounter: social psychological determinants. *Soc Sci Med* 1987; **24**: 351–7.

Meadow R. Difficult and unlikeable parents. *Arch Dis Child* 1992; **67**: 697–702.

P25: The Uncooperative or Difficult Child

Susan Day

One of the keys to seeing children successfully is the ability of the ophthalmologist to gain a child's trust so that all aspects of an eye examination are obtained. In large part, such trust is reflected in the child's co-operation during the examination. It is inappropriate to see a child and to think automatically that an examination under anaesthesia is appropriate. On the contrary, the child's full attentiveness is essential in order to judge one of our most important parameters—vision.

Any child would much rather have fun and play games than go to a stereotypical doctor's office where pain and needles are the anticipated event. Quite possibly, your patient has never been for an eye examination before. If your room looks different than the child's perception of 'doctor', then the child will likely be at greater ease. You may choose not to wear a starched white coat for similar reasons. If the age of your child patients warrants it, a small toy room is invaluable. Magazines suitable for the older child likewise helps set a positive interaction.

Be sure to make contact with the child as you enter the room. After a brief hello, you may wish to ask the child 'And who did you bring with you?' Such an introduction is also beneficial in preventing a blunder on your part such as 'And is this your grandfather?' when in fact it is the child's father! Next, assure the child that you will be playing 'games'. If appropriate, reassure early that there will be no injections. Give the child a sense of control (examples: Would you like to look at letters or numbers? Do you want the stinging drops or the tickling drops?). Save the bright lights for the last portion of the examination. Chit-chat (What did you learn in school today? What are you going to be when you grow up? Can you tell me a joke?) will keep the child's mind occupied as you go about your business. Use age-appropriate toys during the examination, but remember; 'One toy, one look!'

Rarely is it necessary to enter onto the chart, 'uncooperative'. This comment is certainly not to be used as a reflex entry for a particular age. However, if you are unable to perform some portion of the examination, do *not* enter assumed information, as this is basically inaccurate, misleading for future examinations and medicolegally indefensible.

This chapter offers tips that are rather age-specific. My suggestions are ones that have worked *in general* for *me*. There are many ways of handling these situations. This chapter does not provide the definitive answers in the field of managing uncooperative children.

The uncooperative infant

If an infant is unhappy or fussy because he is in some way uncomfortable, hungry, hurting, wet, dirty or left alone, when these problems are addressed and corrected, you are on your way to an easy examination; if you fail to take the time to attend to them, your examination will be infinitely more difficult.

Probably the most difficult portion of the infant examination occurs when lights are shone in the eyes. The retinoscope is usually less uncomfortable, and touching the infant is usually not necessary. In the older baby who has gained some control of the hands, the 'windmill defence' can usually be mastered by gentle restraint by the parents or by placing a toy in each hand. A to-and-fro motion of the head may then ensue or tight squeezing of the eyelids. Quiet humming, clicking noises or whistling may give you enough additional time to complete your refraction. The fundus examination of the infant tests your skills of gaining co-operation. Line up your indirect lens before you bring the light in line. Lower the rheostat for the initial portion of the examination, as this is better tolerated. If the lids are squeezed tightly shut, try having the baby suck on a pacifier, bottle or while breast feeding if the mother is agreeable. The lids usually relax nicely, and the Bell's reflex is lessened. Get information in a montage fashion; it is better to have four or five quick glimpses of separate regions than one prolonged examination marked by a struggling baby.

The uncooperative 2-year-old

Have you ever been tempted to print up business cards saying 'Specializing in children younger than 18 months and older than 4 years'? The manifestations of the terrrible 2s are certainly found in ophthalmologists' offices.

To examine a 2-year-old, think like a 2-year-old. Play games, be slightly mischievous, and surprise the child who is stuck on saying 'no' by saying that word a few times yourself. Consider even a reverse psychology on some portions of the examination ('I bet you can't show me where the bird is'). Keep tasks simple and quick. Rather than asking a child to identify every picture opto-type on a near vision card, ask for one particular object (such as the bird on each line), and block off all lines except the one you are testing. Alter the tempo of the examination, and take breaks (such as asking the child to give you a 'high five'). Use distance fixation objects if these are available in your office.

At times, a child of this age can become totally inconsolable. Don't fight it. Send the child off to the toy room for a break and try again when calm returns. Take a new tack the second time around, perhaps by whistling, or showing a new toy, or starting out with a different portion of the examination. Whatever you do, do not fight stubbornness from this age with your own stubbornness—you will lose every time!

The uncooperative pre-schooler

Major child–parent interplays seem to surface in this very verbal group of children. This can manifest as a clinging behaviour, as apparent (if not feigned) fear, or as a preset notion that cooperation just isn't going to happen. In many ways, these dynamics are some of the most complex ones to judge and to react to in order to proceed with the examination. Gaining the child's interest in something will often magically set things right. Ask the child to touch his or her head, and then with some of your hidden controls, make the room lights dim or raise the examination chair. Such a small ploy will usually delight the child and restore co-operation.

When you sense that the examination is not going in the right direction, it is sometimes appropriate to turn your attention to the parent. Ask the parent if he or she thinks the child would do better alone (sometimes this works wonders) or if the parent wishes to have a talk with the child alone. Sometimes, the child will do better sitting in the parent's lap.

The pre-schooler who has had previous unpleasant eye examinations may have a memory for a particularly difficult portion of the examination. Usually this is related to the use of eye drops. If this information is volunteered, ask the child if the other doctor used the 'stinging' or the 'tickling' drops. When drops are necessary, administer them yourself. It is very possible that the previous instillation was done by actively restraining the child. I would tend to fight that technique myself!

The uncooperative school-aged child

Poor cooperation in the 6–12-year-old child usually takes a very different form. This lack of cooperation is usually one of claiming that the vision is not good. The underlying reasons for failed vision screening tests and visits for glasses reflects the power of peer pressure in this age group. It seems almost invariable that the child who wants glasses does not need them, and that the child set against wearing glasses is in greatest need (see Chapter 56).

Whether the verdict is to advise or not advise glasses, special care must be taken in breaking such unwelcome news to the patient. Expectations have been built up, and what you say may have a very powerful impact. For the child who has no need but wants them, explain that the eyes are still growing and that it is very possible that glasses will be needed in the future. For the reluctant soon-to-be-bespectacled child, emphasize that the glasses will help the eyes grow stronger, or that a role model (perhaps a parent, teacher or sports hero) wears glasses. If the glasses need not be worn full time, stress that point.

The uncooperative teenager

You too would be uncooperative if you were totally cool, came to the appointment with a waiting room of tiny kids, and risked losing your identity because you were maybe going to get glasses!

Above all, it is critical that the teenager realizes that you are interested in him or her. Talk to the teenager. Once a health history has been taken, ask the teenager if he or she wishes the parent to remain or be excused to the waiting room. Try to find an area which interests the teenager and find out what is happening in his or her life.

Finally, look into this person's ophthalmological future. If you have a policy or a preference for only seeing children up to a certain age, raise this issue with the patient. If referral is appropriate, consider the patient's personality in selecting a future ophthalmologist. If the teenager is off to college, provide names of colleagues in that location who can serve the patient well.

The special needs child

A child with multiple handicaps, developmental delay, hearing impairment, speech problems, and so forth is far too often labelled as an 'uncooperative child'. This sad and inappropriate categorization is cruelly unfair to the child and the family. We have seen a child with the Gilles de la Tourette syndrome who was refused an eye examination because he would not sit still!

Several truths must be followed in such a child.

1 Ask the parent for tips on communication and of what the child is capable of doing. For instance, a child with poor motor skills may be able to see an optotype but not be able to point. However, that same child might be able to shake his or her head 'yes' or 'no' if the small letter is an 'E'.

2 Try. You'll be surprised at the information you can gather, even when others have supposedly said it was not possible. Simply be creative and recognize the importance of your diligence.

3 Treat the child and the parent with respect and with dignity. Chances are very high that both parties have become sophisticated in judging a good doctor, and that they have become jaded by some doctors' attitudes towards their children. This child deserves full attention; if you can find a treatable previously unrecognized limitation (such as a substantial refractive error), you may substantially improve this child's life. The child deserves the very best of care that you can offer.

4 Interact directly with the child: talking, touching, praising. Even the most severely handicapped child, who may appear to have little or no communication with anyone that seems to make any sense, should be spoken to directly, touched, and not ignored or only spoken about through a third party. You will be rewarded with the dividends of a more co-operative child. Parents of these children become connoisseurs of good medical communication and are not slow to sing the praises of the successful communicator!

5 Always find a positive twist to what you see. There is nearly always some good news, and one should concentrate on what the child has got not what he hasn't. Parents of such children receive their share of bad news, and your positive words will be remembered.

6 If appropriate, offer references to social agencies, parents groups, disease-specific societies or consider having families of patients with similar stories talk together, remembering the need to respect confidentiality until permission is granted.

7 On follow-up visits, ask how the child is doing in general terms. Include similar enquiries about the parents or siblings. Remind the parents that they need to take care of themselves and have some independent enjoyment if the special needs child is demanding of time and energy.

The child who becomes blind

Many congenitally blind or partially sighted people go through emotionally difficult times in their lives. The cries of 'why me?', 'it's unfair!' or 'it's my parent's fault!' occur in the lives of nearly every such teenager, often accompanied by aggressive outbursts, depression and withdrawal.

The child with acquired blindness may initially suffer shock, bewilderment and withdrawal once it becomes clear that no treatment is possible. This period may last for several months, and little can be done to avoid it completely, although the length of time that the child suffers this problem, and the severity of the long-term effects, can be ameliorated by appropriate action.

1 Emphasize the usefulness of any residual vision. Try to encourage them to focus on what they have got, not what they have not got.

2 Early mobility training will help them to realize that they aren't going to be totally dependent in the long run. This can, in active older children, include taking part in sport, orienteering, walking and tandem bike riding.

3 After the period of withdrawal, it is advantageous to encourage social contacts with both sighted and non-sighted children of an appropriate age.

4 Associated disorders, such as neurological disease, hearing defects or conditions which impair mobility, need to be remedied as far as possible.

5 Depression, behavioural disorders and manipulative behaviour may need expert psychological or psychiatric management.

6 Attention must be paid to education at an early stage; this may require the child to be registered even before it is certain that recovery is not going to occur.

P26: Hand Defects and the Eye

David Taylor

Polydactyly and retinal dystrophy

Laurence–Moon–Biedl syndrome

The Laurence–Moon and the Bardet–Biedl syndromes are similar but polydactyly and obesity are absent in the Laurence–Moon syndrome. Many authors lump them together as the LMB syndrome.

The most common features are (Bell 1958): retinal dystrophy (93%); obesity (91%); mental retardation, often mild (87%); hypogenitalism (74%); and polydactyly (73%).

It is autosomal recessive. Many cases of incomplete forms have been described and many cases have urological or renal abnormalities, deafness is unusual and diabetes has been described (Escallon *et al.* 1989). The retinal dystrophy may be severe in early life (Schachat & Maumenee 1982; Runge *et al.* 1986) but more frequently presents later in life, usually in the teenages or twenties (Campo & Aaberg 1982; Rizzo *et al.* 1986). Both rods and cones are affected (Jacobson *et al.* 1990). In the early stages there is no pigment clumping; the retina has a nearly normal appearance despite a severely abnormal electroretinogram (Runge *et al.* 1986). The prognosis is highly variable and unpredictable, with some cases showing little deterioration over many years (Rizzo *et al.* 1986), others becoming rapidly worse (Runge *et al.* 1986; Fulton *et al.* 1993).

The retinal defect seems to be primarily in the photoreceptor cells (Runge *et al.* 1986). The gene has been linked to 16q (Kwitek-Black *et al.* 1993).

Biemond's syndrome

Biemond described a syndrome similar to LMB with short stature, iris coloboma, mental retardation, obesity, hypogenitalism and polydactyly. Schachat and Maumenee (1982) found four other cases in the literature. It is probably autosomal recessive.

Alström's syndrome

Alström's syndrome (Alström *et al.* 1959) is not usually associated with polydactyly although Alström described an unaffected relative with an extra digit. Alström's syndrome comprises diabetes mellitus, acanthosis nigricans, hypogenitalism, obesity, nerve deafness and a retinal dystrophy that is somewhat different to retinitis pigmentosa (Sebag *et al.* 1984): it may start as a cone dysfunction and progresses to involve the whole retina (Tremblay *et al.* 1993). It is autosomal recessive (see Chapters 44 and P15).

Jeune's syndrome (asphyxiating thoracic dystrophy)

These children are born with hypoplastic lungs and rib cage abnormalities that often lead to asphyxia and death. If they survive they are of moderate short stature with short thumbs. Renal dystrophy (Donaldson *et al.* 1985), hepatic changes and a retinal dystrophy (Bard *et al.* 1978; Allen *et al.* 1979; Phillips *et al.* 1979; Wilson *et al.* 1987) also occur. Postaxial polydactyly is an inconstant feature. It is autosomal recessive.

Ellis–Van Creveld syndrome

In this autosomal recessive disease postaxial polydactyly of the hands and occasionally the feet is a constant feature together with hypoplastic nails, small thorax, heart defect, and short upper lip with multiple frenulae. Cases described as having retinal disease probably represent cases of Jeune's syndrome (Calver *et al.* 1981; Brueton *et al.* 1990).

Albrechtson's syndrome

Albrechtson (1956) described two siblings with ectrodactyly, syndactyly, hypotrichiasis and retinal dystrophy.

Acrocephaly syndactyly syndromes

Apert's syndrome type I

This autosomal dominant syndrome occurs in about 1 in 100 000 live births. They have very shallow orbits, craniosynostosis, optic atrophy, brain defects (Teng *et al.* 1989), eye movement defects (Pollard 1988), strabismus; syndactyly and polydactyly of the toes are characteristic features.

Carpenter's syndrome type II

The main features include preaxial (thumb or big toe side) or postaxial (little finger or little toe side) polydactyly, brachycephaly with synostosis, shallow supraorbital ridges, laterally placed inner canthi, obesity, and mental retardation (Carpenter 1901; Temtamy 1966; Robinson *et al.* 1984; Cohen 1989). It is autosomal recessive.

Pfeiffer's syndrome type V

This dominant syndrome has craniostenosis, broad thumbs and toes, variable syndactyly and occasionally polydactyly or a bifid hallus. Coloboma of the optic nerve, choroid and retina have been described (Pfeiffer & Mayer 1987).

Greig's syndrome

In this autosomal dominant syndrome, a high forehead and frontal bossing are associated with a broad base to the nose and hypertelorism (Baraitser *et al.* 1983). It maps to 7p13 (Brueton *et al.* 1988).

Polydactyly with colobomatous defects

Meckel–Gruber syndrome

This autosomal recessive syndrome includes an occipital encephalocoele, coloboma, microphthalmos, cleft palate, polycystic kidneys and abnormal genitalia with polydactyly (Hsia *et al.* 1971; Altmann *et al.* 1977; Salomen & Norio 1984; various authors 1984).

Goltz syndrome

See Chapter 50.

Sorsby's syndrome

This dominantly inherited syndrome was reported by Sorsby (1935) with a follow-up by Thompson and Baraitser (1988). They have brachydactyly, polydactyly or bifid thumb and macular or optic nerve colobomas.

Buntinx and Majewski's syndrome

This syndrome includes blepharophimosis, iris coloboma, mental retardation, polydactyly, aplasia of the corpus callosum and hydroureter.

Joubert's syndrome

See Chapters 44, 50 and 64. Joubert's syndrome may be associated with postaxial polydactyly, a retinal dystrophy (King *et al.* 1984; Houdou *et al.* 1986) and uveal coloboma (Lindhout *et al.* 1980; Pfeiffer 1981).

Polydactyly with glaucoma

Rubinstein–Taybi syndrome

This probably autosomal recessive syndrome is characterized by broad thumbs and great toes which may occasionally be bifid giving polydactyly. The maxillae are hypoplastic and the palpebral fissures downward slanted. Ocular abnormalities include epicanthic folds, keratoglobus (Nelson & Talbot 1989), strabismus, refractive error, cataract, coloboma (Roy *et al.* 1968; Filippi 1972; Volker & Haase 1975) and glaucoma (Levi 1976). The glaucoma may occur mainly in association with anterior segment dysplasia. It is said that Scoline should be avoided in these children (Stirt 1982).

Oculodentodigital dysplasia syndrome

In this autosomal dominant condition there is anterior segment dysgenesis with glaucoma (Dudgeon & Chisholm 1974; Judisch *et al.* 1979; Traboulsi & Park 1990). The eyes are microphthalmic and they may have cataracts. There is syndactyly of three, four and five digits, and polydactyly of the toes. They have dental enamel hypoplasia, hypotrichosis and a small nose with hypoplastic alae.

Polydactyly with cataract

Smith–Lemli–Opitz syndrome

This not uncommon autosomal recessive syndrome features a broad nasal tip with anteverted nostrils, moderate or severe mental retardation, microcephaly, ptosis, epicanthus, strabismus, cataract (Kretzer *et al.* 1981; Bardelli *et al.* 1985), post-lenticular membrane (Freedman & Baum 1979) and sclerocornea (Harbin *et al.* 1977). Abnormal levels of 7-dehydrocholesterol are the diagnostic feature (Irons *et al.* 1994; Opitz & de la Cruz 1994).

Lenz microphthalmos syndrome

See Chapters 20 and 50 (Van Dorp & Dellenan 1979).

Killian Pallister syndrome

In this syndrome the skin chromosomes are tetrasomic for the short arm of chromosome 12. They have coarse features with a broad forehead, hypertelorism, sagging cheeks and mouth, a bifid hallux or polydactyly, aniridia and catarct.

Martsolf's syndrome

See Chapter 39.

Schachat and Maumenee's patient

Schachat and Maumenee (1982) described a patient with congenital cataracts, mental retardation, obesity, hypogenitalism, skull deformities and polydactyly.

Hand anomalies with miscellaneous conditions with ocular manifestations

Thalidomide embryopathy

Duane's syndrome, gaze palsy, strabismus, coloboma and cataract (Papst 1963; Cullen 1964; Zetterstrom 1966; Treischmann 1973) are the most frequent ocular features of this syndrome with phocomelia, bifid thumbs and polydactyly as well as numerous multisystem manifestations.

Fetal alcohol syndrome

Ectrodactyly (Herrmann *et al.* 1980), congenital hypotonia, low birth weight, microcephaly, short palpebral fissures and a thin, smooth upper lip, heart defects and cleft lip occur in this syndrome which is recognized with increasing frequency.

Duane's syndrome (Holzman *et al.* 1990), optic nerve hypoplasia, Peters' anomaly and chorioretinal atrophy are the ocular features (Stromland 1985, 1987; Chan *et al.* 1991).

Maternal diabetes

Pre- or post-axial polydactyly occurs with a wide variety of neural tube (optic nerve hypoplasia; see Chapter 50), cardiac, renal and intestinal anomalies.

Möbius syndrome

Möbius syndrome has been described with syndactyly, polydactyly and brachydactyly (see Chapter 66).

Acrorenal ocular syndrome

Halil *et al.* (1984) described seven members of a family with acral anomalies, renal ectopia, colobomas and Duane's syndrome.

Papilla nigra

This consists of dermolipoma, cleft palate and an extra thumb (Wolter *et al.* 1971).

LADD syndrome

LADD is an acronym for lacrimo-auriculodentodigital syndrome. These children have autosomal dominantly inherited punctal atresia, cup-shaped ears, deafness, hypoplastic teeth, polydactyly, clinodactyly or finger-like thumbs (Thompson *et al.* 1985).

Basal cell naevus (Gorlin's) syndrome

Medullated nerve fibres in the fundus (De Jong *et al.* 1985) seems to be a frequent feature of this autosomal dominant syndrome with multiple basal cell carcinoma, jaw cysts, and falx calcification: it maps to 9q22.3–q31 (Chevenix-Trench *et al.* 1993). There is pre- or post-axial polydactyly.

Myopia and vitreous veils

Postaxial polydactyly with myopia, vitreous veils, optic atrophy, Fuchs' corneal dystrophy and choroidal atrophy (Cziezel & Brooser 1986).

Fraser's syndrome

See Chapters 20, 21 and 26.

Polydactyly with chromosome defects

Trisomy 13

Polydactyly is a constant feature of the trisomy 13 syndrome. It is a syndrome which is usually fatal in the first days or months of life. Other features are coloboma, microphthalmos, glaucoma and retinal dysplasia (Zimmerman & Font 1966; Hoepner *et al.* 1972; Ginsberg & Bove 1974; Lichter & Schmickel 1975).

Partial trisomy 10q

Although camptodactyly (bent finger) is the more frequent finding, extra digits are a feature of 10q partial trisomy together with severe mental and growth deficiency, and microcephaly. A variety of ocular defects have been described including narrow palpebral fissures, microphthalmos, anti-mongoloid slant and cataract (Jay 1977).

References

Albrechtson B. Hypotrichosis; syndactyly and retinal degeneration. *Acta Dermatol Venereol* 1956; **36**: 96–101.

Allen AW, Moon JB, Hovland KR, Minckler DS. Ocular findings in thoracic-pelvic-phalangeal dystrophy. *Arch Ophthalmol* 1979; **97**: 489–92.

Alström CH, Hallgren B, Nilson LB *et al.* Retinal degeneration combined with obesity, diabetes mellitus and deafness. *Acta Psychiatr Neurol Scand* 1959; **129**: 1–35.

Altmann P, Wegenbichler P, Schaller A. A causistic report on the Gruber or Meckel syndrome. *Hum Genet* 1977; **38**: 357–63.

Baraitser M, Winter R, Brett EM. Greig cephalopolysyndactyly: report of 13 affected individuals in three families. *Clin Genet* 1983; **24**: 257–65.

Bard LA, Bard PA, Owens GW, Hall BD. Retinal involvement in thoracic-pelvic-phalangeal dystrophy. *Arch Ophthalmol* 1978; **96**: 278–81.

Bardelli AM, Lasonella G, Barberi L, Vanni M. Ocular manifestations in Kneist syndrome, Smith–Lemli–Opitz syndrome, Hallermann–Streiff–François syndrome, Rubinstein–Taybi syndrome and median cleft face syndrome. *Ophthalmol Paediatr Genet* 1985; **6**: 343–7.

Bell J. The Laurence–Moon syndrome. In: Enrose LS (ed.) *The Treasury of Human Inheritance*. London: Cambridge University Press, 1958; 51–69.

Brueton LA, Dutton MJ, Winter RM. Ellis van Creveld syndrome, Jeune syndrome and renal-hepatic-pancreatic syndrome: separate entities or disease spectrum? *J Med Genet* 1990; **27**: 252–5.

Brueton L, Huson S, Winter R, Williamson R. Chromosomal localisation of a developmental gene in man: direct DNA analysis demonstrates that Greig cephalopolysyndactyly maps to 7p13. *Am J Med Genet* 1988; **31**: 799–804.

Buntinx I, Majewski F. A new syndrome? Blepharophimosis, iris coloboma, microgenita, hearing loss, postaxial polydactyly, aplasia of the corpus callosum, hydroureter and developmental delay. *Am J Med Genet* 1990; **36**: 273–4.

Calver D, Keast-Butler J, Taylor D. The extra digit. *Trans Ophthalmol Soc UK* 1981; **101**: 35–8.

Campo RV, Aaberg TM. Bardet–Biedl syndrome. *Am J Ophthalmol* 1982; **94**: 750–6.

Carpenter G. Two sisters sharing malformation of the skull and other congenital abnormalities. *Rep Soc Study Dis Child London* 1901; **1**: 110.

Chan J, Bowell R, O'Keefe M, Lanigan B. Ocular manifestations in fetal alcohol syndrome. *Br J Ophthalmol* 1991; **75**: 524–6.

Chevnix-Trench G, Wicking C, Berkman J *et al.* Further localisation of the gene for naevoid basal cell carcinomal syndrome (NBCCS) in 15 Australian families: linkage and loss of heterozygosity. *Am J Hum Genet* 1993; **53**: 760–7.

Cohen MM Jr. A comprehensive and critical assessment of overgrowth and the overgrowth syndromes: Carpenter syndrome. *Adv Hum Genet* 1989; **18**: 282.

Cullen JF. Ocular defects in thalidomide babies. *Br J Ophthalmol* 1964; **48**: 151–5.

Cziezel A, Brooser G. A postaxial polydactyly and progressive myopia syndrome of autosomal dominant origin. *Clin Genet* 1986; **30**: 406–8.

De Jong PTVM, Bistervels B, Cosgrove J, de Grip G, Leys A, Goffin M. Medullated nerve fibres. A sign of multiple basal cell naevi (Gorlin's) syndrome. *Arch Ophthalmol* 1985; **103**: 1833–6.

Donaldson MDC, Wamer AA, Trompeter RS, Haycock CB, Chantler C. Familial juvenile nephronopthisis, Jeune's syndrome, and associated disorders. *Arch Dis Child* 1985; **60**: 426–34.

Dudgeon J, Chisholm JA. Oculo-dento-digital dysplasia. *Trans Ophthalmol Soc UK* 1974; **94**: 203–10.

Escallon F, Traboulsi EI, Infante F. A family with the Bardet–Biedl syndrome and diabetes mellitus. *Arch Ophthalmol* 1989; **107**: 855–8.

Filipi G. The Rubinstein–Taybi syndrome. Report of seven cases. *Clin Genet* 1972; **3**: 303–18.

Freedman RA, Baum JL. Postlenticular membrane associated with Smith–Lemli–Opitz syndrome. *Am J Ophthalmol* 1979; **87**: 675–7.

Fulton A, Hansen R, Glynn R. Natural course of visual functions in the Bardet–Biedl syndrome. *Arch Ophthalmol* 1993; **111**: 1500–6.

Ginsberg J, Bove KE. Ocular pathology of trisomy 13. *Ann Ophthalmol (Chicago)* 1974; **6**: 113–22.

Halil F, Homsy M, Perreault G. Acrorenal ocular syndrome: autosomal dominant thumb hypoplasia, renal ectopia and eye defect. *Am J Med Genet* 1984; **17**: 753–62.

Harbin RL, Katz JI, Frias JL, Rabinowicz IM, Kaufman HE. Sclerocornea associated with the Smith–Lemli–Opitz syndrome. *Am J Ophthalmol* 1977; **84**: 72–4.

Herrmann J, Pallister PD, Opitz JM. Tetraectrodactyly and other skeletal manifestations in the fetal alcohol syndrome. *Eur J Paediatr* 1980; **133**: 221–6.

Hoepner J, Yanoff M. Ocular anomalies in trisomy 13–15. *Am J Ophthalmol* 1972; **74**: 729–37.

Holzman AE, Chrousos GA, Kozma C, Traboulsi E. Duane's retraction syndrome in the fetal alcohol syndrome (letter). *Am J Ophthalmol* 1990; **110**: 565–6.

Houdou S, Ohno K, Takashina S, Takeshita K. Joubert syndrome associated with unilateral ptosis and Leber's congenital amaurosis. *Paediatr Neurol* 1986; **2**: 102–5.

Hsia YE, Bratu M, Herbordt A. Genetics of the Meckel syndrome. *Pediatrics* 1971; **48**: 237–47.

Irons M, Elias ER, Tint GS et al. Abnormal cholesterol metabolism in the Smith–Lemli–Opitz syndrome: report of clinical and biochemical findings in four patients and treatment in one patient. *Am J Med Genet* 1994; **50**: 347–52.

Jacobson SG, Borruat F-X, Apáthy PP. Patterns of rod and cone dysfunction in Bardet–Biedl syndrome. *Am J Ophthalmol* 1990; **109**: 676–89.

Jay M. *The Eye in Chromosome Duplications and Deficiencies.* New York: Marcel Dekker, 1977.

Judisch GF, Martin-Casals A, Hanson JW, Olin WH. Oculodentodigital dysplasia: four new reports and a literature review. *Arch Ophthalmol* 1979; **97**: 878–84.

King MD, Dudgeon J, Stephenson JBP. Joubert's syndrome with retinal dysplasia: neonatal tachypnoea as the clue to a genetic brain–eye malformation. *Arch Dis Child* 1984; **59**: 709–18.

Kretzer FL, Hittner HM, Mehta RS. Ocular manifestations of the Smith–Lemli–Opitz syndrome. *Arch Ophthalmol* 1981; **99**: 2000–6.

Kwitek-Black A, Carmi R, Duyk G et al. Linkage of Bardet–Biedl syndrome to chromosome 16q and evidence for non-allelic heterogeneity. *Nature Genet* 1993; **5**: 392–6.

Levi NS. Juvenile glaucoma in Rubinstein–Taybi syndrome. *J Pediatr Ophthalmol Strabismus* 1976; **13**: 141–3.

Lichter PR, Schmickel RD. Posterior vortex vein and glaucoma in a patient with trisomy 13 syndrome. *Am J Ophthalmol* 1975; **80**: 939–42.

Lindhout D, Barth PG, Volk J, Boen-Tan TN. The Joubert syndrome associated with bilateral chorioretinal colobomas. *Eur J Paediatr* 1980; **134**: 173–6.

Nelson ME, Talbot JF. Keratoglobus in the Rubinstein–Taybi syndrome. *Br J Ophthalmol* 1989; **73**: 385–7.

Opitz JM, de la Cruz F. Cholesterol metabolism in the RSH/Smith–Lemli–Opitz syndrome: summary of an NIHD conference. *Am J Med Genet* 1994; **50**: 326–38.

Papst W. Thalidomid und kongenitale Anomalies der Augen. *Dtsch Ophthalmol Ges* 1963; **65**: 209–15.

Pfeiffer RA. The Joubert syndrome associated with bilateral chorioretinal coloboma (letter). *Eur J Paediatr* 1981; **137**: 101–2.

Pfeiffer RA, Mayer U. Growth retardation, mental deficiency and type I preaxial polydactyly with colobomatous anomalies—a new syndrome. *Klin Mbl Augenheilkd* 1987; **191**: 473–7.

Phillips CI, Stokoe NK, Bartholomew RS. Asphyxiating thoracic dystrophy. *J Pediatr Ophthalmol Strabismus* 1979; **16**: 279–83.

Pollard ZF. Bilateral superior oblique muscle palsy associated with Apert's syndrome. *Am J Ophthalmol* 1988; **186**: 337–40.

Rizzo JF, Berson EL, Lessell S. Retinal and neurologic findings in the Laurence–Moon–Bardet–Biedl phenotype. *Ophthalmology* 1986; **93**: 1452–6.

Robinson LK, James HE, Mubarak S, Allen EJ, Jones KL. Carpenter syndrome: natural history and clinical spectrum. *Am J Med Genet* 1985; **20**: 461–9.

Roy FH, Summitt RL, Hiall RL, Hughes JG. Ocular manifestations of the Rubinstein–Taybi syndrome. *Arch Ophthalmol* 1968; **79**: 292–8.

Runge P, Calver D, Marshall J, Taylor D. Histopathology of mitochondrial cytopathy and the Laurence–Moon–Biedl syndrome. *Br J Ophthalmol* 1986; **70**: 782–96.

Salomen R, Norio R. The Meckel syndrome in Finland. *Am J Med Genet* 1984; **18**: 691–8.

Schachat AP, Maumenee IM. Bardet–Biedl syndrome and related disorders. *Arch Ophthalmol* 1982; **100**: 285–8.

Schinzel A. Syndrome of the month: tetrasomy 12p (Pallister Killian syndrome). *J Med Genet* 1991; **28**: 122–5.

Sebag J, Albert DM, Croft JL. The Alstrom syndrome: ophthalmic histopathology and retinal ultrastructure. *Br J Ophthalmol* 1984; **68**: 494–501.

Sorsby A. Congenital coloboma of the macula, together with an account of the familial occurrence of bilateral macular coloboma in association with apical dystrophy of the hands and feet. *Br J Ophthalmol* 1935; **19**: 65–90.

Stirt JA. Succinylcholine in Rubinstein–Taybi syndrome. *Anaesthesiology* 1982; **57**: 49.

Stromland K. Ocular abnormalities in the fetal alcohol syndrome. *Acta Ophthalmol* 1985; **63** (Suppl.): 171.

Stromland K. Ocular involvement in the fetal alcohol syndrome. *Surv Ophthalmol* 1987; **31**: 277–84.

Temtamy SA. Carpenter's syndrome. *J Pediatr* 1966; **69**: 111–20.

Teng R-J, Wang P-J, Shen Y-Z. Apert syndrome with septooptic dysplasia. *Paediatr Neurol* 1989; **5**: 384–8.

Thompson E, Pembury M, Graham JM. Phenotypic variation in the LADD syndrome. *J Med Genet* 1985; **22**: 382–5.

Thompson EM, Baraitser M. Sorsby syndrome: a report on further generations of the original family. *J Med Genet* 1988; **25**: 313–21.

Traboulsi EI, Parks MM. Glaucoma in oculo-dento-osseous dysplasia. *Am J Ophthalmol* 1990; **109**: 310–13.

Tremblay F, LaRoche R, Shea S, Ludman M. Longitudinal study of the early electroretinographic changes in Alström's syndrome. *Am J Ophthalmol* 1993; **115**: 657–65.

Trieschmann W. Krokodilstränen bei Conterganschäden. *Klin Monatsbl Augenheilk* 1973; **162**: 546–50.

Van Dorp D, Delleman JW. A family with X chromosomal recessive congenital cataracts, microphthalmia, a peculiar form of the ear and dental anomalies. *J Pediatr Ophthalmol Strabismus* 1979; **16**: 166–71.

Various authors. The Meckel symposium. *Am J Med Genet* 1984; **18**: 649–711.

Volker HE, Haase W. Augensymptomatik bein RT syndrome. *Klin Monatsbl Augenheilkd* 1975; **167**: 478–83.

Wilson DJ, Weleber RG, Beals RK. Retinal dystrophy in Jeune's syndrome. *Arch Ophthalmol* 1987; **105**: 651–7.

Wolter JR, Johnson FD, Lewis RA. Papita nigra associated with dermolipoma of the orbit, cleft palate and an extra thumb. *J Pediatr* 1971; **8**: 119–22.

Zetterstrom B. Ocular malformations caused by thalidomide. *Acta Ophthalmol* 1966; **44**: 391–5.

Zimmerman LE, Font RL. Trisomy 13. *J Am Med Assoc* 1966; **196**: 694–7.

P27: Contact Lens Management Problems

Lynne Speedwell

Many conditions in infancy and childhood can benefit from contact lenses for refractive, cosmetic and therapeutic reasons, but all contact lenses are foreign bodies and can induce adverse corneal and conjunctival changes. Extended or overnight wear is therefore not desirable and it is safer to remove lenses where possible overnight. Many parents are nervous of dealing with their children's lenses especially in a resistant infant. With time, however, most overcome their fears.

The care regime needs to be simple and effective and strict hygiene stressed from the outset. Solutions likely to cause an allergic response should be avoided; hence, should a red eye ensue, allergy need not be suspected.

A cardinal rule is that if the eye becomes red, weepy, sore or will not open, then the lens must be removed immediately and the eye examined by an ophthalmologist.

Aphakia

General observations

Aphakia is the most common indication for contact lenses in infancy. It is important when refracting the aphakic infant that care is taken to achieve the correct power of the lens; a +20.00 DS spectacle lens held 16 mm from the eye requires a +29.41 DS in contact lens. Because infants are mainly interested in their immediate environment, they are overcorrected by 2–3 dioptres. The power of the first lens required by the infant aphake is typically +32.00 DS. As the child grows the overcorrection is reduced such that by school age the patient is often wearing a distance contact lens correction with bifocal spectacles for close work.

Spectacles

The high prescriptions needed by an infant aphake make it difficult to centre spectacles on a small face (Fig. P27.1) and the field is greatly reduced.

Contact lenses

Contact lenses may provide a better optical correction than spectacles but the inherent risks incurred are similar to those in an adult: epitheliopathy, chronic hypoxia, contact lens associated papillary conjunctivitis, giant papillary conjunctivitis and endothelial changes (Epstein 1991): the removal of lenses on a daily basis reduces the complications (Neumann *et al.* 1993). Poor hygiene is also a possible cause of infection. Reports of extended wear contact lens complications vary from 14% (Levin *et al.* 1988) to zero (Nelson *et al.* 1985) and differing numbers of lenses are lost or need replacement (Jacobs 1991), varying with the type of lens. Patients are more likely to fail with contact lens wear due to poor vision from amblyopia than due to complications (Moore 1993). Regular aftercare is essential to monitor any changes and alter the contact lenses or solutions accordingly, and it is important to provide back-up spectacles to avoid extended periods without correction.

It is not practical to fit bifocal contact lenses to a young child as most lenses of this type do not provide optimum acuity for both distance and near. This is especially so with soft bifocal lenses, but also applies to gas-permeable lenses (Conklin *et al.* 1992).

Comparison of different forms of aphakic correction

For infants the advantages of contact lenses or spectacles over intraocular lenses or epikeratophakia are substantial.

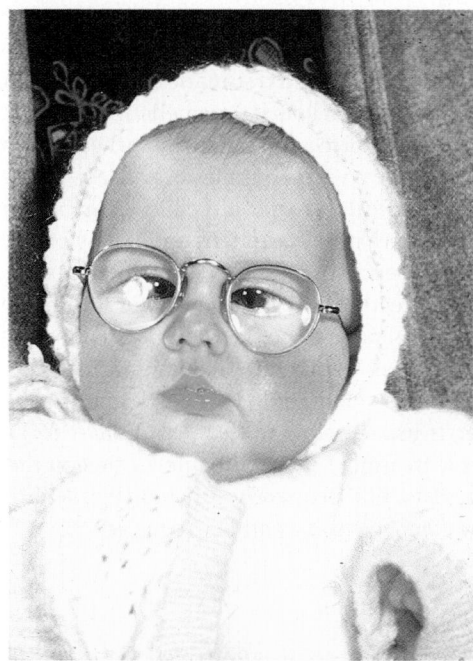

Fig. P27.1 The difficulties of centering aphakic spectacles on a small face.

1 They can both be easily altered as the child's eyes grow. There is a massive reduction in power from the first few weeks of life to that needed by a 2-year-old. Contact lens power can decrease from +34.00 to +18.00 DS during that period (Morris 1979) due to an increasing axial length and flattening corneal curvature (Gordon & Donzis 1985).

2 Emmetropization of the eyes can continue in some children who, were it not for their aphakia, would have been myopic. For example, many phakic children with Down's syndrome are myopic. A prescription for such children who are aphakic can be as little as +5.00 DS; if they had been given an implant as an infant they could develop up to −12.00 dioptres of myopia. (A myopic shift may be a sign of glaucoma.)

3 Aphakes with poor visual acuity derive benefit from the magnifying effects of spectacles; this can enhance an acuity of say, 6/60 vision to 6/36 or even 6/24. Many such aphakes are keen to use their spectacles for school or work and to wear their contact lenses socially. Patients with an intraocular lens lose this advantage.

4 Intraocular lens implantation and epikeratophakia in infants carry risks (Arkin *et al.* 1992) and their long-term safety is still unknown. Epikeratophakia grafts are slow to clear, promoting amblyopia. Baker *et al.* (1990) compared different forms of paediatric aphakic correction: they concluded that contact lenses were the best option and stated that intraocular lenses and epikeratophakias should be reserved for older, unilateral aphakes or for non-compliant contact lens wearers.

5 In traumatic aphakia corrected with an intraocular lens

or epikeratophakia, a cosmetic contact lens may still be necessary.

Specific types of contact lenses

There are three types of lenses: hydrogel (soft) with water contents ranging from 38 to 80%, silicone rubber and rigid gas-permeable (RGP)—both corneal and scleral. The original hard (polymethyl methacrylate, PMMA) lenses are rarely used now as a first option.

Hydrogel lenses are the least expensive and probably the easiest lenses to fit. It is most common, in the initial stages, to fit lenses of high water content (70–80%), as these can be worn during sleep and they have the highest oxygen permeability. They are fitted empirically on known average keratometry readings (Weale 1982; Amaya *et al.* 1990; Speedwell 1996) approximately 2 mm larger than the visible iris diameter. In soft lens form, a +32.00 DS lens is very thick and even in high water content material, extended wear of these lenses can induce corneal hypoxia. Soft lenses are also the most likely of all the types to lead to infection (Epstein 1991) and neovascularization (Arentsen 1986) and this is exacerbated when lenses are worn overnight, especially on microphthalmic or scarred corneas. Although soft lenses are cheap, costs can mount as many lenses are lost or broken in the first 2 years of life.

Silicone rubber lenses are more expensive, but more durable. They are fitted approximately 0.40 mm flatter than average keratometry measurements and 0.70 mm larger than horizontal visible iris diameter. The fit of the lenses is checked using fluorescein and hence any epithelial stain can be seen at the same time. Although the lenses are fitted flat, they rarely cause epithelial damage (Cutler *et al.* 1985). Silicone rubber lenses are much more difficult to rub out and fewer lenses are lost. They have extremely high oxygen permeability (Dk value) allowing almost 100% oxygen transmission, thus the risk of hypoxia is much less than with soft lenses.

Silicone rubber lenses are more complicated to fit and care must be taken to allow them as long as an hour to settle before ordering (Fig. P27.2); a lens that initially fits well may tighten with wear making it difficult to remove. The material itself is hydrophobic; and the surface is coated to make it comfortable. If scratched, it no longer wets properly leading to surface deposits and accumulation of mucus, which is uncomfortable (Harris 1985; Nelson *et al.* 1985). Surface degradation can take several months. Silicone rubber cannot be made with an ultraviolet inhibitor in the polymer. Both soft and RGP lenses can incorporate an ultraviolet inhibitor and this may prove more beneficial in reducing long-term retinal damage.

RGP lenses are able to correct nearly all corneal astigmatism. The amounts of corneal astigmatism are usually small after lensectomy and mostly corrected by the thickness of the material in both soft and silicone rubber lenses.

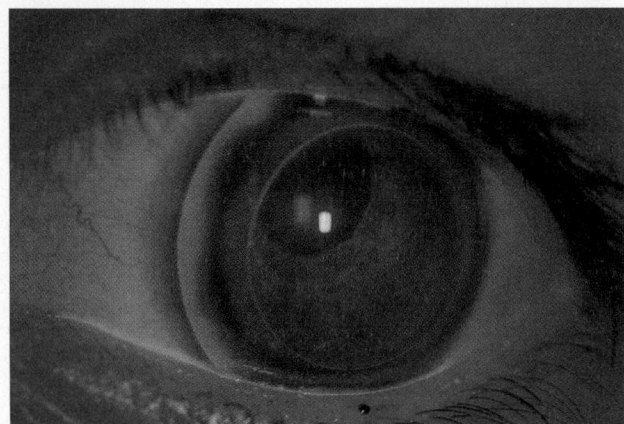

Fig. P27.2 Fluorescein picture of a silicone rubber lens. (Note stand-off at edges and flat central fit.)

Originally, PMMA lenses were fitted (Pratt-Johnson & Tillson 1985) but RGP materials with a high Dk value are now preferred. The initial fitting of these lenses can be difficult and infants are often fitted under general anaesthesia. However, lenses can be fitted empirically, in a similar way to soft lenses, according to age (Saunders & Ellis 1981) or, alternatively, keratometry readings are taken whilst the child is anaesthetized and the lens fitted at follow-up a few days later (Amos *et al.* 1992). With a portable, hand-held, automated keratometer, it is possible to obtain readings on the awake or sleeping child and the fitting can be carried out accordingly (Speedwell 1996). The lens material chosen should have a high Dk and the lens fit should not produce excessive edge clearance so there is less risk of decentration.

Scleral lenses can be fitted by the impression method, which must be done under anaesthetic, or, using pre-formed lenses made up as +30.00 DS in an RGP material, they can be fitted to the awake child and modified to the correct power (Ezekiel 1995). The disadvantages of these lenses are that they are very costly and need specialist equipment and expertise to modify them. However, they are relatively easy for the parents to handle, rarely lost from the eye and they can be polished or modified several times as the prescription alters.

Unilateral aphakia

The aphakic eye is usually densely amblyopic and the phakic eye must be extensively patched to achieve reasonable vision (see Chapters 39 and P28). With early surgery, adequate contact lens correction and a rigorous patching regime, good visual results are achievable (Birch & Stager 1988). Even where the vision is poor, a contact lens may reduce the angle of strabismus (Pollard 1991).

Traumatic aphakia and corneal laceration

In corneal lacerations and traumatic aphakia, scars may be unsightly, requiring a lens for cosmetic and visual reasons. RGP lenses will correct the irregular corneal astigmatism and give optimum vision but they are not always accepted at first. In a typical 2–4-year-old child it can be extremely difficult to insert any type of lens and it may be necessary to prescribe spectacles initially, with a patch over the good eye, and proceed to a contact lens later. If, however, the vision remains poor or contact lens wear impossible, an intraocular lens or epikeratophakia graft may be considered once the eye has settled. The epikeratophakic graft, however, is usually slow to clear (Halliday 1990) making amblyopic treatment more difficult. Occlusion therapy is still necessary but frequently resisted (Elsas 1990) and a cosmetic contact lens may still be required.

Dislocated lenses

Unoperated patients with subluxated lenses usually have a high degree of myopic astigmatism but if the lens has dislocated they may be effectively aphakic. Anisometropia is most easily corrected with contact lenses.

It has been found that after surgery, the vision can slowly improve (Speedwell & Russell-Eggitt 1995).

In patients with Marfan's syndrome, both the corneal diameter and the radius of curvature (mm) are often increased. Horizontal visible iris diameter can be as high as 13.00 mm and it is not uncommon to have keratometry readings flatter than 9.30 mm (Maumenee 1981). As a result, fitting of lenses may be difficult, especially RGP lenses, as all lenses tend to drop down on the cornea. Soft lenses may centre better (Speedwell & Russell-Eggitt 1994).

Corneal transplants

Whilst keratoplasty is not often carried out in young children because of its limited success (Stulting *et al.* 1984), when performed, the postoperative refractive correction is often highly astigmatic and may need to be corrected with a high Dk RGP lens. Aftercare visits should be more frequent than usual, in order to ensure that the transplant is not being compromised by the lens.

High myopia—unilateral and bilateral

Children with high degrees of myopia may benefit from wearing contact lenses. The size of objects is larger with contact lenses than with spectacles and hence the measured visual acuity is better but the field is not enhanced.

Unilateral myopes with a contact lens often require occlusion for amblyopia. Myopia in children is usually axial (Sorsby *et al.* 1962; Grosvenor & Scott 1993) and since aniseikonia is less for both axial and refractive anisometropia when contact lenses are employed (Winn *et al.* 1986), better stereopsis should develop if lenses can be prescribed early. Congenital high myopia is often associated with dense amblyopia and the visual acuity may gradually improve with time.

Soft lenses for myopes are very thin centrally and they can be difficult to insert; rigid lenses may be better. If the child is very upset when trial contact lens fitting is attempted, it may be prudent to delay fitting until they are older.

Other refractive conditions

It is not usual to fit contact lenses to young children who are hypermetropic. Hypermetropic esotropes or children presenting with hypermetropia as part of an ocular condition such as retinal dystrophy have few problems with spectacles. If the child will not wear their glasses, they are unlikely to accept contact lenses. Similarly, parents who are unable to convince their child of the need for glasses are not always the most rigorous at following cleaning instructions.

In microphthalmos with higher refractive errors, contact lenses can be beneficial.

Cosmetic lenses

The child with unsightly anterior segment conditions may derive great benefit from wearing cosmetic lenses which may help parents come to terms with their child's disfigurement, and both the child and the family may be helped (Fig. P27.3). Young children are often resistant to having a cosmetic lens inserted but when older they are more likely to be well motivated.

It is important to differentiate between an eye that is likely to develop useful vision and one that is not. In a stable and comfortable eye that is incapable of any useful sight, it is better to start cosmetic lens fitting as young as possible so that the difficulties likely to be encountered in a more active toddler are avoided and the child is used to having the lens inserted from an early age. For a small blind or phthisical eye, a cosmetic shell is a better choice. If the condition is progressive, it is not always possible to start lens fitting at an early age. In such cases it is safer to wait until the eye has stabilized, at which time the decision should be based on the child's reaction to lens insertion. If the experience is too traumatic, it is better to wait until the child is older.

In an eye that is likely to develop useful vision, extra care must be taken to avoid the undesirable reactions to contact lenses, which tend to occur more frequently in an already compromised cornea: neovascularization, punctate epithelial erosions, and so on. A clear lens should be fitted first and the fit assessed. After about a month of

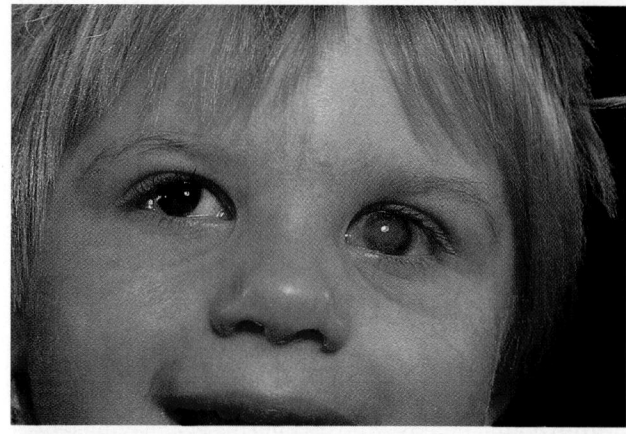
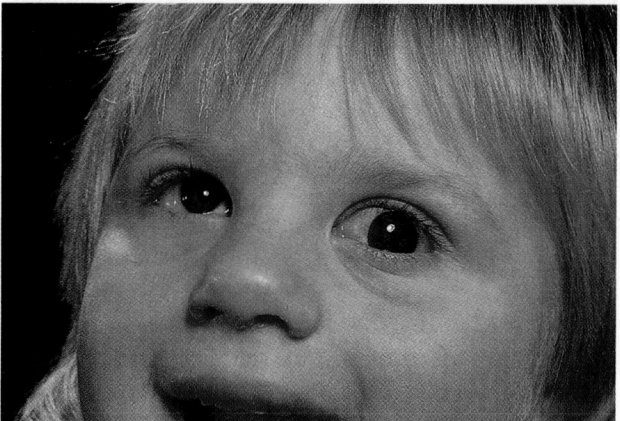

Fig. P27.3 (a) Child with glaucoma and retinal detachment with an ugly phthisical left eye. (b) Same child as in (a) wearing a cosmetic lens.

wearing the clear lens, the cosmetic tinted lens can be ordered. If problems arise during the trial period, an alternative type of lens should be considered.

Tinted lenses

Conditions such as cone dystrophy, albinism, iris coloboma and aniridia may benefit from wearing tinted spectacles. Cosmetically acceptable lenses that are effective against the light can be made either as a high water content soft lens or as an RGP lens. RGP lenses are initially uncomfortable and soft lenses are fragile and thin in low powers and may not stand rough handling. It is not always possible therefore to fit these children with lenses at a young age.

Therapeutic lenses

Therapeutic lenses are occasionally helpful for a child. Keratoplasty and some cases of corneal dystrophy may require such lenses but they are usually only temporarily successful. The lenses needed are thin and soft, difficult to insert into the painful eyes of an awake child and easily rubbed out. Silicone rubber lenses may be useful but their fitting and assessment is difficult.

Some practical tips

Fitting young children with contact lenses always requires more patience than fitting adults, but there are a few practical points that can make management easier.

1 Involve both parents, where possible, from the start in the handling of the lenses. If only one parent is available, there may be a grandparent or friend who can help until the parent is more adept.

2 With young infants, who become upset at having lenses inserted or removed, it can help to wrap them up in a blanket at first until the parent becomes more competent.

3 In a slightly older unco-operative child, it is better to make several short appointments, rather than one long one to help the child become familiar with the surroundings and the practitioner.

4 Many children, having worn lenses since infancy, start to rebel against having them inserted at around the age of 18 months. At that stage they can wear spectacles and return to lenses later.

5 The parents may be reluctant to change their child from contact lenses to spectacles, but they usually find it worthwhile. It is useful to explain, in the early stages, that the form of correction is likely to alter, so that they are not disappointed when a change is suggested later on.

6 Try to involve the older child in the decision to fit contact lenses. The parents may pressurize a reluctant child into having lenses fitted. Lenses fitted for the parents' sake are unlikely to be worn for long!

7 If the child is too scared, the prescription of normal saline drops to instil prior to the fitting appointment may help the child overcome the fear of having something put into the eye.

8 Especially in traumatic aphakes who have already suffered the initial upset, spectacles with patching can be used as an interim step before fitting a contact lens.

References

Amaya LG, Speedwell L, Taylor D. Contact lenses for infant aphakia. *Br J Ophthalmol* 1990; **74**: 150–4.

Amos CF, Lambert SR, Ward MA. Rigid gas-permeable contact lens correction of aphakia following congenital cataract removal during infancy. *J Pediatr Ophthalmol Strabismus* 1992; **29**: 243–5.

Arentsen JJ. Corneal neovascularization in contact lens wearers. *Int Ophthalmol Clin* 1986; **26**: 15–25.

Arkin M, Azar D, Fraioli A. Infantile cataracts. *Int Ophthalmol Clin* 1992; **32**: 107–20.

Baker JD, Hiles DA, Morgan KS. Viewpoint: Visual rehabilitation of aphakic children. *Surv Ophthalmol* 1990; **34**: 366–84.

Birch EE, Stager DR. Prevalence of good visual acuity following surgery for congenital unilateral cataract. *Arch Ophthalmol* 1988; **106**: 40–3.

Conklin JD, Litteral G, Schmeisser E, Van Meter WS. An evaluation of four multifocal contact lenses in young monocular aphakic patients. *CLAO J* 1992; **18**: 92–4.

Cutler SI, Nelson LB, Calhoun JH. Extended wear contact lenses in pediatric aphakia. *J Pediatr Ophthalmol Strabismus* 1985; **22**: 85–91.

Elsas FJ. Visual acuity in monocular pediatric aphakia: does epikeratophakia facilitate occlusion therapy in children intolerant of contact lens or spectacle wear? *J Pediatr Ophthalmol Strabismus* 1990; **27**: 304–9.

Epstein R. Contact lenses for the correction of aphakia. *Int Ophthalmol Clin* 1991; **31**: 53–60.

Ezekiel D. A gas-permeable paediatric aphakic scleral contact lens. *Optician* 1995; **35**(5): 25–7.

Gordon RA, Donzis PB. Refractive development of the human eye. *Arch Ophthalmol* 1985; **103**: 785–9.

Grosvenor T, Scott R. Three-year changes in refraction and its components in youth-onset and early adult-onset myopia. *Optom Vis Sci* 1993; **70**: 677–83.

Halliday BL. Epikeratophakia for aphakia, keratoconus and myopia. *Br J Ophthalmol* 1990; **74**: 667–72.

Harris M. Correction of pediatric aphakia with silicone contact lenses. *CLAO J* 1985; **11**: 343–7.

Jacobs DS. The best contact lens for baby? *Int Ophthalmol Clin* 1991; **31**: 173–9.

Levin AV, Edmonds SA, Nelson LB *et al.* Extended wear contact lenses in pediatric aphakia. *Ophthalmology* 1988; **22**: 86–91.

Maumenee IH. The eye in Marfan syndrome. *Trans Am Ophthalmol Soc* 1981; **79**: 684–733.

Moore BD. Pediatric aphakic contact lens wear: rates of successful wear. *J Pediatr Ophthalmol Strabismus* 1993; **30**: 253–8.

Morris J. Contact lenses in infancy and childhood. *Contact Lens J* 1979; **8**: 15–18.

Nelson LB, Cutler SJ, Calhoun JH *et al.* Silsoft extended wear contact lenses. *Ophthalmology* 1985; **92**: 1529–31.

Neumann D, Weismann BA, Isenberg SJ *et al.* The effectiveness of daily wear contact lenses for the correction of infantile aphakia. *Arch Ophthalmol* 1993; **111**: 927–30.

Pollard ZF. Results of treatment of persistent hyperplastic primary vitreous. *Ophthalmic Surg* 1991; **22**: 48–52.

Pratt-Johnson JA, Tillson G. Hard contact lenses in the management of congenital cataracts. *J Pediatr Ophthalmol Strabismus* 1985; **22**: 94–7.

Saunders RA, Ellis FD. Empirical fitting of hard contact lenses in infants and young children. *Ophthalmology* 1981; **88**: 127–30.

Sorsby A, Leary GA, Richards MJ. The optical components in anisometropia. *Vision Res* 1962; **3**: 43–51.

Speedwell L. Infants and pre-school children. In: Phillips AJ, Speedwell L, eds. *Contact Lenses*, 4th edn, Part 5. London: Butterworth–Heinemann, 1996.

Speedwell L, Russell-Eggitt I. The long and the short and the tall. *J Br Contact Lens Assoc* 1994; **17**: 135–9.

Speedwell L, Russell-Eggitt I. Improvement in visual acuity in children with ectopia lentis. *J Pediatr Ophthalmol Strabismus* 1995; **32**: 94–7.

Stulting RD, Sumers KD, Cavanagh HD *et al.* Penetrating keratoplasty in children. *Ophthalmology* 1984; **91**: 1222–30.

Weale RA. *A Biography of the Eye. Development, Growth, Age*. London: HK Lewis, 1982; 68–78.

Winn B, Ackerley RG, Brown CA *et al.* The superiority of contact lenses in correction of all anisometropia. *Transactions of the British Contact Lens Association Conference*, 1986; 95–100.

P28: Problems with Occlusion Treatment

David Taylor

The purpose of this chapter is to give practical advice to parents on that universally difficult, but wonderfully effective treatment, patching. The section is couched in the sort of language the doctor might use when talking to a parent, because that is exactly who it is intended for. This section is drawn from a booklet that, at Great Ormond Street Hospital, London, we give to parents who are experiencing difficulty in keeping patches on a child.

What is a lazy eye?

A lazy eye (amblyopia) occurs when the vision in one eye is worse than the other during a critical period in development. This can occur because of strabismus or squint (when the eye is pointing in the wrong direction), or anything that gives one eye worse vision than the other to a significant degree, e.g. cataracts, droopy eyelid, and so on. Even a moderate degree of astigmatism or long sight when it occurs in one eye may give rise to a lazy eye.

The purpose of patching

In patching, one eye is relatively disadvantaged by being covered or having its own vision blurred so that the child is forced to use the other eye. Usually of course the 'good' eye is the one that is patched.

There is *no alternative* to patching in one form or another. Squint surgery, glasses or any alternative therapies do not work in amblyopia no matter where you go or how much you pay! The only way to get over a lazy eye is to have the good eye patched to force the bad eye to 'work'. Admittedly, it is very important if there is a refractive error (a need for spectacles), to have that corrected by glasses and obviously more serious conditions such as cataract require their own treatment.

Why is it difficult?

When you patch the good eye, not only is the patch irritating to the child, being sticky and a new and not altogether pleasant sensation, but the child is forced to use the eye with poor vision, which restricts their activities. It is normal for a child not to like being patched but it is remarkable how quickly they get used to it, especially once the vision starts to improve.

Explain it to the child!

As soon as they are capable of understanding they should have the need for patching explained to them. A small treat at the end of the period of patching also never comes amiss!

How to patch

Black patches

You can patch with an ordinary black patch, i.e. a pirate's patch with an elasticated string around the head, but this virtually never works in a small child because they find it too easy to rip off and also it can flick back and cause injury.

Sticky patches

Sticky patches are made by various firms and have different compositions. We prefer one that has just the right amount of stickiness, not too much or too little, and one that completely blocks vision. If the patch is taken on and off very frequently then this can traumatize the skin. These patches are completely fool proof as long as they are put on properly and the sticky part stuck down well and then you know exactly how much patching you are doing.

It is also possible to put a patch on the glasses but this is not as good as patching on the skin itself because most bright children tend to peep over the patch so that they can use their good eye.

Another way of disadvantaging the good eye is to use drops that cause the pupil to dilate and the eye to become out of focus: this only works if there is not very much difference in the vision between the two eyes and it is not usually recommended but it can be very helpful in some forms of squint. The drops have to be prescribed by your ophthalmologist.

1103

There are other methods of patching but on the whole they are not satisfactory but if the worst comes to the worst we are quite happy with anything that disadvantages the good eye and advantages the bad eye.

How do you stop children ripping the patch off?

1 Be firm. Remember that the child is quite likely to be doing it to see whether he can beat you in a battle of will.

2 Explain to the child why he is wearing them.

3 Clean the skin before you put the patch on.

4 Use a stickier patch if he rips them off too frequently, i.e. use Opticlude instead of Coverlet.

5 For a younger child, put the patch on at the end of a sleep or before a meal.

6 Put sticky tape on the top of the patch so that he has to take that off before taking the patch off. This may give you a few valuable moments so that you can distract him before he has done it.

7 Put sticky tape on the tips of the thumb and first two fingers of both hands. This will stop him being able to manipulate his fingers such that he can pull the patch off. Use a sock over the hands taped to the forearm for the same effect.

8 Use elbow restraints made out of a cardboard tube such as a kitchen roll centre or a washing up liquid bottle with the ends cut off (small size). This can be taped to the upper or forearm so that the child can still play but it stops him bringing his hand up to take the patch off.

9 Get elbow restraints made by a physiotherapist.

10 Use large water wings or arm bands, normally used as a swimming aid, placed over elbows before inflation.

11 If the worst comes to the worst we have been known to admit the occasional child to hospital for a day or two. This is only rarely necessary.

The more drastic remedies are usually only necessary for a very short time—enough to demonstrate who is the boss! The main point to make is that you must let your child know that you mean business and that you are not going to be beaten by him! Reward them. Start a 'star' system—put one sticky star on a piece of paper each time they wear the patch well and give them a treat when they have achieved a certain number of stars.

When to patch?

Obviously the best time to patch is when the child is awake, lively and preferably doing detailed work. In an older child reading, writing, drawing or any hand–eye activity is the best. In a younger child just the time of the day when they are most wide awake, often starting a meal helps. The only times that count is when the child is wide awake, i.e. if you are given 3 hours of patching a day to do please don't count his afternoon nap in that! For a young child patching is usually best done at school; after 7 or 8 years they often find it embarrassing and it is best done when doing homework or other 'detailed' work; watching television or playing outdoors is fine, but not as good as detailed work.

What if the patch is irritating?

Allergy to a patch is rare with nearly all patch materials used today, the cause of redness in the area where the patch has been removed is usually the trauma of the patch being removed.

Of course it is irritating to put the patch on but if the patch causes skin irritation then there are two things to do. First, stick the patch on to your hand before you put it on the child then it will come off more easily. The alternative is to use a paper punch to make holes in the patch before the paper backing is removed to substantially reduce the area that is stuck to the skin.

Use a little face or baby cream on the area patched when the patch has come off. If the child complains of itchiness it may very well be that he has become allergic to the patch used.

What are the results?

This depends on the age. The older the child is, the less the effect of patching and the more hours they would have to

1 2 hours 20 mins	2 1 hours 15 mins	3 1 hours 10 mins	4 1 hours 20 mins	5 2 hours 15 mins	6 1 hours 45 mins	7 2 hours
8 2 hours	9 2 hours 40 mins	10 CL	11 CL	12 CL	13 CL	14 CL
15 1 hour 15 mins	16 1 hour	17 2 hour 15 mins	18 1 hour 15 mins	19 15 mins	20	21 1 hour 45 mins
22 3 hour 15 mins	23 15 mins	24	25	26 1 hour 30 mins	27 3 hour 15 mins	28 2 hour 10mins
29 1 hour 30 mins	30 30 mins	31 1 hour 45 mins				

Fig. P28.1 Parents patching/occlusion booklet. Fill in the hours achieved (or minutes if less than 1 hour) in the box corresponding to each day. NB If your child wears a contact lens(es) but has been unable to wear it/them (for any reason), on any day please record that in the relevant box as CL.

patch to get a good result. There is not much point in patching after 10 years of age but even after 6 years of age the results may be poor. In some conditions, such as congenital cataract or glaucoma in one eye, the patching needs to be done very early indeed, i.e. in the first few weeks of life. Another limiting factor is that the amount of patching has to be limited in very young children because of changes that may take place in the good eye and these children need to be watched by the ophthalmologist rather carefully. The amount of patching therefore also depends on the results. If it is possible to measure the vision then we have got a much better way of judging how much patching needs to be done. If we don't, then it is a bit more guess work but there are ways of telling whether the patching has had some effect.

Keeping a log of the patching

It is very useful to use a patching booklet so that you can record how many hours each day and which eye you patch (Fig. P28.1). This booklet contains monthly calendars for you to record how many hours (or minutes) you managed to patch your child each day, and how many hours you were supposed to be patching. It enables the ophthalmologist to judge more accurately how much further patching is needed. It will not be used to criticize you if you have a particularly troublesome month or two with your child's occlusion! Patching can be difficult! It is important, however, that you try to be as honest as possible when filling it in. This will then help us to assess your child's progress accurately.

P29: Non-Accidental Injury/Child Abuse: Child Protection Policy and Procedures

David Taylor

Most of this section is taken with permission from the *Child Protection Policy and Procedures* booklet produced by Great Ormond Street Hospital for Children, London; it is only intended as a series of guidelines, as procedures will vary enormously from hospital to hospital and country to country.

General policy

Responding to and managing suspicions and allegations of child abuse demands much of professionals. They have to recognize that our society embraces a variety of child-rearing practices and be sensitive to, and tolerant of, customs and views which may be held by families, while at the same time distinguishing what is acceptable child care and what is not.

Professionals have to be sensitive both to the child's needs and to the distressing feelings which investigations may arouse in a family and be aware that these may, at times, conflict. In all cases the welfare, well-being and protection of the child has to be paramount.

It is vital that professionals make no lasting assumptions either that abuse must have taken place, or that it never could.

1 The effective management of child abuse demands a multidisciplinary approach with consultation and exchange of information at every stage. No professional should ever intervene on their own. All concerns must be shared with others.

2 A number of agencies, other than the hospital, have key roles. To achieve protection of children and partnership with their families, these agencies must work co-operatively.

3 To ensure this, the social work department of the hospital must immediately be informed of any concern.

4 In order that the child's best interests are served it is important that, whilst any enquiries are being made into possible abuse, discussion within the professional network has priority over that with parents and carers until it is clear that there is not a conflict between the interests of the child and those of the carers.

Where contradictions or inconsistencies, real or apparent, arise between the procedures set out in this document and those for the area in which the child lives, these should be resolved by discussion between appropriate professionals.

Recognition of abuse

While abuse may be identified because of a single sign or symptom, e.g. a particular physical injury, it is common for children who have been abused to show a range or cluster of indicators. Therefore it is essential that when suspicions are aroused by a specific presentation, the child's general physical health, emotional and behavioural state is assessed. A child may have been the subject of more than one type of abuse. In cases of doubt, the guidance of a more experienced professional must be sought.

The following four categories are used to register children's names on Local Authority Child Protection Registers.

1 Neglect. The persistent or severe neglect of a child, or the failure to protect a child from exposure to any kind of danger, including cold or starvation, or extreme failure to carry out important aspects of care resulting in the significant impairment of the child's health or development, including non-organic failure to thrive.

2 Physical injury. Actual or likely physical injury to a child, or a failure to prevent a physical injury (or suffering) to a child including deliberate poisoning, suffocation and Munchausen's syndrome by proxy.

3 Sexual abuse. Actual or likely sexual exploitation of a child or adolescent. The child may be dependent and/or developmentally immature.

4 Emotional abuse. Actual or likely severe adverse effect on the emotional and behavioural development of a child caused by persistent or severe emotional ill-treatment or rejection. All abuse involves some emotional ill-treatment. This category should be used where it is the main or sole form of abuse.

Physical injury

The most serious physical abuse occurs in early childhood because of the inability of the immature child to protect himself.

Presentation of injuries or states which should give rise to concern

The following presentations or parental accounts of injuries or states, should alert concerns.

1 The account of how the injuries occurred being inconsistent with their appearance and nature.

2 Timing of injuries are discrepant with the account given.

3 Injuries of different ages, different stages of healing, indicating a series of injuries.

4 Unexplained injuries noted by others, e.g. school, playgroup.

5 An unusual degree of hostility or over-friendliness towards hospital staff.

6 An unusual lack of concern at the extent and severity of injuries.

Patterns of injuries/states which should give rise to concern

1 Retinal haemorrhages.
2 Subdural and subarachnoid haemorrhages.
3 Head injuries particularly in infants and young children.
4 Multiple fractures at different stages of healing.
5 Unusual fractures, e.g. acromion.
6 Metaphyseal and rib fractures.
7 Cigarette burns, especially if more than one (Fig. P29.1).
8 Human bites.
9 Black eyes.
10 Fingertip bruising.
11 Scalds in the absence of splash marks.
12 Burns, scalds.
13 Bruising on sites not easily injured (Fig. P29.2).
14 Unusual cuts or marks.
15 Any unsatisfactorily explained injury, particularly repeated accidents.

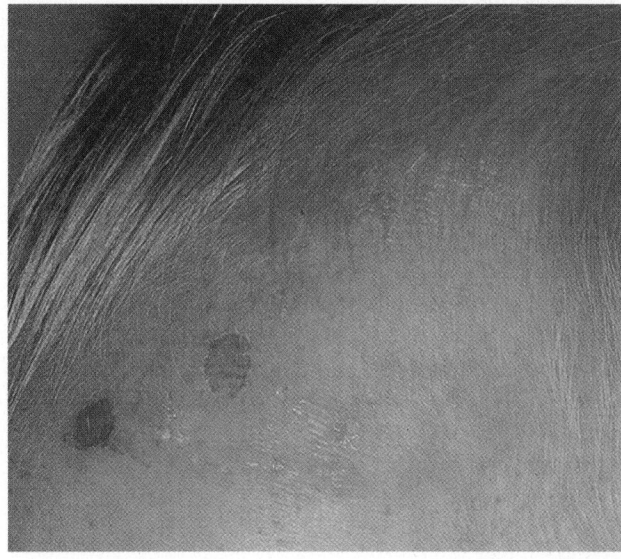

Fig. P29.1 Cigarette burns can be accidental, but two burns are likely to be non-accidental.

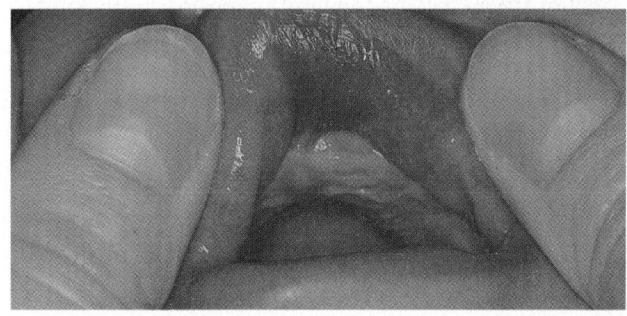

Fig. P29.2 Ripped and bruised frenulum.

Death of a sibling

Where a child is admitted to hospital with an unclear diagnosis and a sibling has died without a satisfactory explanation as to the cause of death.

Behavioural signs which may alert concern

These signs represent the effect on a child of living in a home with an 'abusive' atmosphere.

1 Frozen watchfulness; that is unnatural stillness and watchful observation of those around, extreme anxiety on being approached or touched.

2 Playing-out or acting-out in aggressive, highly active ways.

3 Unusual degrees of closeness or distance between parents and children.

Induced illness—Munchausen syndrome by proxy

Physical injury or suffering can also occur through induction of illness — Munchausen syndrome by proxy is the induction or attribution of illness states.

Presentations which should alert concern

Symptoms which cannot be explained by any medical tests; symptoms never observed by anyone other than the carer; symptoms reported to occur only at home or when a parent visits a child in hospital.

1 High level of demand for investigations of symptoms without any documented physical signs.
2 Unexplained problems with medical treatment such as drips coming out or intravenous lines being interfered with.
3 Presence of unprescribed medication or poisons in the blood/urine.

Neglect

Neglect is characterized in the following ways.
1 Persistent or severe neglect of care.
2 Failure to protect the child from exposure to any kind of danger.
3 Failure of care which is so great that it leads to significant impairment of the child's health or development, including failure to thrive and growth failure.

Alerting signs and symptoms

The characteristic physical appearance of neglect is as follows.
1 Marked drop in height/weight centiles; failure to gain height and weight.
2 Abnormalities of skin and hair.
3 Poor hygiene.
4 Withdrawal or self-isolating behaviour by the child.
5 Food scavenging.
6 Poor intellectual and school performances and failure to achieve potential levels.

Sexual abuse

'The actual or likely sexual exploitation of a child or adolescent under 16 years', this includes the following.
1 Incest — sexual intercourse within prohibited relationships.
2 Any form of sexual activity involving children.
3 Involvement of children in pornographic activities.

Levels of concern

The following levels of concern regarding sexual abuse are noted.

High index of suspicion

1 Semen in vagina, anus or on external genitalia.
2 Pregnancy in a minor where the identity of the father is unknown or concealed.
3 Laceration or scarring of the hymen, attenuation of the hymen with loss of hymeneal tissue in the absence of any other credible explanation.
4 Laceration or scarring of anal mucosa extending beyond the anal verge into the perianal skin in the absence of any other credible explanation.
5 Bruises, scratches or other injuries to the genital or anal areas, or to other 'sexual' areas such as breasts and lips: these injuries may be minor but are inconsistent with accidental injury.
6 Signs of sexually transmitted infections.
7 Repeated and frequent sexualized behaviour.

Medium suspicion

1 Perineal itching, soreness, pain on micturition, discharge.
2 Anal warts.
3 Child hinting that there are secrets that she or he cannot talk about.
4 Psychiatric disturbances, mutism, anorexia nervosa, attempted suicide or self-mutilation.
5 Concern about inappropriate behavioural patterns with other children or adults.

Low suspicion

1 Recurrent urinary tract infections.
2 Recurrent abdominal pain, headaches or other psychosomatic features.
3 Isolated observation of sexualized behaviour.
4 'Eccentric' sexual patterns of family interaction without other observable or reported symptomology.

Emotional abuse

The serious adverse effect on the emotional and behavioural development of a child attributable to persistent or severe emotional ill-treatment or rejection.

Alerting factors

Any form of abuse may involve emotional abuse. The following contexts should be considered.
1 An inability to perceive child's needs objectively, e.g. child labelled as bad.
2 Over compliant and passive behaviour.
3 Restlessness, hyper-vigilance, anxiety, rejection of friendship.
4 Fear, anxiety, depression, no confidence, and learning

and concentration problems.

5 Aggressive conduct, lack of concern, provocativeness.
6 Serious physical or psychiatric illness of a parent, including hospitalization.
7 Breakdown in parental relationships, chronic bitter conflict over contact or residence of the child.
8 Major repeated familial changes, separations, family reconstitution.
9 Parental drug and alcohol addiction.

Referral

If any member of staff has a concern about actual or possible abuse of any kind, whether in an in-patient, out-patient or day-patient, they must follow these guidelines.
1 Inform the consultant or his/her deputy and the senior nurse responsible for the ward/department.
2 Inform the unit social worker or duty social worker at once; this leads to an internal discussion.

Planned admissions where abuse is suspected

A planned admission for medical and psychosocial assessment where abuse is suspected requires careful planning which must include the following.
1 Arrange admission only after internal meetings with psychosocial team to ensure availability of relevant members of clinical team at time of admission.
2 Consider convening a strategy discussion with local agencies prior to admission.
3 A strategy discussion should consider any statutory action which may need to be taken to:
   (a) ensure admission;
   (b) protect the child if abuse is confirmed following assessment; and
   (c) consider appropriate level of parental contact.

Out-patients

If child protection concerns are raised on seeing a child who is an out-patient, inform the unit or duty social worker. In discussion with the social worker consideration should be given to the child's protection. This may require either admitting the child, or arranging for an immediate admission to a local hospital. If the parents/carers are not co-operative, consideration must be given to whether the child requires emergency protection. It may be necessary for the police to be involved.

Gain from the parents/carers in an interview conducted jointly with the social worker, an account of the background and events leading up to admission.

If abuse seems likely but is not spontaneously admitted by a carer or attributed to another carer do not question the parents/carers about the events prior to obtaining the agreement of the social work department and the police.

Keep detailed contemporaneous records.

Check whether there is already salient information about the child in the local social service department and request that they ask for information from the police.

Consult with all other agencies who have direct knowledge of the child and family.

Be prepared to give information to police and local social service department.

The social work manager following consultation with the social worker and other hospital staff, as appropriate, considers all the known information and decides whether there is a need for immediate protection; convening a strategy discussion; specific professionals to undertake further work to gain sufficient information to enable decisions to be made; services to be offered to the child and family; no further action.

If after the initial enquiries and checks, there is no child protection concern, a social work manager must record on the social work file why the decision to proceed no further has been made. The social work manager and social worker will agree what, if any, entry is made on the medical notes.

Immediate protection

Consider whether any emergency statutory protective action is required to ensure the immediate protection of the child. If this is necessary, decide whether it is appropriate to seek an Emergency Protection Order or whether the urgency is such that the police should be asked to consider taking the child into police protection. Where an Emergency Protection Order is sought, consider any directions that might be required regarding contact with family members and significant others.

Consideration should also be given to any supervision/conditions needed, and the resource capacity of hospital staff to provide this.

If there is no need for immediate action but it is considered there is a risk of the parents removing the child from the hospital against either medical advice or in opposition to any immediate protection plan, ensure that:
1 there is a contingency plan written in the medical notes by the social worker;
2 the out of hours social services duty teams are informed;
3 the hospital administration is aware of the situation;
4 ward staff have the telephone number of:
   (a) the police in case of emergency;
   (b) the child's local authority; and
   (c) the out of hours social services duty teams.

If the child is medically fit for discharge but there are unresolved child protection concerns, consider what action needs to be taken to ensure the protection of the child. This may mean keeping the child in hospital longer than medically necessary or transferring to a local hospital until a child protection plan is in place.

Refusal of consent

If the parents refuse to consent to the recommended treatment the following procedures should be followed according to the gravity of the situation.

Acute emergency

This is the situation of the imminent death of the child; the doctor has the right and indeed the duty to administer any treatment deemed to be life-saving.

Less acute emergency

This is where there is a need for rapid treatment (i.e. within hours). The consultant concerned should request a second opinion from another consultant, preferably one on a different team. If both agree on the urgency then a note to that effect must be made in the medical notes and the treatment should be administered.

Elective procedures

If after full discussion there appears to the clinicians to be no alternative to the administration of blood products electively throughout the course of treatment and if the parents still cannot give their consent, consideration should be given by the social work department to whether a Court Order should be obtained.

It is not ethical or satisfactory for doctors to treat repeatedly, throughout a long elective course of treatment, citing only the Department of Health Circular since this is designed to address acute emergencies only.

P30: Support Groups and Resource Centres for the Parent of the Visually Handicapped Child

David Taylor

This chapter is meant to be an aid to ophthalmologists who are trying to help parents who are going abroad from their homeland, or those who have enquiries from parents from abroad. In compiling it, I have been amazed by two things — the generosity of colleagues who have contributed to it, and the wide diversity of aid organizations throughout the world. This diversity is good in some ways, not least because it reflects people reacting locally to local problems, but the lack of uniformity may suggest a lack of international guidance, training and collaboration.

This cannot be a complete list, but I hope it is helpful. Although I have made every effort to be accurate, I would be very grateful if the mistakes could be drawn to my attention!

Antigua, West Indies
Caribbean Council for the Blind, PO Box 1517, 11 Redcliffe Quay, St John's, Antigua, West Indies (Tel: +1 809 4624111, Fax: +1 809 4624111)

Argentina
Helen Keller Institute, Av Velez Sarsfield 2100, Agencia 4, 5000 Cordoba, Argentina (Tel : +54 51 605046)

Australia
Albinism Fellowship and Support Group Inc., PO Box 717, Modbury, SA 5092, Australia

Association for the Blind Ltd, 7 Mair Street, Brighton Beach, Victoria 3186, Australia (Tel: +61 3-5988555, Fax: +61 3-5984158)

Australian Blindness Forum, 87 High Street, Prahran Vic 3181, Australia (Tel: 03 521 3433, Fax: 03 521 3732)

Early Support Services, Townsend House, 24 King George Avenue, Hove, SA 5048, Australia

Institute for the Blind, 557 St Kilda Road, Melbourne Vic 3004, Australia

National Federation for Blind People of Australia, 87 High Street, Prahran Vic 3181, Australia

Royal Blind Society, PO Box 176, Burwood, NSW 2135, Australia

Royal New South Wales Institute for Deaf and Blind Children, 361–365 North Rocks Road, North Rocks, NSW 2151, Australia (Tel: +61 2-8711233, Fax: +61 2-8712196)

Royal Society for the Blind of SA Inc., PO Box 196, Greenacres, SA 5086, Australia

Austria
Bundes-Blindenerziehungstitut, Federal Institute for the Education of the Blind, Wittelsbachstrasse 5, A-1020 Wien, Austria (Tel: +43 222-218 0866/18)

Bahrain
Alnoor Institute for the Arabian Gulf for the Blind, PO Box 33484 Isa Town Bahrain (Tel: +973 780818, Fax: +973 780786)

Bangladesh
Assistance for Blind Children, 167 Green Road, Post Box 5082, Dhaka 1205, Bangladesh (Tel: +880 2-316079, Fax: +880 2-813014)

Belgium
Confederation Belge pour la Promotion des Aveugles et Malvoyants, Belgium Federation for the Welfare of the Blind and Visually Impaired, Rua A Bertulot 21, boite 4, BP276, B-1210 Bruxelles 21, Belgium (Tel: +33332 2-218 5973)

Universitair Ziekenhuis Antwerpen, Wilrijkstraat 10, 2610 Wilrij, Belgium (Tel: 03 829 11 11)

Universitair Ziekenhuis Gent, De Pintelaan 185, 9000 Gent, Belgium (Tel: 09 240 23 06)

Universitair Ziekenhuis Leuven, Kapucijnenvoer 33, 3000 Leuven, Belgium (Tel: 016 33 23 94)

Bolivia
Aprecia Santa Cruz Escuela para Ninos Ciegos y Deficientes Visuales, Centro de Rehabilitacion, School for Blind and Visually Handicapped Children, Rehabilitation Centre, Casilla 3538, 3er Anillo, Detras del Hotel, Los Tajibos, Santa Cruz, Bolivia (Tel: +591 33-9920, Fax: +591 33-1374)

Botswana
Mochudi Resource Centre for the Blind, PO Box 1510, Mochudi, Botswana (Tel: +267 37 478)

Brazil
Associacao Brasileira de Educacao de Deficientes Visuais, Brazilian Association for the Education of the Blind, Rua Rafeel Bandeira 55, 88000 Florianopolis SC, Brazil (Tel: +55 22-4572)

Canada
At Home Program, Ministry of Health, 910 View Street, Main Floor, Victoria, BC, Canada

Canadian National Institute for the Blind, 1931 Bayview Avenue Toronto, Ontario M4G 4C8, Canada (Tel: +1 416 4807580, Fax: +1 416-4807677)

Canadian National Society for the Deaf–Blind, Suite 901, 35 Walmer Road, Toronto, ON M5R 2X3, Canada

Infant Developmental Program, Provincial Office, 2765 Osoyoos

Crescent, Vancouver V6T 1X7, Canada

Support Group Clearinghouse, Family Resource Library, British Columbia Children's Hospital, 4480 Oak Street, Vancouver V6H 3V4, Canada

Chile

Colegio Helen Keller, Rosita Renard 1179, Santiago, Chile

Corporacion Regional para la Integracion Social del Limitado Visual, Patricio Lynch 340, Arica, Chile

Escuela Hogar de Ciegos, Santa Lucia Salesianos 1190, San Miguel, Santiago, Chile

Hospital Guillermo Grant Benavente, Servicio Oftalmologia, Concepcion, Chile

Instituto de Prevencion y Rehabilitacion de la Ceguera, Avda Salvador 943, Providencia, Santiago, Chile

Jardin Infantil La Luciernaga, Bernarda Morin 488, Santiago, Chile

Sociedad Protectora de Ciegos Santa Lucia, Santa Lucia Society for the Protection of the Blind, Salesianos 1190, San Miguel, Santiago, Chile (Tel: +56 2-518222)

Colombia

Instituto Nacional para Ciegos, National Institute for the Blind, Carrera 13 no. 34–91, Santafe de Bogota, Colombia (Tel: +57 1-2329077)

Instituto para Ninos Ciegos y Sordos de Cali, Cali Institute for Blind and Deaf Children, Carrera 38, No. Diagonal 29–39, Cali, Colombia

Costa Rica

Centro Nacional de Educacion Especial 'Fernando Centeno Gueli' Dept de Deficientes Visuales, National Centre of Special Education 'Fernando C. Guell' Dept of the Visually Impaired, Guadalupe, Goiciechea, Costa Rica (Tel: +506 255437)

Cuba

Asociacion Nacional del Ciego, National Association of the Blind, PO Box 4129, Calle 1 no. 201, Municipio Plaza, Havana, Cuba (Tel: +53 7-320449)

Cyprus

Kibris Turk Gormezler Dernegi, Cyprus Turkish Blind Association, PO Box 100, Lefkosa, Mersin-10 via Turkey, Cyprus (Tel: +357 9520 78228)

St Barnabas School for the Blind, PO Box 3511, Nicosia, Cyprus (Tel: +357 2-422131, Fax: +357 2-420256)

Czechoslovakia

Associace Nevidomych a Slabozrakych, Czechoslovakia Association of the Blind and Partially Sighted, Karlinske Namesti c. 12, 186 03 Praha 8, Karlin, Czechoslovakia (Tel: +42 2-2360004)

Denmark

Aalborgskolens Deaf–Blind Department, Kollegievej 1, Postbox 7930, 9210 Aalborg so, Denmark (Tel: +45 98-143066, Fax: +45 98-147177)

Centre for Rare Diseases and Disabilities, Bredgarde 25, Sct Annae Passage opg F, DK 1260, Copenhagen, Denmark (Tel: +45 33 91 4020, Fax: +45 33 01 4019)

Danish Society for Blind Children, Landsforeningen af Foraeldre fil Blinde, og Svagsynede born og Unge, Formand Henrik Behrendt, Vetterslev Bygade 41, 4100 Ringstead, Denmark

Danish Society for the Blind, Dansk Blindesamfund, Formand Svend Jensen, Thoravej 35, DK 2400 Kobenhaun NV, Denmark

Dansk Dovblinde-Forening, The Danish Deaf Blind Association, Theklavej 48, DK-2400 Copenhagen NV, Denmark (Tel: +45 31

199796, Fax: +45 31-197978)

National Eye Clinic for the Visually Impaired, Statens Oienklinik, Rymarks Vej 1, DK 2900 Hellerup, Denmark (Tel: +45 31 62 5022)

Refsnasskolen, Istitut for Blinde og Svagsynede Born og Unge i Danmark, National Institute for Blind and Partially Sighted Children and Youth, Kystvejen 112, DK-4400 Kalundborg, Denmark (Tel: +45 53513300, Fax: +45 53514921)

Ungdomshjem for Dovblinde, Centre for Deaf–Blind Youth, Sohngardsholmsvej 59, 9000 Aalborg, Denmark (Tel: +45 8-981 44577, Fax: +45 8-981 47344)

Dominican Republic

Escuela Nacional de Ciegos, Calle Luis Braille 1, Zona 1, Santo Domingo DN, Dominican Republic (Tel: +1 809-5331210)

Ecuador

Mariana de Jesus, Isla Seymur 1085 y Rio Coca, Quito, Ecuador (Tel: +593 2-240261)

Egypt

Demonstration Centre for Rehabilitation of the Blind/Palace of Light, 184 Aziz El-Masri Street, ex Gessr El-Suess, Cairo, Egypt

El Salvador

Centro de Rehabilitacion para Ciegos 'Eugenia de Duenas', 'Eugenia de Duenas' Centre of Rehabilitation for the Blind, 21a Calle Poniente 240, San Salvador, El Salvador (Tel: +503-258958)

Finland

Nakovammaisten Keskusliitto ry./Synskadades Centralforbund RF, Finnish Federation of the Visually Handicapped, Makelankatu 50, SF-00510, Helsinki, Finland (Tel: +358 0-396041, Fax: +358 0-39604200)

Suomen Kuurosokeat Ry/Finlands Dovblinda RF, The Finnish Deaf–Blind Association, Makelankatu 52a, 00510 Helsinki, Finland (Tel: +358 0-396041, Fax: +358 0-39604678)

France

Association Nationale des Parents d'Enfants Aveugles ou Gravement Deficients Visuels, National Association of Parents of Blind or Seriously Sight-Deficient Children, 12 bis rue de Picpus, 75012 Paris, France (Tel: +33 1-43424040, Fax: +33 1 42731311)

Association Nationale pour les Sourds Aveugles, National Association for the Deaf–Blind, 18 rue Etex, 75018 Paris, France (Tel: +33 1-4624810, Fax: +33 1-4628092)

Federation Nationale des Associations de Parents d'Enfants Deficients Visuels, National Federation of Associations of Parents of Visually Impaired Children, 28 place Saint-Georges, 75009 Paris, France (Tel: +33 1-45267345)

Institut National des Jeunes Aveugles, National Institute for Young Blind, 56 Boulevard des Invalides, 75007 Paris, France (Tel: +33 1-47345744)

Germany

Christoffel-Blindenmission eV, Christian Blind Mission International, Nibelungenstrasse 124, D-614 Bensheim, Germany (Tel: +49 6251-1310, Fax: +49 6251 131165)

Deutsche Blindenstudienanstalt eV, German Institute for the Blind, D-3550, Marburg 1, Am Schlag 8, PO Box 1160, Germany (Tel: +49 6421-6060, Fax: +49 6421-606229)

Deutsche Retinitis-Pigmentosa-Vereinigung e V Ernst-Ludwig-Ring 44, 61231 Bad Nauheim, Germany (Tel: 06032/33499); 52074 Aachen, Vaalser Strasse 108, Germany (Tel: 0241/870018, Fax:

0241/893961)

Deutscher Blindenverband, Bismarckallee 30, 53173, Bonn, Germany

Deutsches Taubblinden-Werk Hannover, Albert-Schweitzer-Hof 27, 30559 Hannover, Germany (Tel: 0511 510080)

Fruhforderung fur Blinde u Sehbehinderte Kinder, Regensburg: Weibenburgstrasse 10, 93055 Regensburg, Germany; Munchen: Romanstrasse 95, 80639 Munchen-Nymphenburg, Germany

NCL-Gruppe Deutschland e V (Neuronale Ceroid Lipofuszinose), Rudolf Nolle, Vierkaten 32 b, 21623 Neu Wulmstorf, Wilma u Djeter Scherberg, Brenkelmannhof 71, 45359 Essen, Germany (Tel: 0201 692916, Fax: 0201 692300)

Von Recklinghausen Gescellschaft EV, AK Ochsenzell, Lanenhorner Chaussee 560, 22419, Hamburg, Germany (Tel: 040 5271 2822)

Ghana

Centre for Deaf–Blind Children, PO Box 33, Mampong-Akwapim, Ghana (Tel: +223 51-34)

Greece

Centre of Education and Rehabilitation of the Blind, 210 El Vemiaelou Avenue, Kallithea, Athens, 176 75, Greece (Tel: +30 1-9582720, Fax: +30 1-958571)

Guatemala

Comite Prociegos y Sordos de Guatemala, Guatemalan Organization for the Blind, 9a calle 3-07, zona 1, Guatemala

Haiti

Ecole St Vincent pour les Enfants Handicapes, St Vincent School for Handicapped Children, PO Box 1319, Port-au-Prince, Haiti (Tel: +509 1-20120)

Hong Kong

Hong Kong Society for the Blind, 248 Nam Cheong Street, Shamshuipo, Kowloon, Hong Kong (Tel: +852 7788332, Fax: +852 7880040)

Hungary

Dr Kettesy Aladar Altalanos Iskola es Diakotton, Dr Kettesy Aladar Elementary Boarding School for the Partially Sighted, 4032 Debrecen, Loverseny u3, Hungary (Tel: +36 52-17945)

Iceland

Blindra Felagid, the Icelandic Association for the Blind, Hamrahlid 17, 105 Reykjavik, Iceland (Tel: +354 1-687333, Fax: +354 1-687336)

India

All India Confederation of the Blind, Institutional area (Near DTC Terminal No. 1), Sector 5, Rohini Delhi 110 085, India (Tel: +91 11-7111372)

Helen Keller Institute for the Deaf and Deaf–Blind, Municipal Secondary School Building, 1st floor South Wing, Near S. Bridge, NM, Joshi Marg, Bycull West, Bombay 400 011, India (Tel: +91 22-397052)

Indonesia

Yayasan Pendidikan Anak-Anak Buta, Association for the Education of Blind Children, 14 Embong Kenongo, Surabaya 60271, Indonesia (Tel: +62 31-41569)

Iran

Sazman Amouzeshi aba Bassir Vigeh Nabinayan, Aba Bassir Educational Organization of the Blind, Dastgerrd Ghaddadeh Road,

Imam Khomeini Avenue, PO Box 81465-774, Isfahan, Iran (Tel: +98 31-60366)

Ireland

Bord Athshlanuchain, National Rehabilitation Board, 25 Clyde Road, Ballsbridge, Dublin 4, Ireland (Tel: +353 1-684181, Fax: +353 1-609935)

Israel

Ministry of Labour and Social Affairs—Services for the Blind, 10 yad Harutzim Street, Talpiot, PO Box 1260, Jerusalem, Israel (Tel: +972 2-708181, Fax: +972 2-731640)

Italy

Associazione delle Famiglie de Bambini Ipotiroidei, Affetti da Sindrome di Turner, Affetti da Sindrome di Prader-Willi, Clinica Pediatrica III, Ospedale S, Raffaele, Via Olgettina 60 20132 Milano, Italy (Tel: 02 2643622)

Associazione Lega del Filo d'Oro per Bambini con Grave Handicap Visivo, Via Montecerno, 1 S. Stefano 60027 Osimo (AN), Italy (Tel: 071 72451)

Associazione Nazionale Italiana fra Genitori di Sordociechi Pluriminorati, National Association for Parents of the Deafblind and Multi-Handicapped, Servizio di Consulenza, PO Box 601, Via Druso 7, 38100 Trento, Italy (Tel: +39 461-239595)

Federazione Nazionale Instituzioni pro Chiechi, National Federation of Institutes for the Blind, Via Gregorio V11 267, 00165 Genoa, Italy (Tel: +39 10-891160)

Fondazione R Hollman per Bambini con Grave Handicap Visivo, Via Oddone Clerici, 6 28051 Cannero (NO), Italy (Tel: 0323 788485)

Unione Italiana Ciechi, Via Borgogna, 38 00100 Roma, Italy (Tel: 06 6784748)

Vividown, Via S Maurilio, 8 20123 Milano, Italy (Tel: 02 8056238)

Jamaica

Jamaica Society for the Blind, 111 1/2 Old Hope Road, Kingston 6, Jamaica (Tel: +809-92 73760)

Japan

National Rehabilitation Centre for the Blind, 4-1 Namiki Tokorozawa 359, Tokyo, Japan (Tel: +81 3-0429953100, Fax: +81 3-0429953102)

Nippon Lighthouse (Welfare Centre for the Blind), 37, 4–2, Imadsunaka, Tsurumi-ku, Osaka 538, Japan (Tel: 06-961-5521)

Tokyo Metropolitan Rehabilitation Centre for the Physically and Mentally Handicapped, 2, 17–3, Toyama, Shinjuku-ku, Tokyo 162, Japan (Tel: 03-3203-6141)

Vocational Develop Centre for the Blind in Japan in INC, 3–10 Honshio-cho, Shinjuku-ku, Tokyo 160, Japan (Tel: 03-3341-0900)

Jordan

Friendship Association for the Blind, PO Box 7063, Amman, Jordan (Tel: +962 6-41570)

Kenya

Kenya Institute for the Blind, Off Langata Road, PO Box 31082, Nairobi, Kenya (Tel: +254 2-501875)

Korea

Chung Ju St Mary's School for the Blind, 1488 Jhihyon-Dong, Chung-Buk, 380-070, Korea (Tel: +82 441-431374, Fax: +82 441-447816)

Seoul National School for the Blind, Chong Ro Ku, Shin Kyo-dong 110-032, Seoul, Korea (Tel: +82 2-7370656)

Kuwait

Blind Institute, PO Box 44006, Cairo Street, Hawalli, Kuwait (Tel: +965-518321)

Lebanon

Lebanese School for the Blind, Box 40021, Baabda, Lebanon (Tel: 961 420601/421024)

Libya

El Nour Association for the Rehabilitation of the Blind, The Light Association for the Rehabilitation of the Blind, PO Box 3770, Tripoli, Libya (Tel: +218 21-71815, Fax: +218 21-71714)

Jamaiet Al Khafif Benghazi, Association for the Blind Benghazi, PO Box 583, Jamaheria, Benghazi, Libya (Tel: +218 61-5831, Fax: +218 61-5831)

Luxembourg

Institut pour Deficients Visuels, 9 rue Pierre Federspiel, L-1512 Luxembourg, Luxembourg (Tel: +352-445455, Fax: +352-457488)

Madagascar

Centre des Aveugles, Centre for the Blind, PO Box 311, Antsirabe 100, Madagascar

Malaysia

International Council for Education of the Visually Handicapped, 4 Taman Jesselton, 10450 Penang, Malaysia (Tel: +60 4-369699, Fax: +60 4-369357)

Persatuan Bagi Orang Buta Malaysia, Malaysian Association for the Blind, No 2, Lorong Utara B, 46200 Petalung Jaya, PO Box 10687 50722 Kuala Lumpur, Malaysia (Tel: +60 3-7577222)

Mauritius

Lois Lagesse Trust Fund, Colonel Maingard Street, Beau Bassin, Mauritis (Tel: +230-543253)

Mexico

Centro de Educacion Especial para la Integracion de Carentes de Vista y Disminuidos Visuales, Centre of Special Education for the Integration of the Visually Impaired, Calle 600 no. 333–35 y Av Colon, CP 97000, Merida, Yucatan, Mexico (Tel: +52 91-99276721)

Montserrat, West Indies

Montserrat Red Cross Society, PO Box 62, Plymouth, Montserrat, West Indies (Tel: +809 491-2699)

Morocco

Organisation Alaouite pour la Protection des Aveugles Marocain, The Alaouite Organisation for the Protection of the Blind of Morocco, Jardin Lalla Aicha, Oujda 00245, Morocco (Tel: +212 68-3645)

Netherlands

Centrum Bartimeushage, Bartimeushage, Centre for Multihandicapped Persons, Oude Arnhemse Bovenweg 3, PO Box 87, 3940 AB Doorn, The Netherlands (Tel: +31 3438-26911, Fax: +31 3438-26798)

Theofaan, Institute of Visually Handicapped, St Elizabethstraat 4, 5361 HK Grave, The Netherlands (Tel: +31 8860-71003, Fax: +31 8860-72441)

Niger

Union Nationale des Aveugles du Niger, National Union of the Blind of Niger, BP Box 2393, Niamey Balafon, Niger (Tel: +227 722601)

Nigeria

Federal Nigeria Society for the Blind, Blind Centre Road, Oshodi, Lagos State, Nigeria (Tel: +234 1-521108)

Norway

Assistanse, Parents' Organisation, Foreldreforeningen for Synshemmede Bbarns Sak, Sporveisgt 10, 0354 Oslo, Norway (Tel: 22 46 69 90)

Foreningen Norges Dovblinde, Norway's Organisation for Deaf/Blind, V/Ola Fjellheim, Eikholtvn 9, 3031 Drammen, Norway (Tel: 32 88 63 64)

Foreningen Norges Dovblinde, Norwegian Association of the Deaf–Blind, Liane 28, 3900 Porsgrunn, Norway (Tel: +47 03-553484)

Hovseter og Huseby Kompetansesenter, Statlig Spesialpedagogisk senter, Gamle Hovseterveg 3, 0768 Oslo, Norway (Tel: 22 02 95 00, Fax: 22 92 15 90)

Norges Blindeforbund, Norway's Organisation for the Blind, Youth Division, Postboks 5900 Majorstua, 0308 Oslo, Norway (Tel: 22 46 69 90)

Statens Sentralteam for Dovblinde, Norway's Deaf/Blind Team, Boks 4370 Torshov, 0402 Oslo, Norway (Tel: 22 71 00 35)

Tambartun Kompetansesenter, Statlig Spesialpedagogisk Senter, 7084 Melhus, Norway (Tel: 72 87 07 00, Fax: 72 87 24 10)

Oman

National Committee for Welfare of the Disabled, Ministry of Social Affairs and Labour, PO Box 560, Muscat, Oman (Tel: +968-601841, Fax: +968-699357)

Pakistan

Al-Faisal Markaz-e-Nabina, Al-Faisal Centre of the Blind, Faisalabad, New Civil Lines, Near Iqbal Stadium, Faisalabad, Pakistan (Tel: +92 411-34526)

Papua New Guinea

Mount Sion Centre for the Blind, PO Box 1068 Goroka EHP, Papua New Guinea (Tel: +675-722850, Fax: +675 722712)

Peru

Centro de Educacion Especial y Rehabilitation Nuestra Senora del Pilar para Ciegos, Our Lady of Pilar Special Education and Rehabilitation Centre for the Blind, Avenida Zamacola 120, Antiquilla AP692, Arequipa, Peru (Tel: +51 54-225389)

San Francisco de Asis, Catholic Organisation Dedicated to Blindness and Low Vision for Children, Educational Centre Marques de Guadalcazar 161, Urb. La Virreyna, Surco, Lima, Peru (Tel: +51 14 449 0210)

Philippines

Philippine National School for the Blind, Galvez Avenue Corner Figueroa Street Pasay City, 1300, Metro Manila, Philippines (Tel: +63 2-8318664)

Poland

Zakilad dla Niewidomych Laski, Institute for the Blind, Laski, PL 05-081 Laski, Warsaw, Poland (Tel: +48 22-345404)

Portugal

Associaco Promotora do Ensino dos Cegos, Promotional Education of Blind Association, Rua Borges Carneiro, 42 1o Dto, 1200 Lisboa, Portugal (Tel: +351 1-3968231)

Romania

Asociatia Nevazatorilor din Romania, Blind Association of Romania, Str Vatra Luminoasa nr. 108 bis, Sectorul 2 cod 73302, Bucuresti, Romania (Tel: +40 0-536525)

Russia

Vserossijskoje Obshchestvo Slepyk, Tsentralnoje Pravlenije, All Russia Association of the Blind, Centre Board, 14 Novaya Ploschad, Moscow 103 672, Russia (Tel: +7 95-923 9149, Fax: +7 95-925 492)

Saudi Arabia

The Regional Bureau of the Middle East Committee for the Affairs of the Blind, Diplomatic Quarter, PO Box 3465, Riyadh 11471, Saudi Arabia

Sierra Leone

Milton Margai School for the Blind, PO Box 533, Wilkinson Road, Freetown, Sierra Leone

Singapore

Singapore Association of the Visually Handicapped, 47 Toa Payoh Rise, Singapore 1129, Singapore (Tel: +65-25114331)

South Africa

Pioneer School for the Visually Impaired, 20 Aderley Street, 6850 Worcester, South Africa (Tel: +27 231-22313)

South African National Council for the Blind, PO Box 11149, Brooklyn, Pretoria 0011, South Africa (Tel: +27 12-3461171, Fax: +27 12-3461177)

Spain

COF Centros de Orientacion Familiar (Centres of Family Advice), Iglesia Santa Maria, Avda Espana 28220, Majadahonda (Madrid), Spain

Concejalia de Servicios Sociales (Social Services Division), Ayuntamiento (Town Hall), Carrera de San Francisco 10, 28025 Madrid, Spain

Consejeria de Integracion Social (Social Integration Counselling), Instituto Madrileno de Atencion a la Infancia, Imain, Orense 11, 28020 Madrid, Spain

Instituto Nacional de Servicios Sociales, National Institute of Social Services, c/Agustin de Foxa 31, 28036 Madrid, Spain (Tel: +34 1-3234353, Fax: +34 1-5331765)

Ministerio de Asuntos Sociales, Ministry of Social Affairs, Direccion General de Proteccion al Menor, C/Condesa de Venadito no. 34, 28027 Madrid, Spain

Sri Lanka

Sri Lanka Council for the Blind, 74A Church Street, Colombo 2, Sri Lanka (Tel: +94 1-29564, Fax: +94 1-545681)

St Lucia, West Indies

St Lucia Blind Welfare Association, PO Box 788, Castries, St Lucia, West Indies (Tel: +1 809-4524691)

Sudan

National Committee for the Care of the Blind, PO Box 915, Khartoum, Sudan (Tel: +249 11-70418)

Swaziland

St Joseph's Resource Centre for the Blind, PO Box 7, Mzimpofu, Swaziland (Tel: +268 53004)

Sweden

Ekeskolan, the State Special School and Resource Centre for Visually Impaired with Additional Disabilities, Box 9024, S-700 09 Orebro, Sweden (Tel: 019 245020, Fax: 019 245 489)

Foreningen Sveriges Dovblinda, Association of the Swedish Deaf–Blind, Sandsborgsvagen 44, S-122 88 Enskede, Sweden (Tel: +46 8-6595042)

Swedish Register of Visually Impaired Children, Krinstina Tornqvist, Low Vision Clinic, University Hospital, S-221 85 Lund, Sweden (Tel: 046 17 21 93, Fax: 046 13 90 45)

Tomtebodaskolans Resurscenter, Tomteboda Resource Centre, Box 1313, S-171 25 Solna, Sweden (Tel: +46 8-151130, Fax: +46 8-305385)

Switzerland

Centre Pedagogique pour Handicapes de la Vue, School for Blind and Partially Sighted Children, Avenue de France 30, CH-1004 Lausanne, Switzerland (Tel: +41 21-241171)

Stiftung fur Blinde und Sehbehinderte Kinder und Jugendloche Zollikofen, Foundation for Blind and Visually Handicapped Children and Youth Zollikofen, Kirchlindachstrasse 49, CH-3052 Zollikofen, Switzerland (Tel: +41 31-9112516, Fax: +41 31-9113041)

Taiwan

St Raphael Opportunity Centre for the Blind, PO Box 4-18, Tainan 70804, Taiwan (Tel: +886 6-226 7131, Fax: +886 6-223 8784)

Taipei Municipal School for the Blind, 76 Lane 155, Tun Hua N Road, Taipei, Taiwan (Tel: +886 2-7133475, Fax: +886 2-7126930)

Tanzania

Tanzania Society for the Blind, PO Box 2254, Dar es Salaam, Tanzania (Tel: +255 51-48695)

Thailand

Foundation for the Blind in Thailand, 420 Rajavidhi Road, Phya Tahi, Bangkok 10400, Thailand (Tel: +66 2-246-0070/1431)

Tunisia

Union Nationale des Aveugles de Tunisie, National Union of the Blind of Tunisia, 21 Boulevard Bab Benet, Tunis 1006, Tunisia (Tel: +216 1-565630)

Turkey

Milli Egitim Bakanligi, Ozel Egitim ve Rehberlik Danima Hismetleri Genel Mudurlugu, Ministry of National Education, Directorate of Special Education Guidance and Counselling Service, Bessevier Egitim Sitesi, A Blok, Kat 1, Behcelievier, Ankara, Turkey (Tel: +90 4-222 8110)

Uganda

Uganda Foundation for the Blind, PO Box 1945, Kampala, Uganda (Tel: +256 41-285458)

United Kingdom

International Association for the Education of Deaf–Blind People, c/o SENSE 311 Gray's Inn Road, London WC1X 8PT, UK (Tel: +44 171-278 1005, Fax: +44 171-837 3267)

Royal London Society for the Blind, 105 Salisbury Road, London, UK (Tel: 0171 6248844, Fax: 0171 328 4353)

Royal National Institute for the Blind, 224 Great Portland Street, London W1N 6AA, UK (Tel: +44 71-3881266, Fax: +44 71-3882034)

United States of America

Blind Children's Center, 4210 Marathon Street, Los Angeles, California 90029, USA (Tel: 213 664 2153/800 222 3566, Fax: 213 665 3828)

Helen Keller International, 15 West 16th Street, New York, New York 10011, USA (Tel: +1 212-8075800, Fax: +1 212-4639341)

Helen Keller National Center for Deaf–Blind Youths and Adults, 111 Middle Neck Road, Sands Point, New York 11050, USA (Tel: +1 516-9448900, Fax: +1 516-9447302)

Uruquay

Escuela No. 198 Especial para Discapacitados Visuales, Special School No. 198 for Visually Impaired, Calle Pabio Zufriategui 990, Montevideo, Uruguay (Tel: +598 2-394378)

Venezuela

Asociacion Zuliana de Ciegos, Association for the Blind of Venezuela, Avenida 3e no. 72-33, Maracaibo, Venezuela

Escuela de Ninas Ciegas, Carretera El Junquito, Kilometro 12, Barrio Luis Hurtado, Sector Monte Verde, Caracas, Venezuela (Fax: +58 33 22609)

Instituto Venezolano de Ciegos, Avenida Luis Braile entre Leoncio, Martinez y Maria Teresa Toro, Las Acacias, Caracas, Venezuela (Fax: +58 2 623330)

Vietnam

School for the Blind, 1 Ngugen Trai, Cholon, Saigon, Vietnam

Yemen Arab Republic

Ministry of Social Welfare and Labour, PO Box 60, Sana'a, Yemen Arab Republic

Zaire

Institut Mama Mobutu pour Aveugles, Mama Mobutu Institute for the Blind, Avenue des Huileries, Quartier Gold, Zone de la Gombe, PO Box 8797, Kinshasa I, Zaire (Tel: +243 24793)

Zambia

National Federation of the Blind, PO Box 32847, Cha Cha Cha Road, Lusaka, Zambia (Tel: +260 1-212260)

Zimbabwe

Council for the Blind, PO Box 506, Bulawayo, Zimbabwe (Tel: +263 (1)9-64940)

The author would be grateful for information to update or correct any of the above entries and to add any addresses. Please write to me at the Eye Department, Great Ormond Street Hospital, London WC1N 3JH, UK.   [D.T.]

Index